CLINICAL
MAGNETIC
RESONANCE
IMAGING

Edited by

ROBERT R. EDELMAN, M.D.

Associate Professor of Radiology, Harvard Medical School;
Director of MRI, Beth Israel Hospital, Boston, Massachusetts

JOHN R. HESSELINK, M.D.

Professor of Radiology and Neurosciences,
University of California, San Diego, School of Medicine,
La Jolla, California; Chief of Neuroradiology and
Magnetic Resonance, UCSD Medical Center/Magnetic Resonance
Institute, San Diego, California

Associate Editors

JEFFREY NEWHOUSE, M.D.

Professor of Radiology, Columbia University College of
Physicians and Surgeons; Director, Body Imaging and Abdominal
Radiology, The Presbyterian Hospital in the City of New York,
New York, New York

DAVID J. SARTORIS, M.D.

Associate Professor of Radiology, University of California,
San Diego, School of Medicine, La Jolla, California;
Chief, Musculoskeletal Imaging, UCSD Medical Center,
San Diego, California

1990

W. B. SAUNDERS COMPANY *Philadelphia, London, Toronto, Montreal, Sydney, Tokyo*
Harcourt Brace Jovanovich, Inc.

W. B. SAUNDERS COMPANY
Harcourt Brace Jovanovich, Inc.

The Curtis Center
Independence Square West
Philadelphia, PA 19106

Library of Congress Cataloging-in-Publication Data

Clinical magnetic resonance imaging / edited by Robert R. Edelman, John R. Hesselink; associate editors, Jeffrey Newhouse, David J. Sartoris.

    p.   cm.

  ISBN 0–7216–2241–0

  1. Magnetic resonance imaging.   I. Edelman, Robert R.
    II. Hesselink, John R.

  [DNLM: 1. Magnetic Resonance Imaging.
    WN 445 C641]

RC78.7.N83C56   1990
616.07′548—dc20

DNLM/DLC   89–70159

Sponsoring editor: Lisette Bralow

Manuscript editors: Keryn Lane, Bonnie Boehme

Production Manager: Frank Polizzano

Designer: Lorraine B. Kilmer

Illustration Coordinator: Joan Sinclair

Page Layout: Joan Sinclair

Indexer: Mark Coyle

CLINICAL MAGNETIC RESONANCE IMAGING   ISBN 0–7216–2241–0

Printed in the United States of America.

Last digit is the print number: 9   8   7   6   5   4   3   2   1

Dedicated to
Susan, Daniel, and Laura
Kay and André

CONTRIBUTORS

JOSEPH J. AHLADIS, C.R.T., A.R.R.T.
MRI Product Specialist, Siemens Medical Systems, Inc., Costa Mesa, California
Practical MRI for the Technologist and Imaging Specialist

DENNIS J. ATKINSON, M.Sc.
Collaborative Scientist, Beth Israel Hospital, Boston, Massachusetts
Basic Principles of Magnetic Resonance Imaging; Clinical Spectroscopy; Pulse Sequence Design; Glossary of MR Terms

DOUGLAS BALLON, M.D.
Assistant Professor of Radiology (Physics), Cornell University Medical College, New York, New York
Clinical Spectroscopy

MARK S. BANKOFF, M.D.
Associate Professor of Radiology, Tufts University School of Medicine; Assistant Radiologist, New England Medical Center, Boston, Massachusetts
Head and Neck

BERNARD A. BIRNBAUM, M.D.
Assistant Professor of Radiology, New York University School of Medicine, New York University Medical Center, New York, New York
Obstetrical MR Imaging

THOMAS J. BRADY, M.D.
Associate Professor, Department of Radiology, Harvard Medical School; Director, NMR, Massachusetts General Hospital, Boston, Massachusetts
Biochemical Basis of the MR Appearance of Cerebral Hemorrhage

MARK A. BROWN, PH.D.
Applications Scientist, Siemens Medical Systems, Inc., Greensboro, North Carolina
Clinical Spectroscopy

C. TYLER BURT, M.D.
Associate Director of Magnetic Resonance Center, University of Illinois College of Medicine, Chicago, Illinois
Clinical Spectroscopy

RICHARD B. BUXTON, PH.D.
Assistant Professor in Residence, Department of Radiological Sciences, University of California at Irvine School of Medicine, Irvine, California
Flow

BARBARA L. CARTER, M.D.
Professor of Radiology and Otolaryngology, Tufts University School of Medicine; Chief of CT Scanning and Chief of ENT Radiology, New England Medical Center, Boston, Massachusetts
Head and Neck

ROLAND CHISIN, M.D.

Senior Lecturer in Nuclear Medicine, Department of Medical Biophysics and Nuclear Medicine, Hadassah University Hospital, Jerusalem, Israel; Otolaryngologist and Nuclear Physician, Hadassah University Hospital, Jerusalem, Israel

MR Imaging of the Musculoskeletal System

KYUNG J. CHUNG, M.D., F.A.C.C.

Associate Professor of Pediatrics, University of California at San Diego School of Medicine, La Jolla; Pediatric Cardiologist, UCSD Medical Center, San Diego, California

Cine MR Imaging of the Heart; Cine MR Imaging of Congenital Heart Disease

EVE K. COHEN, M.D.

Assistant Professor of Radiology, University of Toronto; Diagnostic Radiology, Mount Sinai Hospital, Toronto, Ontario

MR Imaging of the Pelvis

JOHN V. CRUES, M.D.

Director, Magnetic Resonance Imaging, Santa Barbara Cottage Hospital, Santa Barbara, California

MR Imaging of the Knee

KENNETH R. DAVIS, M.D.

Professor, Department of Radiology, Harvard Medical School; Director of Neuroradiology, Massachusetts General Hospital, Boston, Massachusetts

Brain: Neoplasia; Brain: Vascular Diseases; Trauma, Inflammation, Degenerative and Metabolic Disorders

R. DINSMORE, M.D.

Director, Cardiac Radiology Division, Director, Cardiac MRI, Massachusetts General Hospital, Boston, Massachusetts

Examination of the Adult Heart and Great Vessels

J. PAUL FINN, M.D.

Instructor in Radiology, Harvard Medical School; Technical Director, Magnetic Resonance Imaging, New England Deaconess Hospital, Boston, Massachusetts

Glossary of MR Terms

WARREN B. GEFTER, M.D.

Professor of Radiology, University of Pennsylvania School of Medicine; Attending Radiologist, Hospital of the University of Pennsylvania, Philadelphia, Pennsylvania

MR Imaging of Developmental Abnormalities of the Female Pelvis

HARRY K. GENANT, M.D.

Professor of Radiology, Medicine and Orthopaedic Surgery, University of California at San Francisco School of Medicine, San Francisco, California

MR Imaging of the Knee

RENÉE FITZMORRIS GLASS, M.D.

Assistant Clinical Professor, Department of Radiology, University of California at San Diego School of Medicine, La Jolla; Staff Radiologist, Alvarado Hospital Medical Center, San Diego, California

The Brachial Plexus

JEFFREY J. GREENBERG, M.D.

Chief of Neuroradiology, Grant Medical Center; Director of Magnetic Resonance Imaging, Columbus Health Imaging Center, Columbus, Ohio

Brain: Indications, Technique, and Atlas

KATHRYN GRUMBACH, M.D.

Assistant Professor of Radiology, University of Pennsylvania; Attending Radiologist, Hospital of the University of Pennsylvania, Philadelphia, Pennsylvania

MR Imaging of Developmental Abnormalities of the Female Pelvis

BERND HAMM, M.D.

Associate Professor, Medical School, Freie Universität; Chief of Service, Magnetic Resonance, Department of Radiology, Klinikum Steglitz, Freie Universität, Berlin, West Germany

Contrast Agents for MR Imaging

STEVEN E. HARMS, M.D.

Director of Magnetic Resonance, Department of Radiology, Baylor University Medical Center, Dallas, Texas

The Orbit; MR Imaging of the Temporomandibular Joint

ROBERT D. HARRIS, M.D.

Assistant Professor of Radiology, Dartmouth Medical School; Co-Director of MRI, Dartmouth-Hitchcock Medical Center, Hanover, New Hampshire

Artifacts in MR Imaging: Description, Causes, and Solutions

RICHARD J. HICKS, M.D.

Assistant Clinical Professor, Department of Radiology, Tufts University School of Medicine, Boston; Director of Magnetic Resonance Imaging, Baystate Medical Center, Springfield, Massachusetts

Brain: Indications, Technique, and Atlas; Brain: Neoplasia; Brain: Vascular Diseases; Brain: Periventricular White Matter Abnormalities; Brain: Trauma, Inflammation, Degenerative and Metabolic Disorders

KEITH A. JOHNSON, M.D.

Assistant in Neurology, Harvard Medical School; Massachusetts General Hospital, Boston, Massachusetts

Brain: Spontaneous Hemorrhage

HOWARD L. KANTOR, M.D., Ph.D.

Assistant Professor of Medicine, Harvard Medical School; Cardiac Unit, Director of NMR Imaging and Spectroscopy, Massachusetts General Hospital, Boston, Massachusetts

Frontiers in Cardiac Magnetic Resonance

LELAND E. KELLERHOUSE, M.D.

Co-Director, Mercy Magnetic Imaging Center; Staff Radiologist, Radiology Medical Group, Inc., Mercy Hospital and Medical Center, San Diego, California

MR Imaging of the Wrist

JONATHAN KLEEFIELD, M.D.

Assistant Professor, Department of Radiology, Harvard Medical School; Neuroradiologist, Beth Israel Hospital, Boston, Massachusetts

Basic Principles of Magnetic Resonance Imaging; Brain: Indications, Technique, and Atlas

J. BRUCE KNEELAND, M.D.

Associate Professor, Medical College of Wisconsin; Director of Clinical Magnetic Resonance Imaging, Milwaukee County Medical Complex, Milwaukee, Wisconsin

MR Imaging of the Glenohumeral Joint

P. KOENIGSBERG, M.D.

Leading Body MRI Radiologist, MRI Center of Miami and Mercy Hospital, Miami, Florida

Head and Neck

MICHAEL F. KOSKINEN, Sc.D., M.D.
Department of Radiology, New England Deaconess Hospital, Boston, Massachusetts
Site Planning

JASON A. KOUTCHER, M.D., Ph.D.
Assistant Professor of Radiology (Physics), Cornell University Medical College; Chief of Imaging and Spectroscopy Physics, Memorial Sloan-Kettering Cancer Center, New York, New York
Clinical Spectroscopy

HERBERT Y. KRESSEL, M.D.
Professor of Radiology, University of Pennsylvania; Director, David W. Devon Medical Imaging Center, Hospital of the University of Pennsylvania, Philadelphia, Pennsylvania
MR Imaging of the Pelvis

SEVIL KURSUNOGLU-BRAHME, M.D.
Assistant Professor of Radiology, University of Calfornia at San Diego School of Medicine; Department of Radiology, UCSD Medical Center, San Diego, California
MR Imaging of the Wrist

RANDALL B. LAUFFER, Ph.D.
Assistant Professor, Department of Radiology, Harvard Medical School; Director, NMR Contrast Media Laboratory, Massachusetts General Hospital, Boston, Massachusetts
Principles of MR Imaging Contrast Agents

JOEL F. MARTIN, Ph.D.
Assistant Professor, Department of Radiology, University of California at San Diego School of Medicine, San Diego, California
Fast MR Imaging; Clinical Spectroscopy; Cine MR Imaging of the Heart

HEINRICH P. MATTLE, M.D.
Oberarzt, Neurologische Universitätsklinik Inselspital, Bern, Switzerland
Brain: Spontaneous Hemorrhage

ROBERT MATTREY, M.D.
Associate Professor, University of California at San Diego School of Medicine, La Jolla; Director of Research, UCSD Medical Center/MRI Institute, San Diego, California
MR Imaging of the Upper Abdomen and Adrenal Glands; MR Imaging of the Scrotum and Testes

THERESA C. McLOUD, M.D.
Associate Professor, Department of Radiology, Harvard Medical School; Radiologist, Chief of Thoracic Radiology, Massachusetts General Hospital, Boston, Massachusetts
MR Imaging of the Thorax

MICHAEL J. MITCHELL, M.D.
Lecturer, Department of Radiology, Dalhousie University; Staff Radiologist, Victoria General Hospital, Halifax, Nova Scotia.
MR Imaging of the Foot and Ankle

ROBERT W. NEWMAN, M.S., M.B.A.
G.E. Medical Systems, Milwaukee, Wisconsin
Cine MR Imaging of the Heart

GERALD V. O'REILLY, M.D.
Associate Professor, Department of Radiology, Harvard Medical School; Formerly Director of Neuroradiology, Beth Israel Hospital, Boston, Massachusetts
Brain: Spontaneous Hemorrhage

NICHOLAS PAPANICOLAOU, M.D.

Associate Professor, Department of Radiology, Harvard Medical School; Head, Division of Genitourinary Radiology, Massachusetts General Hospital, Boston, Massachusetts

MR Imaging of the Kidney and Retroperitoneum

RICHARD C. PFISTER, M.D.

Former Head, Division of Genitourinary Radiology, Massachusetts General Hospital, Boston, Massachusetts

MR Imaging of the Kidney and Retroperitoneum

GARY A. PRESS, M.D.

Assistant Professor in Residence, Department of Radiology and Magnetic Resonance Institute, University of California at San Diego Medical Center; Neuroradiologist, VA Medical Center, La Jolla, and UCSD Medical Center; Consultant Radiologist, Naval Hospital, San Diego, California

Brain: Congenital Malformations

MARK W. RAGOZZINO, M.D.

Radiologist, Delaney Radiology and New Hanover Memorial Hospital, Wilmington, North Carolina

MR Imaging of the Thorax; MR Imaging of the Musculoskeletal System

MURRAY A. REICHER, M.D.

Co-Director, Mercy Magnetic Imaging Center; Staff Radiologist, Radiology Medical Group, Inc., Mercy Hospital and Medical Center, San Diego, California

MR Imaging of the Wrist

DONALD RESNICK, M.D.

Professor of Radiology, University of California at San Diego School of Medicine; Chief, Radiology Service, VA Medical Center, San Diego, California

MR Imaging of the Foot and Ankle

DANIEL I. ROSENTHAL, M.D.

Associate Professor, Department of Radiology, Harvard Medical School; Director of Bone and Joint Radiology, Massachusetts General Hospital, Boston, Massachusetts

MR Imaging of the Musculoskeletal System

JEREMY B. RUBIN, M.D.

Co-Director, Magnetic Resonance, Department of Diagnostic Imaging, Good Samaritan Hospital, San Jose, California

Flow

VAL M. RUNGE, M.D.

Associate Professor of Radiology, Tufts University School of Medicine; Chief of Service, MRI, New England Medical Center, Boston, Massachusetts

Head and Neck

SANJAY SAINI, M.D.

Assistant Professor, Department of Radiology, Harvard Medical School; Assistant Radiologist, Massachusetts General Hospital, Boston Massachusetts

Contrast Agents for MR Imaging

FRANK G. SHELLOCK, Ph.D.

Assistant Professor of Radiological Sciences, University of California at Los Angeles School of Medicine; Research Scientist-Physiologist, Cedars-Sinai Medical Center, Los Angeles, California

Practical MRI for the Technologist and Imaging Specialist

GREGORY M. SHOUKIMAS, M.D., Ph.D.
Clinical Associate, Massachusetts General Hospital; Clinical Director, West Suburban Imaging Center, Wellesley Hills, Massachusetts
MR Imaging of the Cervical and Thoracic Spine; MR Imaging of the Lumbar Spine

IAIN A. SIMPSON, M.D., M.R.C.P.
Senior Registrar in Cardiology, Department of Cardiological Sciences, St. Georges Hospital, London, England
Cine MR Imaging of the Heart; Cine MR Imaging of Congenital Heart Disease

MARK SLONIM, M.D.
Clinical Instructor, Department of Orthopedics and Rehabilitation, University of San Diego School of Medicine, La Jolla, California
MR Imaging of the Wrist

ECKART STETTER, Ph.D.
Manager, MR Physics (MR Product Development), Siemens Medical Systems, Inc., Erlangen, West Germany
Instrumentation

DAVID W. STOLLER, M.D.
Assistant Clinical Professor of Radiology, Department of Radiology, University of California at San Francisco Medical Center; Director, California Advanced Imaging, San Francisco, California
MR Imaging of the Knee

KEITH R. THULBORN, M.D., Ph.D.
Instructor, Department of Radiology, Harvard Medical School; Assistant Radiologist, Massachusetts General Hospital, Boston, Massachusetts
Biochemical Basis of the MR Appearance of Cerebral Hemorrhage

MICHAEL TRAMBERT, M.D.
Assistant Professor in Residence, University of California at San Diego School of Medicine, La Jolla; Assistant Professor in Residence, UCSD Medical Center, San Diego, California
MR Imaging of the Upper Abdomen and Adrenal Glands; MR Imaging of the Scrotum and Testes

DAVID H. TURKEL, M.D.
Clinical Director of MRI, Cape Cod Hospital, Hyannis, Massachusetts
Brain: Indications, Technique, and Atlas

JEFFREY C. WEINREB, M.D.
Associate Professor of Radiology, New York University School of Medicine; Director of Magnetic Resonance Imaging, New York University Medical Center, New York, New York
Obstetrical MR Imaging

KLAUS U. WENTZ, M.D.
Department of Radiology, Klinikum Mannheim, University of Heidelberg, Mannheim, West Germany
Basic Principles of Magnetic Resonance Imaging

GEORGE E. WESBEY, M.D.
Staff Radiologist and Director, MRI, Scripps Memorial Hospital, La Jolla, California
Artifacts in MR Imaging: Description, Causes, and Solutions

GARY L. WISMER, M.D.

Staff Neuroradiologist, Baptist Medical Center, Jacksonville-Wolfson Childrens Hospital, Jacksonville, Florida

Brain: Neoplasia; Brain: Vascular Diseases; Trauma, Inflammation, Degenerative and Metabolic Disorders

MICHAEL B. ZLATKIN, M.D. F.R.C.P.(L)

Assistant Clinical Professor, Department of Radiology, University of Miami School of Medicine; Staff Radiologist, Hollywood Memorial Hospital, Hollywood, Florida

MR Imaging of the Glenohumeral Joint

FOREWORD

Radiologists of future generations will no doubt consider the end of the twentieth century an exciting and important time in the history of radiology, because it was the period when MR imaging was first introduced into clinical practice. Future radiologists are certain to be impressed by the rapidity with which the technique assumed a vital role in diagnostic radiology, despite the availability of CT, which also was new at the time. Historians will no doubt equate the importance of the invention of MR imaging at the end of the twentieth century with the discovery of the Roentgen ray at the end of the nineteenth century, when radiology itself was born.

Future radiologists are also likely to be sympathetic with the struggles of our generation in defining the proper clinical role of MR imaging in view of the rapid evolution of MR imaging techniques. They will look back at the first journal articles and monographs on MR imaging and be impressed by how quickly they became outdated in rapid sequence, as the field of MR imaging burgeoned and matured.

This work on MR imaging, edited by Drs. Edelman and Hesselink, will no doubt fall prey to the same obsolescence, but fortunately it will be to a lesser extent. This textbook comes at a propitious time, when most of the foreseeable technological advances have already been added to existing MR systems, most of the clinical applications have been evaluated, contrast materials have been introduced, and the role of MR imaging relative to other techniques has been defined, at least in a preliminary manner. At this point much of the initial smoke has cleared, so that this book, which deals with the state of the art, is likely to remain current well into the 1990s.

The editors have been successful in assembling a cadre of experts on MR imaging whose contributions to the field qualify them to write with authority about the subject. The first part of the book offers a complete review of the physics of MR, including two chapters on the fundamentals written for beginners, as well as chapters on specialized topics, such as fast scanning, flow imaging, and spectroscopy, written for the more advanced reader. Chapters in this portion of the book are either coauthored or edited by Robert Edelman, who has a remarkable talent for making complex topics understandable for general readers.

The rest of the book concerns clinical applications of MR imaging and is divided into sections on the central nervous system, the chest and abdomen, the pelvis, and the musculoskeletal system. MR of the brain and spinal cord is the area of expertise of John Hesselink. In this section, each disease is introduced with a paragraph or two on clinical manifestations and pathophysiology, making the book a complete reference rather than a simple collection of illustrations. Emphasis is placed on key facts about specific diseases and on interpretation of the MR images. A differential diagnosis approach is used to help the reader distinguish among lesions, algorithms allow the reader to select pulse sequences logically, and a comprehensive appendix supplies a complete set of MR scanning protocols.

Chapters on MR imaging of the chest, abdomen, and pelvis bring the reader to the frontier of these subjects. All the latest techniques are described, including spin-echo imaging, gating techniques, cine MR, and instant scanning.

The final section on musculoskeletal imaging is another highlight of the book and reflects the importance of this area of MR. In addition to an overview of musculoskeletal MR, chapters are dedicated to individual joints to allow for the most thorough coverage of each topic. Normal anatomy, biomechanics, and disease processes are discussed in detail and are clearly illustrated.

I applaud the editors, authors, and publisher for their masterful work. Radiologists who use MR imaging in their practices, experienced or not, are certain to find in this book everything they need to know to bring them up to date on this powerful new tool and to allow them to perform and interpret MR images with confidence.

ROBERT N. BERK, M.D.

PREFACE

The field of medical imaging has been revolutionized over the past two decades by developments in radionuclide imaging, sonography, and computed tomography. None of these modalities has continued to evoke the same level of excitement and controversy as magnetic resonance imaging. Yet early on many of the spectacular clinical results achieved with this complex technology were unforeseen. When we first became involved with MR, image acquisition was excruciatingly slow, user interfaces were genuinely hostile, sophisticated pulse sequences were nonexistent, and proposals for performing high-resolution imaging of areas such as the spine or knee were greeted, as often as not, with derision.

Rapid advances in the technology have finally unleashed the clinical potential of MR. Magnetic resonance has proved generally superior to other imaging modalities for the study of a variety of disorders involving the central nervous system and the musculoskeletal system and is useful—either as a primary or complementary imaging tool—for studying the abdomen, pelvis, and cardiovascular system. In some cases, such as for the detection of internal derangements in the knee, MR has largely supplanted invasive and less informative methods such as arthrography. Despite these successes, MR has definite limitations: some of these will certainly be overcome with continuing technical improvements, whereas others are absolute.

The clinical applications of MR and its underlying physical principles and technology are presented in this text. In some areas, such as the central nervous system, the clinical indications for MR are clear. In others, such as the upper abdomen and heart, some clinical indications are well defined and others are still tentative or controversial. Certain techniques, such as echo-planar imaging, MR angiography, and in vivo spectroscopy, have finally matured to a degree that the clinical applications can be discussed at some length, although any definitive statements await large-scale clinical studies and further technical developments. We hope that the clinical and technical framework presented here is helpful for choosing appropriate indications for MR imaging, obtaining the best quality images, and deriving the most diagnostic information from the MR examination. In presenting this information, we also wish to convey something of our own excitement and enthusiasm, derived from working in this continually evolving and always interesting field of study.

We would like to thank, first of all, the outstanding group of contributors who made this book a reality. Special thanks go to Thomas Brady, M.D., a pioneer in clinical MR who has been an outstanding teacher and who laid much of the groundwork for this project; to Richard Buxton, Ph.D., who has a special talent for explaining the most complex concepts in the most easily understood terms; to Sven Paulin, M.D., and George Leopold, M.D., for their encouragment and helpful advice; to Kathleen Dupuis, R.T., and Lynne Lord, R.T., who helped develop protocols and maintain high-quality imaging; to Lasaundra Lowe and Vicki Broughton for their assistance with manuscript preparation; to Lisette Bralow and Lorraine Kilmer, whose editorial and publishing expertise are evident on every page; and most of all, to our families, who had the patience of Job from beginning to end.

ROBERT R. EDELMAN, M.D.

JOHN R. HESSELINK, M.D.

CONTENTS

PART I PHYSICS AND INSTRUMENTATION

1
BASIC PRINCIPLES OF MAGNETIC RESONANCE IMAGING 3
Robert R. Edelman, Jonathan Kleefield, Klaus U. Wentz, and Dennis J. Atkinson

2
PRACTICAL MRI FOR THE TECHNOLOGIST AND IMAGING SPECIALIST 39
Robert R. Edelman, Frank G. Shellock, and Joseph Ahladis

3
ARTIFACTS IN MR IMAGING: DESCRIPTION, CAUSES, AND SOLUTIONS 74
George E. Wesbey, Robert R. Edelman, and Robert Harris

4
FLOW 109
Robert R. Edelman, Jeremy B. Rubin, and Richard B. Buxton

5
FAST MR IMAGING 183
Joel F. Martin and Robert R. Edelman

6
PRINCIPLES OF MR IMAGING CONTRAST AGENTS 221
Randall B. Lauffer

7
CONTRAST AGENTS FOR MR IMAGING 237
Sanjay Saini and Bernd Hamm

8
BIOCHEMICAL BASIS OF THE MR APPEARANCE OF CEREBRAL HEMORRHAGE .. 255
Keith R. Thulborn and Thomas J. Brady

9
CLINICAL SPECTROSCOPY 269
Dennis J. Atkinson, Joel F. Martin, Mark A. Brown, Jason A. Koutcher,
C. Tyler Burt, and Douglas Ballon

10
PULSE SEQUENCE DESIGN 313
Dennis J. Atkinson

xvii

11
SITE PLANNING 341
Michael F. Koskinen

12
INSTRUMENTATION 355
Eckart Stetter

PART II   CENTRAL NERVOUS SYSTEM

13
BRAIN: INDICATIONS, TECHNIQUE, AND ATLAS 379
Jeffrey J. Greenberg, David H. Turkel, Jonathan Kleefield, and Richard J. Hicks

14
BRAIN: CONGENITAL MALFORMATIONS 413
Gary A. Press

15
BRAIN: NEOPLASIA 448
Richard J. Hicks, John R. Hesselink, Gary L. Wismer, and Kenneth R. Davis

16
BRAIN: SPONTANEOUS HEMORRHAGE 483
Heinrich P. Mattle, Gerald V. O'Reilly, Robert R. Edelman,
and Keith A. Johnson

17
BRAIN: VASCULAR DISEASES 516
Richard J. Hicks, John R. Hesselink, Gary L. Wismer, and Kenneth R. Davis

18
BRAIN: PERIVENTRICULAR WHITE MATTER ABNORMALITIES 545
John R. Hesselink and Richard J. Hicks

19
BRAIN: TRAUMA, INFLAMMATION, AND DEGENERATIVE AND
METABOLIC DISORDERS 563
Richard J. Hicks, John R. Hesselink, Gary L. Wismer, and Kenneth R. Davis

20
THE ORBIT 598
Steven E. Harms

21
HEAD AND NECK 622
Barbara L. Carter, P. Koenigsberg, Mark S. Bankoff, and Val M. Runge

22

THE BRACHIAL PLEXUS 653
Renée Fitzmorris Glass

23

MR IMAGING OF THE CERVICAL AND THORACIC SPINE 667
Gregory M. Shoukimas and John R. Hesselink

24

MR IMAGING OF THE LUMBAR SPINE 705
John R. Hesselink and Gregory M. Shoukimas

PART III   CHEST AND ABDOMEN

25

MR IMAGING OF THE THORAX 731
Theresa C. McLoud and Mark W. Ragozzino

26

FRONTIERS IN CARDIAC MAGNETIC RESONANCE 745
Howard L. Kantor

27

EXAMINATION OF THE ADULT HEART AND GREAT VESSELS 773
R. Dinsmore

28

CINE MR IMAGING OF THE HEART 810
Iain A. Simpson, Robert W. Newman, Joel F. Martin, and Kyung J. Chung

29

CINE MR IMAGING OF CONGENITAL HEART DISEASE 830
Kyung J. Chung and Iain A. Simpson

30

MR IMAGING OF THE UPPER ABDOMEN AND ADRENAL GLANDS 845
Robert Mattrey, Michael Trambert, and Robert R. Edelman

31

MR IMAGING OF THE KIDNEY AND RETROPERITONEUM 899
Nicholas Papanicolaou and Richard C. Pfister

PART IV   PELVIS

32

MR IMAGING OF THE PELVIS 915
Eve K. Cohen and Herbert Y. Kressel

33
OBSTETRICAL MR IMAGING **938**
Bernard A. Birnbaum and Jeffrey C. Weinreb

34
MR IMAGING OF THE SCROTUM AND TESTES **952**
Robert Mattrey and Michael Trambert

35
MR IMAGING OF DEVELOPMENTAL ABNORMALITIES OF THE FEMALE PELVIS ... **980**
Kathryn Grumbach and Warren B. Gefter

PART V   MUSCULOSKELETAL

36
MR IMAGING OF THE KNEE **989**
David W. Stoller, Harry K. Genant, and John V. Crues

37
MR IMAGING OF THE GLENOHUMERAL JOINT **1010**
Michael B. Zlatkin and J. Bruce Kneeland

38
MR IMAGING OF THE TEMPOROMANDIBULAR JOINT **1031**
Steven E. Harms

39
MR IMAGING OF THE WRIST **1057**
Leland E. Kellerhouse, Murray A. Reicher, Sevil Kursunoglu-Brahme, and Mark Slonim

40
MR IMAGING OF THE FOOT AND ANKLE **1076**
David J. Sartoris, Michael J. Mitchell, and Donald Resnick

41
MR IMAGING OF THE MUSCULOSKELETAL SYSTEM **1097**
Mark W. Ragozzino, Roland Chisin, and Daniel I. Rosenthal

APPENDIX I   MR IMAGING SCAN PROTOCOLS **1132**

APPENDIX II   STAGING SYSTEMS OF PRIMARY MALIGNANCIES **1153**

GLOSSARY OF MR TERMS **1158**
Robert R. Edelman, Dennis Atkinson, and J. Paul Finn

INDEX **1173**

PART I

PHYSICS AND INSTRUMENTATION

1

BASIC PRINCIPLES OF MAGNETIC RESONANCE IMAGING

ROBERT R. EDELMAN, JONATHAN KLEEFIELD, KLAUS U. WENTZ, and DENNIS J. ATKINSON

WHY HYDROGEN IS THE ELEMENT OF CHOICE FOR MR IMAGING

OVERVIEW OF THE MR IMAGING PROCESS

THE ROLE OF MAGNETS IN MR

THE ROLE OF RADIOFREQUENCY PULSES IN PRODUCING THE MR SIGNAL

  SINGLE ATOM (QUANTUM MECHANICAL VIEW)

  GROUP BEHAVIOR OF ATOMS (CLASSIC VIEW)

FACTORS THAT AFFECT THE MR SIGNAL: RELAXATION AND OTHER TISSUE PARAMETERS

  RELAXATION (T_2 AND T_1)

  T_2 Relaxation
  T_1 Relaxation

  MOLECULAR MECHANISMS FOR RELAXATION

  DEPENDENCE OF T_1 RELAXATION TIMES ON FIELD STRENGTH

  CORRELATION OF T_1 AND T_2 RELAXATION TIMES

  PROTON DENSITY

SPATIAL LOCALIZATION OF THE MR SIGNAL

  EFFECT OF A MAGNETIC FIELD GRADIENT

  TWO-DIMENSIONAL IMAGING METHODS

  Slice selection
  Frequency encoding
  Phase encoding
  Fourier transform
  Signal averaging

  THREE-DIMENSIONAL IMAGING

FACTORS THAT AFFECT THE MR SIGNAL: PULSE SEQUENCES

  TYPES OF MR SIGNALS
  SPIN ECHO

  GRADIENT ECHO

  CONVERSION RECOVERY

  Magnitude Reconstruction Versus Phase-Sensitive Reconstruction
  Short Tau Inversion Recovery

  SUMMARY OF PULSE SEQUENCES

DETERMINANTS OF SPATIAL RESOLUTION

CONTRAST AND SIGNAL-TO-NOISE ON SPIN-ECHO IMAGES

  PROTON DENSITY–WEIGHTED IMAGES

  T_1-WEIGHTED IMAGES

  T_2-WEIGHTED IMAGES

  CROSS-OVER

  SIGNAL-TO-NOISE

OTHER FACTORS AFFECTING THE MR IMAGE

  MAGNETIC SUSCEPTIBILITY

  CONTRAST AGENTS

  T_1-Active Agents
  T_2-Active Agents
  Nonproton Agents

  HEMORRHAGE

  FLOW

  CHEMICAL SHIFT

OVERVIEW OF HARDWARE

  MAGNETS

  RADIOFREQUENCY COILS

  Receiver Coils
  Transmitter Coils
  Quadrature (Circularly Polarized) Coils
  Quality

  GRADIENTS

Magnetic resonance (MR) imaging represents a revolution in medical technology. MR imaging provides detailed images of the human body with unprecedented soft tissue contrast. Because of the innate versatility of this modality, tissue anatomy, pathology, metabolism, and flow are all amenable to noninvasive evaluation. Initially, the phenomenon of nuclear magnetic resonance (NMR) was applied to analytical methods in physical chemistry. Nearly four decades passed before MR was successfully employed in medical imaging.

In this chapter, we review the basic principles of

3

MR imaging. This chapter is written for the novice who is interested in a simplified approach to the field. Those interested in more detailed discussions are referred to other chapters within this text and to other references.[1-5]

Magnetic resonance is defined as the enhanced absorption of energy occurring when the nuclei of atoms or molecules within an external magnetic field are exposed to radiofrequency (RF) energy at a specific frequency, called the *Larmor* or *resonance frequency.* The phenomenon was first observed in particle beams by Rabi and coworkers in 1939.[6] Bloch, in 1946, placed his own finger within the probe of an early MR spectrometer and observed a strong signal from hydrogen nuclei. In a sense, this experiment marked the first biologic application of MR. Bloch and Purcell both received the Nobel Prize for elucidating the phenomenon of MR in solids and liquids.[7, 8]

The characteristics of the MR signal arising from a given nucleus were found to depend on the specific molecular environment of that nucleus. This signal dependence proved ideal for both qualitative and quantitative chemical analysis. Furthermore, the RFs involved in MR are nonionizing (Fig. 1–1) and can also penetrate the human body. These features suggested an enormous clinical potential for MR, since it might provide a means for studying the biochemistry of human subjects in vivo. However, the clinical potential of the method was limited by its inability to provide spatial localization of the MR signal, so that it could not be applied as an imaging technique. Lauterbur solved this localization problem by using magnetic field gradients and by 1972 was able to produce the first images of water samples.[9] However, it was not until 1977 that Damadian acquired the first human images using a prototype superconducting magnet.[10] Concurrently, British investigators, including Andrew, Mansfield, and Hinshaw, developed point and line scanning signal localization techniques.[11, 12] Many significant technical innovations followed, such as three-dimensional (3D) data acquisition, two-dimensional (2D) single-slice acquisition using selective irradiation, 2D multislice acquisition, fast scanning with gradient-echo and echo-planar techniques, and the integration of MR imaging and MR spectroscopy (MRS).

WHY HYDROGEN IS THE ELEMENT OF CHOICE FOR MR IMAGING

There are numerous elements that could, in theory, be imaged by MR. Any nucleus with an odd number of either protons or neutrons can produce an MR signal. However, MR is primarily applied to the imaging of hydrogen, for two reasons: (1) high sensitivity for its MR signal and (2) high natural abundance.

The high sensitivity for the signal from the hydrogen nucleus has to do with a number called the *gyromagnetic ratio.* The gyromagnetic ratio (γ), which depends on the size and shape of a nucleus, represents the resonance frequency of that nucleus in a 1-tesla (T) magnetic field. Sensitivity (i.e., the efficiency with which the MR signal is detected) improves with increasing signal (resonance) frequency. Therefore, MR is most sensitive for the signal from hydrogen, which has the highest gyromagnetic ratio of any element. In addition to lower sensitivity, other elements have lower natural abundance than hydrogen (Table 1–1). Although other elements can be imaged, the quality of these images is far inferior to the quality of those obtained from hydrogen.

OVERVIEW OF THE MR IMAGING PROCESS

Several steps are involved in the production of an MR image (Fig. 1–2). These are discussed in greater detail further on but may be summarized as follows:

1. Randomly oriented tissue nuclei are aligned by a powerful, uniform magnetic field.

2. This alignment, or magnetization, is then disrupted by properly tuned RF pulses. As the nuclei recover their alignment by relaxation processes, they produce radio signals that are proportional to the magnitude of the initial alignment. Tissue contrast (i.e., differences in signal) develops as a result of the different rates at which nuclei realign with the magnetic field.

3. The positions of the nuclei are localized during this process by the application of spatially-dependent magnetic fields, called *gradients.*

4. The signals are measured, or read out, after a

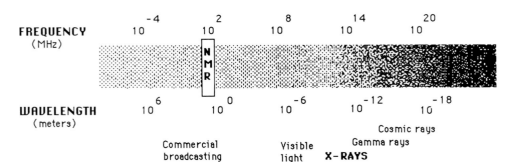

FIGURE 1–1. Electromagnetic spectrum. Unlike conventional radiography, MR uses nonionizing RF energy.

TABLE 1–1. MR CHARACTERISTICS OF VARIOUS ELEMENTS

Nucleus	γ (MHz/T)	Natural Isotopic Abundance (%)	Relative Sensitivity*	Spin
^{1}H	42.576	99.985	1	½
^{2}H	6.536	0.015	0.0096	1
^{13}C	10.705	1.108	0.016	½
^{14}N	3.076	99.635	0.001	1
^{15}N	4.315	0.365	0.001	½
^{17}O	5.772	0.037	0.029	³⁄₂
^{19}F	40.055	100	0.834	½
^{23}Na	11.262	100	0.093	³⁄₂
^{31}P	17.236	100	0.066	½
^{33}S	3.266	0.74	0.0023	³⁄₂
^{39}K	1.987	93.08	0.0005	³⁄₂

*At constant field, with sensitivity of the 1-hydrogen nucleus = 1; 1 gm of material compared with 1 gm of hydrogen.

user-determined time has elapsed from the initial RF excitation.

5. The signal is transformed by the computer into an image using a mathematical process called the *Fourier transform (FT)*.

We now discuss the basic physical principles that underlie the MR imaging process.

THE ROLE OF MAGNETS IN MR

A hydrogen nucleus, being a solitary proton, behaves in certain respects like a tiny bar magnet. This behavior is a consequence of a fundamental physical law: A moving electrical charge possesses a tiny magnetic field. For a structure such as the nucleus, which is spinning, this field is called a *magnetic moment*. Like a bar magnet, the spinning proton has a north and a south magnetic pole. Because of these two magnetic poles, this nucleus can be considered a dipole (spin = 1/2). Certain other nuclei possess more than two alignments. For instance, the sodium nucleus (spin = 3/2) may have four alignments and, unlike the hydrogen nucleus, possesses a quadrupolar moment (see Chapter 9).

When the hydrogen atom is placed within an external magnetic field, experience might dictate that the nucleus, being a dipole, should behave much like the needle of a compass. That is, when placed in the external field, the dipole should align itself parallel to the north-south axis of this field, with the north pole of the dipole opposite the south pole of the external field (Fig. 1–3A). In actuality, according to quantum mechanical principles, the dipole can align itself only either at an angle to this orientation (parallel) or at an angle opposite (antiparallel) to the applied field (Fig. 1–3B). The two alignments correspond, respectively, to lower and higher energy states of the dipole.

Within any externally applied magnetic field, there is always a very small *net excess* of dipoles aligned in the lower energy parallel direction compared with the antiparallel orientation. This excess population is represented by a vector called the *net magnetization* **(M)**.

FIGURE 1–2. Summary of steps involved in the formation of the MR image, starting with the patient entering the magnetic field.

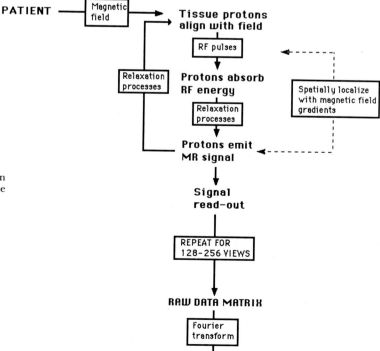

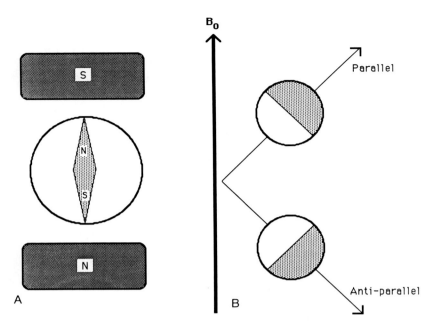

FIGURE 1–3. Comparison of the magnetic properties of a compass and proton. *A,* The compass always points in one direction. S = south; N = north. *B,* The proton may be aligned in either of two directions: parallel to the applied magnetic field (B_0) or antiparallel to the field.

The main reason for using powerful magnets in MR imaging and spectroscopy is to maximize **M,** which results in greater signal strength. In a weak external magnetic field, such as that experienced on earth, the difference in energy (ΔE) between the parallel and antiparallel alignments is minimal. In this environment, there is no significant tendency for dipoles to align in one direction or the other, so that **M** is negligible (Fig. 1–4*A*). However, ΔE increases in direct proportion to the external magnetic field

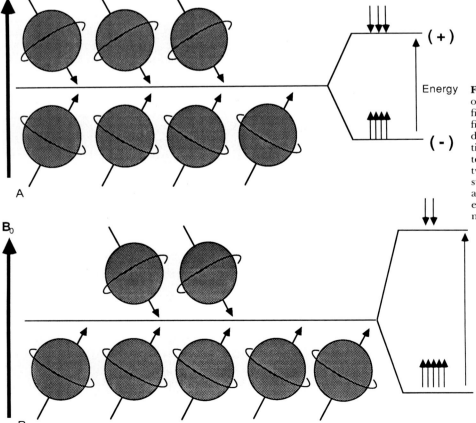

FIGURE 1–4. The degree of alignment of protons with an applied magnetic field depends on the strength of the field. *A,* With a weak field, the energy difference between the parallel and antiparallel states is small, so that protons tend to distribute nearly equally between the two alignments. *B,* With a stronger field, more protons tend to align in the lower energy parallel orientation, resulting in a larger net magnetization **M.**

strength. As a result, a significant excess of dipoles occupy the lower energy (parallel) state (Fig. 1–4*B*). Therefore, **M** also increases in direct proportion to external magnetic field strength.

THE ROLE OF RADIOFREQUENCY PULSES IN PRODUCING THE MR SIGNAL

The RF pulse represents the first step of a process by which **M** begins its transformation into a usable MR signal. There are two ways to look at this process: (1) at the level of an individual atom and (2) at the level of the group behavior of large numbers of atoms.

SINGLE ATOM (QUANTUM MECHANICAL VIEW)

How does the effect of a strong magnetic field tie in with the effect of an RF pulse? First, as discussed above, a magnetic field creates an energy difference (ΔE) between protons aligned with and against the magnetic field. Second, an RF pulse consists of packets of energy, called *photons;* the amount of energy in each packet depends on the frequency of the RF pulse. If the amount of energy in the photon, as determined by its frequency, matches ΔE, then, and only then, can a proton absorb energy from the RF pulse, which causes it to flip from the lower energy to the higher energy state (Fig. 1–5). This special frequency is called the Larmor or resonance frequency. It is a function of field strength and the type of nucleus, as expressed by

$$f_{Larmor} = \gamma B_0 \qquad (1)$$

where f_{Larmor} = resonance frequency (megahertz), B_0 = applied magnetic field strength (tesla), and γ = the gyromagnetic ratio, which can be defined in megahertz per tesla or radians per tesla. For instance, the resonance frequency of the hydrogen nucleus (γ = 42.58 MHz/T) at a field strength of 1 T is approximately 42.6 MHz and at 1.5 T is 64 MHz.

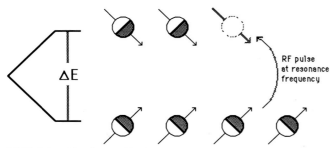

FIGURE 1–5. The application of an RF pulse at the resonance frequency causes some spins to flip from the parallel to antiparallel orientation.

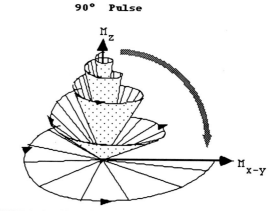

90° Pulse

FIGURE 1–6. Effect of a 90-degree pulse on the net magnetization **M** is to tilt **M** into the transverse plane. The combination of the tilt produced by the RF pulse with the precession of the spins results in a complex spiraling motion. Note that as **M** is rotated by 90 degrees, the M_z component is reduced to zero and M_{x-y} becomes equal to **M**.

GROUP BEHAVIOR OF ATOMS (CLASSIC VIEW)

Unlike an individual spin, which can have only two alignments, **M** may be oriented in any direction. In discussion of this magnetization, convention dictates that the direction of the main field (B_0) is called the *z-axis*. A plane perpendicular to the main field is called the *x-y* or *transverse plane*.

Prior to the application of an RF pulse, the protons are aligned along the z-axis. In the classic view, the RF pulse is an oscillating magnetic field. This magnetic field, called B_1, is produced by a radio antenna called a *transmitter coil*. In an MR system, the transmitter coil is designed and physically oriented so that its B_1 field is in the transverse plane, that is, perpendicular to **M**. When the RF pulse is applied, the effect of its B_1 field is to cause **M** to rotate away from its equilibrium alignment along the z-axis (Fig. 1–6).

The angle by which the RF pulse rotates **M** off the z-axis is called the *flip angle*. The flip angle increases with the amount of voltage or power in the RF pulse, which depends on the strength and duration of the RF pulse. Any flip angle can be applied. The choice of flip angle depends on the particular imaging method. For instance, in spin-echo pulse sequences, described further on, a 90-degree RF pulse is used to excite the protons. Provided that **M** is initially oriented along the z-axis, a 90-degree RF pulse rotates **M** completely into the transverse plane (Fig. 1–7). Small flip angles, used for gradient-echo pulse sequences (see Chapter 5), rotate only a portion of **M** into the transverse plane. As we now discuss, *this transverse component of **M** is responsible for the production of the MR signal.*

At this point, it is useful to introduce the concept of a rotating frame of reference. When viewed from the outside, the motion of the magnetization vectors appears complex because, as they tilt into the transverse plane, the vectors also wobble, or "precess,"

RF Pulses

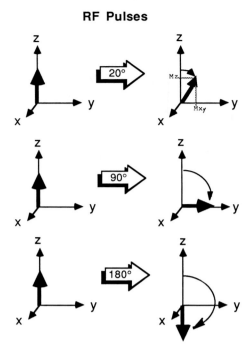

FIGURE 1–7. An RF pulse can be applied to produce any flip angle, depending on the strength and duration of the pulse. Note that in the rotating frame, as shown here, the effect of the RF pulse is to produce a simple tilt of the net magnetization **M,** unlike in Figure 1–6.

around the z-axis. To simplify the motion, one can imagine that the viewer is standing at the origin of the coordinate system, and rotates at the same rate as the magnetization vector as it precesses about the z-axis. As a result, the application of an RF pulse is seen to produce a simple tilt of the magnetization into the transverse plane or beyond (Fig. 1–7), rather than a spiraling motion.

Once the magnetization is in the transverse plane, **M** precesses about the direction of the main field, analogous to the precession of a spinning top that results when it is tilted from the vertical axis. The precession of the component of **M** in the transverse plane induces a voltage across the ends of a properly designed antenna, called a *receiver coil* (see further on) (Fig. 1–8). This voltage constitutes the MR signal.

The concept of *transverse magnetization* introduces an apparent paradox. An individual proton can be aligned in only one of two directions, either with or against the applied magnetic field. If this is so, how can a 90-degree RF pulse tilt the proton magnetization so that it is perpendicular to the magnetic field? This paradox results from attempting to describe the behavior of the macroscopic quantity **(M)** in terms of concepts that apply only to submicroscopic structures (individual protons). The paradox can be resolved by considering the average behavior of a large number of protons. As illustrated in Figure 1–9, the individual magnetization vectors of the protons, whether aligned with or against the magnetic field, are slightly tilted with respect to the z-axis (the direction of the field). Because of this, the

individual magnetization vectors have projections into the transverse plane. However, at equilibrium, there is no *net* magnetization in the x-y plane, because the transverse projections are randomly distributed, that is, lack *phase coherence.* Instead, **M** is aligned *directly* along the z-axis.

Now let us consider the effect of a 90-degree RF pulse. As discussed previously, the RF pulse flips some spins from a parallel to an antiparallel alignment. However, the RF pulse has an additional effect. Like the transaxle of a car, which locks the relative rotational positions of the right and left wheels, the RF pulse locks the phases of the magnetic moments into a coherent relationship. As a result, on the average, the *transverse* components of the individual magnetic moments have the same phase angle and add together to produce an **M** in the x-y plane. Therefore, even though no individual proton is ever aligned in the transverse plane, the **M** of large groups of protons can be.

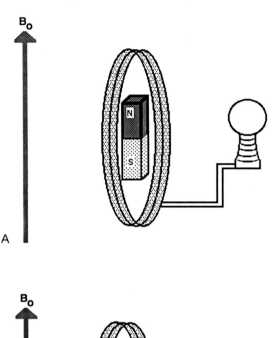

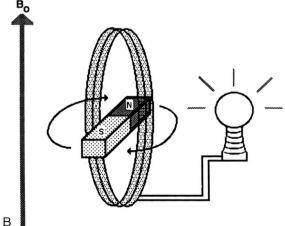

FIGURE 1–8. Production of an MR signal by the proton is analogous to the generation of electricity in a dynamo. *A,* With the net magnetization **M** aligned with B_0, there is no precession and therefore no signal. *B,* After a 90-degree RF pulse, **M** is aligned in the transverse plane. Precession of **M** induces an electrical voltage (MR signal) in a properly oriented antenna.

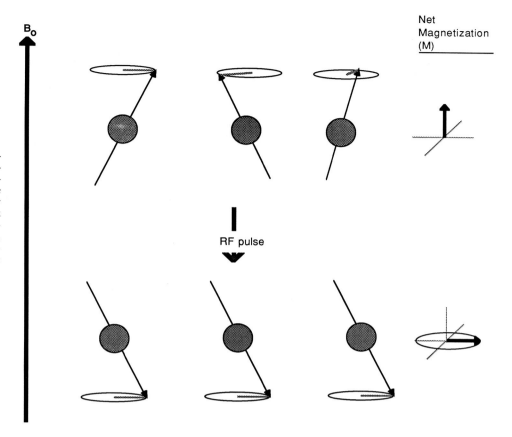

FIGURE 1–9. Prior to the application of an RF pulse, the projections of the individual magnetization vectors into the transverse plane (*stippled lines*) are randomly oriented, so that there is no net transverse magnetization. Immediately after a 90-degree RF pulse, the individual transverse projections have the same phase, so there is a net transverse magnetization.

FACTORS THAT AFFECT THE MR SIGNAL: RELAXATION AND OTHER TISSUE PARAMETERS

Several tissue-related factors influence the strength of the MR signal. The most important factors are the relaxation times, but other factors of importance include proton density, magnetic susceptibility, chemical shift, flow, and contrast agents. These factors are now considered in relation to their influence on the MR image.

RELAXATION (T_2 AND T_1)

Relaxation represents the process by which the spins respond to the perturbing effects of the RF pulse. There are two mechanisms by which this may occur: (1) T_2 relaxation and (2) T_1 relaxation. The duration of these processes, expressed by the T_2 and T_1 relaxation times, is dependent on certain physical and chemical characteristics of the tissue being imaged. Because the signal strength depends more directly on T_2 than T_1, we explain this relaxation mechanism first.

T_2 Relaxation

T_2 *relaxation* relates to the incoherent exchange of energy among neighboring spins. Because of this, it is also called *spin-spin relaxation*. To comprehend the process of T_2 relaxation, we must first consider the concept of *phase*. For this purpose, let us consider a simple analogy between the precession of **M** and the outcome of a track meet (Fig. 1–10).

At the instant immediately following the firing of the starter's gun, the runners are in identical positions at the starting line. As each runner moves around a circular tract, his or her radial position can be represented by the angle between him or her and the starting line; this angle is, in effect, the phase. If the runners are equally swift, they will maintain identical phase angles as they move around the track and are thus said to be phase coherent. However, some runners will usually move faster than others, and the phase angles of the faster runners would increase more rapidly than those of the other contestants. This difference in phase will increase as the race progresses. In MR terminology, this situation is called *dephasing* or *phase dispersion*.

If we liken the firing of the starter's gun to the application of a 90-degree RF pulse, then immediately after the RF pulse the transverse magnetization vectors from different nuclei are expected to have identical phases, resulting in a strong MR signal. However, local magnetic field inhomogeneities cause some nuclei to experience a slightly stronger magnetic field and others to experience a weaker field. By Equation 1, nuclei in the stronger field precess faster, and those in the weaker field, more slowly. As

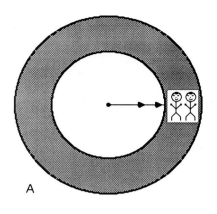

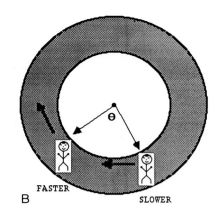

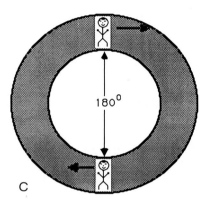

FIGURE 1–10. Analogy between proton phase and a track meet. *A,* At the start of the race, runners have the same phase. *B,* Because one runner is faster than the other, a phase angle (Θ) develops over time (i.e., partial dephasing). *C,* Eventually, the runners will be at opposite ends of the track (i.e., complete dephasing).

a result, the protons dephase, which results in a reduction in the net transverse magnetization. *The reduction in net transverse magnetization causes signal loss* (Figs. 1–11 and 1–12).

The local magnetic field inhomogeneities noted previously are produced by either of two factors: (1) microscopic effects due to magnetic interactions among neighboring molecules or (2) macroscopic effects due to spatial variation of the external magnetic field. Dephasing due to molecular interactions alone is called T_2. Dephasing produced by both factors taken together is termed T_2^*. T_2^* is always much shorter than T_2, resulting in more rapid loss of signal (Fig. 1–13).

T_2 or T_2^* represents a time constant, similar to the half-life used to express radioactive decay. The rate

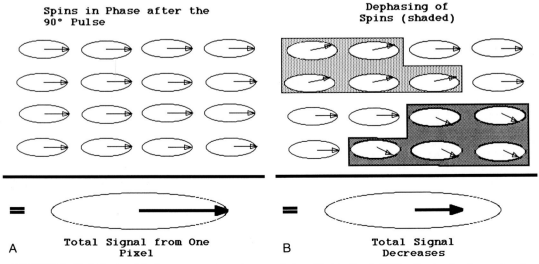

FIGURE 1–11. Relationship between proton phase and signal intensity. *A,* With all spins in phase, signals add to produce a large net signal. *B,* With some spins out of phase, net signal decreases.

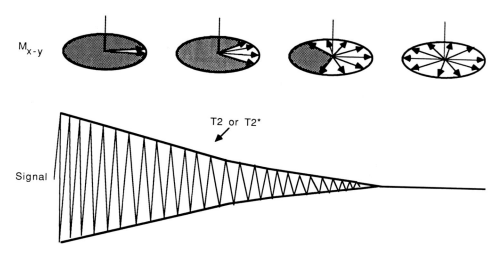

M_{x-y}

T2 or T2*

Signal

FIGURE 1–12. Relationship between signal decay and proton phase. Immediately after an RF pulse, all protons precess in phase, resulting in a strong signal. Over time, the protons dephase, and signal is lost at a rate characterized by T_2^* or, if a spin-echo is used, T_2.

of signal loss is usually an exponential function of time. There is 63 per cent decrease by one T_2 interval, 86 per cent after two T_2 intervals, and so on. The effect of T_2 relaxation time on signal intensity must be considered in the context of the way that the signal is measured. Signal is measured at a certain time interval following RF excitation. This time interval, which is user determined, is called the *echo time (TE)*. As TE is lengthened relative to T_2, more time is available for dephasing to occur and, based on T_2 effects, the signal intensity decreases (Fig. 1–14). For a given TE, the signal intensity of a tissue having a long T_2 will have decreased less than that of a tissue having a short T_2. For instance, the measured signal intensity of water, with a $T_2 > 2$ seconds, changes negligibly as the TE is lengthened from 15 to 30 msec. On the other hand, the signal intensity of liver, with a $T_2 < 50$ msec, decreases by nearly 50 per cent. Differences in T_2 relaxation times can be translated into image contrast by using pulse sequence timing parameters that emphasize T_2 effects. This type of pulse sequence is called T_2 *weighted*.

As will be discussed further on, gradient-echo sequences, which use only one RF pulse, are sensitive to T_2^* effects. However, in spin-echo sequences, the application of an additional 180-degree RF pulse after excitation results in the formation of a signal that is primarily sensitive to T_2 rather than T_2^* effects

(Fig. 1–15). In terms of our track meet analogy, the effect of the 180-degree RF pulse is to turn the runners about face. The result is that the runners arrive at the finish (starting) line nearly at the same time. In vector terminology, the effect of the 180-degree RF pulse is to rotate the vectors about the x- or y-axis, with the net result that the vectors are almost completely rephased at the TE (excluding T_2-related dephasing, which is irreversible).

Dephasing is not the only mechanism for relaxation of the proton magnetization. Because the protons are within a powerful magnetic field, they have a second relaxation mechanism relating to the realignment of the proton magnetization with this field. This is called T_1 relaxation.

T_1 Relaxation

T_1 *relaxation* involves the release of excess energy, absorbed by the spins from the RF pulse, to the molecular environment, or *lattice*. Therefore, it is also called *spin-lattice relaxation*. T_1 relaxation is most easily understood in terms of **M**. Assuming that **M** is initially aligned along the z-axis, a 90-degree RF pulse rotates **M** completely into the transverse plane, so that there is no longer a component of the vector along the z-axis. The T_1 relaxation time is an exponential time constant that relates to the period re-

FIGURE 1–13. Signal loss due to T_2^* decay is much more rapid than that due to T_2 decay.

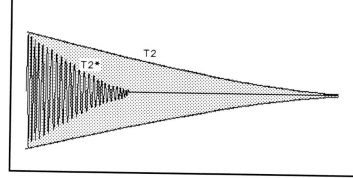

S
I
G
N
A
L

T2

T2*

TIME AFTER RF EXCITATION

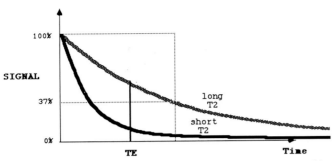

FIGURE 1–14. Signal strength versus time for two tissues with different T_2 relaxation times. Signal decays more slowly for the tissue with the longer T_2. Note that T_2 contrast initially increases and then decreases as the echo time (TE) is lengthened.

quired for the longitudinal, or z, component to recover from zero (its value immediately after the 90-degree RF pulse) to its maximal value (Fig. 1–16). There is 63 per cent recovery of complete alignment after one T_1 interval, 86 per cent after $2 \times T_1$, 95 per cent after $3 \times T_1$, and 99 per cent after $5 \times T_1$ (Fig. 1–17). One should note that this process of T_1 relaxation occurs simultaneously with the faster process of T_2 relaxation (Fig. 1–18).

MR images are not produced from a single excitation of the protons. The protons must be excited multiple times to produce enough data for the image. The time between excitations is called the *repetition time (TR)*. After several excitations, a balance is reached between the rate of T_1 relaxation and TR,

resulting in an equilibrium value for the longitudinal magnetization (Fig. 1–19). This value will be reduced from the maximal value, depending on the ratio of TR to T_1. The strength of the MR signal is proportional to the value of the longitudinal magnetization that existed at the instant before the RF pulse. If the TR is long, then the protons can fully realign between excitations and produce a strong signal (Fig. 1–20A). However, if the TR is short, then there is only partial realignment. Since protons must realign with the magnetic field before they can produce a signal, the signal strength is reduced (Fig. 1–20B). As a result, differences in T_1 relaxation times translate into differences in tissue signal (i.e., contrast).

For instance, fat has a short T_1 (200 to 300 msec). It therefore realigns quickly after an RF pulse and appears bright. Tumors have longer T_1 relaxation times (e.g., 1000 msec). They therefore recover more slowly and appear darker. Tissue contrast based on differences in T_1 relaxation times can be introduced into the image by using pulse sequence timing parameters that emphasize T_1 effects. This type of pulse sequence is called T_1 *weighted*.

MOLECULAR MECHANISMS FOR RELAXATION

T_1 and T_2 relaxation are complex processes that are enhanced by certain magnetic interactions among nuclei and molecules (see Chapter 6). There are several pathways by which T_1 and T_2 relaxation can

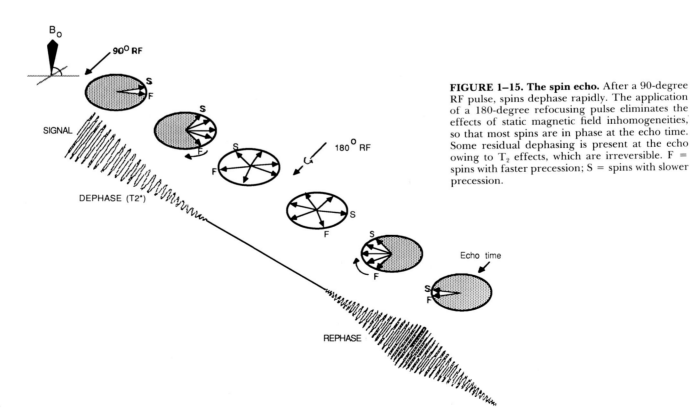

FIGURE 1–15. The spin echo. After a 90-degree RF pulse, spins dephase rapidly. The application of a 180-degree refocusing pulse eliminates the effects of static magnetic field inhomogeneities, so that most spins are in phase at the echo time. Some residual dephasing is present at the echo owing to T_2 effects, which are irreversible. F = spins with faster precession; S = spins with slower precession.

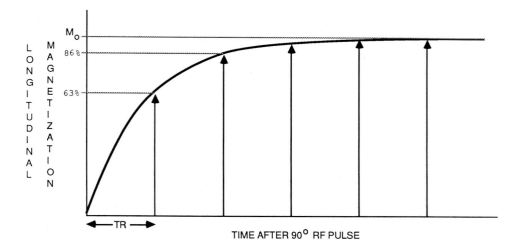

FIGURE 1–16. Longitudinal magnetization versus time after a 90-degree RF pulse. The longitudinal magnetization regrows toward the maximal value (M_0) at a rate determined by the T_1 relaxation time.

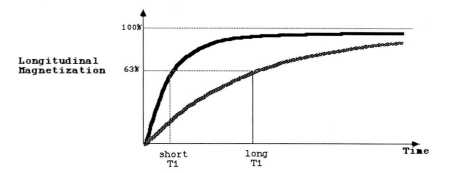

FIGURE 1–17. For two tissues, the longitudinal magnetization of the tissue with the shorter T_1 relaxation times regrows more quickly.

occur. Most of these processes depend on close interactions between water and other molecules.

All molecules, large and small, are in a constant state of motion, tumbling and colliding with other molecules. Each of these molecules has its own minute magnetic field. Intramolecular motion as well as interactions with nearby molecules produce fluctuations in the local magnetic field experienced by a proton. A small molecule such as water moves quickly, so that it produces rapid magnetic fluctuations. A large molecule such as protein moves slower

and produces magnetic fluctuations at a correspondingly low rate.

It turns out that these magnetic interactions can promote both T_1 and T_2 relaxation, but whether they do so depends on the rate at which the magnetic fields fluctuate. Another way of expressing this concept is in terms of the *correlation time* (τ_c), which represents the average time that two molecules remain in close proximity. With rapid molecular motion, the correlation times are short; conversely, with slow motion the correlation times are longer (Fig. 1–

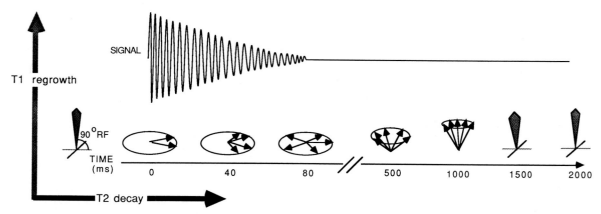

FIGURE 1–18. T_1 relaxation and T_2 relaxation are simultaneous processes. Note that T_2 relaxation is completed much more rapidly than T_1 relaxation.

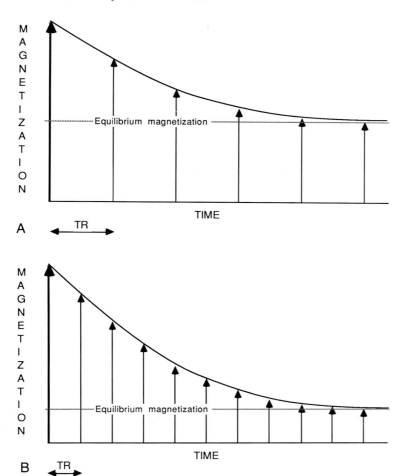

A

B

FIGURE 1–19. Effect of repetition time (TR) on longitudinal magnetization. After several RF pulses, an equilibrium is attained between TR and T_1 relaxation. *A,* With long TR, equilibrium magnetization is large. *B,* With short TR, equilibrium magnetization is smaller.

21). The effects of different rates of molecular motion can be sumarized as follows:

1. If the rate of fluctuation ($1/\tau_c$) is much higher than the resonance frequency of the water protons, then there is only mild enhancement of T_1 and T_2 relaxation. This situation exists in pure water, in which the molecules are moving very rapidly. As a result, both T_1 and T_2 are extremely long (seconds).

2. If the rate of fluctuation is slower, on the same order of magnitude as the resonance frequency, then both T_1 relaxation and T_2 relaxation are strongly promoted. This situation exists in certain proteinaceous solutions, in which the bulky protein molecules

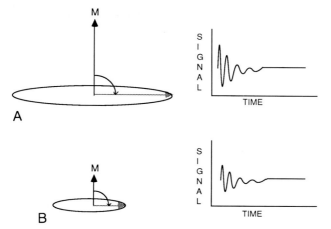

FIGURE 1–20. Longitudinal magnetization is translated by an RF pulse into signal strength. *A,* With a large longitudinal magnetization, signal strength is large. *B,* With a small longitudinal magnetization, signal strength is reduced.

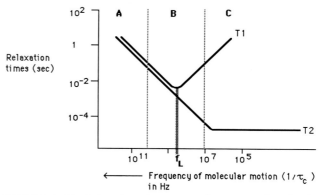

FIGURE 1–21. Relaxation time versus frequency of molecular motion ($1/\tau_c$). Free water has rapid diffusion and long T_1 and T_2 times (*region A*). Bound water associated with restricted motion has shorter T_1 and T_2 times (*region B*). Very restricted motion results in very short T_2 times (*region C*). f_L = Larmor frequency.

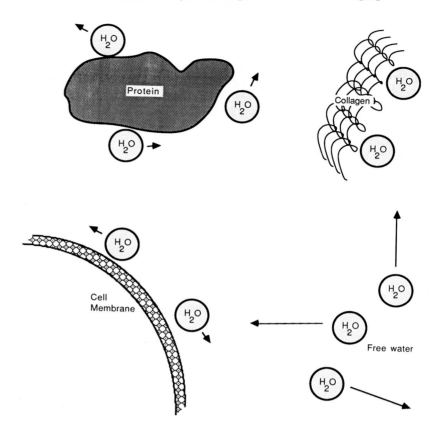

FIGURE 1–22. Effect of molecular motion on relaxation times. "Free" water (H_2O) molecules diffuse rapidly: T_1 and T_2 relaxation times are both long. The motion of "bound" water molecules associated with proteins and cell membranes is restricted; T_1 and T_2 relaxation times are shorter than those of free water. With very restricted motion, as, for example, with water molecules bound to collagen, T_2 relaxation times are very short.

move slowly and restrict the motion of nearby water molecules (Fig. 1–22).

3. If the rate of fluctuation is much lower than the resonance frequency, then only T_2 relaxation is promoted. This situation exists in tendons and chronic scar tissue, in which the motion of water molecules is severely restricted by the highly organized collagen fibrils and other substances.

It should be noted that slow molecular motions promote T_2, but not T_1, relaxation. Because of this additional relaxation mechanism, *T_2 relaxation is always faster than T_1 relaxation.* How much faster depends on the physical and chemical structure of the tissue. In pure water, there are relatively few molecules moving slowly. As a result, relaxation effects due to slow molecular motions are minimal, and T_2 relaxation times are nearly as long as T_1 relaxation times. However, in most tissues, which contain proteins as well as other components that restrict molecular motion, T_2 is much shorter than T_1 (typically tens of milliseconds versus hundreds of milliseconds) (Table 1–2).

Finally, one should note that a single tissue may have more than one T_1 and T_2 relaxation time. Signal decay from such a tissue will not fit a simple exponential. This multiexponential decay results from the complex molecular environment that is present to

TABLE 1–2. PROTON DENSITY, T_1, AND T_2 AS A FUNCTION OF MAGNETIC FIELD STRENGTH

Tissue	T_1				T_2	Proton Density (%)
	0.2 T*	0.3 T†	1.4 T‡	2.4 T§		
Fat	240	—	—	279	60	9.6
Gray matter	—	—	764	—	88	10.6
White matter	—	380	560	—	72	10.6
Cerebrospinal fluid (CSF)	—	1155	1527	—	140	10.8
Liver	380	—	—	570	40	9.7
Muscle	400	—	—	1023	50	9.3
Spleen	420	—	—	701	20	9.8
Pancreas	290	—	—	605	60	9.8
Bone marrow	—	320	—	554	—	—

*From Rupp, Reiser, Stetter: Eur J Radiol 3:68–76, 1983.
†From Wehrli FW, MacFall JR, Newton TH: Parameters determining the appearance of NMR images. *In* Newton TH, Potts DG (eds): Advanced Imaging Techniques. Vol II. San Anselmo, CA, Clavadel Press, 1983.
‡From Wehrli et al: *In* Peterson SB, et al (eds): An Introduction of Biomedical NMR. New York, Thieme, 1985.
§From Damadian R, Zaner K, Hor D, Di Maio T: Human tumors detected by NMR. Proc Natl Acad Sci USA 71:1471, 1974.

some extent in nearly all tissues. In some regions of the tissue, water molecules may be relatively free in solution, whereas in other regions water molecules are bound to proteins, lipids, cell membranes, and so forth. Moreover, these regions may exist within the same voxel (i.e., volume element) or even within the same cell.

DEPENDENCE OF T_1 RELAXATION TIMES ON FIELD STRENGTH

As just discussed, T_1 relaxation depends on the presence of magnetic fields at the molecular level, whose rate of fluctuation approximates the resonance frequency of tissue protons. However, the resonance frequency is proportional to field strength, whereas molecular motions are independent of the magnet. As the resonance frequency increases, fewer molecular collisions produce magnetic field fluctuations at the higher rates required to promote T_1 relaxation. As a result, T_1 relaxation times increase with field strength.

T_2 relaxation depends primarily on molecular interactions that occur at a lower rate than the resonance frequency. Increases in resonance frequency have little effect on this relaxation pathway. As a result, T_2 relaxation times are relatively independent of field strength.

For imaging, the field strength dependence of T_1 relaxation times has an important bearing on choice of pulse sequence and image contrast. Pulse sequences that produce high-contrast images at one field strength may produce images with poor contrast at another field strength. However, if one takes into account the differences in T_1 relaxation times and adjusts the scan parameters accordingly, then it is fair to say that high-contrast images can be obtained at almost any field strength.

Although the T_1 relaxation times of all tissues increase with field strength, the T_1 increase depends on the type of tissue.[13] It is interesting to note that the T_1 relaxation time of fat does not increase as much as that of other tissues, because of the different molecular composition of fat (Table 1–2). Because signal intensity is inversely related to the T_1 relaxation time, *fat appears brighter relative to other tissues as the field strength increases.* This observation would be of little practical importance, except that motion produces certain types of artifacts, called *ghosts*, that degrade image quality. Because the motion of a bright structure typically produces worse artifacts than the motion of a dark one (see Chapter 3), the motion of fat at high field strengths produces worse ghost artifacts than it does at lower field strengths.

CORRELATION OF T_1 AND T_2 RELAXATION TIMES

As just discussed, water molecules can move freely (free water), or their motion can be slowed by protein molecules, cell membranes, or other substances (bound water). Many types of pathology are associated with an increase in the free water content. Moreover, T_1 and T_2 relaxation times tend to be positively correlated, in that they both increase with free water content. This increase results in signal changes that often permit the ready distinction of pathologic from normal tissues (Table 1–3).[14]

Although T_1 and T_2 relaxation times change in the same direction in response to changes in free water content, their effects on image signal intensity are opposite. As T_1 increases, signal intensity *decreases;* however, as T_2 increases, signal intensity also *increases.* If a pulse sequence was selected that produced equal T_1 and T_2 weighting, then, in pathologic tissues, the

TABLE 1–3. SUMMARY OF SIGNAL INTENSITIES ON MR IMAGES

Tissue	T_1 Weighted	T_2 Weighted
Fat	Very bright	Intermediate-dark
Cysts		
Watery fluid	Very dark	Very bright
Proteinaceous fluid	Intermediate-bright	Very bright
Brain		
White matter	Bright	Mod. dark
Gray matter	Mod. dark	Mod. bright
CSF	Very dark	Very bright
Bone marrow		
Yellow	Very bright	Intermediate-dark
Red*	Mod. bright	Mod. dark
Cortical bone	Very dark	Very dark
Cartilage		
Fibrocartilage	Very dark	Very dark
Hyaline†	Intermediate	Intermediate
Intervertebral disk		
Normal†	Intermediate	Bright
Degenerated	Intermediate-dark	Dark
Osteophyte		
Marrow-containing*	Mod. bright	Intermediate-dark
Calcified only	Dark	Dark
Tendons/ligaments	Very dark	Very dark
Muscle	Dark	Dark
Lung	Very dark	Very dark
Liver		
Normal parenchyma	Mod. bright	Dark
Metastasis	Dark	Mod. bright
Hemangioma	Dark	Bright
Pancreas	Mod. bright	Dark
Spleen	Dark	Mod. bright
Contrast-enhanced tissue		
Gadolinium-DTPA		
Low concentration	Very bright	Bright
High concentration	Intermediate-dark	Very dark
Ferrite	Dark	Very dark
Fluosol	Very dark	Very dark
Blood flow	Bright or dark	Bright or dark
Hematoma‡		
Acute	Intermediate-dark	Dark
Subacute	Bright rim	Bright
Chronic	Dark rim, ± bright center	Dark rim, ± bright center

*Dark on phase-contrast proton density–weighted spin-echo or gradient-echo image.
†Bright on proton density–weighted gradient-echo image.
‡Low signal due to magnetic susceptibility effects predominantly seen on high-field images.
Mod. = moderately.

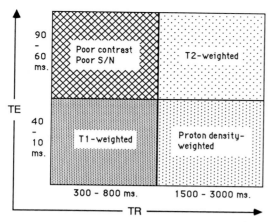

FIGURE 1-23. Simplified representation of image contrast as a function of TR and TE.

signal decrease produced by the long T_1 would be opposed by the signal increase produced by the long T_2, resulting in an intermediate signal that might be difficult to distinguish from the signal of normal tissue (Fig. 1-23).

Therefore, it is prudent to select pulse sequences that are weighted toward *either* T_1 or T_2, to maximize the image contrast between normal and pathologic tissues. With conventional spin-echo imaging methods, a rule of thumb for image interpretation is that T_1-weighted images generally depict pathologic tissues as less bright than normal tissues; on T_2-weighted images, diseased tissue usually appears brighter than normal tissue. Which type of contrast proves most clinically useful depends upon both the organ system and the specific pathologic process being evaluated. Contrast mechanisms are considered further on in greater detail.

PROTON DENSITY

Proton density (ρ or N[H]) contributes significantly to contrast with certain pulse sequences. Proton density represents the number of MR-visible protons in a unit volume of tissue and is usually expressed as a percentage of the proton density of water. Proton density generally increases with water content.

Images can be obtained that are selectively weighted to emphasize the proton density characteristics of a tissue (Fig. 1-23). T_1 and T_2 relaxation times may vary among tissues by tens or hundreds of per cent. On the other hand, proton density, like electron density in computed tomographic (CT) images, varies among different tissues by only a few per cent (Table 1-2). As such, images weighted toward proton density tend to produce only modest levels of tissue contrast.

The quality of being MR visible has great significance in MR imaging. Protons in solid materials, such as cortical bone and dense calcifications, produce no signal on MR images. The reason that solids in general produce no signal is that the protons in these

materials are essentially frozen in position. Each proton is therefore constantly exposed to potent dephasing influences from nearby protons, which are also fixed in position. The end result is that T_2 relaxation times in solids are extremely short, on the order of microseconds. The MR signals from these protons decay too quickly to be observed in a conventional MR imaging experiment. However, although it is generally true that cortical bone and calcifications are not directly observed, they may produce a visible signal when the calcium is hydrated owing to the presence of associated free water.

The fact that cortical bone fails to produce an MR signal does not preclude its being imaged by MR. For example, within a vertebral body, low signal from cortical bone is outlined by contiguous higher signal from medullary bone and adjacent disk material. Many types of bone pathology, including fractures and tumor invasion, are clearly demonstrated by increased signal from soft tissue hemorrhage or edema, which replaces the very low signal of normal cortical bone. However, the fine detail of cortical bone is often inferior to that demonstrated by plain films and CT. Calcifications are also poorly shown by conventional MR imaging methods, although it has recently been demonstrated that the use of gradient-echo pulse sequences can enhance the detection of soft tissue calcification by virtue of magnetic susceptibility effects (see Chapter 5).

SPATIAL LOCALIZATION OF THE MR SIGNAL

With current MR systems, images can be obtained with a spatial resolution competitive with that of CT and ultrasonography. However, it is impossible to collimate radio waves as one can collimate x-rays and sound waves. Furthermore, these other modalities use wavelengths in the submillimeter range, whereas MR imaging uses radio waves with wavelengths on the order of meters. How, then, is submillimeter resolution achieved by MR imaging?

One may consider the uniform B_0 field, in which all nuclei resonate at the same frequency, to be analogous to an untuned harp with all its strings identical in pitch (Fig. 1-24). In listening to such an instrument, one could not tell which harp string was plucked to produce a particular pitch. The situation is different for a properly tuned harp. Just as middle C and concert A have unique, well-defined positions on a harp, so, too, the application of a position-dependent change in the magnetic field, called a gradient, tunes the resonance frequencies according to position along that gradient.

EFFECT OF A MAGNETIC FIELD GRADIENT

A magnetic field gradient is a weak magnetic field, at most a few per cent as strong as the main external

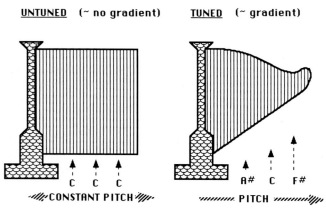

FIGURE 1–24. Application of a magnetic field gradient has a function analogous to the tuning of a harp.

field, that is produced by coils positioned within the magnet bore. For instance, a typical gradient might produce a peak magnetic field difference of 10 milli-tesla (mT) across a distance of 1 meter. This value compares with main field strengths up to 1500 mT. The magnetic field produced by the gradient coils differs in another important respect from the main field. Unlike the highly uniform main field, the magnetic fields produced by the gradient coils are spatially dependent.

The gradient (G) produces a positional change (Δf) in the resonance frequency, expressed as

$$\Delta f = \gamma \, (G \cdot x) \qquad (2a)$$

where x = position along the gradient. When the gradient is superimposed on the main field (Fig. 1–25), the resonance frequencies assume unique values, depending on the position along the gradient, as expressed by

$$f_{Larmor} = \gamma \, B_0 + \gamma \, (G \cdot x) \qquad (2b)$$

There are several methods available for providing spatial localization. The most commonly used methods include two-dimensional Fourier transform (2DFT) and three-dimensional Fourier transform (3DFT) imaging. We consider 2D methods first, since 3D methods are merely an elaboration of 2D techniques.

TWO-DIMENSIONAL IMAGING METHODS

In 2DFT imaging, different methods are employed to localize nuclei along the three orthogonal axes (Fig. 1–26A): (1) one gradient is applied with the RF pulse to choose a slice; (2) a second gradient encodes location along one in-plane dimension in the frequency of the MR signal; and (3) a third gradient encodes location along the other in-plane dimension in the phase of the MR signal. Because of the alteration or so-called "twisting of phase" used for spatial localization in this method, it is also called *spin warp*.

For convenience, we sometimes refer to the slice-selection direction as "z," the frequency-encoding direction as "x," and the phase-encoding direction as "y." However, this designation is arbitrary and is unrelated to the physical orientation of the x, y, and z gradient coils. The x,y,z coordinate system is oriented differently for different planes of section (i.e., axial, sagittal, coronal, and oblique).

Slice Selection

When the slice-selection gradient is applied, the resonance frequencies of the tissue protons become linearly related to position along the z-axis (Fig. 1–27). Individual resonance frequencies correspond to individual planes of nuclei; these planes are oriented perpendicular to the z-axis. If an RF pulse of a specific frequency is applied while the slice-selection gradient is activated, only nuclei in the plane corresponding to that frequency resonate.

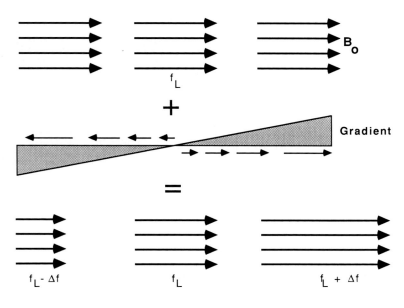

FIGURE 1–25. Gradient magnetic field superimposed on the main field (B_0) produces a positional variation in the local magnetic field strength and resonance frequencies (Δf). As a result, the resonance frequencies of the tissue nuclei depend on position. f_L = resonance frequency without gradient.

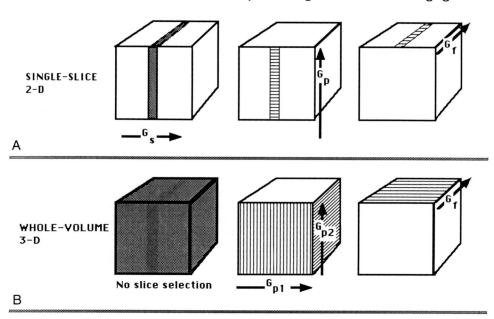

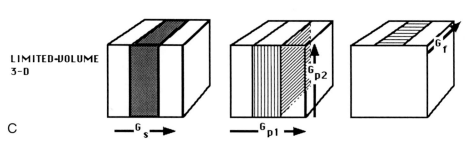

FIGURE 1–26. *A–C,* Comparison between spatial localization methods for 2DFT and 3DFT imaging.

▨▨▨ :	Volume excited by RF pulse(s)
⊪⊪⊪ :	Direction of spatial encoding
G_s :	Slice-selection gradient
G_p :	Phase-encoding gradient
G_f :	Frequency-encoding (read-out) gradient

Slice Position

The location of the center of the excited plane depends on the center frequency of the slice-selecting

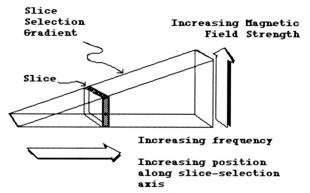

FIGURE 1–27. In the presence of the slice-selection gradient, the application of an RF pulse at a specific frequency excites tissue nuclei in a single slice.

RF pulse. The location of the excited plane can be shifted in the $+z$- or $-z$-direction by increasing or decreasing the frequency of the RF pulse. On commercial MR systems, this frequency shift is produced by a process called *sideband modulation* (see Chapters 10 and 12).

Slice Thickness

An RF pulse actually contains not a single frequency, but a spread of frequencies called the *pulse bandwidth.* As a result, an RF pulse excites a slice of tissue having a finite thickness. The slice thickness depends on the ratio of two factors: (1) the strength of the slice-selection gradient and (2) the bandwidth of the RF pulse (see Chapter 10).

As the slice-selection gradient strength is increased, the range of frequencies across the slice is also increased. As a result, an RF pulse with a fixed bandwidth will excite fewer spins, and the slice thickness is decreased. Conversely, a weak slice-selection gradient and the same RF pulse will produce a thick slice. Another way to alter the slice thickness would be to modify the bandwidth of the RF pulse. Although this is sometimes done, in most systems the slice thickness is primarily adjusted by changing the strength of the slice-selection gradient.

Multislice Imaging

If only a single slice could be excited during each TR interval, the imaging time for a complete examination would be prohibitively long. Fortunately, there is considerable dead-time between each read-out period and the next excitation, during which time the system is idle. Within this idle period, excitation and read-out of additional slices can be performed (Fig. 1–28). The maximal number of slices that can be acquired depends on several variables, as expressed by

$$\text{Number of slices} = \text{TR}/(\text{TE} + \Delta) \qquad (3)$$

where Δ is a lumped, system-dependent factor that is related to the pulse sequence structure and performance constraints of the gradients, RF, and measurement systems.

Frequency Encoding

Spatial localization is performed in one of the two in-plane dimensions during read-out of the MR signal. During the read-out period, spatial position along the x-axis is encoded into the frequency content of the signal by applying the frequency-encoding gradient. The effect of this gradient is to tune the resonance frequencies of the nuclei like the previously mentioned harp strings, and therefore the frequencies of the signals they produce, according to spatial position.

During read-out, the signal is measured as a series of brief samples; the number of samples (typically 256) determines the number of pixels along the x-direction. The read-out period, or *sampling time*, has a duration that can vary widely but typically assumes values from 5 to 30 msec. During this period, the analog-to-digital converter (ADC) is activated, converting the time-varying signal voltage into digital data that can be handled by the computer.

The frequency of the MR signal is in megahertz. However, the hardware used to analyze the MR signal is designed to operate in the kilohertz ("audio") range, just like the components used in home stereo equipment. To convert (demodulate) the MR signal into the proper frequency range, the center frequency of the MR system (e.g., 64 MHz at 1.5 T) is essentially subtracted from the MR signal prior to signal analysis.

Phase Encoding

In any cross-sectional imaging modality such as CT or MR imaging, multiple spatial projections of an object are required to reconstruct an image of that object. In CT, projections are acquired by physically rotating an x-ray fan beam. In MR imaging, two types of projections are acquired: (1) by encoding spatial position in the frequency of the MR signal, as just discussed, and (2) by encoding spatial position in the phase of the signal.

Phase encoding is performed by briefly applying the phase-encoding gradient during the time interval between RF excitation and signal read-out. The phase-encoding gradient imposes a linear relationship between precessional frequency and position (Fig. 1–29). Nuclei accumulate phase shifts (Θ) that are determined by their relative precessional frequencies, as expressed by

$$\Theta = \gamma \, \text{Gyt}$$

where G = magnitude of phase-encoding gradient,

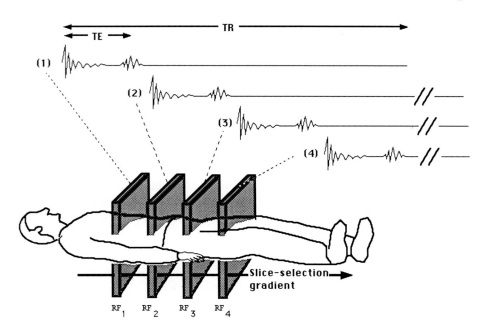

FIGURE 1–28. Sequential application of multiple RF pulses (RF$_1$, RF$_2$, and so on) at different frequencies results in excitation of multiple slices. The number of slices that can be acquired depends on TR, TE, and other factors.

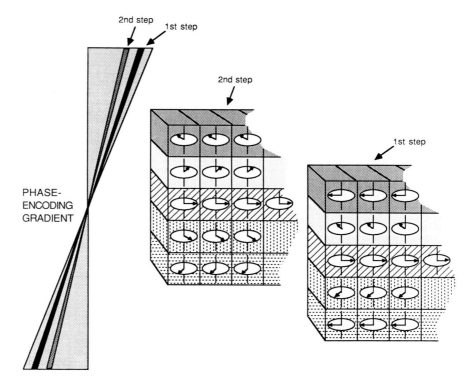

FIGURE 1–29. Principle of phase encoding. The application of a phase-encoding gradient imposes a spatial dependence on proton phase. Different phase-encoding steps use different gradient amplitudes. Note that protons at the center of the gradient experience no phase change.

t = gradient duration, and y = position along the gradient. By the mechanism demonstrated in our track meet analogy, nuclei in a stronger region of the gradient precess faster, and the transverse magnetization of these nuclei accumulates a proportionately larger phase shift, than those in a weaker region of the gradient.

As soon as the phase-encoding gradient is inactivated, the nuclei revert to the resonance frequency determined by the main magnetic field. However, the accumulated phase shifts are retained as a "memory" of their position along the phase-encoding gradient. The spatial variation in phase produces loss of coherence, which is manifested during the read-out period as a reduction in signal intensity and distortion of the signal waveform.

So far, we have considered the effect of a single application of the phase-encoding gradient. However, phase encoding differs from frequency encoding and slice selection in a fundamental way, in that multiple steps are required to encode spatial information fully in the signal phase. After each repetition of the sequence, the strength of the phase-encoding gradient is incremented by an identical amount. Each repetition yields one line of uniquely phase-encoded data, and the combination of these lines of data allows the FT to determine position along the y-direction (Fig. 1–30). The number of phase-encoding steps usually determines the number of pixels along the y-axis; for example, 128 steps produce a matrix with 128 pixels in the y-direction.

In summary, there are three different steps required to resolve 2DFT images spatially in all three dimensions (Fig. 1–31).

Fourier Transform

The measured MR signal represents the sum of the signals from innumerable individual nuclei. This composite signal continuously varies in amplitude as a function of *time*. However, the positions of nuclei are encoded in the *frequency* content of the signal. To extract the individual frequency components (frequency domain) from the time-varying signal (temporal domain), the computer employs a mathematical operation, the FT (Fig. 1–32). The FT performs an operation for the computer in decoding MR signals analogous to that of the basilar membrane of the human cochlea in processing sound.

The FT is applied to each line of data to extract the frequency content of the signal and thereby determine spatial position along the x-axis. After all the phase-encoding steps have been performed, the FT is again applied. Now, however, the transform is applied to all lines of data simultaneously to extract the phase information and thereby determine position along the y-axis.

Signal Averaging

Commonly, it is necessary to average data measured during multiple data acquisitions or excitations to improve signal-to-noise (S/N). S/N improves with $\sqrt{NEX}$, where NEX = number of excitations. Background noise due to certain types of artifacts, such as those resulting from periodic motion, also improves approximately in proportion to $\sqrt{NEX}$.

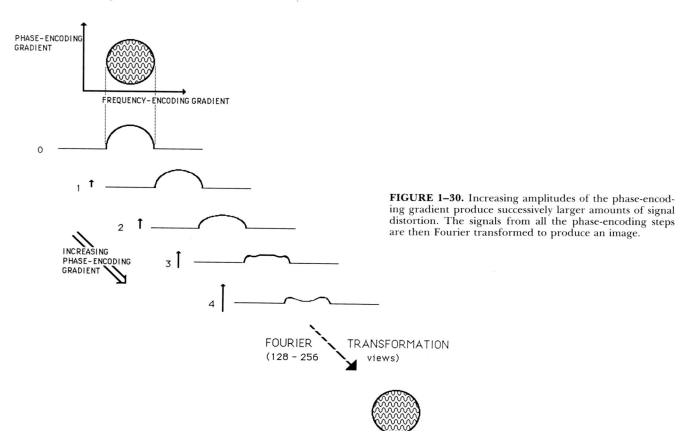

FIGURE 1–30. Increasing amplitudes of the phase-encoding gradient produce successively larger amounts of signal distortion. The signals from all the phase-encoding steps are then Fourier transformed to produce an image.

A penalty must be paid for signal averaging: increased imaging time. This is expressed as

$$\text{Imaging time} = \text{TR} \times \text{N}_\text{y} \times \text{NEX} \qquad (4)$$

where N_y = number of phase-encoding steps. For instance, the imaging time for an image with a TR of 500 msec, 128 phase-encoding steps, and two excitations is 128 seconds; with four excitations, the imaging time would be 256 seconds.

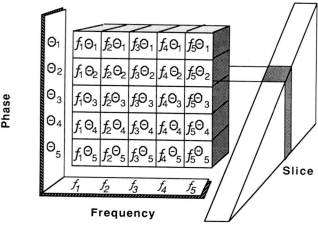

FIGURE 1–31. Summary of spatial localization in 2DFT imaging.

THREE-DIMENSIONAL IMAGING

For most clinical applications, data are acquired using multislice 2DFT methods. In certain applications, it is advantageous to perform a 3D data acquisition. The 3D methods involve excitation and acquisition of data simultaneously from a large volume or slab (see Fig. 1–26B and C), unlike 2D methods, which acquire data from individual slices. Furthermore, 3D methods phase encode spatial information along the slice-selection (z) direction, in addition to the y-direction. As with 2DFT imaging, spatial localization along the x-direction is obtained by frequency encoding during the read-out period. Reconstruction of 3D data requires a 3DFT algorithm, rather than the usual 2DFT method.

The relatively long imaging times for 3D scans generally preclude using conventional spin-echo pulse sequences. However, in conjunction with reduced excitation flip angles, gradient-echo pulse sequences permit much shorter TR to be used (e.g., ≤30 msec), which reduces the imaging time for 3D data to just a few minutes. The 3D gradient-echo acquisitions are finding increasing use in high-resolution imaging of the musculoskeletal system and in MR angiography (see Chapters 4 and 5).

An advantage of 3DFT methods, compared with 2DFT, is that they use a weaker slice-selection gradient for a given slice thickness. This feature permits very thin (e.g., ≤1 mm) sections to be acquired, which

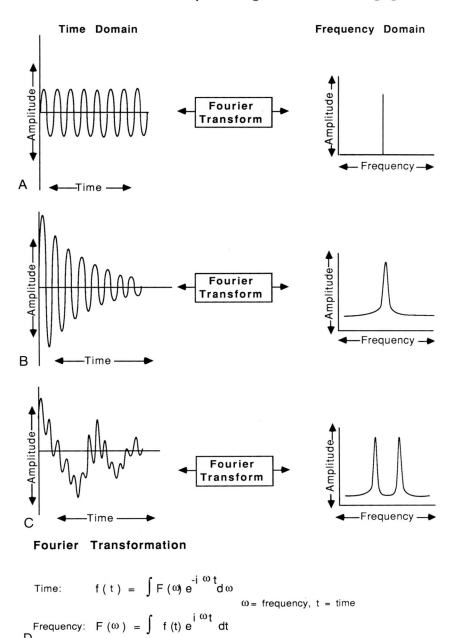

FIGURE 1–32. Fourier transform (FT). *A*, FT of a sine wave yields a single frequency. *B*, FT of an MR signal from a single proton. *C*, FT of an MR signal from two spins in different positions. *D*, Mathematical notation for the FT.

is generally not possible with 2DFT methods owing to limitations of the gradients and RF system. In addition, 3D acquisitions produce essentially contiguous slices, which is often not the case with 2DFT methods because of imperfect slice profiles. Because the images are thin and contiguous, 3D data allow high-quality images to be reconstructed along any arbitrary plane of section.

There are two types of 3DFT acquisitions: (1) *isotropic*, meaning equal spatial resolution along all three dimensions of the volume element (*voxel*), and (2) *anisotropic*, meaning lower spatial resolution along the slice-selection dimension. In both types of 3D methods, a relatively thick slab is initially excited. This slab is then subdivided into a number of thin slices, or *partitions*, by phase encoding along the z-

direction. The number of partitions is equal to the number of phase-encoding steps. The imaging time for a 3D data set increases with the number of partitions, as expressed by

$$\text{Imaging time} = \text{TR} \times N_y \times N_z \times \text{NEX} \qquad (5)$$

where N_z = number of z-phase–encoding steps. Criteria for selecting 3D scan parameters are discussed in Chapter 2.

FACTORS THAT AFFECT THE MR SIGNAL: PULSE SEQUENCES

T_1, T_2, and proton density are intrinsic tissue parameters over which the user has no control.

However, the operator can alter tissue contrast and S/N by the choice of pulse sequence. Pulse sequence design is considered in depth in Chapter 10. Our main concern here is to introduce the various types of pulse sequences and to explain the underlying physical principles and clinical applications.

A pulse sequence represents a series of RF and gradient pulses used to produce a spatially localized signal. Pulse sequences must be repeated multiple times to obtain enough data to form an image. The TR (repetition time) is defined as the time from the center of the first RF pulse in one repetition of the sequence to the center of the first RF pulse in the next repetition of the sequence. The signal is measured over a time interval called the *read-out period*. The time at which the signal is measured is the TE (echo time). The TE is typically defined as the time that elapses between the center of the first RF pulse and the center of the echo.

TYPES OF MR SIGNALS

Different combinations of RF pulses can be used to produce different types of MR signals. Only a few of these are routinely used for imaging. The types of signals are summarized in Table 1–4.

The *free induction decay (FID)* represents the signal that is produced immediately after an RF pulse. This signal is not directly used for MR imaging because time must be allowed for gradients to be applied in order to produce a spatially localized signal.

To produce a useful signal for MR imaging, the signal is actually measured as an echo of the FID. The echo appears at a certain time after the FID, as determined by the pulse sequence. Two strategies are routinely used to create such an echo: (1) application of an additional 180-degree RF pulse to produce a spin echo and (2) application of a gradient reversal, used to produce a gradient echo. Methods for producing these signals, as well as their clinical applications, are now reviewed.

SPIN ECHO

In its most basic form, the *spin-echo pulse sequence* (Fig. 1–33) consists of two RF pulses, 90 degrees and

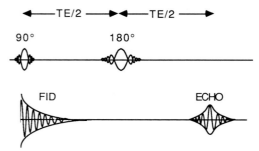

FIGURE 1–33. Simplified diagram of spin-echo pulse sequence.

180 degrees, separated in time by equal intervals of TE/2:

$$90 \text{ degrees -- TE/2 -- } 180 \text{ degrees -- TE/2 --}$$
$$\text{(spin echo)}$$

The 90-degree RF pulse excites the protons and produces an FID signal. The 180-degree RF pulse refocuses the transverse magnetization so that dephasing effects from static magnetic field inhomogeneities, due to the magnet or local differences in magnetic susceptibility, are canceled at the TE. As a result, the image is T_2 weighted, rather than T_2^* weighted.

In a spin-echo pulse sequence, additional 180-degree RF pulses can be applied to generate multiple echoes (Fig. 1–34), with no increase in scanning time unless the TR must be lengthened to accommodate the additional echoes, as expressed by Equation 3. The benefit of multiecho sequences is that the additional echoes provide better image display of T_2 tissue characteristics. For example, a tissue such as liver, which appears bright on an early echo but dark on later echoes, can be inferred to have a short T_2. Conversely, a tissue such as cerebrospinal fluid (CSF), which appears bright on late as well as early echoes, must have a long T_2. Images obtained with long TE can help discriminate between tumor and surrounding edema.

Contrast mechanisms in spin-echo images are discussed further on in detail. Briefly, images can be obtained in which tissue contrast is primarily determined by (i.e., weighted toward) T_1, proton density, or T_2 characteristics. This contrast relationship can be summarized (see Fig. 1–23) as follows:

TABLE 1–4. TYPES OF SIGNALS MEASURED IN MR

Signal	No. of RF Pulses	How Signal is Produced	Comments
Free induction decay	1 (90 degrees)	Magnetization rotated into x-y plane	Very short TE Poorly suited for imaging
Gradient echo	1 (α)	Same as above + gradient reversal	Fast imaging Flow imaging Bad artifacts from B_0 inhomogeneity
Spin echo	2 (90 degrees, 180 degrees)	Same as above + gradient reversal + RF refocusing	Routine clinical use Insensitive to B_0 inhomogeneity

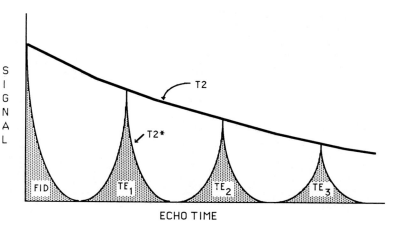

FIGURE 1–34. Signal decay in multiecho spin-echo acquisition.

1. Images acquired with *short TR* (TR $\sim$ T_1) and *short TE* (TE $<$ T_2) are T_1 *weighted* (Fig. 1–35A).

2. Images acquired with *long TR* (TR $>>$ T_1) and *short TE* (TE $<$ T_2) are called *proton density–weighted* or *balanced images* (Fig. 1–35B).

3. Images acquired with *long TR* and *long TE* (TE $\sim$ T_2) are T_2 *weighted* (Fig. 1–35C).

On T_1-weighted images, tissues that have short T_1, such as fat, appear bright, whereas tissues that have long T_1, such as tumors and edema, appear dark. On T_2-weighted images, tissues with long T_2, such as tumors, edema, and cysts, appear bright, whereas tissues that have short T_2, such as muscle and liver, appear dark. On proton density–weighted images, tissues with increased proton density appear moderately bright. Note should be made that both T_1- and T_2-weighted images always are partly weighted toward proton density as well.

GRADIENT ECHO

Gradient-echo pulse sequences bearing abbreviations such as FLASH, GRASS, and FISP use only a single RF pulse, as represented by

$$\alpha \text{ -- TE -- (gradient-echo)}$$

where α is an RF pulse with a flip angle less than 90 degrees. The formation of an echo with these sequences requires the application of two gradient pulses (Fig. 1–36). For instance, the application of the frequency-encoding gradient during the echo immediately dephases the spins along the x-direction. To correct for this dephasing, an inverted gradient pulse is first applied prior to read-out, which produces a compensatory phase shift of opposite sign. The first pulse is called a *dephasing gradient,* and the second pulse a *rephasing gradient.* The pair of dephasing and rephasing gradients constitutes a *gradient reversal,* which results in the formation of a gradient echo at the echo time.

Despite their simple structure, gradient-echo pulse sequences produce images with complex contrast behavior, a phenomenon considered in depth in Chapter 5. We consider only a few of the major features here, those relating to the use of a reduced excitation flip angle and the absence of a 180-degree refocusing RF pulse:

1. Unlike conventional spin-echo pulse sequences, which use a 90-degree flip angle for excitation, the flip angle may be freely varied for gradient-echo imaging. Small flip angles only slightly reduce the longitudinal magnetization (see Fig. 1–7), so that spins can almost fully remagnetize between RF pulses, even with short TR. As a result, faster imaging is possible than with spin-echo sequences. The reduced flip angle also affects contrast. Because T_1 effects are diminished with small flip angles, these images are predominantly weighted toward proton density. Since the effects of T_1 differences on the longitudinal magnetization become more pronounced as the flip angle is increased, gradient-echo images acquired with short TR and large flip angles are predominantly T_1 weighted.

Although the reduced flip angle provides less signal per measurement than a 90-degree RF pulse, when short TRs are used, this is more than compensated for by the larger number of signals that are measured per second. With gradient-echo techniques, high-quality scans can be obtained in as little as 1 second. This feature is useful for the imaging of dynamic processes, such as cardiac motion, contrast enhancement, and blood flow, and for the reduction of motion artifact.

2. Because gradient-echo sequences lack a refocusing RF pulse, images generated with these sequences are sensitive to artifacts from magnetic field inhomogeneities (i.e., T_2^* effects). On the other hand, this sensitivity can be used to advantage. Hemorrhage and calcification can produce variations in local magnetic field homogeneity (magnetic susceptibility effects), leading to localized signal loss on gradient-echo scans. This signal behavior often improves the detectability of these lesions.

3. Signal from flowing blood is increased com-

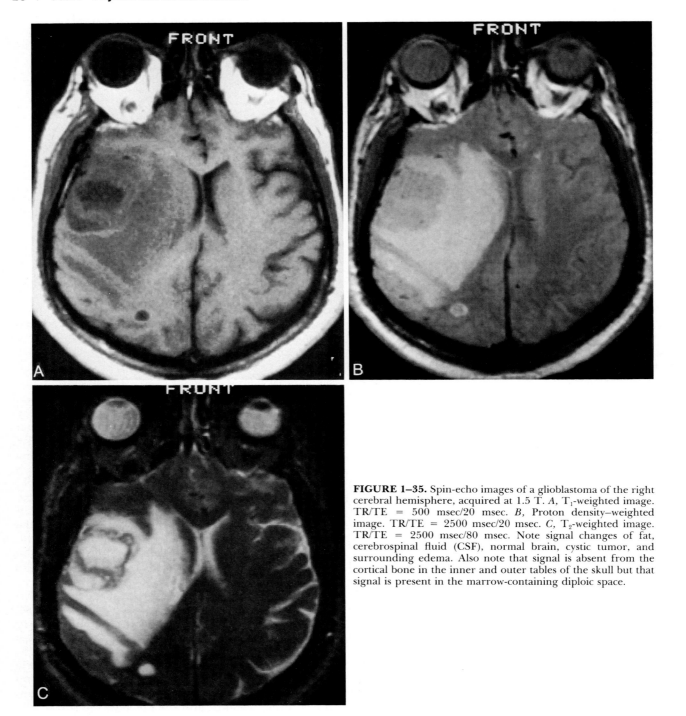

FIGURE 1–35. Spin-echo images of a glioblastoma of the right cerebral hemisphere, acquired at 1.5 T. *A*, T_1-weighted image. TR/TE = 500 msec/20 msec. *B*, Proton density–weighted image. TR/TE = 2500 msec/20 msec. *C*, T_2-weighted image. TR/TE = 2500 msec/80 msec. Note signal changes of fat, cerebrospinal fluid (CSF), normal brain, cystic tumor, and surrounding edema. Also note that signal is absent from the cortical bone in the inner and outer tables of the skull but that signal is present in the marrow-containing diploic space.

pared with that of conventional spin-echo sequences (see Chapter 4). This property is utilized for the production of cardiac cineangiograms and MR angiograms.

INVERSION RECOVERY

The *inversion recovery (IR) sequence* has three RF pulses and basically consists of an initial 180-degree RF pulse followed by a spin-echo sequence:

$$180 \text{ degrees -- TI -- } 90 \text{ degrees -- TE/2 -- } 180 \text{ degrees -- TE/2 -- (spin echo)}$$

The initial 180-degree RF pulse inverts **M.** Then, there is a waiting period called the *inversion time (TI)*, during which the protons remagnetize. After this waiting period, an MR signal is produced using a conventional spin-echo pulse sequence.

Unlike T_1-weighted spin-echo sequences, the IR sequence uses a long TR to allow tissue to remagne-

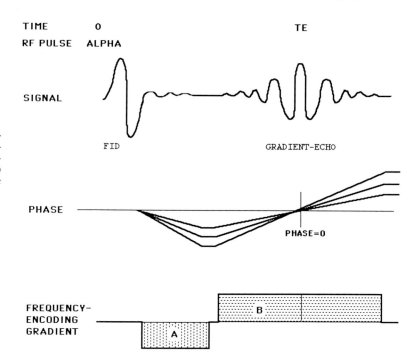

FIGURE 1–36. Principle of the gradient echo. Simplified diagram of pulse sequence showing frequency-encoding gradient. Dephasing gradient pulse (A) produces negative phase shift. Rephasing gradient (B) produces compensatory positive phase shift. At the echo time, phase shifts are precisely canceled. FID = free induction decay.

tize fully between RF pulses. Instead, T_1 contrast develops during the interval TI. Tissues with short T_1 remagnetize quickly and produce a strong signal when the 90-degree RF pulse is applied. However, tissues with long T_1 remagnetize less during the TI interval and, unless TI is very short, produce a weak signal.

Magnitude Reconstruction Versus Phase-Sensitive Reconstruction

The level of T_1 contrast obtained with IR images also depends upon whether or not the images are sensitive to the phase of the MR signal (Fig. 1–37). Some MR systems generate IR images that are insensitive to the phase of the signal. On these *magnitude*

images, information about whether the longitudinal component of **M** is positive or negative is lost. As a result, **M** can vary between 0 and 1. Other systems are able to produce *phase-sensitive images,* which are sensitive to whether **M** is positive or negative. As a result, **M** can vary from − 1 to 0 to 1; that is, the dynamic range for T_1 contrast is doubled (Fig. 1–38). However, phase-sensitive images are more sensitive to image distortions produced by motion or

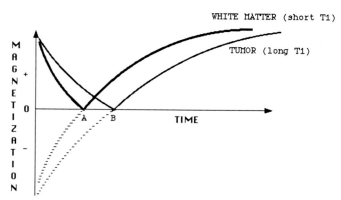

FIGURE 1–37. Longitudinal magnetization versus time after 180-degree RF pulse in an inversion recovery pulse sequence. For each tissue, there is an inversion time (A and B), which results in negligible signal from that tissue. Phase-sensitive image (*dashed line*) retains sign of magnetization and may result in improved tissue contrast.

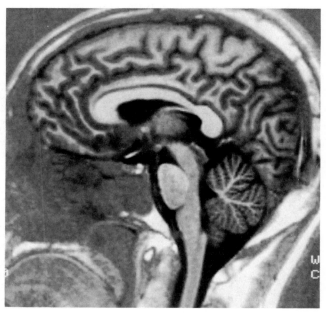

FIGURE 1–38. Sagittal inversion recovery image of a patient with a clivus tumor, using phase-sensitive reconstruction. Note excellent T_1 contrast, as seen in differentiation of gray and white matter. Also note that background (signal near zero) appears gray, CSF (long T_1) appears black, and fat (short T_1) appears bright.

magnetic field inhomogeneity. This problem can be partially eliminated by phase correction algorithms, which are available on some MR systems.

Short Tau Inversion Recovery

One type of IR sequence that has demonstrated clinical utility is the short tau IR (STIR) sequence. This technique relies on the principle that the longitudinal magnetization of any tissue, in crossing from a negative to a positive value, must pass through zero (see Fig. 1–37). If the MR signal is read out when the magnetization is near zero, then little or no signal should be produced. This condition allows signal from a selected tissue to be eliminated based on its T_1 relaxation time. To obtain this result, a short TI must be used. The appropriate choice of TI depends on TR and T_1. At 0.5 T, typical imaging parameters for a fat-suppressed STIR image would be a short TI of approximately 150 to 200 msec and a TR of 1500 msec. Because T_1 is field strength dependent, the appropriate TR and TI for STIR imaging must be optimized for a given magnet field strength. Thus, at 1 T more appropriate parameters would be a TI of 150 msec and a TR of 2000 msec.[15]

STIR methods can be used to suppress the normally intense signal from fat (Fig. 1–39). In the abdomen, the method reduces motion artifacts due to respiratory motion. STIR is also a sensitive method for detecting liver metastases and pathology in the retroperitoneum and pelvis. On these images, tissues with long T_1 relaxation times (e.g., metastases) appear brighter than tissues with shorter T_1 relaxation times (e.g., liver) (see Fig. 1–37). By eliminating fat signal in the orbital cone, STIR sequences can be used to enhance visualization of multiple sclerosis plaques in the optic nerve.

SUMMARY OF PULSE SEQUENCES

Because of the simple contrast behavior of spin-echo pulse sequences and the relative insensitivity to various sources of image artifacts, spin-echo methods are used most commonly in clinical practice. For specific applications, such as fast imaging, flow imaging, and imaging of calcifications and hemorrhage, and for producing an MR myelogram or angiogram, gradient-echo methods can be invaluable. Because they use a long TR, IR methods are inefficient. However, owing to the excellent fat suppression and strong T_1 contrast, at many sites the STIR technique has become a primary method for abdominal and bone marrow imaging.

DETERMINANTS OF SPATIAL RESOLUTION

Spatial resolution, contrast resolution, and S/N are all critical parameters that determine the likelihood of detecting pathology on MR images. In this section, we discuss the factors that determine spatial resolution.

Spatial resolution is determined by slice thickness and pixel size. Pixel size can be expressed in terms of field-of-view (FOV) and matrix size as

$$\text{Pixel} = \text{FOV/matrix} \qquad (6)$$

For instance, with a 25 cm × 25 cm FOV and 256 × 256 matrix, the pixel dimensions would be 1 mm × 1 mm. The FOV represents the horizontal or vertical distance from one side of the image to the opposite side. For body imaging, the typical FOV might be 32 to 50 cm, whereas for head imaging, the

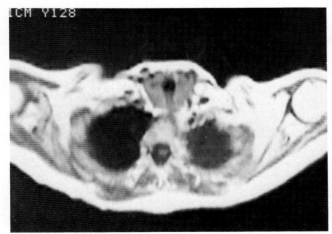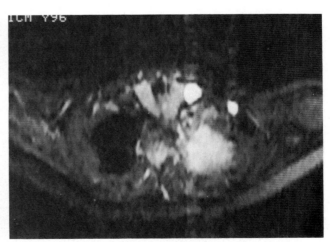

FIGURE 1–39. Patient with neoplasm of left lung apex. Comparison between T_1-weighted spin-echo image, TR/TE = 500 msec/30 msec (*left*), and STIR image, TR/TI/TE = 1500 msec/175 msec/30 msec (*right*), acquired at 0.6 T. Note the effective suppression of fat signal in STIR image, but the reduced S/N compared with SE image. Also note the reversed contrast in the STIR image, with the tumor appearing bright.

FOV would be smaller, on the order of 16 to 24 cm. In some applications, such as imaging of the temporomandibular joints, FOVs $\leq$ 12 cm are preferred. The FOV is typically reduced by increasing the strengths of the phase-encoding and frequency-encoding gradients.

On some MR systems, an asymmetric (rectangular) FOV can be selected. The FOV is reduced asymmetrically by increasing the amplitude of the phase-encoding gradient, without changing the amplitude of the frequency-encoding gradient. The distance across the image is then smaller in the y-direction than in the x-direction. Compared with a symmetric FOV, *the asymmetric FOV provides greater spatial resolution along one direction, because the same number of pixels now spans a smaller distance.*

The matrix size represents the number of pixels in the x- and y-directions. A variety of matrix sizes are available on commercial systems. If the FOV is symmetric in x and y, then equal resolution in both directions is provided by a 256 $\times$ 256 matrix. For the same FOV, spatial resolution can be improved by increasing the matrix (e.g., to 512 $\times$ 512), but this is usually at the expense of longer imaging times. Conversely, to reduce imaging time, the number of phase-encoded projections can be decreased. An image can be acquired with a rectangular 256 $\times$ 128 (x,y) matrix in half the time of a 256 $\times$ 256 matrix; however, the spatial resolution in the y-direction is reduced by half. For instance, the spatial resolution of an image acquired with a 256 (x) $\times$ 128 (y) matrix and a 25-cm FOV would be 1 mm in the x-direction but 2 mm in the y-direction.

It is important to differentiate the acquisition matrix from the display matrix. For instance, images may be interpolated for display onto a 512 $\times$ 512 or 1024 $\times$ 1024 pixel matrix, whether the image is acquired using a 256 $\times$ 256, 256 $\times$ 128, or other matrix size.

Theoretically, the ultimate in-plane spatial resolution that can be obtained on an MR image is very high (<0.1 mm). For human imaging, however, pulse sequence design, gradient limitations, S/N, and patient throughput considerations place the lower limit of spatial resolution at a few tenths of a millimeter.

CONTRAST AND SIGNAL-TO-NOISE ON SPIN-ECHO IMAGES

As noted previously, a tissue's image brightness is directly proportional to the MR signal strength arising from that tissue. Consequently, to distinguish different tissues on an MR image, each must possess differing image brightness. This concept is expressed in the term *contrast*, which represents the difference in signal intensities between two or more tissues.

An argument can be made that S/N should be taken into account directly in contrast curves as "contrast to noise." Unfortunately, the complexities of visual recognition make it difficult to quantify the relative importance of contrast versus S/N. For the sake of clarity, the discussion of contrast in this section will be largely separate from the discussion of S/N.

A number of factors affect MR image contrast. They can be divided into two basic groups: (1) those factors *intrinsic* to tissue and (2) *extrinsic,* operator-dependent factors. Principal intrinsic factors include proton density, T_1, and T_2. Extrinsic factors include the two principal pulse sequence variables: the TR and the TE. Manipulation of these extrinsic parameters is necessary to maximize image contrast.

The signal strength of a given tissue is proportional to the product of three weighting terms: (1) the proton density (ρ); (2) a T_1-weighting term, which is a function of T_1 and TR; and (3) a T_2-weighting term, which is a function of T_2 and TE. By *weighting* is meant the influence of a given term on image contrast, attributable to differences in ρ, T_1, or T_2. This relationship is expressed approximately by the following equation:

$$\text{Signal} = \rho \, [1 - \exp(-TR/T_1)] \times [\exp(-TE/T_2)] \quad (7)$$

PROTON DENSITY–WEIGHTED IMAGES

As previously mentioned, the proton densities (ρ) of various tissues differ by only a few per cent. The best way to produce a proton density–weighted image is to minimize T_1 and T_2 weighting, that is, by using a spin-echo sequence with long TR and short TE or a gradient-echo sequence with low flip angle. Note should be made that, because of the slightly greater ρ of tumors and other pathology, differences in ρ tend to oppose contrast on T_1-weighted images and enhance contrast on T_2-weighted images.

T_1-WEIGHTED IMAGES

The T_1 weighting is increased as the TR is reduced because T_1 differences then have a greater effect on signal intensity (see Fig. 1–17). For T_1-weighted images, the choice of TR is not critical for most tissue comparisons. In general, a choice of TR in the range of 300 to 800 msec will suffice (see Fig. 1–23). However, this will not be true for extreme choices. For instance, if a TR of 50 msec is selected, which is much less than the T_1 of any tissue, then contrast will be poor. On the other hand, if a TR of 4000 msec is used, which is much larger than the T_1 of any tissue except CSF, then T_1 differences become unimportant. Any remaining contrast is then due to differences in proton density and T_2.

Choice of TE is also important. For T_1-weighted images, the TE is minimized to reduce the effects of T_2 weighting. However, it should be understood that a TE of 0 msec is impractical. Therefore, all so-called "T_1-weighted" images contain some degree of T_2 weighting, which increases as the TE is lengthened.

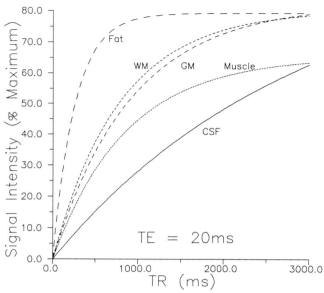

FIGURE 1–40. Calculated signal intensity versus repetition time for spin-echo pulse sequence. WM = white matter; GM = gray matter.

Furthermore, low bandwidth techniques (see Chapters 2 and 10) are commonly used to improve S/N. Although the use of low bandwidth techniques lengthens the minimal TE, the resultant loss of image contrast may be justified by the improvement in image quality, particularly on lower field systems.

The concept of T_1 weighting depends on comparing the signal intensities of two or more tissues (Fig. 1–40). In other words, one cannot say that an image is T_1 weighted for merely one tissue. For instance, one might say that an image obtained with a TR of 2 seconds is poorly T_1 weighted, because most tissues have T_1 relaxation times much less than 2 seconds. This statement might be correct in comparing the signal intensities of gray and white matter, but it would not be valid in comparing the signal intensities of white matter and CSF, since the T_1 relaxation time of CSF is greater than 2 seconds.

T_2-WEIGHTED IMAGES

To understand how T_2 relaxation affects contrast, it must be assumed that T_1 effects can be eliminated (i.e., one must make TR $\gg T_1$ for spin-echo sequences). Then image contrast will be determined solely by the T_2-weighting term. The relationship of tissue signal and contrast to TE is shown in Figure 1–41. We see that although tissue signal is highest at short TE, tissue contrast is poor. As the TE is lengthened, differences in T_2 produce differences in tissue signal intensities. Therefore, tissue contrast improves as TE is lengthened. However, after a certain point, lengthening TE actually worsens tissue contrast, because all tissue signals become small, and their differences may be masked by background

noise. In general, *the best T_2 contrast is obtained when TE is intermediate between the T_2 relaxation times of the tissues.*

It is impractical with most MR imaging systems to obtain a purely T_2-weighted image, since the TR is then so long that imaging times are unacceptable (unless special techniques, such as echo planar, are used; see Chapter 5). In practice, to obtain a T_2-weighted image, a TR is chosen that gives small amounts of T_1 weighting but practical scan times. The choice of TR depends on field strength, since T_1 relaxation times lengthen at higher field strengths. Typical values of TR for a T_2-weighted scan at 0.35 T are 2.0 to 2.5 seconds, and at 1.5 T, typical values are 2.5 to 3.0 seconds.

CROSS-OVER

When practical values for TR and TE are used in double-echo spin-echo sequences, the type of contrast changes or "crosses over" from the first to second echo. Cross-over occurs because the long TR used in T_2-weighted imaging results in contrast curves that are still partly T_1-weighted. At long TEs, T_2 contrast becomes the dominant mechanism (Fig. 1–42).

Cross-over can be useful for image interpretation because two tissues may have similar signal intensities and be difficult to distinguish at one TE but may have quite different intensities at another TE. For instance, on the first echo of a double-echo spin-echo acquisition, a periventricular multiple sclerosis plaque

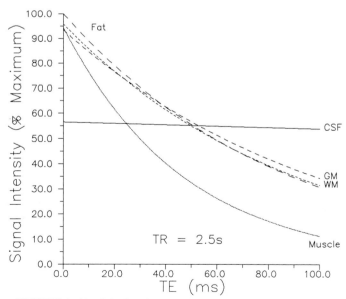

FIGURE 1–41. Calculated signal intensity versus echo time for spin-echo pulse sequence. Note that even with long TR not all tissues start with the same signal intensity, owing primarily to residual T_1 weighting and, to a lesser extent, differences in proton density.

FIGURE 1–42. Cross-over. MR images obtained with practical scan parameters always contain some T_1 weighting, which is most evident at short TR. Note that the cross-over point occurs at relatively long TE in (A) but at shorter TE as the TR is lengthened and T_1 weighting diminishes (B).

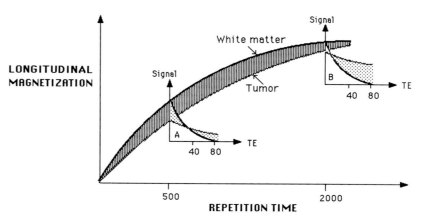

might be readily distinguished from darker CSF (Fig. 1–43A). However, CSF appears bright on the more T_2-weighted second echo and may obscure the plaque (Fig. 1–43B). On the other hand, the second echo may improve the characterization of cystic lesions. Although the optimal choice of TE is seldom known a priori, if one selects a relatively short first TE (e.g., 20 msec) and a relatively long second TE (e.g., 80 msec), one can be reasonably assured that on one or other of the images there will be satisfactory contrast between two tissues.

SIGNAL-TO-NOISE

We have seen that tissue signal is a function of several factors. However, we must also consider the role of noise. In MR imaging there are two major contributions to image noise: (1) the random motion of charged molecules in the body, which produces electromagnetic noise (dominant noise source at high field strengths), and (2) the electrical resistance of the coil itself (dominant noise source at low field strengths). The electrical signal that the MR scanner

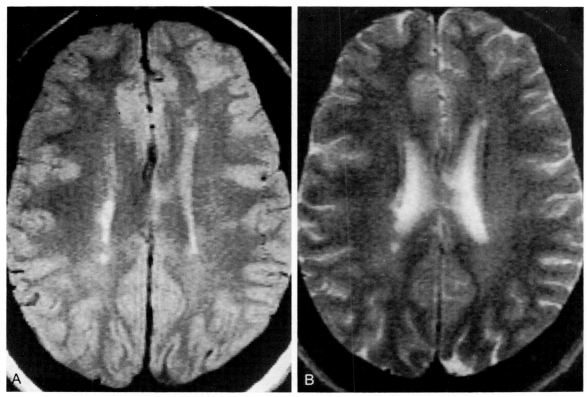

FIGURE 1–43. Spin-echo images acquired at 1.0 T in patient with periventricular multiple sclerosis plaques. A, TR/TE = 2500 msec/30 msec. B, TR/TE = 2500 msec/80 msec. Note that the plaques appear brighter than CSF on the proton density–weighted image but are seen less clearly on the T_2-weighted image because of isointensity with CSF.

then measures is the sum of the actual MR signal plus the unwanted noise. Unfortunately, there is no practical way to reduce the noise in an MR signal. The noise generated in a properly tuned MR coil depends only on the resistance of the coil and the temperature of the patient. For a given coil resistance, there really is no way to change the noise level (freezing the patient in liquid nitrogen is out of the question!). However, the S/N ratio can often be improved by proper selection of a receiver coil (see further on).

The S/N in an MR image depends on the amount of signal from a voxel. The S/N is proportional to the voxel volume. This means that the S/N depends in a straightforward fashion on the FOV of the image, the slice thickness, and the image matrix size. If we denote the matrix size (i.e., number of pixels) as N_p for the phase-encoded direction, and as N_f for the frequency-encoded direction, then the S/N is given by the following proportionality:

$$S/N \sim (\text{voxel volume}) \times \sqrt{NEX}$$
$$= \text{slice thickness} \times$$
$$\left(\frac{FOV_p}{N_p}\right) \times \left(\frac{FOV_f}{N_f}\right) \times \sqrt{NEX \times N_p} \quad (8)$$

This relationship has a number of practical consequences. Improvements in spatial resolution result in a decrease in S/N. If S/N becomes sufficiently low, the perceived spatial resolution in the image may actually deteriorate, despite the use of a thinner slice, larger matrix, or smaller FOV, because small features are obscured by noise.

Provided the patient remains stationary, S/N can always be improved by signal averaging. Both signal and noise increase with the NEX, but the signal increases in proportion to NEX, while the noise, which is random, increases in proportion to $\sqrt{NEX}$, as expressed by

$$S/N \text{ after signal averaging} = (\text{signal} \times NEX)/(\text{noise} \times \sqrt{NEX}) = S/N \times \sqrt{NEX} \quad (9)$$

S/N improves with the NEX, but the penalty in imaging time may be unacceptable; for example, a fourfold increase in NEX results in a fourfold increase in imaging time, but only a twofold increase in S/N.

Signal averaging also reduces another type of image noise, called *ghost artifacts*. These artifacts are commonly produced by respiratory motion and pulsatile flow. Ghost artifacts, like other kinds of image noise, are reduced approximately in proportion to $\sqrt{NEX}$. However, the effectiveness of signal averaging for reduction of ghost artifacts depends on characteristics of the motion and is not effective in all cases (see Chapter 3). In fact, signal averaging, by virtue of increased imaging time, can worsen image quality by increasing the likelihood of gross motion by the patient. Unlike periodic motions, such as flow and respiration, gross motion is not corrected by signal averaging.

One way to improve S/N and reduce imaging time

is to decrease the number of phase-encoding steps. For instance, the voxel volume is doubled when the number of phase-encoding steps is reduced by a factor of 2 (e.g., the matrix is reduced from 256 × 256 to 256 × 128), with a fixed FOV. However, the improvement in S/N is not twofold, as might be expected from the change in voxel volume. As expressed by Equation 8, since fewer signals (i.e., 128 instead of 256) now contribute to the image, image noise is increased. As a result, the S/N is increased by a factor of 2 from the change in voxel, but reduced by a factor of $\sqrt{(256/128)} = \sqrt{2}$ by the change in matrix. The net result is a twofold reduction in imaging time but only a $2/\sqrt{2} = \sqrt{2}$ (41 per cent) improvement in S/N.

In general, if a noisy image is obtained, it is necessary to make one or several of the following changes to the imaging protocol to obtain an adequate S/N: increase NEX, increase slice thickness, increase FOV, decrease matrix size, or use a more appropriate receiver coil. In some cases, it may not be possible to increase the image quality by the above-noted steps because of imaging time constraints, the need to see small structures, the patient's motion, and so forth. The S/N can still be improved by increasing TR or decreasing TE, but not without affecting image contrast. These practical considerations are discussed in more detail in Chapter 2.

MR scan protocols are usually a compromise between a number of factors related to image contrast, S/N, scan time, the patient's motion, and so on. Many standard protocols have been developed through experience. Examples are presented throughout the clinical chapters of this text and in Appendix I at the end of the text.

OTHER FACTORS AFFECTING THE MR IMAGE

MAGNETIC SUSCEPTIBILITY

Magnetic susceptibility represents the tendency of a substance to attract or repel magnetic lines of force. The susceptibility is primarily determined by the magnetic properties of the electrons, which have magnetic moments 1000 times greater than those of protons. There are several types of magnetic susceptibility:

1. *Diamagnetic substances*, which contain paired electrons only, weakly repel magnetic lines of force. Although most tissues are diamagnetic, changes in their signal intensity due to this factor are overwhelmed by much larger effects from other sources, such as relaxation parameters.

2. *Paramagnetic substances*, which contain unpaired electrons, attract magnetic lines of force.

3. *Superparamagnetic substances* more strongly attract magnetic lines of force. These substances have more potent magnetic effects than do paramagnetic

substances. An example of a superparamagnetic substance is hemosiderin.

4. *Ferromagnetic substances* remain permanently magnetized after being removed from a magnetic field. Ferromagnetic substances include a number of iron- and cobalt-containing metal alloys. Both superparamagnetic and ferromagnetic substances strongly attract magnetic lines of force.

Variations in magnetic susceptibilities within a voxel, such as those due to the presence of calcium and water, produce local inhomogeneities in the magnetic field. These field inhomogeneities produce dephasing, which in turn results in signal loss. Signal loss also occurs at the border between two regions with differing magnetic susceptibilities, as, for example, between the brain and air-containing paranasal sinuses (see Chapter 3). Although a source of artifacts, magnetic susceptibility effects can also be useful in delineating certain types of pathology, such as hemorrhage and calcification. Gradient-echo images are more sensitive to these susceptibility effects than are spin-echo images.

Contrast Agents

There are several types of contrast agents in clinical use or under development. These include (1) T_1-active agents (i.e., agents that predominantly shorten T_1); (2) T_2-active agents (i.e., agents that predominantly shorten T_2); and (3) nonproton agents (i.e., agents that contain no hydrogen). These agents are considered in more depth in Chapters 6 and 7.

T_1-Active Agents

Most T_1-active agents in clinical use or under investigation are paramagnetic. The most potent of these is gadolinium, a rare earth element, which contains seven unpaired electrons in its native state. The gadolinium is chelated with diethylenetriaminepentaacetic acid (DTPA) or other ligands to reduce the toxicity of this heavy metal ion. Examples of other paramagnetic substances include manganese, iron, and free radicals. The magnetic fields associated with unpaired electrons in paramagnetic substances have a potent effect on proton relaxation in nearby water molecules. Gadolinium-DTPA is used for many of the same applications for which iodinated contrast agents are used in CT, including screening and characterization of brain tumors and differentiation of postoperative scar from recurrent disk herniation. Although the dominant effect of paramagnetic substances on MR images is T_1 shortening, these substances actually shorten both T_1 and T_2 relaxation times (Fig. 1–44). Enhancement by paramagnetic contrast agents is best seen on T_1-weighted images.

T_2-Active Agents

T_2-active agents produce marked dephasing and result in signal loss on T_2-weighted images. Ferrite, a superparamagnetic substance, is an example of such an agent. These compounds are much more potent than paramagnetic agents such as gadolinium. Because of the large size of the ferrite particles used as contrast agents, they are taken up by the reticuloendothelial system (liver, spleen, and bone marrow). One clinical application of these agents may be to improve lesion detection in the liver, since, unlike normal liver parenchyma, tumors do not contain reticuloendothelial cells and therefore do not take up the agent.

Nonproton Agents

Nonproton agents contain no mobile hydrogen protons. As a result, they appear dark no matter which pulse sequence is used. An example of such a substance is perfluoctylbromide (PFOB), a fluorine-containing molecule that can be used as a contrast agent for the intestine.

Hemorrhage

The biochemistry and MR appearance of hemorrhage are reviewed in detail in Chapters 8 and 16. On CT scans, the appearance of hemorrhage relates only to tissue density. However, on MR images, the appearance of hemorrhage relates to a number of different factors, including the magnetic properties of hemoglobin breakdown products. Native oxyhemoglobin is diamagnetic and has little effect on signal intensity. However, several hemoglobin breakdown products that evolve in a hemorrhage are paramagnetic or superparamagnetic and appear bright on T_1-weighted images or dark on T_2-weighted images, respectively.

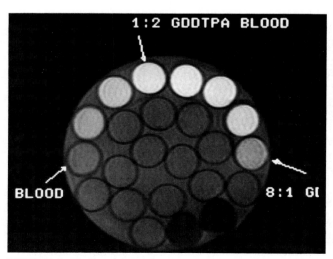

FIGURE 1–44. Signal intensity versus concentration of gadolinium-DTPA in whole blood on T_1-weighted spin-echo image. Note that gadolinium enhances signal at low to moderate concentrations but causes signal loss at high concentrations owing to T_2 shortening.

FLOW

Flow may produce either an increase or a decrease in signal intensity. These effects relate to flow-associated changes in proton phase as well as to longitudinal magnetization (see Chapter 4).

In general, signal intensity decreases as flow velocity increases. However, numerous factors relating to the imaging technique must be considered when interpreting the appearance of flowing blood and CSF. In addition, flow can produce image artifacts. For instance, variation in signal intensity caused by the pulsatile flow of blood or CSF produces mispositioning of the signal within the image, manifested as ghost artifacts. A variety of methods are currently available to suppress these artifacts.

CHEMICAL SHIFT

The electron cloud surrounding the nucleus of an atom shields the nucleus from the applied magnetic field. As a result, the effective local magnetic field experienced by the nucleus (B_{eff}) is altered, and the nuclear resonance frequency is shifted, related to Equation 1. The alteration in resonance frequency produced by the shielding effect of the electron cloud is called the *chemical shift*. The reduction in the local magnetic field caused by the chemical shift (σ) can be expressed as

$$B_{eff} = (1 - \sigma)B_0$$

Chemical shift effects are the basis of MRS and are also responsible for mispositioning of fat signals in MR images, called *chemical shift artifacts* (see Chapters 3 and 10).

OVERVIEW OF HARDWARE

We now present a basic overview of the hardware involved in producing the MR image (Fig. 1–45).

Instrumentation is discussed in greater detail in Chapter 12.

MAGNETS

The magnets used for MR imaging range in strength from <0.06 T to >2.0 T, where 1 T = 10,000 gauss (G). By comparison, the small magnets used to hold notes on refrigerator doors produce a field of approximately 400 G. Several types of magnets are in commercial use. Permanent magnets (Fig. 1–46A), which produce field strengths ≤0.3 T, are made of special rare earth alloys that can retain strong magnetic fields. Such magnets may be massive, weighing as much as 100 tons. However, lower field permanent magnets can be much lighter. Permanent magnets may have significant siting advantages over other types of magnets.

Electromagnets require a constant input of electrical current. The amount of current increases rapidly with magnetic field strength. Currently, such magnets are limited to ≤0.4 T owing to high power consumption.

The most powerful magnets (up to 4 T) employ the principle of superconductivity. When cooled below their so-called critical temperature (a few degrees above absolute zero), certain alloys, such as titanium-niobium, lose all resistance to the flow of electrical current. Superconducting magnets (Fig. 1–46B) consist of miles of titanium-niobium wire wrapped around a cylinder. To maintain superconductivity, the magnet core is encased in an insulating drum (dewar) containing liquid helium (at 4°K). Once energized, the superconducting magnet's field strength is maintained for years. Since conductive and convective losses occur, the liquid helium must be regularly replenished (about once per month in most clinical settings). Failure to do so may cause a sudden loss of superconductivity, called a *quench,* which, although not a significant hazard to the patient, may result in costly boil-off of cryogens.[16]

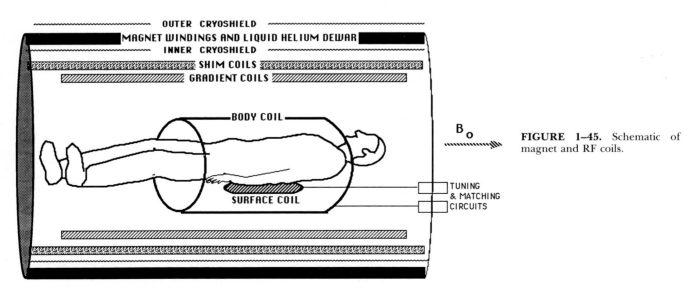

FIGURE 1–45. Schematic of magnet and RF coils.

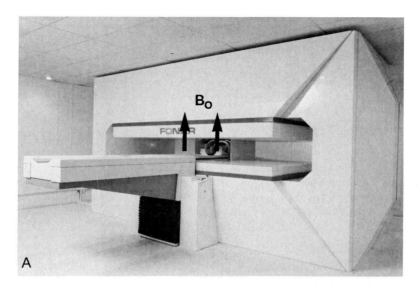

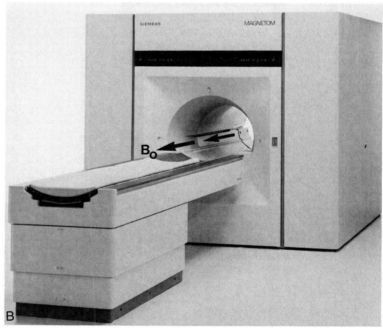

FIGURE 1–46. Main magnet field (B_0) direction is different for (*A*) permanent magnet and (*B*) superconducting magnet.

Each type of magnet has certain advantages. The S/N improves approximately in proportion to magnetic field strength (Fig. 1–47). The high field strengths produced by superconducting magnets yield improved S/N, obviously benefiting both imaging and spectroscopy. However, devices with high field strength create greater siting problems. The stray fields from superconducting magnets extend for dozens of feet in all directions, posing potential risks to electronic equipment and patients with cardiac pacemakers. Large metal objects in the vicinity of the magnet can distort field homogeneity, while smaller metal objects can be attracted into the magnet bore at dangerously high velocities. Solutions for this problem include passive and active magnetic shielding (see Chapter 11).

Unlike a superconducting magnet, whose main magnetic field is oriented along the long axis of the magnet bore, permanent magnets and some electromagnets produce fields that are vertical. The stray fields from these magnets are contained within a few feet, simplifying siting requirements (see Chapter 11).

A homogeneous magnetic field is essential for both MR imaging and spectroscopy. Magnets used for MR imaging must be carefully shimmed to maximize homogeneity. This shimming is accomplished physically by strategic placement of steel plates around the magnet (*passive shimming*), as well as by varying currents into electromagnetic coils (*active shimming*). Homogeneity is especially critical for spectroscopy, in which field uniformity must be an order of magnitude better than for MR imaging; this can be achieved only with superconducting magnets.

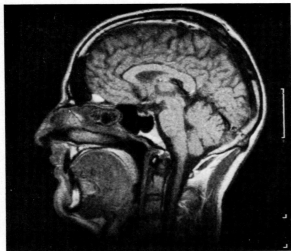

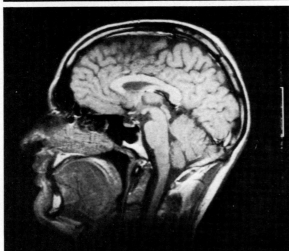

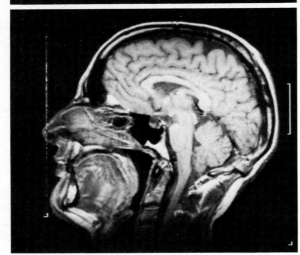

FIGURE 1–47. Comparison of image quality at different field strengths using same pulse sequence and scan parameters. Top = 0.5 T; middle = 1.0 T; bottom = 1.5 T.

RADIOFREQUENCY COILS

Receiver Coils

The receiver coil must be designed to have high sensitivity for the body part being imaged. Sensitivity falls rapidly with distance from the source of the MR signal. As a result, the coil should be placed in proximity to the region of interest. However, the receiver coil is equally sensitive to the MR signal and to the electrical noise produced by thermal motion of ions in the body. Consequently, it is desirable to match the size of the receiver coil, and therefore the sensitive volume of the coil, to the region of interest. Such coils are said to have a high *filling factor*. For instance, the smaller head coil has a higher filling factor and provides better S/N for brain imaging compared with the larger body coil, because it is less sensitive to thermal noise arising from tissues outside the brain.

An application of this principle is the use of *surface coils* (Fig. 1–48). A surface coil is a type of receiver antenna that produces a high signal intensity near the coil owing to the proximity of the tissue. In contrast, a body coil produces a much smaller signal from the same region because that tissue is farther

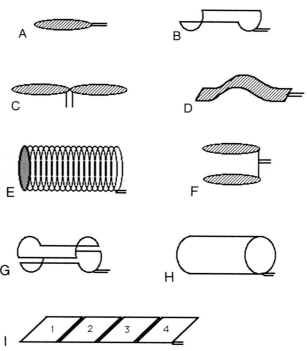

FIGURE 1–48. Schematic drawings of various receiver coils. *A*, Flat surface coil used for spine imaging. Small versions may be used for orbit imaging. *B*, Half-saddle coil used for neck imaging. *C*, Butterfly coil for spine imaging. *D*, Flexible coil for neck imaging. *E*, Solenoid coil used for head and extremity imaging in permanent magnet systems. *F*, Helmholtz pair used for neck and shoulder imaging. *G*, Saddle coil used for head imaging at low to mid field strengths. *H*, Resonator coil used for head and extremity imaging at high field strengths. *I*, Ladder coil for total spine studies.

from the coil and represents only a fraction of the sensitive volume of the coil. In general, surface coils provide better image quality than do body coils when the region of interest is within about a one-coil radius from the antenna.

The MR signal is very weak, on the order of microvolts, and must be amplified prior to analysis using a low-noise preamplifier and amplifier. To exclude extraneous noise sources, such as electrical noise from the thermal motion of ions in the body and from outside radio interference, the receiver must be tuned to the range of frequencies contained in the MR signal, called the bandwidth. To exclude extraneous signal frequencies, the signal detected by the receiver coil is processed by a *bandpass filter.*

Transmitter Coils

The antenna used to deliver the RF pulses is called the transmitter coil. In some cases, the receiver and transmitter coils are identical, but, in general, different coils are used. Usually, the large body coil is used as the transmitter in conjunction with a smaller receiver coil. The reasons for this practice relate to conflicting requirements for reception and transmission of the RF signal. For instance, receiver coils should be kept small for optimal S/N. However, transmitter coils should, in general, be large to produce a uniform field of RF excitation.

Quadrature (Circularly Polarized) Coils

A marked improvement in coil efficacy can be achieved by improving the interaction between the RF coil and the tissue magnetization. Like any vector, the precessing transverse component of the tissue magnetization can be represented as the sum of two other vectors, which have a 90-degree phase difference. A *linear RF coil* has a single magnetic axis and interacts with only one of these two magnetization vectors. However, RF coils that interact with both of these vectors can be designed. These *quadrature* or *circularly polarized coils,* in effect, consist of two distinct RF coils that operate with a 90-degree phase difference, matching the phase difference between the two transverse components of the tissue magnetization. This feature enhances the interaction of the coil with the tissue magnetization, resulting in two significant benefits.

First, because they more fully interact with the tissue magnetization, quadrature coils can, in theory, produce a 90-degree RF pulse with 50 per cent less RF power deposition. Second, when receiving, they can provide a 40 per cent improvement in S/N over the linear mode. In practice, the gain from quadrature operation is less dramatic, in part because the body is not an ideal spherical, homogeneous object. In addition, not all coil designs are suitable for quadrature operation. To maintain the proper phase relationships between the two components of the coil, quadrature coils should possess a high degree of symmetry. As a result, it is easier to design quadrature coils for head and body imaging than for spine imaging. Nevertheless, quadrature surface coils can also be produced.

Quality

The efficiency with which an RF coil converts a radio signal into a measurable electrical voltage is described by the quality (Q) of the coil. A coil with a higher Q factor allows more of the signal it receives to be measured by resonating only at the exact proper frequency. RF coils can have high or low Q. Low-Q coils resonate over a broader range than do high-Q coils.

GRADIENTS

MR imaging systems have three pairs of orthogonal gradient coils, oriented respectively along the x-, y-, and z-axes of the magnet. Activation of an individual gradient coil produces a linear magnetic field gradient along an orthogonal axis. Simultaneous activation of two or three gradient coils produces a linear gradient along a nonorthogonal direction, which is applied for oblique imaging (Fig. 1–49).

Maximal gradient amplitudes, which limit the available slice thickness and FOV, range from 10 to 15 mT/meter, although experimental systems used for echo-planar imaging (EPI) (see Chapter 26) produce peak gradient amplitudes several times as strong. Gradient ramp times—that is, the time required to switch from no gradient to a stable plateau value (rise

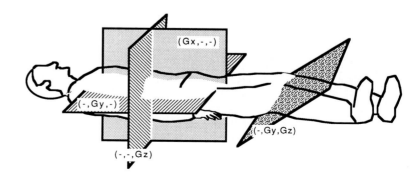

FIGURE 1–49. Oblique imaging uses multiple gradients simultaneously.

time) and vice versa (fall time)—range from a few hundred microseconds to 1.5 msec. EPI systems are different in that the gradients oscillate, rather than plateau, and are capable of very rapid ramping (up to 8000 oscillations per second).

Several problems result from operation of the gradient coils at their maximal capacity:

1. There is a large amount of audible noise generated by the electromechanical torquing of the gradient coils as the magnetic field flux changes rapidly, which can be quite disturbing to the patient lying in the magnet bore.

2. It may be necessary to allow some dead-time for the gradients during the pulse sequence (duty cycle < 100 per cent of the TR).

3. Eddy currents may produce image artifacts (see Chapter 3).

Eddy currents represent undesirable magnetic fields that are induced each time the gradient is pulsed. These magnetic fields, which vary over time and space, occur in conducting structures in proximity to the gradient coil, such as the cryoshield (see Chapter 12). The major effect of eddy currents is to distort the gradient profile, producing unstable gradients. As a result, the dephasing and rephasing lobes of a gradient reversal, used in all gradient-echo and spin-echo pulse sequences, may be unequal, so that the echo is not properly refocused. In addition, the frequency-encoding gradient may be unstable during the read-out period, resulting in image artifacts. The long time constant (up to tens of milliseconds) of some eddy currents is a particular problem for certain spectroscopic experiments. Eddy currents may be compensated for through electronic preadjustment of the gradient waveforms alone or in conjunction with electromagnetic shielding of the gradient coils with an additional coil set (*active gradient shielding*). The effects of eddy currents can also be minimized by attention to pulse sequence design (see Chapter 10).

REFERENCES

1. Abragam A: The Principles of Nuclear Magnetism. London, Oxford University Press, 1961.
2. Slichter CP: Principles of Magnetic Resonance: With Examples from Solid State Physics. 2nd ed. Berlin, Springer-Verlag, 1978.
3. Hinshaw WS, Lent AH: An introduction to NMR imaging: From the Bloch equation to the imaging equation. Proc IEEE 71:338, 1983.
4. Mansfield P, Morris PG: NMR Imaging in Biomedicine. New York, Academic Press, 1982, pp 29–30.
5. Kaufman L, Crooks LE, Margulis AR: NMR Imaging in Medicine. New York, Shoin, 1981.
6. Rabi II, Millman S, Kusch P, et al: The molecular beam resonance method for measuring nuclear magnetic moments. Phys Rev 55:526, 1939.
7. Bloch F, Hansen WW, Packard M: Nuclear induction. Phys Rev 69:127, 1946.
8. Purcell EM, Torrey HC, Pound RV: Resonance absorption by nuclear magnetic moments in a solid. Phys Rev 69:37, 1946.
9. Lauterbur PC: Nature 242:190, 1973.
10. Damadian R, Goldsmith M, Minkoff L: Fonar image of the live human body. Physiol Chem Phys Med NMR 9:97, 1977.
11. Mansfield P, Maudsley AA: Planar spin imaging by NMR. J Magn Res 27:101, 1977.
12. Hinshaw WS, Bottomley PA, Holland GN: Radiographic thin-section image of the human wrist by NMR. Nature 270:722, 1977.
13. Bottomley PA, Hardy CJ, Argersinger RE, Allen-Moore G: A review of 1 H NMR relaxation in pathology: Are T1 and T2 diagnostic? Med Phys 14:1–37, 1987.
14. Damadian R: Tumor detection by NMR. Science 171:1151–1153, 1971.
15. Paling MR, Abbitt PL, Mugler JP, Brookeman JR: Liver metastases: Optimization of MRI pulse sequences at 1.0 T. Radiology 167:695–699, 1988.
16. Bore PJ, Galloway GJ, Styles P, et al: Are quenches dangerous? Magn Reson Med 3:112–117, 1986.

2

PRACTICAL MRI FOR THE TECHNOLOGIST AND IMAGING SPECIALIST

ROBERT R. EDELMAN, FRANK G. SHELLOCK, and JOSEPH AHLADIS

PREPARATION OF THE PATIENT
  CLAUSTROPHOBIA
  MONITORING OF THE PATIENT
  PHYSICAL PREPARATION
  POSITIONING
  PRECAUTIONS
  PREGNANCY
GENERAL PRINCIPLES FOR OPTIMIZING MRI IN THE CLINICAL SETTING
  SIGNAL-TO-NOISE
  CONTRAST
  SPATIAL RESOLUTION
PRESCANNING SYSTEM ADJUSTMENTS
  SET-UP OF RECEIVER COIL
  Selection of Coil
  Restrictions in Receiver Coil Design
  Restrictions in Receiver Coil Positioning
  Coil Centering
  COIL TUNING AND MATCHING
  FREQUENCY ADJUSTMENT
  TRANSMITTER ADJUSTMENT
  RECEIVER ADJUSTMENT
  SPECIFIC ABSORPTION RATE (SAR)
CHOOSING PULSE SEQUENCES AND TIMING PARAMETERS

  SPIN-ECHO SEQUENCES
  T_1 Weighting
  T_2 Weighting
  GRADIENT-ECHO SEQUENCES
  Flow Enhancement
  MR Myelogram
  Steady-State Versus Spoiled Gradient-Echo Sequences
  When Not to Use Gradient-Echo Methods
  OTHER IMAGING PARAMETERS
  Number of Excitations (NEX)
  Slice Thickness
  Interslice Gap and Slice Profile

Field-of-View (FOV)
Matrix
  TRADE-OFFS BETWEEN IMAGING PARAMETERS
SPECIAL TECHNIQUES
  HALF-FOURIER
  FLOW COMPENSATION (BRIGHT BLOOD SEQUENCE)
  PRESATURATION (DARK BLOOD SEQUENCE)
  GRADIENT ROTATION
  REORDERING OF PHASE ENCODING ACCORDING TO RESPIRATORY PHASE
  OVERSAMPLING TO ELIMINATE WRAPAROUND
  ELECTROCARDIOGRAPHIC GATING
  Prospective Cardiac Gating
  Retrospective Cardiac Gating
  LOW BANDWIDTH
  THREE-DIMENSIONAL GRADIENT-ECHO METHODS
  Slice Thickness
  Scan Parameters for Three-Dimensional Methods
  Multislab Three-Dimensional Acquisition
  USE OF CONTRAST AGENTS
IMAGE MEASUREMENT
  PREPARATION SCANS
  MEASUREMENT PERIOD
  BREATH HOLDING
DATA RECONSTRUCTION
PHOTOGRAPHY AND ARCHIVAL
TROUBLESHOOTING
APPENDIX A. SAMPLE CHECKLIST AND WORK-UP SHEET FOR INTERVIEWING PATIENTS
APPENDIX B. CLASSIFICATION OF IMPLANTS FOR MR IMAGING
APPENDIX C. ADVANCED LIFE SUPPORT SYSTEMS FOR MR IMAGING OF UNSTABLE PATIENTS

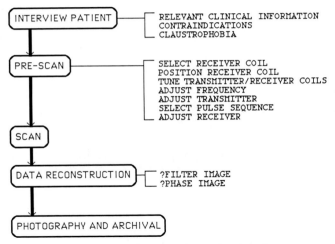

FIGURE 2–1. Flow chart for patient imaging.

The practice of MR imaging (MRI) is, in many ways, an art. Much more so than in CT, it is the technologist's skills that ensure that the highest quality images are routinely obtained. Although advances in software have simplified the operation of MR systems and improved the consistency of the images, it is still necessary for the technologist—and, where possible, the radiologist—to have a working knowledge of the various factors responsible for producing an MR image.

In this chapter, we review, at a very practical level, the steps involved in the scanning of patients (Fig. 2–1). Commercial MR systems differ in both software and hardware; nonetheless, our comments are intended to be as generalizable as possible to current systems and to systems that will be available in the near future.

PREPARATION OF THE PATIENT

The preparation of the patient for MR imaging involves (1) transfer of information and (2) physical preparation. Questioning of the patient should be directed toward obtaining a brief clinical history. It is essential to narrow down the region of interest from information provided by the patient and physician. A simple, concise checklist (Appendix 2–A) can be used to provide consistency in this area. It is also helpful to determine whether the examination will be standardized or will require special set-up. A work-up sheet can be developed to assist the radiologist and technologist in this determination.

CLAUSTROPHOBIA

Claustrophobia is encountered by up to 10 per cent of patients who enter the tunnel of the MR scanner. The following are recommendations for dealing with claustrophobic patients: (1) maintain verbal or physical contact; (2) place patients in a prone position, if possible, so that they may see out of the scanner; (3) use special mirrors or prism glasses; (4) use a blindfold; or (5) use psychologic desensitization techniques.

If these techniques fail, then sedation may be required prior to imaging the patient. The referring physician can prescribe diazepam (Valium), 5 to 10 mg to be taken orally 30 minutes to 1 hour prior to the MR examination. If oral sedation is inadequate, or rapid sedation is desired, then intramuscular or intravenous administration of a short-acting sedative such as midazolam (Versed) is highly effective.

MONITORING OF THE PATIENT

The safe use of MR imaging in sedated, anesthetized, comatose, or critically ill patients requires the use of continuous physiologic monitoring. However, most conventional monitoring systems are not designed to be used in the unique MR imaging environment. Monitoring equipment may be adversely affected by electromagnetic interference produced during the operation of the MR scanner, or the monitors may generate spurious noise that disrupts image quality.[1] In addition, most monitors have ferrous components that are strongly attracted by magnets of mid and high field strength, which poses a potential hazard to the patient and MR scanner. Fortunately, various manufacturers of monitoring devices have recognized these problems and have developed special systems that are compatible with MR imaging.

Several different types of monitors are commercially available to record the following physiologic parameters during MR imaging: (1) heart rate, (2) blood pressure, (3) respiratory rate, (4) temperature, and (5) skin blood flow (see the table in Appendix 2–C for a listing of devices and manufacturers). MR imaging–compatible respirators have also been developed and are now commercially available. In children, measurement of oxygen saturation with a pulse oximeter monitor, as well as respiratory monitoring, is recommended, since it is more difficult to communicate remotely with a child than an adult. Considering the fact that specially modified physiologic monitoring and support equipment exists for use during MR imaging, it is now feasible to perform examinations safely on most high-risk patients.

PHYSICAL PREPARATION

All patients should change into hospital gowns and paper pants if available. Street clothes may harbor unsuspected ferromagnetic objects, which at a minimum produce image degradation and in the worst case can be accelerated to lethal velocities in the magnet bore.[2] In addition, certain clothing or blankets can generate static electricity, which will also degrade image quality, a problem that is worsened by low humidity (e.g., during periods of cold weather). Bras and dentures must be removed. Even small ferromagnetic objects, such as the metallic clips on bra straps, may produce enormous artifacts. Eye makeup, which sometimes contains ferromagnetic iron or cobalt ores, can produce localized artifacts and should be removed prior to scanning.[3] Tattooed eyeliner may also degrade image quality, and some patients have even experienced mild to moderate skin irritation associated with MR imaging. Outpatients should be given the above information at the time their appointments are made.

POSITIONING

The patient should be positioned so that he or she is comfortable. Prone or oblique positioning is generally less comfortable than supine positioning and may increase motion artifacts. Fortunately, most MR systems now have special software capabilities that permit imaging in any plane. This feature obviates placing the patients in an uncomfortable position during MR imaging. Excessive flexion or extension of the neck may be painful and may result in increased motion by the patient, particularly older patients with cervical spondylosis.

Total spine examinations usually require the patient to be moved from his or her original position at least once or twice. Patients who undergo total spine examinations are often neurologically impaired and have difficulty in moving. Because of this, we routinely use a low-friction patient lift to move the patient. To maximize the efficiency of the total spine examination, such devices should allow effortless movement of the patient within the magnet bore and should allow the surface coil to remain near the center of the magnet. Such devices must be nonferromagnetic and should have a diameter of ~1 cm or less, so that the distance between the patient and surface coil is not significantly increased by the device. An example of such a device is a high-pressure air mattress with multiple small holes on the lower surface. The mattress can be transiently inflated by an external pump to provide a frictionless cushion of air when the patient is moved. When the pump is shut off for imaging, the mattress collapses to a few millimeters in diameter. For obvious safety reasons, the pump must be mounted on the floor or wall, at least 6 to 8 feet away from the magnet facade.

PRECAUTIONS

There are few absolute contraindications to MR imaging (Table 2–1, Appendix 2–B).[4–6] Contraindications primarily relate to potential interactions with the static magnetic field or radiofrequency (RF) field.[7–11] Pacemakers are contraindicated, since the magnetic relays contained in pacemakers are susceptible to the effects of magnetic fields as weak as 5

TABLE 2–1. CONTRAINDICATIONS TO MRI*

Absolutely Contraindicated	Relatively Contraindicated	Generally Safe
Pacemaker	Shrapnel in nonvital locations	Nonferromagnetic intracranial aneurysm clips
Ferromagnetic intracranial aneurysm clips	Residual external pacemaker leads	Most cardiac valves
Shrapnel in vital location	Pregnancy	Joint prostheses
Nonremovable neurostimulators		Most surgical clips (including S/P CABG)
Cochlear implants		Most IVC umbrellas‡ (including Mobin-Uddin, Greenfield)
(Hemolytic anemia)†		Infusaid implantable chemotherapy pumps

*Users should always check the current literature, as well as test devices themselves, when there is any concern about a possible hazard. Also see Appendix 2–B for a more complete listing.
†For administration of gadolinium–diethylene triamine pentaacetic acid (DTPA).
‡Exceptions may include birdcage type.
S/P CABG = status post coronary artery bypass graft; IVC = inferior vena cava.

gauss (G). Residual external pacemaker wires left after coronary artery bypass surgery are probably safe, although one cannot completely discount the possibility of current induction in the wires. Certain ferromagnetic intracranial aneurysm clips are contraindicated, since some of these clips are sufficiently deflected or torqued in the presence of a magnetic field to create the potential for vessel rupture. Other intracranial aneurysm clips made of titanium or other nonferromagnetic materials are MR compatible.[12–15] However, if it is not known what kind of aneurysm clip is present, one should err on the side of caution. Most types of surgical clips, including those left following coronary artery bypass surgery, are considered safe, particularly if a sufficient period has elapsed to permit fixation of the clip by fibrosis.

Cochlear implants, certain stapedial implants, and nonremovable neurostimulators are contraindicated. Lens implants and orbital prostheses made entirely of plastic are acceptable. Cardiac valves are safe (with the possible exception of older Starr-Edwards types in patients with valvular dehiscence) but will produce local artifacts.[16, 17] Starr-Edwards valves contain more metal and produce larger artifacts than most other types of valves. Most inferior vena caval umbrellas, including the Greenfield, Mobin-Uddin, and Simon-Nitinol filters, are minimally ferromagnetic or nonferromagnetic, but other types of filters, such as steel birdcage devices, may be more strongly ferromagnetic.[18] Whenever there is any uncertainty, such devices should be tested using ex vivo testing techniques before a decision is made to scan the patient. Hip and knee prostheses, generally made of weakly ferromagnetic or nonferromagnetic metals, can be safely imaged. Patients with Harrington rods can be imaged, but magnetic field distortion produced by the rods and associated surgical paraphernalia generally causes severe local image degradation and may also preclude satisfactory tuning of the RF coils. Halo fixation devices may or may not be MR compatible; information about compatibility may be obtained from the manufacturer. However, even if the halo is MR compatible, other components involved in stabilization, such as cables, fixation pins, or metal weights, may not be.

When there is doubt about the MR compatibility of a device with regard to the risk of displacement, the device should be tested. Testing methods for checking the deflection of an unknown object include suspending it by a string at the opening of the magnet bore and measuring the deflection angle.[14] Devices that produce minimal or no deflection are unlikely to present a risk of displacement from an MR examination. Again, a simple, concise checklist should be used to provide consistency in the screening procedure.

For patients with an occupational history of exposure to, and injury from, shrapnel (e.g., current or former steel workers, carpenters) the decision whether to perform an MR examination may be difficult, and even more so if the shrapnel is near a critical location, such as the globe of the eye. If there is a history of occupational exposure to shrapnel, then an anteroposterior radiograph of the orbits may be an adequate screening procedure. However, small metallic fragments can be missed on plain radiographs. If clinical suspicion is high despite normal plain films, it is reasonable to obtain a limited CT scan of the orbits. Patients with shrapnel in noncritical locations may be scanned, though clinical judgment should be exercised. It may be reasonable to move the patient slowly into the magnet bore to reduce any potential risk of displacing the shrapnel, and the patient should be instructed to remark on any tugging sensations.

The technologist and other personnel who enter the magnet room must exercise caution with respect to metal objects on their persons. Objects such as pens, scissors, keys, and oxygen tanks can be attracted into the magnet bore at high velocities. It is important to be aware that the maximal attraction occurs near the opening of the magnet bore, where the magnetic field strength changes precipitously. This precipitous change in magnetic attraction is even more pronounced in systems with self-contained magnetic shielding. Credit cards, beepers, and such are at risk from the magnetic field and should be excluded from the magnet area. Stationary or portable metal detectors are seldom of value owing to limited sensitivity and may provide a false sense of security.

PREGNANCY

In general, MR imaging is not believed to be harmful to the fetus. However, only a few investigations have examined the teratogenic potential of this imaging modality.[19, 20] A variety of mechanisms exist for possible deleterious effects caused by interactions between electromagnetic fields and the developing embryo. Additional studies are needed in this area to determine if the specific exposure levels of electromagnetic radiation that are used for clinical MR imaging pose a hazard.

MR imaging during pregnancy may be indicated if diagnostic information obtained by ultrasound is inadequate or if the clinician does not want to expose the patient to ionizing radiation. Therefore, patients who are pregnant or suspect that they may be pregnant should be identified prior to MR imaging so that a decision can be made concerning the risks versus the benefits of the examination. Particular caution should be exercised in the first trimester; during this period, there is a high spontaneous abortion rate, with potential medicolegal complications. Similar considerations apply to pregnant technologists, although they are exposed to much lower levels of electromagnetic radiation than are patients.

GENERAL PRINCIPLES FOR OPTIMIZING MRI IN THE CLINICAL SETTING

There are many technical details that are involved in the production of high-quality MR images; these will be discussed in other chapters. However, it is useful to review briefly the features that determine whether an image "looks good."

SIGNAL-TO-NOISE

The signal-to-noise (S/N) represents the graininess of an image. An image with low S/N appears grainy; an image with high S/N appears sharp. It is therefore desirable to maximize S/N, although after a certain point, improvements in S/N are not easily detectable by the human eye. In addition, it is not worthwhile to struggle over technique modifications that produce minimal changes in S/N (e.g., ≤ 10 per cent), since these are barely noticeable in the image.

The S/N depends on several factors, including (1) spatial resolution (slice thickness, field-of-view [FOV], and matrix); (2) receiver coil sensitivity; (3) noise sources, coherent (e.g., ghost artifacts due to the patient's respiration) and incoherent (e.g., RF noise); (4) pulse sequence; and (5) magnetic field strength. There are a number of trade-offs in these factors that one has to consider in choosing an imaging technique. For instance, a high-resolution image will require more imaging time (e.g., more excitations) than a lower resolution image to maintain an adequate level of S/N. Similarly, an image acquired on a low field system with a particular level of spatial resolution will generally require a longer acquisition than will a comparable image on a high field system. In addition, image quality is system dependent, and one must adapt to the capabilities of the individual system to produce consistent, high-quality images.

CONTRAST

Contrast, the difference in tissue signal, is the most critical determinant of one's ability to distinguish pathologic from normal tissues on an MR image. Contrast depends primarily on the choice of pulse sequence and scan parameters, rather than on spatial resolution. To a minor extent, contrast also depends on field strength, since T_1 relaxation times lengthen as the field strength is increased. Good contrast is essential, but not sufficient, for lesion detection; on an image of poor quality, noise will tend to overwhelm the contrast.

SPATIAL RESOLUTION

Spatial resolution represents the ability to distinguish two objects that are close together. High resolution is most essential for head, spine, and joint imaging. However, there is a stiff penalty to be paid for increased spatial resolution: reduced S/N. The loss in S/N can be compensated for by increased imaging time (e.g., more excitations, longer repetition time [TR]).

At most sites, the desire to optimize image quality must be balanced with the need to maintain adequate throughput. Throughput depends, in part, on minimizing the time spent in the magnet room, which in turn depends on good preparation of the patient and choice of efficient imaging techniques. Using a high field system, we generally schedule patients at intervals of 45 minutes, although with faster imaging and reconstruction methods coming into general use, patients might be scheduled more frequently. However, consideration must be given to the possibility of late arrivals, claustrophobic patients, patients who require monitoring, and add-on cases. The last type of patient is most commonly encountered at hospital-based MR imaging sites. Therefore, it may be prudent to schedule cases less frequently than the maximal rate or to leave one or two slots open each day for unscheduled cases.

PRESCANNING SYSTEM ADJUSTMENTS

"Prescan" represents a series of steps required before the measurement process can begin (Fig. 2–1). We now consider these steps in the order in which they are performed.

SET-UP OF RECEIVER COIL

Selection of Coil

The receiver coil is the radio antenna used to detect the MR signal. Prior to positioning of the

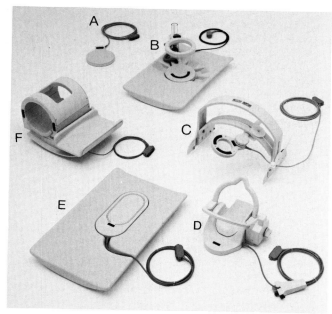

FIGURE 2–2. Examples of surface coils: (a) small circular spine coil; (b) flat Helmholtz pair used for shoulder imaging provides relatively uniform sensitivity, depending on separation of the individual coils; (c) temporomandibular joint (TMJ)/orbit coil; (d) Helmholtz neck coil, which better conforms to anterior neck anatomy than coil (b); (e) large elliptical spine coil; (f) knee resonator coil, which provides uniform sensitivity within the coil volume.

patient, one must choose and position the receiver coil. Whole-volume coils, such as body, head, and most knee coils, are used when the region of interest is relatively large or when a uniform FOV is needed. Surface (local) coils are used to provide improved image quality over a smaller region of interest, at the expense of FOV. *It is important to understand that the receiver coil is a passive device. It does not, per se, change the spatial resolution, which depends on gradient strength and other factors.* The improvement in image quality obtained with surface coils is purely a consequence of better S/N and, to some extent, lesser sensitivity to the motion of distant structures.

Examples of different coil designs are shown in Figure 2–2. Certain types, such as saddle, resonator, and solenoidal configurations, provide relatively uniform image intensity through the FOV. Other types, such as most surface coils, provide greater image intensity near the coil than far from the coil.[21] The bipolar Helmholtz coil, which is composed of a pair of flat or curved loops, provides relatively uniform sensitivity when the separation of the loops is not much greater than the coil radius. Helmholtz coils are particularly useful for imaging of the shoulder and other joints.

In choosing a surface coil, a rule of thumb is to select the smallest coil that can be placed close to (i.e., within one coil radius of) the region of interest. A larger coil provides better depth penetration but also is sensitive to thermal noise from a larger region of the body; a smaller coil provides better S/N for

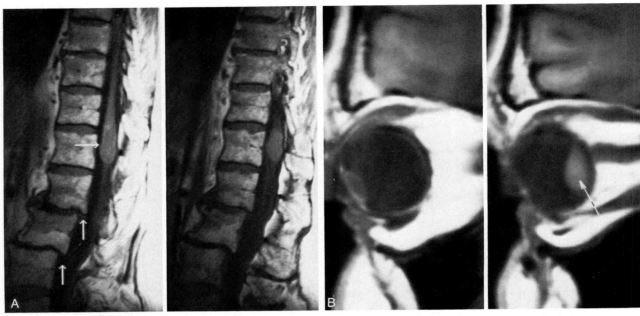

FIGURE 2–3. Examples of surface coil applications. *A,* Ependymoma of conus (*arrows*). Large elliptical spine coil provides adequate sensitivity over a wider field-of-view (FOV) than a small coil, at the expense of reduced S/N. *B,* Retinoblastoma (*arrow*). Smaller coils provide better sensitivity for small FOV applications, such as imaging of the orbit. Note that improved spatial resolution is a direct result of increasing the gradient amplitudes and is not related to the surface coil except insofar as it provides adequate S/N to support imaging with smaller voxels.

superficial tissues (Fig. 2–3). Sometimes, a large coil will be chosen despite inferior S/N because of its larger FOV; this is essential for total spine studies (Fig. 2–4).

Because of the motion sensitivity of coils such as the Helmholtz and solenoid designs, which have uniform sensitivity throughout their FOV, we do not generally use them for cervical spine imaging. Instead, we prefer posteriorly placed coils, such as half-saddle configurations, because they are less sensitive to artifacts and time-dependent variations in coil tuning produced by motion of the anterior neck structures (e.g., swallowing, respiration). Segmented step ladder–type coils, which span a substantial length of the spine, are coming into use for total spine examinations. Such coils markedly expedite the examination by reducing the need to reposition the patient. If a large FOV (e.g., 50 cm) is used with

such coils, then large matrix sizes (e.g., 512 × 512) may be needed to provide adequate in-plane spatial resolution. Alternatively, the body coil may be used for such examinations, though thicker slices and larger FOVs may be needed to provide adequate S/N. For the reasons mentioned previously, motion is typically more problematic in body-coil images than in surface-coil images.

Restrictions in Receiver Coil Design

Optimal coil design depends on field strength. At low to medium field strengths, saddle-shaped and spherical coils can be applied. On high field systems, these coil designs are unsatisfactory because of a phenomenon called *self-resonance,* which prevents tuning of the coil. Therefore, on high field systems, more symmetrically shaped resonator coils are com-

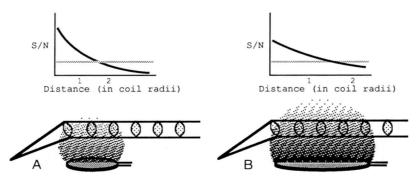

FIGURE 2–4. For spine examinations, the precise positioning of a large coil (*B*) is less critical than for a small coil (*A*). Use of a large coil saves time for extensive spine surveys, as for evaluation of spinal block, for which coverage, rather than spatial resolution, is most important. Solid line in graph is S/N vs. distance from surface coil; speckled line represents S/N for body coil.

COIL ORIENTATIONS   MAGNETIC FIELD ORIENTATIONS

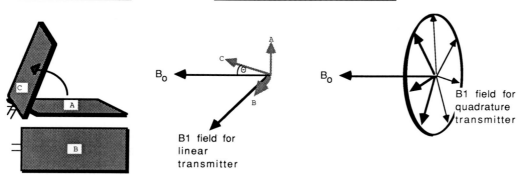

FIGURE 2–5. Positioning of a flat "license plate" receiver coil in a superconducting magnet. *A,* With horizontal positioning of the receiver coil, its B_1 (radiofrequency [RF]) field is perpendicular to the main magnetic field (B_0), resulting in optimal sensitivity for the tissue MR signal. In addition, its B_1 field is perpendicular to that of a linear transmitter coil (i.e., physically decoupled), which is required for safety reasons if the receiver and transmitter coils are not electronically decoupled. Note that the B_1 field of a quadrature (circularly polarized) transmitter coil continually changes (i.e., rotates within the x-y plane). Therefore, it is not possible to decouple the receiver coil physically from the transmitter coil, and electronic decoupling is required. *B,* The receiver coil can be rotated toward a sagittal orientation with no loss of sensitivity. Electronic decoupling of the coils is now required, since the B_1 field of the receiver coil is aligned with that of the transmitter coil. *C,* Tilting of the receiver coil toward a coronal orientation results in a loss of sensitivity because of partial alignment of the B_1 field of the coil with the B_0 field. Optimal sensitivity is attained when the two fields are perpendicular ($\Theta = 90°$), as in *A* or *B*.

monly employed. Moreover, the sensitivity of RF coils depends on the design and orientation of the coil. *Receiver coils have the highest sensitivity for the signal from a sample when the magnetic axis of the coil (B_1) is perpendicular to the direction of the main magnetic field (B_0).* This principle necessitates using different types of RF coils for different main field orientations.

Restrictions in Receiver Coil Positioning

With saddle and resonator designs, B_1 is typically perpendicular to the long axis of the coil. When such coils are oriented in the usual way (long axis of the coil along the length of the magnet), B_1 is also perpendicular to the main field. This is the optimal orientation (Fig. 2–5). For instance, a flat "license plate" receiver coil is usually positioned in a horizontal (coronal) orientation for spine examinations. In this orientation, the coil magnetic field is perpendicular to the main field. If the coil is tilted from a coronal plane toward an axial orientation, then the coil and main magnetic field axes become aligned and S/N declines.

Different coils may be needed for head and body imaging in a magnet with a vertical field orientation. In these systems, coils such as solenoids, whose magnetic field axis is directed along the length of the coil, may be preferred for such applications as head, spine, or knee imaging (Fig. 2–6).

In addition to maintaining the proper orientation of the receiver coil with respect to the main field, it may be important to maintain the proper orientation between the receiver and transmitter coils. In older MR systems without electronic decoupling of the coils, considerations of safety and image quality necessitate keeping the receiver coil in a fixed, prede-

termined orientation (usually horizontal). Failure to maintain orthogonality of the magnetic field axes of the receiver and transmitter coils in such cases can result in damage to the surface coils, or, in the worst case, the patient could suffer burns caused by direct absorption of RF energy from the transmitter into the receiver and subsequent arcing to the patient.[22]

At present, most MR systems use quadrature (circularly polarized) transmitter coils. In these systems, the receiver coil is electronically detuned or decoupled from the transmitter coil. In effect, the receiver coil is deactivated during RF transmission. The re-

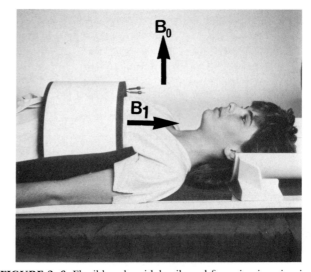

FIGURE 2–6. Flexible solenoidal coil used for spine imaging in a permanent magnet system with a vertical main field (B_0) orientation. Note that the magnetic field of the coil (B_1) is perpendicular to B_0. (Courtesy of Fonar Medical Systems, Inc., Melville, NY.)

ceiver coil may therefore be placed in virtually any position within the center of the magnet. However, decoupling of the coils does not eliminate the need to maintain the proper relationship between the receiver coil and the main field, as addressed previously.

Coil Centering

Centering of the receiver coil with respect to the center of the magnet is important for achieving optimal image quality (Fig. 2–7). Even in the most homogeneous whole-body magnets, field uniformity and gradient linearity decline toward the periphery of the magnet. As a result, extreme positioning of a surface coil with respect to the magnet center (as may be necessary for imaging of the shoulder) may cause a loss of S/N and may produce geometric distortion, which is most apparent on gradient-echo images.

In some cases, it may not be possible to use the optimal receiver coil. For instance, most halos used in neurosurgical fixation are too large for the head coil, a patient with an extreme lordosis might not fit within the neck coil, and the spine coil may be poorly adapted for a patient with an extreme scoliosis. These patients should be imaged within the body coil. Images of good quality can nonetheless be obtained if thicker slices, larger FOVs, and additional excitations are applied.

COIL TUNING AND MATCHING

An RF coil is designed to resonate over a certain frequency range, matching the frequency range contained in the MR signal. However, a coil behaves differently when it is isolated (unloaded) than when it is near a patient (loaded). The loaded coil senses or couples to the electrical properties of the patient's tissues. The additional electrical impedance provided by the patient's tissues changes the effective impedance and resonance frequency of the coil, so that its *quality* (Q) (see Chapter 12) is degraded.

To improve the performance of the coil, it must be tuned again to the resonance frequency of the tissue protons. This tuning is done by adjustment of variable capacitors attached to the coil. In addition, another capacitor is adjusted to improve the match between the impedance of the coil and the preamplifier used to magnify the signal. The ease of tuning an RF coil relates to its Q. In general, low-Q coils are easier to tune than high-Q coils. However, compared with high-Q coils, low-Q coils have the drawback of providing reduced S/N.

During the tuning and matching of the receiver coil, a small amount of RF power is applied continuously by the transmitter coil. A digital display represents the amount of RF power absorbed by the receiver coil. As the tuning and matching of the circuit are improved, the absorbed RF power approaches a maximal value, which corresponds to optimized coil sensitivity (Fig. 2–8). (Alternatively, MR systems may display reflected, rather than absorbed, RF power; in this case, optimal coil sensitivity is obtained when the digital display shows a minimal value.) In some systems the tuning process is automated, whereas in others the tuning is manual.

Tuning of the receiver coil—and, in some systems, the transmitter coil—is necessary every time the loading of the coil changes, that is, if the patient is moved or if a new patient is positioned. However, not all MR systems require tuning of the coils. Some systems use pretuned, low-Q coils that resonate efficiently over a wide range of loading. The time saved in not tuning the coils is at the expense of a mild (10 to 20 per cent) sacrifice in S/N.

In some patients, coil tuning is impossible. These are typically very obese patients or patients with strongly ferromagnetic implants. Although infrequent, this problem is encountered most commonly with high field systems and systems that use RF coils with high-Q factors. In these cases, minor adjustments in the positioning of the patient may make a sufficient difference that coil tuning is possible. In particular, it may be important to avoid having the patient in direct contact with the coil, as this may cause major changes in its tuning characteristics. In very small patients, such as infants, bags of saline may be placed within the receiver coil around the patient to load the coil better and permit tuning.

FREQUENCY ADJUSTMENT

The frequency of the transmitted RF pulse must be matched to the Larmor frequency of the tissue nuclei. Since this matching is determined by the magnetic field strength, frequency adjustment would seem to be an extraneous procedure on superconducting systems, which produce stable magnetic fields. However, frequency variations produced by tissue magnetic susceptibility effects can significantly alter the resonance frequency, requiring an adjustment procedure. Frequency adjustment is particularly important for mobile MR imaging systems, because the main field strength may not be precisely

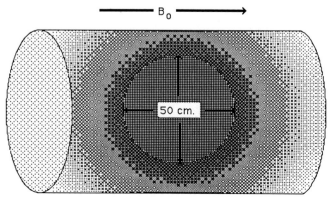

FIGURE 2–7. Image quality is best over a spherical region near the center of the magnet, where there is optimal field homogeneity.

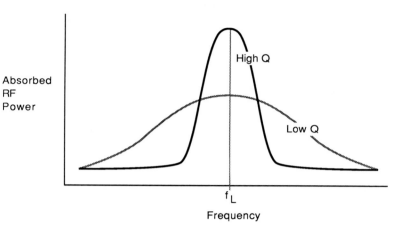

FIGURE 2–8. Sensitivity for the MR signal versus frequency for coils with low- and high-quality factors (Q). The higher Q coil provides better sensitivity over a narrower frequency range. Note that the Q of any coil is lowered when "loaded" (i.e., placed in proximity) to the patient; high Q coils in particular should be tuned after positioning of the patient for optimal performance.

shimmed when the magnet is relocated from site to site.

During the frequency adjustment, a broad bandwidth of frequencies is excited around the nominal tissue resonance frequency, and the received signal is Fourier transformed. The result is a spectrum representing signal intensity versus frequency. On high field systems, both a fat peak and a water peak are seen, with the water peak at higher frequency. Depending on the system, the frequency of the RF pulse may be shifted to match that of the water peak or to an intermediate frequency between the fat and water peaks. Poor magnet homogeneity resulting from improper shimming or ferromagnetic implants may cause broadening and merging of these peaks, precluding accurate frequency adjustment, with resultant loss of S/N.

Transmitter Adjustment

The transmitter adjustment represents the process of determining the amount of RF power necessary to produce a selected flip angle. Transmitter adjustment must be performed each time the patient is moved or a new patient is positioned, because the amount of RF power required to produce a particular flip angle varies with the size of the patient and coil tuning.

Most MR systems go through an iteration procedure to determine the power needed to produce a 90-degree or 180-degree RF pulse and then calculate the power levels needed to produce other flip angles. Several algorithms are in use for transmitter adjustment; one common approach is to increase RF power in stepwise fashion until a signal minimum is produced, representing the 180-degree RF pulse. Two types of transmitter adjustment modes are available. In the nonselective adjustment procedure, the entire imaging volume is excited simultaneously. In the selective adjustment method, RF power levels are determined by measuring signal from a single slice. Transmitter values determined by the selective method are generally more reliable than those of the nonselective method.

Transmitter adjustment may prove impossible in some patients, for a variety of reasons. Transmitter voltages, which increase with the patient's weight, may exceed the capacity of the transmitter tube for large patients. Even in average-sized patients, a failing transmitter tube may not produce the needed voltage. Since transmitter tubes, unlike most other components of the MR system, have a limited lifetime, this potential problem should be kept in mind, requiring evaluation by field service personnel. The transmitter may also fail to adjust properly if the receiver coil is not properly decoupled from the transmitter coil, which may be caused by electronic malfunction or improper coil positioning. Although uncommon on state-of-the-art MR systems, another problem may be that the RF pulse power is incorrectly adjusted to produce a 360-degree, rather than a 180-degree, flip angle. This incorrect adjustment results in increased power deposition and may also produce worsened S/N. This problem may be suspected when transmitter voltages are anomalously high for the weight of the patient.

Receiver Adjustment

In a multislice acquisition, the MR signal is different for each slice. For instance, slices containing large amounts of fat, which has a short T_1 relaxation time, produce higher signal than do slices devoid of fat. However, the analog-to-digital converter (ADC), which converts the MR signal into digital form for computer analysis, has a limited dynamic range. To avoid exceeding the digitization capacity of the ADC, the gain applied to the MR signal is adjusted for each slice during the receiver adjustment procedure.

Improper receiver adjustment, in which the gain setting is too high, is manifested in the image as an abnormally high background intensity and altered tissue contrast (see Chapter 3). This problem is encountered infrequently on state-of-the-art systems. However, for reasons relating to technical considerations or to the patient, this problem may be encountered even when the receiver adjustment is automated. For instance, in determining the receiver gain,

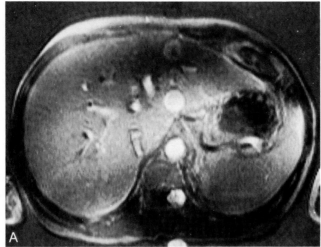

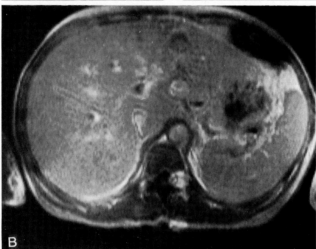

FIGURE 2–9. Bolus administration of gadolinium–diethylene triaminepentaacetic acid (DTPA) breath-hold scanning in a patient with suspected liver metastasis. *A,* Immediate postcontrast scan of upper abdomen. Note the peculiar image contrast and bright background, representing "clipping" of an MR signal that exceeds the dynamic range of the analog-to-digital converter. The receiver gain for this scan was adjusted prior to the administration of contrast agent to avoid any delay before initiating dynamic scanning of the liver. However, there was an overall increase in signal after contrast administration because of the marked enhancement of the liver, spleen, and blood vessels, so that the previously determined receiver gain was too high. *B,* After manual reduction of the receiver gain by 3 dB, image contrast becomes normal.

one assumes that the image signal intensity does not vary over time. However, motion by the patient may occur during data acquisition that did not occur during the brief period when the receiver gain was calculated. Since motion alters signal intensity, the receiver gain setting may prove to be inappropriate. In such cases, manual setting of the receiver gain to a lower value (e.g., −3 dB) than that obtained from the automatic adjustment procedure will usually eliminate the artifact, without altering S/N (Fig. 2–9). However, if the gain is too low, the image may appear dark, with reduced contrast.

SPECIFIC ABSORPTION RATE (SAR)

Specific absorption rate, or SAR, is the mass-normalized rate at which energy from an electromagnetic field is coupled to biologic tissue and is measured in watts per kilogram. The SAR is a complex function of several variables, including (1) the type of RF pulse (e.g., 90 or 180 degrees); (2) the number of RF pulses in a sequence; (3) the pulse width; (4) the TR; (5) the size of the patient; and (6) the type of coil used (i.e., linear, quadrature, and so on).[19, 20] Since the primarily biologic effect of exposure to RF energy is tissue heating and it is possible to produce significant increases in tissue temperature during clinical MR imaging,[23–28] the U.S. Food and Drug Administration has provided guidelines for the safe operation of MR scanners with respect to exposure to RF field. The following are levels that are considered to be safe:

A. If SAR is ≤ 0.4 W/kg, averaged over the whole body, and if SAR is ≤ 8.0 W/kg, averaged over any 1 gm of tissue;

OR

B. If exposure to RF radiation is insufficient to produce a core temperature increase in excess of 1°C and localized heating to greater than 38°C in the head, 39° in the trunk, and 40° in the extremities.

Studies have indicated that individuals with normal heat loss capabilities may safely undergo MR imaging at whole-body averaged SARs as high as 4 W/kg.[28] However, patients who have conditions (e.g., old age, obesity, diabetes, cardiovascular disease, fever-related diseases) associated with heat intolerance or who are taking medications known to affect temperature regulation adversely (e.g., beta blockers, sedatives) should not be subjected to MR imaging procedures that require high SARs (i.e., >2 W/kg).

On low field systems, the selection of pulse sequences is generally not limited by SAR. However, on high field systems, the SAR can limit the number of slices that can be obtained for a particular TR, since power deposition increases with the square of field strength (see Chapter 12). This problem is more of a limitation when the body coil, rather than the head coil, is used as the transmitter. SAR limitations are less significant for brain imaging, since the smaller head coil transmits lower power levels than does the body coil.[26]

There are two approaches to circumvent the SAR limitation:

1. At hospital-based MR sites, permission should be obtained from the hospital institutional review board (IRB) to increase the SAR limit. Outpatient sites must usually be designated by the MR manufacturer as research facilities in order to be permitted to exceed the SAR limit. SAR limits as high as 2 W/kg are in common usage.

2. A pulse sequence that uses longer RF pulses or fewer 180-degree pulses should be chosen. Power deposition decreases as the RF pulse duration is

increased (see Chapter 10). However, choosing a pulse sequence that uses long RF pulses has drawbacks, such as an increase in the minimal echo time (TE) and an increase in chemical shift artifact in the slice-selection direction (not usually a significant problem on lower field systems). It should be noted that newer, computer-optimized RF pulses that permit acquisition of contiguous slices often produce lower RF power absorption than do conventional RF pulses.

CHOOSING PULSE SEQUENCES AND TIMING PARAMETERS

The pulse sequence may be selected according to routine protocols or by the MR physician or technologist in nonroutine cases. Three pulse sequences are commonly used: (1) spin echo (SE), (2) gradient echo (GRE), and (3) inversion recovery (IR). Details of pulse sequence structure, S/N, and contrast are considered in Chapters 1 and 10. The applications of pulse sequences for various clinical problems are discussed in the relevant chapters. Sample protocols are provided in Appendix I at the end of the book. In this section, we consider briefly the unique features of the various pulse sequences and of each sequence parameter and the practical consequence of changing them.

SPIN-ECHO SEQUENCES

SE images remain the mainstay of MR diagnosis, partly because these images are relatively straightforward to interpret and partly because they are less sensitive to certain artifacts than are images produced by other pulse sequences.

T_1-Weighting

SE images obtained with short TR (TR < T_1) and short TE (TE << T_2) are predominantly T_1 weighted. For these images, TR in the range of 300 to 800 msec may be selected. However, it may not be possible to obtain an adequate number of slices within this range of TR. Several options are available in this situation:

1. The minimal TR per slice depends on the pulse sequence. For instance, use of low-bandwidth techniques, flow compensation, or presaturation may reduce the number of slices for a given TR. In addition, for a given TR, GRE sequences may permit more slices to be obtained than with SE techniques.

2. The number of slices can be kept constant, but the slice thickness or interslice gap, or both, may be increased to provide more coverage.

3. The TR may be increased. For most applications, a TR ≤ 1 second may be selected without losing important diagnostic information. However, imaging time increases in proportion to TR.

However, lengthening of the TR generally worsens T_1 contrast. As a result, the choice of TR should be restricted to a more limited range in certain applications, for example, in screening the liver for metastases or the pituitary gland for a microadenoma or in the setting of contrast enhancement with gadolinium–diethylenetriaminepentaacetic acid (DTPA). In addition, on T_1-weighted images of the spine, a lengthened TR increases the signal intensity of cerebrospinal fluid (CSF). This increased signal intensity may result in worsened ghost artifacts from CSF pulsation (see Chapter 3).

In general, for T_1-weighted images, the TE should be kept to a minimum, since longer TEs introduce undesirable amounts of T_2 weighting into the image. However, several factors constrain the free selection of TE. The minimal TE for a given pulse sequence is determined by the sequence structure and cannot be reduced by the operator. Use of flow compensation or low-bandwidth techniques often lengthens the minimal available TE (see further on).

T_2-Weighting

With long TR (TR > 3 × T_1) and long TE (TE ~ T_2), SE images are predominantly T_2 weighted. The degree of T_2 weighting increases, up to a point, as the TE is prolonged. Typically, two echoes are acquired; although both images actually have some degree of T_2 weighting, the first echo image is called proton density weighted, while the second echo image is called T_2 weighted. The precise choice of TE is not critical. Usual sequence parameters include a TE_1 of 20 to 40 msec and a TE_2 of 60 to 90 msec. TEs > 90 msec may produce images that are excessively degraded by low S/N and motion artifacts. However, such long TEs may help characterize lesions with very long T_2 relaxation times, such as cysts and cavernous hemangiomas (see Chapter 29).

For T_2-weighted images, TRs typically vary between 2000 and 3000 msec. T_1 relaxation times increase with field strength. Therefore, for high-field T_2-weighted images, the TR at the upper end of this range should be selected to reduce the amount of T_1 weighting.

GRADIENT-ECHO SEQUENCES

There are several GRE pulse sequences (also called *partial flip* or *field echo*) in common usage, particularly for flow, spine, and three-dimensional (3D) imaging. Commercial acronyms include FLASH, FISP, GRASS, CE-FAST, and PSIF.* Properties of these sequences are considered in depth in Chapter 5.

---

*FLASH = fast low-angle shot; FISP = fast-imaging steady-state precession; GRASS = gradient-recalled acquisition steady state; CE-FAST = contrast-enhanced FAST imaging; PSIF = FISP backward (same as CE-FAST).

Compared with SE methods, GRE techniques permit faster imaging and are more useful for evaluation of flow. Rules for GRE image contrast are as follows: (1) increase the flip angle for T_1 weighting and decrease the flip angle for proton density weighting; (2) keep TEs short to avoid artifacts; and (3) always use flow compensation to maximize signal from blood vessels.

Single-slice GRE acquisitions typically use TRs in the range of 20 to 40 msec; multislice GRE acquisitions must use longer TRs, e.g., between 100 and 300 msec. Multislice techniques are most efficient for routine clinical applications, whereas single-slice techniques are predominantly used for fast imaging and flow imaging applications. Parameter selection depends on the application.

Flow Enhancement

To enhance intravascular signal maximally for flow perpendicular to the plane of section, a single-slice flow-compensated GRE acquisition should be performed with a TR in the range of 20 to 50 msec and a flip angle of 20 to 30 degrees. For flow within the slice, longer TRs and smaller flip angles may improve vascular enhancement (e.g., TR = 70 msec, flip angle = 20 degrees).

MR Myelogram

Multislice, flow-compensated GRE images provide high spinal cord–CSF contrast over a wide range of TRs. In general, TR $\geq$ 100 msec should be selected. We have obtained consistent MR myelograms using a TR of 300 msec and a flip angle of 10 degrees.

Steady-State Versus Spoiled Gradient-Echo Sequences

FISP and GRASS are examples of steady-state GRE pulse sequences, whereas FLASH is an example of a spoiled GRE pulse sequence (see Chapter 5). Unlike FLASH, with a very short TR (e.g., <50 msec), FISP/GRASS types of sequences produce high signal from tissues with markedly prolonged T_2 relaxation times, such as CSF and urine. The short TR effectively limits the acquisition to a single slice. In addition, steady-state effects are limited by motion, which may result in reduced signal intensity and ghost artifacts.

When Not to Use Gradient-Echo Methods

GRE methods should not be used when there is severe magnetic field inhomogeneity, such as that produced by certain metallic implants. In addition, images obtained with most GRE methods do not have enough T_2 contrast to substitute for conventional T_2-weighted SE images in certain applications, such as for detection of subtle tumors or plaques of multiple sclerosis. For imaging of regions such as the chest and abdomen, GRE images should be obtained during periods of suspended respiration.

OTHER IMAGING PARAMETERS

Number of Excitations (NEX)

In general, the number of excitations (NEX) or acquisitions (ACQ) should be kept to a minimum, since imaging time increases with NEX. There are two exceptions: (1) oversampling techniques (see further on; see also Chapters 3 and 10), used to eliminate wraparound in the phase-encoding direction (e.g., NOPHASEWRAP), may require the use of two excitations, though this restriction is eliminated with more recent software versions; and (2) increased NEX may be desirable for reduction of motion and flow artifacts, particularly for imaging of the abdomen and chest.

Slice Thickness

The minimal slice thickness that may be selected is limited by the peak amplitude of the slice-selection gradient and by the characteristics of the RF pulse. The peak gradient amplitude is limited on commercial systems to $\sim$ 10 to 15 mT/meter. In conjunction with an RF pulse short (e.g., 2.5 msec) in duration, this would typically yield a minimal slice thickness of 2 to 3 mm. However, with the same gradient limitations, thinner slices (e.g., 1 mm) may be obtained using RF pulses of longer duration. Thinner slices may also be obtained using 3D techniques (see further on and Chapter 10).

Choice of slice thickness depends on the body part. For head imaging, a slice thickness of 5 mm is adequate for routine screening studies. Thinner slices (2 to 3 mm) should be used for studies of the pituitary gland and internal auditory canals, knees, and temporomandibular joints. However, on low field systems, thicker slices may be necessitated by S/N and throughput considerations. For studies of the chest, abdomen, and pelvis, as well as for musculoskeletal applications, excluding the joints, high spatial resolution is less critical, and slice thicknesses in the range of 5 to 10 mm are commonly selected.

Interslice Gap and Slice Profile[29, 29a]

In theory, contiguous slices (i.e., no gap) should be used for all MR imaging. In practice, it is often necessary to use gaps between slices.

The reason for this practice relates to imperfections in slice profiles. A mathematical function called a *sinc* [sin (x)/x] is commonly used to modulate the waveform of the RF pulse. The Fourier transform of this function is a rectangle. However, a perfectly rectangular slice profile is produced only by a sinc pulse of infinite duration, which is impractical. RF pulses of shorter duration always produce imperfect

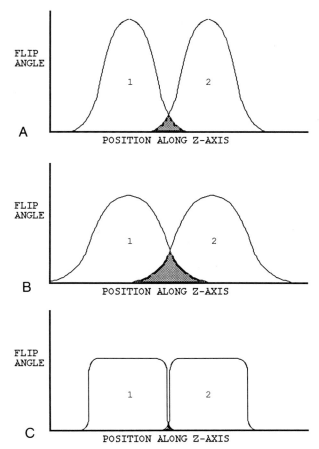

FIGURE 2–10. Slice profiles. *A,* Sinc pulse of moderate duration. *B,* Sinc pulse of shorter duration. Cross-talk between slices (1) and (2) is worse in *B* than *A* owing to the worsened slice profile in the latter case. This necessitates increasing the interslice gap. *C,* Long sinc pulses or computer-optimized RF pulses of shorter duration produce nearly rectangular slice profiles, permitting interslice gaps ≤10 per cent of the nominal slice thickness.

slice profiles, so that the flip angle varies across the width of the slice. If narrow gaps between slices are used, then each slice is contaminated by RF excitations from the edges of the adjacent slices (cross-talk) (Fig. 2–10). The result of these extra excitations is that a slice will have an effective TR less than the nominal TR. On T_2-weighted images, cross-talk is manifested as a reduction in the signal from structures with long T_1 relaxation times, such as CSF and neoplasms (Fig. 2–11). As a result, longer TR and TE are needed to recover the expected T_2 contrast. A gap of at least 50 per cent will eliminate cross-talk in these images. T_1-weighted images are less degraded by cross-talk than are T_2-weighted images, so that slice gaps of 20 to 30 per cent may be adequate.

Cross-talk may be reduced by using sinc pulses of long (e.g., >5 msec) duration. Recently, shorter RF pulses with optimized rectangular slice profiles have been implemented (see Chapter 10). These RF pulses permit imaging with gaps of 10 per cent or less. However, use of small gaps may create a new problem, that of obtaining adequate coverage of the region of interest. Total coverage, defined as the distance between the centers of the outer slices, may be expressed as

$$\text{Coverage} = (\text{number of slices} - 1) \times (\text{slice thickness} + \text{gap})$$

For instance, a 20-slice axial acquisition using 5-mm slices and no gap would produce coverage of 95 mm, which is less than the vertical extent of the average adult brain. Let us further assume that the number of slices is limited by the amount of computer memory available for the storage of raw data, which is the case with certain MR systems. Although the number of slices cannot be increased in this situation, adequate coverage may still be obtained by increasing the slice gap to, for example, 40 per cent.

Field-of-View

The FOV is defined as the horizontal or vertical distance across the image. Typically, FOVs in the range of 8 to 50 cm are used. Decreases in FOV are produced by increasing the strength of the frequency-encoding and phase-encoding gradients; therefore, the minimal FOV is primarily determined by the peak gradient amplitude. Spatial resolution improves as the FOV is decreased, within the constraints of S/N limitations. Whereas reductions in slice thickness produce a proportional decrease in S/N, reductions in FOV produce a more rapid decline in S/N, in proportion to $(\text{FOV})^2$. Therefore, in many applications, adjusting the slice thickness may be a more practical means for reducing partial volume averaging than adjusting the FOV.

Small FOVs are chosen for detailed anatomic evaluation, such as for imaging the temporomandibular joint. Small FOVs may produce wraparound artifacts unless oversampling methods are used (Fig. 2–12). Low-bandwidth techniques, because of the weaker read-out gradient, typically permit smaller FOVs than do higher bandwidth sequences. Larger FOVs (e.g., 32 cm) are used when more spatial coverage is needed, such as in total spine surveys and in abdominal and pelvic imaging.

Matrix

The matrix represents the number of pixels along the frequency-encoding and phase-encoding axes. Imaging time is proportional to the number of phase-encoding steps. Most systems allow the user to select from several matrix sizes. Typically, 256 pixels are selected along the frequency-encoding axis, and from 128 to 256 pixels along the phase-encoding axis. Images acquired with a symmetric FOV and 256 × 256 matrix have equal resolution along both axes.

Images can be acquired using a 256 × 128 (frequency × phase) matrix in half the time of the 256 × 256 matrix, at the expense of a 50 per cent reduction in spatial resolution (see Chapter 5). Because of the lower spatial resolution, S/N improves

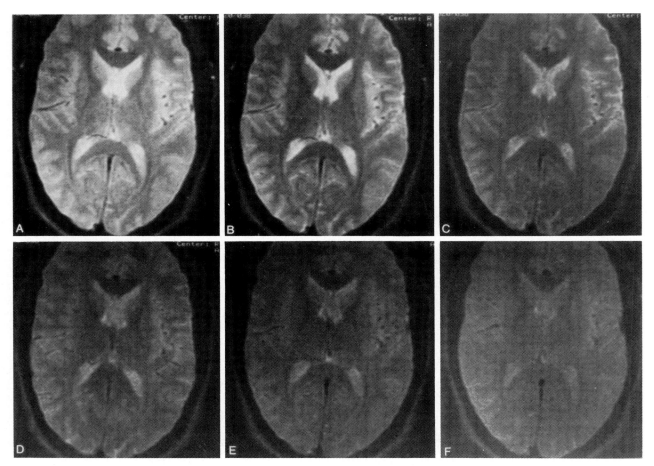

FIGURE 2–11. Effects of cross-talk on image contrast and S/N. T_2-weighted spin-echo (SE) images (*A–F*) and T_1-weighted SE images (*G–L*) with decrease in interslice gap from 100 per cent (*A* and *G*) to 0 per cent (*F* and *L*). Note marked worsening in T_2 contrast and S/N, even with moderate gaps (e.g., 20 per cent in *D*), whereas T_1-weighted images are less severely degraded at the same gap (*J*). (From Kucharczyk W, Crawley AP, Kelly WM, Henkelman RM: Effect of multislice interference on image contrast in T2- and T1-weighted MR images. AJNR 9:443–451, 1988; © by American Roentgen Ray Society.)

with a reduction in matrix size (Table 2–2). However, objectionable ringing artifacts (see Chapter 3) may result from small matrix sizes, so that a compromise may be made between spatial resolution and imaging time by using a 256 × 192 (frequency × phase) matrix.

Ringing artifacts and spatial resolution can also be improved despite a reduced matrix by using an asymmetric (rectangular) FOV. As mentioned in Chapter 1, this technique improves resolution along the phase-encoding axis by increasing the amplitude of the phase-encoding gradient, while keeping constant the number of pixels in the matrix. For instance, one can consider an image acquired with a 256 × 128 matrix and a 30 cm × 30 cm symmetric FOV. In the same amount of time, an image can be acquired with 33 per cent more resolution along the y-axis by using a 30 cm × 20 cm (frequency × phase) FOV. However, compared with the image acquired using the symmetric FOV, this image will have 33

per cent less S/N. In addition, wraparound artifact may limit the application of this method with small FOVs, depending on the dimensions of the body part being imaged.

TRADE-OFFS BETWEEN IMAGING PARAMETERS

It is generally desirable to maximize spatial resolution while minimizing the imaging time. However, it is also necessary to maintain an adequate level of S/N. Changes in slice thickness, FOV, matrix, and NEX produce interdependent changes in spatial resolution and S/N. For instance, a reduction in slice thickness produces a decrease in S/N that may be compensated for by using a slightly larger FOV or smaller matrix. Some examples of the interdependent effects that result from changes in various scan parameters are provided in Table 2–2.

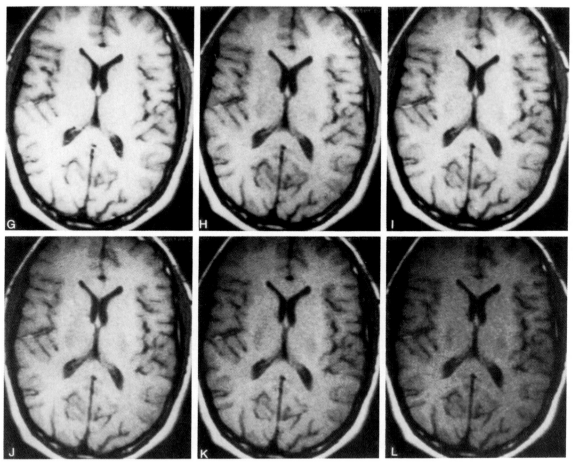

FIGURE 2-11 *Continued*

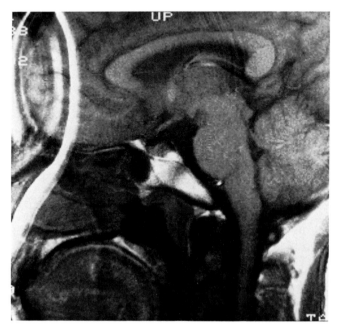

FIGURE 2-12. Head image acquired with 15-cm FOV. Because oversampling was applied only in the frequency-encoding (vertical) direction, the image is degraded only by wraparound artifact in the phase-encoding (horizontal) direction.

SPECIAL TECHNIQUES

HALF-FOURIER[30]

The half-Fourier method reconstructs an image from only half the data, providing a nearly 50 per cent reduction in imaging time (see Chapter 5). However, with the faster acquisition, S/N is reduced by 40 per cent, so the method should be applied only when S/N is not a limiting factor. Moreover, the half-Fourier images are prone to artifacts produced by magnetic field inhomogeneity or motion by the patient. Therefore, this technique should be avoided with GRE pulse sequences. In addition, the extra data manipulations required with half-Fourier imaging may increase reconstruction times as much as twofold.

FLOW COMPENSATION (BRIGHT BLOOD SEQUENCE)[31]

Flow compensation, also called *flow comp, GMR, GMN,* or *MAST**, is a method for reducing flow and

*GMR = gradient motion rephasing; GMN = gradient motion nulling; MAST = motion artifact suppression technique.

**TABLE 2–2. EFFECTS OF CHANGES IN SCAN PARAMETERS ON ACQUISITION TIME, S/N,
AND SPATIAL RESOLUTION**

Matrix	SLT (mm)	FOV (cm)	NEX	ACQ Time* (sec)	S/N†	Resolution (mm)	Voxel (mm³)
256 × 256	5	24	1	128	100	0.9 × 0.9	4.4
256 × 256	5	24	1	64	71	0.9 × 0.9	4.4
Half-Fourier							
256 × 192	5	24	1	96	115	0.9 × 1.3	5.9
256 × 256	5	24 × 30	1	128	125	0.9 × 1.2	5.5
Asymmetric FOV							
256 × 128	5	24	1	64	141	0.9 × 1.8	8.8
256 × 128	5	24	2	128	200	0.9 × 1.8	8.8
256 × 256	5	17	1	128	50	0.7 × 0.7	2.2
256 × 256	5	17	4	512	100	0.7 × 0.7	2.2
256 × 128	5	17	2	128	100	0.7 × 1.3	4.4
256 × 128	7	17	1	64	100	0.7 × 1.3	6.2
256 × 256	3	10	1	128	10	0.4 × 0.4	0.5
256 × 128	3	10	8	512	40	0.4 × 0.8	0.9

*Acquisition time for TR = 500 msec.
†S/N normalized to 100 for 5-mm slice, 256 × 256 matrix, and one excitation.
SLT = slice thickness.

motion artifacts (see Chapter 4). The method incorporates into the pulse sequence additional gradient pulses that reduce motion-related phase shifts. In multiecho pulse sequences used for obtaining T_2-weighted images, the first or second echoes, or both, may be flow compensated, depending on the pulse sequence and MR system.

The effect of flow compensation is to increase signal intensity from flowing blood and CSF. Flow compensation should be used in nearly all clinical applications of T_2-weighted or GRE images. The method is particularly useful for suppressing ghost artifacts arising from CSF pulsation in the brain and spine. When it is used for imaging of the abdomen, signal from moving organs such as the liver is increased, and ghost artifacts are reduced.

The major limitation of flow compensation is that the minimal TE, slice thickness, and FOV may be increased compared with standard pulse sequences. As a result, it may not be possible to use flow compensation in applications that require very high spatial resolution, such as imaging of the temporomandibular joints. In addition, in some patients, flow compensation may not provide adequate suppression of ghost artifacts from CSF pulsation. In these patients, the combination of flow compensation and electrocardiographic (ECG)-gating (see further on) may provide better artifact suppression.

Flow compensation should not be used if it is important for flowing blood or CSF to appear dark. For instance, flow compensation will eliminate the CSF flow void sign in the aqueduct of Sylvius; this sign is occasionally used to characterize hydrocephalus. Similarly, flow compensation may not be desirable on T_1-weighted images of the spine, since it increases the signal from CSF and may reduce contrast between CSF and the spinal cord or cauda equina.

PRESATURATION (DARK BLOOD SEQUENCE)[32, 33]

Presaturation is a method that eliminates ghost artifacts resulting from blood flow or respiratory motion (see Chapter 4). The method incorporates into the pulse sequence additional RF pulses that saturate tissue magnetization over user-defined regions. Presaturation applied along the slice-selection direction eliminates flow artifacts and should be routinely used for imaging of the head and body, wherever flow artifacts may limit image quality. For instance, in head images presaturation will reduce ghost artifacts resulting from pulsatile flow in the intracerebral arteries; it will decrease these artifacts in images of the heart; and, in abdominal images, it will reduce those due to pulsatile flow in the aorta and inferior vena cava.

The effectiveness of flow presaturation depends on the velocity and direction of flow. Therefore, one should not be surprised if the technique fails to eliminate signal completely from CSF within the thecal sac, where the flow is to-and-fro rather than unidirectional, or in certain patterns of blood flow. For instance, presaturation does not typically affect artifacts caused by vascular pulsation in the cerebral venous sinuses, since the effects of the presaturation pulses on arteries do not carry through the capillary system into the veins. It may also fail to suppress intravascular signal adequately within large aortic aneurysms, which have slow flow. Additional limitations of the method include reduced multislice capability and increased RF power deposition.

Some systems offer the capability of applying presaturation along directions other than slice selection. For instance, presaturation applied along the phase-encoding direction may be useful for spine imaging to suppress ghost artifacts arising from vascular pulsation and respiration, particularly if gradient rotation (see below) is not available. Presaturation may also be used to suppress the high signal from subcutaneous fat in the near field of a surface coil.

GRADIENT ROTATION

The orientation of the phase-encoding axis is determined by the user. By reorienting the phase-encoding axis, it may be possible to keep ghost artifacts off the region of interest. For head imaging, the phase-encoding axis is typically oriented horizontally to direct artifacts from eye motion away from the brain. For spine imaging, the phase-encoding axis should parallel the long axis of the spine to prevent ghost artifacts from respiratory motion and vascular pulsation.

A major limitation of gradient rotation is wraparound artifact when the phase-encoding axis is oriented along the long axis of the body. Suppression of wraparound requires concomitant use of oversampling methods. If these are not available, then presaturation should be used for artifact suppression, rather than gradient rotation.

REORDERING OF PHASE ENCODING ACCORDING TO RESPIRATORY PHASE

The order of the phase-encoding steps may be varied according to the respiratory phase, as monitored by a bellows device around the chest or abdomen. This method, which goes by various commercial names or acronyms, such as Exorcist, ROPE, and COPE, provides a substantial reduction in ghost artifacts from respiratory motion. Limitations of the method include difficulty in obtaining adequate sensitivity with the bellows device and increased reconstruction time, since additional data processing is required.

OVERSAMPLING TO ELIMINATE WRAPAROUND

Oversampling methods (e.g., NOPHASEWRAP, EXTENDED MATRIX) acquire an expanded (512 pixel) matrix along either the frequency or the phase direction and then discard the outer 256 pixels to eliminate wraparound along that axis. Limitations of the method include increased reconstruction time. In addition, when the method is used to suppress wraparound along the phase-encoding axis, it may be necessary to acquire a minimum of two excitations, as mentioned previously.

ELECTROCARDIOGRAPHIC GATING

ECG gating involves synchronization of data acquisition to the patient's ECG to suppress flow artifacts, to define cardiac anatomy more precisely, and/or to permit a dynamic display of cardiac function using cine techniques.

There is some confusion of terminology with respect to the terms *triggering* and *gating*. Although these terms are often used synonymously, some manufacturers use the term triggering specifically to refer to prospective methods of cardiac gating.

Prospective Cardiac Gating

For prospective cardiac gating, data acquisition is initiated after a user-determined time interval following the R wave (Fig. 2–13A). This "trigger delay" can

FIGURE 2–13. Comparison of prospective cardiac gating (*A*) and retrospective cardiac gating (*B*) for five-slice acquisition. In prospective gating, the time interval between sequence repetitions is determined by the R-R interval, not TR. The repetition time determines the duration of cardiac cycle during which slices are acquired. In retrospective gating, the time interval between sequence repetitions is determined by the TR, as it would be for an ungated acquisition. Retrospective gating provides more consistent image quality than does prospective gating.

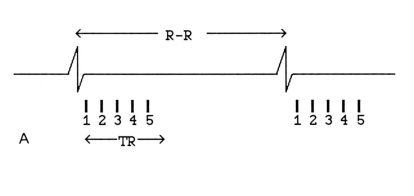

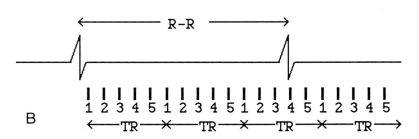

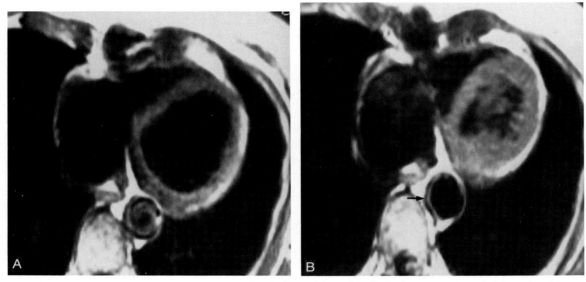

FIGURE 2–14. Axial SE images of heart at level of ventricles. Diastolic SE image (*A*) shows brighter signal in descending aorta, because of slower flow velocity, than does the systolic image (*B*).

be varied so that images are obtained in a particular phase of the cardiac cycle. For instance, triggering with no delay initiates data acquisition at end-diastole, when flow is slow and vascular signal is high (Fig. 2–14*A*). Conversely, a trigger delay on the order of 200 to 300 msec initiates data acquisition during systole, when flow is rapid and vascular signal is low (Fig. 2–14*B*). In a multislice acquisition, the images are acquired over a finite period, corresponding to the user-selected TR. As a result, the images usually span a substantial portion of the cardiac cycle.

ECG gating should be used for cardiac imaging and for imaging of structures directly adjacent to the heart, such as the aortic root and main pulmonary arteries. However, for several reasons, difficulties may be encountered in obtaining a satisfactory ECG tracing:[34]

1. Poor lead contact may result from inadequate skin preparation; the skin should always be cleansed of oil and debris, using an alcohol swab prior to applying the electrodes. In addition, ECG electrodes should contain a minimum of metal, for safety reasons and to reduce local artifacts.

2. Respiratory motion causes a variation in the ECG baseline; this problem may be prevented by attaching the ECG leads to the back of the patient and by using special positioning schemes.[35]

3. Gradient pulsing during imaging induces electrical currents in the ECG leads, which may completely obscure the ECG tracing unless electronic filtering is adequate. Keeping the ECG leads straight along the magnet axis and twisting the leads around one another can help prevent artifacts. Optimal lead placement is shown in Figure 2–15.

4. Another problem is that intense static magnetic fields may alter the ECG by producing an augmented

T wave or other nonspecific ECG changes (see Chapter 4), and these alterations are directly related to the strength of the field. The mechanism responsible for increased T-wave size is postulated to be a superimposition of a low potential on the normally occurring biopotential produced by a magnetohydrodynamic effect, as the blood (i.e., a conductive fluid) flows in the presence of the static magnetic field. The computer may confuse the enlarged T wave with an R wave, resulting in gating twice during each R-R interval. In general, prior to using ECG gating methods, it is wise to consult applications personnel for the manufacturer of the system being used, since gating methods vary widely among different systems.

As mentioned previously, the user-selected TR has a function different from that in ungated acquisitions. In ECG-gated acquisitions, the R-R interval, rather than TR, determines the time between successive excitations of a given slice (Fig. 2–13*A*). The R-R interval may be calculated from the heart rate as follows:

R-R interval = 60 seconds/(number of heartbeats per minute)

Since each R wave triggers the pulse sequence, tissue contrast is determined by the patient-dependent R-R interval, rather than the operator-determined TR. If T_2-weighted images are desired, then data acquisition may be triggered off every third or fourth R wave. However, this practice may produce some inconsistency in data acquisition and worsened image quality, compared with the results obtained with triggering off every R wave.

If data acquisition extends into the subsequent R wave, the system will fail to gate off that R wave. To avoid this problem, the TR should be kept at least

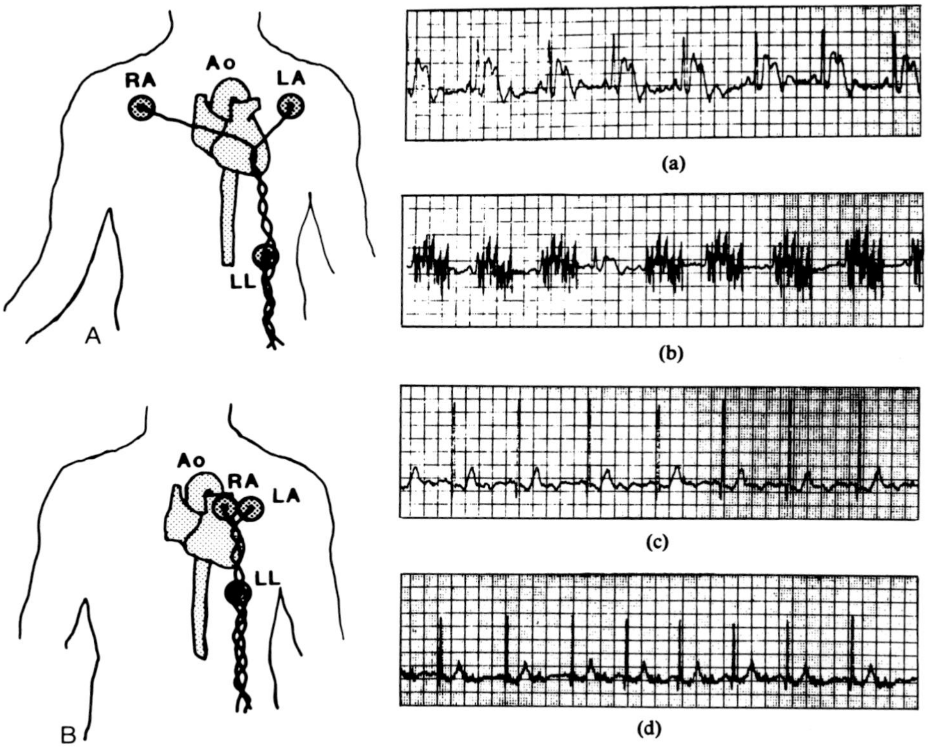

FIGURE 2–15. Examples of cardiac lead placement. *Left*, For optimal results, leads should be twisted, with close placement of limb electrodes (b), rather than placed far apart, as in (a). *Right*, Corresponding ECG tracings for optimal lead placement (c and d) and with limb leads placed apart (a and b). (From Wendt RE, Rokey R, Vick GW, Johnson DL: Electrocardiographic gating and monitoring in NMR imaging. Magn Reson Imaging 6:89–95, 1988; with permission, Pergamon Press, plc.)

30 per cent shorter than the estimated R-R interval, to account for expected physiologic variations in the cardiac rate. Some patients have such a rapid heart rate that a very short TR must be selected, reducing the number of slices that can be obtained.

Scan parameters depend on the particular system. We generally use the following parameters with prospective ECG gating: FOV = 32 to 36 cm, acquisition matrix = 256 × 128, slice thickness = 5 to 10 mm, two to four excitations, and flow presaturation. Although standard orthogonal planes of section may be adequate in many applications, in certain situations it may be preferable to obtain images oriented along the true short and long axes of the heart (see Chapter 26). However, to do this efficiently may require a double oblique acquisition with user-friendly software, which is not universally available.

Retrospective Cardiac Gating

In some patients, conventional ECG triggering fails to produce satisfactory image quality because of physiologic variation of the cardiac rate or because of arrhythmias. In these patients, retrospective cardiac gating is essential. In retrospective gating methods, data are acquired continuously, independently of the R wave (Fig. 2–13*B*). The user-selected TR represents the time between excitations, as it would in an ungated acquisition. To permit subsequent data reconstruction, the patient's ECG is continuously stored in memory. At the end of the acquisition, each line of data is resorted according to the ECG phase in which it was acquired. Errors in the data due to variation in heart rate or, to some extent, respiration can be suppressed during postprocessing of the data (see Chapter 27). Instant imaging methods (e.g., echo planar), which are not yet in routine commercial use, may also prove useful for overcoming arrhythmias (see Chapters 5 and 25).

LOW BANDWIDTH

Low-bandwidth or narrow-bandwidth pulse sequences use a weak frequency-encoding gradient and a prolonged read-out period to improve S/N (see Chapter 10). Matched-bandwidth sequences represent a variation on this technique; the method uses an asymmetric read-out of the echo to shorten the TE in conjunction with a long read-out period. Low-bandwidth methods are particularly useful on low field systems, in which the intrinsic S/N is worse than on high field systems.

Low-bandwidth sequences should not be used when short TEs are desirable (e.g., for obtaining T_1-weighted SE images of the liver), because the prolonged read-out period necessitates an increase in the minimal TE. Images obtained with low-bandwidth methods may also be more susceptible to motion by the patient, magnetic susceptibility artifacts, and any instrument instabilities, such as eddy current effects. Additional drawbacks of low-bandwidth methods include reduced multislice capability and greater chemical shift artifact, which may be troublesome on high field systems. If objectionable, the chemical shift artifact on low-bandwidth images may be decreased by reducing the FOV, at the expense of S/N.

THREE-DIMENSIONAL GRADIENT-ECHO METHODS

These 3D GRE methods permit acquisition of thin (≤ 1 mm), essentially contiguous slices in reasonable amounts of time (Fig. 2–16). It is important to understand that although the data are acquired from a 3D volume, the final result is a set of two-dimensional (2D) images. Furthermore, as with 2D methods, one must select an orientation for the acquisition (e.g., axial, sagittal, coronal, or oblique), and the images are reconstructed in the same plane as the acquisition.

The profiles of the slices acquired by 3D methods are not actually perfectly rectangular. Since the data are phase encoded along the slice-selection direction, ringing (Gibbs or truncation) artifacts occur along this direction, as they occur along the phase- and frequency-encoding directions in 2D images. Despite this, the slices are truly contiguous.

Two types of 3D acquisitions are possible: *isotropic* (i.e., the voxel is a cube) and *anisotropic* (i.e., the voxel is elongated in one dimension, usually the slice-selection axis). In addition, nonselective (i.e., the entire volume is excited by a nonselective RF pulse) or limited-volume (i.e., a thick slab is excited) 3D acquisitions may be performed. The 3D data differ from 2D data in that, if thin slices are acquired, one can perform high-quality multiplanar reconstructions along orientations different from the one in which the data were acquired, particularly if the acquisition is isotropic. The quality of multiplanar reconstructions of anisotropic 3D and 2D images suffers in comparison, because of the larger slice thickness.

Slice Thickness

Three-dimensional acquisitions are performed much like 2D acquisitions; considerations of matrix size and FOV are identical. However, 3D methods are unique in other respects. First, only a single excitation is usually selected. Second, one must define *two* different slice thicknesses. These are the *slab thickness*, representing the thickness of tissue that will be excited by the RF pulse, and the *partition thickness*, representing the thickness of the final images (Fig. 2–16). The partition thickness decreases in proportion to the number of partitions:

$$\text{Partition thickness} = \text{slab thickness}/\text{number of partitions}$$

For instance, four partitions from a slab that is 2 cm thick produces images with a thickness of 5 mm. Although increasing the number of partitions reduces the partition thickness, it also produces a proportional increase in imaging time. For reasons

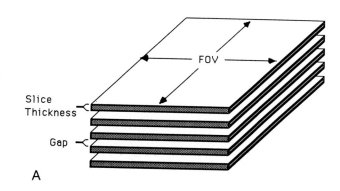

A

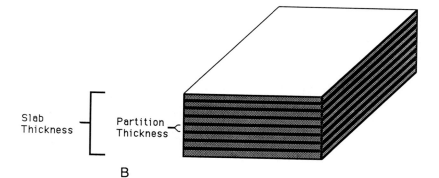

B

FIGURE 2–16. Comparison of (*A*) 2D and (*B*) 3D imaging methods. Note that contiguous slices are directly acquired with 3D methods, unlike with most 2D methods.

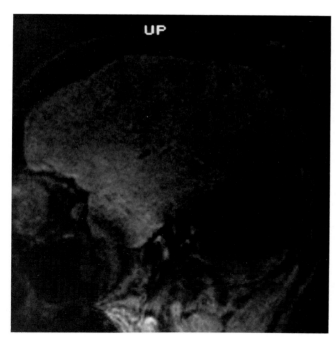

FIGURE 2–17. End slice from 3D acquisition, showing image degradation due to imperfect slab profile and wraparound along slice-selection axis.

relating to the imperfect slab profile produced by the RF pulse, as well as the resulting wraparound across the z-phase–encoding direction, the number of useful images may be at least one fewer than the number of partitions (Fig. 2–17).

Scan Parameters for Three-Dimensional Methods

The choice of TR, TE, and matrix relates to the application. GRE pulse sequences are almost always used, since they permit a shorter TR than do SE sequences. In general, TR should be kept as short as possible (e.g., 20 to 40 msec) to minimize imaging time. The effects of the flip angle are similar to those with 2D GRE methods; that is, large flip angles (e.g., 50 degrees) produce T_1-weighted images, while small flip angles (e.g., 10 degrees) produce proton density–weighted or T_2^*-weighted images or both, depending on the TE. Flow compensation is useful for evaluating blood vessels and for reducing motion artifact.

With 3D methods, one has several options available, which primarily represent trade-offs between faster imaging and higher spatial resolution. For instance, the imaging time for an isotropic 3D data set with a slab thickness of 128 mm, a partition thickness of 1 mm, a TR of 100 msec, a matrix of 128 × 128 × 128, and one excitation is 27 minutes. If the number of partitions is reduced to 32, then the partition thickness increases to 4 mm, resulting in an anisotropic acquisition. However, the advantage is that the imaging time is reduced to 6 minutes. What happens if now, in addition to reducing the number of partitions from 128 to 32, one also reduces

the slab thickness from 128 mm to 32 mm? Then the partition thickness once more becomes 1 mm (resolution is again isotropic), but the imaging time is still only 6 minutes instead of 27 minutes. S/N is proportional to $\sqrt{}$(number of partitions). Therefore, the penalty for maintaining a high level of spatial resolution while reducing the number of partitions in order to image faster is lower S/N.

For technical reasons relating to the use of a 3D Fourier transform for data reconstruction, some MR systems require that the center of a 3D data acquisition be at the center of the magnet (i.e., slab shift = zero) or that the slab shift be an integral multiple of the slab thickness. In this case, it may be necessary to vary the slab thickness to produce an acceptable slab shift. However, this limitation will likely be overcome in most newer software versions.

Clinical applications for 3D methods include evaluation of the cervical spine (Fig. 2–18), anterior cruciate ligaments and menisci, wrist, and other joints for which thin slices are required for optimal assessment; MR angiography (see Chapter 4); and surface modeling (e.g., for radiation therapy planning, reconstructive surgery). Three-dimensional methods are generally not useful in regions such as the chest or abdomen, because they are very sensitive to motion by the patient.

Multislab Three-Dimensional Acquisition

Just as it is possible to perform multislice 2D acquisitions, one can perform multislab 3D acquisition. By multislab, we mean that two or more separate

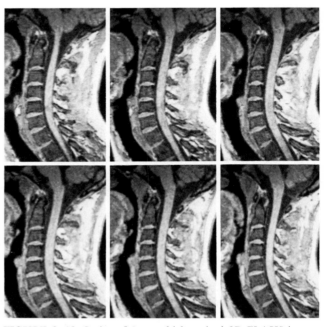

FIGURE 2–18. Series of 1-mm-thick sagittal 3D FLASH images through cervical spine. Note that six slices pass through the spinal cord, which would not be feasible with most 2D methods owing to the larger slice thickness.

tissue volumes are excited. Each of these volumes is then subdivided into thin partitions, as is the case for single-slab 3D acquisition.

Multislab 3D methods have applications similar to those of single-slab 3D methods but are especially useful for imaging two or more regions that are widely separated. For instance, both carotid bifurcations or temporomandibular joints can be imaged simultaneously in a two-slab 3D acquisition. If one attempted to encompass these structures using a single-slab approach, then one would have to excite a much larger volume, which predominantly consists of regions that are of no clinical interest. To obtain a reasonably thin partition thickness from such a wide slab, a large number of z-phase–encoding steps would be required, with a proportionate increase in imaging time.

Using multislab 3D methods does not, per se, increase the imaging time compared with that in single-slice 3D. However, the minimal TR must be increased to accommodate a larger number of slabs. For instance, if the minimal TR for a single-slab 3D acquisition is 30 msec, the minimal TR for a two-slab 3D acquisition is 60 msec, thereby doubling the imaging time. In addition, the slab profiles may be nonrectangular, so that a gap should be left between the slabs.

One major problem with 3D methods, from a practical standpoint, is the large number of images that are generated and that must be viewed by the physician. This problem is compounded when multiplanar reconstructions are performed. Total reconstruction time typically increases in proportion to the number of partitions. Efficient use of 3D methods necessitates having a 3D workstation available for offline data processing. These workstations generally have their own array processor to permit fast multiplanar and surface reconstructions.

USE OF CONTRAST AGENTS

Several contrast agents may be coming into use over the next few years (see Chapter 7). Currently, gadolinium-DTPA (Magnevist, Berlex Imaging, Fairfield, CT) is the most widely used contrast agent for MR imaging. It is primarily applied in the central nervous system (e.g., for detection of brain tumors, including acoustic neuromas and pituitary microadenomas; dropped metastases along the spinal cord; postoperative fibrosis in the spine) but has expanding applications in the body (e.g., for detection of liver metastases). Contraindications to the administration of gadolinium-DTPA include pregnancy and hemolytic anemia.

Contrast studies using gadolinium-DTPA are facilitated by prior placement of an intravenous line with sufficient extension tubing to provide easy access by the physician, thereby eliminating the need to move the patient between precontrast and postcontrast acquisitions. Saline or detrose water solutions can be used to maintain the patency of the line and to flush the injection of contrast agent. Gadolinium-DTPA (0.1 mmol/kg) should be administered intravenously over 1 to 2 minutes.

Although a wide range of imaging techniques may be applied, at least one set of T_1-*weighted* images should be acquired, since proton density–weighted and T_2-weighted images are much less sensitive to the effects of gadolinium-DTPA. For most applications, imaging should be started within a few minutes of contrast administration. Repeated imaging after a suitable delay may be useful for improved characterization of certain lesions, such as cavernous hemangiomas of the liver.

Dynamic imaging may be helpful in certain clinical applications, such as imaging of the pituitary gland or liver. The TR and NEX should be kept to a minimum. In administering a rapid bolus of contrast agent, it may be desirable to follow the injection of contrast agent with a bolus injection of saline, to flush out the several milliliters of contrast agent held in the long extension tubing. Rapid injections are generally without hazard but in some patients may induce nausea (a nonspecific effect resulting from administering a hypertonic solution). One should be aware that nausea is a potentially hazardous condition in the confines of a magnet bore, since the patient's mobility is restricted and vomiting is more likely to result in aspiration than would be the case for CT.

The signal intensities of various tissues in the image may change considerably after the administration of a contrast agent. Owing to T_1 shortening, signal enhancement is especially pronounced in blood vessels, which tends to worsen ghost artifacts from pulsatile flow. These changes are most pronounced when the agent is administered as a concentrated bolus and dynamic imaging is performed. In some situations, the change in signal intensity may result in misadjustment of the receiver gain. The misadjustment occurs because the receiver gain was determined before the contrast agent was administered (necessary for rapid, dynamic imaging studies) or after contrast administration but before the agent had equilibrated. To avoid this problem, the receiver gain may be manually reduced by approximately 3 dB from the value determined automatically by the system, as mentioned previously (see Fig. 2–9).

For certain types of studies, such as evaluation of the cerebellopontine angles for acoustic neuroma, it may not be necessary to acquire precontrast images. For other examinations, comparison of precontrast and postcontrast images may be essential (e.g., for differentiation of postoperative scar from recurrent disk herniation). In this situation, it is important that the same pulse sequence and scan parameters be used for both studies and that the patient remain still.

Oral contrast agents, which are not yet in general use, require no special considerations, being used, for the most part, in the same way as oral contrast agents are used for CT. One exception is that agents producing high signal in the bowel, such as gadolinium-DTPA, may worsen ghost artifacts because of peristalsis over the longer imaging times used in MR. As a result, some investigators administer an agent such as glucagon (1 mg, intramuscularly or subcutaneously) immediately before placing the patient into the magnet bore to suppress peristalsis.

Finally, intravenous contrast agents that predominantly affect T_2 relaxation times, such as ferrite, require different imaging considerations. Such compounds are still in the research phase and are not yet approved for general use. T_2-weighted SE or GRE pulse sequences are most sensitive for signal changes produced by these compounds. In addition, for liver or spleen imaging, certain of these compounds may be administered as much as several hours prior to imaging, because they persist for prolonged periods (e.g., days) in these organ systems.

IMAGE MEASUREMENT

PREPARATION SCANS

After all the prescan adjustments have been made, the measurement process may be commenced. However, data are not actually acquired for several seconds after the nominal start of the measurement. The reason for this relates to the need to establish an equilibrium or steady-state magnetization (see Chapter 1). Before any RF pulses have been applied, the spins are fully magnetized. Therefore, the first RF pulse produces a strong signal. However, each of the next few RF pulses produces less signal owing to incomplete T_1 relaxation between excitations. Only after several excitations is a balance (i.e., equilibrium) reached between the TR and T_1.

To avoid an anomalous change in signal intensity over the first few sequence repetitions, a number of preparation scans (typically eight or more) are applied for the first few seconds of the scan (Fig. 2–19). Some pulse sequences, particularly steady-state GRE techniques such as GRASS or FISP, may require 32 or more preparation scans to establish an equilibrium magnetization.

MEASUREMENT PERIOD

The onset of the image measurement period is indicated by a jackhammer-like knocking sound. This sound represents the mechanical vibrations of the gradient coils produced by changing magnetic fluxes during gradient pulsing. Gradient-produced noise is most severe in pulse sequences that use rapid switching of high-amplitude gradients (e.g., GRE scans with thin slices, small FOV, flow compensation, and short TE and TR). At the start of each measurement, it may be prudent to forewarn the patient of this noise to prevent motion due to involuntary startling. Noises generated by certain MR scanners are sufficiently intense to cause temporary hearing loss in patients, particularly if the duration of exposure is relatively long.[36] Therefore, it is advisable to provide patients with ear plugs or other types of ear protection prior to examination by MR imaging. Ear plugs only partially reduce perceived noise levels, since sound is directly transmitted to the patient from vibration of the table.

Patients may become agitated after the measurement is under way. Several options are then available:

1. On some systems, selection of a "pause" option aborts the acquisition temporarily, until the patient stops moving. However, this option is of limited value, since the patient usually will have moved from his or her original position, necessitating rescanning from the beginning.

2. Some systems can reconstruct images from incomplete data sets if more than 50 per cent of the information has been collected. The quality of such images improves as the percentage of data acquired approaches 100 per cent. If the patient starts to move toward the end of the measurement period, it may be prudent to abort the acquisition prematurely and use these images, which are reconstructed from the incomplete data set.

3. If the patient moves transiently during the acquisition, the resultant image degradation may be

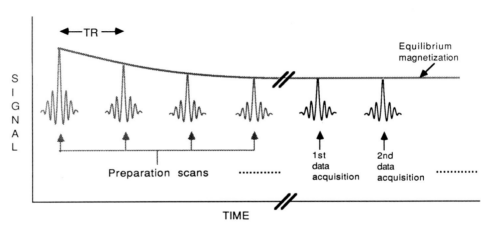

FIGURE 2–19. At the start of the measurement process, a number of preparation scans must be applied to establish an equilibrium magnetization. Data acquisition is started only after the preparation scans are finished.

minimal, particularly if the movement occurs near the beginning or end of the acquisition (i.e., weakest phase-encoding steps). In this case, it may not be necessary to abort the acquisition.

4. The acquisition may be repeated using a smaller matrix, fewer excitations, and shorter TR for faster imaging to improve the likelihood of obtaining a motion-free image. Hybrid or echo planar imaging methods may eventually prove useful in this application.

BREATH-HOLDING

Respiration may be voluntarily suspended for a limited time in certain clinical applications. In particular, breath holding markedly improves the quality of GRE images in the abdomen. These techniques can be used to evaluate vessel patency or to detect metastatic disease in the liver.

In our experience, the most consistent results are obtained when the data acquisition period is kept to a minimum, 10 seconds or less. To maintain the diaphragm at nearly the same position for each scan, images are acquired at end-expiration. The patient is instructed to breathe in (wait ~3 seconds), breathe out (wait ~3 seconds), and stop breathing. Most systems have a slight computational delay between when the user activates the measurement process and when the measurement begins. In addition, preparation scans may add several seconds to the imaging time predicted from the product of TR, matrix, and NEX, so that the prolonged breath-hold period may become unreasonable for the patient. Therefore, the command to stop breathing should be given at the last possible moment, taking into account the intrinsic delays that occur before the start of data acquisition.

DATA RECONSTRUCTION

Reconstruction times depend on matrix size, as well as on the capabilities of the computer and array processor. A 256×128 data matrix will reconstruct in approximately half the time of a 256×256 matrix. Reconstruction times for images obtained with oversampling, which use larger (e.g., 256×512) matrices, are longer than those for standard 256×256 matrix images.

A variety of filters are available for image smoothing and reduction of artifacts. The availability of various filters is system dependent. Some of these filters are applied to the data during reconstruction, whereas others are applied directly to the reconstructed image. Examples of such filters are shown in Figure 2–20. Smoothing filters (e.g., gaussian or Hanning) smooth the appearance of the image by averaging nearby pixels, at the expense of spatial resolution. Noise reduction filters (e.g., sigma) reduce the background noise in the image by determining if the intensity of a pixel exceeds a certain threshold; pixels with lower intensity are assumed to represent background noise and are assigned a zero intensity. Renormalization filters correct for the signal nonuniformity produced by surface coils, either by using an approximate 3D exponential or polynomial correction or by modeling the fall-off in signal from the coil surface based on measurements in phantoms. Edge enhancement and edge detection algorithms consider the difference between the signal intensities of adjacent pixels; if the difference in signal intensities exceeds a certain threshold, indicating an edge, then the pixel intensities are adjusted to accentuate the interface between them.

In addition to standard magnitude reconstructions, phase data may be available for reconstruction of IR images and for evaluation of flow and magnetic susceptibility effects (see Chapter 4).

PHOTOGRAPHY AND ARCHIVAL

MR images are notoriously difficult to photograph, owing to the wide range of tissue contrast, as well as signal inhomogeneity produced by surface coils. Two general goals should be set during photography:

1. To emphasize the region of interest and minimize the conspicuousness of background noise, so that an esthetically pleasing image will be produced.

2. To maximize tissue contrast over the region of interest by using a sufficiently narrow window width, without giving the image a harsh appearance.

With surface coil studies, care must be taken not to choose such a narrow window width that fatty tissues, such as bone marrow, cannot be evaluated (Fig. 2–21A–C). Occasionally, two sets of images with different window settings must be photographed for adequate image evaluation. This practice is particularly useful for knee studies, in which one window setting may be used to evaluate the menisci and another may be used for bone detail (Fig. 2–21D and E).

To improve the visual presentation, images are commonly magnified before being photographed. Two-on-one vertical magnifications are particularly useful for sagittal spine images and reduce the amount of film needed. Magnification is also helpful for evaluating fine meniscal detail in knee studies. However, one must keep in mind that making the image bigger does not improve the in-plane spatial resolution; this can be done only by acquiring the image with a smaller FOV (Fig. 2–22).

Because of the large number of images generated by 3D acquisition methods (as many as 256 from a single acquisition), it may be desirable to preselect images for photography. The large number of images may also be time consuming to archive, since it may be necessary to archive a patient study onto more than one magnetic tape. Data compression will

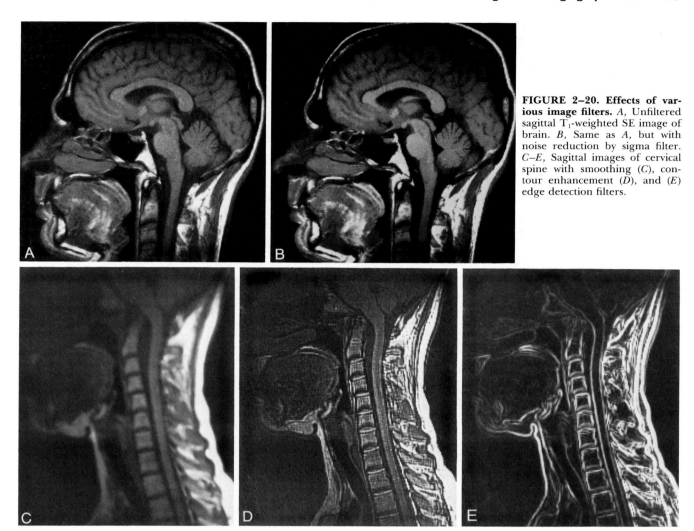

FIGURE 2–20. Effects of various image filters. *A,* Unfiltered sagittal T_1-weighted SE image of brain. *B,* Same as *A,* but with noise reduction by sigma filter. *C–E,* Sagittal images of cervical spine with smoothing (*C*), contour enhancement (*D*), and (*E*) edge detection filters.

permit larger numbers of images per tape, at the expense of additional processing time during archival and retrieval.

Laser cameras produce darker background intensity and more reproducible image quality than standard cameras. In addition, laser cameras allow incorrect exposures to be corrected prior to printing, and duplicate films are easily produced. Digital laser camera interfaces should be preferred to analog interfaces because of their greater flexibility in image formats. Drawbacks of laser cameras include greater initial expense and more costly film, although the extra cost may be deferred by operating them in a multisystem environment.

Archival is usually made on magnetic tape or optical disk. The image storage capacity of a magnetic tape depends on the image matrix size (not related to the acquisition matrix size). For instance, a magnetic tape can typically store approximately 200 uncompressed 256^2 images or fifty 512^2 images. Only a few studies of patients can be placed on a single tape, so that tape storage requirements become considerable. Because of financial and storage space consid-

erations, tapes may have to be recycled periodically. Magnetic tape is a relatively slow medium for archival and retrieval, requiring as much as several seconds for each image. Read-only optical disks are becoming an increasingly attractive option, because of their large storage capacity. An optical disk might contain well over ten thousand 256^2 uncompressed images, with greater storage density available if the data are compressed. Data transfer times may also be reduced.

TROUBLESHOOTING

Quality control is a more complex process for MR imaging systems than for other imaging modalities such as CT. Numerous artifacts may occur in MR images from a variety of causes. These artifacts are reviewed in detail in Chapter 3. Although many of these artifacts require the attention of service personnel, it is helpful to know when image quality problems are related to hardware rather than to inappropriate

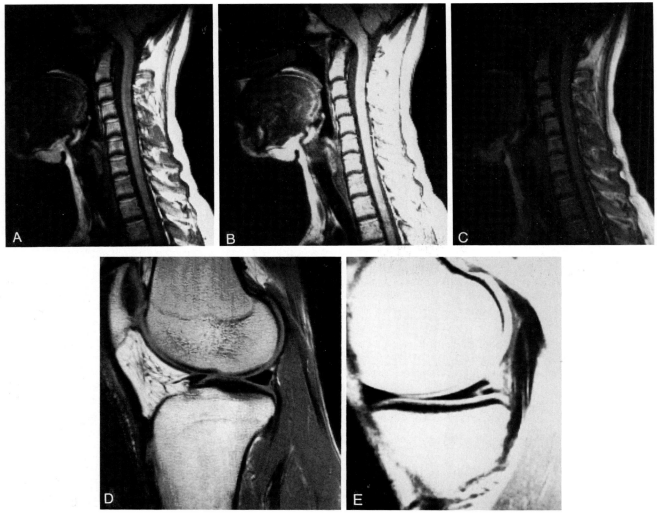

FIGURE 2–21. Adjustment of window settings for photography. *A*, Sagittal T₁-weighted SE image of cervical spine with optimal window settings for spinal cord and vertebra. *B*, Image photographed at narrower window width might be useful for anterior neck structures but is worthless for spinal cord. *C*, Wider window width might be useful for posterior soft tissues, but evaluation of spinal cord is suboptimal. *D*, Sagittal T₁-weighted image of knee, bone windows. Note the good delineation of cartilage, bone marrow, and soft tissues. *E*, Different slice position. With narrower meniscal window and image magnification, there is good delineation of tear of posterior horn of the medial meniscus, but poor representation of other structures.

selection of pulse sequence or scan parameters or to the patient. Therefore, the technologist and physician should be aware of basic troubleshooting procedures.

The most important aspect of quality control is to maintain a daily log of S/N measurements performed on phantoms. Ideally, these measurements should be performed with all receiver coils. However, this practice may be excessively time consuming, so it is reasonable to perform measurements with the various receiver coils on alternate days. S/N measurements with surface coils may be difficult to standardize owing to the depth dependence of coil sensitivity, so service personnel should be consulted with regard to proper procedures. In addition, it is recommended to keep at least a weekly log of transmitter voltages

for various types of patient studies. Significant changes in average transmitter voltages may herald impending failure of the RF tube, excessive magnetic coupling of the RF coils, or other hardware problems.

A consistent downward trend in S/N measurements warrants a call for service. One should note whether the noise has any "structure" to it. For instance, discrete vertical lines oriented perpendicular to the frequency-encoding axis represent RF noise. RF noise may be caused by a defective RF enclosure for the magnet room, and one should check to make sure that the door is tightly closed and that the copper tabs surrounding the door are intact. One should also check for flickering light bulbs within the magnet room. One or more discrete lines oriented perpendicular to the phase-encoding axis may rep-

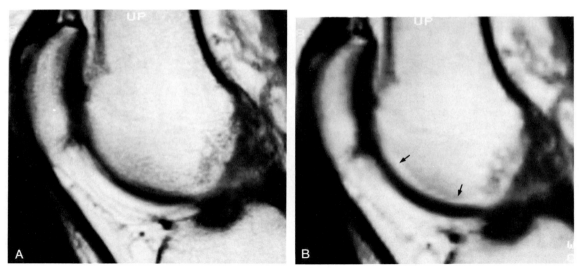

FIGURE 2–22. Sagittal T_1-weighted SE image of knee: comparison between image magnification and gradient zoom. *A,* Gradient zoom shows fine detail. *B,* Magnification of larger FOV image to same size shows less detail and greater chemical shift artifact (*arrows*).

resent ghost artifacts from respiration or pulsatile flow. If this cause is excluded, then the artifacts likely relate to hardware problems, such as RF or gradient instability or inadequate eddy current compensation. Intermittent diagonal lines or "snowstorm" artifacts (Fig. 2–23*A*) may relate to hardware problems or to static discharges, which tend to occur during conditions of low humidity. One should check the humidity levels in both the magnet room and the room containing the gradient subsystems and should consult with service personnel. Artifacts that occur only intermittently may also be caused by temperature in-

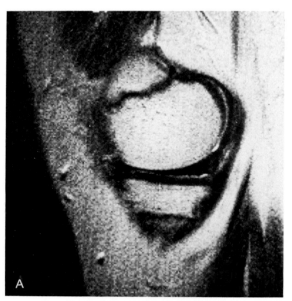

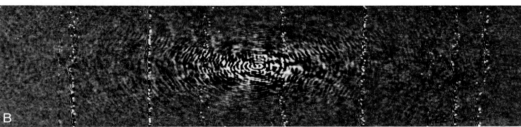

FIGURE 2–23. Diagonal "snowstorm" artifacts usually suggest a hardware problem or static discharges. In this case, the problem was a loose screw in the body coil, resulting in abnormal vibrations and arcing. *A,* Sagittal knee image is degraded by the artifacts. *B,* Raw data set corresponding to *A.* Each column corresponds to a specific time interval or frequency sample; each row, or "line," corresponds to data acquired from one phase-encoding step. The semiperiodic nature of the artifacts, suggesting the presence of abnormal vibrations, is evident in the raw data, but not the image.

stability in the magnet room or the room housing the computer and other hardware. Ambient temperatures >72°F are not usually well tolerated and may result in damage to electronic components. We have also encountered intermittent artifacts from a loose screw or other hardware adjoining the body coil or a gradient coil, which resulted in abnormal mechanical vibration and arcing. These artifacts may be intermittent because the vibrations are problematic only with particular pulse sequences. Direct inspection by service personnel may be required to troubleshoot this problem.

Unstructured noise may be due to a variety of causes. Although service is probably required, one can check the integrity of the connectors and cables for the receiver coils, since these, on occasion, are mangled during handling of the patient. Metallic implants, such as Harrington rods or dental plates, produce localized regions of geometric distortion and may also cause poor S/N owing to improper coil tuning. More generalized evidence of geometric distortion suggests problems with magnet shimming or gradient linearity. If intermittent, this artifact might be caused by the movement of large metal objects, such as cars or elevators, in the vicinity of the magnet.

For any of these artifacts, it is important to save the raw data (Fig. 2–23B), since these often provide additional information about the source of the artifacts. However, in most commercial systems, the raw data must be saved immediately after completion of a scan, since the data may be deleted when the next prescan procedure is initiated.

Finally, either because service personnel are temporarily unavailable or because the schedule of patients cannot be interrupted, it may be necessary to continue scanning despite problems with image quality. In this case, thicker slices, larger FOVs, or more excitations may be used to improve image quality. If artifacts are particularly severe with certain pulse sequences or planes of section, these should obviously be avoided.

In conclusion, we see that there are numerous practical considerations involved in the production of high-quality MR images. Although this chapter offers recommendations for optimizing MR examinations, there are no panaceas. One must experiment with different imaging parameters and decide for oneself what best suits the needs of a particular MR site and the physicians involved there.

REFERENCES

1. Shellock FG: Monitoring during MRI: An evaluation of the effect of high-field MRI on various patient monitors. Med Electron 100:93–97, 1986.
2. Malott JC: Hazards of ferrous materials in MRI: A case report. Radiol Technol 58:233–235, 1987.
3. Sacco DC, Steiger DA, Bellon EM, et al: Artifacts caused by cosmetics in MR imaging of the head. AJR 148:1001–1004, 1987.
4. Laakman RW, Kaufman B, Han JS, et al: MRI in patients with metallic implants. Radiology 157:711–714, 1985.
5. New PFJ, Rosen BR, Brady TJ, et al: Potential hazards and artifacts of ferromagnetic and nonferromagnetic surgical and dental materials and devices in NMR imaging. Radiology 147:138–148, 1983.
6. Pavlicek WA, Weisinger M, Castle L, et al: Effects of NMR on patients with cardiac pacemakers. Radiology 147:149–153, 1983.
7. Bottomley PA, Edelstein WA: Power deposition in whole body NMR imaging. Med Phys 8:510–512, 1981.
8. Budinger TF: NMR in vivo studies: Known thresholds for health effects. J Comput Assist Tomog 5:800–811, 1981.
9. Tenforde TS (ed): Magnetic Field Effects on Biological Systems. New York, Plenum Press, 1979.
10. Bore PJ, Galloway GJ, Styles P, et al: Are quenches dangerous? Magn Reson Med 3:112–117, 1986.
11. Davis PL, Crooks L, Arakawa M, et al: Potential hazards in NMR imaging: Heating effects of changing magnetic fields and RF fields on small metallic implants. AJR 137:857–860, 1981.
12. Becker RL, Norfray JF, Teitelbaum, et al: MR imaging in patients with intracranial aneurysm clips. AJNR 9:885–889, 1988.
13. Holtas S, Olsson M, Romner B, et al: Comparison of MR imaging and CT in patients with intracranial aneurysm clips. AJNR 9:891–897, 1988.
14. Shellock FG, Crues JV: High-field MR imaging of metallic biomedical implants: An ex vivo evaluation of deflection forces. AJR 151:389–392, 1988.
15. Shellock FG: MR imaging of metallic implants and materials: A compilation of the literature. AJR 151:811–814, 1988.
16. Randall PA, Kohman LJ, Scalzetti EM, et al: MR imaging of prosthetic cardiac valves in vitro and in vivo. Am J Cardiol 62:973–976, 1988.
17. Soulen RL, Budinger TF, Higgins CB: MR imaging of prosthetic heart valves. Radiology 154:705–707, 1985.
18. Teitelbaum GP, Bradley WG, Klein BD: MR imaging artifacts, ferromagnetism, and magnetic torque of intravascular filters, stents and coils. Radiology 166:657–664, 1988.
19. Shellock FG: Biological effects of MRI. Diagn Imag 9:96–101, 1987.
20. Shellock FG, Crues JV: MRI: Potential adverse effects and safety considerations. MRI Decis 2:25–30, 1988.
21. Edelman RR, McFarland E, Stark DD, et al: Surface coil MRI of abdominal viscera. Radiology 157:425–430, 1985.
22. Buchill R, Saner M, Meier D, et al: Increased rf power absorption in MRI due to rf coupling between body coil and surface coil. Magn Reson Med 9:105–112, 1989.
23. Shellock FG, Gordon CJ, Shaefer DJ: Thermoregulatory responses to clinical MR imaging of the head at 1.5 Tesla: Lack of evidence for direct effects on the hypothalamus. Acta Radiol [Suppl] 369:512–513, 1986.
24. Shellock FG, Shaefer DJ, Grundfest W, Crues JV: Thermal effects of high-field (1.5 Tesla) MR imaging of the spine: Clinical experience above a specific absorption rate of 0.4 W/kg. Acta Radiol [Suppl] 369:514–516, 1986.
25. Shellock FG, Crues JV: Temperature, heart rate, and blood pressure changes associated with clinical MR imaging at 1.5 Tesla. Radiology 163:259–262, 1987.
26. Shellock FG, Crues JV: Temperature changes caused by clinical MR imaging of the brain at 1.5 Tesla using a head coil. AJNR 9:287–291, 1988.
27. Shellock FG, Crues JV: Corneal temperature changes associated with high-field MR imaging of the brain with a head coil. Radiology 167:809–811, 1988.
28. Shellock FG, Shaefer DJ, Crues JV: Alterations in body and skin temperatures caused by MR imaging: Is the recommended exposure for radiofrequency radiation too conservative? Br J Radiol (in press).
29. Runge VM, Wood ML, Kaufman DM, Silver MS: MRI section profile optimization: Improved contrast and detection of lesions. Radiology 167:831–834, 1988.
29a. Kucharczyk W, Crawley AP, Kelly WM, Henkelman RM: Effect of multislice interference on image contrast in T2- and T1-weighted MR images. AJNR 9:443–451, 1988.
30. Feinberg DA, Hale JD, Watts JC, et al: Halving of MR imaging

time by conjugation: Demonstration at 3.5 kg. Radiology 161:527–531, 1986.

31. Laub GA, Kaiser WA: MR angiography with gradient motion rephasing. J Comput Assist Tomogr 12:377–382, 1988.

32. Edelman RR, Atkinson DJ, Silver MS: FRODO pulses: A new method for elimination of motion, flow, and wraparound artifact. Radiology 166:231–236, 1988.

33. Felmlee JP, Ehman RL: Spatial presaturation: A method for suppressing flow artifacts and improving depiction of vascular anatomy in MRI. Radiology 164:559–564, 1987.

34. Wendt RE, Rokey R, Vick GW, Johnston DL: Electrocardiographic gating and monitoring in NMR imaging. Magn Reson Imaging 6:89–95, 1988.

35. Dimick RN, Hedlund LW, Herfkens R, et al: Optimizing electrocardiograph electrode placement for cardiac-gated MR imaging. Invest Radiol 22:17–22, 1987.

36. Brummett RE, Talbot JM, Charuhas P: Potential hearing loss resulting from MR imaging. Radiology 169:539–540, 1988.

37. Dujovny M, Kossowsky R, Kossowsky N: Aneurysm clip motion during MRI. Neurosurgery 17:543–548, 1985.

38. Barrafato D, Henkelman RM: MRI and surgical clips. Can J Surg 27:509–512, 1984.

39. Matsumoto AH, Teitelbaum GP, Barth KH, et al: Tantalum vascular stents: In vivo evaluation with MRI. Radiology 170:753–755, 1989.

40. Mattucci KF, Setzen M, Hyman R, Chaturvedi G: The effect of NMR imaging on metallic middle ear prostheses. Otolaryngol Head Neck Surg 94:441–443, 1986.

41. Applebaum EL, Valvassori GE: Effects of MRI fields on stapedectomy prostheses. Arch Otolaryngol 111:820–821, 1985.

42. Leon JA, Gabriele OF: Middle ear prosthesis: Significance in MR imaging. Magn Reson Imaging 5:405–406, 1987.

43. Zheutlin JD, Thompson JT, Shofner RS: The safety of MRI with intraorbital metallic objects after retinal reattachment or trauma. Am J Ophthalmol 103:831, 1987.

44. Dekeizer RJW, Le Stake L: Intraocular lens implants (pseudophakoi) and steel wire sutures: A contraindication for MRI? Doc Ophthalmol 61:281–284, 1986.

45. Mark AS, Hricak H: Intrauterine contraceptive devices. Radiology 162:311–314, 1987.

46. Dunn V, Coffman CE, McGowan JE, Ehrhardt JC: Mechanical ventilation during magnetic resonance imaging. Magn Res Imaging 3:169–172, 1985.

Appendix 2–A

SAMPLE CHECKLIST AND WORK-UP SHEET FOR INTERVIEWING PATIENTS*

DATE ____/____/____

NAME _____

SEX _____ AGE _____ PHYSICIAN _____ PATIENT # _____

DATE OF BIRTH ____/____/____ HEIGHT _____ WEIGHT _____

PROCEDURE _____ OUT PATIENT _____ IN PATIENT _____

DIAGNOSIS _____

CLINICAL HISTORY _____

THE FOLLOWING ITEMS MAY INTERFERE WITH MAGNETIC RESONANCE IMAGING AND SOME CAN BE POTENTIALLY HAZARDOUS.
PLEASE INDICATE IF YOU HAVE THE FOLLOWING: ____

Please mark on this drawing the location of any metal inside your body.

cardiac pacemaker .... yes   no
aneurysm clip(s) .... yes   no
implanted insulin pump .... yes   no
implanted drug infusion device .... yes   no
bone growth stimulator .... yes   no
neurostimulator (TENS-Unit) .... yes   no
any type of biostimulator .... yes   no
internal hearing aid .... yes   no
cochlear implant .... yes   no
Gianturco coil (spring embolus coil) .... yes   no

vascular clip(s) .... yes   no
hemostatic clip(s) .... yes   no
any type of surgical clip or staple(s) .... yes   no
heart valve prosthesis .... yes   no
Greenfield vena cava filter .... yes   no
middle ear implant .... yes   no
penile prosthesis .... yes   no
orbital/eye prosthesis .... yes   no
shrapnel or bullet .... yes   no
wire sutures .... yes   no
tattooed eyeliner .... yes   no
any type of dental item held in place
by a magnet .... yes   no
any other implanted item .... yes   no
type: _____

diaphragm .... yes   no
IUD .... yes   no
renal shunt .... yes   no
intraventricular shunt .... yes   no
wire mesh .... yes   no
artificial limb or joint .... yes   no
any orthopedic item(s) (i.e., pins, rods,
screws, nails, clips, plates, wire, etc.) .... yes   no
dentures .... yes   no
dental braces .... yes   no
any type of removable dental item .... yes   no

Right   Left

Have you ever had a surgical procedure or operation of any kind? .... yes   no
Type: _____

*Courtesy of Cedars-Sinai Medical Center, Los Angeles, CA.

68

Have you ever worked in a machine shop or similar environment where you may have been
subjected to small metal slivers? . . . . .yes   no

Have you ever had an injury to your eye involving metal? . . . . .yes   no

Are you pregnant or do you suspect that you are pregnant? . . . . .yes   no

    How many months? _____

    Last menstrual period: _____

    Post menopausal? . . . . .yes   no

If you are having an MRI procedure involving the abdominal area, list what you've eaten last 4 hours: _____

_____

_____

_____

PERTINENT PREVIOUS STUDIES: Diagnostic X-rays _____

    Computed tomography   _____

    Ultrasound   _____

    Radionuclide study   _____

I attest that the above information is correct to the best of my knowledge:

_____
                (Patient's Signature)

MD/RN/RT Signature _____ Date ___/___/___

Print MD/RN/RT Name _____

Appendix 2–B

CLASSIFICATION OF METALLIC IMPLANTS FOR MR IMAGING*

Type of Implant	Deflection?	Maximum Field Strength Tested (Tesla)	Comments

1. *Aneurysm and Hemostatic Clips*[5, 14, 37, 38] (note that certain nominally nonferromagnetic clips may produce substantial image artifacts due to local distortion of the RF field or due to mild ferromagnetism induced by bending of the clips during placement)

Type of Implant	Deflection?	Maximum Field Strength Tested (Tesla)
Drake (SS 301)	Yes	1.50
Drake (DR 14, 24)	Yes	1.44
Drake (DR 16)	Yes	0.15
Drake (DR 20)	Yes	1.50
Downs multipositional (17-7PH)	Yes	1.44
Gastrointestinal anastomosis clip, Auto Suture SGIA (SS)	No	1.50
Heifetz (17-7PH)	Yes	1.89
Heifetz (Elgiloy)	No	1.89
Hemoclip #10 (316L SS)	No	1.50
Hemoclip (Tantalum)	No	1.50
Housepian	Yes	0.15
Kapp straight (SS 404)	Yes	0.15
Kapp curved (SS 404)	Yes	1.44
Kapp (SS 405)	Yes	1.89
Ligaclip #6 (316L SS)	No	1.50
Ligaclip (Tantalum)	No	1.50
Mayfield (SS 301)	Yes	1.50
Mayfield (SS 304)	Yes	1.89
McFadden (SS 301)	Yes	1.50
Olivecrona	No	1.44
Pivot (17-7PH)	Yes	1.89
Scoville (EN-58J)	Yes	1.89
Stevens (50-4190 SS)	No	0.15
Sugita (Elgiloy)	No	1.89
Sundt-Kees (SS 301)	Yes	1.50
Sundt-Kees multiangle (17-7PH)	Yes	1.89
Surgiclip, Auto Suture (M-9.5)	No	1.50
Vari-angle (17-7PH)	Yes	1.89
Vari-angle McFadden (MP35N)	No	1.89
Vari-angle micro (17-7PM)	Yes	0.15
Vari-angle spring (17-7PM)	Yes	0.15
Vari-angle (17-7PH)	Yes	1.89
Yasargil (SS 316)	No	1.89
Yasargil (Phynox)	No	1.89

2. *Heart Valves*[14, 17] (magnetic deflection forces probably not significant compared with mechanical stresses in vivo, with possible exception of older Starr-Edwards models in patients with valvular dehiscence)

Type of Implant	Deflection?	Maximum Field Strength Tested (Tesla)
Beall	Yes	2.35
Björk-Shiley (convexo-concave)	No	1.50
Björk-Shiley (universal/spherical)	Yes	1.50
Björk-Shiley, model MBC	Yes	2.35
Björk-Shiley, model 25 MBRC	Yes	2.35
Carpentier-Edwards, model 2650	Yes	2.35
Carpentier-Edwards (porcine)	Yes	2.35
Hall-Kaster, model A7700	Yes	1.50
Hancock I (porcine)	Yes	1.50
Hancock II (porcine)	Yes	1.50
Hancock extracorporeal, model 242R	Yes	2.35
Hancock extracorporeal, model M 4365-33	Yes	2.35
Hancock Vascor, model 505	No	2.35
Ionescu-Shiley	Yes	2.35
Lillehi-Kaster	Yes	1.50
Medtronic Hall	Yes	2.35
Omnicarbon, model 3523T029	Yes	2.35
Omniscience, model 6522	Yes	2.35
Smeloff-Cutter	Yes	1.50
Starr-Edwards 1260	Yes	2.35

*Magnetic properties of implants. Most implants that demonstrate no deflection in a magnetic field are safe for MR imaging. However, some implants (e.g., pacemakers, cochlear implants, neurostimulators) are still contraindicated because the magnetic field may produce electronic malfunction. Note that the presence of deflection does not necessarily represent a contraindication to MR imaging, particularly if such devices are solidly fixed in position (e.g., by surgical means or fibrosis). However, clinical judgment should be exercised before imaging such implants. In addition, note that absence of deflection at a lower field strength does not preclude deflection at a higher field strength.

Type of Implant	Deflection?	Maximum Field Strength Tested (Tesla)	Comments
Starr-Edwards 2400	No	1.50	
Starr-Edwards pre 6000 (1960–1964)	Yes	1.50	Possibly contraindicated
Starr-Edwards 6520	Yes	2.35	
St. Jude	No	1.50	
St. Jude, model A 101	Yes	2.35	
St. Jude, model M 101	Yes	2.35	
3. Intravascular Devices[14, 18, 39]			
Amplatz filter	No	4.7	
Cragg Nitinol spiral filter	No	4.7	
Simon-Nitinol filter	No	1.5	
Gianturco coil (occluding spring embolus)	Yes	1.5	
Gianturco bird nest filter	Yes	1.5	High magnetic deflection
Gianturco zig-zag stent	Yes	1.5	High magnetic deflection
Greenfield vena cava filter (stainless steel)	Yes	1.5	Minimal magnetic deflection, considered safe
Greenfield vena cava filter (titanium alloy)	No	1.5	
Gunther retrievable filter	Yes	1.5	High magnetic deflection
Maas helical IVC filter	No	1.5	
Maas helical endovascular stent	No	1.5	
Mobin-Uddin filter	No	1.5	
New retrievable IVC filter	Yes	1.5	High magnetic deflection
Palmaz vascular stent	Yes	1.5	Minimal magnetic deflection
Strecker tantalum stent	No	1.5	
4. Orthopedic Materials/Devices[14, 15]			
AML femoral component/bipolar hip prosthesis	No	1.5	
Charnley-Muller hip prosthesis	No	0.3	
Harris hip prosthesis	No	1.5	
Jewett nail	No	1.5	
Kirschner intermedullary rod	No	1.5	
Stainless steel plate (Zimmer)	No	1.5	
Stainless steel screw (Zimmer)	No	1.5	
Stainless steel mesh	No	1.5	
Stainless steel wire	No	1.5	
5. Dental Materials[5, 14]			
Dental amalgam	No	1.44	
Brace band	No	1.50	
Brace wire	Yes	1.50	Probably safe for MRI
Gutta percha points	No	1.50	
Indian head real silver points	No	1.50	
Temporary crown	No	1.50	
Permanent crown amalgam	No	1.50	
6. Prosthetic Ear Implants[41, 42]			
Cody tack	No	0.6	
Cochlear implant (3M/House)	Yes	0.6	Contraindicated
Cochlear implant (3M/Vienna)	Yes	0.6	Contraindicated
House-type incus prosthesis	No	0.6	
McGee stainless steel piston	No	0.6	
Reuter drain tube	No	0.6	
Richards-McGee piston	No	1.5	
Richards-Schuknecht Teflon wire	No	1.5	
Richards plasti-pore with Armstrong-style platinum ribbon	No	1.5	
Richards trapeze platinum ribbon	No	1.5	
Richards House-type wire loop	No	1.5	
Xomed stapes prosthesis, Robinson-style	No	1.5	
Schuknecht gel foam and wire prosthesis, Armstrong-style	No	1.5	
7. Penile Implants			
AMS malleable 600	No	1.5	
AMS 700 CX	No	1.5	
Flexi-flate (Surgitek)	No	1.5	
Flexi-rod (standard) (Surgitek)	No	1.5	
Flexi-rod II (firm) (Surgitek)	No	1.5	
Jonas (Dacomed)	No	1.5	
Mentor flexible	No	1.5	
Mentor inflatable	No	1.5	
Omniphase (Dacomed)	Yes	1.5	

Type of Implant	Deflection?	Maximum Field Strength Tested (Tesla)	Comments
8. *Miscellaneous*[40–45]			
AMS 800, artificial sphincter	No	1.50	
BBs	Yes	1.50	
Bullet (steel tip)	Yes	1.50	
Cerebral ventricular shunt tube connector, Accu-Flow, straight (Codman and Shurtleff)	No	1.50	
Cerebral ventricular shunt tube connector, Accu-Flow, right angle (Codman and Shurtleff)	No	1.50	
Cerebral ventricular shunt tube connector, Accu-Flow, T-connector (Codman and Shurtleff)	No	1.50	
Cerebral ventricular shunt tube connector (type unknown)	Yes	0.15	
Diaphragm (all flex)	Yes	1.50	Probably safe for MRI
Diaphragm (Ortho)	Yes	1.50	Probably safe for MRI
Diaphragm (Koroflex)	Yes	1.50	Probably safe for MRI
Diaphragm (titanium)	No	1.44	
Forceps (titanium)	No	1.44	
Hakim valve and pump	No	1.44	
Infusaid implantable chemotherapy pump	No	1.50	Safe for MRI
Intraocular lens implant, iridocapsular lens, plantium-iridium loop (Binkhorst)	No	1.00	
Intraocular lens implant, iridocapsular lens, titanium loop (Binkhorst)	No	1.00	
Intraocular lens implant, platinum clip lens (Worst)	No	1.00	
IUD copper T	No	1.50	
IUD copper 7	No	1.50	
Tantalum powder	No	1.44	
Thermodilution catheter (Swan-Ganz VIP, 5 Fr, 7 Fr)	No	1.50	May still be unsafe owing to possibility of induced current
Vitallium implant	No	1.50	

Appendix 2–C

ADVANCED LIFE SUPPORT SYSTEMS FOR MR IMAGING OF UNSTABLE PATIENTS

The following is a description of an advanced life support system that has been in use at the Massachusetts General Hospital (MGH) for MR imaging studies of hemorrhage in patients who are medically or neurologically unstable. It is essential that anesthesia personnel should be closely involved in designing the life support system during the initial site planning for any MR system where imaging of sedated or unstable patients is likely to occur. Equipment compatible with MR imaging is listed in Appendix Table 2–1.

APPENDIX TABLE 2–1. EQUIPMENT COMPATIBLE WITH MR IMAGING*

Heart Rate/Blood Pressure Monitor	Temperature Monitor
In Vivo Laboratories	Luxtron
3061 W. Albany	1060 Terra Bella Ave.
Broken Arrow, OK 74012	Mountain View, CA
(918) 250–0566	94043
Respiratory Rate Monitor	(415) 962–8110
Capnometer Monitor	**RESPIRATOR**
Biochem International, Inc.	CMS Medical, Inc.
W238 N1650 Rockwood Drive	702 Jayhawk Tower
Waukesha, WI 53188	700 Jackson
(414) 542–3100	Topeka, KS 66603
Skin Blood Flow Monitor	(913) 234–8199
TSI, Inc.	
500 Cardigan Rd.	
P.O. Box 64394	
St. Paul, MN 64394	
(612) 483–0900	

*Note that each of the devices on this list (with the exception of the respirator) needs certain modifications prior to use with MR imaging. Consult the manufacturer regarding these modifications. In addition, none of the monitors listed above should be positioned closer than 8 feet from the entrance of the bore of a 1.5-T or higher MR scanner.

At MGH, mechanical ventilation is provided by a Monaghan 225 ventilator (Monaghan Medical Corp., Plattsburgh, NY), factory modified to be compatible with MR imaging.[46] Large or critical ferromagnetic parts have been replaced with plastic, stainless steel, or aluminum components. Instead of electricity, the ventilator is powered by oxygen (>50 psi) supplied through high-pressure tubing. Large H oxygen cylinders located outside the scanning suite may be used, but oxygen consumption by the ventilator is sufficiently high to deplete such a tank in less than an hour. Connecting two or more tanks provides a substantial gas reserve during a typical imaging session; however, an oxygen outlet installed in the magnet room eliminates the risk of an exhausted oxygen supply. The patient is connected with the ventilator, and arterial blood gas determinations are made before the patient is placed in the magnet and are repeated midway through the imaging procedure, as well as whenever changes in blood pressure,

pulse, or intracranial pressure (ICP) occur. A Puritan-Bennett ventilator pressure alarm, located outside the MR suite, is connected with the patient's endotracheal tube using a T-piece and high-pressure tubing. Disconnection of the patient or loss of ventilatory pressure can be detected immediately. A full complement of resuscitation equipment and medication is located outside the magnet room.

An electrically shielded extension cable couples the transducer to a physiologic monitor (Spacelabs, Inc., Type 414 Opt 21, Hillsboro, OR 97124) that is located outside the magnet room. Gould DTX physiologic transducers (Gould, Inc., Oxnard, CA 93030) were chosen, as they have minimal metallic components and are familiar to our personnel. Nonmetallic radial artery catheters are inserted prior to imaging. Sixteen feet of heparinized, saline-filled, high-frequency pressure tubing is interposed between the catheter and transducer. Although some signal damping occurs, substantial errors in systolic and diastolic pressure are not observed, as they are when 4 feet of tubing is used. A three-way stopcock is placed 4 feet from the arterial catheter, allowing access to arterial blood during imaging. A standard pressure bag (Sorenson Research, Salt Lake City, UT) produces an infusion of 3 ml/hr through the catheter; the metal and rubber inflator is removed, and a plastic clasp is used to maintain pressure. ICP monitoring is performed using ventricular catheters with nonmetallic components. Twenty feet of saline-filled, high-frequency pressure tubing is used to couple the catheter to the transducer. Metallic subarachnoid bolts are not used.

Transducers are affixed to a nonferromagnetic pole located alongside the magnet at its midpoint to minimize artifact. Care is taken to ensure that the pole and pressure tubing do not contact the imager shell, so that vibration artifact may be avoided. The height of the transducers is set at the level of the right atrium. Cardiac monitoring is performed throughout imaging; cardiac electrodes are placed on each ankle and one wrist. A telemetry system (Hewlett-Packard, model 78100A transmitter and 7803A monitor, Palo Alto, CA) allows continuous monitoring of the ECG during imaging. Medications such as vasopressors, antihypertensives, insulin, and sedatives, routinely administered by motor-driven infusion pumps, are transferred to microdrip burets.

ACKNOWLEDGMENT: We gratefully acknowledge the assistance of Keith Johnson, M.D., in preparation of this appendix.

3

ARTIFACTS IN MR IMAGING: Description, Causes, and Solutions

GEORGE WESBEY, ROBERT R. EDELMAN, and ROBERT HARRIS

STATIC MAGNETIC FIELD ARTIFACTS

MAIN FIELD INHOMOGENEITY

Ferromagnetic Materials
Basis of Ferromagnetism

SUSCEPTIBILITY ARTIFACT

Solutions

RADIOFREQUENCY FIELD ARTIFACTS

EXTERNAL NOISE

Sources
Shielding from Radiofrequency Noise
System Radiofrequency Noise
Room Radiofrequency Noise

SHIELDING THE PATIENT FROM THE RADIOFREQUENCY COIL

SURFACE COIL SENSITIVITY

TIP ANGLE VARIATION

SELECTIVE AND NONSELECTIVE RADIOFREQUENCY PULSES

INTRINSIC PATIENT NOISE

CONTACT ARTIFACT

DIRECT CURRENT INTERFERENCE (CENTRAL POINT ARTIFACT)

CENTRAL LINE ARTIFACT

Zero Frequency Artifact
Zero Phase Artifact

PULSE SEQUENCE DESIGN CONSIDERATIONS FOR MINIMIZING RF ARTIFACTS

DATA ACQUISITION AND GRADIENTS

PARTIAL VOLUME AVERAGING

RECEIVER GAIN ADJUSTMENT (CLIPPING ARTIFACT)

RECEIVER LOW PASS FILTER ADJUSTMENT

LOSS OF DATA

GRADIENT ARTIFACTS

RINGING ARTIFACTS FROM SAMPLING

Phase-Encoding Direction
Frequency-Encoding Direction
Digital Filtering

RINGING ARTIFACTS FROM GRADIENT INSTABILITY

Gradient Peak Power Instability
Gradient Low Power Instability

CHEMICAL SHIFT ARTIFACT

Cause
Solutions

ALIASING

Nature of the Problem
Appearance of Aliasing (Wraparound Artifact)
Solutions

EDDY CURRENTS

Cause
Effects
Solutions

TELESCOPING

MOTION-RELATED ARTIFACTS

SYSTEM CAUSES OF GHOSTING

PATIENT CAUSES OF GHOSTING

Solutions

FLOW ARTIFACTS

PULSE SEQUENCE–RELATED ARTIFACTS

INVERSION RECOVERY

BOUNCE POINT

CHEMICAL SHIFT ETCHING

MOTION-INTERFACE ETCHING (PHASE DISPERSION OR SHEAR ARTIFACT)

The imaging specialist relies on visual impressions in order to make a diagnosis. But in the case of MRI, what one sees can sometimes be a far cry from reality. Images stretch, wrinkle, or distort in ways that are alien to other less complex imaging modalities (radiography, CT, nuclear medicine, ultrasound). Some of these artifacts are due to equipment malfunctions; others are due to improper technique selection or are simply inherent to the MR imaging process. One needs to understand the sources and appearances of MR artifacts, not only to properly interpret the images, but also to be able to eliminate these artifacts so as to obtain the highest quality images. Prerequisite to an understanding of artifacts is a knowledge of the physical principles and instrumentation which form the basis for the infinite variety of signal intensity patterns obtainable in the MR image. We will consider artifacts under several distinct categories, though in reality artifacts arise from an interplay of these factors (Fig. 3–1). Causes and solutions for some of these artifacts are summarized in Table 3–1.

An MR imaging artifact is defined as any signal intensity, or void, that does not have an anatomic basis in the plane of the object being imaged. The classification of artifacts is complicated by the multifactorial basis of production: the interrelationship between software, hardware, and radiofrequency (RF) and static magnetic field components; the pulse sequence parameters; and the system-dependent nature of artifacts relating to static magnetic field strength, magnetic gradient strengths, RF coil type, and body part examined. Bellon and colleagues[1] have categorized artifacts by cause as sequence, recon-

struction algorithm, patient, and system related. In their thorough and comprehensive review article, Henkelman and Bronskill[2] have classified artifacts by both appearance and cause. This chapter is intended to serve as a relatively complete "atlas" of MR imaging artifacts, with an effort toward explanations geared to clinical imaging physicians.

Realizing that any classification of MR imaging artifacts is arbitrary and incomplete, we propose the following general outline based upon the predominant causative agent or affected system component: (1) static magnetic field (B_0), (2) radiofrequency magnetic field (RF or B_1), (3) gradient magnetic field (G_x, G_y, G_z) and data acquisition, (4) motion, and (5) sequence parameters. A brief description of the classic appearance of the artifact, a concise explanation of its origin, and various solutions will accompany examples of more frequently seen MR imaging artifacts. In light of the variability of MR systems from various manufacturers, we have tried to include artifacts common to all systems, including examples from several different vendors.

STATIC MAGNETIC FIELD ARTIFACTS

MAIN FIELD INHOMOGENEITY

A fundamental prerequisite for MR imaging is a homogeneous static magnetic field, B_0. Imperfections in manufacturers' magnet construction or, more commonly, in shimming (the process of compensat-

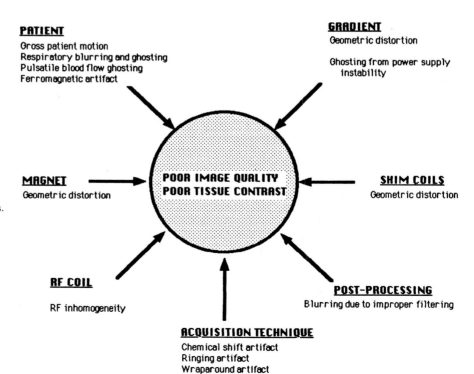

FIGURE 3–1. Summary of artifacts.

TABLE 3–1. SUMMARY OF ARTIFACTS, CAUSES, AND SOLUTIONS

Artifact	Cause	Solution
Blurring	Partial volume averaging	*Reduce slice thickness, FOV
		*Increase matrix
	Eddy currents	Call field service
Center line	Residual transverse magnetization (FID, stimulated echo)	Alternate phase of RF pulse
		Increase spoiler gradient
		Shorten read-out period
Center point	DC offset	Alternate phase of RF pulse
Chemical shift	Difference in Larmor frequencies of fat and water protons	Increase read gradient
		*Reduce FOV (reduces artifact relative to pixel size)
Low S/N, contrast; variation in signal between odd and even images	Cross-talk between slices (depends on order of slice excitation)	*Increase interslice gap
		*Use optimized RF pulses for better slice profiles
Discrete lines perpendicular to frequency-encoding axis	RF noise	*Check integrity of RF shielding
		Call field service
Geometric distortion, signal loss	Susceptibility artifact	*Shorten TE
		Increase read gradient
		*Use spin echo instead of gradient echo
		*Remove external metal objects
		*Check magnet environment
	Bad shimming	Call field service
Ghosting	Variation in signal during acquisition caused by motion	See Table 3–3
	Variation in heart rate during gating	See Table 3–3
	Gradient or transmitter instability	Call field service
	Eddy currents	
No image		*Check patient centering
		*Check coil connections
	Faulty electronics	Call field service
Noisy image	Poor choice of sequence parameters	*Increase signal averages
		*Use thicker slice, larger FOV, smaller matrix
	Body coil plus large patient	*Check for patient contact with body coil
	Surface coil plus large patient	*Use different receiver coil
	Defective electronics	Call field service
	Poor eddy current compensation	Call field service
	Bad coil tuning	*Check coil connections
		*Check for external metal objects, dental plates, etc.
Oblique stripes	Loss of data or anomalous data	*Save raw data
		Call field service
Wraparound	Aliasing of high spatial frequencies	*Oversampling (e.g., NOPHASEWRAP, extended FOV)
		*Presaturate
		*Increase FOV
		Adjust receiver filter

*Can be easily performed by user.

ing for B_0 inhomogeneities) may disrupt the B_0 homogeneity. Areas of image distortion or focal signal loss along the read-out axis are the result (Fig. 3–2). Rarely, B_0 inhomogeneity may present as propagation of signal loss or noise in the phase-encoding direction across the entire image.[3]

For resistive magnets, other causes for B_0 inhomogeneity are temporal fluctuations in the power supply and thermal instability. Resistive magnets are susceptible to accidental power interruption, and images may demonstrate severe artifacts from B_0 inhomogeneity many hours after restoration of power. State-of-the-art superconducting magnets operate with temporal stabilities of 0.1 to 1 ppm over days to weeks.[4]

However, without routine active shimming, the thermal fluctuation of the system can result in accumulated B_0 inhomogeneity that rapidly degrades image quality. Proper magnet design, production, and regular shimming by service personnel will maintain B_0 inhomogeneity at a minimum.

Objects both external and internal to the imaging volume of the MRI system may interfere with static magnetic field linearity. Sizeable ferromagnetic structures in motion near the magnet, such as a truck or elevator, generate magnetic forces of their own. If static field shielding fails to compensate for these forces, these external fields may create B_0 inhomogeneity artifacts.

Ferromagnetic Materials

Magnetic susceptibility is the tendency of a substance to attract magnetic lines of force. Most materials may be classified as ferromagnetic (strongly attracting lines of force), paramagnetic (weakly attracting lines of force), or diamagnetic (weakly repelling lines of force). These three classes of magnetic properties are thus all related by their relative magnetic susceptibilities. Magnetic susceptibility simply represents the ratio of induced magnetization to applied magnetization and is therefore a dimensionless quantity. Diamagnetic substances (e.g., water)

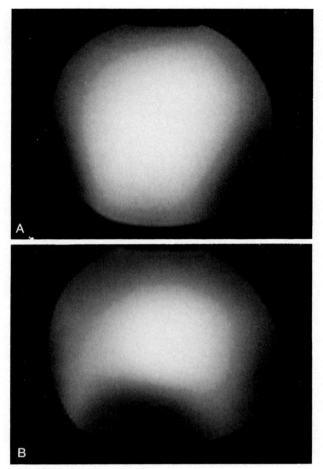

FIGURE 3–2. Transaxial MR image of a homogeneous 28-cm diameter by 40-cm long cylindrical phantom taken at 15 cm superior to z-axis isocenter (*A*) and 15 cm inferior to z-axis isocenter (*B*) reveals focal signal inhomogeneity in the periphery, due to imperfect shimming of the static field in this region. Such inhomogeneity was readily evident in clinical off-isocenter images.

have an induced magnetization that is a million-fold less than the applied field, with opposite polarity (repelling). For example, in a 1.5 T (15,000 gauss) clinical MRI system, water has an induced magnetization of roughly −0.015 gauss (flux lines opposite the direction of magnet). Paramagnetic compounds (e.g., elemental gadolinium) have an induced magnetization four orders of magnitude greater than diamagnetic compounds and are attracted to the applied field (induced magnetization of approximately +150 gauss in above example). Ferromagnetic substances (e.g., iron-containing alloys) have a magnetic susceptibility four orders of magnitude greater than paramagnetic compounds (roughly +1.5 million gauss of induced magnetization in a 1.5 T imager).

Titanium, tantalum, platinum, and aluminum are nonferromagnetic; stainless steel alloys that contain a high content of nickel, such as 304 and 316 L, are nonferromagnetic. However, cold-working of these materials (as when they are bent to form surgical clips) can impart a mild degree of ferromagnetism

(Fig. 3–3).[5] Ferromagnetic artifact may also be encountered from minute metallic particles that wear off surgical instruments, particularly when used to drill through bone.[6] These artifacts are particularly prominent on gradient-echo images (Fig. 3–4), since these are acquired without a refocusing 180-degree RF pulse (see Chapter 5).

Basis of Ferromagnetism

Ferromagnetic materials contain macroscopic magnetic "domains" where the molecules align with the main magnetic field. These materials have very high magnetic susceptibilities, that is, they strongly attract magnetic lines of force and distort magnetic field homogeneity in their vicinity. Since magnetic susceptibility is proportional to magnetic field strength, ferromagnetic artifacts become worse at higher fields.

Appearance of Artifacts Produced by Ferromagnetic Materials

Ferromagnetic artifact has a very specific appearance, consisting of signal abnormality and geometric

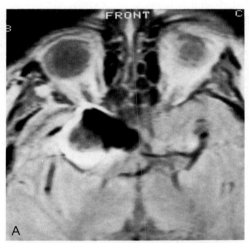

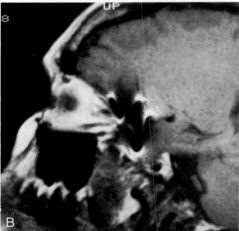

FIGURE 3–3. Cold-working of nonferromagnetic materials can impart a degree of ferromagnetism. Titanium intracerebral aneurysm clip, which is supposed to be nonferromagnetic, demonstrates strong ferromagnetic artifact, a result of bending of the clip.

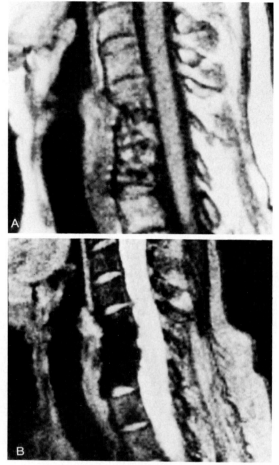

FIGURE 3–4. Ferromagnetic artifact can be caused by metallic particles that wear off surgical devices. *A*, T₁-weighted image of cervical spine after anterior interbody fusion demonstrates signal inhomogeneity due to metallic particles worn off surgical drill. *B*, Gradient-echo image (FLASH 200/13/20 degrees) shows increased artifact, greatly exaggerating the extent of central canal compromise. (Courtesy of M. Modic, M.D.)

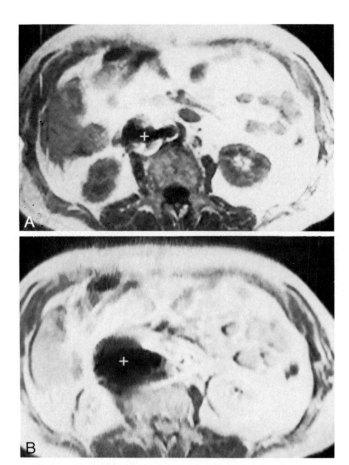

FIGURE 3–5. Ferromagnetic artifact from Gianturco coil. *A*, T₁-weighted image demonstrates central signal void (*cross-mark*) and high intensity curvilinear rim. *B*, T₂-weighted image demonstrates larger artifact since frequency-encoding gradient is reduced (in order to improve S/N, sampling time is increased, same FOV as *A*).

FIGURE 3–6. *A*, **Shunt artifact.** Shunt tube produces minimal artifact (*black arrow*), whereas ferromagnetic connectors produce larger artifact (*white arrow*). *B*, Patient with posttraumatic syrinx (*straight arrow*). Apparent cord deformity (*curved arrow*) above syrinx cavity is caused by ferromagnetic artifact from surgical clips.

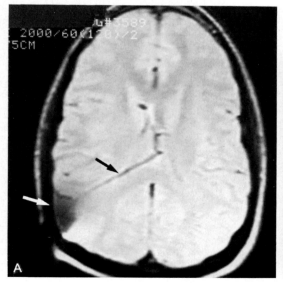

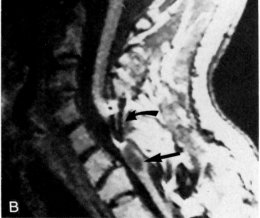

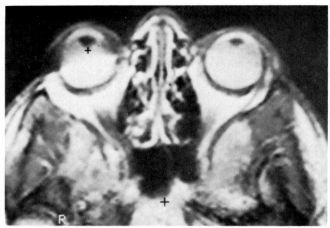

FIGURE 3–7. Mascara artifact (*cross*), caused by ferromagnetic iron ores.

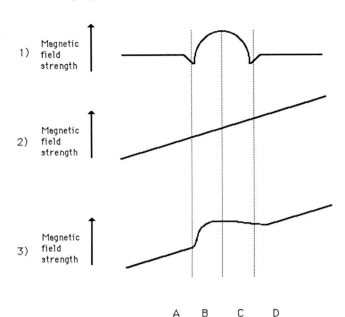

FIGURE 3–9. Explanation of geometric distortion and signal changes caused by a ferromagnetic object. Ferromagnetic object produces localized increase in magnetic field (1). Normally, there is a linear increase in magnetic field strength along the direction of the frequency-encoding gradient (2). In conjunction with the magnetic field gradient, the field distortions caused by the ferromagnetic object cause either stretching and signal loss, due to increased gradient (region B), or increased signal collapsed to a line because of decreased gradient (region C).

distortion: a region of decreased signal intensity abutted on one side by a curvilinear region of marked hyperintensity (Figs. 3–3, 3–5, 3–6, 3–7, and 3–8).

The explanation for this artifact is illustrated in Figure 3–9. Spatial localization for two-dimensional Fourier transform (2DFT) image formation depends on the presence of a highly linear magnetic field gradient. Ferromagnetic objects distort the magnetic field in their vicinity. On one side, the field generated by the ferromagnetic object augments the applied magnetic field gradient, stretching the image as well as causing signal loss. On the other side, the increased field from the ferromagnetic object opposes the applied gradient; the MR signals from the tissue protons, over the region where the gradient is atten-

uated, collapse to a high intensity line. In addition to generating artifacts, larger ferromagnetic objects (such as dental plates) can worsen RF coil performance because they alter the coil tuning; in bad cases,

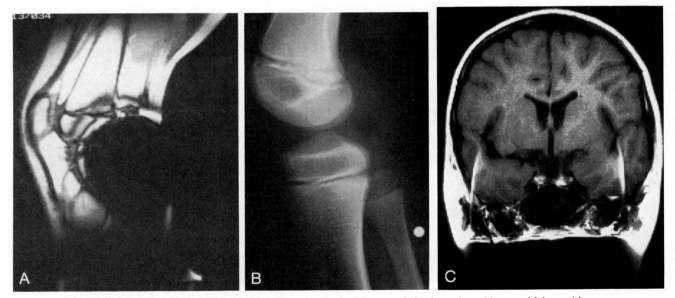

FIGURE 3–8. Ferromagnetic foreign object. *A,* Sagittal image of the knee in a 10-year-old boy with a "BB" pellet in the soft tissues posteroinferior to the joint line. Note the bizarre shape and disproportionate size of the signal void caused by the 5 mm metallic object. *B,* Radiograph image of same knee. *C,* Patient with ferromagnetic dental hardware. Artifactual bright signal overlapping temporal lobes bilaterally represents frequency-shifted signals from mouth.

imaging may be impossible, particularly on systems with high Q coils.

Small ferromagnetic objects in the volume imaged cause characteristic focal MR imaging aberrations. Documented artifact-generating ferromagnetic objects include some types of surgical clips (Fig. 3–6B), interventional radiologic coils (Fig. 3–5), steel implants such as ventriculoperitoneal shunts (Fig. 3–6A), dental steel in orthodontic braces and dentures, hair and safety pins, mascara (Fig. 3–7), and zippers.[5, 7, 8] These artifacts classically consist of a central signal void and asymmetric margins of higher signal intensity in bizarre, nonanatomic configurations (Fig. 3–8). Nonetheless, because of the different acquisition and reconstruction methods employed, MR images are usually more interpretable in the presence of metal than are the "radially streaked" x-ray CT images.

Nonferromagnetic metallic implants, such as some small surgical clips, may be invisible but can also generate artifacts in the form of localized signal voids (Fig. 3–10). The severity of the artifact depends on the shape of the object, since this determines whether closed conducting pathways exist; for instance, a U-shaped clip may generate less artifact than a closed loop. The orientation of the long axis of a surgical nail relative to the read-out gradient axis also influences the degree of artifact present.

SUSCEPTIBILITY ARTIFACT

At the boundary between two tissues with differing magnetic susceptibility, there is local distortion of the magnetic field.[9] Spin dephasing across the slice as well as within the slice results in miscentering of the echo with respect to the read-out period; when severe, this produces signal loss. Geometric distortion is also produced. The geometric distortion can be manifested as a change in shape of the object, as well as by slight mispositioning of the slice. The variation in susceptibility can occur between voxels, resulting in loss of signal at the boundary between tissues, or, if susceptibility varies within the voxel, loss of signal from that voxel.

Ferromagnetic artifact is an extreme example of a susceptibility artifact. Less severe susceptibility artifacts are also commonly seen at the boundary between substances with differing magnetic susceptibility, such as air, bone, brain, and hemorrhage. Signal loss and geometric distortion are present which may mimic partial volume averaging or calcification (Fig. 3–11). They are most prominent on high field systems and on images acquired with gradient-echo, rather than spin-echo, techniques. These artifacts can be seen above the petrous bones and around the paranasal sinuses, as well as around bowel loops on

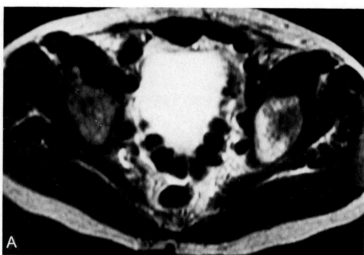

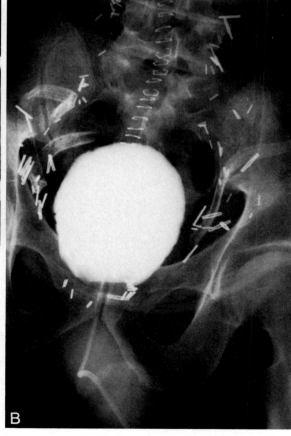

FIGURE 3–10. Apparent loop of colon in pelvis (A) is really a chain of metal surgical staples (radiograph, B).

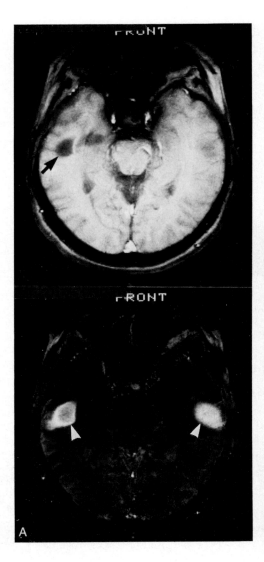

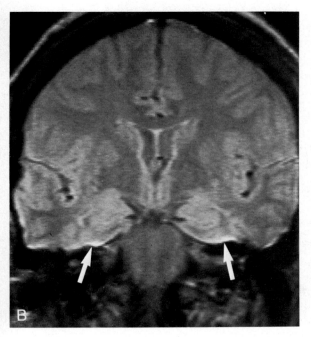

FIGURE 3–11. Magnetic susceptibility artifacts on FLASH images caused by boundary between petrous ridges and brain. *A, Top,* With TE = 13 msec, localized area of decreased signal intensity is seen in right temporal lobe (*arrow*). This does not represent partial volume averaging. Also note decreased signal intensity surrounding maxillary antra. *Bottom,* With longer TE (40 msec) susceptibility artifacts (*arrowheads*) are much worse. *B,* Coronal proton density image of brain, obtained with low bandwidth spin-echo pulse sequence, demonstrates artifactual high signal under temporal lobes (*arrows*), representing susceptibility artifact.

gradient-echo abdominal images. Gradient-echo images obtained remote from magnet isocenter also suffer from these artifacts due to main field inhomogeneity (Fig. 3–12). On gradient-echo images, bone marrow shows lower signal intensity than expected for the echo time. This is also largely a susceptibility effect, representing spin dephasing produced by the presence of substances with differing susceptibility (calcium, water, and fat) within the same voxel.

Presently, there are a few practical solutions to correct susceptibility artifact. (1) In many cases, spurious signal intensities may be decreased with stronger read-out gradients at any given field-of-view (FOV).[9] Ludeke and coworkers[9] demonstrated with constant FOVs that a 2 mT/m read-out gradient (shorter sampling window, larger receiver bandwidth) reduced the magnetic susceptibility artifact at air-water interfaces compared with a 0.8 mT/m read-out gradient (longer sampling window, narrower receiver bandwidth). (2) Short echo times (TE) (see Fig. 3–5A) allow less time for spin dephasing than long TE (Fig. 3–5B), so susceptibility artifact is reduced. (3) Susceptibility artifact can also be minimized by the use of thin slices, which reduces dephasing across the slice.

(4) For gradient-echo images, three-dimensional (3D) volume methods are particularly effective for reducing dephasing across the slice. If enough phase-encoding steps are acquired along the selection axis, then for some of the values of the selection gradient the effects of local magnetic field inhomogeneities will be compensated. As the severity of the susceptibility artifact worsens, more phase-encoding steps are needed to correct for the local field inhomogeneity. Compared with 2D gradient-echo images, 3D gradient-echo images of the head show improved definition of the pituitary gland due to reduced susceptibility effects from the interface between brain and air-containing sphenoid sinus. Three-dimensional gradient-echo images of the spine show increased signal from bone marrow.

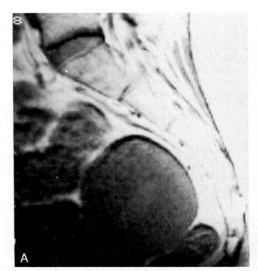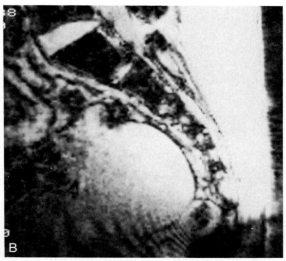

FIGURE 3–12. Gradient-echo images are particularly sensitive to magnetic field inhomogeneity, which worsens with distance from the isocenter of the magnet. *A*, T_1-weighted image of the lower lumbar spine and pelvis demonstrates normal uterine anatomy. Magnetic field inhomogeneity is not apparent. *B*, Gradient-echo (FISP) image acquired with TE = 11 msec demonstrates multiple ringlike artifacts along inferior edge of image, which is distant from the magnet center.

RADIOFREQUENCY FIELD ARTIFACTS

EXTERNAL NOISE

Sources

The radiofrequency pulses utilized to excite protons in MR imaging share frequency ranges with many extraneous RF sources, including fluorescent lights; television and radio broadcasts; distant short-wave broadcasts appearing in the evening; electric motors (particularly direct current) such as in CT scanners, pumps, and floor cleaning equipment; electric trains; forklift trucks; elevator switching gear; defective diodes; bad connections; a leaky magnet room RF-shielding enclosure; patient monitoring devices; typewriters; and computers.[1, 3] Penetration of these extrinsic RF energies into an MRI system results in image noise, with the degree of image degradation dependent upon the frequency range of the noise source and the MR system resonance frequency and bandwidth. Broad band noise may degrade an entire image, whereas extrinsic narrow frequency signal commonly causes linear bands of interference perpendicular to the frequency-encoding axis (Fig. 3–13). The exact location of the artifactual band relates to the difference between the center frequency of the scanner and the frequency of the extraneous signal.

Specifically, amateur radio operators operate within the frequency range of 21.0 to 21.5 MHz. The Larmor frequency for a 0.5 T MRI system of 21.3 MHz falls within this range. A 1.5 T MRI system has a proton resonance frequency of 64.0 MHz, which lies within the frequency domain of 60 to 66 MHz assigned to television channel 3.[1]

Shielding from Radiofrequency Noise

Obviously, shielding from extrinsic RF sources is necessary for preservation of MR images from external noise. The magnet room enclosure should attenuate extrinsic noise by a factor of 80 to 120 dB, depending on the installation. RF leaks can occur through pipes and electrical lines; this can be avoided by enclosing them in waveguides. RF noise will enter

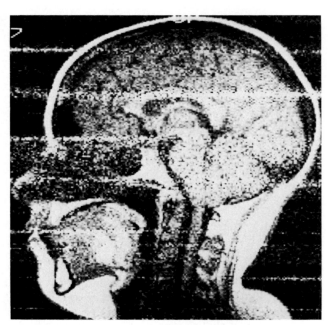

FIGURE 3–13. Radiofrequency interference due to defective magnet room enclosure. Note multiple horizontal lines, oriented perpendicular to the frequency-encoding axis, representing RF interference at multiple frequencies.

if the door is left open, or if the flexible copper tabs along the sides, top, and bottom of some types of door break off. A simple check for room leakage is to play an FM radio within the room with the door open and closed. Closing the door should dramatically decrease reception. If discrete RF noise persists in the image despite all shielding efforts, then field service personnel can always adjust the main field strength and corresponding RF synthesizer frequency up or down to find a "clean" imaging bandwidth.

System Radiofrequency Noise

If linear artifacts are seen along both the frequency-encoding and phase-encoding axes, these artifacts may arise from electrical noise sources intrinsic to the imaging system.[2] These so-called synchronous artifacts are often due to bad system components, as well as poor electrical or RF grounding. In the raw data, these artifacts are manifested as oblique lines which appear through all lines of data. System artifacts are the responsibility of field service personnel.

Room Radiofrequency Noise

Artifacts, similar in appearance on MR images to those from system noise, can also be caused by static electricity due to floor materials with improper conductivity in conjunction with low humidity. Blankets and patient gowns can also be a source of static electricity. Another potential source of noise is 60 Hz interference associated with defective light bulbs or wall sockets. In the raw data, these artifacts are manifested as abnormally high or low intensity data points that occur randomly in the data and are usually not present in all data lines. Changing the environment, for example, by increasing humidity or grounding the floor, may be needed to eliminate these artifacts.

SHIELDING THE PATIENT FROM THE RADIOFREQUENCY COIL

A metallic object between the coil and patient may act as a shield from the transmitted RF pulses, generating local RF field defects and resulting in signal loss and/or distortion.[3] Potential "internal" RF shields are metal-containing dressings, electrode disks, or RF impermeable objects. Removal of the shielding objects will restore RF homogeneity.

SURFACE COIL SENSITIVITY

Artifactual loss of signal is an inherent problem in surface coil imaging due to loss of RF intensity away from the center of the coil (Fig. 3–14). The peripheral drop-off of signal intensity occurs in all possible modes of operation with RF surface coils: transmit-only, receive-only, and transmit-receive. Optimal po-

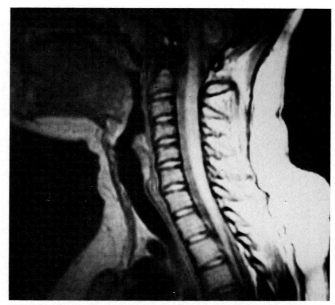

FIGURE 3–14. Surface coil signal loss. Sagittal image of neck obtained with planar surface coil (body coil transmit, surface coil receive). Cervical spinal cord is well visualized, but signal drops off rapidly in adjacent deeper areas.

sitioning of the coil minimizes the loss of diagnostically useful information. Signal inhomogeneity across the image can be improved by appropriate rescaling of the image.[10]

TIP ANGLE VARIATION

Radiofrequency tip angle inhomogeneity may cause asymmetric brightness in an image (Fig. 3–15). This problem may originate in the RF transmitter attenuation setting or RF coil geometry. In the former instance, the RF 90-degree or 180-degree pulse is calibrated to obtain the optimal amount of MR signal in the center slice of the multislice imaging volume. Selected slices of interest away from the center slice may experience more or less attenuation of the RF than the center slice, resulting in RF tip angles greater or lesser than 90 degrees or 180 degrees. Signal intensity of spins in that slice diminishes, corresponding to the decrease in transverse magnetization. Similarly, inhomogeneous energy deposition across the volume of tissue may occur secondary to asymmetric RF coil geometry or off-center patient positioning. The artifactual variation in signal intensity over the image is identical to that caused by RF tip angle inhomogeneity but is correctable by proper patient positioning.

SELECTIVE AND NONSELECTIVE RADIOFREQUENCY PULSES

Radiofrequency pulses may be selective, exciting spins in a discrete volume of finite thickness, or

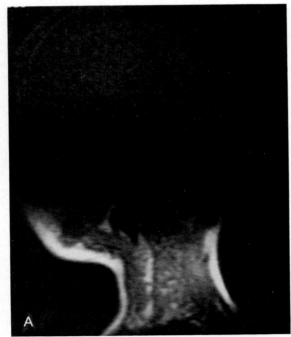

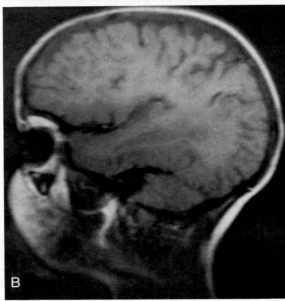

FIGURE 3–15. Incorrect RF attenuation setting. *A,* Sagittal T_1-weighted study of head with RF pulse attenuation erroneously peaked over neck. As a result, the intended 90- to 180-degree RF pulses produced actual tip angles of 180 to 360 degrees in the head, with loss of signal in region of interest. *B,* Correct RF attenuation peaking at the same level yields satisfactory head study.

nonselective, exciting spins in the entire tissue volume. The assumption that a selective RF pulse excites protons in a well-defined geometric slab of tissue is often incorrect, especially with nominal 180-degree RF pulses. Some MR image slice profiles are Gaussian or even M-shaped. Artifactual loss of signal intensity in a stack of multislice images acquired contiguously may occur due to saturation of spins by overlapping,

nonsquare slice profiles in contiguous slice imaging. Interleaving slices in data acquisition, lengthening the repetition time (TR), or increasing the interslice gap will alleviate this "cross-talk" problem. New sophisticated computer-optimized RF excitation pulses resulting in negligible cross-talk with gapless multislice spin-echo imaging are now commercially available. Imperfections in slice profiles refocused by a selective 180-degree RF pulse are not a problem in gradient-echo sequences, where one can routinely obtain gapless, contiguous, multislice sections without significant cross-talk.

INTRINSIC PATIENT NOISE

Random thermal or incoherent noise degrades spatial resolution and contrast over the entire object imaged. Methods of reducing thermal noise are to increase the number of signal averages (excitations) or to use surface coils, thereby limiting detection of thermal noise in more distant tissues not containing the region of interest and thereby increasing the signal-to-noise (S/N) ratio.[12]

CONTACT ARTIFACT

Physical contact between patient and the RF coil produces signal loss and image distortion similar to ferromagnetic artifact. Contact artifact is distinguished by its peripheral location on the image and the bizarre configuration of the anatomic part involved, usually the upper extremity, abdomen, or pelvis. Remedies include patient repositioning or utilizing a smaller FOV. Alternatively, the technique of inner volume imaging of Feinberg and colleagues is able to "focus in" on a central region of interest not affected by peripheral body-coil contact artifact.[13]

DIRECT CURRENT INTERFERENCE (CENTRAL POINT ARTIFACT)

The central point artifact is a central bright or dark area of signal intensity (occasionally with a column of truncation ringing bordering it) and generally occurs in the exact center of the image[3] (Fig. 3–16). It results from a constant direct current (DC) offset in the level of the receiver voltage of each phase-encoding step, which is unavoidable due to factors such as transistor bias voltages. If the DC level of each phase-encoding step is variable, a line parallel to the phase-encoding axis can result (similar to RF feedthrough, see below). This artifact can be reduced to a point by phase alternation of two RF excitation pulses at each phase-encoding step, resulting in cancellation of the two averaged extraneous signals. Also, this artifact can be reduced by calibrating the DC level during the prescan period prior to image data acquisition.

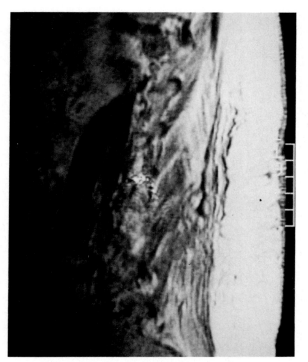

FIGURE 3–16. Central field artifact. Proton density weighted sagittal images of the lumbar spine demonstrate classic central field artifact of bright signal intensity covering several pixels.

CENTRAL LINE ARTIFACT

Central line artifacts can be divided into those parallel to the phase-encoding axis which occur in the center (zero column) of the frequency-encoding axis, which we refer to as zero frequency artifact, and those that occur in the center (zero line) of the phase-encoding axis, which we refer to as zero phase artifact.

Zero Frequency Artifact

Figure 3–17 illustrates this artifact, which results from RF feedthrough[2] detected by the sensitive RF receiver that, by necessity, must reside close to the strong RF transmitter. This artifact can be reduced by alternating the phase of the RF pulses. This artifact can also be eliminated by substitution of the spurious central data point in each phase-encoding step with a point interpolated from adjacent points.[2] This interpolation would take place between the first and second Fourier transformations; so this technique would be ineffective if digital smoothing filters were applied along the read-out axis prior to the first FT (since the filter distributes the RF feedthrough over many frequencies, rendering single point interpolation impossible).[2]

Zero Phase Artifact

Central line artifacts parallel to the frequency-encoding axis can be caused by residual transverse

magnetization, in the form of a free induction decay (FID) or a stimulated echo (STE) signal. These spurious signals arise primarily from imperfections of the 180-degree RF pulses directly preceding the corresponding spin echoes. The imperfections are unavoidable in any practical instrument, especially for multiple slice sequences requiring selective 180-degree RF pulses. For example, a selective pulse must have some finite transition region between its center (where it does its main function) and its exterior (where it is supposed to do nothing). In this transition, a 180-degree pulse passes through lesser values that will generate an FID. In multiecho pulse sequences, additional stimulated echoes can be generated because of imperfections in both the 90- and 180-degree RF pulses (Fig. 3–18A and B). If these stimulated echoes are not phase encoded and if they happen to fall within the read-out period, then a central line ("zipper") can be produced. If the stimulated echoes are phase encoded, then they can also produce an inverted image ghost (as opposed to a 180-degree rotated image from quadrature-phase error), since the phase of the stimulated echo will be opposite in polarity to the Carr-Purcell nth echo ($n > 1$)[2] (Fig. 3–18C).

PULSE SEQUENCE DESIGN CONSIDERATIONS FOR MINIMIZING RF ARTIFACTS

In Figure 3–19, we see a very basic spin-echo pulse sequence. There are the 90-degree and 180-degree RF pulses and three gradient waveforms. Note two potential problems: (1) There is an FID following the 180-degree RF pulse much like the one from the 90-degree RF pulse. (It has been exaggerated in Figure 3–19.) (2) Spatial information in the phase-

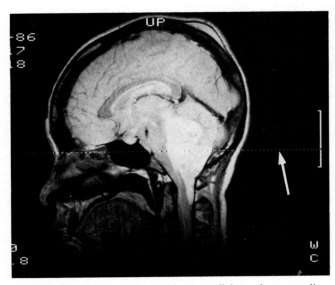

FIGURE 3–17. Center line artifact, parallel to phase-encoding axis, in a proton density image of a patient with an ependymoma.

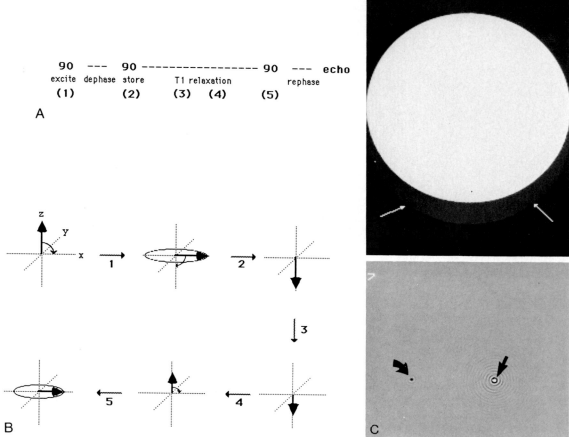

FIGURE 3–18. Stimulated echo artifacts. *A,* Three RF pulses can produce a stimulated echo. *B,* Illustration of how magnetization gets stored and then read out to produce a stimulated echo. *C,* Effect of stimulated echo seen in image of water bottle. *Top,* In addition to normal image, there is a striated inverted ghost image displaced inferiorly along the phase-encoding axis. *Bottom,* Raw data demonstrate normal echo (*black arrow*) as well as lower intensity stimulated echo (*curved arrow*).

encoded direction is imposed before this 180-degree–born FID exists.

The reconstructed image from this sequence will have a thin line of hash through the center of the phase-encoded direction, parallel to the read-out axis (Fig. 3–19*A*). The hash piles up there because it missed being phase encoded and will be treated as a DC component and dumped in the central row along the phase-encoding axis.

A solution to an analogous problem in a different MR application was given in 1977 by Bodenhausen and colleagues.[14] The suggestion was to alternate the phase of the 180-degree RF pulse across phase-encoding steps. Again, the spin echoes are unchanged but the hash from the FID is changing sign, apparently at the Nyquist frequency. The reconstructed image still contains the hash; however, it is no longer in the center of the image, but rather at one edge (Fig. 3–19*B*). Other phase-cycling techniques can be employed as well.[15, 16]

Image artifacts due to spurious FIDs can be limited by using short read-out periods and by adjusting timing parameters within the pulse sequence. In addition, improvement of the slice excitation profile by better RF pulse tailoring should reduce this artifact, but little agreement on the ideal selective pulse has been achieved.[11, 17–22] A commonly employed technique for eliminating residual transverse magnetization is to insert paired pulsed gradients ("crushers") about the 180-degree pulse.[23, 24] The stimulated-echo ghost problem can be eliminated by inversion of the polarity of the second spin-echo signal (relative to the first echo) using an additional phase-encoding gradient between the first echo and the second 180-degree RF pulse.[2]

DATA ACQUISITION AND GRADIENTS

It is impossible to completely separate artifacts relating to data acquisition from those due to the imaging gradients, since they are closely interrelated. We will therefore consider them together.

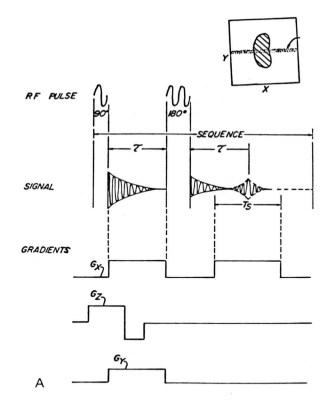

FIGURE 3–19. Explanation of center line artifact. *A,* Without alternating phase of 180-degree RF pulse. Residual transverse magnetization in the form of a free induction decay from the imperfect 180-degree RF pulse spills over into the spin-echo sampling window (T$_s$). Since this spurious signal was created after phase encoding, its multiple frequencies are all dumped into the zeroth phase-encoding column in the image, creating the center line parallel to the phase-encoding axis. *B,* With phase alternation of successive 180-degree pulses, this residual transverse magnetization is shifted to the edge of the image.

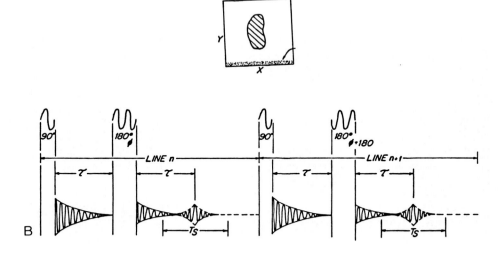

PARTIAL VOLUME AVERAGING

Partial volume averaging occurs when the voxel dimensions are comparable to the dimensions of the object being imaged. Since most MR imaging is performed using anisotropic techniques (i.e., lower resolution in one dimension than in the other two), partial volume averaging is most severe in the direction of slice selection (Figs. 3–20 and 3–21). High contrast structures (e.g., lipid-containing Pantopaque droplets on a T$_1$-weighted image) can be visualized even when they are smaller than the voxel (Fig. 3–22); however, low contrast structures (e.g., small meningiomas) may not be detected.

Partial volume averaging is minimized by improving spatial resolution. This can be accomplished by reducing the section thickness and/or by reducing the FOV. However, this results in a reduction in S/N, which may necessitate increased signal averaging and proportionately increased acquisition time. Because the voxel is usually much larger in the direction of slice selection, a reduction in section thickness

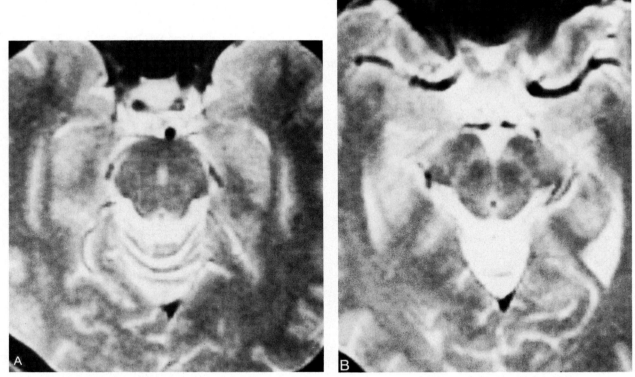

FIGURE 3–20. T₂-weighted image (*A*) with horizontal phase-encoding demonstrates inferior midbrain central high signal intensity (5 mm thick section). Adjacent slice centered 7.5 mm superior (*B*) shows the high-signal interpeduncular cistern as the source for this partial volume averaging artifact.

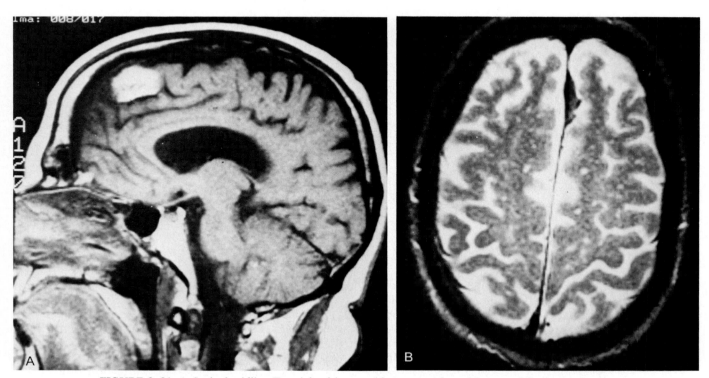

FIGURE 3–21. *A*, Sagittal midline T₁-weighted image with apparent frontal intracranial subacute hemorrhage. *B*, Axial T₂-weighted section shows the short T₂ nature and falx cerebri location, diagnostic of normal bone marrow lipid in an ossified falx.

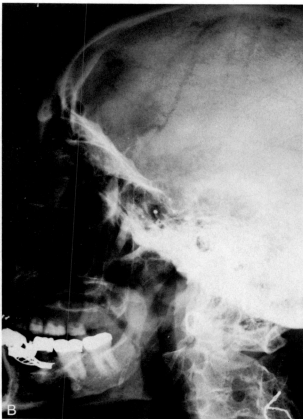

FIGURE 3–22. Sagittal midline T$_1$-weighted image (*A*) illustrates parasellar and olfactory groove hyperintense droplets of intracranial Pantopaque (*B*, radiograph).

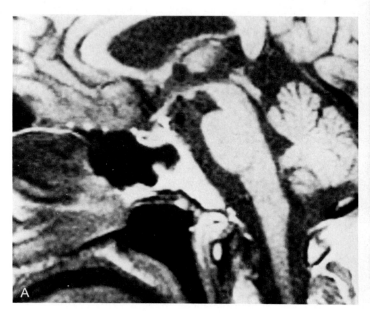

generally provides a greater reduction in partial volume averaging than does a reduced FOV.

typically by a few decibels. However, excessive reductions in receiver gain may worsen image contrast.

RECEIVER GAIN ADJUSTMENT (CLIPPING ARTIFACT)

On occasion one may encounter an image with a peculiar ghostlike quality, a "snowstorm" background, and a loss of contrast between soft tissues (Fig. 3–23). This is a data clipping artifact, resulting from having signal intensity that is outside the digitization range (saturation) of the analog-to-digital converter (ADC). The artifact may be encountered on some sections and not on others in a multisection acquisition. The problem is most severe on surface coil images, where subcutaneous fat contributes high signal, in obese patients, and in techniques that use large numbers of slices or thick sections. Normally, the receiver adjustment is performed using the zero-phase line (i.e., no phase-encoding gradient), since this data line produces the highest signal. However, interactions between the magnetic field of a surface coil and the main field can change which line produces maximal signal. As a result, maximal signal will occur a few lines away from zero, rather than at the zero line.

If the automatic receiver adjustment results in clipping, the receiver gain can be manually reduced,

RECEIVER LOW PASS FILTER ADJUSTMENT

Asymmetric brightness can occur due to low pass filters that are too narrow for the read-out bandwidth. This leads to inappropriate rejection of a portion of the signal emitted by the protons in the section of interest. The characteristic appearance is a uniform decrease in signal intensity on one or both sides of an image. The problem may be corrected by widening the band pass of the frequency filter.

LOSS OF DATA

Loss of one or more lines of data causes a variable degree of artifacts in the image; loss of the central data lines (weakest phase-encoding steps) results in the largest artifacts. Loss of data can result from communication problems, gradient instability, or excessive receiver noise (Fig. 3–24). ADC errors are unavoidable on any MRI system, since over 10 million analog-to-digital conversions take place in a single patient study.[2] An error in the digitization of a *single* data point can result in a uniform background of

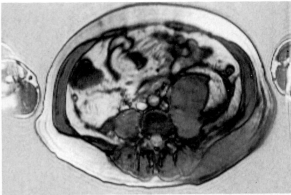

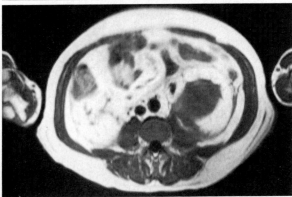

FIGURE 3–23. Data clipping artifact. *Top,* T_1-weighted image of the abdomen demonstrates ghostlike appearance due to incorrect setting of receiver gain. *Bottom,* Lower receiver gain produces normal-appearing image.

vertical, horizontal, or obliquely oriented stripes (Fig. 3–25). The intensity of the stripes can be severe, or barely noticeable, depending on where the bad data point falls in the raw data. Spontaneous occurrence of single data point digitization errors cannot be prevented but can be eliminated by postacquisition processing of the raw image data. It has been suggested that spontaneous discharge of static electricity from patient blankets can result in these single data point errors.[2]

In general, when unusual artifacts suggestive of system problems are seen, it is helpful to save the corresponding raw data set for field service, since the raw data helps define the source of the artifacts. If the raw data is not saved, it is usually automatically deleted prior to the next acquisition.

GRADIENT ARTIFACTS

Magnetic field gradients transform a magnetic resonance signal into the MR image, as they provide the information necessary for slice selection and spatial encoding (see Chapter 1). As a result, even minor gradient problems may render clinical images inaccurate (Fig. 3–26) or uninterpretable. The gradient fields must be designed to switch on and off rapidly,

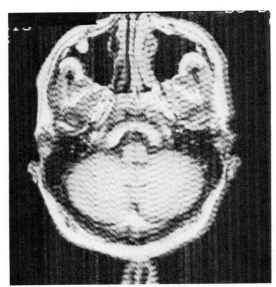

FIGURE 3–24. Moire pattern resulting from loss of line of data during acquisition. In this case, loss of the data line was produced by excessive receiver noise, secondary to a defective service light bulb.

usually within 1 millisecond. This demand exacts strict requirements on gradient coil power supplies and generates mechanical stress on the coil itself, which may lead to malfunction. In addition to gradient coil mechanical problems causing artifacts, the 2DFT reconstruction of gradient-generated spatial-encoding data produces inherent MR artifacts, which will be discussed below.

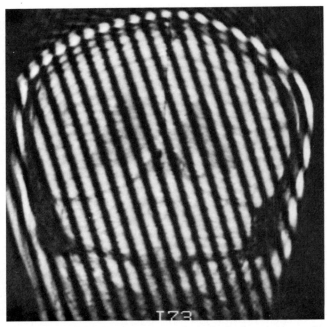

FIGURE 3–25. Digitalization error in a single data point results in an annoying blanket of diagonal stripes in the conventional magnitude reconstruction.

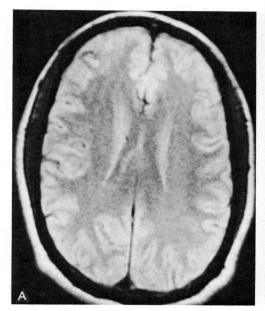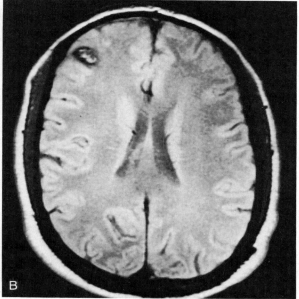

FIGURE 3–26. Gradient power dropoff. *A,* Axial (2000/30) image of the head in a patient with an intracerebral hemorrhage from an AVM. Dolichocephalic appearance of head is due to gradient power dropoff. *B,* Same patient evaluated 7 weeks later on a different MRI system shows normal head configuration and lesion with peripheral rim of low intensity signal secondary to paramagnetic effect of hemosiderin-laden macrophages.

The frequency-encoding gradient is the gradient most sensitive to inherent B_0 static field inhomogeneities.[3] An image obtained with the frequency-encoding gradient selected along the axis of greatest B_0 inhomogeneity, conventionally the z-axis in most systems, may show bands or areas of signal loss corresponding to the areas of B_0 nonuniformity. By exchanging orientation of frequency- and phase-encoding axes, the S/N ratio over the entire image may increase.

RINGING ARTIFACTS FROM SAMPLING

Ringing artifacts (also called Gibbs, edge-ringing, spectral leakage, or truncation artifacts) appear as concentric curvilinear low intensity lines that cross through the entire image. These artifacts arise primarily in two circumstances: (1) due to data interpolation (zero filling), when a smaller acquisition matrix (e.g., 256 × 128) is interpolated into a larger display matrix (e.g., 256 × 256) through the use of sinc or other functions; and (2) near edges where there are abrupt transitions in signal intensity along relatively linear portions of tissue interfaces, for example, between bright scalp fat and dark cortex of the calvarium (Fig. 3–27). On occasion, ringing may mimic motion artifact or a fine structure such as a small syrinx in the spinal cord, muscle bundles, or nerve fibers.[2]

Unlike the other kinds of artifacts we have described, ringing artifacts occur in both the frequency- and phase-encoding directions and are always present to some degree in MR images.

Phase-encoding Direction

Ringing artifacts are clinically most likely to be present along the phase-encoding axis, since throughput and economic pressures often constrain imaging time to the least number of phase-encoding steps possible (e.g., 128). It must be emphasized that with greater sampling of the higher frequencies in k-space (e.g., 256 phase-encoding steps), the spacing of the ringing lines are cut in half, but their amplitude is not diminished.[2] Despite this theoretical lim-

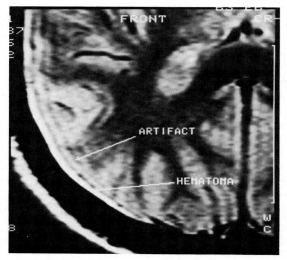

FIGURE 3–27. Patient with small subdural hematoma, 256 × 128 acquisition matrix, no filtering. Note curvilinear lines (ringing artifacts) which parallel the high intensity hematoma along the horizontal phase-encoding axis.

itation of this solution to truncation ringing, it remains the most practical and effective remedy, since the tighter spacing of the ringing lines vastly reduces their conspicuousness.

Frequency-encoding Direction

An artifact similar in appearance to ringing artifacts, but different in etiology and orientation, can be seen on images acquired with marked bandwidth reduction (used to improve S/N). Bandwidth reduction techniques use a weak read-out gradient; ringing artifacts along the read-out axis arise when the gradient is so small that the ratio (duration of read-out period/T_2) approaches unity.[1] So-called matched bandwidth techniques, which employ a long narrow band sampling window asymmetrically displaced earlier in time relative to the center of the echo (in order to achieve earlier minimum TE times for a given bandwidth), also suffer from ringing artifacts along the frequency-encoding axis.

An edge ringing artifact is caused by the sudden truncation of the raw data at the high frequency ends of the spectrum. Another way to reduce this common artifact is to apply a filter that reduces the contribution of the very high frequency components. This has the side effect of reducing the noise content without removing much anatomic information. The result, if done properly, is generally desirable, although there is necessarily a small loss of edge definition (spatial blurring).[25]

Digital Filtering

During the calculation of an image from the raw data, one has the opportunity to introduce some filter functions into the process to improve the image quality with little or no increase in the time required for reconstruction. This is accomplished by a general technique known as digital filtering. A review of the basic applications of digital filters[26] reveals that they are particularly applicable in Fourier transform signal processing.

RINGING ARTIFACTS FROM GRADIENT INSTABILITY

Gradient Peak Power Instability

An artifact similar in appearance to the Gibbs phenomenon can result from inadequate peak power output from the gradient power supply during the strongest phase-encoding steps. This can be corrected by purposely overpowering the gradient during these steps.[2]

Gradient Low Power Instability

Gradient amplifiers can also fail to meet power requirements during the weaker steps of phase encoding, due to dynamic-range problems in the digitization of the gradient, especially for wide FOV acquisitions.[2] *Translated* ghosts (as opposed to *180-degree rotated* or *inverted* ghosts) result from this error in software pulse sequence design. This error can be avoided by ensuring that *all* phase-encoding steps for all possible FOVs have a whole integer value assigned to them by the DAC (digital-to-analog converter), avoiding digital roundoff problems for the lower order phase-encoding steps. This approach may not be feasible for oblique sections and may require interpolation schemes in the reconstruction of the second dimension of the 2DFT.

Sixty Hz electrical noise (from imager or environmental hardware) can result in translated ghosts, as persistent view-to-view errors in the gradient amplifier are introduced. As opposed to gradient-DAC error translated ghosts, these ghosts are reduced by signal averaging[2] or gating the excitation sequence to 60 Hz (TR = a whole integer multiple of 1/60 sec or 16.67 msec). This approach is entirely analogous to averaging and gating with biologic respiratory or cardiac motion (see "Motion-Related Artifacts"). Room lights can be a cause of 60-cycle, noise-induced, translated ghosts.

CHEMICAL SHIFT ARTIFACT

Cause

Chemical shift artifact can occur along either the read-out or slice-selection axes. Along the read-out axis, it is seen at the border between fat-containing tissue (e.g., retroperitoneal fat, bone marrow) and water-containing tissue (e.g., renal cortex, intervertebral disk). As reviewed in Chapter 9, fat protons resonate at approximately 3.5 ppm lower frequency than water protons. However, MR images are usually obtained using the water peak as the central reference frequency. Since frequency is equivalent to position in 2DFT imaging and fat protons resonate at a lower frequency, they appear shifted in position along the frequency-encoding axis to the lower frequency side of the image (Fig. 3–28). As shown in Figure 3–29 for the kidney (which is embedded in fat), when the chemical shift is comparable to or greater than the pixel size, it results in a dark line on the low frequency border of the kidney and a bright line on the high frequency border.[27] Areas in which chemical shift artifact may cause diagnostic problems include the optic nerves, kidneys, pericardium, and vertebral end plates. Note that chemical shift artifact does not usually occur in brain, despite the fat content of myelin, because these fat protons have a very short T_2 and are invisible on MR.

Chemical shift artifact can occur in the head, however, along the slice-selection axis. On an axial section, lipid protons from skull bone marrow can be misregistered (with reference to the same section's water protons) along the z-axis, resulting in bilaterally

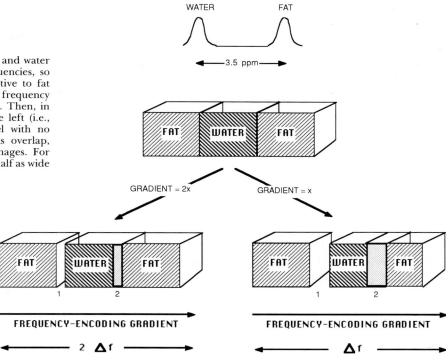

FIGURE 3–28. Chemical shift artifact. Fat and water protons resonate at slightly different frequencies, so water protons appear to be displaced relative to fat protons. Assume that the center (reference) frequency of the system is set to the water resonance. Then, in region 1, fat protons appear shifted to the left (i.e., lower absolute frequency), leaving a pixel with no signal. In region 2, fat and water signals overlap, resulting in high signal on T_2-weighted images. For frequency-encoding gradient-2x, artifact is half as wide as for gradient-x.

symmetric pseudosubdural hematomata.[2] Correction of this artifact may be achieved by reversal of the polarity of the slice-selection gradient between the 90-degree pulse and the 180-degree pulse.

Solutions

Like ferromagnetic artifact, chemical shift artifact worsens in proportion to the magnetic field strength and improves in proportion to the frequency-encoding gradient. Doubling the frequency-encoding gradient (e.g., using a higher bandwidth pulse sequence) reduces chemical shift artifact by a factor of two, but at the expense of a 40 per cent worsening in S/N. Chemical shift artifact can be minimized for certain structures (e.g., optic nerve) by reorienting the frequency-encoding gradient so that it parallels the tissue's long axis. More complex methods are also

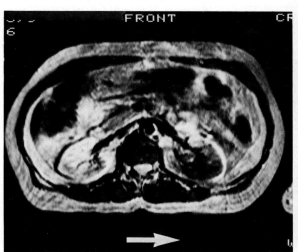

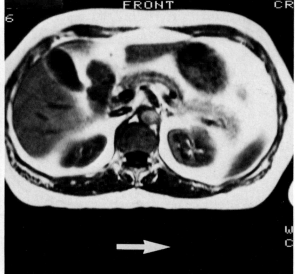

FIGURE 3–29. Chemical shift artifact. White arrow = direction of read-out gradient. *Left,* Note bright curvilinear line along right (high-frequency) side and dark line along the left (low-frequency) side of each kidney representing chemical shift artifact on this T_2-weighted image (SE 2000/60). *Right,* T_1-weighted acquisition, which uses a stronger read-out gradient because of the shorter TE, demonstrates only minimal chemical shift artifact.

under development. For instance, chemical shift-selective imaging (e.g., CHESS) can be used to selectively eliminate signal from fat or water protons. Although a variety of methods are available for reducing chemical shift artifact, we have found that it seldom presents significant diagnostic problems even at high fields with appropriate selection of pulse sequence.

ALIASING

Nature of the Problem

Have you ever watched an old Western on television and noticed how wagon wheels appear to rotate slowly backward when in actuality the wagon is moving rapidly forward? This is an example of aliasing, which arises from insufficiently rapid sampling of a periodic function and causes a high frequency to artifactually appear as a lower frequency. Examples of sampling functions include digital recording of sound, shooting a movie (each frame is one sample), and measuring the MR signal. The Nyquist theorem states that, when sampling a periodic function, one must sample at least twice as fast as the desired frequency:

$$fN > 2 \times fmax$$

where fN is the Nyquist frequency and fmax is the highest desired frequency (Fig. 3–30). In our movie example, a wagon wheel appears to turn the way it does because the movie frames are acquired at less than twice the rotational frequency of the wheel, resulting in aliasing to a slower rate of rotation. This phenomenon is known as "fold over"; frequencies exceeding the Nyquist frequency are assigned a frequency below the Nyquist frequency.

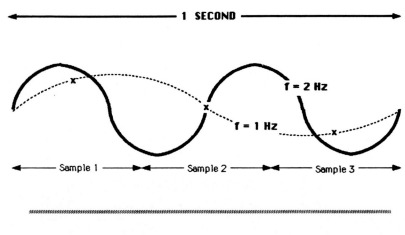

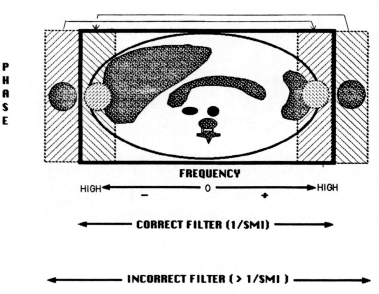

FIGURE 3–30. Aliasing. *Top,* Solid line represents periodic wave with frequency = 2 Hz. If the wave is sampled at less than the Nyquist frequency (4 Hz), an artifactually low-frequency wave is represented (*dotted line*). *Bottom,* Wraparound artifact, an expression of aliasing, causes structures, such as the arms, at the outer edges of the FOV to be folded into the middle of the image (right arm to left side, left arm to right side).

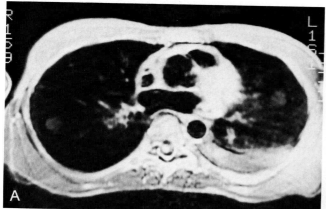

FIGURE 3–31. Aliasing mimicking pulmonary nodules; transverse images from a respiratory and cardiac gated chest study with an FOV of 32 cm demonstrate aliasing of humeral marrow fat bilaterally into the lung parenchyma (A) which disappears on wider FOV acquisition (B).

Appearance of Aliasing (Wraparound Artifact)

One manifestation of aliasing, not encountered in CT, is wraparound. Wraparound can occur on MR images as one reduces the FOV. Objects near the sides of the image (e.g., arms on chest images) overlap structures in the image, creating pseudolesions (Fig. 3–31). The appearance is similar to a piece of paper that has been folded to fit into an envelope. Wraparound occurs because, in reducing the FOV, one increases the precessional frequencies in the object but does not correspondingly increase the number of phase-encoding steps or frequency samples. Mild wraparound is seldom of significance, but severe wraparound renders the images uninterpretable (Fig. 3–32).

Solutions

Wraparound along the frequency-encoding axis can be prevented by matching the receiver band pass filter to the reciprocal of the sampling time and by oversampling along the frequency-encoding axis (e.g., acquiring 512 rather than the usual 256 samples). Wraparound along the phase-encoding axis is a more challenging problem. Reducing the strength of the phase-encoding gradient reduces wraparound but also reduces spatial resolution. Wraparound along the phase-encoding axis can also be reduced by oversampling (e.g., "high sort" *no phase wrap* method).[28, 29] This technique is effective but requires images to be acquired with at least two excitations, so that minimum acquisition time is increased. The inner volume method can eliminate wraparound by limiting the RF excitation to a restricted volume of tissue.[13] With this method, slice selection is performed sequentially along two intersecting planes to define a limited central volume. However, inner volume imaging is essentially a single-slice technique, which

reduces its efficiency for 2DFT imaging. Presaturation of signal from tissues outside the region of interest is a more practical method and does not have any significant drawbacks other than a slight increase in the minimum TR/slice, typically a few milliseconds (Fig. 3–33).[30]

Aliasing can also occur along the slice-selection axis in 3D volume MRI acquisitions from incorrectly tailored selective excitation RF pulses.[2] The appearance of this artifact resembles a bizarre variation of

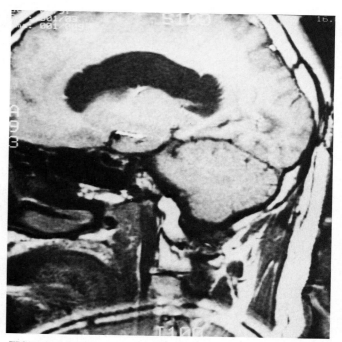

FIGURE 3–32. Aliasing in both phase- and frequency-encoding directions. Sagittal head image (SE 600/25) with FOV of 20 cm demonstrates wraparound posterior and inferior to skull. Region of interest in the pituitary is unaffected by peripheral aliasing. (Frequency gradient is vertical.)

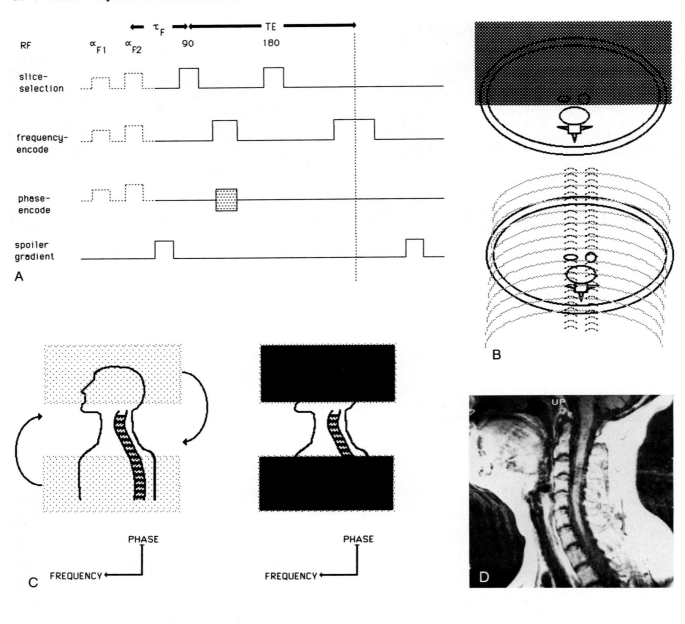

A

B

C

PHASE

FREQUENCY

PHASE

FREQUENCY

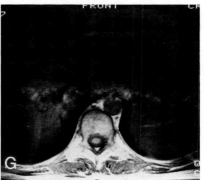

D

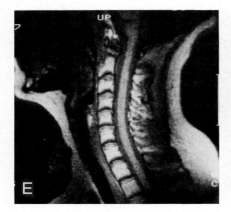

E

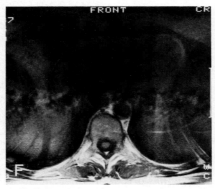

F

G

FIGURE 3–33. *See opposite page for legend.*

partial volume averaging phenomenon (e.g., ear projecting into upper spinal canal of midsagittal cervical spine section).

EDDY CURRENTS

Cause

Eddy currents are residual, undesirable magnetic gradients that persist for a variable time duration after the pulse of electrical current from the gradient power supply is terminated. Eddy currents can be induced in shim coils, other gradient coils, magnet windings, cryostat shields, or RF resonance structures.[2]

Effects

Eddy currents can result in more rapid dephasing of the transverse magnetization, resulting in reduced spin-echo or gradient-echo amplitude (shortening the observed T_2 decay). Eddy current problems are much more noticeable in images obtained "off" magnet z-axis isocenter, because of generally longer time constants of the z-axis gradients than of the x- or y-axis gradients.[2] Longer TE times also bring out these effects on reducing the observed T_2 decay. Residual magnetic gradients can also shift the temporal position of the spin echo from the standard TE time (by introducing a spatially varying phase-shift). This phase-shift can manifest in image artifact ghosting identical to motion-induced phase-shift artifacts (see "Motion-Related Artifacts").

Gradient power supply temporal instability also causes translated phase-axis ghosts, similar in appearance to 60-cycle noise ghosts as well as eddy current ghosting. The key to eliminating motion as the cause of ghosting is to image a stationary phantom. A pattern of dark bands superimposed on the image can also result from eddy currents.[2] The spin-echo signal can be destructively interfered by a stim-ulated-echo signal that has experienced an entirely different gradient pattern. This is most noticeable in later echoes of a multiecho train and in oblique slices.

With short TE times in spin-echo studies, eddy currents from the dephasing lobe of the read-out gradient can interfere with the 180-degree slice-selection gradient, resulting in an oblique plane of 180-degree nutation (despite an orthogonal plane of 90-degree excitation).[2] This results in a major loss of signal from the outer edges of the image along the read-out axis, similar to intentional in-plane presaturation (see "Motion-related Artifacts").

Solutions

Most manufacturers use eddy current compensation circuits in the gradient power supply. This approach does not work for all pulse sequences and for all spatial locations within the magnet, since the spatial and temporal characteristics of the eddy currents vary from sequence to sequence.[2] Other approaches include meticulous physical adjustment of the gradient coils during initial installation. The ultimate approach is elimination of the production of the eddy currents with the use of mirror gradient coils, called active gradient shielding.[31]

TELESCOPING

An MRI artifact that has not been reported in the literature, to our knowledge, is one we call telescoping. The image of the structure under examination, generally the abdomen in a multislice stack of transaxial sections, is reduced in apparent size in all dimensions while maintaining anatomic proportion, with gradual tapering of the dimensions from isocenter to the peripheral-most section (Fig. 3–34). Gradient nonlinearity off from the z-axis isocenter is the cause of this artifact. Software correction algorithms eliminate this artifact.

FIGURE 3–33. **Application of presaturation techniques for reduction of motion artifact.** A, Presaturation pulses can be introduced into any pulse sequence. In this example of a spin-echo sequence, two RF pulses, in conjunction with extra gradient pulses, define two thick slabs where protons are presaturated. No signal is generated within these regions and, therefore, no artifacts. B, Ghost artifacts from swallowing, respiration, and vascular pulsations (*top*) are reduced by applying a presaturation pulse over the offending regions, using the phase-encoding gradient for slab selection (*bottom*). C, With small FOVs, extraneous tissue signal can fold into the region of interest (*left*). Two presaturation pulses, displaced along the phase-encoding axis, can be used to eliminate signal from outside the FOV, and thereby to eliminate wraparound artifact (*right*). D, Surface coil image of the cervical spine in a patient with multiple sclerosis. Ghost artifacts produce a low intensity area in the spinal cord, simulating a syrinx cavity. E, With double presaturation pulses applied over the anterior and posterior soft tissues, ghost artifacts from swallowing and respiration are eliminated. The apparent syrinx has disappeared. F, Axial surface coil image of the cervical spine, obtained with swapping of the frequency-encoding and phase-encoding gradients. Note artifactual variation in signal intensity due to wraparound along the phase-encoding axis. G, Double presaturation slabs, displaced just outside the FOV, reduce wraparound and result in an improved image.

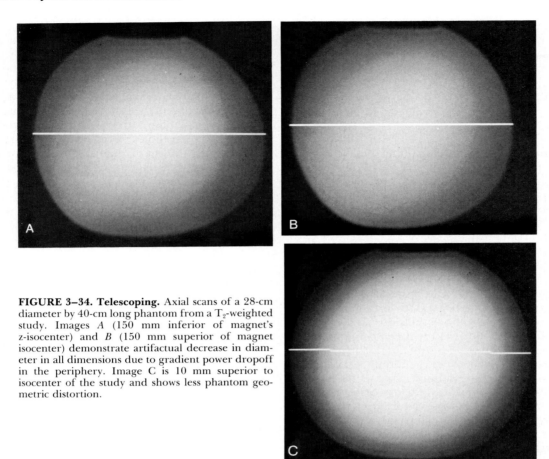

FIGURE 3–34. Telescoping. Axial scans of a 28-cm diameter by 40-cm long phantom from a T_2-weighted study. Images *A* (150 mm inferior of magnet's z-isocenter) and *B* (150 mm superior of magnet isocenter) demonstrate artifactual decrease in diameter in all dimensions due to gradient power dropoff in the periphery. Image C is 10 mm superior to isocenter of the study and shows less phantom geometric distortion.

MOTION-RELATED ARTIFACTS

Motion artifact is a common problem in MR, particularly when imaging the head, spine, chest, abdomen, or pelvis. Two types of artifact are encountered. Motion causes the signal from an object to spread out spatially, producing blurring. Blurring can occur along any axis. In addition to blurring, motion causes ghost artifacts (Fig. 3–35). Unlike blurring, these artifacts, which appear as alternating high and low intensity ghostlike images of a moving object, only occur along the phase-encoding axis.

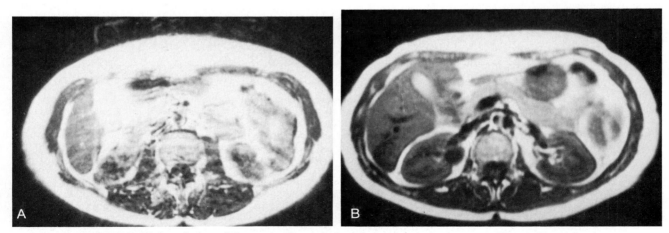

FIGURE 3–35. Reordering of phase-encoding steps in order to reduce respiratory artifact. *A*, T_1-weighted axial image of abdomen obtained with two excitations. Note respiratory ghost artifacts arising primarily from motion of subcutaneous fat, which cause severe image degradation. *B*, By reordering the phase-encoding steps according to the phase of respiratory cycle (EXORCIST method), most of the artifacts can be eliminated. (Courtesy of General Electric Medical Systems, Milwaukee, WI.)

TABLE 3–2. SYSTEM CAUSES OF GHOSTING

Ghost Orientation	Cause	Effect of Averaging
Inverted	STE	None
180-degree rotation	QPD	None
Translated	Gradient DAC	None
Translated	60 Hz noise	Reduced
Translated	Eddy currents	Reduced
Translated	Gradient amplifier instability	Reduced

SYSTEM CAUSES OF GHOSTING

Before discussing biologic ghosting, let us briefly review the various causes and signatures of system-caused ghosting. Before accepting the technologist's plea that patient motion resulted in ghosting, the radiologist should check the daily morning quality assurance phantom for system causes (Table 3–2).

PATIENT CAUSES OF GHOSTING

Ghost artifacts result from temporal variations in signal intensity; the usual culprits are cardiac motion, pulsatile flow of blood or cerebrospinal fluid (CSF), and respiration. The intensity of the ghost artifacts increases with the amplitude of the periodic motion.

The intensity of the ghosts also increases in proportion to the signal intensity of the moving tissue. For instance, ghost artifacts from pulsatile flow will be worst on entrance sections due to the high signal from unsaturated blood protons (see Chapter 4). Ghost artifacts in the abdomen predominantly arise from motion of high intensity structures, such as subcutaneous fat on T_1-weighted images or fluid-filled bowel loops and spleen on T_2-weighted images. Note that nonperiodic motion, such as bowel peristalsis, generates diffuse image noise rather than periodic ghosts along the phase-encoding axis. Ghost artifact conspicuousness can also be a function of the temporal relationship of the motion (e.g., a cough or sneeze or deep sigh) to the phase-encoding cycle (Fig. 3–36).

Solutions

There are a number of effective techniques available for reducing ghost artifacts. These include gating, dynamic reordering of the phase-encoding gradient steps (e.g., ROPE, COPE, EXORCIST) (Fig. 3–35B), variation of the repetition time and number of excitations, and physical restraint of body motion. Techniques also exist for permitting images to be acquired within a breath-holding interval[32] or so rapidly that motion is essentially frozen (e.g., echo planar); these rapid imaging techniques will be cov-

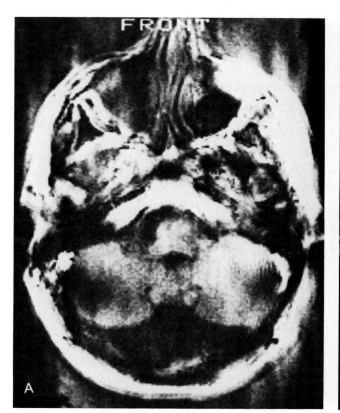
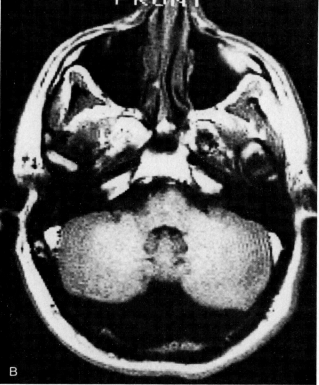

FIGURE 3–36. Images from a volunteer whose head motion was limited to the lower and zeroth order phase-encoding steps in the middle of the scan (A) versus motion limited to the higher order phase-encoding steps at the end of the scan (B). Notice the profoundly greater motion artifacts in A.

TABLE 3–3. SOLUTIONS FOR MOTION ARTIFACT

Method	Reduces Blurring	Reduces Ghosting	Comments
Breathhold*‡	+ + +	+ + +	Limited S/N
Signal average*†‡	–	+ +	Time consuming
Presaturate*†	–	+ + +	Increased RF power deposition, increased minimum TR
Gradient motion rephasing*†	–	+ +	Increased minimum TE
Reorder phase-encoding steps*	–	+ +	Slightly increased imaging time
STIR sequence*‡	–	+ +	Increased ghosts from bowel peristalsis, motion of spleen
Passive restraint of breathing*	+	+	Uncomfortable
ECG-gate†‡	+ +	+ +	Choice of TR inflexible
Respiratory gate*	+ +	+ +	Long imaging time
Pseudogate*†‡	–	+	Limited utility

*Useful for reducing respiratory artifacts
†Useful for reducing flow artifacts
‡Restricts choice of TR

ered in depth in Chapter 5. Most recently, motion compensation using gradient refocusing and presaturation techniques have been efficiently employed, particularly for spine and vascular imaging. Some of the methods for eliminating motion artifact are summarized in Table 3–3.

Gating

Ghost artifacts can be eliminated by ensuring that an object is in the same position and has the same signal intensity during the acquisition of each view. This can be accomplished using physiologic gating techniques, which limit data acquisition to a specific phase of the cardiac or respiratory cycle. Respiratory gating requires measurement of chest wall expansion (e.g., with a mechanical bellows) or air flow (e.g., nasal thermistor); cardiac triggering requires electrocardiographic monitoring or measurement of the peripheral pulse (plethysmography).

Respiratory gating effectively eliminates both ghosting and blurring (Fig. 3–37).[33, 34] However, data collection with respiratory gating is inefficient. Data collected during phases of the respiratory cycle other than the selected phase (usually end-expiration) must be discarded. This inefficiency may typically lead to a two to fourfold increase in acquisition time. Technical difficulties may also be encountered in obtaining consistent gating. Cardiac triggering is also inefficient, since the repetition time is locked to the R-R

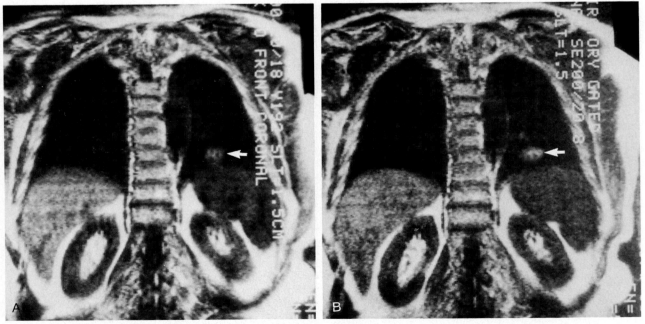

FIGURE 3–37. T_1-weighted coronal images of chest in a patient with a pulmonary hamartoma (*arrow*). *A,* Ungated image obtained with 18 excitations demonstrates blurring of fat-kidney boundary. Hamartoma appears contiguous with left diaphragm. *B,* With respiratory gating and only eight excitations, kidneys and diaphragms are more sharply delineated. Mass is clearly separated from left diaphragm.

interval.[35] Furthermore, cardiac triggering does not completely eliminate ghosting, since variations in signal intensity occur with beat-to-beat variations in the R-R interval and as a result of respiratory motion.

Phase-Reordering Methods

If the patient's respiration is monitored, the periodicity of motion responsible for ghosting can be destroyed by matching the order in which the views are acquired to the appropriate phase of the respiratory cycle.[36] These techniques go by the names of ROPE, COPE, and EXORCIST (Fig. 3–35B). For instance, the COPE method (centrally ordered phase encoding) relies on the fact that motion during phase-encoding steps of high amplitude results in lower amplitude ghosts than motion during the weaker (central) phase-encoding steps (Fig. 3–38). In the COPE method, the phase-encoding gradient is maximized during end-inspiration (maximum displacement of diaphragm) and minimized during end-expiration (minimum displacement of diaphragm) (Fig. 3–38). Unlike respiratory gating, phase-reordering methods are efficient since data from the entire respiratory cycle are used; these techniques typically prolong acquisitions by <15 per cent.

Varying TR and the Number of Signal Excitations

The distance separating ghost artifacts along the phase-encoding axis is a function of the period of the respiratory motion (TB) relative to the time between acquisition of views, represented by TR multiplied by the number of excitations (NEX). For fixed NEX, the spacing of the ghost artifacts increases with TR until

$$TB = 2 \ (TR \times NEX)$$

at which point the ghost artifacts are completely displaced off the body.[37] If TR is further increased, so that TB equals (TR × NEX), then one is effectively gating to respiration and the ghosts disappear completely (pseudogating). However, these techniques do not permit the free selection of TR, which is needed to optimize S/N and tissue contrast, and may be limited by variations in respiratory rate.

Signal Averaging

Rather than displace the ghosts, one can reduce their intensity by signal averaging. Unlike respiratory gating and phase-reordering techniques, signal averaging reduces the intensity of ghost artifacts arising from both respiration and pulsatile flow. Signal averaging does not improve motion-induced blurring. The signal intensity of ghost artifacts, like background noise, is reduced by the square root of the number of NEX. This technique has proved particularly effective in the chest and abdomen.[38] However, signal averaging causes a proportionate increase in acquisition time, rendering it impractical for T_2-weighted acquisitions because of the long TR. The technique of signal averaging can be made more effective by increasing the time interval between averages.[39] This technique of so-called serial averaging, that is, traversing all phase-encoding steps before averaging the data, reduces the likelihood that multiple averages will be acquired at the same point in the respiratory cycle. In other words, spreading out the averages improves the sampling of the respiratory

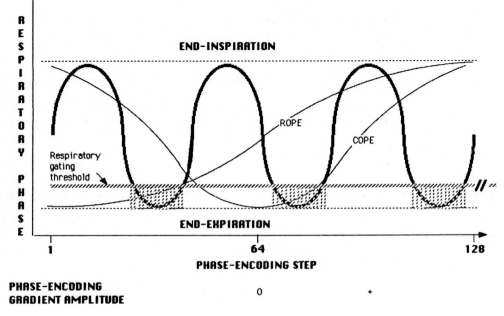

FIGURE 3–38. Methods for reducing respiratory ghost artifacts. Normally, phase-encoding steps are randomly associated with phases of the respiratory cycle (*thick solid line*). COPE and ROPE methods (*thin lines*) reorder the phase-encoding steps so as to reduce the effective periodicity of the respiratory cycle. Respiratory gating is more effective than ROPE or COPE but is inefficient because data are only acquired from a small portion of the respiratory cycle (*shaded areas*).

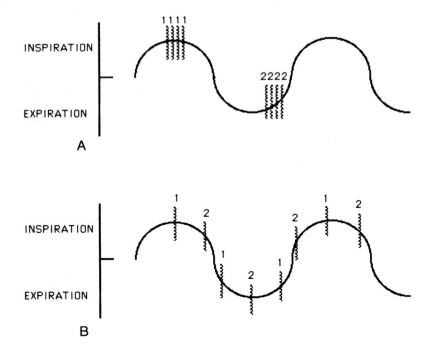

INSPIRATION

EXPIRATION

A

INSPIRATION

EXPIRATION

B

FIGURE 3–39. Signal averaging with short TR but without regard for the order of acquisitions is relatively inefficient (A), because the averaged measurements tend to be obtained in the same part of the respiratory cycle (parallel averaging). By increasing the interval between averaged measurements (serial averaging), a better sampling distribution of the respiratory cycle is obtained with concomitant reduction in ghost artifacts (B). However, this latter approach requires more data processing.

cycle (Fig. 3–39). This is not true for the more usual method of parallel averaging, in which two or more data measurements are averaged in one phase-encoded projection before proceeding to the next projection.

Reducing the Signal Intensity of the Moving Tissue

Still another approach to reducing the intensity of the ghosts is to reduce the intensity of the source tissue. For instance, T_1-weighted images of the spine demonstrate negligible CSF pulsation artifact due to the low intensity of CSF. For imaging of the abdomen, fat signal can be selectively eliminated by the application of lipid frequency-selective RF saturation pulses or by short time inversion recovery (STIR) sequences.[40] STIR sequences have been suggested to be useful for detecting liver masses at both low fields (0.15 T) and high fields (1.5 T). STIR sequences have the drawback of relatively low S/N. Another drawback for abdominal imaging is that, although ghost artifacts from subcutaneous fat are suppressed, ghost artifacts from liver masses and bowel loops are enhanced, since these tissues demonstrate high intensity on STIR images.

Restraining Body Motion

One can also reduce ghosting by splinting the motion of subcutaneous fat. Compression devices are moderately effective but are uncomfortable. In conjunction with surface coil imaging, it can be useful to position the patient so that moving tissue is dependent and restrained by the patient's weight. In order to restrain motion of subcutaneous fat in the near field of a surface coil, supine positioning would be preferred for imaging of the spine, whereas prone positioning would be preferred for the pancreas.

Gradient Reorientation

Ghost artifacts are only detrimental if they cross a region of interest. Since ghost artifacts propagate along the direction of phase-encoding, they can be reoriented away from the region of interest by rotating the phase-encoding axis (Fig. 3–40). However, wraparound along the phase-encoding direction limits the effectiveness of this technique unless oversampling or presaturation techniques are used.

Swapping the phase-encoding and frequency-encoding axes can also be useful for obtaining a better myelogram effect in the cervical and thoracic spine on T_2-weighted images. Normally, the frequency-encoding gradient is oriented along the long axis of the spine, which is also the direction of CSF flow. This results in large phase shifts, associated signal loss, and ghost artifacts which obscure the spinal cord, spondylitic changes, and disk herniations. By orienting the frequency-encoding gradient perpendicular to the direction of flow, signal loss is minimized. An additional benefit of this method is that artifacts arising from motion of subcutaneous fat in the anterior neck, which is prominent with Helmholtz and solenoidal surface coils, are directed off the spine. However, rotating the motion artifacts also rotates chemical shift artifact, which will now be parallel to the axis of the intervertebral disks. Small disk protrusions could be obscured by the chemical shift artifact.[41]

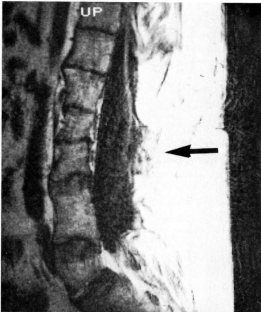

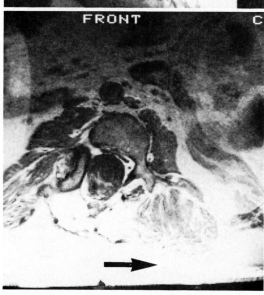

FIGURE 3–40. Reduction of motion artifact by gradient rotation (swapping). *Arrow* = direction of phase-encoding gradient. *Top,* Claustrophobic patient hyperventilated during study despite sedation, resulting in image degradation from ghost artifacts originating in anterior abdomen and posterior subcutaneous fat. *Bottom,* Axial image. Frequency- and phase-encoding axes have been swapped compared with normal orientation so that motion artifacts are kept off the spine. Note absence of artifact over the spine. With smaller FOV, wraparound would degrade image.

Motion Compensation Using Gradient Rephasing

Ghost artifacts are a reflection of phase shifts resulting from motion. This motion may occur between phase-encoding projections or views, as well as during the acquisition of each view. Gating techniques are directed toward elimination of artifacts resulting from motion between views, whereas mo-tion compensation techniques using refocusing gradients are directed toward reducing phase shifts resulting from within-view motion.

Within-view motion results in imperfect rephasing of spins at the echo time, causing signal loss and ghosting artifact. The use of additional gradient pulses within either a spin-echo or gradient-echo pulse sequence, as illustrated in Chapter 4, can be used to correct for phase shifts resulting from within-view motion, resulting in higher, more uniform, signal intensity and reduced ghost artifacts.[42] This effect is similar to that achieved by even-echo re-phasing in a multiecho sequence except that, com-pared with even-echo rephasing, gradient rephasing techniques are more consistently effective. Three gradient pulses can correct for constant velocity mo-tion, regardless of velocity. Four gradient pulses are needed to correct for acceleration and still more to correct for higher order effects such as jerk. Com-pensation may be performed along all three gradient axes but is most important for slice selection and frequency encoding. These methods are considered in greater depth in Chapter 4.

The major clinical application of motion compen-sation using gradient rephasing is the elimination of signal loss and ghost artifacts due to CSF pulsation in the spine (Fig. 3–41) and brain. It is also useful for abdominal imaging, particularly on T_2-weighted images, since the latter use long echo times. Long echo times allow for more within-view motion, mak-ing T_2-weighted images particularly susceptible to motion artifacts.

The use of gradient rephasing for motion compen-sation is not without drawbacks. Because of the stringent timing requirements for the gradient pulses, choice of echo time, FOV, slice thickness, and multiecho capability may be restricted. Finally, gra-dient rephasing does not eliminate ghost artifacts produced by variable flow-related enhancement due to saturation effects (see Chapter 4). These are more effectively suppressed by presaturation methods.

Presaturation

It is obvious that artifacts cannot arise from tissues unless they produce signal. Recently, methods have been developed that use presaturation to eliminate signal over a selected region without affecting other areas. Artifacts arising from tissues in the selected area can thereby be eliminated without affecting tissues in the region of interest.[30]

Presaturation is accomplished by use of special RF pulses inserted prior to the conventional pulse se-quence. An example of such a pulse sequence is given in Figure 3–33. A crafted RF pulse provides a highly rectangular slice profile even when very thick slices are used. Any gradient can be used for defini-tion of the presaturation volume in conjunction with the presaturation pulse, independent of the gradients used for the rest of the pulse sequence. As illustrated by Figure 3–33B and C, presaturation pulses can be

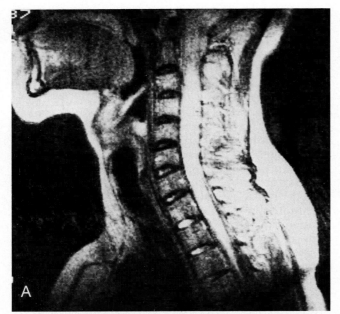

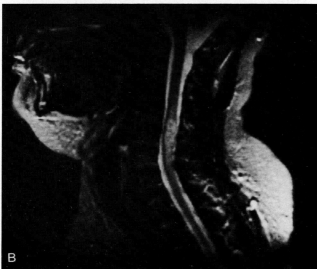

FIGURE 3–41. Sagittal T$_2$-weighted image without ECG gating (*A*) fails to demonstrate intramedullary mass, which is well seen with ECG gating (*B*).

used to eliminate two types of artifact: ghost artifact and wraparound artifact.

As demonstrated in Figure 3–33*D* and *E,* presaturation pulses can be applied along the phase-encoding axis to eliminate ghost artifacts due to swallowing, respiration, and vascular pulsation. This is routinely useful for spine imaging. Alternatively, two presaturation pulses or a single cosine-modulated pulse can be used to eliminate signal from tissues outside of the FOV, thus eliminating wraparound artifact along the phase-encoding axis (Fig. 3–33*F* and *G*). In addition to these two applications, presaturation along the slice-selection direction can be used to selectively eliminate signal from inflowing spins[43]

(Fig. 3–42). With this method, intraluminal flow signal and associated ghost artifacts are vastly reduced. By eliminating intraluminal flow signal, flow presaturation can help avoid confusion between flow-related enhancement and thrombus (see Chapter 4).

FLOW ARTIFACTS

The flow of blood and CSF can generate a variety of artifacts. (1) Flowing blood can demonstrate low or high intensity, depending on the balance of time-of-flight and phase-shift effects. (2) Pulsatile flow generates ghost artifacts that propagate along the phase-encoding axis. (3) Flow signal can be displaced outside of the vessel lumen along the direction of the frequency-encoding axis (Fig. 3–43). Flow signal and associated motion artifacts are most prominent on images acquired with short TE and gradient-echo images. Both cardiac triggering and gradient rephasing help to reduce flow-related ghost artifacts. Flow artifacts and ways to eliminate them are discussed in detail in Chapter 4. Three examples of flow artifacts mimicking anatomic lesions are shown in Figs. 3–44, 3–45, and 3–46.

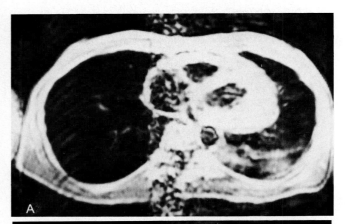

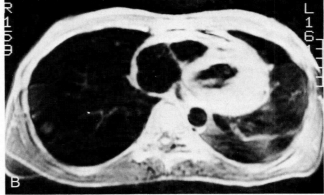

FIGURE 3–42. ECG-gated images with respiratory-ordered phase encoding. *A,* Without z-axis RF presaturation, ghosting from pulsatile blood flow is severe. *B,* With presaturation, the ghosting is markedly reduced.

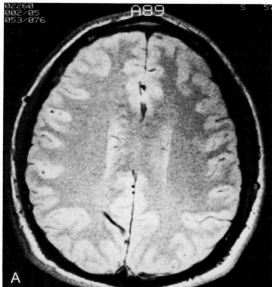

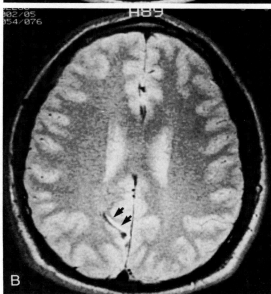

FIGURE 3–43. Flow artifacts. T_2-weighted multiecho study. Image *A* (TE = 20 msec) shows signal void in large feeding vessel to AVM. Image *B* (second echo, TE = 40 msec) demonstrates both even-echo flow rephasing of high signal intensity and artifactual signal shift of obliquely flowing spins (*arrows*) due to phase-encoding gradient spatial misregistration.

PULSE SEQUENCE–RELATED ARTIFACTS

A fourth category of MRI artifacts are pulse sequence–related, that is, they are only observed in studies utilizing specific techniques and timing of RF pulses and data acquisition. In general, these artifacts appear as nonanatomic signal voids, often at the interface between dissimilar tissues or structures. We call this phenomenon *spurious etching* and will review its various forms, causes, and solutions. The common

denominator for all causes of this artifact is its presence in magnitude-reconstructed images and elimination by phase-sensitive reconstruction.

INVERSION RECOVERY BOUNCE POINT

Let us briefly review what happens in an inversion recovery (IR) sequence. The first pulse inverts all of the signals in the slice and the recovery period TI begins. The faster relaxing spins lead the pack and at some point pass through zero on their way to regaining the full positive alignment. The slowest relaxing signals are still pointing in a negative direction. Any two tissues with different spin-lattice relaxation times, T_1, will be in such a state for a period between their respective zero-crossings. The read-out part of the sequence is now applied.

What happens to the image? If full attention is paid to the sign of the signals, the reconstruction will show the longer T_1 tissue as negative image intensity (Fig. 3–47*B*). If the signs are not calculated, as in some MRI systems, then all image intensities are taken to be positive. This will change the appearance of the would-be negative tissue dramatically and will reduce the original contrast. If one were unlucky, the tissue contrast could vanish because two tissues of interest were of opposite sign but equal strength. In the interface between two signals opposite in sign, the image abruptly shoots through zero, hence the dark rim.

This artifact, referred to as IR bounce point, results in an apparent loss of contrast in inversion recovery scans.[44] There is also a thin dark rim, one picture element in width, around some of the features (Fig.

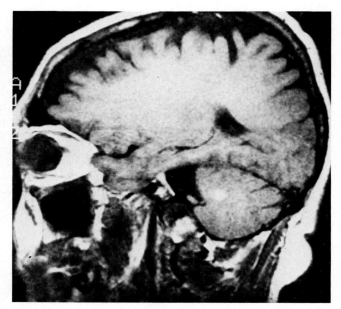

FIGURE 3–44. Left cerebellar "pseudohemorrhage." Mismapping of flow signal from the lateral dural sinus along the phase-encoding axis creates a focus of spurious intracerebellar high signal.

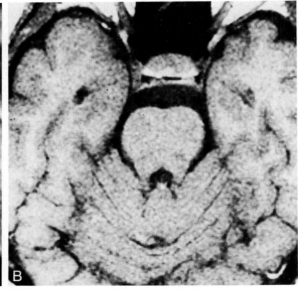

FIGURE 3–45. CSF flow artifact. T_2-weighted image through the basilar cisterns with an apparent mass adjacent to the basilar artery (*A*); the pseudomass disappears on the T_1-weighted image (*B*).

3–47*A*). This is an artifact that can best be described as a display error.

This artifact may simulate the lack of signal seen in calcification, air, or rapidly flowing blood. In the STIR sequence the TI is chosen at the null point (TI = 0.63 × T_1 of fat), taking advantage of the signal void for subcutaneous fat, which reduces the ghosting from body wall motion. The bounce point artifact may be eliminated through phase-sensitive reconstruction, in which image intensities comprise the entire dynamic range from negative to positive values.

CHEMICAL SHIFT ETCHING

Work in proton spectroscopic imaging by Dixon has led to clinically useful MR images of separate water- and fat-containing tissues.[45] The opposed, or out-of-phase, images are obtained with the magnetization vectors of fat and water, which precess at different frequencies due to chemical shift differences of 3 to 4 ppm, pointing in opposite directions. The net transverse magnetization in such an experiment therefore represents water minus fat magnetization, resulting in a minimum signal intensity. If a

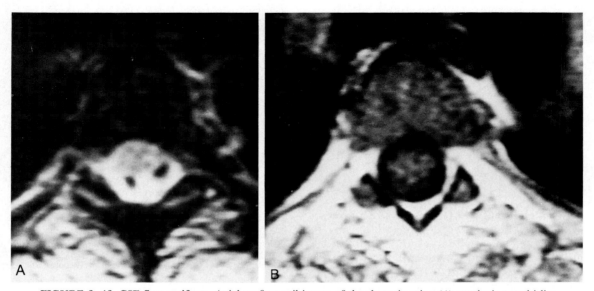

FIGURE 3–46. CSF flow artifacts. Axial surface coil image of the thoracic spine (*A*) employing multislice interleaved gradient echoes (300/15/15°) shows twin filling defects initially confused for a spinal arteriovenous malformation. *B*, Axial T_1-weighted image fails to confirm these findings; normal CT-myelogram.

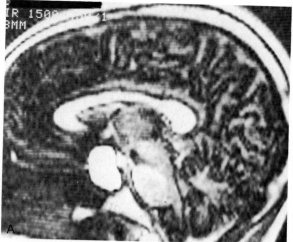

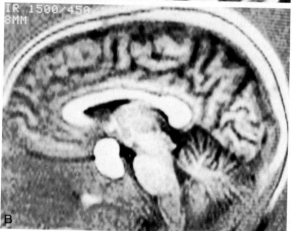

FIGURE 3–47. Inversion recovery bounce point artifact. *A,* Conventional magnitude reconstruction in a patient with a hemorrhagic pituitary adenoma demonstrates artifactual dark line highlighting gray matter–white matter boundary. *B,* Corresponding phase reconstruction demonstrates no artifact.

given voxel contains similar proportions of fat and water protons, the out-of-phase image will register a signal void in the corresponding pixel. This technique contrasts with the standard Hahn spin-echo experiment, in which the echo is obtained at the point where water and fat spins are aligned to produce maximum signal intensity. Clinically, the opposed phase artifact may be seen at any boundary where the voxels at the interface contain both fat and water. This artifact differs from a read-out axis chemical shift artifact by the absence of any orientation along the read-out axis. Swapping the phase and frequency axes has no effect on chemical shift–induced spurious etching.

A similar out-of-phase image may be obtained with gradient echoes. The timing of the TE determines whether the fat and water protons in a voxel of interest are in- or out-of-phase, yielding maximal or minimal spurious etching.[46]

MOTION-INTERFACE ETCHING (PHASE DISPERSION OR SHEAR ARTIFACT)

Spurious etching can also occur at the interface between moving and nonmoving tissues. At the boundary, a spectrum of velocities (and phase angles) can be produced in a single voxel. The distribution of phase angles leads to signal loss in magnitude-reconstructed images. This produces an artifactually "thicker" pericardium in gated cardiac images, as first pointed out by Moran.[47] This artifact can be reduced by using higher in-plane spatial resolution (e.g., 256 phase-encoding steps instead of 128). The presence or absence of the pericardial etching artifact can be used to clinical advantage in assessing the degree of malignant invasion of the pericardium by adjacent neoplasms.

CONCLUSION

MRI artifacts are commonly seen at all clinical imaging sites, and the more frequently encountered ones should be recognized by practitioners in order to avoid diagnostic errors and to maintain image quality. Some artifacts, such as aliasing and motion, are predictable and can be manipulated to reduce their degradation of the image in the anatomic region of interest. Others, for example, RF pulse inhomogeneity and gradient-induced eddy current artifacts, are more sporadic and difficult to diagnose, and correcting them will require field service engineers. The clinical impact of MRI artifacts is minimized by routine preventive maintenance, daily quality control checks, and heightened awareness on the part of the radiologist.

REFERENCES

1. Bellon EM, Haacke EM, Coleman PE, et al: MR artifacts: A review. J Radiol 147:1271–1281, 1986.
2. Henkelman RM, Bronskill MJ: Artifacts in magnetic resonance imaging. Rev Magn Reson Med. 2(1):1–126, 1987.
3. Porter BA, Hastrup W, Richardson ML, et al: Classification and investigation of artifacts in magnetic resonance imaging. Radiographics 7(2):271–287, 1987.
4. Partain CL, Price RR, Patton JA, et al (eds): Nuclear Magnetic Resonance Imaging. 2nd ed. Philadelphia, WB Saunders Company, 1988.
5. New PFJ, Rosen BR, Brady TJ, et al: Potential hazards and artifacts of ferromagnetic and non-ferromagnetic surgical and dental materials and devices in nuclear magnetic resonance imaging. Radiology 147:139–148, 1983.
6. Heindel W, Friedmann G, Bunke J, et al: Artifacts in MRI after surgical intervention. J Comput Assist Tomogr 10:596–599, 1986.
7. Teitelbaum GP, Bradley WG, Klein BD: MR imaging artifacts, ferromagnetism, and magnetic torque of intravascular filters, stents, and coils. Radiology 166:657–664, 1988.
8. Hinshaw DB, Holshouser BA, Engstrom HIM, et al: Dental material artifacts on MR images. Radiology 166:777–779, 1988.
9. Ludeke KM, Roschmann A, Tischler R: Susceptibility artifacts in NMR imaging. Magn Reson Imaging 3:329–343, 1985.

10. Axel L, Costantini J, Listerud J: Intensity correction in surface-coil MR imaging. AJR 148:418–420, 1987.
11. Conolly S, Nishimura D, Macovski A: Optimal control solutions to the magnetic resonance selective excitation problem. IEEE Transactions on Medical Imaging 5:106–115, 1986.
12. White EM, Edelman RR, Stark DD, et al: Surface coil MR imaging of abdominal viscera. Part II. The adrenal glands. Radiology 157:431–436, 1985.
13. Feinberg DA, Hoenninger JC, Crooks LE, et al: Inner volume MR imaging: Technical concepts and their application. Radiology 156:743–747, 1985.
14. Bodenhausen G, Freeman R, Turner D: Suppression of artifacts in 2D J-spectroscopy. J Magn Reson 27:511–514, 1977.
15. Kramer DM, Murdoch JB: Artifact minimization in multislice multiecho MR imaging. Society of Magnetic Resonance in Medicine, 1986, pp 1436–1437 (abstract).
16. Graumann R, Oppelt A, Stetter E: Multiple spin-echo imaging with a 2-D method. Magn Reson Med 3:707–721, 1986.
17. Tycko R, Cho HM, Schneider E, Pines A: Composite pulses without phase distortion. J Magn Reson 6:90–101, 1985.
18. Yan H, Gore JC: Improved selective 180 degree radiofrequency pulses for magnetization inversion and phase reversal. J Magn Reson 71:116–131, 1987.
19. Murdoch JB, Lent AH, Kritzer MR: Computer-optimized narrowband pulses for multislice imaging: Asymmetric amplitude-modulated 180 degree pulses. Society of Magnetic Resonance in Medicine, 1986, pp 1432–1433 (abstract).
20. O'Donnell M, Adams WJ: Selective time-reversal pulses for MR imaging. Magn Reson Imaging 3:377–382, 1985.
21. Lurie DJ: A systematic design procedure for selective pulses in NMR imaging. Magn Reson Imaging 3:235–243, 1985.
22. Silver MS, Joseph RI, Hoult DI: Highly selective 90 and 180 degree pulse generation. J Magn Reson 59:347–351, 1984.
23. Duijn JH, Creyghton JHN, Smidt J: Suppression of artefacts due to imperfect pi pulses in multiple echo Fourier imaging. Society of Magnetic Resonance in Medicine, 1984, pp 197–198 (abstract).
24. Crawley AP, Henkelman RM: A stimulated echo artifact from slice interference in MRI. Med Phys 14:842–848, 1987.
25. Harris FJ: On the use of windows for harmonic analysis with the discrete Fourier transform. Proc IEEE 66:51–83, 1978.
26. Haacke EM: The effects of finite sampling in magnetic resonance imaging. Magn Reson Med 4:407–421, 1987.
27. Soila KP, Viamonte M, Starewicz PM: Chemical shift misregistration effect in MRI. Radiology 153:819–820, 1984.
28. Kurihara N, Kamo O, Umeda M, et al: Applications in one dimensional and two dimensional NMR of a pseudofilter by jittered time averaging. J Magn Reson 65:405–416, 1985.
29. Axel L, Doughterty L: Reduction of aliasing in 2-D FT MRI by pseudofiltering. Magn Reson Imaging 5:63, 1987 (abstract).
30. Edelman RR, Atkinson DJ, Silver MS: FRODO pulses: A new method for elimination of motion, flow, and wraparound artifact. Radiology 166:231–236, 1988.
31. Roemer PB, Edelstein WA, Hickey JS: Self shielded gradient coils. Society of Magnetic Resonance in Medicine, 1986, pp 1067–1068 (abstract).
32. Edelman RR, Hahn P, Buxton R, et al: Rapid magnetic resonance imaging with suspended respiration: Clinical application in the liver. Radiology 161:125–131, 1986.
33. Runge VM, Clanton JA, Partain CL, James AE: Respiratory gating in magnetic resonance imaging at 0.5 Tesla. Radiology 151:521–523, 1984.
34. Ehman RL, McNamara MT, Pallack M, et al: Magnetic resonance imaging with respiratory gating: Techniques and applications. AJR 143:1175–1182, 1984.
35. Lanzer P, Botvinick EH, Schiller NB, et al: Cardiac imaging using gated magnetic resonance. Radiology 150:121–127, 1984.
36. Bailes DR, Gildendale DJ, Bydder GM, et al: Respiratory ordered phase encoding (ROPE): A method for reducing respiratory motion artifacts in MR imaging. J Comput Assist Tomogr 9:835–838, 1985.
37. Axel L, Summers RM, Kressel HY, Charles C: Respiratory effects in two-dimensional Fourier transform imaging. Radiology 160:795–801, 1986.
38. Stark DD, Wittenberg J, Edelman RR, et al: Detection of hepatic metastases by MRI: Analysis of pulse sequence performance. Radiology 159:365–370, 1986.
39. Dixon WT, Brummer ME, Malko JA: Acquisition order and motional artifact reduction in spin warp images. Magn Reson Med 6:74–83, 1988.
40. Bydder GM, Steiner E, Blumgart LH, et al: MR imaging of the liver using short T_1 inversion recovery sequences. J Comput Assist Tomogr 9(6):1084–1089, 1985.
41. Enzmann DR, Griffin C, Rubin JB: Potential false-negative MR images of the thoracic spine in disk disease with switching of phase- and frequency-encoding gradients. Radiology 165:635–637, 1987.
42. Haacke EM, Lenz GW: Improving MR image quality in the presence of motion by using rephasing gradients. AJR 148:1251–1258, 1987.
43. Felmlee JP, Ehman RL: Spatial presaturation: A method for suppressing flow artifacts and improving depiction of vascular anatomy in MR imaging. Radiology 164:559–564, 1987.
44. Hearshen DO, Ellis JH, Carson PL, et al: Boundary effects from opposed magnetization artifacts in IR images. Radiology 160:543–547, 1986.
45. Dixon WT: Simple proton spectroscopic imaging. Radiology 153:189–194, 1984.
46. Wehrli FW, Perkins TG, Shimakawa A, Roberts F: Chemical shift-induced amplitude modulations in images obtained with gradient refocusing. Magn Reson Imaging 5:157–158, 1987.
47. Moran PR, Moran RA: Imaging true motion velocity and higher order motion quantities by phase gradient modulation techniques in NMR scanners. In Esser PD, Johnston RE (eds): Technology of Nuclear Magnetic Resonance. Society of Nuclear Medicine, 1984, pp 149–163.

4

FLOW

ROBERT R. EDELMAN, JEREMY B. RUBIN, and RICHARD B. BUXTON

A—Basic Flow Concepts

TISSUE CHARACTERISTICS OF BLOOD

HEMODYNAMICS

DRIVING FORCE FOR FLOW

EFFECT OF VESSEL DIAMETER ON FLOW VELOCITY

FLOW PROFILES

BASIS OF FLOW EFFECTS

SATURATION

Flow-Related Enhancement
Wash-out Effects

PHASE

BLACK BLOOD

PRESATURATION

PHASE DISPERSION

BRIGHT BLOOD

ENTRANCE SLICE PHENOMENON

PSEUDOGATING

EVEN-ECHO REPHASING

FLOW COMPENSATION/GRADIENT MOTION REPHASING

GRADIENT-ECHO IMAGING

Flow Enhancement
Fast Imaging of Flow

COINCIDENTAL PHASE CANCELLATION (THE "DISAPPEARING" BLOOD VESSEL)

BLOOD IN WRONG LOCATION

DISPLACEMENT ARTIFACT

GHOST ARTIFACTS

MR PSEUDOANEURYSM

DIFFERENTIATION OF INTRAVASCULAR SIGNAL FROM THROMBUS

SIGNAL CHARACTERISTICS OF THROMBUS

PLANE OF SECTION

PRESATURATION

PHASE IMAGING

PULSE SEQUENCE

INTRAVASCULAR DEVICES

B—Advanced Flow Concepts

NATURE OF CEREBROSPINAL FLUID FLOW

MR MYELOGRAM

SOURCES OF ARTIFACTS

SOLUTIONS

Gradient Rotation
Cardiac Gating
Even-Echo Rephasing or Flow Compensation
Gradient-Echo Pulse Sequences

CSF FLOW EFFECTS AND CYSTIC LESIONS IN THE SPINE

MR VENOGRAPHY

MR ANGIOGRAPHY

LIMITATIONS OF CONVENTIONAL TOMOGRAPHIC METHODS

GEOMETRY

Three-dimensional (Volume) Angiography
Maximum Intensity Projection
Sequential 2D Arteriography and Venography
Projection Acquisition
One-dimensional

DISPLAY METHODS

CONTRAST AGENTS

CLINICAL POTENTIAL OF MR ANGIOGRAPHY

Peripheral Vascular Imaging
MR Angiography in the Body
Intracranial and Extracranial Cerebrovascular Disease
Coronary Artery Imaging

MEASUREMENT OF FLOW

SATURATION METHODS

PHASE SHIFT METHODS

Phase Mapping
Zebra Stripes
Flow-Encoding Gradients

DIFFUSION

A—Basic Flow Concepts

Magnetic resonance is a powerful tool for the noninvasive study of flow.[1-5] Computed tomography and conventional angiography require exogenous, potentially hazardous, iodinated contrast media to opacify blood vessels. Furthermore, these imaging modalities are not well suited for flow measurement. Compared with these invasive methods, MR has a significant advantage in that flowing blood has unique characteristics on an MR image; flow is an intrinsic, physiologic contrast medium for MR. Compared with noninvasive modalities such as Doppler ultrasound, MR also has advantages in terms of field-of-view (FOV) and tissue characterization. However, the appearance of flowing blood is complicated by the numerous parameters on which it depends. In addition to the usual dependence on tissue characteristics and on imaging techniques, the signal produced by flowing blood depends on the velocity and direction of flow, flow profile (e.g., parabolic versus plug), plane of section, gradient strength, as well as other factors. Although we tend to think of the "flow void" as the classic manifestation of flow on MR images, flowing blood can have a variety of appearances and produces troublesome artifacts. In addition to blood flow, the motion of cerebrospinal fluid (CSF), which is not detectable by CT, provides useful diagnostic information but also creates artifacts. In addition to bulk flow MR, unlike CT and angiography, is sensitive to the motion of water at the capillary and molecular level, which provides yet another potentially useful parameter of tissue structure and function.

In this chapter, we will first consider the tissue characteristics of blood and the dynamics of blood flow, review the effects of flow on proton saturation and phase (Table 4–1), and illustrate how flow alters the appearance of blood vessels in the context of clinical imaging. Practical approaches for differentiating flow signal from thrombus (Table 4–2) and

TABLE 4–1. SUMMARY OF FLOW EFFECTS

Saturation Effects
- Flow enhancement due to inflow of unsaturated spins
- Flow void due to wash-out of excited spins
- Flow void due to RF presaturation

Spatial Phase Effects
- Flow void due to phase dispersion
- Donut sign due to boundary layer phase dispersion
- Flow enhancement due to EER or flow compensation
- Disappearing blood vessel due to coincidental cancellation of phase effects

Miscellaneous
- Displacement artifact due to time delay between RF excitation and spatial encoding of position
- Pseudoaneurysm due to signal loss produced by transmission of vessel pulsations to surrounding tissues
- Ghost artifacts due to time-dependent variations in signal intensity, produced by pulsatile or turbulent flow

TABLE 4–2. METHODS FOR DIFFERENTIATING FLOW SIGNAL FROM THROMBUS AND FOR ELIMINATING FLOW-RELATED ARTIFACTS

- Flow signal is reduced or eliminated by presaturation; thrombus is unaffected
- Flow signal is particularly intense on fast GRE images, e.g., FLASH with TR/TE/α = 30/10/30° (especially if plane of section is orthogonal to direction of flow), whereas thrombus has moderate or low signal intensity
- Flow signal should have different intensities with different planes of section (e.g., axial/sagittal); thrombus should appear identical
- Comparing T_2- and T_1-weighted images, flow enhancement is less marked on T_2-weighted (i.e., long TE) images; thrombus often has intermediate or bright signal on both T_1- and T_2-weighted images
- For flow perpendicular to plane of section, flow signal should be more intense on entrance slice, whereas signal intensity of thrombus should not vary from slice to slice
- Flow signal may produce ghost artifacts; thrombus does not
- Flowing blood, unlike thrombus, demonstrates a positive or negative phase shift on a phase map and appears brighter or darker than stationary background

for eliminating flow-related artifacts (Table 4–3) will be presented. We will then explore the newer territories of the MR myelogram, the MR arteriogram and venogram, and flow quantification and will consider the principles of perfusion and diffusion imaging.

TISSUE CHARACTERISTICS OF BLOOD

Blood is a complex tissue, with multiple components that have different relaxation properties. Whole blood is 80 per cent water by weight.[6] It has a cellular fraction, approximately 40 to 50 per cent in normal subjects, and a noncellular plasma containing a variety of proteins, organic molecules, and electrolytes. The T_1 relaxation time of whole blood depends on several factors, including field strength, hematocrit, pH, temperature, and storage conditions.[7, 8] Relaxation studies of whole unclotted blood suggest a long T_1 (whole blood = 782 msec, plasma = 1201 msec, serum = 1345 msec at 0.25 T) and a

TABLE 4–3. METHODS FOR ELIMINATING FLOW-RELATED ARTIFACTS

- Use flow compensation and/or cardiac gating to eliminate ghost artifacts from CSF flow crossing brain stem, temporal lobes, and spine on T_2-weighted SE images
- Use GRE (e.g., FISP/GRASS) techniques to obtain myelogram effect in cervical and thoracic spine
- Use RF presaturation techniques to eliminate flow signal and associated ghosting
- Use increased numbers of signal excitations; ghost artifacts are reduced in intensity in proportion to $\sqrt{NEX}$

long T_2.[9] The T_1 relaxation rate of plasma has also been found to depend, in part, on the content of iron bound to one of the major serum proteins, transferrin.[10] Various pathologic states, such as anemia and polycythemia, will alter the cellular and noncellular components and may produce changes in the relaxation times of blood.

The intensity (I) of each *stationary* tissue in an MR image is determined by tissue parameters and operator-determined imaging parameters. This relationship can be expressed as:

$$I = f(PS, TR, TE, T_1, T_2, N(H), \chi, \sigma) \qquad (1)$$

where PS = type of pulse sequence; N(H) = proton density; χ = magnetic susceptibility, which is unimportant to the study of flowing blood but becomes a significant factor for thrombosis; and σ = chemical shift. Based on the relaxation parameters of blood, one would expect blood to appear dark on T_1-weighted images and bright on T_2-weighted images. However, aside from vascular stasis or very slow flow, flow effects preclude seeing these signal characteristics in vivo.

HEMODYNAMICS

In order to understand flow effects on MR images, one must first understand the nature of blood flow. The study of hemodynamics is complex and beyond the scope of this chapter; however, we will consider some of the basic principles.[11-13] A number of factors affect the velocity and profile of blood flow. There are several different types of flow which need to be considered separately. These include: (1) flow through large arteries and veins, (2) flow at the capillary level (perfusion), and (3) molecular level (diffusion) (Fig. 4–1). Perfusion and diffusion, because of their more complex nature, will be addressed at the conclusion of this chapter.

DRIVING FORCE FOR FLOW

Flow (F) represents the quantity of a liquid flowing through a cross-section of a vessel per unit time. As an electrical current is driven by a difference in

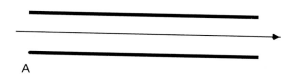

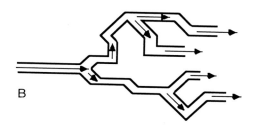

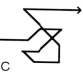

FIGURE 4–1. Flow can be categorized into three subtypes. *A,* Unidirectional bulk flow occurs in medium and large vessels. This is the type of flow most commonly observed in MR images. *B,* Perfusion occurs at the capillary level. Although there is a net direction of flow, within a given voxel the direction of flow is nearly random. *C,* Diffusion represents the random motion of molecules, with no net direction of flow. Perfusion and diffusion require special imaging methods to be observable by MR.

voltage, flow is driven by a difference in pressure (ΔP). For an ideal fluid flowing at a constant rate through a uniform vessel, this relationship can be expressed as:

$$F = \pi R^4 (\Delta P) / 8 \eta L \qquad (2)$$

where η = viscosity, R = vessel radius, and L = vessel length. This pressure difference is generated by the pumping action of the heart and the elasticity of major vessels. In general, the velocity of blood flow is maximal in large diameter vessels, such as the thoracic aorta, and is less in branch vessels, such as the femoral arteries, although flow velocities are very rapid in certain branch vessels supplying low resistance organs such as the brain (e.g., internal carotid arteries) (Tables 4–4 and 4–5).

TABLE 4–4. NORMAL HEMODYNAMIC VALUES FOR 70-KG MAN

Vessel	Velocity (cm/sec)	Reynolds No.	Alpha
Ascending aorta	18 (112/0)	1500	21
Abdominal aorta	14 (75/0)	640	12
Renal artery	40 (73/26)	700	4
Femoral artery	12 (52/2)	200	4
Femoral vein	4	104	7
Superior vena cava	9 (23/0)	550	15
Inferior vena cava	21 (46/0)	1400	17
Main pulmonary artery	19 (96/0)	1600	20
Main pulmonary vein	19 (38/10)	800	10

Velocities are mean values, with systolic/diastolic values in parentheses. Alpha values relate to pulsation frequency and vessel diameter; large alpha suggests plug flow, small alpha suggests laminar flow.
From Milnor WR: Hemodynamics. Baltimore, Williams and Wilkins, 1982.

TABLE 4–5. MEAN MAXIMAL VELOCITIES OF CEREBRAL ARTERIES

Artery	Mean Maximal Velocity (V_m) +/− SD *cm/sec*	Mean Side Difference *cm/sec*	SD of the Side Differences
Common carotid	29.7 +/− 8.0	2.6	3.8
Internal carotid	36.3 +/− 8.6	4.2	5.1
Vertebral	29.2 +/− 9.2	5.0	6.3
Middle cerebral	57.3 +/− 14.8	5.9	8.0
Anterior cerebral	49.2 +/− 15.1	12.0	17.2
Posterior cerebral	37.2 +/− 10.4	5.8	6.3
Basilar	systolic = 58*/60† diastolic = 26*/34†		

*Patients older than 50 years
†Patients younger than 50 years
Adapted from refs. 71–73.

Although flow is the critical parameter in terms of providing essential nutrients to living tissues, in MR it is the direction and rate of flow, that is, the flow *velocity,* which is germane to imaging the vascular system.

In medium to large arteries such as the aorta, there is both a forward and reverse component of flow (again, in arteries supplying low resistance organs, such as brain and thyroid, the flow is forward throughout the cardiac cycle). Whereas the forward component is generated by the pumping action of the heart, the reverse component is generated by the reflection of pulse pressure waves at distal vessel bifurcations, predominantly at the arteriolar level. These reflected waves produce a distinct reversal of flow during diastole. This flow reversal occurs first near the wall of the vessel, where blood flows most slowly and has the least forward momentum (Fig. 4–2A). Flow reversal is minimal or absent in small arteries and also in larger arteries distal to tight stenoses.

EFFECT OF VESSEL DIAMETER ON FLOW VELOCITY

The flow past a point is the product of average velocity and cross-sectional area. Bernoulli's principle states that flow at any two points in a tube must be the same. This can be expressed as:

$$v_1 A_1 = v_2 A_2 \text{ or } v_1 = v_2 (R_2/R_1)^2$$

where v = average velocity, A = area, and R = vessel radius. In other words, velocity is a function of 1/(diameter)². For instance, in a carotid artery that has a twofold reduction in diameter (i.e., 75 per cent stenotic), velocity of blood flow through the stenosis is increased *fourfold.*

FLOW PROFILES

Assuming that blood behaves as a simple fluid and flow is constant, the velocity profile will be *laminar* (Fig. 4–2B). The laminar profile is caused by frictional forces among blood components and between blood and the walls of the vessel which slow the flow of blood; this "boundary layer" effect is maximal toward the wall of the vessel and decreases toward the center. For fully developed laminar flow, the velocity profile is parabolic, and the velocity at any point within the vessel can be expressed as:

$$v = 2v_{av} (1 - r^2/R^2) \qquad (3)$$

where r = radial distance from the central axis of the vessel to the point, R = vessel radius, and v_{av} = average velocity, which for parabolic flow is equal to one half v_{max}.

In fact, blood does not behave like a simple fluid, and arteries do not behave like inflexible tubes. As a result, some interesting hemodynamic phenomena can be observed in vivo.

1. Blood behaves as a non-Newtonian fluid, that is, viscosity is not independent of velocity. At low velocities, the viscosity of blood increases markedly; with blood stasis, thrombus may begin to form. Viscosity also increases with hematocrit. Furthermore, blood does not behave in vivo as a single component fluid; the distribution of blood components within the vessel is not uniform but depends on velocity. Blood demonstrates a phenomenon known as *skimming;* the forward momentum of bulky components, such as red blood cells, keeps them toward the central axis of the vessel, so that toward the periphery of the vessel the blood is plasma-rich and cell-poor. The skimming phenomenon is further enhanced in vessel branches that arise at right angles to the lumen.

2. Laminar flow is typically seen in small arteries and veins. However, several factors, relating to vascular pulsation and to the size and shape of major arteries, tend to produce a plug, rather than laminar, flow profile (Fig. 4–2C). In plug flow, velocities are uniform across the vessel diameter, in contrast to the parabolic profile, which is characteristic of fully developed laminar flow.

Plug flow is most pronounced in large diameter vessels, such as the ascending aorta, where boundary layer effects are minimal. A plug flow profile is further enhanced when fluid from a large diameter tube enters a smaller diameter tube, as occurs when blood flows from the left ventricle into the aorta (Fig.

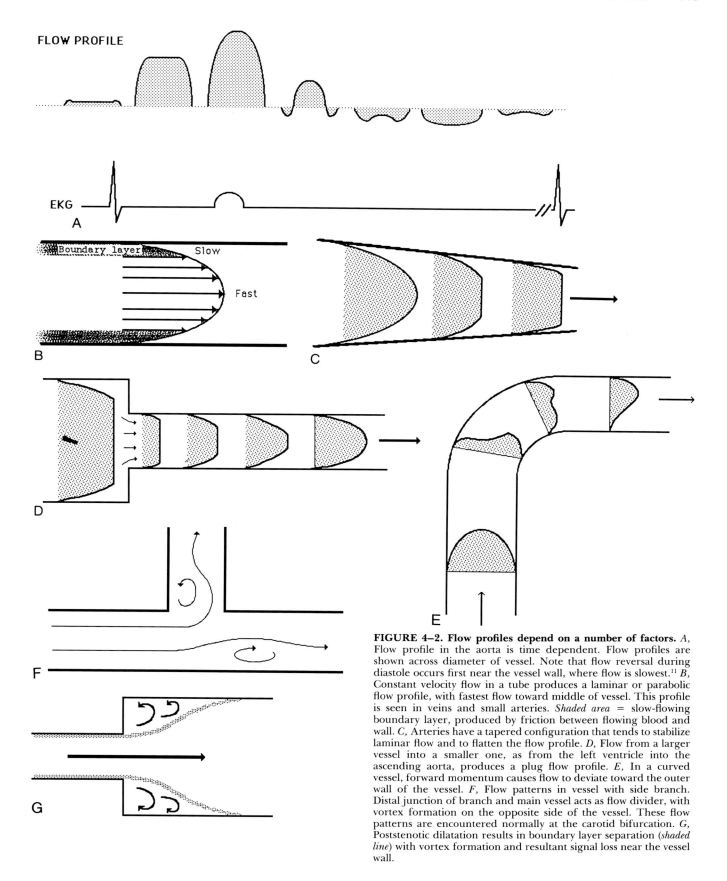

FLOW PROFILE

EKG

FIGURE 4–2. Flow profiles depend on a number of factors. *A,* Flow profile in the aorta is time dependent. Flow profiles are shown across diameter of vessel. Note that flow reversal during diastole occurs first near the vessel wall, where flow is slowest.[11] *B,* Constant velocity flow in a tube produces a laminar or parabolic flow profile, with fastest flow toward middle of vessel. This profile is seen in veins and small arteries. *Shaded area* = slow-flowing boundary layer, produced by friction between flowing blood and wall. *C,* Arteries have a tapered configuration that tends to stabilize laminar flow and to flatten the flow profile. *D,* Flow from a larger vessel into a smaller one, as from the left ventricle into the ascending aorta, produces a plug flow profile. *E,* In a curved vessel, forward momentum causes flow to deviate toward the outer wall of the vessel. *F,* Flow patterns in vessel with side branch. Distal junction of branch and main vessel acts as flow divider, with vortex formation on the opposite side of the vessel. These flow patterns are encountered normally at the carotid bifurcation. *G,* Poststenotic dilatation results in boundary layer separation (*shaded line*) with vortex formation and resultant signal loss near the vessel wall.

4–2D). The tendency to a plug flow profile also depends on the frequency and amplitude of pulsation; rapid, large amplitude pulsation predisposes to plug flow, whereas relatively constant flow predisposes to a parabolic profile.

Flow patterns are altered at curves and at branch points. At curves such as the aortic arch, the highest velocity flow is tilted toward the outer wall (Fig. 4–2E). Flow is also disturbed in proximity to the orifice of a branch (Fig. 4–2F). Secondary flow patterns develop, and retrograde flow may occur along the wall opposite the branch. A typical example of normal retrograde flow is seen in the carotid bulb; this flow pattern can be demonstrated on color Doppler ultrasound studies.

3. The flow profile depends on a number of tissue characteristics: density, viscosity, the radius of the vessel, and average flow velocity. These factors can be lumped together into a unitless number called the Reynolds number (Re), where

$$Re = (\text{density} \times \text{velocity} \times \text{vessel diameter})/\text{viscosity}$$

The Reynolds number determines the velocity threshold at which laminar flow ceases and is replaced by turbulence. For a simple fluid, the laminar profile breaks down when the Reynolds number exceeds 2000 to 2300.

However, unlike a simple fluid, in vivo laminar flow can persist even when the Reynolds number exceeds the critical limit. One reason for this is that arterial flow is pulsatile; fluctuations in flow caused by pulsation interfere with the propagation of minor flow disturbances into turbulence.

Turbulence becomes an important factor with respect to imaging of vascular stenoses. As mentioned previously, velocity increases markedly as the vessel diameter is decreased; in severe stenoses, velocities may exceed several meters per second. Distal to the stenosis, boundary layer separation, caused by the sudden widening of the vessel lumen, results in vortex formation with retrograde flow near the vessel wall progressing to chaotic, turbulent flow as the stenosis worsens (Fig. 4–2G). Signal loss due to turbulence distal to the stenosis produces artifacts on MR images obtained with conventional and angiographic techniques. For instance, on MR angiograms, a vessel may appear artifactually narrowed or even falsely occluded immediately distal to the actual stenosis. These effects have important clinical implications for the study of vascular pathology, such as aortic dissection and carotid stenosis.[14]

ELECTROMAGNETIC EFFECTS OF FLOW

One additional effect relates to the electromagnetic, rather than mechanical, properties of blood flow. According to Faraday's law of induction, the flow of a conductor such as blood across magnetic flux lines induces an electrical current proportional

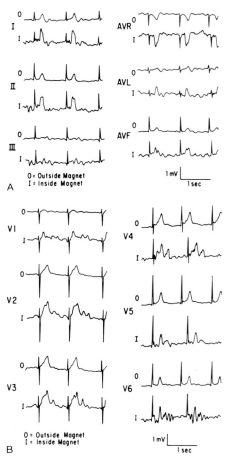

FIGURE 4–3. Twelve-lead ECG tracing in normal volunteer; tracings obtained outside (O) and inside (I) 1.5 tesla magnet. Magnetic field induces peaking of T wave as well as smaller (7 to 10 Hz) voltage potential throughout cardiac cycle. (From Dimick RN, Hedlund LW, Herfkens RJ, et al: Optimizing electrocardiograph electrode placement for cardiac-gated MRI. Invest Radiol 22:17–22, 1987.)

to the velocity of flow and magnetic field strength. At high field strengths a voltage of several millivolts may be induced, depending on the direction of flow with respect to the magnetic field.[15]

Induced voltages cause the appearance of a patient's electrocardiogram (ECG) to change from its normal baseline when the patient is placed within the magnet. One example is peaking of the T wave (Fig. 4–3). However, this effect does not alter the appearance of the MR image. In addition, the induced voltage is too small to represent a significant hazard to the patient. At high field strengths, the alteration in the ECG signal may result in improper cardiac triggering; the large T wave can be mistaken for an R wave, so that triggering occurs twice in some cardiac cycles.

BASIS OF FLOW EFFECTS

Vascular signal depends on *saturation* and *phase* effects. Saturation, or "time-of-flight," effects are produced by changes in longitudinal magnetization, which are a function of applied *radiofrequency* (RF) pulses and T_1 relaxation. Phase effects are produced by changes in transverse magnetization, which are a function of *gradient* pulses and T_2 relaxation (see Chapter 1). Depending on saturation and phase effects, blood can appear bright or dark.

SATURATION

Flow-Related Enhancement

The first observations of flow by MR were made in 1951 by Suryan.[16] He noted that flowing liquid produced a considerably greater MR signal than stationary liquid. This effect, which is now familiar to us as flow-related enhancement (FRE) or paradoxical enhancement, can be explained on the basis of changes in proton saturation. *The key concept for understanding flow-related enhancement is that fresh, unsaturated blood flowing into the imaging volume produces higher signal than stationary tissues within the imaging volume.*

Saturation represents the degree to which the longitudinal magnetization (M) of a collection of protons is reduced from M_0, its maximum value. Before the imaging process begins, all protons, stationary and flowing, are unsaturated, that is, $M = M_0$. During the imaging process, tissue protons are excited by repeated RF pulses, resulting in saturation of these spins. The degree of saturation is important because unsaturated protons produce a large signal, whereas saturated spins produce a smaller signal, which is reduced in proportion to the degree of saturation. For stationary protons within the imaging volume, the degree of saturation during the imaging process depends on a balance of repetition time (TR) and T_1, as expressed by $M = M_0 (1-e^{-TR/T1})$. If TR is long relative to T_1, then the longitudinal magnetization is large, that is, the protons are unsaturated. As TR is shortened, the degree of saturation increases.

If slice-selective RF pulses are used, as is typical, then spins outside the imaging volume escape excitation and remain unsaturated. In the case of blood flow, when fresh spins flow into the imaging volume and are initially excited, they produce a large signal (Fig. 4–4). Although these spins are saturated quickly after entering the imaging volume, they are continually replaced by the inflow of fresh, unsaturated spins. As a result, flowing blood may appear relatively brighter than other tissues, even though the T_1 relaxation time of blood is long. This effect is referred to as flow-related enhancement, since flow produces vascular enhancement similar to that produced by administering an intravenous contrast agent in a conventional angiogram.

Note that FRE is most pronounced for *single slice* imaging, so that blood flows out of the imaging volume immediately after excitation. Flow-related enhancement is less pronounced for multislice im-

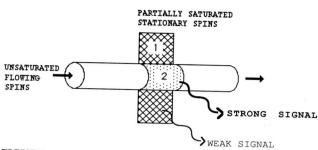

FIGURE 4–4. Explanation of flow-related enhancement. Unsaturated spins flowing into vessel produce a strong signal when first exposed to an RF pulse within the slice (2). These spins are constantly replaced by fresh inflowing spins. In contrast, stationary spins within the slice (1) are partially saturated and produce less signal.

aging and for flow oriented within the plane of section, since blood remains for a longer period of time within the imaging volume. Prolonged transit of blood within the imaging volume increases the likelihood of the blood being exposed to multiple excitations, producing saturation of the spins and reduced signal.

Wash-out Effects

Whereas flow of unsaturated protons into a slice produces increased vascular signal, wash-out effects produce signal loss. The severity of wash-out effects depends on the type of pulse sequence. In a spin-echo (SE) pulse sequence, wash-out effects produce signal loss because protons must be exposed to both the 90-degree and 180-degree RF pulses in order to produce a measurable signal (Fig. 4–5). These RF pulses are separated in time by TE/2. For instance, if echo time (TE) = 30 msec, then the protons would have to remain within the slice for at least 15 msec in order to be exposed to both RF pulses.

For fast flow, a fraction of the protons may move out of the slice during the interval TE/2 and will not produce a measurable signal, resulting in a signal void. For imaging of fast flow using slice-selective SE pulse sequences, we can express the relationship among signal intensity (SI), slice thickness (d), and flow velocity as:

$$SI \sim 1 - (TE/2 * v_p * 1/d) \qquad (4)$$

where v_p = velocity of flow perpendicular to the plane of section.[4, 23] There is, therefore, always a balance between inflow and wash-out effects (Fig. 4–6). As indicated by Equation 4, wash-out effects are reduced and vascular signal is enhanced by increasing the slice thickness, shortening the TE, or using diastolic gating to minimize flow velocity. On the other hand, in certain applications it is useful to maximize wash-out effects in order to make blood appear dark. *With SE pulse sequences, the combination of flow presaturation and very thin (e.g., 2 to 3 mm) slices is an effective method for maximizing the flow void. We*

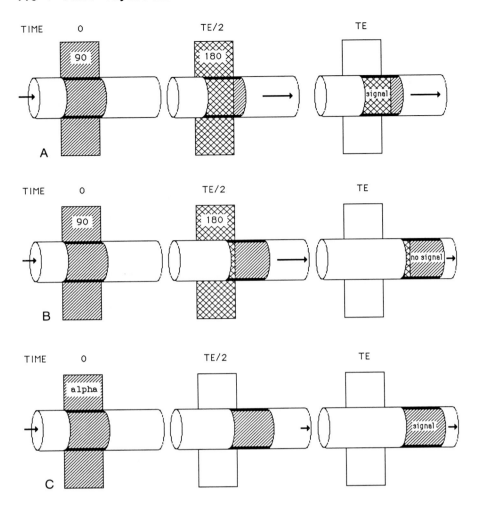

FIGURE 4–5. Wash-out effects in SE and GRE pulse sequences. Direction of blood flow is from left to right. *A,* With slow flow, wash-out effects are minimal. *B,* With fast flow, protons may flow out of the slice before their signal is refocused by the 180-degree pulse. These spins produce no signal. *C,* GRE pulse sequences use a single RF pulse. Since RF refocusing is not used, wash-out of spins from the slice has almost no effect on signal intensity.

call such images, which are designed to make flowing blood appear dark, *black blood images.* Methods for producing them are discussed below.

The wash-out effect can also be minimized for an SE pulse sequence by using a nonselective 180-degree RF pulse, though this limits the acquisition to a single slice. A nonselective 180-degree RF pulse will refocus the MR signal whether the proton is in or out of the slice; however, flow enhancement is actually reduced because, by saturating *all* spins nonselectively, one eliminates inflow effects. The wash-out effect can be minimized without affecting inflow by using gradient-

echo (GRE) pulse sequences (Fig. 4–5*C*), which will be discussed later.

PHASE

Phase shift effects are of primary importance in determining the MR appearance of flow.[17, 18] Phase effects occur whenever there is motion through field gradients. This includes patient motion, bulk flow through a vessel, or the random diffusional motion of water molecules. The nature of these effects was

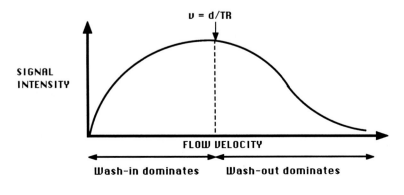

FIGURE 4–6. For SE pulse sequences, the intensity of flow signal depends on a balance of flow enhancement due to inflow of unsaturated protons and signal loss due to wash-out. Maximum signal intensity is obtained when flow velocity (v) is equal to the ratio of slice thickness (d) and TR.

described by Carr and Purcell in 1954 soon after the discovery of nuclear magnetic resonance, but new ways of exploiting these effects are still being developed.

There are two major categories of phase shift effects: (1) spatial effects, due to variations in phase among protons in different radial positions within the blood vessel lumen; and (2) temporal effects, due to time-dependent variations in phase. Spatial phase effects are responsible for several phenomena, including (1) phase dispersion at boundary layers, which decreases signal; and (2) even-echo rephasing (EER), which increases signal. Temporal effects, associated with pulsatile and turbulent flow, produce variations in signal intensity which are responsible for troublesome ghost artifacts. Before trying to understand these effects it is worthwhile to review for a moment the nature of the MR signal and the role of phase.

The MR signal is described by three parameters: magnitude, frequency, and phase. The phase relates to where the peaks and troughs in the MR signal occur relative to a reference signal (see Chapter 1). Two protons can produce signals that have identical magnitude and frequency but nonetheless differ in phase. In vector notation, this phase difference is represented by the *angle* between the two vectors in the x-y plane.

In reality, one is never dealing with just one or two spins, but rather with many trillions of spins. Thus, in discussing flow-related phase effects, a useful concept is the *isochromat*. An isochromat represents a group of spins within a voxel which have identical phase behavior. The signal produced by a voxel is determined by the relative phases of the isochromats within that voxel, which can be significantly altered by the effects of flow. In the discussions that follow, the terms spin and isochromat will be used interchangeably, although it should be understood that it is always the behavior of a large group of protons which is being described.

If all the spins have the same phase, then their signals add together (Fig. 4–7A). However, if the spins have different phase shifts, then destructive interference reduces the measured signal (Fig. 4–7B). This is called phase dispersion. The signal from a voxel decreases as the amount of phase dispersion increases. When the spread in phase equals or exceeds 360 degrees, then all the signal is lost. (One essential point to understand here is that the signals from spins in one voxel are *not* affected by the signals from spins in other voxels, that is, spins must be in the same voxel for a difference in their phases to result in signal loss. However, by enlarging or reducing the voxel, one can include or exclude phase interactions with these other spins and thereby exacerbate or minimize the effects of phase dispersion on flow signal. For instance, in three-dimensional (3D) MR angiography a reduced voxel size is used to minimize phase dispersion and maximize vascular signal.)

Any source of magnetic field inhomogeneity will

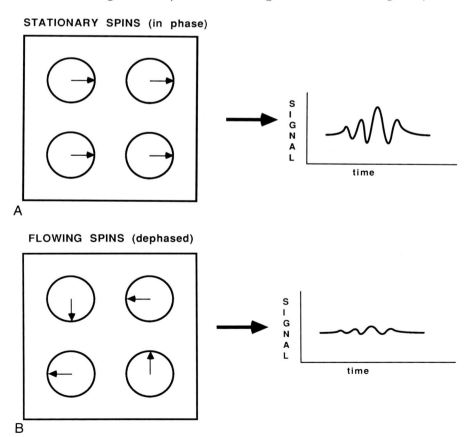

STATIONARY SPINS (in phase)

FLOWING SPINS (dephased)

FIGURE 4–7. Effect of intravoxel phase coherence on signal intensity. *A,* Stationary spins have the same phase, so their signals add together. *B,* Flow across a magnetic field gradient produces phase dispersion. When the spread in phases within a voxel exceeds 360 degrees (2π), the measured signal is nearly zero because of destructive interference.

produce phase dispersion and therefore loss of signal. One may not be accustomed to thinking in these terms, but the linear field gradients used for imaging represent potent magnetic field inhomogeneities. Although essential for imaging, *these gradients also produce phase shifts and are responsible for the phase-related flow effects we observe in MR imaging.*

These flow effects are generally predictable. The amount of flow-related phase shift depends on several factors: gradient strength, duration of gradient pulses, and time between gradient pulses. In order to understand why this is so, consider a simple GRE pulse sequence in which two identical gradient pulses of G and −G are activated, each for a time t. The time between the centers of the two gradient pulses is T (Fig. 4–8A and *B*). Assume that the field is uniform before the gradient is activated, so that all spins are initially in phase. When the first gradient pulse is activated, each *stationary* spin accumulates a phase shift (Θ) as a function of position, expressed as:

$$\Theta = \gamma\, G\, x\, t \tag{5a}$$

where γ = gyromagnetic ratio, G = gradient amplitude, t = gradient duration, and x = position of the spin along the axis of the gradient. Spins in different positions accumulate a difference in phase expressed as a positive phase angle for positive x. The second gradient pulse also causes spins in different positions to accumulate a phase difference, but one that is opposite in sign. For stationary spins, this *negative* phase difference is equal in magnitude to the *positive* phase difference produced by the first gradient pulse. Consequently, at the end of the second gradient pulse, the effects on phase of the first and second gradient pulses cancel, so that net phase shift of stationary spins due to the gradients is *zero* (Fig. 4–8C).

However, if the spins have *moved* during the interval between the gradient pulses, then the phase shifts produced by the first and second gradient pulses are not equal; consequently, a moving spin accumulates a nonzero phase shift (Fig. 4–8C). A spin moving

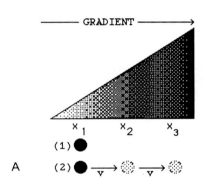

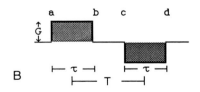

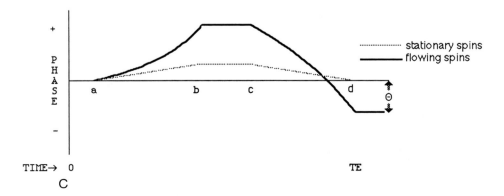

FIGURE 4–8. Effect of flow on proton phase. *A*, Stationary spins (1) experience a constant gradient through the imaging experiment. However, moving spins (2) experience different gradient strengths at different positions (x_1–x_3). *B*, Simplified GRE pulse sequence. The sequence uses two gradient pulses: a compensatory (dephasing) gradient pulse and an imaging (rephasing) gradient pulse. For stationary spins, the compensatory gradient produces a phase shift of opposite sign but of equal magnitude to that produced by the imaging gradient, so that no residual phase shifts are present at the center of the echo (TE). *C*, The phase shifts produced by the compensatory and imaging gradients are unequal for flowing spins due to the inconstant gradient strength experienced by the moving spins. Flowing spins therefore accumulate a nonzero phase shift (Θ) at TE.

with velocity v will move, relative to a stationary spin, a distance x = vT over the time between the gradient pulses. The moving spin will accumulate a phase shift expressed as:

$$\Theta = \gamma \, G \, v \, \tau \, T \qquad (5b)$$

For spins moving at different velocities, we see from Equation 5b that the phase difference will be proportional to the velocity difference. If these spins are located in the same voxel, then this phase dispersion produces signal loss. The signal loss worsens with increased gradient strength, flow velocity, duration of gradient, and time delay between gradient pulses. Note that in the worst case (i.e., gradients on for whole duration of pulse sequence), the phase shift is proportional to the *square* of the TE. The implication is that vascular signal is markedly reduced as TE is lengthened (e.g., for T_2-weighted images).

However, for multiecho pulse sequences, this flow-related phase dispersion can, under certain circumstances, be eliminated. When the identical set of gradient pulses used to produce the first echo is repeated for the second echo, these gradients produce another phase shift in the moving blood equal to the phase shift produced by the first set. However, the second 180-degree pulse flips the sign of the first phase shift, so that the phase shifts produced by the two sets of gradients cancel at the time of the second echo. This phenomenon is called even-echo rephasing, and is discussed further on.

BLACK BLOOD

In addition to wash-out effects, several phenomena can produce low vascular signal.

PRESATURATION

Increased vascular signal produced by FRE may make it impossible to differentiate patent vessels from thrombi or nonvascular structures such as lymph nodes. In addition, ghost artifacts increase with signal intensity and are therefore worse on entrance sections, where FRE is most pronounced.

Fortunately, there are effective methods available on most commercial MRI systems with which one can reduce or eliminate these flow artifacts. Flow-related enhancement and associated flow artifacts result from inflow of *unsaturated* spins. Therefore, saturation of these inflowing spins, prior to excitation and signal acquisition, can be used to suppress these artifacts. This method, called *presaturation*, requires the use of supplementary RF pulses (see Chapters 3 and 10).

Tissue magnetization can be presaturated over large volumes using additional RF pulses that are prefixed to the beginning of any SE or GRE pulse sequence; examples of such techniques are FRODO

(*f*low and *r*espiratory artifact *o*bliteration using *di*rected *o*rthogonal pulses) and FLAK (*f*low *a*rtifact *k*iller).[19, 20] Typically, a 90-degree flip angle provides maximal saturation of inflowing spins, although in certain circumstances smaller or larger flip angles may be more effective.

In order to eliminate the transverse magnetization produced by the presaturation RF pulse, a spoiler gradient is applied immediately afterward to dephase the excited spins. As a result, presaturation pulses, unlike the RF pulses used in the body of the pulse sequence, produce no signal. Immediately after application of the presaturation RF and spoiler pulses, the longitudinal magnetization of the presaturated tissues is zero. Therefore, these tissues produce little or no signal when excited by the RF pulses in the body of the pulse sequence.

The presaturation volume(s) are spatially displaced from the imaging volume in order to affect inflowing spins but not the region of interest. In order to avoid spillover of saturation into the imaging volume, optimized RF pulses have been used which provide highly rectangular slice profiles even with short (e.g., 2.5 msec) pulse duration. Arterial and venous inflow can be presaturated using two RF pulses positioned above and below the imaging volume (Fig. 4–9A). Alternatively, two locations can be saturated simultaneously by using a cosine modulation of the RF waveform, at the expense of increased power deposition. Although the direction of flow presaturation is usually perpendicular to the slice-selection direction, presaturation within the plane of section can sometimes be useful. For instance, on a long axis view of the aorta, presaturation of the arch along a direction perpendicular to the frequency-encoding axis can be used to suppress signal in the descending aorta.

By eliminating the signal from flowing blood, presaturation is almost completely effective for suppressing flow-related ghost artifacts (Fig. 4–9B–D) and, for this purpose, is a more effective technique than flow compensation (discussed further on). However, the effectiveness of presaturation for reduction of flow artifacts is limited by several factors, including the rate and direction of flow, the T_1 relaxation rate of blood, and the TR.

Although presaturation consistently eliminates FRE and ghosting in the entrance slice, once inside the imaging volume, blood is unaffected by additional presaturation pulses (since these are positioned outside the imaging volume) and remagnetizes at a rate determined by its T_1 relaxation time. Because of this, if flowing spins remain within the imaging volume for a sufficiently long time, they can recover a significant portion of their longitudinal magnetization and produce signal in the inner slices. This problem is exacerbated for slow flow velocities (e.g., veins); however, even presaturated arteries may show signal in the inner slices. This can be attributed to slow flow during diastole. Despite this potential problem, in clinical practice presaturation is usually quite effec-

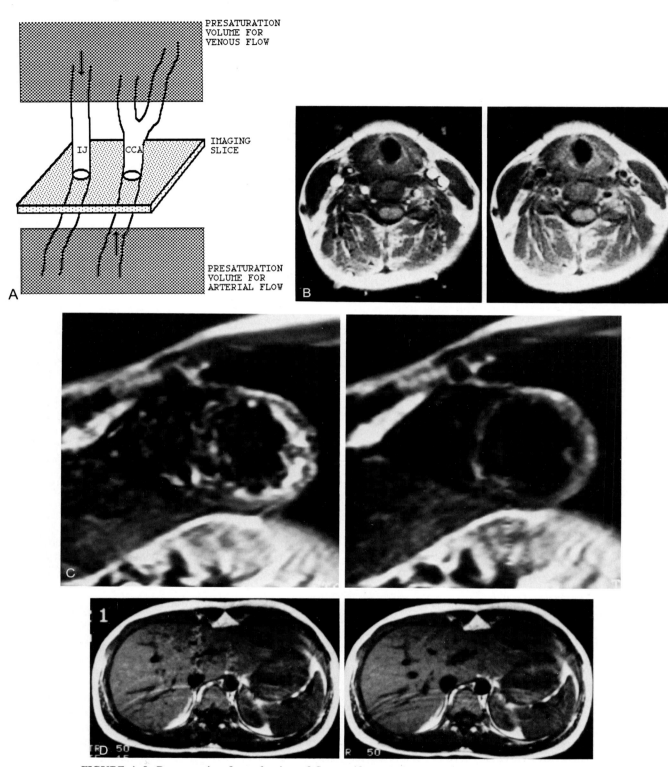

FIGURE 4–9. Presaturation for reduction of flow artifacts. *A,* Presaturation (*dark stippling*) above and below the plane of section can be used to eliminate signal from inflowing spins, illustrated for the carotid artery and jugular vein. *B,* Axial T_1-weighted SE image of neck. *Left,* Without presaturation, there are ghost artifacts, as well as prominent vascular signal, which could mimic thrombus. *Right,* Presaturation eliminates the artifacts. *C,* Short axis T_2-weighted spin-echo images of heart. *Left,* Without presaturation, there is increased signal adjoining the endocardium of the left ventricle, representing flow-related enhancement. This signal may be mistaken for a subendocardial infarction. *Right,* Presaturation eliminates the pseudoinfarct. *D,* Axial T_1-weighted images of abdomen. Ghost artifacts from pulsatile flow in the IVC and aorta obscure left lobe of liver (*top*). With flow presaturation (*bottom*), ghost artifacts are eliminated.

tive. This is because the flowing spins, after entering the imaging volume, are exposed to repeated RF excitations during the multislice imaging process, which further maintain the level of flow saturation independent of the presaturation pulses.

However, there are some circumstances that are unfavorable for flow presaturation. For instance, administration of gadolinium-DTPA reduces the effectiveness of presaturation by shortening the T_1 relaxation time of blood. The effectiveness of flow presaturation is also reduced for spins flowing for long distances within the imaging volume (e.g., on sagittal images of the aorta, axial images of the left ventricle). This limitation can be troublesome when trying to suppress vascular signal in the heart or in imaging aortic aneurysms with slow flow. An additional problem in applying presaturation to the heart is the number of pathways for the inflow of blood: superior and inferior vena cana, pulmonary and coronary veins. For full effect, presaturation may

have to be applied over all these structures, requiring presaturation in all three dimensions.

Using presaturation results in a reduction in multislice capability. The time required to apply the presaturation pulse and spoiler gradient is typically on the order of 5 to 10 msec, which reduces the minimum TR/slice by a corresponding amount of time. Furthermore, power deposition is significantly increased, which becomes a limiting factor on high field systems. Nonetheless, presaturation has proved routinely useful for improving image quality in the head and body. Presaturation may also be used for suppression of motion artifact due to respiration and wraparound artifact (see Chapter 3).

PHASE DISPERSION

Frictional forces between flowing blood and the vessel wall produce a gradient in velocities, or "shear"

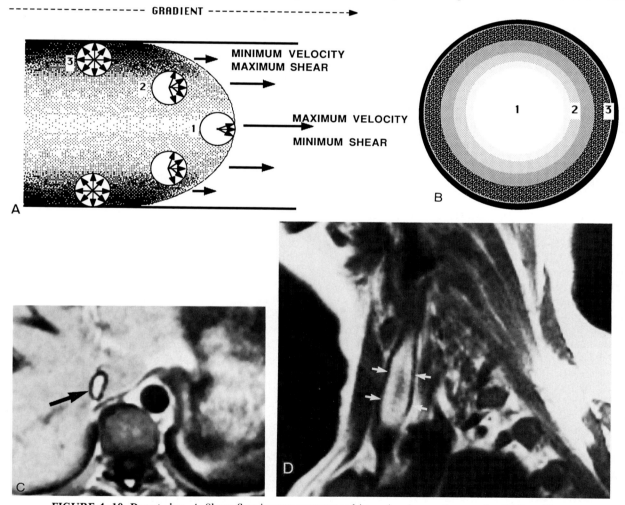

FIGURE 4–10. Donut sign. *A,* Shear flow is most pronounced in region 3 near the vessel wall. Signal loss due to phase dispersion is most pronounced in this region despite slower flow. Signal is greater in region 1 despite faster flow since shear is minimal. *B,* Vessel shown in cross-section shows marked signal loss peripherally in region 3, with higher signal centrally in regions 1 and 2. *C,* Axial image of abdomen shows central high signal in the IVC with peripheral low intensity "donut" sign, representing slow flow rather than vessel wall. *D,* Thrombosis of internal jugular vein due to indwelling catheter. Peripheral low intensity (*arrows*), which could mimic donut sign in patent vessel, represents residual flow around the thrombus.

flow. The velocity gradient within each voxel produces phase dispersion and resultant signal loss, which is most pronounced near the vessel wall (Fig. 4–10A); this distribution of signal loss appears in cross-section as a characteristic "donut" sign (Fig. 4–10B–C).

In addition to phase dispersion, the donut sign represents, in part, a saturation effect. Slower flow in the boundary layer produces less FRE and therefore, lower signal, than faster flow toward the center of the vessel.

The donut sign should not be mistaken for abnormal thickening of the vessel wall or for atherosclerotic plaque. Signal loss due to phase dispersion can be minimized by using short TE, flow compensation, or lower spatial resolution (i.e., weaker gradients). Signal loss due to phase dispersion in the slice-selection direction is minimized by using 3D methods (below). Rarely, thrombosis may mimic the flow-related donut sign because of residual flow near the vessel wall (Fig. 4–10D).

In cardiac imaging, one commonly sees an artifact produced by pericardial motion which is closely related to the phase dispersion effects described above. The artifact is a relatively thick anterior "pericardial" line, sometimes 2 mm or thicker, at the junction between heart and chest wall. This line actually represents artifactual signal loss due to phase dispersion which is produced by the shearing motion of fluid between the more mobile visceral and less mobile parietal pericardium. This artifactual thickening should not be mistaken for pericardial disease.

BRIGHT BLOOD

ENTRANCE SLICE PHENOMENON

Flow-related enhancement due to inflow of unsaturated spins is most pronounced in the entrance slice. Because the direction of flow is opposite in arteries and veins, the entrance slices are on opposite ends of the imaging volume (Fig. 4–11). For instance, on abdominal images the aorta appears brightest in the most cephalad section, and the inferior vena cava appears bright in the most caudal section (Fig. 4–12). Signal intensity is reduced in the inner slices, but the signal intensity in this region depends on a number of factors, including flow velocity, rate of RF pulsing, and order in which the slices are excited (Fig. 4–13). For instance, it is not uncommon for arterial flow to be so fast that some of the flowing spins escape excitation in the first few sections to produce vascular enhancement in the inner slices.

PSEUDOGATING

Because of the pulsatile nature of blood flow in large arteries and veins, these vessels often demonstrate flow patterns that, at first glance, appear to violate the principles we have just set forth. For

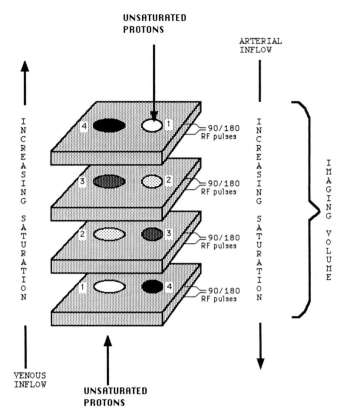

FIGURE 4–11. Entrance slice phenomenon. Unsaturated spins flowing into the entrance slice appear bright. As blood flows through the imaging volume, the likelihood increases that the spins will have been previously saturated by an RF pulse. As a result, vascular signal decreases within the inner slices.

instance, one would expect that the dominant pattern for slow flow is FRE, whereas the dominant pattern for fast flow is the flow void, due to the combination of phase dispersion and wash-out. As an example, consider the aorta. During systole the velocity of blood flow in the aorta approaches 100 cm/second. By Equation 4, an image acquired with a 30-msec TE and 1.5-cm slice thickness will suffer from wash-out effects to the extent that signal intensity is proportional to:

$$[1 - (30 \text{ msec}/2) \times 100 \text{ cm/sec.} \times (1/1.5 \text{ cm})] = 0$$

that is, there should be no signal within the aorta. Yet, we commonly observe high signal in the aorta and other large vessels.

Equation 4 assumes constant velocity flow, whereas arterial flow is pulsatile. Since the TR is independent from, and usually not equal to, the patient's R-R interval, data are acquired randomly throughout the cardiac cycle (Fig. 4–14). Sometimes a particular projection is acquired during systole, when blood is moving rapidly. However, during diastolic acquisitions, blood is moving very slowly, if at all. Random coincidence of data acquisition to slower diastolic flow, called *diastolic pseudogating*, may produce high vascular signal even if peak systolic velocities are

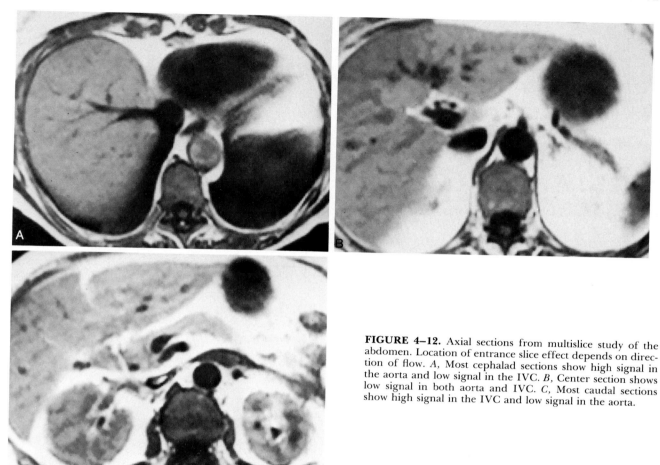

FIGURE 4–12. Axial sections from multislice study of the abdomen. Location of entrance slice effect depends on direction of flow. *A,* Most cephalad sections show high signal in the aorta and low signal in the IVC. *B,* Center section shows low signal in both aorta and IVC. *C,* Most caudal sections show high signal in the IVC and low signal in the aorta.

high. Similarly, random coincidence of data acquisition to fast systolic flow will produce low vascular signal. Therefore, unless data acquisition is limited to one phase of the cardiac cycle by some technique such as ECG gating, arteries may appear bright or dark unpredictably.

In addition, as flow varies over the cardiac cycle, so does vascular signal. This temporal variation in signal intensity is manifested as ghost artifacts (see below).

Sometimes, pseudogating can be deliberately implemented in order to reduce ghost artifacts from

FIGURE 4–13. Illustration showing how flowing spins can escape saturation in the entrance slices. Figure represents flow of a bolus of blood through a vessel, imaged with a three slice acquisition. (*Dark stippling* = saturated blood; *light stippling* = unsaturated blood). *A,* With slow flow, the transit time of the bolus through each slice is relatively long compared with the time between successive excitations of that slice (i.e., TR). These spins are likely to be saturated in slice 1 and produce low signal in subsequent slices (2 and 3). *B,* With rapid flow the transit time is short, and there is a significant likelihood that the flowing spins will pass through slice 1 while data from the other slices are being acquired. These spins may therefore escape excitation in slice 1 and produce high signal in slices 2 or 3. Increasing the repetition time and gap between slices makes this phenomenon more likely.

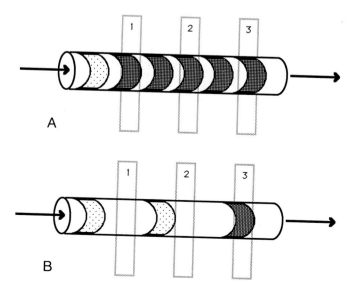

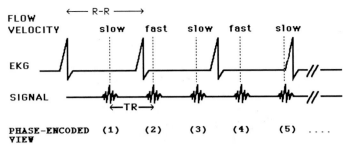

FIGURE 4–14. Pseudogating. Without ECG or pulse gating, data acquisition is independent of the cardiac cycle. As a result, some data are acquired during systole when flow is rapid (views 2, 4), while other data are acquired during diastole when flow is slow (views 1, 3, 5). This random variation in intravascular signal produces ghost artifacts as well as unexpectedly bright signal in arteries.

pulsatile flow. This is accomplished by estimating the R-R interval and setting the TR equal to this value or to a multiple of it. However, with this approach, choice of TR with respect to modifying tissue contrast is obviously limited.

EVEN-ECHO REPHASING

T_2-weighted images are usually acquired using multiple echoes. Compared with the first echo, nearly all tissues show reduced signal intensity on the second echo image, because the longer TE permits more signal loss due to T_2 decay. The only exception is provided by the phenomenon of even-echo rephasing (EER).[21, 22] For the special case of blood flowing at constant velocity; phase dispersion is reduced on the even (e.g., second, fourth) echoes as compared with the odd (e.g., first, third) echoes, resulting in an *absolute* increase in flow signal (Fig. 4–15). Even-echo rephasing is most commonly seen with slow, constant velocity (e.g., venous) flow.

Even-echo rephasing provides one way of differentiating flow from thrombus, since thrombus, like any other stationary tissue, loses signal as TE is increased (Fig. 4–16). However, visual impressions can be misleading, since tissues with long T_2 relaxation times appear *relatively* brighter at the longer TE because other tissues have lost more signal. Therefore, pixel intensities should be quantitated to confirm that EER has really occurred. Alternatively T_2 maps can be generated; on these calculated images, areas of EER are distinguished by a negative T_2 value, a consequence of the absolute increase in signal intensity at the longer TE.[23]

In clinical practice, one finds that real pulse sequences never show complete EER. There are a number of reasons for this: (1) arterial blood does not flow at constant velocity and phase dispersion caused by acceleration and turbulence does not cancel on even echoes; (2) EER does not alter signal loss associated with wash-out of protons from the slice, which is exacerbated by the longer TE of the second echo image; and (3) EER only occurs for gradients

that are symmetric about the 180-degree RF pulse, which is seldom the case in real pulse sequences. A related finding is that images acquired from the second echo of an asymmetric echo train (e.g., TE_1/TE_2 = 20 msec/80 msec) often produce greater flow-related phase shifts than symmetric echoes (e.g.,

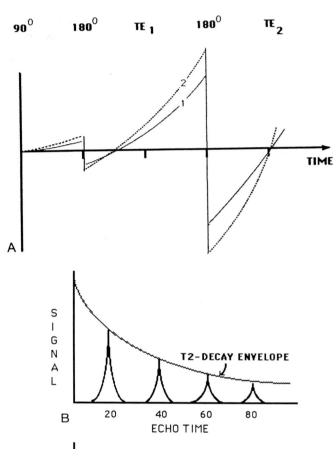

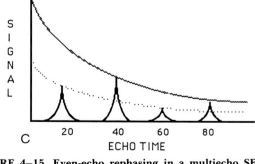

FIGURE 4–15. Even-echo rephasing in a multiecho SE pulse sequence. *A,* During acquisition of the first echo, groups of spins flowing at different velocities (1, 2) within the same voxel accumulate different, nonzero phase shifts at TE_1, resulting in signal loss. If flow velocity is constant and wash-out effects can be ignored, then the phase shifts for both groups are identically zero at TE_2, so that intravascular signal increases. *B,* Signal from stationary spins decreases monotonically due to T_2 decay. *C,* Behavior of flowing spins is more complex, depending on whether the image is acquired with an odd- or even-numbered echo. On odd echoes, signal (*stippled line*) is lost from flow-related phase dispersion as well as T_2 relaxation. On even echoes, signal may be larger because phase dispersion is eliminated.

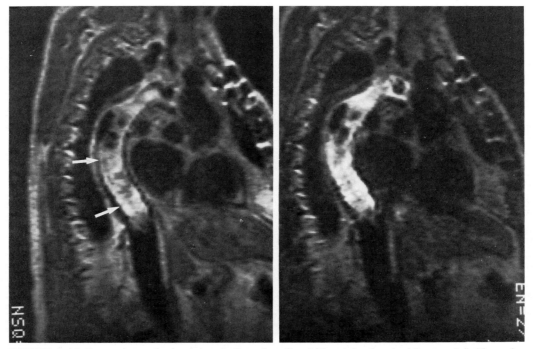

FIGURE 4–16. Even-echo rephasing in aortic dissection. Gated T_2-weighted sagittal images. *Left,* First echo image. Signal intensity in aortic lumen (*arrows*) measures 110. *Right,* Second echo image. Signal intensity measures 130, an absolute increase from first echo. This must represent flow rather than thrombus. (Courtesy R. Felder, M.D.)

TE_1/TE_2 = 30 msec/60 msec), resulting in worse ghost artifacts. However, this depends to a great extent on the particular pulse sequence design, since it is the timing of the gradient pulses, rather than the echo time per se, that determines flow-related phase shifts.

FLOW COMPENSATION/GRADIENT MOTION REPHASING

Even-echo rephasing is an unreliable method for reducing flow artifacts. Much more reliable enhancement of vascular signal and elimination of flow artifacts are accomplished by a method called flow compensation or gradient motion rephasing (GMR).

As just discussed, the magnetic field gradients in a standard SE or GRE pulse sequence induce a flow-related phase shift (Θ_{flow}). Flow compensation uses extra gradient pulses, inserted into the body of the pulse sequence, to produce an opposite flow-related phase shift (Θ_{GMR}). If the timing and amplitudes of the rephasing gradients are properly calibrated (see Chapter 10), so that

$$\Theta_{GMR} = -\Theta_{flow} \qquad (6)$$

then flow-related phase shifts and associated signal loss are eliminated (Fig. 4–17).[24–26] Stationary spins, on the other hand, are unaffected by this pulse sequence modification.

Standard pulse sequences require a minimum of

FIGURE 4–17. Gradient-echo pulse sequence without (*A*) and with (*B*) flow compensation along slice-selection direction. With flow compensation, phase shift (Θ) is zero for both stationary and flowing spins. The integral of the areas under the gradient pulses (*shaded*) must be zero for stationary spins to rephase completely at the echo time.

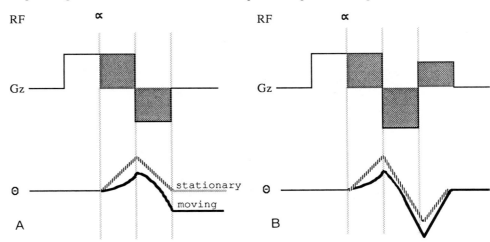

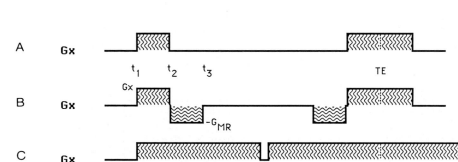

FIGURE 4–18. Diagram of frequency-encoding gradient for various SE pulse sequences. *A*, Conventional sequence without flow compensation. *B*, Sequence (*A*) modified with flow compensation. A pair of extra gradient pulses (*horizontal stippling*) of amplitude ($-G_{MR}$) compensates for residual flow-related phase shifts produced by the compensatory and imaging gradients. *C*, Dephasing sequence for maximizing signal loss.

two gradient pulses (dephase, rephase) (see Chapters 1 and 10). With flow compensation, three gradient pulses are adequate to eliminate phase shifts from constant velocity flow; a minimum of four gradient pulses are needed to compensate for acceleration, and still more gradient pulses are needed to compensate for higher order effects such as jerk and turbulence. In some applications, these additional gradient pulses can be used to increase, rather than decrease, flow-related phase dispersion (Fig. 4–18). These dephasing methods can be useful for MR angiography or can be used in conjunction with presaturation to minimize vascular signal in black blood methods.

The effect achieved by flow compensation is no different from that achieved by EER but is more reliable. Flow compensation reduces ghost artifacts and improves enhancement of intravascular signal in GRE images (Fig. 4–19). By reducing the effects of CSF pulsation, flow compensation is particularly useful for spine imaging in order to improve the mye-

logram effect obtained with T$_2$-weighted SE and GRE images (Fig. 4–20). The improved vascular enhancement obtained with flow compensation is also routinely useful for MR cineangiography, because it improves delineation of the myocardium from the blood pool.

Most commercial systems use first-order (velocity) compensation only. In general, velocity-compensated GMR will produce a satisfactory myelogram effect on T$_2$-weighted SE and GRE images of the spine. With rapid pulsatile flow, as exists in arteries, it might be thought that the combination of velocity and acceleration compensation would be more effective than velocity compensation alone. However, the issue is complicated by the fact that the additional gradient pulses required for acceleration compensation prolong the minimum echo time, which by itself worsens flow-related phase shifts and tends to defeat the purpose of the flow compensation. Because of this, it is easier and usually more effective to implement

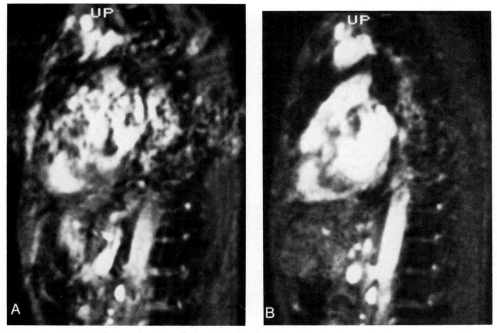

FIGURE 4–19. Sagittal GRE images of chest obtained without (*A*) and with (*B*) flow compensation. Note that flow compensation increases intravascular signal and reduces ghost artifacts.

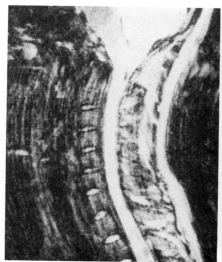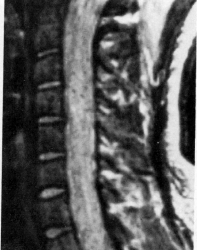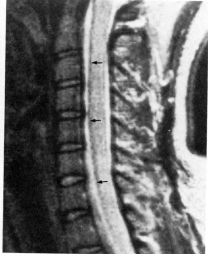

FIGURE 4–20. Effect of flow compensation on T$_2$-weighted sagittal images of cervical spine. *Left,* Without flow compensation, there are extensive ghost artifacts due to CSF pulsation. *Middle,* With improperly calibrated flow compensation, interface between CSF and spinal cord is obscured. *Right,* With properly calibrated flow compensation, CSF interfaces are sharp and ghost artifacts are mostly eliminated. Dark band along anterior surface of cord represents residual boundary layer phase dispersion. (Courtesy M. Modic, M.D.)

velocity compensation only in conjunction with a shorter TE. Flow compensation is also useful for optimizing image quality on T$_2$-weighted images of the upper abdomen, where its salutary effect results from reduction of phase shifts due to respiratory motion.

Flow compensation also has certain limitations.

1. Because time-consuming extra gradient pulses are used, and because flow-compensated sequences are only calibrated for specific timings of the gradient pulses, certain sequence parameters are restricted. In particular, flow compensation requires a longer minimum TE than conventional sequences, due to the time required for the extra gradient pulses. In addition, the minimum slice thickness and FOV may be increased.

2. Certain effects of flow compensation may be undesirable in certain settings. For instance, T$_2$-weighted liver images obtained with flow compensation show increased signal from veins which could be confused with mass lesions. The flow void in the aqueduct of Sylvius is eliminated, which can erroneously suggest the diagnosis of obstructive hydrocephalus.

3. By eliminating flow-related phase dispersion and associated variations in signal intensity, flow compensation reduces ghost artifacts produced by pulsatile flow. However, both phase and saturation effects contribute to flow signal. In systole, there is both faster inflow and faster wash-out than in diastole, with a corresponding variation in signal intensity. Flow compensation does not affect ghost artifacts produced by signal intensity fluctuations from this source, which is often the dominant effect for flow perpendicular to the plane of section. Also, flow compensation as currently implemented fails to com-

pletely eliminate signal loss from turbulence, though more advanced flow compensation schemes (in particular, use of very short TE) are under development to address this problem.

GRADIENT-ECHO IMAGING

Although the contrast behavior of GRE images is complex, the GRE pulse sequence is actually a simplified version of an SE sequence; the major difference is that GRE sequences lack the 180-degree refocusing pulse.[27] Instead of two RF pulses, only a single RF pulse produces the MR signal. Examples of GRE methods include FLASH and its steady-state versions, FISP and GRASS (see Chapter 5).

With conventional SE sequences, the choice of flip angle is independent from TR; a 90-degree excitation is always used. However, with FLASH sequences the choice of flip angle depends on TR; as the TR is shortened, smaller flip angles provide the best signal-to-noise (S/N) ratio. For a rectangular slice profile and stationary spins, maximal S/N is obtained using the Ernst angle (α_{opt}), expressed as:

$$\cos{(\alpha_{opt})} = \exp(-TR/T_1) \qquad (7)$$

Gradient-echo sequences have a number of clinical applications. For flow imaging, the two properties of interest are (1) the marked degree of FRE exhibited on FLASH images, and (2) the reduction in proton saturation produced by small flip angle excitations, which allows use of very short TR. The latter property is particularly useful for fast evaluation of vascular patency and for MR cineangiography. These flow properties may be summarized as follows:

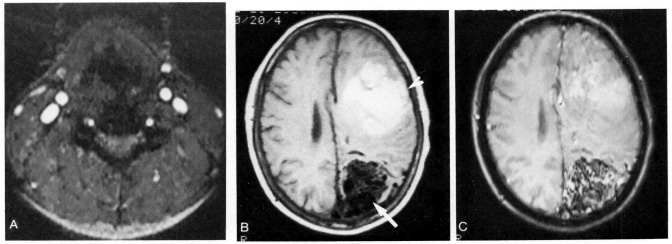

FIGURE 4–21. Intravascular signal is enhanced on GRE images. *A,* Axial FLASH image of neck (TR/TE/flip angle = 100 msec/15 msec/60°) demonstrates high signal in carotid and vertebral arteries and jugular veins. *B,* Patient with arteriovenous malformation. T_1-weighted SE axial image shows anterior cystic component (*arrowhead*) and low intensity vascular component (*arrow*). It is difficult to distinguish calcification from flow void. *C,* FLASH image (TR/TE/flip angle = 100 msec/15 msec/60°) in same patient demonstrates high signal from vascular components and low signal from calcification.

Flow Enhancement

Compared with SE images, FLASH images demonstrate much greater FRE (Fig. 4–21). The reasons for this include (1) unlike SE sequences, FLASH sequences use only a single RF pulse, so there is negligible signal loss from wash-out effects; and (2) because of the simpler structure of the FLASH sequence, shorter TE can be obtained, resulting in less signal loss from phase dispersion.

Using the flip angle given by Equation 7 produces maximal signal for stationary tissues. However, for the case of spins flowing perpendicular to the plane of section, it is usually desirable to use flip angles somewhat larger than the Ernst angle. Compared with small flip angles, large flip angle excitations produce more signal from fresh, inflowing spins, but less signal from stationary spins due to greater saturation. As a result, both flow signal and flow contrast are improved. For flow perpendicular to the plane of section, good flow contrast is usually obtained with TR on the order of 30 to 50 msec in conjunction with flip angles of 20 to 40 degrees.

For in-plane flow, saturation effects become significant for flowing as well as stationary spins. In this case longer TR, on the order of 40 to 100 msec, and smaller flip angles, on the order of 20 to 30 degrees, are sometimes required to improve vascular signal, depending on the velocity and direction of flow, as will be discussed further in the section on MR angiography.

Fast Imaging of Flow

Because small flip angles reduce the amount of proton saturation, high quality FLASH images can be acquired very rapidly. For instance, an image can be obtained in just 5 seconds with TR = 40 msec, 128 projections, and one excitation. Since FLASH images can be acquired in a few seconds, breath holding can be used to suppress motion artifacts in the chest and abdomen.

An additional benefit of these fast imaging techniques is the capability for imaging dynamic processes with high temporal resolution. The most important clinical application of this method is the evaluation of cardiac function, called MR cineangiography.[28, 29] Using a combination of cardiac gating, short TR, and FLASH, one can obtain 32 or more images or "frames" of the heart, each representing a different time point in the cardiac cycle, which can then be played back in a loop to produce a movie of cardiac motion (Fig. 4–22). Flowing blood appears bright on cine images due to the continual inflow of fresh spins into the slice, whereas turbulent flow (e.g., due to valvular regurgitation) appears dark due to phase dispersion (Fig. 4–23). Stasis and thrombosis are characterized on cine acquisitions by constant, medium-to-low signal intensity throughout the cardiac cycle. Cardiac wall motion, valvular regurgitation and stenosis, flow patterns in aneurysms,[30] and other lesions can all be studied by this method (see Chapters 27 and 28).

COINCIDENTAL PHASE CANCELLATION (THE "DISAPPEARING" BLOOD VESSEL)

The frequency-encoding and slice-selection gradients both produce phase shifts for flowing spins. These phase shifts depend on the angle between the

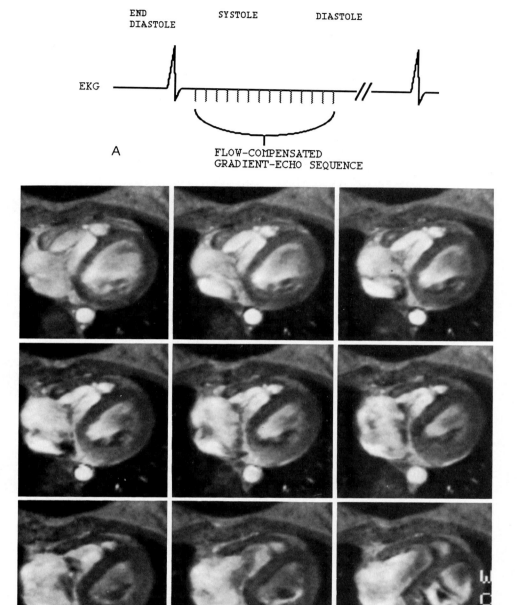

END DIASTOLE　　SYSTOLE　　DIASTOLE

EKG

FLOW-COMPENSATED
GRADIENT-ECHO SEQUENCE

A

FIGURE 4–22. MR cineangiography. *A,* Multiple images or "frames," representing different time points in the cardiac cycle, are acquired at one or more levels using a flow-compensated GRE sequence, short TR, and reduced flip angle. *B,* Nine of 25 frames acquired in 4.7 minutes with TR/TE/flip angle = 30 msec/8 msec/40 degrees. Inflowing spins produce bright signal in heart and great vessels.

direction of flow and the gradient. It is possible for the angle of flow to be such that one gradient produces a positive phase shift and the other a negative phase shift. Although unlikely, in certain vessel orientations and for certain gradient amplitudes the phase shifts produced by the slice-selection and frequency-encoding gradients may cancel, resulting in enhancement of intravascular signal.

This phenomenon may be encountered in MR images of any region of the body. For instance, in pelvic images one occasionally will note that one external iliac artery shows a flow void, but the contralateral artery cannot be identified. Although there are several possible explanations for this appearance, one might be that the first artery appears dark due to flow-related dephasing, but the other artery, which flows at a different angle to the gradients, experiences coincidental phase cancellation. The phase cancellation results in an intermediate signal intensity for the vessel that is nearly indistinguishable from nearby stationary tissues. The vessel therefore "disappears" into the background.

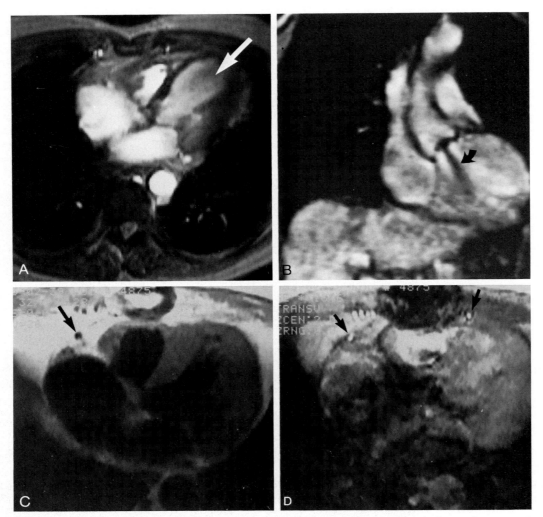

FIGURE 4–23. Signal intensity in MR cineangiograms depends on direction, velocity, and pattern of flow. *A,* True aneurysm of left ventricle. Bright signal is seen in the aorta, right ventricle, and atria. Lack of flow in LV apex (*arrow*) due to akinesis results in increased proton saturation and decreased signal. (Courtesy Dr. G. Laub.) *B,* Moderate aortic regurgitation. Low intensity jet (*arrow*) seen on diastolic frame is caused by turbulence. *C–D,* Cardiac gated axial images of heart obtained with surface coil in patient with angiographically patent right and left coronary bypass grafts. Spin-echo image (*C*) demonstrates only the right graft to be patent (*arrow*). Cine FLASH image (*D*) demonstrates bright signal in both grafts suggesting both are patent. Low intensity region in midanterior chest wall represents ferromagnetic artifact caused by sternal wires, which is more severe on the GRE than on the SE images.

BLOOD IN WRONG LOCATION

DISPLACEMENT ARTIFACT

During data acquisition, spatial information is encoded by the frequency- and phase-encoding gradients. However, the process of spatial encoding is not instantaneous. Blood can flow as far as several centimeters in the time interval between excitation and read-out. Because of this time delay, the position of flowing blood in the image is *always* artifactually displaced from its true position, though the degree of displacement is only significant if it exceeds the dimension of the pixel.[31]

The amount of displacement is dependent on the flow velocity, direction, and pulse sequence structure. The displacement along the frequency-encoding axis (Δx) and phase-encoding axis (Δy) is expressed as:

$$\Delta x = v_x * TE; \Delta y = v_y * t_p \qquad (8)$$

where t_p = time delay between excitation and phase encoding. The amount of displacement increases with TE and therefore tends to be most obvious on heavily T_2-weighted images. For example, with flow along the x-direction at 20 cm/sec and TE = 60 msec, the flow displacement along x would be 1.2 cm. With rapid flow and long TE, vascular signal can be displaced entirely out of the vessel lumen. Flow displacement artifact can mimic or obscure real vascular pathology.

In addition to the absolute positional displacement expressed by Equation 8, there is a *relative* displacement produced by the time delay between phase encoding and frequency encoding. After the y-position is encoded at t_p, blood flows along the frequency-encoding axis for an additional time $t = TE-t_p$ before the x-position is encoded at TE. Because of this additional motion, the apparent positions of flowing spins are displaced further along the frequency-encoding axis than along the phase-encoding axis

(Fig. 4–24A and B). This relative displacement can be minimized by altering the pulse sequence structure so that the phase-encoding gradient is as close as possible to the read-out gradient. Signal patterns suggesting displacement artifact can be mimicked by other conditions such as eccentric thrombus (Fig. 4–24C) or chemical shift artifact (Fig. 4–24D).

One potential benefit of flow displacement artifact is that it can be used to determine the direction of flow. However, the direction of displacement of the flow signal will depend on the pulse sequence structure, in particular on the signs of the gradient pulses

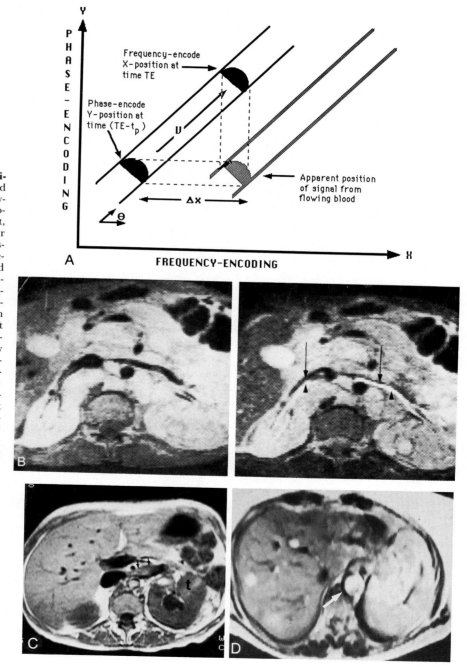

FIGURE 4–24. Flow displacement artifact. *A,* Time delay between excitation and position-encoding causes signal from flowing blood to be displaced from actual position. Because phase-encoding occurs first, the apparent position of the intravascular signal (*shaded semicircle*) appears further displaced along the frequency- than phase-encoding axis. *B,* First (*left*) and second (*right*) echo images of renal veins demonstrate EER on second echo image. Intravascular signal (*arrowheads*) appears displaced out of the vessel lumen (*arrows*) on the second echo image. *C,* Patient with left hypernephroma. Pattern of increased signal (*arrows*) in left renal vein mimics flow displacement artifact but actually represents eccentric tumor thrombus with residual flow seen posteriorly in the vein. T = tumor. *D,* Axial T_2-weighted image in patient with liver metastases. Chemical shift artifact (*arrow*) may be difficult to distinguish from flow displacement artifact. (*B* from von Schulthess GK, Higgins CB: Blood flow imaging with MR: Spin-phase phenomenon. Radiology 157:687–695, 1985.)

and on whether it is an SE or a GRE pulse sequence. Better methods, such as flow presaturation, are available for determining flow directionality.

GHOST ARTIFACTS

Vascular pulsation produces a time-dependent variation in signal intensity. This temporal variation produces an interesting effect after the data undergo a Fourier transformation into the spatial (frequency) domain. In the spatial domain, this periodicity is manifested as a series of ghost images that propagate periodically along the phase-encoding axis, *irrespective of the actual direction of motion* (Fig. 4–25).[32]

The intensity of these ghost images worsens with increasing vascular signal and also with increasing

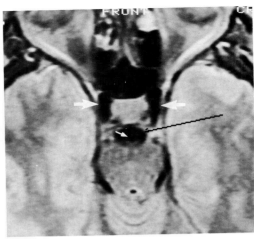

FIGURE 4–26. Vessel size on MR images can be misleading, particularly on images acquired with long TE. Axial T_2-weighted SE image of young male who presented with "worst headache of his life." "Aneurysm" (*black arrow*) of basilar artery represents artifactual signal loss produced by transmission of vessel pulsations to surrounding CSF. Basilar artery (*short white arrow*) is actually normal in size. Note artifactual enlargement of cavernous carotid arteries (*long white arrows*) as well.

amplitude of pulsation. The separation of the ghosts, measured in pixels, is expressed as:

$$\text{Number of pixels} = \text{NEX} \times \text{TR} \times N_y/(\text{R-R interval}) \qquad (9)$$

where N_y = number of pixels across the FOV in the phase-encoding direction, typically 128 or 256, and NEX = number of excitations.

Flow-related ghost artifacts can be suppressed by a variety of means, including cardiac gating, flow compensation, or, most effectively, presaturation. Signal averaging reduces ghost artifact intensity approximately in proportion to $\sqrt{\text{NEX}}$.

MR PSEUDOANEURYSM

Pulsation causes periodic expansion and contraction of the wall of a blood vessel which is transmitted to surrounding tissues, resulting in phase dispersion and associated signal loss. Because of this effect, almost all arteries appear artifactually enlarged on MR images, potentially causing diagnostic confusion as to vessel ectasia or aneurysm (Fig. 4–26).[33] In order to eliminate this artifact, flow-related phase shifts must be reduced, for example, by using flow compensation and short echo times.

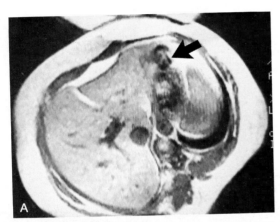

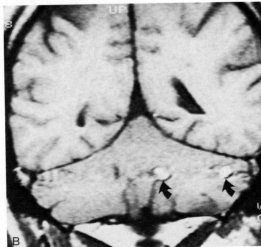

FIGURE 4–25. Pathology can be mimicked by artifacts representing flow signal in the wrong position. *A*, T_1-weighted axial image of abdomen demonstrates alternating high and low intensity ghost artifacts produced by aortic pulsation which propagate along the phase-encoding direction. Low intensity ghost (*arrow*) could be mistaken for mass in left lobe of liver. *B*, T_1-weighted coronal image of brain demonstrates two high intensity foci (*arrows*) in the cerebellum, simulating cryptic arteriovenous malformations. These pseudolesions represent ghost artifacts produced by pulsatile flow in the transverse sinuses.

DIFFERENTIATION OF INTRAVASCULAR SIGNAL FROM THROMBUS

Saturation, phase shift, and flow displacement effects alter the appearance of flowing blood. The dominant effect depends on the flow rate as well as the imaging technique. In veins, slow flow typically produces enhancement of vascular signal, a saturation effect. At moderate flow velocities, there is a balance between FRE and signal loss produced by phase dispersion and wash-out effects. In the limit of high velocity flow, both wash-out effects and phase dispersion produce a signal void. When one considers the varied hemodynamic patterns encountered in normal and diseased vessels, the sometimes disparate effects on signal intensity of saturation and phase, and the various displacement artifacts, it is no surprise that unusual patterns of vascular signal are commonly seen. These should not be confused with vessel occlusion or atherosclerotic plaque. We will now discuss the signal characteristics of thrombus and the means to differentiate it from flow signal.

SIGNAL CHARACTERISTICS OF THROMBUS

In routine clinical practice, one commonly encounters a variety of flow artifacts that can mimic thrombus (Fig. 4–27). Further complicating the process of image interpretation is the variable appearance of thrombus, which depends on the composition and age of the clot. Paramagnetic hemoglobin breakdown products appear to have less influence on the signal intensity of thrombus than on that of hematomas (see Chapter 16). It is also important to differentiate between bland thrombus, which is composed of platelets, fibrin, and trapped blood cells, and tumor thrombus. The signal intensity characteristics of tumor thrombus may mimic those of the primary tumor and, unlike bland thrombus, may enhance following intravenous administration of gadolinium-DTPA.

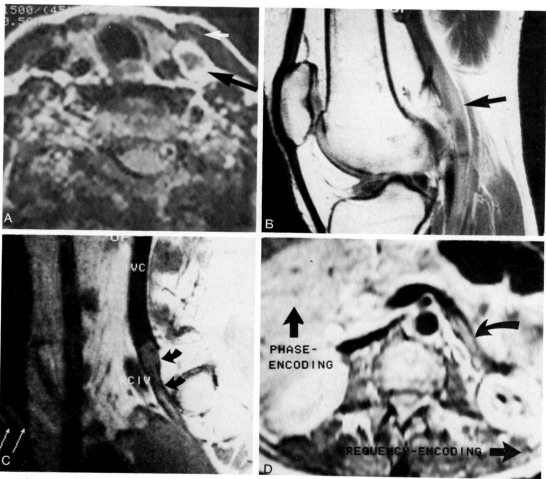

FIGURE 4–27. Flow artifacts simulating thrombus. A, Axial T_2-weighted image of neck demonstrates high signal in left jugular vein (*black arrow*). Presence of subtle ghost artifacts (*white arrows*) confirms that this represents flow signal, not thrombus. B, T_1-weighted sagittal image of knee demonstrates signal in popliteal vein (*arrow*) due to slow flow. This should not be confused with deep venous thrombosis or clot in an aneurysm. C, Sagittal T_1-weighted image of pelvis demonstrates signal (*black arrows*) in right common iliac vein (CIV), but signal void more distally in inferior vena cava (IVC). Both vessels are patent. The bright signal in the CIV comes from this being the entrance slice for venous flow entering from the right. The blood became saturated by the time it entered the IVC. Subtle ghost artifacts (*white arrows*) confirm that signal in CIV represents flow, not thrombus. D, Flow signal in left renal vein (*arrow*) which could be difficult to distinguish from thrombus.

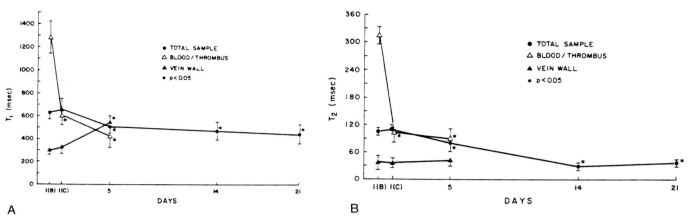

FIGURE 4–28. In vitro relaxation times of stagnant blood and thrombus measured in canine model, plotted as function of time. *A*, T_1 relaxation time of clot is markedly decreased compared with stagnant blood; most of the signal increase occurs over the first few days following thrombosis. *B*, T_2 relaxation time also decreases over time. (From Rapoport S, Sostman HD, Pope C, et al: Venous clots: Evaluation with MRI. Radiology 162:527–530, 1987.)

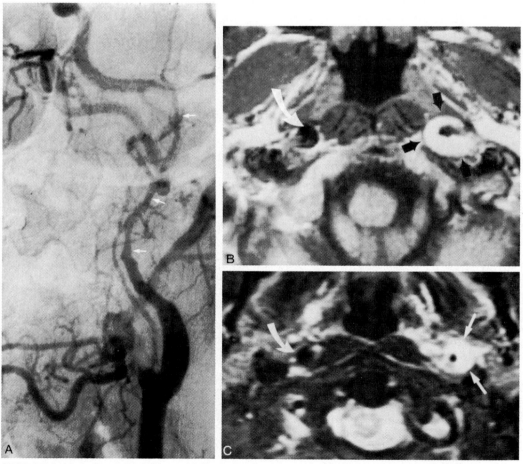

FIGURE 4–29. Patient with left carotid dissection. *A*, Left carotid angiogram shows characteristic irregular narrowing of left ICA (*arrows*), which begins just above bulb and terminates in the skull base. *B*, Intramural thrombus (*arrows*) shows high signal intensity on axial T_1-weighted image. *C*, Thrombus remains intense on T_2-weighted (SE 2500/60) image. Right carotid (*curved arrow*) is normal. (From Goldberg HI, Grossman RI, Gomori JM, et al: Cervical internal carotid artery dissecting hemorrhage: Diagnosis using MR. Radiology 158:157–161, 1986.)

The signal intensity characteristics of bland thrombus are age-dependent, although the time course has not been completely elucidated.[34] In the first few days after thrombosis, an in vitro study showed marked shortening of both the T_1 and T_2 relaxation times of the thrombus (Fig. 4–28). Fresh thrombus may have a variable in vivo appearance, depending on the formation of paramagnetic hemoglobin breakdown products and clot retraction (Fig. 4–29).[35] Over time there is a gradual reduction in signal intensity as the thrombus matures and becomes incorporated into the vessel wall. In our experience, older thrombus has intermediate-to-low signal intensity on both T_1- and T_2-weighted images. Unlike intracerebral hematomas, hemosiderin is not commonly detected. The variable appearance of thrombus and flow signal occasionally causes confusion between the two, and several techniques can be helpful for differentiating them (see Table 4–2).

PLANE OF SECTION

Thrombus does not change in appearance with different planes of section, whereas flow signal usually does. Therefore, imaging of a vessel in multiple planes of section generally allows differentiation of flow signal and thrombus (Figs. 4–30 and 4–31).

PRESATURATION

Application of a presaturation pulse close to the plane of section suppresses FRE. Flow signal disappears with presaturation, while the signal intensity of thrombus should be unaffected, unless the presaturation is so close that there is spillover of saturation into the slice due to a nonrectangular profile of the presaturation slab.

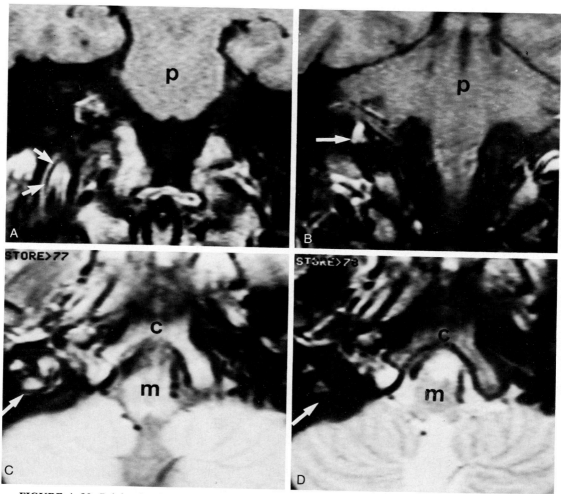

FIGURE 4–30. Bright signal is often seen at base of brain, near the confluence of the inferior petrosal sinus and jugular bulb. This appearance is rarely pathologic and can be eliminated by presaturation. (M = medulla, p = pons, c = clivus.) *A,* Coronal T_1-weighted image of posterior fossa demonstrates signal in right jugular vein (*arrows*). *B,* Next posterior section from (*A*) shows signal in inferior petrosal vein (*arrow*). *C,* Axial proton density (TE = 20 msec) spin-echo image again shows signal in right jugular vein (*arrow*). *D,* Absence of signal in second echo (TE = 80 msec) image confirms patency of jugular bulb and excludes thrombus or tumor.

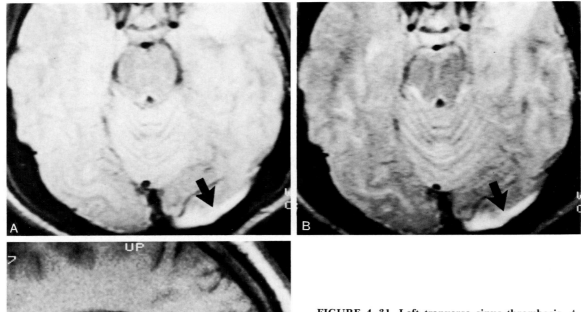

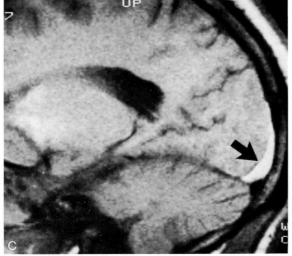

FIGURE 4–31. Left tranverse sinus thrombosis. *A,* SE 2500/22 axial image demonstrates high signal in left transverse sinus (*arrow*), a finding that is not uncommonly seen in normal subjects. *B,* Second echo (SE 2500/80) image also demonstrates high signal in transverse sinus without evidence of flow effects. *C,* Sagittal T_1-weighted image again demonstrates identical appearance of transverse sinus. Persistence of signal on different images suggests thrombosis rather than flow. Presaturation or phase map could also have been used to make the diagnosis.

PHASE IMAGING

Phase imaging, when available, provides reliable differentiation of flow signal from thrombus. Flow produces phase shifts that are apparent on phase maps as bright or dark areas readily distinguishable from the stationary background, which appears gray (Fig. 4–32). However, respiratory motion, chemical shift, and susceptibility variations can all cause non-flow-related phase shifts which can mimic flow.

PULSE SEQUENCE

Use of flow compensated GRE pulse sequences and short TE contributes to vascular enhancement,

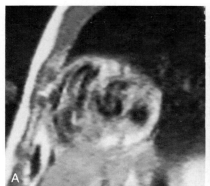
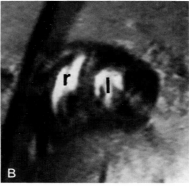

FIGURE 4–32. Short axis gated SE image of heart. *A,* Magnitude reconstruction demonstrates poor contrast between intraventricular signal and ventricular walls. *B,* Phase map demonstrates high signal from flowing blood in right (r) and left (l) ventricles, contrasting with papillary muscles and ventricular walls. Background cancellation is imperfect due to phase shifts caused by patient respiration and cardiac motion.

whereas the combination of SE sequences, presaturation, and long TE contributes to the flow void. The presence of either flow void or ghost artifacts confirms vessel patency. However, vascular pulsation is essential to the production of ghost artifacts; with constant velocity flow (e.g., in small veins), ghost artifacts are not usually seen.

Flow signal can be differentiated from thrombus in just a few seconds by fast GRE acquisitions (Fig. 4–33). However, if the flip angle is too small or the TR is too long, stationary tissues such as thrombus may appear bright and be hard to differentiate from flow (Fig. 4–33*B*).

INTRAVASCULAR DEVICES

Various intravascular devices may be encountered during routine imaging. Devices such as Gianturco coils and Starr-Edwards valves contain ferromagnetic materials and may produce severe local image distortion. Nonferromagnetic devices such as the Simon-Nitinol filter can be demonstrated by MRI with minimal artifact. Their position within the inferior vena cava, vessel patency, and presence of clot are well evaluated using GRE methods (Fig. 4–34).

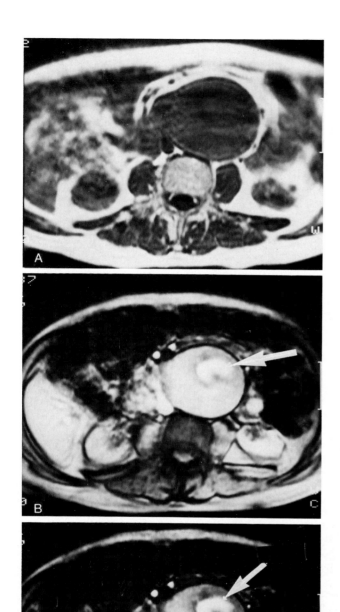

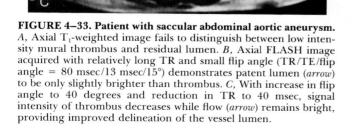

FIGURE 4–33. Patient with saccular abdominal aortic aneurysm. *A,* Axial T_1-weighted image fails to distinguish between low intensity mural thrombus and residual lumen. *B,* Axial FLASH image acquired with relatively long TR and small flip angle (TR/TE/flip angle = 80 msec/13 msec/15°) demonstrates patent lumen (*arrow*) to be only slightly brighter than thrombus. *C,* With increase in flip angle to 40 degrees and reduction in TR to 40 msec, signal intensity of thrombus decreases while flow (*arrow*) remains bright, providing improved delineation of the vessel lumen.

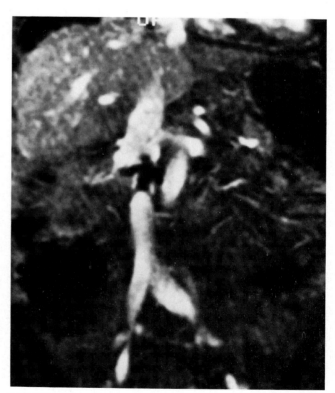

FIGURE 4–34. Simon-Nitinol filter (*dark structure*) positioned within inferior vena cava just below level of renal veins. Coronal flow-compensated FLASH image (TR/TE/NEX = 30 msec/10 msec/1 with flip angle = 30°) acquired during breath-hold is ideal for showing position of these devices.

B—Advanced Flow Concepts

NATURE OF CEREBROSPINAL FLUID FLOW

The diagnosis of spinal and cerebral pathology requires the highest possible tissue contrast and anatomic detail. MR is superior to CT and myelography because it possesses these attributes without requiring exogenous contrast or ionizing radiation. However, until recently MR image quality in the brain and spine on T_2-weighted images has fallen short of its potential because of image degradation caused by CSF motion artifacts.

Cerebrospinal fluid flow effects are routinely exhibited during MR imaging of the brain and spine.[36–38] This is not surprising given that CSF pulsates at velocities up to several centimeters per second.[39–41] In fact, MR angiographic techniques can be used to depict CSF flow, just as they can depict blood flow (Fig. 4–35).[42, 43] CSF flow effects are most obvious when CSF signal intensity is high, which commonly occurs during long TR spin-echo imaging. CSF motion artifacts are clinically important for the following reasons. (1) They degrade image quality by reducing tissue contrast and anatomic detail, thereby potentially obscuring disease (false negative). (2) They may appear similar to pathologic processes from which they must be differentiated (false positive).

The existence of CSF pulsation is well recognized. Although CSF production and circulation produce a slow bulk flow through the ventricular system and cerebrospinal subarachnoid space, during the time course of an MR examination, CSF motion, unlike blood flow, may be considered a form of oscillatory nonpropagating flow. In the past, CSF motion has been quantitatively characterized by manometric and myelographic methods. More recently, flow sensitive MR imaging methods have been employed to quantitatively assess instantaneous CSF velocity.

The characteristics of CSF motion are dependent upon the anatomic region under consideration. CSF within the ventricular system is ejected into the basilar cisterns and cranial subarachnoid space during systolic cerebral perfusion and returns to the ventricular system during the diastolic phase. CSF motion within the spinal subarachnoid space undergoes an oscillatory motion synchronous with cerebral perfusion. Systolic expansion of the brain leads to caudal displacement of CSF within the spinal subarachnoid space. During cerebral venous drainage, reciprocal cranial displacement occurs. It is important to recognize that spinal CSF motion occurs throughout the cardiac cycle and is stationary only briefly at the extremes of its oscillatory excursion in late systole and diastole. The distinction between systolic and diastolic CSF motion is that flow direction reverses between systole and diastole and that flow velocity is lower during diastole than during systole. In the spine, CSF pulsation amplitude is greatest in the cervical spine, less in the thoracic spine, and least in the lumbar spine. However, even in the lumbar spine, CSF flow effects can degrade image quality, particularly on T_2-weighted images.

MR MYELOGRAM

SOURCES OF ARTIFACTS

During long TR spin-echo imaging, stationary CSF appears bright because of its long T_2 relaxation time. Oscillatory motion of CSF under otherwise identical conditions produces signal loss and ghost artifacts.

The magnitude of signal loss is proportional to CSF velocity and inversely proportional to slice thickness during axial imaging. The proximity of the ghost artifacts to the subarachnoid space is dependent upon the relationship between TR and the heart rate. When TR is nearly equal to an integral multiple of the heart rate, the ghost artifacts converge on the pulsatile CSF; overlap of ghost artifacts on CSF interfaces degrades visualization of these interfaces and adjacent neural structures.

Three other manifestations of CSF flow are common. (1) Increased CSF signal may be observed at end slices of a multislice sequence; this artifactual signal can mimic intradural masses (Fig. 4–36). (2) Reduced CSF signal intensity may be observed in regions of rapid or turbulent flow such as the cerebral aqueduct. (3) On systolic gated spine images, bands of decreased signal intensity may silhouette CSF interfaces on sagittal odd echo images (Fig. 4–37).

Although T_1-weighted images often provide a satisfactory view of the CSF–thecal sac interface, there are times when low intensity extradural lesions (osteophytes or discs) are relatively inapparent because of insufficient contrast with the low intensity CSF. In these cases, high signal intensity CSF on T_2-weighted images would be useful to better delineate the CSF interfaces. Unfortunately, CSF motion artifacts, which are common under these conditions, have limited the utility of this approach in the past (Fig. 4–38A).

They also may create difficulty when evaluating the brain stem, basal ganglia, or medial temporal lobes, because these regions are also in proximity to pulsatile CSF (Fig. 4–38B and C).[44] When spatially mismapped CSF signal superimposes upon these low signal intensity neural structures, it may partially obscure real lesions (e.g., multiple sclerosis plaques) or actually simulate a lesion in normal neural structures. CSF pulsations may also create artifactual signal variations within the ventricles (Fig. 4–38D). Artifacts may persist despite use of flow compensation (Fig. 4–38E).

Another manifestation of CSF flow effects is seen

Text continued on page 143

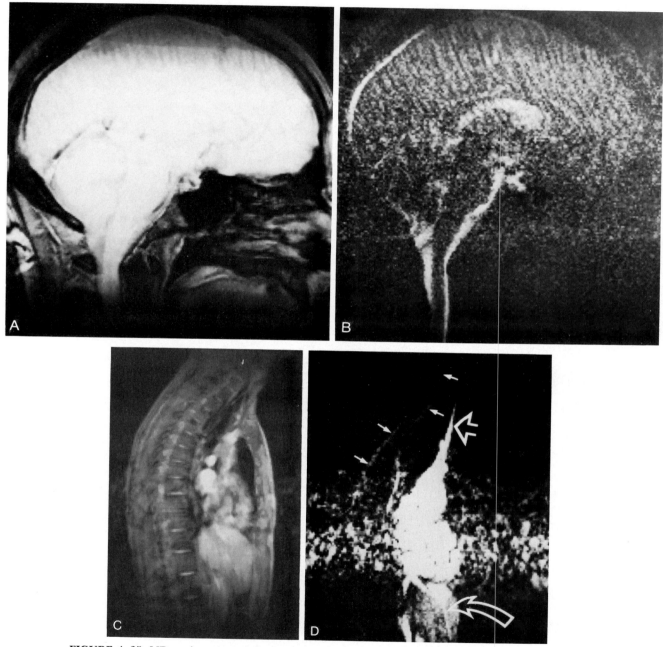

FIGURE 4–35. MR angiograms can be used to demonstrate CSF flow as well as blood flow. Areas of brightest signal represent maximum flow velocity. *A*, Sagittal FLASH image of the head. *B*, Areas of high signal on projection angiogram represent CSF flow in the lateral ventricles, basilar cisterns, and cervical subarachnoid spaces. *C*, Sagittal FLASH image of the chest. *D*, Projection angiogram demonstrates heart, carotid artery (*straight open arrow*), hepatic vein (*curved arrow*), and cerebrospinal fluid within the cervical and thoracic spinal canal (*short arrows*).

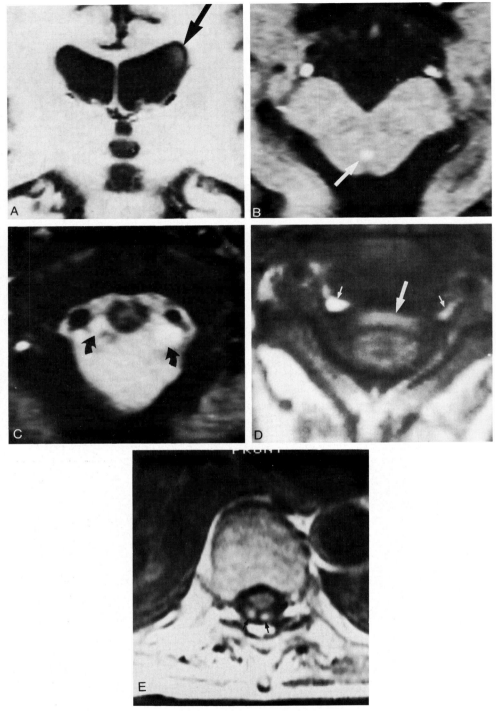

FIGURE 4–36. Flow-related enhancement due to CSF flow is usually seen in the first and last slices from a multislice acquisition. These flow artifacts may simulate pathology. *A,* Most anterior slice from coronal T_1-weighted SE acquisition shows bright signal (*arrow*) due to flow, simulating mass in the anterior horn of left lateral ventricle. *B,* Top slice from axial T_1-weighted SE acquisition shows bright signal (*arrow*) in aqueduct of Sylvius. *C,* Bottom slice from axial T_2-weighted head acquisition demonstrates flow-related enhancement (*arrows*) adjacent to vertebral arteries. *D,* Top slice from axial T_1-weighted SE acquisition shows bright signal in anterior subarachnoid space (*long arrow*), due to inflow of unsaturated spins. This signal could be confused with disk protrusion. Epidural veins (*short arrows*) within neural foramina also appear bright. *E,* On bottom slice, axial T_1-weighted image of thoracic spine demonstrates paired pseudolesions posterior to spinal cord, again representing inflow of unsaturated CSF into slice.

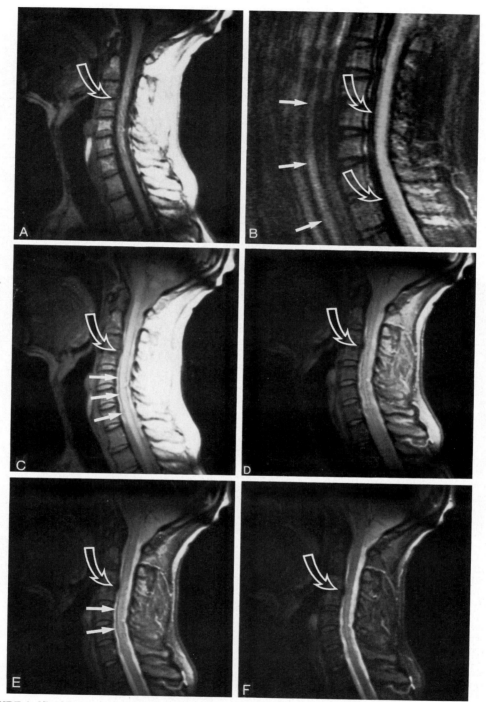

FIGURE 4–37. If flow compensation is unavailable, CSF motion artifacts can be reduced by using cardiac gating and EER. Sagittal images of the cervical spine. *A,* TR/TE 800 msec/20 msec. Degenerative changes at C3/4 are relatively inapparent on T₁-weighted image (*curved open arrow*). *B,* T₂-weighted image without flow compensation demonstrates severe ghost artifacts and low signal in subarachnoid space. *C–F,* Gated on alternate beats, effective TR 1800 msec, consecutive echoes at TE 20, 40, 60, 80 msec. Ghost artifacts are eliminated. There are bands of low CSF signal intensity (*solid straight arrows*) silhouetting CSF interfaces due to boundary layer phase dispersion on odd (C, E) but not even (D, F) echo-gated images. Conspicuity of degenerative changes at C3/4 (*curved open arrow*) is improved on the T₂-weighted images compared to the T₁-weighted image.

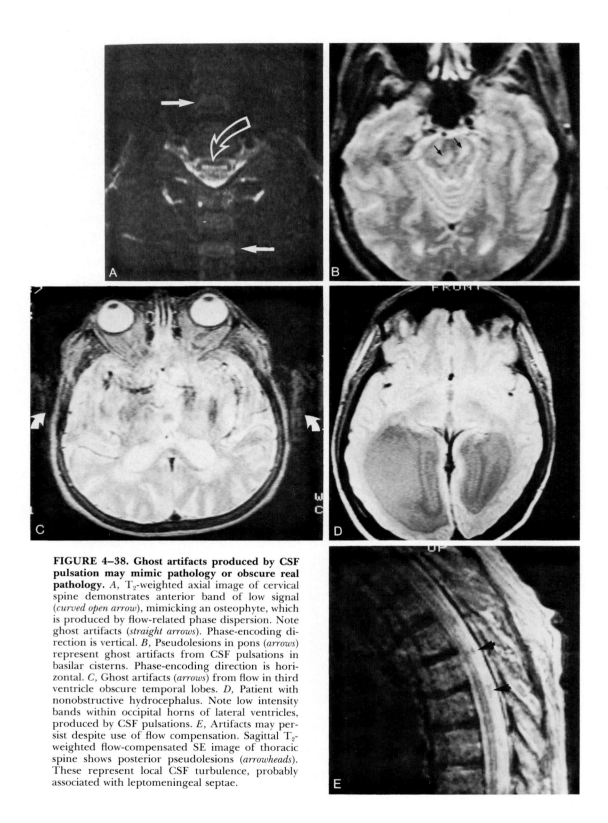

FIGURE 4–38. Ghost artifacts produced by CSF pulsation may mimic pathology or obscure real pathology. *A*, T_2-weighted axial image of cervical spine demonstrates anterior band of low signal (*curved open arrow*), mimicking an osteophyte, which is produced by flow-related phase dispersion. Note ghost artifacts (*straight arrows*). Phase-encoding direction is vertical. *B*, Pseudolesions in pons (*arrows*) represent ghost artifacts from CSF pulsations in basilar cisterns. Phase-encoding direction is horizontal. *C*, Ghost artifacts (*arrows*) from flow in third ventricle obscure temporal lobes. *D*, Patient with nonobstructive hydrocephalus. Note low intensity bands within occipital horns of lateral ventricles, produced by CSF pulsations. *E*, Artifacts may persist despite use of flow compensation. Sagittal T_2-weighted flow-compensated SE image of thoracic spine shows posterior pseudolesions (*arrowheads*). These represent local CSF turbulence, probably associated with leptomeningeal septae.

distal to spinal block. CSF signal intensity may be increased distal to an obstruction due to the decreased amplitude of CSF pulsation, particularly in the cervical and thoracic region. This increase in signal may be seen on T_1- as well as on T_2-weighted images (Fig. 4–39) and should not be confused with pathology such as intradural metastases or purulent meningitis.

SOLUTIONS

There are four general approaches to reducing CSF flow artifacts: (1) gradient rotation, (2) cardiac gating, (3) even-echo rephasing or flow compensation, and (4) GRE pulse sequences.[45, 46]

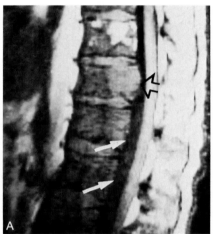

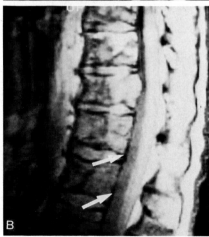

FIGURE 4–39. Signal intensity of CSF can be altered by lesions that reduce the amplitude of CSF pulsation. Sagittal images of thoracic spine in patient with diffuse breast cancer metastases and posterior extrusion of vertebral body into spinal canal (*open arrow*). *A*, T_1-weighted image demonstrates increased CSF signal (*arrows*) distal to the obstruction, representing decreased amplitude of CSF pulsation. The increased CSF signal could be confused with intradural tumor or purulent meningitis. *B*, T_2-weighted image demonstrates same effect.

Gradient Rotation

The relative orientation of the frequency- and phase-encoding axes with respect to the direction of flow has an important bearing on flow artifacts. The process of phase encoding is fundamentally different from slice selection and frequency encoding, since the phase-encoding gradient has a different amplitude after each excitation. Large phase-encoding gradient amplitudes are only encountered for a relatively few excitations. In addition, most phase errors are produced by motion during the time interval between a pair of gradient pulses. These errors are minimal for the phase-encoding gradient, which only uses one gradient pulse. Flow along the phase-encoding gradient produces misregistration but only minimal phase shifts, signal loss, and ghosting. As a result, flow-related signal loss and ghost artifacts can be minimized by orienting the phase-encoding axis along the direction of flow; this is an option available on most MR systems. Because the predominant direction of CSF pulsation is along the length of the spine, the myelogram effect on T_2-weighted images can be enhanced by orienting the phase-encoding axis parallel to the spine.

In practice, there are several limitations to this method. First, in patients with marked lordosis or kyphosis, the long axis of the spine is curved, so that components of CSF flow necessarily parallel both the frequency- and phase-encoding axes. Second, with the phase-encoding axis along the length of the body, wraparound artifact along the phase-encoding axis will degrade image quality unless a method, such as oversampling or presaturation, is available to suppress it (see Chapter 3). Finally, rotating the gradients will also rotate the direction of chemical shift artifact. With chemical shift artifact rotated vertically rather than the usual horizontal orientation, small disk herniations could be obscured, due to overlap of the artifact with the posterior disk and vertebral margins.

Cardiac Gating

Cardiac gating eliminates ghost artifacts by synchronizing successive excitations with the CSF motion. Gating may be accomplished either by direct triggering off the ECG signal or by peripheral gating. The latter may be accomplished using infrared reflective photoplethysmography or peripheral arterial Doppler; these devices can be attached to a finger or ear lobe. Gating is most effective if images are obtained during diastole; during systole, loss of signal at boundaries between CSF and spinal cord or CSF and vertebral body may become prominent.

Even-Echo Rephasing or Flow Compensation

Flow artifacts can be minimized with EER or, more effectively, by flow compensation. If EER is used, then the time interval between successive echos should be minimized for best effect (e.g., use TE 20,

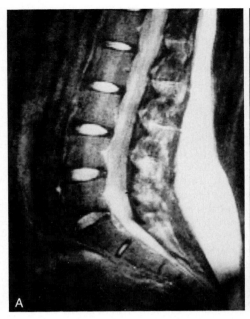
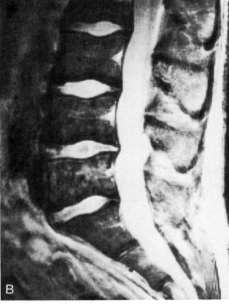

FIGURE 4–40. CSF pulsations are minimal in the lumbar spine but can nonetheless generate significant artifacts. Sagittal T₂-weighted SE images. *A*, CSF pulsations produce ghost artifacts and inhomogeneous signal within spinal canal. *B*, With flow compensation myelogram, effect is enhanced and ghost artifacts are eliminated. (Courtesy M. Modic, M.D.)

40, 60, 80 rather than TE 40, 80) to reduce the effects of higher order motion and wash-out between echoes. Asymmetric multiecho sequences (e.g., TE 20, 80) may exacerbate ghost artifacts unless flow compensation is also used. Flow compensation improves the myelogram effect even in the lumbar region where CSF pulsation is minimal (Fig. 4–40).

In some patients, despite the use of flow compensation, localized CSF turbulence may be produced by tiny leptomeningeal septations that normally cross the spinal canal, as well as osteophytes, disk protrusions, or transmitted vascular pulsations. This localized CSF turbulence may produce focal signal loss that mimics pathology and could be mistaken for vascular malformations (see Fig. 4–38*E*). In these patients, *the combination of flow compensation and dia-* *stolic ECG gating may be more effective than either technique alone* for suppressing the artifacts.

Gradient-Echo Pulse Sequences

Gradient-echo pulse sequences can also be used to produce a myelogram-like effect. Because of shorter TE, these sequences are much less sensitive to the effects of CSF pulsation than SE sequences. The myelogram effect is further enhanced by using flow compensation (Fig. 4–41).

Clinical applications of GRE sequences in the spine are reviewed in depth in Chapter 5. Briefly, a wide range of combinations of TR, TE, and flip angle can be used to produce a satisfactory myelogram effect. As the TR is shortened, the flip angle must be

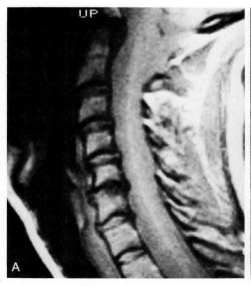
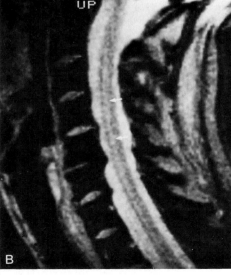

FIGURE 4–41. MR myelogram can be achieved using either flow-compensated SE or FLASH pulse sequences, but images demonstrate markedly dissimilar contrast mechanisms. *A*, SE 2500/22 image shows spondylitic changes at C3/4 to C6/7. Vertebral bodies show moderate signal intensity. Imaging time was 10 minutes. *B*, FLASH image (TR/TE/flip angle = 300 msec/18 msec/10°) demonstrates excellent myelogram effect. Note darker appearance of vertebral bodies and osteophytes due to magnetic susceptibility effects. Imaging time was only four minutes. Note thin band of increased signal (*small arrows*) centrally within spinal cord, which represents truncation artifact rather than syrinx.

reduced in order to maintain satisfactory positive CSF–spinal cord contrast. If TR > 100 msec (multi-slice imaging), either FLASH or its steady-state versions can be used to generate bright CSF. Typical imaging parameters used to obtain the MR myelogram include TR/TE/flip angle = 300 msec/10 msec/10 degrees or 100 msec/10 msec/5 degrees. For TR << 100 msec, steady-state FLASH (e.g., GRASS or FISP) should be used to make CSF bright. However, use of such short TR generally limits two-dimensional (2D) acquisitions to a single slice.

Compared with FLASH, its steady-state versions are much more sensitive to signal loss from CSF pulsation.[47] Steady-state methods rely on maintaining a significant transverse magnetization, which is read out to produce the MR signal. However, motion during the acquisition, from flow or otherwise, produces dephasing. Although use of flow compensation reduces the sensitivity to motion, during steady-state acquisitions even minor dephasing effects accumulate to produce significant signal loss and ghost artifacts. Recently, flow-compensated FISP sequences have been developed in which flow-related phase shifts are completely refocussed at the RF pulse. Unlike conventional FISP/GRASS, these "true" FISP sequences produce an intense myelogram effect with very short TR (e.g., 20 msec). They are also well-suited for 3D acquisitions.

Gradient-echo methods have several limitations for imaging of the spine. Compared with conventional SE images, GRE images are less T_2-weighted and are poorer for showing intrinsic cord pathology such as plaques of multiple sclerosis. Magnetic susceptibility effects, produced by bone–soft tissue interfaces, may make osteophytes appear artifactually large. Artifacts from ferromagnetic implants (e.g., surgical fixation wires) are prominent. Despite these limitations, GRE pulse sequences are routinely used for evaluating spinal pathology, such as radiculopathy, because of their superior sensitivity for osteophytes and lesser sensitivity to flow artifacts.

CSF FLOW EFFECTS AND CYSTIC LESIONS IN THE SPINE

Assuming that flow compensation is *not* used, stationary CSF will appear brighter than pulsatile CSF on T_2-weighted images. This can be useful in differentiating tumor-associated cysts from benign syringohydromyelia (Fig. 4–42).[48, 49] Tumor-associated cysts do not communicate with the ventricular system and therefore contain stationary fluid. The fluid within the cavity will therefore be brighter than the pulsating CSF within the subarachnoid space. In contrast, most actively expanding syringohydromyelic cavities communicate with the fourth ventricle; transmitted CSF pulsations cause the syrinx to have similar signal intensity as surrounding CSF.

However, posttraumatic cavities do not generally

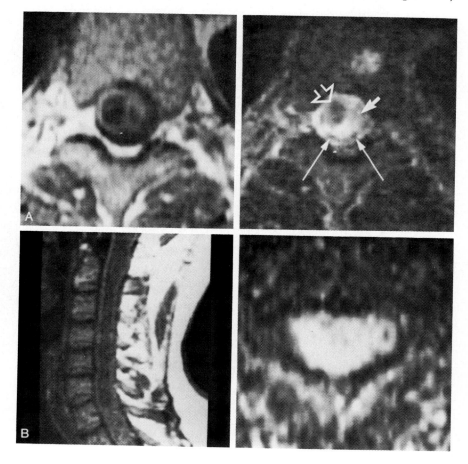

FIGURE 4–42. CSF flow effects can help distinguish among spinal cord cysts associated with benign and malignant lesions. *A,* Traumatic syrinx with pulsatile cyst and nonpulsatile cyst. Left, axial T_1-weighted image demonstrates two cysts of unequal size. Right, T_2-weighted axial image demonstrates signal loss in pulsatile cyst (*open arrow*), but increased signal in smaller nonpulsatile cyst (*short arrow*). Curved black line represents posterior interface between cord and subarachnoid space (*long arrows*). *B,* Cervical spinal cord cyst in association with ependymoma. Left, Sagittal T_1-weighted image shows cord expansion and low intensity cyst. Right, Axial T_2-weighted image shows cyst to have high signal intensity without evidence of CSF pulsation. (From Enzmann DR, O'Donohue J, Rubin JB, et al: CSF pulsations within nonneoplastic spinal cord cysts. AJR 149:149–157, 1987; © by American Roentgen Ray Society.)

communicate with the ventricular system, so that absence of pulsation does not exclude benign syrinx. Successful surgical treatment of syringohydromyelia (e.g., plugging of the obex, shunting of the cyst) results in loss of pulsation within the syrinx. Although evaluation of CSF pulsation is useful, contrast infusion with gadolinium-DTPA provides the most definitive evaluation of spinal cord neoplasia (see Chapter 23).

MR VENOGRAPHY

Deep venous thrombosis (DVT) presents a common diagnostic problem. Several methods have been proposed for diagnosis, including contrast venography, ultrasound, and impedance plethysmography. Although contrast venography remains the gold standard for assessment of DVT, it is an invasive method with potential risks, due to the administration of iodinated contrast, and necessitates radiation exposure, which is particularly undesirable in pregnant patients. Because of these limitations as well as the expense, ultrasound and impedance plethysmography are often used as screening modalities, although they do not precisely delineate the extent of DVT and are less sensitive to calf vein thrombosis. Compared with other noninvasive modalities, MR may be more accurate and has the potential for demonstrating collateral vessels, determining the age of the clot, and demonstrating soft tissue masses which cause extrinsic compression of the veins.

It has been demonstrated that venous patency in the lower extremities can be accurately evaluated using GRE imaging.[50] Axial 5-mm thick sections were obtained sequentially using a flow-compensated GRASS sequence with TR/TE/flip angle of 33 msec/16 msec/30 degrees. Patent veins appear bright due to FRE; thrombosis appears dark (Figs. 4–43 and 4–44). Accurate diagnoses were made in 16 of 17 cases. There was one false-positive case in whom

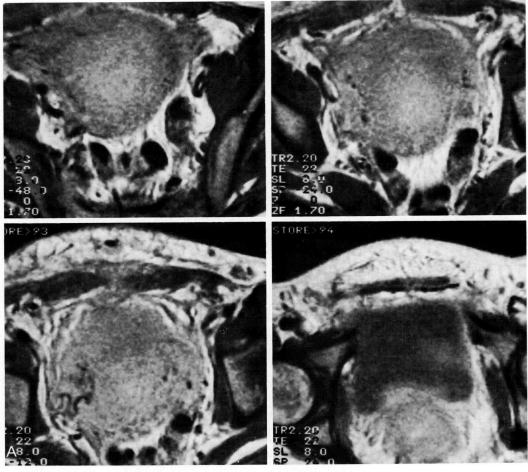

FIGURE 4–43. Postpartum patient with suspicion of pelvic deep venous thrombosis. *A,* Axial proton density-weighted images fail to adequately distinguish blood vessels from bowel loops and lymph nodes. *B,* On FLASH images (TR/TE/flip angle = 60 msec/11 msec/40°) bright signal in veins demonstrates patency.

slow venous flow mimicked clot. By varying the flip angle in questionable cases, further false-positive results were avoided. This method can be extended up into the pelvis to assess pelvic DVT.

Recently, methods have been implemented for producing projection venograms analogous to contrast venograms. These methods produce visualization of the entire venous system in one image rather than in numerous individual slices. These methods will be discussed below.

MR ANGIOGRAPHY

As we have seen, MR is an exquisitely sensitive technique for the detection and characterization of flow. Blood flow is highlighted by flow enhancement and flow void effects as well as by phase-sensitive reconstruction techniques. However, until now we have considered these methods in the context of conventional two-dimensional tomographic imaging, which has significant drawbacks if one is attempting to compete with conventional x-ray angiography.

LIMITATIONS OF CONVENTIONAL TOMOGRAPHIC METHODS

Sometimes conventional MR images demonstrate such striking contrast between blood vessels and background that an angiogram-like display of vascular anatomy is produced (Fig. 4–45). However, in general MR images obtained by standard two-dimensional Fourier transform (2DFT) methods are not well suited for angiography.

There are several reasons why conventional acquisition methods are limited. For instance, whereas some large vessels such as the aorta can often be visualized along their entire length in a single plane of section, this is not true for most blood vessels. If thick sections are used to include more of the vessel, flow contrast is reduced due to partial volume averaging.

Recently, methods have been introduced which overcome these problems. Unlike its radiographic counterpart, MR angiography is noninvasive, with flow-induced contrast substituting for iodinated contrast media. Because MR angiography is in its infancy, a large number of techniques are under active development.[51–54]

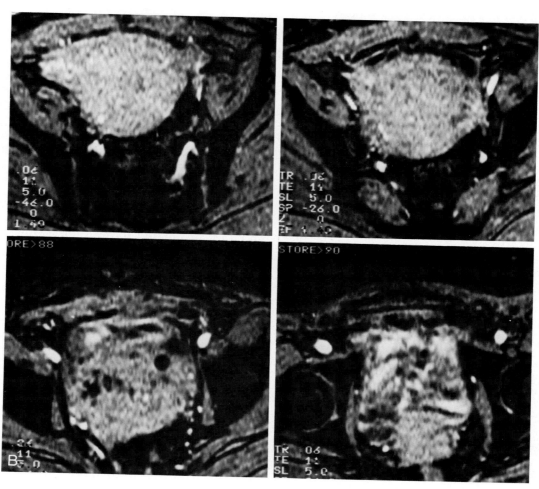

FIGURE 4–43 *Continued*

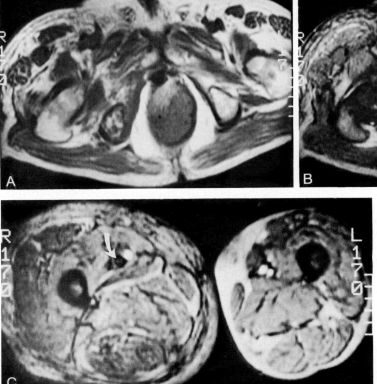

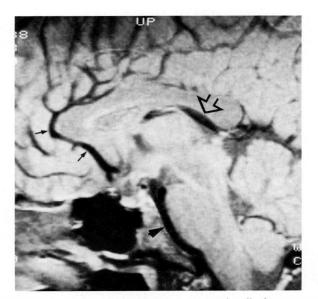

FIGURE 4–44. MR venograms. 40-year-old male S/P abdominal surgery with deep venous thrombosis. *A,* Axial T_1-weighted SE image. Identification of veins is difficult. *B* and *C,* Sequential body coil GRASS images obtained with TR/TE/flip angle = 30/12/30°, slice thickness = 5 or 10 mm, and FOV = 32 cm. Patent veins appear bright, whereas occluded right common and superficial femoral veins (*arrows*) demonstrate low signal intensity. (Compare with Fig. 4–43). (Courtesy C. Spritzer, M.D.)

All of these methods require some way to generate contrast between flowing blood and stationary tissues. This can be accomplished by enhancing vascular signal and/or suppressing background signal. MR angiographic methods can be broadly characterized by the mechanisms used to generate flow contrast and by the geometry of the data acquisition (Table 4–6). For instance, 3D methods acquire a volume of data from which individual thin slices are reconstructed. These slices are then manipulated to produce an angiogram-like image. On the other hand, projection acquisition methods directly produce an angiogram-like image and do not use slices in the conventional sense.

In the next section we will consider the various methodologies for MR angiography and then proceed to current and future clinical applications.

GEOMETRY

Three-dimensional (Volume) Angiography

In 3D or volume acquisition methods, data are acquired from an entire volume simultaneously. In this way, 3D methods differ from 2D methods, which acquire data directly from individual slices (see Chapters 1 and 10). It should be understood, however, that whether the data are acquired by a 2D or 3D method, the images that are initially reconstructed from the data are simply 2D slices.

In 3D methods, a relatively thick slice or slab is excited. The slab is subdivided into thin slices or partitions by phase encoding along the z-direction

FIGURE 4–45. Conventional SE images occasionally demonstrate angiogram-like vascular detail. Short arrows = anterior cerebral artery; arrowhead = basilar artery; open arrow = internal cerebral vein.

TABLE 4–6. METHODS FOR MR ANGIOGRAPHY

Name	Geometry	Flow Contrast	Background Suppression Method	Scan Time	Limitations
Line scan	1D	FRE	Presat	20 msec	*
Projection	2D	Cardiac gated rephased/ dephased	Subtraction	3–10 min	†,‡,¶
Projection	2D	Ungated rephased/ dephased	Subtraction	0.5–3 min	‡,¶,**
Presat	2D	Unsaturated— presaturated or preinverted	Subtraction	3–10 min	†,§
Volume	3D	FRE	None	2–15 min	†,‖
Sequential 2D	2D	FRE	None	< 10 sec/image	

*Low S/N
†Patient motion
‡Incomplete background subtraction due to eddy current effects
§Limited FOV
‖Long reconstruction time
¶Overlap of arteries and veins
**Ghost artifacts suppressed by extensive signal averaging

(in addition to the usual y-direction). With 3D methods the strength of the slice-selection gradient is reduced for a given slice thickness as compared with 2D methods. As a result, limitations in peak gradient amplitude are avoided, and slice thicknesses ≤1 mm can be readily obtained.

High resolution MR angiograms can be obtained using 3D methods in conjunction with GRE pulse sequences. For imaging of flow, 3D FLASH sequences provide certain advantages over 3D SE sequences as well as over 2D FLASH sequences.

Improved Imaging Time

Imaging time for 3D acquisitions is expressed as:

$$\text{Imaging time} = TR \times N_y \times N_z \times NEX \quad (10)$$

where N_y and N_z are the number of phase-encoded views along the y- and z-axes, respectively. With SE sequences, in which TR cannot be reduced much below 200 msec, the imaging time for volume data is prohibitive, typically on the order of one hour. On the other hand, much shorter TR can be used with GRE methods. For instance, the imaging time for a 3D FLASH acquisition using a TR of 20 msec, 128 projections along the y- and z-axes, and a single excitation is only 20 msec × 128 × 128 = 5.5 minutes. By restricting data acquisition to a limited volume such as the carotid bifurcation, imaging is even faster because fewer z-phase–encoding steps are needed to produce the desired slice thickness.

Flow Contrast

Three-dimensional FLASH images demonstrate greater vascular enhancement than 3D SE images. Flow contrast on 3D FLASH images varies with the excitation flip angle, TR, direction, and velocity of flow. Vascular enhancement is prominent when the spins first enter the imaging volume. However, vascular enhancement decreases as the flowing spins are exposed to repeated RF excitations. After several excitations, an equilibrium is reached between saturation and inflow effects. For in-plane flow, flow contrast is best maintained with small-to-moderate flip angles (Fig. 4–46). With TR of 30 to 70 msec, satisfactory results can be obtained with flip angles of 15 to 40 degrees. Larger flip angles can be used for flow perpendicular to the plane of section as long as the 3D slab is not too thick.

An important additional consideration is the geometry of the transmitter coil. Flow contrast is maximized by using a transmitter coil that is large enough to produce a uniform field of excitation over the region of interest, but not so large as to encompass inflowing spins. For instance, certain head coils can be used to image both the carotid bifurcation and intracranial circulation. With these relatively small antennae, spins outside of the coil volume, including the heart and great vessels, are not affected by the RF excitations. When unsaturated blood from these regions flows into the imaging volume of the coil, it produces excellent flow contrast. However, flow contrast is reduced when the body coil is used as transmitter. In this case the heart and great vessels are contained within a larger volume of excitation, and the blood pool becomes saturated. This problem can be ameliorated by orienting the 3D slab so as to avoid the great vessels. Alternatively, an axial RF excitation can be applied to a limited tissue volume (e.g., 10 cm), while read-out is performed in a coronal or sagittal plane. In this way, accidental saturation of the great vessels is avoided.

Susceptibility Artifact

Three-dimensional GRE images demonstrate reduced magnetic susceptibility artifacts compared with 2D GRE images.[55] These artifacts are typically seen near the sphenoid sinus and mastoid air cells. Susceptibility artifacts decrease with slice thickness; thin slices are readily obtained with 3D techniques.

Three-dimensional methods are well suited for

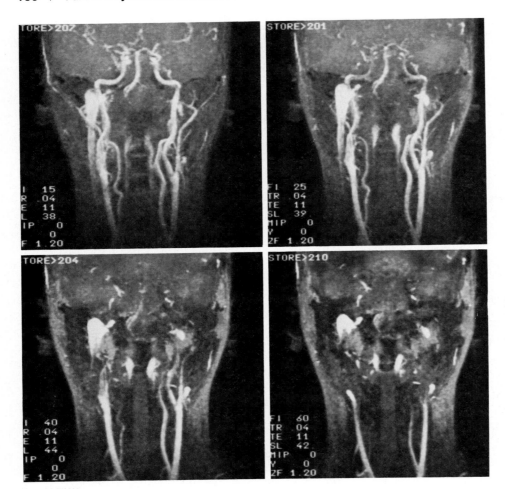

FIGURE 4–46. Effect of flip angle on in-plane flow contrast in 3D FLASH acquisitions. Coronal images through neck vessels obtained with TR = 40 msec, TE = 11 msec. Larger flip angles (40° bottom left, 60° bottom right) produce maximal flow contrast for the proximal carotid arteries, but smaller flip angles (15° top left, 25° top right) produce greater penetration into the imaging volume, allowing visualization of the intracranial circulation.

both small and large FOV applications. Both carotid arteries can be imaged simultaneously using a two slab 3D acquisition in a sagittal orientation, with one slab centered over each carotid bifurcation. Alternatively, a single 3D slab can be imaged in a coronal plane to include both carotid arteries, though in our experience partial volume averaging is then more apparent. Once a 3D data set has been acquired, the images can be manipulated in several ways. Individual images can be viewed to evaluate fine anatomic detail and to eliminate vessel overlap. In addition, angiogram-like images can be produced in any orientation using maximum intensity projection methods.[56]

Maximum Intensity Projection

The maximum intensity projection (MIP) technique processes a series of slices that are acquired by 2D or 3D methods. A straight line (ray) is projected through these slices along a selected orientation (Fig. 4–47). This ray corresponds to a single pixel in the final angiographic image. This pixel is assigned the intensity of the brightest voxel intersected by the ray. Since the brightest voxel should represent flowing blood, only vascular structures are represented in the

final image. The procedure is repeated using parallel rays until a full 2D projection angiogram is generated. Using this technique, angiograms can be reconstructed in multiple projections. Three-dimensional images may be processed using the MIP algorithm to produce exquisite high-resolution angiograms of the carotid bifurcation and intracerebral arteries (Fig. 4–48).

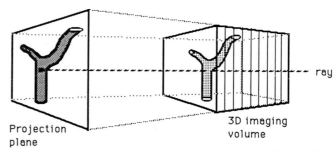

FIGURE 4–47. Maximum intensity projection method. A projection angiogram may be reconstructed from a series of contiguous or overlapping images, along any orientation. A series of rays are projected through the volume in the selected orientation. Along each ray, the voxel with the highest signal intensity is assumed to represent a blood vessel. Each ray is used to determine the intensity of one pixel in the projection image.

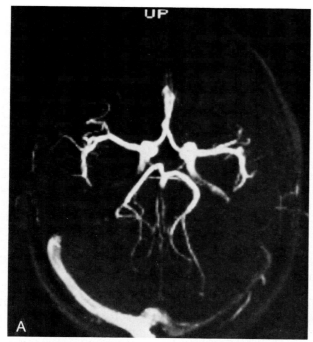

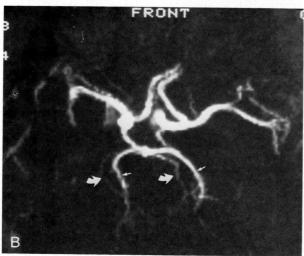

FIGURE 4–48. Axial 3D angiogram demonstrating normal circle of Willis. Scan parameters are: 3D flow-compensated FLASH sequence; TR/TE/NEX = 40 msec/8 msec/1 with flip angle = 20 degrees; slab thickness = 80 mm; 64 partitions with partition thickness = 1.25 mm. Imaging time = 10.7 minutes. *A,* Straight axial projection. *B,* 30-degree oblique projection reconstructed from same data eliminates overlap between superior cerebellar arteries (*curved arrows*) and posterior cerebral arteries (*straight arrows*).

Sometimes, despite proper selection of pulse sequence and timing parameters, flow contrast may not be adequate to permit vessels and background to be distinguished solely on the basis of signal intensity. More elaborate pixel classification schemes can be used in this case.[57] Pixel classification algorithms assign a feature vector to each voxel; this vector contains information about the signal intensity of the voxel and its 3D relationship to adjacent voxels. Certain rules are developed which, in conjunction with the feature vector, allow unambiguous assign-

ment of a voxel as vessel or background. Such rules might include restrictions as to vessel size, shape, and connectivity. Subtraction methods (below) also provide effective identification of vascular structures in situations where flow contrast is modest.

In general, the most severe limitation of 3D imaging is sensitivity to patient motion. This problem is exacerbated because volume images are usually acquired with a single excitation and because ghost artifacts alias along two dimensions instead of just one. However, with anisotropic 3D acquisitions, imaging times have been reduced to as little as 2 to 4 minutes for a carotid angiogram, so that motion is infrequently a problem. Also, because 3D data sets are typically larger than 2D data sets, reconstruction times will be correspondingly longer. The images must then be manipulated to create the projection angiograms, which may also be quite time consuming. Off-line processing on a dedicated 3D workstation can be invaluable if throughput is to be maintained.

Sequential 2D Arteriography and Venography

Although 3D angiograms have yielded excellent results for imaging of the arterial supply to the brain, methods based on 2D acquisitions have proved superior for other applications. An example is sequential 2D angiography, which can be applied when motion precludes using 3D methods.[58] In addition, this method has advantages for imaging of the venous circulation.

Sequential 2D angiography combines several standard techniques to overcome many of the limitations of previously described angiographic methods. The basic principle is similar to the 3D method, in that a series of images are obtained which are then processed to create a projection angiogram. However, rather than use a time-consuming 3D data acquisition, 2D slices are acquired individually using a flow-compensated FLASH sequence. Sample scan parameters are: slice thickness = 5 mm with 1 mm overlap of adjacent slices, TR = 30 msec, NEX = 1, and acquisition matrix = 256 × 256. For this TR, a flip angle of 20 to 30 degrees produces adequate flow contrast independent of the plane of section. However, in small veins with slow flow, which lie predominantly within the plane of section, flow contrast may be decreased. For cerebral venography, this may sometimes necessitate altering the plane of the acquisition in order to maximize flow contrast.

Once a series of 2D images is acquired, spanning the vascular structures of interest, the images are processed by the MIP algorithm to produce a projection angiogram. Like 3D angiograms, a series of different projections can be reconstructed to eliminate overlap between vessels.

There are both advantages and disadvantages for 2D compared with 3D methods. First, because individual slices can be acquired within a breath-hold, this method has been used to produce MR angiograms of the chest, abdomen, and pelvis where 3D methods are not applicable. Second, 2D angiograms show most venous structures better than 3D studies. The reason is that 3D methods use a thick slab for excitation, which increases the likelihood that slowly flowing veins will become saturated as they flow within the plane of section. This is less of a problem for 2D angiograms as long as the slice thickness is reasonably thin (e.g., 5 mm). Finally, another benefit of the method is that it is indifferent to the type of pulse sequence and slice thickness used to produce the individual slices, as long as the FOV and matrix are constant. For instance, one can vary the TR and flip angle so as to maximize flow contrast over selected regions, depending on the direction and velocity of flow. One can even repeat acquisitions at the same slice location and use two images obtained with different slice thicknesses, TRs, and flip angles so as to maximize flow contrast. This is not feasible with 3D methods due to the longer imaging times.

The major disadvantage of 2D angiograms as compared with 3D is that the voxel is larger, resulting in greater signal loss from turbulent flow. There is also the potential for image misregistration, though this has not proved to be a major impediment in practice. Clinical results using these methods will be presented below.

Projection Acquisition

Projection acquisition methods differ fundamentally from 3D and sequential 2D techniques. The former methods acquire discrete slices, each having a finite, thin slice thickness. However, in projection acquisition methods the slice-selection gradient is not applied. As a result, the angiographic image is directly acquired as a true, full-thickness summation of all tissue signal along the direction of the projection (Fig. 4–49). In this sense projection angiograms are like conventional x-ray angiograms. The major advantage of this method compared with conventional MR imaging with tomographic slices is that the full thickness of the blood vessel along with its branches are imaged. Compared with 3D and sequential 2D techniques, direct acquisition of projection images requires less data manipulation. However, practical applications have been limited for reasons discussed below.

On an image obtained with the projection acquisition method, the background signal, which comes from almost all the voxels, will completely overwhelm the much smaller vascular signal, which comes from a relatively few voxels. In order to extract flow signal from the much larger background signal, one can

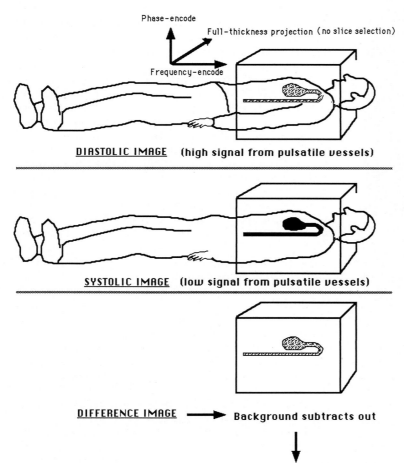

FIGURE 4–49. Principle of subtraction angiography using projection acquisitions. Blood vessels can be made to appear bright using flow compensation and/or diastolic gating. They can be made to appear dark using dephasing gradients, systolic gating, and/or presaturation. The image with low vascular signal (*middle*) is subtracted from the image with high vascular signal (*top*). Difference image only contains blood vessels.

use either of two general approaches: (1) obtain a pair of images with different flow sensitivities; then, like digital subtraction angiography, subtract the images to eliminate signal from stationary tissues; and (2) presaturate stationary tissues so that only inflowing spins produce signal. Examples of subtraction methods include presaturation angiography and phase projection angiography; an example of a method using direct background suppression is line scan angiography.

Image Subtraction Using Presaturation or Preinversion

With this method, two images are acquired. In one of these images the longitudinal magnetization of inflowing spins has been altered in order to reduce vascular signal. Since the two images differ only in the signal from flowing blood but have identical background signal, pairwise subtraction of them produces a pure flow image (Fig. 4–50).

Because of T_1 relaxation, presaturation with a 90-degree RF pulse will only eliminate vascular signal over a limited distance. Saturation effects can be maintained over longer distances by increasing the flip angle, that is, by preinverting the spins, rather than by presaturating them. One method for inverting the spins is *adiabatic fast passage,* which uses continuous, rather than pulsed, RF energy transmitted by a surface coil.[59] More simply, a 180-degree RF pulse can be used to invert the spins.[60] Subtraction of projection images obtained with and without preinversion produces the MR angiogram. Although good results have been obtained for small FOV applications such as carotid angiography, these methods are not well suited for imaging vessels such as the aorta which require a larger FOV.

Image Subtraction Using Phase-Dependent Methods

In phase-dependent methods, a pair of projection images is acquired for the purpose of image subtrac-tion.[61] The flow sensitivities of the two images are modified using cardiac gating, flow compensation and gradient dephasing, or both.

CARDIAC GATING

Phase shifts are velocity dependent, and velocity in turn depends on whether the image is acquired during systole or diastole. In systole, flow is rapid, resulting in large phase shifts and signal loss; in diastole, phase shifts are reduced and vascular signal is higher. Pairwise image subtraction eliminates background signal, which does not vary over the cardiac cycle, thereby producing an angiogram (Fig. 4–51). Major limitations of the technique include relatively long imaging times and the need to know in advance what trigger delays to use in order to maximize flow contrast. It may not be possible to use the same trigger delay for imaging of all parts of the vessel. For instance, in the abdominal aorta, maximal systolic flow contrast is typically obtained with a 200 to 300 msec trigger delay following the R wave. The corresponding trigger delay near the popliteal trifurcation is significantly longer, on the order of 350 to 400 msec. Furthermore, diastolic flow is considerable in vessels with low peripheral resistance such as the internal carotid artery. This results in signal loss, which adversely affects flow contrast. Also, variations in the heart rate between acquisitions will affect the signal intensity of stationary tissues differently in the two projection images, resulting in imperfect image subtraction.

FLOW COMPENSATION AND GRADIENT DEPHASING

The use of flow compensation and dephasing gradients with or without cardiac gating represents a more robust approach for flow imaging than cardiac gating alone. Two images are acquired. In one image, flow signal is maximized by flow compensation; in the other image, flow signal is minimized by gradient dephasing. Pairwise subtraction of the magnitude images produces an angiogram.

Theoretically, a modification of this approach can

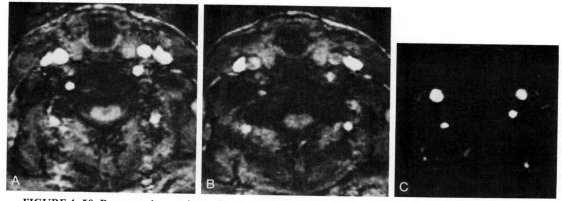

FIGURE 4–50. Presaturation angiography. *A,* Axial FLASH image of neck obtained without presaturation. *B,* Same as (A) but with presaturation below imaging, volume shows reduced signal in carotid and vertebral arteries. *C,* Subtraction (A − B) produces flow image of carotid and vertebral arteries.

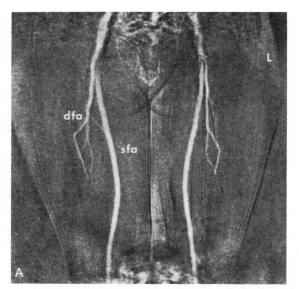

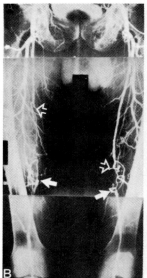

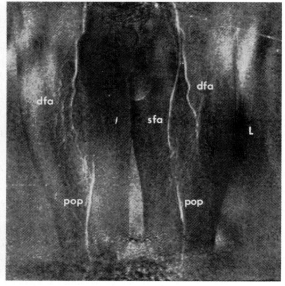

FIGURE 4–51. Angiograms created by pairwise subtraction of systolic and diastolic projection images for evaluation of peripheral arteries. *A,* MR angiogram of thighs in normal subject demonstrates superficial (sfa) and deep (dfa) femoral arteries. Blurring of detail over pelvis is due to bowel peristalsis. Imaging time = 8 minutes; diastolic and systolic trigger delays were 10 msec and 250 msec, respectively. *B,* Patient with vascular occlusions. *Left,* Conventional angiogram demonstrates occlusion of both sfa (*open arrows*) with reconstitution distally (*closed arrows*) via collaterals. *Right,* MR angiogram demonstrates comparable appearance in left leg. In right leg, proximal extent of occlusion is exaggerated because flow contrast is reduced by slow flow. Note imperfect background subtraction because of gradient-induced eddy currents.

be used to enhance flow contrast.[62] Rather than use a pair of rephased/dephased images, both images are acquired with identical flow-sensitizing gradients so that vascular signal is the same for both. However, the second image is acquired with inverted gradients that produce a flow-related phase shift identical in magnitude, but of opposite sign, to that produced by the gradients in the first image (Fig. 4–52). In theory, complex image subtraction could produce flow contrast proportional to $2\sin(\Theta)$. This approach has also been used with 3D acquisitions. However, the need to repeat the acquisition with flow-encoding gradients along each direction prolongs the acquisition time (typically 15 to 30 minutes).[62a]

The subtraction methods described above have significant drawbacks. The extra time required to obtain two sets of images increases the likelihood of patient motion and resultant image misregistration, a familiar problem in digital subtraction angiography.

This problem is minimized by interleaving acquisition of the two data sets. However, misregistration would not be a problem if a method were available for suppressing background signal without the need for

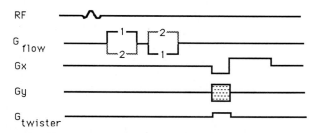

FIGURE 4–52. Compared with a (rephased/dephased) angiogram, increased flow contrast can be extracted using complex subtraction of a pair of rephased images; images differ only in the polarity of the flow-encoding gradients (1 and 2). Note use of twister gradient, which is essential for projection acquisitions in order to avoid dynamic range problems.

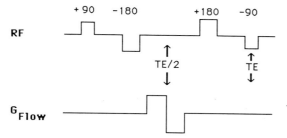

FIGURE 4–53. Signal from stationary spins can be suppressed using a variation of a driven-equilibrium pulse sequence. Four RF pulses rotate the magnetization of stationary spins away from, and then back onto, the z-axis. With their magnetization entirely along the z-axis at the echo time, stationary spins produce no signal. G_{flow} produces a phase shift for flowing spins only. As a result, a portion of the magnetization of flowing spins lies in the transverse plane during read-out to produce a signal.

image subtraction. One such method produces signal from flowing, but not stationary, spins using a modified driven-equilibrium pulse sequence (Fig. 4–53). The modification consists of a bipolar flow-encoding gradient that produces phase shifts only for flowing spins. For stationary spins, the driven-equilibrium sequence eventually returns all magnetization to the z-axis. However, the phase shifts produced by flow interfere with the driven-equilibrium process for flowing blood, so that a portion of their magnetization remains in the transverse plane. If read-out is performed at the end of the sequence, then flowing blood produces a signal; but stationary spins, which are aligned along the z-axis, produce no signal.[63]

There are a number of practical difficulties with projection acquisition methods, including sensitivity to eddy currents, motion, vessel overlap, and dynamic range.

SENSITIVITY TO EDDY CURRENTS. Gradient-induced eddy currents (see Chapters 1 and 12) deform the gradient waveforms. As a result, images acquired with different gradient timings and/or amplitudes (e.g., rephased/dephased) will have different signal intensities and geometric distortions, so that image subtraction is imperfect (Fig. 4–51B). The sensitivity to eddy current effects is particularly severe with methods that use complex subtraction or driven equilibrium. This problem is ameliorated by careful optimization of eddy current compensation, including techniques such as active gradient shielding (see Chapter 12), as well as by attention to pulse sequence design (see Chapter 10).

VESSEL OVERLAP. On projection images, arterial and venous structures may overlap. For instance, in angiograms of the neck, the internal jugular vein may partly obscure the carotid bifurcation. An additional problem is that signals from the carotid artery and jugular vein may cancel if the two structures overlap. The reason for this is that blood flows in opposite directions in the artery and vein; as a result, the phase shifts may have opposite signs. If the artery and vein lie in the same voxel, which will be the case if they overlap in a projection image, then the opposing phase shifts result in signal loss.

Overlap between arteries and veins can be reduced by reorienting the plane of projection or by presaturating venous inflow. Another approach is to obtain an additional image with flow compensation that has been calibrated to enhance signal from slow flow (i.e., veins) only. An angiogram produced from (fully rephased/partially rephased) images shows arterial flow only.[64]

DYNAMIC RANGE. Signal from stationary tissues is very large, since the angiogram represents a full thickness of the body. This large signal can exceed the dynamic range (digitization capacity) of the analog-to-digital converter (ADC) (see Chapter 3). The problem can be overcome by reducing the receiver gain, but this eliminates the much smaller signal contributed by flowing spins. One solution to this problem is to apply a twister gradient.

The twister gradient is simply a weak gradient applied along the projection axis which causes a gradual phase shift along this direction (Fig. 4–52). As may be deduced from Equation 5b, the twister produces a difference in the phases of spins at different positions along the gradient; this difference is proportional to their separation. The most extreme phase differences occur between spins at opposite ends of the voxel, which in a projection acquisition are at opposite sides of the body. Across this large distance, the twister gradient produces more than 360 degrees of phase dispersion, and its effect is to eliminate signal from background spins. However, across the much narrower thickness of a blood vessel, the twister gradient produces only a small amount of phase dispersion so that vascular signal is maintained.

FIELD INHOMOGENEITY. Yet another potential problem for angiograms acquired with projection techniques relates to omnipresent local magnetic field inhomogeneities, which are due to structural imperfections in the magnet and variations in tissue susceptibility. Normally, with 2D and 3D acquisitions, the slice-selection gradient overwhelms these field imperfections. Since projection acquisitions do not use slice selection, these field imperfections may cause loss of spatial resolution, thereby interfering with the depiction of small vessels. The problem is ameliorated by using very short echo times, but this may not be feasible with flow-compensated sequences.

One-Dimensional

Line scan angiograms can be acquired nearly instantaneously in just a few milliseconds.[65] A standard GRE pulse sequence is used; however, rather than acquire the usual 128 to 256 phase encodings, the phase-encoding gradient is not applied. The resulting image is a one-dimensional projection (line). Since the sequence is not repeated, the imaging time is simply the echo time.

Ghost artifacts, due to motion between views, do not occur in these images. Flow contrast is enhanced by presaturating the imaging volume so that only inflowing spins produce signal (Fig. 4–54). Two-dimensional angiograms can be built up from serial

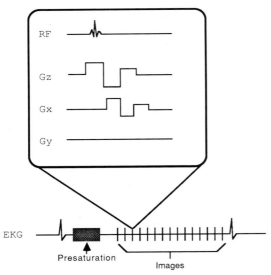

FIGURE 4–54. Gated line scan pulse sequence diagram. Acquisition of flow images with this method is essentially instantaneous (< 20 msec) because only a single projection is obtained; that is, no phase-encoding is performed. Background signal is suppressed by initial in-slice presaturation; signal read-out is performed after a time delay to allow inflow of fresh spins.

line scans. However, image quality is limited, since S/N per unit of time for an N-line image acquired by serial line scanning is only $1/\sqrt{N}$ that of the same image acquired by 2DFT methods.

DISPLAY METHODS

Once 3D or sequential 2D angiograms are reconstructed, they can be viewed by several means. The projections can be displayed on a 3D workstation, which permits smooth rotation of the images to provide a 3D effect. However, the 3D effect can also be reproduced using static displays such as stereoscopy. Using the MIP algorithm, pairs of projection images with different viewing angles can be obtained. If a pair of angiographic images are selected with a difference of approximately 6 degrees in the projection angles, these image pairs provide a 3D aspect of the displayed vascular structures. The images can be viewed either with a stereoscopic viewing device or directly by radiologists with experience in viewing stereo images. This method is often used in conventional angiography but might have a special impact for MR angiography, where arbitrary projections can be created. Even large, complex structures such as arteriovenous malformations (AVM) can be analyzed with this display method (Fig. 4–55). However, individual stereo images do not provide as much information as does the full complement of 3D projection images.

CONTRAST AGENTS

Contrast agents may be classified into three groups: T_1 active, T_2 active, and nonproton (see Chapter 7). T_1-active agents predominantly shorten T_1; T_2-active agents shorten T_2; and nonproton agents contain no hydrogen and therefore appear black on proton images.

An example of a T_1-active agent is gadolinium-DTPA. By shortening the T_1 relaxation time of blood, gadolinium-DTPA produces a marked enhancement of vascular signal (Fig. 4–56). By enhancing vascular signal, T_1-active agents can improve flow contrast on MR angiograms.[65a] However, by increasing vascular signal, these agents also worsen ghost artifacts. In addition, as mentioned earlier, the efficacy of presaturation methods for suppressing flow-related

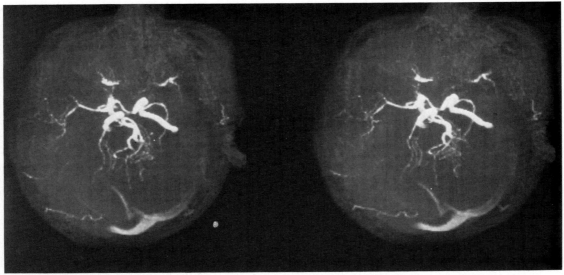

FIGURE 4–55. Stereo images of arteriovenous malformation fed primarily by left posterior choroidal artery. Three-dimensional effect permits determination of relative anteroposterior depth of vessels.

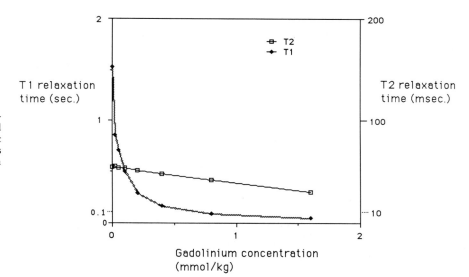

FIGURE 4–56. Effect of gadolinium-DTPA on relaxation times of heparinized whole blood. Over the range of physiologic concentrations of contrast agent, the effects of T_1 shortening dominate, resulting in marked enhancement of vascular signal.

ghost artifacts is reduced because of the shortened T_1 relaxation time of blood.

Alternatively, T_2-active agents such as dysprosium-DTPA and magnetite predominantly shorten T_2 and reduce, rather than enhance, intravascular signal. Dynamic MR imaging following bolus administration of T_1- and T_2-active contrast agents has been used to study organ perfusion (see Chapter 25).

CLINICAL POTENTIAL OF MR ANGIOGRAPHY

Peripheral Vascular Imaging

From a technical point of view, MR angiography of the peripheral vascular system is straightforward. Normally, systolic flow velocities are high and dia-

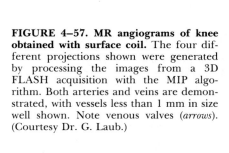

FIGURE 4–57. MR angiograms of knee obtained with surface coil. The four different projections shown were generated by processing the images from a 3D FLASH acquisition with the MIP algorithm. Both arteries and veins are demonstrated, with vessels less than 1 mm in size well shown. Note venous valves (arrows). (Courtesy Dr. G. Laub.)

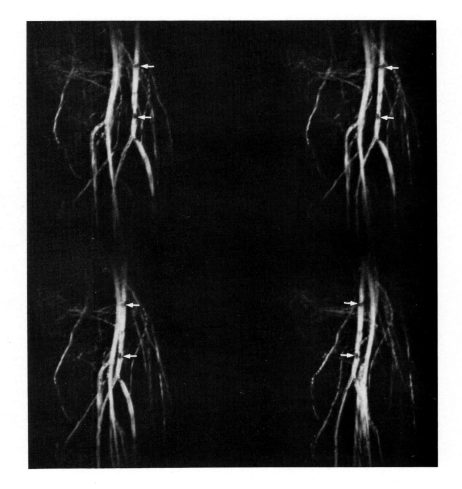

stolic velocities are low, providing good flow contrast on cardiac-gated subtraction images (see Fig. 4–51). Patient motion is not a major problem except in the pelvis, where peristalsis and, to a lesser extent, respiration cause artifacts. Peristalsis can be suppressed by administration of glucagon, 1 mg intramuscularly or subcutaneously. The preferred orientation for image acquisition is the coronal plane, using a large (e.g., 30 to 50 cm) FOV to cover the region of interest. Three-dimensional, sequential 2D, and projection acquisition techniques can be used for peripheral vascular imaging. Demonstration of small branches about the knee is facilitated by use of a surface coil to enhance S/N (Fig. 4–57).

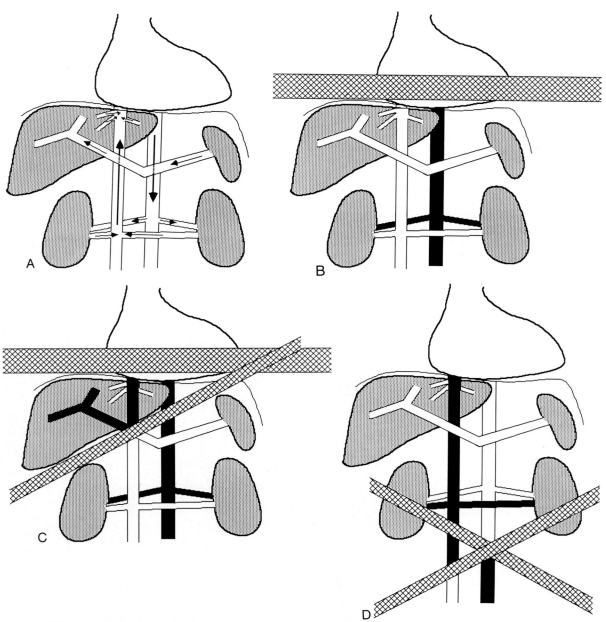

FIGURE 4–58. Illustration of presaturation schemes for selective MR angiography of the various intraabdominal blood vessels (coronal orientation). Presaturation volumes are shown as cross-hatched areas. *A,* Schematic of major intraabdominal arteries and veins showing direction of flow. *B,* In order to eliminate signal from inflowing spins in the aorta, an axial presaturation volume is applied above the diaphragms. Only venous structures are then visualized. *C,* Simultaneous horizontal and oblique presaturations as shown can be combined to eliminate signal from inflowing spins in both the aorta and portal vein. As a result, the hepatic veins are visualized without overlap from the portal veins. *D,* Two presaturation volumes can be applied in crisscross fashion to simultaneously eliminate signal in the inferior vena cava and renal veins. Although the saturation only affects the mid and lower poles of the kidneys, mixing of this dark blood with bright blood from the upper poles is sufficient to eliminate the renal veins from the angiogram. Alternatively, one could apply presaturation of kidneys in a sagittal orientation. However, this would encompass parts of the heart and would thereby reduce signal in the aorta and renal arteries.

At the present time there are major limitations for MR angiography of the lower extremities. Vascular stenoses may produce turbulent flow distal to the lesion, resulting in exaggeration of the apparent extent of the stenosis. This problem may be ameliorated as more effective techniques for flow compensation are developed. Conversely, slow flow proximal to stenoses may also yield inadequate flow contrast. Another problem is that high spatial resolution is essential, since patency of small vessels may be critical for determining vascular runoff and for planning bypass surgery. Although spatial resolution of 300 μ

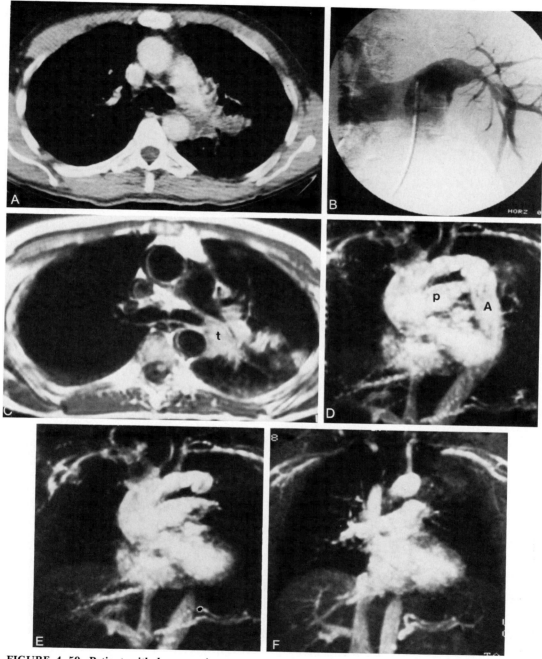

FIGURE 4–59. Patient with lung carcinoma encasing left pulmonary artery. A, Involvement of left pulmonary artery and aorticopulmonary window by tumor is demonstrated by contrast-enhanced CT. B, Pulmonary arteriogram shows constriction of left pulmonary artery. C, Spin-echo image obtained with flow presaturation also shows relationship of tumor (t) to pulmonary artery. D, Left anterior oblique (LAO) projection of MR angiogram shows overlap of aorta (A) with left pulmonary artery (P). E, LAO and (f) coronal projections, reconstructed from a limited set of image data that excludes the aorta, now clearly show the constriction of the left pulmonary artery by the tumor.

can be obtained over small regions using surface coils and 3D methods, it is more difficult to obtain high spatial resolution over larger FOVs.

MR Angiography in the Body

MR angiography of the chest, abdomen, and pelvis has been problematic until recently because of image degradation from respiratory, cardiac, and peristaltic motion. However, high-quality projection angiograms have been obtained in these regions using the sequential 2D technique in conjunction with breath holding. Determination of flow directionality and selective arteriograms or venograms can be obtained by various presaturation schemes (Fig. 4–58).

Potential applications of MR angiography in the chest include evaluation of suspected pulmonary embolism and tumors (Fig. 4–59). In the abdomen, MR venograms delineate the hepatic veins, portal system,

and inferior vena cava (Fig. 4–60 and 4–61). The relationship of hepatic neoplasms to the hepatic veins, which define the segmental anatomy, may be better defined in certain cases than by other imaging techniques (Fig. 4–62). This information may be critical to patients with solitary hepatic neoplasms for whom partial hepatectomy is an option. For patients with cirrhosis of the liver, demonstration of hepatofugal flow in a patient umbilical vein (Fig. 4–63), which has been difficult using SE methods,[66] may have prognostic implications in terms of the likelihood of developing bleeding from esophageal varices.[67] Evaluation of portal flow directionality and collateral circulation in these patients is also straightforward (Fig. 4–64).

Normal renal arteries can be shown (Fig. 4–65). It may eventually prove feasible to screen for renal artery stenosis on the basis of disturbances in flow patterns on MR angiographic images. In a prospec-

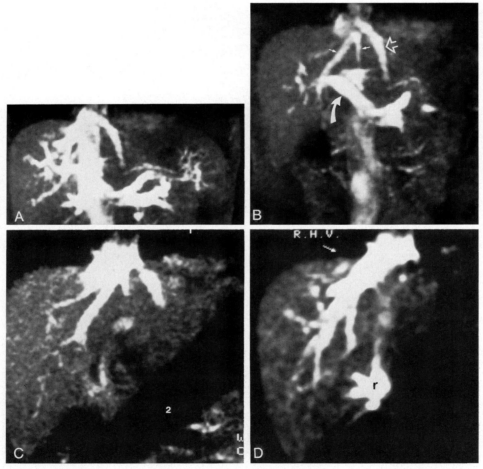

FIGURE 4–60. MR venograms of hepatic and portal venous systems in a normal subject. *A,* Selective saturation of aortic inflow. Full thickness coronal projection shows hepatic, portal, splenic, and renal veins. Precise evaluation is limited by vessel overlap. *B,* Reconstruction of selected slices excluding the inferior vena cava better shows the left hepatic vein (*open arrow*), two branches of the middle hepatic vein (*short arrows*), main portal vein (*curved arrows*) and its branches. *C* and *D,* Tailored presaturation (regions 1 and 2, compare with Fig. 4–58*C*) eliminates signal from the portal veins. The left and middle hepatic veins (*C*) and right hepatic vein (RHV) (*D*) can be shown separately from the portal veins. Portion of right renal vein (r) is also seen.

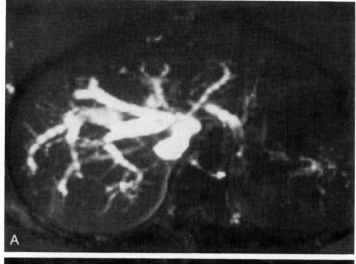

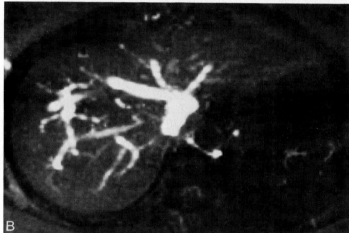

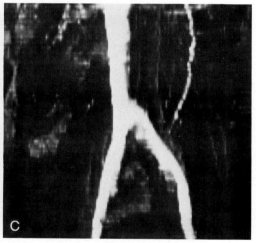

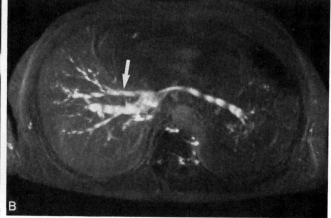

FIGURE 4–61. Projection venograms of abdomen acquired in the axial plane. *A,* Full thickness axial reconstruction shows overlapping hepatic and portal veins. Note visualization of small venous branches. *B,* By excluding the caudal portion of image data from reconstruction, the confluence of the middle and left hepatic veins with the inferior vena cava is better seen. *C,* Multiplanar reconstruction (MPR) techniques can be used to produce projection angiograms in orientations that differ from the original acquisition. Here, coronal MPR was performed on axial image data followed by MIP algorithm. Venogram shows the inferior vena cava and left gonadal vein.

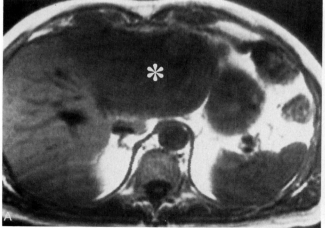

FIGURE 4–62. Metastasis involving left lobe of liver. Presaturation of aorta. *A,* T_1-weighted SE image shows tumor (*asterisk*). *B,* Projection venogram. The middle hepatic vein (*arrow*) is seen to be displaced laterally, confirming that the tumor lies entirely in the left lobe. Note serrations of some of the venous structures, representing partial volume averaging due to the use of relatively thick (7 to 10 mm) slices without overlap and lack of interpolation in the MIP algorithm.

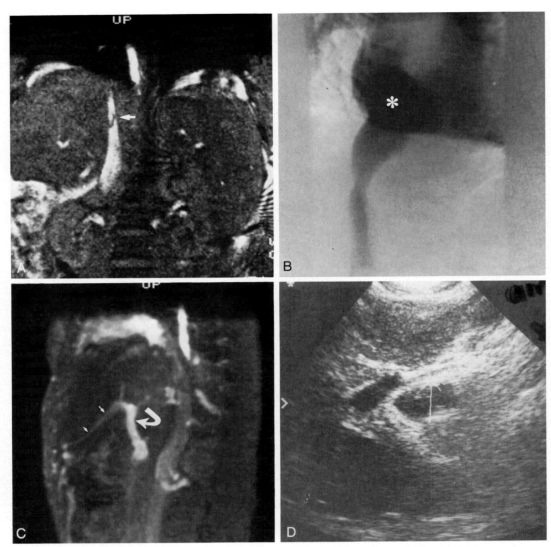

FIGURE 4–63. Budd-Chiari syndrome with patent umbilical vein. *A,* Coronal 2D FLASH image shows weblike constriction (*arrow*) of intrahepatic portion of inferior vena cava. *B,* Lateral digital subtraction venogram of IVC shows corresponding narrowing (*arrow*) (*asterisk* = right atrium). *C,* Sagittal venogram demonstrates a patent umbilical vein (*short arrows*) and collateral vessels in abdominal wall. (*Curved arrow* = left portal vein). *D,* Longitudinal sonogram demonstrates portion of patent umbilical vein (*arrow*).

tive study of 25 patients, we found that MR angiography had an accuracy greater than 90 per cent for detecting and grading the severity of renal artery stenosis and was 100 per cent accurate in determining the number of renal arteries (unpublished data). Mild-to-moderate stenoses were characterized by vessel narrowing, whereas severely stenotic arteries often showed focal or diffuse signal voids (Fig. 4–66). Studies were obtained using coronal and axial slices, 5 mm thick with 1 mm overlap, and a flow compensated FLASH sequence. Atherosclerotic plaque appeared dark and was easily shown in the aorta. However, it will likely prove more difficult to provide exact anatomic definition of the vascular lesion, and conventional angiography will be needed for further evaluation of abnormal MR angiograms. Vascular anatomy in renal transplants can also be shown. MR angiography might prove useful in renal donors and in patients with abdominal aortic aneurysms in determining the anatomy of the renal arteries (Fig. 4–67). It should also be feasible to make projection venograms of the lower extremities in patients with suspected DVT, which may be easier to interpret than on cross-sectional images.

Intracranial and Extracranial Cerebrovascular Disease

Carotid imaging currently represents the most fertile ground for MR angiography. Doppler ultra-

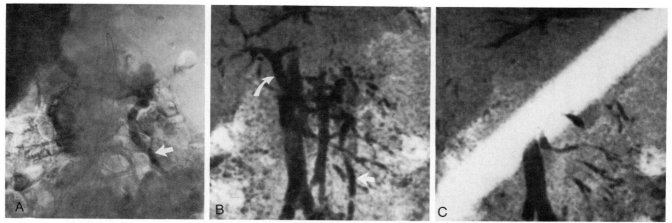

FIGURE 4–64. Patient with cirrhosis, portal hypertension, and mesenteric varices. *A,* Venous phase of a superior mesenteric angiogram. There is abnormal filling of the inferior mesenteric vein (*straight arrow*) consistent with reversed (hepatofugal) flow. However, there is normal filling of the portal vein consistent with normal (hepatocentripetal) direction of flow. *B,* Coronal MR angiogram without presaturation demonstrates inferior mesenteric vein (*straight arrow*) and portal vein (*curved arrow*). *C,* Coronal MR venogram with oblique presaturation (*white stripe*) along liver edge. The portal vein has disappeared, consistent with hepatocentripetal flow (see Fig. 4–1A). However, the inferior mesenteric vein (IMV) has also disappeared, which can only occur if there is hepatofugal flow.

sound, Doppler ultrasound combined with B-mode (duplex), and more recently color-flow Doppler and duplex currently represent the main noninvasive tools for assessment of carotid stenosis.[68] Ultrasound has several limitations, including difficulty in distinguishing occluded from severely stenotic vessels, inability to penetrate calcified plaque, and inability to image high bifurcations. Transcranial Doppler ultrasonography is capable of assessing intracranial hemodynamics, but it cannot image the intracranial vessels.[69] Flow velocities in the intra- and extracranial carotid arteries and other intracranial vessels are high (see Table 4–5). With average flow velocities in the common carotid artery of 30 cm/sec and in the internal carotid artery of 36 cm/sec (see Table 4–5), carefully calibrated flow compensation is essential.[70–73]

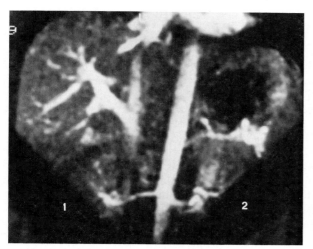

FIGURE 4–65. Coronal MR arteriogram in a normal subject showing renal arteries. Note crisscross pattern of presaturation (regions 1 and 2, see Fig. 4–1D).

Overlap with the internal jugular vein can limit evaluation of the carotid artery, but this problem is easily eliminated by rotating the projection or by presaturating venous inflow. As with digital subtraction angiography (DSA), swallowing and respiration may limit image quality.

In normal patients, a common finding on MR angiograms is signal dropout along the posterior wall, of the carotid bulb opposite the origin of the external carotid artery (Fig. 4–68) due to flow reversal. The common, internal, and external carotid arteries are well shown; external carotid artery branches are sometimes visible (Fig. 4–69).[74] Minor carotid stenoses are well shown (Fig. 4–70). However, distal to high-grade (> 50 per cent diameter) stenoses, turbulence, and vortex formation cause signal loss that may be nonrecoverable with current flow compensation schemes. As a result, the apparent extent of a stenosis can be markedly exaggerated (Fig. 4–71). In critical stenoses (80 to 90 per cent area reduction), velocities may exceed 250 centimeters per second, resulting in complete signal loss suggestive of vascular occlusion. However, carotid occlusion may be excluded by reconstitution of flow signal more distally or by use of black blood methods to anatomically define the vessel[74a] (Fig. 4–72). A preliminary study has shown that 3D MR angiography provides an accurate portrayal of carotid stenoses in most cases.[74b]

Determining whether there is cross-flow between the right and left cerebral hemispheres can be critical for presurgical planning in patients with carotid disease, seizure disorders, and tumors. This can be determined by contrast angiography or transcranial Doppler. MR using flow presaturation represents another method for determining whether cross-flow is present. In the case of unilateral carotid occlusion, this is accomplished by acquiring an axial or coronal

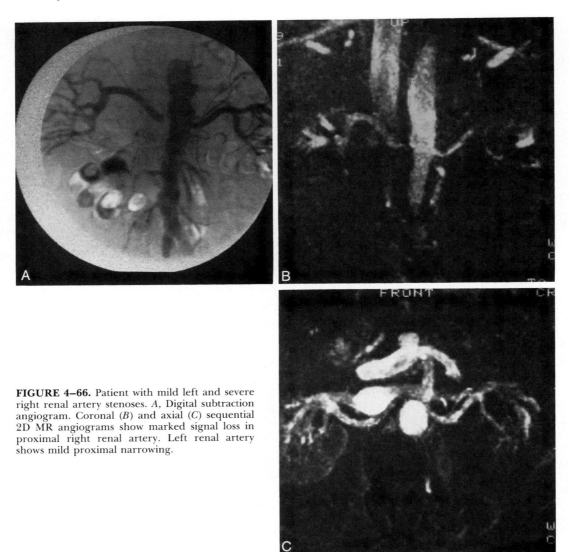

FIGURE 4–66. Patient with mild left and severe right renal artery stenoses. *A,* Digital subtraction angiogram. Coronal (*B*) and axial (*C*) sequential 2D MR angiograms show marked signal loss in proximal right renal artery. Left renal artery shows mild proximal narrowing.

flow-compensated FLASH image through the middle cerebral arteries (Fig. 4–73). Presaturation of the occluded carotid artery has no effect on the signal intensity of the contralateral middle cerebral artery (Fig. 4–73*C*). However, if there is cross-filling, then presaturation of the normal carotid artery will obliterate signal in the contralateral middle cerebral artery that it is supplying (Fig. 4–73*E*). An additional finding in these patients, seen best on 3D angiograms, is that the signal intensity of the middle cerebral artery on the normal side is higher than on the affected side, consistent with higher velocity of flow (Fig. 4–73*B*). (Signal intensities on 3D angiograms may have a complex relationship to flow velocity and flow pattern; however, in general, the flow signal intensity increases with higher velocity flow.) Similarly, presaturation can be used to evaluate filling from other vascular territories. Obviously, in patients with normal carotid arteries, cross-compression must

be performed in conjunction with presaturation to determine the presence of cross-flow.

Vascular malformations can be imaged using 3D angiographic methods, and feeding and draining vessels can be demonstrated (Fig. 4–74). Two- and three-dimensional GRE images allow calcifications within the malformation, which appear dark, to be distinguished from vascular structures, which appear bright. It is even feasible, using presaturation methods, to selectively presaturate individual feeding vessels. The reduction in the signal intensity of the malformation, resulting from presaturation of an individual feeder, might provide information about the relative flow contribution of the feeder and be useful for therapy planning (Fig. 4–74*B* and *C*). Note should be made that turbulent flow within the nidus of the malformation and feeding vessels may produce nonrecoverable signal loss. As a result, the extent of the high flow vascular component of the malforma-

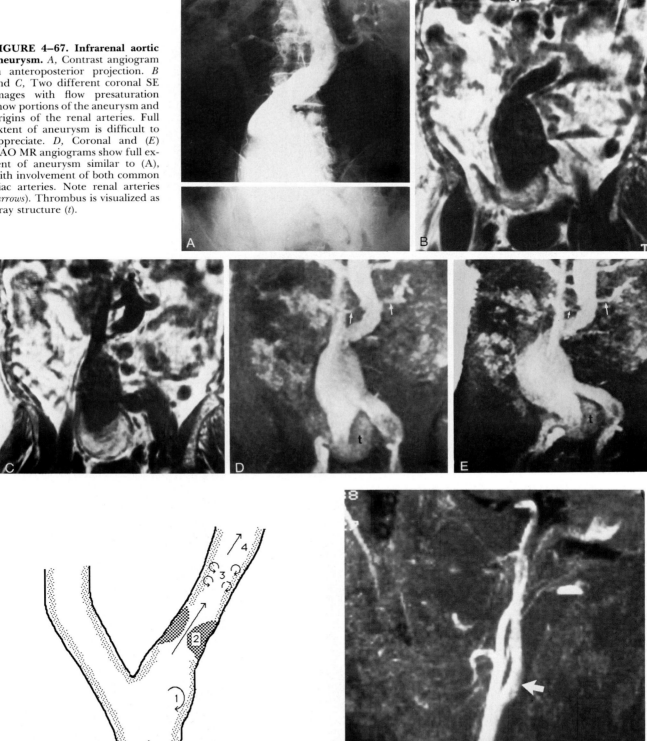

FIGURE 4–67. Infrarenal aortic aneurysm. *A*, Contrast angiogram in anteroposterior projection. *B* and *C*, Two different coronal SE images with flow presaturation show portions of the aneurysm and origins of the renal arteries. Full extent of aneurysm is difficult to appreciate. *D*, Coronal and (*E*) LAO MR angiograms show full extent of aneurysm similar to (A), with involvement of both common iliac arteries. Note renal arteries (*arrows*). Thrombus is visualized as gray structure (*t*).

FIGURE 4–68. Flow patterns in carotid bifurcation with ICA stenosis. (1) Normal vortex formation in carotid bulb opposite origin of ECA. (2) Plaque causes narrowing of lumen with resultant jet formation. (3) Vortex formation and turbulence develop distal to stenosis where lumen widens to normal diameter. (4) Flow pattern returns to normal more distally.

FIGURE 4–69. Normal 3D carotid angiogram. Scan parameters: 3D FLASH; TR/TE/NEX/flip angle = 40 msec/8 msec/1/30°; data acquired from 32 mm thick slab with 32 partitions (partition thickness = 1 mm); field-of-view = 25 cm; imaging time = 4 minutes. Carotid bifurcation and small branches of external carotid artery are shown. Note region of reduced flow signal in carotid bulb (*arrow*), due to normal flow reversal as illustrated in Fig. 4–68.

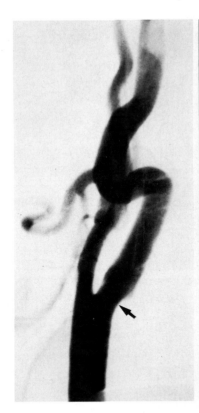

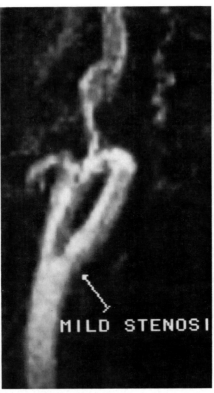

←

FIGURE 4–70. Carotid bifurcation in patient with mild stenosis at origin of internal carotid artery. Both conventional angiogram (*left*) and MR angiogram (*right*) show the stenosis (*arrows*).

→

FIGURE 4–71. Carotid bifurcation in patient with critical stenosis of the right internal carotid artery. Contrast angiogram (*left*) shows faint visualization of patent lumen distal to stenosis (*small arrows*). MR angiogram (*right*) demonstrates an artifactually large flow void, suggesting complete occlusion (*arrow*). This discrepancy can be attributed to reduced flow velocity proximal to the stenosis and turbulence distal to the stenosis.

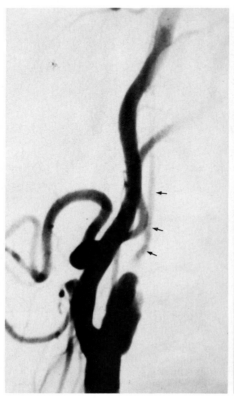

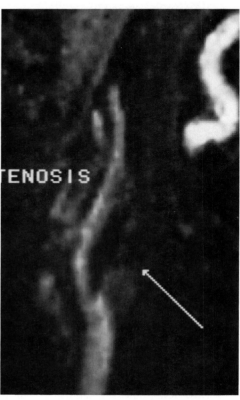

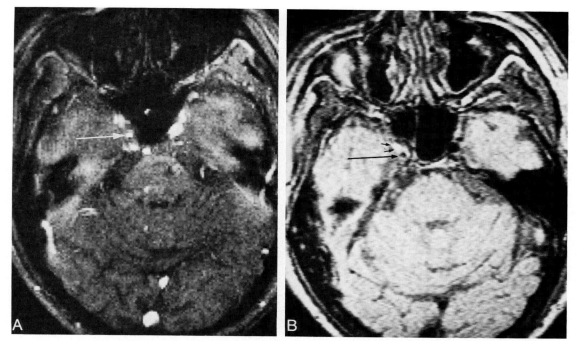

FIGURE 4–72. Same patient as in Figure 4–71. Because of a question of a tandem stenosis involving the right carotid siphon, additional studies of the siphon were performed. MR angiogram failed to demonstrate the right siphon, presumably because of slow flow. To better delineate the flow pattern and anatomy, a bright blood axial FLASH image (*left*) (TR/TE/flip angle = 30 msec/10 msec/40°; slice thickness = 4 mm) and a black blood axial SE image (*right*) (TR/TE = 700 msec/18 msec, using flow presaturation; slice thickness = 2 mm) were acquired. Both images demonstrate narrowing of the right internal carotid artery at the level of the siphon (*long arrows*). On the bright blood image, the vessel narrowing could represent either (1) stenosis or (2) vessel collapse, due to the reduced pressure head distal to the proximal ICA stenosis. However, on the black blood image, the presence of extra soft tissue (*short arrows*) adjoining the narrowed siphon is suggestive of plaque and would make stenosis of the carotid siphon the more likely diagnosis.

tion may be underestimated by bright blood images. Black blood SE images using presaturation should also be obtained for optimal evaluation. It may also be feasible to demonstrate the vascular relationships and supplies of tumors (Fig. 4–75), thereby eliminating the need for preoperative angiography.

3D MR angiography also appears to be sensitive for patent intracranial aneurysms.[75a] However, the sensitivity for very small (e.g., < 5 mm) aneurysms or for aneurysms in the setting of vascular spasm is unknown.

One potential pitfall of angiographic techniques such as 3D is that the MIP algorithm used to process the data assumes that only flowing blood can appear bright. This assumption is not necessarily true in the case of tumor enhancement by gadolinium-DTPA or hemorrhage, since these tissues may also appear bright (Fig. 4–76). Again, the combination of bright blood and dark blood techniques should be helpful to resolve such diagnostic dilemmas.

MR venograms of the intracranial circulation have been demonstrated using 3D and 2D techniques. Arterial signal is eliminated using a presaturation pulse positioned caudal to the brain. Although 3D methods can demonstrate the larger venous sinuses, as previously mentioned small veins with slow in-plane flow become saturated within the thick excitation slab and are poorly visualized. These veins are well seen on sequential 2D venograms. Using this method, one can evaluate suspected slow-flow venous malformations, venous infarction, and sinus thrombosis (Fig. 4–77).

To date, MR has not yet proved competitive with duplex ultrasound and contrast angiography in assessment of the carotid circulation. More precise delineation of plaque ulceration and stenoses is needed. On bright blood images, the surface characteristics of a plaque (e.g., roughness suggesting ulceration) may be invisible due to stasis of blood. Better evaluation in some cases might be provided by black blood techniques (Fig. 4–78). Blood flow can be made to appear dark on SE images by using flow presaturation in combination with a very thin slice (the latter so as to maximize signal loss due to wash-out effects). Black blood images should be superior for demonstrating intraplaque hemorrhage, which may appear bright and be obscured by adjacent flow signal on bright blood images. Fat content of the plaque may be evaluated using chemical shift imaging methods (see Chapters 9 and 10).

As from bright blood images, angiogram-like images could be produced from black blood images

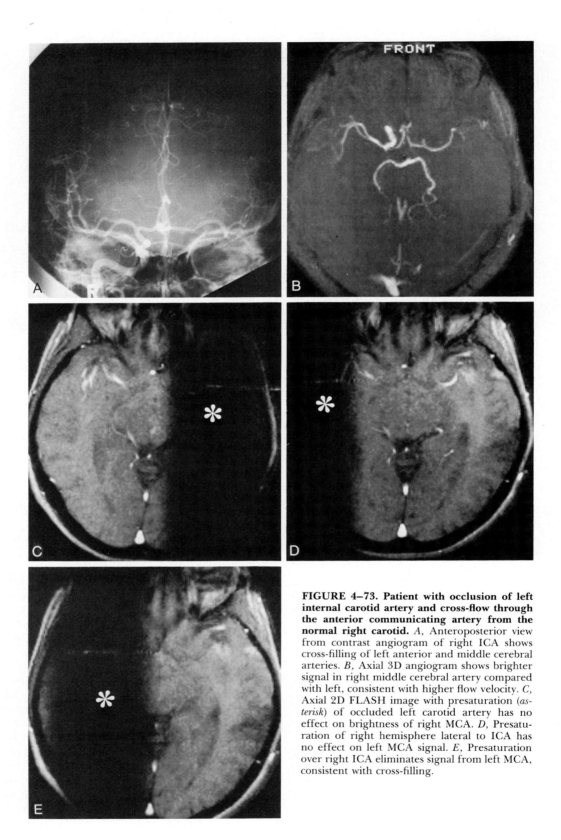

FIGURE 4–73. Patient with occlusion of left internal carotid artery and cross-flow through the anterior communicating artery from the normal right carotid. *A,* Anteroposterior view from contrast angiogram of right ICA shows cross-filling of left anterior and middle cerebral arteries. *B,* Axial 3D angiogram shows brighter signal in right middle cerebral artery compared with left, consistent with higher flow velocity. *C,* Axial 2D FLASH image with presaturation (*asterisk*) of occluded left carotid artery has no effect on brightness of right MCA. *D,* Presaturation of right hemisphere lateral to ICA has no effect on left MCA signal. *E,* Presaturation over right ICA eliminates signal from left MCA, consistent with cross-filling.

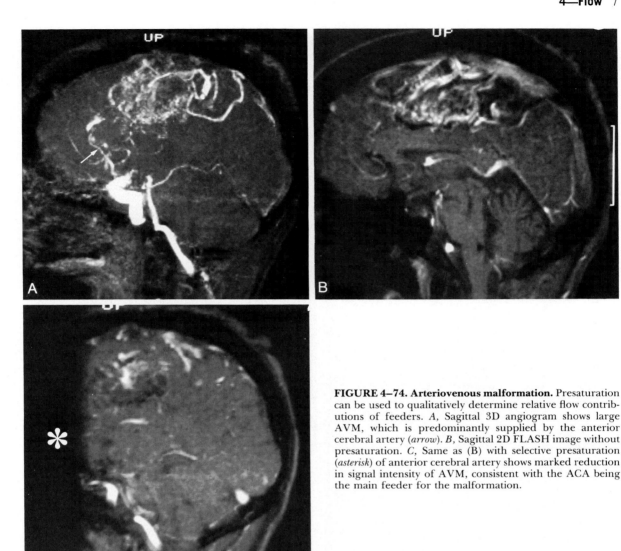

FIGURE 4–74. Arteriovenous malformation. Presaturation can be used to qualitatively determine relative flow contributions of feeders. *A*, Sagittal 3D angiogram shows large AVM, which is predominantly supplied by the anterior cerebral artery (*arrow*). *B*, Sagittal 2D FLASH image without presaturation. *C*, Same as (*B*) with selective presaturation (*asterisk*) of anterior cerebral artery shows marked reduction in signal intensity of AVM, consistent with the ACA being the main feeder for the malformation.

using a ray projection method. However, for black blood images, the signal intensity of each pixel is assigned that of the voxel which has the *minimum*, rather than maximum, signal intensity. Problems with black blood angiograms include poor visibility of calcified plaque and limited S/N.

With further technical development (in particular, the combined use of optimized black blood and bright blood angiographic methods), MR may come to replace other vascular imaging modalities in a substantial proportion of patients, with the benefit of reduced invasiveness. Cost will remain an issue if MR is to become a screening examination.

Coronary Artery Imaging

Imaging of coronary arteries is the most challenging task in MR angiography, and success in this application would have enormous clinical benefit.[75]

Three-dimensional and projection acquisition methods are precluded by respiratory and intrinsic cardiac motion. The small size of the coronary arteries exacerbates the problem.

Proximal coronary arteries and their branches can often be seen as bright structures on cine GRE images or as dark structures on SE images obtained with flow presaturation. One could use a series of these images at different levels, but representing the same phase of the cardiac cycle, to reconstruct a 3D vascular tree. However, this approach is unlikely to produce consistent results due to problems with respiratory motion and variable intrinsic cardiac motion. Ultrafast imaging methods such as echo planar (see Chapter 5) may eventually have potential for coronary artery imaging because they minimize motion effects, but these methods are currently limited in spatial resolution and S/N.[76]

MR angiography of the coronary arteries is unlikely to replace contrast angiography. However,

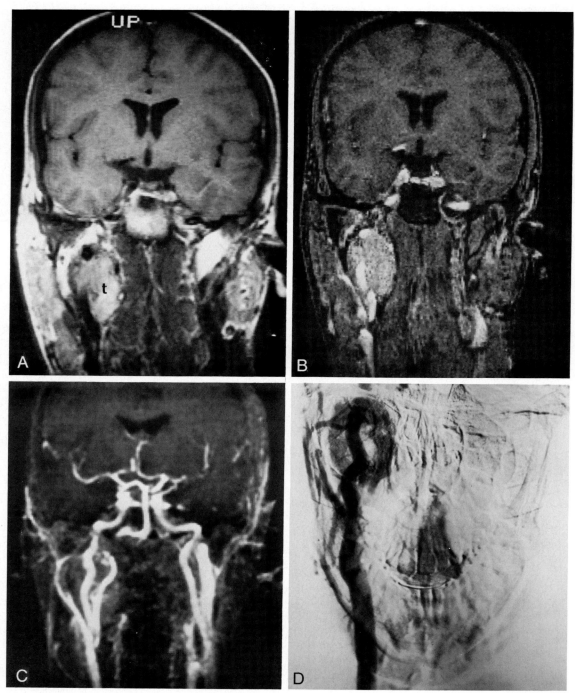

FIGURE 4–75. Glomus tumor involving right carotid sheath. *A,* T₁-weighted SE image obtained with presaturation of arterial inflow, after administration of gadolinium-DTPA. Note tumor (*t*). *B,* Coronal slice from 3D FLASH acquisition shows bright vessels entering and surrounding the tumor. *C,* Coronal 3D angiogram shows intimate relationship of tumor to carotid bifurcation. *D,* Corresponding contrast angiogram.

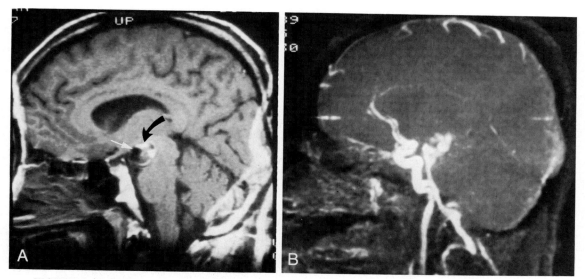

FIGURE 4–76. Basilar tip aneurysm postinsertion of five balloons into the aneurysm. *A,* Spin-echo image with flow presaturation shows signal voids from flowing blood as well as from the balloons (*straight arrow*). Bright signal represents thrombus formation around the balloons (*curved arrow*). *B,* MR angiogram exaggerates the amount of residual flow because both thrombus and flow appear bright.

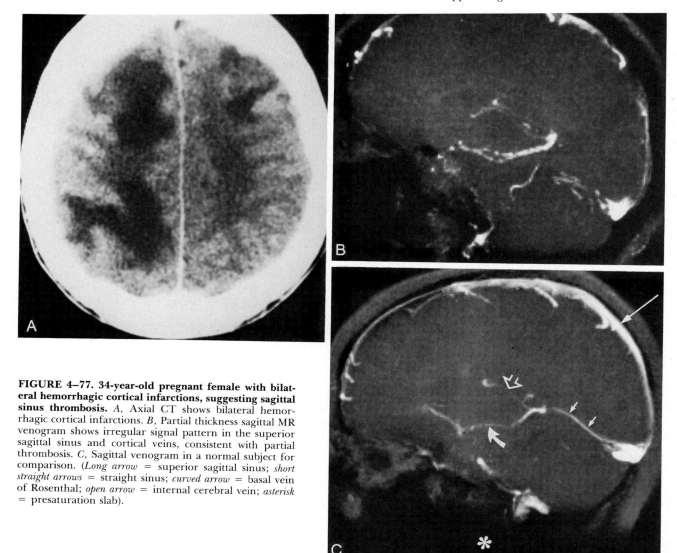

FIGURE 4–77. 34-year-old pregnant female with bilateral hemorrhagic cortical infarctions, suggesting sagittal sinus thrombosis. *A,* Axial CT shows bilateral hemorrhagic cortical infarctions. *B,* Partial thickness sagittal MR venogram shows irregular signal pattern in the superior sagittal sinus and cortical veins, consistent with partial thrombosis. *C,* Sagittal venogram in a normal subject for comparison. (*Long arrow* = superior sagittal sinus; *short straight arrows* = straight sinus; *curved arrow* = basal vein of Rosenthal; *open arrow* = internal cerebral vein; *asterisk* = presaturation slab).

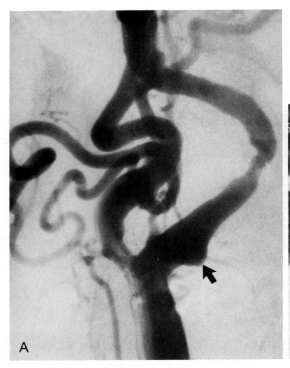

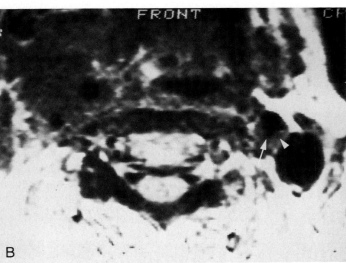

FIGURE 4–78. Ulceration near origin of internal carotid artery. *A,* Conventional angiogram shows ulceration (*arrow*) in plaque at origin of internal carotid artery. *B,* Black blood axial SE image, obtained with slice thickness = 2 mm and flow presaturation, demonstrates the ulceration as dark region (*arrow*). The plaque (*arrowhead*) has intermediate signal intensity.

lower resolution first-pass perfusion studies using ultrafast imaging techniques like echo planar in conjunction with paramagnetic or superparamagnetic contrast agents have great promise for assessing the functional adequacy of the coronary arteries (see Chapter 25). Bolus tracking and phase imaging methods might allow quantification of blood flow, at least in larger vessels such as the left main coronary artery.

Mixed results have been achieved in the assessment of coronary artery bypass grafts. Coronary artery bypass grafts are more easily identified on low flip angle GRE images than conventional SE images because of greater flow enhancement (Fig. 4–23).[77] However, internal mammary grafts are more difficult to evaluate than saphenous vein grafts due to their smaller size. Surface coil imaging may be useful for imaging of grafts due to their anterior, superficial course from the aortic root.

MEASUREMENT OF FLOW

There are numerous methods available for quantitating flow velocity. Flow quantitation methods can be divided into those that use saturation effects and those that use phase shift effects. Accurate quantitation of flow velocity has been demonstrated by both methods.[78–82a]

SATURATION METHODS

For flow perpendicular to the slice, flow signal depends on a balance of wash-in and wash-out ef-

fects. Since this balance is velocity dependent, one could, in theory, measure flow velocity simply by calibrating flow signal as a function of TR, TE, and slice thickness. However, this simple approach is too imprecise. In a better approach, known as bolus tracking, protons are excited in one slice by a 90-degree RF pulse, but the signal is refocused by a 180-degree RF pulse in another slice that is further downstream (Fig. 4–79). By acquiring a series of SE measurements with varying time delays between the excitation and refocusing pulses, the velocity can be

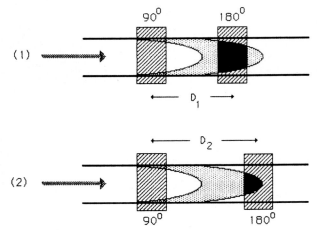

FIGURE 4–79. Flow velocity determination by bolus tracking. Bolus of blood can be "labeled" with a 90-degree RF pulse; signal from this bolus of blood is measured downstream by a 180-degree RF pulse. The velocity of flow can be measured by performing serial experiments with different spatial displacements (D_1, D_2) of the 180-degree RF pulse.

quantitated. However, the need for multiple measurements is time consuming.

Bolus tracking would be more useful if high temporal resolution could be rapidly obtained. This has been accomplished using a technique that combines presaturation with a cine GRE pulse sequence.[83] In this method, a bolus of blood is presaturated by a supplementary 90-degree RF pulse. The motion of the bolus of presaturated blood is imaged at multiple points during the cardiac cycle using a low flip angle GRE pulse sequence. Flowing, untagged blood appears bright; the presaturated bolus appears dark (Fig. 4–80 and 4–81).

This technique is an analog of contrast cineangiography, with presaturation corresponding to bolus injection of iodinated contrast. By measuring the distance (D) travelled by the bolus of blood during each interval (τ), velocity (v) can be calculated simply as:

$$v = D/\tau \tag{11}$$

Flow through the vessel can be calculated as:

$$\text{Flow} = \Sigma_i v_i \cdot A \cdot \tau/(R - R) \tag{12}$$

where A = cross-sectional area of the vessel and v_i = velocity at each time point in the cardiac cycle. This method has a number of potential applications, for example, differentiation of vascular signal from thrombus, evaluation of relative flow in the true and false lumens of a dissecting aortic aneurysm, and

measurement of portal venous flow. Portal vein flow velocity measurements can be obtained within a single breath-hold, since cardiac gating is not required. When applied to the superior sagittal sinus or internal jugular veins, measurements of global cerebral blood flow can be obtained in less than a minute.

The effectiveness of presaturation is limited by the T_i relaxation time of blood. Because contrast between the dark, presaturated bolus and bright, nonpresaturated blood decreases over time, contrast between flowing blood and the tagged bolus becomes inadequate after a few hundred milliseconds. This necessitates the application of a second or third presaturation pulse to image blood flow through the rest of the cardiac cycle.

For this and most other flow measurement techniques, one must know the direction of flow in order to calculate the velocity accurately. Also, for methods that determine in-plane flow velocity, inaccurate results may result from partial volume averaging across the thickness of the vessel. To avoid this problem the slice thickness should be kept small relative to the vessel diameter.

PHASE SHIFT METHODS

Whereas saturation methods track the motion of a bolus of blood, phase methods relate the velocity to

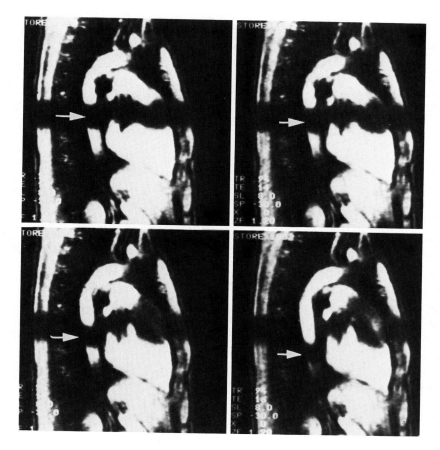

FIGURE 4–80. Dynamic bolus tracking (sagittal images) using presaturation cineangiography of thoracic aorta in normal subject. Bolus of blood is presaturated prior to start of cine sequence and has low intensity. Sequential cine images demonstrate motion of tagged bolus (*arrow*) down the aorta.

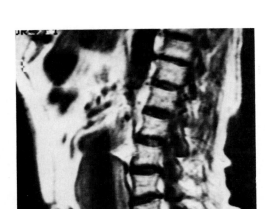

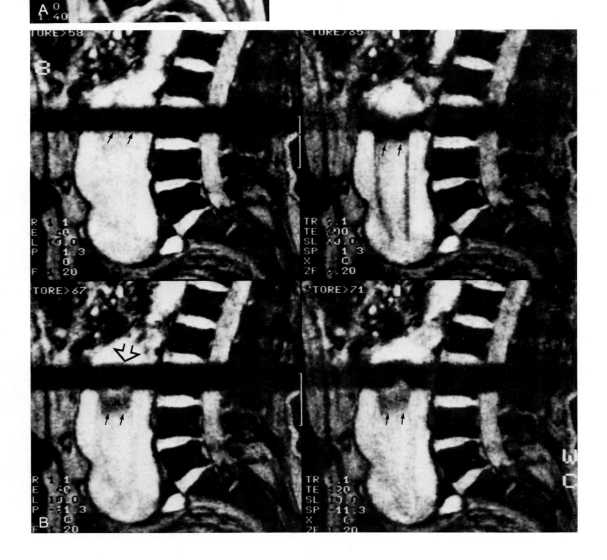

FIGURE 4–81. Dynamic bolus tracking in patient with saccular abdominal aortic aneurysm. Conventional angiogram demonstrated very poor runoff. *A,* Sagittal T_1-weighted image of abdomen demonstrates large aneurysm. *B,* Presaturation cineangiography. Tagged bolus (*small arrows*) is seen to move only a few cm over the cardiac cycle. Because of T_1 relaxation effects, resulting in increased signal intensity of the tagged bolus, flow contrast diminishes by the midportion of the cardiac cycle. To improve flow contrast, a second bolus of blood (*open arrow*) was presaturated near midcycle in order to maintain adequate flow contrast. Note mild flow reversal in diastolic (*lower right*) image.

gradient-induced phase shifts. Just as relaxation parameters are essential to tissue characterization, phase shifts are essential to flow characterization.

MR data are sensitive to phase effects because of quadrature detection; that is, the MR signal is measured in two separate channels (real and imaginary) which are, relative to each other, 90 degrees out of phase (Fig. 4–82A). Images reconstructed from either data channel are sensitive to phase shifts in the data. However, conventional image reconstructions are blind to phase and therefore to the wealth of flow information that exists in the data.

The reason for this is that MR images are usually reconstructed from the magnitude or absolute value of the data, as expressed by:

$$\text{Magnitude data} = (\text{Re}^2 + \text{Im}^2)^{1/2} \quad (13)$$

where Re = real component of data, and Im = imaginary component of data. Phase-sensitive images are less commonly used because they are more sensitive to artifacts caused by magnetic field distortion and gradient-induced eddy currents.

Flow-related phase shifts have been employed in several methods for flow quantitation.

Phase Mapping

The intensity of each pixel on a real or imaginary image is proportional to the cosine(Θ) or sin(Θ), respectively, where Θ is the phase angle. A direct representation of proton phase may be obtained by constructing a phase map, using the relation:

$$\Theta = \text{arctangent (Im/Re)} \quad (14)$$

On a phase map, pixel intensity is proportional to the phase shift (Θ). Since the phase shift is directly proportional to velocity, *the pixel intensity in the phase image is also directly proportional to velocity.*[84, 85]

Flowing blood appears bright or dark depending on the direction of flow and is readily distinguished from stationary spins, which appear a neutral gray (Fig. 4–82B). However, there are other sources than flow for phase shifts; other kinds of motion, static magnetic field inhomogeneity, boundaries between

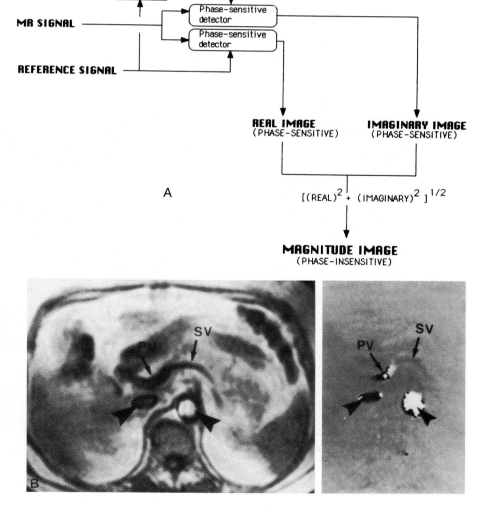

FIGURE 4–82. Phase mapping. *A,* Phase-sensitive quadrature detector splits MR signal into real and imaginary components. The real and imaginary images can be used individually to compute a phase map, or summed to produce a phase-insensitive magnitude image. *B,* Axial T₁-weighted SE image of upper abdomen. *Left,* Magnitude image shows increased signal in aorta, IVC, and portal vein. Vascular signal cannot be distinguished solely on the basis of signal intensity from thrombus. *Right,* On phase map, background appears neutral gray. Vascular signal appears brighter or darker than background, depending on direction of flow. (*B* from Rumancik WM, Naidich DP, Chandra R, et al: Cardiovascular disease: Evaluation with MR phase imaging. Radiology 166:63–68, 1988.)

tissues with differing magnetic susceptibility, chemical shift, and gradient-induced eddy currents are all capable of producing phase shifts. Nonflow-related phase shifts can be eliminated by acquiring two images with different flow sensitivities and then subtracting the images to eliminate stationary background phase shifts, although this introduces additional problems previously discussed in the context of subtraction angiography.

Phase maps provide accurate flow quantitation at low velocities. Fast flow produces larger phase shifts; in order to maintain a linear relationship between phase shift and velocity, these phase shifts must be kept small. If the phase shift exceeds 360 degrees, aliasing will occur and the phase shift becomes ambiguous. For instance, a phase shift of 420 degrees (60 degrees + 360 degrees) is indistinguishable from a phase shift of 60 degrees. The phase shift can be reduced by using short TE, flow compensation, and/or diastolic cardiac gating. Aliasing of phase shifts can also be resolved using the zebra-stripe method.

Zebra Stripes

A useful artifact is produced by off-centering the echo with respect to the middle of the sampling window and then displaying only the real part of the image. This produces a linear variation in the phase of the image which appears as a zig-zag linear variation in signal intensity, called a zebra-stripe pattern,

across the image (Fig. 4–83). Adjacent zebra stripes are separated by a 180-degree phase shift. In regions of constant phase (e.g., no flow), the zebra stripes are vertical.

Flow will cause the zebra stripes to deviate in the direction of flow. By counting the number of vertical stripes crossed, any phase ambiguity can be eliminated, due to the phase shift exceeding 360 degrees.[86] For instance if flow produces a deviation across 2.5 zebra stripes, the phase shift would be 450 degrees. If the slice is thin with respect to the vessel diameter and flow velocity is constant, the deviation of the stripes will be proportional to the velocity of flow. Zebra-stripe reconstructions can be useful for demonstrating flow directionality and for distinguishing flow signal from thrombus (Figs. 4–84 and 4–85).[87–89] However, the zebra-stripe method is not generally available on commercial MR systems. Also, it is more useful for laminar than plug flow.

Flow-Encoding Gradients

Normally, position information along the y-axis is spatially encoded using a time-varying phase-encoding gradient pulse. However, rather than encode position, this gradient pulse can be used to encode flow velocity. One method employs a pair of time-varying flow-encoding gradient pulses that produce a phase shift only for flowing spins (Fig. 4–86).[90] By stepping the flow-encoding gradients through a

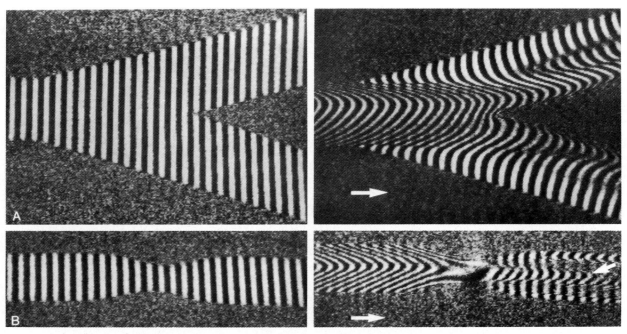

FIGURE 4–83. Flow patterns can be displayed using the phase-sensitive zebra-stripe method. Each pair of zebra stripes is separated by 180-degree phase shift. *A*, Bifurcating flow phantom. Left, Without flow, zebra stripes are vertical. Right, With flow, zebra stripes deviate in proportion to velocity (*arrow* = direction of flow). *B*, Flow phantom simulating vascular obstruction. Left, No flow. Right, With flow in direction of arrow, central high velocity jet (*short arrow*) is present with surrounding signal loss due to vortex formation. These appearances are similar to those seen in vivo with vascular obstruction.

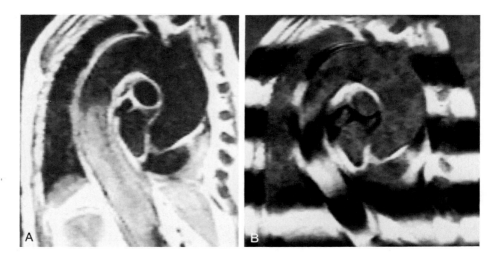

FIGURE 4–84. Diastolic image along long axis of aorta in patient with Marfan's syndrome and aortic root dilatation. Left, Magnitude image shows high signal in descending aorta, which could be mistaken for dissecting hematoma. Right, Zebra-stripe image shows caudal deviation of zebra stripes, consistent with flow.

range of amplitudes, individual velocity components are spatially encoded along the y-axis.

However, this method suffers from a dynamic range problem, because the small flow signal is overwhelmed by the much larger background signal. A variation of the line scan method, called fast Fourier, represents a solution to this problem.[91] In this method, background signal is suppressed by initially presaturating the plane of section; after a suitable interval to allow for inflow of fresh spins, data are acquired. Only fresh spins entering the plane produce signal.

Data from phase projection angiograms can be used to quantify flow.[92] Because it represents a full thickness of the body, like a conventional angiogram, a projection image can be used to measure flow without a significant length of a vessel lying in a single slice. However, since the slice thickness is large relative to the diameter of a vessel, the result is some type of average of flow across the vessel. Accurate flow quantification then depends on knowing the flow profile within the vessel.

DIFFUSION

In addition to bulk flow in vessels, the random diffusional motion of water molecules will also produce phase effects. Water molecules are in constant motion because of their thermal kinetic energy, so that a molecule will migrate over time from its initial position. However, this diffusional motion differs from bulk motion in some basic ways. First, the distance travelled by diffusing water molecules is minute, as discussed below, and is less than the dimension of a voxel. Second, diffusing water molecules move randomly. The effect of this random diffusional motion through magnetic field gradients is signal loss, resulting from phase dispersion.

Let us first consider how diffusion affects the positions of molecules. Because diffusional motion is random, if we were to follow the positions of a group of molecules over a period of time (T), the *average* displacement of all the molecules considered as a group would be zero (as many move in one direction as in the opposite direction).

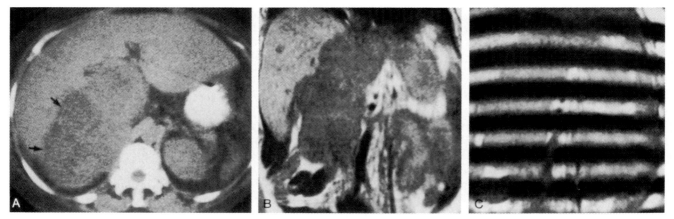

FIGURE 4–85. Primary leiomyosarcoma of IVC. Does any of the signal in the IVC represent flow? *A,* CT shows large retroperitoneal mass (*arrows*). *B,* Coronal MR shows mass following course of IVC. *C,* Zebra-stripe image shows no evidence of residual flow in IVC. (From White EM, Edelman RR, Wedeen VJ, Brady TJ: Intravascular signal in MR imaging: Use of phase display for differentiation of blood flow signal from intraluminal disease. Radiology 161:245–249, 1986.)

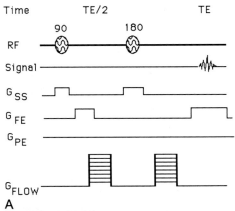

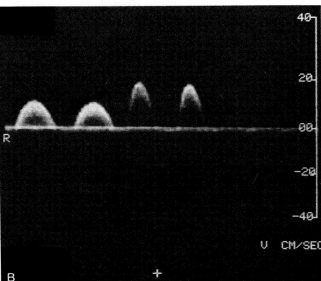

FIGURE 4–86. Flow-encoding gradient pulses can be substituted for the conventional phase-encoding gradient in order to spatially encode fluid flowing at different velocities at different positions in image. A, Pulse sequence diagram demonstrates paired flow-encoding gradient pulses, which produce a phase shift proportional to velocity. Flow-encoding gradient pulses are stepped over a range of amplitudes; velocity resolution increases with number of steps. B, Image obtained with this method demonstrates parabolic flow profiles, measured along y-direction, for four tubes with laminar fluid flow. Image is spatially resolved along z- and x-directions but represents full thickness projections along y-direction. (B from Feinberg DA, Crooks LE, Sheldon P, et al: MR imaging the velocity vector components of fluid flow. Mag Res Med 2:555–566, 1985.)

However, the positions of *individual* molecules do change. For bulk flow this displacement would be directly proportional to T. Diffusion is different. Motion due to diffusion occurs as a "random walk," so the relation between displacement and time is not the same as for bulk flow, where the motion of molecules is essentially unidirectional. As a result, it is the average of the *square* of the distances travelled by an individual molecule, called the mean squared distance $<(\Delta x)^2>$, rather than simply the distance,

which is proportional to time. This may be expressed as:

$$< (\Delta x)^2> = 2 \, DT$$

where D is the diffusion constant.

Molecules travel a much smaller distance due to diffusion than they would due to flow in a blood vessel. For example, compare a water molecule freely diffusing and another one flowing in a capillary with a velocity of 1 millimeter per second. Both molecules will move (on average) about 5 microns in 5 milliseconds, comparable to the diameter of the capillary. However, in 100 milliseconds, the molecule in the capillary will have moved 100 microns, but the diffusing molecule will have moved (on average) only 20 microns. In 1 second the flowing molecule will have moved 1000 microns, comparable to the dimension of a voxel, while the diffusing molecule will have moved only 70 microns.

The diffusion constant of a molecule depends on its configuration and physical environment. A large diffusion constant indicates that the distance moved by the molecules of a solution in a given time interval is relatively large. This is typical, for instance, of small molecules such as water. A typical value for water is $D = 2.3 \times 10^{-5}$ cm²/sec.

Diffusion through a magnetic field gradient produces signal loss due to phase dispersion. The amount of signal loss depends on D and the strength of the gradient; this dependence is expressed in the proportionality:

$$SI \sim e^{(-bD)}$$

where SI = signal intensity, D = diffusion constant, b = a gradient-dependent factor, and e = the base for natural logarithms. Because of this sensitivity, MR has proven to be an accurate and reliable method for measuring diffusion constants in spectrometer studies for many years. With standard pulse sequences using imaging gradients of typical amplitude and duration, the attenuation due to diffusion is usually small (< 10 per cent of the signal intensity). However, with modest increases in the imaging gradients, or by adding additional gradients, images can be made which are sensitive to diffusion.

A diffusion image can be produced by division of two images that have different sensitivities to diffusional effects.[92a] For instance, one could obtain a pair of images using SE pulse sequences with identical gradient amplitudes but different gradient timings (Fig. 4–87). For one image, a pair of diffusion-sensitizing gradient pulses is placed on either side of, but close to, the 180-degree RF pulse. For the second image, the diffusion-sensitizing gradient pulses are placed as far away from the 180-degree RF pulse as possible. With this method, long TE and high gradient amplitudes are needed to provide sensitivity for the effects of diffusion. A typical set of diffusion-imaging parameters might include TE = 100 to 200 msec, and 10 mT/m amplitude for the diffusion-sensitizing gradients. Long TRs are needed to reduce

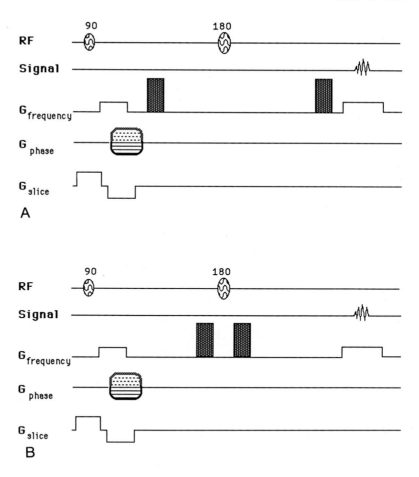

FIGURE 4–87. Example of a diffusion-sensitive pulse sequence. Spin-echo pulse sequence is modified by the addition of a pair of high amplitude diffusion-sensitizing gradient pulses (*stippled areas*), shown along the frequency-encoding axis. Temporal separation of the diffusion-sensitizing gradient pulses (A) produces greater signal loss from diffusion than sequence (B), where the gradient pulses are closely approximated. Because of the symmetry of the diffusion-sensitizing gradient pulses about the 180-degree RF pulse, a tissue would produce nearly identical signal intensity on images obtained with either pulse sequence, if it were not for the effects of diffusion, bulk flow, and other kinds of motion.

the T_1 weighting of the images, so that imaging times are at least several minutes per image.

Fast steady-state GRE methods (such as FISP and CE-FAST [see Chapter 5]), which are very sensitive to the effects of motion, are also being explored for measurement of diffusion.[93] A diffusion-sensitizing gradient can be incorporated into such sequences, with the reduction in signal intensity due to diffusion increasing with gradient amplitude.[93a]

Diffusion-sensitive pulse sequences are sensitive to bulk flow as well as diffusion. However, in the brain, vascular structures make up < 5 per cent of each voxel, whereas diffusing water is present everywhere. As a result, in images obtained with these methods, the signal intensity of each voxel should be strongly related to diffusion. Nevertheless, diffusion-sensitive images are severely degraded by ghost artifacts resulting from CSF pulsation or other kinds of motion. For methods that use a long TR, cardiac gating may improve the accuracy of diffusion measurements.[93b] For methods that use a short TR, signal averaging may prove helpful for artifact reduction. Flow compensation may also be used to reduce ghost artifacts, but this reduces the sensitivity to diffusion.

Perhaps it is not diffusion per se that may be of the greatest biologic interest, but the *restriction* of diffusion. The above equation assumes that there are no physical barriers to molecular motion but, in reality, cell membranes and other constituents of tissue do limit diffusion. The effect of restricted diffusion is that, over a period of time, molecules do not move as far as they would if they were freely diffusing, so the diffusion coefficient appears to be smaller.

The amount of restriction to diffusion may provide useful information about cell size and membrane permeability in normal and disease states. The utility of being able to image diffusion is still being explored, but diffusion-sensitive pulse sequences will at least offer a new tissue parameter that can serve as a source of image contrast between tissues. Recent work has suggested that diffusion measurements may also prove useful in spectroscopy for evaluating the compartment size and mobilization of various metabolites and for measuring tissue temperature.[94]

Diffusion-sensitive imaging is also of interest because of the possibility of imaging tissue perfusion, the flow of blood at the capillary level.[95, 96] The magnitude of capillary motion is somewhat similar to diffusional motion: the distances covered in a typical pulse sequence time (10 to 100 msec) are comparable, and the random orientation of capillaries within a voxel mimics the random directionality of diffusional motions. However, first pass studies with contrast agents offer more immediate potential in this area of study (Fig. 4–88).

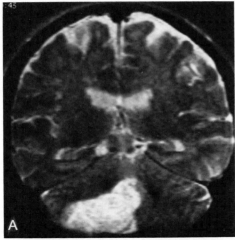

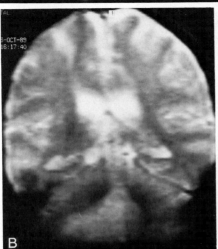

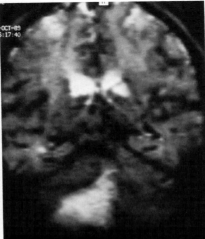

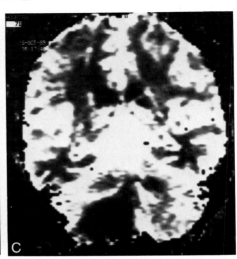

FIGURE 4–88. Regional cerebral perfusion can be assessed by rapid bolus administration of gadolinium-DTPA and dynamic imaging using a T_2^* (susceptibility-weighted) GRE sequence. The sequence is sensitive to T_2^*-shortening produced by the bolus of paramagnetic contrast agent as it passes through the brain capillaries. Although gadolinium-DTPA does not cross an intact blood-brain barrier, the long range T_2^* effect produces marked signal loss in the brain parenchyma nearby the capillaries, to a degree which depends on the amount of perfusion. On the other hand, the T_1 (dipole-dipole) effect of gadolinium-DTPA is short range and produces signal enhancement in vessels but not brain. *A,* Precontrast coronal T_2-weighted SE image in patient with acute cerebellar infarct shows wedge-shaped abnormality in cerebellar hemisphere but gives no information about perfusion. *B,* Series of GRE images obtained during first pass of gadolinium-DTPA bolus (0.1 mmol/kg given IV) through the brain. Scan variables: TR/TE = 42 msec/27 msec, slice thickness = 5 mm. Note darkening of vessels and perfused brain parenchyma but absence of signal change in the infarct since it is not perfused. *C,* Calculated perfusion image obtained by dividing a precontrast image by one obtained during maximum contrast enhancement. Gray matter appears brightest because of high perfusion, white matter shows less perfusion, and the infarct shows no perfusion. (From Edelman RR, Mattle H, Hoogewoud H, et al: Regional cerebral perfusion: assessment by dynamic magnetic resonance imaging (submitted)).

CONCLUSION

An awareness of the various kinds of flow effects is essential in order to properly interpret MR images. Flow-related enhancement, signal loss, misregistration, and ghost artifacts are present in nearly every image. Flow-sensitive pulse sequences are particularly useful for assessing cardiac function and vascular malformations and for differentiating thrombus from flow signal. Cardiac gating and flow compensation can be used to minimize flow-related artifacts. At the present time, problems with reliability limit the clinical application of MR angiography. However, with continued technical development over the next several years, one should expect that MR angiography will come to assume a significant role in clinical diagnosis, replacing current techniques that are more expensive and hazardous than MR.

ACKNOWLEDGMENTS: We would like to thank Dr. Gerald Lenz of Siemens Medical Systems and Dr. Jonathan Kleefield of Beth Israel Hospital for reviewing this manuscript, and Dr. Gerhardt Laub for helpful discussions and for providing several of the images.

REFERENCES

1. Bradley WG, Waluch V, Lai K-S, et al: The appearance of rapidly flowing blood on MR images. AJR 143:1167–1174, 1984.
2. Mills CM, Brant-Zawadzki M, Crooks LE, et al: NMR: Principles of blood flow imaging. AJNR 4:1161–1166, 1983.
3. Arnold DW, Burkhart LE: Spin-echo NMR response from a flowing sample. J Appl Physiol 36:870–871, 1965.
4. Axel L: Blood flow effects in magnetic resonance imaging. AJR 143:1157–1166, 1984.
5. Carr HY, Purcell EM: Effects of diffusion on free precession in NMR experiments. Physiol Rev 94:630–638, 1954.
6. Diem K, Lentner C (eds): Scientific Tables. 7th ed. Ardsley, Geigy Pharmaceuticals, 1970, pp 561–617.
7. Friedman GB, Sandhu HS: NMR in blood. Mag Res Rev 6:247–307, 1981.
8. Lindstrom TR, Koenig SH: Magnetic field dependent water proton spin-lattice relaxation rates of hemoglobin solutions and whole blood. J Mag Res 15:344–353, 1974.

9. Finnie M, Fullerton GD, Cameron IL: Molecular masking and unmasking of the paramagnetic effect of iron on the proton spin-lattice (T_1) relaxation time in blood and blood clots. Mag Res Imag 4:305–310, 1986.

10. Yilmaz A, Chu SC, Osmanoglu S: Dependence of the solvent proton $1/T_1$ on the iron content in normal human serum. Mag Res Med 7:337–339, 1988.

11. Milnor WR: Hemodynamics. Baltimore, Williams and Wilkins, 1982.

12. McDonald DA: Blood Flow in Arteries (2nd ed). Baltimore, Williams and Wilkins, 1974.

13. Caro CG, Pedley JG, Schroter RC, Seed WA: The Mechanics of the Circulation. New York, Oxford University Press, 1978.

14. Harrison MJG, Marshall J: Does the geometry of the carotid bifurcation affect its predisposition to atheroma? Stroke 14:117, 1983.

15. Dimick RN, Hedlund LW, Herfkens RJ, et al: Optimizing electrocardiograph electrode placement for cardiac-gated MRI. Invest Radiol 22:17–22, 1987.

16. Suryan G: Nuclear resonance in flowing liquids. Proc Indian Acad Sci Sect A, 33:107, 1951.

17. Singer JR: NMR diffusion and flow measurements and an introduction to spin-phase graphing. J Physiol 11:281–291, 1978.

18. von Schulthess GK, Higgins CB: Blood flow imaging with MR: Spin-phase phenomenon. Radiology 157:687–695, 1985.

19. Edelman RR, Atkinson DJ, Silver MS: FRODO pulses: A new method for elimination of motion, flow, and wraparound artifact. Radiology 166:231–236, 1988.

20. Felmlee JP, Ehman RL: Spatial presaturation: A method for suppressing flow artifacts and improving depiction of vascular anatomy in MRI. Radiology 164:559–564, 1987.

21. Waluch V, Bradley WG: NMR even echo rephasing in slow laminar flow. J Comput Assist Tomogr 8:594–598, 1984.

22. Alvarez O, Hyman RA: Even echo rephasing in the diagnosis of giant intracranial aneurysm. J Comput Assist Tomogr 10:699–701, 1986.

23. von Schulthess GK, Augustiny N: Calculation of T_2 values versus phase imaging for the distinction between flow and thrombus in MRI. Radiology 164:549–554, 1987.

24. Moran PR: A flow zeugmatographic interlace for NMR imaging in humans. Mag Res Imag 1:197–203, 1983.

25. Moran PR, Moran RA, Karstaedt N: Verification and evaluation of internal flow and motion. Radiology 154:433–441, 1985.

26. Haacke EM, Lenz GW: Improving MR image quality in the presence of motion by using rephasing gradients. AJR 148:1251–1258, 1987.

27. Frahm J, Haase A, Matthaei D: Rapid NMR imaging of dynamic processes using the FLASH technique. Mag Res Med 3:321–327, 1986.

28. Glover GH, Pelc NJ: A rapid gated cine MRI technique. In Kressel H (ed): Magnetic Resonance Annual 1988. New York, Raven Press, 1988.

29. Nayler GL, Firmin DN, Longmore DB: Blood flow imaging by cine MR. J Comput Assist Tomogr 10:715–722, 1986.

30. Tsuruda JS, Halbach VV, Higashida RT, et al: MR evaluation of large intracranial aneurysms using cine low flip angle gradient-refocused imaging. AJNR 9:415–424, 1988.

31. Barth K, Deimling M, Friyschy P, et al: Visualization and measurement of flow with MRI. Biomed Tech 30:12–17, 1985.

32. Perman WH, Moran PR, Moran RA, Bernstein MA: Artifacts from pulsatile flow in MRI. J Comput Assist Tomogr 10:473–484, 1986.

33. Burt TB: MR of CSF flow phenomenon mimicking basilar artery aneurysm. AJNR 8:55–58, 1987.

34. Rapoport S, Sostman HD, Pope C, et al: Venous clots: Evaluation with MRI. Radiology 162:527–530, 1987.

35. Goldberg HI, Grossman RI, Gomori JM, et al: Cervical internal carotid artery dissecting hemorrhage: Diagnosis using MR. Radiology 158:157–161, 1986.

36. Rubin JB, Enzmann DR: Imaging of spinal CSF pulsation by 2DFT MR: Significance during clinical imaging. AJNR 8:297, 1987.

37. Rubin JB, Enzmann DR: Harmonic modulation of proton MR precessional phase by pulsatile motion: Origin of spinal CSF flow phenomenon. AJR 148:983–994, 1987.

38. Bradley WG, Kortmann KE, Burgoyne B, Eng D: Flowing CSF in normal and hydrocephalic states: Appearance on MR images. Radiology 159:611–616, 1986.

39. DuBoulay GH: Pulsatile movements in the CSF pathways. Br J Radiol 39:255–262, 1966.

40. Dardenne G, Dereymaeker A, Lacheron JM: CSF pressure and pulsatility. Eur Neurol 2:192–216, 1969.

41. Lane B, Kricheff I: CSF pulsations at myelography: A videodensitometric study. Radiology 110:579–587, 1974.

42. Ridgway JP, Turnbull LW, Smith MA: Demonstration of pulsatile cerebrospinal fluid flow using MR phase imaging. Br J Radiol 60:423–427, 1987.

43. Edelman RR, Wedeen V, Davis KR, et al: Multiphasic MRI of pulsatile CSF flow. Radiology 161:779–783, 1986.

44. Enzmann DR, Rubin JB, O'Donohue J, et al: Use of CSF gating to improve T_2-weighted images. Radiology 162:768–773, 1987.

45. Rubin JB, Enzmann DR: Optimizing image quality of conventional spin-echo spine MRI. Radiology 163:777, 1987.

46. Rubin JB, Enzmann DR, Wright A: CSF gated spine MRI: Theory and clinical implementation. Radiology 163:784, 1987.

47. Jolesz FA, Patz S, Hawkes RC, Lopez I: Fast imaging of CSF flow/motion patterns using steady-state free precession (SSFP). Invest Radiol 22:761–777, 1987.

48. Enzmann DR, O'Donohue J, Rubin JB, et al: CSF pulsations within nonneoplastic spinal cord cysts. AJR 149:149–157, 1987.

49. Castillo M, Quencer RM, Green BA, Montalvo BM: Syringomyelia as a consequence of compressive extramedullary lesions: Postoperative clinical and radiological manifestations. AJNR 8:973–978, 1987.

50. Spritzer CE, Sussman SK, Blinder RA, et al: DVT evaluation with limited flip angle gradient-refocused MRI: Preliminary experience. Radiology 166:371–375, 1988.

51. Macovski A: Selective projection imaging: Applications to radiology and NMR. IEEE Trans Med Imag 1:42–47, 1982.

52. Axel L, Morton D: MR flow imaging by velocity-compensated/uncompensated difference images. J Comput Assist Tomogr 11:31–34, 1987.

53. Wedeen VJ, Meuli RA, Edelman RR, et al: Projective imaging of pulsatile flow with magnetic resonance. Science 230:946–948, 1985.

54. Hale JD, Valk PE, Watts JC, et al: MRI of blood vessels using three-dimensional reconstruction: Methodology. Radiology 157:727–733, 1985.

55. Haacke EM, Tkach JA, Parrish TB: Reduction of T2* dephasing in gradient field-echo imaging. Radiology 170:457–462, 1989.

56. Laub GA, Kaiser WA: MR angiography with gradient motion rephasing. J Comput Assist Tomogr 12:377–382, 1988.

57. Laub GA, Rossnick S, Braeckle G, et al: Presented at the 6th Annual Meeting of the Society of Magnetic Resonance in Medicine, New York, August 17–21, 1987.

58. Edelman RR, Wentz KU, Mattle H: Projection arteriography and venography: Initial clinical results using MR. Radiology 172:351–357, 1989.

59. Dixon WT, Du LN, Faul DD, et al: Projection angiograms of blood labeled by adiabatic fast passage. Mag Res Med 3:454–462, 1986.

60. Nishimura DG, Macovski A, Pauly JM: Considerations of MR angiography by selective inversion recovery. Mag Res Med 7:472–484, 1988.

61. Dumoulin CL, Souza SP, Walker MF, Yoshitome E: Time-resolved MR angiography. Mag Res Med 6:275–286, 1988.

62. Dumoulin CL, Hart HR: MR angiography. Radiology 161:717–720, 1986.

62a. Dumoulin CL, Souza SP, Walker MF, Wagle W: Three-dimensional phase contrast angiography. Mag Res Med 9:139–149, 1989.

63. Pauly J, Nishimura D, Macovski A: Robust velocity selective excitation. Presented at the 6th Annual Meeting of the Society of Magnetic Resonance in Medicine, New York, August 17–21, 1987.

64. Lenz GW, Haacke EM, Masaryk TJ, Laub G: In-plane vascular imaging: Pulse sequence design and strategy. Radiology 166:875–882, 1988.

65. Pauly J, Nishimura D, Macovski A: Line scan MR angiography. Presented at the 6th Annual Meeting of the Society of Magnetic Resonance in Medicine, New York, August 17–21, 1987.

65a. Moseley ME, White DL, Wang S-C, et al: Vascular mapping using albumin-(Gd-DTPA), an intravascular MR contrast agent, and projection MR imaging. J Comput Assist Tomogr 13:215–221, 1989.

66. Torres WE, Gaylord GM, Whitmire L, et al: The correlation between MR and angiography in portal hypertension. AJR 148:1109–1112, 1987.

67. Mostbeck GH, Wittich GR, Herold C, et al: Hemodynamic significance of the paraumbilical vein in portal hypertension: Assessment with duplex US. Radiology 170:339–342, 1989.

68. Middleton WD, Foley WD, Lawson TL: Color-flow Doppler imaging of carotid artery abnormalities. AJR 150:419–425, 1988.

69. Aaslid R, Markwalder TM, Nornes H: Noninvasive transcranial Doppler ultrasound recording of flow velocity in the basal cerebral arteries. J Neurosurg 57:769–774, 1982.

70. Blackshear WM, Phillips DJ, Chikos PM, et al: Carotid artery velocity patterns in normal and stenotic vessels. Stroke 11:67–71, 1980.

71. Grolimund P, Seiler RW: Age dependence of the flow velocity in the basal cerebral arteries—a transcranial Doppler ultrasound study. Ultrasound Med Biol 14:191–198, 1988.

72. Büdingen HJ, Staudacher T: Die Identifizierung der Arteria basilaris mit der transkraniellen Doppler-Sonographie. Ultraschall 8:95–101, 1987.

73. Mattle H, Schnider A: Extra- and transcranial Doppler sonographic findings in internal carotid artery occlusion. Fourth Toronto Stroke Workshop, Toronto, September 14–16, 1988.

74. Masaryk TJ, Ross JS, Modic MT, et al: Carotid bifurcation: MR imaging. Radiology 166:461–466, 1988.

74a. Katz BH, Quencer RM, Kaplan JO, Hinks RS, Post M: MRI of intracranial carotid occlusion. AJR 10:345–350, 1989.

74b. Masaryk TJ, Modic MT, Ruggieri PM, et al: Three-dimensional gradient-echo imaging of the carotid bifurcation: Preliminary clinical experience. Radiology 171:801–806, 1989.

75. Alfidi RJ, Masaryk TJ, Haacke EM, et al: MR angiography of peripheral, carotid, and coronary arteries. AJR 149:1097–1109, 1987.

75a. Masaryk TJ, Modic MT, Ross JS, et al: Intracranial circulation: Preliminary clinical results with three-dimensional MR angiography. Radiology 171:793–799, 1989.

76. Stehling MJ, Howseman AM, Ordidge RJ, et al: Whole-body echo-planar MRI at 0.5 T. Radiology 170:257–263, 1989.

77. White RD, Pflugfelder PW, Lipton MJ, Higgins CB: Coronary artery bypass grafts: Evaluation of patency with cine MR imaging. AJR 150:1271–1274, 1988.

78. Rumancik WM, Naidich DP, Chandra R, et al: Cardiovascular disease: Evaluation with MR phase imaging. Radiology 166:63–68, 1988.

79. Wehrli FW, Shimakawa A, Gullberg GT, MacFall JR: Time-of-flight MR flow imaging: Selective saturation recovery with gradient refocusing. Radiology 160:781–785, 1986.

80. Wehrli FW, Shimakawa A, MacFall JR, et al: MR imaging of venous and arterial flow by a selective saturation-recovery spin echo (SSRSE) method. J Comput Assist Tomogr 9:537–545, 1985.

81. Feinberg DA, Crooks L, Hoenninger J, et al: Pulsatile blood velocity in human arteries displayed by MR imaging. Radiology 153:177–180, 1984.

82. Singer JR: Blood flow rates by NMR measurements. Science 130:1652, 1959.

82a. Foo TKF, Perman WM, Poon CSO, et al: Projection flow imaging by bolus tracking using stimulated echoes. Mag Res Med 9:203–218, 1989.

83. Edelman RR, Mattle H, Kleefield J, Silver MS: Quantification of blood flow with dynamic MR imaging and presaturation bolus tracking. Radiology 171:551–556, 1989.

84. Bryant DJ, Payne JA, Firmin DN, Longmore DB: Measurement of flow with NMR imaging using a gradient pulse and phase difference technique. J Comput Assist Tomogr 8:588–593, 1984.

85. van Dijk P: Direct cardiac NMR imaging of heart wall and blood flow velocity. J Comput Assist Tomogr 8:429–436, 1984.

86. Wedeen VJ, Rosen BR, Chesler D, Brady TJ: MR velocity imaging by phase display. J Comput Assist Tomogr 9:530–536, 1985.

87. White EM, Edelman RR, Wedeen VJ, Brady TJ: Intravascular signal in MR imaging: Use of phase display for differentiation of blood flow signal from intraluminal disease. Radiology 161:245–249, 1986.

88. Dinsmore RE, Wedeen V, Rosen B, et al: Phase-offset technique to distinguish slow blood flow and thrombus on MR images. AJR 148:634–636, 1987.

89. Dinsmore RE, Wedeen VJ, Miller SW, et al: MRI of dissection of the aorta: Recognition of the intimal tear and differential flow velocities. AJR 146:1286–1288, 1986.

90. Feinberg DA, Crooks LE, Sheldon P, et al: MR imaging the velocity vector components of fluid flow. Mag Res Med 2:555–566, 1985.

91. Hennig J, Muri M, Brunner P, Friedburg H: Quantitative flow measurement with the fast Fourier flow technique. Radiology 166:237–240, 1988.

92. Walker MF, Souza SP, Dumoulin CL: Quantitative flow measurement in phase contrast MR angiography. J Comput Assist Tomogr 12:304–313, 1988.

92a. Ahn CB, Lee SY, Nalcioglu O, Cho ZH: An improved NMR diffusion coefficient imaging method using an optimized pulse sequence. Med Phys 13:789, 1986.

93. Bihan DL: Intravoxel incoherent motion imaging using steady-state free precession. Mag Res Med 7:346–351, 1988.

93a. Merboldt K-D, Bruhn M, Frahm J, et al: MRI of "diffusion" in the human brain: New results using a modified CE-FAST sequence. Mag Res Med 9:423–429, 1989.

93b. Chien D, Buxton RB, Kwong KK, Brady TJ, Rosen BR: Quantitative diffusion imaging in the human brain. Proceedings of the 7th Annual Meeting of the SMRM, San Francisco, 1988, p 218.

94. Moonen CTW, van Zijl P, Bihan DL: In vivo P31 NMR diffusion spectroscopy. Presented at the 7th Annual Meeting of the Society of Magnetic Resonance in Medicine, San Francisco, August 20–26, 1988.

95. LeBihan D, Breton E, Lallemand D, et al: MRI of intravoxel incoherent motions: Applications to diffusion and perfusion in neurologic disorders. Radiology 161:401–407, 1986.

96. Ahn CB, Lee SY, Nalcioglu O, Cho ZM: The effects of random directional distributed flow in NMR imaging. Med Phys 14:43, 1987.

5

FAST MR IMAGING

JOEL F. MARTIN and ROBERT R. EDELMAN

BACKGROUND: SPIN-ECHO METHODS

FAST IMAGING METHODS AND APPLICATIONS

    COLLECTING LESS DATA

    Reduced Number of Excitations
    Reduced Matrix Size
    Half-Fourier Techniques
    Asymmetric Field-of-View

    GRADIENT-ECHO TECHNIQUES

    TYPES OF GRADIENT-ECHO TECHNIQUES

    Spoiled FLASH
    Steady-State FLASH
    Contrast-Enhanced FLASH

    CONTRAST IN GRADIENT-ECHO IMAGING

    Contrast from Tissue Relaxation
    Magnetic Field Effects
    Flow Effects

CLINICAL APPLICATIONS OF GRADIENT-ECHO IMAGING

Abdomen
MR Myelogram
Hemorrhage
Flow
Contrast Agents
Knee
Three-dimensional Imaging (3D GRE)

DRIVEN-EQUILIBRIUM METHODS

STIMULATED-ECHO (STEAM) IMAGING

ALTERNATIVES TO 2DFT IMAGING

Echo-Planar and Single Shot Imaging
Artifacts in Echo-Planar Imaging
Signal-to-Noise in Echo-Planar Imaging
RARE
Hybrid Imaging
Contrast in Echo-Planar Imaging

APPENDIX

Fast MR imaging techniques have become increasingly popular because fast imaging has a number of advantages compared with much slower spin-echo (SE) imaging. Scan time can be a major consideration for severely ill patients, sedated patients, claustrophobic patients, pediatric cases, and patients with involuntary motion. Fast scanning techniques can be useful in reducing a number of artifacts associated with respiration, peristalsis, blood flow, and so forth. In addition, fast MR imaging techniques have the potential for imaging dynamic processes such as joint motion and enhancement from contrast material. Finally, faster techniques can increase patient throughput.

Standard MR scans based on SE techniques have gained rapid acceptance in radiology because these scans show dramatic contrast between different types of soft tissue. This contrast is due to the relaxation properties of the tissue, namely T_1 and T_2. Unfortunately, T_1 and T_2 relaxation also make it difficult to perform rapid imaging. In SE imaging techniques, the need to allow adequate T_1 relaxation after each excitation forces one to wait a relatively long period of time between signal measurements, so that imaging times are correspondingly long. Furthermore, each measured signal disappears rapidly due to T_2 decay. Fast imaging methods must work around these intrinsic limitations.

There are several approaches to fast MR imaging (Table 5–1). The simplest approach is to measure the signal fewer times, either by using fewer phase-encoding steps or fewer excitations. This is represented in the equation for imaging time:

$$\text{Imaging time} = TR \times \text{number of phase-encoding steps} \times NEX \quad (1)$$

where NEX = the number of excitations or acquisitions, and TR = the repetition time. For example,

TABLE 5–1. SUMMARY OF RAPID IMAGING METHODS

Shorten TR
Gradient-echo: Spoiled FLASH
                    Steady-state FLASH
Spin-echo with optimized flip angle: FLAME
Driven equilibrium

Decrease Number of Views
Reduced acquisition matrix (± asymmetric
  FOV half-Fourier)

Acquire Views More Rapidly
Hybrid
Single shot/echo-planar
STEAM
RARE

Decrease Number of Excitations
Single excitation

the imaging time for an image with TR = 0.5 seconds, 128 phase-encoding steps, and two excitations is $(0.5 \times 128 \times 2) = 128$ seconds, but with the same TR, 64 phase-encoding steps, and one excitation, it is only $(0.5 \times 64 \times 1) = 32$ seconds. Although imaging times are reduced by decreases in these scan parameters, the penalty may be compromised image quality and contrast.

A particularly useful method for speeding up the MR imaging process is to work around the T_1 limitations that restrict TR in SE imaging. The T_1 limitation can be avoided by applying a *reduced flip angle* for excitation. Unlike SE methods, in this technique, known as gradient-echo (GRE) imaging, each excitation uses less than the maximum available magnetization to produce the signal. By using this method, one finds that good signal levels can be maintained despite short repetition times.

At first it may seem paradoxical that, by using less of the magnetization to produce the signal, GRE methods give more signal at short TR than do SE methods. The key factor for understanding GRE methods is that, while the signal strength *per measurement* is reduced, *the number of signals measured per second is greatly increased*. On balance, the latter factor dominates at short TR. As a result, GRE methods produce more signal and better image quality with short TR than SE methods and are, therefore, better suited for fast imaging. For instance, it is possible using GRE sequences in conjunction with very short TR (e.g., ≤ 5 msec) to acquire images in as little as half a second.[1a] This method of MR fluoroscopy can be used to image motion in real time, such as with peristalsis or flexion and extension of the neck, to assess spinal cord impingement. In this setting, spin-echo methods would be useless.

Gradient-echo methods produce images that are different from SE images in a number of respects, including contrast, artifacts, and response to imperfections in the MR scanner. For the time being, GRE techniques are the most effective means of performing fast MR imaging. However, there are other techniques that have the potential for much faster MR imaging.

The fastest method of obtaining an MR image is to acquire the entire data matrix within a time less than T_2. This approach, known as single-shot or echo-planar imaging, works by forming a series of echoes, each of which has a different phase-encode value. A single series of echoes is sufficient to reconstruct an entire image. Unfortunately, single-shot imaging places very stringent requirements on the performance of MR scanner hardware. Limitations in current MR imaging equipment make single-shot imaging impractical for most clinical applications, but recent advances in scanner design may make this technique much more useful in the future.

The following sections explain the various techniques used in fast MR scanning, the applicability of these methods, and how fast MR images differ from the more familiar images obtained using SE pulse sequences.

BACKGROUND: SPIN-ECHO METHODS

MR imaging is ordinarily performed using SE pulse sequences. Spin-echo pulse sequences can be represented as:

$$90°\text{--(wait TE/2)--}180°\text{--(wait TE/2)}$$
$$\text{--(signal read-out)}$$

where TE (echo time) defines the center of the SE signal. The pulse sequence is repeated at time intervals equal to TR. The number of times the sequence is repeated is determined by the spatial resolution (specifically, the number of pixels) along the phase-encoding axis and is equal to the number of phase-encoding steps. A large number of phase-encoding steps is needed for high spatial resolution. Furthermore, repetition times must be long with SE methods in order to permit adequate T_1 relaxation between radiofrequency (RF) excitations. Consequently, imaging times with SE methods are long.

The first pulse in the SE sequence, used to excite the spins, is set to 90 degrees in order to completely tip the existing longitudinal magnetization into the transverse plane. This maximizes the amount of signal that can be obtained per measurement. However, immediately after the 90-degree pulse, the remaining longitudinal magnetization is zero. If the spins were again excited at this time, no signal would be produced. Therefore, a time interval (TR) is allowed to elapse between excitations, so that the spins can undergo T_1 relaxation and recover at least part of their longitudinal magnetization.

The next 90-degree pulse produces a signal proportional to this accumulated magnetization, as expressed by:

$$S = S_0 [1 - \exp(-TR/T1)] \qquad (2)$$

where S_0 is the signal that would be produced by a 90-degree pulse when the spins are fully aligned with the magnetic field. The signal (S) depends on the amount of T_1 relaxation that occurs during the interval TR.

The simplest way to speed up an ordinary SE scan would be to drastically reduce the TR interval, thereby obtaining an equivalent increase in speed. From Equation 2 above, it is apparent that this would also result in an unacceptable loss of signal strength. One cannot arbitrarily decrease the TR time for an image, since the quality of conventional SE images produced with very short TR (e.g., <100 msec) is poor.

Nevertheless, several newer SE methods (e.g., FATE, FLAME) offer the potential of substantial improvements in image quality at short TR. These methods are addressed below.

FAST IMAGING METHODS AND APPLICATIONS

COLLECTING LESS DATA

The fact that TR is constrained to fairly long values (e.g., usually >300 msec) in SE imaging leaves open the possibility of speeding up the imaging process by decreasing either the NEX (number of excitations) or the matrix size of the image. There are several ways to take advantage of decreases in these parameters, but there may also be undesirable side effects that need to be understood.

Reduced Number of Excitations

The parameter NEX refers to the number of times the pulse sequence is repeated *in each projection* during the process of acquiring an image. The reason for using more than one excitation is to eliminate certain undesirable features in the image. The features include electrical noise and artifacts from repetitive motion (e.g., ghost artifacts from respiration) (see Chapter 3).

By adding together the signals acquired from multiple excitations, undesirable features tend to be averaged out. This is represented in an improved signal-to-noise (S/N) ratio where

$$S/N \ \alpha \ \sqrt{NEX} \tag{3}$$

Imaging time is proportional to the NEX, so that using a single excitation cuts the imaging time in half compared with two excitations (Fig. 5–1). However, the penalty is 41 per cent reduction (i.e., $\sqrt{2}$) in S/N (i.e., increased graininess of the image).

Single excitation imaging is routinely used on high field MR systems. Even on lower field systems, which have intrinsically less S/N, the loss in S/N resulting from using fewer excitations can be compensated by slight increases in TR. For instance, an image produced with TR = 3000 msec and one excitation may be similar in quality to one acquired with TR = 2000

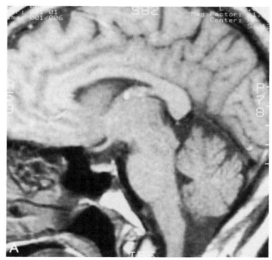

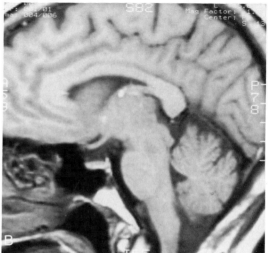

FIGURE 5–1. Comparison of sagittal head images acquired in two minutes with one NEX *(top)* and in four minutes with two NEX *(bottom)*. Despite increased graininess of single NEX image, the diagnostic information on both images is comparable.

msec and two excitations, although the imaging time is less (13 minutes versus 17 minutes for a 256 × 256 matrix).

Signal-to-noise loss is not the only problem with single NEX imaging. Ghost artifacts from respiration and pulsatile flow are decreased by imaging with multiple excitations. The details of this process are quite complex, but if the motion is not correlated with TR, then motion artifacts will average out in much the same fashion as electrical noise (see Chapter 3). Therefore, motion artifacts decrease roughly as $\sqrt{NEX}$.

Ghost artifacts may be objectionable on images acquired with a single excitation. In the abdomen, where motion artifacts are most pronounced, it is usually better to use multiple NEX scans unless a breath-holding study is possible. If an SE image of the abdomen is required, it is almost certainly more productive to decrease imaging time by changing the matrix size, as described below, rather than by using a single excitation.

As a final caveat, it is important to note that single NEX imaging may preclude the use of techniques that eliminate wraparound in the phase-encoding direction. These techniques, commonly known as "no phase wrap" or "extended field-of-view", acquire an image in which the field-of-view (FOV) in the phase-encoding direction is larger than the prescribed FOV. The excess portion of the image which contains the wraparound is discarded, leaving an image with an FOV that is the same as that requested by the user. For a two NEX image, this technique works by obtaining *a one NEX image* with an increased FOV and twice as many projections. Therefore, a minimum of two excitations is needed.

Reduced Matrix Size

Imaging time is proportional to the size of the data matrix, so scan times can be decreased by using a smaller matrix size, that is, fewer phase-encoding steps. As discussed in Chapter 1, each phase-encoding step contains information about the entire image. Each phase-encoding step corresponds to a spatial frequency, which can be loosely translated to resolution. In other words, a higher matrix size improves the definition of sharply defined structures. Decreasing the acquisition matrix size blurs sharp structures and creates multiple ghost images of certain features. This phenomenon, known as truncation artifact, is difficult to discern in most 256 phase-encoded images, but is often seen in images made with 128 phase encodes (see Chapter 3). Truncation artifacts can be reduced by filtering the image, but not without further loss of resolution (see Chapter 2).

For a given FOV, a 256×256 matrix has twice the spatial resolution of a 256×128 matrix in the phase-encoding direction. However, the 256×128 matrix can be acquired in *half the time*. In many applications a 256×128 matrix provides adequate spatial resolution. Furthermore, despite the shorter imaging time, an image acquired with a 256×128 matrix has higher S/N, by 41 per cent, than an image acquired in twice the time using a 256^2 matrix. The reason for this is that, while S/N of the 256×128 image is reduced because of the shorter imaging time, it is improved by a factor of two because of the twofold larger pixel. Several MR systems offer intermediate matrix sizes (e.g., 256×192) which, compared with the 256×128 matrix, are more time consuming but produce substantially fewer truncation artifacts. Intermediate matrix sizes are most useful in imaging the brain and spine, whereas a matrix size of 128 is insufficient for visualizing small structures. S/N comparisons for these different matrix sizes are presented in Chapter 2. Truncation artifacts may also be made less apparent by using an asymmetric FOV (below).

Half-Fourier Techniques

There is an inherent redundancy in the way in which data are acquired for MR images. Positive data are acquired using positive phase-encoding gradient pulses; negative data are acquired using negative phase-encoding gradient pulses. The two halves of the data matrix contain, in principle, the same information. These two sets of data are essentially mirror images of one another (complex conjugates), so it ought to be possible to fill out the entire data matrix by measuring only the positive half of the data and reflecting these data into the other half of the matrix (Fig. 5–2). This would cut imaging time in two. This method is called half-NEX, half-Fourier, or conjugate synthesis.[1] The term half-NEX can be confusing because it really refers to the acquisition of half a *matrix* using one NEX.

In practice, half-Fourier techniques reduce imaging times by slightly less than 50 per cent, because the mirror-image symmetry of the data is only true for a hypothetical "ideal" acquisition. The actual MR data has phase offsets that distort the symmetry of the matrix. Most half-Fourier techniques require the acquisition of some extra negative phase-encoding steps in order to calculate phase corrections for the data.

The first step in the process of image reconstruction is to reflect the positive data so as to generate an entire raw data matrix. The data are then phase-corrected based on a low resolution "phase shift map" generated from the positive and extra negative projections. Finally, the data are processed using ordinary Fourier reconstruction algorithms to produce an image. Unfortunately, the additional data processing steps involved in half-Fourier imaging can easily double reconstruction time.

A variety of effects can distort the phase symmetry of the data. These effects include slice selection, eddy currents, flow, and other kinds of motion. The re-

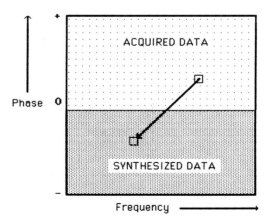

FIGURE 5–2. K-space representation of conjugate synthesis in half-Fourier imaging. Compared with a conventional image, only slightly more than half of the data are acquired. The rest are synthesized from the acquired data, reducing imaging time by a factor of two.

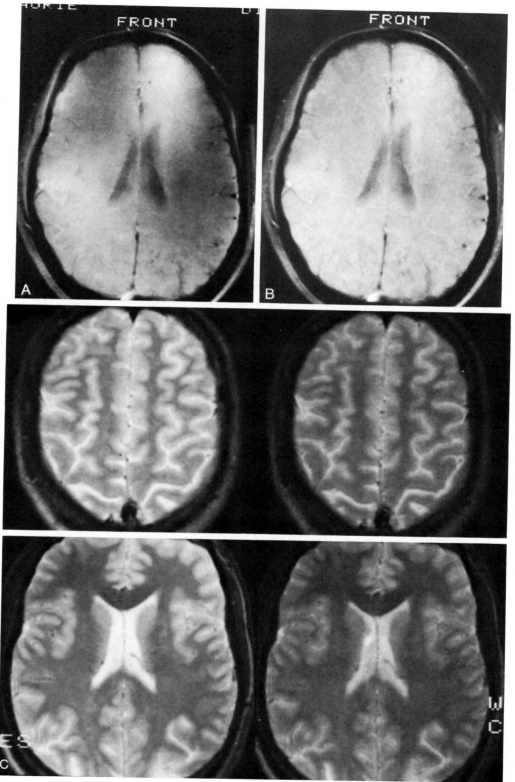

FIGURE 5–3. Half-Fourier GRE images acquired with two extra negative projections *(A)* and 16 extra projections *(B)*. Note signal inhomogeneity in *(A)*, due to spurious phase shifts. This inhomogeneity is reduced by acquiring extra projections *(B)*. C, Comparison of standard SE images *(left)* and half-Fourier images *(right)* acquired in almost half the time (eight extra projections). TR/TE = 3500/60. Image contrast and resolution are identical. Despite lower S/N of half-Fourier images, images have comparable diagnostic utility. (Note that these half-Fourier SE images are less sensitive to spurious phase shifts than are GRE images.)

sulting phase distortions can produce artifacts in half-Fourier images. The problems are worst for GRE methods (Fig. 5–3A and B). Also, as expected from the reduced amount of data used to produce the image, the S/N of a half-Fourier image is reduced by $\sqrt{2}$ compared with a conventional image. However, the resolution and contrast in half-Fourier images are identical to that obtained by standard methods (Fig. 5–3C).

Asymmetric Field-of-View

There is one situation in which the matrix size can be reduced with minimal or no loss in spatial resolution. If the anatomy being imaged is elliptical (e.g., head or abdomen), then an asymmetric or rectangular FOV can be used to recover some or all of the resolution lost by using an asymmetric matrix. These images have equal resolution in the phase and frequency directions except for a subtle increase in truncation artifact (Fig. 5–4).

For instance, consider (1) a 256 × 256 image with a symmetric 24-cm FOV, versus (2) an image with 128 phase-encoding steps and an asymmetric FOV of 24 cm (frequency-encoding direction) × 12 cm (phase-encoding direction). These images have equal pixel resolutions of 0.9 × 0.9 mm, but the image with the smaller matrix is acquired in half the time.

By permitting smaller acquisition matrices to be used without unacceptable compromises of spatial resolution, asymmetric FOVs are routinely useful for reducing imaging time—provided that the FOV will accommodate the anatomy. If the anatomy does not fit in the asymmetric FOV, substantial wraparound artifacts may occur along the phase-encoding direction. This can be a problem, for instance, when imaging the lumbar spine with small FOVs.

In our experience, S/N is not a significant limitation with asymmetric FOVs, as long as the FOV is not too asymmetric. Consider (1) an image acquired with a 256 × 256 matrix and a symmetric 24 × 24 cm FOV, and (2) an image acquired in half the time with a 256 × 128 matrix and a 24 × 17 cm (41 per cent smaller) FOV along the phase-encoding direction. (This degree of asymmetry in the FOV is adequate to minimize truncation artifacts.) Surprisingly, these two images have the same S/N. The loss of S/N resulting from the reduced FOV in the second image is precisely compensated by the gain in S/N from the larger pixel size. Using these parameters, we find that wraparound is seldom a problem for head imaging.

All of the approaches discussed so far are generally applicable to SE pulse sequences. They rely on decreasing the amount of data acquired in the imaging process. These approaches provide modest but useful gains in imaging speed. To image even faster, one

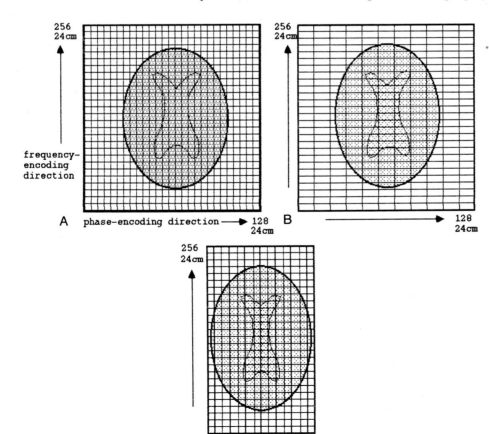

FIGURE 5–4. Schematic comparison of how acquisition with different matrices affects pixel size and image appearance. Note that subtle differences, such as truncation artifacts, are not shown here. A, 256 × 256 (frequency × phase) image has square pixels (0.9 mm × 0.9 mm). B, 256 × 128 image has rectangular pixels (0.9 mm × 1.8 mm) with half the spatial resolution of (A), but image is acquired in half the time. Amplitude of phase-encoding gradient is half that of (A). C, 256 × 128 image acquired using asymmetric FOV with the FOV in the phase-encoding direction one half the FOV in the frequency-encoding direction (24 × 12 cm). The resolution is the same as that in (A), but the image is acquired in one half the amount of time. It may not always be possible to reduce the FOV by 50 per cent in the phase-encoding direction due to wraparound.

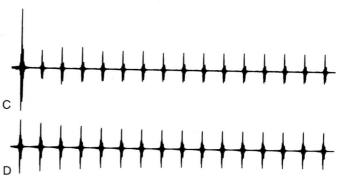

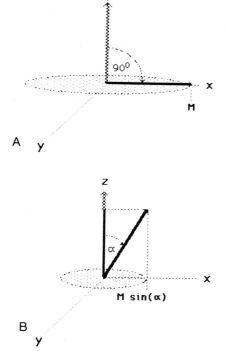

FIGURE 5–5. Comparison of effect on magnetization of *(A)* conventional SE pulse sequence and *(B)* low flip angle FLASH sequence. Transverse magnetization produced by each RF pulse is less with FLASH than SE sequence due to reduced flip angle. However, amount of T_1 relaxation *(stippled arrow)* protons must undergo to remagnetize fully after each RF pulse is markedly reduced with FLASH sequence. As a result, more signals per second can be measured with FLASH technique and the total signal is larger. *C,* A series of echoes produced with TR = 50 msec using 90-degree pulses and *(D)* 28-degree pulses shows that the signal produced by the 90-degree pulse is initially larger. After several excitations, the signal settles to a steady state, and the 28-degree pulse produces a slightly larger amount of signal.

must find ways to acquire data faster, rather than simply acquiring less of it. The following sections describe several means for doing this.

GRADIENT-ECHO TECHNIQUES

Imaging times can be dramatically shortened by reducing TR. In order to maintain adequate image quality despite the reduced TR, it is helpful to abandon conventional SE methods in favor of GRE techniques.

A GRE pulse sequence is actually a simplified version of the SE sequence. To be precise, an SE sequence produces two signals: a spin echo and a gradient echo. The spin echo is produced by the 180-degree pulse and the gradient echo by reversing the magnetic field gradients. These two echoes are used to remove the effects of two very different kinds of magnetic field inhomogeneity; both produce dephasing and signal loss. (1) The spin echo removes the dephasing effects of static magnetic field inhomogeneities. (2) The gradient echo removes the dephasing effects of the pulsed magnetic field gradients (see Chapter 1).

In a properly adjusted SE sequence, these two echoes are coincident in time (see Chapter 10). A GRE pulse sequence is simply an SE sequence that has been modified to eliminate the 180-degree pulse and therefore the SE signal.

Spin-echo methods use a 90-degree excitation in order to maximize the amount of signal produced by each excitation (Fig. 5–5A). This is optimal when TR is long (i.e., TR $\gg$ T_1). However, if the pulse

sequence is repeated quickly, then the spins will not have accumulated enough longitudinal magnetization to produce an adequate signal from the next excitation (Fig. 5–5C).

The key to maintaining image quality at short TR is to use a reduced flip angle for excitation, that is, <90 degrees. With GRE methods, the reduced flip angle actually produces *less* signal from each excitation (Fig. 5–5B), since the signal strength is proportional to the sine of the flip angle. However, because the reduced flip angle preserves more of the longitudinal magnetization after each excitation, the sequence can be repeated rapidly (Fig. 5–5D). Therefore, many more signals can be measured *per second* than with SE methods.

For any combination of TR and T_1 relaxation time, one can determine an optimal flip angle, known as the Ernst angle (θ_{opt}), which provides the maximum amount of signal per second. The Ernst angle is given by:

$$\cos(\theta_{opt}) = \exp(-TR/T_1) \qquad (4)$$

provided TR $\gg$ T_2^*. In essence, this flip angle provides an optimal balance between recovery of the longitudinal magnetization and the production of signal. As an example, if brain has a T_1 = 800 msec, then the optimal flip angle for TR = 2.5 seconds is 87 degrees. Therefore, a conventional 90-degree excitation produces nearly maximal signal. In contrast, if we wish to acquire the image more rapidly, for example, with TR = 100 msec, then the optimal flip angle becomes 28 degrees—far less than the 90 degrees used in an SE sequence.

A small flip angle is precluded for conventional SE

TABLE 5–2. TYPES OF GRADIENT-ECHO METHODS

Sequence Type	Acronyms	Magnetization Component		Contrast Dependence
		Longitudinal	*Transverse*	
Spoiled FLASH	FLASH	yes	no	T_1, proton density
Steady-state FLASH	FISP, GRASS	yes	yes	T_2^*/T_1
Contrast-enhanced FLASH	CE-FAST, PSIF	no	yes	T_2

methods because of the 180-degree RF pulse used to refocus the echo. Consider what happens to the magnetization vector if reduced flip angles were used in an SE sequence. The initial excitation would leave some of the magnetization in the longitudinal direction, such as with GRE methods. The problem is that the 180-degree pulse would then invert this magnetization along the (−z) direction, like an inversion recovery sequence. The resulting steady-state signal would be smaller than that obtained with the usual 90-degree to 180-degree SE sequence. This is why the 180-degree pulse must be eliminated for fast GRE methods.

TYPES OF GRADIENT-ECHO TECHNIQUES

There are several different types of GRE methods in clinical use. Each of these methods relies on using a reduced flip angle to enhance signal with short TR. The techniques differ by relatively small alterations in pulse sequence structure, but these alterations produce dramatic changes in image contrast. These techniques can be best understood by considering the ways in which they affect tissue magnetization and by the ways in which they use this magnetization to produce the MR signal (Table 5–2).

As described in Chapter 1, the tissue magnetization can be split into two parts: (1) a longitudinal component, representing the projection onto the z-axis (direction of main magnetic field); and (2) a transverse component, representing the projection into the x-y plane.

The signal in a GRE image arises from either or both of these components of the tissue magnetization. Part of the signal can be produced by tipping the longitudinal magnetization, and part from the steady-state transverse magnetization. These two contributions can be separated by appropriate manipulations of the pulse sequence.

Spoiled FLASH

The spoiled FLASH sequence (Fig. 5–6), or simply FLASH (*fast low angle shot*), was developed by Frahm and colleagues.[3, 4] Tissue contrast on FLASH images depends solely on the longitudinal component of the tissue magnetization. As a result, of the various GRE methods, FLASH has the simplest contrast behavior and is the most easily understood. Contrast in these images depends primarily on T_1, proton density, or both.

The FLASH sequence employs a gradient pulse called a spoiler at the end of the sequence to destroy any transverse magnetization that persists after signal read-out (see Chapter 10). The spoiler prevents contamination of signal in subsequent excitations by residual transverse magnetization from prior excitations.

Steady-State FLASH

Unlike spoiled FLASH, contrast on steady-state FLASH images represents a mixed contribution from both the longitudinal and transverse components of the tissue magnetization. Steady-state FLASH sequences, also called by several commercial acronyms, such as GRASS (*gradient-recalled acquisition steady state*) and FISP (*fast imaging steady precession*), have an additional gradient pulse placed at the end of the pulse sequence (Fig. 5–7). This gradient pulse, called a rewinder, has a very different purpose than the

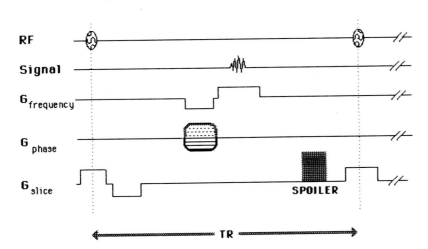

FIGURE 5–6. Spoiled FLASH sequence. This sequence is similar to an SE sequence without a 180-degree RF pulse. In this example, a spoiler gradient pulse along the slice-select direction eliminates residual transverse magnetization (i.e., it eliminates T_2 weighting from subsequent echoes).

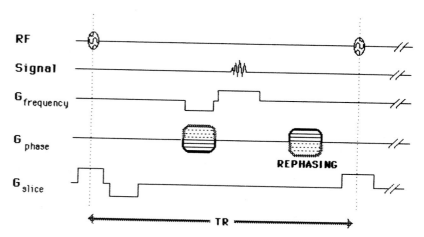

FIGURE 5–7. Steady-state FLASH sequence. This sequence differs from the sequence in Figure 5–6 in that there is no spoiler gradient. Dephasing effects from the phase-encoding gradient are refocused by a "rewinder" gradient applied after signal read-out.

spoiler pulse used in spoiled FLASH. The rewinder gradient serves to eliminate dephasing effects from phase-encoding and enhances, rather than interferes with, persistence of the transverse magnetization. With short TR, signal on subsequent excitations is increased by the persistent transverse magnetization. Contrast in these images depends primarily on the ratio T_2/T_1. Tissues with a large ratio T_2/T_1, such as CSF and edema, tend to appear bright on these images.

Contrast-Enhanced FLASH

As just discussed, in steady-state FLASH sequences, both components of the tissue magnetization contribute to the MR signal. Unfortunately, mixing these components results in reduced image contrast. However, there is a subset of steady-state FLASH methods which produce signals that depend primarily on the transverse component of the tissue magnetization.[5–7] These sequences produce much stronger T_2 contrast than methods such as FISP and GRASS.

With contrast-enhanced FLASH methods (Fig. 5–8), the signals resulting from the longitudinal and transverse components of the tissue magnetization are made to refocus at different times. As a result, these signals can be measured separately. The signal

from the longitudinal component refocuses immediately after the RF pulse. Interestingly, the signal from the transverse component refocuses immediately *before* the subsequent RF pulse. Because the second, more T_2-weighted echo appears before an RF pulse, the term time-reversed has been applied to this echo.

Contrast-enhanced FLASH methods such as CE-FAST and PSIF only measure the second, more T_2-weighted signal. As a result, tissue contrast is no longer confounded by the effects of the signal from the longitudinal component. With contrast-enhanced FLASH methods, T_2 contrast is markedly improved compared with other GRE methods.

CONTRAST IN GRADIENT-ECHO IMAGING

The contrast in GRE imaging is considerably more complex than the contrast in SE imaging.[8–8b] Contrast is a complex function of the user-defined flip angle, magnetic susceptibility, chemical shift, and flow. Fortunately, the complex behavior in fast MR imaging can yield clinically useful information that is difficult to obtain from an SE image. A summary of the effects of changes in flip angle and TE on FLASH images is shown in Figure 5–9, and calculated con-

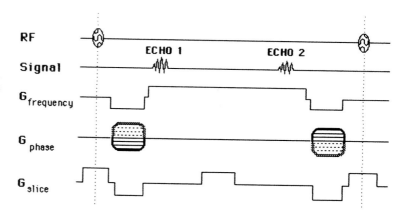

FIGURE 5–8. Contrast-enhanced FLASH sequence. Note that, compared with Figure 5–7, the gradient pulses are unbalanced. This allows temporal separation of the two echoes. Only the second echo is measured in CE-FAST/PSIF methods.

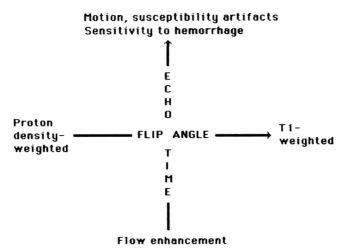

FIGURE 5–9. Rough summary of effects of TE and flip angle on image contrast in GRE imaging. Note that lengthening of TE is not a satisfactory method for producing T_2-weighted images, because image quality is diminished by worsened magnetic susceptibility artifacts.

trast curves for the various GRE techniques are shown in Figure 5–10. The reader should refer to these figures for the following discussion of fast scan contrast.

Contrast from Tissue Relaxation

In SE methods, we do not have the luxury of varying flip angle to alter tissue contrast. Instead, we must vary the TR and TE to produce the desired effects. On the other hand, with fast GRE acquisitions, the TR must be kept short, while the TE must also be kept short for reasons discussed below. Therefore, the flip angle is the primary means for determining tissue contrast.

Slice Profile Effect on Tissue Contrast

Another factor that must be considered before we go into greater depth with specific methods is the effect of slice profile on image contrast (see Chapters 1 and 10). In order to minimize the echo time, which is usually desirable for GRE methods, GRE pulse sequences generally use short RF pulses. These abbreviated RF pulses tend to have imperfect slice profiles, so that flip angles vary across the thickness of the slice. This effect is most severe when short TR and nominally large flip angles are used together. Near the center of the slice, the flip angle will be correct, but the edges of the slice will experience smaller flip angles. For instance, with the spoiled FLASH method, portions of the slice which experience large flip angles show T_1 contrast, whereas portions that experience smaller flip angles show proton density contrast. The combination of these signals results in overall reduced tissue contrast. As a result of this flip angle variation and other effects (e.g., flow and resonance offset), actual tissue contrast

may vary considerably from that predicted below, although general trends will be similar. Even with optimized RF pulses which produce rectangular slice profiles in SE methods, the slice profile may be degraded at short TR.

Spoiled FLASH

With spoiled FLASH methods, the flip angle determines whether the image will be primarily T_1 weighted or proton density weighted. With small flip angles, the longitudinal magnetization remains near its equilibrium value even with short TR. As a result, T_1 relaxation effects are minimal and these images are proton density weighted. However, with increased flip angles, T_1 relaxation effects become important, and the images become T_1 weighted (Figs. 5–10 and 5–11).

In general, to maintain a certain type of tissue contrast with FLASH, flip angles must be scaled with changes in TR. For instance, myelogram-like images can be obtained using a FLASH sequence with TR = 300 msec and flip angle = 10 degrees, but with a shorter TR = 100 msec the flip angle must be reduced to ~ 5 degrees to produce similar contrast. Although the latter image has lower S/N if the NEX is kept constant, both images will have similar S/N if imaging time, rather than NEX, is kept constant. The reason is that, for a given imaging time, more signals can be acquired if the TR is short. The increased number of accumulated signals compensates for the smaller signal per measurement. This latitude in TR (i.e., long TR with few NEX, short TR with more NEX) can be useful in satisfying pulse sequence limitations for multislice GRE imaging or for breath-holding applications.

In a spoiled FLASH image, the transverse magnetization decays in much the same fashion as in an SE sequence. The signal intensity in spoiled FLASH is given by

$$S = S_0 \times [(1 - E_1) \sin\Theta/(1 - E_1\cos\Theta)] \times E_2^* \quad (5)$$

where $E_1 = \exp\{-TR/T_1\}$, $E_2^* = \exp\{-TE/T_2^*\}$, and Θ is the flip angle. S_0 is the maximum obtainable signal, that is, long TR, short TE, and a 90-degree flip angle. The third term, E_2^*, contributes the T_2^* weighting. The T_2^* weighting is somewhat different than T_2 weighting in a spin echo because, as denoted by the asterisk, magnetic field inhomogeneity contributes to the loss of signal. The T_2 and T_2^* weighting increase exponentially with TE. However, artifacts from inhomogeneity and motion worsen with long TE, so heavy T_2 weighting can be difficult to achieve.

Steady-State FLASH

For TR >> T_2, the contrast behavior of steady-state FLASH sequences is identical to spoiled FLASH because the transverse magnetization does not persist between excitations. However, for TR < T_2, a steady-state transverse magnetization develops which

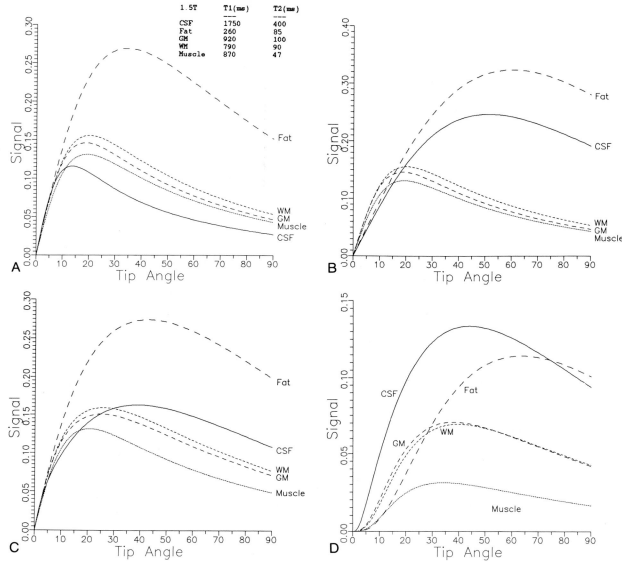

FIGURE 5–10. Simulation of signal strengths from various tissues using different GRE methods. All calculations obtained with TR/TE = 50 msec/12 msec. Vertical axis represents signal strength as a fraction of maximum signal intensity (unweighted image). *A,* Spoiled FLASH. T_1 contrast is highest with large flip angles. However, signal is maximal at smaller flip angles (Ernst angle), here shown to be approximately 15 to 30 degrees. Note that signal curve in region of Ernst angle is relatively flat, suggesting that there is considerable leeway in choice of flip angles. *B,* Steady-state FLASH (FISP, GRASS), obtained with phase alternation of RF pulses. Note marked enhancement of CSF due to its large ratio of T_2/T_1. *C,* Contrast-enhanced FLASH sequence, first echo. Contrast is similar to *(B),* with the exception that CSF has a larger optimal angle. *D,* Contrast-enhanced FLASH sequence, second echo (CE-FAST, PSIF). Note the increased T_2 contrast compared with *A* and *B.* The effective echo time (equals [2TR − TE]) is actually longer than TR.

depends on the ratios T_1/TR and T_2/TR. The steady-state transverse magnetization results in a more complicated expression for the signal intensity than that obtained for spoiled FLASH.[8, 9] The equations for the signal intensity are given in Appendix 5–A. As one would expect, the persistent transverse magnetization favors tissue with a long T_2 (Fig. 5–12). For liquids, such as cerebrospinal fluid (CSF), urine, and blood, the steady-state magnetization is large and

these tissues appear bright. The T_2 of soft tissue (< 100 msec) is shorter than these fluids, so surrounding tissues appear darker. Fat is different from most other soft tissues in having a relatively large ratio T_2/T_1 and appears moderately bright, though darker than liquids.

Steady-state effects tend to dominate at very short TR, on the order of 20 to 50 msec. With a short TR, myelogram-like images of the spine can be acquired

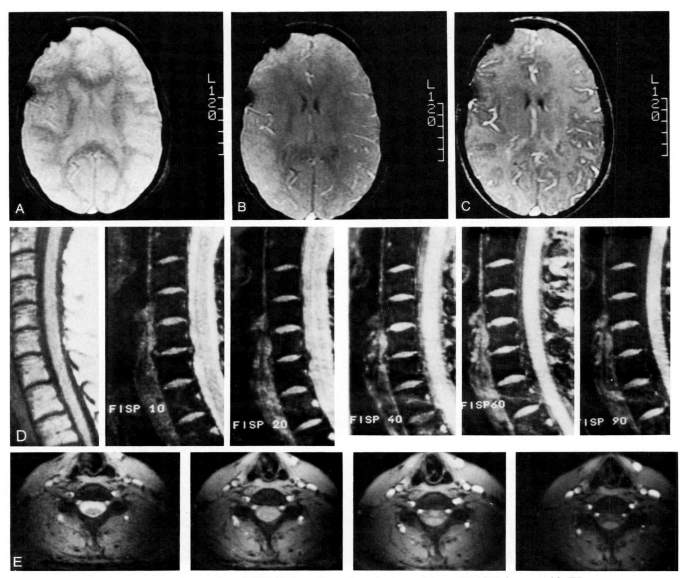

FIGURE 5–11. A–C, A series of GRASS (i.e., alternating phase steady-state FLASH) images with TR = 50 msec, TE = 12 msec, and first order flow compensation. The images were obtained at 1.5 T with tip angles of 8°, 15°, and 40°, for A, B, C, respectively. Note the increase in T_1 weight with increasing tip angle.

D and E, Effect of flip angle on contrast for FLASH imaging of cervical spine. D, Sagittal images. Left to right: SE (TR/TE = 500/17), FISP (TR/TE = 100/18), with flip angles of 10 to 90 degrees. Note maximum CSF enhancement is at smallest flip angles, but maximum S/N is at larger flip angles. (Courtesy M. Modic, M.D.) E, Axial images. FISP (TR/TE = 20/12). Flip angles from left to right = 5°, 10°, 15°, 20°. Although theory predicts maximum CSF enhancement at large flip angles, this example shows that maximum enhancement actually occurs at lower flip angles because of dephasing effects of CSF pulsation.

in just a few seconds; however, *the short TR limits the acquisition to a single slice.* Multiple slices must be acquired sequentially. For stationary fluids such as urine, maximal contrast is obtained with a large flip angle (e.g., 90 degrees). Flow disrupts the steady-state transverse magnetization in CSF and blood, so maximal contrast is obtained at a smaller than expected flip angle. Because of this, flip angles of 5 to 20 degrees produce optimal signal in situations in which there is moderate flow; for example, CSF in the spine.

The exact flip angle used for optimal signal will depend on the scan plane, the direction and velocity of flow, and whether flow compensation is used. Typically, the smallest flip angles are used when the frequency-encoding direction is parallel to the flow. As an example, with a TR of 40 msec, a large flip angle (70 to 90 degrees) would be expected to produce CSF enhancement. This result can be obtained with stationary CSF in the lateral ventricles (Fig. 5–12), but a small flip angle of ~5 degrees is needed to produce the same effect for pulsating CSF in the cervical spine (Fig. 5–11D and E).

A better myelogram effect can be obtained using

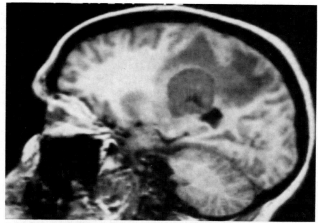

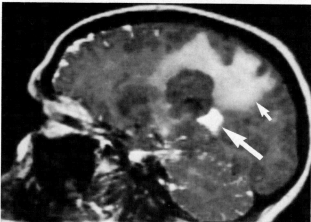

FIGURE 5–12. Spoiled FLASH *(top)* and steady-state FLASH *(bottom)* pulse sequences show markedly divergent contrast behavior with very short TR. Parasagittal images at 1.5 T in patient with brain metastasis. TR/TE/Flip angle = 30/14/90°. Note that spoiled FLASH image appears T_1 weighted, but with same scan parameters the FISP image shows marked enhancement of CSF *(large arrow)* and edema *(small arrow)* (large ratio T_2/T_1).

larger flip angles and a "true" FISP sequence, in which all three gradients are perfectly balanced and flow compensated to produce complete rephasing of the transverse magnetization at the echo time (M. Haake, personal communication). However, this sequence is not yet generally available.

Proton density–weighted images can be obtained from a long TR, steady-state GRE sequence in the same fashion as for spoiled FLASH, that is, with a small flip angle to reduce T_1 weight and a short TE. In fact, *for TR ≥ 100 msec, FLASH and GRASS/FISP have almost identical contrast.* The long TR permits multislice GRE acquisitions, but it also greatly increases imaging time. In addition, just as for spoiled FLASH, the long echo times necessary for T_2^* weight introduce a number of artifacts and are often impractical.

The high signal intensity of CSF on short TR, steady-state GRE images can lead one to erroneously assume that these images are strongly T_2 weighted. In fact, the only tissues that are truly T_2 weighted are those that have very long T_2 values, that is, fluids. Subtle pathology, such as multiple sclerosis plaques, which one would expect to see on a T_2-weighted image, may have poor contrast.

Contrast-Enhanced FLASH

As mentioned earlier, GRE sequences produce signals with two different types of weighting. (1) The echo produced by the steady-state longitudinal magnetization is proton density or T_1 weighted, depending on the flip angle and TR. (2) The echo produced by the persistent steady-state transverse magnetization is heavily T_2 weighted.

In an ordinary steady-state FLASH acquisition, the two echoes are coincident, so that the signal is a complex function of tissue relaxation times and scan parameters. For most tissues that have short or moderate T_2 relaxation times the contrast produced by these sequences is poor. However, in contrast-enhanced FLASH methods, such as CE-FAST/PSIF, only the second echo is measured. The ratio of the signal intensity of the second echo to that of the first is roughly proportional to $\exp(-2TR/T_2)$. As a result, the second echo and resultant images are strongly T_2 weighted.

The effective TE for these sequences is equal to $(2TR - TE)$. We see that the effective TE is actually *longer* than the TR, which at first glance defies common sense. What is happening is that the signal from one excitation is being refocused during a subsequent excitation, resulting in a prolonged TE. The long effective TE permits T_2 contrast effects to develop, unlike GRASS/FISP type images, which have much shorter TE.

A disadvantage of contrast-enhanced FLASH methods is that S/N may be unacceptably low due to the modest amount of steady-state transverse magnetization and the discarding of the longitudinal component. A comparison of SE, FISP, and a strongly T_2-weighted CE-FAST image is shown in Figure 5–13. The signal strength equations for steady-state FLASH and CE-FAST are given in Appendix 5–1. An interesting additional benefit of CE-FAST sequences is lessened sensitivity to magnetic susceptibility artifacts (below) as compared with other GRE methods.

Magnetic Field Effects

Magnetic Field Inhomogeneity

Gradient-echo imaging techniques do not employ RF refocusing to produce a spin echo. The lack of a spin echo means that magnetic field variation (inhomogeneity) influences the strength of the GRE. Any local distortion of the magnetic field results in a loss of signal. The signal loss with increasing TE depends

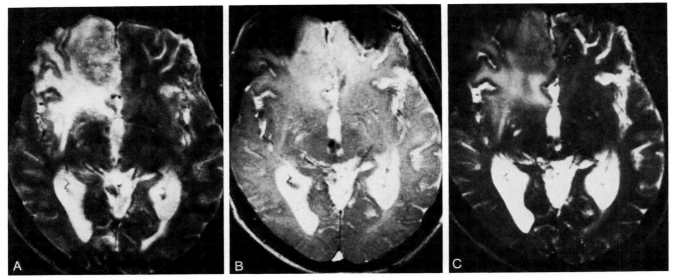

FIGURE 5–13. Images of a patient with a right frontal lobe glioma. *A*, T_2-weighted spin-echo image (TR/TE = 2300/90) with 1 excitation. *B*, FISP flip angle = 60°, TR/TE = 30/6, 8 excitations. Note poor delineation of tumor. Bright areas near frontal sinuses represent susceptibility artifacts near air-brain interface. *C*, CE-FAST flip angle = 60°, TR/TE = 40/9, 8 excitations. CSF is bright on both FISP and CE-FAST images. Note improved T_2 contrast and tumor delineation as well as reduced susceptibility artifacts with CE-FAST. (Courtesy M. Modic, M.D.)

on T_2^* not T_2 alone. The rate at which signal is lost is given by:

$$1/T_2^* = 1/T_2 + \gamma \pi \Delta B_0 \qquad (6)$$

where ΔB_0 is the magnetic field variation across a pixel, and γ is the magnetogyric ratio for hydrogen (42 MHz/T).

Given the strong effect of these field inhomogeneities, what are their causes? First, part of the variation in the magnetic field is due to limitations of the magnet. The magnetic field decreases with the distance from the center of the magnet. This contribution to magnetic field inhomogeneity shows up as a characteristic zebra-stripe effect at the borders of large FOV GRE images, representing severe spatially dependent phase variations (Fig. 5–14). The intrinsic inhomogeneity reduces the useful FOV, but this is not a problem for most scan protocols.

Second, if a substance of any kind is placed in a magnetic field, the magnetic field *within* the substance will have a different strength than the external magnetic field. The effect of the substance can be to enhance or to exclude the external field. Ferromagnetic substances, such as iron, strongly increase the strength of the internal field. As might be expected, these substances form excellent permanent magnets. The effect of a ferromagnetic object, such as an aneurysm clip, in the body is to produce a large magnetic field variation (gradient) in adjacent tissue. Since GRE sequences are particularly sensitive to such variations, a GRE image will have a much larger area of signal loss than an SE image of the same tissue. In addition, since MR images are acquired through the use of carefully calibrated magnetic field gra-

dients, unwanted gradients produced by metal objects will cause a geometric distortion of the image.

Third, when metal objects are not present in the body, the internal magnetic field in tissue is usually shifted only slightly from the external field. Most tissues decrease the magnetic field by a small amount

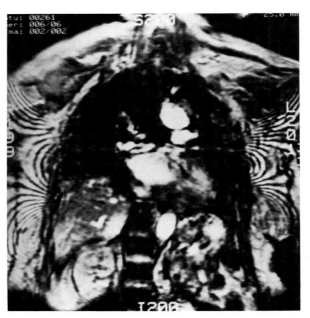

FIGURE 5–14. A coronal GRASS (steady-state FLASH) image obtained with TR = 21 msec, TE = 12 msec, and a 40 cm FOV. Note the zebra-striped patterns of signal loss at the periphery of the FOV due to inhomogeneity of the static magnetic field.

and are called diamagnetic. In some cases, substances that increase the magnetic field can accumulate in the body. These substances are called paramagnetic. Paramagnetic substances include the contrast agent gadolinium-DTPA (Gd-DTPA) and hemoglobin breakdown products in hemorrhage.

The effect of diamagnetic and paramagnetic materials on the internal magnetic field is approximately given by:

$$B_0(\text{tissue}) = B_0(1 + \tfrac{4}{3}\pi k) \qquad (7)$$

where k is the volume magnetic susceptibility of the tissue. The shift in the magnetic field is proportional to k *and* the strength of the external magnetic field. T_2^* signal loss is caused by the *variation* of the magnetic field over a pixel (see Equation 6), so susceptibility effects are greatest when there is a large change in susceptibility over a short distance.

If adjacent regions of tissue have different susceptibilities, there will be a change in the magnetic field at the tissue boundary. If the change is large, T_2^* will be short enough to cause significant signal loss at the border between the two tissues. There are several instances where this effect is noticeable. Air-tissue interfaces, for example, paranasal sinuses, lung, and bowel, produce a moderately wide band of signal loss, which makes it difficult to make GRE images of these structures.

Fortunately, signal loss from susceptibility can also be beneficial. For example, paramagnetic components in hemorrhage can produce a visible border around the hemorrhage which may be diagnostic.[10] In addition, calcification is more easily seen in a GRE image than in an SE image. All of these examples are more pronounced at higher field strengths because the induced magnetic field gradient is proportional to field strength.

There are several ways to minimize susceptibility effects in GRE techniques.

1. The most obvious is to decrease the T_2^* weighting by using the minimum possible TE.

2. T_2^*-related signal loss depends on the amount of magnetic field variation across the voxel. Therefore, susceptibility losses can be minimized by decreasing the voxel, particularly in its largest dimension (i.e., reducing slice thickness).

3. Geometric distortion caused by field inhomogeneity can be minimized by using strong gradients (i.e., large bandwidths). Unfortunately, along the read-out direction this approach reduces S/N, while along the slice-selection direction it results in increased RF power deposition.

4. Finally, three-dimensional (3D) GRE methods reduce T_2^* effects for two reasons. First, thinner slices can be obtained than with two-dimensional (2D) SE methods. Second, if enough z phase-encoding steps (partitions) are used, then for certain strengths of this gradient it may coincidentally cancel local field inhomogeneities produced by susceptibility variations. Nevertheless, some geometric distortion may still occur.[10a]

Chemical Shift Effects

Hydrogen nuclei in different types of tissue have slightly different resonance frequencies. Normally, the frequency differences are small enough that they do not interfere with imaging. The exception is fat and water. Hydrogen nuclei in fat have a chemical environment that is considerably different than that found in the hydrogen nuclei in water. The different chemical environment results in a slightly different local magnetic field and, therefore, a slightly different resonance frequency. The frequency difference between fat and water is: $3.5 \times 10^{-6} \times$ MR frequency. The value typically given for the chemical shift difference between fat and water is 3.5 ppm, or 147 Hz at 1.0 T.

The different resonance frequencies of fat and water result in a slightly displaced image of fat in the frequency-encoding direction. The shift is more pronounced at higher magnetic fields because of the larger frequency difference. The shift between fat and water produces a characteristic bright band and dark band at the fat/water interface. This banding, which appears in both SE and GRE images, is called chemical shift artifact (see Chapters 3 and 10).

In an SE image, the signals of fat and water are normally forced to be the same phase by the formation of a spin echo. The spin echo reverses the effects of both magnetic field inhomogeneity *and* the chemical shift. The RF pulse timings can be changed to produce an out-of-phase SE image.[11] However, in GRE images, there is no spin echo and the fat and water signals will be in- or out-of-phase according to their (magnetic field–dependent) frequency difference and the choice of TE. As with SE, the GRE signals start out in-phase, but they will oscillate in- and out-of-phase during TE (Fig. 5–15). The time required for fat and water to evolve from in-phase to out-of-phase is:

$$\Delta TE = (2 \times 3.5 \times \text{MR frequency in MHz})^{-1} \text{ or}$$
$$\Delta TE = 3.4 \text{ msec}/B_0 \text{ (in tesla)}$$

When TE is equal to an even multiple of ΔTE, the signals are in-phase, whereas images acquired at odd multiples of ΔTE show signal loss due to fat/water phase contrast. For example, at a field strength of 0.6 T, $\Delta TE = 5.5$ msec, so an image with TE = 11 msec is in-phase, while TE = 16 msec shows phase contrast. At 1.5 T, ΔTE is only about 2.1 msec, so small changes in TE can substantially alter the image intensity of tissue containing both fat and water.

Phase-contrast images are useful when it is desired to reduce the signal from tissue that contains both fat and water, for example, bone marrow. *Normal red bone marrow appears dark on a phase-contrast FLASH image* because the fat and water signals nearly cancel. When marrow is replaced by a cellular infiltrate, as occurs with leukemic infiltration and metastatic disease, the increased water content of the marrow is reflected as increased signal intensity on proton density (small flip angle) phase-contrast FLASH images (Fig. 5–15B).

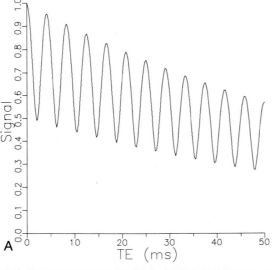

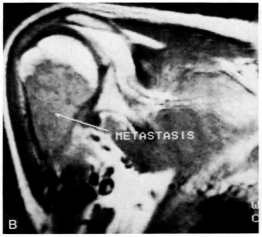

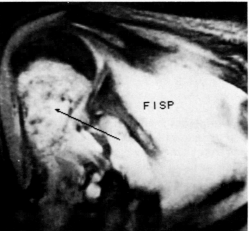

FIGURE 5–15. *A,* Calculated signal intensity versus TE at 1.5 T in a GRE image of simulated marrow consisting of 75 per cent fat and 25 per cent water. The oscillations in the signal intensity are due to a slight difference in the resonance frequency of fat and water (i.e., chemical shift). *B,* Patient with oat cell metastasis to right humeral shaft. Gradient-echo images are sensitive to bone marrow abnormalities such as metastatic lesions. On T_1-weighted SE image *(left),* normal marrow appears bright and metastasis appears dark. On proton density GRE image *(right),* marrow appears dark and metastasis appears bright.

Unfortunately, *bone marrow can appear dark on FLASH images even when the TE is adjusted to produce an in-phase image.* The reason relates to the complex honeycomb structures of cancellous bone; within each voxel, the numerous interfaces produce magnetic susceptibility gradients that shorten the T_2^* of marrow. As TE is lengthened, sensitivity to these susceptibility effects increases, resulting in a decrease in marrow signal regardless of whether the fat and water signal add or cancel. Owing to the RF refocusing pulse, SE phase contrast images are less sensitive to these susceptibility effects.

Flow Effects

Flow effects in MR imaging are discussed in detail in Chapter 4. In this section, we will briefly discuss some of the aspects of flow which are unique to GRE imaging. First, GRE images have enhanced signal intensity for almost all flow rates. This behavior is in contrast to flow enhancement in SE imaging. In SE images, an enhanced signal only occurs if the flowing material does not flow out of the selected slice before the 180-degree pulse, that is, in < TE/2. In GRE images, there is no refocusing pulse, so any unsaturated nuclei moving into the image plane will yield an enhanced signal. To maximize this effect, some GRE sequences image one slice at a time, so all slices show enhancement due to entrance slice effects. In multislice SE imaging, enhancement is usually confined to the outermost slices.

As discussed above, GRE pulse sequences produce a gradient echo by canceling the effect of the magnetic field gradients at the echo time. If material (blood) moves between the start of the pulse sequence and the TE, this cancellation will not be complete, and the signal will have a distorted phase. Constant velocity blood flow produces a phase shift that is proportional to both flow velocity and, more importantly, the square of the duration of the gradient pulse.[11a] The quadratic dependence of the phase distortion on the gradient duration causes the largest flow-dependent phase shift to occur in the frequency-encoding direction, since the read-out gradient has the longest duration in the sequence.

Flow in the body is usually not constant velocity, so the phase shifts produced by flow are slightly different for each acquisition. Pulsatile flow modulates the MR signal with an approximately sinusoidal variation of the phase shift with time. This modulation, in turn, produces a series of ghost images of the vessel. These ghost images are a significant problem in that they can easily obscure the region of interest. Fortunately, there is a solution in that it is possible to substantially reduce ghosting by making a slight modification to GRE pulse sequences.

A GRE sequence can be made less susceptible to flow by the use of additional gradient pulses which cancel out the motion-induced modulation of the signal.[12] This technique, called gradient motion rephasing (GMR), flow compensation (flow comp), or gradient moment nulling, works well with nonturbulent flow (see Chapter 4). For a first order correction, the assumption is made that the flow velocity is constant. This correction removes most but not all of the flow-related ghosting. Corrections for acceleration and higher order flow can be applied to the pulse sequence but tend to extend the TE as gradient pulses are added and generally do not provide noticeable improvements in image quality.

With flow compensation, substantial artifacts and signal loss will still occur in vessels that have highly pulsatile flow, or where there are bends or constrictions in the vessel, that is, where there is significant acceleration. Artifacts and signal loss from large scale turbulent flow cannot be corrected by gradient compensation schemes. However, signal loss due to turbulence may be useful in some situations, for example, in diagnosing a diseased heart valve where stenosis may cause local turbulence and dephasing.

Flow compensation techniques have some disadvantages. The additional compensation pulses take time and therefore increase the minimum TE and TR. The longer TE may then result in susceptibility artifacts. In addition, flow compensation may limit the available FOV, since high amplitude gradient pulses may be used. However, in most imaging protocols, the advantages of flow compensation outweigh its minor shortcomings.

In some commercial MRI systems, flow compensation techniques do not work perfectly, in part because the gradient pulses are distorted by secondary magnetic fields produced by eddy currents in the magnet. A new gradient coil design, known as a shielded gradient, can largely eliminate these disruptive secondary fields. Shielded gradient coils use two sets of concentric gradient coils working in opposite phase. The outer coil protects the magnet from picking up magnetic field gradients and reduces the intensity of any eddy currents. Shielded gradients can substantially improve many applications of GRE imaging, such as angiography and cardiac cinematography, for which flow artifacts are particularly problematic (Fig. 5–16). Similar benefits can be obtained in some systems simply by careful optimization of eddy current precompensation (see Chapter 12).

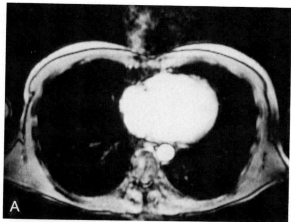
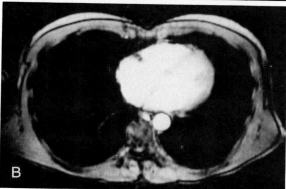

FIGURE 5–16. Gradient-echo cineangiography images of the heart obtained using ordinary gradients *(A)* and shielded gradients *(B)*. The shielded gradients can reduce unwanted magnetic field gradients induced by eddy currents within the magnet. Note the reduction of flow artifacts when shielded gradients are used due to improved flow compensation after eddy currents are reduced (Courtesy of General Electric Medical Systems.)

CLINICAL APPLICATIONS OF GRADIENT-ECHO IMAGING

Gradient-echo methods can be used for several general applications including motion reduction with fast scanning, assessment of a variety of dynamic processes, and utilization of altered contrast mechanisms, such as susceptibility differences and chemical shift information. Table 5–3 summarizes the clinical applications based on imaging time. Typical GRE sequence parameters are summarized in Table 5–4.

TABLE 5–3. CLINICAL APPLICATIONS OF GRADIENT-ECHO IMAGING

1 to 5 sec	0.5 to 3 min
Flow assessment	MR myelogram
Contrast agent dynamics	Hemorrhage assessment
Pediatrics	Calcification assessment
Poor patient compliance	Chemical shift imaging
10 to 20 sec	**5 to 10 min**
Breath-holding abdomen studies	3D surface reconstruction
	MR angiography
	Cardiac cine

TABLE 5–4. SUMMARY OF PARAMETERS FOR RAPID GRADIENT-ECHO IMAGING

Contrast	Sequence Name	TR *(msec)*	TE *(msec)*	Flip Angle
T_1 weighted	FLASH	Short e.g., 100	Short 10	Large 60–90°
T_2 weighted	CE-FAST/PSIF	Very short e.g., 20–40	—	Large 90°
T_2^* weighted	FLASH	Short e.g., 100	Long 30–60	Small 20°
MR myelogram	FLASH	Short e.g., 300	Short 10	Small 10°
MR myelogram (single slice)	FISP/GRASS*	Very short e.g., 20	Short 10	Small 5°
Phase contrast	FLASH or FISP/ GRASS	—	B_0-dependent 2.2, 6.6, 11.0 @ 1.5 T	—

*For "true" FISP with completely balanced, flow-compensated gradients, use large flip angle (e.g., 75 degrees).

Abdomen

Respiratory motion artifacts are a significant obstacle to using MR as a routine tool to screen the liver for metastatic disease. Blurring and ghost artifacts routinely reduce lesion detectability. Gradient-echo imaging provides an attractive solution to the problem of respiratory motion because it provides a method for obtaining images within a breath-holding interval (10 to 20 seconds).[13] Screening of the liver can be performed using T_1-weighted FLASH images in a multislice mode (Fig. 5–17). The multislice capability varies from system to system. Although S/N may not be as good when compared with longer SE acquisitions, the absence of respiratory ghost artifacts in conjunction with strong T_1 weighting allows satisfactory liver/lesion contrast to be obtained. Furthermore, the short imaging time permits dynamic imaging with contrast agents such as Gd-DTPA. Since Gd-DTPA equilibrates between tumor and liver after several minutes, dynamic imaging can be used to observe changes in liver/lesion contrast (Fig. 5–18A–D). Preliminary experience on high field systems suggest that breath-hold T_1-weighted GRE images using ultrashort TE may replace standard T_1-weighted SE images for liver imaging.[14]

Peristalsis can be imaged using sequential one-second acquisitions, permitting differentiation of the head of pancreas and duodenum without an oral contrast agent. Magnetic susceptibility artifacts, caused by bowel gas, help identify bowel loops but may also reduce image quality, particularly on high field systems. These susceptibility artifacts can be reduced using very short echo times (e.g., TE = 5 msec), which are now becoming available on commercial MR systems.

T_2- and T_2^*-weighted GRE images can also be obtained with breath-holding. It may be possible to distinguish cavernous hemangiomas, which have markedly prolonged T_2^* relaxation times, from malignant tumors using these fast images. However, additional clinical experience must be accumulated with these techniques. At the present time, contrast and S/N limitations preclude using T_2-weighted FLASH methods to supplant SE methods for lesion detection and characterization. However, with continued technical improvements, rapid MR imaging may prove useful for T_2- and T_2^*-weighted imaging of the liver. Some of the single-shot imaging techniques described below may allow strongly T_2-weighted images to be obtained within a breath-holding interval. Contrast-enhanced FLASH may also have potential applications for characterization of cavernous hemangiomas (Fig. 5–18E and F).[14]

MR Myelogram

Cerebrospinal fluid–enhanced (proton density) GRE images are particularly useful for demonstrating degenerative disk and spondylotic changes in the spine (Fig. 5–19). GRE images have several advantages over SE images for assessment of radiculopathy: (1) improved S/N for equal imaging time, (2) reduced sensitivity to CSF motion, and (3) better delineation of osteophytes. Disk herniations and marrow-containing osteophytes have a variable appearance on T_2-weighted SE images; herniated disks and osteophytes may both appear bright or dark. Because FLASH images are less sensitive to T_2 shortening from disk degeneration, disk protrusions almost always appear bright, whereas osteophytes appear dark due to susceptibility effects, providing more reliable differentiation between these two types of pathology (Fig. 5–19). One caveat in using GRE methods clinically is that mild degrees of lumbar disk degeneration may be missed on FLASH images (Fig. 5–20).

Both T_1- and proton density–weighted GRE images can be obtained (Fig. 5–21). Because of the shorter acquisition time (30 seconds to 3 minutes) compared with T_2-weighted SE images (> 10 minutes), FLASH methods can reduce image degradation from patient motion and improve throughput. Reduced acquisition time is particularly useful for total spine surveys in patients with spinal block. Because of lower T_2 contrast, GRE methods in our experience cannot supplant SE methods for assessment of myelopathy, for which sensitivity to subtle inflammatory lesions is important. However, one study has shown similar sensitivity to cord lesions for SE or GRE techniques.[14a] Contrast-enhanced FLASH techniques may improve applications of GRE imaging in this area, though their extreme sensitivity to motion artifact, such as produced by CSF pulsation, currently limits their application.

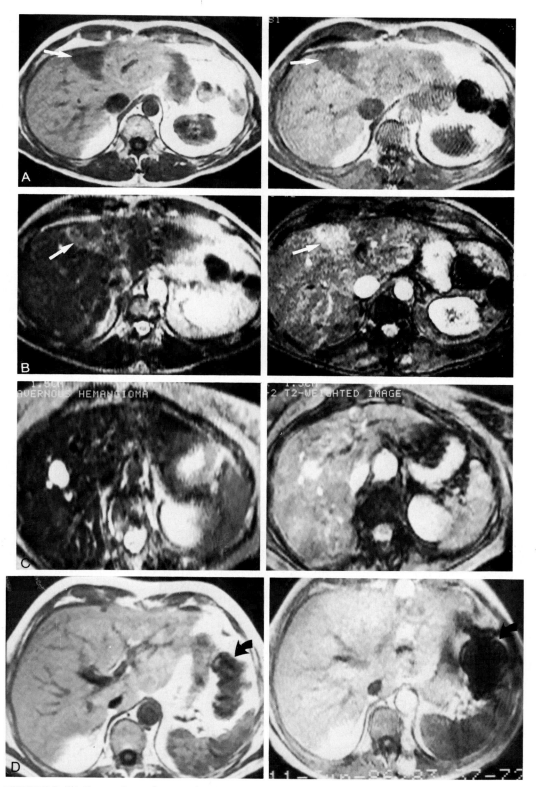

FIGURE 5–17. Comparison of conventional SE images *(left column)*, acquired in 10 to 15 minutes, with fast FLASH images *(right column)*, acquired in 10 to 20 seconds, during a single breath-hold at 0.6 tesla. *A*, Both SE (300/14) image *(left)* and T_1-weighted FLASH (200/11/90°) image *(right)* show hepatic metastasis as low intensity lesion *(arrow)*. Note that, at 0.6 T, TE = 11 msec an in-phase GRE image is produced. *B*, In same patient as *(A)*, T_2-weighted FLASH (200/30/20°) image *(right)* shows lesion better than SE (2350/120) image, perhaps due to reduced motion artifact. Note much greater flow-related enhancement on FLASH image, as well as low intensity rings surrounding abdominal viscera, due to fat-water phase contrast effects. *C*, Cavernous hemangioma of liver is comparably demonstrated on SE 2000/180 image *(left)* and FLASH 100/20/20° image *(right)*. *D*, Note artifactually increased diameter of air-containing bowel loop *(arrow)* on FLASH image *(right)* compared with SE image *(left)* due to magnetic susceptibility effect.

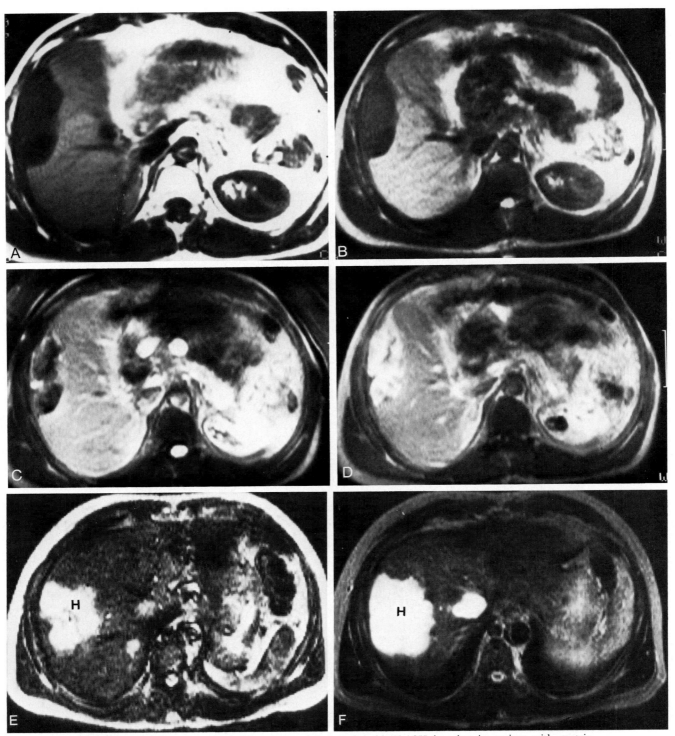

FIGURE 5–18. *A–D,* Standard SE and dynamic breath-hold FLASH imaging in patient with gastric leiomyosarcoma metastatic to liver. All images acquired with 256 × 128 matrix at 1.5 tesla. *A,* Conventional 8-minute SE sequence with TR/TE/NEX = 450 msec/12 msec/8 excitations. Because of the long acquisition time, dynamic imaging is not possible with this sequence. *B,* Precontrast FLASH image acquired during 10-second breath-hold (one of nine images) using TR/TE/flip angle = 100 msec/5 msec/80° and one excitation. Note excellent T_1 contrast between lesion and liver, comparable to *(A).* Flow artifacts are suppressed by presaturation. *C,* Immediate postcontrast FLASH image acquired as in *(B),* following administration of 0.1 mmol/kg Gd-DTPA over 30 seconds, demonstrates enhancement of liver with only minimal enhancement of edge of lesion. (Vascular pulsation artifacts are worsened, despite presaturation, due to shortened T_1 relaxation time of blood.) *D,* Delayed postcontrast FLASH image demonstrates partial filling in of lesion.

E and *F,* Different patient with three cavernous hemangiomas in the liver. CE-FAST image *(E)* obtained with TR = 30 msec in <10 seconds provides comparable evaluation of hemangioma (H) to that obtained in 10 minutes using T_2-weighted SE image (slightly different slice position) *(F).*

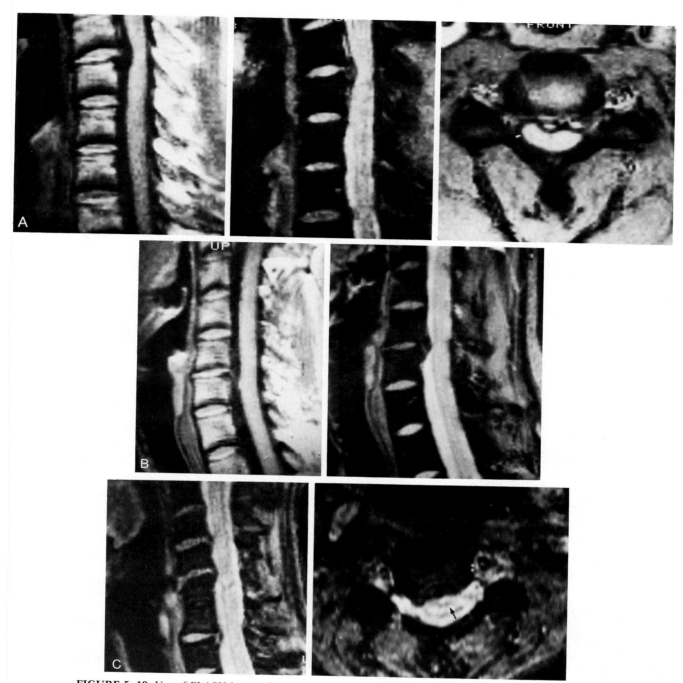

FIGURE 5–19. Use of FLASH images for evaluation of cervical spine disease in three patients at 1.5 T.

A, Patient with bilateral arm pain and weakness. Left to right, SE (500/20) image demonstrates cord impingement but fails to clearly show disk protrusion; sagittal proton density FLASH (TR/TE/flip angle = 300/18/15°) shows disk protrusion; degree of cord impingement is best shown on 3 mm thick T_1-weighted FLASH axial image (300/18/60°). Note improvement in S/N and decreased intensity of CSF with larger flip angle.

B, Patient with neck pain. Left, Sagittal T_1-weighted SE image fails to demonstrate full extent of disk pathology; right, proton density FLASH image sharply demonstrates osteophyte abutting cord. Note low intensity of osteophyte as compared with higher disk intensity in *(A).*

C, Patient with multiple disk bulges and osteophytes. Left, Sagittal proton density FLASH image. Right, 3-mm axial proton density FLASH image shows encroachment on right neural foramen by osteophyte. High intensity within cord *(arrow)* represents truncation artifact from cord-CSF interface.

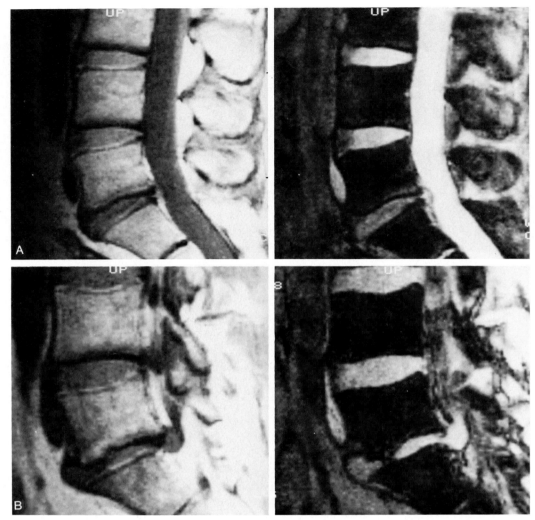

FIGURE 5–20. FLASH can provide rapid myelographic images in lumbar spine but is insensitive to disk degeneration. *A, left,* SE 500/20; *right,* proton density FLASH 300/18/15°. Degenerated disk at L5/S1 level has decreased signal intensity. *B, left,* SE 500/20 image demonstrates herniated disk at L5/S1; *right,* on proton density FLASH 300/18/15° image herniated disk appears bright. On T_2-weighted SE images, herniated disks usually appear dark due to disk degeneration.

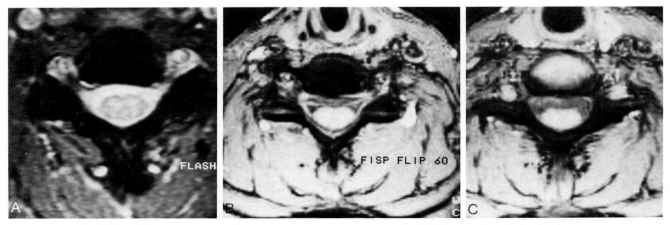

FIGURE 5–21. Comparison of T_1- and proton density–weighted FLASH for axial cervical spine images. *Left to right,* Proton density FLASH (300/18/15°) demonstrates excellent gray-white matter differentiation in cord and myelogram effect; T_1-weighted FLASH (300/18/60°) demonstrates dorsal and ventral nerve rootlets entering the neural foramina; T_1-weighted FLASH image at level of interspace demonstrates bright disk, whereas disk would appear darker on T_1-weighted SE image.

Hemorrhage

Acute and chronic hemorrhage produce magnetic susceptibility changes that are easily detected with SE imaging on high field systems (see Chapters 8 and 16).[15] These changes, which are attributed to the presence of paramagnetic deoxyhemoglobin (acute) and ferritin and hemosiderin (chronic), produce signal loss that is not usually detected with low or intermediate magnetic field strength systems on SE images. T_2^*-weighted GRE images are very sensitive to bulk magnetic susceptibility variation from tissue iron and can detect both acute and chronic hemorrhage at field strengths as low as 0.15 T even in the absence of methemoglobin (Fig. 5–22). GRE images, which can be obtained quickly, should improve the diagnostic specificity for hemorrhage on low and intermediate field systems.

On high field systems, GRE images enhance detection of hemorrhagic lesions. However, the specificity of GRE images may be less than that of SE images. Both SE and FLASH images often demonstrate a ring of decreased signal intensity surrounding a hemorrhagic lesion. On an SE image, a low intensity ring would suggest the presence of hemosiderin and would indicate a subacute or old hemorrhage. On GRE images the dark ring can appear because of a much smaller change in susceptibility at the junction

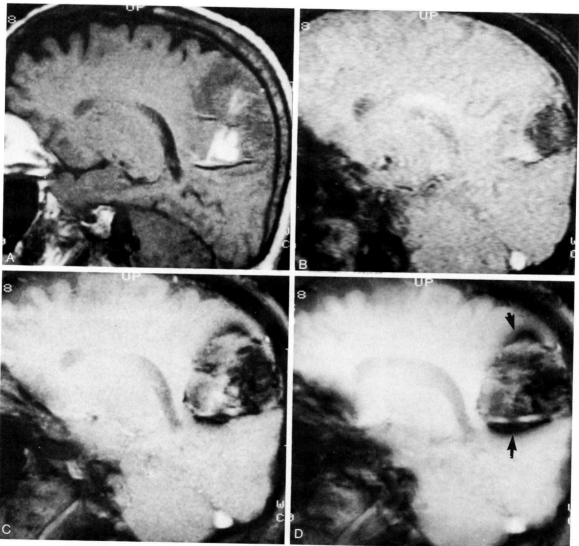

FIGURE 5–22. Sensitivity of GRE images to magnetic susceptibility effects from hemorrhage increases with echo time and slice thickness. Patient with hemorrhagic parietal infarct. Frequency encoding gradient is vertical. *A*, Parasagittal T_1-weighted SE image demonstrates increased signal from extracellular methemoglobin. *B*, FLASH image acquired with TR/TE/flip angle = 60/11/30° demonstrates relatively small region of decreased signal due to susceptibility effects. *C*, With longer TE (22 msec), the low intensity region has markedly increased in size. The low intensity lesion falsely appears larger than the actual region of hemorrhage due to the marked sensitivity of the image to susceptibility effects. *D*, With doubling of slice thickness, extent of signal loss is still greater. Note rim of low signal intensity *(arrows)*, which represents a boundary effect between two regions of differing magnetic susceptibility (normal brain and hemorrhage).

TABLE 5–5. CAUSES OF LOW INTENSITY ON GRADIENT-ECHO IMAGES

1. Hemorrhage: deoxyhemoglobin
   intracellular methemoglobin
   hemosiderin
2. Calcification
3. Ferritin
4. Air (e.g., paranasal sinuses)
5. Contrast agents: superparamagnetic
   paramagnetic in high concentration, long TE
6. Flow turbulence/shear flow
7. Susceptibility borders

of two regions with differing magnetic susceptibility (i.e., hemorrhage and normal brain).[10] Other causes of low signal intensity on GRE images must also be considered in the differential (Table 5–5).

Flow

Even very rapidly flowing blood produces a signal in fast GRE images. Vessels that would show a flow void in an SE image usually have a very intense signal in a GRE image, particularly when flow compensation is used. The bright signal from flowing blood can be used to advantage in a number of ways. For example, flow can be distinguished from calcification in arteriovenous malformations (Fig. 5–23). As another example, GRE sequences that have been modified to selectively cancel out signal from stationary tissue can be used to produce MR projection angiograms[16] (Fig. 5–24). Angiographic images or ordinary fast GRE images can be used to confirm the presence of flowing blood within vessels (see Chapter 4).

Another use for GRE imaging is in MR cineangiography.[17] Fast scan MR techniques can be used to

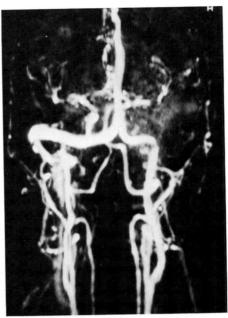

FIGURE 5–24. MR projection acquisition angiogram using complex subtraction method (see Chapter 4). This image was generated using magnetic gradients to create a deliberate phase shift for flowing blood. The signal from surrounding tissue was removed by subtracting images with opposite amounts of flow encoding, resulting in the cancellation of stationary tissue. (Courtesy of General Electric Medical Systems.)

perform MR cineangiography by acquiring multiphase data synchronized to the cardiac cycle during the course of 128 or 256 heartbeats. Cine images of the heart can be used to evaluate ejection fraction, valve function, and congenital defects. Flow and cineangiographic imaging via GRE techniques will

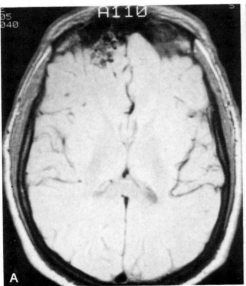 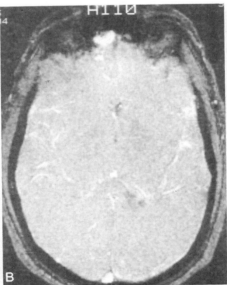 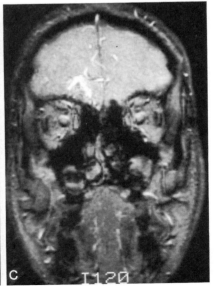

FIGURE 5–23. Flow-compensated FLASH images are useful for differentiating calcification and thrombus from patent blood vessels. Patient with right frontal arteriovenous malformation (AVM). *A*, AVM appears uniformly dark on T₁-weighted SE image. *B*, Axial steady-state FLASH (GRASS) 21/12/30° image demonstrates marked flow enhancement in patent vessels. *C*, Coronal GRASS image shows similar findings.

improve with new hardware, pulse sequences, and reconstruction techniques. These applications will be discussed in more detail in later chapters devoted to these topics.

Contrast Agents

The assessment of tissue perfusion with contrast agents like Gd-DTPA requires rapid image acquisition (Fig. 5–25). However, one must be aware that GRE images are more sensitive than SE images to susceptibility effects that occur with high concentrations of paramagnetic contrast agents; this can cause unexpected loss of signal. For instance, this effect is seen in the renal pelvis following administration of Gd-DTPA due to the high concentration of the paramagnetic agent (Fig. 5–26). In the future, sensitivity to susceptibility effects may be useful in conjunction with susceptibility agents such as dysprosium-DTPA for imaging of brain and cardiac perfusion (see Chapter 25).

The Knee

On proton density FLASH images (e.g., TR/TE/flip angle = 40 msec/10 msec/30 degrees), normal knee menisci appear dark; meniscal tears appear bright. Effusions and Baker's cysts are well demon-

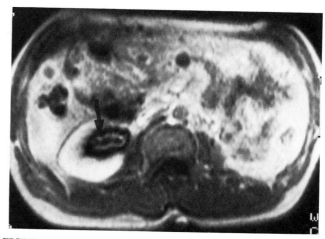

FIGURE 5–26. FLASH image of right kidney following administration of Gd-DTPA demonstrates loss of signal in renal pelvis *(arrow)* due to susceptibility effect (T_2^* shortening) of concentrated paramagnetic agent.

strated. Cartilage appears bright, particularly on FLASH images acquired with small flip angles; the cartilage enhancement is useful for detection of subtle chondral irregularities. However, contrast between fluid and cartilage is lower than on T_2-weighted SE images, which can limit cartilage evaluation in the presence of an effusion.

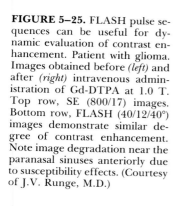

FIGURE 5–25. FLASH pulse sequences can be useful for dynamic evaluation of contrast enhancement. Patient with glioma. Images obtained before *(left)* and after *(right)* intravenous administration of Gd-DTPA at 1.0 T. Top row, SE (800/17) images. Bottom row, FLASH (40/12/40°) images demonstrate similar degree of contrast enhancement. Note image degradation near the paranasal sinuses anteriorly due to susceptibility effects. (Courtesy of J.V. Runge, M.D.)

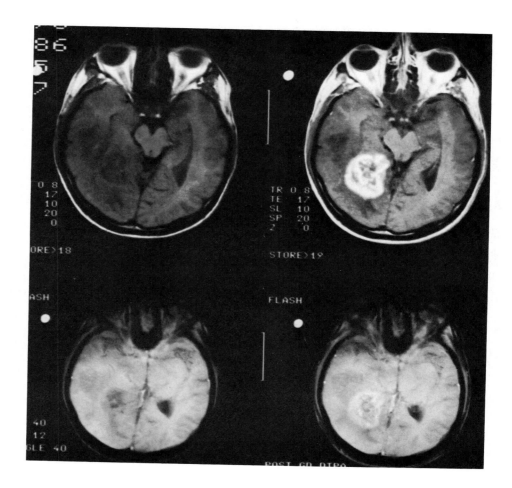

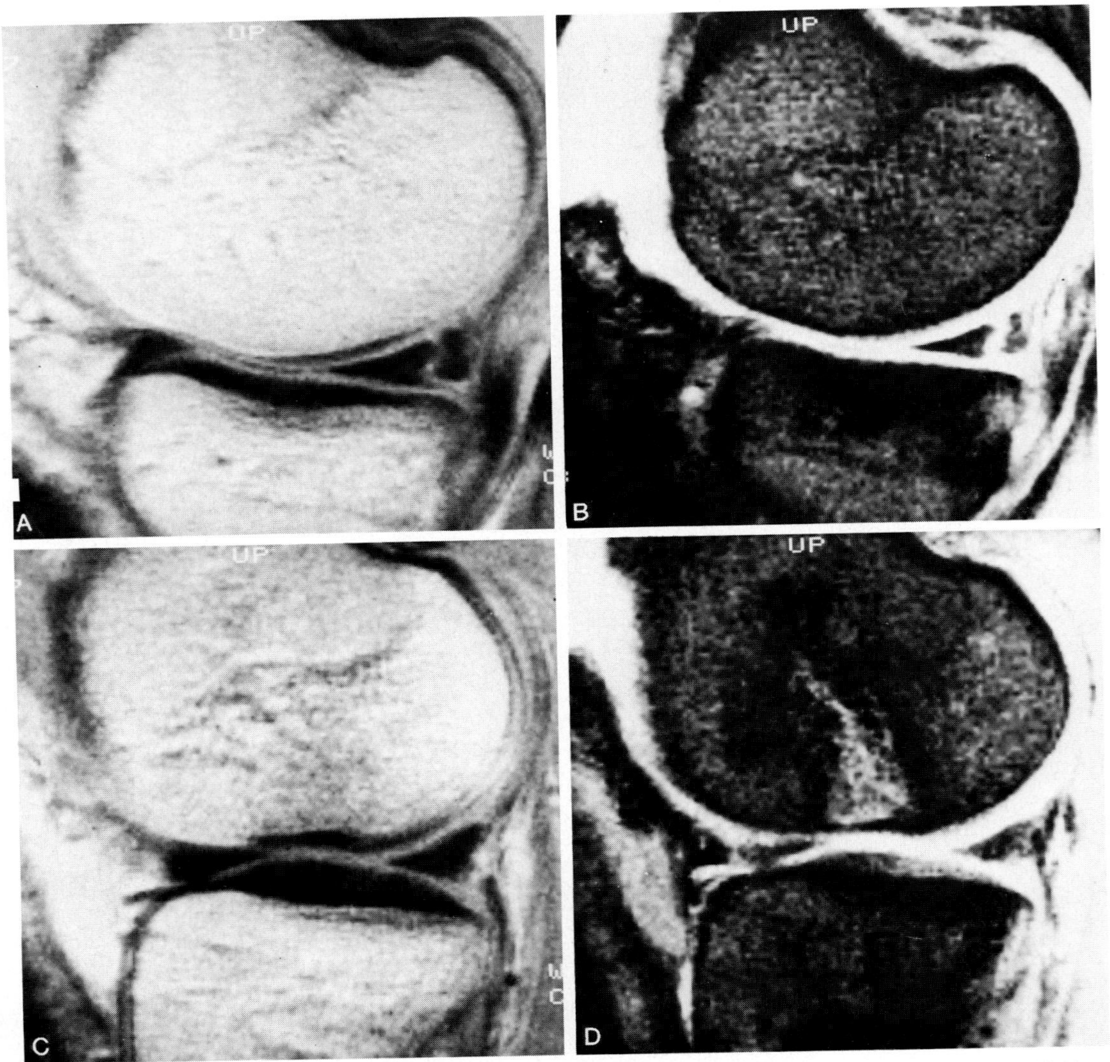

FIGURE 5–27. Comparison of spin-echo (TR/TE = 1200/26) and FLASH (TR/TE/flip angle = 600/18/15°) images of patient with torn posterior horn of medial meniscus and osteochondral fracture at 1.5 T. *A,* SE image shows meniscal tear and articular cartilage as moderate signal intensity. *B,* FLASH image shows meniscal tear and articular cartilage as high intensity. Note decreased signal intensity of bone marrow relative to SE image, in part due to phase contrast effects between fat and water signals, and in part due to local magnetic field inhomogeneity produced by the honeycomb structure of cancellous bone. *C,* SE image poorly demonstrates subchondral fracture. *D,* On FLASH image subchondral fracture appears bright due to bone marrow edema and is better seen.

Short imaging times permit dynamic assessment of joint motion, such as assessing patellar tracking abnormalities during knee flexion. Three-dimensional GRE methods (discussed below) permit rapid acquisition (5 to 10 minutes) of contiguous thin slices, which may be beneficial for imaging small structures such as the menisci and cruciate ligaments of the knee (Figs. 5–27 and 5–28).[18]

Three-Dimensional Imaging (3D GRE)

Three-dimensional MR imaging has some obvious advantages over a multislice acquisition (see Chapters 1 and 2). For example, (1) 3D data acquisition may allow one to reconstruct images in arbitrary orientations. (2) A 3D data set typically has a much smaller pixel volume than a 2D acquisition, thus limiting partial volume effects. (3) Three-dimensional acquisitions also generate truly contiguous slices, something difficult to accomplish with 2D slice-selective techniques. Unfortunately, a 3D data set of even modest resolution requires extremely long acquisition times if a long TR is used. For example, a 128^3, 1 NEX, T_1-weighted 3D image would require nearly three hours to acquire. In contrast, a 3D proton density GRE image of the same resolution could be acquired in as little as 5 to 10 minutes (Fig. 5–29).

There are many applications for 3D GRE images, such as imaging joints, reduction of susceptibility effects, and modeling volumes or surfaces. The po-

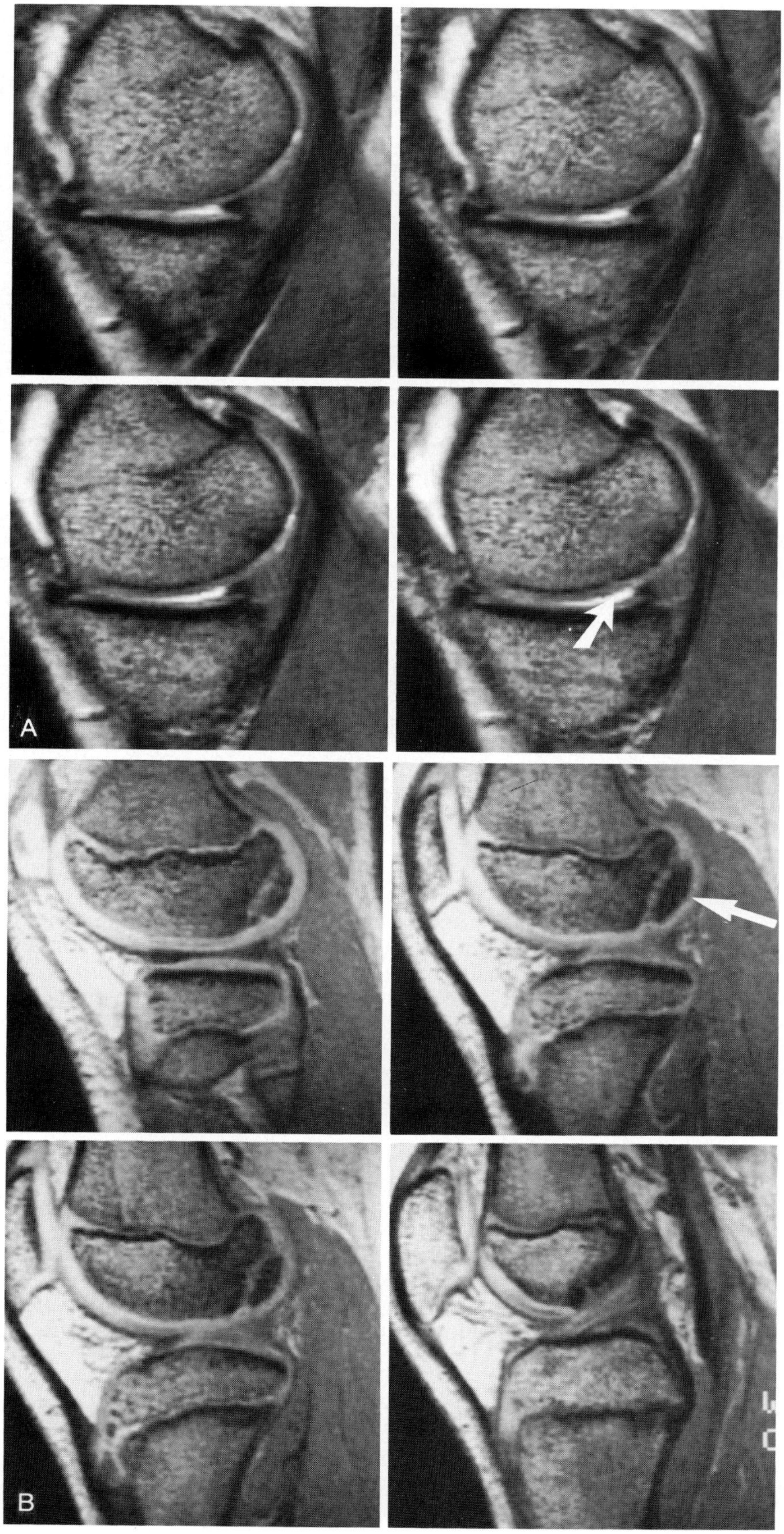

FIGURE 5–28. Examples of contiguous 1.7 mm knee images obtained at 1.0 T from 3D FLASH acquisitions in two different patients (TR/TE/flip angle = 30/14/40°). Imaging time < 10 minutes for 64 slices. *A*, Truncated posterior horn of medial meniscus *(arrow)*. *B*, Osteochondral fragment *(arrow)*. Note high signal intensity of cartilage. (Courtesy of R. Tyrell, M.D.)

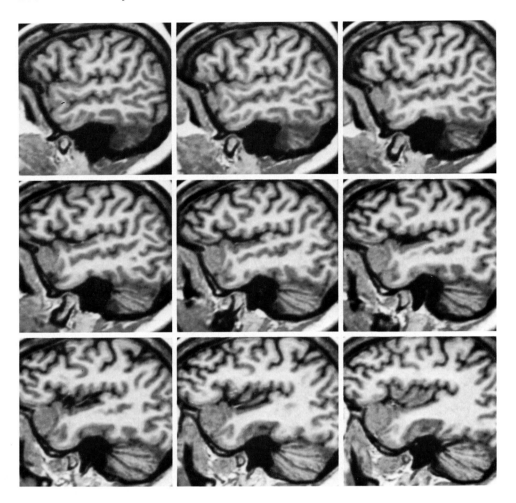

FIGURE 5–29. Three-dimensional FLASH acquisitions permit thin, contiguous slices to be obtained in a reasonable amount of time. Patient with meningioma; 9 of 126 contiguous images acquired at 1.5 T in 20 minutes using 3D FLASH (40/15/40°) with slice thickness of 1.5 mm, FOV = 28 cm. (Courtesy of P. Ruggieri, M.D.)

tential for resolving the surfaces of specific features is exciting because such information could prove useful in planning surgery or radiation therapy. Many algorithms have been developed for extracting surfaces from 3D data. In one such algorithm, a "seed" voxel is manually chosen within the surface of interest. The other voxels are then characterized by their intensity and their relationship to neighboring voxels. This information is used to distinguish between features that represent the surface of interest and those that do not. The voxels that represent the surface of interest are automatically joined. When combined with the automated addition of perspective and shading, a surface image is easily obtained. In addition to viewing the external features of the surface, the images can be separated (segmented) to reveal internal details and the spatial relationship between normal and pathologic tissues (Fig. 5–30).

DRIVEN-EQUILIBRIUM METHODS

Gradient-echo imaging is faster than SE imaging because the TRs are much shorter—a benefit of using reduced flip angles. As pointed out earlier, a small flip angle will not work with a conventional SE

sequence because the 180-degree refocusing pulse would invert the magnetization, resulting in a loss of signal. In principle, there is a method for avoiding this problem. Following read-out of the MR signal, a combination of RF and gradient pulses could be used to realign the tissue magnetization with the magnetic field. *The tissue magnetization would then be immediately available for additional excitations and signal measurements, without the need to wait for a long time to allow T_1 relaxation to occur.* Such methods are generally categorized as driven equilibrium Fourier transform (DEFT) techniques.

An SE analog of a reduced flip angle GRE pulse sequence may be obtained by incorporating a second 180-degree pulse at the end of an SE pulse sequence. Now the tissue magnetization winds up along the direction of the main field. The pulse sequence works as follows. The initial small flip angle tips some of the longitudinal magnetization into the transverse plane where it begins to dephase. However, most of the magnetization remains along the direction of the magnetic field. The 180-degree refocusing pulse occurs at a time TE/2 after the initial pulse and serves to produce a spin echo from the transverse magnetization. The refocusing pulse has the secondary effect of placing the longitudinal magnetization in a direc-

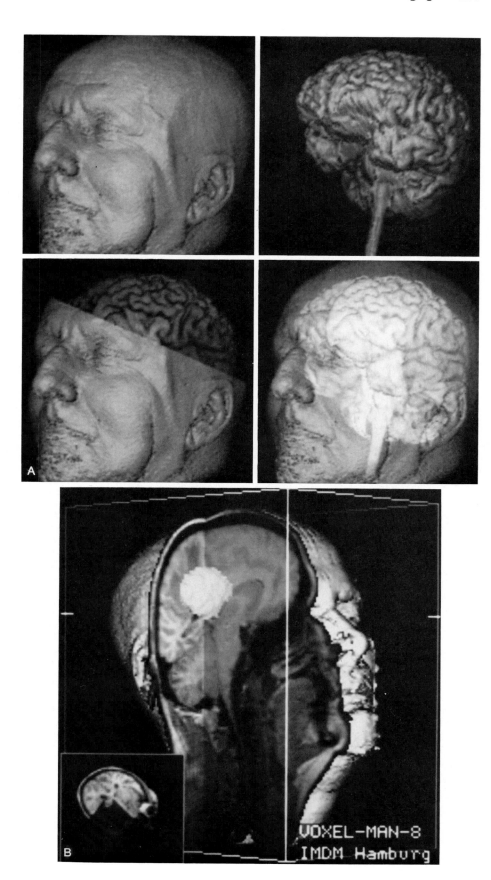

FIGURE 5–30. Surface images can be reconstructed in an arbitrary orientation from a 3D data acquisition. 3D FLASH (40/15/40°), slice thickness = 1.4 mm. *A,* Surface images of face and brain. *B,* Surface image of head in patient with brain tumor. A wedge of brain and overlying tissues has been "removed" to reveal tumor. (Courtesy of H. Koenig, Ph.D., Siemens Medical Systems.)

tion opposing the magnetic field ($-z$). A second 180-degree pulse is used, at the conclusion of the sequence, to return the inverted magnetization to its original longitudinal ($+z$) orientation. Pulse sequences based on this idea include FLAME[19, 19a] and FATE[20] (Figs. 5–31 and 5–32).

In an SE pulse sequence, it is possible to restore both the longitudinal *and* transverse components of the magnetization to the longitudinal direction. This is accomplished by adding both a 180-degree pulse and a (-90-degree) pulse to the end of the SE sequence. In principle, the second two pulses undo the effect of the first two pulses. This highly symmetric pulse sequence is the one classically referred to as driven-equilibrium, though the term is sometimes applied to sequences such as FLAME. The driven-equilibrium sequence leaves the magnetization along the longitudinal direction except during the echo time TE.

T_2 relaxation occurs during the driven-equilibrium sequence. Since dephased spins cannot be tipped back along the z-axis, the effect of T_2 relaxation is to oppose the driven-equilibrium effect. As a result, fluids that have a very long T_2, such as CSF, will produce an intense signal on short TR DEFT images, but other tissues appear darker (Fig. 5–32B).

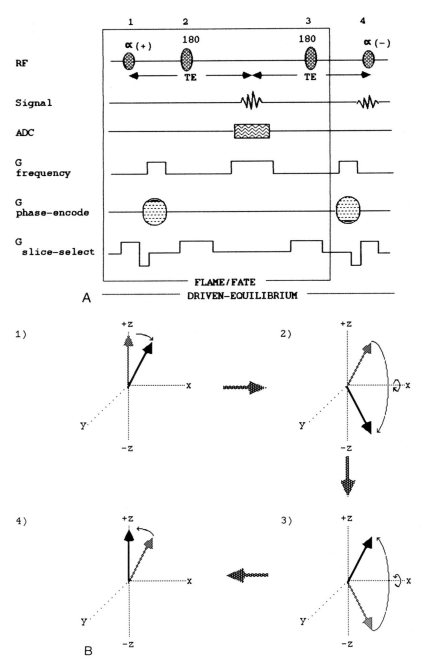

FIGURE 5–31. Driven equilibrium methods are modified SE sequences that realign the magnetization along the magnetic field after signal read-out. *A*, Pulse sequence diagram for driven equilibrium—type sequences. Sequences 1 through 3 correspond to FLAME and FATE methods; sequences 1 through 4 correspond to classic DEFT method. In theory, these sequences exhibit similar behavior to reduced flip angle FLASH methods, except that the effects of magnetic field inhomogeneities have been eliminated by the addition of an RF refocusing pulse. Driven equilibrium sequences produce maximal signal enhancement for tissues with large ratio T_2/T_1, such as CSF.

B, Path of magnetization vector with these methods. (1) Reduced flip angle excitation tips part of longitudinal magnetization ($+z$ direction) into transverse (x-y) plane. (2) First 180-degree RF pulse tips transverse magnetization around x-axis to ($-z$) direction. (3) Second 180-degree RF tips magnetization back to ($+z$) direction. (4) Additional RF pulse, used in classic DEFT method, tips magnetization into alignment with main magnetic field.

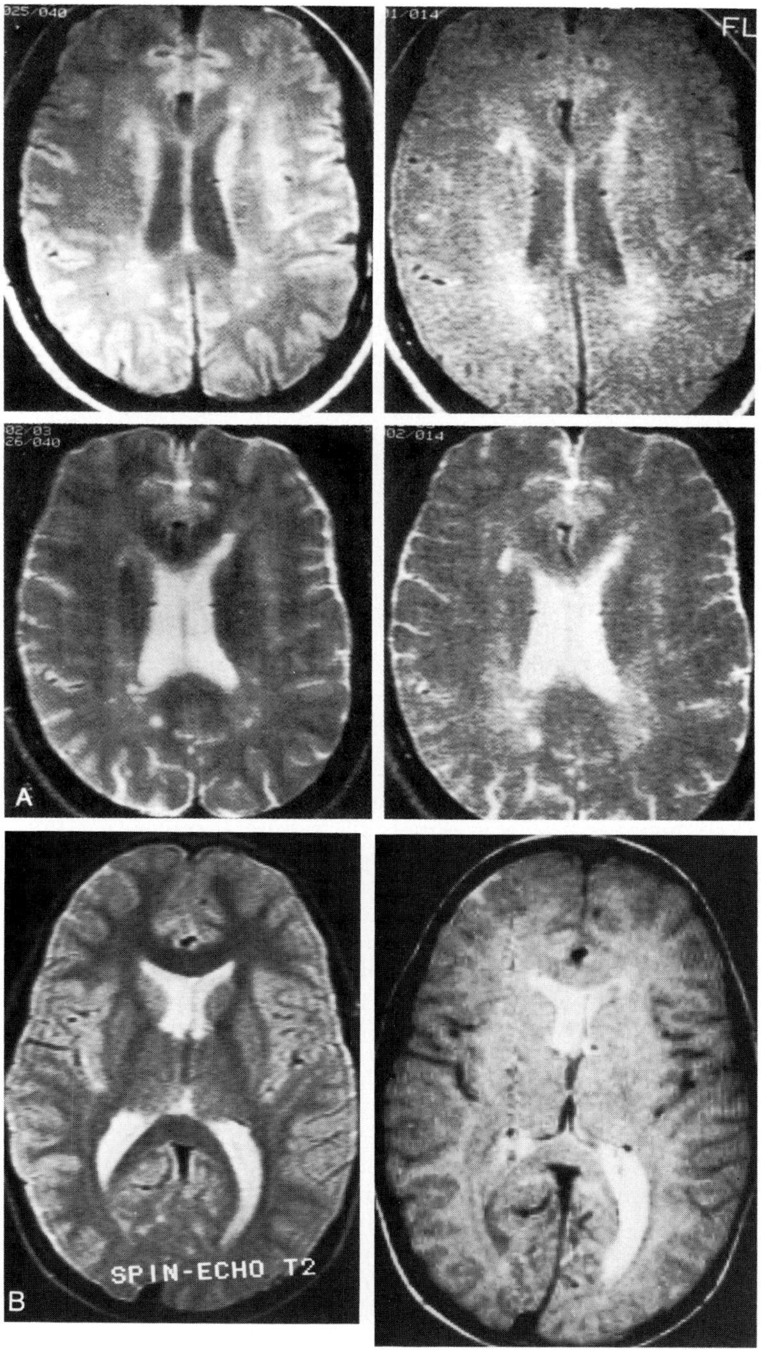

FIGURE 5–32. Comparisons of head studies obtained with SE and driven equilibrium–type methods. *A*, Comparison of conventional SE and FLAME methods in patient with multiple sclerosis. Upper left, lower left, SE (2500/20), SE (2500/80). Imaging time = 11 minutes. Upper right, lower right, FLAME images with TR/TE/flip angle = (750/30/30°), (750/80/30°). Imaging time = 3.3 minutes. Although S/N is reduced in the FLAME images, the white matter plaques are well shown. *B*, Comparison of head images in normal subject obtained with SE and classic DEFT methods. Left, SE (2500/80). Imaging time = 11 minutes. Right, DEFT with TR/TE/flip angle = (500/30/80°). Imaging time = 2.2 minutes. CSF appears bright in both images. However, SE image shows improved gray matter–white matter contrast, suggesting that T_2 contrast is better with SE method than with DEFT.

In theory, the combination of a spin echo with restoration of the magnetization combines the best features of SE and GRE sequences. Thus, fast imaging may be conducted without undo sensitivity to magnetic susceptibility effects. Unfortunately, all of the sequences described above are more sensitive to instrument imperfections than are SE or GRE sequences. This sensitivity arises because the driven-equilibrium sequences rely on undoing the effect of one pulse with another. Problems occur because flip angles are never exact, and slice profiles depend on the flip angles of the pulses. In addition, other imperfections such as patient motion, eddy currents, the precision of the gradient amplitudes, RF phase stability, and a host of similar limitations can cause a cumulative loss of signal. These problems severely limit the use of driven equilibrium–type sequences. Future improvements in instrumentation, such as shielded gradients, self-correcting pulses, and enhancements to the pulse sequences themselves, may make these techniques more practical for clinical use, though the applications are likely to be limited in scope.

STIMULATED-ECHO (STEAM) IMAGING

Stimulated echoes, like spin echoes, consist of transverse magnetization which refocuses some period of time after an RF pulse (see Chapter 3). Unlike spin echoes, stimulated echoes work by storing transverse magnetization temporarily along the ($-z$) longitudinal direction (i.e., opposite to the direction of the main magnetic field). This stored magnetization is reconverted back to a precessing transverse magnetization by an RF pulse applied at some later time. The restored transverse magnetization then refocuses to produce a "stimulated" echo. A simple stimulated echo (STE) pulse sequence is: 90 degrees —— (let the nuclei precess for a time t_1) —— 90 degrees (store transverse magnetization along the negative z-axis) —— (let T_1 relaxation occur for some period of time) —— 90 degrees (transfer stored magnetization to transverse magnetization) —— (let nuclei precess for a time t_1 at which point they will form an echo) —— measure the MR signal. By adding the usual assortment of gradient pulses to this sequence, STE sequences can be used for imaging. Imaging by stimulated echoes is usually referred to by the acronym STEAM for *st*imulated *e*cho *a*cquisition *m*ode.[21, 22]

STEAM imaging can be modified to function as a fast scan technique. The modification is to use small flip angle pulses to read out a series of stimulated echoes. The resulting sequence is: 90 degrees —— 90 degrees —— [α —— read] —— [α —— read] —— [α —— read] . . . . The α pulses each transfer a small amount of the stored magnetization into the transverse plane. By separately phase encoding each one of the stimulated echoes, an entire image can be built up in the course of a few applications of the pulse sequence. Imaging time is on the order of seconds.

The contrast of STEAM images is essentially reversed compared with T_1-weighted SE images. During the period the magnetization is stored along the longitudinal axis, T_1 relaxation occurs which reduces the intensity of the stimulated echoes. Because of this, tissues with a long T_1, such as tumor, lose less signal and appear bright, whereas tissues with a short T_1, such as fat, lose more signal and appear dark. This reversal of the normal contrast relationships could prove useful in certain circumstances, such as visualizing an orbital tumor embedded in fat. However, the clinical applications of this technique have not yet been defined. One drawback is that STEAM images have lower S/N than SE or GRE images, since only a small portion of the tissue magnetization contributes to the signal.

ALTERNATIVES TO 2DFT IMAGING

Almost all clinical MR imaging is performed using variations of the two-dimensional Fourier transform (2DFT) (spin warp) technique.[23] In spin-warp imaging, a 2D image is formed by acquiring many (e.g., 128 to 512) 1D frequency-encoded "images" of the sample, each of which has slightly different amounts of phase encoding. As discussed in Chapter 1, the resulting 2D signal matrix can be analyzed by Fourier transformation to yield frequencies in both the phase- and frequency-encoding directions. The 2D frequency map forms a picture because the magnetic field gradients ensure that the frequency and rate of phase change of each pixel is proportional to its position.

An example of a spin-warp data set is shown in Figure 5–33. The raw MR data are mapped in what is called k-space.[24] The name k-space refers to the wave nature of the measured data. Each point in k-space refers to a spatial frequency. Spatial frequency in turn corresponds to the number of features in a given distance. Structures that have sharp borders are described by high spatial frequencies, less detailed structures by lower spatial frequencies. The point in the center of k-space corresponds to mean intensity of the image. As an example, suppose each letter on a page of text could emit an MR signal. If we made an MR image of the text, the intensity of the center point of the unprocessed MR data would be proportional to the number of letters on the page. The intensity of the other points in k-space would be difficult to predict given the irregular shapes of the letters. However, certain spatial frequencies would be much more intense than others. Looking down a page of text, one can see that there is a very regular spatial frequency (k_y) corresponding to the number of lines of text per inch. Looking across the page, there is obviously another strong signal at a spatial frequency (k_x) equal to the number of characters per inch on the page. A 2DFT of the k-space data would reproduce the original text.

In spin-warp imaging, the data in k-space are sampled one line per phase encode. This sampling scheme has proved to be a very effective one, but it is not the only way to measure the data. Any pattern for measuring the points in k-space will provide enough information to reconstruct the image. The measurement pattern, or k-space trajectory, is determined by the details of the pulse sequence. Many different pulse sequences for scanning k-space have been proposed, including spiral, diagonal, sinusoidal, and rectangular trajectories. Any pattern that scans more of k-space per unit of time than the line-by-line method used in spin-warp imaging has the potential to decrease image acquisition time.

Echo-Planar and Single Shot Imaging

The fastest methods for MR imaging are those that measure all of the k-space in one single acquisi-

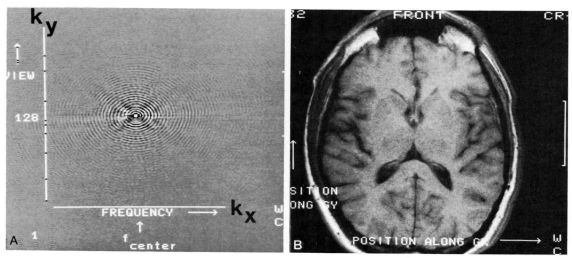

FIGURE 5–33. Image space and k-space are equivalent via the two-dimensional Fourier transform. The raw data *(left)* represent 2D display of signal amplitudes for a 256 × 256 pixel image. There are 256 samples of frequency-encoded data along the horizontal axis, with the center column representing the center of the read-out period. There are 256 lines of phase-encoded data (vertical axis). Two-dimensional Fourier transform converts data to an image with x-axis (horizontal) and y-axis (vertical). Star pattern represents raw data of head image *(right)*, prior to Fourier transformation.

tion. The idea is to incorporate the entire spatial information in the MR signal before it decays away through T_2^* relaxation. The first technique to exploit this idea was echo-planar imaging (EPI).[25] Newer techniques, sometimes referred to as single shot imaging, have improved on the echo-planar concept by using more efficient scans of k-space and improved instrumentation.

Recently, a one shot scanning technique was used to acquire snap shot images of a human heart with a temporal resolution of 40 milliseconds[21] (Fig. 5–34). Images are acquired by forming a series of separately phase-encoded gradient echoes, each formed by a rapid reversal of the frequency-encoding gradient, within the envelope of a traditional spin echo. The signal traces a path through k-space which is similar to the path in spin-warp imaging but which scans the entire k-space region in one TE interval (Fig. 5–35C). Because the entire k-space must be scanned in a very short period of time, the resolution of the technique (128 × 64) is somewhat less than typical spin-warp image resolution, though recently 128 × 128 matrix images have been shown and still larger matrices may be feasible.[26, 27] Many different types of dynamic studies may be conducted using EPI. For example, the peristaltic motion of the gastrointestinal tract may be shown.[27a]

One shot techniques are much more demanding, in terms of instrument performance, than are spin-warp style sequences. Extremely fast switching times (< 500 microseconds) are required of the magnetic field gradients in order to rapidly refocus gradient echoes. Typically, sinusoidally oscillating rather than trapezoidal gradient waveforms are used to permit rapid switching. A typical peak amplitude for the oscillating gradient would be 40 mT/m, roughly four times larger than used for standard 2DFT imaging. Large peak amplitudes and rapid gradient oscillations of thousands of cycles per second result in large dB/dt (e.g., > 50 T/sec); potentially the induction of hazardous electrical currents will ultimately be a limiting factor for spatial resolution. Not only must the gradients be fast, but they must also be largely free of eddy current effects. The data acquisition hardware must be capable of measuring and storing data at an astonishing rate. In addition, nonlinear sampling of the signal is needed if the gradients are not constant during read-out (e.g., as is the case for sinusoidal gradients). These extreme requirements may limit one shot imaging techniques to MR systems that have been designed specifically for this purpose.

Artifacts in Echo-Planar Imaging

The extreme demands in one shot imaging result in image artifacts and S/N limitations that are somewhat different from those encountered in SE or GRE imaging. For example, eddy current effects, which can never be entirely eliminated, dephase the gradient-echo train resulting in signal and resolution loss. In addition, the echo envelope, which decays with a time constant T_2^*, acts as a filter to remove high spatial frequencies in the phase-encoding direction. Many artifacts seen in SE imaging, such as flow void and susceptibility and chemical shift effects, are also observed in one shot imaging, though the details of these artifacts will differ from those seen in SE images due to the markedly different data acquisition scheme.

Chemical shift artifacts in one shot imaging can be severe. The problem is that chemical shift phase distortion accumulates during the course of scanning

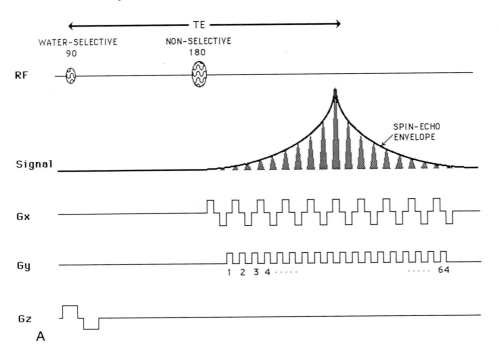

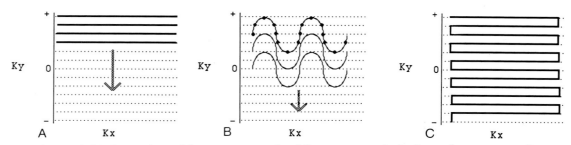

FIGURE 5–34. *A*, Water-selective single shot imaging technique represents a modification of an SE pulse sequence. A train of GREs *(shaded areas)* is obtained during the SE by rapidly oscillating the frequency-encoding gradient. Each GRE is individually phase-encoded by a brief ("blipped") y-gradient pulse. A water-selective 90-degree RF pulse is used to suppress fat signal and eliminate chemical shift artifact, which would otherwise be unacceptably large. Alternatively, fat could be saturated with a 90-degree prepulse. Note that, unlike the diagram, it is usually more practical to implement a sinusoidal rather than trapezoidal profile for the oscillating frequency-encoding gradient. *B*, Diastolic *(left)* and systolic *(right)* single shot images. Each image is acquired with a 128 × 64 matrix in < 50 msec. Because images are acquired from a single excitation, the TR is essentially infinite; tissues such as CSF *(arrow)* appear bright despite long T_1 relaxation time. Note absence of fat signal due to use of water-selective RF pulse. (Courtesy of Ian Pykett, Ph.D.)

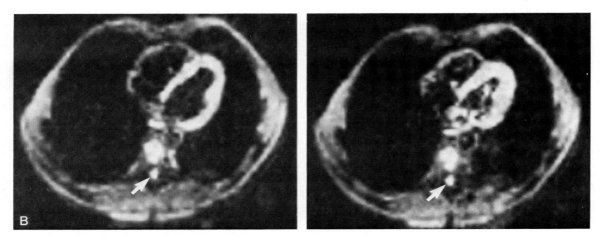

FIGURE 5–35. Comparison of k-space coverage by different scan methods. Kx = frequency-encoding axis, Ky = phase-encoding axis. *A*, In standard 2DFT imaging, one line of data is acquired after each excitation (i.e., one line per TR interval). *B*, Hybrid imaging represents compromise between *A* and *C*. Hybrid imaging is faster than standard 2DFT. It is slower than EPI *(C)*, but rate of gradient oscillation and corresponding special hardware requirements are less. *C*, Echo-planar or "instant scan" imaging. A series of separately phase-encoded GREs are acquired within the time period of a single SE signal. One line of data is acquired with each GRE. All lines of data (64 to 128) are obtained after a single excitation (e.g., imaging time < 50 msec).

k-space. Each point in the raw MR data set has a different phase offset which depends on the exact trajectory in k-space. This in turn causes unacceptable image degradation. These artifacts may be eliminated by selectively imaging water or fat (rather than both water and fat) by using chemical shift-selective pulses such as CHESS.[28]

Signal-to-Noise in Echo-Planar Imaging

Based on the number of signal acquisitions, it would seem that single shot images would have very poor S/N ratios. After all, for the same matrix size (N), there would be at least N acquisitions of the MR signal versus just one for the single shot. Given our previous arguments regarding S/N, one might expect that the S/N for the SE would be $\sqrt{128}$ times greater than the single shot image. Fortunately, this is not the case. If one could ignore instrument imperfections and run the scanner fast enough, then all of the data could be measured before there was an appreciable decay in the MR signal, and the acquired signal would be as strong as that obtained via an SE sequence. The limitation in this approach is that, because the data must be acquired at a rapid rate (i.e., high data bandwidth), more noise is allowed into the system and the S/N is degraded. In practice, the S/N is also reduced by eddy current effects, T_2^* signal loss, and magnetic field inhomogeneity. The lower sensitivity of single shot imaging necessitates the use of medium-high magnetic field strengths to obtain adequate S/N. Also, the short time available for application of the magnetic field gradients makes use of flow compensation methods problematical.

RARE

A different type of single shot image can be obtained using a multiecho pulse sequence known as RARE.[29] In RARE, each spin echo is individually phase encoded, so an entire image can be formed by a single string of (64 to 128) spin echoes. As with any multiecho sequence, the later echoes are heavily T_2 weighted; only tissue with a *very* long T_2, such as CSF, will contribute to the image. Nonetheless, RARE can be used to produce rapid images similar to contrast myelograms. Considerations of RF power deposit preclude using the RARE method on high field systems.

Hybrid Imaging

There are many possible ways to sample raw k-space MR data. The signal can be measured by one phase encode per acquisition, the entire k-space in one acquisition, or any technique in between. Intermediate schemes are called hybrid imaging.[30] In hybrid imaging, several phase encodes are obtained for each acquisition; for example, an oscillating gradient applied during the signal read-out can be employed to scan multiple phases (Fig. 5–35*B*). As

expected, hybrid techniques are considerably faster than spin-warp acquisitions, but significantly slower than single shot acquisitions. The advantage of hybrid imaging is that the instrument requirements are not too severe, so hybrid scans can be conducted on most MR systems without extensive modifications. MR data acquired by hybrid imaging require some preprocessing prior to image reconstruction; this may substantially increase the overall reconstruction time. Despite the S/N reduction expected from the shorter scan time, image contrast is identical to standard acquisitions (Fig. 5–36). Coherent noise (i.e., ghost artifacts) due to flow and respiration tend to be redistributed throughout the image, making these artifacts less intense.

Contrast in Echo-Planar Imaging

The single shot technique shown in Figure 5–34 produces images that are not T_1 weighted, because they have essentially an infinite TR. The strong T_2 weighting in these scans may be useful in characterizing cavernous hemangiomas and cysts. By introducing a 90-degree pulse followed by a TR interval *prior* to the start of a single shot acquisition, T_1 weighting can be added to single shot images. The 90-degree pulse destroys the longitudinal magnetization just as in an SE image. The signal then recovers during the TR interval as given by Equation 1. Thus, single shot images can be produced which have essentially the same contrast as SE images. In conjunction with reduced flip angles, single shot methods can also be used to produce FLASH-type images.

Hybrid techniques built around an SE sequence will also produce images that have the same contrast as an SE sequence with the same TE. There are many possible implementations of single shot or hybrid imaging sequences. The contrast in images generated using these techniques generally depends on the precise implementation of the corresponding pulse sequences.

CONCLUSION

The motivations for faster MR imaging techniques are obvious. Unfortunately, faster imaging techniques are usually accompanied by decreases in resolution or S/N ratio. Nonetheless, many techniques provide a reasonable compromise between speed and image quality. The simplest methods to increase imaging speed are those that make fewer measurements of the MR signal, by reducing the image matrix size or the number of averages. Although the increase in speed produced by these approaches is modest, they are very general and can be applied to most MR imaging sequences. In some instances, for example, an asymmetric FOV, reducing the amount of data acquired will decrease acquisition time without a substantial reduction in image quality.

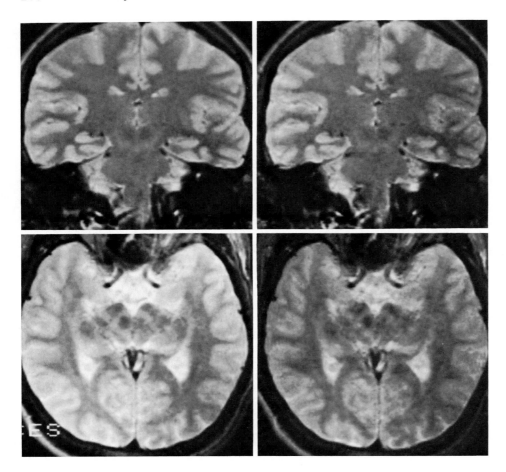

FIGURE 5–36. Comparison of standard SE images *(left)* and hybrid images *(right)* acquired in half the time. Aside from lower S/N, hybrid images appear comparable to standard images. (Courtesy Picker International Medical Systems, Inc.)

To obtain images at very high speed, it is necessary to make more efficient use of the available MR signal. For the time being, the most practical methods of fast MR scanning are those that use only a small portion of the magnetization. These techniques are usually small flip angle GRE pulse sequences known by a variety of acronyms such as FLASH, GRASS, FISP, and FATE. These techniques are useful for a variety of situations that require short imaging times, for example, cardiac cineangiography, blood flow imaging, eliminating respiratory artifacts, and so forth. Gradient-echo imaging has a secondary benefit in that GRE images have much different contrast than SE images.

To obtain extremely fast MR images, it is necessary to employ single shot pulse sequences that measure the entire image from a single excitation. Single shot techniques are the only means of obtaining true stop action images of cardiac motion. Unfortunately, single shot imaging is very demanding of instrumentation and requires dedicated scanning hardware.

All of the fast scan pulse sequences will become more useful with improvements in scanner hardware. Advances, such as shielded gradients and/or better eddy current compensation schemes, may improve both GRE and single shot images. Single shot imaging, in particular, should become much more practical as instrumentation improves.

APPENDIX 5–A

The contrast equations for steady-state FLASH and CE-FAST are considerably more complex than the corresponding equation for spoiled FLASH. This additional complexity results from the persistence of transverse magnetization from one TR interval to the next. The equations given below assume a steady-state longitudinal *and* transverse magnetization. If there is appreciable motion of any kind, actual image intensities may be substantially different than those predicted by the contrast equations. In particular, the signals from blood and CSF are usually considerably different than their predicted values.

The signal intensity for a steady-state FLASH sequence with an alternating phase RF pulse is given by[8, 9]:

$$S = S_0 \times \frac{(1 - E_1) \sin\theta}{1 - (E_1 - E_2) \cos\theta - E_1 E_2} \times E_2^*$$

where $E_1 = \exp\{-TR/T_1\}$, $E_2 = \exp\{-TR/T_2\}$, and $E_2^* = \exp\{-TE/T_2^*\}$. Note that T_2 contrast arises from decay of the transverse magnetization during TE (E_2^*) and decay of the transverse magnetization during TR (E_2). This equation also gives the contrast for the GRASS pulse sequence.

In all of the steady-state GRE sequences, the signal intensity arises from contributions from the steady-state transverse and longitudinal components of the magnetization. Two distinct signals occur: the FID produced by tipping the steady-state longitudinal magnetization, and the so called time reversed FID produced by refocusing of the steady-state transverse magnetization. For a pulse sequence with constant RF phase, the FID portion of the signal is given by[8]:

$$S = \frac{\sin\theta \; E_2^*}{1 + \cos\theta} \times (1 - [E_1 - \cos\theta] \; \Theta \; [\theta, E_1, E_2])$$

and the time-reversed FID portion is given by:

$$S = \frac{-\sin\theta \; E_2^*}{(1 + \cos\theta) \; E_2} \times (1 - [1 - E_1 \cos\theta] \; \Theta \; [\theta, E_1, E_2])$$

Where the weighting factor Θ is given by:

$$\Theta = \left[\frac{1 - E_2^2}{1 - E_1^2 E_2^2 - 2E_1 (1 - E_2^2) \cos\theta + (E_1^2 - E_2^2) \cos^2\theta} \right]^{1/2}$$

If an alternating phase steady-state sequence is used, the sign of the time-reversed FID is changed. Note that, in general, the value of E_2^* is different for the FID and time-reversed FID, since these signal components do not necessarily have the same TE. In sequences such as CE-FAST, the time-reversed portion of the signal can be measured without the FID portion. Since the time-reversed FID has much more

T_2 weight than the FID, images generated by CE-FAST and FATE typically have much more T_2 contrast than FLASH, GRASS, or FISP images.

REFERENCES

1. Feinberg DA, Hale JD, Watts JC, et al: Halving MR imaging time by conjugation: Demonstration at 3.5 kG. Radiology 161:527–531, 1986.
1a. Farzaneh F, Riederer SJ, Lee JN, et al: MR fluoroscopy: Initial clinical studies. Radiology 171:545–549, 1989.
2. Becker ED, Ferretti JA, Gambhir PN: Selection of optimum parameters for pulse Fourier transform nuclear magnetic resonance. Anal Chem 51:1413–1420, 1979.
3. Haase A, Frahm J, Matthaei D, et al: Rapid NMR imaging using low flip-angle pulses. J Magn Reson 67:258–266, 1986.
4. Frahm J, Haase A, Matthaei D: Rapid NMR imaging of dynamic processes using the FLASH technique. Magn Reson Med 3:321–327, 1986.
5. Gyngell ML, Palmer ND, Eastwood LM: Proceedings of the Fifth Annual Meeting of the Society of Magnetic Resonance in Medicine. Montreal, August 1986, p. 666.
6. Redpath TW, Jones RA: FADE—a new fast imaging sequence. Magn Reson Med 6:224–234, 1988.
7. Bruder H, Fischer H, Graumann R, Deimling M: A new steady-state imaging sequence for simultaneous acquisition of two MR images with clearly different contrasts. Magn Reson Med 7:35–42, 1988.
8. Zur Y, Stokar S, Bendel P: An analysis of fast imaging sequences with steady-state magnetization refocusing. Magn Reson Med 6:175–193, 1988.
8a. Edelman RR, Buxton RB, Brady TJ: Rapid MR imaging. *In* Kressel H (ed): Magnetic Resonance Annual 1988. New York, Raven Press, 1988 pp 189–216.
8b. Winkler ML, Ortendahl DA, Mills TC, et al: Characteristics of partial flip angle and gradient-reversal MRI. Radiology 166:17–26, 1988.
9. Buxton RB, Edelman RR, Rosen BR, et al: Contrast in rapid MR imaging: T1- and T2-weighted imaging. J Comput Assist Tomogr 11:7–16, 1987.
10. Edelman RR, Johnson K, Buxton R, et al: MR of hemorrhage: A new approach. AJNR 7:751–756, 1986.
10a. Haacke EM, Tkach JA, Parrish TB: Reduction of T2* dephasing in gradient field-echo imaging. Radiology 170:457–462, 1989.
11. Dixon WT: Simple proton spectroscopic imaging. Radiology 153:189–194, 1984.
11a. Bradley WG, Waluch V: Blood flow: Magnetic resonance imaging. Radiology 154:443–450, 1985.
12. Pattany PM, Marino R, McNally JM: Velocity and acceleration desensitization in 2DFT MR imaging. Magn Reson Imaging 4:154–155, 1986.
13. Edelman RR, Hahn PF, Buxton R, et al: Rapid MR imaging with suspended respiration: Clinical application in the liver. Radiology 161:125–131, 1986.
14. Edelman RR, Singer A, Longmead B, et al: Fast MRI of liver cancer: Improved methods for lesion detection and characterization at 1.5 Tesla. Radiology (in press).
14a. Katz BH, Quencer RM, Hinks RS: Comparison of gradient-recalled-echo and T2-weighted spin-echo pulse sequences in intramedullary spinal lesions. AJNR 10:815–822, 1989.
15. Young IR, Khenia S, Thomas DGT, et al: Clinical magnetic susceptibility mapping of the brain. J Comput Assist Tomogr 11:2–6, 1987.

16. Dumoulin CL, Hart HR: Magnetic resonance angiography. Radiology 161:717–720, 1986.

17. Glover GH, Pelc NJ: A rapid-gated cine MRI technique. *In* Kressel H (ed): Magnetic Resonance Annual 1988. New York, Raven Press, 1988.

18. Tyrrell RL, Gluckert K, Pathria M, Modic MT: Fast 3D MRI of the knee: Comparison with arthroscopy. Radiology 166:865–872, 1988.

19. Hackney DB, Lenkinski RE, Grossman RI, et al: Initial experience with fast low angle multi-echo (FLAME) imaging of the central nervous system. J Comput Assist Tomogr 12:171–174, 1988.

19a. Mitchell DG, Vinitski S, Burk DL, et al: Variable flip angle SE MR imaging of the pelvis: More versatile T2-weighted images. Radiology 171:525–529, 1989.

20. Tkach J, Haacke M: FATE. Presented at the 6th Annual Meeting of the Society of Magnetic Resonance in Medicine. New York, August 1987.

21. Frahm J, Merboldt KD, Hanicke W, et al: Stimulated echo imaging. J Magn Reson 64:81–93, 1985.

22. Haase A, Frahm J, Matthaei, et al: MR imaging using stimulated echoes (STEAM). Radiology 160:787–790, 1986.

23. Edelstein WA, Hutchison JM, Johnson G, Redpath T: Spin warp imaging and applications to human whole-body imaging. Phys Med Biol 25:751–756, 1980.

24. Tweig DB: The k-trajectory formulation of the NMR imaging process with applications in analysis and synthesis of imaging methods. Med Phys 10:610–621, 1983.

25. Mansfield P, Maudsley AA, Baines T: Fast scan proton density imaging by NMR. J Phys E 9:271–278, 1976.

26. Stehling MJ, Howseman AM, Ordidge RJ, et al: Whole-body echo-planar MRI at 0.5 T. Radiology 170:257–263, 1989.

27. Crooks LE, Arakawa M, Mylton NM, et al: Echo planar pediatric imager. Radiology 166:157–163, 1988.

27a. Stehling MK, Evans DF, Lamont G, et al: Gastrointestinal tract: Dynamic MR studies with echo planar imaging. Radiology 171:41–46, 1989.

28. Haase A, Frahm J: Multiple chemical-shift-selective NMR imaging using stimulated echoes. J Magn Reson 64:94–102, 1985.

29. Hennig J, Nauerth A, Friedburg H: RARE imaging: A fast imaging method for clinical MR. Magn Reson Med 3:823–833, 1986.

30. Haacke EM, Bearden FH, Clayton JR, Linga NR: Reduction of MR imaging time by the HYBRID fast-scan technique. Radiology 158:521–530, 1986.

6

PRINCIPLES OF MR IMAGING CONTRAST AGENTS*

RANDALL B. LAUFFER

HISTORICAL BACKGROUND

PARAMAGNETIC SUBSTANCES AND NUCLEAR RELAXATION

DEPENDENCE OF MR IMAGE INTENSITY ON TISSUE RELAXATION TIMES

DISTINCTION BETWEEN T_1 and T_2 AGENTS

GENERAL REQUIREMENTS FOR MR CONTRAST AGENTS

   RELAXIVITY

   SPECIFIC IN VIVO DISTRIBUTION

   IN VIVO STABILITY, EXCRETABILITY, AND LACK OF TOXICITY

T_1 AGENTS

   RELAXIVITY

   Theory
   Relaxivity in Solution
   Relaxivity in Tissue

   TOXICITY AND THE STABILITY OF METAL COMPLEXES

   IN VIVO TARGETING

   Extracellular Distribution: Renal Excretion
   Extracellular Distribution: Hepatobiliary Excretion
   Intravascular Distribution
   Tumor-Localizing Agents

T_2 AGENTS

The development of MR imaging techniques as a clinical diagnostic modality has prompted the need for a new class of pharmaceuticals. These drugs would be administered to a patient to (1) enhance the image contrast between normal and diseased tissue and/or (2) indicate the status of organ function or blood flow. The image intensity in ^1H MR imaging, largely composed of the MR signal of water protons, is dependent on nuclear relaxation times. Paramagnetic substances, which possess large magnetic moments and can decrease the relaxation times of nearby nuclei, have received the most attention as potential contrast agents.

The extension of MR to in vivo tissue characterization, including both imaging and spectroscopy of metabolites, has brought new chemistry into diagnostic medicine. Paramagnetic contrast agents are an integral part of this trend; they are unique among diagnostic agents. In tissue, these agents are not visualized directly on the MR image but are detected indirectly by virtue of changes in proton relaxation behavior. In contrast, other diagnostic agents, such as the iodine-containing radiographic contrast agents (which absorb and scatter x-rays) and radiopharmaceuticals, are directly visualized. The lack of ionizing radiation in MR imaging and in its new contrast media is attractive to physicians (and patients) as well as investigators.

The need for MR contrast agents and the interesting research problems associated with their development have produced an active research area. Over the past 3 years, roughly 140 reports related to contrast agents have appeared in the literature, and the rate of publication is steadily increasing. The purpose of this chapter is to review the basic principles of MR contrast agents and to discuss new applications. A more detailed scientific account of the chemical and biophysical facets of contrast agent design is given in Reference 1.

---

*Portions of this chapter are reprinted with permission from Lauffer RB: Paramagnetic metal complexes as water proton relaxation agents for NMR imaging: Theory and design. Chem Rev 87:901–927, 1987. Copyright 1987 American Chemical Society.

HISTORICAL BACKGROUND

Fundamental investigations leading to the new area of MR contrast agents are briefly discussed here. Bloch first described the use of a paramagnetic salt, ferric nitrate, to enhance the relaxation rates of water protons.[2] The standard theory relating solvent nuclear relaxation rates in the presence of dissolved paramagnetic substances was developed by Bloembergen, Solomon, and others.[3–6] Eisinger, Shulman, and Blumberg demonstrated that binding of a paramagnetic metal ion to a macromolecule—in their case, DNA—enhances the water proton relaxation efficiency via lengthening of the rotational correlation time.[7] This phenomenon, which came to be known as proton relaxation enhancement (PRE), has been utilized extensively to study hydration and structure of metalloenzymes.[8–10]

The pioneering 1973 work of Lauterbur[11] in imaging with MR was extended to human imaging in 1977.[12–14] Lauterbur, Mendonca-Dias, and Rudin were first to show the feasibility of paramagnetic agents for tissue discrimination on the basis of differential water proton relaxation times.[15] In their experiments, a salt of manganese (Mn) (II), a cation known to localize in normal myocardial tissue in preference to infarcted regions, was injected into dogs with an occluded coronary artery. The longitudinal proton relaxation rates ($1/T_1$) of tissue samples correlated with Mn(II) concentration, and thus normal myocardium could be distinguished from the infarcted zone by relaxation behavior alone. Brady, Goldman, and colleagues subsequently confirmed the feasibility of paramagnetic agents in imaging studies of excised dog hearts treated in a similar fashion.[16, 17] Normal myocardium, containing Mn(II), exhibited greater signal intensity than did infarcted regions on MR images; no contrast was present without Mn(II).

The first human MR imaging study involving a paramagnetic agent was performed by Young and associates; orally administered ferric chloride was used to enhance the gastrointestinal tract.[18] The diagnostic potential of paramagnetic agents was first demonstrated in patients by Carr and coworkers.[19] Gadolinium (III)–diethylenetriaminepentaacetate ($[Gd(DTPA)]^{2-}$) was administered intravenously to patients with cerebral tumors, providing enhancement of the lesion in the region of cerebral capillary breakdown. This is currently the only agent approved for clinical use.

PARAMAGNETIC SUBSTANCES AND NUCLEAR RELAXATION

Paramagnetic species affect nuclear relaxation rates because they possess electrons whose spins are unpaired. Electron spin is analogous to the quantum-mechanical property of spin possessed by nuclei. For most molecules, electrons are distributed in pairs into various *orbitals* (an orbital defines a region in space

where an electron has some probability of residing). The two electrons in a given orbital must have opposite spins (one up and one down), as described by the Pauli exclusion principle. Since these two spins cancel, there is no net electron spin associated with the molecule, and it is said to be *diamagnetic*.

Some substances, however, have several orbitals at identical (or very similar) energy levels. In this case, only one electron may be placed into each orbital, all with parallel spins. A net electron spin results, and the substance is said to be *paramagnetic. The unpaired electrons of paramagnetic substances generate strong, fluctuating magnetic fields at nearby nuclei, thus stimulating nuclear relaxation.*

The most common paramagnetic species in nature are metal ions, which usually possess incompletely filled *d* or *f* orbitals. These ions possess between one and seven unpaired electrons, as shown in Table 6–1. For the transition metal ions and Gd(III), the strength of the magnetic moment of the ion (which is one factor that determines the efficiency of nuclear relaxation enhancement) is roughly proportional to the number of unpaired electrons. For the lanthanide ions other than Gd(III), the orbital motion of the unpaired electrons adds to the angular momentum from their respective spins to create magnetic moments larger than that predicted by the number of unpaired electrons.

Other paramagnetic substances include organic free radicals (e.g., nitroxides) and molecular oxygen. These have rather low magnetic moments and thus have received less attention as MR contrast agents.

DEPENDENCE OF MR IMAGE INTENSITY ON TISSUE RELAXATION TIMES

For a detailed description of MR imaging techniques, the reader is referred to other chapters in

TABLE 6–1. MAGNETIC MOMENTS OF SELECTED PARAMAGNETIC METAL IONS

Ion	Number of Unpaired Electrons	Magnetic Moment (Bohr Magnetons)
Transition Metal Ions		
Copper (II)	1	1.7–2.2
Nickel (II) (high spin)*	2	2.8–4.0
Chromium (III)	3	3.8
Iron (II) (high spin)	4	5.1–5.5
Manganese (II), iron (III)	5	5.9
Lanthanide Metal Ions		
Praseodymium (III)	2	3.5
Gadolinium (III)	7	8.0
Dysprosium (III)	5	10.6
Holmium (III)	4	10.6

*The number of unpaired electrons depends on the chemical environment around the metal ion. The table shows the maximal number of unpaired electrons, that is, the high spin state. Under some conditions, electrons can pair, giving a low spin state; for instance, Fe (II) in the low spin state has no unpaired electrons.

this text. The simplest form of MR imaging involves the application of a linear magnetic field gradient in addition to the main static field to "spatially encode" nuclei in the subject with different resonance frequencies. The free induction decay signal following a radiofrequency (RF) pulse is Fourier transformed to yield a one-dimensional projection of signal amplitude along a particular line through the subject. With the aid of algorithms used in x-ray CT and other imaging applications, a series of such projections can be reconstructed into two-dimensional images of MR signal intensity.

The dependence of ^1H MR image intensity on tissue relaxation times (which is the basis of image enhancement using paramagnetic agents) is inherent in the basic principles of pulse MR.[20] Briefly, the net macroscopic magnetization of proton spins, which is aligned parallel with the applied field along the z-axis, is perturbed by application of one or more RF pulses. The component of the magnetization along the z-axis "relaxes" back to its equilibrium value with an exponential time constant, T_1, the longitudinal (or spin-lattice) relaxation time. The time dependence of the magnetization perpendicular to the z-axis is characterized similarly by T_2, the transverse (or spin-spin) relaxation time, which measures the time for the decay of the transverse magnetization to its equilibrium value of zero. In image data acquisition, the pulses are rapidly repeated for each projection. Tissues with short T_1 values generally yield greater image intensity than those with longer values, since the steady-state magnetization along the z-axis is greater in the tissue with the fastest relaxation. On the other hand, short T_2 values are always associated with lower signal intensity, since this diminishes the net transverse magnetization available for detection.

DISTINCTION BETWEEN T_1 AND T_2 AGENTS

For the purposes of this discussion, it is useful to classify MR contrast agents into two broad groups based on whether the substance increases the $1/T_2$ of water protons roughly the same amount that it increases $1/T_1$ or whether the transverse relaxation rate ($1/T_2$) is altered to a much greater extent. (Relaxation rates, the reciprocals of relaxation times, are additive and thus much more useful in quantitative discussions.) We can refer to the first category as T_1 agents, since, on a percentage basis, these generally alter the $1/T_1$ of tissue more than $1/T_2$ owing to the fast endogenous transverse relaxation in tissue. With most conventional pulse sequences, this dominant T_1-lowering effect gives rise to increases in MR signal intensity; thus, these are positive contrast agents. On the other hand, T_2 agents largely increase the $1/T_2$ of tissue rather selectively; this leads to decreases in signal intensity, and thus these represent negative contrast agents. Contrast agents, constituting a third

class—nonproton agents, such as certain perfluorocarbons—do not affect relaxation rates but produce low signal by virtue of the absence of hydrogen; these agents are not considered in this chapter.

GENERAL REQUIREMENTS FOR MR CONTRAST AGENTS

MR imaging contrast agents must be biocompatible pharmaceuticals in addition to nuclear relaxation probes. Aside from standard pharmaceutical features, such as water solubility and shelf stability, the requirements relevant for metal ion–based agents can be classified into three general categories.

RELAXIVITY

The efficiency by which the agent enhances the proton relaxation rates of water, referred to as *relaxivity*, must be sufficient to increase significantly the relaxation rates of the target tissue. The dose of the agent at which such alteration of tissue relaxation rates occurs must, of course, be nontoxic. Increases in $1/T_1$ as small as 10 to 20 per cent could be detected by MR imaging.

SPECIFIC IN VIVO DISTRIBUTION

Ideally, to be of diagnostic value, the agent should localize for a period in a target tissue or tissue compartment in preference to nontarget regions. This is a basic tenet in any agent-based imaging procedure, in which detection of the agent is usually a simple function of its tissue concentration. For MR relaxation agents, however, this requirement should be qualified: It is sufficient *only* that the relaxation rates of the target tissue be enhanced in preference to the rates of other tissues. This goal might be accomplished by means other than concentration differences if the agent has a higher relaxivity in the environment of one tissue.

IN VIVO STABILITY, EXCRETABILITY, AND LACK OF TOXICITY

The acute and chronic toxicity of an intravenously administered metal complex is related in part to its stability in vivo and its tissue clearance behavior. The transition metal and lanthanide ions are relatively toxic at doses required for MR relaxation rate changes, and thus the dissociation of the complex cannot occur to any significant degree. (The toxicity of the free ligand also becomes a factor in the event of dissociation.) In addition, a diagnostic agent should be excreted within hours of administration.

T_1 AGENTS

RELAXIVITY

Theory

The addition of a paramagnetic solute causes an increase in the $1/T_1$ and $1/T_2$ of solvent nuclei. The diamagnetic and paramagnetic contributions to the relaxation rates of such solutions are additive and given by

$$(1/T_i)_{obs} = (1/T_i)_d + (1/T_i)_p \qquad i = 1,2 \quad (1)$$

where $(1/T_i)_{obs}$ is the observed solvent relaxation rate in the presence of a paramagnetic species, $(1/T_i)_d$ is the (diamagnetic) solvent relaxation rate in the absence of a paramagnetic species, and $(1/T_i)_p$ represents the additional paramagnetic contribution. In the absence of solute-solute interactions, the solvent relaxation rates are linearly dependent on the concentration of the paramagnetic species ([M]); relaxivity, R_i, is defined as the slope of this dependence in units of $M^{-1}sec^{-1}$ or, more commonly, $mM^{-1}sec^{-1}$:

$$(1/T_i)_{obs} = (1/T_i)_d + R_i[M] \qquad i = 1,2 \quad (2)$$

The large and fluctuating local magnetic field in the vicinity of a paramagnetic center provides this additional relaxation pathway for solvent nuclei. Since these fields fall off rapidly with distance, random translational diffusion of solvent molecules and the complex as well as specific chemical interactions that bring the solvent molecules near the metal ion (e.g., within 5 Å) are important in transmitting the paramagnetic effect. Each type of chemical interaction can yield different relaxation efficiencies, as governed by the distance and time scale of the interaction; the sum of these contributions and that due to translational diffusion gives the total relaxivity of the paramagnetic species.

For the discussion that follows, it is useful to classify the relevant contributions to water proton relaxivity with respect to three distinct types of interactions, as shown in Figure 6–1. In case A, a water molecule binds in the primary coordination sphere of the metal ion and exchanges with the bulk solvent. The term *inner sphere relaxation* is often applied loosely to this type of relaxation mechanism. Case B represents hydrogen-bonded waters in the second coordination sphere. Because of the lack of understanding of

second coordination sphere interactions, investigators often do not distinguish between this relaxation mechanism (case B) and that due to translational diffusion of the water molecule past the chelate (case C), referring simply to *outer sphere relaxation*. The total relaxivity of a paramagnetic agent is therefore generally given by

$$(1/T_i)_p = (1/T)_{inner\ sphere} + (1/T_i)_{outer\ sphere} \qquad i = 1,2 \quad (3)$$

The longitudinal relaxation contribution from the inner sphere mechanism results from a chemical exchange of the water molecule between the primary coordination sphere of the paramagnetic metal ion (or any hydration site near the metal) and the bulk solvent, as shown in Figure 6–2, yielding the following expression:

$$\left[\frac{1}{T_1}\right]_{inner\ sphere} = \frac{P_M q}{T_{1M} + \tau_M} \quad (4)$$

Here P_M is the mole fraction of metal ion, q is the number of water molecules bound per metal ion, T_{1M} is the relaxation time of the bound water protons, and τ_M is the residence lifetime of the bound water. The value of T_{1M} is in turn given by the Solomon-Bloembergen equation[4, 6]:

$$\frac{1}{T_{1M}} = \frac{2}{15} \frac{\gamma_I^2 g^2 S (S+1) \beta^2}{r^6} \left[\frac{7\tau_c}{(1+\omega_S^2\tau_c^2)} + \frac{3\tau_c}{(1+\omega_I^2\tau_c^2)}\right] \quad (5)$$

where γ_I is the proton gyromagnetic ratio, g is the electronic g-factor, S is the total electron spin of the metal ion, β is the Bohr magneton, r is the proton–metal ion distance, and ω_S and ω_I are the electronic and proton Larmor precession frequencies, respectively. The dependence on the last two quantities makes relaxivity a function of magnetic field as well as other physical and chemical properties. (The above equation includes only the dipolar ["through space"] contribution to relaxivity; the scalar, or contact ["through bonds"] contribution is rarely significant for metal ion species used as contrast agents.)

The key feature of paramagnetically induced nuclear relaxation is that the local magnetic field from the electron spin must fluctuate at proper frequencies to stimulate nuclear relaxation. The time scale of these fluctuations is characterized by the overall correlation time τ_c; the characteristic rate of these fluctuations, $1/\tau_c$, is dominated by the fastest of three processes:

$$\frac{1}{\tau_c} = \frac{1}{T_{1e}} + \frac{1}{\tau_M} + \frac{1}{\tau_R} \quad (6)$$

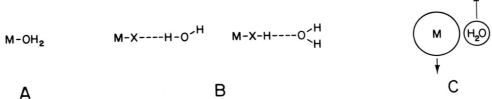

FIGURE 6–1. Interactions between water and metal complexes (*M*). *A*, Inner sphere relaxation due to binding of water molecules to primary coordination sphere of metal ion. *B* and *C*, Outer sphere relaxation due to hydrogen-bonded water in outer coordination sphere (*B*) and motion of water past the metal ion (*C*).

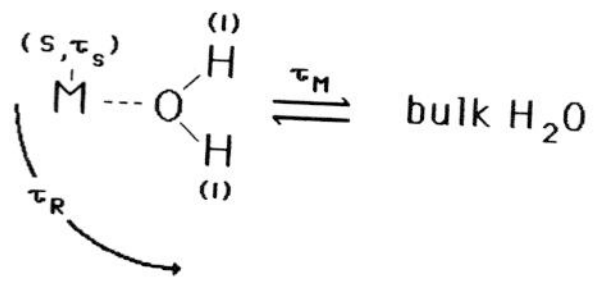

FIGURE 6–2. Proton relaxation by paramagnetic metal ions. The proton spin I on a metal-bound water molecule experiences the fluctuating magnetic field of the electron spin S; this water exchanges with the bulk solvent. The rates of water exchange (τ_M^{-1}), rotation of the paramagnetic complex (τ_R^{-1}), and electron spin relaxation (τ_s^{-1}) determine the relaxation rate ($1/T_1$) of the bound water, as expressed by the Solomon-Bloembergen equations.

where T_{1e} (also called τ_S) is the *longitudinal electron spin relaxation time;* τ_M is the *water residence time,* as mentioned above; and τ_R is the *rotational tumbling time* of the entire metal-water unit. These processes, all of which alter the magnetic field at the nucleus, are shown in Figure 6–2.

Similar theories exist for outer sphere relaxation. It should be pointed out, however, that the quantitative understanding of both inner and outer sphere relaxivities of metal complexes is still at an early stage (see Reference 1).

Relaxivity in Solution

Table 6–2 lists the 20-MHz longitudinal relaxivities for various simple metal complexes; structures of selected ligands are shown in Figure 6–3. Relaxivity is proportional to the number of inner sphere water molecules (q), which decreases when large ligands (e.g., DTPA) are bound to the metal ion to ensure stability of the complex. For example, chelation of Gd(III) with DTPA decreases q from 8 or 9 to 1; the structure of the resulting complex is shown in Figure 6–4. When q = 0, relaxation is limited to outer sphere mechanisms; from Table 6–2 one can see that outer sphere relaxivities are quite sizable. In the design of MR contrast agents, the use of multidentate

TABLE 6–2. LONGITUDINAL RELAXIVITIES (R_1) AT 20 MHz AND THE NUMBER OF COORDINATED WATER MOLECULES (q) FOR SELECTED METAL COMPLEXES*

Complex	q	R_1 (mM^{-1} s^{-1})
Gd (III)		
Aquo ion	8,9	9.1
EDTA	2,3	6.6
DOTA	1	3.4
DTPA	1	3.7
TETA	0	2.1
TTHA	0	2.0
Mn (II)		
Aquo ion	6	8.0
EDTA	1	2.0
DTPA	0	1.1
Fe (III)		
Aquo ion	6	8.0
EDTA	1	1.8
EHPG	0	0.95
DTPA	0	0.73
Cr (III)		
Aquo ion	6	5.8
EDTA	1	0.2
Cu (II)		
Aquo ion	6	0.84
Dy (III)		
Aquo ion	8,9	0.56
EDTA	2,3	0.17
DTPA	1 (?)	0.096

*Relaxivity values given for the temperature range of 35 to 39° C.
Reprinted with permission from Lauffer RB: Paramagnetic metal complexes as water proton relaxation agents for NMR imaging: Theory and design. Chem Rev 87: 901–927, 1987. Copyright 1987 American Chemical Society.

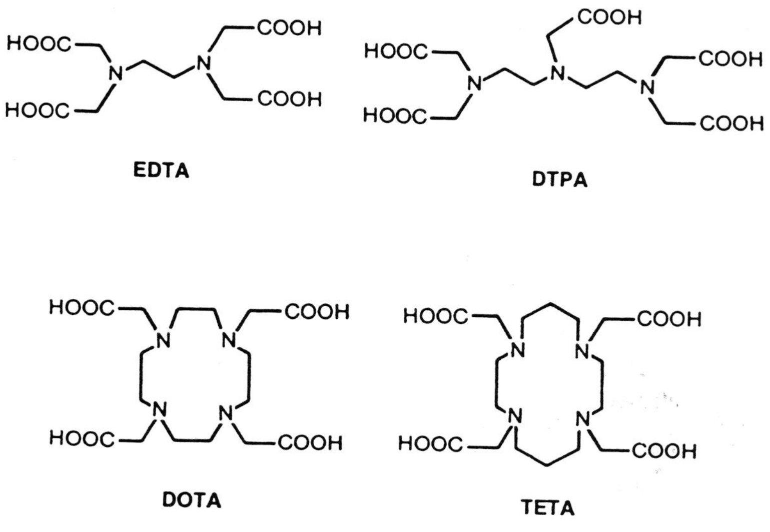

ligands to ensure in vivo stability of the complexes reduces the number of coordinated water molecules; the outer sphere contribution to these low molecular weight complexes thus becomes a significant fraction (if not all) of the total relaxivity.

In general, relaxivities are also proportional to the magnetic moment of the metal ion. However, we can

FIGURE 6–3. Structures of selected chelating agents.

EDTA

DTPA

DOTA

TETA

Coordination of Gd³⁺ with DTPA · H₂O

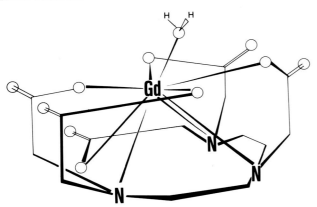

FIGURE 6–4. Structure of gadolinium-DTPA. (Courtesy of Schering AG.)

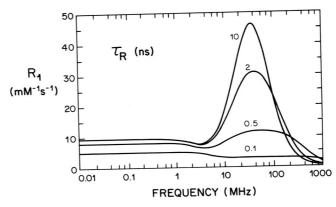

FIGURE 6–5. Calculated inner sphere longitudinal relaxivities versus Larmor frequency, or NMRD profiles, as a function of different values of the rotational correlation time, τ_R, of a metal complex. Values chosen are typical of a Gd(III) complex with q = 1. The lowest value of τ_R chosen, 0.1 nsec, is roughly that of low molecular weight complexes such as [Gd(DTPA)]²⁻; the single dispersion at ~ 5 MHz is that of the $7\tau_c$ term in Equation 5 (the $3\tau_c$ term does not disperse under these conditions until ~1000 MHz). Increasing τ_R (e.g., by increasing size of complex) allows the frequency dependence of T_{1e} to be expressed; T_{1e} is thought to rise dramatically with increasing frequency beginning at 10 MHz, creating the peak characteristic of slowly rotating paramagnetic ions. The increase in τ_c pushes the $7\tau_c$ dispersion to lower frequency (~2 MHz) and brings the $3\tau_c$ dispersion down to ~100 MHz. With the parameters used here, raising τ_R above 10 nsec does not increase relaxivity further, since T_{1e} or τ_M or both become the dominant correlation times. (Reprinted with permission from Lauffer RB; Paramagnetic metal complexes as water proton relaxation agents for NMR imaging: Theory and design. Chem Rev 87: 901–927, 1987. Copyright, 1987 American Chemical Society.)

see from Table 6–2 that dysprosium(III) with DTPA has a much lower relaxivity than the analogous Gd(III) complex despite the larger magnetic moment of Dy(III). As it turns out, for all of the lanthanide(III) ions except Gd(III) and for certain transition metal ions, electron spin relaxation occurs so rapidly (T_{1e} ~ 1 psec) that fluctuations at the proper frequencies for nuclear relaxation are less probable and thus relaxivities are low. (This is equivalent to saying that a short T_{1e} leads to a small value of τ_c [$\tau_c = T_{1e}$ in this case], which, in turn, leads to low relaxivity, as shown in Equation 5.)

For metal ions with relatively long T_{1e}'s—Gd(III), Mn(II), and iron(III) are good examples—alteration of the rotational tumbling time τ_R is the single most important source of relaxivity enhancement. The degree of enhancement possible, which is limited by the values of T_{1e} and τ_M according to Equation 6, exceeds that which is realistically available from optimizing any of the other relevant parameters. Figure 6–5 shows the magnetic field dependence of relaxivity (also known as nuclear magnetic relaxation dispersion profiles, or NMRD) as a function of τ_R calculated from the Solomon-Bloembergen equation. Parameters typical of Gd(III) complexes are utilized. The enhancement in R_1 predicted at longer τ_R values (the PRE effect) has been experimentally observed for metal ions bound to DNA or proteins. One can see from Figure 6–5 that both the magnitude of relaxivity and the functional form of its field dependence are altered when the rotation rate is decreased. The prominent peak that forms is noteworthy, since it is predicted to occur over the clinically relevant field range.

The PRE effect has been shown to be operative when intact chelates are covalently attached to protein amino acid residues. The ligands ethylenediamine tetraacetic acid (EDTA) and DTPA were attached to amino groups on bovine serum albumin (BSA) and bovine immunoglobulins using cyclic anhydride forms of the ligands.[21, 22] The structure of the bound ligands, shown in Figure 6–6, most likely involves an amide linkage between a ligand carboxylate and the lysine or terminal amino groups. Metal ions can be titrated selectively into the chelating sites on the proteins. Figure 6–7 displays the complete NMRD profiles of the free and bound Gd(III) chelates. Binding is generally accompanied by an increase in the amplitudes of the curves and a change in their functional form, resembling that calculated from theory and observed in slowly rotating metalloenzyme systems. This finding implies that despite the potentially flexible linkage to the protein the chelates appear to be fairly immobilized. The magnitudes of the relaxivities most likely relate to the average number of coordinated waters in each case, which is greater for the EDTA conjugates than for the DTPA conjugates.

Relaxivity in Tissue

The efficiency by which a metal complex influences tissue relaxation rates is dependent on two factors:

1. The chemical environment (or environments) encountered by the complex in vivo. By far the greatest effect is exerted by binding of the agent to macromolecular structures, which can potentially cause significant relaxivity enhancement.

2. Compartmentalization of the complex in tissue. Generally, tissue water is compartmentalized into

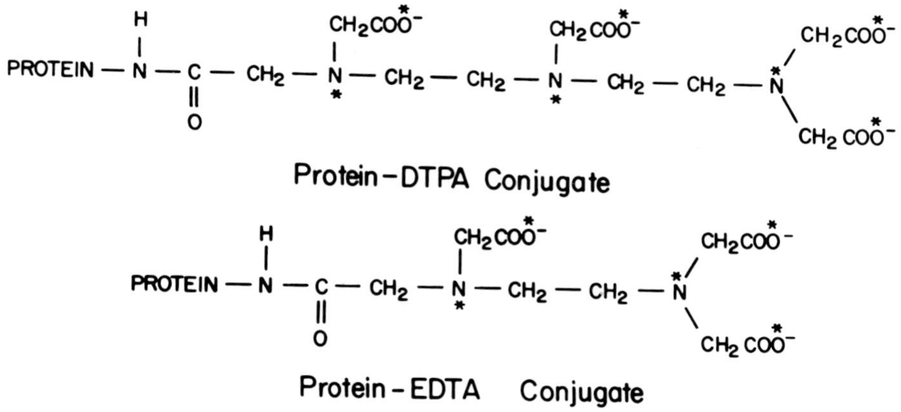

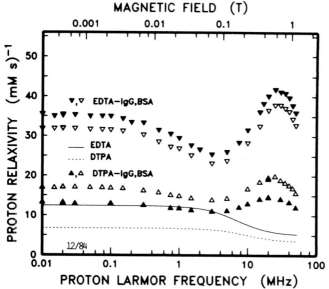

FIGURE 6–6. Anticipated structure of the DTPA and EDTA ligands when covalently attached to protein amino groups. Heteroatoms most likely involved in Mn(II) or Gd(III) binding are denoted with asterisks. These protein-bound complexes can be used to slow molecular rotation and thereby enhance relaxivity. (From Lauffer RB, Brady TJ, Brown RD, et al: 1/T1 NMRD profiles of solutions of Mn + 2 and Gd + 3 protein-chelate complexes. Magn Reson Med 3:541–548, 1986; with permission.)

intravascular, interstitial (fluid space between cells and capillaries), and intracellular space constituting roughly 5, 15, and 80 per cent of the total water, respectively. Cellular organelles further subdivide the intracellular component. If water exchange between any of these compartments is slow relative to the relaxation rate in the compartment with the longest T_1, multiexponential longitudinal relaxation may result. This can decrease the effective tissue relaxivity of an agent because all of the tissue water is not encountering the paramagnetic center.

Estimates of tissue relaxivities of metal complexes require the measurements of excised tissue T_1's from

FIGURE 6–7. NMRD profiles of Gd(III) chelates covalently attached to protein amino groups. Data are shown for Gd-EDTA attached to bovine immunoglobulins (IgG,▼) and bovine serum albumin (BSA,▽) and the corresponding Gd-DTPA conjugates (▲,△). The solid and dashed curves in the lower portion of the figure indicate data for the free chelates Gd(EDTA)⁻ and Gd(DTPA)²⁻, respectively. (From Lauffer RB, Brady TJ, Brown RD, et al: 1/T1 NMRD profiles of solutions of Mn + 2 and Gd + 3 protein-chelate complexes. Magn Reson Med 3:541–548, 1986; with permission.)

two groups of animals: those receiving the agent and a control group. The tissue concentration of the complex should be determined by analysis of the tissue for metal content or by use of a suitable radioactive tracer. The largest source of error in these determinations is the animal-to-animal variation in baseline relaxation rates.

For low molecular weight, hydrophilic metal complexes, the available data show clearly that the relaxivity in blood and soft tissue is within experimental error of that in aqueous solution; this has been shown, for example, for [Gd(DTPA)]²⁻ and [Gd(DOTA)]⁻ (DOTA = 1,4,7,10-tetraaza cyclodo-decane N, N', N'', N''' tetraacetate) by Tweedle and colleagues.[23, 24] This observation suggests that no binding interactions between the chelate and proteins or membrane structures are taking place. The early use of cobalt(II) EDTA as an extracellular marker suggests that the distribution of these Gd(III) complexes is the same.[25] The hydrophilic nature of the complexes as well as their extracellular localization (where protein concentrations are lower relative to intracellular environments) apparently results in unhindered rotational mobility.

Koenig and associates have measured NMRD profiles for blood containing [Gd(DTPA)]²⁻.[26] The single exponential decay of the longitudinal relaxation in these samples indicates that water exchange between erythrocytes and plasma must be fast relative to the relaxation rates. It is interesting that the NMRD difference curves obtained after subtracting out the diamagnetic contribution to the observed rates were identical in amplitude and functional form with that of the complex in aqueous solution.

Compartmentalization effects have been noted for the kidney by Koenig, Wolf, and coworkers in another study of [Gd(DTPA)]²⁻.[27] Longitudinal relaxation in the renal medulla was found to be biexponential in the presence of the paramagnetic agent, resulting from concentration of the agent in the collecting tubules.

The most prominent evidence for a paramagnetic agent binding in vivo and generating greater relaxivity is that of the Mn(II) ion. Though not relevant as a contrast agent owing to its toxicity, Mn(II) has both a historical and an instructive importance. Lauterbur, Mendonca-Dias, and Rudin, in their landmark 1978 paper, noted an approximately 50 per cent increase in relaxivity for Mn(II) in heart tissue at 4 MHz.[15] Kang and Gore measured enhancement factors (relative to the aquo ion in aqueous solution) of 4 to 6 at 20 MHz for Mn(II) in heart, liver, spleen, and kidney.[28] Kang and colleagues found that Mn(II) binding to serum albumin in blood induces a 10-fold enhancement in relaxivity.[29] Koenig and colleagues measured NMRD profiles of liver and kidney tissue after injection of Mn(II) (or weakly chelated complexes) and found peaks in relaxation rate centered at approximately 10 to 20 MHz indicative of Mn(II) in slowly tumbling environments, possibly bound to proteins or membrane surfaces.[30] The field dependence of relaxation is thus valuable in that it can qualitatively indicate binding interactions in tissue without independent determinations of agent concentration.

TOXICITY AND THE STABILITY OF METAL COMPLEXES

The acute and chronic toxic effects of paramagnetic metal complexes will be important to understand in view of the likely possibility of routine intravenous administration of such compounds for MR imaging examinations in the future. The required doses of such compounds (roughly 0.5 to 5.0 gm per patient) greatly exceeds those of metal ions or complexes used in radioscintigraphy. However, iodine-containing contrast agents are used in CT and other radiologic procedures at much higher doses than MR agents (~50 to 200 gm per patient). With the development of relatively nontoxic chelates, the contrast-enhanced MR examination is likely to be safer than similar CT procedures.

Toxicity and stability are discussed together here to emphasize the historical importance of metal complex stability in determining toxicity in early evaluations of MR agents. The dissociation of a complex generally leads to a higher degree of toxicity stemming from the free metal ion or free chelating ligand.

Toxic effects from a metal complex can arise from (1) free metal ion, released by dissociation; (2) free ligand, which also arises from dissociation; and (3) the intact metal complex. In the last two cases, one may also have to consider metabolites, which may be more toxic than the parent compound.

The available toxicologic data point to the importance of metal complex dissociation as an important source of toxicity. Table 6–3 lists acute LD_{50} values (interpolated dose at which 50 per cent of the animals would die) determined for metal ions, complexes, and ligands. Both metal ions and free ligands tend to be more toxic than metal chelates. This finding is reasonable if one considers that complexation itself "neutralizes" the coordinating properties of both the

ligand and the metal ion to some degree, decreasing their avidity for binding to proteins, enzymes, or membranes via electrostatic or hydrogen-bonding interactions or covalent bonds.

In the simplest view, the degree of toxicity of a metal chelate is related to its degree of dissociation in vivo before excretion. A good example of how toxicity and in vivo stability depend on the chelating ligand is the comparison between [Gd(EDTA)]⁻ and [Gd(DTPA)]²⁻. The latter is a very stable complex (metal-ligand formation constant, log K_{ML} = 22.5) that is excreted intact readily by the kidneys, exhibiting a very low degree of toxicity (LD_{50} ~ 10 to 20 mmol/kg).[31] [Gd(EDTA)]⁻, on the other hand, has a toxicity comparable to that of GdCl₃ (LD_{50} ~ 0.5 mmol/kg), despite its apparently high thermodynamic stability (log K_{ML} = 17.4). The straightforward interpretation is that the latter complex quantitatively dissociates in vivo, yielding the toxicity of the free ion.

The toxicity of metal ions has been extensively reviewed.[32] The coordination of ions to oxygen, nitrogen, or sulfur heteroatoms in macromolecules and membranes alters the dynamic equilibria necessary

TABLE 6–3. ACUTE LD_{50} VALUES FOR METAL SALTS, METAL COMPLEXES, AND FREE LIGANDS

Compound	LD_{50} (mmol/kg)	Animal	Administration*
GdCl₃	0.5	Rat	IV
	0.4	Mouse	IV
	0.26	Rat	IV
	1.4	Mouse	IP
Gd (OH)₃	0.1	Mouse	IV
(MEG) [Gd(EDTA) (H₂O)ₙ]	0.3	Rat	IV
	0.62	Mouse	IP
MEG[Gd(CDTA)(H₂O)ₙ]	<2.5	Rat	IV
MEG[Gd(EGTA) (H₂O)ₙ]	<2.5	Rat	IV
(MEG)² [Gd(DTPA) (H₂O)]	10	Rat	IV
	>10	Mouse	IV
Na²[Gd(DTPA) (H₂O)]	>10	Mouse	IV
	20	Rat	IV
(MEG)[Gd(DOTA) (H₂O)]	>10	Mouse	IV
Na[Gd(DOTA) (H₂O)]	>10	Mouse	IV
(MEG)₃[Gd(TTHA)]	6	Rat	IV
MnCl₂	0.22	Rat	IV
	1.5	Mouse	IP
Na₂[Mn(EDTA) (H₂O)]	7.0	Rat	IV
	5.9	Mouse	IP
Na₃[Mn(DTPA)]	1.9	Rat	IV
FeCl₃	1.6	Mouse	IP
Na[Fe(EDTA) (H₂O)]	3.4	Mouse	IV
	1.7	Mouse	IP
Na₃[Ca(DTPA)]	5.0	Rat	IV
	3.5	Mouse	IV
(MEG)₃H₂DTPA	0.15	Mouse	IV
Na₂H₃DTPA	0.1	Mouse	IV
Na₂[Ca(DOTA)]	>7.0	Mouse	IV
(MEG)₂H₂DOTA	0.18	Mouse	IV

*IV = intravenous; IP = intraperitoneal.
MEG = N-methylglucamine; CDTA = trans-1,2-cyclohexylenedinitrilotetraacetic acid; EGTA = ethylene glycol(2-aminoethylether)tetraacetic acid; TTHA = triethylenetetraamine hexaacetic acid.
Reprinted with permission from Lauffer RB: Paramagnetic metal complexes as water proton relaxation agents for NMR imaging: Theory and design. Chem Rev 87:90–927, 1987. Copyright 1987 American Chemical Society.

to sustain life. *Gd(III), for example, can bind to calcium (Ca)(II) binding sites, often with higher affinity owing to its greater charge-radius ratio.*

The toxicity of free ligands, which is less understood, can stem from the sequestration of essential metal ions, such as Ca(II), in addition to "organic" toxicity.

The toxicity of intact metal complexes can stem from a wide variety of specific and nonspecific effects. At the high doses required in LD_{50} determinations of relatively nontoxic hydrophilic chelates like $[Gd(DTPA)]^{2-}$, the nonspecific hypertonic effect is thought to be important. A difference in osmolality between intracellular and extracellular compartments is established after injection of large quantities of the ionic complexes and appropriate counter-ions. Water is drawn out of cells as a result of the osmotic gradient, causing cellular and circulatory damage. Current efforts are now directed to the development of neutral (nonionic) derivatives that may lessen this effect and improve tolerability.

Other possible mechanisms of chelate toxicity include enzyme inhibition, nonspecific protein conformational effects, and alteration of membrane potentials. The interactions between metal chelates and biologic macromolecular structures, which are not well understood, represent an important area of investigation relevant to understanding toxicity on a molecular basis.

IN VIVO TARGETING

Targeting a paramagnetic agent to a particular site within the body is one of the most challenging aspects of MR contrast agent design. The diagnostic utility of a contrast-enhanced MR imaging examination will depend on the absolute concentration of the agent in the desired tissue and the selectivity of the distribution relative to other tissues. True targeting is rarely achieved. After administration, the agent equilibrates in several body compartments prior to excretion; preferential distribution of the agent to the desired site is all that can be expected in most circumstances. MR imaging agents are similar to radiopharmaceuticals or iodinated CT agents in that the MR image enhancement depends on the concentration of a paramagnetic metal complex. The principles of distribution governing these other agents are directly applicable to MR agents.

However, the dependence of relaxivity on the chemical environment of a paramagnetic complex alters this simple view. What is directly relevant to MR imaging is not the actual distribution of the agent but the distribution of the relaxation rate changes induced by the agent. The enhancement in relaxivity induced by binding the agent to a macromolecule (the PRE effect) is of central importance. By targeting a complex to desired sites where such binding interactions occur, the target-nontarget ratio in terms of relaxation rate changes may be increased above that

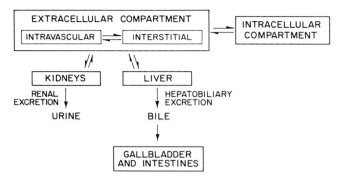

FIGURE 6–8. Principal distribution sites and excretion pathways for intravenously administered soluble metal complexes.

in terms of concentration. Little has been done to reduce this "binding-enhancement" concept to practice.

Figure 6–8 illustrates potential distribution sites and excretion pathways relevant for soluble metal complexes. An intravenously administered chelate rapidly equilibrates in the intravascular and interstitial (space between cells) fluid compartments; these collectively are referred to as the extracellular compartment. Depending on its structure, the complex may also be distributed into various intracellular environments (including that of liver and kidney) by passive diffusion or specific uptake processes.

The structure of the complex determines its excretion pathway. Most commonly, small molecular weight hydrophilic chelates that do not bind to plasma proteins are nonspecifically filtered out in the kidneys (glomerular filtration).[33] If the molecule possesses a balance between hydrophobic and hydrophilic character, particularly if it contains aromatic rings, some fraction of the complex is taken up by liver cells and excreted into the bile (hepatobiliary excretion).[34] Such molecules often exhibit some degree of plasma protein binding, particularly to albumin, which reduces the free fraction available for glomerular filtration. The hepatobiliary and renal pathways can thus be competitive. Generally, the greater the degree of lipophilicity a molecule possesses, the greater the hepatobiliary excretion. The complete clearance of the agent from the body by either route is, of course, desirable to minimize toxicity. If, however, the complex is very lipophilic, it can (1) distribute into fat storage sites or membranes or (2) precipitate in blood and be taken up by reticuloendothelial cells in the liver and spleen. Both possibilities lead to long-term retention of the agent, which may be associated with chronic toxicity.

The following is a discussion of the various classes of metal complexes under investigation as MR imaging agents. Owing to the relatively high concentration of a paramagnetic agent required for image enhancement, the targeting of low-concentration receptor sites (<1 μM), as in traditional radioscintigraphy or positron emission tomography,[35] is not feasible for MR imaging. Therefore, the diagnostic utility of most of the complexes under examination is linked to their general distribution or excretion pathway, or both, and this fact is reflected in the classifications that follow.

Extracellular Distribution: Renal Excretion

$[Gd(DTPA)]^{2-}$ and, more recently, $[Gd(DOTA)]^{-}$ are prototype complexes of this class of agents.[23, 31, 36] Compared with other substances discussed further on, these agents are nonspecific in reference to their nonselective extracellular distribution. Their localization in tissues does not usually reflect specific cellular processes. They nevertheless form an important class of potential MR agents that resemble iodinated CT contrast media as well as more analogous radiopharmaceuticals, such as the DTPA complexes of technetium-99m (^{99m}Tc) or indium-113 (^{113}In).[35]

The structural requirements for these agents are satisfied by simple metal complexes. The presence of charged or hydrogen-bonding groups such as carboxylates and the lack of large hydrophobic groups ensure minimal interaction with plasma proteins, other macromolecules, and membranes. This situation allows for the equilibration of the complex in the extracellular space and efficient renal excretion. The stereochemistry of the complex or other subtle structural features are not likely to be important. Most members of this class are anionic.

The above requirements, as well as others discussed in this chapter, are satisfactorily met by $[Gd(DTPA)]^{2-}$ and $[Gd(DOTA)]^{-}$. Further developments toward lowering toxicity even more may take place (as mentioned previously, to decrease the osmolality of injected solutions), but the more interesting challenge is to develop more specific agents, as is discussed in the following sections.

The renal excretion of these agents yields the obvious application of imaging the kidneys, both for structural and for functional information.[36, 37] The status of blood flow to a tissue (perfusion) may be another application of these agents[38]; this requires the development of fast imaging techniques to follow the rapid passage through the tissue.

The major use of these nonspecific agents is in the detection of cerebral capillary breakdown or the enhancement of tissues with an increased extracellular volume. Both applications stem from the dependence of the bulk tissue $1/T_1$ on the volume of distribution of the paramagnetic agent. If we assume that water exchange between the extracellular and intracellular compartments is fast relative to their T_1's, then the bulk tissue $1/T_1$ before injection of the agent is given by

$$(1/T_1)_{pre\ inj} = f_{ex}(1/T_1)_{ex,\ pre} + f_{in}(1/T_1)_{in} \quad (7)$$

where f_{ex} is the fraction of water protons in the extracellular space, $(1/T_1)_{ex,\ pre}$ is the extracellular relaxation rate in the absence of the paramagnetic species, and f_{in} is the intracellular fraction characterized by $(1/T_1)_{in}$. The extracellularly localized agent increases $(1/T_1)_{ex}$ directly, and the net change in the overall tissue $1/T_1$ is given by

$$\begin{aligned}
\Delta(1/T_1) &= (1/T_1)_{post\ inj} - (1/T_1)_{pre\ inj} \\
&= f_{ex}(1/T_1)_{ex,\ post} + f_{in}(1/T_1)_{in} \\
&\quad - f_{ex}(1/T_1)_{ex,\ pre} - f_{in}(1/T_1)_{in} \quad (8) \\
&= f_{ex}[(1/T_1)_{ex,\ post} - (1/T_1)_{ex,pre}]
\end{aligned}$$

If an agent equilibrates to roughly the same concentration in the extracellular space, and therefore $(1/T_1)_{ex,\ post}$ is relatively constant in different tissues, then those tissues with the greatest fraction of extracellular space will yield the greatest MR signal intensity changes. This finding has been observed for tumors and abscesses, which often exhibit increased interstitial volume.[23, 37]

The most dramatic enhancement of lesions with these agents is seen in the brain (Fig. 6–9), where normal tissue exhibits little enhancement because of the impermeable nature of brain capillaries (the blood-brain barrier) and the small intravascular volume of distribution (5 per cent) of the agent. The capillaries of tumors, however, do allow the passage of the complex into the interstitial space, allowing very selective enhancement.

Extracellular Distribution: Hepatobiliary Excretion

Hepatobiliary agents are the second most important class of potential MR contrast agents. By virtue of their efficient excretion from the body, the development of safe derivatives of this class seems likely. In addition, in contrast to the nonspecific renal agents, hepatobiliary agents may give an indication of the status of specific cellular function: that of the hepatocytes of the liver.

The potential diagnostic utility of this class of MR agents includes the following:

1. Selective enhancement of normal, functioning liver tissue to aid in the detection of small lesions, such as metastatic tumors (focal liver disease).

2. Indication of the status of liver function to detect diffuse liver disease such as cirrhosis.

3. High-resolution visualization of bile ducts and the gallbladder.

Other forms of diagnostic hepatobiliary agents are radioactive ^{99m}Tc complexes[35, 39] and iodinated CT agents.[40, 41] Currently, various substituted ^{99m}Tc–acetanilidoiminodiacetic acid (^{99m}Tc-IDA) complexes are used in scintigraphic imaging to detect obstruction of bile ducts. However, the image resolution is very low compared with that in MR, limiting biliary visualization. Further, the detection of small lesions in the liver by these complexes or other radiopharmaceuticals is not possible. The hepatobiliary agents for CT that have been evaluated are not used clinically owing to their toxicity and high dose requirements.[41]

The mechanisms by which the hepatocytes of the

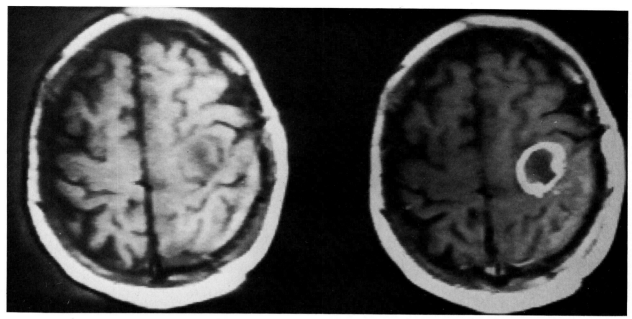

FIGURE 6–9. Transverse MR images (0.6 T, 24 MHz) through the brain of a patient before (*left*) and 3 minutes after (*right*) intravenous injection of [Gd(DTPA)]$^{2-}$ (dimeglumine salt); (Berlex Laboratories, Wayne, NJ) at a dose of 0.1 mmol/kg. Characteristic ring enhancement of a tumor (high-grade astrocytoma) is seen in the postinjection image. Pulse sequence: spin-echo (SE), repetition time (TR) = 500 and echo time (TE) = 20 msec. (Courtesy of Dr. Thomas Brady, Massachusetts General Hospital, Boston, MA.)

liver extract certain molecules from the blood and secrete them into bile have not been refined.[34, 42] Diagnostic hepatobiliary agents are generally anionic and are therefore thought to be taken up by the same carrier system that transports bilirubin, the dicarboxylic acid breakdown product of heme, and various anionic dyes, such as sulfobromophthalein sodium (bromosulfophthalein, or BSP). Membrane proteins that are thought to play a crucial role in the uptake of these compounds have been identified, and it is likely that some type of carrier-mediated transport is at work. Separate anionic transport systems for fatty acids and bile acids apparently exist in addition to that for bilirubin. However, Berk and coworkers have recently suggested that anionic compounds such as the ^{99m}Tc-IDA chelates may actually be taken up by more than one of the three carriers.[43] Alternatively, a single, complex system for all three types of anionic compounds may exist. An additional unsolved problem in hepatocellular uptake is how the molecules are extracted efficiently despite the tight binding by albumin in the blood, which these molecules often exhibit. It is thought that some form of facilitated diffusion of the albumin-ligand complex may occur at or near the hepatocyte surface.

The structural and physicochemical properties required for hepatocellular uptake are poorly defined.[34] It is generally believed that high molecular weight (>300 for rats and >500 for humans) as well as the presence of both hydrophilic and lipophilic moieties will direct a compound to the bile in preference to the urine. The molecular weight require-

ment probably reflects the need for large lipophilic groups, especially aromatic rings, which may interact favorably with hydrophobic regions of the membrane receptor or other transport proteins. The ^{99m}Tc-IDA complexes, bilirubin, and various cholephilic dyes (such as BSP) possess at least two delocalized ring systems. The more polar moieties, especially ionized groups, are probably required for water solubility; molecules lacking these might precipitate in blood or become deposited in fat tissue or membranes. It is also likely that these groups, especially anionic residues, are important for electrostatic or hydrogen-bonding interactions at macromolecular binding sites.

Our group chose to evaluate iron(III)ethylene-bis-(2-hydroxyphenylglycine (Fe[EHPG]$^-$) as a prototype MR hepatobiliary agent in view of these overall requirements and on the basis of early reports showing that EHPG induced the biliary excretion of Fe(III).[44] The complex contains coordinated carboxylates, two phenyl rings, net anionic charge, and octahedral coordination to the metal center.[45] These features are common to the suspected structures of the ^{99m}Tc-IDA agents as octahedral bis-IDA complexes with a −1 charge.[35, 39]

The fact that Fe(EHPG)$^-$ is coordinatively saturated and therefore relaxes water protons only via outer sphere mechanisms did not dissuade us from evaluating it. The longitudinal relaxivity was found to be ~1 mM^{-1}sec^{-1}, roughly four times less than [Gd(DTPA)]$^{2-}$, but nevertheless sufficient if the complex localizes in the liver and bile.[46]

The initial MR imaging and biodistribution studies

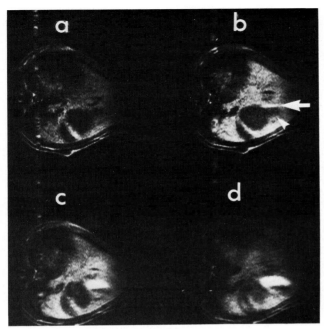

FIGURE 6–10. Transverse MR images (0.6 T, 24 MHz) of the dog abdomen before (*A*) and 14, 50, and 60 minutes after (*B* to *D*, respectively) intravenous injection of Fe(EHPG)$^-$ (0.2 mmol/kg). Enhancement of the liver and gallbladder is evident. Bile in the gallbladder prior to injection of the agent appears dark (*arrowhead*), whereas newly formed bile containing the paramagnetic agent appears bright (*arrow*) and layers on top. (From Lauffer RB, Greif WL, Stark DD, et al: Iron-EHPG as an hepatobiliary MR contrast agent: Initial imaging and biodistribution studies. J Comput Assist Tomogr 9:431–438, 1985; with permission.)

of Fe(EHPG)$^-$ were encouraging.[46] At a dose of 0.2 mmol/kg, the complex increases the $1/T_1$ of rat liver from approximately 3.2 to 4.3 sec^{-1} (20 MHz, 37°) at 10 minutes after injection, corresponding to ~1 mM concentration in the water space of the tissue. This localization yields a 200 per cent increase in MR image signal intensity on a 60-MHz system. (We demonstrated later that the degree of enhancement is dependent on the choice of pulse sequence parameters in accordance with theoretical expectations.[47]) The biliary clearance of the intact agent from the liver was noted for rats, rabbits, and dogs (Fig. 6–10).

Recent studies with Fe(EHPG)$^-$ in a mouse model of liver metastasis have revealed that even this prototype agent is capable of enhancing contrast between normal liver and tumors (Fig. 6–11).[48]

The biliary excretion of ^{99m}Tc-IDA derivatives has been observed to be sensitive to simple chemical substitutions on the aromatic rings, stemming presumably from alterations in lipophilicity and binding affinity to albumin, receptor proteins, and/or cytosolic proteins.[49] Substituents in the *para* positions seem to be most effective, perhaps owing to their penetration into hydrophobic binding sites.[50] Thus, in a recent study, we chose to compare Fe(EHPG)$^-$ with the 5-Me, 5-Cl, and 5-Br derivatives shown in Figure 6–12 to explore the structural basis for biodistribution and imaging characteristics.[51] These particular *para* substituents were selected to study the effect of gradually increasing the lipophilicity of the complexes in the order H < Me < Cl < Br, as predicted by additive π constants.[52] The three new derivatives exhibit higher degrees of lipophilicity (as measured by octanol-buffer partition coefficients) and human serum albumin (HSA) binding affinity, as well as varying degrees of improvement in liver-blood and bile-liver concentration ratios measured 30 minutes after injection. MR imaging of the injected animals over 3-hour periods revealed that the more lipophilic derivatives exhibit slower excretion from the liver.[51]

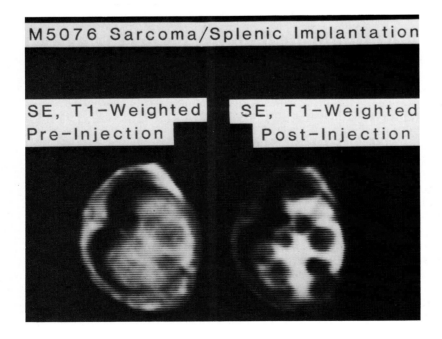

FIGURE 6–11. MR images (SE 200/15) of a mouse exhibiting multiple liver metastases. M5076 sarcoma cells were implanted in the spleen and allowed to metastasize to the liver. Figure shows enhancement of normal liver parenchyma with 0.1 mmol/kg iron-EHPG, facilitating the detection of the lesions (image at right was obtained 15 minutes after injection). (Courtesy of Drs. Faina Shtern and Thomas Brady, Massachusetts General Hospital, Boston, MA.)

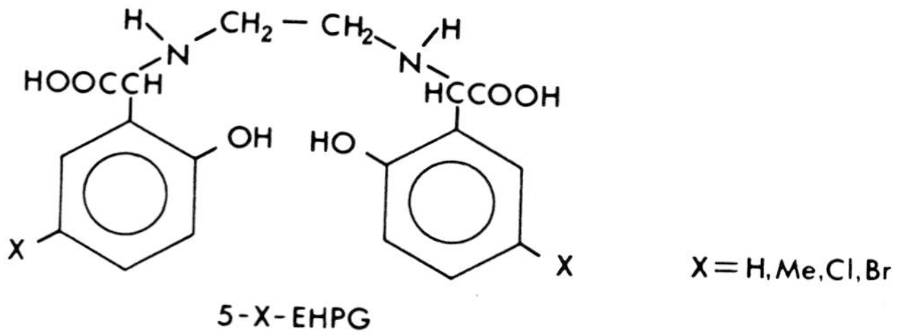

FIGURE 6–12. Structure of the ring-substituted EHPG derivatives.

The sensitivity of the biodistribution behavior to changes in ring substituents is related to alterations in lipophilicity and protein or receptor binding affinity. Our results reveal a correlation between lipophilicity and albumin binding,[51] and one might expect similar behavior with binding to hepatocyte membrane receptors or cytosolic proteins. From the point of view of hepatobiliary agent design, the importance of these multiple binding events is that their net effect determines the pharmacokinetic rate constants that control relative tissue ratios. For example, a high affinity for serum albumin will decrease the rate of liver uptake, whereas strong binding to hepatocyte cytosol proteins will decrease the excretion rate. In the Fe(5-X-EHPG)$^-$ series, liver-blood and intestine-liver ratios appeared optimal for the 5-Cl and 5-Me complexes, with intermediate lipophilicity. Apparently, although some degree of lipophilicity (or protein binding affinity) is necessary for liver uptake, complexes of higher lipophilicity exhibit slower kinetics, most likely because of greater protein binding affinity. This parabolic dependence of biologic behavior with increasing lipophilicity has been well documented for other homologous series of molecules.[53] Its importance here is that it may be possible to adjust the biodistribution properties of each new prototype hepatobiliary agent with appropriate substitutiions.

Intravascular Distribution

A paramagnetic agent that would be confined in the intravascular space by molecular size or by binding to plasma proteins may have potential for the enhancement of normal, perfused tissues in preference to tissue with decreased blood supply. In addition, these agents may be useful in enhancing smaller blood vessels using the novel MR angiography techniques recently developed.[54]

An intravascular agent could be composed of a paramagnetically labeled protein or polymer with a molecular weight greater than 60,000. Alternatively, a small molecular weight chelate could be designed to bind strongly to HSA. Both the noncovalent and covalent attachments would yield relaxivity enhancement.

HSA labeled heavily with multiple Gd-DTPA groups has been evaluated as an intravascular contrast agent.[55] The authors did not, however, address the possibility that Gd(III) may be released from such conjugates during proteolytic degradation.

Tumor-Localizing Agents

Two groups have described the use of synthetic paramagnetic metalloporphyrins to decrease the proton relaxation times of tumors.[56, 57] The properties of these complexes are somewhat different compared with those of the free porphyrin ligand mixture, known as hematoporphyrin derivative, which localizes in tumors and is used in phototherapy.[58] Nevertheless, some degree of retention of synthetic complexes, such as Mn(III) tetrakis(4-sulfonatophenyl) porphyrin, in tumors has been observed. The mechanism for this retention is not known, and this prevents a rational approach to the design of these agents. However, the stability and high relaxivity of these complexes, in addition to their unexplained tumor localization, do make them attractive prototype contrast agents.

An alternative approach to tumor imaging involves the use of labeled monoclonal antibodies specific to a particular tumor line. Though greeted initially with enthusiasm, this method is likely to be useful only in radioimaging, in which only minuscule concentrations of the label are needed. For MR imaging, the required concentration of paramagnetic species is roughly 10 to 100 μM, whereas the concentration of antigenic sites in tumors is 0.1 μM or less (e.g., see Reference 59). Even if these sites could be saturated with paramagnetically labeled antibody molecules, such conjugates would require 100 to 1000 chelates per molecule for significant relaxation time differences. Because of this factor, coupled with the obvious problems of the potential toxicity and lower antigenic affinity of these conjugates, this approach is not likely to be clinically feasible. Perhaps other diagnostically useful target sites of higher concentration exist for magnetoimmunoimaging.

T$_2$ AGENTS

T$_2$ agents are also referred to as *homogeneity spoilers.* An early example of this class of agents is ferromagnetic (or superparamagnetic) particles, such as ferrite (Fe$_3$O$_4$). When water molecules diffuse through the microscopic magnetic field gradients around such particles, the protons experience efficient spin dephasing and transverse relaxation, leading to *decreases in signal intensity.* Since particulates are efficiently scavenged by reticuloendothelial cells, various compositions incorporating such particles are being evaluated as "negative" contrast agents for the liver and spleen.[60, 61] The metabolism or retention of these intravenously injected agents, however, is an important concern in their clinical evaluation. The oral use of such agents for the elimination of bowel signal is more likely to achieve approval.

It has recently been shown that soluble metal chelates such as Gd-DTPA can also be used as T$_2$

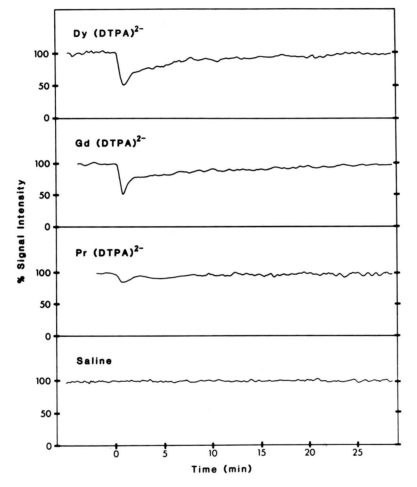

FIGURE 6–13. Effect of different lanthanide chelates on rat brain signal intensity using a one-dimensional rapid imaging technique designed to isolate the brain intensity with 8-second temporal resolution; (SE 1000/120). In each case, 1 mmol/kg of the agent was injected intravenously. The selected complexes exhibit varying magnetic moments: dysprosium (Dy) (III), 10.6 Bohr magnetons; gadolinium (Gd) (III), 8.0; and praseodymium (Pr) (III), 3.5. The percentage decrease in signal intensity was found to correlate with the magnetic moment of the ion. (From Villringer A, Rosen BR, Belliveau JW, et al: Dynamic imaging with lanthanide chelates in normal brain: Contrast due to magnetic susceptibility effects. Magn Reson Med 6:164–174, 1988; with permission.)

contrast agents. If present in sufficient concentration in the blood or extracellular space (such as immediately after injection), paramagnetic substances increase the bulk magnetic susceptibility of a given tissue compartment, leading (apparently) to field gradients at compartment interfaces and enhanced transverse relaxation. Early studies showed that injection of Dy-DTPA causes a very transient decrease in rat liver image intensity using conventional spin-echo pulse sequences (RB Lauffer, S Saini, and TJ Brady, unpublished results). Further work using different lanthanide DTPA chelates confirmed the effect on rat brain signal intensity and showed that the degree of signal loss correlated with the magnetic moment of the metal ion (Fig. 6–13).[62] It is thought that this type of contrast agent will be especially useful in examining cardiac and brain perfusion, particularly when combined with recently developed fast imaging techniques (echo planar or gradient echo).

REFERENCES

1. Lauffer RB: Paramagnetic metal complexes as water proton relaxation agents for NMR imaging: Theory and design. Chem Rev 87:901–927, 1987.
2. Bloch F, Hansen WW, Packard M: The nuclear induction experiment. Phys Rev 70:474, 1948.
3. Bloembergen N, Purcell EM, Pound RV: Relaxation effects in nuclear magnetic resonance absorption. Phys Rev 73:679, 1948.
4. Bloembergen N: Proton relaxation times in paramagnetic solutions. J Chem Phys 27:572, 1957.
5. Kubo R, Tomita K: Paramagnetic relaxation. J Phys Soc Jpn 9:888, 1954.
6. Solomon I: Relaxation processes in a system of two spins. Phys Rev 99:559, 1955.
7. Eisinger J, Shulman RG, Blumberg WE: Relaxation enhancement by paramagnetic iron binding in deoxyribonucleic acid solutions. Nature 192:963, 1961.
8. Dwek RA: Nuclear Magnetic Resonance in Biochemistry: Applications to Enzyme Systems. Oxford, Clarendon Press, 1973, Chapters 9–11.
9. Mildvan AS: Proton relaxation enhancement. Annu Rev Biochem 43:357, 1974.
10. Burton DR, Forsen S, Karlstrom G, Dwek RA: Proton relaxation enhancement (PRE) in biochemistry: A critical survey. Prog NMR Spectroscopy 13:1, 1979.
11. Lauterbur PC: Image formation by induced local interactions: Examples employing nuclear magnetic resonance. Nature 242:190, 1973.
12. Hinshaw WS, Bottomley PA, Holland GN: Radiographic thin-section image of the human wrist by nuclear magnetic resonance. Nature 270:722, 1977.
13. Andrew ER, Bottomley PA, Hinshaw WS, et al: NMR images by the multiple sensitive point method: Application to larger biological systems. Phys Med Biol 22:971, 1977.
14. Damadian R, Goldsmith M, Minkoff L: NMR in cancer. XVI. Fonar image of the live human body. Physiol Chem Phys 9:97, 1977.
15. Lauterbur PC, Mendonca-Dias MH, Rudin AM: Augmentation of tissue water proton spin-lattice relaxation rates by in vivo addition of paramagnetic ions. In Dutton PL, Leigh LS, Scarpaa A (eds): Frontier of Biological Energetics. New York, Academic Press, 1978, p 752.
16. Brady TJ, Goldman MR, Pykett IL, et al: Proton nuclear magnetic resonance imaging of regionally ischemic canine hearts: Effect of paramagnetic proton signal enhancement. Radiology 144:343, 1982.
17. Goldman MR, Brady TJ, Pykett IL, et al: Quantification of experimental myocardial infarction using nuclear magnetic resonance imaging and paramagnetic ion contrast enhancement in excised canine hearts. Circulation 66:1012, 1982.
18. Young IR, Clarke GJ, Gailes DR, et al: Enhancement of relaxation rate with paramagnetic contrast agents in NMR imaging. Comput Tomogr 5:534, 1981.
19. Carr DH, Brown J, Bydder GM, et al: Intravenous chelated gadolinium as a contrast agent in NMR imaging of cerebral tumors. Lancet 1:484, 1984.
20. Farrar TC, Becker ED: Pulse and Fourier Transform NMR. New York, Academic Press, 1971.
21. Lauffer RB, Brady TJ: Preparation and water relaxation properties of proteins labeled with paramagnetic metal chelates. Magn Reson Imaging 3:11, 1985.
22. Lauffer RB, Brady TJ, Brown RD, et al: 1/T1 NMRD profiles of solutions of Mn+2 and Gd+3 protein-chelate complexes. Magn Reson Med 3:541, 1986.
23. Tweedle MF, Brittain HG, Eckelman WC: Principles of contrast-enhanced MRI. In Partain CL, Price RR, Patton JA, et al (eds): Magnetic Resonance Imaging. 2nd ed. Philadelphia, WB Saunders Company, 1988.
24. Tweedle MF, Gaughan GT, Hagan J, et al: Considerations involving paramagnetic coordination compounds as useful NMR contrast agents. Nucl Med Biol 15:31, 1988.
25. Brading AF, Jones AW: Distribution and kinetics of CoEDTA in smooth muscle and its use as an extracellular marker. J Physiol 200:387, 1969.
26. Koenig SH, Spiller M, Brown RD III, Wolf GL: Relaxation of water protons in the intra- and extracellular regions of blood containing Gd(DTPA). Magn Reson Med 3:791, 1986.
27. Spiller M, Koenig SH, Wolf GL, Brown RD III: Presented at the 4th Annual Meeting of the Society of Magnetic Resonance in Medicine, London, 1985.
28. Kang YS, Gore JC: Studies of tissue NMR relaxation enhancement by manganese. Dose and time dependences. Invest Radiol 19:399, 1984.
29. Kang YS, Gore JC, Armitage IM: Studies of factors affecting the design of NMR contrast agents: Manganese in blood as a model system. Magn Reson Med 1:396, 1984.
30. Koenig SH, Brown RD III, Goldstein EJ, et al: Magnetic field dependence of tissue proton relaxation rates with added Mn2+: Rabbit liver and kidney. Magn Reson Med 2:159, 1985.
31. Weinmann H-J, Brasch RC, Press RC, Wesbey GE: Characteristics of gadolinium-DTPA complex: A potential NMR contrast agent. AJR 142:619, 1984.
32. Luckey TD, Venugopal B: Metal Toxicity in Mammals. Vol 1. New York, Plenum Press, 1977.
33. Venkatachalam MA, Rennke HG: The structural and molecular basis of glomerular filtration. Circ Res 43:337, 1978.
34. Klaassen CD, Watkins JB III: Mechanisms of bile formation, hepatic uptake, and biliary formation. Pharmacol Rev 36:1, 1984.
35. Heindel ND, Burns HD, Honda T, Brady LW: The Chemistry of Radiopharmaceuticals. New York, Masson, 1978.
36. Wolf GL, Fobben ES: The tissue proton T1 response to gadolinium DTPA injection in rabbits: A potential renal contrast agent for NMR imaging. Invest Radiol 19:324, 1984.
37. Brasch RC, Weinmann H-J, Wesbey GE: Contrast-enhanced NMR imaging: Animal studies using gadolinium-DTPA complex. AJR 142:625, 1984.
38. McNamara MT, Tscholakoff D, Revel D, et al: Use of gadolinium DTPA in assessing myocardial perfusion. Radiology 158:765, 1986.
39. Chervu LR, Nunn AD, Loberg MD: Radiopharmaceuticals for hepatobiliary imaging. Semin Nucl Med 12:5, 1984.
40. Koehler RE, Stanley RJ, Evans RG: Isofemate meglumine: An iodinated contrast agent for hepatic computed tomography scanning. Radiology 132:115, 1979.
41. Moss AA: Computed tomography of the hepatobiliary system. In Moss AA, Gamsu G, Genant HK (eds): Computed Tomog-

raphy of the Body. Philadelphia, WB Saunders Company, 1983, p 615.

42. Berk PD, Stremmel W: Hepatocellular uptake of organic anions. *In* Popper H, Schaffner F (eds): Progress in Liver Disease. Vol VIII. Orlando, FL, Grune & Stratton, 1985, pp 125–144.
43. Okuda H, Nunes R, Vallabhajosula S, et al: Studies of the hepatocellular uptake of the hepatobiliary scintiscanning agent Tc-DISIDA. J Hepatol 3:251, 1986.
44. Haddock EP, Zapolski EJ, Rubin M: Biliary excretion of chelated iron. Proc Soc Exp Biol Med 120:663, 1965.
45. Bailey NA, Cummins D, McKenzie ED, Worthington JM: The crystal and molecular structure of iron(III) compounds of the sexadentate ligand *N,N'*-ethylene-bis-(*o*-hydroxyphenylglycine). Inorg Chim Acta 50:111, 1981.
46. Lauffer RB, Greif WL, Stark DD, et al: Iron-EHPG as an hepatobiliary MR contrast agent: Initial imaging and biodistribution studies. J Comput Assist Tomogr 9:431, 1985.
47. Greif WL, Buxton RB, Lauffer RB, et al: Pulse sequence optimization for MR imaging using a paramagnetic hepatobiliary contrast agent. Radiology 157:461, 1985.
48. Shtern F, Garrido L, Compton C, et al: Comparison of Fe-EHPG, a new prototype hepatobiliary agent, with Gd-DTPA in MR imaging of blood-borne metastasis in mice. Presented at the 73rd Scientific Assembly of the Radiological Society of North America, Chicago, 1987.
49. Nunn AD, Loberg MD, Conley RA: A structure-distribution-relationship approach leading to the development of Tc-99m Mebrofenin: An improved cholescintigraphic agent. J Nucl Med 24:423, 1983.
50. Nunn AD: Preliminary structure distribution relationships of Tc-99m hepatobiliary agents. J Labeled Compnds Radiopharm 18:155, 1981.
51. Lauffer RB, Vincent AC, Padmanabhan S, et al: New hepatobiliary MR contrast agents: 5-Substituted iron-EHPG derivatives. Magn Reson Med 4:582–590, 1987.
52. Hansch C, Leo A: Substituent Constants for Correlation Analysis in Chemistry and Biology. New York, Wiley, 1979.
53. Kubinyi H: Lipophilicity and biological activity: Drug transport and drug distribution in model systems and in biological systems. Drug Res 29:1067, 1979.
54. Wedeen VJ, Meuli RA, Edelman RR, et al: Projective imaging of pulsatile flow with magnetic resonance. Science 230:946–948, 1985.
55. Schmeidl U, Ogan M, Paajanen H, et al: Albumin labeled with Gd-DTPA as an intravascular, blood-pool–enhancing agent for MR imaging: Biodistribution and imaging studies. Radiology 162:205, 1987.
56. Lyon RC, Faustino PJ, Cohen JS, et al: Tissue distribution and stability of metalloporphyrin MRI contrast agents. Magn Reson Med 4:24, 1987.
57. Fiel RJ, Button TM, Gilani S, et al: Proton relaxation enhancement by manganese(III)TPPS4 in a model tumor system. Magn Reson Imaging 5:149, 1987.
58. Doiron DR, Gomer CJ (eds): Porphyrin Localization and Treatment of Tumors. New York, Alan R Liss, 1984.
59. Unger EC, Totty WG, Neufeld DM, et al: Magnetic resonance imaging using gadolinium labeled monoclonal antibody. Invest Radiol 20:693, 1985.
60. Mendonca-Dias MH, Lauterbur LH: Ferromagnetic particles as contrast agents for magnetic resonance imaging of the liver and spleen. Magn Reson Med 3:328–330, 1986.
61. Saini S, Stark DD, Hahn PF, et al: Ferrite particles: A superparamagnetic MR contrast agent for enhanced detection of liver carcinoma. Radiology 162:217–222, 1987.
62. Villringer A, Rosen BR, Belliveau JW, et al: Dynamic imaging with lanthanide chelates in normal brain: Contrast due to magnetic susceptibility effects. Magn Reson Med 6:164–174, 1988.

7

CONTRAST AGENTS FOR MR IMAGING

SANJAY SAINI and BERND HAMM

MAGNETISM
    BASIC MAGNETIC PROPERTIES
    MAGNETIC STATES OF MATTER
        Diamagnetism
        Paramagnetism
        Ferromagnetism
        Antiferromagnetic and Ferrimagnetic
          Materials
        Superparamagnetism
RELAXOMETRY
EFFECT OF DOSE AND PULSE
SEQUENCES ON SIGNAL INTENSITY
GADOLINIUM-DTPA

DOSE AND RISKS
CLINICAL APPLICATIONS
Central Nervous System
Liver
Gastrointestinal Tract
Miscellaneous
NEW CONTRAST AGENTS
GADOLINIUM-DOTA
FERRITES
FERIOXAMINE METHANE SULFONATE
MISCELLANEOUS
CONCLUSION

The alteration of signal intensity in diseased tissue forms the basis for MR imaging in diagnostic radiology. Tissue signal intensity observed in MR images is the result of a complex interaction of numerous factors.[1, 2] These factors are classified into those that reflect intrinsic properties of biologic tissues (tissue relaxation times [T_1 and T_2] and proton density) and those that are instrument dependent (pulse sequences, timing parameters, and field strength). Soft tissue contrast in MR images is obtained by selecting instrument-dependent parameters so that signal intensities in various tissues will differ owing to differences in their intrinsic properties. Thus, in malignant tissue an increase in tissue water content is associated with a prolongation in T_1 and T_2 times, and at MR imaging, tumor masses, when compared with normal tissue, appear hypointense on T_1-weighted pulse sequences and hyperintense on T_2-weighted pulse sequences. However, MR imaging performed with routine screening pulse sequences has many inherent limitations. For example, because of wide biologic variation, relaxation times of normal and abnormal tissues overlap, and standard pulse sequences are unable to detect many pathologic processes. Histo-logic characterization of abnormal tissues that are detected (benign versus malignant) is even more difficult. Some of these shortcomings can be overcome by imaging with additional specialized pulse sequences. However, this solution is impractical, as it unpredictably increases examination times.

MR contrast agents provide an alternative solution to overcome some of the limitations of plain MR imaging. MR contrast agents alter tissue relaxation times and can therefore be used to manipulate their signal intensity. Owing to vast flexibility in their design, these magnetopharmaceuticals may be utilized to enhance soft tissue contrast (Fig. 7–1), characterize tissue noninvasively, portray physiologic processes in vivo, and reduce imaging times. Already, a large number of naturally occurring as well as synthetic materials have been investigated in animal studies, and newer formulations are continually being proposed for the diagnosis of a variety of clinical conditions. The eventual role for these materials will certainly broaden as the capabilities and limitations of MR imaging are recognized and as newer magnetopharmaceuticals are formulated.

This chapter summarizes the principles of phar-

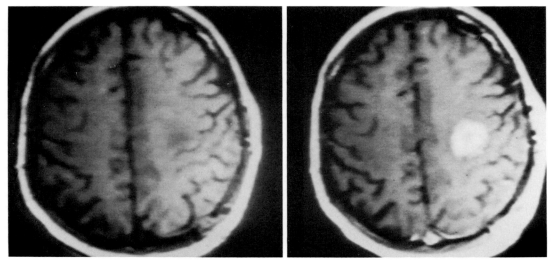

FIGURE 7–1. Enhancement of tumor brain contrast after administration of gadolinium-diethylenetriamine-pentaacetate (Gd-DTPA); 30 minutes after injection, 0.1 mM/kg; spin echo (SE) 500/32. *Left,* Before Gd-DTPA, the glioma appears as a faintly hypointense area. *Right,* After Gd-DTPA, there is marked enhancement of the tumor, producing striking increase in signal difference between the lesion and normal brain tissue. There is a hypointense rim around the tumor nodule representing perifocal edema that does not enhance with Gd-DTPA. Also note the enhancement of the superior sagittal sinus.

macologic manipulation of MR contrast and the current role of MR contrast agents that are available for clinical investigation.

MAGNETISM

BASIC MAGNETIC PROPERTIES

The chemical alteration of proton relaxation time was first described in 1946, when the T_1 time of water was shown to be reduced after the addition of ferric nitrate.[3] Because of their unique magnetic properties, certain chemical compounds, such as ferric iron (Fe^{3+}), enhance proton relaxation rates. These magnetic properties are based in atomic structure and arise from the motion of electrically charged particles (electrons, protons, and neutrons) that are basic to all materials.[4, 5]

Nuclear magnetism originates from the gyroscopic spin and orbital movement of protons and neutrons within atomic nuclei. The nuclear magnetic moment is the vector sum of the magnetic moments on each nuclear particle. When protons or neutrons exist in pairs, their magnetic moments will orient in opposite directions and cancel. Thus, atoms with an even number of protons and neutrons possess no net nuclear magnetic moment. However, nuclei with an odd number of protons, neutrons, or both have a nonzero net nuclear magnetic moment, which leads to the phenomenon of MR.

When placed in an external magnetic field, nuclear magnetic moments precess at the Larmor frequency. However, nuclei are surrounded by electrons, which also respond magnetically to the applied field (Fig. 7–2A). The magnetic dipole moments that arise owing to the gyroscopic spin and orbital movement of electrons are considerably larger than the nuclear magnetic moments. Thus, if atoms, ions, or molecules with large electronic magnetic dipole moments are placed adjacent to hydrogen nuclei (also referred to as protons), their magnetic dipole moments can interact to enhance relaxation of protons and alter tissue signal intensity. Therefore, compounds with large electronic magnetic dipole moments may be utilized as contrast agents in MR imaging (Table 7–1).

MAGNETIC STATES OF MATTER

Diamagnetism

There are several magnetic states in which chemical species can exist (Table 7–2). Most chemical species have a negligibly small electronic magnetic dipole moment. In these compounds, electrons in orbital shells are paired (the preferred low-energy state). The magnetic dipole moments in paired electrons align opposite to each other and cancel. In the presence of an external magnetic field, there is a very slight asymmetric alteration in the orbital motion of paired electrons, and a small net magnetic dipole moment can then be detected. This induced magnetization (i.e., a magnetic moment induced by the applied magnetic field) is extremely weak and points opposite to the direction of the external magnetic field (antiparallel) (Fig. 7–2B). This behavior is termed *diamagnetism* and is necessarily present in all materials. Diamagnetism is generally too weak to alter relaxation rates significantly and therefore is not a useful source for developing MR contrast agents. In

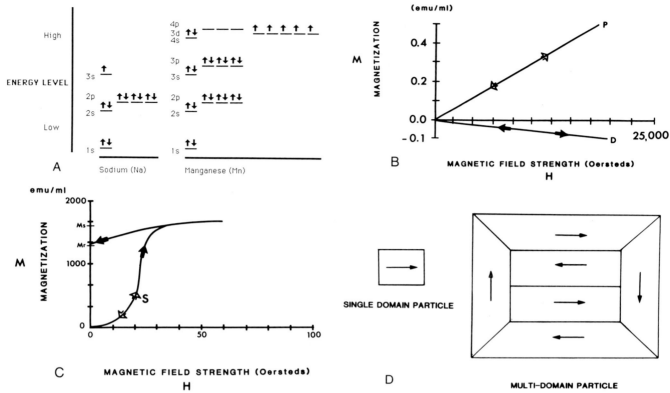

FIGURE 7–2. *A*, Electron distribution in energy levels. Each arrow denotes the magnetic dipole moment of a single electron. Electrons orbit in shells of prescribed energy level around atomic nuclei and preferentially occupy shells of lowest energy level. In each subshell, electrons pair with those having opposite magnetic dipole moment. Thus the total magnetic dipole moment in filled shells and subshells is zero. In unfilled shells, electrons remain unpaired until the shell is half full. Electron distribution around nuclei of sodium and manganese atoms is illustrated.

B and *C*, Magnetic behavior of matter. Induced magnetization (emu/ml) versus applied magnetic field (oersteds).[8] *B* shows that diamagnetic materials (D) have a small, negative (oriented opposite to the applied field) magnetic susceptibility. In comparison, the induced magnetization in paramagnetic materials (P) is much larger and positive. Net magnetization (**M**) in both materials is linear and directly proportional to the strength of the applied field. *C* Shows that superparamagnetic (S; *open arrow*) and ferromagnetic *(closed arrow)* materials have enormously large magnetic susceptibilities that are nonlinear and saturate even in the presence of relatively weak magnetic fields. Arrowheads indicate direction of magnetization as field strength is varied. Initially, ferromagnetic materials become magnetized, similar to superparamagnetic materials. Once magnetized, only ferromagnetic materials retain their magnetization even when the external field is removed. Note that a group of superparamagnetic, paramagnetic, and diamagnetic materials does not possess any magnetization in the absence of an external field.

D, In ferromagnetic particles *(right)*, multiple magnetic domains exist, whereas in superparamagnetic particles *(left)*, there is only a single magnetic domain.

(*A–C* from Saini S, Frankel RB, Stark DD, Ferrucci JT: Magnetism: A primer and review. AJR 150:735–743, 1988; © by American Roentgen Ray Society.)

many substances, however, diamagnetism is accompanied by more powerful paramagnetism, or superparamagnetism, or by ferromagnetism. These forms of magnetism are characterized by relatively larger magnetic dipole moments and are highly effective in manipulating tissue relaxation times and therefore MR signal intensity.

Paramagnetism

Paramagnetism arises in atoms that have unpaired electrons. Since the magnetic dipole moments of these electrons do not pair and cancel, individual paramagnetic atoms possess intrinsic magnetic dipole moments even in the absence of an external magnetic field. A collection of paramagnetic ions or atoms, however, will not show any *net* magnetization because of random orientation of the paramagnetic dipole moments on each atom or ion. However, when these paramagnetic ions or atoms are placed in an external magnetic field, a significant net magnetization can be observed because there is preferential orientation of the component paramagnetic dipole moments parallel to (in the same direction as) the applied magnetic field, and its magnitude is proportional to the magnitude of the external magnetic field (Fig. 7–2*B*).

The major chemical subgroups of paramagnetic species relevant to MR imaging include (1) metal ions of the lanthanide series and the first transition series, (2) nitroxide free radicals, and (3) molecular oxygen.

TABLE 7–1. EFFECTIVE ATOMIC MAGNETIC DIPOLE MOMENTS FOR 3d AND 4f TRANSITION METAL IONS

Ion	3d Electrons	4f Electrons	Unpaired Electrons	Effective Magnetic Dipole Moment/ Ion (Bohr Magnetons)
Cr^{2+}	4	0	4	4.90
Mn^{2+}, Fe^{3+}	5	0	5	5.92
Fe^{2+}	6	0	4	4.90
Co^{2+}	7	0	3	3.87
Cu^{2+}	9	0	1	1.73
Gd^{3+}	10 (full)	7	7	7.90
Dy^{3+}	10 (full)	9	5	10.50[a]

Note—3d and 4f are energy levels that electrons of higher energy occupy.

[a] Dy^{3+} has a larger magnetic moment than Gd^{3+} does, even though there are fewer unpaired electrons, because of a larger contribution by the orbital angular momentum.

From Saini S, Frankel RB, Stark DD, Ferrucci JT: Magnetism: A primer and review. AJR 150:735–743, 1988; © by American Roentgen Ray Society.

Molecular oxygen is paramagnetic, even though it has an even number of electrons, because for the two bonding electrons, the preferred low-energy state is one of parallel alignment.[6] The rare earth transition element of the lanthanide series, gadolinium (Gd), is one of the strongest paramagnetic substances because it has seven unpaired electrons in its outermost shell and possesses an effective magnetic dipole moment of 7.9 Bohr magnetons (the effective magnetic dipole moment of a single atom is expressed in units of Bohr magnetons). As gadolinium-diethylenetriaminepentaacetate (DTPA), chelated to reduce biologic toxicity, it is the only contrast agent widely available for clinical use. Other potential paramagnetic metal ions, such as manganese (II) (Mn^{2+}) and Fe^{3+}, both possessing five unpaired electrons, and chromium (III) (Cr^{3+}), with three unpaired electrons, have also been investigated, but only in animals.[7-10]

Ferromagnetism

Permanent magnets are made of *ferromagnetic* materials, such as iron, nickel, cobalt, ferrite (Fe_3O_4), and so on. Whereas diamagnetism and paramagnetism are properties of individual atoms, ions, or molecules, ferromagnetism is a property of a group of atoms or molecules in a solid crystal. When atoms with paramagnetic properties are packed closely, their magnetic dipole moments will spontaneously interact with those of their neighbors and will preferentially align parallel to each other. These materials are magnetically ordered and contain regions or domains that are always (spontaneously) magnetized. Unmagnetized ferromagnetic samples contain multiple domains whose magnetic dipole moments are oriented randomly to produce zero net magnetization. These samples can be easily magnetized when placed in an external magnetic field because the magnetic moments of individual domains will readily orient parallel to an applied magnetic field. Owing to cooperative interaction, these materials can be magnetized to saturation (maximal magnetization) even when exposed to relatively weak external magnetic fields (Fig. 7–2C). When the external magnetic field is removed, ferromagnets retain some of this magnetization (Fig. 7–2C). Permanent magnets are materials in which this remanent magnetization approaches the saturation magnetization.

Antiferromagnetic and Ferrimagnetic Materials

As noted earlier, ferromagnets belong to a class of materials that are magnetically ordered because their component paramagnetic dipole moments are oriented in an orderly parallel fashion. There are two other classes of magnetically ordered substances. In *antiferromagnetic* materials, neighboring paramagnetic dipole moments are ordered antiparallel to each other, so that no net spontaneous magnetization is present. These materials show complex temperature-dependent magnetization curves. *Ferrimagnetic* materials have both parallel and antiparallel ordering of their constituent paramagnetic dipole moments. Because there is an excess of parallel over antiparallel magnetic dipole moments or because the parallel magnetic dipole moments are larger than the antiparallel magnetic dipole moments, a net spontaneous magnetization can also be present in ferrimagnets. Materials with spinel and garnet crystal structures have ferrimagnetic ordering. Spinel crystals containing iron are known as ferrites, of which Fe_3O_4 is the most common in the earth's crust. Fe_3O_4 is also the

TABLE 7–2. PROPERTIES OF DIFFERENT FORMS OF MAGNETISM

Type of Magnetism	Net Alignment to the External Field	Relative Magnetic Susceptibility	Saturation Magnetization	Remanent Magnetization	Temperature Dependence	Cooperative Interaction	Structure
Diamagnetism	Antiparallel	−1	No	No	No	No	All materials
Paramagnetism	Parallel	+10	No	No	Yes	No	Ions, atoms, molecules
Superparamagnetism	Parallel	+5,000	Yes	No	Yes	Yes	Small crystal solids
Ferromagnetism	Parallel	+25,000	Yes	Yes	Yes	Yes	Large crystal solids

From Saini S, Frankel RB, Stark DD, Ferrucci JT: Magnetism: A primer and review. AJR 150:735–743, 1988; © by American Roentgen Ray Society.

only ferrimagnetic material known to occur in living cells.[11]

Superparamagnetism

When the size of multidomain ferromagnetic or ferrimagnetic particles is decreased (e.g., to 350 Å for Fe_3O_4), a particle consisting of a single magnetic domain is eventually formed (Fig. 7–2D). These single-domain particles have a unique magnetic property known as *superparamagnetism*.[12] When placed in an external magnetic field, a sample containing many of these particles will behave like ferromagnets and show saturation magnetization even in weak external magnetic fields (Fig. 7–2C). However, when the external field is removed, magnetic dipole moments of individual superparamagnetic particles become oriented randomly because of thermal agitation, and the sample will not retain any net magnetization. Thus, its magnetization curve will be like that of paramagnetic materials, but with a much stronger response, so that saturation magnetization is readily attained. Since the magnetic dipole moments of these compounds are greater than those of paramagnetic species, these materials are highly efficient in promoting proton relaxation. Superparamagnetic particles have been used as tissue-specific contrast agents by incorporation into vesicles that are < 1 μm in size (by way of comparison, erythrocytes are 5 μm in diameter). These small vesicles can readily traverse the body's capillary network and are cleared from the circulation by the phagocytic function of the reticuloendothelial system.[13, 14]

RELAXOMETRY

The relaxation of protons following excitation by a radiofrequency (RF) pulse is highly complex and is modulated by a number of factors.[15] Of these, the most important ones relate to the species promoting relaxation, including (1) the magnitude of its magnetic moment, (2) its concentration in tissue, and (3) its proximity to protons undergoing relaxation. The design of a clinically useful magnetopharmaceutical must not only consider the relaxation efficiency (relaxivity) of a paramagnetic compound but also pay attention to potential in vivo toxicity of the drug. For example, paramagnetic Gd^{3+} ions, while very efficient relaxation agents, are quite toxic.[16] Complexation of the ion with suitable organic ligands, such as DTPA, dramatically reduces toxicity but leads to diminished relaxivity, since the ligand prevents close interaction between the protons and the paramagnetic ion.[10, 17, 18] Such trade-offs are necessary in the development of clinically suitable contrast, and other, even more subtle, effects on relaxivity, such as that due to binding and immobilization of the paramagnetic species, can become important.[7, 19]

The T_1 relaxation time describes the return to equilibrium by the bulk magnetization vector that has been perturbed by an RF pulse. Proton T_1 relaxation is most efficient when there are neighboring magnetic dipole moments whose rotational frequency (a phenomenon arising from thermal agitation and molecular tumbling) matches the proton's nuclear Larmor frequency. For this situation to occur, species promoting T_1 relaxation must be small enough to be able to come close to the hydrogen nucleus and to be able to tumble rapidly in solution (approximately 10^8 to 10^{11} sec^{-1}). The resultant T_1 shortening increases tissue signal intensity on T_1-weighted images.

The T_2 relaxation time refers to the component of the bulk magnetization vector that is in the plane perpendicular (x-y plane) to the direction of the external magnetic field. Immediately after a 90-degree RF pulse, nuclear magnetic dipole moments of protons lie in the x-y plane and are oriented parallel to each other. However, because of local magnetic field inhomogeneities, individual nuclear magnetic dipole moments precess at slightly different frequencies. The T_2 relaxation time describes the time taken to produce dephasing in the x-y plane. At MR imaging, materials with large magnetic susceptibilities produce inhomogeneities in the local magnetic field, which accelerates proton dephasing and results in T_2 shortening of tissues in which these materials are located. This shortening results in signal loss on T_2-weighted images. This effect is modulated by the tissue concentration of these materials, the magnitude of the external field, and the ability of protons to approach closely the protons' nuclear magnetic dipole moments.[20, 21] This phenomenon is referred to as the *magnetic susceptibility effect*.

Paramagnetic ions are highly effective in promoting T_1 relaxation, principally because of their large magnetic moments, rapid molecular tumbling, and close interaction with protons. This effect forms the basis of Gd-DTPA–enhanced MR imaging. Diamagnetic susceptibility can also produce small changes in the T_1 relaxation rate and is given as the explanation for the high signal intensity sometimes seen in certain protein-rich body fluids (e.g., that of the gallbladder) on T_1-weighted images. This phenomenon is largely the result of molecular tumbling rates, and the magnitude of induced diamagnetic magnetization is of much lesser importance. Large molecules, such as ferrites, that do not tumble rapidly *do not produce T_1 shortening and are known to enhance primarily T_2 relaxation rates (i.e., $1/T_2$)*. The large magnetic dipole moments associated with superparamagnetic ferrite particles create inhomogeneities in the proton's local magnetic field. The diffusion of protons through these local field disturbances produces rapid proton dephasing, which results in the shortening of T_2. Since the dephasing effects of water diffusion through an inhomogeneous field are not constant over time, a refocusing 180-degree pulse cannot recover the signal loss. Thus, ferrites reduce signal intensity on both T_1- and T_2-weighted pulse sequences.[14]

EFFECT OF DOSE AND PULSE SEQUENCES ON SIGNAL INTENSITY

Because of the greater effect that superparamagnetic contrast agents have on T_2 times, MR imaging after the use of these agents is best done with pulse sequences having T_2-dependent contrast. Maximal effects are seen with gradient-echo (GRE) pulse sequences that are particularly sensitive to magnetic susceptibility effects. With T_1-weighted pulse sequences, the expected effect on signal intensity will be blunted. The dose-related effect on signal intensity with these materials is also simple. Larger doses make tissues progressively more hypointense until background noise levels are reached (Fig. 7–3). With exceptionally large doses, metallic-type artifacts can arise, a situation reported only in MR images of the gut.

The effect of drug concentration and pulse sequences on tissue signal intensity with paramagnetic contrast agents is much more complex. *Paramagnetic contrast agents have a relatively larger effect on T_1 relaxation times, and therefore imaging is best done with T_1-weighted pulse sequences.* However, their dose-related effect on signal intensity is *biphasic* (Fig. 7–3), and an increase in tissue signal intensity is observed only at low tissue concentrations of paramagnetic contrast agents. With increasing tissue concentrations shortening of the T_2 relaxation time becomes progressively more important. Eventually, it will obscure the effect of T_1 relaxation time shortening, and paramagnetic compounds will then decrease tissue signal intensity. This effect will be most apparent on T_2-weighted GRE pulse sequences and least apparent on spin-echo (SE) T_1-weighted pulse sequences. Large tissue

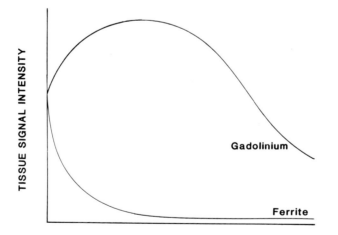

FIGURE 7–3. Dose-related effect of MR contrast agents on tissue signal intensity. Paramagnetic gadolinium affects both T_1 and T_2 times. At low doses of Gd-DTPA, there is an increase in signal intensity as effects of T_1 shortening predominate and T_2 shortening is minimal. With higher doses, T_2 effects also become important and tissue signal intensity begins to decrease. Superparamagnetic ferrite particles mainly affect T_2 times and thus reduce only tissue signal intensity.

TABLE 7–3. EFFECTS OF MRI CONTRAST AGENTS ON SIGNAL INTENSITY OF T_1-WEIGHTED IMAGES (T_1 SIGNAL) AND T_2-WEIGHTED IMAGES (T_2 SIGNAL)

Class of Contrast Agent	Example	T_1 Signal	T_2 Signal
1. T_1 active* (paramagnetic)	Gd-DTPA† Gd-DOTA Gd-albumin‡ Ferric ammonium citrate (Geritol)†	+ + +	+
2. T_2 active (superparamagnetic)	Magnetite microspheres§	−	−
3. Nonproton	PFHB† Fluosol Effervescent†	−	−
4. Fat containing	Mineral oil Milkshake†	+ +	±
5. Diamagnetic	Kaolin (Kaopectate)†	−	−

*High concentration of agent (e.g., in renal medulla) produces decreased signal.
†Applications include use as gut contrast agent.
‡Intravascular agent.
§Specific uptake by reticuloendothelial system (e.g., liver, spleen, bone marrow).
Gd-DTPA = gadolinium-diethylenetriaminepentaacetate; Gd-DOTA = gadolinium with 1,4,7,10-tetraazacyclododecane N,N',N'',N''' tetraacetate; PFHB = perfluorohexylbromide.

concentrations may result from inadvertently large dose administration or from compact bolus injection or may be due to physiologic hyperconcentration in tissues, as in the renal medulla.

Thus, in summary, to capture the tissue signal–enhancing effects of paramagnetic contrast agents, heavily T_1-weighted SE or inversion recovery (IR) pulse sequences must be employed. On the other hand, the signal-depleting effects of superparamagnetic and paramagnetic contrast agents will be best seen on T_2-weighted GRE pulse sequences. These effects are summarized in Table 7–3.

GADOLINIUM-DTPA

DOSE AND RISKS

Gadolinium-DTPA (Berlex Laboratories, Cedar Knolls, NJ, United States; and Schering AG, Federal Republic of Germany) is currently the only intravenous MR contrast agent approved for routine clinical use, albeit limited to imaging diseases of the central nervous system. Gd-DTPA has a biodistribution entirely analogous to that of the iodinated intravenous contrast media used in x-ray radiography.[17, 22] It has an extracellular distribution and undergoes rapid renal excretion by glomerular filtration. In humans, it has a plasma half-life of 90 minutes, and more than 90 per cent of it can be recovered in the urine within 3 hours following administration. It increases signal intensity on MR images at doses of 0.1 to 0.2 mM/kg and has an LD_{50} (dose at which 50 per cent of animals die) of approximately 10 mM/kg.[18] This feature produces a safety factor of approximately 50 to 100. In comparison, the safety factor of iodinated compounds is only 15. In more than 7000 clinical studies to date, no fatal reactions have been associated with Gd-DTPA.[23] Minor reactions requiring no treatment (headache, local burning, urticaria) occur in approximately 0.14 per cent of cases. Since the agent is hypertonic, rapid bolus injection can induce nausea on the basis of osmotic effects, similar to that induced by iodinated contrast agents used for CT and intravenous pyelography. In patients and volunteers, transient elevations in serum iron and bilirubin levels have been noted. However, these return to normal within 4 hours of drug administration. No electrocardiographic (ECG) or vital sign aberrations have been reported. In patients with brain tumors, there may be a small incidence of seizure activity. Current contraindications include hemolytic anemia and pregnancy.

The role of Gd-DTPA in imaging human disease is still evolving. In distinction to contrast media used in conventional radiography, considerations in proper application include not just the dose injected but also the pulse sequences utilized, as well as the time following injection at which imaging is performed. Since investigations have been done in a number of centers worldwide, the pulse sequences employed have been quite variable, and the degree of T_1 weighting and the time at which imaging is done following injection have not always been optimal. Although there is a general consensus on the clinical role of these contrast agents, particularly in imaging of central nervous system pathology, the literature contains many conflicting reports, which often arise because of limitations in operator-controlled variables.

In areas outside the central nervous system, the indicators for Gd-DTPA are even less well defined. Very few clinical studies have been completed, and most of these have been undertaken in a small number of patients. Thus, the findings reported are inconclusive, are often confusing, and need confirmation in larger series. As of this writing, in the United States, no contrast agent has been approved for routine evaluation of diseases outside the central nervous system.

CLINICAL APPLICATIONS

Central Nervous System

The effects of Gd-DTPA on MR images are similar to those of iodinated contrast media used in x-ray CT studies. Because of its extracellular distribution, it highlights the breakdown of the blood-brain barrier as well as enhances vascular tissues. Human studies to date have employed a dose of 0.1 mM/kg of body weight injected as a slow bolus (over about 1 minute).

In normal individuals, Gd-DTPA routinely enhances the structures that lack a blood-brain barrier, such as the pituitary stalk; the choroid plexus; the nasal mucosa; the cavernous sinus, including its walls; the area around the intracavernous portions of cra-

nial nerves III to VI; the gasserian ganglion; and the second and third divisions of cranial nerve V at the base of the skull.[24] Peak enhancement occurs shortly after injection and persists for up to 1 hour. The falx and tentorium, however, do not enhance consistently. Similarly, the enhancement of signal in vessels is most obvious when there is slow flow (e.g., veins). No enhancement is detectable in the cerebrospinal fluid, gray and white matter, cerebellar hemispheres, brain stem, structures of the inner ear, and the cisternal segments of the fifth, seventh, and eighth nerves. In the orbit, enhancement is evident in the retinal choroid but not in the optic nerve, the retroorbital fat, or the rectus muscles.

Pathologic conditions evaluated with Gd-DTPA include primary and secondary malignancies, infectious processes, and the white matter diseases. Owing to its ability to identify breakdown in the blood-brain barrier, Gd-DTPA has been useful in delineating intraaxial tumor masses from peritumoral edema (see Fig. 7–1). Thus, after Gd-DTPA infusion, rim enhancement of tumors is seen. Tissue enhancement occurs within 5 minutes of contrast infusion, peaks at approximately 30 minutes, and then decreases as the contrast agent is eliminated from the interstitial space. However, because of the large size of the Gd-DTPA molecule, leakage into regions of blood-brain barrier breakdown is inconsistent and, even if present, may not necessarily demarcate the tumor-edema boundary.[25] This is particularly true for low-grade gliomas. Gd-DTPA is also unable to discriminate necrosis in tumor from necrosis in abscesses. Gd-DTPA should be routinely used for detection of intracerebral metastases, due to the improvement in sensitivity compared with nonenhanced MRI.[25a]

Similarly, spinal lesions, particularly occult metastases, are better seen after Gd-DTPA (Fig. 7–4) and, because of tumor enhancement, may be distinguished more easily from adjoining edema. Gd-DTPA has also been helpful in differentiating intramedullary from extramedullary lesions.[25b]

Gd-DTPA is also useful in evaluating extraaxial mass lesions. Meningiomas, which often are isointense with surrounding brain on plain MR images, are better seen after Gd-DTPA. Owing to the high tumor vascularity, meningiomas become markedly hyperintense on T_1-weighted images.[26, 27] This enhancement pattern is entirely analogous to that of meningiomas on contrast-enhanced CT—namely, intense and prolonged increase in tumor signal intensity (Fig. 7–5). This phenomenon is also true for schwannomas, tumors arising from nerve cells; but unlike meningiomas, these lesions are also hyperintense on plain T_2-weighted images. Similarly, Gd-DTPA has proved to be of considerable value in detecting intracanalicular and recurrent acoustic neuromas.[28] These tumors may be otherwise missed because of volume averaging or postoperative scarring.

Lesions arising in the sella have unique enhancement patterns after Gd-DTPA infusion.[26] With large pituitary adenomas, enhancement characteristics

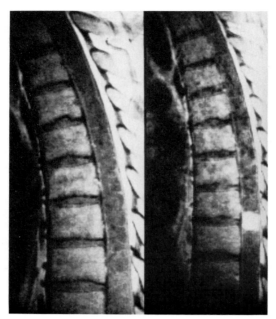

FIGURE 7–4. Improved visualization of a spinal cord metastasis after administration of Gd-DTPA, 0.1 mM/kg; SE 500/15. *Left*, Noncontrast. *Right*, After Gd-DTPA.

after Gd-DTPA are similar to those of other extraaxial masses described previously (intense and prolonged enhancement). Gd-DTPA, however, is most useful in enhancing soft tissue contrast for improved detection of pituitary microadenomas. Following contrast injection, normal pituitary enhances early (3 minutes), and microadenomas appear hypointense (Fig. 7–6). Later, tumor tissue enhances, which decreases tumor-pituitary signal differences. On delayed images, adenomas appear hyperintense because of slower wash-out of Gd-DTPA from the abnormal tissue.

Gd-DTPA may also be useful for imaging patients with white matter diseases, particularly multiple sclerosis. Although T_2-weighted MR images are highly sensitive in detecting lesions (especially when compared with CT), on plain MR both active and inactive multiple sclerosis plaques have an identical appearance. Gd-DTPA may be able to distinguish the two, as it will enhance only the active foci (Fig. 7–7). Furthermore, Gd-DTPA–enhanced MR imaging is more sensitive in showing lesion enhancement than even high-iodine CT. Most lesions enhance as early as 3 minutes, but a few may enhance as late as 55 minutes after injection.[29] At low field strengths (0.5 T), these effects may be less pronounced.[30]

Thus, in summary, Gd-DTPA may be useful in improving the ability of MR to detect and characterize lesions of the central nervous system. However, because of cost considerations, it is likely that noncontrast T_2-weighted MR imaging will remain the screening modality. Patients with normal screening T_2-weighted images may not need a T_1-weighted examination (enhanced with Gd-DTPA or unenhanced). However, in patients with equivocal examinations or abnormal findings, a Gd-DTPA–enhanced T_1-weighted study may be added to increase sensitivity or to characterize pathologic processes.

Liver

Imaging neoplastic disease of the liver with Gd-DTPA requires rapid scan times. Since this contrast agent lacks tissue specificity, differential enhancement between tumor and normal liver occurs only in the first 2 or 3 minutes after bolus injection of Gd-DTPA (Fig. 7–8).[31–33] This behavior is analogous to that of diatrizoates used in x-ray CT. On delayed images or on images acquired with long scan times, Gd-DTPA may actually obscure lesions.[34]

The current approach to imaging focal lesions

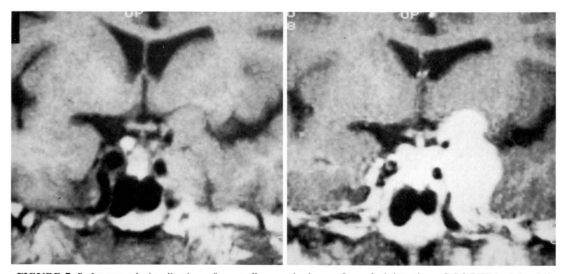

FIGURE 7–5. Improved visualization of parasellar meningioma after administration of Gd-DTPA, 0.1 mM/kg; SE 500/15. *Left*, Before contrast, the tumor is isointense to normal brain parenchyma. *Right*, After Gd-DTPA, there is intense enhancement of the meningioma.

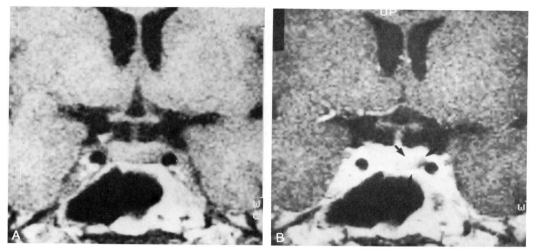

FIGURE 7–6. Effect of Gd-DTPA on pituitary microadenoma, 0.1 mM/kg; SE 500/15. *A,* Before Gd-DTPA. *B,* Two minutes after Gd-DTPA. Note the lesion remains hypointense *(arrows)* as the extraaxial pituitary gland enhances after Gd-DTPA administration. The confidence in the diagnosis of a microadenoma is increased, even though soft tissue contrast is not significantly increased after Gd-DTPA.

requires T_1-weighted SE (short repetition time [TR] and short echo time [TE] with one or two acquisitions) or GRE pulse sequences with short scan times (Fig. 7–9).[35] A dose of 0.2 mM/kg produces greater tissue enhancement than 0.1 mM/kg. Lesions that are slightly hypointense or isointense on noncontrast images appear markedly hypointense in the immediate postinfusion period, as Gd-DTPA enhances only normal liver tissue. Rim enhancement is also

routinely identified, allowing easier lesion detection and improved delineation of lesion boundaries (Fig. 7–9).[35] Later, as Gd-DTPA passively diffuses into cancer nodules, their signal intensity increases, rendering them isointense with normal liver. On even more delayed images, these nodules become hyperintense owing to the slow wash-out of Gd-DTPA from tumor tissue (Fig. 7–10). The tumor-liver signal difference on these delayed images, however, is less

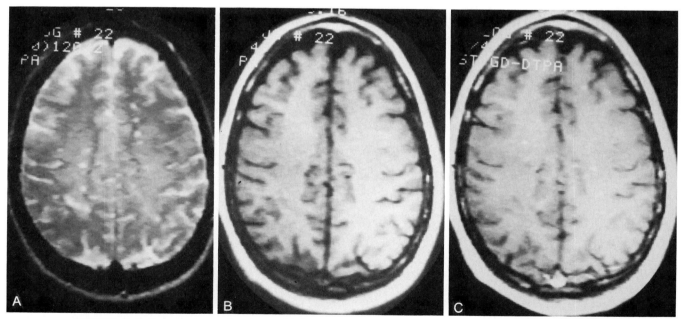

FIGURE 7–7. Enhancement of active multiple sclerosis plaques after administration of Gd-DTPA. *A,* SE 2000/120. Precontrast. *B,* SE 500/32. Precontrast. *C,* SE 500/32. Thirty minutes post contrast. On the T_2-weighted image, numerous periventricular foci of high signal intensity are seen. It is well known that T_2-weighted images are more sensitive in depicting these lesions, and therefore only a few of these plaques are seen on the accompanying T_1-weighted image. After Gd-DTPA, there is enhancement of two or three plaques, which presumably represent the active foci of multiple sclerosis.

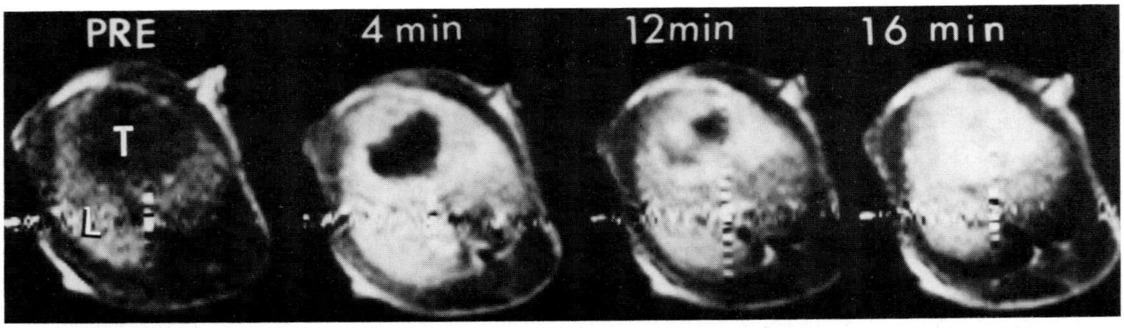

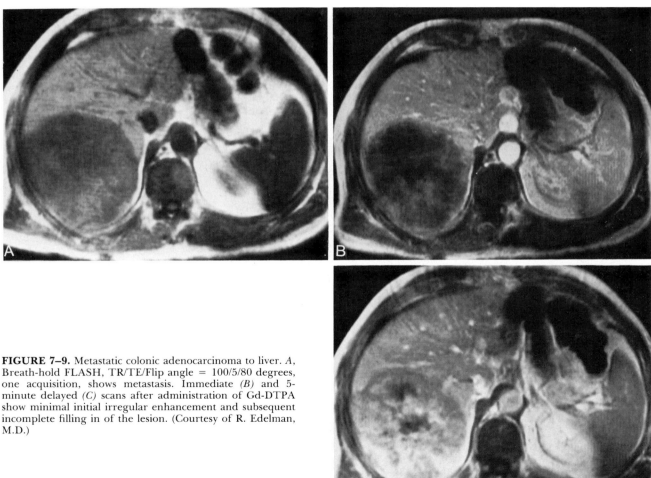

FIGURE 7–8. Effect of Gd-DTPA on liver cancer. SE 250/15/1 (36-second scan). Precontrast, the tumor nodule appears hypointense. In the immediate post-Gd-DTPA infusion period, there is preferential enhancement of liver tissue, resulting in increased tumor-liver signal differences. Later, as Gd-DTPA diffuses into tumor tissue, the tumor-liver signal differences decrease. Thus, maximal benefits of Gd-DTPA for tumor-liver contrast occur in the first 2 to 3 minutes after infusion. (From Saini S, Stark DD, Brady TJ, et al: Dynamic spin echo MRI of liver cancer using gadolinium-DTPA: Animal investigation. AJR 147:357–362, 1986; © by American Roentgen Ray Society.)

than that observed on noncontrast T_1-weighted images. Hypervascular lesions (e.g., carcinoid metastases) have not been extensively evaluated but will certainly have enhancement patterns distinct from those of the usual hypovascular metastases as well as cavernous hemangiomas. These lesions will manifest the effects of early perfusion and rapid wash-out. Thus, such lesions may appear hyperintense early

FIGURE 7–9. Metastatic colonic adenocarcinoma to liver. *A,* Breath-hold FLASH, TR/TE/Flip angle = 100/5/80 degrees, one acquisition, shows metastasis. Immediate *(B)* and 5-minute delayed *(C)* scans after administration of Gd-DTPA show minimal initial irregular enhancement and subsequent incomplete filling in of the lesion. (Courtesy of R. Edelman, M.D.)

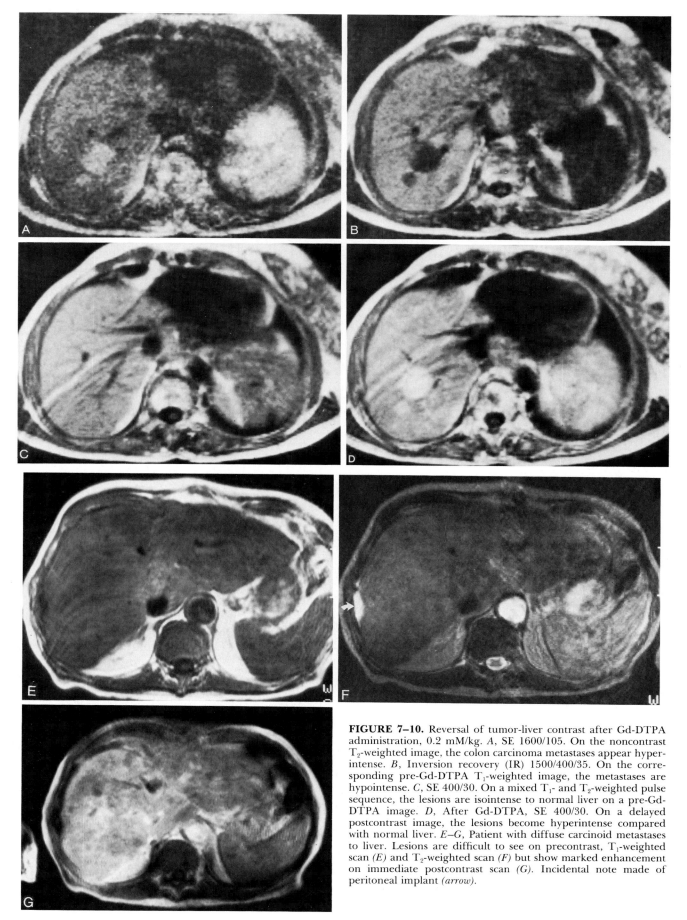

FIGURE 7–10. Reversal of tumor-liver contrast after Gd-DTPA administration, 0.2 mM/kg. *A*, SE 1600/105. On the noncontrast T_2-weighted image, the colon carcinoma metastases appear hyperintense. *B*, Inversion recovery (IR) 1500/400/35. On the corresponding pre-Gd-DTPA T_1-weighted image, the metastases are hypointense. *C*, SE 400/30. On a mixed T_1- and T_2-weighted pulse sequence, the lesions are isointense to normal liver on a pre-Gd-DTPA image. *D*, After Gd-DTPA, SE 400/30. On a delayed postcontrast image, the lesions become hyperintense compared with normal liver. *E–G*, Patient with diffuse carcinoid metastases to liver. Lesions are difficult to see on precontrast, T_1-weighted scan *(E)* and T_2-weighted scan *(F)* but show marked enhancement on immediate postcontrast scan *(G)*. Incidental note made of peritoneal implant *(arrow)*.

247

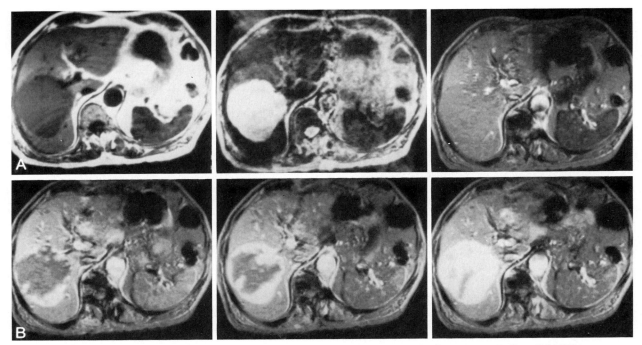

FIGURE 7–11. Dynamic imaging of hemangioma after administration of Gd-DTPA. *A,* Before Gd-DTPA. Compared with normal liver, the hemangioma appears hypointense on the T_1-weighted image (*left:* SE 500/15), hyperintense on the T_2-weighted image (*center:* SE 2000/80), and isointense on the T_1-weighted gradient-echo (GRE) image (*right,* GRE TR:40/TE:10/angle 30 degrees). *B,* Dynamic imaging after Gd-DTPA, with the T_1-weighted gradient echo pulse sequence showing intense rim enhancement at 2 minutes (*left*), progressive fill-in of the tumor from the periphery at 6 minutes (*center*), and nearly complete enhancement by 10 minutes (*right*). This pattern follows the contrast enhancement characteristics of hemangiomas on CT.

(within 1 minute of infusion) and hypointense later (>5 minutes after infusion) (Fig. 7–10*E–G*).

Differentiation between hemangiomas and liver metastases is also possible after Gd-DTPA administration. The contrast agent fills in hemangiomas from the periphery and produces intense lesion enhancement on delayed T_1-weighted images (Fig. 7–11). This enhancement is greater and more prolonged than that present in metastases and is useful in characterizing lesions that have an atypical appearance on noncontrast T_2-weighted MR images.

Faster imaging, improved tumor-liver signal differences, and increased tumor detection following Gd-DTPA have given considerable impetus to the routine MR imaging of liver. Such an examination may soon become a screening study for evaluating patients with suspected hepatic metastases.

Gastrointestinal Tract

As with x-ray CT, interpretation of abdominal MR images will be considerably easier once a suitable bowel contrast agent is available that will allow the loops of bowel to be distinguished from visceral organs, such as the pancreas, and from retroperitoneal lymph nodes. Without a bowel marker, the appearance of bowel loops can be quite variable and confusing. Areas containing air appear hypointense on both T_1- and T_2-weighted pulse sequences, while fluid-containing loops are hyperintense only on T_2-weighted images. Occasionally, ingested paramagnetic materials may cause bowel loops to appear hyperintense even on T_1-weighted images. Furthermore, because of peristalsis and long imaging times associated with currently available clinical pulse sequences, areas may contain air on one image and fluid on another.

Initial attempts at opacifying the bowel involved using commercially available paramagnetic ferric ammonium citrate (Geritol) or solutions containing fat (mineral oil).[36, 37] These compounds were helpful in opacifying the stomach and identifying the duodenum, but, perhaps because of dilution, delineation of the entire small bowel was not possible. Furthermore, acceptability by the patient was extremely poor, since these materials caused diarrhea resulting from bowel irritation. More recently, Gd-DTPA has been shown to be more promising in marking both the proximal and the distal small bowel (Figs. 7–12 and 7–13).[38] Clinical studies have reported routine opacification of the entire small bowel when a 0.1 mM/kg oral dose is administered with 15 gm of mannitol. The hypertonic effect of mannitol causes water to be retained within the bowel, thereby allowing the Gd-DTPA to make the bowel appear hyperintense on T_1-weighted images. No degradation in image quality has been noted when short TR and short TE T_1-weighted pulse sequences are utilized.

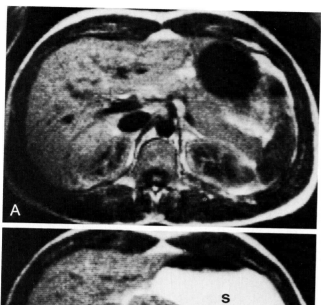

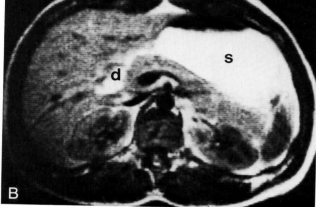

FIGURE 7–12. *A* and *B*, Enhancement of stomach (s) and duodenum (d) with Gd-DTPA, 0.1 mM/kg; SE 400/35. Oral Gd-DTPA makes fluid-filled bowel appear hyperintense. Note the improved delineation of the pancreas after Gd-DTPA.

Miscellaneous

HEART

Imaging myocardial infarct has been largely limited to animal models. In one clinical study (26 patients), investigators from Germany evaluated the enhancement pattern of infarcted myocardium (acute, subacute, and chronic) after administration of Gd-DTPA (0.1 mM/kg) and compared it with that of healthy myocardium.[39] The location of infarcts was confirmed on noncontrast T_2-weighted images, on which infarcts appeared as areas of high signal intensity. Results showed that normal tissue enhanced by approximately 20 per cent. Seven-day-old acute infarcts appeared "hot" and enhanced much more (70 per cent), while chronic infarcts (> 21 days) appeared "cold" and did not enhance. Subacute infarcts, however, enhanced like normal myocardium. A limitation of the study was that cardiac imaging requires gated studies. Thus, the TR values are dictated by the pulse rate. A T_1-weighted SE pulse sequence was not routinely possible, as the TR in these patients varied from 0.4 second to 1 second and the TE minimum utilized was 35 msec. Appro-

priate application will require more T_1-weighted pulse sequences, perhaps with images acquired in a few milliseconds, such as those with echo planar techniques.

LUNG CANCER

Bronchogenic carcinoma has also been evaluated (10 patients) after Gd-DTPA infusion (0.1 to 0.2 mM/kg).[40] Enhancement of tumor masses was noted to be heterogeneous, while collapsed lung (usually distal to the tumor) enhanced uniformly and had sharp margins. This finding suggests a potential for distinguishing tumor masses from normal lung. Furthermore, the peak enhancement of neoplastic tissue occurred at 5 minutes, while the peak enhancement of atelectatic lung was slightly later, between 5 and 10 minutes. It is interesting that malignant pleural effusion also enhanced after Gd-DTPA, and peak enhancement was noted 10 to 15 minutes after infusion. This study also showed that metastatic lymph nodes did not enhance, allowing distinction of these masses from adjacent enhancing structures.

BREAST CANCER

In patients with breast masses, Gd-DTPA (0.2 mM/kg) added diagnostic information in 12 of 35 cases examined.[41] In all patients, pathologic proof was available following biopsy. Benign fibroadenomas

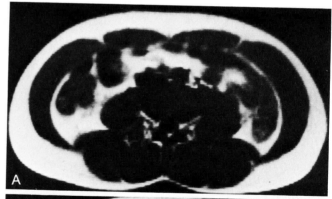

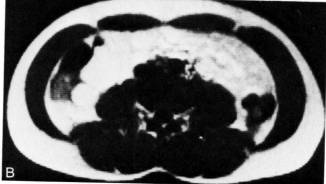

FIGURE 7–13. *A* and *B*, Enhancement of small bowel with Gd-DTPA, 0.1 mM/kg and 15 gm mannitol; SE 400/35. Oral Gd-DTPA makes fluid-filled bowel appear hyperintense. Note that the entire small bowel is demarcated and no increase in motion-related artifacts is present.

and cancer nodules enhanced considerably more than dysplastic breast tissue. However, scars and fatty lesions enhanced slightly or not at all. Peak enhancement was noted at 6 to 7 minutes for fibroadenomas and carcinomas and between 9 and 11 minutes for dysplastic tissue. The authors concluded that masses that enhance greater than 200 units on their system require biopsy, while those that enhance minimally may be left alone. The potential for evaluating patients with surgical scars was emphasized.

KIDNEY AND ADRENAL GLAND

Despite the fact that Gd-DTPA has tissue specificity for the kidney, Gd-enhanced renal MR imaging has not received much attention. This lack of attention is probably due to the high diagnostic standards set by x-ray CT and the less favorable early results of Gd-DTPA–enhanced renal imaging. In one study involving 34 patients, it was suggested that the delineation of tumor margins was better after 0.1 mM/kg of Gd-DTPA in only half the patients (see Fig. 7–15).[42] The enhancement of tumor masses was variable—some (hypervascular lesions) enhancing more than normal renal tissue, others (hypovascular masses) enhancing less, and others enhancing equally. The signal difference between normal tissue and renal tumors was not always improved after Gd-DTPA administration. With the advent of more rapid imaging techniques (subminute imaging times), the differential blood flow between tumor and kidneys may be better depicted and the results of contrast enhancement more useful.[43, 44] The renal pelvis was noted to have variable signal intensity, sometimes appearing hyperintense and sometimes appearing hypointense, a sequela of concentration of Gd-DTPA and associated T_2 shortening. This feature was thought to limit the interpretation of images.

Adrenal masses have also been evaluated and enhanced after Gd-DTPA and may be therefore distinguished from normal adrenal tissue. As a result, nodules less than 1 cm can be demonstrated.[44]

PELVIS

Twenty-two patients with pelvic tumors (11 cervical carcinomas, 8 uterine carcinomas, 3 ovarian carcinomas) were evaluated with Gd-DTPA (0.1 mM/kg) in the only clinical study to date.[45] Necrotic and cystic areas could be identified because of the absence of enhancement. Uterine leiomyomas enhanced identically with normal myometrium and could not be differentiated. However, leiomyomas and normal myometrium could be distinguished from tumor masses, since the latter enhanced less than normal tissue.

MUSCULOSKELETAL LESIONS

Use of Gd-DTPA to differentiate postsurgical fibrosis from recurrent disk herniation is considered in Chapter 24. Fibrosis usually shows generalized enhancement, whereas a herniated disk shows no enhancement or enhancement only along the disk margin.[45a] In the evaluation of 52 patients with inflammatory lesions of bones, joints, and soft tissues, the paraosseous extension of inflammation appeared as high signal intensity on unenhanced T_2-weighted images, and this signal intensity increased even more on T_2-weighted images after Gd-DTPA administration.[46] However, on Gd-DTPA (0.1 mM/kg)–enhanced T_1-weighted images, paraspinal subligamentous extension of infection was better delineated and could be differentiated from cerebrospinal fluid and intervertebral disks. Similarly, soft tissue abscesses had rim enhancement and could be distinguished from normal muscle.

In 29 patients with bone and soft tissue tumors, Gd-DTPA decreased contrast between abnormal and normal bone marrow on both T_1- and T_2-weighted images.[46] However, the extent of soft tissue tumor was better depicted after Gd-DTPA owing to tumor enhancement. This agent may potentially play an important role in distinguishing tumor from adjacent soft tissue edema, which has recently been documented on MR imaging of musculoskeletal lesions.[47, 47a]

NEW CONTRAST AGENTS

GADOLINIUM-DOTA

Recently, formulations other than Gd-DTPA have undergone clinical investigations. These include Gd-DOTA (1,4,7,10-tetraazacyclododecane N,N',N'',N'''' tetraacetate; Laboratorie Guerbet, France), ferrite (Advanced Magnetics, Cambridge, MA), and ferioxamine methane sulfonate (Salutar, Sunnyvale, CA).

The physiologic and MR image effect of Gd-DOTA is identical with that of Gd-DTPA.[18] Its major advantage is that it has a stronger ion-chelate bond and dissociation kinetics. Since no significant side effects have been reported from any of the clinical Gd-DTPA studies to date, the benefits of Gd-DOTA with current dose recommendations are hypothetical.

FERRITES

A more exciting formulation is ferrite. This contrast agent is targeted to the reticuloendothelial system (liver, spleen, and bone marrow).[14] It is a superparamagnetic particulate agent that dramatically decreases liver, spleen, and bone marrow signal intensity in 10 to 20 μmol/kg doses.[48, 49] This effect is seen on all pulse sequences but best on T_2-weighted GRE pulse sequences. The significant advantage with this formulation is that it alters signal intensity selectively in one of two tissues being compared (e.g., liver and cancer). Ferrites have a blood half-life of less

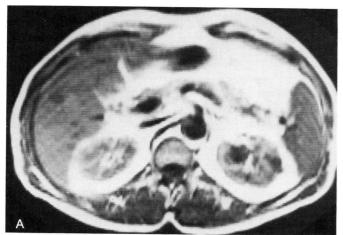

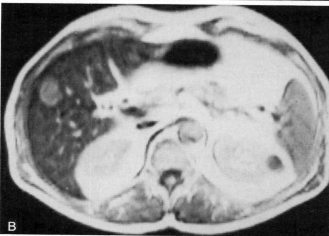

FIGURE 7–14. Ferrite-enhanced liver MR scan in patient with small hepatic metastasis. *A*, SE 300/14. Noncontrast scan. A small hypointense lesion is seen in the liver. *B*, SE 500/30. Postferrite (10 μmol/kg) scan. The normal liver becomes hypointense, and the tumor nodule is now better seen as a larger mass that is hyperintense relative to the liver. Note that persistent signal in or around blood vessels may mimic small lesions.

than 30 minutes and are cleared from the liver within 7 days.[50] After administration of ferrites, dynamic MR imaging reveals signal loss in liver, spleen, bone marrow, and all vascular structures. This feature has relevance for discriminating vessels from other structures and for characterizing hemangiomas. Postferrite MR images show marked increases in tumor-liver contrast (Figs. 7–14 and 7–15). When the liver is affected by diffuse diseases such as lymphoma, a smaller than expected decrease in signal intensity occurs, although the spared segments of liver will become markedly hypointense because the ferrite will be concentrated in a smaller volume of tissue. Evaluation of splenic metastases and lymphomatous infiltration is also dramatically improved after ferrite administration (Fig. 7–16).[51, 52] However, subtle degrees of lymphomatous involvement might still be difficult to detect. The principal disadvantage of ferrite is that fat adjoining vessels can simulate small metastases. Data on toxicity are limited. Animal studies have shown no acute or chronic liver injury.[53] In clinical studies, transient hypotension occurs if the dose is administered too rapidly. No clinical evaluation of bone marrow diseases has been reported to date. Because the agent is rapidly taken up by liver and spleen, bone marrow signal changes are small after ferrite administration. Better evaluation might be achieved after reticuloendothelial liver blockade, for example, using empty liposomes.[53a]

FERIOXAMINE METHANE SULFONATE

Ferioxamine methane sulfonate is a paramagnetic compound that utilizes iron as its paramagnetic moiety. Since iron is not as strong a paramagnetic substance as gadolinium and because the recommended doses of this drug are smaller (5 mg/kg), little enhancement in soft tissues is seen. Since the contrast agent is eliminated via the kidneys, urinary enhancement is routinely seen (Fig. 7–17). Thus,

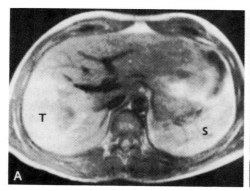

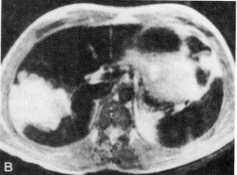

FIGURE 7–15. Patient with liver tumor and normal spleen, imaged before and after administration of ferrite (40 μmol/kg AMI-25). SE 1500/42. *A*, Precontrast scan. There is only modest tumor-liver contrast. The spleen appears hyperintense. *B*, Postcontrast scan. Note that the spleen and normal regions of the liver become dark owing to uptake of ferrite by phagocytic cells in the reticuloendothelial system. Since the liver tumor lacks these cells, its signal intensity is not markedly altered by the contrast agent. (From Weissleder R, Elizondo G, Stark DD, et al: The diagnosis of splenic lymphoma by MRI: Value of superparamagnetic iron oxide. AJR 152:175–180, 1989; © by American Roentgen Ray Society.)

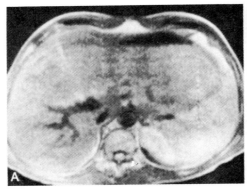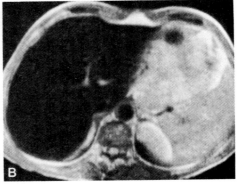

FIGURE 7–16. Patient with diffuse infiltration of spleen by Hodgkin's lymphoma, imaged before and after administration of ferrite (40 μmol/kg, AMI-25). *A*, Precontrast scan. Presence of lymphomatous infiltration in spleen is difficult to detect. *B*, Postcontrast scan. Although a normal spleen should appear black, there is only a modest decrease in splenic signal intensity, suggesting diffuse infiltration by tumor. Compare with Figure 7–15. (From Weissleder R, Elizondo G, Stark DD, et al: The diagnosis of splenic lymphoma by MRI: Value of superparamagnetic iron oxide. AJR 152:175–180, 1989; © by American Roentgen Ray Society.)

ferioxamine methane sulfonate has been shown to be useful in imaging tumors of the bladder (Fig. 7–18).

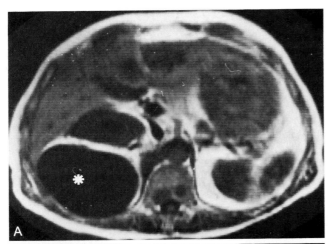

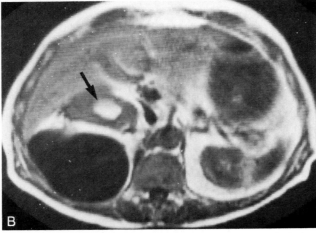

FIGURE 7–17. Enhancement of urine after paramagnetic ferioxamine methane sulfonate, 5 mg/kg. *A*, Precontrast scan; SE 300/14. A large urinoma *(asterisk)* is seen posterior to the right kidney. *B*, Postcontrast scan; there is enhancement of the renal pelvis *(arrow)*. The signal intensity of the urinoma remained unchanged, suggesting lack of communication with the urinary collecting system.

MISCELLANEOUS

Research into even newer drug formulations is under way. These formulations include hepatobiliary agents such as iron (III) ethylene-bis-(2-hydroxyphenylglycine) (Fe-EHPG), in which paramagnetic ferric iron is bound to an analog of hepatic iminodiacetic acid complexes used in cholescintigraphy and is partially excreted in bile.[10] Reticuloendothelial system–targeted liposomes containing gadolinium and manganese chelates have been formulated.[54] Gadolinium-DTPA bound to albumin macromolecules remains in the intravascular compartment and may be utilized for investigations on tissue vascularity.[19] At 2 T, it produces greater tumor-liver contrast than Gd-DTPA in one tenth of the dose.[55] Furthermore, the effect is longer, lasting for more than 15 minutes. Monoclonal antibodies and porphyrins tagged with potent magnetopharmaceuticals have also been investigated in animals, with an aim toward disease-specific localization.[56] However, limited sensitivity remains a significant problem with antibody studies.

For gastrointestinal tract imaging, effervescent agents and ferrites have been investigated in humans.[57, 58] These materials not only allow ready identification of bowel loops owing to signal elimination but also permit evaluation of the bowel wall. Further, in conjunction with glucagon, they also reduce motion artifacts; since these loops of bowel are devoid of signal (air contains few protons), peristaltic motion will not produce ghost artifacts even if long imaging times are utilized. A disadvantage, of course, is that accompanying signal void in blood vessels will be difficult to distinguish from bowel loops. Nonproton agents produce a signal void because they do not contain any hydrogen atoms. Initial clinical investigations with one such agent (perfluorohexylbromide [PFHB]) has shown acceptability by patients as well as clinical usefulness.[56]

Clay minerals, such as kaolin (used in Kaopectate) and bentonite, also reduce the signal intensity of gut. This effect has a relatively weak field strength de-

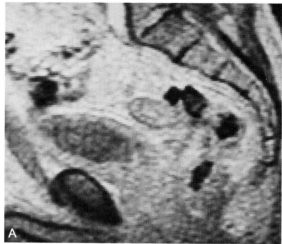
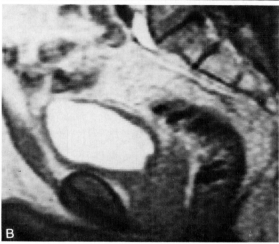

FIGURE 7–18. Enhancement of the urinary bladder after administration of ferioxamine methane sulfonate, 5 mg/kg. *A*, Precontrast scan; SE 300/14. *B*, Postcontrast scan; SE 300/14. A slight asymmetry is present in the bladder wall thickness that was radiation induced and not appreciated prior to bladder distention and opacification.

pendence. The proposed mechanism of action of these agents is that they strongly absorb water molecules, reducing their mobility and thereby shortening T_2 relaxation times.[59]

CONCLUSION

Contrast-enhanced MR is in its infancy. This chapter has summarized the current understanding of only one contrast agent, namely, Gd-DTPA. Even with this agent, our concepts are very rudimentary and stand to undergo considerable revision with greater experience and new imaging techniques. The availability of each new compound only adds to the complexity.

Early reports on MR emphasized the tremendous intrinsic soft tissue contrast between tissues and touted the lack of need for a contrast agent as an advantage of this imaging technique. Current think-

ing, however, has radically changed. Contrast agents are being developed not just to enhance soft tissue contrast but also to depict in vivo physiologic processes. Contrast media will therefore play an integral role in MR imaging of all parts of the body, just as it does today in cardiac and vascular studies.

REFERENCES

1. Gadian DG: Nuclear Magnetic Resonance and Its Application to Living Systems. New York, Oxford, 1982.
2. Wehrli FW, MacFall JR, Glover GH, Grigsby N: The dependence of nuclear magnetic resonance image contrast on intrinsic and pulse sequence timing parameters. Magn Reson Imaging 2:3–16, 1983.
3. Bloch F, Hansen WW, Packard P: The nuclear induction experiment. Phys Rev 70:474–485, 1946.
4. Cullity BD: Introduction to Magnetic Materials. Reading, MA., Addison-Wesley, 1972.
5. Saini S, Frankel RB, Stark DD, Ferrucci JT: Magnetism: A primer and review. AJR 150:735–743, 1988.
6. Koutcher JA, Tyler CT, Lauffer RB, Brady TJ: Contrast agents and spectroscopic probes in NMR. J Nucl Med 25:506–513, 1984.
7. Lauffer RB, Brady TJ: Preparation and water relaxation properties of proteins labelled with paramagnetic metal chelates. Magn Reson Imaging 3:11–16, 1985.
8. Kany YS, Gore JC: Studies of tissue NMR relaxation enhancement by manganese. Invest Radiol 19:399–407, 1984.
9. Chilton HM, Jackels SC, Hinson WH, Ekstrand KE: Use of paramagnetic substance, colloidal manganese sulfide, as an NMR contrast material in rats. J Nucl Med 25:604–607, 1984.
10. Lauffer RB, Greif WL, Stark DD, et al: Iron-EHPG as an hepatobiliary MR contrast agent: Initial imaging and biodistribution studies. J Comput Assist Tomogr 9:431–438, 1985.
11. Blakemore RP, Frankel RB: Magnetic navigation in bacteria. Sci Am 246:58–65, 1981.
12. Bean CP, Livingston JD: Superparamagnetism. J Appl Phys 30:120S–129S, 1959.
13. Renshaw PF, Owen CS, McLauglin AC, et al: Ferromagnetic contrast agents: A new approach. Magn Reson Med 3:217–225, 1986.
14. Saini S, Stark DD, Hahn PF, et al: Ferrite particles: A superparamagnetic MR contrast agent for the reticuloendothelial system. Radiology 162:211–216, 1987.
15. Burton DR, Forsen S, Karlstrom G: Proton relaxation enhancement (PRE) in biochemistry: A critical survey. Prog NMR Spectroscopy 13:1–45, 1979.
16. Wolf GL, Baum L: Cardiovascular toxicity and tissue proton response to manganese injection in the dog and rabbit. AJR 141:193–197, 1983.
17. Weinmann H-J, Brasch RC, Press W-R, Wesbey GE: Characteristics of gadolinium-DTPA complex: A potential NMR contrast agent. AJR 142:619–629, 1984.
18. Bousquet J-C, Saini S, Stark DD, et al: Gadolinium DOTA: Characterization of a new paramagnetic complex. Radiology 166:693–698, 1988.
19. Schmiedl U, Ogan M, Peajanen H, et al: Albumin labeled with Gd-DTPA as an intravascular, blood pool enhancing agent for MR imaging: Biodistribution and imaging studies. Radiology 162:205–210, 1987.
20. Koenig SH, Brown RD: Relaxometry of ferriting solutions and the influence of Fe^{3+} cores. Magn Reson Med 3:755–767, 1986.
21. Thulborn KR, Waterton JC, Matthews PM, Radda GK: Oxygenation dependence of the transverse relaxation time of water protons in whole blood at high field. Biochim Biophys Acta 714:265–270, 1982.
22. Wolf GL, Fobben S: Tissue proton T_1 and T_2 response to Gd-DTPA injection in rabbits: A potential renal contrast agent for NMR imaging. Invest Radiol 19:324–328, 1984.

23. Niendorf HP, Ezumi K: Magnevist (Gd-DTPA): Tolerance and safety after four years of clinical trials in more than 7000 patients. *In* Abstracts of the 2nd European Congress of NMR in Medicine and Biology. Berlin, 1988.

24. Kilgore DP, Breger RK, Daniels DL, et al: Cranial tissues: Normal MR appearance after intravenous injection of Gd-DTPA. Radiology 160:757–762, 1986.

25. Brant-Zawadski M, Berry I, Osaki L, et al: Gd-DTPA in clinical MR of the brain: 1. Intraaxial lesions. AJNR 7:781–188, 1986.

25a. Healy ME, Messelink JR, Press GA, Middleton MS: Increased detection of intracranial metastases with Gd-DTPA. Radiology 165:619–624, 1987.

25b. Parizel PM, Baleriaux D, Rodesch G, et al: Gd-DTPA–enhanced MR imaging of spinal tumors. AJNR 10:249–258, 1989.

26. Berry I, Brant-Zawadski M, Osaki L, et al: Gd-DTPA in clinical MR of the brain. 2. Extraaxial lesions and normal structures. AJNR 7:789–793, 1986.

27. Zimmerman RD, Fleming CA, Saint-Louis LA, et al: MR imaging of meningiomas. AJNR 6:149–157, 1985.

28. Curati WL, Graif M, Kingsley DPE, et al: Acoustic neuromas: Gd-DTPA enhancement in MR imaging. Radiology 158:447–451, 1986.

29. Grossman RI, Gonzalez-Scaranof, Atlas SW, et al: Multiple sclerosis: Gadolinium enhancement in MR imaging. Radiology 161:721–726, 1986.

30. Beyer HK, Uhlenbrock D: Use of Gd-DTPA enhanced magnetic resonance imaging in multiple sclerosis. *In* Runge VM, Claussen C, Felix R, James AE (eds): Contrast Agents in Magnetic Resonance Imaging. Princeton, NJ, Excerpta Medica, 1986, pp 141–146.

31. Stark DD, Wittenberg J, Edelman RR: Detection of hepatic metastases: Analysis of pulse sequence performance in MR imaging. Radiology 158:327–332, 1986.

32. Reinig JW, Dwyer AJ, Miller DL, et al: Liver metastases detection: Comparison studies of MR imaging and CT scanning. Radiology 162:43–48, 1987.

33. Saini S, Stark DD, Brady TJ, et al: Dynamic spin echo MRI of liver cancer using gadolinium-DTPA: Animal investigation. AJR 147:357–362, 1986.

34. Carr DH, Brown J, Bydder GM, et al: Gd-DTPA a contrast agent in MRI: Initial clinical experience in 20 patients. AJR 143:215–224, 1984.

35. Hamm B, Wolf K-J, Felix R: Conventional and rapid MR imaging of the liver with gadolinium-DTPA in clinical use. Radiology 164:313–319, 1987.

36. Wesby GE, Brasch RC, Engelstad BL, et al: NMR contrast enhancement study of the GI tract of rats and a human volunteer using nontoxic oral iron solutions. Radiology 149:175–180, 1983.

37. Mano I, Yoshida H, Nakabayashi K, et al: Fast spin echo imaging with suspended respiration: Gadolinium enhanced MR imaging of liver tumors. J Comput Assist Tomogr 11:73–80, 1987.

38. Kornmesser W, Laniado M, Hamm B, et al: First clinical use of Gd-DTPA for gastrointestinal contrast enhancement in man. Presented at the 87th Annual Meeting of the American Roentgen Ray Society, Miami, FL, April 28, 1987.

39. Eichstaedt H, Felix R: Use of Gd-DTPA enhanced magnetic resonance imaging for diagnosis of acute myocardial infarction. *In* Runge VM, Claussen C, Felix R, James AE (eds): Contrast Agents in Magnetic Resonance Imaging. Princeton, NJ, Excerpta Medica, 1986, pp 150–154.

40. Zeitler E, Kaiser W, Feyrer R, Holik B: Magnetic resonance imaging with and without Gd-DTPA of bronchial carcinoma. *In* Runge VM, Claussen C, Felix R, James AE (eds): Contrast Agents in Magnetic Resonance Imaging. Princeton, NJ, Excerpta Medica, 1986, pp 147–149.

41. Heywang SH, Fenzl G, Eirmann W, et al: Magnetic resonance imaging of the breast with Gd-DTPA: Development of diagnostic criteria. *In* Runge VM, Claussen C, Felix R, James AE (eds): Contrast Agents in Magnetic Resonance Imaging. Princeton, NJ, Excerpta Medica, 1986, pp 155–158.

42. Lanaido M, Kornmesser W, Nagel R, et al: Spin echo, inversion recovery, and fast imaging sequences with Gd-DTPA enhanced magnetic resonance imaging of renal tumors. *In* Runge VM, Claussen C, Felix R, James AE (eds): Contrast Agents in Magnetic Resonance Imaging. Princeton, NJ, Excerpta Medica, 1986, pp 162–166.

43. Pettigrew RI, Avrich L, Darrels W, et al: Fast-field-echo MR imaging with Gd-DTPA: Physiologic evaluation of the kidneys and liver. Radiology 160:561–563, 1986.

44. Bluemm RG, Doornbos J, Koops W, et al: Gd-DTPA in fast field echo MR imaging. *In* Runge VM, Claussen C, Felix R, James AE (eds): Contrast Agents in Magnetic Resonance Imaging. Princeton, NJ, Excerpta Medica, 1986, pp 177–182.

45. Roth G: Experience with Gd-DTPA enhanced magnetic resonance imaging of gynecologic tumors. *In* Runge VM, Claussen C, Felix R, James AE (eds): Contrast Agents in Magnetic Resonance Imaging. Princeton, NJ, Excerpta Medica, 1986, pp 167–169.

45a. Mueftle MG, Modic MT, Ross JS, et al: Lumbar spine: Post-operative MRI with Gd-DTPA. Radiology 167:817–824, 1988.

46. Reiser MF, Erhardt W, Bauer R, et al: Gd-DTPA enhanced magnetic resonance imaging of the diagnosis of inflammatory and neoplastic musculoskeletal lesions. *In* Runge VM, Claussen C, Felix R, James AE (eds): Contrast Agents in Magnetic Resonance Imaging. Princeton, NJ, Excerpta Medica, 1986, pp 170–176.

47. Beltran J, Simon DC, Katz W, Weis L: Increased MR signal intensity in skeletal muscle adjacent to malignant tumors. Radiology 162:251–255, 1987.

47a. Erlemann R, Reiser MF, Peters PE, et al: Musculoskeletal neoplasms: Static and dynamic Gd-DTPA–enhanced MR imaging. Radiology 171:767–773, 1989.

48. Saini S, Stark DD, Hahn PF, et al: Ferrite particles: A superparamagnetic MR contrast agent for enhanced detection of liver carcinoma. Radiology 162:217–222, 1987.

49. Stark DD, Weissleder R, Elizondo G, et al: Superparamagnetic iron oxide: Clinical application as a contrast agent for MR imaging of the liver. Radiology 168:297–302, 1988.

50. Weissleder R, Stark DD, Engelstad BL, et al: Superparamagnetic iron oxide: Pharmacokinetics and toxicity. AJR 152:167–173, 1989.

51. Weissleder R, Hahn PF, Stark DD, et al: MR imaging of splenic metastases: Ferrite enhanced detection in rats. AJR 149:723–726, 1987.

52. Weissleder R, Elizondo G, Stark DD, et al: The diagnosis of splenic lymphoma by MRI: Value of superparamagnetic iron oxide. AJR 152:175–180, 1989.

53. Bacon B, Stark DD, Park CH, Saini S, et al: Ferrite particles: A new MRI contrast agent: Lack of acute and chronic hepatotoxicity following intravenous administration. J Lab Clin Med 110:164–171, 1987.

53a. Federico M, Iannone A, Chan MC, Magin RL: Bone marrow uptake of liposome-entrapped spin label after liver blockade with empty liposomes. Mag Res Med 10:418–425, 1989.

54. Cardide VJ, Sostman HD, Winchell RJ, Gore JC: Relaxation enhancement using liposomes carrying paramagnetic species. Magn Reson Imaging 2:107–112, 1984.

55. Hamm B, Taupitz M, Wienmann H-J, Bauer H: Comparison of Gd-DTPA and Gd-DTPA–albumin in MRI of liver tumors. Presented at the 88th Annual Meeting of the American Roentgen Ray Society, San Francisco, CA, May 1988.

56. Renshaw PF, Owen CS, Evans AE, Leigh JS: Immunospecific NMR contrast agents. Magn Reson Imaging 4:351–357, 1986.

57. Mattrey RF, Hajek P, Baker L, et al: Perfluorohexylbromide (PFHB) as an MRI gastrointestinal contrast agent for proton imaging. SMRM Abstr 4:1516–1517, 1986.

58. Widder DJ, Grief WL, Widder KJ, et al: Magnetite albumin microspheres: A new MR contrast material. AJR 148:399–404, 1987.

59. Listinsky JJ, Bryant RG: Gastrointestinal contrast agents: A diamagnetic approach. Magn Reson Med 8:285–292, 1988.

8

BIOCHEMICAL BASIS OF THE MR APPEARANCE OF CEREBRAL HEMORRHAGE

KEITH R. THULBORN and THOMAS J. BRADY

BIOCHEMICAL EVOLUTION OF IRON IN CEREBRAL HEMATOMA

IRON METABOLISM IN HEMORRHAGE

Arterial Blood
Deoxygenation
Erythrocyte Lysis
Extracellular Iron-Binding Proteins
Intracellular Iron Processing

INTEGRITY OF THE BLOOD-BRAIN BARRIER

EDEMA

COAGULATION

RELAXATION MECHANISMS

SENSITIVITIES OF MR PULSE SEQUENCES

SPIN-ECHO PULSE SEQUENCE

ASYMMETRIC SPIN-ECHO PULSE SEQUENCE

GRADIENT-ECHO PULSE GRADIENT

FIELD STRENGTH DEPENDENCE

MR IMAGING OF HEMORRHAGE

THE ROLE OF IRON PRODUCTS

Oxyhemoglobin
Deoxygenated Hemoglobin
Erythrocyte Lysis
Extracellular Iron-Binding Proteins
Intracellular Iron Storage

IMAGES OF EVOLVING CEREBRAL HEMATOMA

CONCLUSION

APPENDIX

The highly variable appearance of MR images for resolving cerebral hemorrhage holds a wealth of information about the underlying biochemical processes. This information is often neglected in the MR evaluation of hemorrhagic pathology. A complete analysis utilizing the full information content of such images requires an understanding of the biochemical processes influencing the relaxation mechanisms controlling signal intensity.

Extrapolating from in vitro studies and clinical observations, hypotheses have been proposed to explain the evolution of the MR features of cerebral hematomas.[1-6] The explanations have emphasized the role of iron from hemoglobin in determining relaxation mechanisms of these variable patterns. This is based on the high concentration and changing magnetic properties of iron as the biochemical form, oxidation state, and spatial distribution change with time. Other pathophysiologic processes such as changes in integrity of the blood-brain barrier with alteration of the degree of edema and protein concentration have explained other features of these images. This chapter reviews the physiochemical principles of the magnetic properties of biologic systems, discusses the biochemical pathways of iron metabolism in resolving hematoma, and presents a nonmathematical scheme for relating these biochemical aspects to the relaxation phenomena which produce the variable signal contrast observed in MR images of hemorrhage. Clinical aspects involved in the MR imaging of hemorrhage will be considered separately in Chapter 16.

BIOCHEMICAL EVOLUTION OF IRON IN CEREBRAL HEMATOMA

Hemorrhage is a complex process, biochemically and pathologically, evolving over many months. The pattern of evolution of hemorrhage described for computed tomography is relatively simple, reflecting the protein content of the tissues at the site of the lesion,[7, 8] as compared with the richness of information content reflected in the variability reported for MR images of the same process.[3–6] The rate of the many biochemical changes[9] will depend on the location and size of the lesion and on the physiologic status of the patient. Better vascularized areas would be expected to show more rapid repair. The integrity of the blood-brain barrier will make intraparenchymal repair and clearance processes different from subarachnoid and subdural hemorrhages. Such variability in hematoma-induced repair response has been reported also from biochemical studies of hemorrhage at different sites outside the central nervous system.[10]

Iron Metabolism in Hemorrhage

Iron is a transition metal with an atomic number of 26 and an electronic configuration described as:

$$1s^2\ 2s^2\ 2p^6\ 3s^2\ 3p^6\ 3d^6\ 4s^2$$

The distribution of electrons in the outer 3d electronic orbital is dependent on the number of electrons. As the oxidation state increases, outer electrons are lost, leaving the ferrous ion (Fe^{2+}) with six 3d electrons and the ferric ion (Fe^{3+}) with five 3d electrons. Unpaired electrons within the outer 3d orbitals of iron are of critical importance in determining the magnetic properties of this atom.

As the most abundant transition metal in the human body, iron is vital for oxygen transport by hemoglobin in the erythrocyte of blood, oxygen storage by myoglobin in the tissues, and multiple catalytic functions in enzyme systems throughout the body. In contrast to its functional chelated form, free iron is toxic as is evident from toxic ingestions and iron overload states.[11–13] Toxicity is believed to be due to enhanced catalysis of free radical production by unchelated iron.[14] Hemorrhage can be thought of as a tightly controlled iron salvage pathway, in which iron from the extravasated erythrocytes is mobilized from hemoglobin, detoxified by chelation to short-term iron transport proteins for transfer back to the reticuloendothelial system, or converted to long-term storage proteins for local deposition.[12, 15, 16] The different forms of iron in this still incompletely understood pathway have different magnetic properties that can influence the magnetic relaxation properties of the proton spin system used to form the MR image.

The iron salvage pathway of arterial hemorrhage is now examined stepwise in terms of the magnetic properties of the iron (Fig. 8–1). No time scale is

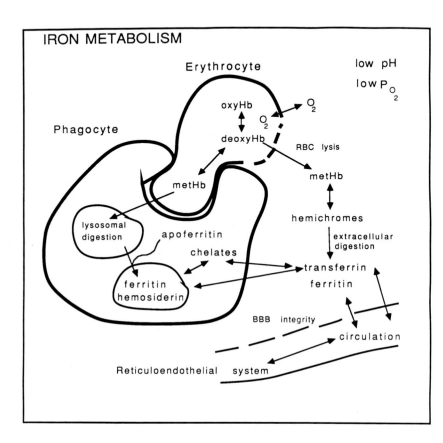

FIGURE 8–1. Schematic depiction of iron metabolism in a hematoma showing simplified iron salvage pathways in the erythrocyte, phagocyte, and extracellular space. *Abbreviations:* oxyHb = oxyhemoglobin; deoxyHb = deoxyhemoglobin; metHb = methemoglobin; BBB = blood-brain barrier; p_{O2} = partial pressure of oxygen.

given as this can only be misleading, given the multiple factors that determine rate of repair as described above.

Arterial Blood

In an arterial hemorrhage, the freshly extravasated erythrocytes contain fully oxygenated hemoglobin. Hemoglobin is a tetramer of polypeptide chains, with each polypeptide chain having considerable ordered secondary and tertiary structure.[11] Each chain has a prosthetic heme group bound within a hydrophobic cleft. The heme group is protoporphyrin IX with a centrally chelated ferrous ion. Initially, in arterial blood, iron is bound in octahedral geometry with six ligands. The tetrapyrole nitrogens of the protoporphyrin constitute four ligands in a plane around the iron. The imidazole group of a histidine from the polypeptide chain is the axial ligand below the protoporphyrin plane, while molecular oxygen is the sixth exchangeable ligand above the plane. The interaction of the six ligands with the metal center in oxyhemoglobin causes the six outer electrons of the ferrous ion to pair in the t_{2g} group of 3d orbitals of the lowest energy (Fig. 8–2). As all the electrons of the iron and other atoms that constitute hemoglobin are paired, oxygenated blood is diamagnetic ($\chi < 0$).

Deoxygenation

In tissues undergoing aerobic respiration, the partial pressure of dissolved oxygen is lower than that required to fully saturate the oxygen-binding sites of hemoglobin. The binding equilibrium is reversed, and molecular oxygen is delivered to the tissues. A cerebral hematoma has a mass effect compressing surrounding tissue, thereby reducing perfusion to these regions. A gradient in the partial pressure of oxygen from the hematoma to the compromised surrounding tissue results in hemoglobin desaturation. Additionally, there is reduced wash-out of by-products, such as CO_2 from remaining aerobic respiration and lactate from anaerobic glycolysis, which results in a decline in pH as the buffering capacity of the tissue is exceeded. This leads to further deoxygenation of the hemoglobin by displacement of the hemoglobin oxygen-binding equilibrium toward dissociation (Bohr effect). The removal of molecular oxygen changes the coordinate geometry of the heme ferrous ion to a five ligand system of deoxyhemoglobin, which decreases the energy separation between the e_g and t_{2g} groups of electronic orbitals. The six 3d electrons redistribute among the five 3d orbitals, leaving four unpaired electrons of parallel spin (Fig. 8–2). These unpaired electrons confer deoxyhemoglobin with its paramagnetic properties ($\chi > 0$). Because the paramagnetic ferrous ion is bound to the heme group in the hydrophobic cleft of the globin protein, water molecules are unable to approach the iron center. This restricts relaxivity effects (Fig. 8–3). *As the deoxyhemoglobin is packaged in erythrocytes, the magnetic susceptibility of the interior of the red blood cell is different from the suspending fluid, resulting in susceptibility variations within the hematoma* (Fig. 8–4). The importance of the integrity of the red blood cell membrane has been demonstrated in vitro[18, 19] but remains to be verified in vivo.

Erythrocyte Lysis

The tissue damage elicits an inflammatory repair response within the surrounding tissue, with phagocytes, such as macrophages, infiltrating the boundaries of the hematoma to clear extravasated materials and damaged tissues. Glial cells also show phagocytic activity. Red blood cells may be phagocytosed entirely, partially, or lysed by enzymes released into the region by the inflammatory cells.[8, 9] Loss of red blood cell membrane integrity releases hemoglobin. In the absence of the functional reductase enzyme systems of the red blood cell (NADH-cytochrome b_5 reductase, NADPH-flavin reductase),[17] hemoglobin is rapidly converted to methemoglobin in which the iron, still bound to the heme moiety within the globin protein, is oxidized to the ferric state with five 3d electrons. Once in the ferric oxidation state, the iron is paramagnetic ($\chi > 0$). The protein undergoes a number of changes, ultimately irreversible, in secondary, tertiary, and quaternary structure in which the ferric iron is no longer protected from the surrounding solvent.[20] The electronic configuration of the iron changes from initially five unpaired electrons, one in each of the five 3d suborbitals, to one unpaired electron as the weak sixth ligand of water

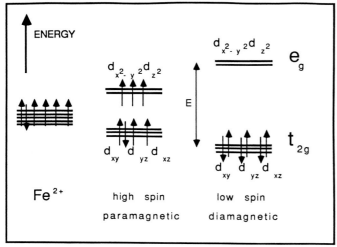

FIGURE 8–2. Energy diagram of the 3d electronic orbitals of the ferrous form of iron with different ligands. In the absence of ligands, all 3d orbitals have the same energy. In deoxyhemoglobin, the five ligands produce little energy separation between the e_g and t_{2g} groups of 3d orbitals, allowing the six electrons to distribute such that four electrons are unpaired (i.e., paramagnetic). In oxyhemoglobin, the six ligands produce marked energy difference E between the e_g and t_{2g} groups of 3d orbitals, causing electron pairing in the lowest energy state of the t_{2g} orbitals (i.e., diamagnetic).

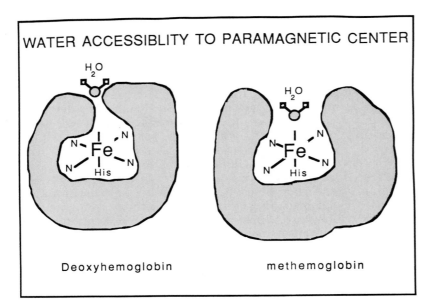

FIGURE 8–3. Schematic representation of the exclusion of water from the paramagnetic iron of deoxyhemoglobin by the surrounding globin protein until the protein undergoes conformational changes that lead to access of water to the heme cleft and oxidation of the ferrous iron to ferric iron in methemoglobin. Water access explains relaxivity effects of methemoglobin and the absence of such effects for deoxyhemoglobin, although both are paramagnetic.

is exchanged for a hydroxide and then another imidazole nitrogen of a histidyl residue of the protein. These changes define the hemichromes as described by electron paramagnetic resonance spectroscopy.[21] The time course of these processes in vivo are unknown, as yet.

Extracellular Iron-Binding Proteins

Extracellular protein is further degraded with release of the iron to localized extracellular binding proteins such as lactoferrin and transferrin. Some extracellular ferritin is also present. These binding proteins detoxify free iron for recycling to the reticuloendothelial system via the circulation and for local storage by glial cells and macrophages. The chelated iron remains paramagnetic.[22–24]

Intracellular Iron Processing

Erythrocytes and hemoglobin, phagocytosed by macrophages and glial elements of the central nervous system, are digested by the lysosomal system, with the iron being stored as ferric oxyhydroxide in the hydrophobic center of the major iron storage protein called *ferritin.*[15, 25] Ferritin is a water soluble protein of about 450,000 MW with 24 polypeptide subunits surrounding a core of as many as 4500 ferric ions. If the quantity of available iron exceeds the capacity of the cell to synthesize apoferritin,

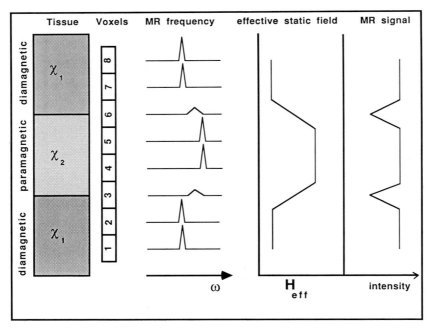

FIGURE 8–4. Schematic representation of the different effective magnetic fields H_{eff} produced by tissues of different magnetic susceptibilities $\chi_1 < 0$, and $\chi_2 < 0$ in an applied field H_0. The signal frequency ω and intensity of the magnetization in voxels across the tissues 1 to 8 are plotted to show frequency changes and signal loss at the boundaries of tissue of different susceptibility.

excess iron is stored as hemosiderin.[16] Hemosiderin is an insoluble larger aggregation of ferric oxyhydroxide with less protein than ferritin and, as yet, with a poorly characterized biochemical structure. These storage forms with large aggregates of iron behave antiferromagnetically and ferromagnetically, sometimes with superparamagnetic properties ($\chi > 0$).[26–28] *These aggregates of iron are inaccessible to surrounding water, thereby minimizing relaxivity effects. However, magnetic susceptibility variations can be expected in tissues containing such materials.* The iron storage processes occur throughout resolution of hemorrhage but become significant later, presumably reflecting concentration changes and the cessation of other relaxation processes. Much of the ferritin is intracellular within both macrophages and astrocytes, whereas the hemosiderin is in macrophages.[29] The process of redistribution of the storage forms has not been elucidated.

INTEGRITY OF THE BLOOD-BRAIN BARRIER

EDEMA

The loss of the blood-brain barrier around the site of hemorrhage causes vasogenic edema. The damage to the tissue in and around the site from mass effect, reduced perfusion, and inflammation worsen the edema. Although such changes do not affect the magnetic properties of the tissues which remain diamagnetic ($\chi < 0$), other magnetic relaxation phenomena occur to alter the MR image. These mechanisms are discussed below.

COAGULATION

The extravasated blood initiates the coagulation cascade leading to clot formation to limit further bleeding. The protein network of the clot with trapped red blood cells is expected to undergo a number of changes, including clot contraction with changes in the concentration and distribution of blood products, which can change magnetic properties of the tissue and thus the MR imaging characteristics. This has not been systematically studied in vivo.[30, 31]

RELAXATION MECHANISMS

For totally diamagnetic tissues, the most important relaxation mechanism for both longitudinal and transverse relaxation is attributed to dipole-dipole interactions.[32, 33] Other mechanisms of scalar-spin coupling, chemical shift anisotropy, and quadrupolar and spin-rotational effects are usually less important

in proton MR imaging and are described elsewhere.[32–37] Paramagnetic substances have several effects of much greater magnitude than diamagnetic substances, as discussed in Appendix 8–A and in Chapter 6. These effects include (1) relaxivity effects due to dipole-dipole interactions, which produce T_1 and T_2 relaxation, generally with T_1 effects dominating to produce increased signal intensity; and (2) susceptibility effects, which produce only T_2 relaxation and signal loss on MR images.

The dipole-dipole effects of paramagnetic substances are discussed in Appendix 8–A, but consideration must be given to other exchange processes not involving paramagnetic species.

Changes in the protein content within the hematoma also occur as clot formation, clot contraction, and necrosis occur. From in vitro studies,[37] increasing protein concentration would be expected to promote T_1 and T_2 relaxation rates, although rigorous in vivo studies have not been reported. It is possible that the exchange of water between bulk and protein bound phases may be a significant relaxation process in some situations. Increasing edema has been suggested to allow increased diffusion by removing diffusional barriers such as macromolecules and cell membranes, thereby promoting T_2 relaxation. In areas of necrosis, diffusional barriers may not be removed to the same degree as in vasogenic edema in intact, albeit damaged, tissue. The relative influences of diffusion and protein exchange on in vivo relaxation processes cannot be predicted as yet.

SENSITIVITIES OF MR PULSE SEQUENCES

The basic principles of imaging pulse sequences have been presented in numerous excellent texts,[38–42] and only features pertaining to hemorrhage will be elaborated upon here.

SPIN-ECHO PULSE SEQUENCE

The spin-echo (SE) sequence, shown in Figure 8–5, uses a 180-degree radiofrequency (RF) pulse centered between the initial 90-degree RF pulse and the center of the acquisition time period to refocus nuclear spins of variable Larmor frequencies into an echo, producing the MR signal. This minimizes the effect of static H_0 inhomogeneities on transverse relaxation which would otherwise reduce the signal intensity. By selecting appropriate timing parameters for the pulse sequence, the MR image can be made selectively sensitive to relaxivity and magnetic susceptibility effects. If significant diffusion through field inhomogeneities occurs during the echo time (TE), signal loss occurs as discussed in Appendix 8–A. As TE is made longer relative to the diffusional correlation time, the pulse sequence becomes more sensi-

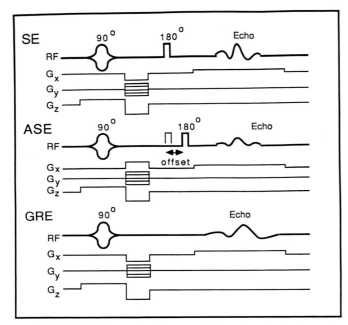

FIGURE 8–5. Schematic diagrams of the spin-echo (SE), asymmetric spin-echo (ASE), and gradient-echo (GRE) imaging pulse sequences showing slice selection and compensation using G_z, data acquisition with frequency encoding and compensation using G_x, and phase encoding using G_y. RF is the radiofrequency pulse train with shaped 90-degree and rectangular 180-degree pulses. Echoes are labeled.

ity heterogeneity, can be altered by varying the size of the offset. Comparison with ASE and SE images of the same TE allows calculation of T_2^* and has been suggested as a means of quantifying the iron content of tissue.[44]

GRADIENT-ECHO PULSE SEQUENCE

The GRE sequence does not use a 180-degree refocusing pulse and is thus sensitive to both static magnetic field inhomogeneities (magnet imperfections and tissue susceptibility heterogeneity) as well as the effects of diffusion.[43] Magnet imperfections over the volume of the imaging voxel have become less important with improved magnet technology, allowing detection of tissue susceptibility variations via the diffusional effects. Even without diffusion, signal cancellation occurs due to the range of Larmor frequencies caused by susceptibility variations within a voxel, as is also the case for the ASE sequence. This makes the GRE sequence useful for enhancing detection of susceptibility effects that may be less clearly identified on SE images. The artifacts from unwanted susceptibility effects, such as from the paranasal sinuses on intracranial lesions close to the base of the skull,[45] make the GRE sequence less useful for initial clinical screening examinations.

tive to these inhomogeneities. *As susceptibility differences are a source of field nonuniformity, increasing TE increases sensitivity of SE images* to processes such as hemorrhage which generate such susceptibility variation. The effect is readily recognized as *signal loss on T_2-weighted images* which is not present on T_1-weighted images.

Two other imaging sequences can be used to enhance detection of the susceptibility effects on T_2 relaxation. These are the gradient or field echo (GRE) and the asymmetric spin-echo (ASE) sequences that have been described in detail elsewhere[43, 44] (Fig. 8–5).

ASYMMETRIC SPIN-ECHO PULSE SEQUENCE

The ASE sequence offsets the 180-degree refocusing pulse by a time interval that can be varied to alter the amount of signal refocusing. This sequence is sensitive not only to the effects of diffusion through magnetic field gradients as used by the SE sequence, but also to variations of Larmor frequencies within a single voxel due to nonuniform magnetic susceptibility (Fig. 8–6). This results in rapid loss of phase coherence among the nuclear spins within the voxel and hence rapid signal loss. The amount of signal loss, and thus the sensitivity to intravoxel susceptibil-

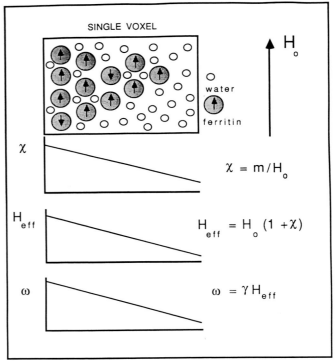

FIGURE 8–6. Schematic representation of the effects of nondiamagnetic substances on the intravoxel distribution of susceptibility χ, H_{eff}, and resonance frequency ω. Variation of resonance frequencies within the voxel produces signal loss.

FIELD STRENGTH DEPENDENCE

The variation of $1/T_1$ and $1/T_2$ with magnetic field strength is termed nuclear magnetic relaxation dispersion (NMRD). As the mathematical treatment of NMRD is beyond the scope of this chapter, the interested reader is referred to a recent article for a more formal introduction.[26] Only the observations relevant to hemorrhage are discussed here. At the limit of zero field, $1/T_1 = 1/T_2$. As field strength changes, the efficiency of relaxation is dependent on matching correlation times of local fluctuating magnetic fields generated by diffusional processes to the Larmor frequency. This occurs over a wide range (10^{-10} to 10^{-11} seconds) corresponding to low imaging field strengths, and the effects on T_1 and T_2 relaxation rates are comparable. In contrast, at higher fields, $1/T_1$ tends toward zero and $1/T_2$ tends to a nonzero value termed the "secular" contribution to T_2 relaxation. Therefore higher magnetic field strengths emphasize susceptibility effects. In vitro studies of deoxygenated erythrocytes indicate *a quadratic dependence of $1/T_2$ on magnetic field strength over a range of 2 to 5 tesla.*[18] Although the theoretical treatment is incomplete for susceptibility effects induced by ferritin and hemosiderin (speculated to be due to antiferromagnetic and ferromagnetic properties of these iron aggregates), it is clear that *higher imaging magnetic field strengths increase sensitivity of MR images to susceptibility-induced relaxation mechanisms, irrespective of the source of the susceptibility variation.*[26, 27]

MR IMAGING OF HEMORRHAGE

THE ROLE OF IRON PRODUCTS

The magnetic properties of the iron products of resolving hematoma have been discussed earlier. Although deoxygenated hemoglobin and all the products containing iron in the ferric oxidation state are paramagnetic (methemoglobin, hemichromes, transferrin, lactoferrin, low molecular weight iron chelates) or ferromagnetic (ferritin, hemosiderin), the production of relaxivity effects is dependent on close approach of water protons to the iron, and the production of the susceptibility effects is dependent on the distribution of the iron. The relaxation properties and the imaging characteristics are discussed and summarized in Table 8–1.

Oxyhemoglobin

The MR image of the center of an acute hematoma is essentially a collection of protein-rich diamagnetic fluid. Relaxivity and susceptibility effects are not observed for the diamagnetic iron of oxygenated hemoglobin. Image intensity is determined by other dipole-dipole mechanisms as operating in normal surrounding tissue. This means a variably long T_1 (isointense to dark on T_1-weighted images) and relatively long T_2 (bright on T_2-weighted images). The change in water content and distribution is clearly evident as areas of long T_1 (dark on T_1-weighted SE images) and long T_2 (bright on T_2-weighted SE images) in the areas bordering the hematoma.[46] Changes in the protein content within the hematoma also occur as clot formation, clot contraction, and necrosis occur. From in vitro studies,[47] increasing protein concentration would be expected to promote T_1 and T_2 relaxation rates, although rigorous in vivo studies have not been reported. Exchange of water between bulk phase and protein bound phases may provide an explanation for small modulations in image intensity.

Deoxygenated Hemoglobin

The paramagnetic iron of deoxygenated hemoglobin is held within a hydrophobic cleft. The exclusion of water from close approach to the paramagnetic center prevents relaxivity effects. T_1 relaxation is not affected so that the hematoma remains dark on T_1-weighted images. The packaging of the paramagnetic centers within the erythrocytes produces susceptibility variations that produce transverse relaxation. This explains the loss of signal on T_2-weighted SE and GRE images (dark on T_2-weighted images).

TABLE 8–1. THE INFLUENCE OF IRON METABOLISM ON THE MR APPEARANCE OF HEMORRHAGE

Stage	Biochemical Form	Location	Magnetic Property	Relaxation Mechanism		MR Intensity	
				R	χ	T_1w	T_2w
Oxyhemoglobin	Fe(II) oxyHb	RBC	Diamag	–	–	Dark	Bright
Deoxygenation	Fe(II) dexoyHb	RBC	Paramag	–	+	Dark	Dark
RBC lysis	Fe(III) metHb, hemichromes	Extracellular	Paramag	+	–	Bright	Bright
Extracellular Fe processing	Fe(III) transferrin, lactoferrin	Extracellular	Paramag	+	–	Bright	Bright
Intracellular Fe storage	Fe(III) ferritin, hemosiderin	Phagocytes	Superpar	–	+	Iso	Dark

MR signal intensities are estimated relative to cerebral cortex.
Abbreviations: paramag = paramagnetic; diamag = diamagnetic; superpar = superparamagnetic; oxyHb = oxyhemoglobin; deoxyHb = deoxyhemoglobin; RBC = red blood cell; R = relaxivity; χ = susceptibility; T_1w = T_1 weighted; T_2w = T_2 weighted; iso = isointense.

Erythrocyte Lysis

Loss of integrity of the red blood cells homogenizes the distribution of paramagnetic iron to minimize the susceptibility variations and reduces transverse relaxation. As the enzyme systems employed within the erythrocyte to maintain the ferrous oxidation state of the iron become nonfunctional, methemoglobin and other hemichromes are formed. These proteins allow water access to the paramagnetic iron to induce the relaxivity effects that shorten T_1 and to a lesser degree T_2. Thus, a hematoma at this stage shows increasing brightness on T_1-weighted SE images. Although the concomitant shortening of T_2 from relaxivity effects may suggest further loss of brightness on T_2-weighted SE and GRE images, the loss of red blood cell integrity removes the paramagnetic aggregation responsible for susceptibility-induced relaxation effects. As this is the dominant T_2 relaxation process, loss of this mechanism means that

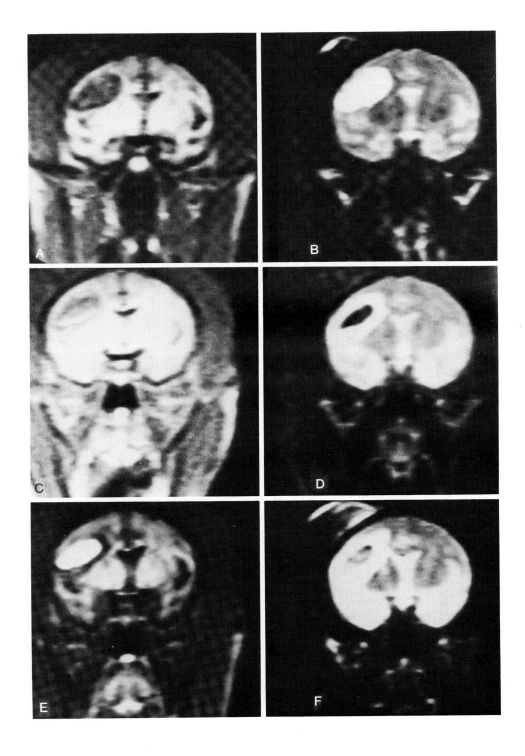

FIGURE 8–7. Longitudinal study, using inversion recovery (T_1-weighted) SE (A,C,E,I) and T_2-weighted SE coronal images B,D,F,J, of a monkey following injection of 3 ml venous blood injected into the right cerebral hemisphere. Images were selected at 2 hours (A,B), 2 days (C,D), 6 days (E,F), 10 days (G,H), and 2 months (I,J) from a more complete study published by Di Chiro G, Brooks RA, Girton ME, et al: Sequential MR studies of intracerebral hematomas in monkeys. AJNR 7:193–199, © by American Society of Neuroradiology 1986.

the effective T_2 is still longer than with intact red blood cells. Hence T_2-weighted SE and GRE images appear brighter after erythrocyte lysis has occurred.

Extracellular Iron-Binding Proteins

The specific relaxivity and susceptibility effects of ferric ions chelated to these proteins described in vitro[22-24] remain unknown for resolving in vivo hemorrhage. The concentration of these substances may be too low to have a significant role in determining signal intensity within an MR image.

Intracellular Iron Storage

The structure of iron storage proteins such as ferritin excludes water from close approach to the paramagnetic ferric ion eliminating relaxivity effects. The ferromagnetic properties of these crystalline aggregates of ferric oxyhydroxide induce susceptibility variations from surrounding tissue. The implications for imaging of old resolving hematomas are that T_1-weighted MR images are isointense with surrounding tissue due to the absence of relaxivity effects and that T_2-weighted and GRE images show

signal loss due to susceptibility effects. If the T_2 is significantly shortened below the TE used for T_1-weighted images, then the susceptibility effect will be observed on these images. This is not a relaxivity effect. Rather, the term "T_1 weighted" is inappropriate under these conditions.

IMAGES OF EVOLVING CEREBRAL HEMATOMA

The best controlled longitudinal study of resolving intraparenchymal hematoma was reported for an experimental model of hemorrhage in the monkey[46] in which venous blood was injected into the right cerebral hemisphere and followed by MR imaging over several months. Selected images from this study are reproduced with permission for discussion.

At 2 hours after injection of blood (Fig. 8–7A and B), the acute hematoma has low signal intensity on the T_1-weighted and high signal intensity on the T_2-weighted images relative to normal cortex. This is consistent with the absence of significant relaxivity and susceptibility relaxation mechanisms in the acute setting. Although the injection used venous blood, marked susceptibility effects are not observed, sug-

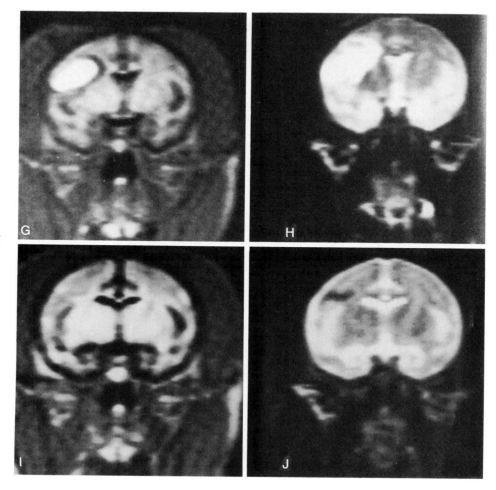

FIGURE 8–7 *Continued*

gesting that greater deoxygenation is required. The T_1-weighted image shows greater signal loss in the periphery consistent with edema in surrounding tissue having slightly different relaxation phenomena from the center of the hematoma. Over the next 2 days (Fig. 8–7C and D), the signal intensity of the center of the hematoma on the T_1-weighted image increases, presumably from the relaxivity mechanism of methemoglobin, hemichromes, and other paramagnetic centers allowing close approach of water protons. The signal intensity from the surrounding edematous zone shows little change. In contrast, the same area of hematoma on the T_2-weighted image displays decreased signal intensity, presumably from susceptibility-induced relaxation mechanisms as the intact erythrocytes become increasingly deoxygenated and from any intracellular methemoglobin that may form as the energy status of the cells declines. It is not clear if the methemoglobin and hemichromes form intracellularly or that the hematoma is a mixture of intact deoxygenated cells suspended within a solution of hemoglobin degradation products. Over 6 to 10 days (Fig. 8–7E–H), the T_1-weighted images show increasing signal intensity due to relaxivity effects from increasing concentrations of hemoglobin degradation products. The T_2-weighted images show increasing signal intensity when susceptibility effects diminish as red blood cell integrity is lost within the hematoma. The edematous periphery of the lesion shows minimal changes over this time interval. After 2 months (Fig. 8–7I and J), the T_1-weighted image shows little evidence of the lesion, whereas an area of decreased signal remains on the T_2-weighted image. This can be attributed to the susceptibility-induced relaxation mechanism of the iron storage products.

CONCLUSION

The basis of the highly variable MR appearance of resolving intraparenchymal cerebral hematoma reported clinically can be rationalized largely in terms of a model encompassing current concepts of iron metabolism and integrity of the blood-brain barrier. The time scale is dependent on the size of the lesion, its location with respect to both vascular supply and white and gray matter, and the physiologic status of the patient. The model should be regarded as a working hypothesis. The delineation of the in vivo biochemistry of iron metabolism and water balance remains to be performed. It is unlikely that descriptive analysis of the MR appearance of cerebral hemorrhage can be verified with biochemical studies in patients, making animal models a necessary vehicle for further detailed studies.

Appendix 8–A

MAGNETIC PROPERTIES OF BIOLOGIC TISSUES

ORIGIN OF MAGNETIC PROPERTIES

A magnetic field is generated by a moving electric charge, that is, an electric charge with momentum.[48] The strength of the magnetic field is determined by the magnitude of both the charge and momentum. Such a charge with a magnetic field is termed a *magnetic dipole*. Electrons and protons moving in an orbital about a nucleus represent moving charges with both orbital angular momentum and spin angular momentum and generate a magnetic field. However, as the magnetic moment of the charged particle is inversely proportional to its mass, and the mass of the nucleus is three orders of magnitude greater than that of the electron, the contribution of the nucleus to the magnetic properties of the atom is much less than that of the electrons. Hence, although nuclear magnetic interactions occur and nuclear magnetization is the source of the signal in the MR image, the magnetic properties of tissue are predominantly determined by the electronic configuration of the atoms and molecules. The dominant effects encountered on MR images are discussed below.

DIAMAGNETISM

Most biologic materials consist of low atomic weight elements such as carbon and hydrogen in which the electrons are paired in atomic and molecular suborbitals. When the electrons are paired, the spin angular momentum is cancelled and no magnetic dipole is observed. However, the paired electrons still have orbital angular momentum which produces a magnetic field (termed a Lenz field) opposing the applied magnetic field. The resultant field within such a material is less than that of the original applied magnetic field. Such materials are termed *diamagnetic*.

PARAMAGNETISM

Some biologic substances have atomic or molecular structures in which some of the electrons are unpaired. Transition metal ions, such as iron with the ferrous and ferric oxidation states, are important examples in which the number of unpaired electrons varies with the biochemical state of the metal ion. An unpaired electron has a spin angular momentum and therefore a magnetic moment that is not canceled as in the paired state. At physiologic temperatures, more electrons align parallel to the applied field, resulting in an enhancement of that applied field.

Materials that have no magnetic field in the absence of an applied magnetic field but that respond to enhance an applied magnetic field are termed *paramagnetic*. Examples of paramagnetic substances include gadolinium, used as an MR contrast agent, and ferrous and ferric iron. On T_1-weighted images, uniform distributions of such species produce increased signal intensity. However, nonuniform distributions of such species alter the MR image by producing a range of effective magnetic fields within the sample and therefore a range of resonance frequencies of the MR signal. Depending on the type of imaging pulse sequence used, the frequency dispersion can be manipulated to decrease signal in the area of the paramagnetic species (see "Sensitivities of MR Pulse Sequences").

OTHER FORMS OF MAGNETISM

There are other biologically important closely packed ensembles of atoms, such as crystalline structures, in which unpaired electrons of neighboring atoms interact to minimize the magnetic forces outside the material in the absence of an applied magnetic field. The magnetic forces producing preferred patterns of spin alignments to reach magnetic equilibrium are termed *exchange forces*.

Antiferromagnetism (Individual Opposition)

If unpaired electrons of neighboring atoms interact to align with opposing spins, the magnetic forces are minimized. In an applied magnetic field, spin pairing must be disrupted for realignment. Thus, the response to the applied field is less than that of a paramagnetic substance, but the effective field is still enhanced. Such materials are termed *antiferromagnetic*. The alignment pattern can be disrupted if the thermal energy is increased, and initially the response to an applied field is enhanced as the temperature is increased. Above a critical temperature, known as the Neel temperature, adjacent spin pairing is disrupted and the substance becomes paramagnetic. The effects of antiferromagnetic substances on MR images are similar to those of paramagnetic substances although reduced in magnitude and with a different temperature dependence.

Ferromagnetism (Group Opposition)

If the unpaired electrons of a group of atoms can align in domains, each domain has a net magnetic field. Adjacent domains can then interact via these magnetic fields to minimize, although not completely cancel, the field outside the material. If that material is immersed in a high magnetic field, domains respond to both the applied field and neighboring domain fields to markedly enhance the field. Such materials show a magnetic field in the absence of an applied magnetic field and are termed *ferromagnetic*. The effect of such substances on the MR image is of greater magnitude than for paramagnetic substances.

If a ferromagnetic crystal is reduced in size to that of a single domain, this single-domain particle has a net magnetic dipole equivalent to that of a domain. If a collection of such particles is free to rotate in an applied magnetic field on a time scale that is shorter than the observation time, the magnetic dipoles behave as expected for paramagnetism discussed above. However, the larger magnetic moments of the particles produce a greater enhancement of the applied magnetic field. Such particles are termed *superparamagnetic*.[49, 50]

If the size of the particles, usually containing many domains, is reduced *below* the size of a single domain, the aligning exchange forces and disaligning thermal forces become comparable. If the time scale of the observation is longer than the switching rate of the equilibrium between the aligned and disordered states, then the magnetic properties of the particles are dependent on the temperature-volume relationships that determine the switching frequency. An aggregate of such particles behaves paramagnetically but with a greater magnetic dipole than if no domain formed at all and thus is termed *supermagnetic*.[48] Thus, the effects of superparamagnetic and supermagnetic substances on the MR image are similar to paramagnetic substances but of a magnitude between that of paramagnetic and ferromagnetic species.

MAGNETIC SUSCEPTIBILITY

As all biologic materials have at least one of the above magnetic properties, they interact with a static magnetic field, H_0, to produce a magnetization, m, that reduces (diamagnetism) or enhances (paramagnetism, antiferromagnetism, ferromagnetism) the effective magnetic field, H_{eff}, established within the material. Note that m in this sense is usually referring to the effects of electronic configurations, not nuclear magnetization M. This effect can be expressed in terms of the magnetic susceptibility χ of the material in which

$$H_{eff} = H_0 + m = H_0(1 + \chi) \qquad (1)$$
$$\text{where } \chi = m/H_0$$

Thus $\chi < 0$ for diamagnetic materials, $\chi > 0$ for paramagnetic materials, and $\chi = 0$ for a vacuum.

When placed in a static magnetic field of the imaging magnet, tissues of different magnetic susceptibility establish different effective magnetic fields

experienced by the nucleus under observation. Thus, the response of the nuclear magnetization generated in the MR study is altered with resultant changes in the MR image. Susceptibility-induced field variations within a voxel broaden the Larmor frequency range (see Fig. 8–6). SE imaging minimizes this effect by using a 180-degree RF pulse to refocus the dispersion that occurs in the transverse magnetization M_{xy}, during the pulse sequence. If significant molecular diffusion occurs during TE (time from initial 90-degree RF pulse to formation of the echo) through regions of variable H_{eff}, due to either magnet imperfections or susceptibility variations in the tissue, incomplete refocusing results in loss of transverse magnetization and thus signal loss in the MR image. The effect becomes more apparent as the TE exceeds the diffusional correlation time (time taken for a proton to move from one position to the next position). Spins diffusing in the x-y plane experience these variations in H_{eff} as a fluctuating magnetic field h_z, with resultant transverse but not longitudinal relaxation. This effect is well known in MR spectroscopy,[33–35] in which a known magnetic field gradient (G) can be applied to a sample in order to measure the diffusion coefficient (D) of protons through a solvent. The signal intensity (S) for a Hahn spin echo at TE is given as:

$$S = S_0 \exp ([TE/T_2 + \text{}^{1}/12 \cdot \gamma^2 \cdot G^2 \cdot D \cdot TE^3]) \qquad (2)$$

Hence, differences in susceptibilities at the boundary of a hematoma containing paramagnetic blood products and surrounding normal diamagnetic tissue produce T_2 relaxation if sufficient diffusion is permitted to occur during the imaging sequence. Such effects cause signal loss at these boundaries on T_2-weighted MR images of sufficiently long TE without corresponding signal loss on T_1-weighted MR images.

RELAXIVITY

The relative rotational and translational motions of water molecules and paramagnetic entities in biologic systems occur on a time scale that produces an apparent isotropically fluctuating magnetic field in the range of the Larmor frequencies for protons at current imaging field strengths. If the water molecules are able to approach the paramagnetic center, then magnetic interactions allow efficient energy exchange to occur and the magnetically perturbed water proton spin system can relax to its equilibrium state.[51] The phenomenologic equation for intermolecular relaxation interactions of a paramagnetic agent (P) in bulk solution is:

$$\text{}^{1}/T_{i(obs)} = \text{}^{1}/T_{i(dia)} + \text{}^{1}/T_{i(para)} \qquad (3)$$

$$\text{}^{1}/T_{i(para)} = R[P] \qquad (4)$$

where i = 1,2; R is the relaxivity constant ($s^{-1}mM^{-1}$); and [P] is the concentration (mM) of the paramagnetic substance P. $\text{}^{1}/T_{i(dia)}$ is the rate attributable to diamagnetic relaxation processes and $^1/T_{i(para)}$ is the relaxation rate in the presence of P. In the presence of a suitable paramagnetic substance, the paramagnetic term dominates over the diamagnetic term of Equation 3. The same equation applies for both longitudinal and transverse relaxation. Because T_1 is generally longer than T_2, $^1/T_1$ is smaller than $^1/T_2$, and so the constant term R[P] contributes a greater proportion to the longitudinal relaxation rate ($^1/T_1$) than transverse relaxation rate ($^1/T_2$). The implication to MR imaging is that the relaxivity effects of paramagnetic substances are detected with greater sensitivity on T_1-weighted images than on T_2-weighted images. The paramagnetic relaxation rate can be further analyzed mechanistically as "inner-sphere" (ligand exchange in which water molecules are in the first coordination sphere of P) and "outer-sphere" (diffusion with close approach of water near to but without coordination to P) contributions, but it is not the purpose of this review to describe the more mechanistic Solomon-Bloembergen equations that are presented in detail elsewhere.[51] Application of Equation 3 in biologic systems as complex as cerebral hematomas can only be approximate because of the heterogeneity in type and distribution of the various paramagnetic substances involved. When water is unable to approach the paramagnetic center, no magnetic interaction and therefore no relaxation occurs by relaxivity mechanisms (see Fig. 8–3). However, susceptibility effects can still be manifested so that, whereas T_1 is unaffected, T_2 is shortened and the MR signal is decreased.

REFERENCES

1. Sipponen JT, Sepponen RE, Sivula A: Nuclear magnetic resonance (NMR) imaging of intracranial hemorrhage in the acute and resolving phases. J Comput Assist Tomogr 7:954–959, 1983.
2. DeLaPaz RL, New PFJ, Buonanno FS, et al: NMR imaging of intracranial hemorrhage. J Comput Assist Tomogr 8:599–607, 1984.
3. Gomori JM, Grossman RI, Goldberg HI, et al: Intracranial hematomas: Imaging by high-field MR. Radiology 157:87–93, 1985.
4. Gomori JM, Grossman RI: Head and neck hemorrhage. In Kressel HY (ed): Magnetic Resonance Annual 1987. New York, Raven Press, 1987, pp 71–112.
5. Gomori JM, Grossman RI, Hackney DB, et al: Variable appearances of subacute intracranial hematomas on high-field spin-echo MR. AJNR 8:1019–1026, 1987.
6. Zimmerman RD, Heier LA, Snow RB, et al: Acute intracranial hemorrhage: Intensity changes on sequential MR scans at 0.5 T. AJNR 9:47–57, 1988.
7. New PFJ, Scott WR: Blood. In New PFJ, Scott WR (eds): Computed Tomography of the Brain and Orbit (EMI Scanning). Baltimore, Williams & Wilkins, 1975, pp 263–267.
8. Enzmann DR, Britt RH, Lyons BE, et al: Natural history of experimental intracerebral hemorrhage: Sonography, computed tomography and neuropathology. AJNR 2:517–526, 1981.
9. Kreindler A, Marcovici G, Florescu I: Histoenzymologic and biochemical investigations into the nervous tissue round an experimentally-induced cerebral hemorrhagic focus. Rev Roum Neurol 9:313–319, 1972.
10. Lalonde JMA, Ghadially FN, Massey KL: Ultrastructure of intramuscular haematomas and electron-probe X-ray analysis of extracellular and intracellular iron deposits. J Pathol 125:17–23, 1978.
11. Finch CA, Huebers HA: Iron metabolism. Clin Physiol Biochem 4:5–10, 1986.
12. Trump BF, Valigorsky JM, Arstila AU, et al: The relationship of intracellular pathways of iron metabolism to cellular iron overload and the iron storage diseases. Am J Pathol 72:295–324, 1973.
13. Weinberg ED: Iron, infection and neoplasia. Clin Physiol Biochem 4:50–60, 1986.
14. Southern PA, Powis G: Free radicals in medicine. I. Chemical nature and biologic reactions. II. Involvement in human disease. Mayo Clin Proc 63:390–408, 1988.
15. Munro HN, Linder MC: Ferritin: Structure, biosynthesis and role in iron metabolism. Physiol Rev 58:317–396, 1978.
16. Wixon RL, Prutkin L, Munro HN: Hemosiderin: Nature, formation and significance. Int Rev Exp Pathol 22:193–225, 1980.
17. Bunn HF, Forget BG (eds): Hemoglobin: Molecular, Genetic and Clinical Aspects. Philadelphia, WB Saunders Company, 1986, pp 13–35, 634–662.
18. Thulborn KR, Wateron JC, Matthews PM, Radda GK: Oxygenation dependence of the transverse relaxation time of water protons in whole blood at high field. Biochim Biophys Acta 714:265–270, 1982.
19. Brindle KM, Brown FF, Campbell ID, et al: Application of spin-echo nuclear magnetic resonance to whole cell systems: Membrane transport. Biochem J 180:37–44, 1979.
20. Koenig SH, Brown RD, Lindstrom TR: Interactions of solvent with the heme region of methemoglobin and fluoro-met-hemoglobin. Biophys J 34:397–408, 1981.
21. Blumberg WE: Spectroscopic properties of hemoglobins: The study of hemoglobin by electron paramagnetic resonance spectroscopy. In Ho C (ed): Methods in Enzymology. New York, Academic Press, 1981, pp 312–329.
22. Windle JJ, Weirsema AK, Clarke JR, Feeney RE: Investigation of the iron and copper complexes of avian conalbumins and human transferrins by electron paramagnetic resonance. Biochemistry 2:1341–1345, 1963.
23. Aasa R, Aisen P: An electron paramagnetic resonance study of the iron and copper complexes of transferrin. J Biol Chem 243:2399–2404, 1968.
24. Koenig SH, Schillinger WE: Nuclear magnetic relaxation dispersion in protein solutions. II. Transferrin. J Biol Chem 244:6520–6526, 1969.
25. Harrison PM, Fischbach FA, Hoy TG, Haggis GH: Ferric oxyhydroxide core of ferritin. Nature 216:1188–1190, 1967.
26. Koenig SH, Brown RD: Relaxometry of magnetic resonance imaging contrast agents. In Kressel HY (ed): Magnetic Resonance Annual 1987. New York, Raven Press, 1987, pp 263–286.
27. Gillis P, Koenig SH: Transverse relaxation of solvent protons induced by magnetized spheres: Application to ferritin, erythrocytes and magnetite. Mag Res Med 5:323–345, 1987.
28. Weir MP, Peters TJ, Gibson JF: Electron spin resonance studies of splenic ferritin and haemosiderin. Biochim Biophys Acta 828:298–305, 1985.
29. Boas JF, Troup GJ: Electron spin resonance and Mossbauer effect studies of ferritin. Biochim Biophys Acta 229:68–74, 1971.
30. Darrow YC, Alvord EC, Hodson WA: Histological evolution of the reactions to hemorrhage in the premature human infant's brain: A combined autopsy study and a comparison with the reaction in adults. Am J Pathol 130:44–58, 1988.
31. Cohen MD, McGuire W, Cory DA, Smith JA: MR appearance of blood and blood products: An in vitro study. AJR 146:1293–1297, 1986.
32. Hayman LA, Ford JJ, Taber KH, et al: T2 effect of hemoglobin concentration: Assessment with in vitro spectroscopy. Radiology 168:489–491, 1988.
33. Abragam A: Principles of Nuclear Magnetism. Oxford, Clarendon Press, 1985.

34. Becker ED: High Resolution NMR. Theory and Chemical Applications. New York, Academic Press, 1980.

35. Farrar TC, Becker ED: Pulse and Fourier Transform NMR. New York, Academic Press, 1971, pp 2–15.

36. Fukushima E, Roeder SBW: Experimental Pulse NMR. A Nuts and Bolts Approach. London, Addison-Wesley Publishing Company, 1981, pp 1–125.

37. Yoder CH, Schaeffer CD Jr: Introduction to Multinuclear NMR. Menlo Park, Benjamin/Cummings Publishing Company, 1987.

38. Fullerton GD: Basic concepts for nuclear magnetic resonance imaging. Mag Res Imaging 1:39–53, 1982.

39. Bottomley PA: NMR imaging techniques and applications. Rev Sci Instrum 53:1319–1337, 1982.

40. Brant-Zawadzki M, Norman D: Magnetic Resonance Imaging of the Central Nervous System. New York, Raven Press, 1987.

41. Pykett IL, Newhouse JH, Buonanno FS, et al: Principles of nuclear magnetic resonance imaging. Radiology 143:157–168, 1982.

42. Wehrli FW: Principles of magnetic resonance. *In* Stark DD, Bradley WG (eds): Magnetic Resonance Imaging. St. Louis, C. V. Mosby, 1988, pp 1–23.

43. Edelman RR, Buxton RB, Brady TJ: Rapid MR imaging. *In* Kressel HY (ed): Magnetic Resonance Annual 1988. New York, Raven Press, 1988, pp 189–216.

44. Wismer GL, Buxton RB, Rosen BR, et al: Susceptibility induced magnetic resonance line broadening: Applications to brain iron mapping. J Comput Assist Tomogr 12:259–265, 1988.

45. Ludeke KM, Roschmann P, Tischler R: Susceptibility artefacts in NMR imaging. Mag Res Imaging 3:329–343, 1985.

46. Di Chiro G, Brooks RA, Girton ME, et al: Sequential MR studies of intracerebral hematomas in monkeys. AJNR 7:193–199, 1986.

47. Kamman RL, Go KG, Brouwer W, Berendsen HJC: Nuclear magnetic resonance relaxation in experimental brain edema: Effects of water concentration, protein concentration and temperature. Magn Reson Med 6:265–274, 1988.

48. Burke HE: Handbook of Magnetic Phenomena. New York, Van Nostrand Reinhold Company, 1986, pp 9–57.

49. Bean CP, Livingston JD: Superparamagnetism. J Appl Phys 30:120S–129S, 1959.

50. Bean CP: Hysteresis loops of mixtures of ferromagnetic micropowders. J Appl Phys 26:1381–1383, 1955.

51. Lauffer RB: Paramagnetic metal complexes as water proton relaxation agents for NMR imaging: Theory and design. Chem Rev 87:901–927, 1987.

9

CLINICAL SPECTROSCOPY

DENNIS J. ATKINSON, JOEL F. MARTIN, MARK A. BROWN,
JASON A. KOUTCHER, C. TYLER BURT, and DOUGLAS BALLON

A—Clinical Applications and Techniques

INTRODUCTION TO CLINICAL SPECTROSCOPY

INTRODUCTION TO THE INTERPRETATION OF MR DATA

CLINICAL RESULTS

  PHOSPHORUS-31 SPECTROSCOPIC STUDIES

  Musculoskeletal Physiology
  Brain
  Heart
  Tumor Studies

  PROTON SPECTROSCOPIC STUDIES

  Fat/Water Separation
  High-Resolution Studies

  CARBON-13 SPECTROSCOPY

  SODIUM IMAGING

  FLUORINE SPECTROSCOPIC STUDIES

  OTHER NUCLEI

  CONCLUSION

LOCALIZED SPECTROSCOPY

  B_0 METHODS

  Topical Magnetic Resonance
  Stimulated-Echo Acquisition Method
  Image Selected In Vivo Spectroscopy
  Spatially Resolved Spectroscopy
  Chemical Shift Imaging

  B_1 METHODS

  Surface Coil Localization
  Rotating Frame Zeugmatography
  DEPTH Pulses

  COMBINED B_0 AND B_1 METHODS

  Depth Resolved Surface Coil Spectroscopy
  Fast Rotating Gradient Spectroscopy

  SUMMARY OF LOCALIZATION METHODS

FAT/WATER IMAGING

  PHASE CONTRAST USING A SPIN-ECHO SEQUENCE

  PHASE CONTRAST USING A GRADIENT-ECHO SEQUENCE

  FREQUENCY-SELECTIVE PULSES

B—Practical Considerations and MR Theory

PRACTICAL IMPLEMENTATION OF CLINICAL SPECTROSCOPY

  INSTRUMENTATION AND S/N CONSIDERATIONS

  Resonance Frequencies
  Magnetic Field Strength
  Shimming
  Sequence Design
  Computer Resources

  PATIENT PREPARATION

  DATA ACQUISITION

  DATA POSTPROCESSING

MR SPECTROSCOPIC THEORY

  HIGH-RESOLUTION MR

  Magnetic Resonance Effect
  Characteristics of the MR Spectrum
  Chemical Shift of the Resonance Frequency
  J-Coupling, Source of Fine Spectral Details
  Chemical Exchange

  RELAXATION TIME MEASUREMENT

  MAGNETIZATION TRANSFER— SATURATION AND INVERSION

  DIFFUSION

  TEMPERATURE MEASUREMENT

  TWO-DIMENSIONAL FOURIER TRANSFORM SPECTROSCOPY

  QUADRUPOLAR NUCLEI

  SOLVENT SUPPRESSION FOR RESOLVING ^{1}H SPECTRA

  T_2 Decay
  Binomial Suppression
  Selective Saturation
  Multiple Quantum Filtering

A—Clinical Applications and Techniques

INTRODUCTION TO CLINICAL SPECTROSCOPY

Magnetic resonance has been one of the most powerful analytical tools available to the chemist. Until the early 1970s, its primary use was in elucidating the structure of organic molecules. More recently, the application of MR spectroscopy to biochemical problems has been made possible by numerous technologic advances. Fourier transform MR spectroscopy and new electronic components such as mini-computers with extended memories, high power, programmable pulse controllers, and wide bore, very high field superconducting magnets with excellent stability and homogeneity have increased the sensitivity of MR by several orders of magnitude. These advances also have helped extend the capability of MR to medical imaging over the past 10 years.

Before discussing clinical MR spectroscopy, certain terms require definition.

1. Magnetic resonance imaging (MRI) involves obtaining an image without attention to molecular composition. Because of the high abundance of hydrogen and sensitivity to its signal, clinical applications rely almost exclusively on proton MRI. In earlier work this was also referred to as nuclear magnetic resonance (NMR) imaging.

2. Magnetic resonance spectroscopy (MRS) is the term generically used to describe the study of chemical information from a given sample. Typically, information is obtained from the entire sample, with no definition of the spatial source of the signal.

3. Localized spectroscopy involves obtaining this same type of spectroscopy (chemical) information, but from a defined localized region of the sample.

4. Spectroscopic imaging involves displaying spectral information from a region that is spatially resolved in two or three dimensions. When applied to proton imaging to demonstrate the presence or absence of fat or water, this may be referred to as fat/water imaging.

The clinical application of spectroscopy necessitates the use of either localized spectroscopy or spectroscopic imaging to be effective, since the human body is composed of many metabolically different regions. These studies will no doubt draw heavily from the large knowledge base of in vitro spectroscopic studies or spectroscopic results from in vivo animal models. In addition, while certain spectroscopic studies may not yet be feasible for routine clinical application, the rapid advances in technology hold promise for their application in the near future. Therefore, while this chapter is primarily involved with clinical spectro-scopic results, mention will also be made of results of previous nonclinical studies and potential future applications.

INTRODUCTION TO THE INTERPRETATION OF MR DATA

Proper interpretation of MR data requires a basic understanding of the MR effect and the physical basis for obtaining clinically important information.

In Chapter 1, the basic concepts of magnetic resonance were introduced. An important concept is that of *spin*, which is closely related to the angular momentum of the nucleus. To be observable by MR, a nucleus must have a nonzero spin. When there is only one unpaired nucleon (neutron or proton) the spin is half-integral (e.g., 1/2, 3/2). Examples of nuclei with half-integral spin include ^1H, ^{13}C, ^{19}F, ^{23}Na, and ^{31}P. When two unpaired nucleons exist, the spin is integral (e.g., ^2H and ^{14}N) (Fig. 9–1). Nuclei with spin greater than 1/2 have a characteristic called *quadrupole moment* which can make it difficult to study them in a clinical setting. The most vexing problem in studying a quadrupolar nucleus is that its relaxation time is very short (e.g., T_2 times on the order of a few milliseconds), so its signal decays before it can be measured. (An exception is heavy water, ^2H_2O, which has reasonably long relaxation times and can be studied quite readily.)

The interpretation of spectra is simplified by the separation of the resonances from different nuclei. This separation results from the relationship between resonance frequency and local magnetic field strength. Interactions between nuclei and their local environment (i.e., chemical bonds) result in a shift in resonance frequency, called the *chemical shift* (Fig. 9–2). The chemical shift often enables different chemical species to be uniquely identified.

A more subtle, and complex, frequency shift may result from spin interactions between nuclei in close proximity. This effect, called *scalar* or *J-coupling*, is seen with bonding of ^{13}C to ^1H. A proton has a spin of 1/2, indicating that the angular momentum allows it to have one of two possible orientations: up or down (see Chapter 1). The proton will produce a subtly different shift in the ^{13}C resonance frequency depending on its orientation, so that the ^{13}C resonance is split in two. If the ^{13}C is bound to multiple ^1H nuclei, then the carbon resonance is split into multiple peaks. For ease of interpretation, these complex spectra may be simplified by saturating the ^1H–^{13}C coupled resonances with radiofrequency (RF) pulses through a process called *decoupling* (Fig. 9–3).

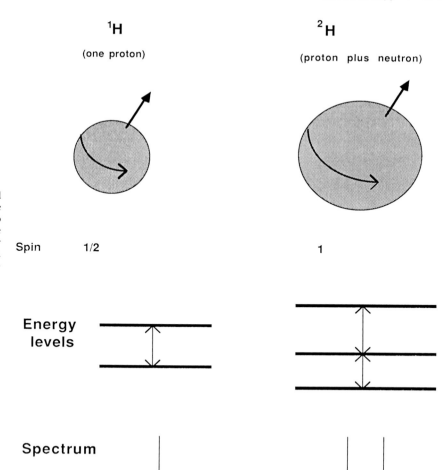

FIGURE 9–1. Schematic diagram of a ^{1}H and ^{2}H atom. Since ^{1}H has a spin of 1/2, the number of energy levels will be $2I + 1$ or two and the number of resonances is one. In the case of a higher spin number where $I = 1$ (for ^{2}H), three levels now exist, thus allowing a more complex relaxation pattern and two resonances are theoretically possible. This complex relaxation is called *quadrupolar* relaxation and is characterized by short T_2 times.

The typical manner for displaying MR data is to plot signal intensity values along a frequency axis using a standard chemical compound as the reference frequency. The positions of individual peaks could be displayed as a function of frequency (in Hz).

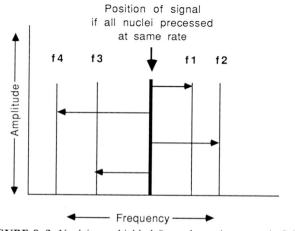

FIGURE 9–2. Nuclei are shielded from the main magnetic field by their local chemical environment, producing a chemical shift (*horizontal arrows*) off the central resonance. The degree of shift is a function of the chemical species studied.

Normally, shifts in resonance frequency are displayed in parts per million (ppm), that is, frequency shift $\times 10^6$/resonance frequency.[1] When expressed in ppm, chemical shifts do not depend on the field strength of the magnet. In addition to frequency shift, other characteristics of the spectra can be used to provide additional information. For instance, the relative concentration of nuclei can be determined by comparing the areas under each spectral peak. In addition, the *linewidth* (defined as the distance, in Hz or ppm, across a peak at one-half its maximum amplitude) relates to the T_2^* of the nucleus (Fig. 9–4). For best results, T_2^* should be maximized (i.e., minimal linewidth). This requires *shimming* of the magnetic field over the volume of interest in order to improve field homogeneity (Fig. 9–5). Field homogeneity for in vivo studies of 0.1 ppm or less is possible.

In addition to determining chemical structure, spectroscopy permits dynamic information about chemical reactions to be obtained. An example of this process is called *magnetization transfer* and is discussed in section B. This method applies RF pulses which eliminate or invert signal from the nuclei in a particular compound, which is involved in an exchange with other, nondisturbed compounds. The exchange of a chemical group, for example, phos-

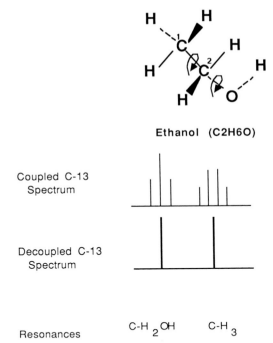

Ethanol (C2H6O)

Coupled C-13
Spectrum

Decoupled C-13
Spectrum

Resonances   C-H₂OH   C-H₃

FIGURE 9–3. Upper diagram, schematic representation of ethanol (C_2H_6O) with freely rotating molecular bonds. Lower diagram, since both ^{13}C resonances are in differing environments, there exists two resonance frequencies, one for each environment. However, in observing finer detail, the C-H₂OH resonance is split into three peaks while the C-H₃ resonance has four. This splitting of the resonances is due to the *coupling* effect of the protons and may be eliminated through a process called *decoupling*. The resulting spectra from decoupling will "collapse" back to a single resonance (bottom spectrum).

phate, between one compound and another will result in a change in MR signal intensity. By measuring the relative signal changes in the different compounds as a function of time, chemical reaction rates can be determined.

CLINICAL RESULTS

PHOSPHORUS-31 SPECTROSCOPIC STUDIES

The widespread use of phosphorus-31 (^{31}P) for in vivo NMR studies reflects a combination of factors including the central importance of high energy phosphate compounds in the regulation of cellular metabolism, the relative ease of interpretation of the ^{31}P MR spectra due to the small number of visible phosphorus compounds present in tissue, the 100 per cent abundance of the ^{31}P isotope, and its favorable sensitivity for MR detection.

Adenosine triphosphate (ATP) and phosphocreatine (PCr) are high energy metabolites present in healthy, oxygenated cells (Fig. 9–6). Cells use these metabolites to perform work and replenish them under conditions of normal aerobic activity by catabolizing glucose or other nutrients. This process,

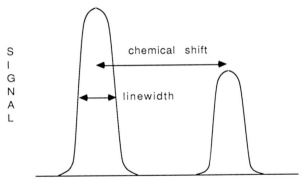

Frequency (Hz or ppm)

FIGURE 9–4. Diagram showing the relationship between the resonance frequency and a chemical shift of a nearby peak. The integrated area under the peak is proportional to the concentration. From this relationship, characterization of relative concentration ratios between substances is possible. Unfortunately, the proportionality constant is often a function of the pulse sequence parameters. This fact is often ignored, resulting in measurements of dubious accuracy. The ability of a spectrum to resolve fine details depends on its linewidth (the frequency range at half the peak amplitude, or *FWHM*), that is, broad spectral peaks, will not allow resolution of finer resonances.

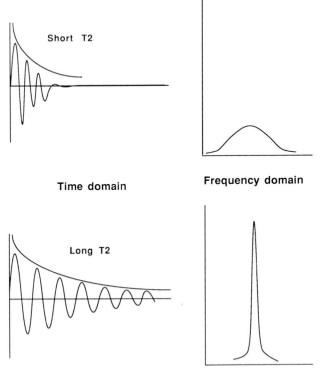

Short T2

Time domain   Frequency domain

Long T2

FIGURE 9–5. A simple illustration of the effects of shimming to obtain a longer T₂*. *In the upper figure, a short* T₂* *in the time domain results in a very broad linewidth and a reduced peak amplitude in the frequency domain. Shimming to extend the* T₂* *significantly longer dramatically reduces the linewidth and, since the area under the curve is constant, increases the peak amplitude.*

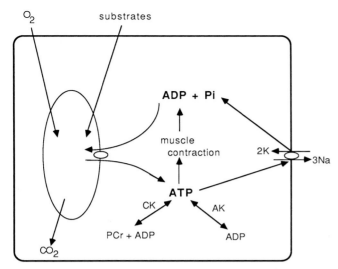

FIGURE 9–6. A simplified illustration of the high-energy phosphate reactions within a muscle cell. ADP = adenosine diphosphate; ATP = adenosine triphosphate; AK = adenylate kinase; CK = creatine kinase; Pi = inorganic phosphate.

which takes place within mitochondria, is called oxidative phosphorylation or aerobic respiration. Long-term aerobic sources of energy are:

$$\text{Glycogen/glucose} + ADP + Pi + O_2 \rightarrow H_2O + CO_2 + ATP$$

$$\text{Free fatty acids} + ADP + Pi + O_2 \rightarrow H_2O + CO_2 + ATP$$

The ^{31}P spectrum (Fig. 9–7) shows three ATP peaks, representing the three different phosphate groups (γ, α, and β). The lower energy metabolite adenosine diphosphate (ADP) has only two peaks (α and β). The ADP spectrum overlaps ATP at the γ (−2.7 ppm relative to PCr) and α (−7.8 ppm) peaks,

so assessment of ATP concentration is typically made using the β peak (−16.3 ppm).

When oxygen is unavailable, cells will replenish ATP by less efficient anerobic processes. Short-term reactions involved in cellular energetics include:[2]

Reaction 1: $PCr + ADP + H^+ \rightleftharpoons ATP + Cr$

Reaction 2: $ATP \rightarrow ADP + Pi + \text{work}$

Reaction 3: $\text{glucose} + Pi + ADP \rightarrow ATP + \text{lactic acid}$

Reaction 1 is catalyzed by creatine kinase (CK). If adequate reserves of PCr and CK are present, the equilibrium in Reaction 1 will maintain ATP levels. ADP levels are normally very low in healthy tissues. With ischemic stress, the rate of utilization of ATP for cell work (Reaction 2) may exceed the rate of production. This leads to the accumulation of ADP, a stimulant for glycolysis, and additional lactate formation and metabolic acidosis (Reaction 3). When most of the PCr has been exhausted, a drop in ATP signal will be observed. Therefore, careful monitoring of ADP and inorganic phosphate in relation to PCr (i.e., the PCr/Pi ratio) gives a valuable index about the stress response of the cell.

Ischemia produces a drop in intracellular pH (Reaction 3). A common method for measuring pH is to calibrate the chemical shift of Pi relative to PCr.[3] Inorganic phosphate exists as H_2PO4^- and $HPO4^{-2}$ at a neutral pH, with the resonances from these two species separated by approximately 2.4 ppm. However, in solution the two species exchange rapidly and are observed as a single resonance. When the pH changes, the ratio of $HPO4^{-2}$ to H_2PO4^- also changes and thus alters the position of the Pi peak, which is referenced to a known standard (i.e., PCr). This method of pH calibration has several potential

FIGURE 9–7. Normal ^{31}P MR spectrum demonstrating the association of molecular bonding sites and their specific resonances, that is, β-, α-, and γ-phosphates of ATP. The chemical shift is specified relative to PCr, since the resonance frequency of PCr is relatively insensitive to changes in pH.

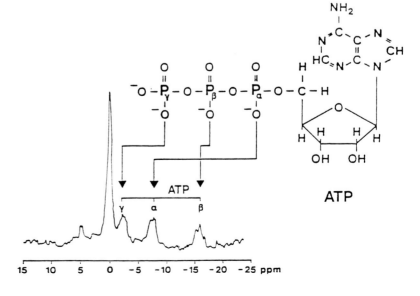

sources of error (e.g., temperature variations, metal ion binding, low pH, and cellular compartmentalization) but has nonetheless gained wide acceptance.

Musculoskeletal Physiology

The bulk of ^{31}P MR studies has focused on the study of muscle bioenergetics. MR is unsurpassed in being able to monitor normal musculoskeletal physiology. For instance, it can be used to study the effect of exercise on high energy phosphates and intracellular pH in normal muscle.[4] The resting muscle spectrum consists of large PCr and ATP peaks, along with a weak Pi peak (PCr/Pi = 10 to 20).[5] In one study, moderate exercise produced a decrease in PCr, while Pi increased (PCr/Pi = 3) and pH dropped (−0.4 unit). After exercise ceased, recovery of PCr and Pi occurred within 5 minutes. There was no change in ATP concentration during the study. With more vigorous exercise, the PCr/Pi ratio dropped to 1, while the change in pH was similar to that from moderate exercise. The authors concluded that the PCr/Pi ratio is a more sensitive indicator of muscle energy metabolism during vigorous exercise than is intracellular pH.[6] Other studies have shown an excessive depletion of PCr and acidosis in patients with peripheral vascular disease.[7] In studies of aging, ^{31}P MR has not shown any significant differences either at rest or with exercise between younger and older patients.[8]

Hereditary skeletal muscle myopathies are rare, but ^{31}P MR offers promise as a noninvasive tool for studying these diseases. For instance, McArdle's syndrome is a disease caused by a lack of glycogen phosphorylase in skeletal muscle (Fig. 9–8).[9] Diagnosis is confirmed by muscle biopsy, which demonstrates excess glycogen content and absent phosphorylase activity. Because these patients are unable to metabolize glycogen, glucose reserves are rapidly depleted (Reaction 3, above) and the patients are unable to sustain exercise. In response to exercise, they fail to generate lactic acid and no pH change is exhibited. In one study, the baseline spectrum of a patient was compared with a control volunteer (Fig. 9–9). With aerobic exercise, the pH of the patient changed minimally (7.19 to 7.09), while that of the volunteer dropped significantly (7.04 to 6.67). The decrease in PCr and rise in Pi was greater in the patient than in the normal volunteer. With ischemic exercise (i.e., exercise with arterial occlusion) (Fig. 9–10), the muscle pH of the patient rose (7.04 to 7.23), while that of the normal volunteer dropped (7.04 to 6.43).[10]

Other kinds of hereditary myopathies can be differentiated based on ^{31}P studies.[11] Patients with Type IX glycogen storage disease (phosphofructokinase

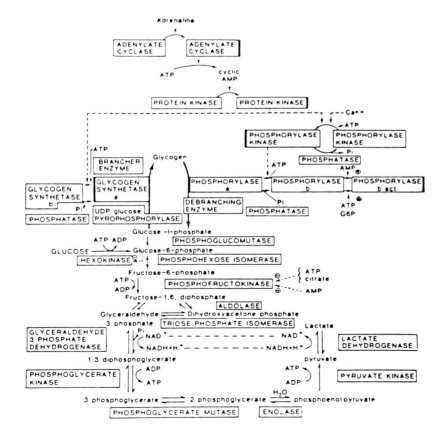

FIGURE 9–8. Schematic representation of the main biochemical pathways involved in glycogen synthesis and utilization in skeletal muscle. (From Griffiths RD, Edwards RHT: The biochemical applications of spectroscopy and spectrally resolved imaging. *In* Wehrli FW, Shaw D, Kneeland JB (eds): Biomedical MR Imaging. Principles, Methodology and Applications. New York, VCH Publishers, 1988, p 526; with permission.)

FIGURE 9–9. *Top,* Phosphorus-31 MRS spectra of McArdle's patient showing the effect of aerobic exercise (i.e., exercise with muscular blood flow uninhibited). The signal areas assigned as follows: 1, 2, and 3: the β, α, and γ-phosphates of ATP; 4, phosphocreatine (PCr); and 5, inorganic phosphate (Pi). The pH values given above each Pi signal were determined from the frequency shift of the Pi and PCr signals. The first spectrum (A) was recorded at rest before exercise; subsequent spectra (B to D) were recorded during the periods labeled (zero represents the start of exercise). Exercise was maintained only during the period from zero to one minute, and an unhindered aerobic recovery followed. All measurements used a TR of 2.0 seconds. Resting spectrum was acquired with 64 acquisitions; subsequent spectra represent 32 acquisitions.

Bottom, Phosphorus-31 MRS spectra in a control subject, showing the normal effects of aerobic exercise. Acquisition parameters are the same as above in the McArdle's patient, but note that where the pH of the control patient dropped only minimally (7.19 to 7.09) with aerobic exercise, the McArdle's patient showed significant change (7.03 to 6.67). (From Ross BD, Radda GK, Gadian DG, et al: Examination of a case of suspected McArdle's syndrome by ^{31}P NMR. N Engl J Med 304:1338, 1981; reprinted by permission of the New England Journal of Medicine.)

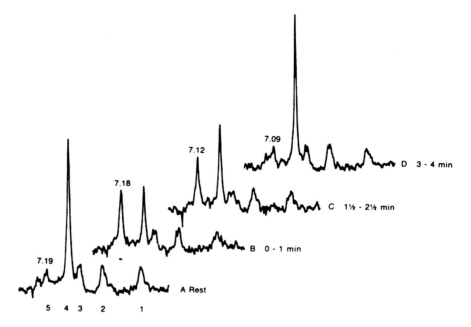

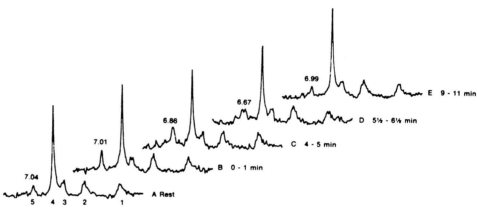

[PFK] deficiency) have normal resting muscle spectra. However, unlike McArdle's syndrome, after exercise Pi levels remain low and sugar phosphate levels increase 50-fold.[12]

Patients with deficiency of NADH-CoQ reductase (an enzyme involved in synthesis of ATP through electron transport in mitochondria) had decreased PCr/Pi at rest.[13] During exercise, they demonstrated a more rapid drop in the PCr/Pi ratio and pH than did normal controls. The most marked abnormality seen in these patients was the extremely slow return of PCr and Pi to their initial values after exercise ceased. The slow rate of recovery of PCr is consistent with a decreased rate of oxidative metabolism.

Phosphorus-31 spectroscopy has also been applied to other muscular disorders. For instance, patients with Duchenne's or Becker's muscular dystrophy demonstrate an unusually alkaline resting pH, reduced PCr/ATP and PCr/Pi, and generally low concentrations of metabolites. [31]P studies of patients suffering from prolonged exhaustion after a viral illness demonstrated premature and rapid pH changes after exercise.[14]

Brain

In vivo ^{31}P MR has been used to study cerebral metabolism in newborn infants and adults with impaired cerebral function. In studies of brain development in humans, PCr increases with maturity, while the phosphomonoesters decrease relative to the nucleoside triphosphate concentration.[15] In the normal adult brain, concentration of Pi is less than half that of PCr (PCr/Pi > 2), and PCr/ATP = 1.93 ± 0.12. In general, the PCr/Pi ratio appears to be a more sensitive indicator of metabolic derangement than ATP, since a reduction in ATP has been observed only when there is a depletion of more than 50 per cent of the PCr.[16, 16a, 17]

Most of the early ^{31}P MR studies of brain metabolism focused on babies since they could fit into

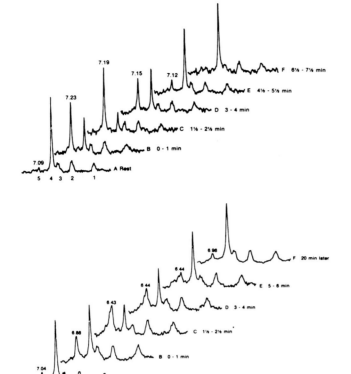

FIGURE 9–10. *Top,* Phosphorus-31 MRS spectra in a patient with McArdle's syndrome showing the effects of ischemic exercise. The patient exercised from time zero to 0.75 minutes, and arterial occlusion was maintained for a period up to 3 minutes. Normal arterial flow was restored after this period.

Bottom, Phosphorus-31 MRS of a normal control subject demonstrating the effects of ischemic exercise. Data acquisition methods used are identical to those used in the top spectrum, except that exercise was extended to 1.5 minutes before normal arterial flow was allowed. Note that the pH increases by 0.19 unit for the McArdle's patient while the normal patient shows a 0.6 unit decrease. (From Ross BD, Radda GK, Gadian DG, et al: Examination of a case of suspected McArdle's syndrome by ^{31}P NMR. N Engl J Med 304:1338, 1981; reprinted by permission of the New England Journal of Medicine.)

smaller-bore, high field magnets. The ratio of PCr/Pi was found to be abnormally low in infants who had severe asphyxia at birth but who tended to recover as their clinical condition improved. It appeared that in birth-asphyxia patients, the lower the PCr/Pi ratio, the worse the prognosis.[18] Patients with PCr/Pi ratios above 0.8 progressed normally (Fig. 9–11). No pH changes were noted in this patient population. Other studies have shown a latency period of a day or so when the PCr/Pi ratio was near normal before deteriorating.[19, 20] This deterioration predated any morphologic changes on ultrasound and may suggest a role for MRI in early diagnosis. Comparative studies using animal models have demonstrated that the neonate appears more resistant to ischemic and/or hypoxic insult than the adult.[21]

The PCr/Pi ratio was also a sensitive indicator for other pathology. A low ratio was found in infants with meningitis and atrophy; the ratio was depressed

as much as two to fourfold, yet without significant reduction in pH. Acidemic infants demonstrate a very low pH (6.4) along with a gross distortion of spectra (i.e., no ATP, PCr, PD, or Pi resonances).[22]

Studies of adult cerebral metabolism with ^{31}P spectroscopy have not been as promising to date. For instance, one study followed patients 18 hours to 15 years after a stroke. PCr/Pi reductions were seen only within the first 7 days with complete recovery thereafter, even when persistent clinical neurologic problems were present.[23] Another study focused on this problem by comparing PCr/Pi ratios with electroencephalogram (EEG) signals in an animal model. EEG signal strength and PCr/Pi were both directly related to metabolic changes; however, it appeared that PCr/Pi recovered more quickly after a cerebral insult.[24]

The relationship between brain glucose stores and ischemic response to stroke has long been an area of active clinical research.[25] Unfortunately, most clinical studies have investigated only systemic glucose changes and have found a poor correlation between neurologic outcome and systemic glucose concentra-

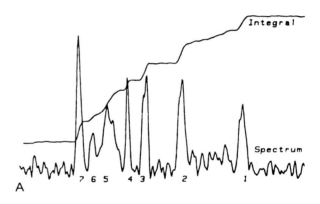

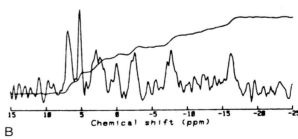

FIGURE 9–11. *A,* Phosphorus-31 MRS brain spectrum from a 17-day-old infant with hypotonia due to congenital muscular dystrophy. The PCr/Pi ratio was 1.7 and the pH was 7.0. Note that an integral is calculated over the frequency range to better delineate small peak amplitude changes and to assess differences in overall concentration (the area under the peaks is proportional to the number of nuclei observed).

B, Phosphorus-31 MRS spectrum from a 5-day-old infant suffering from severe brain asphyxiation. In this case, the PCr/Pi ratio was 0.3 and the pH was 7.0. (From Hope PL, de L. Costello AM, Cady EB, et al: Cerebral energy metabolism studied with phosphorous NMR spectroscopy in normal and birth-asphyxiated infants. Lancet 2:366–370, 1984; with permission.)

tions in patients with stroke.[26] Using pH and high energy phosphates as indicators, ^{31}P MRS has been used in an animal (cat) model to study global cerebral changes with ischemia and reperfusion.[27] Over a two-hour period following a 16-minute ischemic event, the authors reported a significant drop in pH during ischemia and a subsequent recovery to near normal values within an hour of the initial onset. The reduction of pH level correlated well with glycemic condition prior to the stroke. Under conditions of hyperglycemia induced prior to ischemia, cats became significantly more acidotic than under conditions of hypoglycemia.

Heart

Cardiac spectroscopy presents numerous technical problems. First, it is difficult to precisely separate the myocardial signal from that of the nearby blood pool. As a result, cardiac spectra tend to be contaminated by 2,3-diphosphoglycerate (2,3-DPG) signals from the blood in the ventricles. These resonances fall in the Pi–phosphomonoester (PME) region, making interpretation of in vivo data difficult. To circumvent this problem, localized surface coils have been used in perfused animal models. Second, cardiac and respiratory motion require that gating techniques be used not only for obtaining the measurement spectra but in order to do the shimming as well. Third, poor sensitivity is a serious limitation, since surface coils only provide adequate surface-to-noise (S/N) ratio for superficial portions of the right ventricle, which is of less clinical importance than the left ventricle. Clinical applications of MRS in the heart are discussed in depth in Chapter 26 and will be reviewed here briefly.

Spectra from the heart are similar to those of skeletal muscle, except that the PCr/Pi and PCr/ATP ratios appear to be lower. The reduced steady-state level of PCr may reflect the fact that the cardiac muscle is continually active. In one study, ATP and PCr concentrations were found to decrease and Pi increased during systole.[28] However, another study failed to duplicate this finding.[29]

Analogous to the above studies of cerebral metabolic studies, some early studies investigated the use of the PCr/Pi ratio as an indicator of cardiac metabolism in the neonate. Due to rapid and variable heart rates, some of the studies have been done without cardiac gating and represent an average of systolic and diastolic spectra. In an 8-month-old patient with cardiomyopathy, MRS showed a reduced PCr/Pi ratio.[30] In another study, a child with an organic aciduria similar to glutaric aciduria type II was found to have a cardiac PCr/Pi ratio of 1.0, compared with an asymptomatic twin's value of 1.5. The affected twin was treated with dietary therapy and riboflavin and, after 6 months of treatment, was found to have a normal PCr/Pi ratio of 1.5. In quantitatively evaluating both cases, the authors noted that signals from the 2,3-DPG in the ventricular erythrocytes probably contributed to the Pi peak, so that the actual changes in Pi were underestimated.[31]

MRS studies of cardiac ischemia have centered on the PCr, Pi, pH, and ATP levels. In almost all studies, complete ischemia produced rapid cessation of myocardial contraction, followed by a fall in PCr, a rise in Pi, and a reduction of pH over the next few minutes. ATP levels are maintained until PCr is exhausted.[32]

Tumor Studies

Owing to the ease of access by surface coils and minimal requirements for localization techniques, most early ^{31}P MRS studies of neoplasms were applied to extremity tumors. More recent MRS has been applied to the study of brain, abdominal, and thoracic tumors. However, much more needs to be done in terms of basic cell and animal models (as well as localization methods and instrumentation) in order to begin to systematically identify tumor types and stage their progress using phosphorus spectroscopy. At this point, ^{31}P MRS is just beginning to have a defined clinical role in the initial diagnosis and follow-up of cancer.

To date, ^{31}P MRS has been disappointing in its ability to consistently identify and characterize tumors.[33] One fairly consistent finding, particularly among extracerebral neoplasms, is an increase in phosphomonoesters (PME) and phosphodiesters (PDE). These substances are intermediate and breakdown products of phospholipid synthesis and may be indicative of cellular proliferation. One study of eight patients (including lymphomas, sarcomas, and carcinoma) showed high PME/ATP ratios in tumors, with an average reduction of 55 per cent when tumors responded to treatment and a 50 per cent increase when they did not.[34] In a study of 23 patients with superficial extremity tumors of varying histology (including osteosarcoma, Ewing's sarcoma, squamous cell carcinoma, rhabdomyosarcoma, malignant melanoma, and benign pleomorphic adenoma), it was found that tumors contained elevated amounts of Pi, PME, and PDE and decreased PCr peaks relative to normal muscle. In monitoring the patients' responses to treatment (chemotherapy and radiation), changes were noted in the PCr/Pi ratio and PCr + Pi sum.[35]

Another study of 43 patients with intracranial tumors used a combination of proton and phosphorus spectroscopy. Meningiomas demonstrated the strongest differences: PCr decreased to below ATP, PDE decreased, and PME increased in some cases (Fig. 9–12). Malignant gliomas showed less distinct changes: the PDE peak was reduced and split in some cases, and PCr was reduced. In this study, nonmalignant astrocytomas could not be differentiated from normal tissue.[36] Another study (Table 9–1) of intracranial tumors had comparable PDE results but was able to more clearly characterize lesions based on changes in PME, PCr, and Pi.[37]

In assessing the effect of radiation treatment, ^{31}P MRS studies have demonstrated spectral changes in brain tumors after therapy. Treatment of an intracranial lymphoma resulted in an increase in the PCr

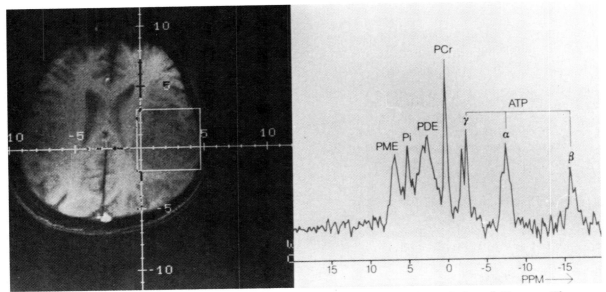

FIGURE 9–12. A localized 5 cm x 5 cm x 5 cm MRS study demonstrating the ^{31}P peaks in a glioblastoma. The spectrum is similar to that of a normal spectrum with the exception of an increased phosphomonoester (PME) concentration. (Courtesy of the University of Innsbruck, Innsbruck, Austria.)

resonance. Treatment of a Grade II astrocytoma resulted in a relative decrease in PDE and an increase in PCr and PME. The pH level was 7.08 prior to radiation, 6.95 during treatment, and recovered to 7.06 as the patient progressed.[38] Another study of the effects of radiation treatment on the metabolism of a non-Hodgkin's lymphoma showed transient changes in the PCr resonance within 3 hours of treatment. It was found that the PDE peak was the most sensitive indicator of response to radiation therapy (Fig. 9–13).[39] A study of infants with intraabdominal neuroblastoma showed a correlation between the PME–ATP ratio and tumor growth or regression (Fig. 9–14).[40]

PROTON SPECTROSCOPIC STUDIES

Fat/Water Separation

The clinical application of these methods is primarily for the evaluation of disorders of structures that contain fat and water, such as red bone marrow. For instance, it can be difficult to detect diffuse leukemic infiltration of the marrow on conventional T_1-weighted spin-echo images.[41] However, a water-only chemical shift image obtained with proton density weighting shows abnormally high signal, resulting from replacement of fatty marrow with water-containing leukemic cells. The simplest way to obtain this kind of information is by a method called phase-contrast gradient-echo imaging (see Chapter 5). For instance, a normal vertebral body appears dark on an opposed gradient-echo image obtained with a small flip angle, due to signal cancellation from fat and water (Fig. 9–15A). However, with increased water content, as in metastatic disease or diffuse leukemic infiltration, the marrow appears bright.[42] This technique may have other applications, particularly in the investigation of suspected fatty infiltration of the liver (Fig. 9–15B).

High-Resolution Studies

Proton (^{1}H) MRS methods have only gradually been introduced into the clinical arena. One problem is that water is present in many thousand times the concentration of the metabolites of interest. As a result, the water resonance dominates the ^{1}H spectra and masks other resonances. In fat-containing tissue, there are also significant proton peaks arising from the -CH_2- and -CH_3 lipid groups which mask other resonances. In order to circumvent these problems, methods known as solvent suppression have been developed to reduce these unwanted signals. An advantage of proton MRS over MRS of other nuclei is that standard receiver coils, used for imaging, may also be used to obtain spectra. As for clinical appli-

TABLE 9–1. METABOLITE CHANGES IN INTRACRANIAL TUMORS, RELATIVE TO NORMAL VOLUNTEERS, BY ^{31}P SPECTROSCOPY

Tumor Type	PDE	PME	pH	PCr	Pi
Glioblastoma	↓ ↓ ↓		↑ ↑		
Low grade glioma	↓ ↓ ↓		↑ ↑		
Low grade astrocytoma		↓ ↓ ↓			
Pituitary adenoma	↓ ↓ ↓	↑ ↑ ↑	↑ ↑	↓ ↓ ↓	↓ ↓ ↓
Meningioma	↓ ↓ ↓		↑ ↑		

Adapted from Karczmar GS, Poole J, Boska MD, et al: ^{31}P MRS Study of response of human tumors to therapy. Abstracts of the Society for Magnetic Resonance in Medicine. San Francisco, 1988, p 615.

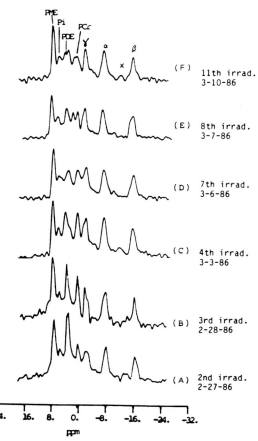

FIGURE 9–13. Serial study of MRS ³¹P brain spectra of a non-Hodgkin's lymphoma (NHL) tumor obtained over multiple irradiation treatments. Note the changes in peak intensity of PCr and phosphodiesters (PDE). (From Ng TC, Vijaya Kumar S, Majors AW, et al: Response of non-Hodgkin's lymphoma to Co-60 therapy monitored by ³¹P in situ. Int J Radiat Oncol Biol Phys 13:1545–1551, 1987; with permission, Pergamon Press, plc.)

Cr/PCr ratio. Surprisingly, the ¹H resonances of ATP frequently do not show up well in these spectra, suggesting that the sensitivity achieved to date is well below the theoretical maximum.[44]

In normal brain, *N*-acetylaspartate (NAA) is the most prominent peak. One MRS study demonstrated that NAA is completely depleted 4 days after stroke, while in parallel there is a dramatic increase in the concentration of lactic acid (Fig. 9–17). This finding is due to anaerobic respiration and eventual cell death. Concominant brain edema may dilute the concentration of various metabolites, resulting in a further decrease in their spectral peaks.[45]

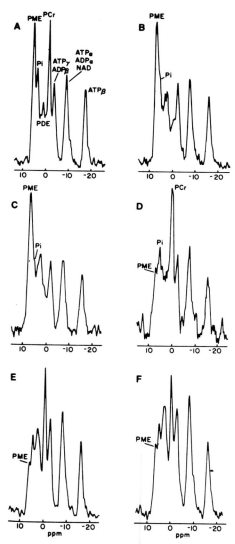

FIGURE 9–14. Serial study of an infant with an intraabdominal neuroblastoma. The initial study *(A)* was performed prior to treatment response. Successive studies *(B–D)* show the response to treatment 4, 8, and 16 weeks later. Studies *(E)* (at the edge of the liver) and *(F)* (anterolateral to the edge) were made 24 weeks after the initial response. (From Maris JM, Evans AE, McLaughlin AC, et al: ³¹P NMR spectroscopic investigation of human neuroblastoma in situ. N Engl J Med 312:1500–1505, 1985; with permission, Pergamon Press, plc.)

cations, ¹H MRS can, in principle, be used to study the metabolism of amino acids, neurotransmitters, and fatty acids, as well as the substrates involved in energy metabolism.

The STEAM (stimulated-echo acquisition method) sequence in combination with CHESS (chemically shift-selective) pulses for water suppression has proved useful for obtaining localized proton spectra. One advantage of using the STEAM method for data acquisition is the capability for rapid, interactive shimming on an accurately selected tissue volume. For example, within 5 minutes, field homogeneities on the order of 0.25 ppm over the entire brain can be achieved. Similarly, on the same system, a 64 ml volume of interest was shimmed with a minimum water linewidth of 3 Hz (0.05 ppm) (Fig. 9–16).[43]

In muscle cells, proton MRS can identify lactate, taurine, creatine (Cr), phosphocreatine lipid resonances and the histidine-containing peptides. The ¹H chemical shifts of these species can be used to monitor the intracellular pH value and to determine the

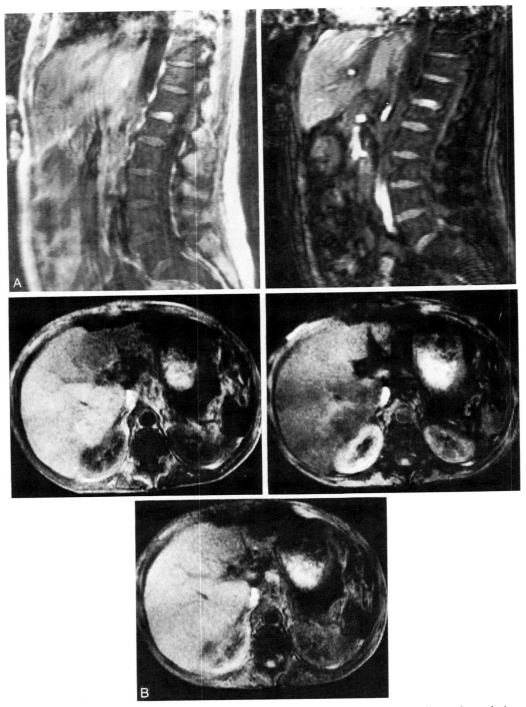

FIGURE 9–15. *A*, A simple demonstration of the fat/water phase contrast using a gradient-echo technique. The fat and water differ in frequency and at 1.5 tesla, these vectors modulate in and out of phase every 2.38 msec. Left, at TE = 5 msec, the fat and water signals within the red bone marrow mostly add. Right, at TE = 7 msec, the fat and water signals cancel, resulting in lower signal.

B, Clinical demonstration of fatty infiltration of the liver using gradient-echo fat/water phase cycling. Upper left, TE = 5 msec; the fat/water vectors in-phase (bright liver), upper right, TE = 7 msec: out-of-phase image (dark liver); bottom, TE = 9 msec: in-phase image (bright liver).

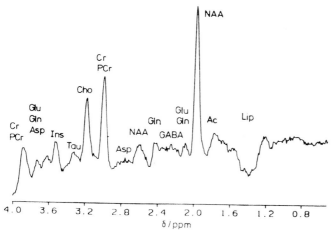

FIGURE 9–16. Water-suppressed proton spectrum from a normal volunteer brain at 64 MHz with a TR of 6000 msec and a TE of 50 msec. Detailed resonances are listed (from right to left): lipids (Lip), acetate (Ac), N-acetyl-aspartate (NAA), γ-aminobutyric acid (GABA), glutamine (Gln), glutamate (Glu), aspartate (Asp), creatine (Cr), and phosphocreatine (PCr), choline-containing compounds (Cho), taurine (Tau), and inositol phosphates (Ins). (From Frahm J, Bruhn H, Gyngell ML, et al: Localized high-resolution proton NMR spectroscopy using stimulated echos: Initial application to human brain in vivo. Magn Reson Med 9:79–93, 1989; with permission.)

Cerebral metastases and primary tumors demonstrated a reduction or absence of NAA and Cr/PCr and a stable level of choline and glutamine.[46] Lactate levels may be elevated due to higher metabolic activity. Research is proceeding into histologic differences associated with changes in concentrations of lactate, adenine nucleotides, as well as malignancy-associated lipoproteins (MAL).[47, 48]

An intriguing proton MRS study of nine large brain tumors, using STEAM to obtain localized spectra, showed similar spectral features among tumors of the same histologic type, but significant spectral differences among tumors of different histologic type.[48a] For instance, spectra from these astrocytomas showed an absence of resonances from NAA (which is predominantly localized in neurons and is therefore not seen in tumors) and creatine/phosphocreatine, and a prominent resonance from lactate (indicating increased anaerobic glycolysis). Increased resonances from mobile fatty acids and adenine nucleotides suggested an increased phospholipid synthesis and an increased nucleotide or purine pool. Lactate was not increased in other tumor types. Prominent choline resonances were seen in an oligodendroglioma and two meningiomas, consistent

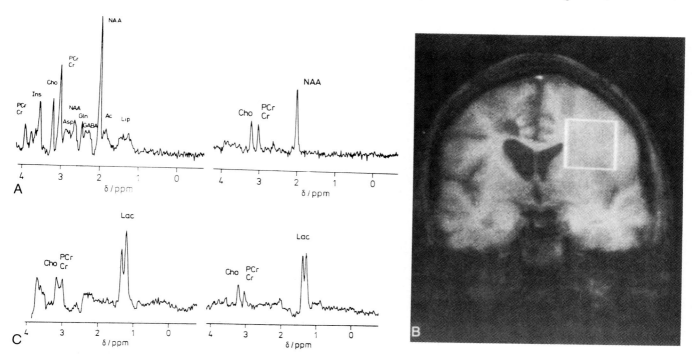

FIGURE 9–17. A, 1.5 tesla proton MRS spectra of normal human brain from a 3 x 3 x 3 cm volume of interest (VOI) localized in the insular area of a healthy volunteer using a STEAM sequence (TM = 30 msec, TR = 1500 msec, with 512 acquistions). Spectra were recorded at TE of 50 msec and 270 msec. Intensities are directly comparable.

B, FLASH MR image of a 42-year-old patient four days after presenting with an acute stroke in the left frontodorsal area. Imaging was at 1.5 tesla with TR = 100 msec, TE = 10 msec, and the RF flip angle was 70 degrees. The rectangle illustrates the 3 x 3 x 3 cm VOI for localized proton MRS in C.

C, MRS study of the infarcted area with intensities multiplied by a factor of two from A. Note the absence of NAA and reduction of Cr/PCr and Cho compounds as well as a strong contribution from lactic acid (Lac). Left, TE = 50 msec; Right, TE = 270 msec. (From Bruhn H, Frahm J, Gyngell ML, et al: Cerebral metabolism in man after acute stroke: New observations using localized proton NMR spectroscopy. Magn Reson Med 9:126–131, 1989; with permission.)

with a relatively high content of choline phosphoglycerides. An unassigned resonance in the 3.4 to 3.8 ppm range from a breast cancer metastasis was attributed to carbohydrate residues that in vitro studies have previously shown are present on the surface of phospholipid membranes in malignant cells.

In addition to compound identification, the ease of detecting ^1H signals allows relaxation times to be measured. Usually the water resonance is examined since it is the most abundant. On a molecular level, the tissue water may be in more than one environment, for example, compartmentalized or exchanging between a free and bound state. Under these conditions, the observed relaxation times may be composites of more than one value (i.e., multiexponential decay). In vitro tissue studies have the added problem that tissue preparation is critical for obtaining accurate results. Sample contamination from metal scalpels, evaporation of tissue fluids, and measurement of temperature make accurate comparison of in vivo and in vitro relaxation times difficult. Nonetheless, relaxation time measurements continue to be explored as a method to characterize normal and pathologic tissues.[49]

In one study of breast tissue specimens (including samples of normal tissue, fibroadenoma, fibrocystic disease, and adenocarcinoma), there was a marked difference in relaxation times between adenocarcinoma and normal samples. The mean T_1 times were 874 msec for adenocarcinoma and 682 msec for normal tissues, with fibroadenoma tissue having a T_1 time of 980 versus 655 for fibrocystic tissue. The T_2 times for the two groups differed as well. The T_2 times for normal, fibroadenomatoid, fibrocystic, and adenocarcinomatoid tissues were 35, 37, 62, and 68 msec, respectively.[50, 51]

High field proton MRS has been used to analyze human plasma as a potential diagnostic test for cancer. Attention has been focused on the methylene and methyl groups of plasma lipids in comparison to the higher field component of the methyl proton resonance of the lactate molecule (Fig. 9–18).[52] Changes in the linewidth, chemical shift, and relaxation times have been observed in the blood of patients with malignant tumors. Initially, it was hoped that this test would provide a fast, low-cost cancer screening tool, but succeeding studies have proved inconclusive to date.[53, 54] Further study is required to validate this technique.

CARBON-13 SPECTROSCOPY

Although present in low natural abundance, ^{13}C has several advantages when compared with proton or phosphorus spectroscopy. The peaks are widely separated over a large chemical shift range (200 ppm versus 12 ppm for proton MRS) and are fairly specific,[55] so that a large amount of metabolites can be distinguished and measured in a single spectrum. There are numerous metabolic pathways where carbon is involved. For instance, it is possible to identify

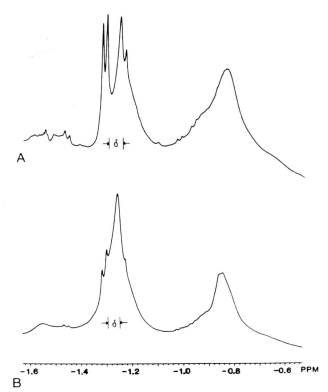

FIGURE 9–18. Demonstration of the methyl and methylene regions of the 400 MHz proton MR spectra recorded from the blood plasma of (A) a neonate and (B) an adult with a malignant tumor. The chemical shift values on the scale at the bottom are referenced to the external tetramethylsilane (TMS) resonance. (From Eskelinen S, Hiltunen Y, Jokisaari J, et al: ^1H NMR studies of human plasma from newborn infants, healthy adults and adults with tumors. Magn Reson Med 9:35–38, 1989; with permission.)

glycine, taurine, alanine, lactate, aspartate, creatine, γ-aminobutyrate, inositol, glutamate, glutamine, N-acetylaspartate, phosphoryletholamine, and glycerol phosphorylcholine. Storage compounds (e.g., glycogen and triacylglycerols) can have high intracelluar concentrations and are easier to detect.

However, limited S/N represents a barrier to routine clinical application in that the sensitivity for ^{13}C is only 1.6 per cent of hydrogen and the natural abundance is only 1.1 per cent. Enrichment of the abundance is possible, but this approach may find only limited clinical application given its currently high cost (e.g., $1000 for a dose of enriched glucose sufficient for a ^{13}C MRS study).[56]

An important feature with ^{13}C spectroscopy is the spin-spin or J-coupling between neighboring carbon-hydrogen nuclei on the same molecule. This spin-spin coupling splits the ^{13}C resonances, reducing the S/N but also further complicating the spectra. The solution for simplifying the spectrum is to decouple the carbon spins from the proton spins with an extra RF pulse. This decoupling pulse is centered at the hydrogen resonance frequency and has an adequate bandwidth to reduce or eliminate ^{13}C–^1H interactions. Full decoupling makes the carbon resonance appear as a singlet, while partial decoupling may be used to determine the number of hydrogen nuclei attached to the carbon. In addition, decoupling can markedly increase carbon sensitivity via the nuclear Overhauser effect (NOE). Unfortunately, the decoupling RF pulse produces increased power deposition.

High-resolution studies (e.g., 100 MHz) have suggested specific molecular parameters that might differentiate neoplastic from nonneoplastic tissues. In particular, prostatic carcinoma and colon carcinoma have been differentiated from adjacent hyperplastic tissue. Compared with normal parenchyma, prostatic tumors showed (1) larger concentrations of triacylglycerols, (2) smaller amounts of citrate, and (3) acidic mucins. The colon tumors demonstrated (1) smaller amounts of triacylglycerols, (2) higher concentrations of phospholipids and lactate, and (3) decreased lipid fatty acyl chain saturation. In another study of a poorly differentiated lung carcinoma, there appeared to be smaller ^{13}C signals from mucins and other proteins along with changes in the triacylglycerol levels.[57]

SODIUM IMAGING

Sodium has several characteristics that make it a potentially useful nucleus for imaging. It is 100 per cent naturally abundant and occurs in extracellular fluids in a relatively high concentration of 0.14 molar. Unlike the hydrogen nucleus, the sodium nucleus is quadrupolar. The quadrupole magnetic moment of sodium interacts with local electric fields. This interaction results in very short relaxation times, on the order of 50 msec or less.

In order to take advantage of the very short T_1 times, ^{23}Na imaging is usually performed using correspondingly short TR times (e.g., 50 to 100 msec) and three-dimensional (3D) acquisition methods. Coarse acquisition matrices are used to limit imaging time, which is nonetheless quite prolonged (30 to 60

minutes) due to the need for extensive signal averaging to compensate for poor sensitivity and concentration. This coarse matrix typically produces in-plane spatial resolution of several millimeters compared with submillimeter resolution for proton MRI.

Interpretation of sodium images is complicated by the fact that the sodium nucleus is quadrupolar with spin = 3/2. As a result, there are four different energy levels and three possible nuclear transitions or resonances (Fig. 9–19A and B). An additional issue is that the separation of the energy levels depends on the orientation of the sodium nucleus with respect to the external magnetic field. Static interactions with the molecular environment cause the outer resonances to broaden to the point of being undetectable (Fig. 9–19C). This effect is called *heterogeneous broadening*. Molecular motion complicates the linewidths further. This dynamic effect is called *homogeneous broadening*. Because of broadening of the outer resonances, three discrete peaks are never observed in vivo. Instead, only a single peak at the resonance frequency of the central transition is observed. The degree of line broadening will determine how much of the sodium is actually observed spectroscopically, since very broad resonances may not be detectable. Early reports have suggested that as much as 60 per cent (the contribution of the outer resonances) of the sodium may be "MR invisible."[58] More recent work suggests that the amount of MR-invisible sodium is actually much smaller. The reason is that rapid molecular motions tend to average the two outer resonances to a fairly sharp, and therefore observable, single resonance, which overlaps the resonance from the central transition (Fig. 9–19D). Unfortunately, it appears that much of the signal intensity is lost during the TE interval due to complicated differential relaxation.

For clinical studies, it is important to differentiate intracellular from extracellular sodium. The sodium-

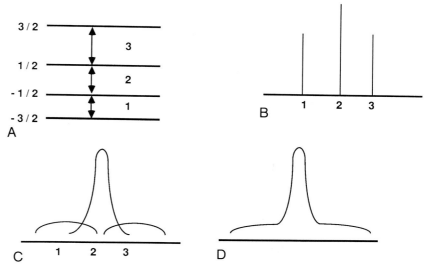

FIGURE 9–19. Diagram of the effects of quadrupolar coupling on the sodium resonance. *A,* With quadrupolar nuclei of spin = 3/2, four energy levels exist and three transitions take place (3/2 to 1/2, 1/2 to −1/2, and −1/2 to −3/2). *B,* A schematic diagram of an ideal environment where the three resonances are at a constant angle to the magnetic field. Quantum mechanical calculations assign 40 per cent of the total intensity to the central peak with 30 per cent assigned to each of the outer lines. *C,* A more typical case in which the resonances 1, 2, and 3 in *B* have broadened. Due to random orientations and other effects, the outer resonances are broad (and have a short T_2^*) with the result that their peak height is diminished. Under these circumstances, the outer resonances may be broadened beyond detection so that only the central 40 per cent of the signal is observable. *D,* A diagram of a typical observed spectrum in which further molecular motions have averaged the outer resonances toward a central peak.

potassium ATPase continually pumps sodium out of the cell, so that intracellular sodium is present in a concentration less than 0.02 molar. As a result, sodium is present in highest concentration in the extracellular space. Impairment of the function of the sodium pump, for example, as a result of ischemia, is reflected in an increase in intracellular sodium. An elevated intracellular to extracellular sodium concentration ratio is an indicator of cell death. Sodium imaging has been used to differentiate ischemia from infarction and to grade malignancies.

Several methods have been proposed for differentiating intracellular from extracellular sodium. In one study, sodium T_2 relaxation times were used to differentiate the two cellular compartments. T_2 relaxation of sodium has two components. The slow component has relaxation that is dominated by the central resonance and has a T_2 of about 40 msec. The faster component has a T_2 of much less than 10 msec and is more a measure of the outer resonances. The fast component would not be observed unless either a very short TE time (e.g., less than 10 msec) or free induction decay (FID) were used. By selecting an echo time greater than 10 msec, the slow component is preferentially imaged.[59] It has been proposed that the fast and slow relaxation components correspond roughly to the extracellular and intracellular compartments, respectively. Unfortunately, more recent work has cast doubt on this two-compartment model[60] and has shown overlap between relaxation times of intracellular and extracellular sodium.

Another approach for separating the signals from intracellular and extracellular sodium is to use compounds known as shift reagents, which change the resonance frequency of sodium. Shift reagents include lanthanide chelate complexes similar to gadolinium-DTPA, but with dysprosium (Dy) as the metal ion. The useful characteristic of these reagents is that they do not penetrate into the cell, so that only the resonance frequency of extracellular sodium is altered[61, 62] (Fig. 9–20). This preferential shifting of only the extracellular component allows a more direct means of quantifying the ratio of intracellular to extracellular sodium. However, application of shift reagents to sodium imaging of the brain is limited by the inability of these agents to penetrate through an intact blood-brain barrier. Furthermore, clinical application of these shift reagents has been limited by the toxicity of these compounds. Superparamagnetic compounds, such as dextran-magnetite, have also been used as sodium MR contrast agents. This intravascular agent shortens T_2 and thereby eliminates signal from blood.[64]

Clinical applications of sodium imaging are still in their infancy. Preliminary clinical studies suggest a potential role for sodium MRI in the study of brain ischemia and infarction (Fig. 9–21). One study of vasogenic edema in dogs and humans showed elevated sodium levels in the edematous tissue. This was consistent with breakdown of the blood-brain barrier

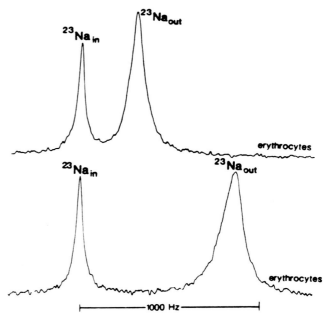

FIGURE 9–20. The [23]Na spectrum of packed suspension of human erythrocytes at a constant concentration of NaCl but differing levels of shift reagent (SR) [Dy (PPP)₂][7]. Top = low concentration of shift reagent; bottom = high concentration. The [23]Na on the left represents the intracellular sodium, unaffected by the large molecules of the shift reagent, which cannot enter the cell. However, the extracellular component (right peak) demonstrates a 1000 Hz shift away from the intracellular resonance when exposed to high shift reagent concentrations. (From Narayana PA, Kulkarni MV, Mehta SD: NMR of [23]Na in biological systems. *In* Partain CL, Price RR, Patton JA, et al (eds): Magnetic Resonance Imaging. Vol II. Philadelphia, WB Saunders Company, 1988, pp 1553–1561.)

and leakage of plasma electrolytes.[65] Sodium images are more sensitive than proton images to subtle changes in water content, so that sodium MRI may be a more sensitive indicator of early infarction.[66] However, the long acquisition time for sodium MRI studies may limit the application of this technique in acute stroke patients who are often agitated. Furthermore, poor spatial resolution precludes visualization of small lesions such as lacunar infarcts. Brain tumors, gliosis, encephalomalacia, and inflammatory disorders increased extracellular fluids with high-sodium content that may be observed by sodium MRI. Tumors, unlike necrosis or edema, show high-sodium signal on images acquired with short TE compared with images acquired with long TE. Therefore, sodium MRI may provide a means of differentiating tumor recurrence from radiation necrosis, which can be difficult using proton MRI. The explanation for this result is not entirely clear, given the demonstrated overlap between relaxation times of intracellular and extracellular sodium.

Another area of research is focused on the extracellular sodium present in the eyes. The formation of cataracts has been biochemically correlated with increased lens sodium concentration. In one study of

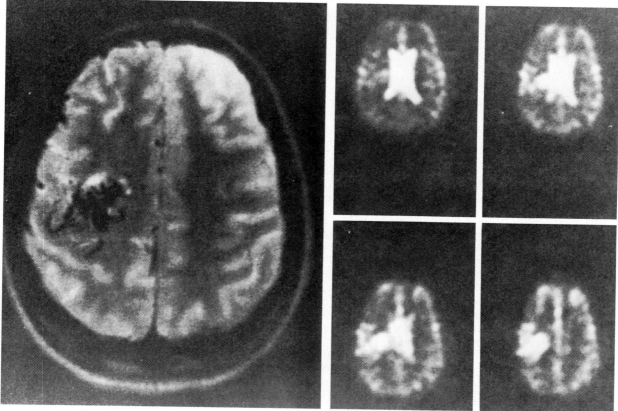

FIGURE 9–21. Proton *(left)* and sodium *(right)* MR images of a patient with an arteriovenous malformation and a history of recent hemorrhage and spasm. The proton image (TR = 4.0 seconds, TE = 80 msec) demonstrates increased signal from a recent hemorrhage. The sodium images demonstrate the same focal lesion, but also reveal associated changes in the convexity. (From Hilal SK, Maudsleu AA, Ra JB, et al: Imaging of Sodium-23 in the human head. J Comput Assist Tomogr 9:1–7, 1985; with permission.)

normal bovine eyes, sodium imaging showed high correlation with the biochemical analyses of the respective tissues: high signal from the vitreous body and anterior chamber with minimal signal from the lens, sclera, cornea, zonular fibers, and ciliary body.[67]

FLUORINE SPECTROSCOPIC STUDIES

Fluorine does not occur naturally in the human body in significant concentrations. This lack of a systemic background signal makes ^{19}F MR attractive in conjunction with the administration of fluorine-containing contrast agents. Promising areas of research include monitoring the distribution and effects of fluorinated chemotherapeutic agents and fluorinated hydrocarbons.

5-Fluorouracil (5-FU) is a chemotherapeutic agent primarily used in the treatment of breast, rectal, and colon cancer. However, its pharmacodynamics are poorly understood and about 70 per cent of patients do not respond. Metabolism and distribution of 5-FU can be studied by localized fluorine MRS. 5-FU is anabolized to 5-fluorouridine-5′-monophosphate (FUMP) and 5-fluorodeoxyuridine-5′-monophos-

phate (FdUMP), or is catabolized in the liver to α-fluoro-β-alanine (FBAL). ^{19}F MRS studies of 5-FU and its breakdown products have shown a correlation between pooling of 5-FU in target tissues and response to therapy (Fig. 9–22).[68, 69] These studies are simplified by the lack of background signal, the broad spectral range (FBAL and FUMP are separated by

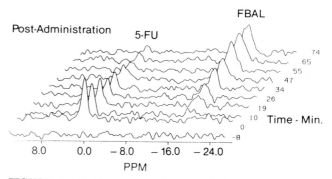

FIGURE 9–22. Time, or stack, plot of the breakdown of 5-fluorouracil into fluoro-β-alanine. The axis along the right side of the plot indicates the time since the injection of the fluorinated chemotherapy agent, with (−8) minutes as the baseline measurement.

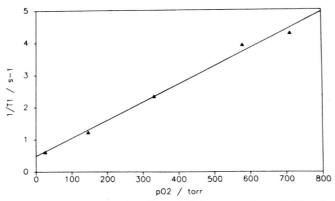

FIGURE 9–23. Calibration line of $1/T_1$ versus pO_2 at 37°C and 0.5 tesla for 19-F resonance of a perfluorocarbon (RFC) compound (a perfluorotributylamine emulsion). The straight line shows the relationship $1/T_1 = 0.47 + 0.0055 \, pO_2$ demonstrating a dependency on oxygen tension. (From Eidelberg D, Johnson G, Barnes D, et al: ^{19}F NMR imaging of blood oxygenation in the brain. Magn Reson Med 6:344–352, 1988; with permission.)

approximately 25 ppm), and high sensitivity for the fluorine signal (86 per cent of hydrogen).

Perfluorocarbons (PFCs) (e.g., Fluosol DA and Oxypherol ET) are excellent solvents of oxygen and are used in the manufacture of blood substitutes. One interesting characteristic of these agents is that the ^{19}F T_1 relaxation rates ($1/T_1$) increase in linear proportion to the partial pressure of oxygen, permitting evaluation of brain oxygenation (Fig. 9–23).[70] Other potential applications include use as a bowel contrast agent[71] and for lung imaging.[72] Practical difficulties with using PFCs include long T_1 and short T_2 relaxation times and the presence of several peaks at different resonance frequencies, resulting in severe chemical shift artifacts.

OTHER NUCLEI

Potassium MRI might be a useful adjunct to sodium MRI for studying the function of Na-K ATPase. ^{39}K is 93.1 per cent abundant and, like sodium, is a quadrupolar nuclei (spin = 3/2). Because potassium is predominantly intracellular, the MR-visible concentration is small, making clinical imaging impractical at the current time. Short TE sequences with nonselective excitation have been used to study tissue samples in vitro, but the method has not been applied in vivo.[73]

^{17}O might prove useful for evaluation of ischemia and to estimate capillary permeability in the central nervous system. Unfortunately, it has low natural abundance (requiring enriched studies) and relatively poor sensitivity. However, ^{17}O compounds such as $H_2^{17}O$ can be administered as contrast agents. This agent causes reductions in tissue T_2 relaxation rates which are linearly dependent on its concentration up to 5 per cent enrichment. The reduction in T_2 is a result of proton exchange processes and is affected

by factors, such as pH, which control the rate of exchange. This effect is unrelated to the T_1 shortening observed with administration of high concentrations of paramagnetic O_2, and in fact the T_1 relaxation times are not affected by administration of $H_2^{17}O$.[74]

Lithium has been used as a pharmacologic agent and as a sodium substitute in electrophysiologic studies. Lithium MRS has been used to monitor patients in antidepression therapy.[75]

^{15}N MRS studies have been limited to date. The method has been used to demonstrate specific peaks for urea, ammonium, trimethylamines, and amino acids in rat kidneys. However, the poor sensitivity and poor natural abundance may limit its eventual clinical utility.[76]

CONCLUSION

At its current stage of development, MRS has not been shown to be a significantly useful clinical modality. Methodologic difficulties have previously slowed the pace of development in this field. Now that these problems have been substantially overcome and a sizable data base has been accumulated in animal models, it is necessary to accumulate spectroscopic data in normal and disease states in human subjects. One promising application for MRS is to study the effects of chemotherapy on neoplasms and thereby to predict which chemotherapeutic regimens are most likely to be beneficial. In conjunction with MR angiography (see Chapter 4) and perfusion imaging (see Chapter 26), another application of MRS would be for the study of brain ischemia. MRS could be used to study vascular lesions that are responsible for ischemia and to determine whether the reduction in flow is causing deleterious effects on brain function. MRS may prove to be of benefit in studying the heart as well. However, substantial methodologic hurdles remain to be overcome before MRS will have routine clinical application in this organ system.

LOCALIZED SPECTROSCOPY

Methods for obtaining localized spectra from a defined volume of interest are under active development. These methods must deal with problems of line broadening, diffusion, overlapping spectra, patient motion, low spin densities, limited examination time, limitations in RF power deposition, and imperfections in magnetic field gradients. Imperfect spatial localization results in unwanted contamination of spectra by signals from tissues outside of the region of interest. For example, ^{31}P spectra from liver, which does not normally exhibit a PCr resonance, may nonetheless demonstrate a prominent PCr peak due to imperfect spatial localization and contamination by signals from skeletal muscle.

Spatial localization techniques may be classified by whether they require shaping of the main magnetic field (B_0), the radiofrequency field (B_1), or a combination of both. Like conventional MRI, B_0 methods generally rely on the application of magnetic field gradients for spatial localization. B_1 methods do not use magnetic field gradients but rely instead on using special transmitter coils and/or combinations of RF pulses to provide the needed spatial selectivity. The combination of the two methods provides increased flexibility at the expense of other problems.

B_0 METHODS

B_0 techniques allow precise selection of the volume of interest. Most of these techniques use magnetic field gradients in some manner to select this volume. One difficulty in employing these methods is that application of the gradient pulses is time consuming so that echo times are prolonged. As a result, several of these methods are not optimal for the study of metabolites with short T_2 relaxation times.

Topical Magnetic Resonance

A conceptually simple method for obtaining volume-localized spectra is to maximize the B_0 field homogeneity in one region and make the rest of the field very inhomogeneous. In the inhomogeneous region, spins either are off resonance or produce signals that decay rapidly and therefore should not contaminate the signal from the area of interest. This is essentially the scheme utilized initially by Damadian and colleagues—field focused NMR (FONAR)[77]—for obtaining early human body images. A modification of this method for spectroscopy was later developed and is called topical magnetic resonance (TMR).[78] This technique is relatively easy to implement but suffers from problems with signal spillover from undesired regions and generates signal from only a single location at a time. As a result, this method is of limited value.

Like TMR, STEAM, ISIS, and SPARS are all methods for defining a single region from which spectral information will be obtained. The underlying principle is that the process of slice selection (i.e., applying an RF pulse and gradient pulse simultaneously) can be used to ensure that MR signals are only produced by a single slice of tissue. Sequential excitation of three perpendicular slices defines a single volume of tissue. Spectra are measured after completion of the spatial localization process. As a result, no gradients are applied during signal measurement; otherwise the spectrum would be severely distorted.

Stimulated-Echo Acquisition Method

STEAM (*st*imulated-*e*cho *a*cquisition *m*ethod) (Fig. 9–24) derives its spatial selectivity from the application of three RF pulses that intersect at a single cubic volume. The STEAM sequence may be represented as:

$$90°\text{--}wait_1\text{--}90°\text{--}wait_2\text{--}90°\text{--}wait_1\text{--}measure$$

where $wait_1$ is a short period of time, and $wait_2$ is a long period of time. The first RF pulse rotates the longitudinal magnetization into the x-y plane and the second RF pulse stores a portion of it along the z-direction. During the second time interval ($wait_2$), T_1 relaxation occurs. Finally, a third RF pulse rotates the stored magnetization back into the x-y plane, and the signal, called a stimulated echo, is measured. This signal appears at a specific time interval after the third RF pulse equal to $wait_1$, the time interval between the first and second RF pulses.[79, 80]

This technique takes advantage of the fact that the stimulated echo occurs well after the FIDs and spin echos from the first two RF pulses have decayed. As a result, the STEAM sequence measures only signals produced by tissues at the intersection of the three planes defined by the RF pulses. The spectrum is well localized and has rectangular slice profiles with little contamination from regions outside the volume of interest. For in vivo spectroscopy, the two main advantages of STEAM are that (1) it does not require any subtraction of spectra, and (2) it can be used with solvent suppression methods (discussed in Section B).

The main disadvantage of STEAM is its relatively low S/N, since at most half the available nuclear magnetization goes into the production of the stimulated-echo signal. Also, resonances with short T_2 values dephase too quickly to be observed. Nonetheless, STEAM is proving to be one of the more useful

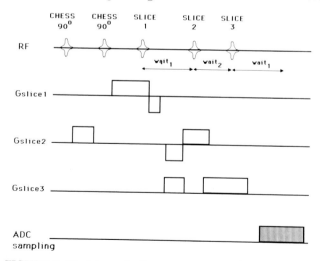

FIGURE 9–24. Schematic diagram of a 3D STEAM localization sequence. The narrow bandwidth, CHESS 90-degree RF pulses suppress the fat signal across the volume of interest. The two subsequent gradients (slice$_1$ and slice$_2$) ensure proper elimination of the transverse vectors prior to the localization sequence. A slice-selective 90-degree RF pulse defines one plane, while two additional RF pulses define the remainder of the volume to be the intersection of three planes.

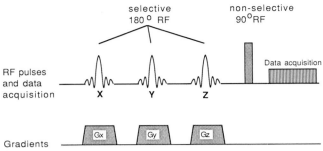

FIGURE 9–25. Schematic diagram of the ISIS sequence. The process of isolating a volume is predicated on measuring the differences in signals between a nonlocalized acquisition and a localized measurement. For example, to localize along a plane, two FID measurements may be used. In one, the FID is preceded by a selective 180-degree RF pulse applied to invert the nuclei along the axis. In the other measurement, no prior 180-degree pulse is applied. The difference in signals then defines a spectrum localized to only those nuclei within the plane. Further definition of the volume requires additional RF pulses and a more complicated data separation method.

methods for producing localized spectra particularly for ¹H studies.[81]

Image Selected In Vivo Spectroscopy

The ISIS (*image selected in vivo spectroscopy*) sequence consists of a series of spatially selective 180-degree pulses that resolve spectra by acquiring FIDs with and without inversion of spins (Fig. 9–25).[82] By selectively processing data after the entire series of acquisitions it is possible to resolve spectra within the selected volume. For example, to resolve along one plane, two measurements are made—one with the in-plane spins inverted prior to an observation pulse, the second without inversion. Data are then subtracted and only in-plane spins are demonstrated. In

performing ISIS localization, two acquisitions are needed to define a plane, four for a column of data, and eight to define a cube (Fig. 9–26). ISIS can be combined with various conventional MR spectroscopic sequences such as solvent suppression, inversion recovery, and spin echo.

An advantage of the ISIS technique is its applicability to ³¹P MRS,[83] because it requires minimal delays before data acquisition, and therefore signals with short T_2 times (10 to 20 msec) can be measured. However, practical drawbacks include the large number of 180-degree RF pulses (with their high-power deposition) and the fact that these 180-degree pulses have imperfect (nonrectangular) slice profiles. Another problem is that the method is motion-sensitive because of the need to repeat the sequence multiple times. Finally, the large number of acquisitions necessary to achieve proper volume selection makes the technique unusable for shimming procedures. Shimming must be done using a different technique, with the potential for misregistration of the shimmed volume and of the volume used for spectroscopic measurements.

Dynamic range can be a problem. In ISIS, all of the tissue is sampled with each pulse, resulting in a very large signal. This signal can overwhelm the digital resolution of the sampling circuitry, resulting in loss of the spectrum for the sampled volume. One variation of the ISIS method (OSIRIS) saturates (or, more precisely, randomizes) spins outside the volume of interest in order to provide better spatial localization.[84]

Spatially Resolved Spectroscopy

SPARS (*spatially resolved spectroscopy*) is another method that uses multiple RF pulses and gradients in orthogonal planes to define a cubic volume. The

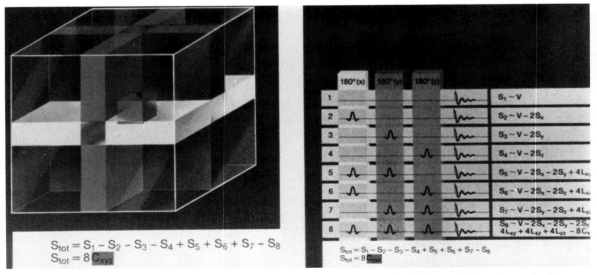

FIGURE 9–26. An overview of the number of steps required to properly define an ISIS volume. In this example, eight steps were used to define the three intersecting planes and isolate a cube.

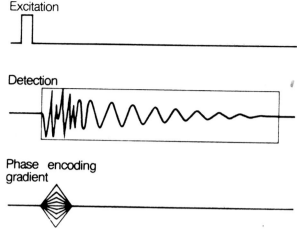

Excitation

Detection

Phase encoding gradient

FIGURE 9–27. In a process analogous to 2DFT imaging, CSI (chemical shift imaging) uses phase-encoding principles to localize spectra along an axis. In this example of a surface coil localized 1D CSI experiment, an RF excitation pulse is used to create a signal, then a phase-encoding gradient is used to localize along one axis, and finally the data are sampled. During successive measurements, the phase-encoding gradient steps through a series of (n) values, where n ultimately determines the acquired resolution. Before the data can be presented it must be Fourier transformed in a manner similar to the normal MR imaging process.

process attempts to maintain longitudinal magnetization within this volume while destroying it elsewhere. To simplify the discussion of SPARS, we shall first consider spatial localization along a single axis. Initially, a broadband RF pulse tips the spins 90 degrees, followed by a gradient to dephase them. The subsequent application of a 180-degree pulse (typically nonselective) followed by an identical but complementary gradient produces an echo. If a selective 90-degree pulse is then applied to the plane

of interest, only those spins should recover their longitudinal magnetization, while the remainder of spins will dephase under the applied gradient. Following spatial localization, the restored longitudinal magnetization is then measured. The advantage of SPARS over, for example, ISIS is that the data acquisition is completed in one experiment, reducing its sensitivity to motion.[85] However, the method requires that the tissues have long T_2 times, so it has limited value for ^{31}P MRS.

Chemical Shift Imaging

Chemical shift imaging (CSI) is not imaging in the traditional sense in that a map of modulated intensities is produced. Instead, it is a spectroscopic method that allows simultaneous acquisition of spectra from multiple regions.[86] The simplest implementation of this technique works by phase-encoding the FID or echo, then Fourier transforming the data to resolve the location of individual spectra along one axis (one-dimensional CSI—Figs. 9–27 and 9–28). One attraction for this method is the lack of a read-out gradient which would distort the spectrum. In expanding CSI methods into two dimensions, data are obtained from a single slice using standard slice-selection (selective irradiation) methods. The two in-plane dimensions of the image are then spatially resolved by phase encoding (Fig. 9–29). Three-dimensional methods phase encode in all three dimensions.[87] Long measurement times and voluminous amounts of data unfortunately limit the practical application of volumetric 3D methods to short TR and coarse matrix acquisitions.[88]

Since spatial resolution is a function of the number of phase-encoding steps, one advantage of CSI is its ability to resolve fine spatial details. Also, as discussed

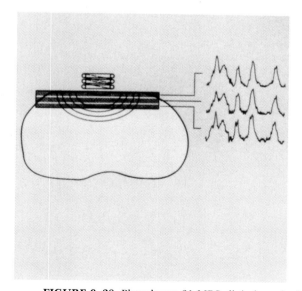

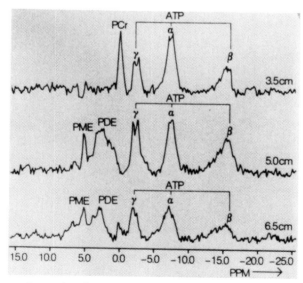

FIGURE 9–28. Phosphorus-31 MRS clinical results from a liver using the 1D CSI method and a surface coil. In this example, the one-dimension localization is along a "depth" axis. Note that localized planes in the liver do not demonstrate a PCr peak. The one plane outside the liver and near the surface does exhibit a high PCr peak associated with the normal skeletal muscle.

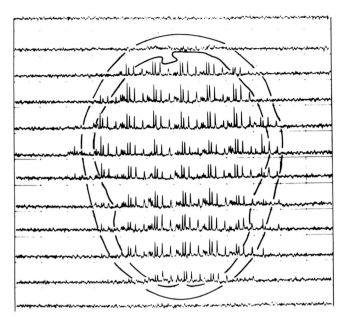

FIGURE 9–29. Phosphorus-31 MRS study of the human head using 3D CSI. In this example, the dimensions of the pixels are 2 cm x 2 cm with a slice thickness of 5 cm. (From Bottomly PA: Human in vivo NMR spectroscopy in diagnostic medicine: Clinical tool or research probe? Radiology 170:1–15, 1989; with permission.)

in Chapter 1, for a given volume of interest and a specified number of acquisitions, S/N is a function of the number of signal measurements (in this case, equal to the number of phase-encoding steps), so the CSI process has inherently more signal than line- or point-scanning techniques such as ISIS or STEAM.

One promising application of CSI is for ^{31}P studies,[89, 90] despite its low sensitivity (7 per cent of proton signal) and low concentrations (millimolar versus 110 molar for H atoms in H_2O). However, the short T_2 of many of the ^{31}P-containing metabolites (T_2 times of 10 to 20 msec as opposed to typical proton tissue T_2 values of 70 to 2000 msec) restrict the choice of TE.

B_1 METHODS

B_1 methods rely on the use of surface coils with a very inhomogeneous B_1 field. The surface coil is typically one or two loops of wire placed adjacent to the patient or phantom sample. Since the coil is placed onto the patient or sample and does not surround it, the RF excitation profile is not uniform. This causes the effective flip angle to vary as a function of distance from the coil across the sample and provides some opportunities to develop strategies for spatial localization (Fig. 9–30).

The main advantage of techniques that rely on B_1 is that they retain chemical shift information, since the frequency content of the MR signal is not distorted by magnetic field gradients. Disadvantages to their use in a clinical environment include difficulty

in precisely defining the desired volume of interest, coil-specific geometry, and the potential limit of RF power in more complex measurements.

Surface Coil Localization

Owing to the limited volume of excitation, one of the simplest methods for localizing a spectrum is to use a surface coil for RF excitation and signal reception. This method confines data collection to only the region nearest the coil (Fig. 9–30). This has an advantage in that rapid nonselective RF excitation pulses are possible, a method that may be essential when measuring short T_2 times. This method also simplifies the measurement process for measuring surface or near surface spectra since the sequences and set up times are limited. Unfortunately, this method suffers from a lack of discrimination in that it integrates all signals within its volume.

Rotating Frame Zeugmatography

One way to utilize the inhomogeneity of surface coil transmission is to observe the changes in spectra when pulses with successively larger RF power levels are applied. Those spins closest to the coil experience the most rapid change in flip angle, while those distant may experience only minor changes in excitation. By performing a series of experiments in which the pulse length (or RF power) is varied, and then performing a 2D Fourier transform (2DFT) on the data, one can obtain a spatially resolved chemical shift spectrum from a region beneath the coil (Fig. 9–31). The technique, called *rotating frame zeugmatography* (RFZ), was first suggested by Hoult.[91]

While modeling the B_1 inhomogeneity throughout the adjacent volume may be straightforward, in clinical practice quantitation may be difficult. Not only does the excitation angle vary with depth, but sensitivity also drops exponentially,[92] reaching an effective minimum beyond a distance equal to the radius of the coil. Furthermore, strong surface or side volume signals may contaminate and/or alias back onto signals from more remote tissue.[93] Implementation of

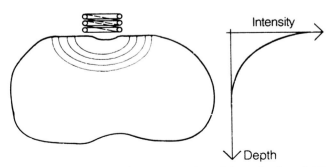

FIGURE 9–30. Schematic representation of the reduction of RF excitation intensity at increased distances from a solenoidal surface coil. The received signal intensity for a surface coil varies as a function of depth, such that strong surface signals may overwhelm smaller, deeper signals.

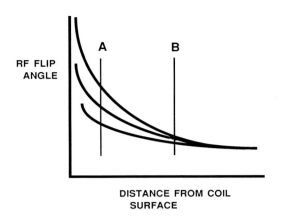

RF FLIP ANGLE

A   B

DISTANCE FROM COIL SURFACE

FIGURE 9–31. Schematic representation of the underlying principle in rotating frame zeumatography (RFZ). Position A is closer to the surface coil, which should expose it to more RF power than position B. However, position A also will experience a larger change in flip angle with changes in the transmitter power level (or higher RF flux) than position B. By successive measurements with progressive changes in the RF flip angle, this flux difference between A and B, results in spatial localization through subsequent Fourier transform of the data.

practical calibration procedures for this method is an area of active research, including development of better simulation phantoms or attempting to use calibration standards during the acquisition of data.[94]

DEPTH Pulses

An alternative approach for volume localization uses DEPTH pulses, which have been developed by Bendall and Gordon.[95] This technique uses multiple RF pulses (also called phase cycled pulses) along differing axes and having different flip angles, with the goal of canceling signal at all volumes except the desired location. The signal that is detected is at a positive maximum when the pulse angle is 90 degrees, zero when the angle is 180 degrees (or 360 degrees), and a negative maximum when the angle is 270 degrees. In addition, surface coils have a basic inhomogeneity of the B_1 field, where the pulse angle varies as a function of depth. Combining these two concepts, a localization method can be constructed in which a series of measurements combining a complex sequence of RF pulses will produce a spectrum from a user-defined volume.

Unfortunately, this technique requires large numbers of pulses (e.g., to discriminate ± 16 degrees of the desired flip angle necessitates 24 acquisitions) and produces a sensitive volume strongly dependent on the coil geometry.[96] In addition, it can be very difficult to adjust the phase of the spectra. Practical problems in a clinical setting include the potential of high RF power deposition, poor B_0 homogeneity (the long minimum acquisition time makes it impractical for shimming operations, necessitating other techniques that will not have identical sensitive volumes), and the fact that the sequence requires precise calibration of the initial RF flip angle.[97]

COMBINED B_0 AND B_1 METHODS

It is possible to combine B_0 and B_1 localization techniques to provide additional methods to select a localized volume of tissue. For example, when a surface coil is placed parallel to the x-y plane, the excitation profile of the surface coil provides proximal volume localization along both x- and y-axes. Combining this with the use of localizing gradients allows a simple method to localize a volume along all three axes.

Depth Resolved Surface Coil Spectroscopy

One method to select a particular plane parallel to the plane of the coil involves applying a slice-selective magnetic field gradient perpendicular to the coil surface and then exciting the region with a selective RF pulse. By adjusting this gradient and the width of the RF pulse, the location and thickness of the slice can be selected by the user. This simple technique called DRESS (*d*epth *r*esolved *s*urface coil *s*pectroscopy) was developed by Bottomley and colleagues and has been used to obtain ^{31}P MR spectra of muscle, heart, tumors, and so forth.[98]

Some of its current limitations include the limited spatial selectivity of the method within the section, given that it depends on imperfections in surface coil sensitivity. For instance, in spectroscopy of the myocardium, spectral contamination from the blood pool and epicardium are inevitable. Like other techniques that require gradients for spatial localization, the long pulse widths necessary to define a particular slice, gradient-induced eddy currents, and delays prior to acquiring data caused by the presence of refocusing gradients may introduce spectral artifacts. Delays between excitation and signal measurement result in distortions of the baseline of the spectrum, which can necessitate difficult phase corrections of the data.

Fast Rotating Gradient Spectroscopy

One of the difficulties with surface coil methods is the contamination of spectra by strong signals from superficial tissues. One technique for eliminating this artifact is called FROGS (*f*ast *ro*tating *g*radient *s*pectroscopy) and relies on a presaturating pulse prior to data acquisition (Figs. 9–32 and 9–33).[99] This saturating pulse is spatially located using a gradient in a manner similar to the B_0 methods above and is immediately followed by two spoiler pulses to eliminate any residual transverse magnetization. The advantages of this method is that it allows volume selection in a single acquisition, it is simple to implement with a transmit/receive surface coil, and it provides a method to reduce spectral artifacts (Fig. 9–34).

SUMMARY OF LOCALIZATION METHODS

Localization methods must be tailored to the tissue and nucleus of interest. For instance, the relaxation

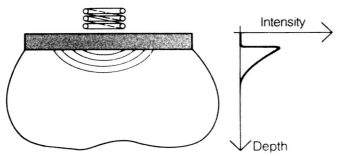

FIGURE 9–32. Schematic representation of the coil set up and coil sensitivity with a FROGS technique. The coil has a typical exponential sensitivity plot; however, the strong surface signal is removed through the use of a saturating slab near the coil. The result is less surface contamination from skeletal muscle and allows an expanded dynamic range for the deeper tissues.

times of a particular nucleus may not be compatible with long, complicated pulse sequences. Using a 140-msec saturation period in a FROGS method on a tissue with a 2200-msec T_1 time will result in a suppression of 1:100, but if the T_1 is only 220 msec then suppression drops to 1:10.[100] CSI is an attractive alternative, but experience has shown that it requires stable gradients with little or no eddy currents along with gradients that can encode rapidly to allow fast sampling of short T_2 species. Also, for reasons of efficient application in a clinical setting, techniques should allow compatibility between the imaging process and spectral localization.

Physiologic motion may require gating methods to shim the B_0 field and acquire data optimally. For example, the beating heart makes it very difficult for a long sequence like ISIS to acquire data, but a

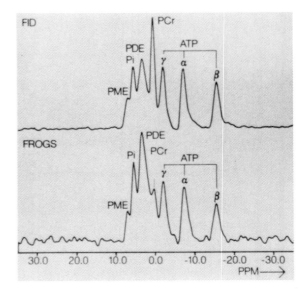

FIGURE 9–34. Clinical demonstration of the FROGS method using surface coil localization on the liver. As expected, the ^{31}P spectrum using the FID technique without saturation demonstrates "contamination" from surface skeletal muscle as there is a pronounced PCr peak. When the FROGS method is used to eliminate this skeletal muscle signal, the ^{31}P spectrum shows a diminished PCr peak.

shorter, simpler method (e.g., FROGS) may provide better results.

The field of spatial localization is an evolving one. It is important when analyzing a clinical problem to survey the current methods (and their many variants) for the strategies that offer the best promise of success.

FAT/WATER IMAGING

The hydrogen nuclei in fat and water have resonance frequencies that differ by approximately 3.3 ppm (Fig. 9–35). As a result, it is possible to construct images that represent the spatial distribution of either fat or water nuclei, or images that demonstrate the presence of both.[101] There are three general approaches for fat/water imaging.

PHASE CONTRAST USING A SPIN-ECHO SEQUENCE

This method uses a spin-echo pulse sequence with a 180-degree RF pulse that is shifted from the middle of the sequence. This method, originally described by Dixon[102] and Sepponen and coworkers,[103] utilizes the fact that fat and water signals can either add (in-phase image) or subtract (out-of-phase or opposed image) depending on the phase of the signal. The difference in signal phase results from the difference in resonance frequencies between fat and water. In a conventional spin-echo pulse sequence, the signals

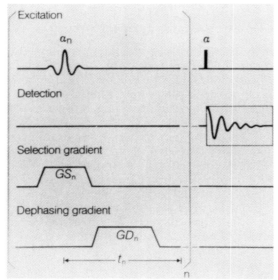

FIGURE 9–33. FROGS pulse sequence showing a typical RF excitation and sampling period prefaced by a presaturating selective pulse.

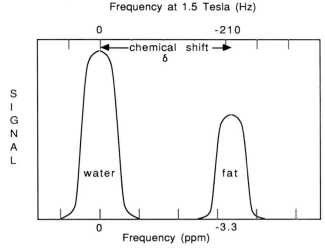

Frequency at 1.5 Tesla (Hz)

FIGURE 9–35. Simplified display of the water and lipid resonances. The water peak in this example is larger due to a higher concentration of nuclei. The lipid resonance is shifted about 3.3 ppm (it is a broad resonance, so that it may be listed in the literature between 3.7 and 3.2). At 1.5 tesla, this frequency (chemical) shift represents about 210 Hz separation between the two.

from fat and water are in phase at the time of signal measurement and add. However, if the 180-degree RF pulse is moved by a time (t), the signals evolve a 180-degree phase difference at the echo time. If fat and water are both present in the voxel, their signals cancel. This value of time (t) depends on the resonance frequency, or field strength, and can be expressed as:

$$t = 1/(2\Delta f)$$

where Δf = difference in resonance frequencies between fat and water. By combining phase and magnitude data from images in which the signals add and subtract, specific water and/or fat images can be produced. However, this method is sensitive to phase errors produced by RF or magnetic field inhomogeneity and can require elaborate schemes to correct for this problem.

Phase Contrast Using a Gradient-Echo Sequence

This method employs a gradient-echo pulse sequence with an echo time selected to cause signals from fat and water protons to either add or cancel (Fig. 9–36).[104] Combinations of gradient-echo images in which these signals add or subtract can be used to produce selective fat or water images.[105]

The basis for this method is given by the chemical shift difference between lipid and water precessional frequencies. At 63 MHz, these lipid and water vectors oscillate with a frequency difference of 210 Hz (63 MHz * 3.3 ppm). Conversely, the period of in-phase and out-of-phase addition and cancellation is 1/210 Hz or 4.77 msec. By varying the TE by one half of a

period (2.38 msec), an in-phase image can be altered to an out-of-phase one, or vice versa.

Frequency-Selective Pulses

The third possibility is to introduce frequency-selective RF pulses to selectively excite or saturate nuclei according to their chemical shift (a method referred to as *che*mically *s*hift *s*elective [CHESS][106] saturation. This sequence works by preceding an imaging sequence with a single frequency saturation pulse to eliminate signals from either fat or water. For proper suppression, this method requires precise alignment of the basic resonance frequency with either the fat or water resonance, as well as requiring a basic main magnetic field with a homogeneity better than 3.3 ppm.

Because they rely on reductions in signal intensity produced by the difference in signal phase between fat and water protons, the first two methods are also called phase-contrast methods. The advantage that fat/water imaging has over other spectroscopic techniques is that fat and water are present in abundant quantities in most tissues. This, in conjunction with the intrinsically high sensitivity provided by the hydrogen nucleus, permits images to be rapidly obtained with high spatial resolution and adequate S/N.

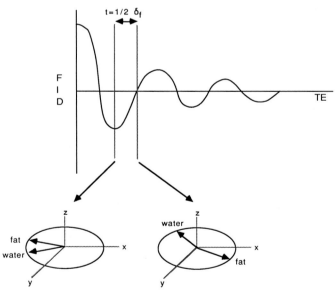

FIGURE 9–36. Schematic representation of the phenomenon of fat/water phase cycling. At time zero (TE = 0), both the fat and water vectors are synchronized in-phase *(bottom diagram)*. At a slightly later time (left hash mark), the two vectors have rotated in the x-y plane such that they are both along the negative direction and they basically add. This results in the strong negative signal at this point in the FID *(top diagram)*. At a time later (right hash mark), the vectors have rotated further along this rotating frame, such that the fat vector is now 180 degrees in opposition to the water vector (i.e., opposed). If both vectors have identical amplitudes, they cancel and a node is produced in the modulation of the FID above. This modulation due to phase addition and cancellation is called phase cycling.

B—Practical Considerations and MR Theory

PRACTICAL IMPLEMENTATION OF CLINICAL SPECTROSCOPY

This section is intended to address practical issues in obtaining clinical spectra on a typical high field MR imaging system. While the actual mechanics and theory for operating a given system are best addressed by that manufacturer's applications and research personnel, a number of topics are generically relevant.

INSTRUMENTATION AND S/N CONSIDERATIONS

In order to use a typical MRI whole body scanner for clinical spectroscopy, most vendors require the installation of additional instrumentation, usually configured as a "spectroscopy" package.

The basic MR imaging system is capable of transmitting and receiving RF pulses, applying gradient pulses, sampling, and Fourier transforming data. However, to study multiple nuclei, different transmitter and receiver frequencies must be available. The same holds true for surface coils. Local (i.e., patient-caused) magnetic field inhomogeneities must be rapidly compensated by shimming. Additionally, specialized pulse sequences and data processing algorithms are needed. And finally, postprocessing of the data requires different filtering and display methods for spectroscopy.

Resonance Frequencies

There is a wide range of gyromagnetic ratios associated with various clinically relevant nuclei. This results in a wide range of resonance frequencies, requiring hardware that can easily switch from proton, for example, to phosphorus. At a typical 1.5-tesla field strength, this means switching between 63 MHz (proton) and 26 MHz (phosphorus) for imaging and spectroscopy. Rapid switching helps in two ways. By quickly alternating between two frequencies, essential steps (i.e., coil tuning and shimming) can proceed rapidly and provide more time for patient data acquisition. Other applications, such as decoupling, require that the system instantaneously switch frequencies (or provide two frequencies).

Multiple resonance frequencies require specific hardware options. The RF transmitter is typically designed to operate over a broad range (10 to 84 MHz) of frequencies. On the receiver side of the RF system, multiple resonance frequencies may not be compatible with high Q coils or narrow bandwidth preamplifiers. To alleviate this limitation, most manufacturers of MR equipment offer coils and preamplifiers tuned to specific resonances (e.g., a sodium head coil or a phosphorus surface coil). These coils are then typically connected to a switching network that ensures a proper signal path between the specific coil and preamplifier. In this configuration, the local, or surface, coil may be used for obtaining spectra, while the larger body coil is used for imaging and aligning the localized volume. Of course, when doing ^1H spectroscopy on an MR imaging system, no additional resonance frequencies are necessary.

Unfortunately, when one coil is used to image or localize and another coil is used for data collection, their respective user-defined volumes of interest can be misaligned. To circumvent this problem, proton images can be made using the spectroscopy coil if the resonances are close (e.g., ^{19}F). More typically, a dual resonance or doubly tuned coil package is used. This package may consist of two coils fixed in relation to each other, each with its own tuning and matching network. Other configurations are possible with this package, including sophisticated electronic switching for rapid frequency changes. In cases in which decoupling is performed, dual resonance coil sets are essential. The usual configuration is that the decoupling coil encompasses a larger volume of interest to ensure a complete decoupling over the measured volume. Since the time between decoupling and measurement is so brief, decoupling experiments normally require a second RF transmitter channel.

Magnetic Field Strength

Given the poor sensitivity, low concentration and low natural abundance of most nuclei of interest for spectroscopy, obtaining adequate S/N becomes a major problem. Similar to MR imaging, increasing the main magnetic field increases the S/N of the spectra. This has been one of the primary reasons for the abundance of clinical studies performed at field strengths of 1.5 tesla and above.

The other primary reason has been that the higher field strengths spread the chemical shift resonances farther apart (in absolute terms), making discrimination easier between nearby resonances (Fig. 9–37). For example, the chemical shift between PCr and PDE is about 3 ppm. At 1.5 tesla this corresponds to a 7.7 Hz shift, while at 4 tesla this is about a 20.6 Hz shift. So, although the shift is constant in ppm, in absolute terms the larger (i.e., 20.6 Hz) difference is easier to discriminate, based on certain sampling constraints (below).

Shimming

Merely increasing magnetic field strength is usually not sufficient to ensure adequate S/N for clinical spectroscopy; care must be taken that field inhomo-

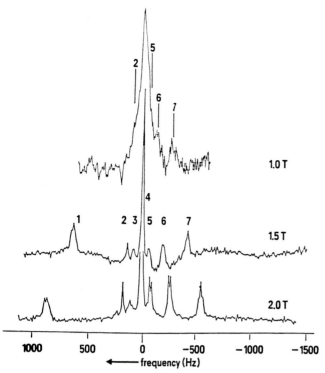

FIGURE 9–37. A comparison of a normal ^{31}P spectrum taken at different field strengths, 1.0, 1.5, and 2.0 T. Note that with the higher field strength, the finer spectral detail is more apparent, and in absolute terms the chemical shift of resonances becomes more separated. Peaks are assigned as: 1, a reference standard; 2, inorganic phosphates (Pi); 3, phosphodiesters (PDE); 4, phosphocreatine (PCr); and 5, 6, 7 are the γ, α, and β-phosphates of ATP.

geneities do not cancel out any improvements. As discussed in greater detail in Equations 5 and 6 further on, field inhomogeneity acts to rapidly disperse the transverse magnetization vectors. The more inhomogeneous the magnetic field, the faster the dispersal occurs and the shorter the effective transverse relaxation time (T_2^*). This shortening of the relaxation time acts on the spectra to broaden the linewidth and reduce the peak height.

As mentioned in Chapter 1, the main field is distorted by the introduction of tissues and their susceptibility properties (e.g., homogeneity of 5 ppm in an empty magnet may worsen to 10 ppm when the patient is introduced). To correct for this problem, the local magnetic field is adjusted to the patient by methodically varying shim settings along the orthogonal axes and along combinations of the axes. This is typically done prior to any measurement of spectra. Since the sensitivity and population of spins other than hydrogen are relatively low, most shimming procedures rely on leaving the frequency of interest and switching to hydrogen (after all, hydrogen and all other nuclei within the sample of interest should be experiencing the same B_0 field). By taking advantage of this very strong signal, shimming is typically done with no averaging of data and may

proceed very rapidly by maximizing the duration of integral of the FID envelope or using Fourier-transformed FIDs (monitoring the peaks directly). The lower limit of B_0 homogeneity is about 0.01 ppm, but in clinical practice patient motion and time constraints may necessitate accepting a lesser level of homogeneity.

Adjustment of the local magnetic field is normally accomplished through varying current amplitudes to a shim coil set within the magnet bore. These shim coils are wound to correct for linear errors along the three orthogonal axes (called first order corrections), for higher order inhomogeneity along the longitudinal (z) axis, and for correction of off axis problems (e.g. x-z, y-z, x-y, or x^2-y^2). The typical commercial shim coil sets available in whole body MR systems contain 13 coil options in all. The simplest, most straightforward, and useful corrections are made using linear corrections along with some z^2 adjustment. These adjustments are made through software controls at the operator's console. This direct software control has made the automation of the shimming procedure an attractive research area.

Finally, in order to compensate for normal physiologic motion during the shimming and data acquisition periods, gating of the spectroscopy sequences is normally available. These gating procedures operate identically to the normal imaging mode, allowing the optimization of the field for specific point(s) during normal physiologic cycles. Gating, when possible, is important when doing studies on the heart, the upper abdomen, or the thorax.

Given that B_0 homogeneity is not perfect and that the excitation pulse may therefore be slightly off-resonance in some parts of the region of interest, another way to improve S/N is by sweeping the excitation over a range or bandwidth of frequencies during the pulse. The process of sweeping the spin frequencies through resonance and back is called *adiabatic fast passage* (AFP)[107] and was originally required for continuous wave MR due to the poor main field stability. Fortunately, with modern spectrometers it is not necessary to fully sweep through resonance and then go back.

Using a slightly more complicated RF pulse, it is possible to rotate the longitudinal magnetization until it precesses primarily along one axis. Once in this position, rotating the B_1 field to align along this axis provides a consistent synchronization of the magnetization. This *spin lock* of the magnetization effectively holds spins in their positions invariant of normal transverse relaxation processes. In practice, this process of modulating the RF excitation has the potential to rotate spins to a similar effective flip angle over a wide range of inhomogeneities. When used to flip spins 90 degrees this process is called *adiabatic half passage* (AHP).[108] AHP pulses are used to produce better S/N in the presence of intrinsic B_1 (e.g., surface coil excitation profiles) and B_0 inhomogeneities. However, the clinical use of these pulses may be limited by RF power deposition restrictions.

Sequence Design

Analogous to MR imaging, the process of designing a spectroscopic measurement requires certain programming capabilities on the spectrometer. Programming functions that would prove useful in spectroscopy include tailoring of the RF pulses, modification of the sampling timing and data processing, and adjustment of gradient timings and amplitudes.

Computer Resources

In MR imaging, there typically is little postprocessing (e.g., filtering, spatial corrections, and so forth) on the acquired data, and a relatively large amount of data (i.e., megabytes) is stored for a complete study. In clinical spectroscopy, the requirements are reversed. Little data are stored (one scan typically represents 1/256 or one line of a high-resolution image), but the postprocessing demands may be high. These demands are not so much for computing power in terms of speed but rather for flexibility and the ability to present data in a number of different formats. Also, since there may be many complicated ways of postprocessing the data, a typical system may have the option to program a procedure, or macro, to repeat a redundant set of instructions.

PATIENT PREPARATION

The physical preparation of the patient for a clinical spectroscopy examination, and the contraindications, are identical to those of MR imaging. Since the spectroscopic examination may be very sensitive to field inhomogeneity, certain prosthetic devices may eliminate a patient from a spectroscopy study when an MR imaging study would be acceptable. In fact, it is a good practice to have prospective MRS patients studied with MRI prior to their spectroscopy examination.

Before entering the patient onto the system, some advance planning may prove beneficial. If the examination requires use of a surface coil, the coil should be placed where its limited volume of coverage will best encompass the suspected lesion. When gravity might prove helpful, the patient's weight can be used to ensure the coil's proximity, for example, having the patient lie prone on a horizontally aligned coil to access the liver.

Once the patient is properly centered in the isocenter and the respective coils are properly tuned and matched, the spectroscopic examination may require additional images. This *base image* localizing procedure is normally accomplished with protons using the larger body coil in a normal imaging mode. Localization may also be part of a complete MR imaging study prior to any spectroscopy testing. Given the wider latitude in magnet homogeneity for imaging, this process may be done before any shimming is necessary.

Since the best homogeneity is near the magnet isocenter, placement of the suspected lesion at this location should give a good initial shim. Also, since the shims tend to act around this isocenter, the process of shimming will proceed more rapidly with the lesion there. Finally, the shimming process may progress more rapidly if previous settings can be recalled from prior examinations using an identical coil on a similar patient location. If no previous settings were saved, a simple shimming optimization prior to studying the patient by using a volunteer may be a propitious use of time.

The procedures used in shimming a volume may vary with systems and operators but are based on the concept of iteratively stepping through shim values along one axis, or option, until a system optimum is achieved. For example, given the variation in patient length, the z-axis shim would be the logical first axis to test. Optimizing the shim along this axis may be accomplished by monitoring the FID waveform as a series of test shim values are sent to the z-axis coils. Since the inhomogeneity will make the FID decay rapidly, one method to monitor this process is by maximizing either the length of FID or the integral under the FID curve.

Unfortunately, this process is complicated by the fact that not all of the nuclei in the area of interest will resonate at precisely the same frequency, so that the FID will appear modulated in its decaying exponential.

Alternatively, a Fourier transform may constantly be applied to the FID stream and the shimming procedure may monitor changes in the peak height and linewidth.

Having optimized along the z-axis, the x-axis, y-axis, or z^2 shim would be a next logical choice. Iteration for these axes would proceed the same as for the z-axis: changing a current value and monitoring the result until an optimized FID or linewidth is found. One important consideration in optimizing these axes when using a B_0 and B_1 localization sequence is that any nonisocenter volume location will change if the RF center frequency is not readjusted to account for the local change in field. This could lead to poor spectral results as the volume of interest is not matched to the area specified in the imaging procedure.

In theory, there should be no interaction between the three orthogonal axes, and there should be no need to constantly recheck the optimization when shimming. However, in practice there is some interaction between shim coils, and so the FIDs (or lineshapes) should be periodically rechecked when altering shim values. Hysteresis of the shim coils may also influence the iteration if identical FIDs (or lines) cannot be reproduced with identical shim coil values. In addition, when higher order shim options or multiaxis parameters are adjusted, the direct interaction between the coils will require even further rechecking and adjustment. For example, if the second, third, or fourth order z-axis shims are adjusted, the first order z-axis shim must be rechecked. Because of this multiparameter optimization, shimming can be a long, tedious procedure or may be patient-limited to a readjustment of only the lower order values. Despite the potential time-consuming nature of the task, optimization of the shim is essential to producing high-quality spectra.

DATA ACQUISITION

As discussed earlier, there are a number of methods to define a volume of interest. Each of the methods in turn requires different sequences for proper application. The selection of a spectroscopy sequence on most commercial MR imaging systems is very similar to the selection of an imaging sequence, allowing a broad range of experiments.

Generic to these sequences are a number of parameters similar to imaging. Items common to both imaging and spectroscopy include repetition time (TR); number of acquisitions or excitations (thousands may sometimes be required for adequate S/N); slice data (including location, size, orientation, angulation, and so forth); echo time (if applicable); along with software switches for gating and automated adjustment of frequency, transmitter power, and receiver gain.

However, additional parameters are used for MRS. For example, when using FIDs with surface coil localization, there needs to be some time between the application of the RF pulse and the initiation of the sampling. Delays in MRS are usually implemented because of the eddy currents or the need for gradient refocusing.

In imaging, the matrix defines the spatial resolution. Similarly, spectroscopy software allows the operator to set the number of points to be sampled. The rate and duration of the sampling have a direct bearing on the resolution of the acquired spectrum. To properly and unambiguously resolve a band of frequencies, one must sample at a rate equal to or exceeding the inverse of the width of the entire spectrum. One half of the total spectral width is referred to as the Nyquist frequency. For example, on a quadrature detection system, to resolve a ± 2.5 kHz (5 kHz total) bandwidth of a ^{13}C spectrum, the time per sample point (dwell time) is the reciprocal of the sampled frequency ($1/5000$ s^{-1}), resulting in a dwell time of 200 microseconds. Owing to a more crowded spectrum, the same system when using protons may require a ± 0.5 kHz bandwidth, or a 1 kHz sampled frequency. In this case, the dwell time would be 1000 microseconds.

Once the digitization rate has been calculated, it is the sampling time (or window) that determines the final resolution of the spectrum. The dwell time multiplied by the number of sample points gives the length of the sampling window. For example, if the FID is digitized for 1 second, this should allow resolution down to 1 Hz. The combination of mod-

erately fast sampling times and the requirement of a reasonably wide sampling window can result in large data sets. Fortunately, the relatively wide lines encountered in in vivo spectroscopy do not have a stringent demand for digital resolution. Therefore, data sets of 1024 or fewer points are usually sufficient.

Of course, it is rare that the signal of the FID will last for even 1 second, so that the late portions of an FID consist primarily of electronic noise. One solution to this problem is to apply a weighting function to the data which takes into account the gradual decay of the FID. Such a matched filter or apodization improves S/N and results in some loss of resolution. If an insufficient number of data points was acquired in the original data, the data may be extended with zeros (zero filling). Zero filling results in a smoother interpolated spectrum. Unfortunately, zero filling does not improve resolution.

Finally, since surface coils are typically used in multinuclear spectroscopy, adjustment of the transmitter is usually done manually, as the automated routines used for imaging may make some improper assumptions. One such assumption is that the system is using a volume coil for excitation. When using a surface coil, those areas nearest the surface will experience a greater change in flip angle than those lying deeper. Therefore, one method of setting the transmitter power levels is to use an anatomic phantom and place the sample of interest at the appropriate distance from the surface of the coil. In this method, power may be adjusted to achieve optimal results at the level of the suspected lesion. Iterative variation of the power level should demonstrate a peak value when the phantom sample experiences a 90-degree flip angle. Of course, it is impossible to duplicate anatomic conditions, so suboptimal flip angles often result from this approach.

DATA POSTPROCESSING

The processing of the acquired signal may be either a simple application of a 1DFT or a complicated one with multiple filtering and correction options. The typical flow of processing for the acquired data proceeds from averaging the acquisitions, to data storage, to filtering of the raw data, through a Fourier transform, and finally, some data analyses and presentation functions. The result of these operations is usually plotted out as a series of processed spectra. The unprocessed data are typically archived along with the results of any further processing.

While improving S/N, the choice of filters for apodization of the data may limit the resolution of the spectra. For example, if an exponential weighting function is used, the elimination of the later higher order components of the time domain signal will reduce the final resolution in the frequency domain. In the case where an exponential function is used which has a decay constant of 36 msec, this would correspond to a line broadening of 9 Hz (i.e., 1/[3.14 times 0.036 seconds]), so that details finer than 9 Hz cannot be resolved.

Since spectroscopy represents the study of RF absorption at specific energies, the data are displayed as *absorption mode* spectra. In this mode, the peak areas are proportional to the number of nuclei generating the peak (assuming equal T_1 and T_2 times). The spectrum is displayed as a series of peaks versus resonance frequencies. The phase of the signal (i.e., sine wave versus cosine wave) is arbitrary. The result is that the Fourier transform is a mixture of the absorption mode and a second mode, known as the *dispersion mode*. To separate these two modes, the transformed spectra are phase corrected to project the spectrum onto the "real" axis. This phase correction may be a simple scalar multiplication (also called zero order correction) or more complex, such as making the phase correction linearly dependent on frequency (known as first order correction). Further corrections are possible to alleviate baseline problems or unwanted noise artifacts. The display of FID signals is also available, but the majority of studies are presented as amplitude/frequency (in ppm or Hz) plots.

When the time course of events is important (for example, studying spectra pre- and postinjection of a flourinated chemotherapy agent), multiple 1DFT spectra may be displayed on one graph. On this graph, successive plots are offset slightly and are stacked along a time axis. These stack plots are useful to demonstrate spectra changes over time (e.g., peak intensities of breakdown products from 5-FU on ^{19}F spectra) and are demonstrated in the preceding clinical section.

MR SPECTROSCOPIC THEORY

HIGH-RESOLUTION MR

The basic theory of MR has been presented in Chapter 1. A brief review will be presented here, with special reference to those ideas pertinent to MRS.

Magnetic Resonance Effect

The study of MR involves interactions with atomic nuclei. Nuclei are composed of protons and neutrons. The hydrogen nucleus, which is the simplest atomic nucleus, consists solely of a proton. Electrons, protons, and neutrons have an inherent angular momentum or spin, which was first suggested by Pauli in the case of electrons and was subsequently verified by Stern and Gerlach. Since these subatomic particles also have a charge distribution in addition to rotational movement, the net result is a magnetic vector, or moment (μ). The maximum observable magnetic moment is given by:

$$\mu = \gamma \, (h/2\pi)I \qquad (1)$$

In this equation, γ is the gyromagnetic ratio, h is a fundamental unit of angular momentum, called Planck's constant, and I is the quantum spin number, or spin. The quantum spin number may vary depending on the nucleus and the isotope measured. In general, a nuclear configuration consisting of an upaired nucleon (a proton or neutron) will have a half-integral spin (^1H, ^{13}C, ^{15}N, ^{19}F, ^{23}Na, ^{39}K, ^{31}P). If there are no unpaired nucleons, a net spin of zero may result (as with the most common isotopes of carbon and oxygen, ^{12}C, ^{16}O), or if there are two or more unpaired nucleons, an integral spin is observed (^2H, ^{14}N).

A nucleus must have a net spin to be observable by MR. Nuclei with a net spin of zero have no net magnetic moment and, therefore, do not give rise to an MR signal. All other nuclei can be observed by MR, although some are more easily examined than others.

In the absence of a magnetic field, all nuclei in the sample will be oriented randomly and there will be no net magnetization. However, if the sample is placed in a magnetic field, B_0 (by convention, the field is aligned with the z-axis of a 3D Cartesian coordinate system), the nuclei will orient themselves relative to the magnetic field (nuclear Zeeman effect). Nuclei precess or revolve about the magnetic field. At any moment in time, the x and y components (those perpendicular to B_0) of the magnetic moment vector for a given nucleus will be nonzero. However, for the sample, the x and y components will be randomly distributed and will generate no net magnetization in these directions. The z (B_0) component of the magnetic moment vector for each nucleus will have a discrete number of orientations that can be observed.

Spin 1/2 nuclei may orient themselves in one of two different orientations, which correspond to two different states (parallel versus antiparallel—i.e., spin up versus spin down, or spin + 1/2 versus spin − 1/2), each of which has a slightly different energy (Fig. 9–38). The energy difference (ΔE) between the two levels is given by:

$$\Delta E = \gamma \, B_0 \, h/2\pi = h\nu \qquad (2)$$

where ν is the frequency of nuclear transition, or resonance frequency, and h is Planck's constant (note that B_0 may be expressed as H_0 in some references).

Several important points arise from Figure 9–38. The energy difference (ΔE) between the two states is very small. The distribution of nuclei between the two states is determined by the Boltzmann equation, which dictates that the relative populations are dependent in an exponential manner on the energy difference between the two states.

$$N_{up}/N_{down} = e^{-\Delta E/kT} \qquad (3)$$

where N_{up} is the number of spins in the upper energy state and N_{down} is the number in the lower energy

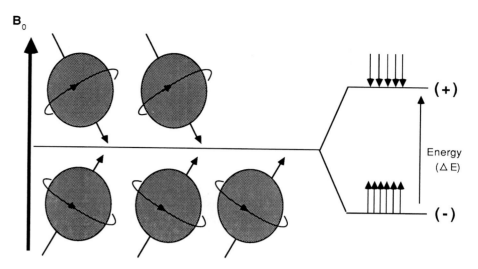

FIGURE 9–38. Nuclei with spin 1/2 (e.g., protons), the magnetic vectors align parallel *(bottom)* or antiparallel *(top)* to the main magnetic field. At higher field strengths, the energy difference between states (ΔE) increases, resulting in a more highly populated parallel state. This quantitatively higher difference in population gives rise to a higher net magnetization and a higher S/N ratio.

state, k is Boltzmann's constant, and T is the sample temperature.

For example, at room temperature with a magnetic field of 10,000 gauss (G) (= 1 tesla), the difference in population between the two spin states corresponds to approximately seven nuclei per two million—a very small difference. Since the MR signal is dependent upon the net difference in nuclei populating the two spin states, it becomes clear that MR is inherently an insensitive technique. Similarly, the energy difference (ΔE) is proportional to B_0, the applied static magnetic field. Increasing the magnetic field strength will result in a larger energy separation between the two spin states and an increased asymmetry in the population, which gives rise to a stronger MR signal.

The third important point that arises from Figure 9–38 is that the energy required to cause the transition, that is, ΔE, is different for each nucleus (i.e., ^1H, ^2H, ^{13}C, and so forth). Table 1–1 demonstrated that in their simplest form, the listed nuclei have unique resonances and provide the possibility of differentiating spins based on frequencies.

The frequency corresponding to the energy difference (ΔE) in Equation 2 is called the resonance or Larmor frequency (ω_L) and represents the frequency that will induce nuclear transitions between the parallel and antiparallel alignments. Equation 2 can therefore be put into a form that is more immediately useful for MR:

$$\omega_L = \gamma B_0 \qquad (4)$$

Taking into account that f (cycles/second) = $\omega/2\pi$ (radians/second), the proton resonance frequency will be 42.6 MHz at a magnetic field of 1.0 tesla.

In and of itself, the steady-state ratio of populations in differing energy states provides no useful information. In order to measure the resonance frequency of a sample and the population of spins at resonance, the equilibrium steady state must be disturbed by applying energy (RF pulses) at the resonance fre-

quencies. Frequencies too far off this resonance will not induce these transitions and thus will not affect the alignment of spins.

The RF energy is supplied to the sample by applying a small oscillating magnetic field, B_1, oriented in the x-y plane perpendicular to the large field, B_0, and, to satisfy Equation 3, oscillating at the Larmor frequency. The RF power (typically a short 5- to 10-msec pulse) is generated in the RF power amplifier and transmitted to a coil surrounding the sample. The coil transmits the RF pulse to the nuclei, which are perturbed from their equilibrium positions along B_0. The same coil, or a different antenna such as a surface coil, can also function as a receiver coil to detect the signals.

Characteristics of the MR Spectrum

The signal obtained from the experiment just described is referred to as an FID (free induction decay) and represents the signal of the nuclei as they return to their steady-state configurations in the magnetic field (the time signal in Fig. 9–39). If a Fourier transformation is applied to the echo or FID signal, an MR spectrum is obtained, as shown by the amplitude versus frequency plot (Fig. 9–39). This MR spectrum is composed of multiple resonance peaks or lines and has three important features:

1. Frequency of the resonance
2. Area under the resonance peak
3. Width of the resonance peak (linewidth)

The resonance frequency is proportional to the gyromagnetic ratio and the local magnetic field experienced by the nucleus. The area under the resonance is proportional to the number of nuclei observed by the coil. The linewidth is inversely proportional to the time constant of decay of the FID (i.e., T_2^*).

The shape of the resonance peak also depends on the shape of the decay of the FID or echo signal. If an exponential decay is observed in the time domain, the lineshape of the resulting resonance in the frequency domain is known

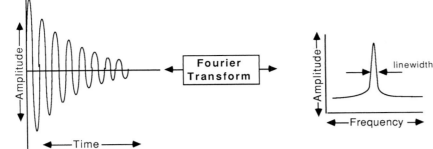

FIGURE 9–39. The process of Fourier transforming an FID into a frequency peak.

as **Lorentzian**. This is the most common lineshape observed in MR spectra.

The relationship between T_2^* and linewidth is:

$$1/T_2^* = \pi\Delta f_{1/2} \qquad (5)$$

where $\Delta f_{1/2}$ is the frequency difference (bandwidth) at one half the peak amplitude. Thus, nuclei in which signals decay rapidly (short T_2^*) are represented by broad lines in the spectrum, whereas more slowly decaying signals produce sharp lines. For example, given a constant number of spins, a T_2^* of 1 msec yields a $\Delta f_{1/2}$ of 300 Hz and a reduced peak amplitude when compared with a slower decaying signal with a T_2^* of 1 sec which has a $\Delta f_{1/2}$ of 0.3 Hz.

Broad linewidths can cause difficulties in measuring spectra because they reduce the peak signal amplitude (remember that the area under the peak depends only on the number of nuclei), making it difficult to distinguish from background noise. Also, with crowded spectral resonances, the line broadening may overlap with data from other nuclear species. One method to reduce line broadening is to locally correct, or shim, for B_0 inhomogeneities that can cause the short T_2^*:

$$1/T_2^* = 1/T_2 + \gamma\Delta B_0 \qquad (6)$$

Equation 6 implies then that as ΔB_0 is reduced toward zero (main field differences over the region of interest reduced to a few ppm or less), the T_2^* should begin to lengthen toward the actual T_2 time, with consequential less line broadening.

Chemical Shift of the Resonance Frequency

Equation 2 suggests that all species of a given nucleus resonate at exactly the same frequency (e.g., protons in water should have the same resonance frequency as protons in fat). However, the strength of the MR technique lies in its ability to determine molecular structure based on subtle differences in resonance frequencies, which are very sensitive to variations in the electronic and nuclear environment of the nucleus being studied. One important way in which this is manifested is by small differences in

resonance frequencies between identical nuclei in slightly different chemical environments. These small differences in resonance frequencies are called *chemical shifts*. One example of this chemical shift is the different resonance frequencies of the protons in water and those in fat (see Fig. 9–35). Another important example is that of the different resonance frequencies of the phosphorus atoms found in ATP.

All atoms contain clouds of electrons surrounding the nucleus. Because the electrons possess a negative charge, they interact with the main magnetic field, B_0. The electron cloud generates a small local magnetic field which subtracts from B_0. Different chemical groups give rise to different electron distributions, so that their nuclei experience slightly different local magnetic fields. These fields are effective only over a short range and affect only nuclei in close proximity to the electron cloud generating the field. Because of the subtractive nature of this magnetic field, the nucleus does not experience B_0, the full magnetic field. B_{eff}, the effective magnetic field felt by the nucleus, can then be written as

$$B_{eff} = B_0 - \sigma B_0 \qquad (7)$$

where B_0 is the induced field arising from the circulating electrons and σ is the shielding constant. Different values of σ are generated by different electron cloud configurations and cause nuclei in different chemical compounds, as well as those at different positions within the same compound, to resonate at slightly different frequencies. These frequencies are determined by replacing B_0 in Equation 4 with B_{eff}.

In order to study and identify the resonances, a reference frequency is established using a substance usually contained within the bandwidth of frequencies and in the selected volume of interest. In high resolution ^{1}H and ^{13}C spectroscopy, a common reference is tetramethylsilane (TMS) (Figs. 9–40 and 9–41), while for ^{31}P biologic samples, the PCr resonance is used (Fig. 9–42). Internal references are preferred because the main B_0 field at the sample may be different from that of an external phantom a short distance away (depending on homogeneity and susceptibility). By using reference compounds, quantitative analysis of these chemical shifts is possible.

The chemical shift of a resonance is defined as the frequency difference between the peak in question (ω_s) and the reference peak (ω_r). There are two ways

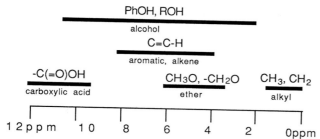

FIGURE 9–40. H-1 chemical shifts of selected function groups referenced to tetramethylsilane (TMS).

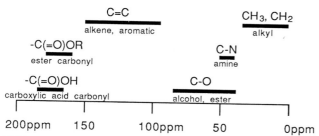

FIGURE 9–41. C-13 chemical shifts of selected function groups referenced to TMS.

to express this frequency difference. One is a direct difference in Hz. For example, the frequency difference between the β-ATP and PCr at 1.0 tesla is 280 Hz. Unfortunately, this frequency difference is field strength dependent, making it difficult to easily compare results from different systems. Alternatively, the chemical shift can be expressed invariant of field strength:

$$\delta = (\omega_s - \omega_r)/\omega_r * 10^6 \qquad (8)$$

This converts the chemical shift (δ) from Hz into a dimensionless scale, parts per million, or ppm. There are several advantages to using the ppm scale, but the primary one is that the δ scale does not depend on the field strength or frequency used. For instance, the β-ATP resonance occurs at −16.3 ppm relative to PCr, at 1.5, 2.0, or 4.0 tesla. It is for this reason that tabulations of chemical shift use ppm.

In addition to being important for adequate S/N, strong magnetic fields are essential for sharp sepa-

ration of the individual spectral lines produced by nuclei with different chemical shifts. If B_0 is doubled, the separation between peaks (chemical shift) also doubles (Equation 7), opening up a crowded spectrum where many compounds may overlap.

J-Coupling, Source of Fine Spectral Details

Under low resolution, the ¹H (proton) MR spectrum of 5 per cent water/95 per cent ethanol consists of three peaks in an area ratio of 1:2:3 corresponding to the OH, CH_2, and CH_3 protons. Under higher resolution, the number of spectral peaks changes. Now the methylene (-CH_2-) and methyl (-CH_3) proton peaks appear as a quartet (four peaks) and a triplet (three peaks) (see Fig. 9–3). Unlike separations due to chemical shift differences, the splitting is found to be *independent* of field strength. The observation of these splitting patterns is explained by assuming that the magnetic field at the nucleus is influenced by the spin arrangements of the protons in adjacent groups. Certain arrangements will slightly increase B_{eff}, whereas others decrease it. This effect, which produces subtle changes in the resonance frequency, is called coupling or J-coupling (where J is a coupling constant of a few Hz, described below).

As discussed above, each proton can have one of two possible alignments with respect to the magnetic field, alignments that will affect the resonances of any bound nuclei. For example, two protons bound to ¹³C can have four possible combinations of spin orientation: ↑↑, ↓↓, ↑↓, ↓↑ (Fig. 9–43A). Two of

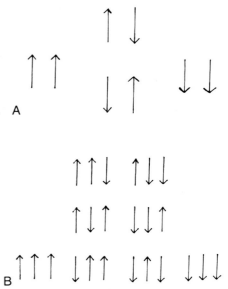

FIGURE 9–43. *A*, Possible spin combinations for the protons of CH_2 group. Note that the middle state is twice as likely to occur since there are two possible spin combinations that give rise to it. The adjacent CH_3 will, therefore, be split into three peaks with area intensities of 1:2:1. *B*, Possible spin combinations for the CH_3 group. There will be four peaks with an area ratio of 1:3:3:1.

FIGURE 9–42. Phosphorus-31 chemical shifts of biologically relevant compounds referenced to phosphocreatine.

these combinations (↑↓   ↓↑) have no net effect and cause no shift in the ^{13}C resonance. The other two states (↑↑ , ↓↓) alter the effective field sensed by the ^{13}C nucleus and shift its resonance by ± J. Given equal probabilities of proton spin orientation, the combination having no net effect should be twice as prevalent as the others. This higher population is observed in the spectra where the central, unshifted resonance is twice as intense as either side resonances, that is, a 1:2:1 intensity ratio.

However, more complex combinations are the rule. For example, ethanol is a two carbon molecule consisting of a methylene group (-CH_2-), a methyl group (-CH_3), and an -OH group. In looking at the methyl group and the effect of its protons on the neighboring methylene group, this peak is divided into three peaks in the same manner discussed above (i.e., 1:2:1). Similarly, the methylene resonance is split into four peaks by the four different spin arrangements possible for the protons on the neighboring methyl group (Fig. 9–43B). The relative intensities of the four methylene peaks are in the ratio of 1:3:3:1. The -OH proton does not cause a splitting, because it is in rapid chemical exchange with the water molecules.

In generalizing for other groups, if a resonance peak undergoes spin-spin splitting due to a number of identical neighboring nuclei, the peak will be split into multiple peaks (or a multiplet).

$$\text{Number of peaks} = 2 N I + 1 \qquad (9)$$

Therefore, from the example above, the hydrogen nuclei attached to the (-CH_3) group will be influenced by the two hydrogen spins on (-CH_2-), so that N (the number of equivalent spins) will be 2, I is 1/2, and the number of lines demonstrated will be three, or a triplet. The intensity ratios of these peaks will be 1:2:1. Similarly, the protons on the methylene group (-CH_2-) will "see" three equivalent spins with I = 1/2 and will be split into four lines (a quartet). The ratios of peak intensities for singlets, doublets, triplets, quartets, and higher numbers of lines with spins of 1/2 can be predicted using Pascal's triangle (Fig. 9–44).

The above example illustrates that from a simple excitation of the sample and some data processing, a great deal of chemical information can be obtained. In addition, specialized pulse sequences have been developed to yield additional information, including relaxation time measurements, saturation transfer experiments, diffusion experiments, and 2D experiments.

Chemical Exchange

If instead of 5 per cent water/95 per cent ethanol, a sample of 100 per cent ethanol is examined, the ^1H spectrum would be different. The -CH_2- resonance would be an octet (eight peaks), or more precisely, a doublet of quartets. This further splitting is due to J-coupling between the -OH and -CH_2- protons. The reason this additional splitting is not

Pascal's Triangle

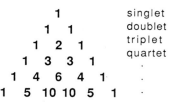

FIGURE 9–44. Pascal's triangle predicts the intensity of each peak within a multiplet. For example, if a single peak splits into a triplet, the three peak intensities will be in a ratio of 1:2:1. Each successive line in the triangle is formed by adding the two numbers found directly above it. However, this system only works for spin 1/2 nuclei.

observed in the 100 per cent ethanol sample is the phenomenon known as chemical exchange.

If a molecule that contains labile or relatively weakly bound protons is placed in aqueous solution, these labile protons will exchange with the water protons:

$$HOH + H^*O\text{-}CH_2\text{-}CH_3 \rightleftharpoons HOH^* + HO\text{-}CH_2\text{-}CH_3$$

Thus, the original hydroxyl proton (H*) now resides on the water molecule and experiences a different chemical shift. Likewise, the original water proton (H) moves to the ethanol molecule where it too experiences a different chemical shift (Fig. 9–45). If the rate of proton transfer or exchange is slow relative to the difference in frequency of the resonances, two separate signals are observed. If the exchange occurs faster than the frequency difference (known as fast exchange), a single resonance is observed. This central resonance occurs at a frequency that is a mean position of the two separate signals. The exact position of this average signal is the weighted average of the two:

$$\omega_a = (\omega_{H2O} N_{H2O} + \omega_{OH} N_{OH}) / (N_{H2O} + N_{OH}) \quad (10)$$

where ω_{H2O} (ω_{OH}) is the frequency of the normal water (OH) resonance, and N_{H2O} (N_{OH}) is the number

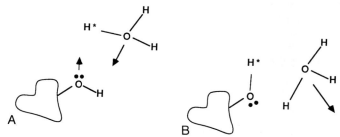

FIGURE 9–45. A simplified view of hydrogen exchange involving alcohol and water. Under acidic conditions (excess H^+), some fraction of water exists as H_3O^+. In this state, one of the hydrogen atoms may be attracted (H* in A) to the oxygen on an alcohol molecule. An exchange ensues, which then frees another hydrogen as the water molecule drifts away. This process is greatly slowed down in nonaqueous systems. This process may be observed in the coupling of hydrogen to a given molecule. In nonaqueous systems, slow exchange leads to coupling as the hydrogen stays in residence longer, and so observed resonances tend to be sharper. In aqueous solutions, faster exchanges occur so the resonances are smeared or shifted depending on the pH.

of water (OH) protons undergoing exchange. At intermediate exchange rates, the two resonances will occur at intermediate positions, depending on the exchange rate and the original separation.

Another effect of the chemical exchange is a variation in the resonance linewidth. At slow exchange rates, an increase in the exchange rate will cause the lines to broaden as they move together. When the resonances merge, an increase in the exchange rate causes the lines to narrow.

In the example of 5 per cent water/95 per cent ethanol, the proton exchange rate is rapid enough so that the water and -OH protons emit a single, narrow resonance. In the case of 100 per cent ethanol, there are no water protons to exchange with, so that the exchange of -OH protons occurs only with other -OH protons on other ethanol molecules. Not only do these protons have the same chemical shift, but the exchange rate is slow enough so that the -OH couples with the $-CH_2-$ protons to induce a doublet of quartets (every combination of $-CH_3$ protons which generates the quartet can see the -OH proton either spin up or spin down). Likewise, the $-CH_2$ protons split the -OH resonance into a triplet.

Two examples of chemical exchange are important in biologic MR. The Pi used as a pH indicator in ^{31}P spectra described above in in vivo studies is actually an exchange narrowed resonance of the $HPO_4^{-2}/H_2PO_4^-$ species:

$$HPO_4^{-2} + H^+ \rightleftharpoons H_2PO_4^-$$

The resonance frequency depends on the exact concentration of HPO_4^{-2} and $H_2PO_4^-$. These depend on the exact pH as described by the equilibrium reaction above. Increasing the pH (decreasing the H^+ concentration) generates more HPO_4^{-2} at the expense of $H_2PO_4^-$ and shifts the Pi resonance away from the PCr resonance. Decreasing the pH increases the $H_2PO_4^-$ concentration and shifts the Pi resonance toward PCr.

The second example involves shortening the relaxation times of water in ^1H spectroscopy or imaging studies. MR imaging contrast agents are molecules that contain unpaired electrons and provide mechanisms for water protons to relax following excitation. In order for these molecules to be effective, the water must be near the unpaired electrons. Once a water molecule relaxes, it must move away so that another molecule can move in and relax. This exchange process must occur fast enough so that a significant fraction of the water protons are relaxed when the signal is detected. Because of the nature of the metal ions used (e.g., Gd^{+3} or Mn^{+2}), the water resonance frequency does not change, but the change in relaxation times can be observed.

RELAXATION TIME MEASUREMENT

After excitation by an RF pulse, the nuclei return to equilibrium at a rate described by two time constants, T_1 and T_2. Because the nuclei return to equilibrium by interacting with their surroundings, the measurement of relaxation times yields information regarding the local interactions of these nuclei. Measurement of T_1 and T_2 time constants is typically done through a series of experiments. The details of these experiments can be found in standard MR textbooks.

T_1 can be measured by a series of inversion recovery experiments (180-degree RF pulse, delay time, 90-degree RF pulse, measure signal) or through a series of saturation recovery sequences (e.g., 90-degree RF pulse, delay time, measure signal, then repeat with varying time delays). Precise measurement of T_1 can be compromised by a number of factors. For example, imperfect RF pulses may produce flip angle variations across the sample. The result will be an incorrect inversion of spins, out-of-plane contamination from adjacent planes, and an unreliable T_1 calibration. Alternately, patient motion or partial volume averaging of multiple tissues may strongly influence T_1 calibrations.

T_2 is typically measured with a long TR, multiecho pulse sequence, for example, CPMG sequence (90-degree RF pulse, wait and encode data, 180-degree RF pulse, measure signal, 180-degree RF pulse, measure signal). Unfortunately, not all T_2 times are sufficiently long to allow multiple spin echos to form before a significant signal loss. For these cases, gradient echo sequences in conjunction with varying RF tip angles may be useful. The use of short TE sequences may allow the study of multiexponential T_2 decay.

Multiexponential decay is observed where multiple spin-spin processes influence the dephasing, so that the measured T_2 is comprised of different components. The ability to separate these components is attractive in that it may offer insight into fast/slow exchange mechanisms and hydration states of proteins. Unfortunately, the study of multiexponential decay requires multiple data points in order to properly resolve the individual time constants. These points may be difficult to obtain when the sample contains very short T_2 times (i.e., less than 5 msec). In addition, unless the short and long T_2 components differ by a factor of 10 or more, it is generally impossible to separate the two components.

MAGNETIZATION TRANSFER— SATURATION AND INVERSION

One important application for biologic MR studies is the measurement of the rate at which different molecules react. If the reacting molecules in question have significantly different chemical shifts, then irradiation of one of the reactants will affect the spin population of the other reactant. Comparison of the unirradiated and irradiated spectra allows the reaction rate to be measured.

Measurement of reaction rates is accomplished

through magnetization transfer experiments. In these, an RF pulse is applied at a precise resonance frequency to excite a single resonance in a spectrum. A clinical example is the study of the ATP reactions. Two types of transfer experiments are possible, depending on the nature of the RF pulse applied.

Saturated nuclei with a random distribution of phase do not produce a signal. If a chemical reaction takes place between a saturated chemical species and another, then the saturated spins are gradually transferred from the first species to the second. As this happens, the amount of signal from the second species or, more specifically, the area under its spectral line decreases. The rate at which the signal decreases is therefore a gauge of the reaction rate between the two species. This technique, known as *saturation transfer*, has been used extensively to measure the reaction rates of phosphorus compounds during metabolic processes[109] (Fig. 9–46).

One problem with saturation transfer is that the measurement of exchange rates is difficult when the T_1 of the peak is very short. When this is true, the peak relaxes before significant change occurs. An improved approach is to use a large flip angle (i.e., 180 degrees) RF pulse to invert one of the peaks. This produces a negative signal for that resonance and provides more range for the exchange measurement. This technique is known as *inversion transfer*.

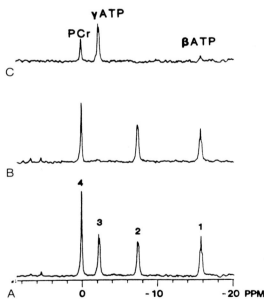

FIGURE 9–46. Phosphorus-31 MR saturation transfer of creatine kinase reaction. Spectra were obtained at 97.2 MHz and represent the sum of 16 acquisitions using a 90-degree pulse (22 msec) and an 8-second cycle time. During the delay between pulses the selective RF irradiation was left on. *A,* A control spectrum with the selective irradiation at 2.5 ppm. *B,* A spectrum with the α-ATP saturated. *C,* The difference of A minus B. Peak assignments are 1, β-ATP; 2, α-ATP; 3, γ-ATP; 4, PCr. (From Koretsky AP, Basus VJ, James TI, et al: Detection of exchange reactions involving small metabolite pools using NMR magnetization transfer techniques: Relevance to subcellular compartmentalization of creatine kinase. Magn Reson Med 2:587–594, 1985.)

In clinical studies, this method is seriously limited by magnetic field inhomogeneity.

DIFFUSION

Diffusion represents the random motion of molecules (also called Brownian motion). In general, small molecules such as water diffuse rapidly, while large molecules such as protein diffuse more slowly. Unlike flow in blood vessels, which is unidirectional, the random nature of diffusional flow produces much smaller average displacements of a molecule. For instance, in one second a water molecule might travel tens of centimeters in a blood vessel, but in the same time would only diffuse a few microns (roughly the diameter of a red blood cell).

Diffusion has been discussed previously in Chapter 4. Briefly, diffusion through a magnetic field gradient produces signal loss due to dephasing. The rate of signal loss depends on the duration and strength of the field gradients as well as on a number called the *diffusion constant*, which relates to how far a molecule will travel on average in one second. For instance, water has a relatively large diffusion constant (10^{-5} to 10^{-6} cm²/sec), and a bulky protein molecule will have a small diffusion constant (e.g., 10^{-6} cm²/sec).[110] The effect of these factors on signal intensity can be expressed as:

$$S \propto exp^{(-bD)} \qquad (11)$$

where D = diffusion constant and b is a factor that depends on the strength of the magnetic field gradients.

Early researchers in this field sought to measure diffusion constants through modification of existing measurement methods. For example, Stejskal and Tanner[111] modified a basic Hahn[112] spin-echo sequence. In this experiment, the diffusion constant calculated was based on the effective T_2, or dephasing, primarily due to diffusion. The sequence was designed such that the observed T_2 had a first order dependence on diffusion and a second order relationship to both the TE and gradient amplitude. Then, through a succession of experiments with differing TEs and/or gradient amplitudes, their effects could be removed and a diffusion constant could be calibrated.

The major clinical relevance of diffusion measurements relates to the restriction of diffusion produced by structures such as protein molecules and cell membranes. Such measurements can characterize the physical environment of a molecule such as water and might prove useful for evaluating disorders in which the physical environment of water molecules is altered, such as edema, neoplasm, and stroke.[113, 114] Unfortunately, in vivo diffusion measurements are extremely sensitive to other kinds of motion, such as blood flow and cerebrospinal fluid (CSF) pulsation. The large, bulk motions produce much larger displacements with correspondingly large phase shifts and associated signal loss, which may preclude obtaining accurate measurements of the diffusion coefficient. Strategies such as flow compensation and cardiac gating are useful for reducing the effects of these bulk motions.[115]

TEMPERATURE MEASUREMENT

Over the range of temperature found in vivo, there is an approximately linear relationship between absolute temperature and tissue T_1 relaxation times. Rapid sequential T_1 measurements provide a potential means for in vivo monitoring of temperature changes during diathermy.[116, 117] However, the method has limited practical application, since inaccuracies in T_1 measurements overwhelm the subtle temperature-dependent changes in T_1. Alternatively, temperature-dependent changes in diffusion coefficients can be evaluated.[117]

TWO-DIMENSIONAL FOURIER TRANSFORM SPECTROSCOPY

Sometimes it can be difficult to distinguish the spectral lines of different nuclear species which have similar resonance frequencies, especially in a crowded spectra. One approach to overcome this is to use higher magnetic field strengths. Another is to use a technique called two-dimensional spectroscopy.

Two-dimensional FT spectroscopy may be simplified to three stages (preparation, evolution, and mixing) leading up to a final detection period. Data are detected over a period t_2 (no relation to the relaxation time T_2), analogous to the sampling period for most spectroscopy sequences. However, prior to the acquisition a perturbation of some sort is applied. This perturbation starts with a preparation period during which an RF pulse creates transverse magnetization. Subsequently, a period of delay (t_1, again no relation to T_1) allows the transverse magnetization to evolve, then a mixing period with a second RF pulse allows transfer of related spins. For a constant t_1, the observed FID over t_2 will produce a spectrum similar to that obtained through ordinary FT spectroscopy. However, if the t_1 is varied as well, then a second FT may be employed to plot a two-dimensional spectrum.[118] The axes for this 2DFT spectrum are plotted as two independent frequencies (v_1, v_2).

In order to reduce confusion between the evolution and detection times and relaxation times, t_1 and t_2 are sometimes referred to as "time 1" and "time 2." A common 2DFT technique is called *correlation spectroscopy* (COSY).[119] Other variants (e.g., NOESY, TOCSY)[120] employ similar data acquisition and processing strategies in combination with different pulse schemes in order to measure other physical quantities.

To illustrate the use of this technique, a ^{13}C decoupling sequence provides a good example. Without any decoupling, the preparation period uses a 90-degree pulse to rotate the magnetization into the transverse plane. Over the evolution period t_1, this magnetization precesses under the influence of the ^{13}C-^1H J-couplings. The mixing period then applies a proton decoupling pulse to remove the proton-caused multiplets. Finally, a simple detection period samples the FID over t_2, and a Fourier transform of the data provides one line of the spectra. Subsequent changes in the t_1 times allow monitoring of further changes in the transverse magnetization over the evolution period (Fig. 9–47).

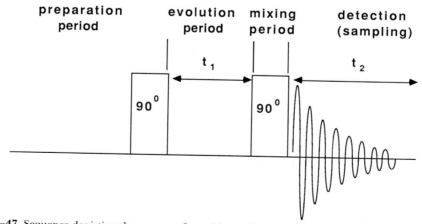

FIGURE 9–47. Sequence depicting the process of acquiring a 2DFT spectrum. During the preparation period, the nuclei are allowed to reach an equilibrium state appropriate for the measurement. This period ends with an RF preparation pulse. The purpose of the pulse is to create transverse magnetization that may "evolve" over the evolution period (t_1). During the evolution period, couplings and other interactions will take place. The mixing period stops this process by applying a second RF pulse to initiate a measurement. Measurement of the signal is accomplished over the detection period (t_2) in a manner similar to sampling for FIDs. The 2D nature of the measurement, which allows separation of chemical shift effects from dipolar effects, is achieved by varying the evolution time over multiple acquisitions.

When plotted, a projection of resonances along the ν_1 axis appears the same as an ordinary coupled spectrum, while a projection of spectra onto the ν_2 axis will look identical to a completely decoupled spectrum. Plotting of the 2DFT spectra may be either a series of stacked plots along the ν_1 axis or a "vertical view" of these stacked plots showing a 2D map with the resonances encircled (a contour plot as demonstrated in Figure 9–48). Projections along either the ν_1 or ν_1 axes are also available. Unfortunately, 2D methods are impractical for clinical MRS at the present time.

QUADRUPOLAR NUCLEI

Several nuclei of physiologic interest have spin greater than 1/2. These nuclei are referred to as *quadrupolar*, meaning that the nucleus has an electric

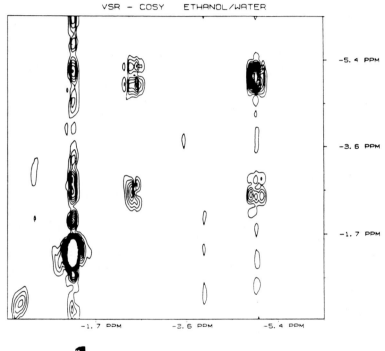

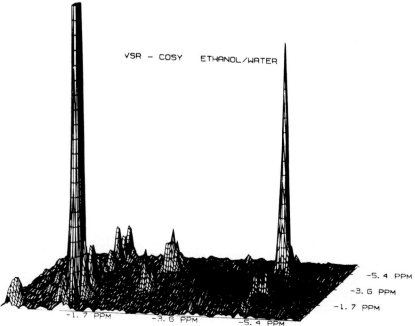

FIGURE 9–48. Two methods for displaying a 2D contour plot from an analysis of ethanol and water using a localized correlation spectroscopy experiment (COSY). Prominent features are a water peak at $(-1.47, -1.47)$, a CH_2 peak at $(-2.46, -2.46)$, and a CH_3 peak at $(-5.03, -5.03)$. (From McKinnon GC, Boisiger P: Localized double-quantum filter and correlation spectroscopy experiments. Magn Reson Med 6:334–343; with permission.)

quadupole moment, as well as a magnetic dipole. There are two main effects observed with the higher spin numbers. The first effect is that the nuclear energy states have three or more possibilities; in the case of spins of 1/2, only two states (up and down) are possible. The relationship between I, the spin number, and the number of energy states may be generalized to state that the possible energy states produced is $2I + 1$. There are two consequences of having multiple energy states. First, there may be multiple resonance frequencies for a given nucleus and environment. These resonances depend on the energy of transition between different levels, which may or may not be equally spaced. For instance, sodium has the possibility of multiple resonance frequencies. However, these have never been observed in physiologic conditions and may be ignored. The second consequence is the possibility that multiple relaxation times may exist (nonexponential relaxation), even when that system is a homogeneous pool of nuclei. In contrast, with protons, which have spins of 1/2, multiple relaxation times imply multiple states of the protons.

The second main effect of the quadrupolar moment of the nuclei is the presence of a strong mechanism for relaxation. This mechanism is the interaction of the quadrupolar moment with the local electric field gradients and tends to be a much stronger mechanism than the dipolar relaxation observed in proton MR. Therefore, quadrupolar nuclei, such as sodium, tend to have very short relaxation times (on the order of a few milliseconds), while the dipolar nuclei (e.g., protons) may have relaxation times of several hundred milliseconds to several seconds. This fast relaxation leads to technical difficulties, primarily in the ability to rapidly acquire data before the signal has decayed. Also, the short T2s for these nuclei cause the linewidth to be much broader than for dipolar nuclei (Equation 6). If the relaxation time is so fast that the nuclei are relaxed before data acquisition, or if the signal is acquired but the resulting resonance is so broad that it is lost in the spectrum, the signal is referred to as being MR invisible, as mentioned previously for intracellular sodium.

The problem of short relaxation times is exacerbated in localized spectroscopy or imaging studies in which multiple pulses are used (i.e., allowing more time for nuclei to relax) and/or where physical gradient eddy current limitations restrict the time available for data acquisition. However, these shorter relaxation times (specifically the T_1 time) have a distinct advantage in that they allow very rapid repetition times with minimal saturation of the signal (e.g., 100 msec). This high data acquisition rate may help compensate for the intrinsic lower sensitivity of these nuclei. In addition, because the T_2^* is a function of this short T_2 time, the linewidth is less sensitive to the magnet inhomogeneity. This means that the shim is not quite as critical for sodium as for high resolution hydrogen or phosphorus spectroscopy.

SOLVENT SUPPRESSION FOR RESOLVING ^{1}H SPECTRA

In examining weak proton signals, for example, from amino acids or lactic acid, the signal of interest may be hundreds or thousands of times smaller than that of water or fat. In fact, the difference in signal strength between water and the metabolites may be as great as 10,000 to one. This presents a problem in clinical setting, since most systems cannot discriminate the small signals, given that the digital conversion in the receiver may be limited to one part in 4000 (See Chapters 10 and 11). The accepted solution to this limitation involves eliminating the unnecessary large signals (i.e., fat and water) in order to better resolve small signals. These methods may take advantage of the chemical shift difference between signals of interest and use a sharp resonance frequency to first saturate, or remove, the large signals. At that point, a measurement sequence is used to detect the remaining small signals. This process of eliminating the large, unnecessary signals is typically called solvent suppression and has various alternate strategies.

T_2 Decay

The simplest technique exploits the short T_2 of water protons in tissues relative to certain other metabolites such as lactate (30 to 60 msec compared with more than 100 msec) to separate the signals of water from others. Collection of a signal after a long echo delay (80 msec), by which time most of the water signal has decayed, leads to spectra with appreciable signal from metabolites and a much reduced water signal.

Binomial Suppression

An alternative technique is to selectively avoid exciting the water resonance. The transmitter frequency is set at the water resonance frequency, and the pulse sequence delivers a tailored pulse that avoids exciting the water resonance. The net effect is that resonances to the low- and high-frequency sides of water will be excited but not water (Fig. 9–49A versus Fig. 9–49B). These pulse sequences consist of a series of pulses of duration equal to the coefficients of binomial expansion (i.e., $1\bar{1}$ and $1\bar{3}3\bar{1}$ where the bar refers to a 180-degree phase shift). Generally, the total pulse length of $1\bar{3}3\bar{1}$ is chosen such that the total of pulse lengths $(1 + 3 + 3 + 1)$ adds up to a 90-degree pulse. A $2\bar{6}6\bar{2}$ that is a 180-degree pulse can also be used so that selective excitation can be coupled with the spin-echo technique.

Selective Saturation

Selective saturation, analogous to the CHESS method for in vivo fat/water separation, employs an RF pulse with a frequency exactly equal to that of

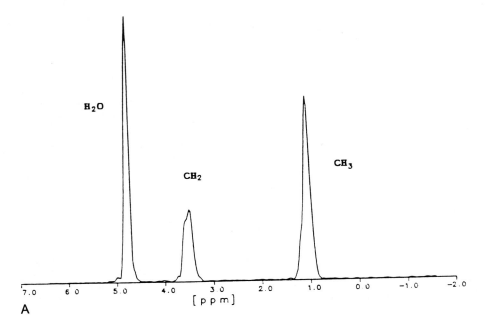

A

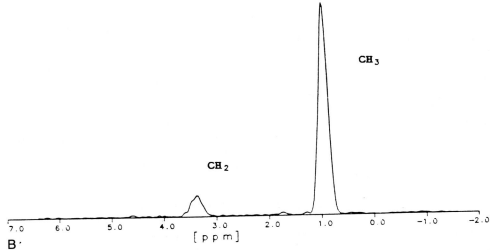

B

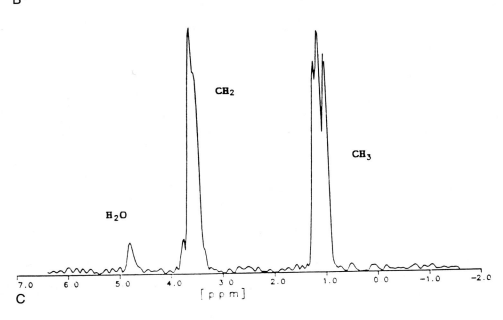

C

FIGURE 9–49. *A,* Localized spectrum obtained with a block excitation 90-degree RF pulse at 1.5 tesla, on a 200 ml phantom of 20 per cent ethanol and 80 per cent water. Note the presence of a very strong water peak. *B,* Localized spectrum obtained with a binomial ($1\bar{3}3\bar{1}$) excitation pulse on the same phantom. Note the ability of the pulse to suppress the water resonance (on the order of 400), but at the expense of also reducing the peak amplitude of nearby resonances, that is, CH_2. *C,* Localized spectrum obtained with a double-quantum filter excitation sequence with identical conditions as *B.* Note that the water signal has been suppressed by a factor of 100, while the nearby CH_2 resonance is not suppressed. (From McKinnon GC, Boisiger P: Localized double-quantum filter and correlation spectroscopy experiments. Magn Reson Med 6:334–343, 1988; with permission.)

water. However, in this case, a low energy pulse lasting a few milliseconds is used. This pulse excites a relatively narrow spectral region (i.e., the bandwidth is proportional to the inverse of the pulse length), and the low power helps limit local heating. Since water takes milliseconds to regain magnetization, this pulse saturates the water protons and allows a subsequent short duration, high bandwidth pulse to excite all other protons. This method is effective because the second pulse is applied before water regains its equilibrium magnetization and contributes to the measured signal.

Multiple Quantum Filtering

The peaks from different proton species are so crowded that in vivo ^1H MR spectra can become very complex. Furthermore, the chemical shift range in proton spectra is relatively limited, unlike ^{31}P and ^{13}C spectra (see Figs. 9–40 to 9–42), and the spectrum is further complicated by the fact that complex molecular interactions in vivo widen the widths of peaks relative to those obtained in typical solution MR. These problems lead to a significant limitation on the information content of the spectra. The use of spectral editing techniques and multiple quantum filters, which allows one to selectively monitor specific peaks, will limit the number of peaks that can be monitored but yields better defined spectra (Fig. 9–49C). The multiple quantum filtering technique relies on the J-coupling that occurs between different proton species. By applying multiple RF pulses with appropriate timings (analogous to the COSY experiment above) and appropriate cycling of the phases of the RF pulses, only signal from proton species that have certain J-coupling interactions, called double quantum coherence, is maintained. Lacking J-coupling, that is, without double quantum coherences, signal from water is suppressed.

REFERENCES

1. Spectroscopy Labeling Guidelines—Draft Standard 1989. Washington, DC, National Electrical Manufacturers Association (NEMA), 1989.
2. Edwards RHT, Dawson MJ, Wilkie DR, et al: Clinical use of NMR in the investigation of myopathy. Lancet 1:725–731, 1982.
3. Moon RB, Richards JH: Determination of intracellular pH by ^{31}P magnetic resonance. J Biol Chem 248:7226, 1973.
4. Chance B, Eleff S, Bank W, et al: ^{31}P NMR studies of control of mitochondrial function in phosphofructokinase-deficient human skeletal muscle. Proc Natl Acad Sci USA 79:7714–7718, 1982.
5. Radda GK, Bore PJ, Rajagopalan B: Clinical aspects of ^{31}P NMR spectroscopy. Br Med Bull 40:15–159, 1983.
6. Radda GK, Taylor DJ, Arnold DL: Investigation of human mitochondrial myopathies by phosphorous MRS. Biochem Soc Trans 13:654, 1985.
7. Hands L, Bore P, Galloway G, et al: ^{31}P NMR of calf muscle in peripheral vascular disease. Abstracts of the Society for Magnetic Resonance in Medicine. New York, 1984, pp 297–298.
8. Taylor DJ, Crow M, Bore PJ, et al: Examination of the

energetics of aging skeletal muscle using NMR. Gerontology 30:2–7, 1984.
9. Griffiths RD, Edwards RHT: The biomedical applications of spectroscopy and spectrally resolved imaging. In Wehrli FW, Shaw D, Kneeland JB (eds): Biomedical MR Imaging, Principles, Methodology and Applications. New York, VCH Publishers, 1988, p 526.
10. Ross BD, Radda GK, Gadian DG, et al: Examination of a case of suspected McArdle's syndrome by ^{31}P NMR. N Engl J Med 304:1338, 1981.
11. Edwards RHT, Dawson MJ, Wilkie DR, et al: Clinical use of NMR in the investigation of myopathy. Lancet 1:725, 1982.
12. Ross BD, Radda GK: Application of ^{31}P NMR to inborn errors of metabolism. Biochem Soc Trans 11:627, 1983.
13. Radda GK, Bore PJ, Gadian DG, et al: ^{31}P NMR examination of 2 patients with NADH-CoQ reductase deficiency. Nature 295:608, 1982.
14. Radda GK: The use of NMR spectroscopy for the understanding of disease. Science 233:640–645, 1986.
15. Donlon E, Lawson B, Guillet R, et al: ^{31}P NMR studies of cerebral metabolism in healthy human neonates. Abstracts of the Society for Magnetic Resonance in Medicine. London, 1985, pp 713–714.
16. Ackerman JJH, Grove TH, Wong GG, et al: Mapping of metabolites in whole animals by ^{31}P NMR using surface coils. Nature 283:167–170, 1980.
16a. Delpy DT, Gordon PE, Hope PL, et al: Noninvasive investigation of cerebral ischemia by phosphorus NMR. Pediatrics 70:310–313, 1982.
17. Behar KL, Prichard JW, Petroff OAC, et al: Acid-base disturbances in the brain and their relationship to the creatine kinase reaction. An in-vivo ^{31}P NMR study. Magn Reson Med 1:101–102, 1984.
18. Hope PL, de L Costello AM, Cady EB, et al: Cerebral energy metabolism studied with phosphorous NMR spectroscopy in normal and birth-asphyxiated infants. Lancet 2:366–370, 1984.
19. Younkin DP, Delivora-Papadopoulis M, Leonard JC, et al: Unique aspects of human cerebral metabolism evaluated with phosphorous NMR spectroscopy. Ann Neurol 16:581–586, 1984.
20. Chance B, Leigh JS, Nioka S, et al: An approach to the problem of metabolic heterogeneity in brain. Ann NY Acad Sci 508:309–320, 1987.
21. Wyrwicz AM, McNeil A, Gregory GA, et al: Effects of severe hypoxia on cerebral phosphate levels in neonatal rabbits. Abstracts of the Society for Magnetic Resonance in Medicine. London, 1985, pp 297–298.
22. Cady EB, de L Costello Am, Dawson JM, et al: Non-invasive investigation of cerebral metabolism in newborn infants by phosphorous NMR. Lancet 1:1059–1062, 1984.
23. Levine SR, Welch KMA, Helpern JA, et al: Clinical investigation of ischemic stroke by serial ^{31}P NMR spectroscopy. Abstracts of the Society for Magnetic Resonance in Medicine. New York, 1987, p 536.
24. Smith DS, Kioka S, Subramanian HV: Brain high energy metabolites and EEG power during and after an episode of profound hypoxia. Abstracts of the Society for Magnetic Resonance in Medicine. New York, 1984, pp 546–547.
25. Melamed E: Reactive hyperglycemia in patients with acute stroke. J Neurol Sci 29:267–275, 1976.
26. Woo E, Ma JTC, Robinson JD, et al: Hyperglycemia is a stress response in acute stroke. Stroke 19:1359–1363, 1988.
27. Chopp M, Welch KMA, Tidwell CD, Helpern JA: Global cerebral ischemia and intracellular pH during hyperglycemia and hypoglycemia in cats. Stroke 19:1383–1386, 1988.
28. Fossel ET, Morgan HE, Ingwall JS: Measurements of changes in high-energy phosphates in the cardiac cycle by using ^{31}P NMR. Proc Natl Acad Sci USA 77:3654, 1980.
29. Koretsky AP, Wang S, Murphy-Boesch J, et al: ^{31}P NMR spectroscopy of rat organs, in situ, using chronically implanted radiofrequency coils. Proc Natl Acad Sci USA 80:7491, 1983.

30. Whitman GJ, Chance B, Bode H, et al: Diagnosis and therapeutic evaluation of a pediatric cardiomyopathy using ^{31}P NMR. J Am Coll Cardiol 5:745–749, 1985.

31. Ingwall JS, Kobayashi K, Bittl JA: Phosphorous NMR of cardiac and skeletal muscles. Am J Physiol 242:H729, 1982.

32. Bottomley PA, Smith LS, Brazzamano S, et al: The fate of inorganic phosphate and pH in regional myocardial ischemia and infarction: A noninvasive ^{31}P NMR study. Magn Reson Med 5:129–142, 1987.

33. Ross BD, Higgins RJ, Conley FK, et al: ^{31}P NMR spectroscopy of an experimentally induced intracerebral tumor in mice. Magn Reson Med 4:323–332, 1987.

34. Karczmar GS, Poole J, Boska MD, et al: ^{31}P MRS study of response of human tumors to therapy. Abstracts of the Society for Magnetic Resonance in Medicine. San Francisco, 1988, p 615.

35. Semmler W, Gademan G, Bachert-Bauman P, et al: Monitoring human tumor response to therapy by means of ^{31}P MRS. Radiology 166:533–539, 1988.

36. Heindel W, Bunke J, Glathe S, et al: Combined ^{1}H MR imaging and localized ^{31}P spectroscopy of intracranial tumors in 43 patients. J Comput Assist Tomogr 12:907–916, 1988.

37. Shoubridge EA, Arnold DL, Emrich JF, et al: Phosphorous MRS and characterization of astrocytomas, meningiomas and pituitary adenomas. Abstracts of the Society for Magnetic Resonance in Medicine. San Francisco, 1988, p 616.

38. Seegbarth CM, Baleriaux DF, Arnold DL, et al: Image guided ^{31}P spectroscopy in the evaluation of brain tumor treatment. Radiology 165:215–219, 1987.

39. Ng TC, Vijayakumar S, Majors AW, et al: Response of non-Hodgkins lymphoma to Co-60 therapy monitored by ^{31}P in situ. Int J Radiat Oncol Biol Phys 13:1545–1551, 1987.

40. Maris JM, Evans AE, McLaughlin AC, et al: ^{31}P NMR spectroscopic investigation of human neuroblastoma in situ. N Engl J Med 312:1500–1505, 1985.

41. Wismer GL, Rosen BR, Buxton R, et al: Chemical shift imaging of bone marrow: Preliminary experience. AJR 145:1031–1037, 1985.

42. Paling MR, Brookeman JR, Mugler JP: Tumor detection with phase contrast imaging: An evaluation of the clinical potential. Radiology 162:199–203, 1987.

43. Frahm J, Bruhn H, Gyngell ML, et al: Localized high-resolution proton NMR spectroscopy using stimulated echos: Initial application to human brain in vivo. Magn Reson Med 9:79–93, 1989.

44. William SR, Gadian DG, Prouter E, et al: Proton NMR studies of muscle metabolites in vivo. J Magn Reson 63:406–412, 1985.

45. Bruhn H, Frahm J, Gyngell ML, et al: Cerebral metabolism in man after acute stroke: New observations using localized proton NMR spectroscopy. Magn Reson Med 9:126–131, 1989.

46. Bruhn H, Frahm J, Gyngell ML, et al: Localized proton spectroscopy of tumors in vivo: Patients with primary and secondary cerebral tumors. Abstracts of the Society for Magnetic Resonance in Medicine. San Francisco, 1988, p 253.

47. Mountford CE, Saunders JK, May GL, et al: Classification of human tumors by high-resolution MR. Lancet 1:651–653, 1986.

48. Luyten PR, Segebarth C, Baleriaux D, den Hollander JA: ^{1}H NMR spectroscopic examination of human brain tumors in situ at 1.5 T. Abstracts of the Society for Magnetic Resonance in Medicine. San Francisco, 1988, p 971.

48a. Bruhn H, Frahm J, Gyngell ML, et al: Noninvasive differentiation of tumors with use of localized H-1 MR spectroscopy in vivo: Initial experience in patients with cerebral tumors. Radiology 172:541–548, 1989.

48b. Mountford CE, Wright LC: Organization of lipids in the plasma membranes of malignant and stimulated cells: A new model. Trends Biochem Sci 13:172–177, 1988.

49. Mariappan SVS, Subramanian S, Chandrakumar N, et al: Proton relaxation times in cancer diagnosis. Magn Reson Med 8:119–128, 1988.

50. Medina D, Hazelwood CF, Cleveland GG, et al: NMR studies on human breast dysplasias and neoplasms. J Natl Cancer Inst 54:813, 1975.

51. Beall PR, Hazelwood CF: Distinction of the normal, preneoplastic and neoplastic states by water proton NMR relaxation times. In Partain CL, Price RR, Patton JA, et al (eds): MRI: Physical Principles and Instrumentation. Philadelphia, WB Saunders Company, 1988.

52. Fossel ET, Carr JM, McDonagh J: Detection of malignant tumors. Water-suppressed proton nuclear magnetic resonance spectroscopy of plasma. N Engl J Med 315:1369, 1986.

53. Eskelinen S, Hiltunen Y, Jokisaari J, et al: ^{1}H NMR studies of human plasma from newborn infants, healthy adults and adults with tumors. Magn Reson Med 9:35–38, 1989.

54. Chmurny GN, Hilton BD, Halverson D: An NMR blood test for cancer: A critical assessment. NMR Biomed 3:136–150, 1988.

55. Cohen SM: C-13: NMR spectroscopy. In Partain CL, Price RR, Patton JA, et al (eds): Magnetic Resonance Imaging: Physical Principles and Instrumentation. Philadelphia, WB Saunders Company, 1988, p 1521.

56. Jue T, Shulman GI, Alger JR, et al: Future applications of high resolution NMR to liver metabolism. Abstracts of the Society for Magnetic Resonance in Medicine. London, 1985, pp 6–7.

57. Sillerud LO, Halliday KR, Griffey RH, et al: In vivo ^{13}C NMR spectroscopy of the human prostate. Magn Reson Med 8:224–230, 1988.

58. Cope FW: NMR evidence for complexing of sodium ions in muscle. Proc Natl Acad Sci USA 54:225–227, 1965.

59. Ra JB, Hilal SK, Cho ZH: A method for in vivo MRI of the short T2 component of sodium-23. Magn Reson Med 3:296–392, 1986.

60. Foy B, Burstein D: Measurement of interstitial ^{23}Na relaxation in perfused rat hearts. (Submitted.)

61. Chu SC, Pike MM, Fossel ET, et al: Aqueous shift reagents for high resolution cationic nuclear magnetic resonance III Dy (TTHA)$^{3-}$, TM (TTHA)$^{3-}$, and Tm (PPP)$_2$$^{7-}$. J Magn Reson 56:33–47, 1984.

62. Hilal SK, Fabry M, Segebarth C, et al: In vivo and in vitro chemical shift imaging of sodium. Proc Soc Magn Reson Med 1984, p 322.

63. Narayana PA, Kulkarni MV, Mehta SD: NMR of 23Na in biological systems. In Partain CL, Price RR, Patton JA, et al (eds): Magnetic Resonance Imaging. Vol II. Philadelphia, WB Saunders Company, 1988, pp 1553–1561.

64. Summers RM, Joseph PM, Renshaw PF, Kundel HL: Dextran-magnetite: A contrast agent for sodium-23 MRI. Magn Reson Med 8:427–439, 1988.

65. Turski P, Perman WH, Halt JK, et al: Clinical and experimental vasogenic edema: In vivo sodium MR imaging. Work in progress. Radiology 160:821–825, 1986.

66. Hilal SK, Maudsleu AA, Ra JB, et al: Imaging of sodium-23 in the human head. J Comput Assist Tomogr 9:1–7, 1985.

67. Garner WH, Hillal SK, Lee S, Spector A: Na-23 MRI of the eye and lens. Proc Natl Acad Sci USA 83:1901–1905, 1986.

68. Semmler W, Bachert-Bauman P, Guckel F, et al: Noninvasive monitoring of the 5-fluorouracil catabolism and anabolism in patients by means of ^{19}F MRS: Comparison of intraarterial and intravenous administration. Abstracts of the Society for Magnetic Resonance in Medicine. San Francisco, 1988, p 258.

69. Wolf W, Presant CA, Albright MJ, et al: ^{19}F NMR of 5-FU as a method for noninvasive monitoring of drug targeting and delivery. Abstracts of the Radiological Society of North America. Chicago, 1988, p 84.

70. Eidelberg D, Johnson G, Barnes D, et al: ^{19}F NMR imaging

of blood oxygenation in the brain. Magn Reson Med 6:344–352, 1988.

71. McFarland E, Koutcher JA, Rosen BR, et al: In vivo ^{19}F NMR imaging. J Comput Assist Tomogr 9:8–15, 1985.

72. Thomas SR, Clark LC, Ackerman JL, et al: MRI of the lung using liquid perfluorocarbons. J Comput Assist Tomogr 10:1–9, 1986.

73. Burstein D, Litt HI, Fossel ET: NMR characterization of "visible" intracellular myocardial potassium in perfused rat hearts. Magn Reson Med 9:66–78, 1989.

74. Hopkins AL, Haacke EM, Barr RG, et al: Oxygen-17 alteration of brain contrast: Rapid sequential monitoring with FISP. Abstracts of the Society for Magnetic Resonance in Medicine. San Francisco, 1988, p 224.

75. Komoroski RA, Newton J, Walker E, et al: Lithium-7 in vivo NMR spectroscopy of rats and humans. Abstracts of the Society for Magnetic Resonance in Medicine. San Francisco, 1988, p 57.

76. Balaban RS, Knepper MA: Nitrogen-14 NMR spectroscopy of mammalian tissues. Am J Physiol 245:C439, 1983.

77. Damadian R, Minkoff L, Goldsmith M, et al: Field focusing NMR (FONAR): Visualization of a tumor in a live animal. Science 194:1430–1432, 1976.

78. Gordon RE, Hanley PE, Shaw D, et al: Localization of metabolites in animals using P-31 topical magnetic resonance. Nature 287:367–368, 1980.

79. Hahn EL: Spin echoes. Physiol Rev 80:580, 1950.

80. Frahm J, Merboldt KD, Hanicke W: German patent offenlegunggschrift P 34 45 689.9. (Priority: December 14, 1984.)

81. Frahm J, Bruhn H, Gyngell ML, et al: Localized high-resolution proton NMR spectroscopy using stimulated echos: Initial application to human brain in vivo. Magn Reson Med 9:79–93, 1989.

82. Ordidge RJ: Localized chemical shift measurements in phosphorous and protons. Abstracts of the Society for Magnetic Resonance in Medicine. London, 1985, pp 131–132.

83. Matson GB, Twieg DB, Karczmar GS, et al: Application of image-guided surface coil P-31 MR spectroscopy to human liver, heart, and kidney. Radiology 169:541–547, 1988.

84. Connelly A, Counsell C, Lohman JAB: Outer volume suppressed image related in vivo spectroscopy (OSIRIS), a high sensitivity localization technique. Magn Reson Med 78:519–522, 1988.

85. Luyten PR, den Hollander JA: ^{1}H MR spatially resolved spectroscopy of human tissues in situ. Magn Reson Imaging 4:237, 1986.

86. Brown TR, Kincaid B, Ugurbil K: NMR chemical shift imaging in three dimensions. Proc Natl Acad Sci USA 79:3523, 1982.

87. Bottomley PA: Human in vivo NMR spectroscopy in diagnostic medicine: Clinical tool or research probe? Radiology 170:1–15, 1989.

88. Cox IJ, Sargentoni J, Calam J, et al: Four-dimensional phosphorous-31 chemical shift imaging of carcinoid metastases in the liver. NMR Biomed 1:56–60, 1988.

89. Brown TR, Buchthal SD, Murphy-Boesch J, et al: Chemical shift imaging at 1.5 tesla. Abstracts of the Society for Magnetic Resonance in Medicine. San Francisco, 1988, p 707.

90. Bottomley PA, Charles HC, Roemer PB, et al: Human in vivo phosphate metabolism imaging with ^{31}P. Magn Reson Med 7:319–336, 1988.

91. Hoult DI: Rotating frame zeumatography. J Magn Reson 33:183–197, 1979.

92. Ackerman JJH, Grove TH, Wong, GG, et al: Mapping of metabolites in whole animals by P-31 using surface coils. Nature 283:167–170, 1980.

93. Hanstock CC, Lunt JA, Allen PS: The modification of the RF field distribution of surface coils by weakly conducting saline samples. Magn Reson Med 7:204–209, 1988.

94. Thulborn KR, Ackerman JJH: Absolute molar concentrations by NMR in inhomogeneous B1. A scheme for analysis of in vivo metabolites. J Magn Reson 55:357–371, 1983.

95. Bendall MR, Gordon RE: Depth and refocusing designed for multipulse NMR with surface coils. J Magn Reson 53:365–385, 1983.

96. Aue WP: Localization methods for in vivo NMR spectroscopy. Rev MR Med 1:21–72, 1986.

97. Bendall MR, Gordon RE: Depth and refocusing pulses designed for multipurpose NMR using surface coils. J Magn Reson 53:365, 1983.

98. Bottomley PA, Foster TB, Darrow RD: Depth resolved surface coil spectroscopy (DRESS) for in-vivo ^{1}H, ^{31}P, and ^{13}C NMR. J Magn Reson 59:338–342, 1984.

99. Sauter R, Mueller S, Weber H: Localization in in vivo ^{31}P NMR spectroscopy by combining surface coils and slice-selective saturation. J Magn Reson 75:167–173, 1987.

100. Sauter R, Mueller S, Weber H: Localization in in vivo ^{31}P NMR spectroscopy by combining surface coils and slice-selective saturation. J Magn Reson 75:167–173, 1987.

101. Haacke EM, Patrick JL, Lenz GW, Parrish TR: The separation of water and lipid components in the presence of field inhomogeneities. Rev Magn Reson Med 1:123–154, 1986.

102. Dixon WT: Simple proton spectroscopic imaging. Radiology 153:189, 1984.

103. Sepponen RE, Sipponen JT, Tanttu JI: A method for chemical shift imaging: Demonstration of bone marrow involvement with proton chemical shift imaging. J Comput Assist Tomogr 8:585, 1984.

104. Edelman RR, Buxton RB, Brady TJ: Rapid MR imaging. In Kressel HY (ed): Magnetic Resonance Annual 1988. New York, Raven Press, 1988, pp 189–216.

105. Szummowski J, Plewes DB: Fat suppression in the time domain in fast MR imaging. Magn Reson Med 8:345–354, 1988.

106. Haase A, Frahm J, Haenicke W, Matthei D: ^{1}H NMR chemical shift selective (CHESS) imaging. Phys Med Biol 30:341–344, 1985.

107. Silver MS, Joseph RI, Hoult DI: Highly selective $\pi/2$ and π pulse generation. J Magn Reson 59:347, 1984.

108. Bendall MR, Pegg D: Uniform sample excitation with surface coils for in vivo spectroscopy by adiabatic rapid half passage. J Magn Reson 67:376–381, 1986.

109. Koretsky AP, Basus VJ, James TI, et al: Detection of exchange reactions involving small metabolite pools using NMR magnetization transfer techniques: Relevance to subcellular compartmentalization of creatine kinase. Magn Reson Med 2:587–594, 1985.

110. Mansfield P, Morris PG: NMR imaging in biomedicine. In Waugh JS (ed): Advances in MR. New York, Academic Press, 1982.

111. Stejskal EO, Tanner JE: Spin diffusion measurement: Spin echoes in the presence of time-dependent field gradient. J Chem Phys 42:288, 1965.

112. Carr HY, Purcell EM: Effects of diffusion on free precession in nuclear magnetic resonance experiments. Phys Rev 94:630, 1954.

113. Bydder GM, Thomas DGT, Gill SS, Young IR: Assessment of intravoxel incoherent motion in patients with intracerebral tumors. Abstracts of the Society for Magnetic Resonance in Medicine. San Francisco, 1988, p 217.

114. LeBihan D, Breton E, Lallemand D, et al: MRI of intravoxel incoherent motions: Applications to diffusion and perfusion in neurologic disorders. Radiology 161:401–407, 1986.

115. Merboldt KD, Gyngell ML, Hanicke W, et al: Rapid NMR imaging of diffusion using a modified CE-FAST sequence. Abstracts of the Society for Magnetic Resonance in Medicine. San Francisco, 1988, p 604.

116. Dickinson RJ, Hall AS, Hind AJ, Young IR: Measurement of changes in tissue temperature using MRI. J Comput Assist Tomogr 10:468–472, 1986.

117. Parker DL, Smith V, Sheldon P, et al: Temperature distribution measurements in two-dimensional NMR imaging. Med Phys 10:321–325, 1983.

117a. LeBihan D, Delannoy J, Levin RL: Temperature mapping with MR imaging of molecular diffusion: Application to hyperthermia. Radiology 171:853–857, 1989.

118. Jeener J: Pulse pair techniques in high resolution NMR. Abstracts of the Second Ampere International Summer School on Pulsed Magnetic and Optical Resonances. Basko Polje, 1971.

119. Mckinnon GC, Boisiger P: Localized double-quantum filter and correlation spectroscopy experiments. Magn Reson Med 6:334–343, 1988.

120. Ernst RR, Bodenhausen G, Wokaun A: Principles of NMR in One and Two Dimensions. Oxford, Clarendon Press, 1987.

Suggested Readings

Becker ED: High Resolution NMR—Theory and Chemical Applications. New York, Academic Press, 1969.

Farrar TC, Becker ED: Pulse and Fourier Transform NMR—Introduction to Theory and Methods. New York, Academic Press, 1971.

Fukishima E, Roeder SBW: Experimental Pulse NMR, Reading, MA, Addison-Wesley Press, 1981.

Gadian DG: NMR and Application to Living Systems, Oxford, Clarendon Press, 1982.

Mansfield P, Morris PG: NMR in Biomedicine, New York, Academic Press, 1982.

Morris PG: NMR Imaging in Medicine and Biology. London, Oxford Press, 1986.

Partain CL, Price RR, Patton JA, et al: Magnetic Resonance Imaging. Vol II. Physical Principles and Instrumentation. Philadelphia, WB Saunders Company, 1988.

10

PULSE SEQUENCE DESIGN

DENNIS J. ATKINSON

SEQUENCE DESIGN OVERVIEW

THE TWO-DIMENSIONAL FOURIER TRANSFORM SPIN-ECHO SEQUENCE

Slice Selection
Radiofrequency Pulses
Phase Encoding
Frequency Encoding and Data Read-out
Eliminating Residual Magnetization

OTHER MR IMAGING METHODS

Gradient Reversal and Gradient-Echo Sequences
Gradient Motion Rephasing
Three-Dimensional Fourier Transform or Volume Acquisition Techniques

TECHNICAL CONSIDERATIONS IN THE DESIGN OF AN MRI SEQUENCE

MRI INSTRUMENTATION, SYSTEM, AND PATIENT CONSIDERATIONS

RADIOFREQUENCY PULSES

Radiofrequency Instrumentation
Nonselective Radiofrequency Pulses
Selective Radiofrequency Pulses
Sinc Pulses
Crafted Radiofrequency Pulses
Radiofrequency Pulse Synthesis
Refocusing of Transverse Magnetization
Selective 180-Degree Pulses
Rotational Axis for Refocusing
Rephasing Slice Magnetization
Slice Offsets

MAGNETIC FIELD GRADIENTS

Gradient System Overview and Gradient System Controls

Gradient Coils
Gradient Waveforms
Gradient Strength

DATA ACQUISITION AND IMAGE-PROCESSING SYSTEMS

Data Acquisition Instrumentation
Image Calculation

READ-OUT OF THE ACQUISITION DATA

Radiofrequency and Gradient Refocusing
Data Sampling
Chemical Shift Effects
Sampling Bandwidth and Signal-to-Noise Ratios
Reduced-Bandwidth Methods
Undersampling Artifacts
Alignment of Sampling and Echo Times

SPOILER PULSES

OFF-CENTER AND OBLIQUE IMAGING

ARTIFACT REDUCTION THROUGH THE USE OF SATURATION PULSES

MOTION REDUCTION THROUGH GRADIENT MOTION REPHASING

INVERSION RECOVERY

SEQUENCE CALIBRATION

VARIATIONS ON TWO-DIMENSIONAL FOURIER TRANSFORM METHODS

Projection Reconstruction
Half-Fourier Data Reconstruction
Fat-Water Separation Techniques

MRI CONTROL SYSTEMS

Control Instrumentation
Control Systems in Sequence Design

SEQUENCE EDITOR AND PROGRAMMER

SEQUENCE DESIGN OVERVIEW

The process of producing an image in MR is the result of a series of compromises involving the physics of the spinning protons; the physical, economic, and computational limits of the MR system; safety constraints concerning the patient; image quality; and clinical efficacy. Where possible, the manufacturers of these MRI systems are seeking to remove the system boundaries and allow the clinical user the flexibility in pulse sequence design to achieve a broad range of imaging possibilities, efficiently and with optimal image quality.

In this chapter, we first review the basic building blocks of a pulse sequence. We then delve into more technical considerations, which are required for understanding and designing pulse sequences.

THE TWO-DIMENSIONAL FOURIER TRANSFORM SPIN-ECHO SEQUENCE

The MR signal is produced by the application of a series of RF pulses and gradients, called a *pulse sequence*. The most widely used MRI sequence is the two RF pulse *spin-echo (SE)* sequence. Data are spatially encoded using the *two-dimensional Fourier transform (2DFT)* method. This method uses a mathematical transformation, called the *Fourier transform*, to convert a time-varying signal into its individual frequency, and therefore spatial, components. The 2DFT SE pulse sequence provides a good model for study of the MR imaging sequence design process, since it requires the basic building blocks for most other sequence methods. As demonstrated schematically in Figure 10–1, the sequence consists of a number of events occurring from an initial excitation pulse to a signal read-out to a final dephasing of spins. Repeated applications of this sequence with different values for the phase-encoding gradient and a subsequent 2DFT give the MR image. Some specific

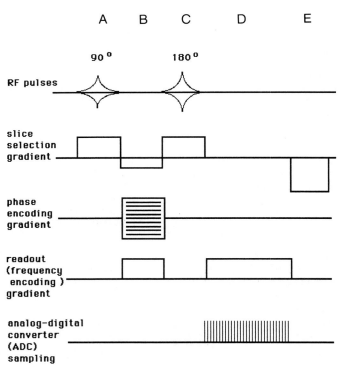

FIGURE 10–1. Simplified SE sequence. The five phases of a typical SE sequence: (A) slice selection—application of slice-selection gradient simultaneous with a selective RF pulse; (B) phase encoding—applying a succession of phase-encoding steps, starting at first with the maximal positive amplitude, stepping through zero, and finishing with the maximal negative amplitude. The dephasing gradient pulse in the frequency-encoding direction is also applied; (C) refocusing spins—applying 180-degree RF pulse simultaneously with slice-selection gradient to refocus spins within the slice; (D) frequency encoding and data read-out—applying the read-out gradient to encode data over a bandwidth of frequencies while simultaneously sampling the data; (E) eliminating residual magnetization—using the slice selection gradient as a spoiler to dephase spins completely across the slice.

TABLE 10–1. LIMITATIONS IN PULSE SEQUENCE DESIGN

Parameter	Sequence Limitations
Minimum repetition time (TR)	RF pulse duration, read-out period, TE, gradient duty cycle, number of slices, RF power deposition, presaturation RF pulses
Minimum echo time (TE)	RF pulse duration, read-out period, peak gradient strength, duration of gradient motion rephasing (GMR) gradient pulses
Minimum slice thickness	RF pulse duration and shape, maximal gradient amplitude
Minimum field-of-view (FOV)	Read-out period, maximal gradient amplitude

limitations in pulse sequence design are listed in Table 10–1.

Slice Selection

To separate the plane of protons to be imaged from the remainder of the patient volume, a slice-selective RF pulse is used. Protons resonate at a frequency determined by the local magnetic field. That local magnetic field can be determined by the application of the slice-selection gradient. For instance, given a field gradient of 1 mT/meter, there would be a 0.01-mT difference from one edge of a 10-mm slice to the other side. This field gradient then translates into a difference in precessional frequencies from one edge to the other of about 420 Hz (cycles per second). This range of frequencies is called the *bandwidth*. An RF pulse also contains a range or bandwidth of frequencies, as discussed further on. Once the bandwidth of a particular plane is defined using the slice-selection gradient, all that remains is to define an RF pulse so that its bandwidth matches that of the slice, and with the appropriate power to tip the proton magnetization the desired amount.

Radiofrequency Pulses

Ideally, an RF pulse should produce uniform power levels (or uniform *flip angles*) across the slice bandwidth and then sharply drop off to zero power outside this bandwidth, so that protons outside the slice remain unaffected. To understand better what this pulse should look like, we may use the Fourier transform process to translate between time functions and frequency functions. This step is necessary because the RF pulse is produced by an oscillator and is a time-varying function, but its spatial effect on the image depends on frequency. A sharply defined bandwidth with a uniform power level translates into the mathematical form *sin (x)/x*, or a *sinc* time function. Graphically, this function has a large central lobe and a number of smaller amplitude oscillations symmetrically radiating outward from it along a time line. These oscillations cross the zero amplitude line a number of times before finally decaying to zero amplitude themselves.

Unfortunately, a sinc RF pulse would have to contain an infinite number of zero crossings and thus be almost infinitely long to produce a perfectly rectangular slice profile. A long RF pulse, in turn, increases the minimal echo time (TE) and repetition time (TR) of the pulse sequence, so the decay of the RF pulse is generally expedited via an exponential weighting function, *at the expense of a worsened slice profile.* The worsened slice profile results in *cross-talk* contamination of adjacent slices. *This cross-talk artifact effectively reduces the TR on the wings of the slice and has the clinical result of reducing overall contrast and making an image more T_1-like.*

Solutions to this problem are being researched, including optimal design of the RF pulses to correct these artifacts (Fig. 10–2). These *optimized* or *crafted RF pulses* are tailored to accommodate short pulse lengths, reduce RF power deposition, and allow minimal slice gaps or spacings without cross-talk effects.

Phase Encoding

Thus far, we have seen how to select a given plane of tissues through an application of a gradient and a specialized RF pulse. Next we consider how data are spatially localized within the plane along one axis by the process of phase encoding. Phase encoding is unique in that it relies on spins retaining a phase memory of a previous event. It is also unique because the amplitude of the phase-encoding gradient changes as each new projection is acquired, whereas the slice-selection and frequency-encoding gradients do not vary during the entire data acquisition.

When a gradient is applied, spins near the center of the gradient are largely unaffected, whereas spins at one end of the gradient will precess relatively faster and at the other, relatively more slowly (Fig. 10–3). If this gradient is applied for a brief, but definite, time interval, spins retain a phase memory of the local field. Spins at the center will have no phase distortion, but away from the center, spins experiencing an additive gradient will precess slightly faster and have a positive phase distortion relative to the center. Conversely, those on the opposite end of the gradient will have a subtractive effect and thus a negative phase distortion. In principle, then, by looking at phase memory we have a way of encoding location.

Unfortunately, there is no practical way specifically to test a local area's phase distortion, since the signal received is from spins throughout the entire selected plane. Therefore, to determine where along the phase-encoding axis tissues lie, we need to make multiple tests. For example, in Figure 10–3, the gradient advances spins in the positive direction 90 degrees and in the negative direction −90 degrees. As a result, the phases of the spins are 180 degrees apart, and their signals cancel, leaving only the cen-

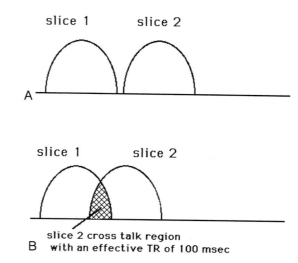

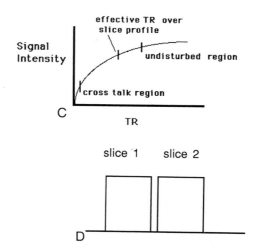

FIGURE 10–2. Cross-talk effects with gaussian and optimized RF pulse profiles. *A,* Schematic representation of two nonrectangular slice profiles spaced by a distance that is 100 per cent of the slice thickness. *B,* Representation of these profiles with interslice distance reduced to 20 per cent. If the time difference between the slices is 100 msec, the protons in the cross-talk region experience a TR of only 100 msec, while the remainder of the slice has an effective TR equal to the sequence TR. *C,* A comparison of signal intensity versus TR showing the effect of integrating a cross-talk region into a slice profile. In *B,* the majority of the slice profile experiences the desired TR, as shown on the right. However, the region experiencing a very short TR, on the left, must also be integrated so that the total effective TR is something less than the desired TR. In this case, the result is a loss of signal intensity, or a more "T_1" appearance to the image. *D,* Slice thickness and spacing similar to that in *B,* but replacing the gaussian pulses with optimized rectangular slice profiles. Problems of T_1 weighting are significantly reduced or eliminated with these pulses, since the entire slice experiences the same TR.

tral portion generating a signal. With a different amplitude for the phase-encoding gradient, the signals will add or subtract differently, depending on position. By using a number of different gradient strengths, spins can be spatially resolved along one axis.

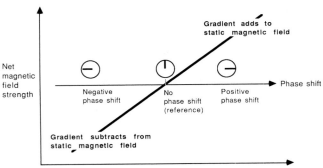

FIGURE 10–3. The process of encoding spin phase for local areas of spins. In the center, the gradient neither adds or subtracts from the base magnetic field, so that the rate at which these spins resonate forms a reference phase by which other phases may be measured. On the right, the gradient adds to the base magnetic field, so that the phase of the spins advances slightly farther (i.e., goes in a more clockwise direction) than the spin phase at the center. On the left, the gradient subtracts from the base magnetic field, so that the phase of the spins is slightly behind the spin phase at the center.

The pixel resolution depends on the number of phase-encoding steps. If we wish to resolve 128 pixels across the phase-encoding direction of a slice, we need 128 different, independent pieces of information. The way we get them is by varying the phase-encoding gradient in 128 steps (typically changing amplitude from a positive maximum to a negative maximum in equal steps).

Frequency Encoding and Data Read-out

Having found a method to select a given plane and encode data along one axis, we need now to encode data along the other axis to produce a 2D map of tissue intensities. This step is done by applying a gradient during signal read-out along the remaining axis (Fig. 10–4). The gradient tunes the resonance frequencies according to position. The spread in resonance frequencies, or bandwidth, is proportional to the strength of the frequency-encoding gradient.

The MR system uses a receiver filter to exclude signals, including thermal noise, that lie outside this bandwidth. If the MR signal is read out over a short interval (which is necessary, for instance, to obtain short TE), then the frequency-encoding gradient strength must be increased to maintain spatial resolution. The stronger gradient increases the signal bandwidth and necessitates the use of a larger receiver filter to avoid cutting off image information. However, as the receiver bandwidth is increased, more noise is allowed into the image. As a result, it is a common practice to reduce noise (and thus increase the signal-to-noise ratio, or S/N) by using a reduced receiver bandwidth; this technique is widely available on most commercial MR imaging systems under a variety of names ("matched bandwidth," "optimized bandwidth," "low-noise bandwidth," and others).

Eliminating Residual Magnetization

Typically, data are acquired before the dephasing of spins from previous application of the pulse sequence is complete. In most cases, the TR is less than the time for more than 90 per cent of the spins to dephase (three times the T_2 time). Therefore, we accelerate this dephasing by applying an additional "spoiler" gradient. This high-amplitude, long-duration gradient ruins, or spoils, the residual transverse magnetization by disturbing the local magnetic field homogeneity. The best results occur when the spoiler gradient is applied across the slice-selection direction.

OTHER MR IMAGING METHODS

We saw in the previous example how a single-echo, single-slice, single-acquisition SE sequence is designed. A variety of other pulse sequences can also be generated.

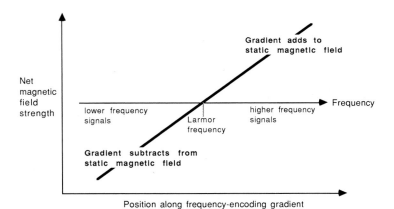

FIGURE 10–4. The process of frequency encoding. As shown in Figure 10–3, the gradient neither adds nor subtracts at the center, providing reference frequency. On the right, the gradient strength adds to the base magnetic field, so spins resonate faster than those at the center. On the left, the gradient strength subtracts from the base magnetic field, so spins resonate more slowly than those at the center. Overall, the difference between the fastest and slowest spins then gives a bandwidth of frequencies over which to encode the data. Actual resolution along this axis depends on the degree of resolving frequency differences in these locations.

Gradient Reversal and Gradient-Echo Sequences

As discussed previously, it is necessary to apply magnetic field gradients for imaging. However, a gradient represents a marked magnetic field inhomogeneity, which produces rapid dephasing of spins. As a result, for the slice-selection and frequency-encoding gradients, it is necessary to apply an extra gradient pulse that has an area equal to that of the imaging gradient but that has an amplitude of opposite sign. The first gradient pulse dephases the spins, and the second pulse rephases the spins to produce maximal signal at the center of the read-out interval. This signal produced by gradient reversal is called a *gradient echo (GRE)* and is used to produce the signal in GRE (e.g., FLASH, GRASS) pulse sequences (Fig. 10–5). However, gradient reversal is an equally essential part of SE pulse sequences. In SE sequences, the signal represents a combination of the GRE and an SE produced by the 180-degree RF pulse.

In SE imaging, tissue contrast may be manipulated by changes in the TR and TE. By removing the 180-degree RF pulse and using a GRE sequence, we have additional control over contrast in the way we vary the excitation flip angle, as discussed in Chapter 5. Because of their simpler structure, GRE sequences permit shorter TE (10 msec or less) than the SE method (TE of 15 msec or less).

In general, the GRE sequences may be further divided into two categories according to how they handle the residual magnetization after the data acquisition: those that attempt to maintain it in a steady-state condition and those that eliminate it. Those that eliminate it (e.g., FLASH* sequences) typically use a spoiler pulse in a manner similar to that described earlier. The other methods (e.g., FISP or GRASS†) rephase spins along one or more axes prior to reapplication of the next RF pulse.

Gradient Motion Rephasing

Unlike stationary spins, moving spins do not rephase properly at the TE. Furthermore, they may move during the application of a gradient and thus experience a slight undesired phase distortion. Evidence of this distortion and dephasing can be found on MR images in which flowing fluids may produce ghost artifact along the phase-encoding direction.

One solution to this problem is to change the gradient timing so that flowing spins will optimally rephase at the center of the read-out period. Unfortunately, simply changing the timing is not sufficient, since the stationary spins are then not optimally rephased and image quality will suffer. However, if we add a second set of gradients, we may be able to handle both problems. This technique is called *gradient motion rephasing (GMR)* or *flow compensation*. Since this dephasing occurs along any axis where gradients are used, an optimally rephased sequence will contain GMR pulses on multiple axes.

Three-Dimensional Fourier Transform or Volume Acquisition Techniques

In addition to slice-selection approaches, images can be produced using *volume acquisition* or *three-dimensional Fourier transform (3DFT)* techniques. Covering a volume of tissues with a 3D sequence requires one modification to the 2D method described previously, the addition of a phase-encoding gradient across the slice-selection direction. In a manner similar to the phase-encoding gradient steps discussed earlier, by applying a series of gradients across the slice-selection direction, the volume is divided into a number of individual slices. This additional slice-selection encoding process will extend the acquisition time. As a result, the total acquisition time is as follows: TR × number of acquisitions × number of phase-encoding steps in the imaging plane × number of partitions or slices across the volume. Because of the need for long TR, T_2 weighting on 3D images is not practical. But for GRE imaging with TR of 30 msec or less, a complete set of high-resolution images for a volume may be produced in just a few minutes.

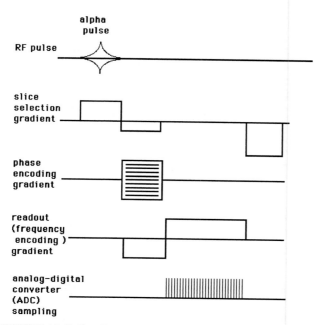

FIGURE 10–5. Simplified GRE technique. This sequence is similar to the SE diagram in Figure 10–1, except for a few modifications: The 90-degree pulse is made variable (alpha pulse) to allow additional contrast control; the 180-degree pulse is removed; and the minimal TE and TR times are reduced.

---

*FLASH = fast low angle shot.

†FISP = fast imaging with steady-state precession; GRASS = gradient-recalled acquisition steady state.

TECHNICAL CONSIDERATIONS IN THE DESIGN OF AN MRI SEQUENCE

This section of the chapter explores the process and technical considerations involved in designing an MR imaging sequence.

MRI INSTRUMENTATION, SYSTEM, AND PATIENT CONSIDERATIONS

The limiting factors in the design of any MR imaging sequence are the basic physics of the MR experiment and those limitations imposed by the individual system. Other considerations in designing sequences for clinical imaging systems include RF power deposition and time-varying gradient limits as indicated by Food and Drug Administration (FDA) guidelines, patient-to-patient variability, physiologic motion, acceptable image quality, and an overall ease of operation.

RADIOFREQUENCY PULSES

Radiofrequency Instrumentation

Typical instrumentation for the transmission of RF pulses consists of a number of stages, beginning first with a digital computer to synthesize points for the RF waveforms. This series of digital values is converted to an analog signal, filtered to remove conversion artifacts, mixed with a resonance frequency, and amplified to the desired power. Throughout the imaging process, the RF system remains locked in phase to the original pulse so that subsequent pulses have the same phase information (or *rotating frame of reference*) as the initial pulse.

Sequence design techniques incorporate awareness of the process of RF waveform generation and setting of requisite power levels but rarely need to delve into the more basic functions, such as digital-to-analog conversion, filtering, or RF modulation and demodulation.

Nonselective Radiofrequency Pulses

One of the simplest RF pulses to produce is merely a burst of RF power at the resonance frequency. This is accomplished by a rectangular modulation of the RF power. In the absence of a magnetic field gradient, this has the effect of exciting resonance spins throughout the RF coil volume and is referred to as a *nonselective pulse*. Nonselective RF pulses are typically used in certain volume-imaging methods, in which it is desirable to excite a large volume of tissue with a single RF pulse.[1]

The duration of the nonselective pulse (t_p) is inversely proportional to the effective bandwidth of the pulse (Δf):

$$\Delta f = 1 / t_p \text{ (seconds)} \qquad (1)$$

For example, an RF pulse of 10 msec duration has a bandwidth of 100 Hz. As is explained later, bandwidth is only one consideration in a discussion of RF pulses; required RF power, RF coil design, coverage, and flip angles also factor into the design of a sequence.

The static field produced by the main magnet is typically referred to as B_0 (in units of gauss or tesla). B_1 refers to the strength of the RF pulse. The B_1 field is linearly related to the amount of rotation or flip angle (θ) of the spins from the B_0 field alignment:

$$\theta = \gamma B_1 t_p \qquad (2)$$

That is, the angle of rotation is determined by the strength of the RF pulse multiplied by its duration. This means that protons may be excited by weak pulses of long duration or by those of shorter duration, with higher RF power.

The amount of power required to generate a given flip angle depends on the amount of RF coil loading by the patient and varies for the individual patient. Typically, the amount of RF power needed for a 180-degree flip angle, as well as for other flip angles, is calculated from this value. The 180-degree flip-angle adjustment is accomplished during the prescanning phase by increasing the RF power level so that the signal increases to a maximum (90 degrees) and then decreases to a minimum (180 degrees). Calibration may be done with either nonselective or selective excitation pulses.[2]

Selective Radiofrequency Pulses

To perform slice selection, a magnetic field gradient is produced simultaneously with the RF pulse so that only one portion of the volume will resonate at the excitation frequency. The size and location of this slice depend upon the RF bandwidth and frequency modulation of the resonance frequency.[3] Application of a selective RF pulse is shown in Figure 10–6, where the frequency bandwidth, or range of frequencies, is demonstrated.

The bandwidth of the RF pulse is determined according to the formula

$$\Delta f = \gamma G_{ss} d \qquad (3)$$

where d is the slice thickness, G_{ss} is the slice-selection gradient strength, and γ is the gyromagnetic ratio (for protons, about 42 MHz/T). For example, the selection of a 3-mm slice using a slice-selection gradient strength of 10 mT/meter will require a frequency bandwidth of 1260 Hz. From the formula, we see that there is a linear relationship between the gradient strength, RF bandwidth, and slice thickness; thinner slices require either a smaller bandwidth or stronger slice-selection gradients or both. Inevitably, these parameter trade-offs necessitate a set of compromises, which will be discussed further in the sequence design.

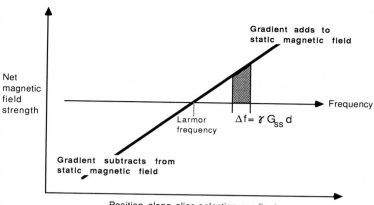

FIGURE 10–6. Diagram comparing slice (*shaded area*) thickness with slice-selection gradient amplitude. All else being held constant, the following holds true: (1) if the gradient strength is increased, a constant RF bandwidth will produce a thinner slice; (2) conversely, if the gradient amplitude is reduced, a wider slice thickness results; (3) if a narrower RF bandwidth is chosen, a thinner slice is produced; conversely, a wider bandwidth produces a thicker slice.

There are several techniques under development which overcome some of the limitations of standard selective RF pulses in 2D and 3D imaging. One method called "POMP" (phase-ordered multiplanar) increases the number of slices that may be acquired within a given TR.[3a] It does so by applying an RF pulse containing multiple frequencies, which excite multiple slices simultaneously. Multifrequency RF waveforms can be constructed by simply adding together the waveforms of several single frequency RF pulses. The slice positions are encoded in the phases of the MR signals by phase modulating the RF pulse. This imparts a phase shift, which depends on the position along the slice-selection gradient, to the signal from each slice. The method requires multiple excitations: at least n NEX are needed to spatially resolve n slices. After data reconstruction, the images appear displaced within the field-of-view (FOV) along the phase-encoding axis. Compared with a standard multislice acquisition, the FOV must be increased to avoid overlap of the images.

Another variation on slice-selective techniques permits an excitation to be applied to a nonstandard volume.[3b] For instance, one can, in principle, excite a cylindrical volume of tissue (as opposed to a 2D slice or a rectangular 3D volume) by applying a specially modulated RF pulse while two gradients are simultaneously oscillated. Volume-selective excitations might be particularly useful for MR angiography and localized spectroscopy.

Sinc Pulses

Uniform excitation of a slice of tissues requires an RF pulse containing equal energy within a narrow band of frequencies. To excite a rectangular distribution of resonance frequencies uniformly, a sinc function (the inverse Fourier transform of a square wave) is typically used to modulate the RF signal:

$$A(t) = \sin(t) / t \qquad (4)$$

where A(t) is the amplitude of the modulation function at time t.

This function will produce a bandwidth of frequencies that evenly excite the protons over the selected slice; that is, a sinc pulse with a gradient will cause only the selected slice to resonate, and all other locations outside the slice will have resonance frequencies outside the RF bandwidth and will not resonate. In practice, however, a practical RF pulse duration requires that the sinc function be truncated before its constituent infinite series is accurately represented. It is this truncation that presents problems.

To truncate the RF pulse—that is, to reduce its value to zero—a weighting filter is applied to the sinc function to reduce the amplitude without an abrupt transition. Many types of filters have been researched for the qualities they impart in the truncation, or *apodization* (from the Greek, "cutting off the feet"), of the RF pulse. On commercial MR imaging scanners, a variety of truncation functions are possible. Frequently, an exponentially decaying envelope or Hanning window is used (see Equation 8, further on).

One simple indication of the degree of truncation is a count of the number of zero crossings made by the RF pulse before reaching a steady-state zero amplitude. Reasonable approximations to sinc functions of an infinite length can be made in 8 to 12 zero crossings. However, as a practical consideration, the additional zero crossings make the RF pulse (and minimal TEs) longer.[4] The time between zero crossings is related to the bandwidth used in the slice selection (see Equation 3),

$$T = 1 / \Delta f \qquad (5)$$

Thus, generation of an optimal sinc RF pulse with 8 zero crossings on each side of a central lobe and having an excitation bandwidth of 1260 Hz would require 16 (8 zero crossings on either side) × 0.794 msec (from 1/1260 Hz), or about 13 msec. However, 13 msec per RF pulse is not acceptable for most MR imaging.

Crafted Radiofrequency Pulses

Given the compromises necessary in working with sinc functions, some commercial MR imaging systems use selective RF pulses that resemble gaussian functions. Their advantages over the truncated sinc functions are reduced power deposition (gaussian functions require only about 70 per cent of the power of a sinc pulse), better excitation profiles at shorter RF pulse lengths, and their ability to be realized with fewer digitization points for a given slice shift. However, with adequate time and number of points, the sinc function will produce a more rectangular excitation profile.

Improvement in slice profiles with selective RF pulses having other than a gaussian or sinc modulation is one of the active areas of MR imaging research[5] (Fig. 10–7). Criteria for improving selective pulses include a more rectangular excitation profile, minimization of phase shifts across the slice, and

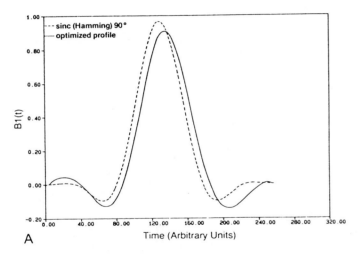

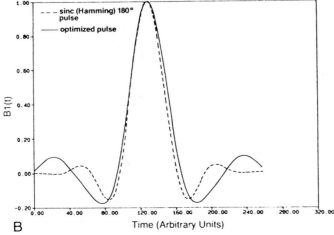

FIGURE 10–7. A comparison of RF pulses. *A*, Comparison of typical apodized sinc function and a crafted RF pulse optimized for a 90-degree flip angle. *B*, Comparison of a Hamming weighted sinc pulse with an optimized RF pulse for a 180-degree flip angle.

excitation outside the slice, while retaining good S/N, contrast, and multislice capability. Also being investigated are improvements for reduction of RF pulse lengths, RF power deposition, and B_1 field inhomogeneity.

What about using a high bandwidth, with its shorter time per crossing, to produce a better slice profile with a shorter duration? By Equation 4, the peak RF amplitude occurs when it is zero (the center of the echo). If we analyze changes in this peak amplitude with a wider excitation bandwidth, we find that an increasing bandwidth requires a higher peak amplitude. By L'Hospital's rule, a twofold increase in excitation bandwidth doubles the peak amplitude, and therefore current, required. Furthermore, power is proportional to the square of the current used (I):

$$P = I^2R \qquad (6)$$

where P is RF power and R is the coil impedance. Generation of these high power requirements is limited by hardware considerations for the transmitter and by FDA power deposition limits. For these reasons, optimal slice profiles may not always be achievable for all sequences and in all slice positions.

Radiofrequency Pulse Synthesis

The basic equation for the digital synthesis of sinc pulses may take the following form[6]:

$$W(t) = [\sin (\gamma\ G_{ss}\ d\ F\ t_s)\ /\ (\gamma\ G_{ss}\ d\ F\ t_s)] \\ \times \text{(envelope function)} \qquad (7)$$

where γ is the gyromagnetic ratio (42 MHz / T), G_{ss} is the strength of the slice-selection gradient, d is the slice thickness (full width at half the maximal amplitude [FWHM]), F is a shaping factor (approximately $\Delta f_{pulse}\ /\ \Delta f_{slice}$), and t_s is the time per point value.

The digital sampling points, k, of a simple Hanning window, used to truncate the sinc pulse waveform, are of the following form:

$$\text{Envelope(k)} = [1\ +\ \cos (2\ \pi\ k\ /\ N)]\ /\ 2 \qquad (8)$$

where N is the total number of points defining the RF envelope. More precise definition of the waveform is possible as N is increased; typically, 512 points is adequate in most applications.

Since the final stage of the RF amplifier may be nonlinear, the RF pulse envelope may require a further correction factor. If this is the case, tests at varying power levels are necessary to calculate a modulation correction function having the proper transfer characteristic.

Refocusing of Transverse Magnetization

Once a slice is selected and the longitudinal magnetization is tipped into the transverse plane with a 90-degree RF pulse, another RF pulse must be applied to help refocus transverse magnetization. In the SE sequence, this pulse has a flip angle of 180 degrees and is typically slice selective to facilitate multislice acquisitions. In using the 180-degree pulse to help refocus the transverse magnetization, some concerns need to be addressed.

Selective 180-Degree Pulses

Slice-selective 180-degree RF pulses are produced in much the same fashion as the excitation pulse described previously. However, their use in this application presents some problems as well as opportunities. In general, it is much more difficult to produce even excitation profiles with 180-degree pulses. Whereas truncation effects may slightly misshape a 90-degree pulse, the effects on a 180-degree pulse will be much more severe. The overall SE slice profile is largely dependent upon this refocusing pulse. Uncorrected RF amplifier nonlinearities, profile phase errors, and even patient loading variances may also add to slice profile errors. To correct for some of the anticipated errors, the 180-degree pulse will typically use a slightly larger shaping constant (excitation bandwidth–pulse bandwidth ratio) in the sinc equation given earlier (Equation 7).

A potential solution is to extend the pulse length or increase the gradient amplitude, as described previously. However, increased gradient amplitude in conjunction with increased RF amplitudes results in increased power deposition, which can be problematic, since overall power deposition is largely defined by the 180-degree pulse.

Rotational Axis for Refocusing

In using 180-degree pulses to refocus spins, the choice of axis about which to rotate the magnetization vector will affect the eventual strength and location of the refocused vector. Specifically, if we assume that the delivered 180-degree RF pulse will have flip-angle variations, how can we best minimize their effects?

One technique, the Carr-Purcell (CP) SE sequence, rotates the magnetization with the 180-pulse about the same axis as the original 90-degree pulse. This technique is effective for those protons that experience both the 90- and the 180-degree pulses. However, flip-angle variations about the 90- and 180-degree pulses will result in magnetization both above and below the transverse plane. This off-plane refocusing will cause a reduced signal, as only a projection of the echo is received. In any whole-body imaging system, RF inhomogeneity and slice profile imperfections exist, so that this technique will result in degraded (shortened) T_2 values.

To circumvent this problem, one commonly used variation is the Carr-Purcell-Meiboom-Gill (CPMG) sequence. In CPMG, there is a 90-degree phase shift between the 90- and 180-degree pulses. The resulting signal from a CPMG sequence tends to be less influenced by RF inhomogeneities.[7]

Rephasing Slice Magnetization

There is another complicating factor in the use of selective RF pulses that has not been mentioned; this is the problem of phase distortion across the slice profile. Given a selective RF pulse, there is a frequency difference between opposite sides of a slice (see earlier discussion of bandwidths); that is, spins precess at different rates across the slice while the slice-selection gradient is on. Therefore, after the gradient is off, a phase difference will exist within the selected slice. This phase difference will cause a self-cancellation of spin vectors within the slice unless it is corrected. Aligning spins within the slice is usually accomplished by applying the slice-selection gradient in the opposite direction to increase the precessional rates on one side and decrease them on the other. The integral value for this rephasing step is equal to a significant fraction (50 to 70 per cent) of the integral for the gradient used in the slice selection. This rephasing may be done immediately after the pulse or, if ramping times are a problem, adjacent to the 180-degree pulse gradient (the refocusing pulse acts like a sign change for gradient amplitude values). Failure to refocus magnetization properly across the slice typically results in reduced S/N, as the signals cancel when sufficiently out of phase. Final adjustment of this refocusing is usually performed by a series of experiments with differing refocusing integral values, a method that tends to converge to a value that offers a maximal signal. Intensity shading artifacts may also result with improper slice rephasing, since out-of-plane magnetization may be selectively refocusing over the slice.

Gradient compensation for 180-degree pulses is not typically a concern, since by their symmetric nature, selective 180-degree pulses are considered to be self-compensating for these phase distortions.

Recently, RF pulses have been designed that are self-refocusing (i.e., dispense with the gradient reversal). Two approaches have been proposed for self-refocusing pulses: (1) use of a gaussian 270-degree pulse[7a] or (2) use of complex amplitude and/or phase modulated pulses.[7b, 7c] By eliminating the need for the gradient reversal, self-refocusing pulses might shorten the minimum echo time and eliminate signal loss from imperfect gradient refocusing.

Slice Offsets

The ability to offset a given slice position allows MR scanning at arbitrary positions as well as affording the opportunity to do multislice examinations.[8] Shifting of a slice in MR imaging is accomplished by changing the RF excitation frequency with a constant gradient (Fig. 10–8). Typically, the RF pulse is modulated by the desired offset frequency and then transmitted at the resonance frequency (sideband modulation). This method has the advantages of not requiring additional hardware and not being as

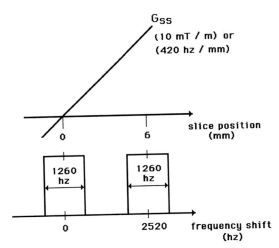

FIGURE 10–8. Diagram of slice excitation bandwidth and offset frequency. Given the slice-selection gradient strength of 10 mT/meter, the excitation bandwidth is 420 Hz/mm, or a 1260-Hz bandwidth selects a slice that is 3 mm thick. Furthermore, a frequency shift or modulation of +2560 Hz produces a shift of +6 mm for the selected slice (i.e., 2560 / 420, or 6 mm) while still maintaining a slice thickness of 3 mm. Conversely, a frequency shift of −2560 Hz would achieve the same offset value and thickness, but the slice would then be shifted to the left (or negative) direction.

prone to frequency misadjustments. One potential drawback to this method, however, is that a large number of data points may be necessary when generating large frequency shifts (i.e., large offsets with restricted bandwidth pulses).

MAGNETIC FIELD GRADIENTS

Gradient System Overview and Gradient System Controls

Gradient hardware consists of a set of gradient coils affixed within the main magnetic field and aligned orthogonally to one another, along with a sophisticated amplifier to energize, or drive, the required currents. The coil set is made up of multiple conductor windings fixed to a form and optimized to produce linear field gradients over a wide range of distances and directions. To produce the driving current for these coils, a series of high-current, audio bandwidth amplifiers are used. In state-of-the-art commercial systems, control signals for these amplifiers are digitally synthesized. Translation of the synthesized data to precise gradient amplitudes is accomplished by *digital-to-analog converters (DACs)*, with 12 bits (or 4096 levels) being sufficient for routine imaging applications. As these gradient systems are aligned to produce field gradients along the x-, y-, and z-axes, they are normally referred to as G_x, G_y, and G_z.

Control of the timing and amplitude of these field gradients is crucial to the success of spatial localiza-

tion and echo production, since the gradients are used both to locate RF pulses spatially and to encode information spatially for MR imaging.[9]

Gradient Coils

Physical placement of the gradient coils on clinical imaging systems leads to another complicating factor. When a strong time-varying magnetic field gradient is produced near a conducting surface, *eddy currents* are induced in the adjacent surface. These induced currents then follow local pathways of differing resistances within that conductor, thus producing multiple current loops. These induced current loops or series of loops will then produce an associated magnetic field that is opposed to the original time-varying gradient. The interaction between the two time-varying fields will produce a nonlinear gradient response that can alter image intensity. The duration of these eddy currents is in a range from milliseconds to seconds. These currents are induced only when there is little distance between the coil set and a conductor, but eddy currents are a significant problem in clinical MR imaging systems in which the gradient coil set is located within the bore of the main magnet and only slightly separated from the metallic inner linings of the cryogen dewar. The effects of distant objects, such as external magnetic shielding or the external pressure vessel, are negligible.

The tight confines of the patient bore limit further separation of the coil set and the magnet itself, so what else can be done? One solution is to take advantage of the magnet-coil geometric symmetry and rely on symmetric counterdirectional currents to cancel out the effects of these induced currents. This method necessarily entails precise mechanical alignment of components in magnet construction, gradient coil assembly, and support structures and may have a limited effect on local, short time-constant currents.

An alternate solution is to assume some asymmetry and electronically alter the driving current so that the desired time-varying gradient field is produced. This overdriving or underdriving of the coil then produces a spatially linear field gradient with the required amplitude and duration. In overdriving the amplifier, though, there is an increase in the peak current used; a peak current may exceed 150 per cent of the steady-state current. This method also requires compensation characteristics that are precisely matched to the final imaging settings with regard to timing, gradient amplitudes, and possible gradient interactions.[10] Since these and other methods seek to minimize eddy current effects, these techniques are referred to as *eddy current compensation* methods.

To minimize the disturbance of the eddy currents, another solution being researched is to shield the magnet from the gradient coil magnetically. This method uses another localized gradient system between the main gradient coil and the magnet to minimize the time-varying field at the cryogen shields. Since the second localized gradient is active only when the main gradient system is driven, this method is referred to as *active shielding* of gradients. This system uses an additional coil set that may reduce the inner diameter of the patient bore and requires a more complex power supply to drive both coil sets.

An additional focus of research in this area concerns the redesigning of the metallic inner linings of the cryogen dewars. Metallurgic and geometric alterations to the inner lining of the cryogen dewar may limit eddy current effects by precisely defining current paths. This delineation of current paths may be accomplished either by a further separation or by establishing defined eddy currents with extremely short settling times.

Gradient Waveforms

The gradient waveforms used in typical MR imaging are of two types, sinusoidal and trapezoidal. Sinusoidal gradient waveforms produce amplitudes that vary approximately as a sine function, typically operating in a range of 100 Hz to 8 kHz. Trapezoidal waveforms have a finite rise time slew rate, a relatively stable peak value, and a finite fall time back to a zero level. For systems with a predefined constant rise time, it typically equals the fall time and ranges from 0.1 msec to 2.0 msec. In those cases in which the rise time is a function of the final amplitude, the slew rate (in milliteslas per millisecond or teslas per second) is the limiting factor in the time necessary for switching. For example, given a maximal slew rate of 10 T/sec, a stable amplitude of 2 mT is possible in 0.2 msec.

Uncompensated eddy currents will distort gradient pulses by extending rise and fall times and may cause the peak plateau to be unstable and oscillate. Properly compensated, the waveforms approximate the ideal shape and timing (Fig. 10–9). At the present time, most commercial systems rely upon trapezoidal wave-

forms; however, some allow direct digital control of the waveform for further research purposes.[11]

Gradient Strength

In determining the strength of the encoding, the read-out, and, to some extent, the slice-selection gradients, one factor to consider is the overall magnetic field (B_0) inhomogeneity. To overcome the pixel-to-pixel variations in field, gradient strength should be adjusted accordingly:

$$(\gamma \, G \, \Delta x) > f_0 \, (\Delta B_0 \, / \, B_0) \qquad (9)$$

where Δx is the pixel dimension, f_0 is the Larmor frequency, and $\Delta B_0 \, / \, B_0$ is the magnetic field inhomogeneity (pixel-to-pixel variation). This inhomogeneity may be from the magnet, the patient's prostheses, or tissue susceptibility differences. Modern superconducting magnets produce stable fields with variations of 15 ppm or less over a 50-cm sphere; main field distortion does not present problems with typical SE imaging. However, as discussed later, susceptibility may be a serious consideration in GRE techniques and when using low-bandwidth sequences.

To obtain short TE sequences, gradient usage needs to be optimized along the slice-selection and phase- and frequency-encoding axes. This process is elaborated later in the discussion of sequence design and requires taking into account system limits, safety restrictions for the patient, and typical clinical protocols. For example, the slice-selection gradients may be limited on the basis of RF power deposition to the patient, as well as peak RF power considerations (Equation 6). In general, short TE sequences require large encoding gradient amplitudes along with a large percentage of on-time, or a *high duty cycle*, during the sequence. Caution should be observed in the design of sequences in which large-amplitude gradients are necessary for long periods. Extended duty cycles may cause resistive heating of the coil set and a reduction (or *derating*) of the available amplifier output. All systems have physical limitations on the

FIGURE 10–9. Plot of time versus gradient amplitude showing a 1-msec rise time and a 1-msec fall time. Proper compensation for the eddy current effects results in the ideal case of a trapezoidal waveform with stable on and off values reached in 1 msec. Overcompensation tends to overshoot the desired stable level, causing a slight oscillation in the gradient after 1 msec. Conversely, undercompensation does the opposite, causing the gradient to take longer to stabilize at the on or off level.

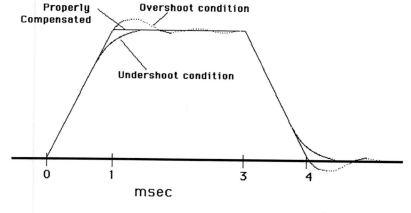

peak available gradient strength; thus, care should be taken in any sequence test so that excessive currents do not cause an unprotected amplifier system to be overdriven.

DATA ACQUISITION AND IMAGE-PROCESSING SYSTEMS

Data Acquisition Instrumentation

Data acquisition systems on MR scanners are substantially different from those used in CT. In MR imaging, the emitted low signals from the tissues are detected using single or multiple receiver coils tuned to the specific resonance frequency. This low-level signal proceeds through a preamplifier and is demodulated into amplitude and phase, or *real* and *imaginary* (sine and cosine) *waveforms*. These audio range signals are then low-pass filtered to limit spectral bandwidth and are finally digitized using high-speed *analog-to-digital converters (ADCs)*. Appropriate ADC discrimination depends on S/N considerations. For clinical MR imaging systems, 16 bits per channel is adequate. Typical digitizing speeds for these systems are from 3 to 25 kHz, and on most commercial MR scanners this rate remains fixed throughout a sampling interval. Multipole (sharp cut-off) analog *low-pass filters* are used to reduce overall noise and prevent aliasing of nonessential frequencies. Typical filters range from 1 to 130 kHz and are usually settable through software control. Once digitized, the signal progresses into a data processing computer that removes any signal offset and averages successive samples to improve the S/N ratio.

Because MR imaging scans generate tremendous amounts of information very rapidly, data storage is usually handled by one or more magnetic disks connected with the data acquisition computer. For example, a typical clinical scan with 20 slice positions, two echoes, 256×256 matrices, and both real and imaginary data axes, each with 16 bits resolution, will produce more than 83 million bits of data—an amount of information beyond the capacity for internal storage on most current computer systems.

These unprocessed acquisition data are typically available to research or service personnel in formats that include display of the digitized values in numerical form or as a modulated gray-scale image. These raw data images can display data from the real or imaginary axes, or the combined magnitude, in a form in which intensity is a linear function of ADC value (Fig. 10–10A). On these images, one axis is the read-out time period, scaled from one edge of the image to the other, and the other axis is the phase-encoding magnitude (in 2DFT imaging). Thus, these images provide a time map of acquisition data over the course of the scan and may be useful in troubleshooting transient data problems or in pulse sequence calibration (Fig. 10–10B).

To reduce overall system costs, most commercial MR scanners will use the data acquisition computer for image processing. Therefore, acquisition data are routed through the central computer to the raw data disk, where they are stored until the acquisition is complete, when they are recalled, Fourier transformed into images, and sent to the mass storage device as complete image frames. From this mass storage device, the images are then made available to the operator. Since raw data are of little use once

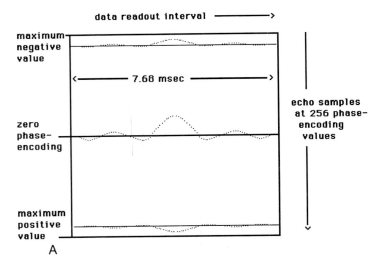

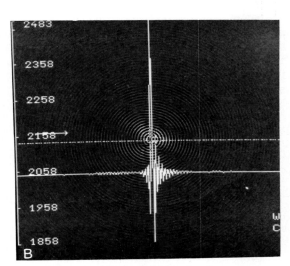

FIGURE 10–10. Two-dimensional map of acquisition data. *A*, Map of the process of data acquisition showing read-out samples horizontally versus changes in phase-encoding gradient amplitude vertically. Typically, the phase-encoding value traverses linearly from a maximal negative to maximal positive amplitude, with the low and zero values represented centrally. *B*, Map of raw data values as outlined in *A*, in which image intensities are linearly scaled to sample amplitude values. A profile of signal intensities along the zero phase encoding is demonstrated. In this example, the data read-out period is 7.68 msec for 256 points (30 μsec per point), with 256 phase-encoding steps. In the case of multiple acquisitions, each data line is averaged using identical gradient values, before being stored as raw data.

the image is calculated, they are typically not archived and their disk space is reused on the subsequent scan.

Image Calculation

Image calculation in MR imaging is accomplished through a Fourier transform along two directions (2DFT) and pixel scaling to produce a magnitude image. Pixels are scaled so that lower numerical values correspond to minimal signal (e.g., background air signal) and the highest values to the maximal expected intensity. (Unfortunately, at this point there does not exist a well-defined standard for pixel values analogous to CT Hounsfield units.) An image of phase variations is also possible from this 2DFT. Currently, these phase data are utilized in investigations of flow or motion and in research on local magnetic field variations.

Unlike CT, most MR scanners do not typically apply elaborate correction filters to remove artifacts, although some do allow the user to invoke a choice of spatial filters, when appropriate. Various filters can be used to eliminate background noise. An example is the sigma filter, which evaluates local regions in the image to determine if pixel intensities exceed a preset threshold. Regions with pixel intensities that are below the threshold are assumed to be noise, and the pixel value is set to zero; other regions are unaffected. Other filters, such as sinc and Hamming filters, suppress certain artifacts, such as truncation artifacts on 256×128 matrix acquisitions, although at the expense of blurring of image detail.

READ-OUT OF THE ACQUISITION DATA

Radiofrequency and Gradient Refocusing

The echo portion of the SE sequence is actually composed of two components, the refocusing caused by the RF pulse and that caused by compensating gradient integrals. RF refocused echoes, sometimes called *Hahn echoes*, will occur at a time after the midpoint of the 90-degree pulse equal to twice the time between the 90-degree pulse and the 180-degree pulse. In addition, as discussed earlier, the combination of a dephasing gradient and rephasing gradient produces a GRE, which is a distinctly separate echo from the Hahn echo. The GRE occurs when the integral of the dephasing gradient is compensated for by an opposite rephasing integral and may or may not be in synchrony with the RF refocused echo. A misalignment of these echoes may degrade the signal quality as spin vectors cancel each other or, as used in the Dixon technique discussed further on, may produce images containing useful chemical shift information.

Data Sampling

MR imaging data acquisition differs from that in CT in that resolution is not determined by the

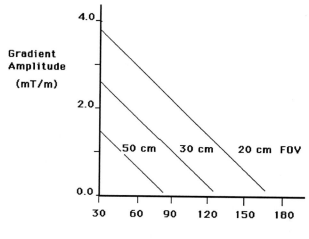

FIGURE 10–11. Plot of required gradient amplitude versus sampling time for a constant FOV. Constant FOVs of 50, 30, and 20 cm are displayed to demonstrate the increased demand on the gradient amplitude in obtaining a smaller FOV while maintaining a constant sampling rate. Note that although small FOVs may be obtained with relatively small gradients, the increased sampling time may make the compromise prohibitive.

number of detectors or detecting positions. Pixel size (Δx) is linearly related to read-out gradient strength (G_{RO}), number of sample points (N), and sampling interval (Δt):

$$\Delta x = 2\pi / (\gamma \, G_{RO} \, N \, \Delta t) \qquad (10)$$

As a practical concern, this means increased resolution may be obtained with a longer read-out period (and longer TE), more samples, or a higher read-out gradient. An illustration of this parameter trade-off is shown in Figure 10–11, comparing gradient amplitudes with sampling times for different FOVs.[12] In revising the gradient amplitudes or sampling times for a given system, it is again essential that changes are consistent with those used to scale distances and FOVs for display purposes. Variations on sampling techniques, with their advantages and limitations, are given in Table 10–2.

TABLE 10–2. ADVANTAGES AND DISADVANTAGES OF VARIATIONS ON STANDARD SAMPLING TECHNIQUES

Technique	Description	Advantage	Limitation
Low band width	Reduced read-out gradient, increased read-out time	Improved S/N	Increased TE Reduced spatial resolution if poor B_0 homogeneity Increased potential for chemical shift artifacts
Asymmetric sampling	Echo asymmetrically centered in sampling	Shorter TE for given bandwidth window	Increased potential for truncation artifacts
Half-Fourier	Use of half of phase-encoding steps	Reduction in acquisition time	Reduced S/N Not useful for GRE sequences

Chemical Shift Effects

In concerning ourselves with the sampling bandwidth, one potential problem is that of the chemical shift of fat relative to water and its influence on read-out gradient and sampling choices.

Water and fat resonate at frequencies roughly 3.5 ppm apart (i.e., 140 Hz at 1.0 T and 225 Hz at 1.5 T). A per pixel bandwidth less than the fat-water frequency difference will result in a misregistration of their signals into adjacent pixels (Fig. 10–12), called a *chemical shift artifact*. This artifact is manifested by sharp high intensity–low intensity bands at fat-water interfaces.[13] The width of these bands will vary, depending on the ratio of pixel bandwidth to chemical shift differences. For the effect to be made negligible, the misregistration must be reduced to less than one pixel along the read-out or frequency-encoding direction; that is, the per pixel bandwidth must be increased (Fig. 10–13). This can be accom-

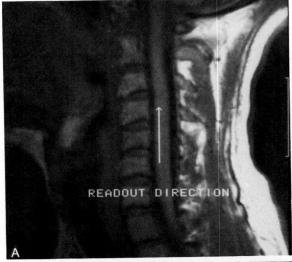

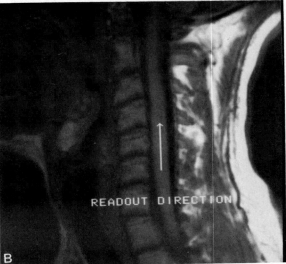

FIGURE 10–13. Sagittal image of a subject showing the effects of sampling bandwidth. The read-out direction (where the artifact is demonstrated) is vertical in the image, while the horizontal direction is used for phase encoding. *A*, A value of 16.7 kHz (about 65 Hz per pixel). *B*, A value of 8.3 kHz (about 32 Hz per pixel). Note the increase in signal intensity banding around the disk–vertebral body interfaces, resulting from chemical shift.

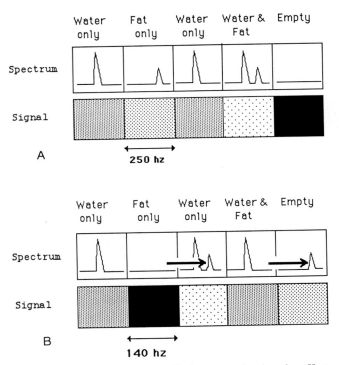

FIGURE 10–12. Chemical shift displacement showing the effect of changing the read-out bandwidth on misregistration of fat-water spins. This example demonstrates the effect at 1 T, at which an expected chemical shift of 3.5 ppm translates into a 140-Hz resonant frequency difference between fat and water. In these schematic matrices, the assumption is that the system has adjusted the frequency to the water peak signal (the larger of the two). The upper image in each pair represents the spectrum (signal intensity versus frequency) for fat and water protons; the lower image represents the resultant signal intensity in each pixel. *A*, In this example, the bandwidth per pixel is 250 Hz. Because the bandwidth of each pixel is relatively large compared with the frequency changes produced by chemical shift differences, there is no observable chemical shift artifact. *B*, In the lower example, the bandwidth per pixel is reduced to 140 Hz. The fat signals now appear in the wrong pixels, resulting in significant alterations in the observed signal intensities.

plished by increasing the amplitude of the read-out gradient, although at the expense of S/N.

The expression for the sampling bandwidth (BW) is:

$$BW = (1 / \Delta t_s) \qquad (11)$$

where Δt_s is time per sample. For example, a read-out period of 5.12 msec for 256 points will have a sampling time of 20 μsec per point and thus a per pixel bandwidth of 50 Hz (or an overall bandwidth of 12.8 kHz for 256 points). It is this per pixel bandwidth that is compared with the relevant chemical shift (δ, in parts per million) and operating frequency (f_o, in megahertz) to assess the potential for chemical shift artifacts.

Number of pixels shifted = $(\delta f_o) / (BW)$ (12)

For example, with a 1-T magnet, the fat-water chemical shift is 140 Hz, and with a bandwidth of 50 Hz, the image will have a shift artifact of about three pixels. To eliminate this effect, the bandwidth must be increased to 140 Hz or more; that is, the time per sample will have to be reduced (in this case down to about 7 μsec per point). In addition, we see from Equation 10 that to keep resolution constant the product of the time per sample and the read-out gradient must be constant. In principle, then, a reduced time per sample requires both a higher read-out gradient strength and an increase in sampling bandwidth.

The location of the chemical shift banding is also dependent on the sign of the gradient used. If the gradient is reversed, the fat-water chemical shift is reversed and the position of dark and light bands will be interchanged. Chemical shift artifacts may also be a problem when using low slice-selection gradients, on which fat-water signals may be selected or refocused outside the imaging plane.

Sampling Bandwidth and Signal-to-Noise Ratios

In choosing the sampling bandwidth, we must also consider the sources of noise in the MR imaging signal and how best to minimize their effect.[14] Uncorrelated background noise comes primarily from the patient and from the RF system, with the patient's noise dominating on the higher field systems. This interference tends to be spectrally broad or *white noise*, affecting equally signals across a wide spectrum of frequencies. Therefore, if a broad bandwidth of read-out frequencies is chosen, more of this background noise is encoded into the signal. Conversely, if a narrow sampling bandwidth is chosen, proportionally less noise per pixel bandwidth will result (Fig. 10–14).

On a per pixel basis, then, S/N is related to pixel size, bandwidth, and averaging of signals

$$\text{Pixel S/N} = k \, V \, \sqrt{N \, \Delta t} \qquad (13)$$

where k is a constant related to system factors (field

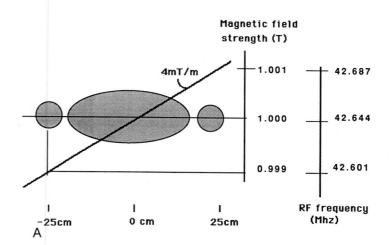

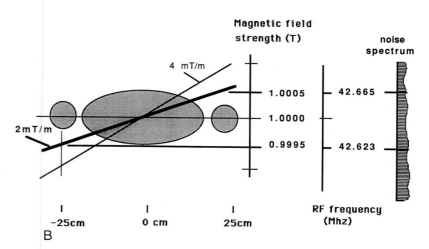

FIGURE 10–14. A comparison of read-out gradient strength with signal bandwidth. *A,* Schematic representation of an axial body scan using a read-out gradient amplitude of 4 mT/meter over a ±25-cm axis. In this example, the main field is 1.000 T, and the gradient field produced covers a range of 2 mT (or about 85 kHz) over a 50-cm FOV. Over 85 kHz, the FT process will assess the 256 or 512 columns of data and localize them for the image. *B,* Comparison of the use of 2 mT/meter versus 4 mT/meter for reading out data. The 2 mT/meter sequence produces the same 256 or 512 columns of data, but over a smaller field range of 1 mT (or 42 kHz). In assuming that a background, "white" noise is inherent in imaging (shaded area on right), this method of reduced gradient strength will produce comparable images with reduced noise (i.e., an increase in the S/N).

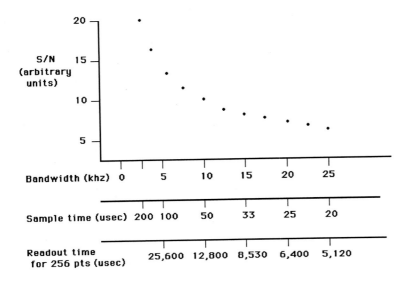

Bandwidth (khz)

Sample time (usec)

Readout time for 256 pts (usec)

FIGURE 10–15. A comparison of S/N versus sampling bandwidth (ignoring consideration of signal decay with extended TEs and other potential compromising factors). With use of an arbitrary S/N standard, a reduction of the sampling bandwidth by 50 per cent shows an increase of S/N by 40 per cent. However, this plot also shows that this reduction in bandwidth requires an increase in the signal sampling times by 100 per cent and that for low bandwidths sampling times may begin to exceed 25 msec.

strength, coil design, and so forth) and sample signal, V is pixel volume, Δt is the time per sample, and N is number of acquisitions or excitations.

Thus, decreasing the read-out bandwidth results in an overall S/N improvement (Fig. 10–15). Assuming white noise sources, there is an improvement of about $\sqrt{2}$ (or 40 per cent), with a reduction in bandwidth of 50 per cent (ignoring for a moment all other effects). Actual S/N gains from bandwidth reduction strategies may be compromised by T_2 decay because of a longer TE and T_2^* decay during the extended read-out period. T_2^* decay over the expanded read-out period may cause a loss of resolution resulting from a loss of the higher frequency components at the tails of the echo.[15]

Reduced-Bandwidth Methods

Sequences incorporating *reduced-bandwidth* or *narrow-bandwidth* techniques have become relatively common on commercial MR imaging systems and, for certain applications, have significant advantages. (As a general rule, any sequence that has a chemical shift of greater than one pixel is considered to be low bandwidth.) These low-bandwidth techniques are amenable to all field strengths; however, their use at higher field strengths is potentially limited by chemical shift artifacts, since the chemical shift is linearly related to field. In this regard, then, the higher field systems may, for some applications, be constrained to using a broader bandwidth read-out than that used by a lower field system. Fat suppression techniques (e.g., CHESS or STIR) can be used to eliminate chemical shift artifact and may enhance the usefulness of low bandwidths on high field systems.[15a]

The use of one bandwidth for both a first and a second echo in a sequence may not produce optimal results. Higher bandwidths have a lower S/N but allow a shorter minimal TE. This feature, therefore, makes a high bandwidth appealing for a first echo, since S/N is typically not as much of a problem. Low

bandwidths produce better S/N, but the minimal TEs tend to get longer. One solution to this is a *mixed-bandwidth* approach; in this method, the combination of a high bandwidth and shorter sampling time allows a rapid first TE, but the S/N may be improved on a second echo by using a low bandwidth.

Finally, when using extended read-out periods to allow reduced bandwidths, artifacts may be encountered owing to gradient instabilities. Unstable peak trapezoidal gradient values over the read-out period will result in bandwidth variations during the sampling time that produce artifacts in the frequency-encoding directions. (These artifacts may vary from geometric distortion to intensity banding over the image.) These gradient instabilities may be due to eddy current compensation methods not suited for prolonged gradient on-times or to hardware duty cycle limits. Reduced-bandwidth techniques will also require increased attention to the main field homogeneity (Equation 9), as it may vary with position in the bore or with local changes in the susceptibility of the patient.

Undersampling Artifacts

Another consideration in determining data read-out parameters is the existence of artifacts resulting from an improper or incomplete sampling. Such faulty sampling will result in image artifacts sometimes referred to as *truncation artifacts*. One common MR imaging problem is an undersampling artifact (or *Gibbs phenomenon*)[16] that manifests itself with a "ringing" or intensity modulation at high-contrast borders. As discussed earlier with selective RF pulses, the time domain truncation of a signal causes a modulation of the frequencies associated with the signal. It is a similar truncation of read-out data that results in this loss of edge definition and a ringing artifact near high-contrast edges. Recalling that these edge definitions in an image are representations of frequency amplitudes at specific locations, sampling to high frequencies is therefore necessary for the edges to be well defined by the Fourier transform. Unfortunately, limited sampling time and data truncation make exact edge definition impossible. As a practical matter, additional sampling (at a constant FOV) will reduce, but not totally remove, these oscillations. Smoothing filters may be of some use for this problem, although at the expense of spatial resolution. Computer modeling methods[17] are being researched for solutions to this problem. Current research is investigating the possibilities of predictive and correlative models that may afford increased resolution from a limited, finite data set.

The *aliasing artifact* unique to MR imaging is also a result of undersampling. When the sampling frequency is less than twice that of the measured signal, there will not be sufficient data for accurate signal representation. This limit of sampling at a minimum of twice the measured frequency is called the *Nyquist criterion*. In other words, to define a 2-kHz signal accurately, samples must be taken at 4 kHz or higher. Failure to sample adequately will result in artifacts, since the data represent, or are a model for, both the original waveform and a nonexistent or aliased waveform. For practical purposes, an undersampled set of data cannot discriminate between the original and aliased waveform and will result in the display of two data sets (main FOV plus the aliased higher frequencies outside the FOV) (Fig. 10–16A).

Aliasing is a problem in both the read-out and the phase-encoding directions. Along the read-out axis, problems will arise when signal outside the FOV (at higher frequencies in read-out, for example) cannot be discriminated from that inside the FOV. This artifact has the appearance of data beyond the edges folding back onto the image; thus, aliasing is sometimes called a *foldover* or *wraparound artifact*.

One solution to this problem, as discussed earlier, is to use low-pass filters to eliminate nonessential frequencies along the read-out direction. Another solution is to oversample data along the read-out and expand the acquisition FOV along that axis, but not expand the displayed FOV. For example, the FOV should be sampled as though it were 50 cm instead of 25 cm, but then after the image reconstruction only a 25-cm FOV should be displayed (Fig. 10–16B). This expanded FOV may still contain foldover artifacts; however, their effect is minimized, since the foldover of nonessential data occurs outside the displayed image. Because the overall sampling interval may remain constant while the digitizing rate increases, this technique may not require further acquisition time.

This oversampling technique is also possible along the phase-encoding axis; however, additional samples along this direction will result in longer acquisition times. Therefore, one proposed solution is to oversample selectively (primarily near the zero phase line) and remove the majority of the large-feature ghost artifacts. This problem could potentially be resolved

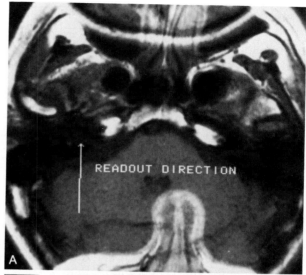

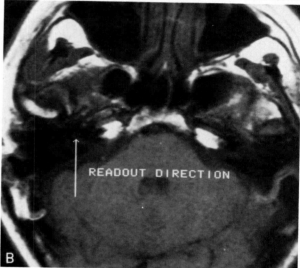

FIGURE 10–16. Effect of undersampling with small FOVs. *A*, Clinical example of a 256 × 256 matrix with a reduced FOV, so that signals outside the imaging FOV wrap around into the image because of undersampling along the read-out direction. *B*, Example identical with (*A*) except that the matrix was extended to 256 × 512 and the FOV was extended, so that the aliased tissues do not appear in the displayed image FOV.

by using one or more slice-selection pulses across the image and eliminating areas that would normally wrap around onto it. This method and its variations are often referred to as *inner-volume techniques*.

Alignment of Sampling and Echo Times

When aligning the timing of the Hahn (RF) and the gradient-refocused echoes with the sampling window, several options are available. The first is to move the center of the sampling window from the center of the refocused echo, a technique known as *asymmetrically sampling* the echo. By moving the center

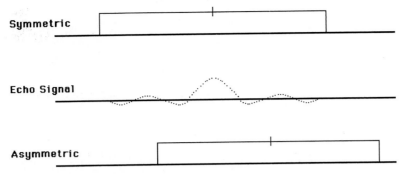

Symmetric

Echo Signal

Asymmetric

(showing 1:3 sampling ratio)

FIGURE 10–17. A comparison of symmetric and asymmetric sampling of the same echo signal. The above read-out shows the received echo centered symmetrically in the sampling interval. The lower example demonstrates the ability to shift the sampling window so that one third of the samples are taken prior to the center of the echo. This asymmetry allows longer read-out periods for low-bandwidth methods or may be used to generate shorter TEs, sometimes at the expense of ringing artifacts in the frequency-encoding direction.

of the sampling window later in the echo, the benefits of a longer sampling time (i.e., lower bandwidth read-out) are achieved while maintaining shorter TEs (Fig. 10–17). Typically, the ratios between the sample time before and after the echo range from 1:1 to 1:3. Since the Fourier transform treats an echo as two free induction decay (FID) signals with a relative phase shift, excessive asymmetry will truncate the sampling of one FID and give an erroneous phase value. Thus, asymmetric sampling beyond about a 1:3 (or 3:1) ratio will tend to produce images with truncation artifacts.

A further option when aligning TEs is to misalign the Hahn and GRE times. The typical use for this technique is to incorporate the difference in precessional frequencies between fat and water and to produce echoes in which the fat-water vectors are in alignment (*in-phase imaging*) or out of alignment (*opposed imaging*). This technique, called the *Dixon method* or *fat-water separation*, is clinically useful when pixel contents cannot be discerned by intensity differences due to tissue T_1, T_2, or proton density (see discussion further on for details).

SPOILER PULSES

Should the T_2 values begin to approach or exceed TR values, problems may result from residual transverse magnetization not completely dephased during the read-out period. This residual magnetization vector may not be in phase with subsequent RF pulses and will result in refocusing of secondary echoes not coherent with the intended measurement. Incoherence of this type may cause a signal loss, a banding artifact across the image, or ghosts superimposed on the images (see Chapter 3). These artifacts or ghost images result when extraneous echoes occur during subsequent slice-selection or read-out periods.

Elimination of the artifact may take many forms; however, the typical manner is to apply a gradient at maximal strength for an extended time. Since the intent is to spoil the remaining magnetization, these are sometimes referred to as *spoiler* or *homospoil gradients*.

In designing dephasing pulses, care should be taken to avoid a situation in which use of this gradient in later data collection will result in gradient refocusing of this magnetization. Therefore, the slice-selection gradient is typically used as one of the spoiler gradients, since it dephases uniformly across the slice and may remain at a constant level during all acquisitions. Furthermore, because the voxel is largest across the slice-selection dimension, a gradient pulse will produce more dephasing when applied in the slice-selection direction than in the phase-encoding or frequency-encoding direction. An alternate method for spoiling the transverse magnetic vector is through a table of steps that decrease from a large maximum to zero.[18] However, this method is most effective when an additional, constant-amplitude gradient is used (e.g., in the frequency-encoding direction); otherwise, when the spoiler gradient table reaches zero, there will be no spoiler gradient and an artifact will be produced owing to the nondispersed transverse magnetization. Use of other gradients may also be indicated when time, as well as limitations in peak gradient amplitude, does not allow the slice-selection direction to have an adequate dephasing gradient integral.

One may estimate the amplitude needed for the spoiler gradient as follows. To disperse the transverse magnetization completely, it must be dephased over at least 360 degrees (2π). Assuming a uniform object, the phase shift (θ) produced by a slice-selection gradient of constant amplitude G and duration t, over a slice with thickness Δz, may be expressed as

$$\theta = 2\pi * \Delta f * t \tag{14}$$

where Δf = bandwidth across the slice. If we substitute $\Delta f = \gamma G \, \Delta z$ into this expression, we obtain

$$t = (\gamma G \, \Delta z)^{-1} \tag{15}$$

In reality, objects are not uniform, so that a larger spoiler gradient might be needed in some instances. On the other hand, in certain multislice applications, sufficient dephasing may occur as a result of subsequent gradient usage. In those cases, these dephasing gradient integrals may be reduced or eliminated to allow more slices within a given TR. Alternatively, *RF spoiling* may be used instead of gradient spoiling (especially for fast 3D sequences). In this method, the phases of successive RF excitations are randomized to prevent the steady-state build-up of transverse magnetization.

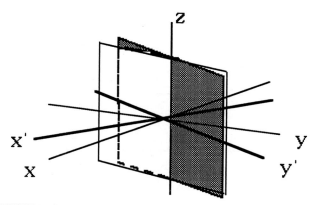

FIGURE 10–18. Diagram showing the process of rotating a plane (x-y to x′-y′) about one axis (z) through the use of multiple slice-selection gradients. The rotation angle for this oblique plane is a trigonometric relationship between the physical gradients and their use as slice-selection and encoding amplitudes.

OFF-CENTER AND OBLIQUE IMAGING

In high-resolution clinical imaging, one of the problems is that of how to move the FOV to a more lateral location. Another question is how to rotate a plane in space so that imaging does not require a precise alignment between the patient's body plane and the orthogonal axes of the gradients.

As discussed in the preceding sections, the location of an object is determined in the read-out direction by assigning a frequency range to the imaged FOV.[19] Therefore, it is possible to vary the location being imaged by shifting the imaging frequency. For example, given that the frequency encoding of data covers a range of +10 kHz to −10 kHz, a basic shift of the imaging frequency by +5 kHz will move the center of the image to one side by 25 per cent (5/20 kHz). Of course, if uncorrected, this will also alter the slice position, since it, too, is frequency dependent. Therefore, a comprehensive off-center high-resolution method must account for changes in both read-out gradient and slice-selection gradient strength, when making imaging frequency adjustments.

The proper implementation of *off-center FOV imaging* therefore requires a basic shift in the imaging frequency, a correction to the slice-shift calculation, and a proper calibration of the image with the display software for directions, legends, and so on.

One significant advantage of MR imaging over CT or other modalities is its ability to image multiple slices at off-center locations with arbitrary angulation for imaging. As discussed previously, imaging to one of the orthogonal gradient directions—that is, sagittal, axial, and coronal—requires only proper assignments between the physical gradients and their logical gradient usage in a sequence. However, imaging along oblique planes is also possible by applying two or more gradients simultaneously during slice selection, phase encoding, and read-out.

Figure 10–18 shows the relationship of a rotated

coordinate system, rotated about one axis (z) by an angle (θ) from its initial orientation. The oblique gradient values are generated from the primary gradients (G_x, G_y, G_z) by the following equations:

$$G_x' = G_x \cos(\theta - G_y \sin(\theta)) \qquad (16)$$

$$G_y' = G_x \sin(\theta) + G_y \cos(\theta) \qquad (17)$$

$$G_z' = G_z \qquad (18)$$

where G_x', G_y', G_z' are the oblique gradients used in typical sequence, and they may be used for slice selection, phase encoding, or read-out.[20]

Semantic variations by commercial vendors for this oblique imaging method include *paracoronal* (rotation of the coronal plane), *parasagittal* (rotation of the sagittal plane), and *paraaxial* (rotation of the axial plane). Paraaxial may also be used as a generic term to indicate oblique imaging. Rotation of the imaging plane about two axes is typically referred to as *double oblique imaging*.

There are certain potential limitations to oblique imaging. Because more than one gradient must be used simultaneously, the pulse sequence timing may need to be altered to accommodate oblique imaging; that is, the minimal TE is increased.

ARTIFACT REDUCTION THROUGH THE USE OF SATURATION PULSES

Motion of objects in the imaging field during the process of data acquisition results in smearing or ghosting artifacts or both. One simple solution for removing these artifacts employs additional RF pulses to eliminate the signal from nonessential objects within the imaging FOV (Fig. 10–19). These pulses

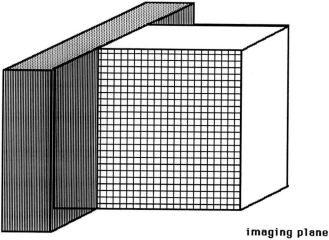

imaging plane

saturation plane

FIGURE 10–19. Diagram showing the use of a presaturation slab to eliminate signal selectively from an area of the imaging plane. In this example, a plane of protons is saturated orthogonal to the imaging. These protons are typically saturated with 90- to 180-degree pulses prior to imaging to prevent motion artifacts from potentially moving structures.

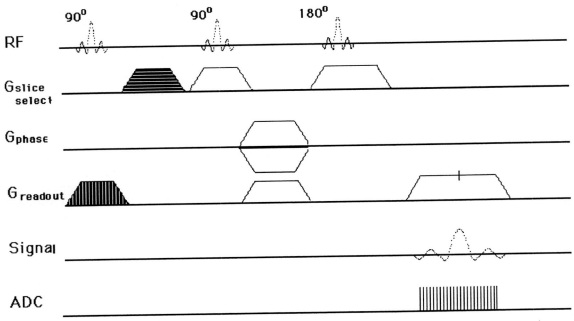

FIGURE 10–20. Sequence used to produce the diagram in Figure 10–19, showing the addition of a saturating selective 90-degree pulse prior to a standard SE sequence. In this example, the presaturating FRODO pulse is oriented along the read-out axis *(vertical bars)*, and the slice-selection gradient *(horizontal bars)* is used to dephase spins prior to the imaging sequence.

may also be used to remove signal from adjacent planes that may introduce artifacts by later moving into the imaging field.[21]

Application of these pulses to saturate signal is most effective when they are immediately prior to the imaging sequence. A typical clinical problem for these saturation pulses involves an axial slice of the abdominal area, where the lumbar spine information is compromised by aortic pulsation, abdominal peristaltic motion, and linear excursions of anterior subcutaneous fat. In this case, a saturating RF pulse of 90 degrees may be applied over the anterior portion of the abdomen (similar to a coronal slice orientation) in such a way that the spinal area is undisturbed yet almost all signal is removed from the offending region. Actual implementation of this technique should also include a dephasing (spoiler) gradient to remove any residual transverse vector after the RF pulse (Fig. 10–20). Because this technique gives, in essence, an image of the saturation profile, optimization of the saturation slice profile is necessary (i.e., a bad profile may partially saturate the area of interest).

Further applications of presaturation methods include anti-aliasing for small FOV imaging, flow signal removal, and flow quantification. Another application of saturation pulses is to label a segment of myocardium in order to better assess regional wall motion.[21a] More precise evaluation of wall motion is obtained using a two-dimensional grid of presaturation stripes.[21b] The grid is created by the sequential application of nonselective RF pulses, separated by gradient pulses that modulate the phases of the excited spins. The relative RF amplitudes are proportional to the binomial coefficients (e.g., 1-4-6-4-1). The spacing of the stripes is determined by the gradient G and is equal to $(1/\gamma Gdt)$, where γ is the gyromagnetic ratio. With this method, the presaturation grid can be applied in as little as 9 msec.

MOTION REDUCTION THROUGH GRADIENT MOTION REPHASING

As discussed previously, it is possible to design and test imaging sequences that will routinely refocus stationary spins so that their net phase at the center of the echo is zero. However, for moving spins this situation becomes more complex.

In assessing stationary spins, we assume that at a given location complementary gradient integrals will refocus transverse magnetization; that is, the net phase for those spins is zero. This was the principle discussed in, for example, the dephasing and rephasing of spins along the read-out axis so that they refocus at the center of the echo. This assumption proves faulty in relation to moving spins, since their location is not constant for all of the gradient pulses. Thus, if moving blood receives a dephasing gradient at one location, it is almost certain not to be in the same location when a complementary refocusing gradient is applied. Furthermore, as blood moves along an axis defined by a gradient, the phase evolution

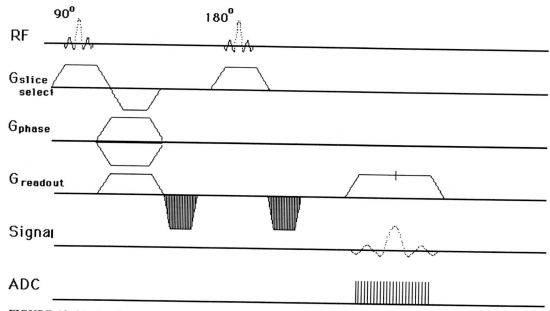

FIGURE 10–21. Gradient motion refocusing (GMR) sequence timing for rephasing along the read-out axis (SE pulse sequence). Additional gradients *(shaded areas)* were added to rephase both stationary and moving spins properly along the frequency-encoding axis. However, in doing so, the minimal TE is extended to incorporate the additional gradient pulses.

for those spins begins to react nonlinearly for the duration of that gradient pulse. Therefore, the problem is that moving fluids are not in the same position for the rephasing gradient and that the longer the duration of the gradient pulses or the interval between pulses, the more nonlinear becomes the phase response of the moving spins.

One solution to this problem lies in adding an extra set of refocusing gradients for motion, while maintaining the original set of refocusing values (Fig. 10–21).[22–25] Commercial variants of this technique are referred to as *bipolar gradient pulses, gradient motion refocusing (GMR), gradient moment nulling (GMN), flow compensation,* or others. These rephasing gradients may be added to the read-out, slice-selecting, and phase-encoding gradients independently to compensate for motion along any or all of these directions. Motion refocusing techniques may be applied to SE (including multiple echo sequences) or GRE sequences. Improper compensation, as with a typical SE sequence, will demonstrate smearing along the phase-encoding direction, as spins are not rephased and thus have a phase (misregistration) artifact. The flow within the vessel demonstrates diminished signal as its intensity is distributed over the image.

Analytical solutions for the proper refocusing pulses are based upon the integral used to calculate the accumulated phase (θ) for spins along one axis:

$$\theta = \gamma \int G\,(t)\,x\,dt \qquad (19)$$

in the case of stationary spins. For the case of a constant velocity v (i.e., x is a function of time t), another phase term is introduced (θ_v):

$$\theta_v = \gamma \int G\,(t)\,vt\,dt$$
$$\text{or}$$
$$= 1/2\,(\gamma\,G\,\mathcal{T}^2\,v) \qquad (20)$$

where $\mathcal{T}$ represents the gradient duration. Linear combination of the cumulative phase evaluation is possible for both stationary spins and protons with a velocity v. A simplified example of the linear combination is shown in Figure 10–22, where the read-out gradient rephases both moving and stationary spins midpoint in the read-out interval (a typical situation for GRE sequences).

$$\theta_v = \gamma \int G_1\,vtdt \text{ (for time 0 to } \mathcal{T}) + \qquad (21)$$
$$\gamma \int G_2\,vtdt \text{ (for time } \mathcal{T} \text{ to } 2\mathcal{T}) +$$
$$\gamma \int G_3\,vtdt \text{ (for time } 2\mathcal{T} \text{ to } 3\mathcal{T})$$
$$= \gamma/2\,(G_1\,\mathcal{T}^2\,v) +$$
$$\gamma/2\,(4G_2\,\mathcal{T}^2\,v - G_2\,\mathcal{T}^2\,v) +$$
$$\gamma/2\,(9G_3\,\mathcal{T}^2\,v - 4G_3\,\mathcal{T}^2\,v)$$

where if $G_1 = G_3 = 1$ (unit amplitude) and $G_2 = -2$, then Equation 21 simplifies to $\Theta_v = 0$; similarly, the phase of stationary spins (Equation 19) rephases to a net phase value of 0.

In practice, an analytical solution for both stationary and a constant-velocity compensation along a given direction may be derived from the preceding equations. However, before implementing these techniques, a final calibration of these sequences should be done using a flow or motion phantom that can simulate conditions found in clinical imaging. Final adjustment techniques will vary with commercial sys-

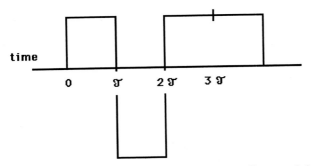

FIGURE 10–22. An example of a rephasing gradient sandwich used to refocus spins along the read-out axis (GRE pulse sequence). In this case, moving and stationary spins rephase at $3\mathcal{T}$ at the middle of the sampling window.

tems and calibration phantoms, but the majority of the methods vary gradient amplitudes in a systematic manner to converge upon an optimal result through a series of experiments.

In designing an adjustment protocol, the symmetry about the 180-degree pulse allows amplitudes of the compensation pulse pair to vary but still maintain refocusing for stationary spins. In the case of adjusting these gradient amplitudes for compensation along the read-out axis, we would align the slice-selection and read-out axes so that the flow pattern parallels the read-out axis. One protocol for adjustment proceeds through a pattern of gradient amplitudes to produce an image with minimal smearing and maximal signal from the flowing liquid. An alternate method is to program the amplitudes to

pass through a pattern of values and then evaluate the raw data to search for a signal maximum at the optimal value. Assuming there is little interaction between gradients, adjustment of this sequence may proceed by independently optimizing each gradient amplitude. As with all sequences destined for clinical use, these rephasing sequences should be tested in a clinical setting on volunteers before being used in trials with patients.

Further expansion of the integrals given in the preceding equations is required for the case in which velocity is not constant and some acceleration is assumed. A proper compensation for the effects of acceleration or higher order motion terms requires additional rephasing gradients (and a further increase in the minimal TE). In clinical practice, the compromise necessary in increasing the minimal TE by adding these extra gradients has not made its use as widely accepted as the velocity rephasing method.

INVERSION RECOVERY

Inversion recovery (IR) was more widely used on many earlier MR imaging systems, as the technique offers excellent T_1 contrast and a larger dynamic range of pixel values. However, higher field strengths (with their associated lengthening of T_1 values) and the requirement of long TR values for a limited number of images have reduced this method's role in routine clinical imaging.

The basic IR sequence is much the same as a SE sequence, with the exception of a prefacing 180-

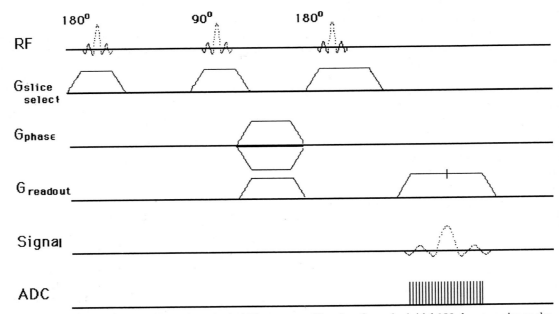

FIGURE 10–23. Sequence timing for a typical IR sequence. The time from the initial 180-degree pulse to the 90-degree pulse is the inversion time and is typically variable to emphasize or de-emphasize image features. The subsequent 90- and 180-degree pulses represent a typical SE sequence used to read out the recovered longitudinal magnetization of the inverted spins.

degree pulse to invert the spins (Fig. 10–23).[26] In fact, some early users of the technique referred to it as an "inversion spin-echo" technique.

The IR sequences available on most commercial systems today can be divided into two methods: magnitude reconstruction and phase reconstruction. In magnitude reconstruction, the phase of the echo is ignored and only an absolute amplitude is used in scaling the image. This method is limited in that it is unable to differentiate whether the magnetization vector has traversed the x-y plane. This inability to differentiate presents a potential problem in that both short and long T_1 values will have the same absolute value and will be scaled to the same intensity. The artifact associated with this technique is sometimes referred to as a *bounce point artifact* (see Chapter 3), since increases in TR will produce a high intensity that is reduced (bounces) when the zero signal line is traversed and then increases again with a longer TR. To circumvent this problem, the phase reconstruction method uses the phase of the returning echo to indicate the sign of the vector (+ or −) and thus give a dynamic range of values twice as large as that given by the magnitude method. However, this method requires additional hardware so that a phase signal can be measured and calculated from the RF demodulator and may not be available on all commercial systems.

As in SE methods, flip-angle variations (as found with an imperfect slice profile) will cause difficulties in the proper refocusing of magnetization. However, IR is different in that imperfect 180-degree inversions will cause variations in how the magnetization vectors then refocus and realign with the main field. For example, if an RF pulse contains 120-, 180-, and 240-degree components, only the 180-degree pulse will properly invert the spins, while the 120- and 240-degree pulse will actually rotate them toward the x-y plane. Thus, the vectors from the 120- and 240-degree pulses will not properly represent the longitudinal relaxation and will produce erroneous refocusing of signals above and below the plane.

To avoid this situation, either RF pulses with better slice profiles are used or, more commonly, a broader bandwidth for the 180-degree pulse is incorporated. This method then uses the 90-degree pulse to refocus only the central, more completely inverted section. Having a broad slice-selection pulse, of course, limits the multislice capability because successive slices must be widely separated.

SEQUENCE CALIBRATION

Most commercial MR scanners offer SE as well as GRE techniques. GRE methods may be categorized into two types: those that maintain steady-state transverse magnetization (e.g., FISP, GRASS) and those that do not (e.g., FLASH).

Calibration of these sequences consists primarily of a series of gradient integral (i.e., duration × amplitude) adjustments:

1. To compensate for dephasing across the slice-selection direction, a negative gradient integral is applied. The product of amplitude and duration is about 50 to 70 per cent of the initial slice-selection integral, with the exact calibration being dependent on local gradient capabilities and selective RF pulse shape. A series of test values should converge quickly to a value producing a maximal S/N and minimal artifacts. Improper adjustment results in reduced S/N.

2. To compensate for dephasing along the read-out direction, the integral is altered until the echo is centered onto the desired portion of the sampling period (TE for symmetric data sampling). Although the magnitude image is relatively tolerant of moderate misadjustments, severe misadjustments result in truncation artifacts along the read-out direction as well as reduced S/N and, for SE images, Dixon-type chemical shift effects. Misadjusted GRE images demonstrate zebra stripe artifacts.

3. Final adjustment of phase and read-out gradients should also be made to correct for any geometric distortion.

The adjustment of RF pulse angles is automated on most modern commercial imaging systems, taking the initial calibration of the patient and making the necessary trigonometric calculations for various flip angles. Since contrast patterns are directly related to RF excitation, small variations in flip angle across a slice may produce an image whose contrast is not accurate. In other words, a poor slice profile that has a peak flip angle of 70 degrees and wide tails with flip angles of 20 degrees will produce an image that is a composite of differing contrast patterns over the slice. Proper attention to improving the slice profiles and a rechecking of clinical contrast patterns are necessary to produce the most consistent image quality.

Calibration of the 2D FISP sequence is much the same except that care must be taken in trying to maintain the optimal steady-state conditions. Given an optimized 2D FLASH imaging sequence, the slice-selection gradient pulse following read-out should be adjusted for the best refocusing of spins during the subsequent RF pulse. Improper refocusing may produce secondary vectors that are not in phase with the excitation pulse. These vectors may then refocus out of phase with the primary echo and may cancel the signal or add to it to produce artifacts.

VARIATIONS ON TWO-DIMENSIONAL FOURIER TRANSFORM METHODS

Projection Reconstruction

The earliest MR image was made by Paul Lauterbur, using a projection reconstruction technique he named *Zeugmatography*.[27] In this technique, the initial read-out gradient is gradually rotated into one of the orthogonal axes through successive acquisitions.[28] During each of the steps, the projection of the slice is taken by the rotating read-out gradient. These data are then transformed from a time-based sampling to a gradient-specified frequency projection of the object; that is, the FID is converted into amplitude projection at each angle. A series of projections is then filtered and back-projected using standard tomography algorithms. Because this method used off-the-shelf tomography techniques and equipment, it was the method of choice for earlier systems. Unfortunately, imaging artifacts from magnetic field inhomogeneity, physiologic motion, metallic artifacts, and other problems limited its utility.

At the present time, this method is used for research and when short read-out (FID) images are needed (i.e., flow studies and multinuclear imaging). This method is compatible with both the SE and the GRE techniques.

Half-Fourier Data Reconstruction

The data from a standard 2DFT sequence are redundant because data acquired during the initial half of the phase-encoding process are the phase-shifted *complex conjugate* of those obtained from the second half. In other words, there exists some redundancy between the data received during the first and second halves of an acquisition. Therefore, given proper phase definition up to the midpoint, it is possible to Fourier transform this data and construct a full-resolution image from only half of the data (*half-Fourier imaging*).[29] However, though this method will produce an image in half the time of standard 2DFT methods with identical resolution, its S/N will be significantly less (about 40 per cent) and may be susceptible to artifacts (especially with GRE sequences).

An important variation on this method is *conjugate synthesis*. This method uses only slightly more than 50 per cent of the phase-encoding process to produce a database. From these data, a complete full-Fourier data set is synthesized, using the additional zero transition phase-encoding lines to eliminate ghosting artifacts. This synthesized full data set is then transformed using the same image-processing algorithms.

An innovative variation on this technique produces images, should the operator have to abort imaging. In those clinical cases in which the patient requires immediate attention, the scanning series may be halted and images will be produced if more than 50 per cent of the scanning was completed.

Fat-Water Separation Techniques

When it is difficult to determine whether a voxel contains protons bound primarily in fat or water, or in both, on the basis of variations in TR, TE, and signal intensities, MR imaging may offer other possibilities. Since fat and water have two slightly differ-

ent resonance frequencies (about 3.5 ppm difference), it is possible to design sequences that take advantage of this additional characteristic to specify a voxel's contents more precisely. The two most widely known on commercial MR scanners are the *Dixon* or *phase-cycling technique* and the *chemical shift selective saturation (CHESS) technique*.

Because of their resonance frequency difference, fat and water spins begin to dephase immediately after the slice-selection RF pulse. They continue to dephase until the 180-degree pulse is applied, at which time their spins are inverted. This refocusing pulse reverses the dephasing so that by the middle of the read-out interval both fat and water are in phase. The typical SE sequence also symmetrically rephases the spins along the read-out gradient so that they are in phase at the same time as the RF-refocused or Hahn echo.

The Dixon technique[30] differs in that the 180-degree pulse is advanced in time so that fat and water spins are opposed, or 180 degrees apart, during the sampling interval. Application of this method to a single-echo SE sequence is demonstrated in Figure 10–24, where the TE for the GRE is offset from the RF echo by a time t:

$$t = 1 / 2 (f_{water} - f_{fat}) \qquad (22)$$

where the precessional frequency difference is a linear function of field strength. Given a 3.5 ppm

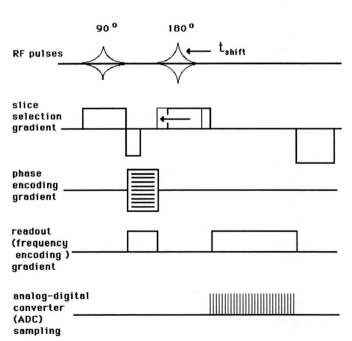

FIGURE 10–24. Modification of SE sequence (Fig. 10–1) to perform a phase-contrast (opposed) image using the Dixon technique. In this example, the 180-degree pulse is moved in the sequence so that the refocusing from the RF pulses should refocus the spins with a slightly shorter TE. However, the read-out gradients have not been altered, so that the spins from the Hahn echo and the gradient-rephasing echo should produce fat-water vectors that are in opposition (180 degrees) to each other.

chemical shift between water and lipid peaks, we may then expect a difference of 147 Hz on a 42-MHz (or 1-T) MR system. An opposed image should be produced when the GRE (or RF echo) is shifted 3 msec.

Proper clinical application of this method to specify the fat and water content of a voxel requires, then, both an in-phase and an opposed image, as well as some additional phase information. For example, if a voxel contains both fat and water, the in-phase minus the opposed image should show a high intensity, whereas if the voxel is mostly fat or water, the subtraction should produce a low intensity (i.e., no internal self-cancellation of signal). However, there is some difficulty with whether a voxel is mostly fat or mostly water, since we have only two pieces of information with the magnitude reconstructed images. Since fat spins should be rotated 180 degrees and water 0 degrees when sampled, for example, a complex reconstruction method is required to specify the voxel's contents completely.

In practice, it is difficult to determine with absolute certainty the phase, since field inhomogeneities will cause local distortions. Various solutions have been proposed to map these disturbances using phantoms and to correct for timing phase misadjustments through additional mathematical processing of the data.[31]

In routine clinical operation, a number of physicians have opted not to do a complete fat-water specificity test but rather to rely on the opposed images to highlight areas of encroachment of fat or water into otherwise homogeneous structures.

CHESS techniques are based on tailoring the frequency of an RF pulse to one species of protons so that signals from those protons are removed from a subsequent imaging sequence.[32, 33] A typical sequence might begin with a narrow-bandwidth, nonselective pulse that selectively excites only the water-bound protons throughout the volume. If we then apply a dephasing gradient, the water-bound protons will not contribute signals until rephased or normal relaxation processes reestablish a net magnetic vector. Thus, if we initiate a normal SE sequence immediately after the dephasing pulse, only the non–water-bound (i.e., fat-bound) protons will be imaged (Fig. 10–25). To produce a water-only image, the selective excitation frequency needs only to be shifted slightly so that the fat-bound protons will be preselected and removed from the imaging sequence.

MRI Control Systems

Control Instrumentation

Run-time control of most commercial MR imaging systems begins with the user's selection of operating parameters. These choices are stored by a central computer and then are translated into individual timing and control commands for each of the subsystems.

During the preimaging loading procedure, each of the subsystems is set up for the particular sequence. During this stage, the RF pulses are calculated, there is a translation of orientation to specific gradients, timing calibrations are made, and a general consistency and safety check is made of the sequence. The second phase of the sequence loading procedure is a downloading of information through a communications device to control computers in each of the subsystems. This information includes sequence programs to be executed by the controlling computers or data sets to control the operation of these programs. It will also notify the image-processing computer of the algorithm to be used in data acquisition and image calculation.

Run-time control begins when the operator initiates the sequence and a central computer takes over the coordination of the timing, subsystem integrity, and data collection. Once execution has finished, this computer then initiates image processing, checks for subsystem errors, and notifies the operator of the completion of sequence and image processing.

Control Systems in Sequence Design

In designing sequences, control is usually handled through this central computer system and rarely through direct regulation of individual subsystems. The format for the sequence control editor is discussed in the next section, but in most modern MR imaging systems, it is a stand-alone program that takes sequence design parameters and translates them into an executable form.

Sequence Editor and Programmer

Depending on the particular clinical MR imaging system, capabilities for editing and programming changes into sequences may vary from none at all to those that are user friendly with power to operate at a number of different levels. One example of a commercially available sequence editor output is included in part in Figure 10–26. In reviewing sequence editing and programming capabilities on various commercial clinical systems, the following features should be considered.

Language-Based Feature. Editing should proceed using a self-explanatory, easily formated language. It should require little user education to make trivial changes and should check user responses for consistency and safety. In the interest of user friendliness, the time to change and the time from change to test should be minimized.

Dialogue Control. To communicate better with the MR imaging operator, the editor should allow direct control of dialogue choices. For example, the sequence editor would be able to define a working range of TR, TE, slice thickness, and so forth.

Commenting Capability. A useful feature for

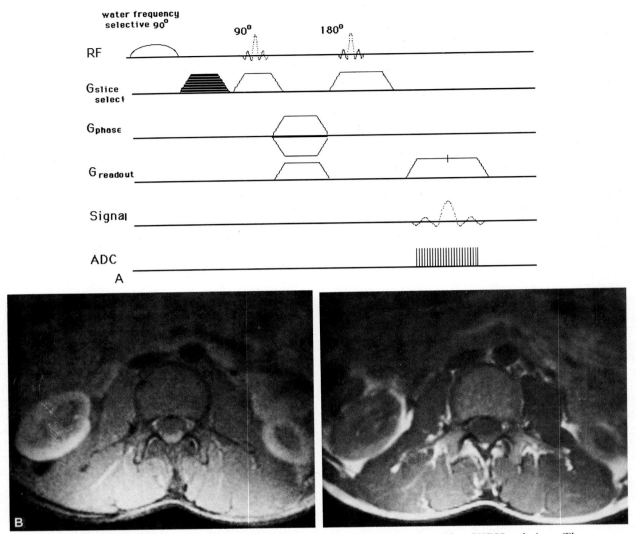

FIGURE 10-25. CHESS technique. *A,* Sequence design for 2DFT SE imaging with a CHESS technique. The water frequency–selective 90-degree pulse tips water-bound spins only. Then the slice-selection gradient *(shaded area)* dephases the spins so that only the non–water-bound (i.e., fat-bound) protons will be imaged (in this case, by a typical 2DFT SE sequence). *B,* Results from a CHESS method to eliminate fat signal. The right image represents a typical axial section through the lumbar region using a SE method to image both fat and water. The left image demonstrates that by the elimination of the fat signal through a fat-selective RF pulse, the subsequent SE sequence is able to image primarily the water-bound protons through the same section.

setting up multiple sequences with different capabilities is the ability to comment on the specifics of operation. These comments are useful to explain overall sequence characteristics as well as individual timing events.

TIMING CONTROL. Control of the event timing is key to working with the potential of MR imaging sequences. Some features essential to achieving this potential are as follows:

1. Independent control of RF pulses (nonselective and selective), gradient amplitudes and durations, and sampling.
2. Automatic calculation of variables such as RF

pulses (including flip angles, power levels, slice offsets, and so on), gradient scaling factors and orientations, and internal timing controls.
3. Loop programmability for averaging, imaging lines, and 3D planes, that is, progressing through a sequence via a loop while having automatic calculation of the incremental values.
4. Graphic display of each timing event.
5. Control of both local and global values, such as gradient amplitudes for slice, phase encoding, and read-out.
6. Independent control of preparation scans, such as looping through a GRE sequence n times to approximate steady-state behavior.

EVENT DURATION (msec)	RF PULSE	ADC	LOGICAL GRADIENT PHASE	READOUT	SLICE
1.000					1.000
2.560	PULSE1				1.000
1.400			TABLE1	1.200	
1.140			TABLE1	1.200	
1.300			TABLE1	1.200	-1.000
0.100				1.200	
1.000					1.000
2.560	PULSE2				1.000
0.480					1.000
0.400					
1.500				1.000	
7.680		ON		1.000	
15.000					-10.000
2.000					

------------- RF PULSE TABLE -------------------

RF PULSE	FLIP ANGLE
PULSE1	90
PULSE2	180

------------- PHASE ENCODING TABLE ------------------

PHASE TABLE	CALCULATION METHOD
TABLE1	2D PROGRESSION -

FROM MAXIMUM NEGATIVE TO MAXIMUM POSITIVE

FIGURE 10–26. Sequence editor output from a commercially available MR scanner. An abbreviated example of a typical sequence controller timing program is shown. In this short TR SE example, the design rules used 1-msec rise and fall time for the gradient pulses and 2.56 msec for the RF pulses. Only logical gradients are shown, on the assumption that the physical gradient selection will be made at execution time. Also at execution time calculations will be made, based upon chosen FOV, slice thickness, and other variables, to set individual gradient amplitudes and ADC timing intervals. The flow of this sequence example is that of a loop structure in which a phase-encoding gradient is progressively stepped through a table of amplitudes.

ABILITY TO CREATE MULTIPLE SEQUENCE VARIATIONS. Each sequence should exist as a separate computer file to allow multiple versions to be made during testing and eventual use. If possible, the file size should be minimized so as not to detract from image storage space.

CONTROL OF IMAGE PROCESSING. Control should be given to select data and image-processing algorithms, such as 3D, IR, multiple SEs, half-Fourier, or others.

DEBUGGING CAPABILITY. Given that sequences may require some problem-solving tools, an attractive sequence programmer will contain the ability to check for errors upon editing, upon loading of the subsystem commands, and upon the inevitable failure when executing.

REFERENCES

1. Faul DD: An Overview of MR System Design: Technology of NMR. New York, Society of Nuclear Medicine, 1984, pp 3–14.

2. Young IA, Payne JA, Bryant DJ, et al: Artifacts in the Measurement of T1 and T2. *In* Partain CL, Price RR, Patton JA, et al (eds): Magnetic Resonance Imaging. Philadelphia, WB Saunders Co., 1988, pp 1321–1334.
3. Garroway AN, Grannell PK, Mansfield P: Image formation in NMR by a selective irradiative process. J Phys 7:457, 1974.
3a. Glover GH, Shimakawa A: POMP (phase-offset multiplanar imaging): A new high efficiency technique. Proceedings of the Society of Magnetic Resonance in Medicine, 7th Annual Meeting. San Francisco, August 20–26, 1988, p 241.
3b. Pauly J, Nishimura D, Macovski; A: Multi-dimensional selective excitation. Proceedings of the Society of Magnetic Resonance in Medicine, 7th Annual Meeting. San Francisco, August 20–26, 1988, p 654.
4. Feinberg DA, Crooks LE, Hoenninger JC, et al: Contiguous thin multisection MRI by two-dimensional Fourier transform techniques. Radiology 158:811–817, 1986.
5. Loaiza F, Lim K-T, Warren WS, et al: Crafted pulses and pulse sequences for MR imaging. Health Care Instrum 1:188–195, 1986.
6. Warren WS, Silver MS: The Art of Pulse Crafting: Advances in Magnetic Resonance. New York, Academic Press, 1988, pp 284–384.
7. Thomas SR, Dixon RL (eds): NMR in Medicine: The Instrumentation and Clinical Applications. Portland, OR, AAPM Summer School, 1985.
7a. Emsley L, Bodenhausen G: Self-refocusing 270° Gaussian pulses for slice selection without gradient reversal in MRI. Magn Res Med 10:273–281, 1989.
7b. Morris PG, Rourke D, Ngo JT, McIntyre DJO: 7th Annual Meeting of the Society of Magnetic Resonance in Medicine, San Francisco, August 1988.
7c. Hardy CJ, Bottomley PA: 7th Annual Meeting of the Society of Magnetic Resonance in Medicine, San Francisco, August 1988.
8. Budinger TF, Margulis AR (eds): Medical MRI and Spectroscopy. Berkeley, CA, Society for Magnetic Resonance in Medicine, 1986.
9. Mansfield P, Morris PG: NMR Imaging in Medicine. New York, Academic Press, 1982.
10. Heubes P: Evaluation of Gradient Pulse Shapes by MR. Siemens Medical Systems, Iselin, NJ, 1984, pp 1–7.
11. Partain CL, James AE, Rollo FD, Price RR (eds): NMR Imaging. Philadelphia, WB Saunders Company, 1983.
12. Crooks LE, Hoenninger J, Arakawa M, et al: High-resolution MRI. Radiology 150:163–171, 1984.
13. Viamonte M, Soila KP, Starewicz PM: Chemical misregistration effects in MRI. Radiology 153:819, 1984.
14. Mugler JP, Brookeman JR: The optimum symmetry and duration of data sampling for maximum image signal-to-noise ratio. Proceedings of the Society of Magnetic Resonance, San Francisco, 1988, p 1038.
15. King KF, Moran PR: A unified description of NMR imaging, data-collection strategies, and reconstruction. Med Phys 11:1–14, 1984.
15a. Mitchell DG, Vinitski S, Rifkin MD, Burk DL: Sampling bandwidth and fat suppression: Effects on long TR/TE MR imaging of the abdomen and pelvis at 1.5 T. AJR 153:419–425, 1989.
16. Bracewell RN: The Fourier Transform and its Application. New York, McGraw-Hill, 1978.
17. Wood ML, Henkelman, RM: Truncation artifacts in magnetic resonance imaging. Magn Reson Med 2:517–526, 1985.
18. Wood ML, Silver MS, Runge VM: Optimization of spoiler gradients in FLASH MRI. Magn Reson Imaging 5:455–463, 1987.
19. Edelstein W, Hutchison J, Johnson G, Redpath T: Spin warp NMR imaging and applications to human whole-body imaging. Phys Med Biol 25:751–756, 1980.
20. Huber DJ, Mueller E, Heubes P: Oblique MRI of normal structures. AJR 145:843–846, 1985.
21. Edelman RR, Atkinson DJ, Silver MS, et al: FRODO pulse sequences: A new means of eliminating motion, flow and wraparound artifacts. Radiology 166:231–236, 1988.

21a. Zerhouni EA, Parish DM, Rogers WJ, et al: Human heart: Tagging with MR imaging–a method for noninvasive assessment of myocardial motion. Radiology 169:59–74, 1988.

21b. Axel L, Dougherty L: Heart wall motion: Improved method of spatial modulation of magnetization for MR imaging. Radiology 172:349–350, 1989.

22. Moran PR: A flow velocity Zeugmatographic interface for NMR imaging in humans. Magn Reson Imaging 1:197–203, 1982.

23. Bryant DJ, Payne JA: Measurement of flow with NMR imaging using a gradient pulse and phase difference technique. J Comput Assist Tomogr 8:588–593, 1984.

24. Deimling M, Mueller E, Lenz G, et al: Description of flow phenomena in MRI. Diagn Imag Clin Med 55:37–51, 1986.

25. Haacke EM, Lenz GW: Improving MR image quality in the presence of motion by using rephasing gradients. AJR 148:1251–1258, 1987.

26. Stroebel B: Fundamentals of MR tomography. Bruker Med Rep 1:7–12, 1985.

27. Lauterbur PC: Image formation by induced local interactions: Examples employing nuclear magnetic resonance. Nature 242:190–191, 1973.

28. Kumar A, Welti D, Ernst R: NMR Fourier Zeugmatography. J Magn Reson 18:69–83, 1975.

29. Margozian P: Faster MR imaging—imaging with half the data. Proceedings of the Society of Magnetic Resonance in Medicine, London, 1985, p 1024.

30. Dixon WT: Simple proton spectroscopic imaging. Radiology 153:189–194, 1984.

31. Sauter R, Margozian P, Koenig H, Weber H: Proton chemical shift imaging: An improvement in the specificity of MRI. Health Care Instrum 1:205–211, 1986.

32. Rosen BR, Wedeen VJ, Brady TJ: Selective saturation NMR imaging. J Comput Assist Tomogr 8:813–818, 1984.

33. Haase A, Frahm J, Haenicke W, Matthei D: 1H NMR chemical shift selective (CHESS) imaging. Phy Med Biol 30:341–344, 1985.

11

SITE PLANNING

MICHAEL F. KOSKINEN

MAGNETS
QUENCHES
RADIOFREQUENCY INTERFERENCE

FRINGE FIELDS
SAFETY

Site planning for an MR imaging facility involves the same primary issues as planning for a CT suite or other imaging facility. Some of these considerations are listed in Table 11–1. In addition to these familiar issues, MR imaging site planning involves some special concerns not seen in other types of imaging. These are primarily related to the very weak MR signal, which must be protected from electrical interference, and to the interactions of the magnetic field with the environment. If a supercon-

ducting magnet is used, there are some special issues related to cryogens and superconduction.

Site planning for an imaging facility is done by a professional, skilled in this discipline, in cooperation with the eventual users of the site and the site planning staff of the MR imaging manufacturer. This chapter is designed to provide an overview of the major issues that are unique to MR imaging site planning and to describe some of the main physical phenomena that influence these issues. A few related procedural considerations are also discussed. It is hoped that this background will allow radiologists and other medical professionals to make better contributions to the site planning process. Somewhat more technical presentations are also available.[1] Information for the participating medical physicist can be found in more detail in a report from the American Association of Physicists in Medicine (AAPM).[2]

TABLE 11–1. SOME OF THE ISSUES THAT MUST BE ADDRESSED IN SITE PLANNING

Patients' access and comfort	Lounges
Changing facilities	Traffic patterns of radiologists
Lavatories	Referring clinicians
Types of cases expected	House officer teams
Health and ambulatory status of expected patients	Students
	Professional visitors
Waiting areas	Access to patients' records and previous imaging studies
Stretcher and wheelchair parking	Access to recent cases
Nursing support	Discussion and teaching areas
Reception	Reporting facilities
Patient flow	Transcription facilities
Booking	Equipment weight
Registration	Power
Record keeping	Power conditioning
Education of the patient	Cooling water
Answering questions	Heating, ventilating, and air conditioning
Preparation of patients	Delivery paths and rigging
Traffic pattern of technologists	Construction staging
Film development	Impact on adjacent areas
Staff changing facilities	

MAGNETS

Imaging magnets are built according to any of several basic designs. Chapter 12 describes them in detail. The selection of an MR imaging system depends primarily on the uses to which it will be put, such as clinical imaging, spectroscopy, research, and so on. The siting requirements of a system, however, will depend strongly on the type of magnet that the selected system employs.[3]

Superconducting magnets[4] are the most common type of imaging magnet in use today. The advantages of superconducting magnets include highest available magnetic field strength, high homogeneity, and excellent field stability. These features make them well suited for fast imaging, as well as high signal-to-noise (S/N), spin-echo (SE) imaging. Field strengths, ranging from about 0.35 T up to 1.5 to 2.0 T, are commercially available. Whole-body magnets up to 4 T have been produced and used experimentally.

Once the magnetic field is energized (ramped up), superconducting magnets remain on, day and night, without interruption. This constant high field requires special considerations, which are discussed in the "Safety" section of this chapter.

Superconducting magnets require cryogens. Cryogens can be supplied in one of two forms. The most common method is the weekly delivery to the site of liquid cryogens in large, insulated containers, called dewars. Dewars are available in nonmagnetic stainless steel. Liquid nitrogen is typically delivered every week, and helium is included in the order once a month. Depending on their capacity, dewars can range from 2 to 4 feet in diameter, stand 5 to 6 feet high, and weigh from 400 to 1000 pounds, when filled with cryogens. A delivery path and a storage area for these dewars, preferably in or near the MR imaging suite, must be provided. Dewars also need to be brought up next to the magnet during the filling of cryogens. They are mounted on small casters and roll reasonably easily on smooth floors but can damage mat switches for automatic doors. Refilling liquid nitrogen typically requires about 1 to 1.5 hours each week. This time increases to about 3 to 5 hours for the monthly fill when liquid helium is also supplied. Patients are not usually scanned while cryogens are being filled. The ceiling height above many magnets cooled by liquid cryogens must be about 10 feet, to permit access for filling cryogens.

The other method of meeting the cryogenic requirements of a superconducting magnet is to fit it with its own cryogenic refrigerator. Usually, this device directly cools the "nitrogen" shield in the magnet, making the delivery of liquid nitrogen unnecessary. It also reliquefies much of the helium vapor that evaporates from the helium reservoir. The reliquefied helium is returned to its reservoir in the magnet, thus greatly extending the intervals between helium fillings. The selection between these two methods is usually made on economic grounds: liquid gases and associated space and service costs for cryogens versus capital cost and cost of electrical power for a refrigerator. Refrigerators are often more economical in mobile systems, where special logistics and storage space represent problems with additional costs for liquid gas delivery.

A typical superconducting magnet may weigh up to 10 tons with a full charge of cryogens. Although this is moderately heavy, most existing buildings can carry this load without much difficulty. Some buildings, however, may require the spreading of this load over an increased floor area.

Superconducting magnets have magnetic fields, called "fringe fields," which extend beyond the magnet for rather large distances. These fringe fields have many important effects on the site design. These are dealt with in a section of their own and in the "Safety" section of this chapter.

Superconducting magnets in mobile systems are ramped down to a very low field before the trailer is moved. On arrival at the next site, they are ramped up to full field again, and the shims are reset to predetermined values that have been established for the specific site. This procedure sometimes requires accurate placement of the trailer to ensure reproducible conditions for the magnet. After reaching full field, the magnet requires some time for the field to stabilize adequately before starting to image. Ramping down, ramping up, and stabilization each can require about an hour.

The imaging bore of a superconducting magnet is rather narrow and can cause claustrophobic reactions in a significant number of patients, even ones who had not previously experienced claustrophobia. In addition to good rapport with the patient, a warm, nonthreatening architectural design of the scan room and patient route to the magnet can be helpful. Good lighting in the magnet bore is also recommended.

Resistive magnets are the predecessors of superconducting magnets. They produce a magnetic field, similar to that produced by a superconducting magnet, generally along the length of the patient. The electrical current, flowing in the heavy copper windings, produces a large amount of heat, which is carried away by water flowing inside these copper wires. The copper "wires" can be copper tubing, about a quarter of an inch in diameter. The difficulty in cooling the copper windings and the large amount of power (about 100 kW) required to drive the electrical current through the windings put a limit of about 0 to 0.15 T on the imaging field of these magnets.

A more recent commercial system, designed to be very economical, operates in the range of 0.01 to 0.02 T and uses a resistive magnet, which does not require special cooling. This is possible because the amount of power required to drive a resistive magnet, as well as the resulting cooling load, varies with the square of the imaging field. This feature makes the electrical and cooling requirements of this ultralow field magnet quite modest.

The fringe fields of these resistive magnets are similar to those of superconducting magnets, but because of the lower field strengths of resistive magnets, the fringe fields are proportionally less intense. Resistive magnets also have the advantage that they can be turned off with no difficulty.

Another variation of the resistive magnet design uses iron around the outside of the magnet. This iron guides the magnetic flux lines along a much shorter path back to the magnet bore, rather than allowing them to take the long route of the usual fringe fields. This has the effect of concentrating the flux lines in the imaging bore, thereby producing a more intense imaging field with no increase in magnet power. This iron flux return path also reduces the extent of the fringe fields. Imaging systems using magnets of this type operate at field strengths up to 0.4 T.

Permanent magnets form the third major category of imaging magnets. The structure is made of soft iron to guide the magnet flux in an efficient manner. The pole pieces are assembled from blocks of permanent magnetic material, which produce the required magnetic field. One important advantage of this design is that the magnet can be transported to the site in pieces and assembled on site. This eliminates the need for a moderately high and wide delivery path, as is required for a superconducting magnet. The almost complete lack of fringe fields is another advantage. Such a magnet, however, can be impractical in some locations because of its weight. A commercial imaging system, using this type of magnet at 0.3 T, weighs 100 tons. This weight is actually supported economically on grade or in new construction, which is designed for this weight. It can become a problem at sites one or more floors above the foundation level, where reinforcement of the building structure can become expensive, as well as disruptive of activities on the floors below.

Modern, high-performance magnetic materials (samarium-cobalt) have been used to build an imaging magnet of novel design, which is lighter than a superconducting magnet.[5] The component magnets are attached to a horizontal cylinder in a so-called two-theta distribution of orientations. This arrangement produces a uniform, vertical magnetic field within the horizontal imaging tube and almost perfect cancellation of the fringe fields outside the imaging tube. Imaging fields of 0.2 to 0.3 T were produced in this way, but the imaging system, of which it was a part, did not develop past early clinical testing.

QUENCHES

Superconducting magnets have currents from a few hundred to a thousand or more amperes flowing in relatively thin wires. These electrically conducting wires, which have absolutely zero electrical resistance, are called superconductors. More details are available in Chapter 12. These wires maintain their superconducting properties only at temperatures within a few degrees of absolute zero.

The superconducting wire is maintained at an adequately low temperature by being immersed in a container of liquid helium within the magnet. Helium boils at 4.2° above absolute zero. The tiny amount of heat that slowly leaks into the highly insulated region of the electrical windings is carried away with the vapor produced in the boiling of the helium, thus keeping the temperature of the wires at 4.2° K. This process normally takes place with no difficulty in well-designed modern magnets, and the imaging field remains highly stable.

On the other hand, one may imagine that something warms a small region of the superconducting wire. The temperature of the superconductor could be raised above its critical temperature, which means that this region of the wire will develop normal resistance. A very large current is then flowing through a region of normal resistance, which will generate additional heat. This ohmic heating can cause the region of nonsuperconduction to grow larger, which in turn would lead to an even more rapid production of heat. This cycle, once started, will continue until the entire energy of the magnetic field is converted into heat in the windings of the magnet. This process is called a "quench." A quench may require from less than a minute to several tens of minutes to go to completion. Although quenches are now fairly rare events, they usually occur with little or no warning, and provisions must be in place ahead of time if they are to be dealt with safely, when they do occur.

The heat produced during a quench can be sufficiently concentrated to melt wires in the coil windings. Such a catastrophic event is called a "destructive quench," and it necessitates the replacement of the magnet, a very expensive process. The design of recent magnets distributes the thermal energy of most quenches sufficiently uniformly that the destruction of the magnet is usually prevented. As unlikely as it is, it might be prudent, in designing an MR imaging site, to consider the route for magnet removal if such a destructive quench were to occur.

The full energy of the magnetic field is dissipated within the liquid helium container. The amount of this energy is rather large, being on the order of a megajoule. A megajoule equals the amount of energy needed to keep a 100-W light bulb burning for more than 2.5 hours. The amount of energy released is greatest at high imaging fields, increasing as the square of the operating magnetic field. The energy liberated in the helium reservoir is enough to vaporize most or all of the liquid helium, which can amount to 1000 liters. The enormous amount of gaseous helium produced could not be contained within the helium vessel without severe damage to the internal structure of the magnet. The helium is, therefore, allowed to escape as rapidly as it builds up.

The volume of escaping gas is often so great that it is capable of entirely displacing the air from a scan room. This situation could lead to the asphyxiation of patients and staff and, possibly, damage to the building, owing to the development of overpressure. For these reasons, the port on the magnet, from which the gaseous helium rushes, is connected with a large duct. This duct conducts the helium to an area where it can be diluted with an adequate amount of ambient air, usually out of doors. This duct, which is called a "quench vent," might be 12 inches in diameter in some installations. The actual diameter depends on the length of the duct, the number of corners that the duct must go around, other impediments to flow that may be present, as well as safety margins established by the MR imaging system manufacturer.

The escaping helium is very cold and can cause oxygen from the ambient air to start condensing on and dripping from the outside of the quench vent. This liquid oxygen might present a danger of fire or explosion, similar to that of 100 per cent gaseous oxygen. For this reason, some manufacturers recommend thermal insulation of the quench vent ot minimize the accumulation of liquid oxygen during a quench.

There are several potential causes of quenches. The magnet windings, carrying large currents, are located in regions of high magnetic fields. This current causes large forces to be placed on these wires. When a magnet is brought up to field (ramped) for the first time, these wires may shift their positions slightly in response to the forces to which they are subjected. The friction produced by the movement of a wire can generate enough heat to initiate a quench. The next attempt to bring the magnet up to full strength will allow the field to attain a higher value, since all movements of wires caused by lower fields will have already taken place. These quenches, occurring during initial ramping of the magnet, are called "training quenches" and normally do not occur after the magnet has been tested at the factory.

A process similar to a training quench can occur if a large piece of magnetic material (iron or steel) becomes stuck to the magnet. The magnetic material distorts the magnetic field felt by the coil windings and thereby changes the forces on the individual wires. These new forces can cause the wires of the coil windings to shift position, generating heat and initiating a quench. Pulling a large, stuck piece of metal off a magnet can initiate a quench by again changing the forces seen by the coil windings. If a large piece of metal becomes attached to the magnet and there is no danger to life or limb requiring immediate action, the MR imaging system manufacturer should be consulted before attempting to remove the piece of stuck metal from the magnet.

A quench can occur during periodic replenishment of the liquid helium. Just before filling, liquid helium is allowed to flow through the helium transfer tube and out into the room, until the tube is cooled sufficiently. Only when liquid helium is coming from the end of the tube will it be introduced into the helium reservoir, in which the magnet windings are located, to begin helium filling. Failure to execute this step properly can lead to relatively warm helium gas (perhaps 50° above absolute zero) blowing on the coil winding and initiating a quench. Because of the risks of a quench and the risk of severe frostbite from coming in contact with cryogenic vapors, only well-trained and properly equipped personnel should attempt filling of cryogens. Allowing the liquid helium level to get too low can lead to a slight increase in the temperature of the windings, thereby leading to a quench.

Because large volumes of cryogens could be spilled in the scan room, there is a potential risk of asphyxiation. For this reason, oxygen sensors, connected with an alarm, are often installed in the scan room. The heating and ventilating duct openings are often located both near the floor and near the ceiling. The low return will quickly remove cold nitrogen vapor, which sinks to the floor. The high return takes up helium, which rises to the ceiling.

The costs of a quench include replacement of the liquid helium, perhaps at a premium price for emergency service, specially trained personnel and equipment to restart and test the magnet, and lost operating time. During the installation process, the MR imaging system manufacturer should be responsible for any costs of a quench. After the system is turned over to the user, a service and cryogen contract should include "quench insurance." The limits of this "insurance" should be made clear at the outset.

Some MR imaging system manufacturers may recommend or require specific procedures immediately following a quench to prevent the incurring of further costs. This procedure might be the closing of a valve, or similar action, to prevent back-flow of ambient air into the helium reservoir. There it would form "ice" (frozen air), which could prevent immediate restarting of the magnet. Procedures for all other quench-related activities should also be in place, such as immediately removing the patient from the scan room.

The manufacturer normally provides an emergency run-down switch for the magnet, for use in case of threat to life or limb, such as an injured person pinned to the magnet by a large piece of metal. The run-down switch simply initiates a controlled quench on command. It should be located in a clearly visible position near the magnet but should be protected from accidental activation. The MR imaging staff should know how to operate this switch and under what conditions it should be used.

RADIOFREQUENCY INTERFERENCE

The electrical signal received from the patient's body during MR imaging is very weak. It must be protected from contamination by extraneous signals, which could drown out the signal containing the image information. The sources of these interfering signals are manifold. They include television transmitters; commercial radio stations; police, fire, taxi, and other two-way radios; beeper paging systems; and many types of electrical equipment, especially computers. If not screened out, this interference reaches the MR imaging system by means of radio waves that are emitted by the interfering equipment. Although the MR imaging receiving coil is not really an antenna, it still will pick up any radio waves that reach it. Extraneous signals, via radio waves, mixed with the MR imaging signal, can lead to unacceptable image degradation.

This interference is dealt with by blocking the objectionable radio waves before they reach the MR receiving coil. Very often, the scanning room is located inside a radiofrequency (RF)–shielded enclosure. The enclosure's main feature is an electrically continuous sheet of metal in its walls, floor, and ceiling, completely surrounding the scan room. A continuous sheet of metal such as this will block incoming radio waves to any required degree, if it is thick enough. A good electrical conductor, such as copper, needs to be only a fraction of a millimeter thick to provide the required shielding. The RF enclosure is electrically insulated from other structures and is grounded at a single point to prevent circulating currents (ground loops). This continuous shell is appropriately modified at various points to allow entry of people, electrical wires, ventilation ducts, and so forth. Other designs of the metal RF barrier, which do not completely surround the magnet and scan room, are also discussed.

Some MR imaging system manufacturers do an RF site survey before recommending a detailed method of excluding these environmental RF signals. The site survey is conducted by placing an antenna, in various orientations, at the proposed MR imaging site and measuring the received RF signal. This procedure is done in a range of appropriate frequencies with a special receiver, called a "spectrum analyzer." The selection of frequencies depends on several factors, some of which are system specific. The frequencies at, and near, all Larmor frequencies that are envisioned for use are always important. MR receivers often internally convert the Larmor frequency that they receive to an intermediate frequency (IF) for internal processing. The process used for converting the Larmor frequency to the IF involves the production of two frequencies, only one of which is normally used. A side effect of this process can be to create, for each Larmor frequency, a second frequency at which RF interference can be received. The values in this second group of frequencies depend on the design details of each specific system.

RF site surveys are often conducted over a relatively brief period (a few hours). Since some sources of RF interference may be intermittent, the results of the survey do not necessarily represent the worst case conditions under which imaging must be done. The study does, however, indicate the general level of RF interference that must be dealt with. It does not, of course, detect any future sources of interference. Some MR imaging system manufacturers simply specify a strength of RF shielding that is adequate for all reasonable situations. This specification is typically an attenuation of 90 to 110 dB. That is, the interfering signals must be attenuated enough to reduce their amplitudes by a factor of about 100,000.

RF-shielded rooms are commercially available and are used for many diverse purposes besides screening out RF interference for MR imaging such as housing delicate electrical experiments or preventing detectable RF radiation from escaping from spy-proof computer systems. These rooms are typically lightweight structures that are assembled inside a normal room within a building. Only a narrow gap needs to be left, for assembly purposes, between the walls of the RF-shielded room and the conventional walls of the building. These rooms are available from several shielding manufacturers, who assemble them from standardized, prefabricated components, plus a few special components as required for each installation.

One manufacturer uses 4- by 8-foot panels of particle board as the main wall, ceiling, and floor components. The panels are covered with heavy copper foil bonded to one side to provide the RF shielding. An architectural finish can be bonded to the other side. These panels are joined together by special hardware, which holds the panels together and also makes the electrical connections between the panels. They can be assembled from inside the RF room, without access to the often confined space just outside the room.

Another manufacturer uses heavy copper foil stretched over the outside of lightweight wooden frames made of two-by-two's. These panels are then bolted together through the two-by-two's. The electrical contact between the panels is made by clamping the respective foils between the adjacent pieces of wood. The RF-shielded floor is made by laying long sheets of copper side by side, to cover the existing floor, and soldering them together into a single sheet.

Still another system uses stainless steel (nonmagnetic) panels instead of heavy copper foil on a support. These panels are bolted together at flanged edges. This arrangement provides the mechanical structure for the room and the electrical continuity between the panels to ensure that radio waves are well excluded. If necessary, these panels can be disassembled and reassembled. Another company combines an RF-shielded room with an iron, magnetically shielded room, where the thick iron walls provide RF shielding, in place of the heavy copper foil.

RF-shielded doors are manufactured with a sheet of heavy copper foil within them. A continuous electrical connection is required between the foil in the door and the foil in the adjacent walls and floors. This connection is made by many small, adjacent wiper springs, which bridge the gap between the door and its jam and threshold. Even short stretches of noncontact can allow significant amounts of RF interference to leak into the room. The wiper spring contacts are moderately delicate and need to be protected, especially from objects on the floor when the door is opened or closed. Carpeting is best avoided under the swing area of the door.

Although each wiper spring is rather soft, the several hundred springs around the periphery of the door can result in the need for a moderately large force to close the door. Because of this force, many RF-shielded doors use roller cams in place of a conventional latch and a long lever in place of a door knob. This mechanism makes opening and closing the door easier, but it also gives the door a rather vaultlike appearance. This appearance can be a source of concern for patients if they incorrectly assume that the door is to protect the staff from some danger in the scan room, as the door to an x-ray room does. A warmer, more inviting architectural treatment of the scan room and door area or good prescan education for the patient, or both, can avoid this problem.

Good magnetic safety practice dictates being able to restrict the access to the magnet when it is unattended. This is often best done by locking the door to the scan room. Many RF-shielded doors do not have locks included in their design. The mounting of a lock or hasp on an RF door or its jam, or both, should be done in cooperation with the manufacturer of the door. This practice is to ensure that the integrity of the RF shielding is not breached, for example, by a mounting bolt that penetrates the copper foil.

RF-shielded windows allow the operator to see inside the scan room. The shielding is accomplished by stretching copper screen or finely perforated sheet copper across the window opening in the RF barrier wall and electrically connecting the two along their peripheries. One sheet of screen does not provide an adequate barrier to interfering RF, so two layers are used. Both sides of the RF window are usually covered with glass to protect the screens from mechanical damage and to prevent conversations in the control room from being heard in the scan room. An intercom system, specially designed to work in high magnetic fields, is often used to communicate with the patient. Sliding glass panes can be used to have periodic, direct voice communication with the patient.

RF windows do not often provide as clear a view into the scan room as one would want. Distracting reflections from the copper screens can be minimized if they are colored flat black. Since the holes in both layers of screen are almost equally spaced, broad optical interference bands, called "moire patterns," are seen. They are prominent and can interfere significantly with the view into the scan room. This problem can be minimized by good lighting in the scan room. An additional improvement in viewing quality can be obtained by a modification of the window design, which some suppliers can make.

If, instead of orienting the wires of both screens parallel to each other, they are each rotated 10 to 20 degrees in opposite directions, the moire bands of dark and light will become very narrow and closely spaced. These narrow bands will not be well resolved by an operator in the control room, and the view into the scan room will look as if the moire bands had disappeared. A video system can also be used to improve the view into the magnet bore. Charge-coupled device (CCD) cameras can operate in higher magnetic fields than do ordinary, electron-beam cameras.

Penetrations for pipes and ducts through the RF shielding must be constructed to prevent RF leakages at these points of entry. Even a small hole in the copper foil—for example, to allow the passage of an oxygen line—would allow the entry of so much unwanted RF that the overall performance of the room would be seriously degraded. A simple electrical wire penetrating the RF barrier would act as an antenna outside the RF room, picking up unwanted interference. It would then conduct the interference into the RF enclosure and reradiate it from that portion of the wiring inside the room, where it could seriously interfere with image acquisition. To avoid these problems, special wall penetrations are used.

For a hole to be acceptable in the RF-shielded wall, the hole can be fitted with a closely fitting piece of copper tubing, which is soldered to the RF barrier wall (Fig. 11–1). If the length of the tube is five or six times its diameter, radio waves from outside will not penetrate the tube sufficiently to cause a problem. An additional condition for this method to work properly is that the diameter of the tube must be small compared with the wavelength of the radio waves that are to be excluded. Since the wavelength, corresponding to the Larmor frequency of H-1 at 1.5 T, is 4.7 meters, this last condition is easily met. The physical process, which excludes the external RF interference, is the same process that occurs in a wave guide operating at a frequency lower than its lowest transmission frequency. This type of RF shield penetration is, therefore, usually called a wave guide.

If the tubing, which passes through the wave guide, and its contents are not electrically conducting, nothing further needs to be done for this simple penetration. It could be used without modification, for example, to bring a polyvinyl chloride (PVC) line carrying a gas into the RF-shielded room.

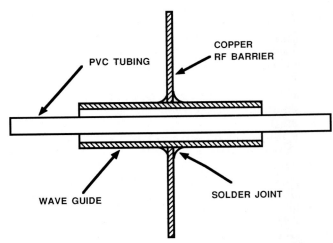

FIGURE 11–1. Typical wave guide penetration through the wall of an RF-shielded room. The tubing is not electrically conductive.

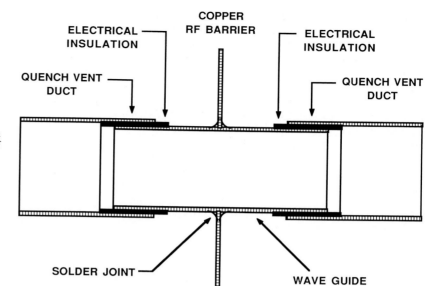

FIGURE 11–2. Wave guide penetration, for a large-diameter quench vent, through the wall of an RF-shielded room.

Even a quench vent 12 inches in diameter can be led out of the RF enclosure by means of a large wave guide. For this application, the wave guide can serve directly as part of the ducting (Fig. 11–2). Since the quench vent ducts, both inside and outside the RF enclosure, are usually made of metal, an electrically insulating segment is often introduced between each of these duct segments and the wave guide. This insulation prevents electrical ground loops through the RF shielding. Although a 6-foot-long wave guide is somewhat awkward to construct and install, it is often a good choice for a quench vent because of its relative lack of resistance to the rapid flow of gas.

Heating and ventilating ducts can be led through the wall of the RF enclosure by a modification of the simple wave guide. Instead of a single tube that is six times longer than its diameter, several parallel tubes of smaller diameter can be used. Since each of these tubes is narrower than a single tube would be, they can also be proportionately shorter. This configuration can be created inexpensively by folding sheet metal to make a honeycomb consisting of many parallel hexagonal ducts of quarter-inch diameter, which are each about an inch and a half long (Fig. 11–3). The honeycomb is mounted in the RF-shielded wall, and normal ventilating ducts are connected on either side of the honeycomb by means of standard cloth duct couplings. These couplings are electrically insulating and thereby interrupt potential ground loops. Although the pressure drop through the honeycomb wave guide is greater than that through a simple wave guide, a heating and ventilating system can easily handle the pressure associated with typical flows.

All of these wave guides are available from the manufacturers of RF-shielded rooms. They are typically supplied premounted on flanges, ready to be bolted into the wall of an RF enclosure. Several penetrations may be mounted on a single flange.

Pipes that carry water present a special problem. Water is somewhat electrically conductive and will tend to short out the insulating segments at each end of a wave guide. This problem is easily solved for a sprinkler system by supplying pressurized air to the portion of the system inside the RF enclosure. This practice excludes water from the penetration and prevents any possibility of a resulting ground loop. Sprinkler systems of this type, called "dry systems," are standard products that are typically used when there is danger of the sprinkler pipes freezing.

Sink drains are normally dry enough where they penetrate normal walls that they could easily be handled with simple wave guides. The hot and cold water lines for a sink, however, would be difficult to keep dry where they would pass through a wave guide. RF enclosures have been built with sinks inside the scan room, using simple penetrations, with no

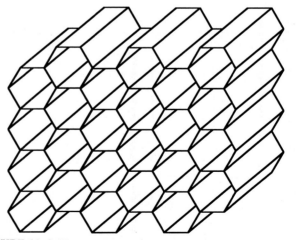

FIGURE 11–3. Honeycomb wave guide for mounting in the wall of an RF-shielded room. This type of penetration can be used for heating and ventilating ducts.

apparent detrimental effect. Before going ahead with such an installation, assurances need to be obtained from both the RF shielding supplier and the MR imaging system manufacturer that the degree of shielding will be adequate and that any ground loop problems can be dealt with. The same caveat applies to nondry sprinkler systems.

Electrical penetrations need to prevent any RF interference that is picked up by the wires outside the RF enclosure from entering the RF-shielded room. This is done by adding a circuit, called a "low-pass filter." A low-pass filter allows direct current and low-frequency alternating current to pass through it, while blocking the very high frequencies against which the MR imaging signal must be protected.

Low-pass filters are available as standard components from manufacturers of screened rooms. They are available in a variety of voltages and currents to meet most needs. Low-pass filters are typically housed in an RF-shielded metal box, which is mounted on the outside wall of the RF enclosure (Fig. 11–4). Wires pass from the low-pass filter in the box through a hole in the screening wall and into the RF enclosure. The metal case of the low-pass filter covers the hole in the shielding wall to prevent RF leakage into the room. On the outside of the room, wires extend from the low-pass filter out through the metal case, where they can be connected with the external circuit.

MR imaging system manufacturers normally supply all the electrical penetrations that are specific to the imager. They are often mounted on one or more large panels, which in turn mount in the wall of the shielded room. Most shielded room manufacturers work with the MR imaging system manufacturers to provide a good installation for these panels.

Low-pass filters are also used for other equipment within the RF-screened room. They are used for electrical lighting, electrical wall outlets, smoke detectors, oxygen sensors, emergency call buttons, and so forth. These filters are generally mounted directly on the wall of the screened room.

Another method of transmission through the RF barrier is to convert the electrical signal to a fiber-optics signal. The optical fiber can be passed to the other side of the RF wall, via a wave guide, and can then be converted back to an electrical signal on the far side of the RF barrier.

Alternative RF shielding methods have been developed to reduce the costs that would normally be associated with a full RF-shielded room of the type described previously.

One MR imaging system manufacturer provides a semitubular cover that pulls out of the magnet bore and covers the patient and the half of the patient's table closest to the magnet. The cover is electrically connected with the magnet housing and with an RF barrier beneath the surface of the patient's table. The magnet housing and this tubular extension of its bore prevent radio waves from reaching the receiver coil by means of the same process that occurs in wave guide RF penetrations. The far end of the magnet bore is provided with an RF barrier and appropriate penetrations for circuits within the magnet bore. The RF shielding is partially spoiled by conduction of RF interference within the patient's body into the region of the receiver coil. Although this shielding is not as strong as that provided by a conventional RF-shielded room, the manufacturer feels that it is adequate to deal with moderate RF interference.

An experimental method uses a smaller than normal RF-shielded room that houses only the patient's table and associated areas (Fig. 11–5). The magnet is located outside this room, but its bore abuts the wall, toward which the patient's table is directed from inside the room. The magnet's bore mates with an opening in the wall of the RF-shielded room. The patient's table extends through this hole in the RF shielding and into the bore of the magnet, as it normally does. The magnet housing is electrically connected with the wall of the RF shielding. The far end of the magnet bore is covered with an RF barrier. This arrangement completes the RF shielding, which is made up of the small RF-shielded room and the housing of the magnet. The shielded room and the RF barrier, at the far end of the bore, are fitted with penetrations as required.

The financial savings potentially available from this design are not just from the use of an RF enclosure of smaller than normal floor area. The RF room does not require the high ceiling height, often required

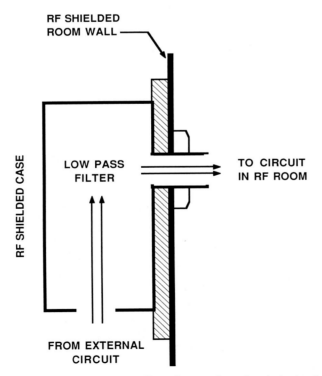

FIGURE 11–4. Low-pass filter for passing electrical signals through the wall of an RF-shielded room.

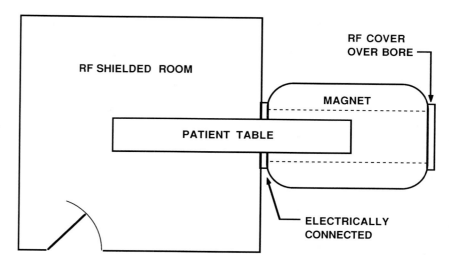

FIGURE 11–5. A method of using a smaller than normal RF-shielded room.

above the magnet, to allow for cryogen access. A magnet housing with a fitting around the bore, designed to make an RF-tight seal to an RF-shielded room, is not yet commercially available.

FRINGE FIELDS

The current flowing through the windings of a superconducting magnet causes the magnetic field lines to come through the bore of the magnet in a dense parallel bundle and thereby produce the imaging magnetic field. But magnetic field lines always form closed loops. Therefore, they loop around the outside of the magnet in a wide arc and rejoin themselves where they first entered the bore, forming smooth, continuous, closed curves. This arrangement leads to additional magnetic fields (fringe fields), which extend outside the bore of the magnet for rather large distances.

These fringe fields are associated, to some degree, with all imaging magnets. The fringe fields of air-core resistive magnets are very similar to those of superconducting magnets. The difference is that their fringe fields are much lower in strength, in proportion to the lower field strength of resistive magnets. Iron-core resistive, permanent, and hybrid magnets have significantly reduced fringe fields. This is because their iron yokes conduct the return magnetic flux back to where it reenters the imaging region, rather than allowing it to spread freely throughout the surrounding space. For these reasons, this discussion is primarily addressed to the siting of superconducting magnets, for which fringe field considerations are most important.

Fringe fields of superconducting magnets spread widely in all three dimensions. Figure 11–6 shows the extent of these fields, in the form of iso-gauss contours, for a typical 1-T magnet. The fringe fields are primarily dipolar in nature, which leads to some approximate rules of thumb for estimating the fringe

fields of other unshielded magnets. The fringe field strength at any fixed point varies in direct proportion to the imaging field strength. That is, if a similar magnet were operated at 1.5 T, its 15-G line would be located where the 10-G line is located in Figure 11–6. The strength of the fringe field varies inversely proportionally with the cube of the distance to the magnet's center. The volume within any iso-gauss contour varies in direct proportion to the strength of the imaging field.

The extent of fringe fields leads to a number of siting considerations that are unique to MR imaging. The main areas to be considered are physical forces on metal objects, caused by the fringe field; magnetic interference with the operation of nearby equipment, including components of the imager itself; magnetization of environmental iron objects by the fringe field, affecting the operation of the MR imager; and magnetic shielding to control the extent of these fields.

Physical forces on ferromagnetic objects, caused by the fringe fields of the magnet, can lead to rather dramatic and unexpected effects. These forces have important safety considerations, which are discussed in the "Safety" section of this chapter, together with other safety issues.

Ferromagnetism refers to the property of a material that becomes strongly magnetized when placed in a magnetic field, as iron does. Most steels are little more than iron that has been purified by reducing its carbon content and also, perhaps, by adding small amounts of other alloying elements. These common steels, like iron, are ferromagnetic and are strongly affected by magnets. Iron and steel, however, are not the only ferromagnetic materials. Nickel and cobalt are also ferromagnetic, as are ferrites and ceramic magnets. Stainless steels, on the other hand, often contain large proportions of chromium and nickel, which cause them to retain the crystalline structure (austenite) associated with their high-temperature, nonmagnetic state. Although many com-

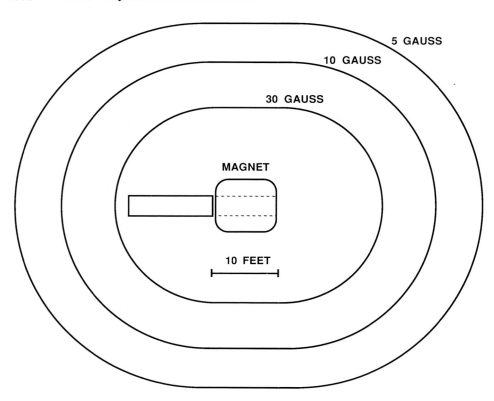

FIGURE 11–6. The extent of the fringe fields of a typical 1-T superconducting magnet, displayed as iso-Gauss lines.

mon stainless steels are not ferromagnetic, some are, and caution must be exercised in each new situation.

When a ferromagnetic object is placed in a magnetic field, it develops an average dipole moment much like the development of a nuclear dipole moment by water-containing tissues in a magnetic field. There are two major differences that account for ferromagnetism's being many millions of times stronger than nuclear magnetism. The first is that the source of the average dipole moment is the alignment of electronic dipoles of unpaired inner shell electrons. There may be several of these electrons per atom, and each is a thousand times stronger than a nuclear dipole. The second difference is that by means of a poorly understood quantum mechanical effect all of the unpaired, inner shell electrons are constrained to point in the same direction. That is, their total potential dipole moment is not disrupted by thermal agitation the way nuclear magnetism and, for that matter, paramagnetism, is. This quantum mechanical effect depends on the crystalline structure of the material, which is why some predominantly iron-containing substances are ferromagnetic and others are not.

If a spherical ferromagnetic object is placed in a magnetic field, some of the tiny regions of uniform magnetization, called "domains," will reorient themselves to align with the magnetic field. The object thereby becomes partially magnetized. As the applied magnetic field becomes stronger, more domains are aligned with the field, and the average magnetization of the object becomes stronger. Eventually, most of the domains become aligned with the magnetic field, and the magnetization of the object stops increasing. This condition, in which the object is fully magnetized, is called "saturation."

The pull on a ferromagnetic object by the fringe field of a magnet increases very rapidly with distance as the object approaches the magnet. This force can vary approximately inversely as the seventh power of distance. The greatest pull on a ferromagnetic object in the fringe field of a magnet is in the neighborhood of the mouth of the magnet bore, where the strength of the magnetic field varies most rapidly with position. There is no pull on a ferromagnetic object in a region of uniform magnetic field, such as in the central imaging region in the bore of a magnet.

Slender objects, such as screwdrivers, the tubular frames of stretchers, or the cylindrical walls of oxygen bottles, are more fully magnetized than would be a sphere of the same material. This is especially true if the long axis of the object is aligned with the fringe magnetic field. The magnetic moment of a slender object tends to align along the axis of the object. If the object is not aligned with the field, it will experience a strong torque, which will tend to align it, and its dipole moment, with the fringe field. This alignment, if allowed to occur, will ensure that the object is maximally magnetized for any given magnetic field. In the uniform imaging region of the magnet, there will be a very strong torque on any nonspherical ferromagnetic object, even though there is no translation force.

If a light bulb is lit in a high magnetic field, the alternating current passing through its filament interacts with the magnetic field to produce a rapidly alternating force on the filament (no *ferro*magnetism in this case). These 60-Hz alternating forces can lead to burn-out of the light bulbs every few hours. Direct current is often used in the lighting of scan rooms to avoid this problem.

Magnetic interference with the operation of nearby equipment falls into several categories: deflection of electron beams, saturation of transformer and other iron, physical forces on equipment components, erasure of magnetic media, and effect on cardiac pacemakers or other implanted devices. Some typical allowable field limits are tabulated in Chapter 12. The actual limits for any specific piece of equipment should be determined from its manufacturer or from the manufacturer of the MR imaging system being installed. These limits can sometimes be overstepped if some degradation in performance can be tolerated.

Electron beams are bent in circular arcs by magnetic fields. This bending can produce a rotation or displacement of the image on the screen of a monochrome computer monitor or an oscilloscope. These effects become noticeable in the range of 5 to 10 G. Some of these instruments have adjustments that allow correction for these effects. If the magnetic field is nonuniform, the image may also be distorted. Video-based image printers, which are monochrome but have a higher standard of performance than computer monitors, may tolerate only 3 G for acceptable results. But the steel case of a printer may provide enough magnetic shielding to allow a unit to operate in 10 G. Laser image printers can generally tolerate much higher fields. They do not use an electron beam. One manufacturer specifies that its unit will function properly in 30 G.

The hue seen on a color monitor or color television is controlled by the angle at which the electron beam comes through the mask and strikes the phosphors. The bending of the electron beam by the fringe field also changes the beam's angle of incidence on the mask. Color distortion of this type can usually be avoided below about 3 G. The effect of magnetic fields on cathode ray tubes can easily be demonstrated with a simple refrigerator magnet.

The electron beams of x-ray tubes can tolerate up to about 10 G. Image intensifiers show a shift of their images when their orientation in the magnetic field is changed (the fluoro table is tilted) in a field of 1 or 2 G. The electronic cascades of photomultiplier tubes (PMTs) are deflected by magnetic fields above 1 G. This situation changes the gains of the PMTs, which can produce artifacts in moving detector CT scanners, if photomultipliers are used. Similar problems occur in single photon emission computed tomography (SPECT) scanners. These values are strongly dependent on any internal magnetic shielding, which may be present by design or fortuitously. The electron beams of electron microscopes and the ion beams of mass spectrometers can operate satisfactorily below 1 G.

Transformer iron can concentrate enough flux that its magnetic properties are significantly distorted. Power transformers and conditioners for the imaging system generally operate satisfactorily in 30 G. Alternating current–powered test equipment can be damaged at high fields. If the transformer iron is saturated, proper inductive voltages are not produced, and excessive primary currents can burn out the power transformer. Heat guns (hair dryers), used to warm magnet parts during cryogen servicing, may have their motor iron saturated, leading the motors to slow or stop. This can lead to the burn-out of the fan motor if corrective action is not promptly taken. Changing the orientation of the motor is often enough to get it going again and protect the motor. Magnetic disk drives can usually operate properly in fields up to 10 G. At higher fields, their read-write heads can become magnetically saturated enough to harm performance.

The physical force and permanent magnetization of internal parts of mechanical watches, by the field near the magnet, can lead to complete failure of these watches. There is anecdotal evidence that quartz-driven analog watches usually stop running near a high field magnet but spontaneously resume operation when they leave the magnetic environment (no guarantees). Digital watches seem to function properly, even within high field magnets, except that the alarm function becomes muted, presumably because of demagnetization of an enunciator field magnet. Beepers seem to suffer a similar fate.

Magnetic media are erased at high magnetic fields. These include computer tapes, floppy disks and other demountable media, magnetic strips in credit cards, employee badges, parking garage tickets, prepaid dormitory meal cards, and so forth. These media are safe behind the 30-G line.

The magnetically operated switches in cardiac pacemakers can be actuated in magnetic fields as low as 10 or 20 G for the most sensitive units oriented in their most sensitive directions. For this reason, the Food and Drug Administration (FDA) has recommended that warning signs be placed in the vicinity of the 5-G line to warn pacemaker wearers. This restriction has been extended by apparently excessive administrative caution and, in at least one case, state regulation, to a requirement of completely controlling the entire region within the 5-G line. This region is often a large area, and its control can be expensive. This limit should probably be evaluated by relevant medical and scientific professional groups, together with a proposal for placing this limit at, perhaps, the 15- or 30-G line. Until that happens, sites may have to treat the 5-G line as an absolute barrier for the general public and for pacemaker wearers, unless the pacemaker wearer has a physician's permission to enter this region.

Environmental iron can be magnetized by the fringe

field. These environmental objects then create a magnetic field of their own, which distorts the imaging field in the bore of the magnet. As part of an MR imaging site evaluation, the potential supplier computes the field distortions that will be produced by the fringe field acting through the environmental iron and determines whether the distortions are within the shim capabilities of the magnet. These estimates require a large, complex computer program for their computation. Differences in estimates from different potential suppliers are to be expected. Stationary environmental iron includes structural steel, floor decking, concrete reinforcing rods, piping, iron-bearing soil, buried pipes, and so on. During the installation of the system, extraneous iron in the region of the magnet must be removed before shimming is carried out.

Small amounts of steel close to the magnet can sometimes have a more important effect than larger pieces that are farther away. Beams that run parallel to the local fringe field will be more fully magnetized than those perpendicular to the field and will, thereby, have a much larger effect on magnet homogeneity. Placement of large pieces of iron in a symmetric position, relative to the magnet, tends to reduce the adverse effects of the iron. In new construction, nonmagnetic materials can be substituted for conventional materials, when required. Examples include a stainless steel or fiberglass reinforcing rod in the floor under the magnet, no steel decking under this floor, and the use of beams directly under the magnet, fabricated from conventional stainless steel shapes.

Nonstationary environmental iron presents a special problem. Since its distorting fields vary too rapidly with time to be shimmed out, steps must be taken to ensure that these items do not have a significant effect on the imaging volume. Alternatively, if the moving iron is present only for short periods—for example, a large truck picks up a dumpster early every morning—one can elect to exclude those times for scanning. Movable iron includes elevators (especially their counterweights), parking lots and vehicles (lift trucks, cars, trucks, trains), cranes, construction scaffolding, and so forth. Larger objects need to be kept farther away from the magnet than smaller ones. Cars need to be kept about 40 feet away, while trucks need to be kept at 50 feet. These distances can be significantly shortened by magnetic shielding.

Time-varying magnetic fields can also be produced by large, stationary electrical equipment, such as power transformers or emergency generators. Electrically powered trains can interfere with MR imaging by means of its moving mass of metal and by the large magnetic fields that it generates.

Magnetic shielding can be used to confine the fringe fields of an imaging magnet to a more compact volume or to direct the field away from selected areas.[6] The design of magnetic shielding is a complex field and requires the assistance of a highly skilled and experienced professional. Incorrectly placed shielding can actually increase the magnetic field in an area where it is desired to reduce it.

One method, sometimes called "self-shielding," places standard, carefully designed, large pieces of iron around the outside of the magnet housing. This arrangement provides a short flux return path for the fringe field and can reduce the linear extent of any given degree of field intensity by about a factor of 2. One such shield, weighing 21 tons, is shown in Chapter 12. This standard shield has been carefully studied, and its effects on magnet homogeneity are well understood.

Another method of shielding at the magnet is called "active shielding." It involves the incorporation of additional superconducting coils within the magnet, which are arranged to cancel much of the fringe field. This practice can provide a high degree of shielding for relatively little additional weight. A commercially available, superconducting, self-shielded magnet brings the 5-G line to within 8 feet of the axis of the magnet. This will usually keep the 5-G line above the heads of people on the floor below and below the floor's surface on the floor above. Magnets of this type have been incorporated into some commercially available MR imaging systems.

Another form of shielding involves placing carefully designed sheets of iron on the scan room walls and/or ceiling and floors. This again provides a shortened flux return path, with the net effect of confining the extent of the fringe field. Such a shield might be made of many thin sheets of transformer iron or single full-thickness sheets of low-carbon steel. In either case, the total thickness of the shield might be 1 inch and have a weight of around 50 tons. Structural considerations for self-shielding and for room shielding are obviously important.

One manufacturer provides a magnetic shield, which looks something like an open-ended small barn made of thick steel plates, which is placed over the magnet. Another supplier can provide a double-walled, heavy steel garage for the magnet end of a semitrailer, used for mobile MR imaging.

If only a small area needs to be shielded, partial shielding might be appropriate. For example, if the 5-G line only needs to be pulled out of an adjacent public corridor, a single, correctly placed plate of steel may solve the problem. In any case, the adequacy of the shielding and the effect of the shielding on magnet homogeneity need to be carefully analyzed with the aid of a well-tested computer program.

Isolated magnetic interference with a limited number of small instruments can sometimes best be dealt with by installing shielding around, or built into, the instrument. A good candidate for this approach might be a computer monitor, for which it would be desirable to reduce the distortion due to the fringe fields. Some MR imaging system manufacturers do this for the cathode ray tubes (CRTs) on the MR operator's console. Individual PMTs are often easily shielded, sometimes with commercially available shields.

SAFETY

Personal safety issues present some unique problems in siting and operating an MR system.[7] The dangers to patients, visitors, and staff who are in the fringe field of an MR system or are being scanned are generally less severe than dangers faced in many everyday hospital situations. Safety procedures related to MR imaging, however, are significantly different from those employed in most of medical practice. Because of these differences, we cannot rely as heavily on the general training and experience of medical personnel to behave in a safe manner, as we do in the general medical environment. It is prudent, therefore, to give safety in MR imaging special emphasis so that avoidable accidents, and even deaths, can be prevented. The procedures used to operate an MR imaging facility safely can be made easier, more effective, and less intrusive by considering them early in the architectural planning stage.

Ferromagnetic objects are pulled toward an imaging magnet by its fringe field, as previously described. For high field, superconducting magnets, the region of significant physical pull extends for several feet in all directions from the sides and ends of the magnet. These forces range from ones near the magnet, which would overpower anyone, to ones farther away, which could be easily resisted by an attentive person. These latter, gentler forces in many ways probably represent the greatest danger for injury to people and equipment because one can become complacent about them. A superconducting magnet remains constantly on, day and night, which means that safety procedures cannot be relaxed at any time.

The attractive force on an object increases rapidly as the object approaches the magnet, sometimes as rapidly as inversely proportional to the seventh power of distance. In approaching the magnet, the pull can increase significantly in a short distance, causing the object to leap out of one's hand before there is time to react. As the now uncontrolled object moves closer to the magnet, it accelerates at an ever-increasing rate, until it hits the magnet with great force, if it does not hit someone or some other object first. This is the so-called "missile effect."

Next to the magnet, the attractive forces can be impressive, many times the weight of an object that is pinned there. A stretcher or a tank of oxygen cannot simply be pulled away from the magnet housing by one person. At a distance of 3 or 4 feet from a 1-T magnet housing, the pull on a typical ferromagnetic object would be about equal to its weight. If it is not restrained, the object can literally take off and fly toward the magnet. From a distance of 10, 20, or more feet, an unrestrained ferromagnetic object will start sliding toward the magnet, the exact distance depending on the friction with the floor. In other words, if it is not restrained, a ferromagnetic object can "taxi" from almost anywhere in a typical scan room to a point where it can take off and fly toward the magnet, hitting with high impact.

Outside most scan rooms, if the magnet is not too close to one of the walls, the pull of the fringe field may be very noticeable, but probably not dangerous from the missile effect. This is true even though there may be more pull on objects than there is in dangerous locations inside the scan room. The difference is that outside the scan room an architectural wall restrains all loose ferromagnetic objects, except near the doorway into the room. It is desirable if the architectural plan aids the total plan for keeping unrestrained ferromagnetic objects out of the scan room.

A design that requires anyone entering the scan room to pass by the on-duty staff is helpful. It is easier to control the scan room if there is a single entrance to the suite and the scan room is the farthest room from the entrance. A means of easily locking the scan room door, when the area in not staffed, is desirable. Some groups prefer to make the scan room key not part of the local master key system to avoid curiosity problems from, for example, night staff. In this case, a method for emergency access needs to be developed and should be considered in the architectural plan. The solution might be as simple as keeping a scan room key in a breakable glass front box, mounted near the scan room. Perhaps such a box requires connection with an alarm system to notify security when it is used.

All ferromagnetic objects should be kept out of the scan room. Small objects may not represent a severe threat from the missile effect, except perhaps to eyes. But if lost in the bore of the magnet, they can seriously degrade image quality by means of hurting the magnetic field's homogeneity. If the technologist and others are to change into scrubs, signifying they are carrying no ferromagnetic objects, changing facilities and lockers are needed.

Since visitors will enter the scan room at times, a secure place to leave one's keys, watch, credit cards, beeper, purse, brief case, hair pins, clip-on bow tie, and so on, is desirable. One good solution is a set of conveniently placed, lockable cabinets, hopefully with nonmagnetic keys on wrist bands. Some sites then have visitors put on disposable jump suits over their street clothes, to try to confine any loose ferromagnetic objects that may have been overlooked by their owner. If this is to be done, space for putting on the jump suits is required, perhaps near the watch and wallet cabinets.

Small bits of metal on the patient's person can cause serious imaging artifacts, as well as the problems described previously. Patients need to be screened for contraindications to MR scanning, such as pacemakers, aneurysm clips, orbital metallic foreign bodies, and so forth. The place where this is done needs to be provided for in the plan.

Metal detectors cannot be adjusted to an adequately sensitive setting to detect all the small objects that should be excluded from the scan room, without causing many false alarms, which leads to ignoring the detector. Relying on a metal detector, instead of good procedures and training, can lead to a false sense of security. Metal detectors do not discriminate between ferromagnetic and nonmagnetic metals. A hand-held metal detector may be useful, at times, in screening patients who are not able to cooperate.

Special nonmagnetic medical equipment (e.g., stretcher, wheelchair, intravenous pole, oxygen bottle, stethoscope) is necessary and needs a place to be stored. The same holds for the required nonmagnetic housekeeping equipment. The scan room floor material should be selected with the knowledge that the usual hospital floor power buffers, for example, cannot be used. A built-in vacuum system with plastic hoses and plastic implements might be a good solution. The MR imaging service team has nonmagnetic hand tools, ladders, and transfer lines that it uses in the scan room, as well as documentation, spare parts, and test equipment, which need to be stored.

Cardiopulmonary resuscitation cannot be carried out properly in the scan room under emergency conditions. An electrocardiograph (ECG) machine or defibrillator can fly toward the magnet or burn out. ECG tracings are unlikely to be correct. The magnetic pull on the batteries of a laryngoscope can make a difficult intubation impossible. No time is available to screen the responding cardiopulmonary resuscitation (CPR) team for other ferromagnetic objects. A special set of emergency medical procedures needs to be developed for use in, and near, the scan room. Many sites station a nonmagnetic stretcher close by so that a patient may be removed quickly to a special resuscitation area outside the high field. This precaution has the virtue of quickly converting an unusual emergency, in a high magnetic field, into a standard emergency, for which normal procedures apply. In addition to space for CPR equipment storage, the access route of the responding CPR team and the method of keeping any superfluous responders out of the scan room should be considered in the architectural design.

The procedures and equipment for providing scheduled life support or general anesthesia while a patient is being scanned are being developed and are used at a few centers.[8] The space and special services such as an anesthesia exhaust, should be considered if these procedures are envisioned. If young children are to be scanned, sedation and recovery areas may be required.

Pacemaker wearers probably have to be kept behind the 5-G line until higher fields are definitively declared as safe. Although the low field concerns of pacemakers have probably been overemphasized, there are real dangers in being close to the magnet or, worse, in being scanned. Other people have "implants," which should exclude them, or at least raise the question of whether they should be excluded, from the scan room. These objects include aneurysm clips, artificial cochleas, biostimulators, artificial heart valves, shrapnel (especially in the orbit), surgical clips, and orthopedic prostheses. Since all of these objects are believed to be safe outside the 5-G line, the screening for these objects should probably take place at, or outside, the 5-G line, together with the screening for pacemakers. This precaution may mean that everyone, including medical staff, must be screened even to enter consultation areas that are inside the 5-G line.

To enforce this screening procedure, it is probably necessary to have some sort of barrier at the screening point. A scheduler/secretary/receptionist might do the screening. The design of this reception area can be used to aid the receptionist in ensuring that everyone is screened, even busy people who feel they do not have time to stop for screening. An electrically activated, remote control lock on the access door might be useful. The relationship of the reception desk to the access door can affect how smoothly this screening takes place.

REFERENCES

1. Steidley WS, Coil JD, Einstein SG: [Site] planning and preparation. *In* Partain CL, Price RR, Patton JA, et al (eds): Magnetic Resonance Imaging. 2nd ed. Vol II: Physical Principles and Instrumentation. Philadelphia, WB Saunders Company, 1988.
2. Bronskill MJ, Carson PL, Einstein S, et al: Site Planning for Magnetic Resonance Imaging Systems. AAPM Report No. 20. American Association of Physicists in Medicine. New York, American Institute of Physics, 1987.
3. Oldendorf WH: A comparison of resistive, superconductive, and permanent magnets. *In* Partain CL, Price RR, Patton JA, et al (eds): Magnetic Resonance Imaging. 2nd ed. Vol II: Physical Principles and Instrumentation. Philadelphia, WB Saunders Company, 1988.
4. Roos CE, Coffey HT, Efferson KR: Principles of superconducting magnets. *In* Partain CL, Price RR, Patton JA, et al (eds): Magnetic Resonance Imaging. 2nd ed. Vol II: Physical Principles and Instrumentation, Philadelphia, WB Saunders Company, 1988.
5. Holsinger RF, Lown RR, Remillard PA, et al: Novel lightweight permanent ring magnet MR imaging system: Design, installation, and clinical experience. Presented at Fifth Annual Meeting, Society of Magnetic Resonance in Medicine, Montreal, August 1986.
6. Oxford Magnet Technology: Magnets in Clinical Use, Site Planning Guide. Oxford, England, Oxford Magnet Technology, 1983.
7. Pavlicek W: Safety considerations. *In* Stark DD, Bradley WG Jr: Magnetic Resonance Imaging. St. Louis, CV Mosby, 1988.
8. Karlik SJ: Patient anesthesia and monitoring at a 1.5-T MRI installation. Magn Reson Med 7:210–221, 1988.

12

INSTRUMENTATION

ECKART STETTER

SYSTEM OVERVIEW

MAGNETS

    TYPES OF MAGNETS

    Field Strength
    Homogeneity
    Field Stability

    SUPERCONDUCTING MAGNETS

    Construction, Field Strength, and
       Homogeneity
    Cryostat
    Ramping and Quenching
    Fringe Field Shielding
    Shimming

    CRITERIA FOR SELECTING MAGNETIC
       FIELD STRENGTH

    Chemical Shift Artifact
    Main Field Inhomogeneity
    Radiofrequency Power Deposition
    Radiofrequency Penetration
    T_1 Relaxation
    Safety

GRADIENTS

    POWER SUPPLY

    EDDY CURRENTS

    ACTIVE GRADIENT SHIELDING

    EDDY CURRENT CORRECTION BY
       PRECOMPENSATION OF THE DRIVING
       CURRENT

    CRITERIA FOR REQUIRED GRADIENT
       STRENGTH

RADIOFREQUENCY SYSTEM

    COILS AND RESONATORS

    Antenna Characteristics
    Matching
    Noise Sources
    The Optimal MR Antenna

    ANTENNAS WITH HOMOGENEOUS FIELD
       DISTRIBUTION

    Quadrature (Circularly Polarized) Coils

    SURFACE COILS

    Decoupling

    TRANSMIT AND RECEIVE SYSTEM

    Transmit Path
    Radiofrequency Power Transmitter
    Receive Path
    Demodulator
    Signal Levels
    Dynamic Range
    Transmit/Receive Switch

    RADIOFREQUENCY ROOM SHIELDING

SUBJECT-DEPENDENT SYSTEM
CALIBRATIONS

    ANTENNA ADJUSTMENT (COIL TUNING)

    SETTING THE CENTER FREQUENCY
       (FREQUENCY ADJUSTMENT)

    PULSE AMPLITUDE CALIBRATION
       (TRANSMITTER ADJUSTMENT)

    RECEIVER GAIN (RECEIVER ADJUSTMENT)

    APPENDIX A. MATHEMATICAL DETAILS OF
       SHIM PROCEDURE

    APPENDIX B. MATHEMATICAL DETAILS OF
       THE MODULAR AND DEMODULAR

SYSTEM OVERVIEW

In principle, an MR imaging system is quite simple, consisting of a large main magnet and smaller auxiliary field coils (gradient coils), radio frequency antennas (transmitter and receiver coils), associated electronics, and a computer to process the data from the imaging experiment. However, in practice, MR imaging systems are quite complex, and careful attention must be paid to the design of all components to ensure consistent, high-quality images.

In this chapter, we attempt to present a balanced view of MR imaging instrumentation, giving an overview of the various components as well as more technical details essential to a full understanding of the system.*

*Some portions of this chapter have been modified from Krestel E (ed): Bildgebende Systeme für die medizinische Diagnostik. Siemens Verlag, München, 1988, Chapter 10. Figs. 12–17, 12–18, and 12–24 have been taken from Hutten, H (ed): Biomedizinische Technik (Vol. 1), Springer Verlag, Berlin, Heidelberg and Verlag TÜV-Rheinland, Köln, in press.

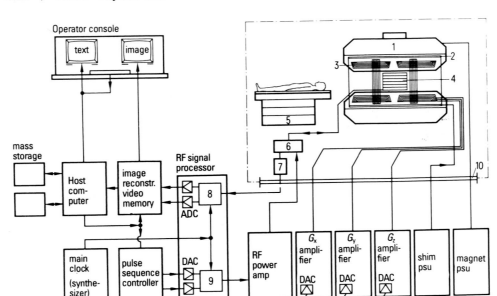

FIGURE 12–1. Overview of an MR imaging system: 1, magnet with cryostat and cryoshield; 2, shim coil system; 3, gradient coil system; 4, radiofrequency (RF) resonator (antenna); 5, patient table; 6, transmit/receive switch; 7, preamplifier; 8, quadrature demodulator with two low-pass filters and analog-to-digital converters (ADCs); 9, single sideband (SSB) modulator with two digital-to-analog converters (DACs) and low-pass filters; 10, feed-through filters.

An MR imaging system has many similarities to the NMR spectrometers, applied to chemical analysis, which have been in use for decades. In addition, MR imaging systems use magnetic field gradient coils and associated power supplies, as well as an image processor for reconstruction and display of images. The system must obviously be scaled to the size of a patient, rather than of test tubes, as are most spectrometers. The basic components of an MR imaging system using a superconducting magnet are shown in Figure 12–1. These components can be summarized as follows.

MAIN MAGNET. The main magnet generates a stable magnetic field to align the nuclei in the patient's tissues. This magnet has a large opening, called the *bore*, containing additional hardware (shim, gradient, radiofrequency [RF] coils). The open bore that remains after placement of this hardware must be large enough to hold the patient comfortably.

SHIM COILS. The shim coils, placed within the magnet bore, guarantee the homogeneity of the main magnetic field throughout the imaging volume. Additional iron plates placed inside and outside the magnet further improve the homogeneity.

GRADIENT COILS. The gradient coils are mounted on a cylinder that is concentrically placed within the magnet bore. There are three sets of windings, designed to generate a linear magnetic field gradient along three orthogonal axes (x,y,z). The strength of the gradient field is proportional to the strength of the applied electrical current.

RADIOFREQUENCY COILS. The RF coils are placed inside the gradient coils. The RF transmitter coil converts the electrical power from a power transmitter into an oscillating magnetic field (the RF pulse) to excite the tissue nuclei. A receiver coil detects the minute MR signal, which is then amplified by preamplifiers and amplifiers and forwarded to the receiver.

PULSE SEQUENCE CONTROLLER. The pulse sequence controller acts as the chief operating officer for the MR system. It uses the user-defined pulse sequence as a blueprint for running the signal measurement procedure. It ensures the correct timing and amplitudes of the gradient pulses using digital-to-analog converters (DACs) and generates an RF pulse with the correct amplitude and phase using a *modulator*. A *synthesizer* acts as a central clock. The analog-to-digital converter (ADC) translates the MR signal into digital numbers that can be used directly by the computer.

IMAGE PROCESSOR. Data acquired during the imaging process are fed into the image processor, which reconstructs them as two-dimensional (2D) images. The images are copied into the video memory of the console monitor.

HOST PROCESSOR. The host processor manages interactions between the various subsystems.

MAGNETS

TYPES OF MAGNETS

Several types of magnets are in routine clinical use. These can be categorized as *permanent, resistive,* and *superconducting.* Permanent magnets consist of material that can be strongly magnetized. Such materials are said to have a high *magnetic remanence.* Resistive magnets are electromagnets, consisting of an air core or iron yoke wrapped with loops of wire in a configuration that produces a uniform magnetic field. Commercial permanent and resistive yoke-type magnets usually have a vertical magnetic field. Like electromagnets, superconducting magnets consist of loops of wire wrapped around a support structure.

FIGURE 12–2. Construction of several types of magnets. *A*, Resistive magnet (air core). *B*, Superconductive magnet. *C*, Permanent magnet (yoke type).

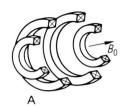
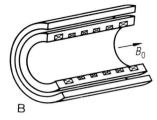
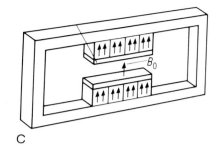

However, once powered up by an electrical current, these magnets remain at full strength without any additional input of electrical power. These are illustrated in Figure 12–2, and their characteristics are summarized in Table 12–1. There are significant differences in attainable field strength, homogeneity, field stability, and siting requirements for the different types of magnets.

Field Strength

For a permanent magnet, the attainable field strength within the imaging volume is determined by the amount of energy needed to produce the desired field versus the amount of energy that can be stored in the permanent magnetic material. Practical permanent magnet design is a compromise between an extremely large amount of a fairly inexpensive material with a modest magnetic remanence and a smaller amount of more expensive material having a high remanence.

Resistive magnets are limited in field strength by electrical power requirements. The available power in most clinical installations does not usually exceed 100 kW, which currently limits the maximal field strength for whole-body systems to 0.3 to 0.4 T. On the other hand, superconducting whole-body MR systems have been constructed with field strengths up to 4 T. The attainable field strength of superconducting magnets is limited by the current-carrying capacity of the superconducting wire and by the physical forces generated at these large field strengths.

Homogeneity

The usable imaging volume in a magnet is determined by magnetic field homogeneity over this region. A large magnet is required to produce a homogeneous field over a large region. This is best accomplished with superconducting magnets, which can produce usable fields-of-view (FOVs) up to 50 cm. The usable imaging volume for permanent and resistive magnets is usually smaller than that for superconducting magnets. The Fourier transform (2DFT) imaging process is much more tolerant of main field inhomogeneities than is spectroscopy. In most in vivo spectroscopy, the magnet is reshimmed

TABLE 12–1. COMPARISON OF MAGNET TYPES FOR MR SYSTEMS

	Superconductor	Resistive	Permanent Magnet
Technical characteristics			
Field strength	Very high field possible (to 4 T)	Relatively small (to 0.4 T)	To 0.3 T
Effective volume and typical homogeneity	Large (15 ppm/50 cm)	Sufficient (40 ppm/40 cm)	Sufficient (40 ppm/40 cm)
Field stability	Very good	Moderate, dependent upon power supply (0.3 to 1 ppm)	Very good
Shielding of external interfering fields	Significant	Extensive shielding with (iron yoke); no shielding without (iron yoke)	Good shielding
Eddy currents due to pulsed gradients	Extensive compensation measures needed	Few (retroactive to power supply)	Few, anisotropic
Field orientation	z	z (or y)	y
Fringe field	Very large	Small (owing to small B_0)	Negligible
Emergency shutdown	Relatively slow because of quench	Can be shut down	Cannot be shut down
Dimensions	Large (1.8 meters × 2 meters)	Average (1.5 meters × 1.6 meters)	Very large (4.2 meters × 2.5 meters × 2.3 meters)
Mass	Average (6 tons)	Relatively low (2 tons)	Very large (yoke type) (80 tons)*
Costs			
Initial price	High	Low	High
Energy usage	None	Very high, to 100 kW ($\sim B_0^2$)	None
Cooling	Cryogens—0.5 liter of liquid helium per hour	Large amount of cooling water needed	None

*Ultra-low field systems (e.g., 0.06 tesla) can be substantially less heavy and less expensive.

to optimize homogeneity for each individual volme of interest (e.g., brain, kidney). This reshimming is not necessary for imaging.

Field Stability

MR imaging requires a very stable main magnetic field. Any temporal variation in the field will produce phase errors and result in image artifacts. Simulations show that field variations having a magnitude of only a few ten billionths of a tesla, resulting in phase errors as small as 3 degrees, can produce visible artifacts. Because of fluctuations in the power supply, resistive magnets have difficulty producing the required level of stability. In contrast, this degree of stability is readily achieved by superconducting magnets and by permanent magnets, especially if the latter are in a temperature-stabilized environment.

Superconducting magnets have an additional benefit in that they intrinsically shield against external magnetic field interference, such as that produced by moving cars or alternating current (AC) power lines. These magnets can tolerate external field interference of up to one millionth of a Tesla (1μT) without significantly affecting image quality.

SUPERCONDUCTING MAGNETS

We now consider in depth the technical factors involved in the construction and operation of superconducting magnets used for MR imaging. Further details on the construction and basic physics of superconducting magnets are available elsewhere.[1]

Construction, Field Strength, and Homogeneity

Superconductors have no resistance to electrical current. By constructing magnets from these materials, large, stable magnetic fields can be generated. There are several important considerations in the choice of superconducting material. First, the superconducting wire material must be capable of carrying large currents needed to produce strong magnetic fields. In addition, it must be possible to keep the material in a superconducting state. Therefore, the critical temperature of the material (i.e., the temperature above which the material develops resistance and is no longer superconducting) must be higher than the boiling point of liquid helium, the primary coolant used for superconducting magnets, which is 4.2° above absolute zero at atmospheric pressure. Finally, the material must have the appropriate physical properties (e.g., ductility, flexibility) to permit it to be drawn out as a wire and formed into the correct configuration.

A suitable material is titanium-niobium. A multifilament wire composed of 30 titanium-niobium strands, of 0.1-mm diameter each, is embedded in a copper matrix (2 mm diameter) for stability. Such a wire can carry currents of up to 500 amperes (A). The wire is wound around a cylindrical core, and the number of windings is determined by the required field strength. A 2-T magnet typically uses nearly 40 miles of wire.

The magnet is divided into six subcoils, and the number of windings in each is calculated to maximize homogeneity in a central spherical volume of 50-cm diameter. The best possible homogeneity that can be achieved over a 50-cm central sphere is approximately 5 ppm and in practice is typically much worse, for example, 150 ppm, due to unavoidable tolerances in the construction of the magnet. Therefore, the magnet must be shimmed, as described further on. To avoid spatial distortion, the magnet homogeneity over the imaging region should be better than 15 ppm.

Cryostat

The superconducting windings are bathed in liquid helium. To insulate these windings from the higher temperature of the outside environment and prevent boil-off of the helium, the magnet is contained within a dewar, called the *cryostat*.

The cryostat must have excellent thermal-insulating characteristics. The amount of insulation can be calculated, based on the allowable rate of evaporation and the surface area of the helium tank. A cross-section of a cryostat is shown in Figure 12–3, which illustrates the measures that must be taken to ensure low heat transfer between the outside environment and the magnet windings. Care must be taken to prevent any kind of thermal energy from penetrating to the helium. This protection is accomplished by a heat radiation shield and superinsulating foil. Convection of heat energy is avoided by maintaining the entire dewar in a high vacuum. The components of the cryostat are suspended on thin, strong plastic rods that are poor conductors of heat. A final protective measure is that the helium tank is suspended within a tank filled with liquid nitrogen, which boils off at a much faster rate than the helium but is also quite inexpensive. Typically, the liquid nitrogen is topped off once a week, and the more expensive liquid helium only once a month. At the top of the cryostat, there is an insulated service access that allows cryogens (N_2, He) to be refilled and power cables to be attached. Some systems are designed to reliquefy cryogen boil-off and require no additional input of cryogens.

Ramping and Quenching

Superconducting magnets must be initially powered up *(ramped)* to full field strength but then maintain the magnetic field for years without additional power input. For the initial ramping procedure, the magnet is first cooled to the point that the windings become superconducting, and then an elec-

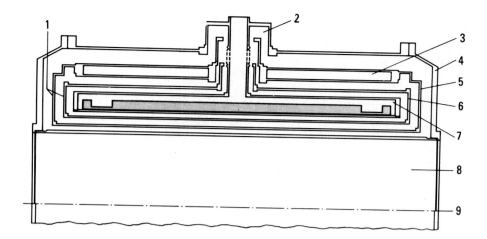

FIGURE 12–3. Construction of the cryostat of a superconducting magnet (longitudinal cross-section): 1, superinsulating foil is located both inside and outside the 77-K shield; 2, service turret; 3, nitrogen vessel; 4, vacuum vessel; 5, 77-K shield; 6, 20-K shield (cooled by helium exhaust); 7, helium vessel with coils; 8, magnet bore; 9, magnet axis.

trical current is induced within the windings by connecting them with a power supply. This procedure is explained by the circuit diagram shown in Figure 12–4. S_L is a superconducting switch, which, when cooled to the temperature of liquid helium, short-circuits the magnet windings. To bring the magnet to full field strength, this switch is first inactivated by heating it above its critical temperature so that it develops electrical resistance. It is then possible to induce a current in the magnet windings by applying a voltage across the terminals of this switch. Once the desired magnet field strength is attained, the power supply and heater are shut off, so that the switch returns to being a superconductor. As a result, the current can now flow through the magnet windings, including the switch, without any resistance. Controlled discharging of the energy stored in the magnetic field (approximately 7 megawatts for a 2-T magnet), which might be needed for servicing, is performed by reversing the above procedure.

A *quench* represents the sudden loss of superconductivity, either spontaneous or due to external influences. The magnet can be quenched in an emergency by heating the superconducting switch. More often, quenches result from negligence, as, for ex-

ample, when liquid helium levels are allowed to drop too low. The quench may begin in one region of the windings but rapidly spreads to other regions as the no longer superconducting portions of the windings generate heat because of electrical resistance. The rate of loss of magnetic field strength is determined by the resistance, self-inductance, and mutual inductance of the coil windings. To slow the quench, so-called *quench protection resistors* (R_Q) are connected in parallel with the windings to provide an alternative low-resistance pathway for the rapidly discharging electrical current and thereby reduce the voltage across the windings, which might destroy the insulation of the wires. The heat produced by the quench causes the liquid helium to boil off. To prevent asphyxiation in the magnet enclosure from release of gaseous helium, the helium gas is vented to the outside environment.

Fringe Field Shielding

If limited space is available for siting, then it is necessary to provide adequate shielding from the fringe field of the magnet. Siting considerations are discussed in more detail in Chapter 11.

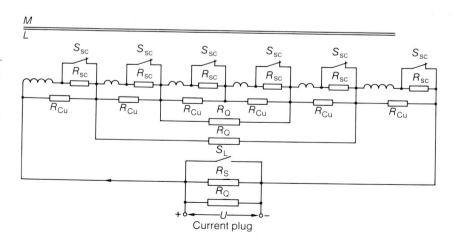

FIGURE 12–4. Equivalent circuit diagram of a superconductive (SC) magnet; inductive coupling (M) between the coils with winding inductance (L).

S_{SC} = closed during SC state; S_L = SC switch (open during ramping); R_{SC} = distributed ohmic resistance of the SC; R_{Cu} = distributed resistance of the copper matrix; R_Q = quench protection resistors; R_S = SC switch resistor while S_L is open; U = voltage across coil during ramp.

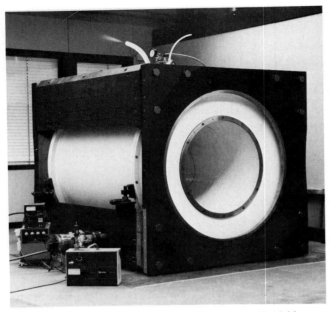

FIGURE 12–5. A 1-T magnet with an iron self-shield.

Magnetic shielding using ferromagnetic iron plates can be placed around the magnet room[2] or directly on the magnet (*self-shielding*). In either case, a large mass of iron is necessary for effective shielding. One may assume that the required mass of iron is similar in both cases; although the required thickness of shielding material is less for room shielding, the surface area to be shielded is larger than that for self-shielding.

Magnetic shielding affects the homogeneity of the magnet. The tighter and more eccentric the distribution of the shielding, the more difficult it is to shim the magnet properly. Room shielding has the drawback of being dependent on the structure of the building and is seldom positioned symmetrically around the magnet. Self-shielding has the advantage of being highly symmetric and decreases fringe fields near the magnet. The major disadvantage of self-shielding is the required weight-bearing capacity of the floor. Figure 12–5 illustrates a 1-T magnet in a 21-ton self-shield. Sometimes, an incomplete magnetic shield will be adequate—for instance, to shield an adjoining waiting area from the 5-G cardiac pacemaker zone.

The fringe field can also be reduced by *active shielding*. This method uses an opposing current-carrying winding that is external to the magnet to decrease fringe fields. Superconducting active shields are incorporated directly into the cryostat. Although active shielding increases the physical size of the magnet, the weight is much reduced compared with the weight involved in shielding with ferromagnetic materials. Active shields compensate the so-called "dipole" field of the magnet; without the shield, the dipole magnetic field decreases only by the cube of the distance and extends many feet in each direction

from the magnet. With active shielding, the dipole field is eliminated, leaving only a quadrupole field. This latter magnetic field decreases by the fifth power of distance and therefore extends for only a few feet from the magnet.

Shimming

Shimming is the process by which magnetic field inhomogeneities are eliminated. These inhomogeneities may arise from imperfections in the magnet itself or may be due to ferromagnetic materials in the magnet environment. Correction of these magnetic field inhomogeneities may be accomplished by active shimming, using special coil windings that act as electromagnets, and by passive shimming, using iron plates placed inside and/or outside the magnet.

Shimming is accomplished by using a special probe to measure the magnetic field strength at multiple points along the spherical surface of the 50-cm imaging volume. A mathematical method, called a spherical harmonics expansion, is used to determine the shim coefficients needed to correct the magnetic field inhomogeneities (Appendix 12–A).

ACTIVE MAGNETIC FIELD SHIMMING. There are 12 current-carrying windings arranged on a cylindrical tube within the magnet bore, as illustrated by Figure 12–6. These windings are configured so that each generates a magnetic field correction approximating one of the shim coefficients. These windings must be designed to avoid magnetic interactions between

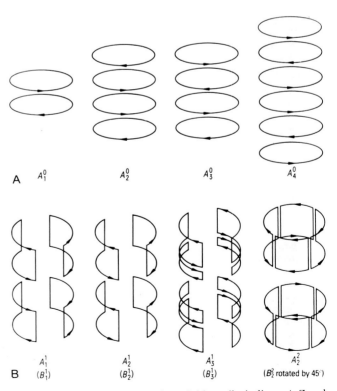

FIGURE 12–6. Schematic drawing of shim coil windings. *A*, Zonal windings. *B*, Tesseral windings.

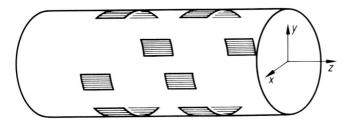

FIGURE 12–7. Position of iron plates (passive shim) of the $A_4{}^4$ term.

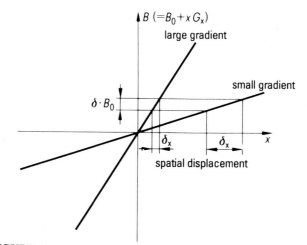

FIGURE 12–8. Fat-water shifts as a function of the field gradient.

them, as well as between them and the magnet and gradient coils.

PASSIVE SHIMMING. Field inhomogeneity can also be corrected by placing sheets of iron inside the magnet bore or on the outside of the cryostat (Fig. 12–7).[3] Preferably one uses a standard configuration of iron plate positions. The number of iron sheets to be placed at each location is computed by a special shim program. Shimming with iron has the advantage that the iron can be placed in a large number of different configurations, which allows for correction of higher order magnetic field inhomogeneities.

CRITERA FOR SELECTING MAGNETIC FIELD STRENGTH

It has been shown that the signal-to-noise (S/N) ratio increases linearly with the strength of the main magnetic field (B_0).[4] One might therefore assume that image quality would continue to improve at arbitrarily high magnetic field strengths. However, other factors, some of which we now review, limit the improvement in image quality at high fields.[5] These factors relate to chemical shift artifact, RF characteristics such as power deposition, T_1 relaxation times, and safety (Table 12–2).

Chemical Shift Artifact

Chemical shift represents the shift in resonance frequency due to the magnetic shielding effect of the

TABLE 12–2. FACTORS IN THE SELECTION OF FIELD STRENGTH IN ¹H MRI

Cause	Effect
Chemical shift	Image shift between tissue containing water and that containing fat
Inhomogeneity of the main field	Spatial distortion
RF eddy currents (skin effect)	Lack of image uniformity
RF loss	Rise in patient's temperature
T_1 time dependence on field	Changed contrast-to-noise ratio
Fringe field	Attraction of ferromagnetic objects at a given distance from the main magnet, interference with cardiac pacemakers and other devices

electron cloud that surrounds the nucleus. In MR images, this magnetic shielding, which is different for fat and water protons, produces a difference in their resonance frequencies of approximately 3.5 ppm (parts per million) of the resonance frequency. As a result, as discussed in more detail in Chapters 3 and 10, the effect of chemical shift is to produce an artifactual shift in the position of fat relative to water along both the slice-selection and the frequency-encoding directions. Since chemical shift is proportional to magnetic field strength, chemical shift artifact is most serious on high field systems.

Along the frequency-encoding axis, chemical shift artifact can be compensated for by using a stronger read-out gradient (Fig. 12–8). However, this solution results in an increased signal bandwidth and, consequently, more image noise. Along the slice-selection axis, chemical shift artifact is more easily controlled. The slice-selection gradient can be increased, resulting in a proportional reduction in chemical shift artifact. To maintain the slice thickness, the increase in gradient strength necessitates an increase in the bandwidth of the RF pulse, which can be accomplished by reducing the RF pulse duration. The main drawback of this approach is greater peak and average RF power deposition.

Main Field Inhomogeneity

Like chemical shift, magnetic field inhomogeneities increase with field strength. These inhomogeneities produce signal loss because of dephasing (T_2^* effect) as well as geometric distortion. Field distortions due to variations in the magnetic susceptibility of the patient (e.g., at air-tissue interfaces) also increase with field strength. To overcome the distortions caused by main field inhomogeneities, the magnetic field gradients used on higher field systems must be stronger than those used on lower field systems.

Radiofrequency Power Deposition

Disregarding the frequency dependence of tissue conductivity and power loss in the RF coil, the amount of transmitted RF power required to produce a given flip-angle excitation increases as the square of the resonance frequency. Therefore, RF power deposition increases with field strength. The problem is worsened by the larger RF pulse bandwidths generally used at high field strengths. RF power deposition heats the body much as a microwave oven heats a frozen dinner.

For safety reasons, some countries have established regulations for power deposition, represented by the specific absorption rate (SAR). The SAR is the allowable amount of RF power deposition per kilogram of body weight (see Chapter 2). Figure 12–9 shows the experimentally determined RF power deposition for an average patient as a function of field strength. Within these guidelines, one finds that excess power deposition can limit the repetition time (TR) at field strengths of 1.5 T, for example, for a two-echo spin-echo (SE) pulse sequence using RF pulses of 1 msec duration.

Radiofrequency Penetration

The RF (B_1) field induces electrical currents within the patient's tissues. These RF-induced *eddy currents* (to be differentiated from gradient-induced eddy currents in the cryoshield, discussed further on) oppose the RF field and reduce penetration of the RF pulse into deep tissues. This so-called "skin effect,"[6] which is frequency dependent, causes the RF excitation to be nonuniform throughout the imaging volume and can result in prominent shading artifacts at high field strengths.

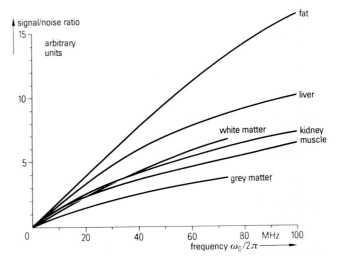

FIGURE 12–10. Signal-to-noise (S/N) ratio as a function of B_0 (constant receiver bandwidth assumed). Increase in the S/N ratio with the field, taking into consideration the dependence of the T_1 relaxation time on the field strength B_0 for a constant repetition time (TR).

T_1 Relaxation

As discussed in Chapter 1, T_1 relaxation times increase with field strength.[7] For a given TR, this increase results in greater saturation of the nuclear magnetization and therefore reduced signal. Consequently, the actual increase in S/N is less than proportional to field strength (Fig. 12–10).

Safety

High field magnets have several potential safety problems. Because the energy stored in the magnetic field increases with the square of the field strength, it must be possible to dissipate this efficiently (quench) in case of emergency. Furthermore, large magnets exert strong forces on ferromagnetic objects inadvertently brought near the magnet. If these objects are fully saturated (fully magnetized), which depends on the shape and composition of the object, the attractive forces increase linearly with field strength. Finally, fringe fields increase with field strength (Chapter 11). Table 12–3 shows the distance of the 5-G line (pacemaker restriction) for magnets

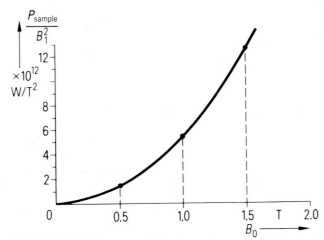

FIGURE 12–9. Pulse power (P_{sample}) require per B_1 field squared for a given field strength B_0. (B_1 field—circular component—for a linear polarized resonator; average patient at 75 kg.)

TABLE 12–3. RECOMMEND SAFETY DISTANCE FROM CENTER OF MAGNET*

B_0	0.5 mT-Line (Radial)	0.5 mT-Line (Axial)
0.5 T	6.5 meters	8.3 meters
1.0 T	8.2 meters	10.5 meters
1.5 T	9.4 meters	12.0 meters
2.0 T	10.3 meters	13.1 meters

*Valid for nonshielded magnets having a 1.05-meter bore and a length of 2.30 meters.

TABLE 12–4. SENSITIVITY OF VARIOUS DEVICES TO STATIC MAGNETIC FIELDS

Magnetic data storage devices (disks, tapes, and so on)	3 mT
Screened video monitors	3 mT
Video monitors (monochrome)	1 mT
Cardiac pacemakers and other electronic implants	0.5 mT
X-ray equipment	0.2 mT
Image intensifiers	50 μT
Photo multipliers	50 μT
Earth's magnetic field (for comparison)	50 μT

of the same size but different field strengths. Various electronic devices are also sensitive to weak magnetic fields (Table 12–4). Magnetic shielding can reduce siting problems considerably.

GRADIENTS

The gradient coils are configured to produce highly linear magnetic field gradients within the imaging volume. An example of a gradient coil system is shown in Figure 12–11. In most applications, the gradient waveform is trapezoidal. A trapezoidal gradient is designed to increase (ramp up) from zero to a plateau value determined by the pulse sequence. The gradient stays at the plateau value for a certain time and then rapidly decreases (ramps down) to zero. The coils and power supply are designed for strong amplitudes and rapid ramping. Echo-planar and hybrid imaging systems sometimes use oscillating, sinusoidal gradients, which permit more rapid switching and require large power supplies (see Chapter 5).

POWER SUPPLY

The power supply imposes severe constraints on maximal gradient amplitude. The gradient power requirements depend on a number of design assumptions but in general increase by the fourth to fifth power of the gradient coil radius. Although current requirements can be reduced by increasing the number of windings in the gradient coil, this increases the coil inductance and requires a correspondingly high voltage to allow rapid switching. Typical current requirements are in the range of 120 to 150 A, including eddy current compensation (see further on). To meet this requirement with rapid gradient switching, the power supply must be able to support current changes at rates of 150 kA/sec. In addition, the power supply must be extremely precise, have minimal electronic noise, and have minimal voltage instability (ripple). High gradient stability (less than a few hundred thousandths of maximal gradient strength) is essential because the gradient determines the sampled point in the spatial frequency domain,[8] and instabilities lead to image artifacts such as smearing in the phase-encoding direction.

EDDY CURRENTS

As the gradients switch amplitudes during the imaging process, the changing magnetic field induces time-varying currents in nearby conducting materials. In particular, they induce electrical currents in the wall of the magnet dewar (cryoshield). These eddy currents themselves create a time-varying magnetic field in the same distribution as that produced by the gradient coils, but with opposite direction (Fig. 12–12). The net effect of the gradient-induced eddy currents is to oppose and weaken the gradient magnetic field.

Eddy currents increase with the gradient amplitude and the rate of change of that amplitude. Once the gradient reaches a stable, plateau value, the eddy currents begin to decay. The decay of the eddy

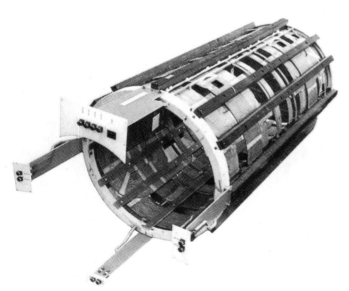

FIGURE 12–11. Gradient coil system with 72-cm diameter for 6 mT/meter at 100 A.

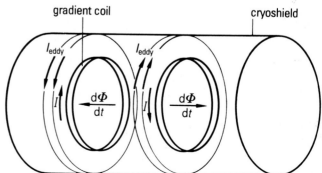

FIGURE 12–12. Eddy currents generated by a pulsed gradient field.

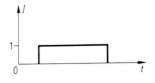

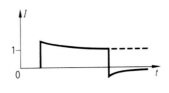

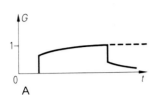

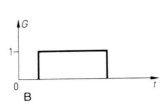

A

B

FIGURE 12–13. Current and gradient pulse form. *A*, Without eddy current compensation. *B*, With eddy current compensation.

currents can be approximated mathematically by an exponential function, with a time constant that is generally determined by the conductivity and effective inductance of the cryoshield.

Without any compensation for eddy currents, a square current pulse produces a distorted gradient waveform, rather than the expected trapezoidal waveform (Fig. 12–13*A*). The distorted gradient pulse produces image artifacts, such as blurring and spatial misregistration.

ACTIVE GRADIENT SHIELDING

Eddy current effects can be largely eliminated by imposing shielding coils between the gradient coil and cryostat (active shielding). In effect, the active shield is a second set of gradient coils mounted concentrically around the imaging gradient coils.[9] Current flow in the active shield is opposite to that of the imaging gradient coils; this shielding current is switched on and off in synchrony with the imaging gradients. The effect of the active shield is to counteract the magnetic field of the imaging gradient in the vicinity of the cryoshield and thereby to eliminate eddy currents.

Active gradient shielding has proved effective on MR systems but also has significant drawbacks. By counteracting the gradient magnetic field, active shielding may reduce the effective amplitude of the imaging gradients. Stronger power supplies are therefore necessary. Active shielding also adds to the size, weight, and cost of the gradient system. Finally, despite the use of active shielding, some degree of precompensation of the driving current (see the following section) must also be used for best results.

EDDY CURRENT CORRECTION BY PRECOMPENSATION OF THE DRIVING CURRENT

Good eddy current suppression can be obtained without active shielding by precompensating the driving current for the gradients (Fig. 12–13*B*). Basically, the driving current is dynamically modified so that the gradient magnetic field, when added to the opposing field generated by the eddy currents, always produces a net magnetic field of the proper strength and pulse shape.

However, as shown in Figure 12–12, the distribution of the eddy currents differs from the gradient coil current distribution. This deviation is primarily along the radial direction but also occurs along the long axis of the magnet. Because the spatial distribution of the eddy current–induced magnetic fields differs slightly from that of the gradient-induced magnetic fields, precompensation of the driving current does not perfectly eliminate eddy fields at every point in space. This problem can be minimized by proper consideration of the design of the gradient coil. However, the eddy currents decay over time, and this *dynamic nonlinearity* cannot be completely compensated for in the design of the gradient coil or in precompensation of the driving for the gradients.

The net result is that the effectiveness of eddy current compensation has a slight spatial dependence. This problem can be overcome by using a highly conductive material for the cryoshield, which reduces the rate of decay of the eddy currents. By making the decay time constants for the eddy currents long relative to the duration of the gradient pulses, the field nonlinearities produced by the eddy currents can be considered essentially static during the read-out, slice-selection, and phase-encoding periods. As a result, the effect of the eddy current–induced inhomogeneity is like that of a main magnetic field inhomogeneity. For most superconducting MR imaging systems with magnet bores larger than 1 meter, using typical gradient amplitudes, these eddy current–induced field inhomogeneities are well below 10 per cent of the nominal gradient within the imaging volume. The spatial distortions resulting from eddy current–induced dynamic nonlinearity are therefore less than those resulting from main field inhomogeneity.

CRITERIA FOR REQUIRED GRADIENT STRENGTH

The cost of a gradient system increases considerably with the level of performance capability. In particular, power requirements become a limitation at higher gradient amplitudes. Therefore, a compromise must be reached between unlimited, expensive gradient capabilities and practical requirements for MR imaging. The essential question is as follows: How strong a gradient is needed to achieve the desired level of spatial resolution and contrast, which depend on pulse sequence timing parameters,[10] and also permit use of newer techniques, such as flow compensation with MR angiography?

Spatial resolution depends strongly on the duration of the gradient and its amplitude (i.e., the area under the gradient pulse). Different pulse sequences have different requirements in this regard. For instance, low-bandwidth methods use a long sampling time (T_s) and weak gradients. The benefit of low-bandwidth methods is reduced image noise (N), since

$$N \sim 1/\sqrt{T_s} \quad (1)$$

Use of a long T_s necessitates an increase in echo time (TE), which in turn affects S/N and contrast. The relationship between TE and T_s is dependent on the pulse sequence structure. For conventional SE pulse sequences (Fig. 12–14), TE may be expressed as

$$TE = T_s + 2T_p + 3t_g \quad (2)$$

where t_g represents the ramp times of the gradients and T_p represents the duration of the RF pulses (typically 2 to 5 msec). The image noise can be expressed as a function of the pulse sequence structure,

$$N \sim 1/(TE - 2T_p - 3t_g)^{1/2} \quad (3)$$

With use of this relationship, contrast-to-noise ratios can be calculated as a function of TE and RF pulse duration for various pairs of materials (Figs. 12–15 and 12–16).[11]

It can be seen that short RF pulses and ramp times, in conjunction with low-bandwidth methods, gener-

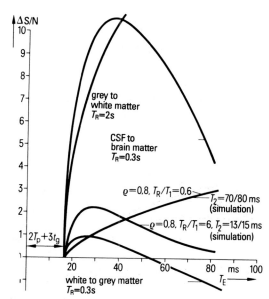

FIGURE 12–15. Contrast-to-noise ratio as a function of the echo time (TE) for various tissue parameters. CSF = cerebrospinal fluid.

ally produce optimal contrast-to-noise. The implication for gradient design is that strong, fast gradients are needed. There are additional limiting factors that increase the gradient requirements. Bandwidth reduction is limited by chemical shift displacement, which should not be much greater than the pixel dimension. The minimal duration of the RF pulses is also limited by considerations of slice profile, which worsens as the pulse duration is decreased, and by the fact that such a decrease causes a quadratic increase in peak pulse power and a linear increase in power deposition into the patient.

Strong gradients are also needed for high spatial resolution, as expressed by the following:

$$\Delta x = 2\pi/\gamma G_x T_s \quad (4)$$
$$\Delta y = 2\pi/\gamma G_y T_s \quad (5)$$
$$\Delta z = \Delta\omega_p/\gamma G_z \quad (6)$$

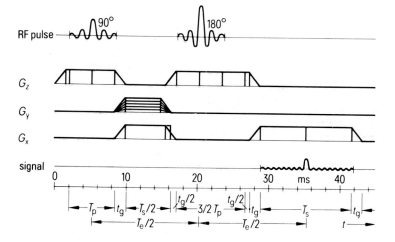

FIGURE 12–14. Multislice spin-echo (SE) pulse sequence.

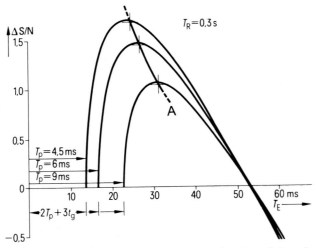

FIGURE 12–16. Contrast-to-noise ratio as a function of the echo time (TE) for gray and white brain matter at various pulse times. A = peak contrast-to-noise.

where $\Delta\omega_p$ represents the RF pulse bandwidth. For example, using a 2.5-msec sinc RF pulse and a minimal slice thickness of 3 mm, one can estimate that a gradient of 6 mT/meter should be sufficient.

However, still stronger gradients are needed for techniques such as flow compensation. Furthermore, newer methods, such as the use of ultrashort TEs for breath-hold liver studies, may require gradient strengths of 10 mT/meter or greater.

RADIOFREQUENCY SYSTEM

In this section, we consider some rather technical aspects involved in the design of the RF system. Clinical imaging specialists interested in a more basic discussion of the RF system are referred to Chapter 1 and, for considerations related to pulse sequence design, Chapter 10.

The coils used to transform electrical signals to high-frequency magnetic (B_1) fields (transmit coils) or to convert these fields to electrical signals (receive coils) represent the heart of the RF system.

COILS AND RESONATORS

Coils and resonators, types of RF antennas, are components of the MR system that directly interact with the object to be imaged.

Antenna Characteristics

A coil can be characterized by the spatial distribution of the magnetic field per current through the coil winding $B_i(r)$. Because of reciprocity rules, the peak output voltage ($\hat{u}$) induced by a sample with magnetization rotating with ω_0[12] can be written as

$$\hat{u} = \omega_o \int_{v_{sample}} \vec{M}\,\vec{B}_i\,dV \tag{7}$$

As a result, the received output power (short circuit at the coil outputs) is

$$P = \tfrac{1}{2}\,\hat{u}^2/R \tag{8}$$

Matching

The term *matching* may have multiple connotations in MR instrumentation. For example, a maximum of only half the output is available when the coil has been matched to subsequent components; hence a matching circuit (employing impedance transformers) is typically used (Fig. 12–17). Additionally, the useful signal output rises with the matching of the spatial coil field distribution to the distribution of the magnetization and falls with the resistive loss (R). This expression of matching is to be understood in a very general manner, that is, not only that the sample volume should correspond to the sensitive volume of the antenna but also that the vectors $\vec{M}$ and $\vec{B}_i$ should be parallel. Given an antenna whose B_1 field is perpendicular to B_0 and is circularly polarized, it should theoretically be superior to any other configuration because of the nuclear magnetization precession $\vec{M}$ about the B_0 direction.

Noise Sources

In addition to signal loss, resistance (R) may also be the source of undesirable noise. The resistance may be divided into the resistance induced by the sample and that caused by the coil:

$$R = R_{sample} + R_{coil} \tag{9}$$

The loss in useful signal caused by the subject of measurement and the noise it generates is unavoidable. The R_{sample} is strongly dependent on the shape of the object to be measured and the distribution of conductive material therein. For simple and homogeneously conductive objects, R_{sample} can be derived as follows:

$$R_{sample} = \tfrac{1}{4}\,\sigma\,\omega_0^2 B_i^2\theta \tag{10}$$

where

$$\theta = \int_{v_{sample}} r\perp\,dV \tag{10a}$$

is some kind of momentum of inertia with respect to the B_1 axis, $r\perp$ is the radius perpendicular to B_1, σ is the conductivity of the object. In the case of a cylinder

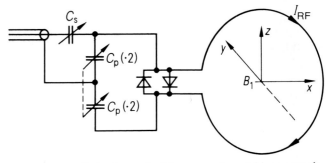

FIGURE 12–17. Surface coil with symmetric matching network.

(diameter D, length L) with the axis parallel to B_0, the integral (θ) is

$$\theta = (D^4L + \tfrac{4}{3}D^2L^3)\ \pi/64 \qquad (11)$$

R_{coil}, on the other hand, can be optimized:

$$R_{coil} = \frac{\omega_0\int_{vcoil}B_i^2dV}{2\ \mu_0Q_0} \qquad (12)$$

With the definition of the filling factor (η),

$$\eta = \int_{vsample}B_i^2dV/\int_{vcoil}B_i^2dV \qquad (13)$$

that is, the fraction of the field energy penetrating the sample in relation to total field energy produced, it follows that

$$R_{coil} = \omega_0\int_{vsample}B_i^2dV/(2\ \mu_0\eta Q_0) \qquad (14)$$

Coil losses therefore increase with sample volume and decrease with the (unloaded) Q_0 and the filling factor.

The Optimal MR Antenna

In summary, the following goals are set for an optimized MR antenna:

1. Field distribution should be homogeneous across the measurement volume to ensure spatially uniform excitation.

2. The filling factor (volume of the sample/volume of the coil) should be large.

3. The direction of polarization should be perpendicular to the main field and (if possible) circular.

4. Coil losses should be minimal compared with the losses induced by the subject to be measured; that is, the unloaded Q_0 should be high.

Goals 1 and 2 may occasionally prove counterproductive in medical practice, namely, when a portion of the body that cannot be surrounded by a coil is to be imaged. For these cases, surface coils are used; that is, the homogeneity of the B_1 field is sacrificed in favor of a large filling factor.

ANTENNAS WITH HOMOGENEOUS FIELD DISTRIBUTION

Coils and resonators must surround the subject to be measured to generate a homogeneous B_1 field within it.

A suitable configuration would be a solenoid arranged coaxially to the axis of the body. Given that B_1 and B_0 should ideally be perpendicular to each other, this type of coil configuration is limited to use with yoke magnets (see Fig. 12–2). In addition, the eigen resonance frequency of a solenoid having a diameter corresponding to the size of a human body is substantially lower than the MR frequency normally used. Therefore, at high frequencies, it is necessary to find cylindrical structures that generate a homogeneous field that is polarized in the direction perpendicular to the axis of the magnet. A sufficiently long tube, subjected to a constant current distribution J (ϕ),

$$J(\phi) = \hat{J}\sin(\phi) \qquad (15)$$

as shown in Figure 12–18A and B, will generate the desired field distribution.[13] Implementing this current distribution is not a simple matter. The current density is simulated for several angles with discrete conductor paths (Fig. 12–18C and D). The conductors at $\phi = 0$ and 2π may be eliminated, since they do not carry any current. If the wire rods are connected in the manner shown in Figure 12–19, the result is a saddle coil that can be used in situations in which the frequency is not too high nor the diameter too large (up to 30 cm at approximately 25 MHz).

At higher frequencies and larger diameters (whole-body antennas), the length of the conductors is no longer short compared with the RF wavelength, so that the desired current distribution can no longer be achieved with a saddle coil.

At this point, the $\lambda/2$ transmission line resonator

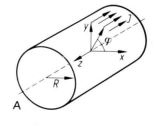
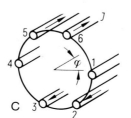
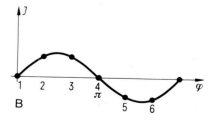
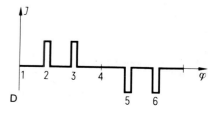

FIGURE 12–18. RF antenna with homogeneous B_1 field. *A*, Hollow tube with current density distribution in longitudinal direction. *B*, Ideal current distribution. *C*, Resonant conductors arranged as a discrete hollow tube. *D*, Current distribution in a discrete hollow tube for a nearly homogeneous B_1 field.

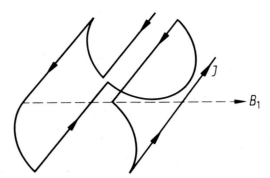

FIGURE 12–19. Saddle coil for low frequencies and small coil dimensions.

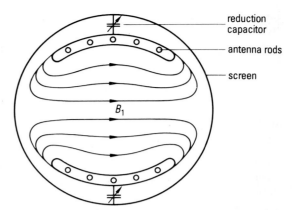

FIGURE 12–21. Cross-section of a whole-body antenna using the transmission line resonance principle suitable for high frequencies.

principle becomes of interest. If a wave having the length $\lambda = 2\pi c/\omega_0$ (c is the velocity of wave propagation) is generated on a double transmission line (Fig. 12–20A) and the line is $\lambda/2$ long, a resonance or standing wave is produced. Its current distribution is shown in Figure 12–20B, which results in the corresponding B_1 field distribution. The circuit can be shortened symmetrically by adding capacitances, so that a nearly uniform current distribution is created in the longitudinal direction (Fig. 12–20C and D). Such resonance conductors can be configured as a hollow tube. A cross-section of such a configuration is shown in Figure 12–21. The sections of the conductors are composed of rods having adjustable capacitors connected between the antenna and ground (exterior shielding). This $\lambda/2$ resonator[14] can be used as a transmit/receive antenna for whole-body MR imaging up to more than 63 MHz.

Alderman and Grant have developed a variation of this principle (Fig. 12–22).[15] It is used primarily for head imaging antennas, since the structure is open on two sides and is therefore more pleasant for the patient.

Quadrature (Circularly Polarized) Coils

A circularly polarized B_1 field can be generated with the antennas described in the preceding para-

graphs by joining pairs of resonators via a power divider and a phase shifter in such a way that a rotating high-frequency field is generated within the antenna. Inversely, the voltages, induced in the resonators by the precessing magnetization and shifted by 90 degrees, are forwarded to the preamplifier via a summation network. This configuration requires only half the RF output to generate a rotating B_1 field and results in S/N that is improved by the $\sqrt{2}$ (40 per cent)[16] if the Q of the antenna under load conditions corresponds to that of a comparable, linearly polarized configuration. Unfortunately, since a cross-section of the human body is more elliptical in shape (i.e., the coils are not evenly loaded), the advantages of circular polarization may not be fully realized in practice.

SURFACE COILS

As the name indicates, these coils are used for imaging organs that are located close to the surface of the patient's body. They are placed on the patient directly over the position in which the organ is located. The coil must be oriented so that the B_1 field

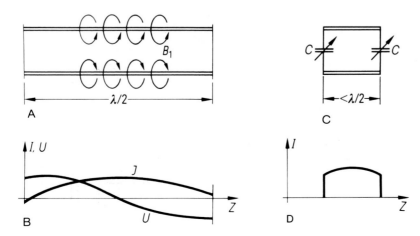

FIGURE 12–20. A $\lambda/2$ (½ wavelength) resonator (antenna). *A*, Conductor configuration. *B*, Current distribution. *C*, Electrically shortening the conductors by applying a capacitance load to the ends. *D*, Current distribution with shortened conductors.

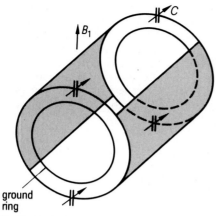

FIGURE 12–22. Variation of the conductor resonance principle according to Aldermann and Grant.

is perpendicular to B_0. In the simplest case, the coil comprises a single wire ring that is tuned to resonance at ω_0 via variable capacitors (see Fig. 12–17). The field distribution of a current-carrying circular loop with a radius of r is described along the y-axis of the coil by the following equation:

$$B_i(y) = \mu_0 r^2/[2(r^2 + y^2)^{3/2}] \tag{16}$$

Figure 12–23 demonstrates the decay of sensitivity along the coil axis with increasing distance from the coil plane. The maximal sensitivity and the effective penetration depth ("break-even" distance when comparing the S/N of a surface coil with that of a volume coil) depends strongly on the radius of the surface coil. Depending upon the imaging objective, it is possible to trade sensitivity for the magnitude of the useful volume by varying the dimensions of the coil.

The configuration of the coil windings can also be adapted to the surface of the human body. Surface coils are generally used only to receive MR signals because of the inhomogeneity of the field distribution; for instance, a 180-degree excitation may be generated near the surface while at some distance away the tissues experience only a 90-degree flip. For this reason, the typical MR imaging configuration uses the whole-body resonators for more uniform excitation and uses the surface coil for a receiving antenna.

Decoupling

When using the body resonator for excitation, the surface coil must not oscillate during the transmit phase, or the distribution of the transmitter field will be distorted. This interaction between the transmit and receive coils is called *coupling*. Complete decoupling through the appropriate orientation of the surface coil to the direction of polarization of the transmission antenna is not usually possible, even on linearly polarized systems. Decoupling is therefore forced via "dentuning" diodes, which are illustrated in Figure 12–24. These diodes are switched into the conductive state by the induced voltage during RF transmission and thus detune the coil off resonance.

TRANSMIT AND RECEIVE SYSTEM

The RF electronics of an MR system are designed to generate the pulsed RF output needed for MR and to prepare the signals picked up by the antenna

FIGURE 12–23. Effectivity of a surface coil relative to a volume (body) coil.

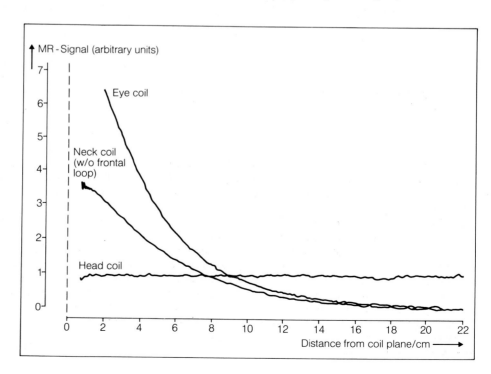

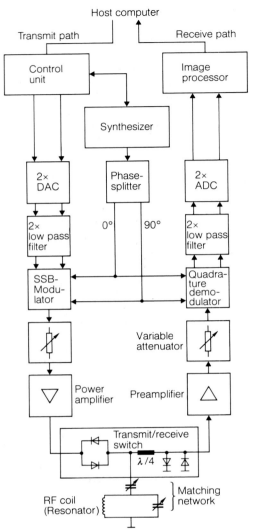

FIGURE 12–24. Circuit diagram of the RF system.

formation from the rotating coordinate system (the phase at the resonance frequency) to the laboratory coordinate system (what the coil actually "sees"). It multiplies the complex pulse form (the audio frequency signal) $F(t)$ by the complex carrier signal $e^{i\omega_0 t}$. The real portion of the product appears at the output of the modulator and is fed to the RF power transmitter. More details of the modulator are presented in Appendix 12–B.

Radiofrequency Power Transmitter

The RF final stage must amplify the pulse so that a B_1 field is generated in the subject surrounded by the resonator. This field must fulfill the following requirements:

$$B_1 = \alpha/(\gamma t_p) \tag{17}$$

where α is the tip angle of magnetization and t_p is the effective time for the B_1 field.

This expression applies to a circularly polarized B_1 field. If the RF field is linearly polarized, twice the B_1 amplitude is required for the same tip angle. The power needed depends on the losses in the object being measured as well as in the resonator and its connecting lines. For a cylinder whose axis is parallel to the main field and therefore perpendicular to the B_1 field, the power required to generate a certain B_1 field can be approximated using Equations 10 and 11 for R_{sample} multiplied by $\frac{1}{2}\hat{I}^2$

$$P_{sample} = (\pi/512)\ \omega_0^2 \sigma B_1^2 (D^4 L + \tfrac{1}{3} D^2 L^3) \tag{18}$$

One may insert the following values, for example: cylinder dimension $D = 1 = 40$ cm; conductivity $\sigma = 0.5/\Omega m$ (equivalent of physiologic NaCl solution); tip angle $= 180$ degrees at an effective time of $t_p = 1.0$ msec, thus resulting in a linearly oscillating field; $B_1 = 23.5\ \mu T$; and a center frequency $= 42.576$ MHz. The P_{sample} then equals approximately 2.8 kW.

Under experimental conditions using a patient of average weight (approximately 75 kg), 1.3 kW of power can be measured at the input of the antenna. As was determined by the measurement of loaded and unloaded Q, approximately 20 per cent of power is lost in the resonator. In this case, only slightly more than 1 kW was absorbed by the patient; experimentally, it appears that the cylinder-shaped model exaggerates the required power. This observation can be explained by the inhomogeneity of conductivity and the shape of the human body.

In designing a practical RF system, further considerations are necessary. The cables and components of the transmit/receive switch attenuate the RF output by approximately 1 dB. The final stage, therefore, must be able to provide a minimum of 2 kW of pulse power. To provide some reserve for shorter pulses and for a greater degree of attenuation caused by heavier patients, the final stage at 42 MHz should be designed for approximately 8 kW. A 63-MHz final stage should be made possible for a pulse output of 15 kW to allow for the rise in loss proportional to

for image processing. The signal paths are illustrated in Figure 12–24.

Transmit Path

The RF pulses required for MR are first digitally synthesized as a series of complex numbers by the sequence controlling unit. The magnitude of a complex numerical value represents the momentary amplitude, and the phase determines the direction of the B_1 field in the rotating coordinate system.

The series of complex numbers is converted to voltages by two DACs. The bandwidth and the length of the programmed pulse form are determined by the sample clock and the number of data points. The signals are fed into the modulator via two low-pass filters, which suppress any undesirable harmonics caused by the digital generation of the pulse. The function of the modulator corresponds to the trans-

$\omega_0{}^2$ within the measured object; however, the average available output power may be considerably lower than that figure.

Output power is governed by how much the patient's safety will be affected by the absorbed RF power (heating effect) and is enforced through local regulations for medical equipment. Thermal dimensioning and the power supply for the final stage are designed for the continuous-output power needs, while the energy for a high-output pulse or series of pulses may be taken from a capacitor battery that is recharged during off-times.

Receive Path

The receiving channel is shown in the right half of Figure 12–24. The MR signals coming from the receiver coil are raised to a sufficient level by the preamplifier so that line attenuation and input noise from the following stage are negligible. After further amplification, the signal is demodulated.

Demodulator

The function of the demodulator is complementary to that of the modulator, namely, the transformation of the laboratory coordinate system into the coordinate system that rotates with ω_0. A more detailed description of the demodulator is given in Appendix 12–B. At the two outputs, signals representing the magnetization components in the rotating frame $\mathbf{M}_x$ and $\mathbf{M}_y$ appear. This type of circuit is called a quadrature demodulator. It can distinguish between frequencies greater and smaller than ω_0 (upper and lower sidebands); therefore, the output bandwidth is half of the input bandwidth. This feature improves the S/N ratio by $\sqrt{2}$ in comparison with simple phase-sensitive rectifiers.[17]

The output signals of the demodulator pass through a pair of low-pass filters that cut off all frequencies that exceed half the sampling (Nyquist) frequency. Finally, two ADCs convert them into a sequence of complex numbers suitable for digital image processing.

Signal Levels

To specify the necessary total receiver gain and dynamic range—that is, the signal limit divided by noise—the expected S/N and input voltage at the preamplifier should be known. As discussed in the section on pulse output, any assumption is valid only to a certain extent because the human body cannot be described by a simple mathematical model. Similarly, coil characteristics cannot be calculated exactly. Therefore, one must rely on the results of empirical studies to design a practical receiver system. If the antenna impedance is always matched to the actual line impedance R_L (50Ω) via tuning circuits, the noise voltage (U_N) at the input of the preamplifier (input

impedance Z) is always the same regardless of the coil load.

$$U_n = (4kTR_L\Delta\omega_s /2\pi 10^{F/10dB})^{1/2} | Z_i | (R_L + | Z_i |) \quad (19)$$

F is the noise figure of the preamplifier in decibels. The total gain of the receive channel consists of the gain of the individual components minus the attenuation values of both the attenuator and the cables. The antenna and preamplifier noise, which is dependent upon the input bandwidth $\Delta\omega_s$ should be sufficiently higher than the frequency-independent ADC quantization noise. For the smallest commonly used bandwidth, the gain U_o/U_i must be greater than

$$U_o /U_i > \frac{U_{LSB}}{\sqrt{12}\ U_N} \quad (20)$$

Dynamic Range

The size of a useful signal depends largely on the type of MR imaging sequence performed, especially on the volume excited. At 63 MHz, the dynamic range of the MR signal may be substantially higher than 100 dB. This means that the S/N gain resulting from the excitation of a large volume (e.g., for three-dimensional [3D] imaging) cannot be fully realized with conventional 16-bit ADCs. The adaptability of the preamplifier, as well as the variable attenuation elements in the intermediate amplifier, still allows the processing of high input signals, for example, with thick slices and with nonselective excitation, as well as low input signals with thin slices or low flip-angle sequence even if the MR signal dynamic range exceeds the capabilities of the ADC.

Transmit/Receive Switch

The transmit/receive switch is the link between the RF resonator and the RF pulse transmitter or the preamplifier. It must make possible the path from the transmitter to the antenna during the RF pulse and at the same time protect the sensitive preamplifier from the high pulse power. In the receive mode, the weak MR signal must reach the preamplifier with as little attenuation as possible, and the noise of the final stage must be kept out of the antenna circuit. Figure 12–24 (bottom) shows a simplified diagram of the switch, which automatically switches between transmit and receive without additional control circuitry. The antiparallel pair of diodes in the transmit cable does not conduct during the receive mode. This feature prevents noise generated by the power section from reaching the preamplifier while preventing the MR signal from disappearing into the transmitter. In the transmit mode, the voltages are high enough to switch on the diodes, so that the power reaches the antenna (resonator) with practically no loss. The pair of diodes at the preamplifier input also conducts. The quarter-wavelength cable connected in front of the diodes transforms the short circuit to a high impedance at the input of the antenna. In the receive mode, the impedance of the diodes is high, and the signal reaches the preamplifier virtually unattenuated by the $\lambda/4$ line. The circuit contains other adjustable components that neutralize the diode capacitance.

RADIOFREQUENCY ROOM SHIELDING

Effective antenna shielding against RF interference is essential because of the extreme sensitivity of the receiving system to high-frequency fields. Antenna sensitivity, self-shielding capacity (a function of the length and diameter of the antenna resonator relative to wavelength λ), and estimates of the intensity of possible RF interference (e.g., short-wave broadcasting stations) must all be included in the calculation of the required attenuation factor.

Experience has shown that the shielding factor must be greater than 100 dB to prevent interference from a 5-kW monofrequency transmitter at a distance of 10 km. To accomplish such shielding, the receiving antenna must be inside a metal housing, which is, for all practical purposes, completely closed. An extension of the shielding tube in which the antenna is located, a practice that is seen occasionally, can be effective only in areas completely free of interference and only when using low frequencies. Since high-frequency magnetic fields can hardly penetrate conductive material because of the skin effect, electrostatic shielding of a thickness several times skin depth is sufficient, for example, 0.5 mm of copper foil. Gaps in the shielding are to be avoided if possible. If necessary, however, the linear dimensions of such gaps must be clearly smaller than those of the wavelength corresponding to the MR frequency. Doors must be constructed so that they are RF sealed when closed. In most cases, the entire field generation system—that is, the magnet, the shim, the gradient and RF coils, and the table for the patient—must all be set up inside the shielded room (see Fig. 12–1). This means that all the cables for these components must be routed through appropriately dimensioned suppression filters. Otherwise, these cables, which are excellent antennas for high-frequency interference, would conduct RF noise into the shielded room. If even these extensive measures are insufficient (in the case of a high-powered short-wave transmitter in the area), the main field must be changed to provide for sufficient distance between the frequency band used for MR imaging and that of the interference.

SUBJECT-DEPENDENT SYSTEM CALIBRATIONS

After the patient has been positioned, the parameters that are influenced by the subject to be measured must be calibrated before the measurement can be started. Calibration procedures for an MR examination are performed as follows:

1. Positioning the patient
2. Adjustment of antennas (coil tuning)
3. Checking and setting the MR center frequency (frequency adjustment)
4. Pulse amplitude calibration (transmitter adjustment)
5. Selection of measurement parameters (or pulse sequence)
6. Setting of the receiver gain (receiver adjustment)
7. Starting measurement
8. Image reconstruction, image retrieval

Steps 2 to 4 must be repeated only if the patient has moved. The selection of measurement parameters (Step 5) may initially be performed earlier in this sequence but will require a receiver adjustment when subsequent sequence parameters are changed.

ANTENNA ADJUSTMENT (COIL TUNING)

The transmit/receive coil impedance, which is dependent on the size and position of the patient, must first be matched to the impedance of the transmission line. With the help of a fully automatic control system, the capacitors of the matching network are set so that there is practically no reflection of the RF power fed into the antenna. After the desired measurement parameters have been selected, the following procedures are normally performed automatically by the system.

SETTING THE CENTER FREQUENCY (FREQUENCY ADJUSTMENT)

The next step is the determination of the MR frequency. This would seem to be a superfluous step when dealing with the stability of supercoding magnets, but the frequency will change by tens of hertz from patient to patient because of varying susceptibility. A variation in resonance, as shown in Equation 1, would cause a noticeable shift in the image corresponding to the gradient strength employed. Resonance frequency can be determined by a simple MR experiment, namely, the excitation and read-out of a free induction decay (FID). The synthesizer is then readjusted accordingly.

PULSE AMPLITUDE CALIBRATION (TRANSMITTER ADJUSTMENT)

Since the degree of efficiency of the transmission antenna, expressed in generated B_1 field per square

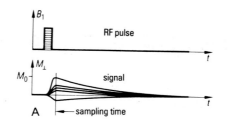 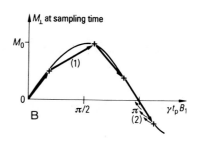

FIGURE 12–25. Pulse amplitude calibration procedure. The $\gamma\, t_p B_1 = 180°$ condition is reached first in large steps (1) up to the sign reversal of $M_\perp$, and then in fine steps (2) to the signal minimum. *A*, Measurement sequence for pulse amplitude calibration. *B*, MR signal as a function of the B_1 amplitude.

root of the RF power input, is strongly dependent on the subject of the examination, the pulse amplitude must be adjusted. This adjustment determines the RF output necessary to tip the nuclear magnetization by an angle of α by using a pulse of the length t_p. A practical method makes use of the following relationship between transverse magnetization $\mathbf{M}_\perp$, which is proportional to the MR signal, and the $\overline{B}_1$ amplitude (Fig. 12–25):

$$\mathbf{M}_\perp = \mathbf{M}_0 \sin (\gamma\, t_p\, B_1) \qquad (21)$$

With this expression, the first signal minimum corresponds to a nutation angle of 180 degrees. Therefore, the first zero passage of the MR signal directly after the RF pulse is sought by increasing the pulse amplitude in a series of FID excitations, first in larger steps and then in finer steps. With use of the pulse length t_p and the amplitude determined during calibration, any flip angle for any other pulse form may be calculated.

RECEIVER GAIN (RECEIVER ADJUSTMENT)

The last step in the calibration process is the adjustment of receiver gain with respect of the maximal MR signal occurring during imaging. This adjustment, discussed in Chapter 3, is important because inappropriate signal levels may introduce image distortion if the ADC is overloaded or increased noise if the ADC is underloaded. The same pulse sequence is used for the receiver adjustment as for imaging, except that the phase-encoding gradient is not switched on so as to find the MR signal is at its maximum. For this reason, the pulse sequence parameters must be selected prior to this step. If no overload has occurred, the resulting measurement data can be used to calculate the amplifier settings necessary for proper modulation of the receiving components. If this is not the case, the calibration measurement must be repeated using reduced total gain.

Appendix 12–A

MATHEMATICAL DETAILS OF SHIM PROCEDURE

Spherical Harmonics Expansion

The characteristics of the magnetic field can be described by the Laplace equation:

$$\vec{\nabla}^2 \ (Bx, By, By) = 0$$

As long as the field is sufficiently homogeneous, the field magnitude most important for MR frequency is equal to the field component $B_z = B_0$. The following spherical harmonic expansion is a solution of the Laplace equation in spherical coordinates with the center of the magnet as the origin:

$$B_0 \ (r, \theta, \phi) = \sum_{n=0}^{N} \sum_{m=0}^{M \leq N} \frac{r^n}{R^n} P_n^m \ (\cos\theta)$$
$$[A_n^m \cos m\phi \ + \ B_n^m \sin m\phi]$$

The coordinate system is illustrated in Figure 12–26A. The P_n^m functions are designated as associated Legendre polynomials of the n degree and m order.[18] The A_n^m and B_n^m coefficients are the so-called spectrum of the spherical harmonics expansion. They are expressed either as absolute field units (in T) or as relative field deviations (B $(r,\theta,\phi) - B_0)/B_0$ (in ppm), each normalized to the radius R. The goal of the spherical harmonics expansion is the evaluation of the spectrum from the field measurements across the surface of the sphere with radius R (the analysis). Using the coefficients, the reverse is also possible: calculation of the field at any point within the sphere (the synthesis). A simple interpretation of spherical harmonics expansion is possible for the special case of m = 0:

$$B_0(r,\theta) \ = \ \sum_{n=0}^{N} \frac{r^n}{R^n} \ P_n(\cos\theta)A_n^0$$

On the surface of the sphere, the field is not dependent upon the angle ϕ. The A_n^0 coefficients are also called zonal terms; terms where m is not equal to 0 are called tesseral terms. The P_n functions are Legendre polynomials of the n degree. P_0 is the constant 1, so the A_0^0 coefficient can be interpreted as the strength of the main field without deviation and all other terms can be interpreted as deviations. P_1 describes a linear change in the field in z direction. A_1^0 is then the z gradient. The tesseral coefficients, A_1^1 and B_1^1, correspond to the linear gradients in the x and y directions. The factors $(r/R)^n$ show that for small radii, substantial field deviations at higher degrees are only effective at the edges of the spherical volume. The magnitudes of the coefficients decrease with increasing degree. For this reason expansion can be terminated beyond a certain degree.

Measurement and Determination of Shim Coefficients

In order to calculate the spectral term to the n degree and the order m from measurement values, the field must be measured to n + 1 circles parallel to the x-y plane in 2m points. The sampling points are equidistant in θ and ϕ, that is, the distances from the circles to the origin are like $R\cos\theta$. Field measurement is performed by using a small MR probe attached to positioning gear that allows the coordinates $r = R\sin\theta$, and $z = R\cos\theta$ to be adjusted. The field spectrum is calculated from the values acquired at the measurement points.

Appendix 12–B

MATHEMATICAL DETAILS OF THE MODULATOR AND DEMODULATOR

SSB MODULATOR

The modulator multiplies the complex pulse form $F(t)$ with the complex carrier signal $e^{i\omega_0 t}$. The real part of the product appears at the output of the modulator (see Fig. 12–26B):

$$\text{Re}\{F(t)e^{i\omega_0 t}\} = \text{Re}\{F(t)\}\cos\omega_0 t - \text{Im}\{F(t)\}\sin\omega_0 t$$

If the LF signal is:

$$\cos(\omega_z t + \phi) + i\sin(\omega_z t + \phi) = e^{i\omega_z t + \phi}$$

the output signal is:

$$\text{Re}\{e^{i(\omega_0 t + \omega_z t + \phi)}\} = \cos(\omega_0 + \omega_z + \phi)$$

By introducing the factors $e^{i(\omega_z t + \phi)}$ into the low frequency (LF) pulse signal, the frequency and phase of the high frequency excitation pulse can be shifted as desired. When feeding the modulator with $e^{i\omega_z t}$, only one frequency $\omega_0 + \omega_z$ appears at the output. Since the carrier frequency ω_0 as well as the mirror frequency $\omega_0 - \omega_z$ are suppressed, the configuration is referred to as a single sideband modulator (SSB). Programming a frequency offset is a simple method for achieving a shift z of the slice excited with the help of a selective pulse in the gradient:

$$z = \omega_z/(\gamma G_z)$$

The modulator is composed of a pair of ring mixers that are supplied with the carrier signals shifted in phase by zero degrees or 90 degrees. The most important characteristic data are the linearity (i.e., the absence of spurious signals and harmonics), which determines the fidelity of the pulse form, and the suppression of carrier and unwanted sideband signals. Insufficient suppression of undesirable frequencies results in MR excitation at locations other than the slice selected and therefore leads to artifacts. A constant DC voltage on the LF side generates a carrier signal at the modulator output. A signal from the unwanted sideband is generated if the two ring mixers are not precisely balanced or when the carrier signals are not shifted by exactly 90 degrees.

QUADRATURE DEMODULATOR

The input voltage to the demodulator represents the transversal magnetization as:

$$M_x\cos\omega_0 t + M_y\sin\omega_0 t$$

with

$$M_x + iM_y = M_\perp e^{i(\omega_0 t + \phi)}$$

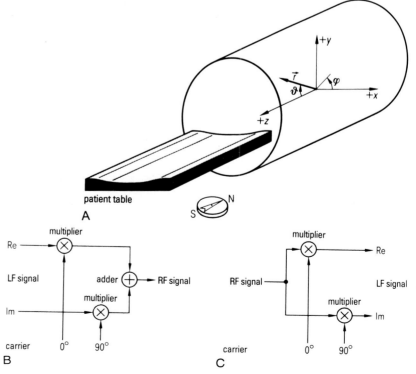

FIGURE 12–26. *A,* Coordinate system (Cartesian and spherical coordinates) of the gradient coils; definition of field polarity. *B,* Single sideband modulator, and *C,* quadrature demodulator. Re = real part; Im = imaginary part; LF = low frequency.

The demodulator multiplies the complex carrier signal with the input signal as follows (see Fig. 12–26C).

$$(M_x\cos\omega_0 t + M_y\sin\omega_0 t)\cos\omega_0 t =$$
$$\tfrac{1}{2}M_x + \tfrac{1}{2}M_x\cos 2\omega_0 t - \tfrac{1}{2}M_y\sin 2\omega_0 t$$

$$(M_x\cos\omega_0 t + M_y\sin\omega_0 t)\sin\omega_0 t =$$
$$\tfrac{1}{2}M_y + \tfrac{1}{2}M_y\sin 2\omega_0 t - \tfrac{1}{2}M_x\cos 2\omega_0 t$$

With exemption of terms having twice the carrier frequency, signals representing the M_x and M_y components of the magnetization are reaching the demodulator outputs. Such a device is called a quadrature detector. Since it can distinguish frequencies $>\omega_0$ and $<\omega_0$ (upper and lower sidebands), the output bandwidth is only half of the input bandwidth. Therefore the signal-to-noise is $\sqrt{2}$ larger than compared with normal phase sensitive detectors. In addition, only half the conversion rate is necessary for the analog-to-digital conversion. On the other hand, there must be two of each of the components after the demodulator. The quadrature demodulator is set up by using balanced ring mixers. The frequency responses and the phases of the ring mixers, filters, and ADCs must be in exactly equal pairs, and the two carrier signals for the quadrature demodulator must be shifted by exactly 90 degrees. If these conditions are not met, the result will be artifacts such as mirror images corresponding to the incomplete separation of the upper and lower sidebands.

REFERENCES

1. Wilson MN: Superconducting Magnets. Oxford, United Kingdom, Clarington Press, 1983.
2. Oxford Magnet Technology: Magnets in Clinical Use. Oxford, United Kingdom, OMT Publishing, 1983.
3. Hoult DI, Lee D: Shimming a superconducting imaging magnet with steel. Rev Sci Instrum 56:131, 1985.
4. Hoult DI, Chen CN, Sank VJ: The field dependence of NMR imaging. II. Arguments concerning an optimal field strength. Magn Reson Med 3:730, 1986.
5. Loeffler W, Oppelt A, von Wulfen H, Zimmermann B: An approach for selecting the best field strength for proton imaging. In Proceedings of the SMRM, 1984, 483.
6. Bottomley PA, Andrew ER: RF Magnetic field penetration, phase shift and power dissipation in biological tissue: Implications for NMR imaging. Phys Med Biol 23:630, 1978.
7. Bottomley PA, Foster TH, Argersinger RE, Pfeifer LM: A review of normal tissue hydrogen NMR relaxation times and relaxation mechanisms from 1–100 MHz: Dependence on tissue type, NMR frequency, temperature, species, excision, and age. Med Phys 11:425, 1984.
8. Ljunggren S: A simple graphical representation of Fourier based imaging methods. J Magn Reson 54:33, 1983.
9. Mansfield P, Chapman B: Active magnetic screening of gradient coils in NMR imaging. J Magn Res 66:573, 1986.
10. Stetter E, Oppelt A: Image quality in NMR tomography. In Proceedings of the World Congress on Medicine, Physics and Biomedical Engineering, 1982, paper 24.10.
11. Wehrli FW, McFall JR, Glover GH, et al: The dependence of nuclear magnetic resonance (NMR) image contrast on intrinsic and pulse sequence timing parameters. Magn Reson Imaging 2:3, 1984.
12. Hoult DI, Lauterbur PC: The sensitivity of the Fungmatographic experiment involving human samples. J Magn Reson 34:425, 1979.
13. Hayes CE: Radiofrequency coil for NMR. European Patent Application No. 0 151 745, 1985.
14. Krause N: Hodifrequentfeld einrichtung in eine Vernrasonant apparatur. German Patent Application No. 32 33 432, 1983.
15. Alderman D, Grant D: An efficient decoupler coil design which reduces heating in conductive samples in superconducting spectrometers. J Magn Reson 36:447, 1979.
16. Hoult DI, Chen CN, Sank VJ: Quadratur detection in the laboratory frame. Magn Reson Med 1:339, 1984.
17. Hoult DI: The NMR receiver: A description and analysis of design. Progress in NMR Spectroscopy. 2:4, 1978, Chapter 6.4.
18. Jahnke E, Emde F: Tafeln nöherer Funktionen. Leipzig, Taubner Verlag, 1952.

PART II

CENTRAL NERVOUS SYSTEM

13

BRAIN: Indications, Technique, and Atlas

JEFFREY J. GREENBERG, DAVID H. TURKEL, JONATHAN KLEEFIELD, and RICHARD J. HICKS

CLINICAL INDICATIONS
IMAGING TECHNIQUES
ATLAS

Because of its geometric shape and size, its relative lack of inherent cardiac or respiratory variation, and the variety of pathologic processes affecting it, the head was the first anatomic area for which both CT and MR were extensively applied. More experience has been acquired imaging the central nervous system with MR than any other area of the body, and its clinical utility has been proved beyond a doubt. However, debates about the relative merits of MR and CT and the exact indications for MR as the primary imaging procedure will continue for some time. With the availability of gadopentetate dimeglumine or Gd-DTPA (Magnevist, Berlex Laboratories, Wayne, NJ) as a contrast agent, indications for enhanced MR are being clarified. Further experience with this agent may show that one of the much touted advantages of MR—the lack of a need for intravenous contrast—is less of a relative advantage over CT than first thought.

MR of the brain remains a dynamic technology that is striving to go beyond "*what* do we see" to "*why* do we see." With its dependence on the more biologically variable parameters of proton density, longitudinal relaxation time (T_1), and transverse relaxation time (T_2), the possibilities for "why" become much greater than with CT and its dependence on x-ray attenuation. Moreover, MR spectroscopy has enormous but yet unrealized potential for providing information about the biochemistry and metabolism

of tissues. It will be some time before we learn to take full advantage of the capabilities of MR.

The general consensus has been that MR is more sensitive but less specific than CT in neuroimaging, with few exceptions. While not specifically addressing relative sensitivities, in a retrospective study of 212 patients Zimmerman and colleagues[1] found MR to give more clinically useful information about pathology in 56.5 per cent of patients. MR was more specific in 29.5 per cent, equally specific in 64.9 per cent, and less specific in 1.9 per cent. MR revealed additional lesions in 12.5 per cent of patients and changed the diagnosis in 8.7 per cent. The advantages of multiplanar capabilities, superior contrast resolution, and increased specificity for subacute hematomas and flowing blood were cited for MR; while CT maintained a clear edge for detection of calcification. Franken and coworkers,[2] in a prospective study of 189 patients, found the suspected diagnosis was refined or changed in 16 per cent after MR. Referring physicians indicated that in two thirds of cases the treatment or estimated prognosis was altered. In 65 of 120 brain studies, there were new findings on MR not revealed by CT, while CT revealed findings missed by MR in 16 cases. Different results were reported by Haughton and colleagues[3] in a study of 61 patients. In this study CT not only had better specificity than MR (90 per cent versus 81 per cent), but it also had better sensitivity (91 per cent versus

82 per cent). However, the difference in sensitivity was related to small, benign calcified lesions, and when those were excluded the difference between sensitivities of MR and CT was not statistically significant.

In any case, most comparative studies between MR and CT have been unfairly skewed toward CT, because noncontrast MR was compared with plain and contrast-enhanced CT. There is little doubt that noncontrast MR is far superior to noncontrast CT in both sensitivity and specificity. The superiority of MR over CT will be further clarified with additional comparative studies of contrast-enhanced scans from the two competitive imaging modalities.

CLINICAL INDICATIONS

There is a general consensus about many applications for MR of the brain, but owing to the relative newness of the field and the variety of imaging systems in use, other indications are more controversial and may in part be field dependent. Because of its extreme sensitivity for white matter disease, many of the white matter processes are superbly imaged by MR and constitute obvious indications for its use. The demyelinating plaques of multiple sclerosis (MS) are well demonstrated by MR,[4, 5] but its utility in older patients is somewhat limited by the presence of asymptomatic white matter lesions related to chronic ischemia.[6, 7] Contrast-enhanced MR can help detect the acute MS plaques. When MR of the brain is normal in patients with suspected MS, T_1-weighted sagittal images of the craniocervical junction may reveal a lesion of the foramen magnum, which at times can mimic the signs and symptoms of MS. Hypertensive encephalopathy, vasculitis, herpes encephalitis, postinfectious encephalitis,[8, 9] and progressive multifocal leukoencephalopathy[10] are other good indications for MR.

History of a seizure disorder is a suitable indication for MR, as MR has been shown to detect more abnormalities than CT in seizure patients.[11–14] Partial complex seizures constitute the most common adult form, and the seizure focus is frequently in the temporal lobe, an area obscured on CT scans by streaking artifacts from the skull base. Coronal T_2-weighted MR gives exquisite pictures of the temporal lobes. On the other hand, if small calcifications are the only parenchymal abnormality, the MR may be normal.[15, 16] Positron emission tomography (PET) has revealed more lesions in patients with partial complex seizures than either MR or CT, and in a significant number of cases there is poor correlation of PET, EEG, and MR findings.[14, 17] Since at this time only a few cases have had pathologic correlation, the significance of positive MR findings has yet to be proved.

The value of MR for defining congenital malformations is unquestioned. The multiplanar display of anatomy gives important information about the corpus callosum and posterior fossa structures. The superior gray/white contrast allows accurate assessment of myelination.[18, 19]

If the primary concern is a lesion of the posterior fossa—whether due to neoplasm,[20] infarct,[21] MS,[22] or a vascular malformation[23]—MR is preferable owing to the lack of interpetrous bone artifacts that are invariably present on CT. Multiple studies have shown noncontrast MR to be equivalent to air CT–cisternography for the evaluation of acoustic neuromas,[24–26] so that many patients with suspected acoustic neuroma are now being studied with MR rather than CT. Gd-DTPA increases the sensitivity of MR for intracanalicular lesions even further.

The role of MR as the first imaging procedure in patients with suspected pituitary adenomas is controversial. Reports in the literature on the sensitivity of MR for microadenomas have varied from 54 per cent[27] to 90 per cent.[28] Both of these studies were performed with 1.3 to 1.5 tesla MR systems. It is known that the thin sections necessary for pituitary imaging may result in excessively noisy images, especially at lower field strengths.[29] Gd-DTPA augments the MR diagnosis, but CT will remain competitive until MR technology can achieve comparable spatial resolution. On the other hand, for suspected macroadenomas, MR has proven superior to CT for assessment of involvement of perisellar structures.[28, 30, 31]

Along with the function of MR as a primary imaging procedure, there are indications for MR as a secondary procedure after the pathology has already been demonstrated by CT. As mentioned above, since MR nicely delineates the extent of sellar and perisellar lesions, it can often add useful information in these cases. If the diagnosis of a vascular malformation is suggested by CT, MR may show evidence of flow voids, subacute or chronic hemorrhage, and hemosiderin deposition to further support the diagnosis.[23, 32] This information becomes particularly important in cases in which the angiogram fails to demonstrate a cryptic or thrombosed vascular malformation or a cavernous angioma. In patients with solitary lesions by CT, in whom the diagnosis of metastatic disease or MS would be strengthened by the finding of additional lesions, MR may resolve the issue. Similarly, in a patient with brain metastases, in whom none of the lesions account for the patient's signs or symptoms, MR can help evaluate the particular anatomic area of interest. A potential problem in both of these circumstances is the nonspecificity of white matter hyperintensities, and contrast MR may be necessary to clarify the situation.

As a prelude to surgery or radiation therapy or to aid in prognosis, MR can be helpful to define the full extent of lesions. Although MR is hampered by difficulties in identifying tumor-edema boundaries, some radiation therapists will treat the full extent of abnormal signal, knowing that edema is a potential site of microscopic tumor infiltration.[33, 34]

The role of MR in acute head trauma remains limited by problems with identification of acute hemorrhage, fractures, and displaced bone fragments, as well as the inherent problems of imaging acutely ill, uncooperative patients. In subacute trauma, however, MR can help when there is discordance between clinical and CT findings. MR is more sensitive than CT for nonhemorrhagic deep white matter shear injuries that may have important prognostic implications.[35] The full extent of subacute extracerebral collections is also well demonstrated by MR, even when these collections are isointense by CT.[36] The multiplanar capability of MR is of great help in this setting.

IMAGING TECHNIQUES

MR imaging of the brain has evolved to a point where standard protocols can be set to handle most clinical situations (see Appendix I). Nonetheless, protocols need to be modified in special cases and as software upgrades and new imaging capabilities are added to MR systems. In order to properly select a technique, an understanding of the interrelationships of the imaging parameters is required. Signal-to-noise (S/N) and spatial resolution must be balanced against scan time, and compromises must often be made. In addition to the standard parameters, multiple options are available for motion and artifact reduction, and one must know when to use them and be aware of how they limit other parameters. Gradient-echo techniques allow for fast scanning and flow imaging. Finally, decisions must be made about the use of Gd-DTPA, a contrast agent for MR. The principles of MR contrast, pulse sequence design, fast scanning, MR artifacts, and paramagnetic enhancement are covered in detail in Part I of this textbook. The following overview is intended to guide the physician with MR scanning techniques.

The scan parameters include repetition time (TR), echo time (TE), matrix size, field-of-view (FOV), slice thickness, and number of excitations (NEX). The TR and TE are the only parameters that affect the T_1 and T_2 weighting of the image. A long TR and long TE (TR > 1500 msec, TE > 60 msec) provides T_2 weighting, whereas a short TR and short TE (TR < 1000 msec, TE < 30 msec) results in T_1-weighted images. The T_2-weighted sequence is usually employed as a dual-echo sequence. The first or shorter echo (TE < 30 msec) is proton density weighted or a mixture of T_1 and T_2. In the literature the proton density–weighted image is also referred to as mixed T_1/T_2 weighted, the balanced image, or simply as the first echo image. This image is very helpful for evaluating periventricular pathology, such as multiple sclerosis, because the hyperintense plaques are contrasted against the lower signal cerebrospinal fluid (CSF).

The TR, matrix size, and NEX are the only parameters that affect scan time. Increasing any one of these parameters increases the minimum scan time. Spatial resolution is determined by matrix size, FOV, and slice thickness. Increasing matrix size or decreasing FOV and slice thickness increases spatial resolution but at the expense of either decreased S/N or increased scan time. To obtain images of high resolution with a high S/N ratio requires longer scan times. All of the scan parameters affect S/N. The signal within an image can be improved by increasing TR, FOV, slice thickness, and NEX or by decreasing TE and matrix size. The most direct way to increase signal is by increasing NEX, but one must keep in mind that increasing NEX from two to four, for example, doubles the scan time but increases the signal by only the square root of two.[37, 38] Finally, TE does not affect scan time; however, it does determine the maximal number of slices in multislice mode. Increasing the TE or shortening TR decreases the number of slices that can be obtained with one pulse sequence.

Since studies have shown that T_2-weighted images are most sensitive for detecting brain pathology, patients with suspected intracranial disease should be screened with a T_2-weighted spin-echo sequence (TR 3000 msec, TE 30/80 msec). The axial plane is commonly used because of our familiarity with the anatomy from CT. As outlined in Appendix I, the other scan parameters include a 192 x 192 matrix, 1 NEX, 20-cm FOV, and 5-mm slice thickness for a scan time of 10.5 minutes and a voxel size of 5 x 1.04 x 1.04 mm. A 2.5-mm interslice gap prevents radiofrequency (RF) interference between slices.[39]

If an abnormality is found, additional scans help characterize the lesion. Noncontrast T_1-weighted images are needed only if the preliminary scans suggest hemorrhage, lipoma, or dermoid. Otherwise, contrast-enhanced scans are recommended. Gadopentetate dimeglumine or Gd-DTPA, a paramagnetic contrast agent for brain imaging, has demonstrated excellent biologic tolerance. No significant complications or side effects have been reported. It is injected intravenously at a dose rate of 0.1 mmol/kg. Gd-DTPA does not cross the intact blood-brain barrier (BBB). If the BBB is disrupted by a disease process, the contrast agent diffuses into the interstitial space and shortens the T_1 relaxation time of the tissue, resulting in increased signal intensity on T_1-weighted images.[40] The scans should be acquired between 3 and 30 minutes postinjection for optimal results.

Contrast enhancement is especially helpful for extraaxial tumors because they tend to be isointense to brain on plain scans, but it also identifies areas of BBB breakdown associated with intraaxial lesions. Gd-DTPA is essential for detecting leptomeningeal inflammatory and neoplastic processes. Contrast scans are obtained routinely in patients with symptoms of pituitary adenoma (elevated prolactin, growth hormone, and so forth) or acoustic neuroma (sensorineural hearing loss). To screen for brain metastases in patients with a known primary, contrast-enhanced T_1-weighted scans alone are probably sufficient.[41]

Gd-DTPA does not enhance rapidly flowing blood. If vascular structures are not adequately seen on plain scan, the positive contrast provided by gradient-echo techniques may be helpful to confirm or disprove a suspected carotid occlusion or cerebral aneurysm, to evaluate the integrity of the venous sinuses, and to assess the vascularity of lesions. Gradient-echo imaging also enhances the magnetic susceptibility effects of acute and chronic hemorrhage, making them easily observable, even on low and mid-field MR systems. Finally, using lower flip angles, gradient-echo sequences are an efficient method for obtaining a few T_2-weighted images of a focal area.

Although the axial plane is the primary plane for imaging the brain, the multiplanar capability of MR allows one to select the optimal plane to visualize the anatomy of interest. Coronal views are good for parasagittal lesions near the vertex and lesions immediately above or below the lateral ventricles (corpus callosum or thalamus), temporal lobes, sella, and internal auditory canals. The coronal plane can be used as the primary plane of imaging in patients with temporal lobe seizures. Sagittal views are useful for midline lesions (sella, third ventricle, corpus callosum, pineal region) and those of the brain stem and cerebellar vermis.[39]

As outlined in the protocols, scan techniques are slightly different for the sella and cerebellopontine angle. For the sella, the plain and contrast-enhanced scans are obtained in the coronal and sagittal planes using a smaller FOV and thin (3 mm or less) contiguous or overlapping sections. For patients with a sensorineural hearing loss or suspected acoustic neuroma, contrast-enhanced scans with T_1 weighting are obtained through the internal auditory canals, again using thin overlapping sections.

Specialized techniques for reducing motion and artifacts on the images also have applications for brain imaging. Gradient motion rephasing or flow compensation techniques effectively reduce ghost artifacts resulting from CSF flow. They should be used for T_2-weighted spin-echo and gradient-echo acquisitions, but not with T_1-weighted imaging because they increase the signal from CSF. Flow compensation techniques do not contribute to SAR (a measure of power deposition), but the extra gradient pulses lengthen the minimum TE, and gradient heating may limit the number of slices, the minimum FOV, and the slice thickness.[42] Cardiac gating also reduces artifacts from CSF pulsations, resulting in superior object contrast and resolving power in the temporal lobes, basal ganglia, and brain stem.[43]

Saturation (SAT) techniques use extra RF pulses to eliminate artifacts from moving tissues outside the imaging volume, such as from swallowing or respiratory motion, and from unsaturated protons that enter the imaging volume through vascular channels.[44] SAT should be used for T_1-weighted imaging of the sella and internal auditory canals. The extra RF pulses cost SAR and take time, lengthening the minimum TR or decreasing the maximum number of slices in a multislice mode.

Methods for eliminating wraparound or aliasing should be prescribed when imaging small anatomic areas, such as the sella and internal auditory canals, with smaller FOVs. The "no phase wrap" option is most effective in the anteroposterior direction for sagittal and axial scans.[39]

MR imaging represents a major advance in the delineation of anatomy and pathologic processes affecting the central nervous system. MR possesses significant advantages over CT: (1) the ability to image directly in multiple planes without sacrificing spatial resolution due to the reformation process, (2) visualization of vascular structures without the need for injection of potentially hazardous iodinated contrast agents, and (3) no ionizing radiation. Additionally, by employing various pulse sequences, MR can provide soft tissue characterization not readily obtainable by CT. These attributes create new interpretative challenges, especially considering changes in image appearance caused by the selection of a given pulse sequence. Therefore, an MR atlas considered useful for clinical practice must take into account this variability. However, as MR has matured there has been a proliferation of pulse sequences, some of which have yielded dramatic changes in image appearance. As a consequence, an atlas of practical size must, of necessity, represent a compromise. Therefore, the authors have chosen to illustrate brain anatomy using both T_1- and T_2-weighted pulse sequences in the most commonly employed axial planar orientation. The axial T_1 and T_2 images were matched as closely as possible with respect to anatomic location and are positioned on opposing pages. Complementary sagittal and coronal image series of the brain are also displayed using a T_1-weighted pulse sequence.

The brain images were obtained using a 1.5 tesla MR scanner (Signa, General Electric Company, Milwaukee, WI). Pulse sequences and other pertinent scan parameters were as follows:

1. *Axial T_1 scan:* TR 800 msec; TE 20 msec; 5 mm interleaved sections; 2 excitations; 256 × 256 acquisition matrix.

2. *Axial T_2 scan:* TR 2000 msec; TE 80 msec; 5 mm interleaved sections; 2 excitations; 256 × 256 acquisition matrix.

3. *Sagittal T_1 scan:* TR 800 msec; TE 20 msec; 5 mm interleaved sections; 1 excitation; 256 × 256 acquisition matrix.

4. *Coronal T_1 scan:* Same parameters as for sagittal T_1 scan.

MR Atlas
of the
Normal Brain

T₁ AXIAL

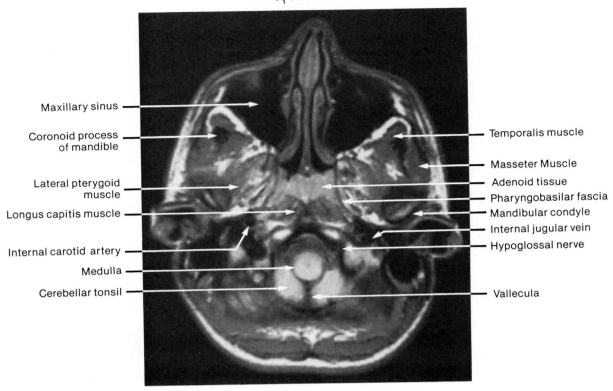

Maxillary sinus

Coronoid process
of mandible

Lateral pterygoid
muscle

Longus capitis muscle

Internal carotid artery

Medulla

Cerebellar tonsil

Temporalis muscle

Masseter Muscle

Adenoid tissue

Pharyngobasilar fascia

Mandibular condyle

Internal jugular vein

Hypoglossal nerve

Vallecula

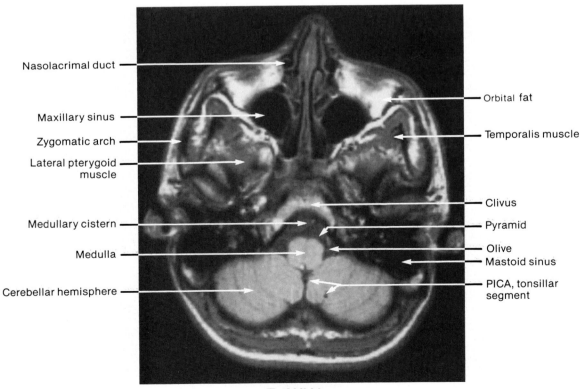

Nasolacrimal duct

Maxillary sinus

Zygomatic arch

Lateral pterygoid
muscle

Medullary cistern

Medulla

Cerebellar hemisphere

Orbital fat

Temporalis muscle

Clivus

Pyramid

Olive

Mastoid sinus

PICA, tonsillar
segment

T₁ AXIAL

T₂ AXIAL

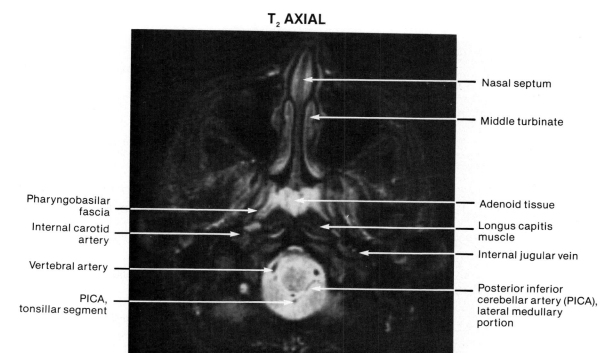

Nasal septum

Middle turbinate

Pharyngobasilar fascia

Adenoid tissue

Internal carotid artery

Longus capitis muscle

Internal jugular vein

Vertebral artery

PICA, tonsillar segment

Posterior inferior cerebellar artery (PICA), lateral medullary portion

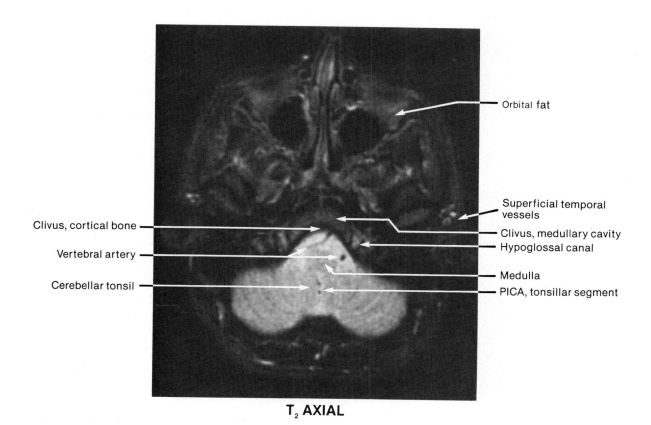

Orbital fat

Superficial temporal vessels

Clivus, cortical bone

Clivus, medullary cavity

Vertebral artery

Hypoglossal canal

Cerebellar tonsil

Medulla

PICA, tonsillar segment

T₂ AXIAL

T₁ AXIAL

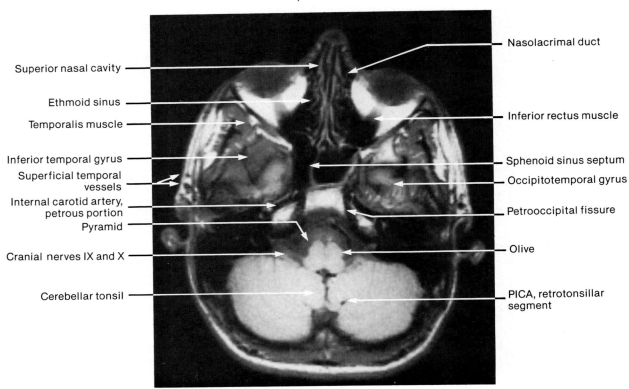

Superior nasal cavity

Ethmoid sinus

Temporalis muscle

Inferior temporal gyrus

Superficial temporal vessels

Internal carotid artery, petrous portion

Pyramid

Cranial nerves IX and X

Cerebellar tonsil

Nasolacrimal duct

Inferior rectus muscle

Sphenoid sinus septum

Occipitotemporal gyrus

Petrooccipital fissure

Olive

PICA, retrotonsillar segment

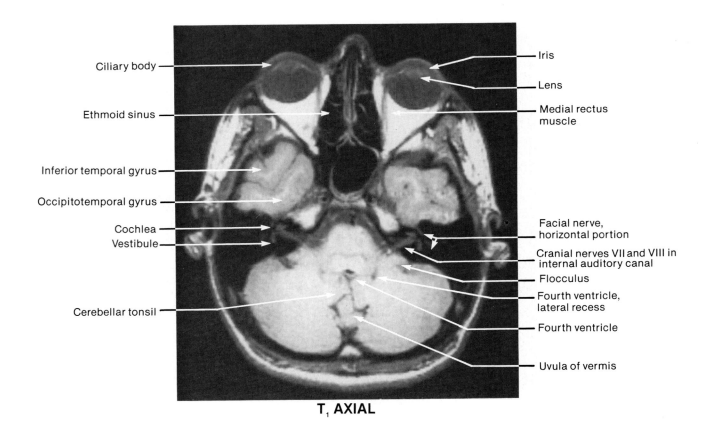

Ciliary body

Ethmoid sinus

Inferior temporal gyrus

Occipitotemporal gyrus

Cochlea

Vestibule

Cerebellar tonsil

Iris

Lens

Medial rectus muscle

Facial nerve, horizontal portion

Cranial nerves VII and VIII in internal auditory canal

Flocculus

Fourth ventricle, lateral recess

Fourth ventricle

Uvula of vermis

T₁ AXIAL

T$_2$ AXIAL

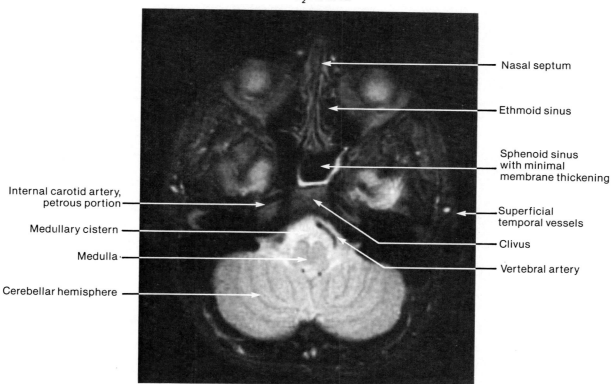

Nasal septum

Ethmoid sinus

Sphenoid sinus with minimal membrane thickening

Internal carotid artery, petrous portion

Superficial temporal vessels

Medullary cistern

Clivus

Medulla

Vertebral artery

Cerebellar hemisphere

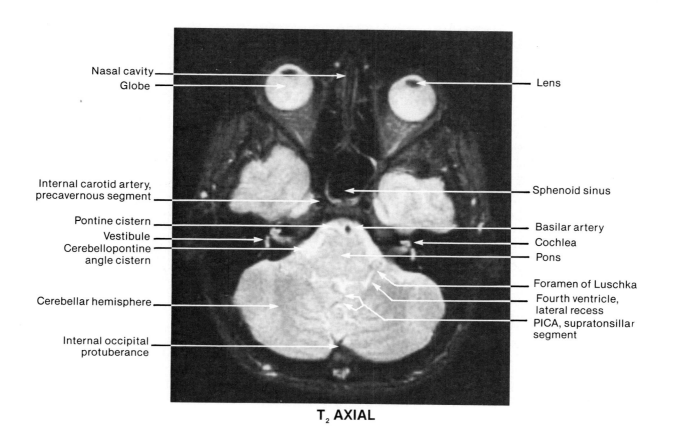

Nasal cavity

Globe

Lens

Internal carotid artery, precavernous segment

Sphenoid sinus

Pontine cistern

Basilar artery

Vestibule

Cochlea

Cerebellopontine angle cistern

Pons

Foramen of Luschka

Cerebellar hemisphere

Fourth ventricle, lateral recess

PICA, supratonsillar segment

Internal occipital protuberance

T$_2$ AXIAL

T₁ AXIAL

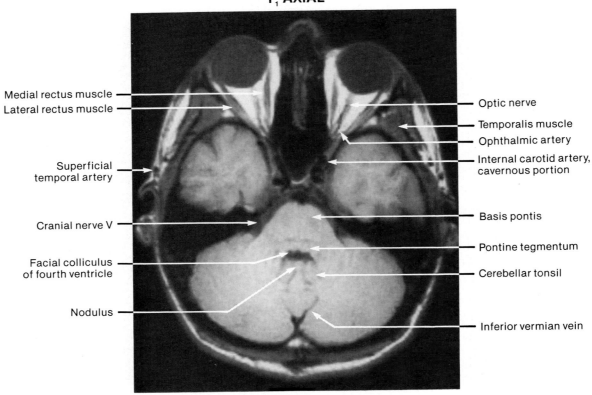

Medial rectus muscle

Lateral rectus muscle

Superficial
temporal artery

Cranial nerve V

Facial colliculus
of fourth ventricle

Nodulus

Optic nerve

Temporalis muscle

Ophthalmic artery

Internal carotid artery,
cavernous portion

Basis pontis

Pontine tegmentum

Cerebellar tonsil

Inferior vermian vein

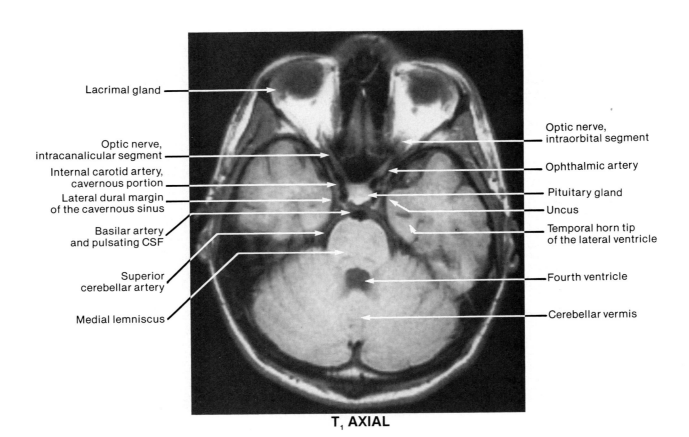

Lacrimal gland

Optic nerve,
intracanalicular segment

Internal carotid artery,
cavernous portion

Lateral dural margin
of the cavernous sinus

Basilar artery
and pulsating CSF

Superior
cerebellar artery

Medial lemniscus

Optic nerve,
intraorbital segment

Ophthalmic artery

Pituitary gland

Uncus

Temporal horn tip
of the lateral ventricle

Fourth ventricle

Cerebellar vermis

T₁ AXIAL

T$_2$ AXIAL

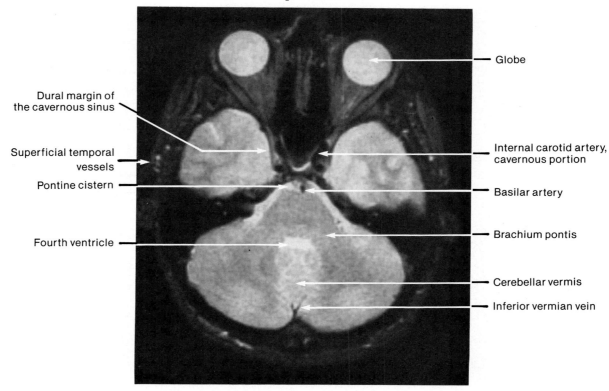

Globe

Dural margin of
the cavernous sinus

Superficial temporal
vessels

Pontine cistern

Fourth ventricle

Internal carotid artery,
cavernous portion

Basilar artery

Brachium pontis

Cerebellar vermis

Inferior vermian vein

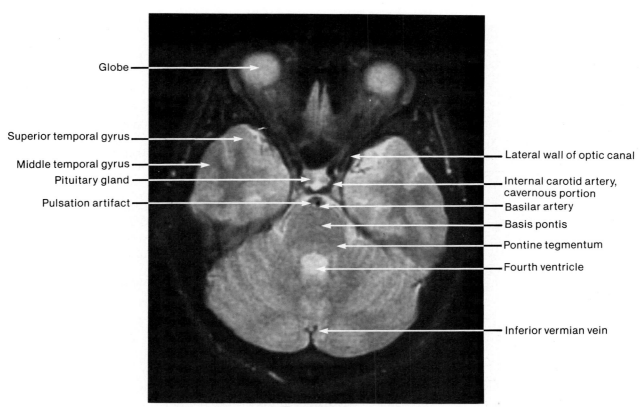

Globe

Superior temporal gyrus

Middle temporal gyrus

Pituitary gland

Pulsation artifact

Lateral wall of optic canal

Internal carotid artery,
cavernous portion

Basilar artery

Basis pontis

Pontine tegmentum

Fourth ventricle

Inferior vermian vein

T$_2$ AXIAL

T₁ AXIAL

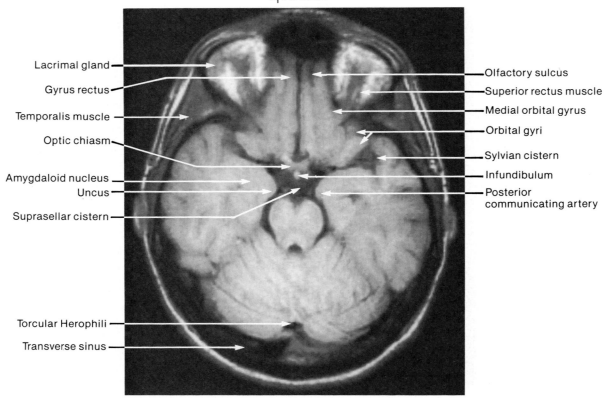

Lacrimal gland
Gyrus rectus
Temporalis muscle
Optic chiasm
Amygdaloid nucleus
Uncus
Suprasellar cistern
Torcular Herophili
Transverse sinus

Olfactory sulcus
Superior rectus muscle
Medial orbital gyrus
Orbital gyri
Sylvian cistern
Infundibulum
Posterior communicating artery

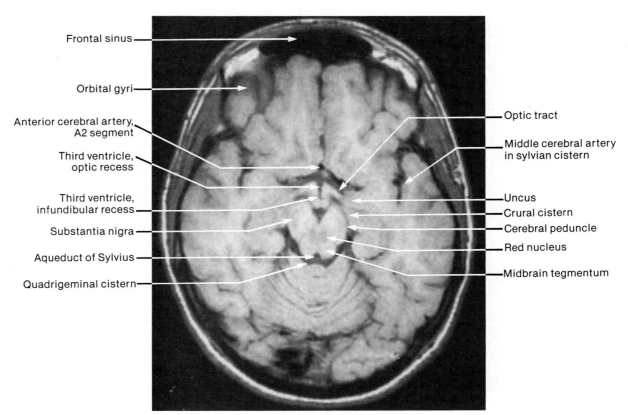

Frontal sinus
Orbital gyri
Anterior cerebral artery, A2 segment
Third ventricle, optic recess
Third ventricle, infundibular recess
Substantia nigra
Aqueduct of Sylvius
Quadrigeminal cistern

Optic tract
Middle cerebral artery in sylvian cistern
Uncus
Crural cistern
Cerebral peduncle
Red nucleus
Midbrain tegmentum

T₁ AXIAL

T$_2$ AXIAL

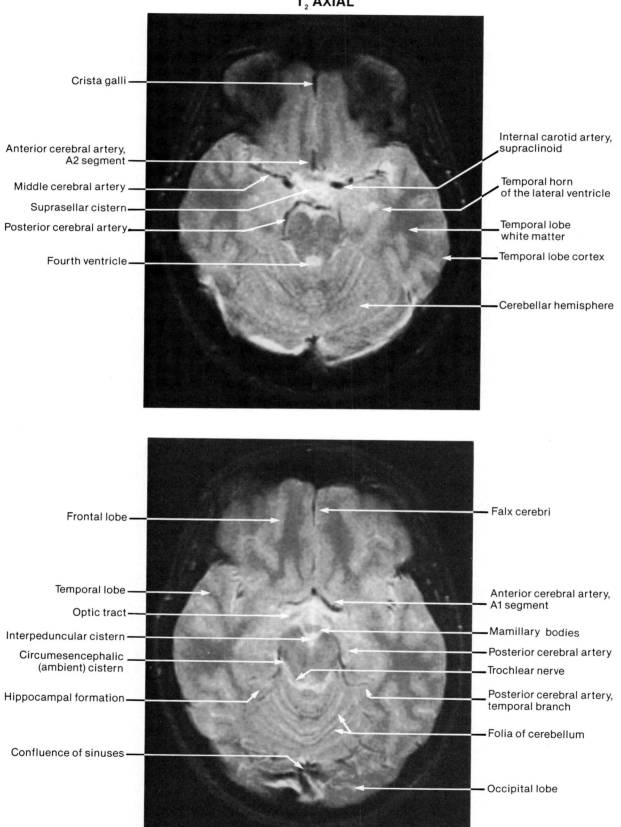

Crista galli

Anterior cerebral artery,
A2 segment

Middle cerebral artery

Suprasellar cistern

Posterior cerebral artery

Fourth ventricle

Internal carotid artery,
supraclinoid

Temporal horn
of the lateral ventricle

Temporal lobe
white matter

Temporal lobe cortex

Cerebellar hemisphere

Frontal lobe

Temporal lobe

Optic tract

Interpeduncular cistern

Circumesencephalic
(ambient) cistern

Hippocampal formation

Confluence of sinuses

Falx cerebri

Anterior cerebral artery,
A1 segment

Mamillary bodies

Posterior cerebral artery

Trochlear nerve

Posterior cerebral artery,
temporal branch

Folia of cerebellum

Occipital lobe

T$_2$ AXIAL

T₁ AXIAL

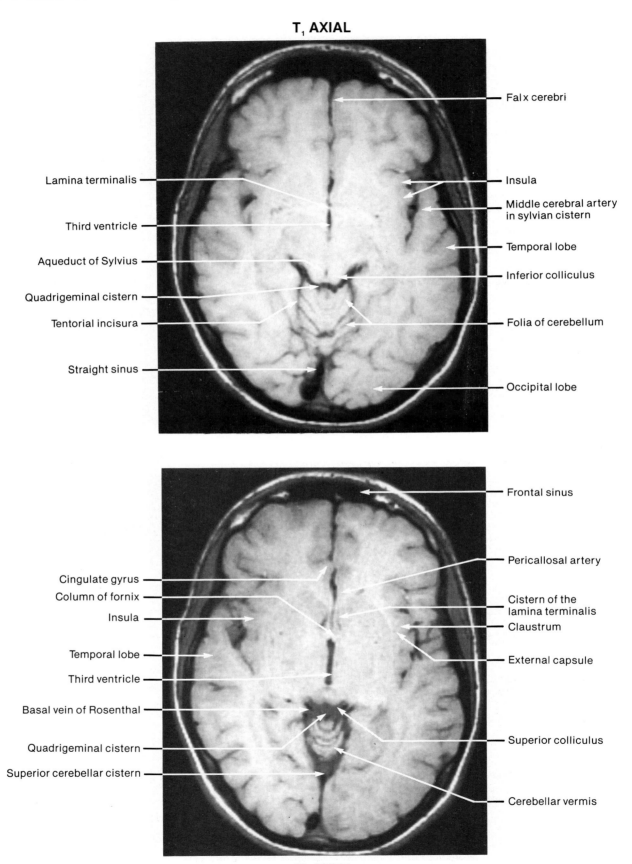

Falx cerebri

Lamina terminalis

Insula

Middle cerebral artery in sylvian cistern

Third ventricle

Aqueduct of Sylvius

Temporal lobe

Quadrigeminal cistern

Inferior colliculus

Tentorial incisura

Folia of cerebellum

Straight sinus

Occipital lobe

Frontal sinus

Cingulate gyrus

Pericallosal artery

Column of fornix

Insula

Cistern of the lamina terminalis

Claustrum

Temporal lobe

External capsule

Third ventricle

Basal vein of Rosenthal

Superior colliculus

Quadrigeminal cistern

Superior cerebellar cistern

Cerebellar vermis

T₁ AXIAL

T₂ AXIAL

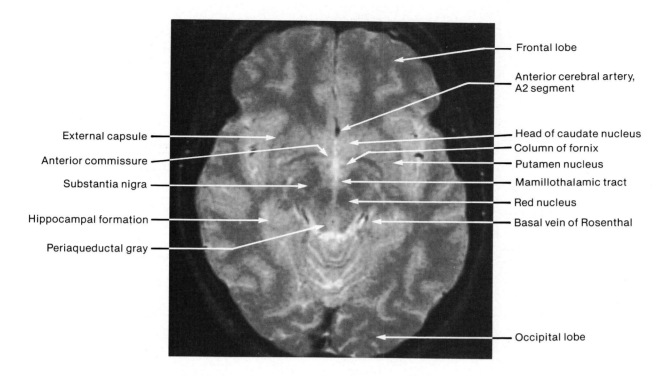

External capsule

Anterior commissure

Substantia nigra

Hippocampal formation

Periaqueductal gray

Frontal lobe

Anterior cerebral artery, A2 segment

Head of caudate nucleus

Column of fornix

Putamen nucleus

Mamillothalamic tract

Red nucleus

Basal vein of Rosenthal

Occipital lobe

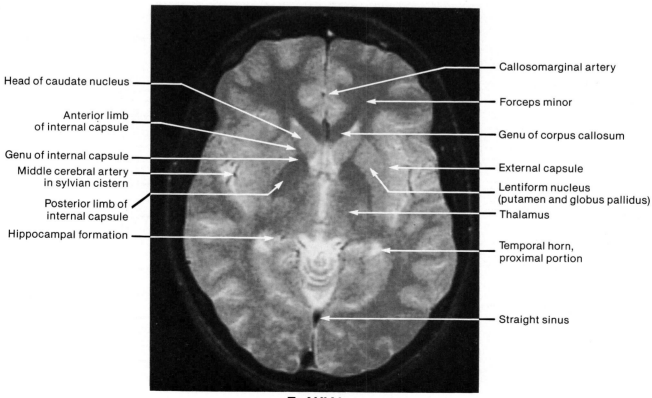

Head of caudate nucleus

Anterior limb of internal capsule

Genu of internal capsule

Middle cerebral artery in sylvian cistern

Posterior limb of internal capsule

Hippocampal formation

Callosomarginal artery

Forceps minor

Genu of corpus callosum

External capsule

Lentiform nucleus (putamen and globus pallidus)

Thalamus

Temporal horn, proximal portion

Straight sinus

T₂ AXIAL

T₁ AXIAL

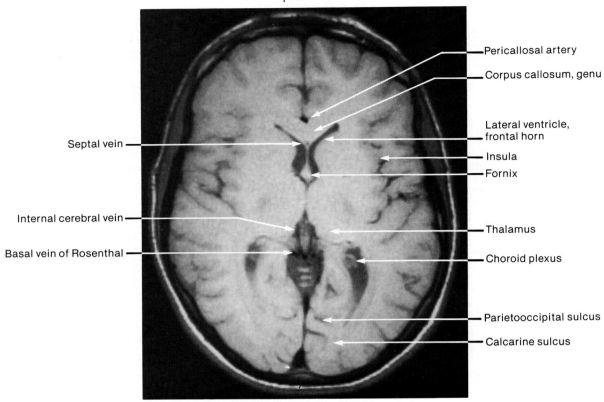

Pericallosal artery

Corpus callosum, genu

Lateral ventricle, frontal horn

Insula

Fornix

Thalamus

Choroid plexus

Parietooccipital sulcus

Calcarine sulcus

Septal vein

Internal cerebral vein

Basal vein of Rosenthal

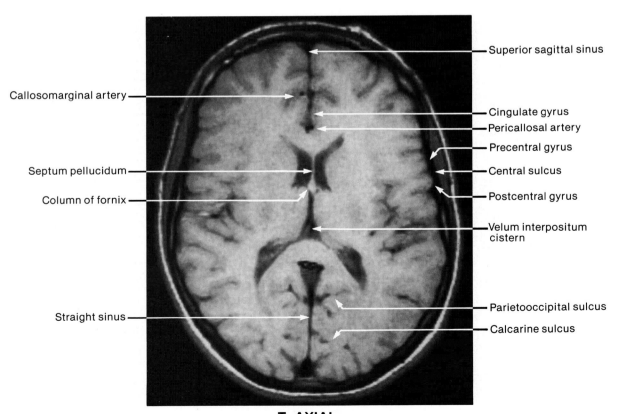

Callosomarginal artery

Septum pellucidum

Column of fornix

Straight sinus

Superior sagittal sinus

Cingulate gyrus

Pericallosal artery

Precentral gyrus

Central sulcus

Postcentral gyrus

Velum interpositum cistern

Parietooccipital sulcus

Calcarine sulcus

T₁ AXIAL

T₂ AXIAL

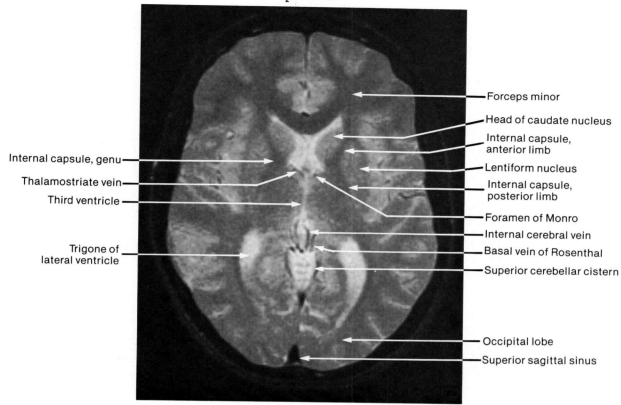

Internal capsule, genu —

Thalamostriate vein —

Third ventricle —

Trigone of
lateral ventricle —

— Forceps minor

— Head of caudate nucleus

— Internal capsule,
anterior limb

— Lentiform nucleus

— Internal capsule,
posterior limb

— Foramen of Monro

— Internal cerebral vein

— Basal vein of Rosenthal

— Superior cerebellar cistern

— Occipital lobe

— Superior sagittal sinus

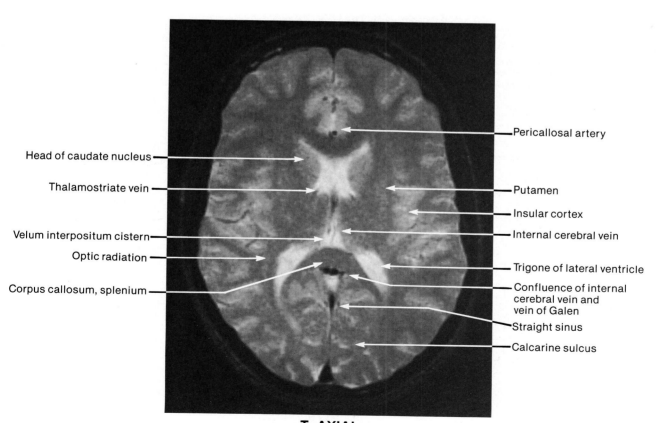

Head of caudate nucleus —

Thalamostriate vein —

Velum interpositum cistern —

Optic radiation —

Corpus callosum, splenium —

— Pericallosal artery

— Putamen

— Insular cortex

— Internal cerebral vein

— Trigone of lateral ventricle

— Confluence of internal
cerebral vein and
vein of Galen

— Straight sinus

— Calcarine sulcus

T₂ AXIAL

T₁ AXIAL

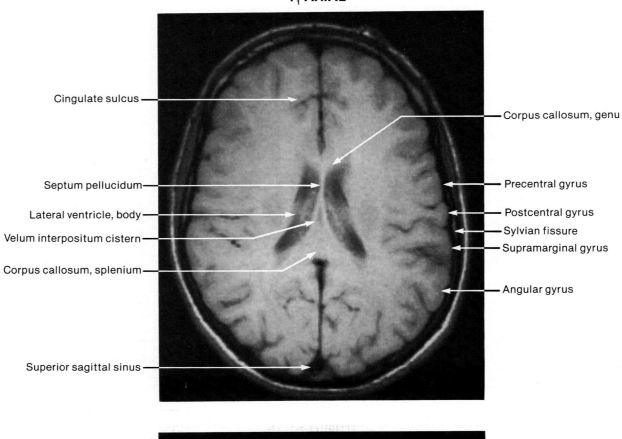

Cingulate sulcus

Corpus callosum, genu

Septum pellucidum

Precentral gyrus

Lateral ventricle, body

Postcentral gyrus

Velum interpositum cistern

Sylvian fissure

Supramarginal gyrus

Corpus callosum, splenium

Angular gyrus

Superior sagittal sinus

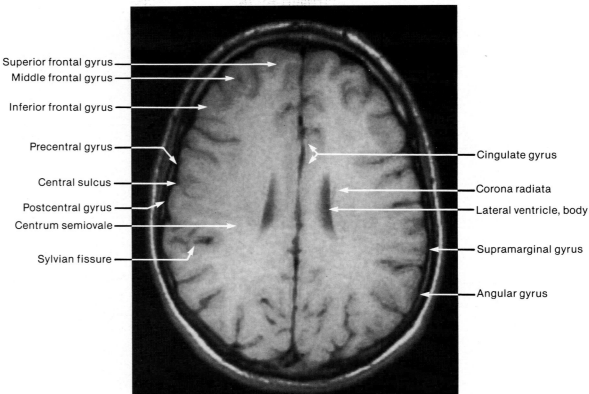

Superior frontal gyrus

Middle frontal gyrus

Inferior frontal gyrus

Precentral gyrus

Cingulate gyrus

Central sulcus

Corona radiata

Postcentral gyrus

Lateral ventricle, body

Centrum semiovale

Supramarginal gyrus

Sylvian fissure

Angular gyrus

T₁ AXIAL

T₂ AXIAL

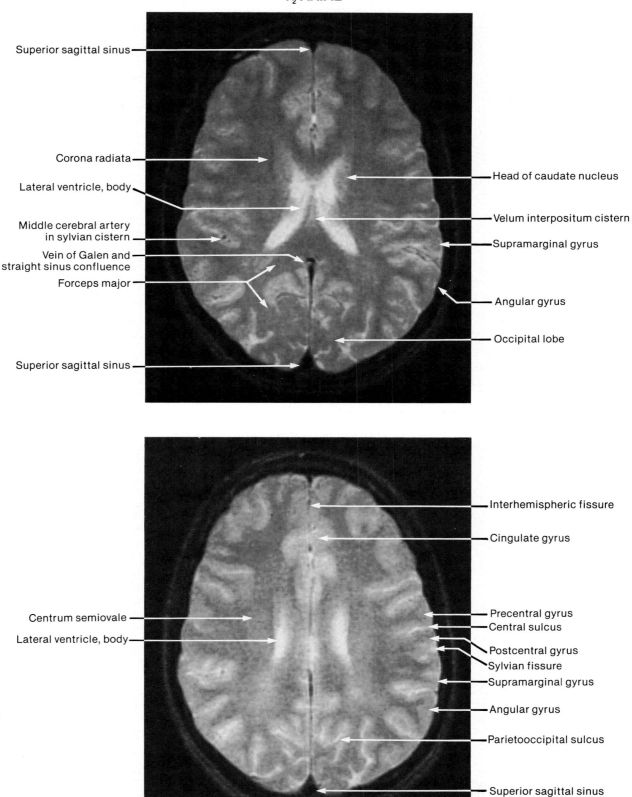

Superior sagittal sinus

Corona radiata

Lateral ventricle, body

Middle cerebral artery in sylvian cistern

Vein of Galen and straight sinus confluence

Forceps major

Superior sagittal sinus

Head of caudate nucleus

Velum interpositum cistern

Supramarginal gyrus

Angular gyrus

Occipital lobe

Interhemispheric fissure

Cingulate gyrus

Centrum semiovale

Lateral ventricle, body

Precentral gyrus

Central sulcus

Postcentral gyrus

Sylvian fissure

Supramarginal gyrus

Angular gyrus

Parietooccipital sulcus

Superior sagittal sinus

T₂ AXIAL

T₁ AXIAL

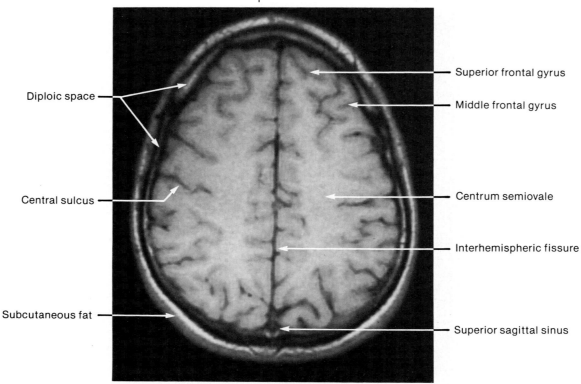

Diploic space

Central sulcus

Subcutaneous fat

Superior frontal gyrus

Middle frontal gyrus

Centrum semiovale

Interhemispheric fissure

Superior sagittal sinus

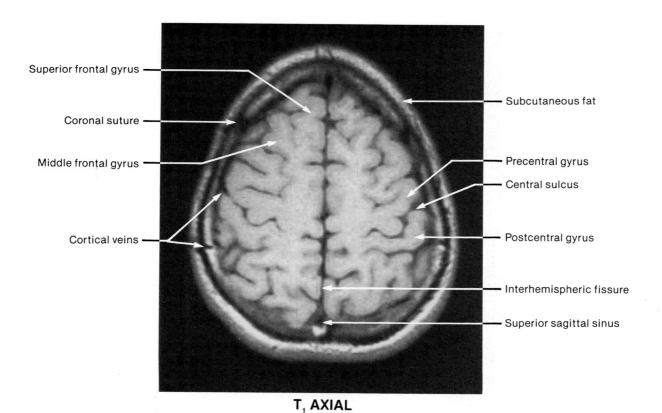

Superior frontal gyrus

Coronal suture

Middle frontal gyrus

Cortical veins

Subcutaneous fat

Precentral gyrus

Central sulcus

Postcentral gyrus

Interhemispheric fissure

Superior sagittal sinus

T₁ AXIAL

T₂ AXIAL

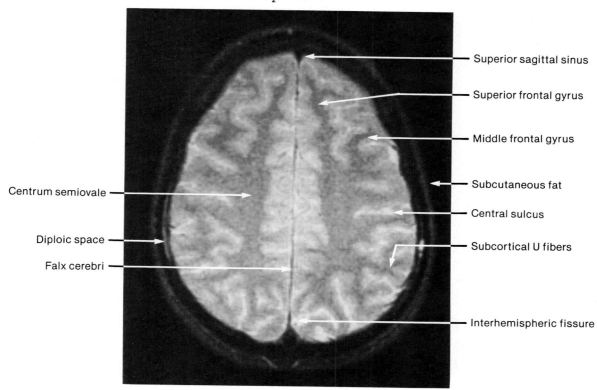

Superior sagittal sinus

Superior frontal gyrus

Middle frontal gyrus

Subcutaneous fat

Central sulcus

Subcortical U fibers

Interhemispheric fissure

Centrum semiovale

Diploic space

Falx cerebri

Superior frontal gyrus

Middle frontal gyrus

Subcortical U fibers

Cortical veins

Falx cerebri

Subcutaneous fat

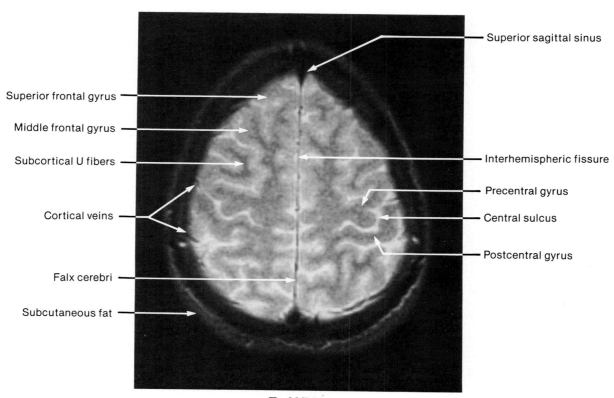

Superior sagittal sinus

Interhemispheric fissure

Precentral gyrus

Central sulcus

Postcentral gyrus

T₂ AXIAL

T₁ CORONAL

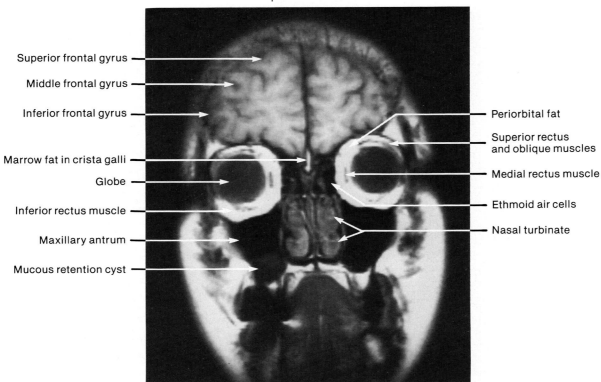

Superior frontal gyrus

Middle frontal gyrus

Inferior frontal gyrus

Marrow fat in crista galli

Globe

Inferior rectus muscle

Maxillary antrum

Mucous retention cyst

Periorbital fat

Superior rectus and oblique muscles

Medial rectus muscle

Ethmoid air cells

Nasal turbinate

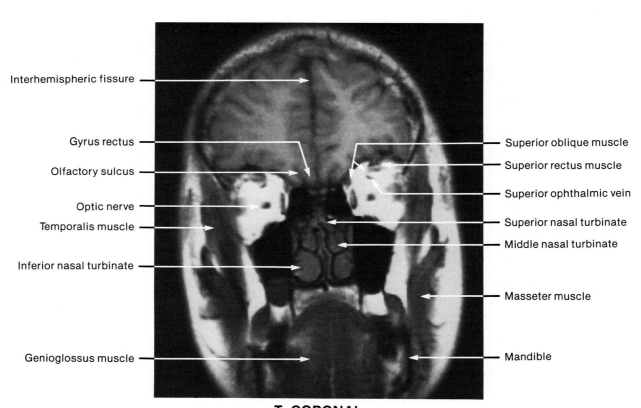

Interhemispheric fissure

Gyrus rectus

Olfactory sulcus

Optic nerve

Temporalis muscle

Inferior nasal turbinate

Genioglossus muscle

Superior oblique muscle

Superior rectus muscle

Superior ophthalmic vein

Superior nasal turbinate

Middle nasal turbinate

Masseter muscle

Mandible

T₁ CORONAL

T₁ CORONAL

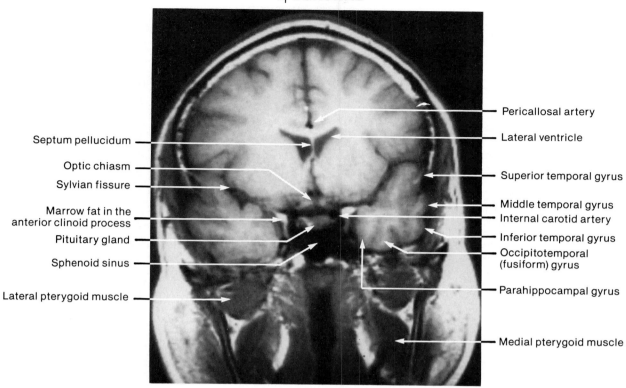

Septum pellucidum —

Optic chiasm —

Sylvian fissure —

Marrow fat in the anterior clinoid process —

Pituitary gland —

Sphenoid sinus —

Lateral pterygoid muscle —

— Pericallosal artery

— Lateral ventricle

— Superior temporal gyrus

— Middle temporal gyrus
— Internal carotid artery

— Inferior temporal gyrus

— Occipitotemporal (fusiform) gyrus

— Parahippocampal gyrus

— Medial pterygoid muscle

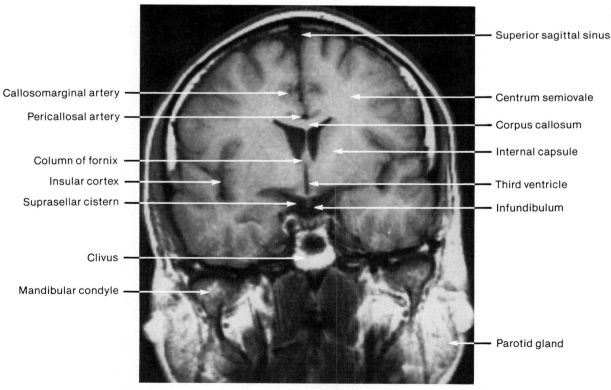

Callosomarginal artery —

Pericallosal artery —

Column of fornix —

Insular cortex —

Suprasellar cistern —

Clivus —

Mandibular condyle —

— Superior sagittal sinus

— Centrum semiovale

— Corpus callosum

— Internal capsule

— Third ventricle

— Infundibulum

— Parotid gland

T₁ CORONAL

T₁ CORONAL

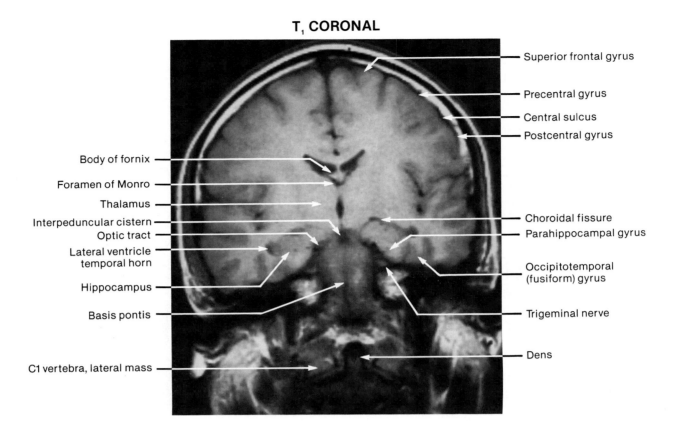

Superior frontal gyrus

Precentral gyrus

Central sulcus

Postcentral gyrus

Body of fornix

Foramen of Monro

Thalamus

Interpeduncular cistern

Optic tract

Lateral ventricle temporal horn

Hippocampus

Basis pontis

Choroidal fissure

Parahippocampal gyrus

Occipitotemporal (fusiform) gyrus

Trigeminal nerve

Dens

C1 vertebra, lateral mass

T₁ CORONAL

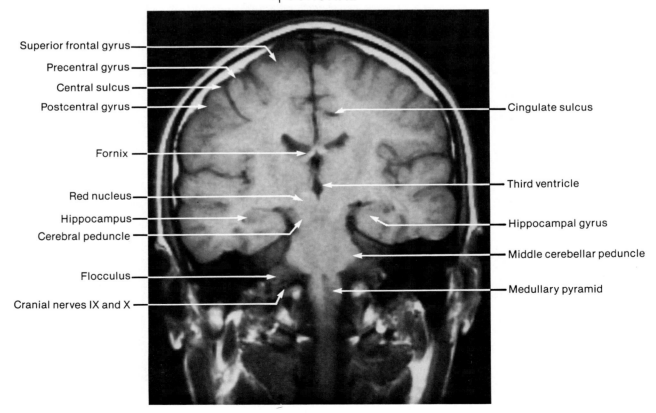

Superior frontal gyrus

Precentral gyrus

Central sulcus

Postcentral gyrus

Fornix

Red nucleus

Hippocampus

Cerebral peduncle

Flocculus

Cranial nerves IX and X

Cingulate sulcus

Third ventricle

Hippocampal gyrus

Middle cerebellar peduncle

Medullary pyramid

T₁ CORONAL

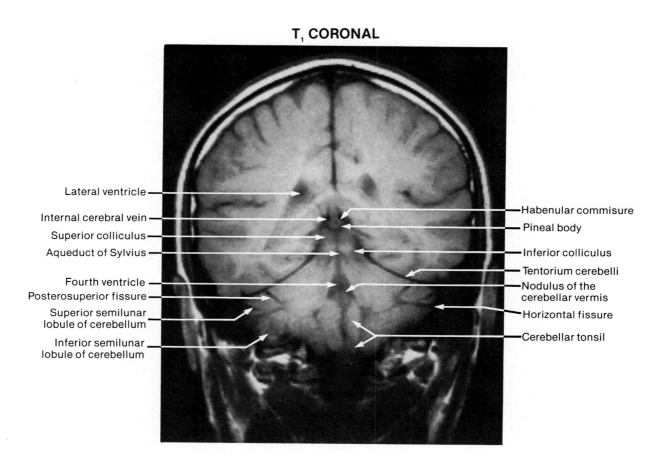

Lateral ventricle

Internal cerebral vein

Superior colliculus

Aqueduct of Sylvius

Fourth ventricle

Posterosuperior fissure

Superior semilunar
lobule of cerebellum

Inferior semilunar
lobule of cerebellum

Habenular commisure

Pineal body

Inferior colliculus

Tentorium cerebelli

Nodulus of the
cerebellar vermis

Horizontal fissure

Cerebellar tonsil

SAGITTAL T₁

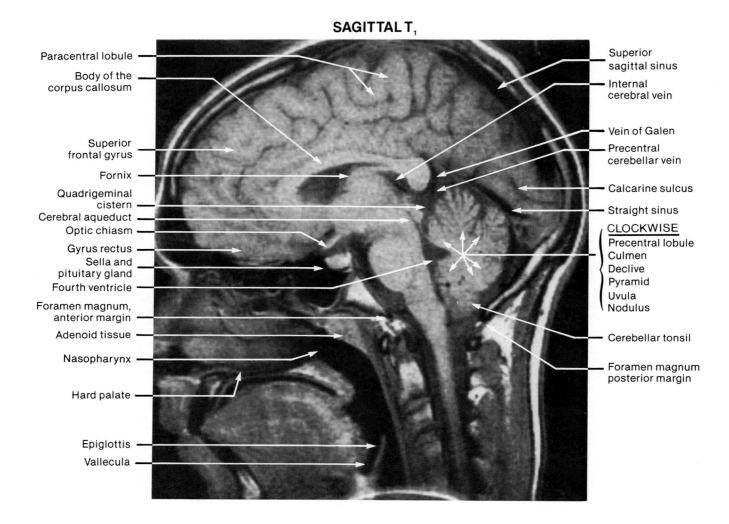

Paracentral lobule

Body of the
corpus callosum

Superior
frontal gyrus

Fornix

Quadrigeminal
cistern

Cerebral aqueduct

Optic chiasm

Gyrus rectus

Sella and
pituitary gland

Fourth ventricle

Foramen magnum,
anterior margin

Adenoid tissue

Nasopharynx

Hard palate

Epiglottis

Vallecula

Superior
sagittal sinus

Internal
cerebral vein

Vein of Galen

Precentral
cerebellar vein

Calcarine sulcus

Straight sinus

CLOCKWISE
Precentral lobule
Culmen
Declive
Pyramid
Uvula
Nodulus

Cerebellar tonsil

Foramen magnum
posterior margin

SAGITTAL T₁

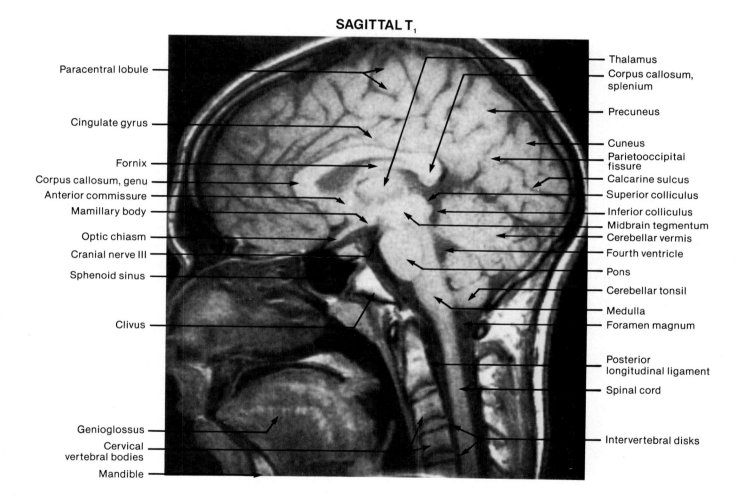

Paracentral lobule

Cingulate gyrus

Fornix

Corpus callosum, genu

Anterior commissure

Mamillary body

Optic chiasm

Cranial nerve III

Sphenoid sinus

Clivus

Genioglossus

Cervical vertebral bodies

Mandible

Thalamus

Corpus callosum, splenium

Precuneus

Cuneus

Parietooccipital fissure

Calcarine sulcus

Superior colliculus

Inferior colliculus

Midbrain tegmentum

Cerebellar vermis

Fourth ventricle

Pons

Cerebellar tonsil

Medulla

Foramen magnum

Posterior longitudinal ligament

Spinal cord

Intervertebral disks

SAGITTAL T$_1$

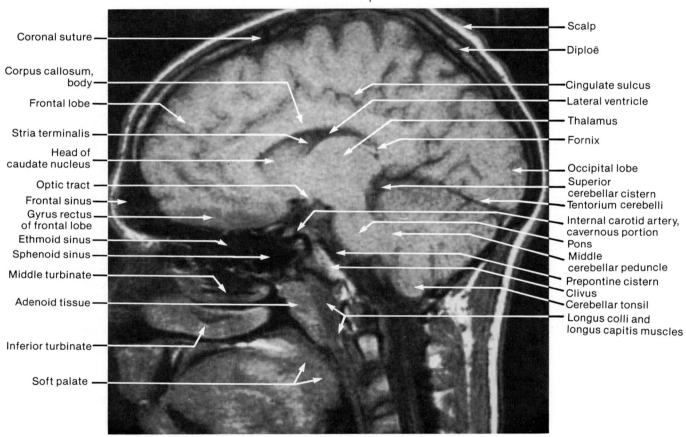

Coronal suture

Corpus callosum, body

Frontal lobe

Stria terminalis

Head of caudate nucleus

Optic tract

Frontal sinus

Gyrus rectus of frontal lobe

Ethmoid sinus

Sphenoid sinus

Middle turbinate

Adenoid tissue

Inferior turbinate

Soft palate

Scalp

Diploë

Cingulate sulcus

Lateral ventricle

Thalamus

Fornix

Occipital lobe

Superior cerebellar cistern

Tentorium cerebelli

Internal carotid artery, cavernous portion

Pons

Middle cerebellar peduncle

Prepontine cistern

Clivus

Cerebellar tonsil

Longus colli and longus capitis muscles

SAGITTAL T₁

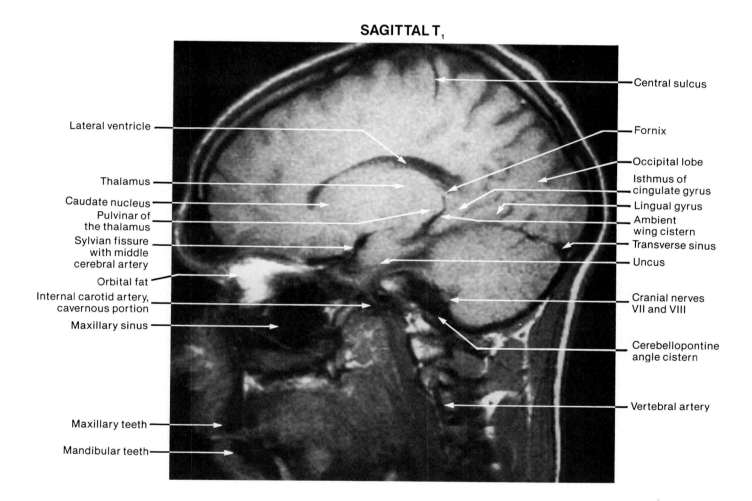

Lateral ventricle

Thalamus

Caudate nucleus

Pulvinar of the thalamus

Sylvian fissure with middle cerebral artery

Orbital fat

Internal carotid artery, cavernous portion

Maxillary sinus

Maxillary teeth

Mandibular teeth

Central sulcus

Fornix

Occipital lobe

Isthmus of cingulate gyrus

Lingual gyrus

Ambient wing cistern

Transverse sinus

Uncus

Cranial nerves VII and VIII

Cerebellopontine angle cistern

Vertebral artery

SAGITTAL T₁

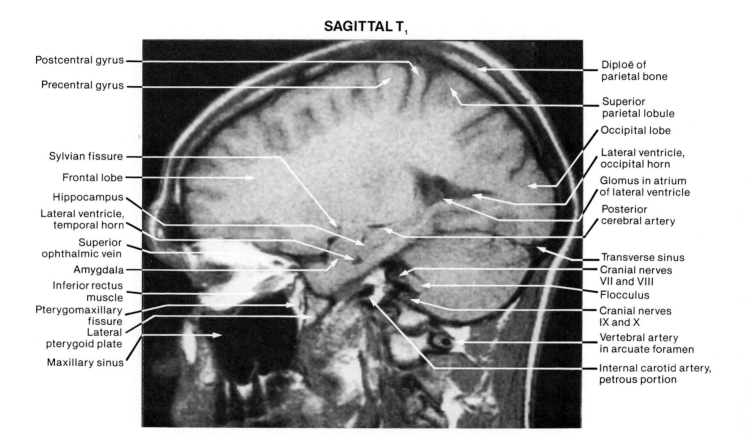

Postcentral gyrus

Precentral gyrus

Sylvian fissure

Frontal lobe

Hippocampus

Lateral ventricle, temporal horn

Superior ophthalmic vein

Amygdala

Inferior rectus muscle

Pterygomaxillary fissure

Lateral pterygoid plate

Maxillary sinus

Diploë of parietal bone

Superior parietal lobule

Occipital lobe

Lateral ventricle, occipital horn

Glomus in atrium of lateral ventricle

Posterior cerebral artery

Transverse sinus

Cranial nerves VII and VIII

Flocculus

Cranial nerves IX and X

Vertebral artery in arcuate foramen

Internal carotid artery, petrous portion

SAGITTAL T₁

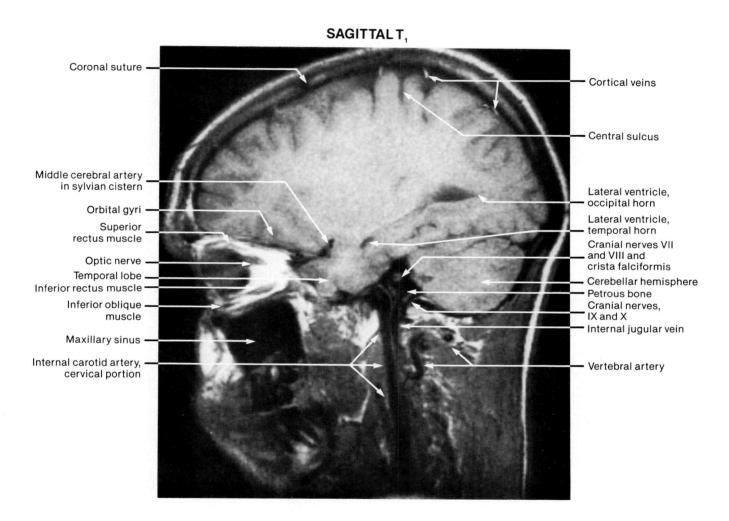

Coronal suture

Cortical veins

Central sulcus

Middle cerebral artery in sylvian cistern

Lateral ventricle, occipital horn

Orbital gyri

Lateral ventricle, temporal horn

Superior rectus muscle

Cranial nerves VII and VIII and crista falciformis

Optic nerve

Temporal lobe

Cerebellar hemisphere

Inferior rectus muscle

Petrous bone

Inferior oblique muscle

Cranial nerves, IX and X

Internal jugular vein

Maxillary sinus

Internal carotid artery, cervical portion

Vertebral artery

SAGITTAL T₁

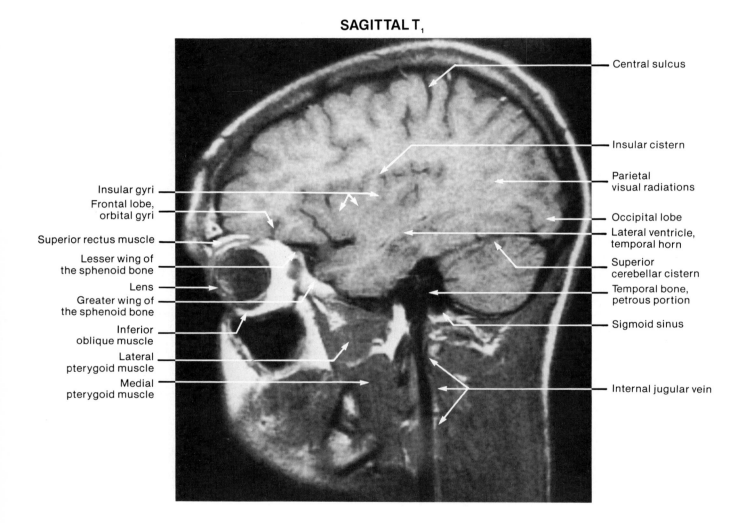

Central sulcus

Insular cistern

Parietal
visual radiations

Occipital lobe

Lateral ventricle,
temporal horn

Superior
cerebellar cistern

Temporal bone,
petrous portion

Sigmoid sinus

Internal jugular vein

Insular gyri

Frontal lobe,
orbital gyri

Superior rectus muscle

Lesser wing of
the sphenoid bone

Lens

Greater wing of
the sphenoid bone

Inferior
oblique muscle

Lateral
pterygoid muscle

Medial
pterygoid muscle

SAGITTAL T₁

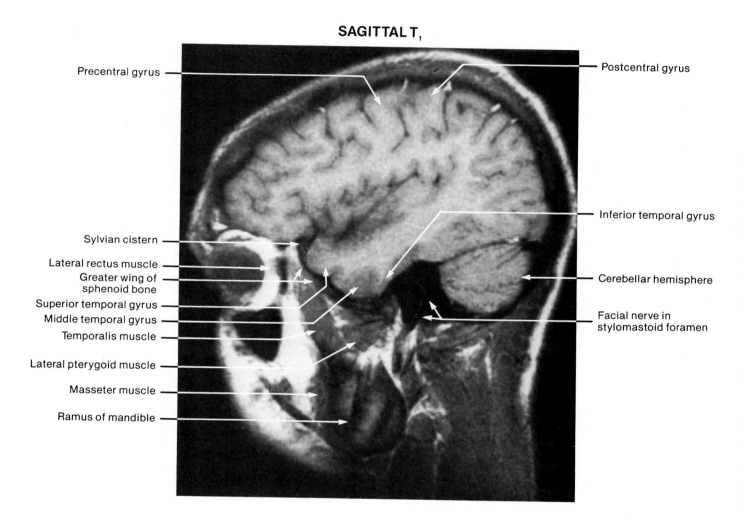

Precentral gyrus

Postcentral gyrus

Sylvian cistern

Lateral rectus muscle

Greater wing of sphenoid bone

Superior temporal gyrus

Middle temporal gyrus

Temporalis muscle

Lateral pterygoid muscle

Masseter muscle

Ramus of mandible

Inferior temporal gyrus

Cerebellar hemisphere

Facial nerve in stylomastoid foramen

REFERENCES

1. Zimmerman RA, Bilaniuk LT, Johnson MH, et al: MRI of the central nervous system: Early clinical results. AJNR 7:587–594, 1986.
2. Franken EA, Berbaum KS, Dunn V, et al: Impact of MR imaging on clinical diagnosis and management: A clinical study. Radiology 161:377–380, 1986.
3. Haughton VM, Rimm AA, Sobocinski KA, et al: A blinded clinical comparison of MR imaging and CT in neuroradiology. Radiology 160:751–755, 1986.
4. Sheldon JJ, Siddharthan R, Tobias J, et al: MR imaging of multiple sclerosis: Comparison with clinical and CT examinations in 74 patients. AJNR 6:683–690, 1985.
5. Jacobs L, Kinkel PR, Kinkel WR: Impact of nuclear magnetic resonance imaging on the assessment of multiple sclerosis patients. Semin Neurol 6:24–32, 1986.
6. Brant-Zawadzki M, Fein G, VanDyke C, et al: MR imaging of the aging brain: Patchy white-matter lesions and dementia. AJNR 6:675–682, 1985.
7. George AE, de Leon MJ, Kalnin A, et al: Leukoencephalopathy in normal and pathologic aging: 2. MRI of brain lucencies. AJNR 7:567–570, 1986.
8. Dunn V, Bale JF, Zimmerman RA, et al: MR in children with post-infectious disseminated encephalomyelitis. Magn Reson Imaging 4:25–32, 1986.
9. Atlas SW, Grossman RI, Goldberg RI, et al: MR diagnosis of acute disseminated encephalomyelitis. J Comput Assist Tomogr 10:798–801, 1986.
10. Guilleaux M-H, Steiner RE, Young IR: MR imaging in progressive multifocal leukoencephalopathy. AJNR 7:1033–1035, 1986.
11. Ormson MJ, Kispert DB, Sharbrough FW, et al: Cryptic structural lesions in refractory partial epilepsy: MR imaging and CT studies. Radiology 160:215–219, 1986.
12. Laster DW, Penry JK, Moody DM, et al: Chronic seizure disorders: Contribution of MR imaging when CT is normal. AJNR 6:177–180, 1985.
13. Aaron J, New PFJ, Strand R, et al: NMR imaging in temporal lobe epilepsy due to gliomas. J Comput Assist Tomogr 8:608–613, 1984.
14. Lateck JT, Abou-Khalil BW, Siegel GJ, et al: Patients with partial seizures: Evaluation by MR, CT and PET imaging. Radiology 159:159–163, 1986.
15. Oot RF, Pile-Spellman J, Rosen BR, et al: The detection of intracranial calcification by MR. AJNR 7:801–810, 1986.
16. Holland BA, Kucharczyk W, Brant-Zawadzki M, et al: MR imaging of calcified intracranial lesions. Radiology 157:353–356, 1985.
17. Theodore WH, Dorwart R, Holmes M, et al: Neuroimaging in refractory seizures: Comparison of PET, CT and MRI. Neurology 36:750–759, 1986.
18. Atlas SW, Zimmerman RA, Bilaniuk LT, et al: Corpus callosum and limbic system: Neuroanatomic MR evaluation of developmental anomalies. Radiology 160:355–362, 1986.
19. Curnes JT, Laster DW, Koubek TD, et al: MRI of corpus callosal syndromes. AJNR 7:617–622, 1986.
20. Bonstelle CT, Kaufman B, Benson JE, et al: Magnetic resonance imaging in the evaluation of the brainstem. Radiology 150:705–712, 1984.
21. Fox AJ, Bogousslavsky J, Carey LS, et al: Magnetic resonance imaging of small medullary infarctions. AJNR 7:229–233, 1986.
22. Bogousslavsky J, Fox AJ, Carey LS, et al: Correlates of brainstem oculomotor disorders in multiple sclerosis: Magnetic resonance imaging. Arch Neurol 43:460–463, 1986.
23. New PFJ, Ojemann RG, Davis KR, et al: MR and CT of occult vascular malformations of the brain. AJNR 7:771–779, 1986.
24. Kingsley DPE, Brooks GB, Leving AW-L, Johnson MA: Acoustic neuromas: Evaluation by magnetic resonance imaging. AJNR 6:1–5, 1985.
25. New PFJ, Bachow TB, Wismer GL, et al: MR imaging of the acoustic nerves and small neuromas at 0.6 T: Prospective study. AJNR 6:165–170, 1985.
26. Cuarti WL, Graif M, Kingsley DPE, et al: MRI in acoustic neuroma: A review of 35 patients. Neuroradiology 28:208–214, 1986.
27. Pojunas KW, Daniels DL, Williams AL, Haughton VM: MR imaging of prolactin secreting microadenomas. AJNR 7:209–213, 1986.
28. Kucharczyk W, Davis DO, Kelly WM, et al: Pituitary adenomas: High resolution MR imaging at 1.5 T. Radiology 161:761–765, 1986.
29. Bradley WG, Kortman KE, Erves JL: Central nervous system high-resolution magnetic resonance imaging: Effect of increasing spatial resolution on resolving power. Radiology 156:93–98, 1985.
30. Davis PC, Hoffman JC, Spencer T, et al: MR imaging of pituitary adenoma: CT, clinical and surgical considerations. AJNR 8:107–112, 1987.
31. Karnaze MG, Sartor K, Winthrop JD, et al: Suprasellar lesions: Evaluation with MR imaging. Radiology 161:77–82, 1986.
32. Kucharczyk W, Lemme-Pleghos L, Uske A, et al: Intracranial vascular malformations: MR and CT imaging. Radiology 156:383–389, 1985.
33. Shuman WP, Griffin BR, Haynor DK, et al: The utility of MR in planning the radiation therapy of oligodendroglioma. AJNR 8:93–98, 1987.
34. Shuman WP, Griffin BR, Haynor DR, et al: MR imaging in radiation therapy planning. Radiology 156:143–147, 1986.
35. Zimmerman RA, Bilaniuk LT, Hackney DB, et al: Head injury: Early results of comparing CT and high-field MR. AJNR 7:757–764, 1986.
36. Snow RB, Zimmerman RD, Gandy SE, Deck MDF: Comparison of magnetic resonance imaging and computed tomography in the evaluation of head injury. Neurosurgery 18:45–52, 1986.
37. Wehrli FW, MacFall JR, Glover GH, et al: The dependence of nuclear magnetic resonance (NMR) image contrast in intrinsic and pulse sequence timing parameters. Magn Reson Imaging 2:3–16, 1984.
38. Wehrli FW, MacFall JR, Newton TH: Parameters determining the appearance of NMR images. In Newton TH, Potts DG (eds): Modern Neuroradiology. Vol 2. Advanced Imaging Techniques. San Anselmo, CA, Clavadel Press, 1983, p 81.
39. Hesselink JR, Berthoty DP: MR parameters must be chosen judiciously to optimize brain studies. Diagn Imag 10:163, 1988.
40. Carr DH, Brown J, Bydder GM et al: Intravenous chelated gadolinium as a contrast agent in NMR imaging of cerebral tumors. Lancet 1:484–486, 1984.
41. Hesselink JR, Healy ME, Press GA, Brahme FJ: Benefits of Gd-DTPA for MR imaging of intracranial abnormalities. J Comput Assist Tomogr 12:266–274, 1988.
42. Haacke EM, Lenz GW: Improving MR image quality in the presence of motion by using rephasing gradients. AJR 148:1251–1255, 1987.
43. Enzmann DR, Rubin JB, O'Donahue JO, et al: Use of cerebrospinal fluid gating to improve T_2-weighted images. Part 2. Temporal lobes, basal ganglia and brain stem. Radiology 162:768–773, 1987.
44. Frahm J, Merboldt K-D, Hanicke W, Haase A: Flow suppression in rapid FLASH NMR images. Magn Reson Med 4:372–377, 1987.

14

BRAIN: Congenital Malformations

GARY A. PRESS

TECHNIQUE

STAGES OF BRAIN DEVELOPMENT
DORSAL INDUCTION
VENTRAL INDUCTION
NEURONAL PROLIFERATION,
    DIFFERENTIATION, AND HISTOGENESIS
MIGRATION
MYELINATION

DEVELOPMENTAL ANOMALIES
DISORDERS OF DORSAL INDUCTION
Cephaloceles
Chiari Malformations
DISORDERS OF VENTRAL INDUCTION
Holoprosencephaly

Septooptic Dysplasia
Dysplasias of the Cerebellum
DISORDERS OF NEURONAL
    PROLIFERATION, DIFFERENTIATION,
    AND HISTOGENESIS
Neurofibromatosis
Sturge-Weber Syndrome
Tuberous Sclerosis
Hippel-Lindau Disease
DISORDERS OF MIGRATION
Lissencephaly
Pachygyria
Polymicrogyria
Heterotopic Gray Matter
Schizencephaly
Anomalies of the Corpus Callosum
DISORDERS OF MYELINATION

As a rule, the different categories of congenital malformations of the CNS reflect the *time* at which a noxious agent disrupted the normal sequence of neural development rather than the nature of the noxious agent itself. Accordingly, Volpe[1] arranged many congenital central nervous system (CNS) disorders according to the time of onset of the morphologic derangement. This classification was later expanded to include several important conditions formerly omitted: cerebellar malformations, congenital vascular malformations, congenital tumors, and secondarily acquired congenital abnormalities.[2] A portion of the complete classification including all of the primary brain malformations is presented in Table 14–1. We emphasize that the etiology and time of insult of several congenital deformities (e.g., corpus callosum dysgenesis, schizencephaly) remain controversial. We have tried to present the most up-to-date information available for each of them.

TECHNIQUE

At no other time are we made more acutely aware of the need to minimize patient motion than when an MR examination is performed in the pediatric age group. During the second through fourth years of life, patients tend to be especially uncooperative and will require sedation. Younger infants may often be examined merely by employing a pacifier, or by withholding food until they are quite hungry, feeding them, and then performing the MR examination during a postprandial nap. Older children may be surprisingly cooperative, especially following a brief, nonthreatening introduction to the machine. Parental presence by or partly in the scanner during the examination is most helpful.

When pharmacologic restraint is required, chloral hydrate 30 to 50 mg/kg PO 30 minutes prior to the examination is most effective. Pentobarbital 5 mg/kg

TABLE 14–1. CLASSIFICATION OF CONGENITAL CEREBRAL AND CEREBELLAR MALFORMATIONS

Disorder	Time of Onset (Gestational Age)
Dorsal induction, primary neurulation/ neural tube defects	(3–4 wks)
Craniorachischisis totalis	3 wks
Anencephaly	4 wks
Myeloschisis	4 wks
Encephalocele	4 wks
Myelomeningocele	4 wks
Chiari malformation	4 wks
Hydromyelia	4 wks
Ventral induction	(5–10 wks)
Atelencephaly	5 wks
Holoprosencephaly	5–6 wks
Septooptic dysplasia	6–7 wks
Agenesis of the septum pellucidum	6 wks
Diencephalic cyst	6 wks
Cerebral hemihypoplasia/aplasia	6 wks
Lobar hypoplasia/aplasia	6 wks
Hypoplasia/aplasia of the cerebellar hemispheres	6–8 wks
Hypoplasia/aplasia of the vermis	6–10 wks
Dandy-Walker syndrome/variant	7–10 wks
Craniosynostosis	6–8 wks
Neuronal proliferation, differentiation, and histogenesis	(2–5 mos)
Micrencephaly	2–4 mos
Megalencephaly	2–4 mos or later
Unilateral megalencephaly	2–4 mos or later
Neurofibromatosis	5 wks–6 mos
Tuberous sclerosis	5 wks–6 mos
Sturge-Weber syndrome	5 wks–6 mos
Hippel-Lindau disease	5 wks–6 mos
Ataxia telangiectasia	5 wks–6 mos
Other neurocutaneous syndromes	5 wks–6 mos
Congenital vascular malformations	2–3 mos
Congenital tumors of the nervous system	2–5 mos
Aqueduct stenosis	4 mos
Colpocephaly	2–6 mos
Porencephaly	3–4 mos
Multicystic encephalopathy	3–4 mos
Hydranencephaly	3 mos or later
Migration	(2–5 mos)
Schizencephaly	2 mos
Lissencephaly	3 mos
Pachygyria	3–4 mos
Polymicrogyria	5 mos
Neuronal heterotopias	5 mos
Anomalies of the corpus callosum	3–5 mos
Myelination	(7 mos gestation– 18 mos of age)
Hypomyelination	Variable
Retarded myelination	Variable
Accelerated myelination	Variable

Modified from van der Knapp MS, Valk J: Classification of congenital abnormalities of the CNS. AJNR 9:315–326, 1988.

IM is a good alternative, as is Nembutal 2 to 6 mg/kg IV, infused slowly.

Rarely, a pediatric patient will require general anesthesia during an MR study. Considerable effort and coordination between the anesthesiologists and the MR staff is required in such instances. At our institution, a respirator without ferrous components is placed immediately adjacent to the scanner (1.5 T); connecting the respirator to the patient are six-foot-long plastic hoses introduced into the bore of the magnet from the foot of the scanning table. The patient is closely monitored during the study by two anesthesiologists, one of whom remains in the scanning room at all times. All monitoring is performed with nonferrous devices.

Selection of imaging parameters for evaluation of congenital CNS malformations is straightforward.[3] Since morphologic information is often paramount, T_1-weighted sequences that provide excellent parenchyma–cerebrospinal fluid (CSF) contrast can be employed alone for most patients. Assessing the progress of myelination is best performed using T_1-weighted (or inversion recovery [IR]) images for patients from 29 weeks gestation to 6 months of age (see "Myelination" below). Above this age, T_2-weighted images must be employed. T_2-weighted images are also useful for the detection of parenchymal abnormalities (tumors, heterotopias) associated with the neurocutaneous syndromes.

STAGES OF BRAIN DEVELOPMENT[2, 4]

A brief review of the stages of *normal* development of the CNS will facilitate understanding the MR appearance of congenital CNS malformations. The developmental stages occur serially or concurrently at well-defined fetal and postnatal ages; unique patterns of congenital abnormalities may result from disruption of any one of the stages.

DORSAL INDUCTION

Dorsal induction occurs during the third and fourth weeks of gestation. This stage has three phases, only the first of which concerns us in this discussion. During the first (neurulation) phase the neural tube is formed, which ultimately gives rise to the brain and spinal cord. The second (canalization) and third (retrogressive differentiation) phases apply only to the caudal neural tube and will not be further described in this chapter.

During the neurulation phase, the embryonic ectoderm dorsal to the cellular notochord is induced to thicken and form a neural plate. The ectoderm of the plate (neuroectoderm) invaginates along its central axis to form the neural groove with neural folds created along each side of the groove. Fusion of the neural folds in the midline begins in the thoracic region and then progresses toward both ends to form the neural tube. The interaction between the forming neural tube and the adjacent mesoderm produces the meningeal coverings, vertebrae, and skull.

VENTRAL INDUCTION

Occurring between the fifth and tenth weeks of gestation, the major events of ventral induction result in formation of the brain and the face. Initially, the prechordal mesoderm at the cephalic end of the embryo induces the formation of the prosencephalon, mesencephalon, rhombencephalon, and facial structures. The prosencephalon divides into the telencephalon and diencephalon, while the rhombencephalon divides into the metencephalon and myelencephalon. By dividing into two halves, the telencephalon forms two hemispheres and two lateral ventricles. Subsequent opercularization results in formation of the sylvian fissures and temporal lobes. The two hemispheres are then joined by the corpus callosum. The cerebellum forms also during this stage from the dorsal part of the metencephalon. The successful completion of the first two stages of cerebral development results in the brain lying within an intact calvarium with a complete face. Hereafter, the brain grows by neuronal proliferation.

NEURONAL PROLIFERATION, DIFFERENTIATION, AND HISTOGENESIS

Following the successful formation of the external form of the brain by ventral induction, three processes (neuronal proliferation, differentiation, and histogenesis) become operative simultaneously between 8 and 20 weeks of gestation and continue into the postnatal period. In the normal embryo, beginning at the seventh week of gestation, neuroblasts are generated in the proliferative zones situated along the ependymal surface of the developing brain (germinal matrix). Shortly after the beginning of this stage, the germinal matrix separates from the more superficial cellular layer so that an intervening zone of low cell density is formed which will become the future white matter of the brain.

Derangements of neuronal proliferation, differentiation, and histogenesis result in tumors of remains of embryonic neural cells, for example, hamartomas, craniopharyngiomas, and medulloblastomas. Moreover, although the precise origin and onset of the various neurocutaneous syndromes remain unknown, several authors believe that abnormal neuronal proliferation, differentiation, and histogenesis may be responsible.[2]

MIGRATION

This highly complex and lengthy (8 to 20 weeks of gestation) stage is vulnerable to many possible insults. During this period, neuroblasts formed in the germinal matrix migrate from the ventricular wall through the white matter to form the superficial cortex and deep nuclei of the basal ganglia. More-

TABLE 14-2. SEQUENCE OF APPEARANCE OF CEREBRAL SULCI

Name of Sulcus	Time of Appearance (Gestational Week)
Sylvian fissure	14
Calcarine, rolandic	16–20
Superior temporal and pre- and postcentral	23–25
Remainder of sulci	26–30

From Larroche JC: Development of the nervous system in early life. Part II: The development of the central nervous system during intrauterine life. *In* Falkner F (ed): Human Development. Philadelphia, WB Saunders Company, 1966, pp 257–276.

over, in this stage, the cerebellar cortex and nuclei are formed. The sequence of appearance of the surface sulci is provided in Table 14–2.[5]

By 28 to 32 weeks of gestation, the surface of the cerebral cortex amounts to 10 to 11 per cent (180 sq cm) of that of the adult brain.[6] The further vast increase in cortical surface area is accomplished by an increase in the size and complexity of the gyri. By 8 to 16 weeks *postnatal* age, the surface of the cortex measures 44 per cent (724 sq cm) that of the adult, whereas at two years postnatal age, it lies within the limits of variation observed in adults (1635 sq cm). In the adult, the intrasulcal component of the surface of the cortex is approximately 65 per cent.[6]

MYELINATION

The process of normal myelination as visualized on MR images has been described in detail (Table 14–3; Figs. 14–1 through 14–7).[7-9] The initial phase of myelination is detected most sensitively on T_1-weighted and IR pulse sequences; increased signal intensity of the myelinating white matter is possibly due to T_1 shortening by the components of the

TABLE 14-3. AGES WHEN CHANGES OF MYELINATION APPEAR

Anatomic Region	T_1-weighted Images	T_2-weighted Images
Mid. cerebellar peduncle	Birth	Birth–2 mos
Cerebellar white matter	Birth–4 mos	3–5 mos
Posterior limb int. capsule		
Anterior portion	Birth	4–7 mos
Posterior portion	Birth	Birth–2 mos
Anterior limb int. capsule	2–3 mos	7–11 mos
Genu corpus callosum	4–6 mos	5–8 mos
Splenium corpus callosum	3–4 mos	4–6 mos
Occipital white matter		
Central	3–5 mos	9–14 mos
Peripheral	4–7 mos	11–15 mos
Frontal white matter		
Central	3–6 mos	11–16 mos
Peripheral	7–11 mos	14–18 mos
Centrum semiovale	2–4 mos	7–11 mos

Note: Observations were made at 1.5 T using T_1-weighted sequence (600/20) and T_2-weighted sequence (2500/70).

From Barkovich AJ, Kjos BO, Jackson DE Jr, Norman D: Normal maturation of the neonatal and infant brain: MR imaging at 1.5 T. Radiology 166:173–180, 1988; with permission.

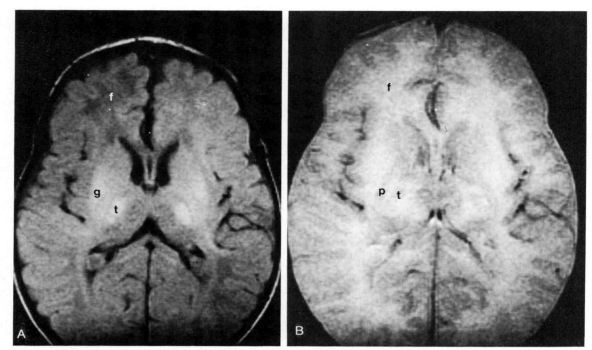

FIGURE 14–1. Normal myelination; 15-day-old male. Axial T_1-weighted image *(A)* demonstrates normal early myelination as high signal intensity within the basal ganglia (g) and ventrolateral thalami (t) at this level. Low signal intensity persists in the nonmyelinated forceps minor (f). On corresponding T_2-weighted image *(B)*, the maturation of the white matter is manifested as a decrease in signal intensity. In this subject, subtle low signal intensity is seen in the posterior limb of the internal capsule (p) and ventrolateral thalami (t) only. The remainder of the white matter including the forceps minor (f) retains high signal intensity at this level.

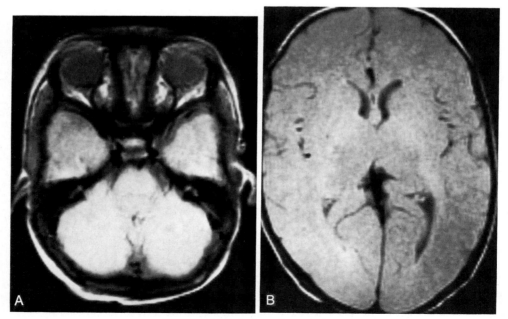

FIGURE 14–2 *See legend on opposite page*

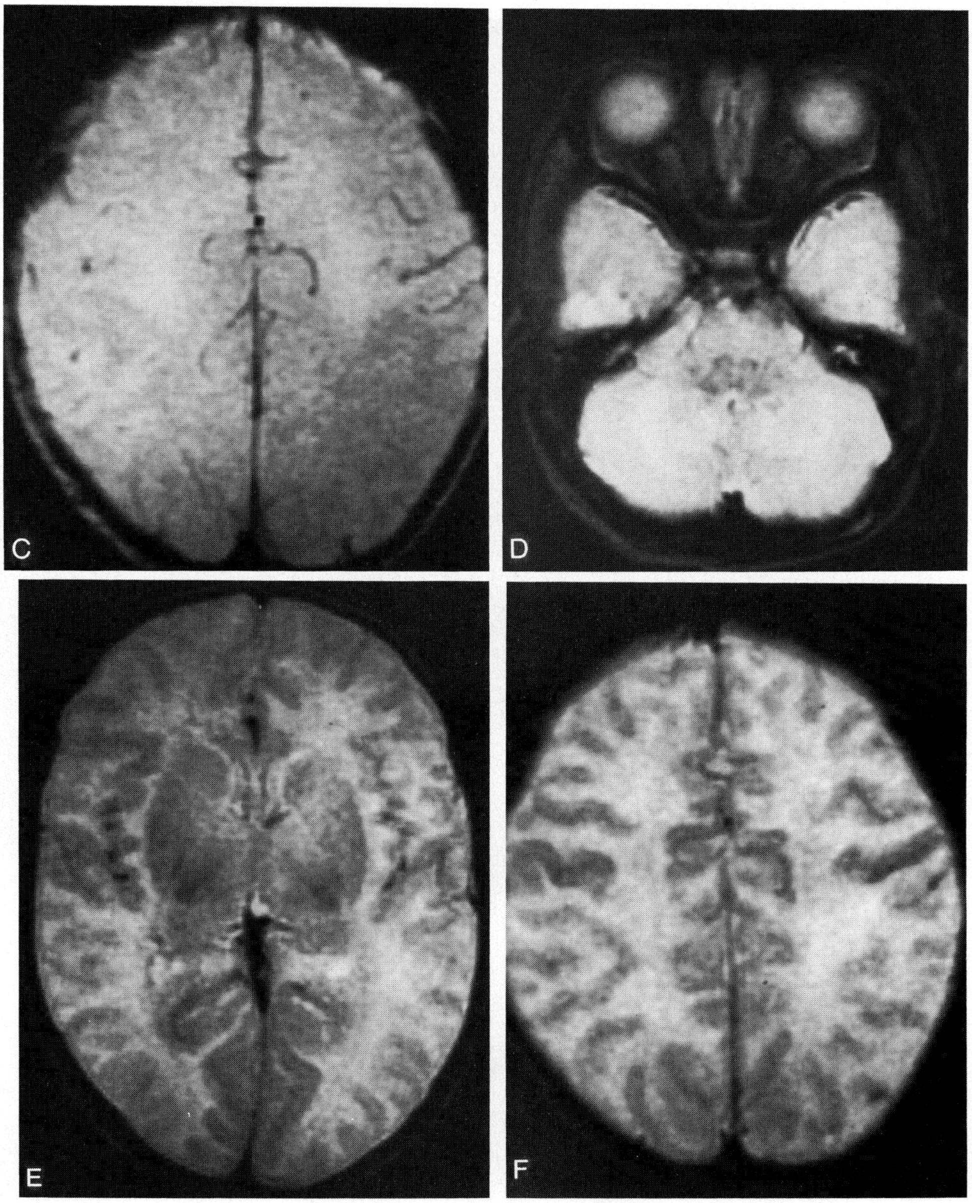

FIGURE 14–2. Normal myelination; 15-day-old male. Axial T$_1$-weighted (A–C) and T$_2$-weighted (D–F) images. Mild hyperintensity within the dorsal pons, posterior limbs of the internal capsule, optic radiations, and centrum semiovale (A–C) represents normal early myelination. Subcortical white matter remains hypointense (nonmyelinated). T$_2$-weighted images (D–F) at same levels demonstrate that hypointensity is restricted to the dorsal pons, the posterior limb of the internal capsule, the ventrolateral region of the thalamus, and the paracentral region of the cortex corresponding to mature myelin in these areas.

developing myelin sheaths.[7–9] This early phase of myelination occurs from 29 weeks of gestation to 6 months postnatal age. Beyond this age, the further maturation of myelin may be followed on T$_2$-weighted images. On these images, mature myelinated white matter has decreased signal intensity explained by the decrease in water content of the brain over the first two years of life. T$_2$-weighted images correlate best with the development of myelination as demonstrated with histochemical methods.[9]

Normal CNS myelination begins during the fifth fetal month with the myelination of the cranial nerves and continues throughout life.[9] On T$_1$-weighted or IR images, at 29 weeks postconception, immature (early) myelin is found in the brain stem and cerebral peduncles. Between 29 and 36 weeks, myelination progresses to the level of the posterior limb of the internal capsule. Early myelin is seen in the corona radiata by 37 weeks and in the centrum semiovale by 42 weeks.

At birth in normal infants, only the dorsal pons, portions of the superior and inferior cerebellar peduncles, and the ventrolateral thalamus have mature myelin and appear as regions of relatively decreased signal intensity on T$_2$-weighted images. Mature myelin is present within the precentral gyrus within the first two postnatal months. Mature myelin may be detected within the deep white matter of the cerebellar hemispheres between three and five months postnatally on T$_2$-weighted images. Myelin within the white matter of the corpus callosum, internal capsule,

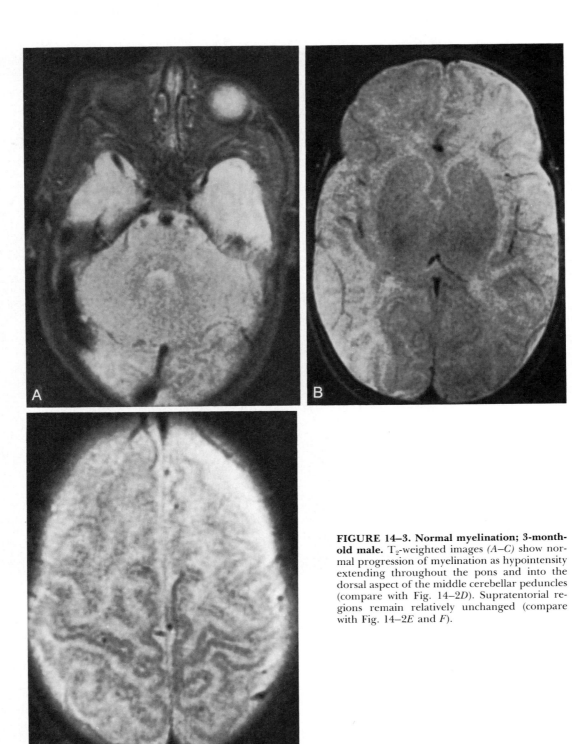

FIGURE 14–3. Normal myelination; 3-month-old male. T$_2$-weighted images *(A–C)* show normal progression of myelination as hypointensity extending throughout the pons and into the dorsal aspect of the middle cerebellar peduncles (compare with Fig. 14–2D). Supratentorial regions remain relatively unchanged (compare with Fig. 14–2E and F).

FIGURE 14–4. Normal myelination; 5-month-old female. T_1-weighted images *(A–C)* show hyperintensity within deep white matter of cerebellar hemipheres, genu and splenium of the corpus callosum, internal and external capsules, and forceps major and minor. There is increased arborization within the centrum semiovale and subcortical white matter, most notably in the occipital and paracentral regions (compare with Fig. 14–1A and 14–2A–C). On T_2-weighted images at the corresponding levels *(D–F)*, maturation of myelin is seen as hypointensity within deep white matter of the cerebellum, entire posterior limb of the internal capsule, and splenium of the corpus callosum (compare with Fig. 14–1B, 14–2D–F, and 14–3A–C). Centrum semiovale and subcortical white matter are normally hyperintense at this age. Overall, the progress of normal myelination from birth to 6 months may be followed best on T_1-weighted images.[7–9]

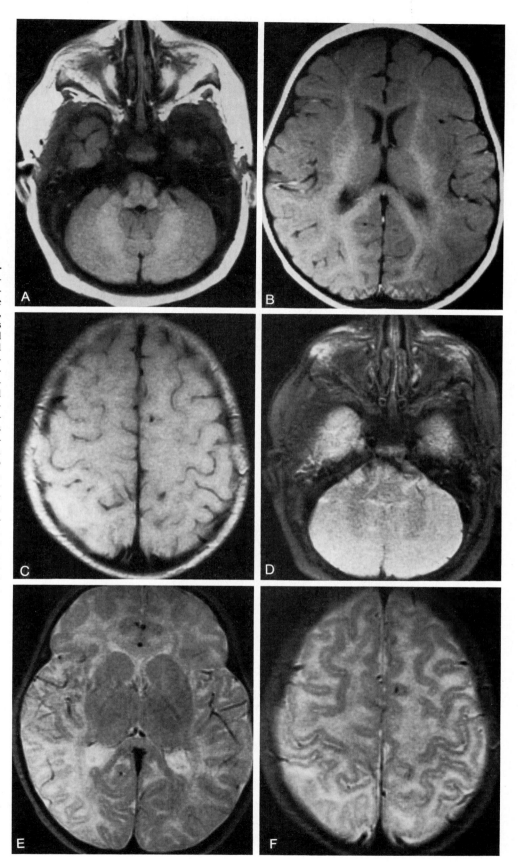

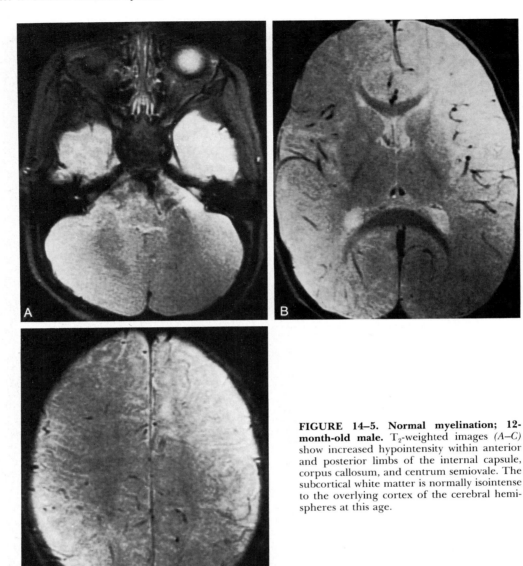

FIGURE 14–5. Normal myelination; 12-month-old male. T_2-weighted images *(A–C)* show increased hypointensity within anterior and posterior limbs of the internal capsule, corpus callosum, and centrum semiovale. The subcortical white matter is normally isointense to the overlying cortex of the cerebral hemispheres at this age.

corona radiata, and centrum semiovale matures during the first 4 to 11 months postnatally. The subcortical white matter matures last, with myelination proceeding from the occipital region anteriorly to the frontal lobes from 11 to 18 months postnatally.[9]

DEVELOPMENTAL ANOMALIES

DISORDERS OF DORSAL INDUCTION

These disorders include malformation of the meningeal coverings, vertebrae, and skull. Cephaloceles, anencephaly, and myelomeningoceles are manifestations of aberrant dorsal induction.

Cephaloceles

A defect in the dura and cranium with associated extracranial herniation of intracranial structures is known as a cephalocele. When only the leptomeninges (pia and arachnoid) and cerebrospinal fluid (CSF) herniate extracranially, a meningocele is formed. Parenchymal herniation together with the meninges creates an encephalocele (Fig. 14–8). Herniation of meninges, brain, and ventricles together is called an encephalocystomeningocele.[10]

In North America and Europe, the large majority (71 per cent) of cephaloceles occur in the occipital region (Fig. 14–8). Other common locations include the parietal (10 per cent), frontal (9 per cent), nasal

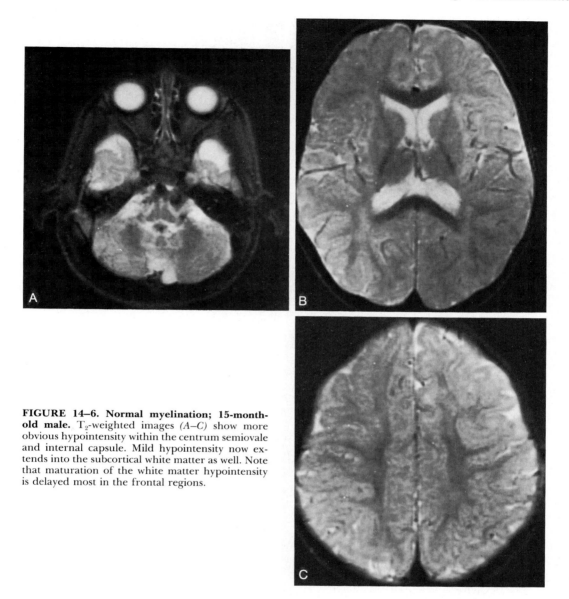

FIGURE 14–6. Normal myelination; 15-month-old male. T_2-weighted images *(A–C)* show more obvious hypointensity within the centrum semiovale and internal capsule. Mild hypointensity now extends into the subcortical white matter as well. Note that maturation of the white matter hypointensity is delayed most in the frontal regions.

(9 per cent) (Fig. 14–9), and nasopharyngeal (1 per cent) regions. Interestingly, nasal cephaloceles are reported to be the most common form in Southeast Asia.[11] The incidence of cephaloceles is between 1 to 3 for every 10,000 births.[11]

Cephaloceles may result from defective tissue induction (simultaneously causing both parenchymal and calvarial abnormalities), defective formation of the endochondral portion of the calvarium, or constriction of the fetal head by in utero bands. The latter etiology usually results in a "nonanatomic" site of presentation (e.g., lateral parietal bone).

Patients with cephaloceles may present with microcephaly and a skin-covered sac protruding from the skull.[3] Symptoms depend on the location of the cephalocele and the volume of protruding brain. Poor motor coordination may be seen in patients with low occipital encephaloceles; visual problems may be detected in those with high occipital encephaloceles; sensory and speech disturbances may be present in patients with parietal encephaloceles. An association with facial anomalies is a unique feature of sphenoethmoidal cephaloceles. Midline clefts of the upper lips and nose, optic nerve dysplasias, and dysgenesis of the corpus callosum occur in 40 to 60 per cent of patients with sphenoethmoidal cephaloceles.

Typical MR findings in patients with cephaloceles include (Figs. 14–8 and 14–9):

1. Microcephaly and a cranial defect through which protrudes a variable amount of meninges, CSF, and brain, contained by a skin-covered sac. The subcutaneous fat of the sac lining is continuous with that of the scalp (Fig. 14–8).

2. There may be torquing and displacement of the

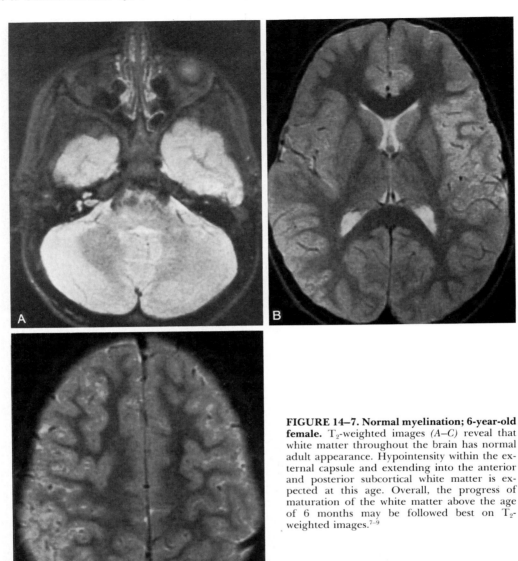

FIGURE 14–7. Normal myelination; 6-year-old female. T$_2$-weighted images *(A–C)* reveal that white matter throughout the brain has normal adult appearance. Hypointensity within the external capsule and extending into the anterior and posterior subcortical white matter is expected at this age. Overall, the progress of maturation of the white matter above the age of 6 months may be followed best on T$_2$-weighted images.[7–9]

parenchyma within both the cranium and the hernia sac. Portions of the ventricles within the sac are commonly more dilated than those that remain within the cranial cavity. Arterial supply herniates along with the brain into the sac. Azygous anterior cerebral arteries may accompany a frontal encephalocele. Large veins drain blood through the cranial defect from the sac contents to the intracranial sinuses.

3. Nests of disorganized neuroglial tissue may line the walls of the sac.

Chiari Malformations

Controversy exists in the classification of Chiari malformations. Since myelomeningoceles, Chiari malformations, and hydromyelia are so often associated with one another, they are considered by some to be different components of a single clinical syndrome;[2, 12] others consider them to be unrelated anomalies of the hindbrain.[10, 13]

Chiari I

This malformation combines cervicomedullary and craniovertebral anomalies. In such patients, MR reveals low position of the cerebellar tonsils, which protrude through the foramen magnum to reach the level of the arch of C1 or C2 (Figs. 14–10 and 14–11). The inferior aspect of the cerebellar hemispheres may be drawn slightly toward the foramen magnum; the fourth ventricle may be normal or

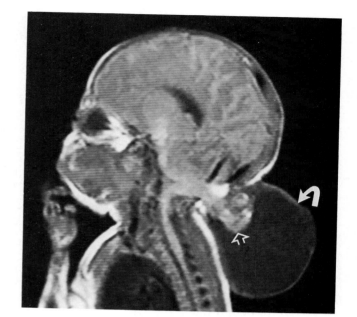

FIGURE 14–8. Inferior occipital myelomeningoencephalocele; neonate. T₁-weighted sagittal image demonstrates the inferior cerebellum, medulla, and high cervical spinal cord *(open arrow)* protrude through a cranial defect into a skin-covered, CSF-filled sac *(curved arrow).*

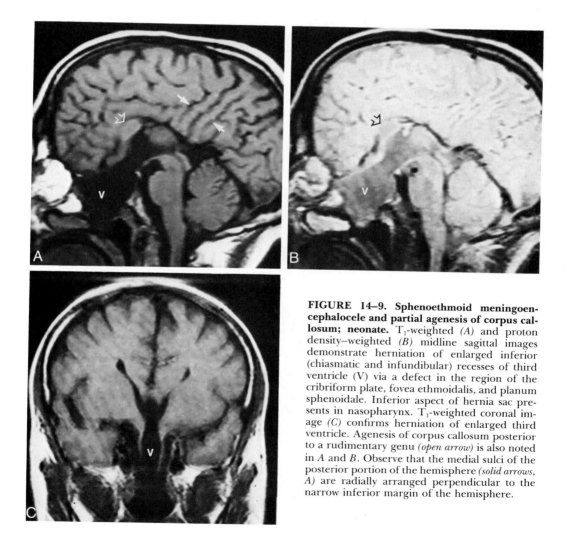

FIGURE 14–9. Sphenoethmoid meningoencephalocele and partial agenesis of corpus callosum; neonate. T₁-weighted *(A)* and proton density–weighted *(B)* midline sagittal images demonstrate herniation of enlarged inferior (chiasmatic and infundibular) recesses of third ventricle (V) via a defect in the region of the cribriform plate, fovea ethmoidalis, and planum sphenoidale. Inferior aspect of hernia sac presents in nasopharynx. T₁-weighted coronal image *(C)* confirms herniation of enlarged third ventricle. Agenesis of corpus callosum posterior to a rudimentary genu *(open arrow)* is also noted in *A* and *B*. Observe that the medial sulci of the posterior portion of the hemisphere *(solid arrows, A)* are radially arranged perpendicular to the narrow inferior margin of the hemisphere.

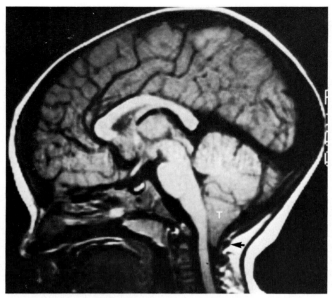

FIGURE 14–10. Chiari I malformation; 2-year-old male. Midline sagittal T$_1$-weighted image demonstrates low position of peglike tonsils (T). The inferior aspect of the tonsils reaches the level of the posterior arch of C1 *(arrow).* The cisterna magna is effaced.

slightly elongated craniocaudally. The cisterna magna is extremely small or nonexistent. This abnormality presents in adolescents and young adults with manifestations related to cerebellar, spinal cord, or brain stem compression or due to hydromyelia, which is associated in 20 to 73 per cent of cases (Fig. 14–11).[3, 14] Associated craniovertebral anomalies include basilar impression (25 per cent), atlantooccipital fusion (10 per cent), and Klippel-Feil anomaly (10 per cent).[10] Recently,[15] it was determined that MR

demonstration of less than 2 mm of tonsillar ectopia is probably of no clinical significance.

Chiari II (Arnold-Chiari malformation)

This complex deformity is characterized by an elongated, small cerebellum and brain stem and caudal displacement of the medulla, parts of the cerebellum, and pons through an enlarged foramen magnum into the cervical spinal canal. The Arnold-Chiari malformation is nearly always accompanied by a meningomyelocele and hydrocephalus[16] and occurs in 2 to 3 per 1000 births.[3] Although most cases are sporadic, a higher incidence is encountered in families with a history of neural tube defects. Maldevelopment of the telencephalon, diencephalon, mesencephalon, and upper cervical canal often accompany the rhombencephalic deformity of Chiari II malformation.

Patients present with sensory and motor deficits of the lower extremities owing to the accompanying myelomeningocele. Hydrocephalus may cause raised intracranial pressure and requires shunting in 90 per cent of patients. Nevertheless, normal intelligence is also present in 90 per cent of patients.

In a review of 24 patients with Chiari II malformations,[16] characteristic MR manifestations were delineated (Figs. 14–12 through 14–14).

RHOMBENCEPHALON AND SPINAL CORD. The surface of the cerebellar vermis was unusually smooth on sagittal images owing to dorsocaudal angulation of the surface sulci and fissures (Fig. 14–12). Both inferior and superior lobules were so affected. The cerebellar dysplasia accompanying Chiari II represents a spectrum varying from heterotopias and heterotaxias to marked cerebellar and brain stem dys-

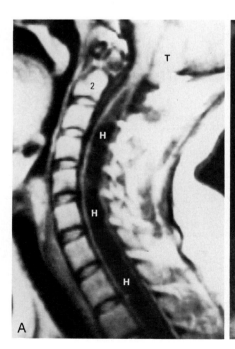

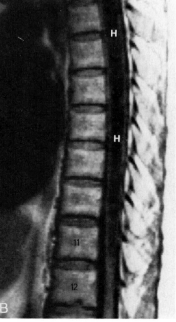

FIGURE 14–11. Chiari I malformation and hydromyelia; 12-year-old female. Midline sagittal T$_1$-weighted images at the level of the cervical *(A)* and low thoracic *(B)* spine. Tonsillar (T) herniation below the level of the foramen magnum is evident *(A).* Hydromyelia (H) expands the spinal cord from C2 *(A)* through T11 and T12 *(B).*

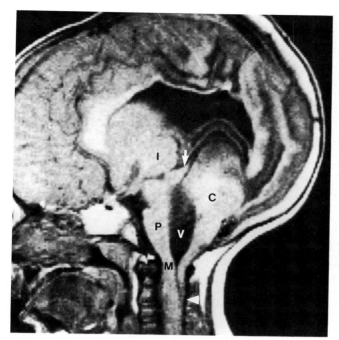

FIGURE 14–12. Chiari II (Arnold-Chiari) malformation; 6-year-old female. Midline sagittal T₁-weighted image demonstrates marked elongation of the cerebellum (C) and fourth ventricle (V). The surface of the inferior vermis is very smooth. There is caudal displacement of the medulla (M), vermis, and tonsils into the cervical spinal canal (*arrowhead*) through an enlarged foramen magnum. The superior and inferior colliculi (*arrow*) are fused and form a peak posteriorly. Sylvian aqueduct is not seen. The massa intermedia (I) is large and the posterior aspect of the corpus callosum is very thin. (P = pons).

genesis. Upward bulging of the cerebellum occurs through a wide tentorial incisura which inserts low near the foramen magnum (Fig. 14–13). Medial portions of the cerebellar hemispheres migrate forward into the prepontine or premedullary cisterns,

enveloping the brain stem (Fig. 14–14). The fourth ventricle elongates and descends into the spinal canal along the posterior surface of the medulla. Varying amounts of the inferior cerebellar hemispheres and the tonsils herniate through the wide foramen magnum and appear as a peg or tongue of tissue below the C1 ring, behind the spinal cord and medulla. From posterior to anterior in a sagittal MR image one sees a sequence of protrusions: of cerebellum behind fourth ventricle, ventricle behind medulla, and medulla behind spinal cord. In 20 to 83 per cent of patients with Chiari II, hydromyelia is seen also.[16]

TELENCEPHALON. Small, closely spaced gyral folds, or stenogyria, may be seen in the cerebral hemispheres. This histologically normal cerebral cortex is different from polymicrogyria in which the cellular layers of the cortex are deficient. Anteroinferior pointing of the frontal horns may be noted often in the coronal plane. Partial agenesis of the corpus callosum was seen in one third of the patients in this series.[16] Severe callosal dysplasia may be associated with mental retardation.

DIENCEPHALON. Enlargement of the massa intermedia may be identified in 75 to 90 per cent of patients (Fig. 14–12). The third ventricle is most often normal or mildly dilated in patients with Chiari II.

MESENCEPHALON. Nonvisualization of the sylvian aqueduct on sagittal images occurs in the majority of patients with Chiari II (Fig. 14–12). The explanation—whether aqueduct occlusion is present and whether it is primary or secondary due to external compression—remains controversial. The two inferior colliculi may be elongated sagittally, or the superior and inferior colliculi may be fused into a single collicular mass. Some authors[17] believe that there is an association between the degree of tectal elongation, compression of the brain stem by the dilated ventricles, and narrowing of the aqueduct.

FIGURE 14–13. Chiari II (Arnold-Chiari) malformation; 10-year-old male. Coronal T₁-weighted (*A*) and axial proton density–weighted (*B*) images demonstrate the posterior fossa is small and the tentorial leaves (*arrows*) are hypoplastic, inserting low, near the foramen magnum. Upward bulging of the cerebellar vermis (Ve) through the wide tentorial incisura forms a pseudomass between the temporal lobes (T).

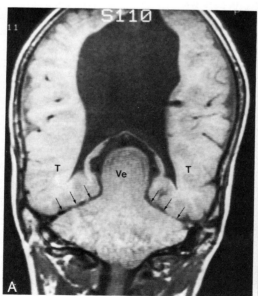
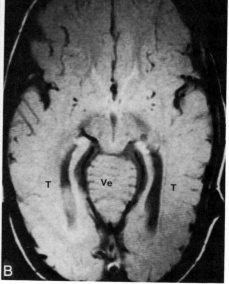

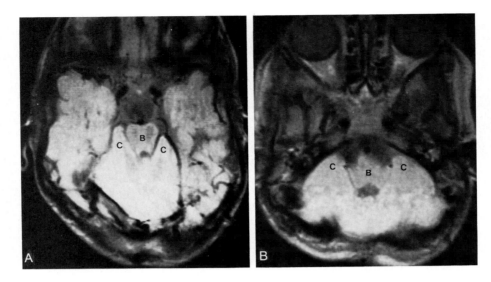

FIGURE 14–14. Chiari II malformation; 5-year-old male. Axial proton density–weighted images (A and B) demonstrate that the medial portions of the cerebellar hemispheres (C) migrate forward into the prepontine and premedullary cisterns enveloping the brain stem (B).

MESODERM. Scalloping of the clivus (basiocciput only) and of the petrous bone was seen in 79 per cent of patients in one series.[16] These changes are, however, a result from pressure by the adjacent cerebellum.

DISORDERS OF VENTRAL INDUCTION

Holoprosencephaly

The disorders of ventral induction affect formation of the forebrain and face; variable failure of normal separation of the primitive forebrain into individual cerebral hemispheres is associated with typical facial anomalies. Three points along the spectrum of disease from most to least severe are alobar, semilobar, and lobar holoprosencephaly.

In alobar holoprosencephaly, MR reveals a single, unlobed holoprosencephalon with a monoventricle (Fig. 14–15).[18] No interhemispheric fissure, falx, septum pellucidum, or corpus callosum is present. The thalami are fused into a single midline mass. This central gray matter mass indents the inferior aspect of the monoventricle, imparting a horseshoe shape. The membranous roof of the third ventricle may

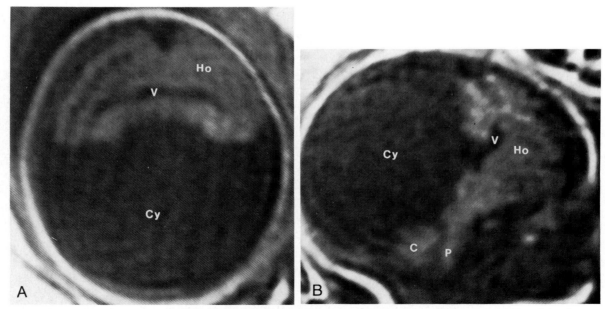

FIGURE 14–15. Alobar holoprosencephaly seen by MR at 33 weeks gestation (in utero). Axial T_1-weighted image (A) shows single, unlobed holoprosencephalon (Ho) with monoventricle (V) anterior to a large dorsal cyst (Cy). Falx cerebri, septum pellucidum, and corpus callosum are absent. Sagittal T_1-weighted image (B) shows dorsal cyst communicates with ventricle. (P = pons, C = cerebellum).

balloon into a dorsal cyst or saclike structure that lies either above or above and below the tentorial incisura (Fig. 14–15). There is absence of the straight, superior, and inferior sagittal sinuses and internal cerebral veins. Increased incidence of azygous anterior cerebral arteries and of hypoplastic middle cerebral arteries accompanies alobar holoprosencephaly.

In semilobar holoprosencephaly (Fig. 14–16), MR reveals partial development of the posterior interhemispheric fissure, falx, and associated dural sinuses. There may be partial separation of the occipitotemporal lobes and partial differentiation of the temporooccipital horns from the monoventricle (Fig. 14–16). There is often partial cleavage of the diencephalon into two thalami with formation of a rudimentary third ventricle. A rudimentary corpus callosum may also be present.

In lobar holoprosencepaly, MR reveals more normal cerebral hemispheres and thalami. There remains only partial fusion of the two frontal lobes with local continuity of the gyri and underlying white matter across the midline beneath a shallow interhemispheric fissure.[3] The temporal and occipital horns are well formed, and the bodies of the lateral ventricles are narrow. The septum pellucidum remains absent, and the frontal horns maintain a squared-off appearance.

The incidence of holoprosencephaly is approximately 1 in 16,000 births. Most cases are sporadic. Most patients with alobar and semilobar forms present at birth with characteristic facial anomalies, including microcephaly, hypotelorism, and one of cyclopia, ethmocephaly, cebocephaly, or absent premaxillary segment.[10] Poikilothermia, apneic spells, motor and mental retardation, and reduced life expectancy are part of the clinical spectrum.

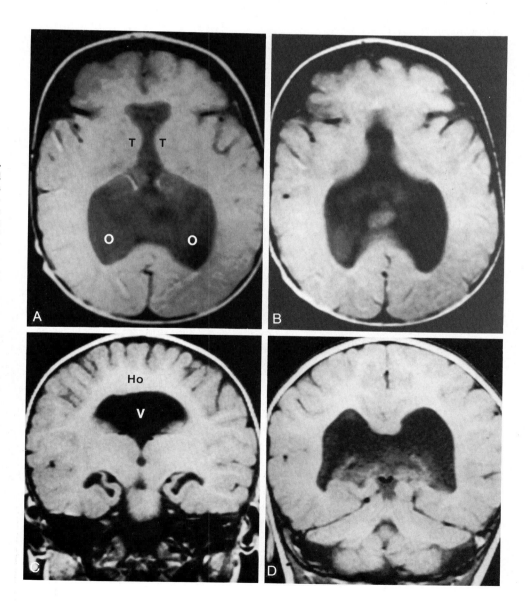

FIGURE 14–16. Semilobar holoprosencephaly; 10-month-old male. Axial T_1-weighted images show absence of the septum pellucidum *(A and B)* and absence of the anterior interhemispheric fissure superiorly *(B)*. Continuity of the gray and white matter across the midline is seen *(B)*. Nevertheless, partial formation of separate hemispheres is evident, with presence of interhemispheric fissure posteriorly *and* anteriorly at the level of the frontal horns *(A)*, partial formation of occipital horns (O), and separate thalami (T). Coronal T_1-weighted sections *(C and D)* emphasize the continuity of the holoprosencephalon (Ho) and the ventricle (V) across the midline. There is partial formation of the temporal horns as well *(C)*.

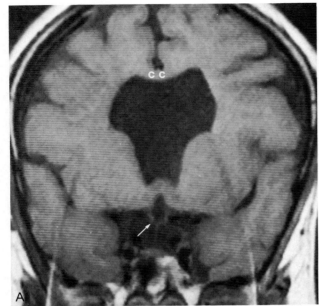

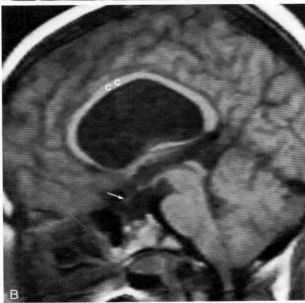

FIGURE 14–17. Septooptic dysplasia in a child. Coronal *(A)* and midline sagittal *(B)* T₁-weighted images demonstrate absence of the septum pellucidum, dilatation of the suprasellar cistern, and hypoplasia of the optic chiasm and optic tracts *(arrow)*. Moderate dilatation of the lateral ventricles and thinning of the corpus callosum (cc) are evident.

Septooptic Dysplasia

In this disorder (also known as De Morsier's syndrome) development of the midline telencephalic structures is defective. The etiologic insult may occur during the fifth to seventh weeks of gestation at the time of differentiation of the optic vesicle and of the commissural plate (necessary for the subsequent development of the septum pellucidum and the midline anterior hippocampal and callosal structures). MR may reveal optic nerve hypoplasia, dilatation of the suprasellar cistern and anterior third ventricle, absence of the septum pellucidum, flattening of the roof of the frontal horns, and dysplasia of the corpus callosum and fornix (Fig. 14–17). Additional features reported in patients with septooptic dysplasia include mild to moderate lateral ventricular dilatation, schizencephalic defects, and falx hypoplasia.[19] Pituitary/hypothalamic insufficiency is recognized clinically in these patients.

Dysplasias of the Cerebellum

Posterior Fossa Cystic Malformations

The common finding in this group of hindbrain malformations is the presence of a large CSF space situated posterior to the cerebellum. The Dandy-Walker cyst, Dandy-Walker variant, and the retrocerebellar arachnoid pouch (Blake's pouch of the cisterna magna) are the most important members of this group.

In patients with Dandy-Walker malformation, MR reveals partial agenesis of the vermis (inferior lobules), hypoplasia of the cerebellar hemispheres, and marked dilatation of the fourth ventricle, which forms a cyst posterior to the cerebellar hemispheres

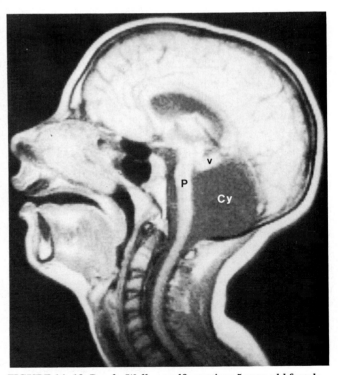

FIGURE 14–18. Dandy-Walker malformation; 5-year-old female. Midline sagittal T₁-weighted image demonstrates near complete agenesis of the vermis; only the superior lobules (v) are preserved and displaced upward to lie posterior to the tectal plate. There is continuity between the fourth ventricle and the large posterior fossa cyst (Cy). Sagittal diameter of the pons (P) is abnormally small in this patient. Hydrocephalus was relieved by placement of a CSF shunt catheter (not shown) prior to MR examination.

that are displaced anteriorly (Fig. 14–18). The cyst expands the posterior fossa causing scaphocephaly and pressure erosion of the petrous pyramids. The tentorium inserts above the lambdoid suture (the reverse of the normal situation), and the superior vermis may be displaced upward into the cistern of the velum interpositum or may lie posterior to the tectal plate (Fig. 14–18). No falx cerebelli is present. Hydrocephalus may or may not be present for unknown reasons.[10] The foramen of Magendie is absent in this disorder.

In patients with the Dandy-Walker variant, MR reveals that the fourth ventricle is smaller and better formed, the retrocerebellar cyst is smaller, and midline or paired paramedian retrocerebellar septae are present. There is milder vermal agenesis. The foramen of Magendie is present in this form, allowing free communication between the fourth ventricular cyst and the basal cistern. Nevertheless, hydrocephalus may be present.

The Dandy-Walker malformation and its variant account for 2 to 4 per cent of patients with hydrocephalus. The variant is believed to be far more common than the true Dandy-Walker malformation. Most cases are sporadic.[10]

Clinically, patients with the Dandy-Walker malformation and its variant present with macrocephaly and high pressure hydrocephalus requiring shunting. Mental retardation is common in affected patients. There is an association between Dandy-Walker malformation and other cerebral anomalies, including dysplasia of the cerebral and cerebellar hemispheres (20 to 25 per cent), dysgenesis of the corpus callosum (15 to 25 per cent), and holoprosencephaly (10 to 25 per cent).

Collections of CSF which lie posterior to *intact* cerebellar hemispheres and vermis have traditionally been considered to be unrelated to the Dandy-Walker malformation and its variant forms. Such a retrocerebellar arachnoid pouch may occur when the retrocerebellar and supracerebellar CSF spaces are divided by a transverse meningeal fold; a bifid falx cerebelli, and a defective tentorium that allows superior extension of a CSF cyst or pouch into the intradural compartment between the leaves of the falx cerebri are seen often (Fig. 14–19).[13] Such pouches are believed to arise when the tela choroidea evaginates posterior to and above the vermis. The cyst may be noncompressive and, therefore, asymptomatic (mega cisterna magna); alternatively, a ball-valve effect may result in expansion of the cyst and in symptomatic compression of the cerebellar hemispheres and vermis (arachnoid cyst).

Recently,[20] a new classification of posterior fossa cystic malformations that "connect in some way with the fourth ventricle" has been proposed on the basis of a review of mainly sagittal and coronal MR images obtained in 29 patients. These authors contend that the Dandy-Walker cyst, the Dandy-Walker variant, and the mega cisterna magna represent three points on a continuum for which appearance depends pri-

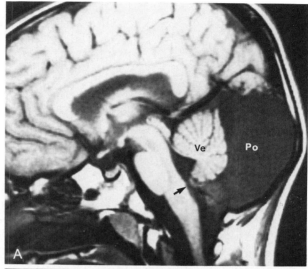

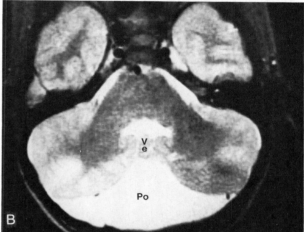

FIGURE 14–19. Retrocerebellar arachnoid pouch; 11-year-old male. Sagittal T₁-weighted *(A)* and axial T₂-weighted *(B)* images demonstrate a large CSF space (Po) posterior to an intact but small (possibly hypoplastic) vermis (Ve) and hemispheres of the cerebellum. The fourth ventricle and CSF space appear to communicate via the foramen of Magendie *(arrow).* The superior aspect of the cyst lies at or above the level of the torcular Herophili.

marily on varying degrees of vermian hypoplasia, rotation, or displacement. A possible embryologic basis for this continuum is offered.[20] The authors mention two additional unrelated causes of large posterior fossa CSF collections: (1) posterior cerebellar and vermal atrophy, often associated with degenerative disorders; and (2) discrete posterior fossa CSF collections clearly separated from and not in communication with the fourth ventricle or vallecula (Fig. 14–20). Such cysts generally require surgical intervention.

Cerebellar Agenesis/Hypoplasia

Agenesis of the cerebellum is most uncommon and has been described in a heterogeneous group of patients. Other severe anomalies may be associated

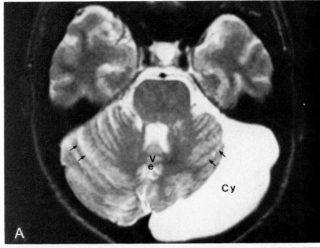

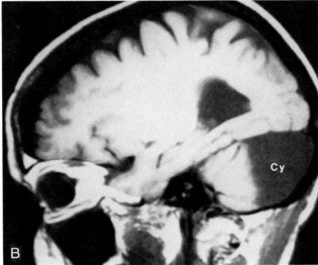

FIGURE 14–20. Arachnoid cyst; 45-year-old female. Axial T₂-weighted *(A)* and paramidline sagittal T₁-weighted *(B)* images demonstrate that unilateral posterior fossa CSF collection (Cy) displaces cerebellar hemispheres and vermis (Ve) from left to right. Sulci *(arrows)* of left cerebellar hemisphere are effaced when compared with those on the right side. Subtle thinning of overlying left occipital bone is evident.

terosuperior portion of the vermis is preserved, presumably because fusion of the vermis proceeds from rostral to caudal during the second month of gestation.[24]

Hypoplasia of the vermis may be regionally localized (e.g., posterior vermis in autism)[25] or diffuse (e.g., Down syndrome).[26] There are no reports of hypoplasia involving *only* anterosuperior vermal regions. In all reported cases, vermal hypoplasia is accompanied also by hypoplasia of the cerebellar hemispheres.

In patients with cerebellar or vermal agenesis/hypoplasia, MR reveals variable-sized remnants of cerebellar tissue associated with hypoplastic or absent

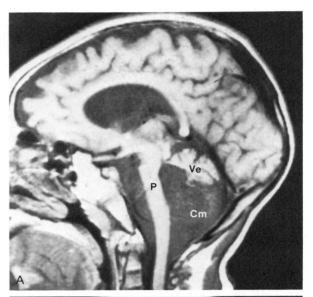

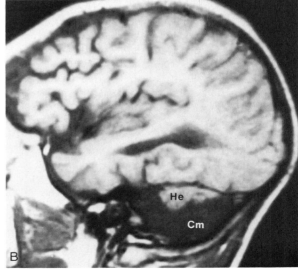

FIGURE 14–21. Marked generalized cerebellar hypoplasia; 6-year-old female. Sagittal T₁-weighted images *(A* and *B)* demonstrate that cerebellar vermis and hemispheres are very small with a relatively smooth surface suggesting hypoplasia. Brain stem is diminutive also. Ex vacuo dilatation of the cisterna magna (Cm) is seen. (P = pons).

(anencephaly, amyelia). A survey of twelve cases of "agenesis of the cerebellum"[21] revealed small remnants of cerebellar tissue in several instances. In affected patients, related structures, including the pontine nuclei, inferior olives, and cerebellar peduncles, are either hypoplastic or malformed. Absence of one cerebellar hemisphere occurs more frequently; anomalies of the contralateral inferior olive and pons may take the form of atrophy rather than maldevelopment.

Total or partial agenesis of the vermis may also occur. The cerebellar hemispheres may be fused to one another[22] or separated by a wide CSF-filled cleft[23] in the region of absent vermal parenchyma.

The most common lesion is partial agenesis of the vermis. In all instances of partial agenesis, the an-

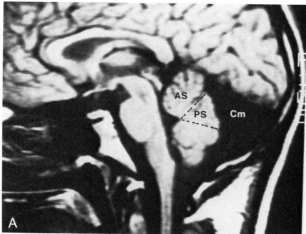

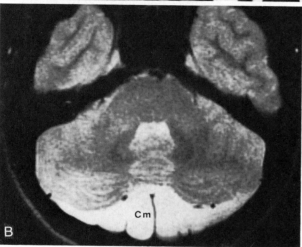

FIGURE 14—22. Focal hypoplasia of cerebellar vermis in autism; 22-year-old male. Sagittal T_1-weighted (A) and axial T_2-weighted (B) images demonstrate focal hypoplasia of posterosuperior (PS) lobules (declive, folium, and tuber) of the vermis. Anterosuperior (AS) vermal lobules are normal in size. Ex vacuo dilatation of the cisterna magna (Cm) is seen.

cerebellar peduncles and brain stem (Figs. 14—21 and 14—22). Ex vacuo dilatation of the retrocerebellar CSF space usually accompanies these deformities.

DISORDERS OF NEURONAL PROLIFERATION, DIFFERENTIATION, AND HISTOGENESIS

Neurofibromatosis

Two elements are operative in this disorder: *neuroectodermal* (Schwann cell) *neoplasia* surrounded by reactive *mesenchymal hyperplasia* of varying degree. In 50 per cent of cases, neurofibromatosis is transmitted with autosomal dominant inheritance; an additional 50 per cent are caused by a mutation of the dominant gene. The incidence of neurofibromatosis is approximately 1 in 2500 to 3300 births.[27] The disorder has been divided into categories featuring different clin-

ical or pathologic manifestations including CNS, peripheral, central, and mixed peripheral forms. More recently, the designation of neurofibromatosis I (or von Recklinghausen neurofibromatosis), neurofibromatosis II (or bilateral acoustic neurofibromatosis), and other forms has been utilized by several investigators.[28, 29]

Cutaneous signs of neurofibromatosis include café au lait spots, axillary freckles (33 per cent), and subcutaneous nodules. These are less common in patients with the CNS (central) form of the disease. Mental retardation accompanies the diagnosis of neurofibromatosis in 10 to 30 per cent of patients.[30]

A review of MR images obtained in 53 patients with neurofibromatosis revealed the following manifestations.[31]

HETEROTOPIAS (Fig. 14—23). Small, focal areas of abnormally increased signal intensity were noted primarily within the basal ganglia, internal capsule, midbrain, cerebellum, and subcortical white matter on T_2-weighted images of 23 patients. Although the exact nature of these lesions remains unclear, they most likely represent focal areas of heterotopic or possibly dysplastic tissue. The pathologic varieties of heterotopias in neurofibromatosis include meningioangiomatous malformations, atypical glial cell nests, subependymal glial nodules, ependymal ectopias, and intramedullary schwannosis. CT and T_1-weighted images revealed few or no abnormalities in corresponding locations. Sixteen of the patients were asymptomatic; the remaining seven patients were studied for other known lesions or symptoms.

OPTIC NERVE AND CHIASMAL GLIOMAS. Optic nerve enlargement accompanied optic nerve glioma in two patients; however, signal intensity of the enlarged optic nerve remained normal. On the other hand, in eight patients with chiasmal gliomas, T_2-weighted images consistently revealed abnormally high signal within the region of the primary chiasmal neoplasm and in the areas of gliomatous extension into the optic tracts.

PARENCHYMAL GLIOMAS. MR features of nine parenchymal gliomas included homogeneous increased signal in tumor cysts and slightly inhomogeneous increased signal from the solid tumors on T_2-weighted images. Decreased signal was occasionally noted in the tumor nidus on T_1-weighted images. A variable degree of white matter edema was noted to surround the tumors.

ACOUSTIC NEURINOMAS AND MENINGIOMAS. Acoustic tumors appeared as mass lesions in the cerebellopontine angles extending from widened internal auditory canals (Figs. 14—24 through 14—26). Bilateral acoustic tumors are seen commonly in neurofibromatosis.[32] Multiple meningiomas also occur frequently.

OTHER NEURINOMAS. Bilateral trigeminal neurinomas were reported in three patients with bilateral acoustic neurinomas and neurofibromatosis (Figs. 14—24 and 14—25).[32] Trigeminal neurinomas caused fusiform enlargement of the cisternal portion of the

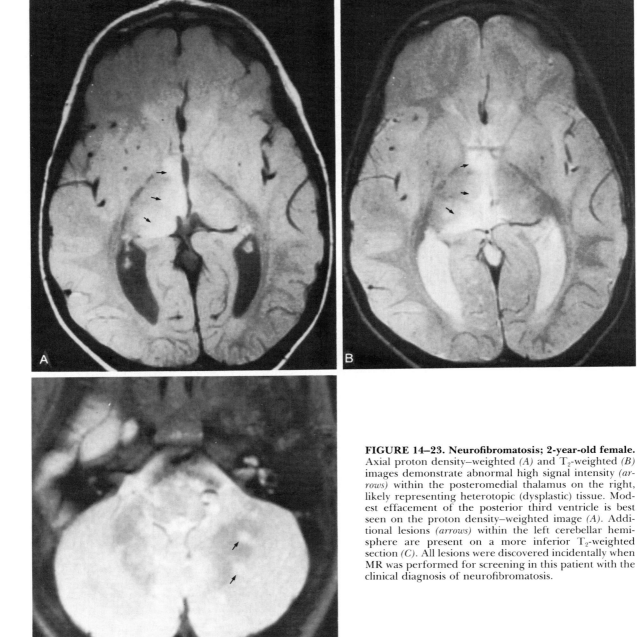

FIGURE 14–23. Neurofibromatosis; 2-year-old female.
Axial proton density–weighted *(A)* and T₂-weighted *(B)* images demonstrate abnormal high signal intensity *(arrows)* within the posteromedial thalamus on the right, likely representing heterotopic (dysplastic) tissue. Modest effacement of the posterior third ventricle is best seen on the proton density–weighted image *(A)*. Additional lesions *(arrows)* within the left cerebellar hemisphere are present on a more inferior T₂-weighted section *(C)*. All lesions were discovered incidentally when MR was performed for screening in this patient with the clinical diagnosis of neurofibromatosis.

nerve in all cases. In several instances, the normal CSF signal within Meckel cave was completely replaced by signal intensity identical to that of tumor. Extension of neoplasm from the gasserian ganglion to involve the cisternal portion of the fifth nerve was diagnosed in those cases. Coronal sequences helped demonstrate the medial margin of the roof of the internal auditory canal (IAC) separating the fifth nerve tumor above the petrous bone from the eighth nerve tumor within the IAC.[32]

Sturge-Weber Syndrome

Encephalotrigeminal angiomatosis is a phakomatosis that includes the following clinical characteristics: a facial vascular nevus in the territory of the ophthalmic division of the trigeminal nerve, seizures, dementia, hemiplegia, hemianopsia, and buphthalmos or glaucoma.[33] Intraparenchymal calcification, parenchymal volume loss, engorgement of deep veins, and leptomeningeal and choroid plexus an-

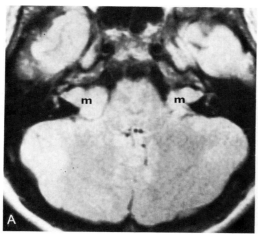

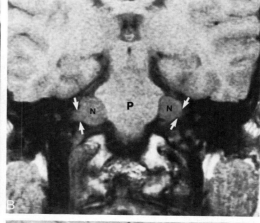

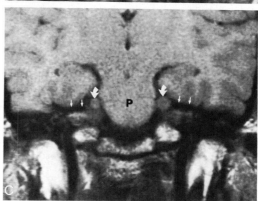

FIGURE 14–24. Neurofibromatosis; 17-year-old female. Axial proton density–weighted image (A) demonstrates bilateral fifth and eighth nerve neurinomas seen as single large masses (m) within both cerebellopontine angle cisterns. Coronal T_1-weighted images (B and C) distinguish hypointense (B) eighth nerve tumors (N) widening internal auditory canals (large straight arrows) and compressing pons (P) from slightly hypointense (C) neurinomas of cisternal portions of fifth nerves (curved arrows), cut in cross-section above roofs of internal auditory canals (small straight arrows) on slightly more anterior section.

giomata are seen at pathology.[12] The incidence of Sturge-Weber syndrome is 1 per 1000 patients in mental institutions. It appears sporadically.[3]

In patients with Sturge-Weber syndrome, MR reveals the following (Figs. 14–27 and 14–28).

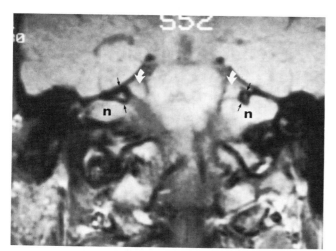

FIGURE 14–25. Neurofibromatosis; 19-year-old male. Coronal proton density–weighted image distinguishes bilateral isointense fifth nerve tumors (curved arrows) above roofs of internal auditory canals (straight arrows) from bilateral eighth nerve tumors (n) within enlarged internal auditory canals. Acoustic tumor on left extends into cerebellopontine angle cistern.

ATROPHY. Uni- or bilateral parenchymal volume loss may be associated with hemicranial atrophy (Fig. 14–27).[33] Thickened cortex and decreased convolutions in regions of parenchymal atrophy may represent disturbed neuronal proliferation and migration as a consequence of abnormal cerebral venous blood flow (Figs. 14–27 and 14–28).[33]

CALCIFICATION. Regions of hypointensity on T_2-weighted images were seen at the cortical-subcortical junction in areas of known parenchymal calcification detected by CT (Fig. 14–27). MR with spin-echo sequences continually underestimated the severity and extent of parenchymal calcification in this[33] and other[34] disorders. Recently, MR with gradient-echo acquisition proved to be more sensitive than spin-echo MR for the detection of intraparenchymal calcification.[35]

VASCULAR ANOMALIES. In one small series[33] no superficial regions of flow-related signal void, thrombosis, or other direct evidence suggested the presence of leptomeningeal angiomas. Nevertheless, a paucity of superficial cortical veins and engorgement and tortuosity of subependymal and medullary veins were seen on the affected side, providing important indirect evidence of abnormal cerebral hemodynamics (Fig. 14–27). Enlarged and calcified choroid plexus lesions, hyperintense on T_2-weighted images, are reported to represent angiomatous involvement.[33, 36]

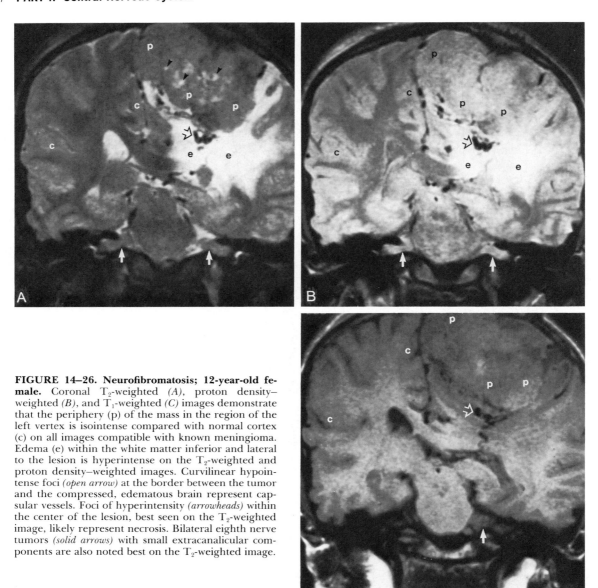

FIGURE 14–26. Neurofibromatosis; 12-year-old female. Coronal T$_2$-weighted *(A)*, proton density–weighted *(B)*, and T$_1$-weighted *(C)* images demonstrate that the periphery (p) of the mass in the region of the left vertex is isointense compared with normal cortex (c) on all images compatible with known meningioma. Edema (e) within the white matter inferior and lateral to the lesion is hyperintense on the T$_2$-weighted and proton density–weighted images. Curvilinear hypointense foci *(open arrow)* at the border between the tumor and the compressed, edematous brain represent capsular vessels. Foci of hyperintensity *(arrowheads)* within the center of the lesion, best seen on the T$_2$-weighted image, likely represent necrosis. Bilateral eighth nerve tumors *(solid arrows)* with small extracanalicular components are also noted best on the T$_2$-weighted image.

ACCELERATED MYELINATION. In three infants under the age of nine months, MR demonstrated accelerated myelination; affected white matter had prematurely decreased signal intensity on T$_2$-weighted images[33, 37] and had increased signal intensity on IR images (Fig. 14–28).[37] It is possible that ischemia of the brain parenchyma underlying the leptomeningeal angioma may lead to a hypermyelinative state once myelin begins to be laid down.[37]

Tuberous Sclerosis

This is a rare heredofamilial disease with the classic clinical triad of adenoma sebaceum (30 to 85 per cent of cases), seizures (80 per cent), and mental retardation (50 to 80 per cent). Hyperpigmented nevi (83 per cent), shagreen patches, subungual fibromas, rhabdomyomas and sarcomas of the heart, and angiomyolipomas of the kidney (80 per cent) may also be seen.[3] Its incidence varies from 1 in 20,000 to 1 in 500,000 persons.[27] The disorder is inherited in autosomal dominant fashion in 20 to 50 per cent of cases; a genetic mutation is believed to be responsible for the remainder.

In the CNS, tubers containing hamartomatous overgrowth of astrocytes and giant cells, and fibrillary gliosis may be seen in the cortex, white matter, or in a subependymal location. Tubers in a subependymal location have a greater tendency to calcify.[27] Subependymal and intraventricular giant cell astrocytoma occurs in 1.7 to 10 per cent of patients. These neoplasms, arising from the giant astrocytes within

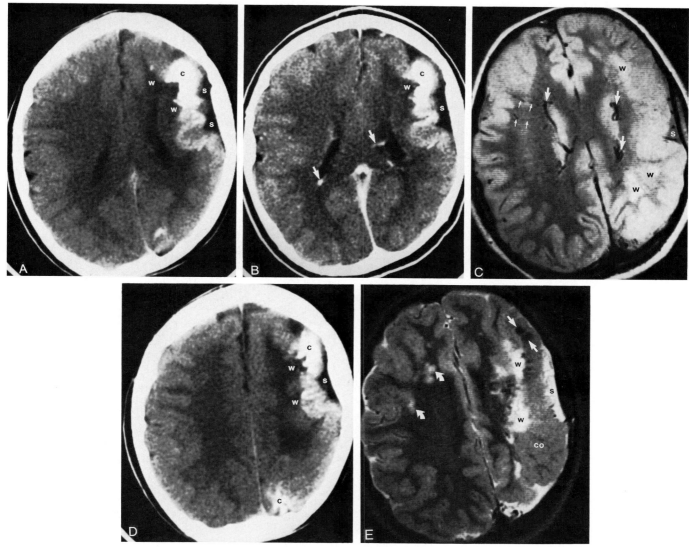

FIGURE 14–27. Sturge-Weber syndrome; 6-year-old male. Noncontrast *(A)* and postcontrast *(B)*, axial CT sections demonstrate prominent subarachnoid spaces (s) overlying atrophic left frontal lobe. Cortical calcification (c) and hypodense white matter (w) of the forceps minor are well shown. Proton density–weighted axial MR section *(C)* at the same level shows high signal intensity within the subcortical and periventricular white matter of the left frontal and parietal lobes (w). In addition, dilated medullary veins *(small arrows, C)* and subependymal veins *(large arrows, B and C)* are more obvious on MR. A paucity of superficial cortical veins is seen overlying the left hemisphere. No evidence of calcification is detected on MR examination at this level.

Noncontrast CT section *(D)* at a slightly higher level detects calcification (c) within the left occipital and frontal cortex. On corresponding T_2-weighted MR section *(E)*, two nonspecific foci of hypointensity measuring < 5 mm in diameter *(arrows)* are the only findings suggesting calcification. MR, however, shows best the thickened cortex (co) overlying the left parietal lobe (compare with *D*). MR also demonstrates abnormally high signal intensity within the white matter of the right frontal lobe *(curved arrows)* which appeared normal on CT (compare with *D*). Dilated subarachnoid spaces (s) and abnormal white matter (w) within the left centrum semiovale are also seen.

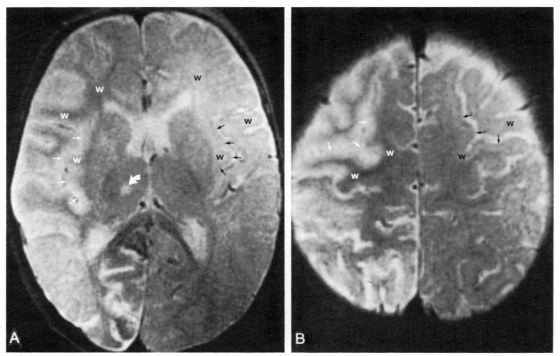

FIGURE 14–28. Sturge-Weber syndrome; 5-month-old female. Axial T_2-weighted MR images show abnormal thickening and high signal intensity affecting the insular cortex (*white arrows, A*) and cortex of the high right frontal lobe (*white arrows, B*). Compare with the normal cortex (*black arrows, A and B*) on the left side. White matter within the right forceps minor and beneath the thickened cortex (*white w, A and B*) has low signal intensity, unusual in a patient only five months in age. Compare with normal white matter (*black w, A and B*) on left side. A focal lesion (*curved arrow, A*) is also detected within the right thalamus.

subependymal nodules, are most frequently located adjacent to the foramen of Monro.

In patients with tuberous sclerosis, MR reveals the following (Fig. 14–29).

TUBERS. These lesions may be visualized as bilateral asymmetrical foci with central low signal and irregular ringlike borders of high signal on T_2-weighted images; they may be found in cortical, subcortical, white matter, and subependymal locations (Fig. 14–29).

CORTICAL HETEROTOPIAS. Owing to deranged neuroblast migration, focal islands of gray matter with cortexlike signal intensity on T_1- and T_2-weighted images may remain within the white matter of the hemispheres.

GIANT CELL ASTROCYTOMAS. These tumors are most frequently seen in the region of the foramen of Monro.

HYDROCEPHALUS. Tubers (or giant cell astrocytomas) located subependymally may restrict egress of CSF from the lateral or third ventricles by compressing the foramen of Monro or the aqueduct of Sylvius, respectively.

Hippel-Lindau Disease

This syndrome comprises disseminated capillary angiomas in the skin and viscera with, at times, cyst formation. The tumors in the CNS are called capil-

lary hemangioblastomas; lesions are found most frequently in the cerebellum (36 to 60 per cent of cases),[38] brain stem, or spinal cord (< 5 per cent). Tumors of the retina are also characteristic (> 50 per cent). Hemangioblastomas rarely occur in the cerebral hemispheres. Associated visceral lesions include renal cell carcinoma (25 to 38 per cent) and pheochromocytoma (> 10 per cent). The disease has autosomal dominant inheritance with nearly 100 per cent penetrance. Both sexes are affected equally.[12, 27, 38]

Clinical manifestations of patients with Hippel-Lindau disease include increased intracranial pressure, cerebellar dysfunction, subarachnoid hemorrhage, and polycythemia (secondary to hemangioblastoma, renal cell carcinoma, or pheochromocytoma).[27] The most common causes of death are cerebellar hemangioblastoma and renal cell carcinoma.

During a two-year study,[38] MR of the head, spine, and abdomen was used for screening and follow-up of 26 members of nine families with the disease. Lesions causing significant morbidity and mortality (cerebellar and spinal cord hemangioblastomas, renal cell carcinoma, and pheochromocytoma) were correctly depicted with MR imaging, sometimes before the lesions could be seen with other imaging modalities.

In most cases the intracranial tumor consists of a

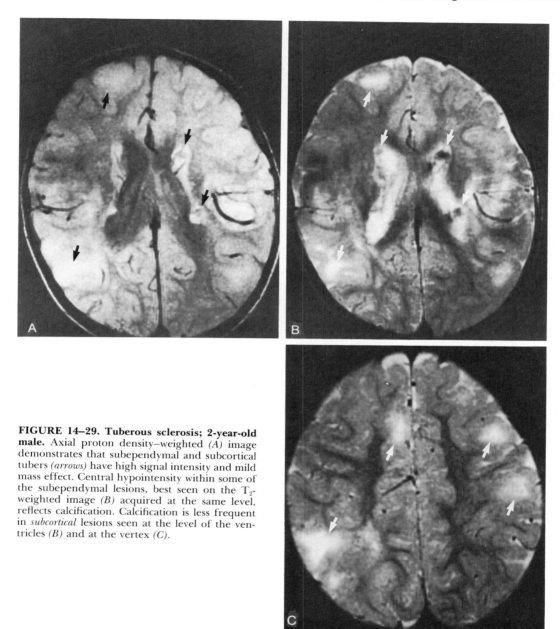

FIGURE 14–29. Tuberous sclerosis; 2-year-old male. Axial proton density–weighted *(A)* image demonstrates that subependymal and subcortical tubers *(arrows)* have high signal intensity and mild mass effect. Central hypointensity within some of the subependymal lesions, best seen on the T_2-weighted image *(B)* acquired at the same level, reflects calcification. Calcification is less frequent in *subcortical* lesions seen at the level of the ventricles *(B)* and at the vertex *(C)*.

vascular nodule incorporated into the wall of a cyst situated at the surface of the cerebellum (Fig. 14–30). The tumor may be completely solid in 20 per cent of cases. The tumor is often within the posterolateral aspect of the cerebellar hemisphere; the vermis may also be involved on occasion.

Cerebellar and spinal cord hemangioblastomas have a characteristic appearance on MR (Fig. 14–30). The vascular mural nodule is hyperintense compared with normal parenchyma on T_2-weighted images and hypo- to isointense on T_1-weighted images. The tumoral cyst has a relatively high protein content[27] and, therefore, often appears slightly hyperintense compared with normal CSF on both T_1- and T_2-weighted images. Detection of associated tumoral vessels as

regions of serpentine signal void may help to differentiate hemangioblastomas from other cystic neoplasms, such as cystic astrocytoma and medulloblastoma.

DISORDERS OF MIGRATION

Such disorders are characterized by abnormalities of the cerebral cortex: the cortical mantle may appear too thick, too flat, or too folded.[18] Often bilateral and symmetric, the neuronal migration abnormalities may be distinguished from the predominantly unilateral, acquired intrauterine insults caused by infection or infarction. The earlier the disturbance of

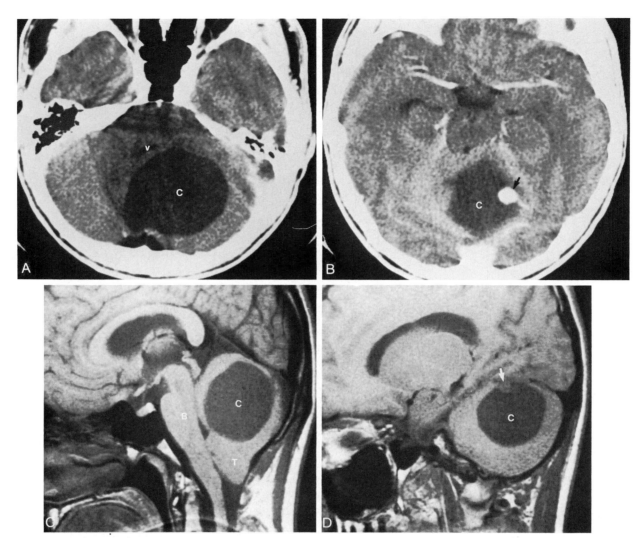

FIGURE 14–30. Hippel-Lindau disease and cerebellar hemangioblastoma; 32-year-old male. Axial postcontrast CT images *(A* and *B)* demonstrate a large cyst (C) within the left cerebellar hemisphere at the level of the fourth ventricle (v, *A)*, which is partially effaced. Highest section *(B)* shows enhancing mural tumor nodule *(arrow)*. T$_1$-weighted midline sagittal image *(C)* shows brain stem (B) flattened against the clivus, and tonsillar (T) herniation caused by large cystic component of tumor. Paramidline sagittal T$_1$-weighted image *(D)* sections through tumor nodule *(arrow)* situated along superior wall of the cyst. Nodule is isointense with cortex on this image. Proton density–weighted axial images *(E* and *F)* at levels similar to CT (compare with *A* and *B)* demonstrate mural tumor nodule *(arrow)* is slightly hyperintense relative to cortex in this pulse sequence *(F)*, whereas the cystic portion (C) is hypointense to cortex. *G* and *H*, Anteroposterior and lateral subtraction views of left vertebral artery injection demonstrate well the vascular tumor nodule (n) and stretching of cerebellar arteries *(arrowheads)* around the avascular mass (cyst on MR and CT).

Illustration continued on opposite page.

neuroblast migration, the more severe and generalized is the resulting cerebral deformity.

Lissencephaly

The most severe form of migrational disorder is associated with a smooth brain having no gyri. In most cases, however, regions of broad, flattened gyri (pachygyria) may be seen in the same hemisphere.[39] Lissencephaly occurs in association with abnormalities in other parts of the body as part of a syndrome (e.g., Miller-Dieker) or as an isolated abnormality.[40]

It may be inherited (autosomal recessive) or may occur spontaneously. The most severely affected patients with lissencephaly are decerebrate. All have mental retardation. Seizures develop by the age of one year; death ensues by the age of two years. Microscopically, the cortex has only four layers; in contrast, normal cortex has six layers. The cortex is thickened in this disorder due to arrest of the later waves of migrating neuroblasts. Accordingly, the white matter becomes reduced in size, and the cortical surface remains devoid of gyri.

On axial MR images, there is micrencephaly, with

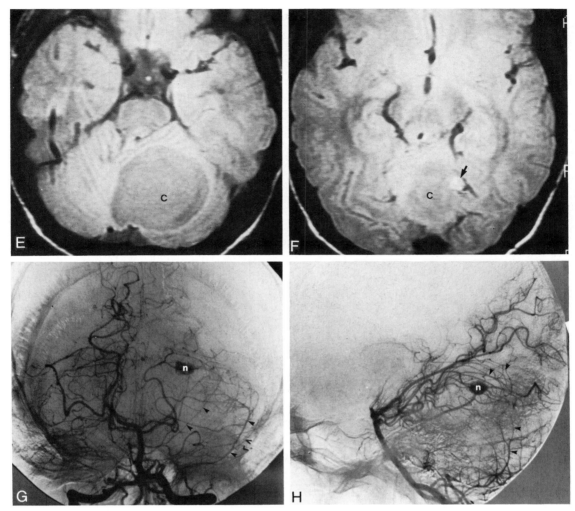

FIGURE 14–30 *Continued*

the cerebral hemispheres taking on an hourglass contour because the brain fails to develop opercula (Fig. 14–31). The insular cortex remains superficial, and the middle cerebral arteries course within shallow sylvian grooves. The claustrum and the extreme capsule are often absent. Other findings include atrophy of the corpus callosum, heterotopic nodules of gray matter near the lateral ventricles, and mild dilatation of the lateral ventricles with accentuation in the region of the atria and occipital horns (colpocephaly).[3, 39, 40]

Pachygyria

Pachygyria is a rare disorder occurring sporadically. The severity of clinical symptoms varies with the degree of morphologic derangement. The most severely affected patients may have a lack of awareness of the environment and severe mental retardation. Seizures may develop in childhood. Patients with pachygyria have a longer survival than those with lissencephaly. This anomaly may occur without associated agyria.

MR demonstrates abnormally broad and thickened gyri separated by shallow sulci (Fig. 14–32). All or only a part of the brain may be involved. The gray matter/white matter interface is abnormally smooth with incomplete digitations.[3]

Polymicrogyria

The final waves of neurons migrate to the cortex during the fifth to sixth month of fetal gestation; these neurons form the most superficial cortical layers. If these migrating neurons do not distribute normally at their final destination, an imbalance of growth rates may occur between cortical layers. Such an imbalance causes the formation of numerous small gyri—polymicrogyria.[12] The affected gyri may involve large areas of both hemispheres or be restricted to smaller regions in one or both hemispheres. Even at autopsy, polymicrogyria may be mistaken for pachygyria because the multiple small gyri have fused surfaces that are not exteriorized by sulci. This is a potential pitfall in imaging diagnosis.

Patients with small foci of polymicrogyria may be

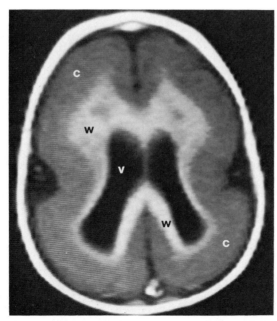

FIGURE 14–31. Lissencephaly; neonate. Axial T$_1$-weighted image demonstrates smooth brain surface has hourglass configuration. The white matter (w) is reduced in thickness due to premature arrest of later waves of migrating neuroblasts. Accordingly, the cortex (c) is thickened. Mild dilatation of the lateral ventricles (v) with posterior predominance is seen.

asymptomatic, but those with extensive regions are often retarded and have other neurologic deficits.

Heterotopic Gray Matter

Such lesions are islands of neurons located anywhere from the subependymal region to the cortex which result from arrested neuroblast migration. Heterotopias are a recognized focus of seizures.[41] They typically form nodular masses from 1 to 2 mm in size but may be considerably larger (Fig. 14–33). They may occur as isolated derangements or in association with other migrational abnormalities.[18] MR demonstrates heterotopias as nests of nerve cells within the white matter which have the same signal intensity as gray matter on T$_2$- and T$_1$-weighted or IR images (Fig. 14–33).[41] MR may detect heterotopias missed by CT before and after intravenous contrast administration.[41]

Schizencephaly

This term refers to full-thickness clefts within the cerebral hemispheres. At pathology, there is an infolding of gray matter along the cleft from the cortex to the ventricles and a fusion of the cortical pia and ventricular ependyma forming a pial-ependymal seam (Fig. 14–34). An ischemic episode occurring during the seventh week of gestation has been proposed as the underlying cause of these anomalies.[42] Two varieties of schizencephaly may be encountered: type I with fusion of the cleft lips and type II with open clefts allowing communication between the sylvian subarachnoid space and the lateral ventricles. Associated findings include (1) abnormal cortex (pachygyria) flanking and lining the cleft, (2) lateral ventricular diverticulum subjacent to the cleft, (3) hypoplastic sylvian vessels ipsilateral to the cleft, (4) absence of the septum pellucidum, (5) thinning of the corpus callosum, and (6) small pyramidal tracts owing to axonal loss.[43] MR proved to be more accurate than cranial ultrasonography and CT in the depiction of the pathoanatomy in two neonates with schizencephaly.[43]

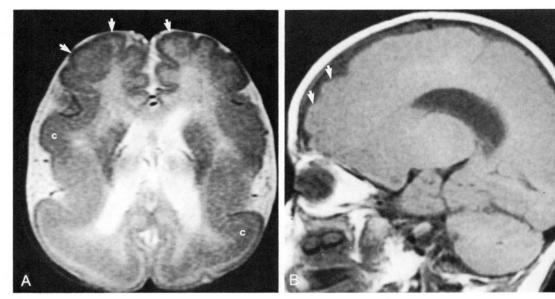

FIGURE 14–32. Pachygyria; neonate. Axial T$_2$-weighted *(A)* and sagittal T$_1$-weighted *(B)* images demonstrate frontal gyri *(arrows)* are abnormally broad and separated by shallow sulci. Posterior hemispheres are nearly agyric. Cortex (c) is abnormally thick, especially posteriorly, best seen on the T$_2$-weighted image *(A)*.

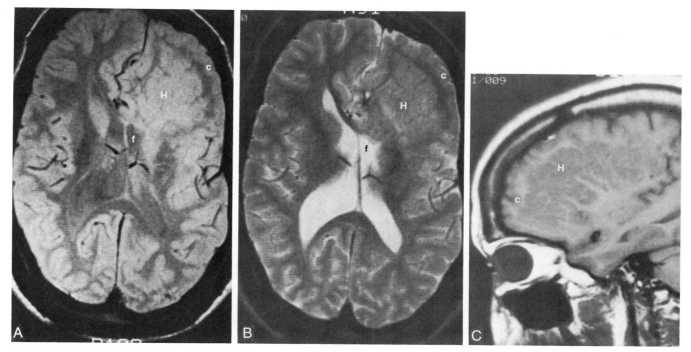

FIGURE 14–33. Heterotopic cortex; 22-year-old female. Large focus of nerve cells (H) within the white matter of the left frontal lobe has the same signal intensity as cortex (c) on proton density–weighted *(A)* and T$_2$-weighted *(B)* axial, and T$_1$-weighted *(C)* sagittal images. Cortical mantle (c) overlying the left frontal lobe is thinned. Left frontal horn (f, *A* and *B*) is effaced by mass effect.

FIGURE 14–34. Schizencephaly; 4-month-old. Proton density–weighted *(A)* axial image shows full thickness clefts (Cl) within both hemispheres. T$_2$-weighted image *(B)* at slightly higher level shows cortex (c) lining both clefts has lower signal intensity than underlying white matter (w) as expected in a subject of this age.

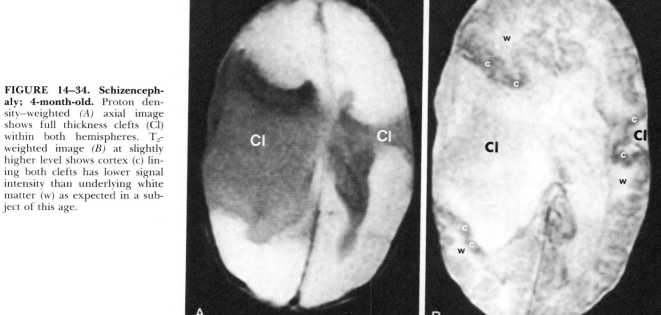

Anomalies of the Corpus Callosum

The numerous disorders of formation of the corpus callosum include partial or complete callosal agenesis, lipomas of the interhemispheric fissure, and callosal atrophy or "hypoplasia." Recent evidence[44] suggests that partial or complete callosal agenesis is caused by insults that arrest formation of callosal embryologic precursors (lamina reuniens, sulcus medianus telencephali medii, massa commissuralis) between eight and 13 weeks of gestation. Lipomas and sphenoidal encephaloceles probably occur as a result of faulty dysjunction of neuroectoderm and cutaneous ectoderm at the anterior neuropore.[44] A complete but atrophic corpus callosum results from an insult to the cortex or white matter after formation of the corpus callosum is complete (18 to 20 weeks of gestation).

The incidence of callosal agenesis is not known. It has been observed in 0.7 per cent of pneumoencephalograms. Most cases are sporadic; males and females are affected with equal frequency. Clinically, most patients with complete agenesis are asymptomatic. Careful examination may reveal that learning and memory are not shared between the hemispheres (cerebral disconnection syndrome).[3] When symptoms (seizures, developmental delay) are present, they are often related to concurrent migrational disorders, not the callosal anomaly itself.

In patients with callosal agenesis, MR demonstrates the following (Figs. 14–35 and 14–36).

PARENCHYMAL AND VASCULAR ANOMALIES. Midline sagittal images reveal the partial or complete absence of the corpus callosum and, possibly, the concurrent absence of the hippocampal and anterior commissures (Fig. 14–35). Since the axons from the

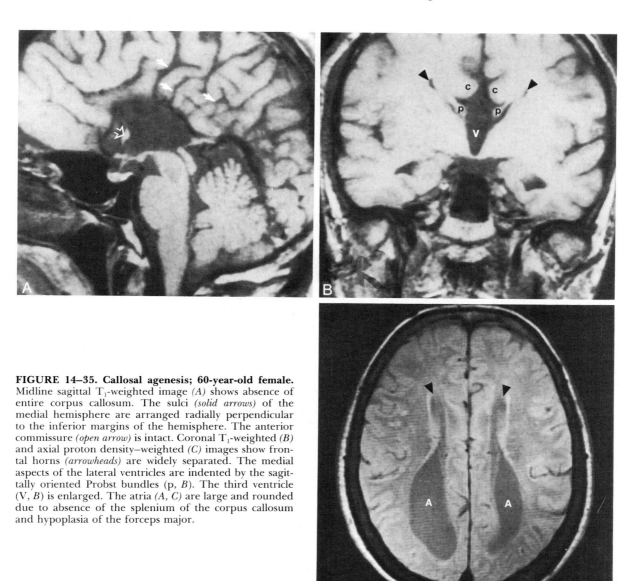

FIGURE 14–35. Callosal agenesis; 60-year-old female. Midline sagittal T₁-weighted image *(A)* shows absence of entire corpus callosum. The sulci *(solid arrows)* of the medial hemisphere are arranged radially perpendicular to the inferior margins of the hemisphere. The anterior commissure *(open arrow)* is intact. Coronal T₁-weighted *(B)* and axial proton density–weighted *(C)* images show frontal horns *(arrowheads)* are widely separated. The medial aspects of the lateral ventricles are indented by the sagittally oriented Probst bundles (p, *B*). The third ventricle (V, *B*) is enlarged. The atria (A, *C*) are large and rounded due to absence of the splenium of the corpus callosum and hypoplasia of the forceps major.

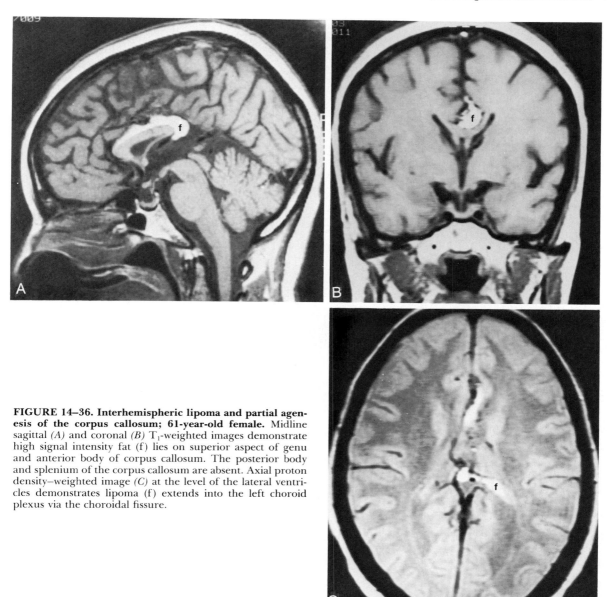

FIGURE 14–36. Interhemispheric lipoma and partial agenesis of the corpus callosum; 61-year-old female. Midline sagittal *(A)* and coronal *(B)* T_1-weighted images demonstrate high signal intensity fat (f) lies on superior aspect of genu and anterior body of corpus callosum. The posterior body and splenium of the corpus callosum are absent. Axial proton density–weighted image *(C)* at the level of the lateral ventricles demonstrates lipoma (f) extends into the left choroid plexus via the choroidal fissure.

hemispheres do not cross in the commissure, they course sagittally instead to establish paired bundles along the medial aspects of the lateral ventricles known as the bundles of Probst (Fig. 14–35). The parietooccipital and calcarine sulci fail to intersect. Like the other sulci of the medial hemisphere, they become radially oriented perpendicular to the narrow inferior margin of the hemisphere (Fig. 14–35). Abnormal formation of the cerebral cortex with agyria, pachygyria, polymicrogyria, and gray matter heterotopias may be seen. Lateral separation of the pericallosal arteries and internal cerebral veins may be caused by a high third ventricle and/or interhemispheric cyst. Azygous anterior cerebral arteries may be seen.

VENTRICULAR AND CSF-SPACE ANOMALIES. The small frontal horns are widely separated with concave medial borders and sharply angled lateral peaks (Fig. 14–35). The medial walls of the frontal horns diverge, forming an angle that opens anteriorly. The third ventricle is large in size and may have a high position. A variably large interhemispheric cyst may spread the hemispheres; the cyst may communicate freely with the third ventricle or may consist of multiple poorly or noncommunicating lobules. The atria are large and rounded secondary to absence of the splenium and hypoplasia of the forceps major.

INTERHEMISPHERIC LIPOMAS (Fig. 14–36).[45] Forty per cent of patients with these rare lesions have callosal agenesis. Lipomas appear as variably asymmetric masses of fat within the interhemispheric fissure, usually adjacent to the genu. The lesion may

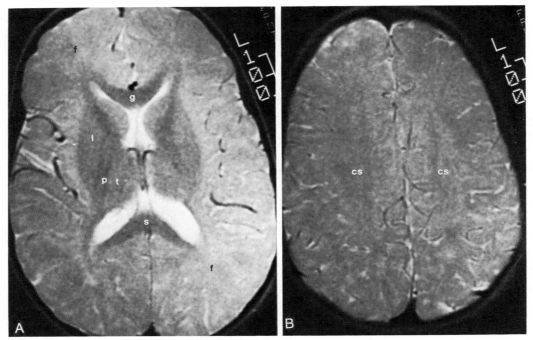

FIGURE 14–37. Delayed myelination in a patient with development and speech delay; 4-year-old female. Axial T₂-weighted images (A and B) demonstrate that mature myelin within the genu (g) and splenium (s) of the corpus callosum, posterior limb of the internal capsule (p), and lentiform nucleus (l) has decreased signal intensity. White matter of the forceps minor and major (f) and centrum semiovale (cs) remains isointense with the cortex indicating delayed myelination in these areas. (Myelination of all white matter tracts should be completed by two years postnatally.⁹)

extend to the choroid plexus uni- or bilaterally through the choroidal fissure. The pericallosal arteries course through the lipoma.

DISORDERS OF MYELINATION

The early landmarks of normal myelination have been discussed (see "Myelination" above and Figs. 14–1 through 14–7). Many reports have described delayed myelination in association with hydrocephalus,⁴⁶ presumed rubella infection,⁴⁴ periventricular leukomalacia,⁴⁸, ⁴⁹ and cerebral palsy.⁴⁴ In one series including 33 infants⁵⁰ with delayed myelination, hydrocephalus was detected also in 9, bronchopulmo-

nary dysplasia in 14, infarction and/or cerebral atrophy in 18, and respiratory insufficiency requiring assisted ventilation in 25 infants. In a group with normal myelination, no infants with these problems were seen.

Preliminary results indicate that delay in myelination observed by MR methods may have prognostic implications.⁵⁰ In a small series of 13 infants with initial delayed myelination who had a repeat MR examination in the first year of life, the condition persisted in 11 infants. Seven infants proceeded to have developmental delay (Fig. 14–37).⁵⁰

Myelination delay has been reported also in patients with nonketotic hyperglycinemia (NKH), a heritable disorder of amino acid metabolism in which

FIGURE 14–38. Patient with nonketotic hyperglycinemia and abnormal progress of myelination. *A–C,* Initial (8 days postnatal) axial T₂-weighted MR images demonstrate normal myelination of the brain as decreased signal intensity limited to the dorsal brain stem (b), ventrolateral thalami (t), and paracentral gyri of the cortex (g). The forceps major and minor (f), internal capsule (i), and centrum semiovale (cs) are not myelinated at this age and appear hyperintense relative to the cortex, as expected.⁹

D–F, Follow-up (10 months postnatal) axial T₂-weighted MR images demonstrate interval dilatation of ventricles (v) and subarachnoid spaces overlying the hemispheres (s) compatible with moderate volume loss (compare with *B* and *C*). Decreased signal intensity within the entire brain stem, middle cerebellar peduncles (p), and deep white matter of the cerebellum reflects normal interval progression of myelination in these regions *(D).* However, white matter within forceps major and minor (f), external capsule (e), and centrum semiovale (cs) remains distinctly brighter than the cortex and basal ganglia *(E and F),* indicating delayed myelination in these areas. (The cortex, underlying white matter, and basal ganglia regions should appear essentially isointense in a normal 10-month-old.⁹)

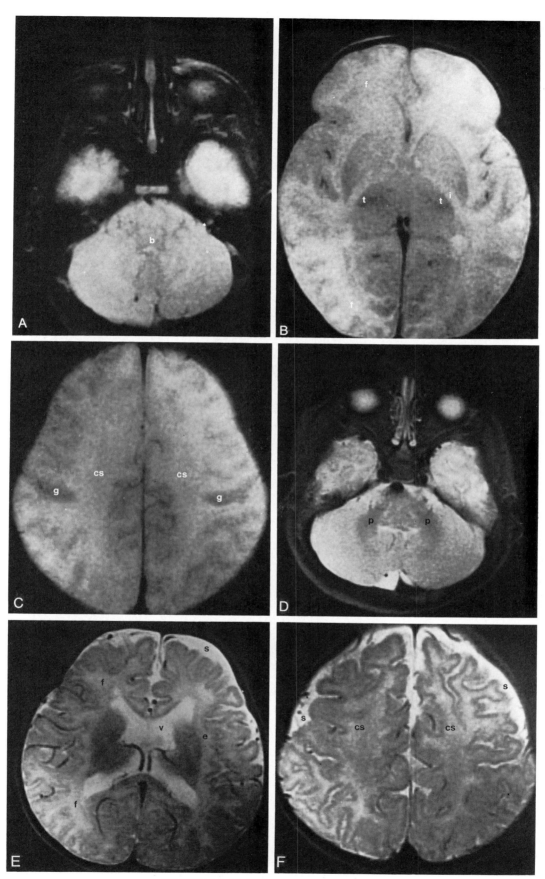

FIGURE 14–38 *See legend on opposite page*

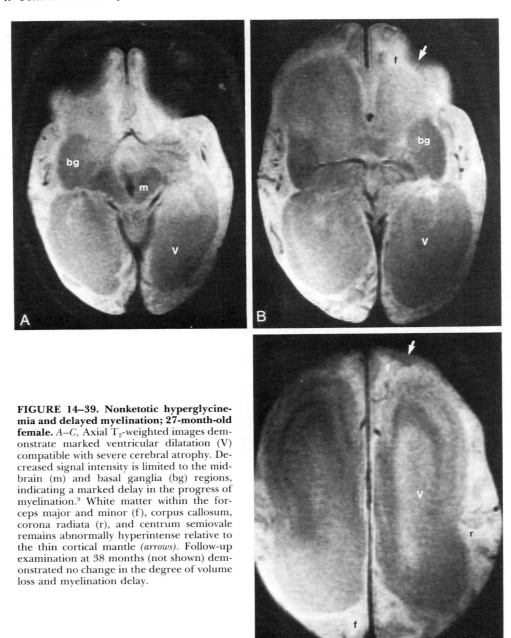

FIGURE 14–39. Nonketotic hyperglycinemia and delayed myelination; 27-month-old female. *A–C,* Axial T$_2$-weighted images demonstrate marked ventricular dilatation (V) compatible with severe cerebral atrophy. Decreased signal intensity is limited to the midbrain (m) and basal ganglia (bg) regions, indicating a marked delay in the progress of myelination.[9] White matter within the forceps major and minor (f), corpus callosum, corona radiata (r), and centrum semiovale remains abnormally hyperintense relative to the thin cortical mantle *(arrows).* Follow-up examination at 38 months (not shown) demonstrated no change in the degree of volume loss and myelination delay.

large quantities of glycine accumulate in plasma, urine, and CSF.[51] Onset of this disease occurs most often in early infancy. Clinical manifestations include seizures, abnormal muscle tone and reflexes, and pronounced developmental delay. Death ensues usually before the age of five years.[51] When assessed using T$_2$-weighted images, decreased or absent myelination within supratentorial white matter tracts was detected in four NKH patients greater than 10 months in age. Myelination of the brain stem and cerebellum was normal (Figs. 14–38 and 14–39). Abnormalities shown by MR correlate well with known pathologic findings in patients with NKH.

Accelerated myelination has been detected on MR in three infants under the age of five months with Sturge-Weber syndrome.[33, 37] MR findings in such patients are described earlier in this chapter (see Fig. 14–28).

REFERENCES

1. Volpe JJ: Neurology of the Newborn. 2nd ed. Vol 22. Major Problems in Clinical Pediatrics. Philadelphia, WB Saunders Company, 1987.
2. van der Knapp MS, Valk J: Classification of congenital abnormalities of the CNS. AJNR 9:315–326, 1988.

3. Naidich TP, Zimmerman RA: Common congenital malformations of the brain. *In* Brant-Zawadzki M, Norman D (eds): Magnetic Resonance Imaging of the Central Nervous System. New York, Raven Press, 1987, pp 131–150.

4. Volpe JJ: Normal and abnormal human brain development. Clin Perinatol 4:3–30, 1977.

5. Larroche JC: Development of the nervous system in early life. Part II: The development of the central nervous system during intrauterine life. *In* Falkner F (ed): Human Development. Philadelphia, WB Saunders Company, 1966, pp 257–276.

6. Scammon RE, Hesdorffer MB: Growth of the human nervous system; indices of relation of cerebral volume to surface in developmental period. Proc Soc Exp Biol Med 33:418–421, 1935.

7. McArdle CB, Richardson CJ, Nicholas DA, et al: Developmental features: MR imaging. I. Gray-white matter differentiation and myelination. Radiology 162:223–229, 1987.

8. McArdle CB, Richardson CJ, Hayden CK, et al: Abnormalities of the neonatal brain: MR imaging. II. Hypoxic-ischemic brain injury. Radiology 163:395–403, 1987.

9. Barkovich AJ, Kjos BO, Jackson DE Jr, Norman D: Normal maturation of the neonatal and infant brain: MR imaging at 1.5 T. Radiology 166:173–180, 1988.

10. Byrd S, Naidich TP: Common congenital brain abnormalities. Radiol Clin North Am 26:755–772, 1988.

11. Friede RL: Developmental Neuropathology. New York, Springer-Verlag, 1975.

12. Larroche JC: Malformations of the nervous system. *In* Adams JH, Carsellis JAN, Ducken LW (eds): Greenfield's Neuropathology. 4th ed. New York, John Wiley & Sons, 1985.

13. Zimmerman RA, Bilaniuk LT: Pediatric central nervous system. *In* Stark DD, Bradley WG Jr (eds): Magnetic Resonance Imaging. St. Louis, CV Mosby, 1988, pp 683–714.

14. Spinos E, Lasler DW, Moody DM, et al: MR evaluation of Chiari I malformations at 0.15 T. AJNR 6:203–208, 1985.

15. Barkovich AJ, Wippold FJ, Sherman JL, et al: Significance of cerebellar tonsillar position on MR. AJNR 7:795–799, 1986.

16. Wolpert SM, Anderson M, Scott RM, et al: Chiari II malformation: MR imaging evaluation. AJNR 8:783–792, 1987.

17. Emery JL: Deformity of the aqueduct of Sylvius in children with hydrocephalus and meningomyelocele. Dev Med Child Neurol (Suppl) 16(32):40–48, 1974.

18. Zimmerman RA: Congenital abnormalities. Syllabus for the Categorical Course on MR, 1985. The American College of Radiology.

19. Arrington JA, Martinez CR, Kaffenberger DA, et al: Associated intracranial abnormalities with septo-optic dysplasia: Evaluation with CT and MRI. AJNR 8:951, 1987 (abstract).

20. Barkovich AJ, Kjos BO, Edwards MS, Norman D: New concepts in posterior fossa cysts in children. Presented at the 26th Annual Meeting of the American Society of Neuroradiology, Chicago, May 15–20, 1988.

21. Macchi G, Bentivoglio M: Agenesis or hypoplasia of cerebellar structures. *In* Vinkin PJ, Bruyn GW (eds): Congenital Malformations of the Brain and Skull. Amsterdam, North Holland Publishing Company, 1977, pp 367–393.

22. DeMorsier G: Études sur les dysraphies cranio-encephaliques. II. Agenesie du vermis cerebelleux-dysraphie rhombocephalique mediane (rhomboschisis). Monatsschr Psychiatr Neurol 129:321–344, 1955.

23. Joubert M, Eisenring JJ, Robb JP, Andermann F: Familial agenesis of the cerebellar vermis. A syndrome of episodic hyperpnea, abnormal eye movements, ataxia and retardation. Neurology 19:813–825, 1969.

24. Press GA, Murakami J, Courchesne E, et al: The cerebellum in sagittal plane: Anatomic-MR correlation. Part II. The cerebellar hemispheres. AJNR 10:667–676, 1989.

25. Courchesne E, Yeung-Courchesne R, Press GA, et al: Hypoplasia of cerebellar vermal lobules VI and VII in infantile autism. N Engl J Med 318:1349–1954, 1988.

26. Benda CE: Down's Syndrome. Mongolism and its Management. New York, Grune and Stratton, 1969, pp 134–166.

27. Braffman BH, Bilaniuk LT, Zimmerman RA: The central nervous system manifestations of the phakomatoses on MR. Radiol Clin North Am 26:773–800, 1988.

28. Mulvihill JJ: Tentative definitions of neurofibromatosis. Neurofibromatosis Research Newsletter 2(2):1, 1986.

29. Riccardi VM: Alternative forms of neurofibromatosis. *In* Neurofibromatosis: Program and Abstracts. NIH Consensus Development Conference, July 1987, pp 32–35.

30. Goodman RM, Gorlin RJ: Atlas of the Face in Genetic Disorders. 2nd ed. St Louis, CV Mosby, 1977.

31. Bognanno JR, Edwards MK, Lee TA, et al: Cranial MR imaging in neurofibromatosis. AJNR 9:461–468, 1988.

32. Press GA, Hesselink JR: MR imaging of cerebellopontine angle and internal auditory canal lesions at 1.5 T. AJNR 9:241–251, 1988.

33. Chamberlain MC, Press GA, Hesselink JR: MR and CT in three cases of Sturge-Weber syndrome: A prospective comparison. AJNR 10:491–496, 1989.

34. Oot RF, New PJF, Pile-Spellman J, et al: The detection of intracranial calcifications by MR. AJNR 7:801–809, 1986.

35. Atlas SW, Grossman RI, Hackney DB, et al: Calcified intracranial lesions: Detection with gradient-echo acquisition rapid MR imaging. AJNR 9:253–259, 1988.

36. Stimac GK, Solomon MA, Newton TH: CT and MR of angiomatous malformations of the choroid plexus in patients with Sturge-Weber disease. AJNR 7:629–632, 1986.

37. Jacoby CG, Yuh WTC, Afifi AK, et al: Accelerated myelination in early Sturge-Weber syndrome demonstrated by MR imaging. J Comput Assist Tomogr 11:226–231, 1987.

38. Sato Y, Waziri M, Smith W, et al: Hippel-Lindau disease: MR imaging. Radiology 166:241–246, 1988.

39. Byrd SE, Bohan TP, Osborn RE, Naidich TP: The CT and MR evaluation of lissencephaly. AJNR 9:923–927, 1988.

40. Lee BCP, Engel M: MR of lissencephaly. AJNR 9:804, 1988.

41. Dunn V, Mock T, Bell WE, Smith W: Detection of heterotopic grey matter in children by magnetic resonance imaging. Magn Reson Imaging 4:33–39, 1986.

42. Barkovich AJ, Norman D: MR imaging of schizencephaly. AJNR 9:297–302, 1988.

43. Chamberlain MC, Press GA, Bejar RF, Hesselink JR: Neonatal schizencephaly: Comparison of MR, CT and US in two patients. J Child Neurol (submitted for publication).

44. Barkovich AJ, Norman D: Anomalies of the corpus callosum: Correlation with further anomalies of the brain. AJNR 9:493–501, 1988.

45. Dean B, Drayer BP, Beresini DC, Bird CR: MR imaging of pericallosal lipoma. AJNR 9:929–931, 1988.

46. Johnson MA, Pennock JM, Bydder GM, et al: Clinical NMR imaging of the brain in children: Normal and neurologic disease. AJR 141:1005–1018, 1983.

47. Levene MI, Whitelaw A, Dubowitz V, et al: Nuclear magnetic resonance imaging of the brain in children. Br Med J 285:774–776, 1982.

48. Dubowitz LM, Bydder GM, Mushin J: Developmental sequence of periventricular leukomalacia: Correlation of ultrasound, clinical and nuclear magnetic resonance functions. Arch Dis Child 60:349–355, 1985.

49. Wilson DA, Steiner RE: Periventricular leukomalacia: Evaluation with MR imaging. Radiology 160:507–511, 1986.

50. McArdle CB: MRI helps detect injury in neonatal, infant brain. Diagn Imaging 9:272–278, 1987.

51. Press GA, Barshop BA, Haas RH, et al: Abnormalities of the brain in nonketotic hyperglycinemia: MR manifestations. AJNR 10:315–321, 1989.

15

BRAIN: Neoplasia

RICHARD J. HICKS, JOHN R. HESSELINK, GARY L. WISMER,
and KENNETH R. DAVIS

CEREBRAL GLIOMAS
   ASTROCYTOMA
   OLIGODENDROGLIOMA
   MR FEATURES OF GLIOMAS
LYMPHOMA
METASTATIC DISEASE
MENINGIOMA
PINEAL REGION TUMORS
SELLAR AND PERISELLAR LESIONS
   PITUITARY ADENOMA
   CHIASMATIC/HYPOTHALAMIC GLIOMAS
   CRANIOPHARYNGIOMA
   DIFFERENTIAL DIAGNOSIS

BENIGN CYSTIC MASSES
   ARACHNOID CYST
   EPIDERMOID CYST
   GIANT CHOLESTEROL CYST
   DERMOID CYST

COLLOID CYST
DIFFERENTIAL DIAGNOSIS
NERVE SHEATH TUMORS
   ACOUSTIC NEUROMA
   OTHER CRANIAL NERVE NEUROMAS
BRAIN STEM AND CEREBELLUM
   BRAIN STEM GLIOMA
   EPENDYMOMA
   CHOROID PLEXUS PAPILLOMA
   CEREBELLAR ASTROCYTOMA
   MEDULLOBLASTOMA
   HEMANGIOBLASTOMA
   DIFFERENTIAL DIAGNOSIS
SKULL BASE LESIONS
   CHORDOMA
   CHONDROMA AND CHONDROSARCOMA
   MR FEATURES
   PARAGANGLIOMA
   DIFFERENTIAL DIAGNOSIS

In the diagnostic work-up of intracranial tumors, the primary goals of the imaging studies are to detect the abnormality, localize and determine its extent, characterize the lesion, and provide a list of differential diagnoses or, if possible, the specific diagnosis. Correlative studies have proved that MR is more sensitive than CT for detecting intracranial masses.[1, 2] Moreover, the multiplanar capability of MR is very helpful to determine the anatomic site of origin of lesions and to demarcate extension into adjacent compartments and brain structures. The superior contrast resolution of MR displays the different components of lesions more clearly. In particular, MR elucidates cystic lesions, as it appears to be better than CT in distinguishing arachnoid cysts, hemorrhagic cysts, tumoral cysts, and postoperative cysts.[3] High signal intensity on T_1- and T_2-weighted images has been noted in hemorrhagic cysts as well as in colloid cysts. In the latter this has been attributed to very high protein content. Collections that were nearly isointense with cerebrospinal fluid (CSF) on T_1-weighted images but which became brighter than CSF on T_2-weighted images correlated with tumoral and inflammatory cysts, but this has also been noted in some cases of arachnoid and postoperative cysts, perhaps related to diminished CSF pulsations in these collections.[4] MR can assess the vascularity of lesions without contrast infusion. On the other hand, CT detects calcification far better than MR, a useful finding for differential diagnosis.[5] Gradient-echo techniques improve MR detection of calcification by accentuating the diamagnetic susceptibility properties of calcium salts, but the observed low signal on T_2-weighted images is nonspecific, in that any accompanying paramagnetic ions would produce the same effect.[6] Nevertheless, at least the gradient-echo image detects the probable calcification, and if that information is important, CT can be done to confirm or disprove the MR finding.

A disappointing feature of MR has been the lack of specificity. Initial hopes of precise tissue characterization by T_1 and T_2 values have proven unrealistic. Although T_1 and T_2 relaxation times vary among different pathologic tissues, the numbers overlap and are not helpful.[7, 8]

When going through the exercise of differential diagnosis, localization of the mass to a specific region of the intracranial cavity is very important, because most tumors occur in certain places and not in others. First, is the lesion intraaxial or extraaxial? If extraaxial, for example, is it in the sella turcica, the pineal region, or a parasagittal location? Is it a solitary lesion or a multifocal process? Once the location of a solitary mass has been determined, then the internal texture and enhancement features help narrow the list of differential possibilities further.

Gadolinium–diethylene triamine pentaacetic acid (Gd-DTPA) or gadopentetate dimeglumine (Magnevist, Berlex Laboratories, Wayne, NJ) increases both the sensitivity and the specificity of MR.[9] Gd-DTPA is a blood-brain barrier (BBB) contrast agent like iodinated agents for CT. It does not cross the intact BBB, but when the BBB is absent or deficient, Gd-DTPA enters the interstitial space to produce enhancement (increased signal) on T_1-weighted images. All the collective knowledge learned from contrast-enhanced CT can be applied directly to the Gd-DTPA–enhanced MR images. The mechanisms of paramagnetic enhancement and contrast agents for MR are discussed in Chapters 6 and 7, respectively. The dosage for Gd-DTPA and pulse sequence selection are covered in Chapter 13.

Although the enhancement patterns are not tumor specific, the additional information is often helpful for diagnosis. Lesions can be classified as homogeneous or heterogeneous, and necrotic and cystic components are seen more clearly. The margins of enhancement provide a gross measure of tumor extension.[10–12] Contrast MR is particularly valuable for extraaxial tumors because they tend to be isointense to the brain on plain scan.[13, 14]

Any intracranial structures that do not have a BBB will enhance and should not be confused with pathology. Enhancement is routinely seen in the choroid plexus, pituitary gland, infundibulum, dura, cavernous sinuses, cortical veins, and sinus mucosa. Enhancement is more variable in the superior sagittal and transverse sinuses. Rapid-flowing arteries do not enhance.[15]

CEREBRAL GLIOMAS

Gliomas are malignant tumors of the glial cells of the brain and account for 30 to 40 per cent of all primary intracranial tumors. They occur predomi-

nantly in the cerebral hemispheres, but the brain stem and cerebellum are frequent locations in children (see "Brain Stem and Cerebellum"), and they are also found in the spinal cord (see Chapter 23). The peak incidence is during middle adult life, when patients present with seizures or symptoms related to the location of the gliomas and the brain structures involved.

ASTROCYTOMA

Astrocytomas are graded according to their histologic appearance. The higher Grades 3 and 4, also called glioblastomas, are very cellular and pleomorphic. They are very aggressive tumors, readily infiltrate adjacent brain structures, and have a uniformly poor prognosis. The lower grade astrocytomas (Grades 1 and 2) have more well-differentiated astrocytes, and the clinical course often proceeds over many years. These tumors often have cystic components, and calcification is not uncommon. Unfortunately, with time the histology frequently changes to a more malignant grade.[16]

OLIGODENDROGLIOMA

Oligodendrogliomas are the most benign of the gliomas. Calcification is common, and they occur predominantly in the frontal lobes. Ependymomas originate from the ependymal lining of the ventricles; they are discussed in the section on brain stem and cerebellar lesions.

MR FEATURES OF GLIOMAS

The common signal characteristics of intraaxial tumors include high signal intensity on T_2-weighted images and low signal on T_1-weighted images, unless fat or hemorrhage is present. Fat and subacute hemorrhages (methemoglobin) exhibit high signal on T_1-weighted images, and acute hemorrhage (deoxyhemoglobin) and chronic hemorrhage (hemosiderin/ferritin) show low signal intensity on T_2-weighted scans (see Chapter 16). Gliomas have poorly defined margins on plain MR. They infiltrate along white matter fiber tracts, and the deeper lesions have a propensity to extend across the corpus callosum into the opposite hemisphere (Fig. 15–1). They are often quite large by the time of clinical presentation.

The higher grade gliomas appear heterogeneous due to central necrosis with cellular debris, fluid, and hemorrhage. Peritumoral edema and mass effect are common features (Fig. 15–2). Following injection of Gd-DTPA, T_1-weighted images show irregular ring enhancement, with nodularity and nonenhancing necrotic foci.[17] As mentioned above, gliomas are infiltrative lesions, and microscopic fingers of tumor usually extend beyond the margin of enhancement.[18]

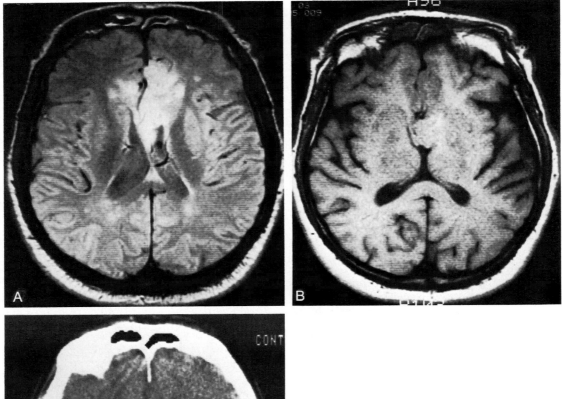

FIGURE 15–1. 40-year-old man with a low grade astrocytoma. *A,* Proton density–weighted image (SE 3000/20) shows a hyperintense mass within the anterior body and genu of the corpus callosum which compresses the lateral ventricles. The tumor extends into both medial frontal lobes. *B,* On a T$_1$-weighted image (SE 600/20) the glioma is primarily isointense to brain tissue. *C,* Contrast-enhanced CT scan reveals two foci of calcification which are not evident on the MR scans. The tumor does not enhance.

Enhanced scans are particularly helpful to outline subependymal spread of tumor along a ventricular surface, as well as leptomeningeal involvement.

The lower grade astrocytomas tend to be more homogeneous without central necrosis. Large cystic components may be present. The cysts have smooth walls, and the fluid is of uniform signal, to distinguish them from necrosis.[12] Enhancement is variable, depending on the integrity of the BBB (Fig. 15–3). Preliminary data suggest that a higher percentage of gliomas, but not all, will enhance on MR than CT.[10] The nonenhancing lesions will remain a challenge for diagnosis and for directing therapeutic measures.

Radiotherapists are beginning to rely more on MR for radiation treatment planning. The advantages of MR are its multiplanar capabilities and better visualization of brain stem and posterior fossa lesions. Although the margins between tumor and edema are not clearly depicted, in most cases the interface is seen better with MR than CT. In cases of oligodendrogliomas, measurements of tumor volumes were found to be more accurate with MR.[19] The possibility of microscopic infiltration of tumor into areas of edema has influenced some radiotherapists to include the entire extent of the signal abnormality on MR in the radiation field for gliomas.[20]

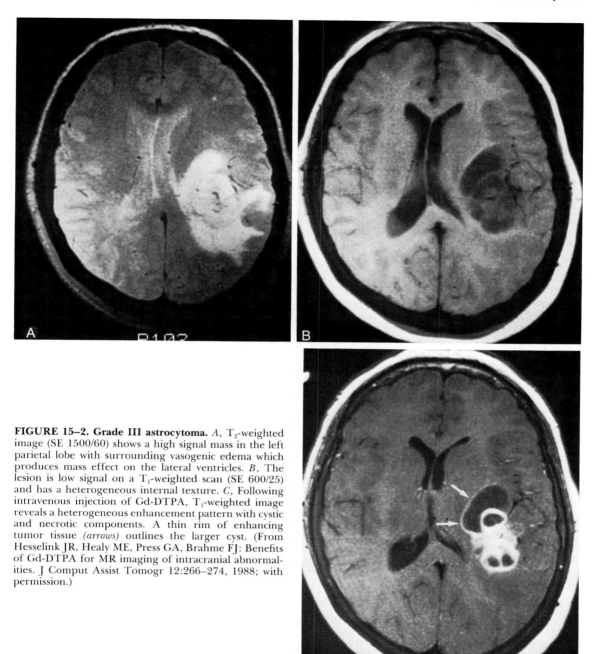

FIGURE 15–2. Grade III astrocytoma. *A*, T$_2$-weighted image (SE 1500/60) shows a high signal mass in the left parietal lobe with surrounding vasogenic edema which produces mass effect on the lateral ventricles. *B*, The lesion is low signal on a T$_1$-weighted scan (SE 600/25) and has a heterogeneous internal texture. *C*, Following intravenous injection of Gd-DTPA, T$_1$-weighted image reveals a heterogeneous enhancement pattern with cystic and necrotic components. A thin rim of enhancing tumor tissue *(arrows)* outlines the larger cyst. (From Hesselink JR, Healy ME, Press GA, Brahme FJ: Benefits of Gd-DTPA for MR imaging of intracranial abnormalities. J Comput Assist Tomogr 12:266–274, 1988; with permission.)

LYMPHOMA

Primary malignant lymphoma, formerly called reticulum cell sarcoma, histiocytic lymphoma, and microglioma, is a non-Hodgkin's lymphoma that occurs in the brain in the absence of systemic involvement. These tumors are highly cellular and grow rapidly. About 70 per cent represent large-cell variants of the B-cell type. Favorite sites include the deeper parts of the frontal and parietal lobes, basal ganglia, and hypothalamus. Most occur in patients who are immunocompromised secondary to chemotherapy or acquired immunodeficiency syndrome (AIDS) or in organ transplant recipients who are on immunosuppressant drugs.[21] Cerebral lymphomas are very radiosensitive and respond dramatically to steroid therapy.

Lymphomas typically appear as homogeneous, slightly high signal to isointense masses deep within the brain on T$_2$-weighted images (Fig. 15–4). The observed mild T$_2$ prolongation is probably related to dense cell packing within these tumors, leaving rela-

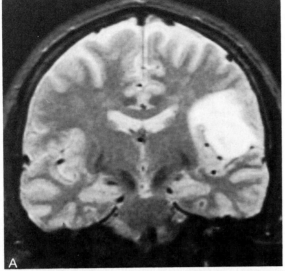

FIGURE 15–3. A low grade astrocytoma in a 42-year-old man with seizures. *A*, T₂-weighted coronal scan (SE 2000/70) demonstrates a hyperintense mass in the left posterior frontal lobe which expands the operculum and deforms the adjacent sylvian fissure. *B*, The mass is hypointense and slightly heterogeneous on the T₁-weighted image (SE 600/25). *C*, The postcontrast image (SE 600/25) shows enhancement in the superior portion of the tumor, indicating only partial breakdown of the blood-brain barrier.

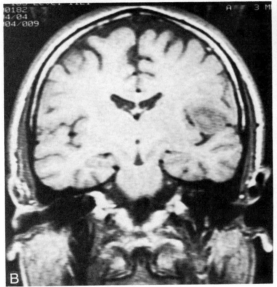

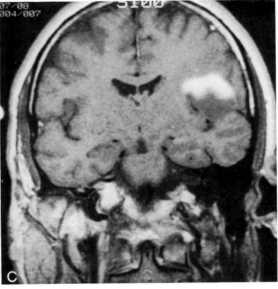

tively little interstitial space for accumulation of water. They are frequently found in close proximity to the corpus callosum and have a propensity to extend across the corpus callosum into the opposite hemisphere, a feature that mimics glioblastoma. Multiple lesions are present in as many as 50 per cent.[22] Despite their rapid growth, central necrosis is uncommon. They are associated with only a mild or moderate amount of peritumoral edema. Lymphomas are infiltrative tumors. By time of presentation they can be quite large and yet produce relatively little mass effect, a feature that sets lymphoma apart from glioblastoma and metastases. Intratumoral cysts and hemorrhage are unusual. Most lymphomas show bright homogeneous contrast enhancement.

The pattern is modified somewhat in AIDS patients. Multiplicity seems to be more common. Moreover, the lymphomas exhibit more aggressive behav-

ior and readily outgrow their blood supply. As a result, central necrosis and ring enhancement are often seen in lymphomatous masses in AIDS patients.

METASTATIC DISEASE

Metastases to the head can occur in three different patterns or locations, including the skull and dura, brain parenchyma, and meninges (carcinomatous meningitis). Any tumors that metastasize to bone are also prone to involve the skull. Breast and prostate are the most common primary sites, and skull metastases often occur without associated brain lesions. If the skull base is involved, cranial nerve deficits may result. Skull metastases are clearly demonstrated on T₂- and proton density–weighted images as slightly

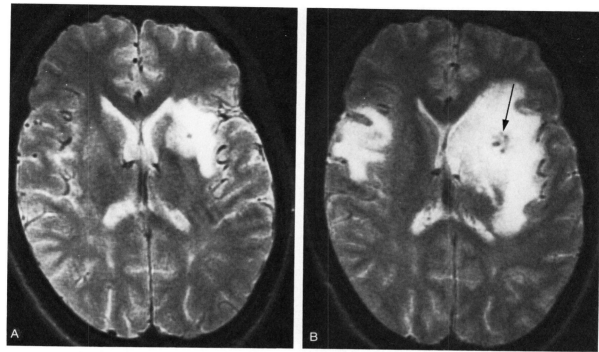

FIGURE 15–4. Primary malignant lymphoma in a 22-year-old man with AIDS. *A*, Preliminary T₂-weighted scan (SE 3000/70) reveals a deep mass in the left anterior basal ganglia. The lesion is hyperintense but slightly lower in signal compared with the adjacent edema. *B*, A follow-up scan one month later shows marked enlargement of the mass in the interval, a feature consistent with lymphoma, and a second lesion in the right hemisphere. The primary lesion is relatively homogeneous except for a few focal hypointense areas *(arrow)* that probably represent enlarged vascular structures. Mass effect is rather modest considering the size of the tumor.

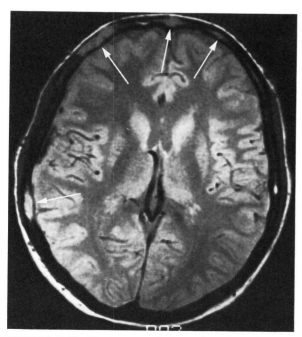

FIGURE 15–5. Skull metastases from breast carcinoma. Proton density–weighted scan demonstrates multiple metastases *(arrows)* to the skull.

hyperintense masses that have replaced the lower signal diploic space and cortical bone (Fig. 15–5). They can also be seen on T₁-weighted images because the lower signal metastases replace the higher signal marrow fat. The coronal and sagittal planes are helpful for evaluating the skull base.

Metastases to the brain parenchyma occur by hematogenous spread, and multiple lesions are found in 70 per cent of cases. The most common primaries are lung (Fig. 15–6), breast, and melanoma, in that order of frequency. Other potential sources include the gastrointestinal tract (Fig. 15–7), kidney, and thyroid. Metastases from other locations are uncommon. Clinical symptoms are nonspecific and no different from primary brain tumors. If a parenchymal lesion breaks through the cortex, tumor can extend and seed along the leptomeninges.[16]

Metastatic lesions can be found anywhere in the brain, but a favorite site is near the brain surface at the corticomedullary junction of both the cerebrum and cerebellum. They are hyperintense on plain T₂-weighted images (Fig. 15–6A). Areas of necrosis are prevalent in the larger lesions, accounting for their heterogeneous internal texture. Peritumoral edema is a prominent feature, but multiplicity is the most helpful sign to suggest metastatic disease as the likely

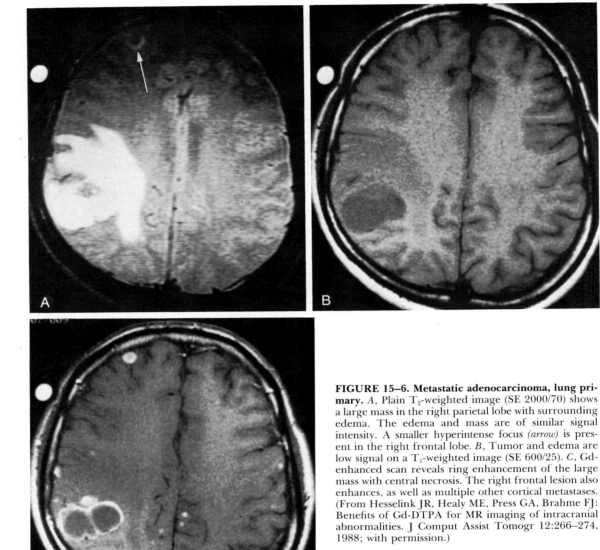

FIGURE 15–6. Metastatic adenocarcinoma, lung primary. *A*, Plain T_2-weighted image (SE 2000/70) shows a large mass in the right parietal lobe with surrounding edema. The edema and mass are of similar signal intensity. A smaller hyperintense focus *(arrow)* is present in the right frontal lobe. *B*, Tumor and edema are low signal on a T_1-weighted image (SE 600/25). *C*, Gd-enhanced scan reveals ring enhancement of the large mass with central necrosis. The right frontal lesion also enhances, as well as multiple other cortical metastases. (From Hesselink JR, Healy ME, Press GA, Brahme FJ: Benefits of Gd-DTPA for MR imaging of intracranial abnormalities. J Comput Assist Tomogr 12:266–274, 1988; with permission.)

diagnosis. Correlative studies have shown MR to be more sensitive than CT for detecting metastases,[5] particularly lesions near the base of the brain and in the posterior fossa (Fig. 15–7). One limitation of plain MR is the frequency of periventricular white matter hyperintensities found in the same older age group at risk for metastatic disease.

Gd-DTPA–enhanced MR has resulted in improved delineation of metastatic disease compared with nonenhanced scans.[17] Moderate to marked enhancement is the rule, nodular for the smaller lesions and ringlike with central nonenhancing areas for the larger ones (Fig. 15–6C). Controlled clinical trials have also shown that contrast-enhanced MR is more

sensitive than both plain MR and contrast-enhanced CT for detecting cerebral metastases.[23, 24] In patients with a known primary, T_1-weighted enhanced MR is probably sufficient to screen the brain for metastatic disease.

Hemorrhage is present in 3 to 14 per cent of brain metastases, mainly in melanoma, choriocarcinoma, renal cell carcinoma, bronchogenic carcinoma, and thyroid carcinoma. Atlas and colleagues[25] noted some distinctive features of tumoral hemorrhage compared with nonneoplastic hemorrhage. First, they observed delayed evolution, which they postulate is due to relative hypoxia within tumors and slower conversion of deoxyhemoglobin to methemoglobin.

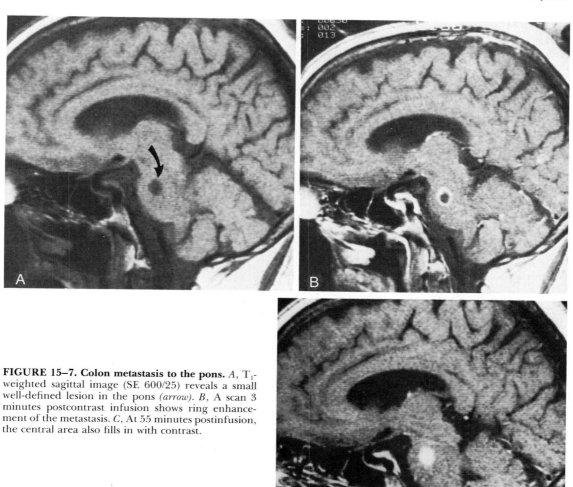

FIGURE 15–7. Colon metastasis to the pons. *A*, T$_1$-weighted sagittal image (SE 600/25) reveals a small well-defined lesion in the pons *(arrow)*. *B*, A scan 3 minutes postcontrast infusion shows ring enhancement of the metastasis. *C*, At 55 minutes postinfusion, the central area also fills in with contrast.

Second, despite evidence of multiphasic hemorrhage, deposition of hemosiderin was spotty, and in some cases absent. This lack of a well-developed hemosiderin ring could be related to breakdown of the BBB and more efficient removal of the hemosiderin, or erosion by tumor growth. The presence of nonhemorrhagic tissue and pronounced surrounding vasogenic edema are other clues to the underlying neoplasm (see Chapter 16).

Metastatic melanoma has been a topic of special interest in the MR literature because of the presence of paramagnetic, stable free radicals within melanin. The MR appearance is variable depending on the histology of the melanoma and the components of hemoglobin. Most are hyperintense to white matter on T$_1$-weighted scans and hypointense on T$_2$-weighted scans.[26] Atlas and coworkers[27] observed three distinct signal intensity patterns. Nonhemorrhagic melanotic melanoma was markedly hyperintense on T$_1$-weighted images and isointense or mildly hypointense on T$_2$-weighted images. Nonhemorrhagic amelanotic melanoma appeared isointense or slightly hypointense on T$_1$-weighted scans and isointense or slightly hyperintense on T$_2$-weighted scans. The signal pattern for hemorrhagic melanoma was variable depending on the components of hemoglobin. Some uncertainty remains as to whether the predominant effect on signal intensity within melanomas is due to stable free radicals, chelated metal ions, or hemoglobin.

MENINGIOMA

Meningiomas account for 15 per cent of all intracranial tumors and are the most common extraaxial tumors. They originate from the dura or arachnoid and occur in middle-aged adults. Women are affected twice as often as men. Clinical symptoms consist of seizures, or focal weakness or numbness in an opposite extremity if the mass compresses the brain around the Rolandic fissure.[16]

Meningiomas are well-differentiated, benign, and

encapsulated lesions that indent the brain as they enlarge. They grow slowly and may be present for many years before producing symptoms. The histologic picture shows cells of uniform size which tend to form whorls or psammoma bodies. On rare occasions, a meningioma will exhibit malignant and invasive features of a hemangiopericytoma.[21]

The parasagittal region (Fig. 15–8) is the most frequent site for meningiomas, followed by the sphenoid wings, parasellar region (Fig. 15–9; [also see Fig. 15–20]), olfactory groove, cerebellopontine angle (Fig. 15–10), and rarely the intraventricular region. Meningiomas often induce an osteoblastic reaction in the adjacent bone, resulting in a characteristic focal hyperostosis. They are also hypervascular, receiving their blood supply predominantly from dural vessels. A prominent and persistent vascular stain is a classic sign on angiography. Those that are accessible can be completely cured with surgical excision. The ones at the skull base may invade the bone and adjacent

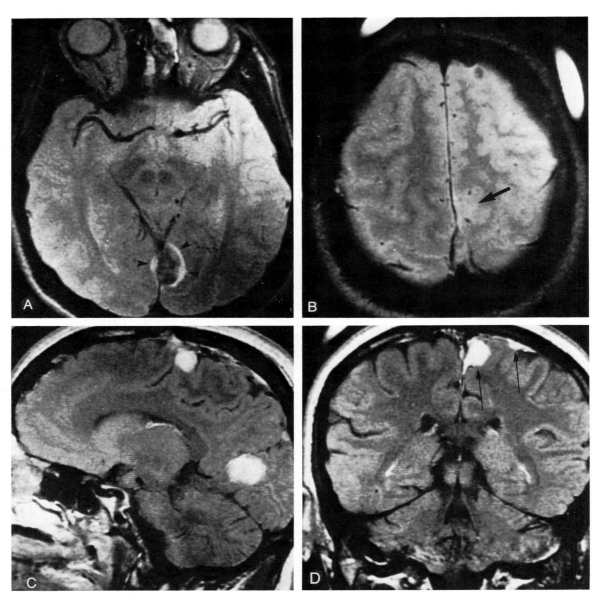

FIGURE 15–8. Multiple meningiomas. *A* and *B*, T$_2$-weighted plain scans demonstrate two parafalcine lesions, one posteriorly *(arrowheads)* and another near the vertex *(arrow)*. The posterior mass is heterogeneous and outlined by high signal edema, but the parasagittal lesion is isointense to gray matter and difficult to visualize. *C*, Following Gd-DTPA injection, both lesions enhance on a sagittal proton density–weighted image (SE 1500/25). *D*, A coronal-enhanced scan reveals two areas of enhancement *(arrows)*—the parasagittal lesion and a second mass along the high convexity of the left hemisphere. Both lesions exhibit bright homogeneous enhancement and have a broad base against the dura, features of meningioma. (From Hesselink JR, Press GA: MR contrast enhancement of intracranial lesions with Gd-DTPA. Radiol Clin North Am 26:873–887, 1988.)

cavernous sinuses and incorporate cranial nerves and major vascular structures as they grow, rendering them unresectable.

Initially there was great concern that MR would miss many significant meningiomas, but with more experience and the use of multiple imaging sequences this has not proved to be the case. Comparing studies performed at or below 0.5 T[1, 28] with higher field strength (1.5 T) images,[29] there appears to be an advantage for the higher field systems in meningioma detection. For evaluation with noncontrast scans alone, T_1-weighted images are essential at all field strengths, providing the best depiction of anatomic distortion and white matter buckling indicative of an extraaxial mass. Inversion recovery T_1-weighted images have some advantages over spin-echo T_1-weighted scans, particularly at intermediate field strengths. At 0.15 and 0.5 T, slightly greater than 50 per cent of meningiomas were isointense with cortex on T_1- and T_2-weighted images,[28] but at 1.5 T all lesions were hyperintense to white matter on T_2-weighted images (Fig. 15–8B) and almost all were hypointense to white matter on T_1-weighted images (Fig. 15–9).[29] In the same study, a heterogeneous internal texture was noted in all but the smallest meningiomas. The mottled pattern is likely due to a combination of flow void from vascularity, focal calcification, small cystic foci, and entrapped CSF spaces. Hemorrhage is not a common feature. An interface between the brain and lesion was often identified, and at 1.5 T this could be characterized as representing a CSF cleft, a vascular rim, or a dural margin. MR has special advantages over CT in assessing venous sinus involvement and arterial encase-

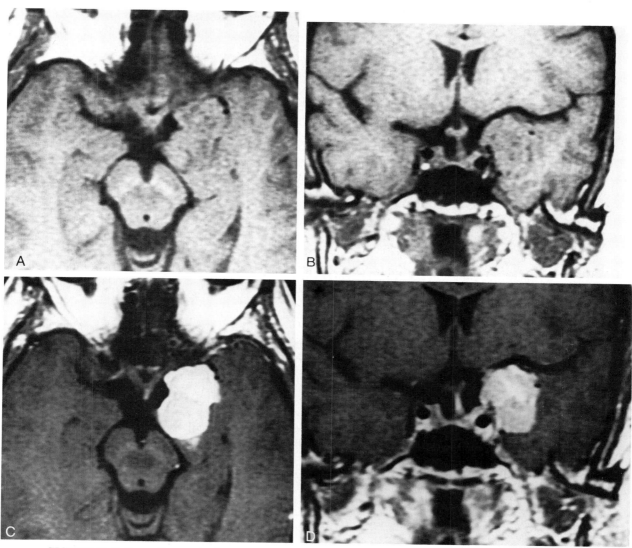

FIGURE 15–9. Parasellar meningioma. *A* and *B*, Axial and coronal noncontrast T_1-weighted scans (SE 600/20) show a mass in the left parasellar region. The mass is isointense to gray matter, but slightly hypointense to white matter in the adjacent temporal lobe. *C* and *D*, Corresponding contrast-enhanced scans (SE 600/20) disclose a dural-based mass along the superolateral aspect of the cavernous sinus, consistent with a meningioma.

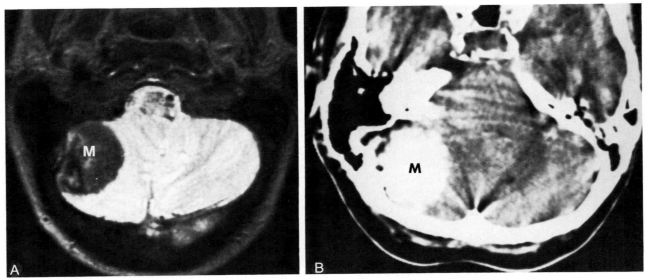

FIGURE 15–10. Heavily calcified meningioma. *A,* Axial T_2-weighted image (TR 3000/70) reveals a markedly hypointense mass (M) within the posterior fossa. *B,* Unenhanced CT scan confirms a densely calcified mass (> 150 H units), based against the dura, suggesting meningioma. (From Press GA, Hesselink JR: MR imaging of cerebellopontine angle and internal auditory canal lesions at 1.5 T. AJNR 9:241–252, 1988; © by American Society of Neuroradiology.)

ment.[28, 29] Occasionally, a densely calcified meningioma is encountered which is distinctly hypointense on all pulse sequences (Fig. 15–10).

Meningiomas show intense enhancement with Gd-DTPA (Figs. 15–8 and 15–9) and are sharply circumscribed.[30] They have a characteristic broad base of attachment against a dural surface. Associated hyperostosis may result in thickening of low signal bone (Fig. 15–20C) as well as diminished signal from the diploic spaces. Although meningiomas are not invasive, vasogenic edema is present in the adjacent brain in 30 per cent of cases. Contrast scans are especially helpful for imaging the en plaque meningiomas that occur at the skull base.[13, 14]

Ossification or bony metaplasia of the falx has a distinctive MR appearance that should not be misinterpreted as a meningioma. Ossification has a central area of fatty marrow that is high signal on T_1-weighted images and isointense or low signal on T_2-weighted images. The peripheral rim of cortical bone is low signal on both pulse sequences.[31] Since hemorrhage is rare in meningiomas, high signal is not normally seen on T_1-weighted images. Moreover, on contrast scans, although both would be bright on T_1-weighted images, the enhancing meningioma would remain bright on T_2-weighted scans, but the falx ossification does not enhance and would be isointense or low signal.

PINEAL REGION TUMORS

Tumors in the pineal region can be classified into three major groups based on their origin: germ cell, pineal parenchyma, and parapineal. *Germinoma* is the least differentiated of the germ-cell group. It occurs in children and young adults and accounts for more than 50 per cent of all pineal region tumors. The other germ-cell tumors include *embryonal carcinoma, yolk-sac tumor,* and *choriocarcinoma.* Differentiation along three germ layers results in a *teratoma.* The true pinealomas consist of pineoblastoma and pineocytoma. *Pineoblastoma* is an embryonal tumor of neuroectoderm, related to neuroblastoma and medulloblastoma, which is found primarily in young children. *Pineocytomas* are less cellular and exhibit benign behavior. The parapineal lesions include *gliomas* of the tectum and posterior third ventricle, *meningiomas* arising within the quadrigeminal cistern, and *developmental cysts* (epidermoid, dermoid, arachnoid cyst).[32]

The clinical expression of these tumors is usually related to mass effect upon adjacent brain structures. Hydrocephalus secondary to aqueductal obstruction is a common presentation. Compression of the tectum of the midbrain can produce paralysis of upward gaze, the classic Parinaud's syndrome. Germinomas and gliomas have a propensity to grow into the third ventricle and compress the hypothalamus, resulting in endocrine dysfunction. Dissemination through the CSF pathways is a known complication of pineoblastoma and germinoma.[16]

Pineal germinomas and primary pineal tumors are most often isointense with the brain on T_1- and T_2-weighted images (Fig. 15–11). A few lesions exhibit long T_1 and T_2, which may correlate with embryonal cell elements. Despite this relative lack of contrast, with multiplanar imaging plain MR delineates pineal region masses better than CT, showing the relationships of the tumor to the posterior third ventricle, vein of Galen, and aqueduct.[33] These tumors are well

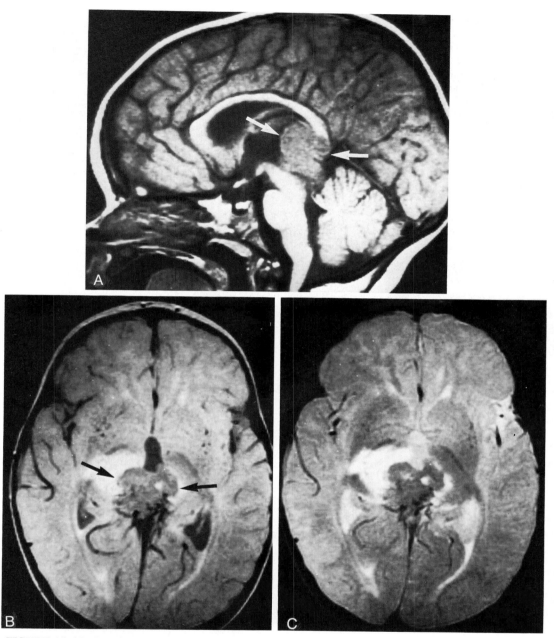

FIGURE 15–11. Germinoma. *A*, T_1-weighted scan (SE 600/25) demonstrates a hypointense mass *(arrows)* in the pineal region which compresses the midbrain and elevates the splenium of the corpus callosum. *B* and *C*, The tumor *(arrows)* is essentially isointense to brain on proton density and T_2-weighted images (SE 2000/25,70) and is associated with some peritumoral edema.

defined and enhance to a moderate degree, usually without central necrosis, cystic change, or hemorrhage. Enhanced scans are essential to assess CSF spread of tumor.[34] In young patients with germinoma, the difficulty of visualizing calcium is a disadvantage of MR, as this may be the only evidence of tumor. For this reason and because identification of calcification assists with differential diagnosis, CT may maintain a role in evaluating these patients.[35]

Meningiomas can appear very similar on plain scan, but their intense enhancement may set them apart from other lesions. Gliomas infiltrate the tectum and posterior walls of the third ventricle (Fig. 15–12). They tend to be poorly circumscribed and produce symptoms earlier. Edema is not a consistent finding, and enhancement is variable. Larger gliomas in the splenium of the corpus callosum may present as pineal region masses (see "Cerebral Gliomas" and "Meningioma").

Teratomas are of mixed signal intensity, frequently with calcification. They may also have cystic components and fat. Arachnoid cysts and epidermoid and

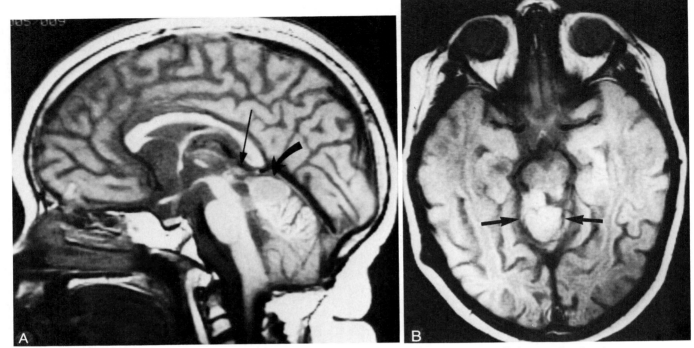

FIGURE 15–12. Exophytic tectal glioma. *A*, T_1-weighted sagittal image (SE 600/25) discloses a pineal region mass *(curved arrow)* that is distinct from a normal pineal gland *(long arrow)*. *B*, The lesion *(arrows)* is slightly hyperintense on a proton density–weighted image (SE 2000/70). Surgery revealed a glioma arising from the quadrigeminal plate with a large exophytic component occupying the quadrigeminal cistern.

dermoid tumors can usually be distinguished from other pineal region tumors by their increased signal on T_2-weighted images (see "Benign Cystic Masses").

Pineal cysts were visualized in 4.3 per cent of normal patients in one MR study.[36] These apparently benign lesions are seen best as areas of high signal on intermediate T_2-weighted images. They are not associated with hydrocephalus or a pineal mass and are not clinically significant (Fig. 15–13).

SELLAR AND PERISELLAR LESIONS

PITUITARY ADENOMA

Pituitary adenomas arise within the anterior lobe of the gland (adenohypophysis). Clinical symptoms depend on whether the tumor is secreting or nonsecreting. Secreting adenomas manifest with specific endocrine syndromes. Prolactinomas present with amenorrhea and galactorrhea. Serum prolactin levels are increased, usually in excess of 100 ng/ml. Tumors that secrete growth hormone produce gigantism before puberty and the classic syndrome of acromegaly after puberty. Cushing's disease develops with adrenocorticotropic hormone–secreting tumors. Although less common, pituitary adenomas may also secrete thyroid-stimulating hormone, beta-lipotropin,

luteinizing hormone, or follicle-stimulating hormone.[16] Secreting tumors present earlier and are often smaller and confined to the gland. Tumors less than 1 cm are called microadenomas (Fig. 15–14).

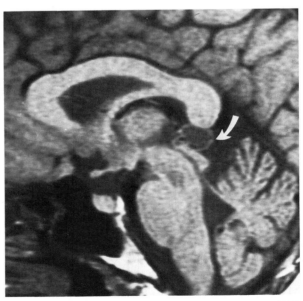

FIGURE 15–13. Pineal cyst. T_1-weighted sagittal scan (SE 600/20) demonstrates a low signal lesion *(curved arrow)* within the pineal gland. Its homogeneous texture and smooth margins suggest a benign cyst.

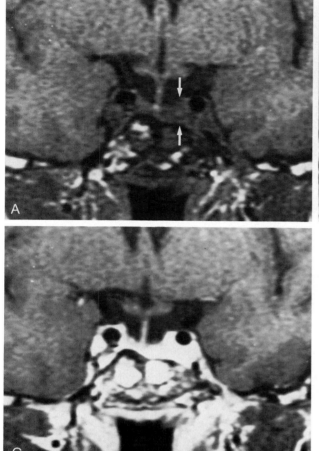

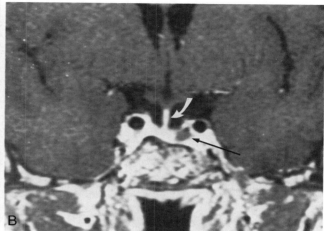

FIGURE 15–14. Pituitary microadenoma. *A*, T_1-weighted coronal scan (SE 600/20) reveals enlargement of the left side of the pituitary gland *(arrows)*. *B*, Contrast-enhanced scan (SE 600/20) shows a 5 mm mass *(arrow)* on the left. On this 3-minute postcontrast scan, the normal gland enhances brightly to give improved contrast between the gland and microadenoma. The enhancing pituitary stalk *(curved arrow)* is deviated to the right. Note that the cavernous sinuses also enhance, but the carotid arteries do not. *C*, A 30-minute postcontrast scan demonstrates delayed enhancement of the microadenoma, making the tumor isointense to the normal gland.

Nonsecreting adenomas grow and compress adjacent structures. Superior extension through the diaphragma sellae into the suprasellar region can result in chiasmal compression and a bitemporal hemianopia (Fig. 15–15). Lateral growth and involvement of the cavernous sinuses lead to cranial nerve deficits.

Pituitary apoplexy is an acute clinical syndrome consisting of ophthalmoplegia, bilateral amaurosis, and decreased level of consciousness related to sudden hemorrhagic necrosis of an adenoma (Fig. 15–16). The symptoms result from mass effect caused by the hematoma or infarction and acute swelling of the tumor. Postpartum pituitary necrosis, also called Sheehan's syndrome, represents an acute pituitary deficiency secondary to infarction of the gland. It is thought to be due to a hypercoagulable state during the postpartum period and compromise of the vascular supply to the pituitary.[16]

The "empty sella" is caused by a defect in the diaphragma sellae and bulging of arachnoid into the sella turcica (Fig. 15–17). The accompanying subarachnoid space gradually expands from CSF pulsations and enlarges the sella. Although the gland may be flattened against the floor of the sella, pituitary function is preserved. In fact, the empty sella is usually asymptomatic unless downward herniation of the optic chiasm results in a visual disturbance.

The reported sensitivity of noncontrast MR for detecting pituitary microadenomas has been variable. This relates in part to field strength, as higher field strengths provide better signal-to-noise (S/N) ratios for the thin sections required for pituitary imaging.[37] Sensitivities ranging from 54 per cent[38] to 90 per cent[39] have been reported with higher field imaging using a 3-mm slice thickness.

On plain T_1-weighted images, microadenomas are usually hypointense compared with the normal gland. They may be slightly hyperintense on T_2-weighted images, but more often the contrast is better on T_1-weighted scans.[37, 38, 40] Secondary signs of microadenoma include asymmetric upward convexity of the gland surface, deviation of the infundibulum (Fig. 15–14), and focal erosion of the sellar floor.[41] Coronal and sagittal are the preferred imaging planes for pituitary adenomas.

The macroadenomas are more or less isointense to the normal gland and brain parenchyma (Fig. 15–15), unless cystic or hemorrhagic components are

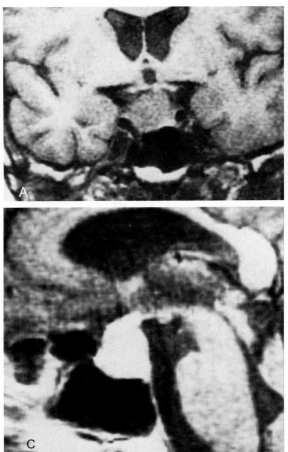

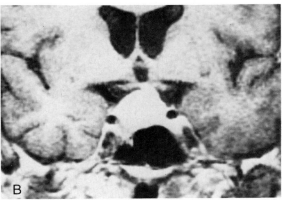

FIGURE 15–15. Pituitary macroadenoma. *A*, Coronal T₁-weighted scan (SE 600/25) reveals an intrasellar mass with suprasellar extension. *B* and *C*, Following Gd-DTPA injection, the tumor exhibits bright homogeneous enhancement. On the coronal view, flow void persists in the carotid arteries, but the cavernous sinuses enhance to obscure margins between the sinus and tumor. (From Hesselink JR, Press GA: MR contrast enhancement of intracranial lesions with Gd-DTPA. Radiol Clin North Am 26:873–887, 1988.)

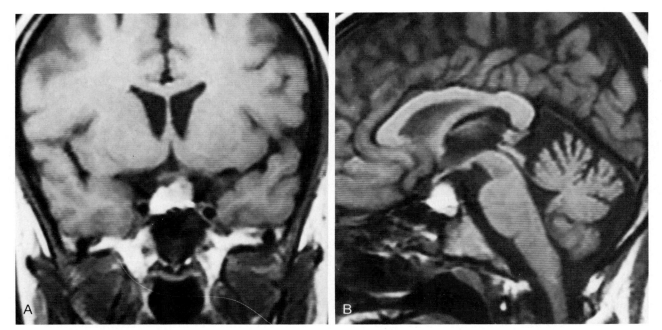

FIGURE 15–16. Pituitary apoplexy. *A* and *B*, Coronal and sagittal T₁-weighted images show high signal intensity within the sella, consistent with subacute hemorrhage (methemoglobin). The left side of the lesion abuts the optic chiasm.

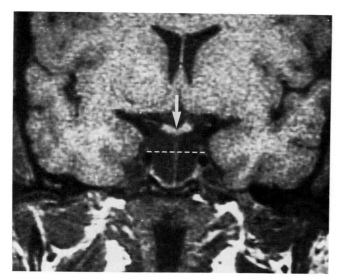

FIGURE 15–17. Empty sella. The dashed line indicates the normal position of the diaphragma sellae. Low signal CSF occupies much of the sellar volume. A thin gland lines the floor of the sella, and an elongated infundibulum extends from the gland up to the level of the optic chiasm *(arrow)*.

present. Hemorrhage is depicted better by MR than CT, and the signal characteristics suggest the age of the hemorrhage. Central necrosis is not common until the tumors become quite large or pituitary apoplexy develops (Fig. 15–16).

Multiplanar MR accurately defines suprasellar and parasellar extension. Upward growth into the suprasellar cistern is outlined by the lower signal CSF on T_1-weighted scans.[39, 42] Deformity of the optic chiasm, the inferior recesses of the third ventricle, and the hypothalamus can be clearly seen.[43] With high-resolution scans, the diaphragma sellae can be visualized as a thin band of low signal, and its position can be used to differentiate intrasellar lesions with suprasellar extension from purely suprasellar lesions.[44] The ability to visualize the lateral dural margin of the cavernous sinus as a thin band of low signal is helpful in assessing parasellar extension. The medial margin is not reliably seen as a discrete structure;[38] however, any invading tumor is outlined by the flow void within the cavernous sinuses. For the same reason, encasement of the carotid arteries is clearly demonstrated by MR.[45] Erosion of the dorsum sellae and adjacent clivus is shown best on T_1-weighted images as low signal tumor replacing the higher signal bone marrow.

The enhancement characteristics of pituitary adenomas followed those observed with CT. With microadenomas, the normal gland enhances more than the tumor to increase the conspicuity of the small lesions (Fig. 15–14*B*). Gd-DTPA significantly increases the sensitivity of MR for detecting microadenomas.[46] If scanning is delayed more than 30 minutes after injection of the Gd-DTPA, the microadenoma may become isointense to the normal gland (Fig. 15–14*C*). The macroadenomas exhibit homogeneous enhancement and are clearly demar-

cated from normal suprasellar structures (Fig. 15–15). Cavernous sinus extension is seen better on plain scans because the tumor tissue is contrasted against the flow void within the sinuses. On Gd-DTPA–enhanced scans, the flow void is maintained within the carotid arteries, but both the cavernous sinuses and the macroadenoma enhance and they cannot be easily separated.[12]

On plain T_1-weighted scans, increased signal is present in the posterior sella, immediately in front of the dorsum sellae, in 90 per cent of normal patients. This was initially called the pituitary "fat pad"; however, the signal intensity does not follow ordinary fat in that it becomes isointense rather than hypointense on T_2-weighted images.[47, 48] Studies by Colombo and colleagues[49] have localized the signal to the posterior lobe of the pituitary gland and the likely source to be intracellular lipid. They also noted that the hyperintensity was evident in only 43 per cent of patients with macroadenomas and in 12 per cent of empty sellas because of associated compression of posterior lobe. Absence of the signal in diabetes insipidus suggests a relationship between the hyperintensity and functional status of the hypothalamic-hypophyseal axis.[50] An abnormal superior position of the posterior lobe at the base of the infundibulum has been associated with pituitary dysfunction.[51]

CHIASMATIC/HYPOTHALAMIC GLIOMAS

Chiasmatic gliomas occur primarily in children and young adults. Girls are afflicted more often than boys. Patients with neurofibromatosis are particularly at risk for developing optic and chiasmatic gliomas. These tumors are usually low grade but have a propensity to infiltrate along the visual pathways. *Hypothalamic gliomas* tend to behave more aggressively and produce symptoms earlier. They present with hypothalamic syndromes, such as diabetes insipidus, inappropriate antidiuretic hormone secretion, Fröhlich's syndrome, or disturbances of temperature, appetite, or metabolism.

Chiasmatic gliomas are usually isointense or slightly hypointense on T_1-weighted images and hyperintense on T_2-weighted images (Fig. 15–18).[41] Expansion of the chiasm and optic tracts is seen best on coronal T_1-weighted scans. The sagittal plane often provides a longitudinal view of the proximal optic nerves.[42] Posterior extension to the lateral geniculate body and beyond into the optic radiations is displayed best as areas of increased signal on axial T_2-weighted images.[52] Cystic components may be present, and occasionally exophytic growth extends into the suprasellar and intrapeduncular cisterns.

MR is especially good for detecting and delineating hypothalamic gliomas.[42] Subtle deformity of the inferior recesses of the third ventricle can be visualized on coronal views. These tumors have a tendency to infiltrate the adjacent thalamus and upper brain stem. Signal characteristics are similar to the chias-

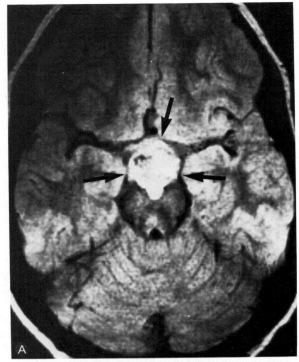

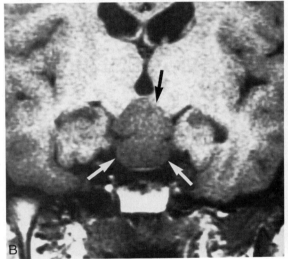

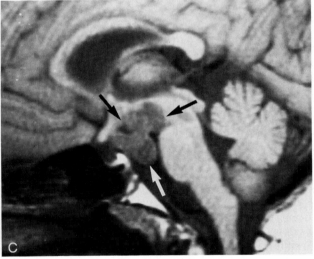

FIGURE 15–18. Chiasmatic/hypothalamic glioma in a 14-year-old girl with neurofibromatosis. *A*, Axial proton weighted–image (SE 2000/25) shows a hyperintense mass *(arrows)* within the suprasellar cistern. *B* and *C*, On T₁-weighted scans (SE 600/25) the tumor *(arrows)* deforms the inferior third ventricle and extends posteriorly into the interpeduncular and prepontine cisterns.

matic gliomas, and they may also exhibit exophytic features (Fig. 15–18). As a rule, both tumors enhance to a moderate degree and in a homogeneous fashion, except for the cystic portions.

CRANIOPHARYNGIOMA

Craniopharyngiomas originate from epithelial remnants of Rathke's pouch, usually at the junction of the infundibulum and the pituitary gland. Although primarily tumors of children, some have a delayed presentation in middle age or older. Symptoms vary from pituitary to hypothalamic-chiasmal dysfunction. A suprasellar location is certainly the rule, but occasionally they are found below the diaphragma sellae. They are benign slow-growing tumors composed of both solid epithelial tissue and cystic components. The cysts contain variable amounts of cholesterol, keratin, necrotic debris, proteinaceous fluid, and hemorrhage. Calcification is present in 75 to 85 per cent of cases.[16]

Craniopharyngiomas have a variable appearance on MR, depending on their solid or cystic nature and the specific cyst contents (Fig. 15–19). The solid lesions are hypointense on T₁-weighted images and hyperintense of T₂-weighted images.[41, 42] The cysts also have a long T₂, but if they have a high cholesterol

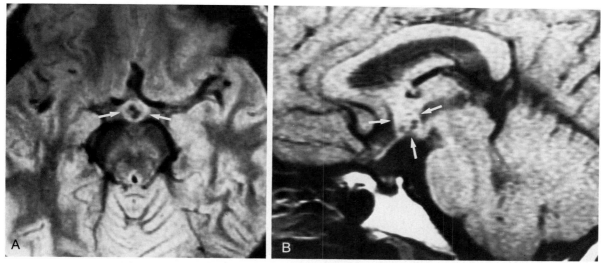

FIGURE 15–19. Craniopharyngioma. *A* and *B*, Axial proton density (SE 3000/30) and sagittal T$_1$-weighted (SE 600/20) scans disclose a small suprasellar mass *(arrows)* adjacent to the optic chiasm which effaces the inferior recesses of the third ventricle. The mass has a heterogeneous internal texture, and the discrete low signal areas present on both scans likely represent calcification.

content or methemoglobin shortening of T$_1$ results in high signal intensity on T$_1$-weighted images.[53] Other features of craniopharyngioma include truncation of the dorsum sellae and upward growth into the third ventricle. Calcification is not reliably detected with MR, a disadvantage for differential diagnosis.[54]

DIFFERENTIAL DIAGNOSIS

The differential list of diseases that can be found in the sella and perisellar region is exceedingly long. To make the correct diagnosis requires accurate localization of the lesion and careful analysis of the signal and enhancement features. The four primary locations are intrasellar, suprasellar cistern, optic chiasm-hypothalamus, and parasellar. Separation of intraaxial from extraaxial masses in the suprasellar region is not always possible; however, multiplanar MR facilitates localization. If it can be determined that a mass is within the sella or originates from the sella, then it very likely is a pituitary adenoma. As mentioned above, occasionally a craniopharyngioma will arise below the diaphragma sellae. Rathke's cleft cysts are rare lesions found in either the anterior sella or the suprasellar cistern.[55]

The suprasellar cisternal group includes craniopharyngioma, arachnoid cyst, dermoid, epidermoid, teratoma, and germinoma. These lesions are discussed under "Benign Cystic Masses" and "Pineal Region Tumors." Briefly, the signal characteristics provide clues about the solid or cystic nature of the abnormality. Arachnoid cysts have no solid components and should follow CSF signal (see Fig. 15–21).

Epidermoids often follow CSF signal as well, but they appear more heterogeneous (see Fig. 15–23). Both teratomas and dermoids (see Fig. 15–24) may have fat components; some pathologists classify dermoids as cystic teratomas. Calcification is a feature of craniopharyngioma, teratoma, and dermoid, and CT is often helpful in the differential diagnosis of suprasellar masses. Germinomas have signal attributes similar to brain tissue and exhibit more uniform enhancement than the other lesions.

The differential for chiasmal-hypothalamic masses consists of glioma, lymphoma, metastasis, hamartoma, abscess, granuloma, and reticuloendothelial diseases.[53, 56] Glioma is the most common tumor, but it is a popular site for lymphoma as well. Hamartomas of the tuber cinereum are one of the important causes of precocious puberty. Infectious and granulomatous diseases have a nondescript appearance but are usually multifocal, and the patients have evidence of other CNS involvement or systemic disease (see Chapter 19).

The parasellar area is the site for meningioma, neuroma, and aneurysm, rarely a chordoma or chondromatous tumor. Also, it can be secondarily involved by tumors and inflammatory processes in the sphenoid sinus and orbits.[57] The two more common lesions—meningioma and aneurysm—can be readily distinguished in most cases. Meningiomas show bright homogeneous enhancement (Fig. 15–20) (also see "Meningioma" and Fig. 15–9). Aneurysms are heterogeneous, with more or less concentric layers of fibrosis, calcification and clot of different ages about the periphery, and areas of flow void or even flow enhancement in the center (see Chapter 17). The patent lumen of an aneurysm can be demonstrated more clearly with gradient-echo imaging.[58]

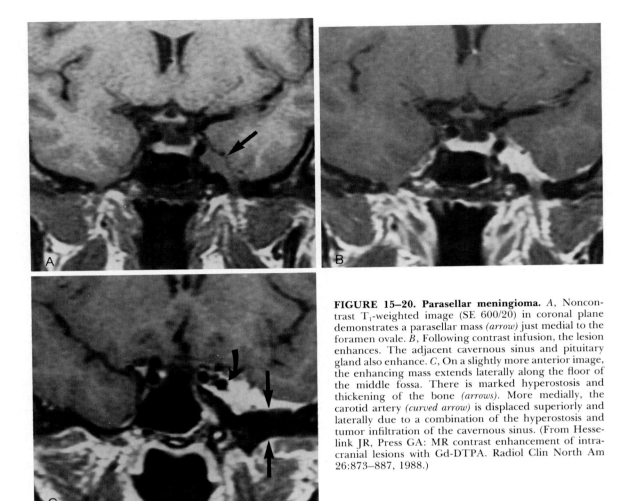

FIGURE 15–20. Parasellar meningioma. *A,* Noncontrast T_1-weighted image (SE 600/20) in coronal plane demonstrates a parasellar mass *(arrow)* just medial to the foramen ovale. *B,* Following contrast infusion, the lesion enhances. The adjacent cavernous sinus and pituitary gland also enhance. *C,* On a slightly more anterior image, the enhancing mass extends laterally along the floor of the middle fossa. There is marked hyperostosis and thickening of the bone *(arrows).* More medially, the carotid artery *(curved arrow)* is displaced superiorly and laterally due to a combination of the hyperostosis and tumor infiltration of the cavernous sinus. (From Hesselink JR, Press GA: MR contrast enhancement of intracranial lesions with Gd-DTPA. Radiol Clin North Am 26:873–887, 1988.)

BENIGN CYSTIC MASSES

Cystic lesions occur most often in the basal cisterns, a midline location, or within the ventricular system. They include arachnoid cyst and dermoid, epidermoid, and neuroepithelial cysts, including colloid cyst. These lesions are interesting in that their MR appearance is quite distinct from solid masses. Their signal characteristics depend to a large extent on the cyst contents, but associated solid components may also have specific features.

ARACHNOID CYST

Arachnoid cysts are CSF-containing cysts that are found in the middle fossa, posterior fossa, suprasellar cistern, or near the vertex. The anterior middle fossa and sylvian fissure are particularly favorite sites for these lesions. They may be congenital or can develop from adhesions within the subarachnoid space. They are benign but slowly grow as they accumulate fluid,

compressing normal brain structures. Remodeling of the adjacent skull is an important clue for a benign expansile process.

Arachnoid cysts are smoothly marginated and homogeneous. They are not calcified and do not enhance. The multiplanar capability of MR is particularly helpful in establishing the exact location, and the diagnosis is supported by the cyst fluid being isointense with CSF on all pulse sequences (Figs. 15–21 and 15–22).[59] The cysts may appear higher signal than CSF on intermediate T_2-weighted images. The exact reason for this is uncertain, although it may reflect dampening of the CSF pulsations which normally results in signal loss in the ventricles and cisterns.[4] This effect will be less apparent with pulse sequences that incorporate flow compensation techniques.

It is important to distinguish arachnoid cysts from porencephaly and encephalomalacia, because they require different therapies. Porencephalic cysts can be decompressed with a ventricular shunt. Arachnoid cysts do not communicate with the ventricle and must

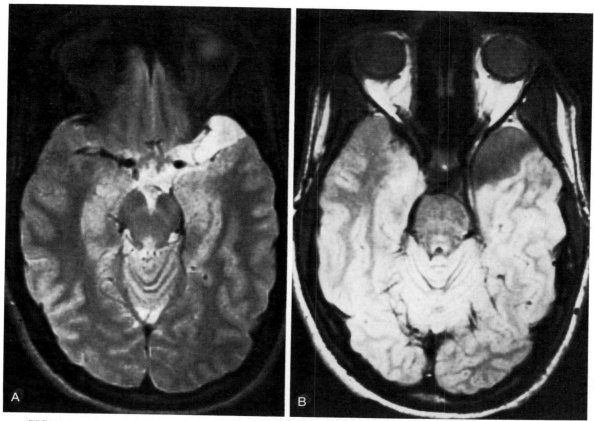

FIGURE 15–21. Arachnoid cyst. *A*, On a T$_2$-weighted scan (SE 2000/70), a hyperintense mass in the middle cranial fossa compresses the temporal lobe, but gray/white matter contrast is preserved. The mass is homogeneous and isointense to CSF. *B*, On a proton density–weighted image (SE 2000/25), the lesion is low signal and isointense to CSF, confirming a fluid-containing arachnoid cyst.

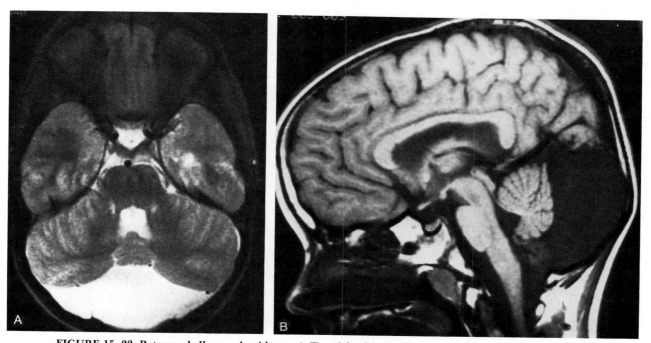

FIGURE 15–22. Retrocerebellar arachnoid cyst. *A*, T$_2$-weighted image (SE 2000/70) discloses a homogeneous hyperintense mass behind the cerebellar hemispheres which is similar in signal to CSF. *B*, On a T$_1$-weighted sagittal image (SE 600/25), the lesion follows CSF signal, compresses the vermis, and has enlarged the posterior fossa.

be resected or marsupialized. In most cases, brain tissue separates the extraaxial cyst from the ventricle. With the very large congenital variety, occasionally intrathecal contrast is required to establish the diagnosis. The presence of mass effect and the lack of adjacent brain reaction are usually sufficient to differentiate an arachnoid cyst from encephalomalacia, which is an atrophic process associated with gliosis. No therapy is indicated for encephalomalacia.

EPIDERMOID CYST

Epidermoid cysts are referred to as "pearly tumors" because of their glistening white appearance at surgery. They arise from epithelial cell rests in the basal cisterns. They are benign and grow slowly along the subarachnoid spaces and into the various crevices found at the base of the brain. The tumor or cyst wall is lined by simple stratified squamous epithelium supported by a tough outer layer of collagenous tissue. The cyst contents, formed by desquamation of the tumor wall, are composed chiefly of keratin and cholesterol crystals having a soft, white waxy or flaky consistency.[32]

Epidermoids can be intradural or extradural, but certainly the majority are intradural within the basal cisterns and middle cranial fossa. They often compress adjacent brain structures but do not induce any brain reaction or edema. The extradural type is an intradiploic lesion found primarily in the temporal bone.

The intradural epidermoids are usually quite large with lobulated outer margins and an insinuating pattern of growth. They have a heterogeneous texture and variable signal intensity on MR.[60, 61] Most are slightly higher signal than CSF on both T_1- and T_2-weighted images (Fig. 15–23). An occasional epidermoid will have a very short T_1 and will appear bright on T_1-weighted images (see Fig. 21–4). The

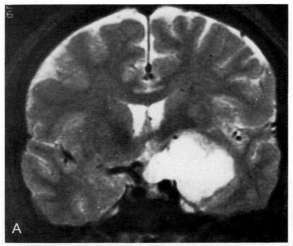

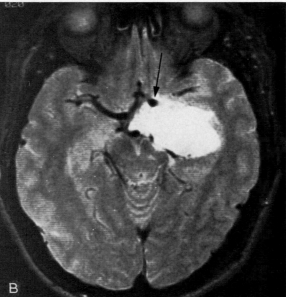

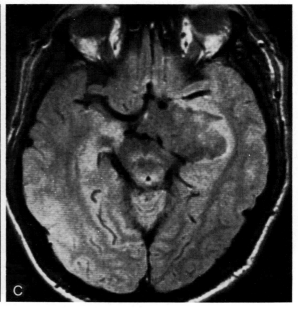

FIGURE 15–23. Epidermoid cyst. *A* and *B*, Coronal and axial T_2-weighted scans (SE 3000/70) show a hyperintense lesion within the basal cisterns. The left temporal lobe is compressed, but the cortical gray matter is preserved. The mass indents the cerebral peduncle and surrounds the carotid artery *(arrow)*. *C*, On a proton density–weighted scan (SE 3000/25), the mass is slightly higher signal than CSF and is heterogeneous. The lack of edema in the temporal lobe favors a benign extraaxial lesion, and the signal characteristics are most compatible with an epidermoid.

heterogeneous signal pattern is likely related to varying concentrations of keratin, cholesterol, and water within the cyst, as well as the proportion of cholesterol and keratin in crystalline form.[62] Calcification is sometimes present. Epidermoid tumors do not enhance with contrast.

GIANT CHOLESTEROL CYST

Giant cholesterol cysts (cholesterol granulomas) appear as areas of bright signal on T_1- and T_2-weighted images because the semiliquid cyst material contains both blood degradation products and cholesterol. The bright T_1 signal may cause some confusion with acquired cholesteatomas, but the petrous apex location of giant cholesterol cysts and their generally brighter T_1 appearance are helpful distinguishing features.[63] Prior to clarification by MR, these lesions were called extradural epidermoids.

DERMOID CYST

Dermoid cysts have both dermal and epidermal derivatives, accounting for their more varied histologic and MR appearance. They are primarily midline lesions, occurring in the pineal and suprasellar regions. Dermoids have some distinctive features on MR (Fig. 15–24). They tend to be heterogeneous owing to the multiple cell types within them. Fatty components are common, producing high signal on T_1-weighted images.[64] On axial and sagittal scans, a fat-fluid level may be seen, or a level between fat and matted hair within the cyst.[65] Rupture of a dermoid and leakage of cyst contents into a ventricle or subarachnoid space may produce an ependymitis or meningitis, respectively.

Lipomas are also midline lesions and are often associated with partial or complete agenesis of the corpus callosum (see Chapter 14). Occasionally, an incidental lipoma will be found in the region of the quadrigeminal plate or cerebellopontine angle.

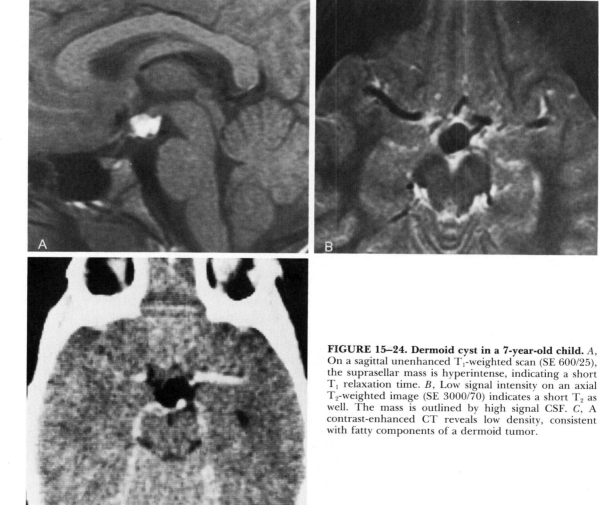

FIGURE 15–24. Dermoid cyst in a 7-year-old child. *A,* On a sagittal unenhanced T_1-weighted scan (SE 600/25), the suprasellar mass is hyperintense, indicating a short T_1 relaxation time. *B,* Low signal intensity on an axial T_2-weighted image (SE 3000/70) indicates a short T_2 as well. The mass is outlined by high signal CSF. *C,* A contrast-enhanced CT reveals low density, consistent with fatty components of a dermoid tumor.

COLLOID CYST

Colloid cysts originate from primitive neuroepithelium within the roof of the anterior third ventricle. They are positioned just posterior to the foramina of Monro between the columns of the fornix. Histologically, they consist of a thin, fibrous capsule with an epithelial lining. The cysts contain a mucinous fluid with variable amounts of proteinaceous debris, blood components, and desquamated cells.[32] The classic symptoms are positional headaches related to intermittent obstruction of the foramina of Monro. Most present during adult life and are relatively small (less than 2 cm) at the time of presentation.

Colloid cysts are smoothly marginated spherical lesions without surrounding brain reaction (Fig. 15–25). Two signal patterns have been reported on MR scans and correlated with their CT features. Those that are low density on CT are isointense on T_1-weighted images and hyperintense on T_2-weighted images, probably indicating a fluid composition similar to CSF. Most colloid cysts are isodense or slightly hyperdense on CT. The MR counterpart is a high signal capsule and a hypointense center on T_2-weighted images.[66, 67] The low signal center has been attributed to high concentrations of metal ions, such as sodium, calcium, magnesium, copper, and iron, within the cyst fluid.[68]

Dilatation of the lateral ventricles is a common finding, and the enlargement may be unequal owing to asymmetric positioning of the cyst at the foramina of Monro. The expanding cyst also enlarges the anterior third ventricle, but the posterior third, aqueduct, and fourth ventricle should be normal. Following contrast infusion, colloid cysts may show ring enhancement owing to either enhancement of the cyst wall or choroid plexus draped around the cyst. In some cases, delayed scans will reveal enhancement of the cyst contents.

DIFFERENTIAL DIAGNOSIS

The differential diagnosis of an intracranial cystic lesion includes the entities described above, other tumoral cysts, encephalomalacia, porencephaly, inflammatory cysts, and postoperative cysts. In most cases, the diagnosis can be narrowed down to one of three categories based on the signal characteristics. Arachnoid cysts, encephalomalacia, porencephaly, and postoperative cysts are isointense to CSF. Methods for distinguishing these lesions have been outlined above. Inflammatory cysts, such as cysticercosis and nonhemorrhagic tumoral cysts, often have more proteinaceous fluid and demonstrate an intermediate signal intensity pattern—hypointense to brain on T_1-weighted images and higher signal than CSF on T_2-weighted scans.[3] Moreover, these cysts have thicker walls and the tumors exhibit nodularity. They also induce a response of vasogenic edema in the surrounding brain parenchyma. The third category is represented by hemorrhagic cysts that contain methemoglobin and are hyperintense on all pulse sequences. Hemorrhage is a feature of more aggressively growing tumors. Cysts containing cholesterol may show similar properties if sufficient water is also present to prolong T_2 relaxation time.

NERVE SHEATH TUMORS

Included in this group are *schwannoma* and *neurofibroma*. Schwannomas arise from the Schwann cells that cover the cranial nerves. They are benign encapsulated tumors, whitish in color, with a smooth, firm texture. Their distinct histologic pattern consists of spindle-shaped cells, arranged in bundles and palisades and intermingled with looser hypocellular areas. These tumors tend to adhere to the nerve fibers rather than infiltrate them. Hemorrhage and necrosis are common, but malignant transformation is rare.[21]

The most common site for schwannoma is the eighth cranial nerve, followed by the fifth and then the other cranial nerves. Eighth-nerve schwannomas, better known as acoustic neuroma, are identified with neurofibromatosis. In these patients the tumors occur at an earlier age, are often bilateral, and are associated with other neuromas and multiple meningiomas (see Chapter 14).

Intracranial neurofibromas are rare except in patients with neurofibromatosis. There is some debate about the precise cell of origin, but the tumors arise from either perineural cells or neoplastic proliferation of the Schwann cells. Unlike schwannomas, neurofibromas tend to grow within the nerve and entangle the nerve fibers, making resection difficult. They also have a more disorganized histologic pattern and are more prone to malignant degeneration.[21]

ACOUSTIC NEUROMA

Acoustic neuromas originate on the vestibular division of the eighth cranial nerve just within the internal auditory canal. They usually present in middle-aged adults with a sensorineural hearing loss, but other symptoms include headache, vertigo, tinnitus, unsteady gait, and facial weakness. Large tumors may fill the cerebellopontine angle cistern and compress adjacent brain structures, producing additional symptoms.

Noncontrast MR has proven to be better than enhanced CT and as accurate or better than air-contrast CT cisternography for detecting and delineating acoustic neuromas.[69, 70] The relative signal intensities of brain and acoustic neuromas are variable, but generally neuromas have a slightly longer T_1 and T_2 than the adjacent brain (Figs. 15–26 and 15–27). As a rule, the differences are small, rendering these tumors more or less isointense to the brain.

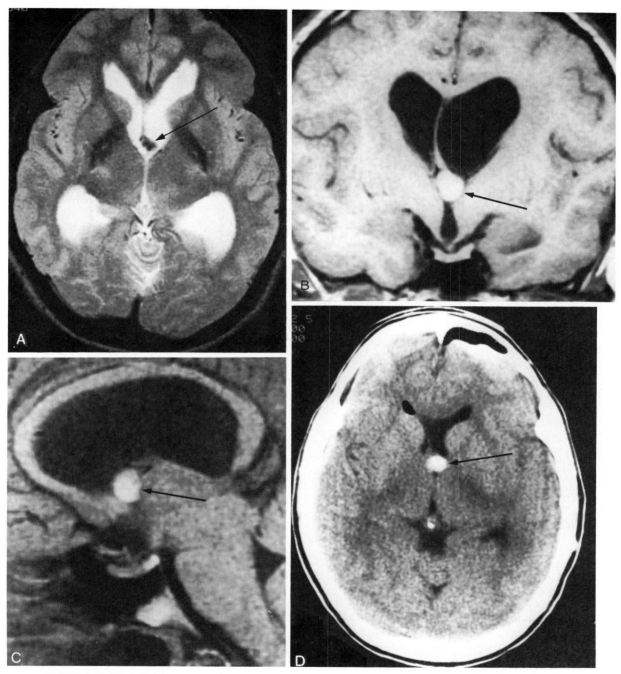

FIGURE 15–25. Colloid cyst. *A,* Axial T$_2$-weighted scan (SE 2800/80) reveals a small hypointense mass *(arrow).* The lateral ventricles are moderately enlarged, but the third ventricle is normal, indicating obstruction at the level of the foramina of Monro. *B* and *C,* Coronal and sagittal T$_1$-weighted images (SE 600/20) confirm the mass *(arrow)* positioned at the foramina of Monro. The mass is slightly higher signal than brain. The left lateral ventricle is larger as a result of asymmetric obstruction of the two foramina. *D,* On a noncontrast CT scan, obtained after a ventricular shunting procedure, the colloid cyst *(arrow)* is hyperdense to brain parenchyma. (Courtesy of George Wesbey, Scripps Memorial Hospital, LaJolla, CA.)

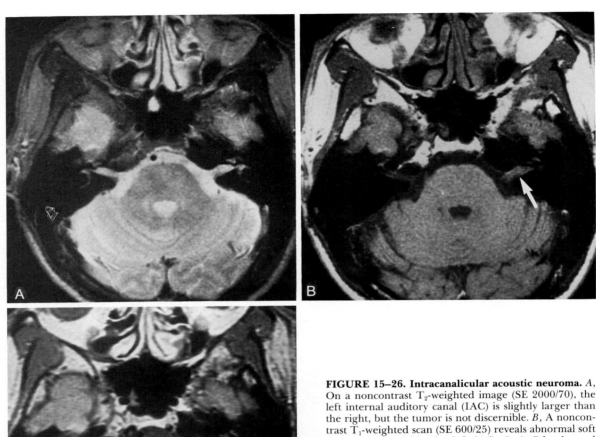

FIGURE 15–26. Intracanalicular acoustic neuroma. *A,* On a noncontrast T$_2$-weighted image (SE 2000/70), the left internal auditory canal (IAC) is slightly larger than the right, but the tumor is not discernible. *B,* A noncontrast T$_1$-weighted scan (SE 600/25) reveals abnormal soft tissue *(arrow)* within the left IAC. *C,* A Gd-enhanced scan shows marked enhancement of the intracanalicular acoustic neuroma. (From Hesselink JR, Healy ME, Press GA, Brahme FJ: Benefits of Gd-DTPA for MR imaging of intracranial abnormalities. J Comput Assist Tomogr 12:266–274, 1988; with permission.)

Occasionally, an acoustic neuroma will be hyperintense on T$_1$-weighted images or, less often, have a mixed pattern owing to foci of hemorrhage. They may be heterogeneous on T$_2$-weighted images as well, particularly the larger ones, due to necrosis, hemorrhagic components, and occasional calcification.[70, 71] With small intracanalicular tumors, partial voluming effects may result in uneven signal intensity.

T$_1$-weighted sequences provide the best contrast between the tumor and surrounding CSF. A slice thickness of 3 mm or less in conjunction with a small field-of-view (< 20 cm) is important to give adequate spatial resolution. With this technique, bony erosion and widening of the internal auditory meatus can be reliably identified. Other signs of acoustic neuroma include obscuration of the margins of the seventh and eighth nerves and displacement of CSF signal from the internal auditory canal. In about one half of cases, a hypointense vascular rim is present, which is attributed to posterior and lateral displacement of the petrosal veins and their tributaries (Fig. 15–27).[72]

Gd-DTPA causes approximately 50 per cent shortening of the T$_1$ relaxation time of acoustic neuromas, making them appear very bright on T$_1$-weighted images (Fig. 15–26C).[73] Contrast enhancement is greater at 3 minutes postcontrast injection than on delayed scans of 25 or 55 minutes.[14] Those lesions that are heterogeneous on plain scan will likely exhibit heterogeneous enhancement as well. Most acoustics, even the intracanalicular lesions, are readily detected on noncontrast MR; however, Gd-DTPA markedly increases the conspicuity of the smaller tumors.[74] Also, a potential problem exists when the internal auditory canals are obstructed, as changes in

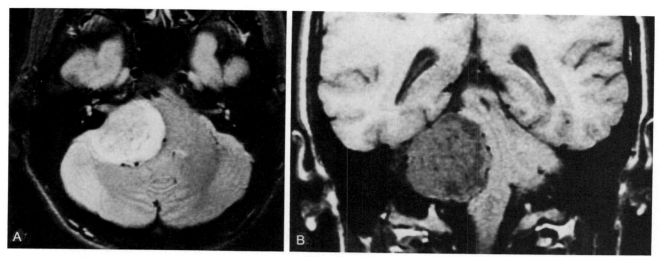

FIGURE 15–27. Acoustic neuroma. *A*, Unenhanced T_2-weighted scan (SE 2000/70) demonstrates a large hyperintense mass in the right cerebellopontine angle, adjacent to the internal auditory meatus. The low signal structures about the periphery represent capsular veins. *B*, The tumor is slightly lower signal than brain on a T_1-weighted image (SE 600/25).

the CSF may lead to abnormally high signal on intermediate T_2-weighted images.[70] Contrast-enhanced MR more accurately delineates the lateral extent of tumor growth within the canal—important information for the surgeon.

The ability to differentiate between acoustic neuroma and meningioma, the second most common cerebellopontine angle lesion, is important. Acoustic neuromas tend to be slightly lower signal on T_1-weighted images and higher signal on T_2-weighted images compared with meningiomas, but this is not constant enough to be a distinguishing feature. Acoustic neuromas enhance more than meningiomas; homogeneous enhancement is a feature of meningioma.[63, 75] Diagnostic judgment also depends on location, and MR has an advantage over CT in depicting the precise relationships of the tumor to the seventh and eighth cranial nerves and the tentorium cerebelli.

OTHER CRANIAL NERVE NEUROMAS

Other cranial nerve neuromas have signal characteristics similar to acoustic neuroma and must be differentiated by location and the specific nerve of origin. Trigeminal neuromas are situated more anteriorly at the petrous apex (Fig. 15–28). The usual site of origin is between the ganglion and the nerve root. For the more anterior lesions, the differential must include other parasellar masses. Replacement of the normal CSF signal within Meckel's cave is an early sign of trigeminal neuroma. Erosion of the petrous apex and involvement of both the middle and posterior fossa are other diagnostic clues.[76]

Seventh nerve neuromas occur most often along the descending portion of the facial canal within the petrous bone but are also found about the geniculate ganglion (see Figs. 21–8 and 21–9). Neuromas of the ninth, tenth, and eleventh cranial nerves cannot be separated and are grouped together. They are located posterior and inferior to the internal auditory

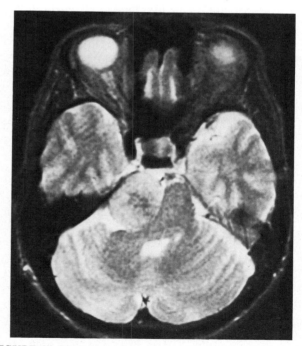

FIGURE 15–28. Trigeminal neuroma. Unenhanced T_2-weighted scan (SE 3000/70) shows a large cerebellopontine angle tumor that compresses the adjacent pons. The tumor is essentially isointense to gray matter and is located more anterior and superior than the usual acoustic neuroma.

canal in the region of the jugular foramen. The coronal and sagittal planes effectively display the anatomy of this area.[77] Also, gradient-echo sequences are helpful for assessing patency of the internal jugular vein (see "Skull Base Lesions").

BRAIN STEM AND CEREBELLUM

MR is particularly well suited for imaging the posterior fossa. The lack of bone-induced artifacts results in a clear depiction of the anatomy of the brain stem and cerebellum. Multiplanar imaging allows for accurate delineation of lesion margins, showing their relationships to the fourth ventricle, tentorial incisura, and foramen magnum. In general, the axial and sagittal planes are preferable for midline lesions; hemispheric cerebellar masses are shown best with axial and coronal scans.

Except for hemangioblastoma and metastatic disease, the majority of intraaxial posterior fossa tumors occur in children. Cerebellar astrocytoma accounts for 33 per cent of these childhood tumors; medulloblastoma, 26 per cent; brain stem glioma, 21 per cent; ependymoma, 14 per cent; and choroid plexus papilloma, only 2 per cent. Clinical findings reflect obstruction of the ventricles (listlessness, projectile vomiting, morning headaches, papilledema) or involvement of cranial nerve nuclei (cranial nerve palsies), long white matter fiber tracts (extremity weakness or sensory disturbance), and cerebellar structures (ataxia, unsteady gait).[16] Intraaxial lesions are more likely to obstruct the ventricles than are extraaxial lesions. Most of these tumors have a higher water content than normal brain, resulting in nonspecific prolongation of T_1 and T_2 relaxation times,[78, 79] but individual MR features also exist as outlined below.

BRAIN STEM GLIOMA

Brain stem gliomas are relatively benign initially but frequently evolve to a higher grade. They usually present with a cranial nerve palsy, most often involving the sixth or seventh nerves. The pons is the common location, but they also occur in the medulla and midbrain (see Fig. 15–12). Histologic features were discussed in the section on cerebral gliomas.

These tumors infiltrate the brain stem and induce surrounding vasogenic edema in the brain parenchyma (Fig. 15–29). Since both the tumor and edema are hyperintense on T_2-weighted images, tumor margins tend to be indistinct and poorly defined. In any case, signal characteristics and margin definition are not accurate predictors of clinical behavior. Brain stem gliomas are relatively homogeneous masses without much cystic change, necrosis, vascularity, or calcification.[80, 81] About 50 per cent of cases will show mild enhancement on contrast CT.[82] Very little MR data are available on enhancement of childhood tumors, but based on adult experience, MR enhancement with Gd-DTPA will probably occur in a higher percentage and to a slightly greater degree than is observed with contrast-enhanced CT.

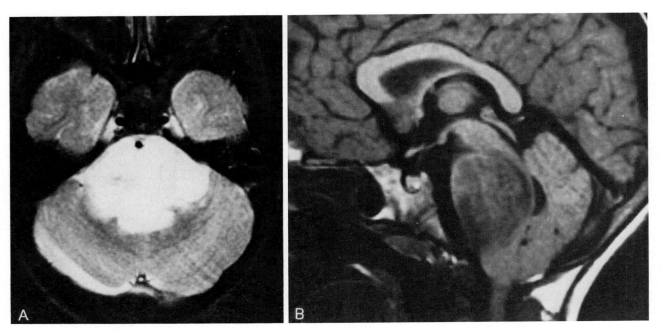

FIGURE 15–29. Brain stem glioma in a 5-year-old boy. *A*, T_2-weighted image (SE 3000/70) discloses a hyperintense mass involving the pons and adjacent middle cerebellar peduncles. *B*, On a T_1-weighted sagittal image (SE 600/20), the pons is markedly enlarged by the tumor, and the fourth ventricle and aqueduct are bowed posteriorly.

As the gliomas grow, they enlarge the brain stem, producing effacement of the basal cisterns, anterior displacement of the basilar artery against the clivus, and compression and posterior bowing of the fourth ventricle (Fig. 15–29). Hydrocephalus is often present. Exophytic growth is a well-known feature of these tumors. Tumor may extend laterally into the cerebellopontine angle or anteriorly into the prepontine cistern, encasing the basilar artery and pushing both the artery and pons posteriorly.

EPENDYMOMA

About 70 per cent of ependymomas are found in the fourth ventricle. The atria of the lateral ventricles is another common site. Males are affected twice as often as females. The cellular structure is organized into canals and rosettes to give them a distinctive histologic appearance. They originate from the ependyma of the ventricles but may grow either into the ventricle or into the brain substance. Ependymomas are slow-growing, but malignant, tumors and grow by expansion and infiltration. Ventricular and subarachnoid seeding are not infrequent. Their more aggressive, malignant counterpart is the ependymoblastoma.[21]

A related tumor, the subependymoma, is derived from cells lying just beneath the ependyma. Histologically, it has features of both ependymal cells and astrocytes.

Most ependymomas arise in the floor of the fourth ventricle. They have a propensity to extend through the foramina of Luschka and Magendie into the basal cisterns. They tend to be well defined, particularly if they are marginated by CSF within a ventricle or cistern. Calcification is present in 50 per cent, cysts and necrotic areas are common, and most are moderately vascular (Fig. 15–30). These properties account for their heterogeneous internal texture on both plain and contrast scans.[83]

CHOROID PLEXUS PAPILLOMA

Choroid plexus papillomas are rare tumors that arise from cells of the choroid plexus. They are slightly more common in the lateral ventricles but are discussed in this section with other pediatric brain tumors. Their histologic picture is strikingly similar to normal choroid plexus. These lesions are benign and expand within a ventricle, eventually leading to obstruction of CSF pathways. Moreover, they may be associated with increased CSF production, another factor contributing to hydrocephalus. Parenchymal invasion is uncommon and should suggest malignant degeneration to choroid plexus carcinoma.[21]

Choroid plexus papillomas usually have well-defined margins, with parts of the tumor outlined by CSF. On T_2-weighted scans they are only mildly hyperintense because their T_2 relaxation times are not as prolonged as in parenchymal tumors. They are relatively homogeneous, but hypervascularity can result in areas of flow void or flow enhancement. Choroid plexus papillomas demonstrate intense homogeneous contrast enhancement.

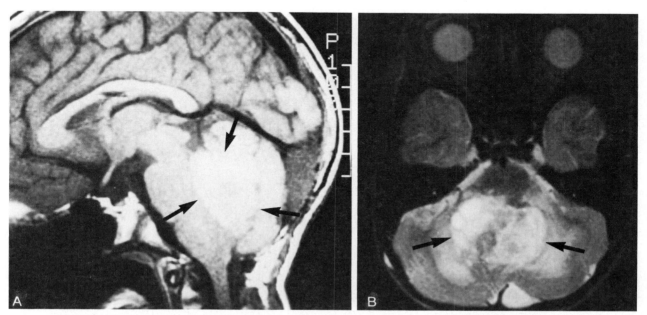

FIGURE 15–30. Ependymoma of the fourth ventricle. *A,* Sagittal T_1-weighted scan (SE 600/25) shows a large mass *(arrows)* within the fourth ventricle. *B,* The mass is hyperintense on a T_2-weighted scan (SE 3000/70) and has a heterogeneous character. Some peritumoral edema is present in the adjacent cerebellar hemispheres. (From Press GA, Hesselink JR: MR imaging of cerebellopontine angle and internal auditory canal lesions at 1.5 T. AJNR 9:241–252, 1988; © by American Society of Neuroradiology.)

CEREBELLAR ASTROCYTOMA

Cerebellar astrocytoma is the most common CNS tumor in children. Histology was discussed in the section on cerebral gliomas. They tend to be lower grade than the supratentorial variety found in adults and are often quite large by time of presentation. The majority are hemispheric in location, a helpful but not absolute criterion to distinguish them from medulloblastoma.

More than 50 per cent of cerebellar astrocytomas are cystic, and the cyst contents often have elevated protein, making them slightly higher signal than CSF but lower signal than brain on T_1-weighted images. The solid components are hyperintense to brain on proton density–weighted images. Both solid tumors and cysts are bright on T_2-weighted scans (Fig. 15–31). Calcification is occasionally present. Peritumoral edema is not pronounced, and in general their margins are better defined than in supratentorial gliomas. Cerebellar astrocytomas exhibit nodular or ringlike enhancement. Since these tumors are frequently large, mass effect is a prominent feature. Anterior and lateral displacement of the fourth ventricle is common. Upward herniation of the superior vermis and downward herniation of the cerebellar tonsils can also occur.[83]

MEDULLOBLASTOMA

The majority of medulloblastomas occur in children between four and eight years old, and males outnumber females three to one. These patients usually present with symptoms of hydrocephalus.

Medulloblastomas arise from remnants of primitive neuroectoderm in the roof of the fourth ventricle. Histologic sections show undifferentiated small cells, closely packed with hyperchromatic nuclei, scanty cytoplasm, and many mitoses. These tumors are very malignant and exhibit an aggressive biologic behavior, commonly invading the adjacent brain stem and leptomeninges. Widespread dissemination through the ventricular system and distant seeding to other area of the neuraxis occur in as high as 30 per cent. Metastases outside the central nervous system to the bones, cervical lymph nodes, and peritoneum have also been reported.[21]

Medulloblastomas are primarily midline vermian lesions, but hemispheric locations are also possible. Since they arise close to the fourth ventricle, growth predominantly into the ventricle may make them simulate an intraventricular mass. Necrosis, hemorrhage, and cavitation are common features, giving these tumors a slightly heterogeneous appearance on MR but not to the same degree as seen with ependymomas. Calcification is rare in medulloblastomas.[84, 85] As a result of the dense cell packing, there is relatively little extracellular water, so these tumors are only mildly hyperintense to brain on T_2-weighted images (Fig. 15–32). They are hypervascular lesions and show moderate contrast enhancement.

HEMANGIOBLASTOMA

Hemangioblastoma is a benign tumor of middle age. In fact, it is the most common primary intraaxial tumor of the posterior fossa in adults. About 20 per cent are associated with Hippel-Lindau disease, and

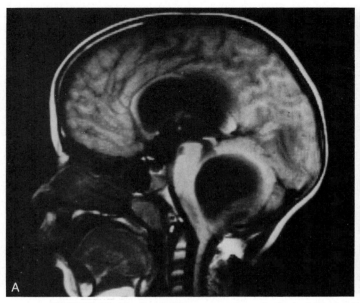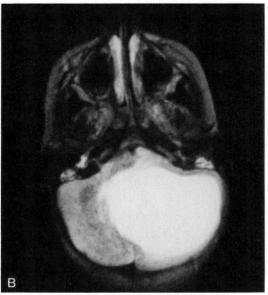

FIGURE 15–31. Cerebellar astrocytoma. *A*, Sagittal T_1-weighted image discloses a large hypointense mass within the posterior fossa which compresses the fourth ventricle and displaces the brain stem against the clivus. *B*, The mass is hyperintense on an axial T_2-weighted image and is centered in the left cerebellar hemisphere. It has smooth margins and is relatively homogeneous on both images, consistent with a cystic lesion.

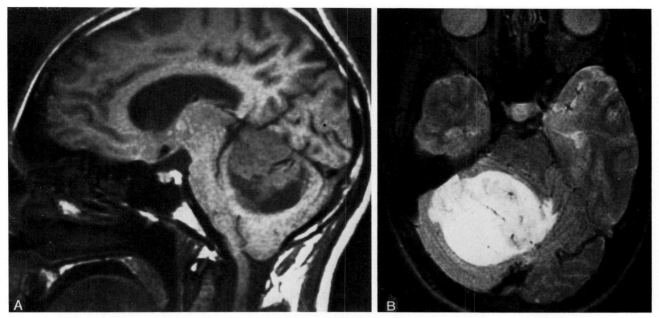

FIGURE 15–32. Medulloblastoma. *A*, Sagittal T$_1$-weighted scan (SE 600/20) demonstrates a lesion in the superior vermis. The fourth ventricle is compressed, and the brain stem is displaced anteriorly. *B*, On a T$_2$-weighted axial scan (SE 3000/70), the tumor is hyperintense and has extended into the right cerebellar hemisphere. The low signal vessels within the lesion indicate the hypervascular nature of the tumor.

hereditary factors have been implicated in another 20 per cent. The cerebellum and vermis are the common sites, but hemangioblastomas can also be found in the medulla and cervical spinal cord. Multiplicity is a well-known feature but is present in only about 10 per cent of cases. Histologic examination reveals a meshwork of capillaries and small vessels.[21]

The classic MR appearance of hemangioblastoma is a cystic mass with a brightly enhancing nodule (Fig. 15–33). About 60 per cent are cystic, so solid lesions are not uncommon. Calcification is rare. Hemangioblastomas are sharply marginated and induce minimal surrounding parenchymal reaction. The tumor nodules are hypervascular, and the vascular pedicle often produces a characteristic flow void on MR.[9, 85]

DIFFERENTIAL DIAGNOSIS

Differential diagnosis of brain stem and cerebellar lesions can be accomplished by a stepwise analysis of the images and clinical information. First, the intraaxial location must be established, which usually can be readily determined with multiplanar MR. Occasionally, predominantly exophytic growth of an intraaxial lesion may lead to confusion. Next, the mass should be localized to the brain stem, ventricle, or cerebellum. With this information and a knowledge of the patient's age, one can often arrive at a specific diagnosis. For example, a metastasis may simulate a brain stem glioma, or a cystic astrocytoma may look a lot like a hemangioblastoma, but they

occur in different age groups. Specific features of metastatic disease are discussed in a separate section. Signal intensity, internal texture, and enhancement patterns also assist in differential diagnosis.

SKULL BASE LESIONS

The skull base can be involved by primary, secondary, and metastatic tumors. The primary tumors include chordoma, chondroma and chondrosarcoma, plasmacytoma, paraganglioma, neuroma/neurofibroma, and cholesteatoma. Secondary tumors are most often carcinomas from the nasopharynx and paranasal sinuses, pituitary tumors, or more aggressive meningiomas. The common metastases are from lung and breast carcinoma, but other tumors can also metastasize to the skull. Also included in the differential are fibrous dysplasia and hyperostosis secondary to meningioma. This section is devoted to the primary group of tumors. Cholesteatoma was discussed under the section of benign cystic masses.

CHORDOMA

Chordoma is a rare neoplasm, but it is the most common primary of the clivus. These lesions arise from notochordal remnants in the clivus, meninges along the prepontine cistern, sphenoid, or nasopharynx. The most common site is near the sphenooccipital synchondrosis. Chordomas are slow growing and

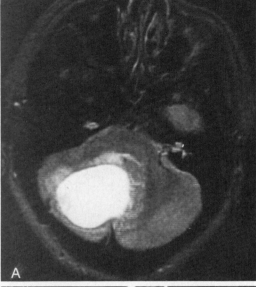

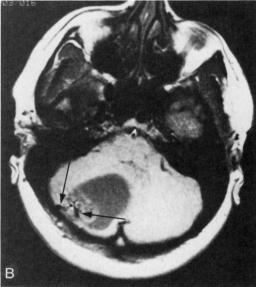

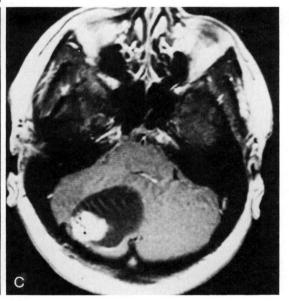

FIGURE 15–33. Hemangioblastoma. *A,* Noncontrast T₂-weighted image (SE 3000/80) shows a high signal mass within the right cerebellar hemisphere with a small amount of surrounding edema. *B,* The mass is hypointense on a plain T₁-weighted image (SE 600/20). The lower signal structures *(arrows)* are vessels within the vascular pedicle of the tumor. *C,* A Gd-enhanced scan discloses an enhancing nodule and a large cystic component.

erode bone by direct extension. The soft tissue mass readily extends into the sella, perisellar region, prepontine cistern, sphenoid sinus, and middle fossa. Cartilaginous foci, bone fragments, and calcifications are interspersed within the tumor matrix.[86]

CHONDROMA AND CHONDROSARCOMA

Chondroma is a benign tumor that arises from cartilage cell rests at the skull base. Chondrosarcoma is the malignant counterpart that often originates from a preexisting benign lesion. Calcification is common in both tumors. *Plasmacytoma* is another rare tumor of the skull base which is derived from plasma cells. With time, many evolve to multiple myeloma.

MR FEATURES

Chordomas and chondrosarcomas have been studied by MR and compared with CT.[87] MR was found to define more clearly the relationships of the tumors to the brain stem, optic chiasm, nasopharynx, and cavernous sinus, as well as to show arterial encasement. CT is better for precise determination of the extent of bone destruction. Separation of the two lesions is difficult on the basis of MR findings, each exhibiting long T₁ and long T₂. Both lesions can be difficult to identify on T₁-weighted axial images alone due to low contrast with the adjacent low signal cortical bone and CSF, but alteration of the normal high signal clival fat is a sensitive indicator of disease on T₁-weighted images (Fig. 15–34) (also see Fig. 21–

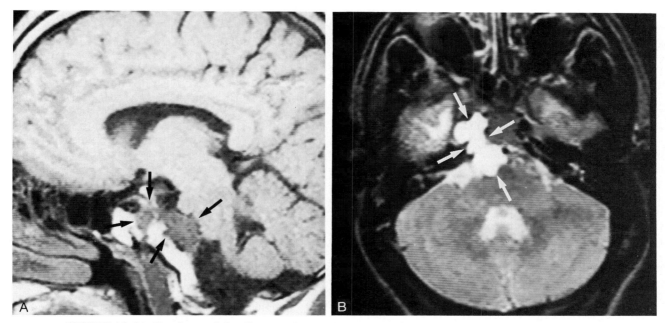

FIGURE 15–34. Chordoma of the clivus. *A*, On a sagittal T$_1$-weighted image, a soft tissue mass *(arrows)* has eroded the clivus and has extended into the prepontine cistern. *B*, The tumor is high signal intensity on a T$_2$-weighted scan and indents the pons.

14). Plasmacytoma also has no distinctive MR features to allow for a definitive diagnosis. Enhancement with Gd-DTPA is helpful to assess the intracranial components of these tumors, but it is not as useful in the extracranial compartments, due to the lack of a BBB in extracranial tissues and because the enhancing tumor blends in with the high signal fatty tissue on T$_1$-weighted images.

PARAGANGLIOMA

Paragangliomas, also referred to as chemodectomas, include glomus tympanicum and glomus jugulare tumors, so called because of their respective sites of origin. They arise from paraganglionic glomus tissue within the middle ear and jugular fossa. They are benign lesions that slowly erode into adjacent areas

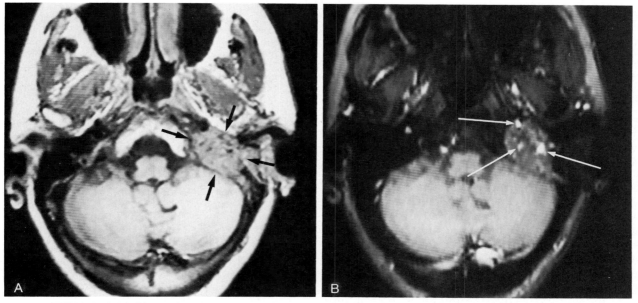

FIGURE 15–35. Glomus jugulare tumor. *A*, Axial T$_1$-weighted scan (SE 600/25) through the skull base reveals a heterogeneous soft tissue mass *(arrows)* that fills the left jugular foramen and has eroded the inferior aspect of the temporal bone. *B*, Gradient-echo image (GRE 100/16) demonstrates high signal foci *(arrows)* within the tumor, indicating its hypervascular nature.

of the skull base and posterior fossa. Most present with pulsatile tinnitus or neurologic deficits secondary to involvement of the seventh, ninth, tenth, and eleventh cranial nerves. A normal multiplicity rate of 3 per cent increases to 26 per cent if familial factors are present.

Paragangliomas (glomus tumors) have a unique MR appearance related to their extreme hypervascularity (Fig. 15–35). Serpiginous areas of signal void from blood flow are interspersed among areas of higher signal intensity representing flow-related enhancement and more isointense tumor cells.[88] They are of variable signal intensity but are usually hyperintense to the surrounding muscles on T_2-weighted images. Even-echo rephasing may be noted within the tumor and any remaining patent portions of the jugular vein. Vascular flow effects are particularly well displayed with gradient-echo sequences.[89] MR is more helpful than CT in determining involvement of the carotid artery and jugular vein.[77] MR can show bony erosion, but subtle erosions are better visualized with CT (also see Figs. 21–6 and 21–7).

DIFFERENTIAL DIAGNOSIS

Neuromas are the other major tumor in the differential of masses within the jugular foramen. They arise from the ninth, tenth, or eleventh cranial nerves and are uncommon except in patients with neurofibromatosis. They tend to be isointense to brain and are more homogeneous than glomus tumors. Histologic and MR features of neuromas were covered in a separate section.

CONCLUSION

Since many brain tumors exhibit similar signal characteristics, owing to prolonged T_1 and T_2 compared with brain, it might be helpful to quickly review those lesions that appear different. The reader is referred back to the individual sections that discuss the following lesions for further information and references. Hyperintensity within masses on T_1-weighted images usually represents fat (dermoid, lipoma, teratoma), hemorrhage (including necrotic gliomas and metastases), or paramagnetic effects (gadolinium enhancement, possibly metastatic melanoma). A few colloid cysts have been described with a bright T_1 and bright T_2 appearance, possibly related to a very high protein content. Secondary (acquired) cholesteatomas may also exhibit a short T_1. Hypointense lesions on T_2-weighted scans include calcified meningiomas, hemorrhage (acute and chronic stages), lipomas, and fibroosseous lesions of the skull base. Tumors that are often isointense with brain on T_1- and T_2-weighted images are germinoma, pituitary adenoma, meningioma, hamartoma, and acoustic neuroma. Any highly cellular tumors with relatively little interstitial fluid space also tend to be isointense to brain parenchyma, such as lymphoma, medulloblastoma, and an occasional metastasis. Hypothalamic/chiasmal gliomas are usually isointense with brain on T_1-weighted images but are hyperintense on T_2-weighted images. Epidermoids must be kept in mind as being isointense with CSF on T_1-weighted images, and while these lesions are usually hyperintense on T_2, they may be isointense with CSF on this sequence as well. Hypervascular tumors are likely to show a mixed signal intensity due to foci of flow void and flow enhancement.

REFERENCES

1. Bradley WG Jr, Waluch V, Yadley RA, Wycoff RR: Comparison of CT and MR in 400 patients with suspected disease of the brain and cervical spinal canal. Radiology 152:695–702, 1984.
2. Brant-Zawadzki M, Davis PL, Crooks LE, et al: NMR demonstration of cerebral abnormalities: Comparison with CT. AJR 140:847–854, 1983.
3. Kjos BO, Brant-Zawadzki M, Kucharczyk W, et al: Cystic intracranial lesions: Magnetic resonance imaging. Radiology 155:363–369, 1985.
4. Enzmann DR, Rubin JR, DeLaPaz R, Wright A: Cerebrospinal fluid pulsation: Benefits and pitfalls in MR imaging. Radiology 161:773–778, 1986.
5. Lee BCP, Kneeland JB, Cahill P, Deck MDFD: MR recognition of supratentorial tumors. AJNR 6:871–878, 1985.
6. Atlas SW, Grossman RI, Hackney DB, et al: Calcified intracranial lesions: Detection with gradient-echo acquisition rapid MR imaging. AJNR 9:253–260, 1988.
7. Komiyama M, Yagura H, Baba M, et al: MR imaging: The possibility of tissue characterization of brain tumors using T1 and T2 values. AJNR 8:65–70, 1987.
8. Rinck PA, Meindl S, Higer HP, et al: Brain tumors: Detection and typing by use of CPMG sequences and in vivo T2 measurements. Radiology 157:103–106, 1985.
9. Hesselink JR, Healy ME, Press GA, Brahme FJ: Benefits of Gd-DTPA for MR imaging of intracranial abnormalities. J Comput Assist Tomogr 12:266–274, 1988.
10. Graif M, Bydder GM, Steiner RE, et al: Contrast-enhanced MR imaging of malignant brain tumors. AJNR 6:855–862, 1985.
11. Schorner W, Laniado M, Niendorf HP, et al: Brain tumors: Imaging with gadolinium-DTPA. Radiology 156:681–688, 1985.
12. Hesselink JR, Press GA: MR contrast enhancement of intracranial lesions with Gd-DTPA. Radiol Clin North Am 26:873–887, 1988.
13. Berry I, Brant-Zawadzki M, Osaki L, et al: Gadolinium-DTPA in clinical MR of the brain: 2. Extraaxial lesions and normal structures. AJNR 7:789–793, 1986.
14. Breger RK, Papke RA, Pojunas KW, et al: Benign extraaxial tumors: Contrast enhancement with Gd-DTPA. Radiology 163:427–429, 1987.
15. Kilgore DP, Breger RK, Daniels DL, et al: Cranial tissues: Normal MR appearance after intravenous injection of Gd-DTPA. Radiology 160:757–761, 1986.
16. Adams RD, Victor M: Principles of Neurology. 2nd ed. New York, McGraw-Hill Book Company, 1981, pp 440–474.
17. Claussen C, Laniado M, Schorner W, et al: Gadolinium-DTPA in MR imaging of glioblastomas and intracranial metastases. AJNR 6:669–674, 1985.
18. Brant-Zawadzki M, Berry I, Brasch R, et al: Gadolinium-DTPA in clinical MR of the brain: 1. Intraaxial lesions. AJNR 7:781–788, 1986.
19. Shuman WP, Griffin BR, Haynor DK, et al: The utility of MR

in planning the radiation therapy of oligodendroglioma. AJNR 8:93–98, 1987.

20. Shuman WP, Griffin BR, Haynor DR, et al: MR imaging in radiation therapy planning. Radiology 156:143–147, 1986.

21. Bonnin JM, Garcia JH: Histology and growth characteristics of brain neoplasms. In Taveras JM, Ferrucci JT (eds): Radiology: Diagnosis, Imaging, Intervention. Vol 3. Philadelphia, JB Lippincott Company, 1988, pp 1–11.

22. Tadmor R, Davis KR, Roberson HG, Kleinman GM: Computed tomography in primary malignant lymphoma of the brain. J Comput Assist Tomogr 2:135–140, 1978.

23. Healy ME, Hesselink JR, Press GA, Middleton MS: Increased detection of intracranial metastases with intravenous Gd-DTPA. Radiology 165:619–624, 1987.

24. Russell EJ, Geremia GK, Johnson CE, et al: Multiple cerebral metastases: Detectability with Gd-DTPA–enhanced MR imaging. Radiology 165:609–617, 1987.

25. Atlas SW, Grossman RI, Gomori JM, et al: Hemorrhagic intracranial malignant neoplasms: Spin-echo MR imaging. Radiology 164:71–77, 1987.

26. Woodruff WW Jr, Djang WT, McLendon RE, et al: Intracerebral malignant melanoma: High-field-strength MR imaging. Radiology 165:209–213, 1987.

27. Atlas SW, Grossman RI, Gomori JM, et al: MR imaging of intracranial metastatic melanoma. J Comput Assist Tomogr 11:577–582, 1987.

28. Zimmerman RD, Fleming CA, Saint-Louis CA, et al: Magnetic resonance imaging of meningiomas. AJNR 6:149–157, 1985.

29. Spagnoli MV, Goldberg HI, Grossman RI, et al: Intracranial meningiomas: High-field MR imaging. Radiology 161:369–375, 1986.

30. Bydder GM, Kingsley DPE, Brown J, et al: MR imaging of meningiomas including studies with and without gadolinium-DTPA. J Comput Assist Tomogr 9:690–697, 1985.

31. Sands SF, Farmer P, Alvarez O, et al: Fat within the falx: MR demonstration of falcine bony metaplasia with marrow formation. J Comput Assist Tomogr 11:602–605, 1987.

32. Russell DS, Rubinstein LF: Pathology of Tumors of the Nervous System. 4th ed. Baltimore, Williams & Wilkins, 1977.

33. Kilgore DP, Strother CM, Starshak RJ, Haughton VM: Pineal germinoma: MR imaging. Radiology 158:435–438, 1986.

34. Muller-Forell W, Schroth G, Egan PJ: MR imaging in tumors of the pineal region. Neuroradiology 30:224–231, 1988.

35. Zimmerman RA, Bilaniuk LT, Wood JH, et al: Computed tomography of pineal, parapineal, and histologically related tumors. Radiology 137:669–677, 1980.

36. Mamourian AC, Towfighi J: Pineal cysts: MR imaging. AJNR 7:1081–1086, 1986.

37. Bradley WG, Kortman KE, Erves JL: Central nervous system high-resolution magnetic resonance imaging: Effect of increasing spatial resolution on resolving power. Radiology 156:93–98, 1985.

38. Pojunas KW, Daniels DL, Williams AL, Haughton VM: MR imaging of prolactin secreting microadenomas. AJNR 7:209–213, 1986.

39. Kucharczyk W, Davis DO, Kelly WM, et al: Pituitary adenomas: High resolution MR imaging at 1.5 T. Radiology 161:761–765, 1986.

40. Davis PC, Hoffman JC, Spencer T, et al: MR imaging of pituitary adenoma: CT, clinical, and surgical considerations. AJNR 8:107–112, 1987.

41. Kulkarni MV, Lee KF, McArdle CB, et al: 1.5 T MR imaging of pituitary microadenomas: Technical considerations and CT correlation. AJNR 9:5–12, 1988.

42. Karnaze MG, Sartor K, Winthrop JD, et al: Suprasellar lesions: Evaluation with MR imaging. Radiology 161:77–82, 1986.

43. Lee BCP, Deck MDF: Sellar and juxtasellar lesion detection with MR. Radiology 157:143–147, 1985.

44. Daniels DL, Pojunas KW, Kilgore DP, et al: MR of the diaphragma sellae. AJNR 7:765–769, 1986.

45. Daniels DL, Pech P, Mark L, et al: Magnetic resonance imaging of the cavernous sinus. AJNR 6:187–192, 1985.

46. Dwyer AJ, Frank JA, Doppman JL, et al: Pituitary adenomas in patients with Cushing disease: Initial experience with Gd-DTPA–enhanced MR imaging. Radiology 163:421–426, 1987.

47. Mark L, Pech P, Daniels DL, et al: The pituitary fossa: A correlative anatomic and MR study. Radiology 153:453–457, 1984.

48. Fukisawa I, Asato R, Nishimura K, et al: Anterior and posterior lobes of the pituitary gland: Assessment by MR imaging. J Comput Assist Tomogr 11:214–220, 1987.

49. Colombo N, Berry I, Kucharczyk J, et al: Posterior pituitary gland: Appearance on MR images in normal and pathologic states. Radiology 165:481–485, 1987.

50. Fukisawa I, Nishimura K, Asato R, et al: Posterior lobe of the pituitary in diabetes insipidus: MR findings. J Comput Assist Tomogr 11:221–225, 1987.

51. Fujisawa I, Kikuchi K, Nishimura K, et al: Transection of the pituitary stalk: Development of an ectopic posterior lobe assessed with MR imaging. Radiology 165:487–489, 1987.

52. Albert A, Lee BCP, Saint-Louis L, Deck MDF: MR of optic chiasm and optic pathways. AJNR 7:255–258, 1986.

53. Pusey E, Kortman KE, Flannigan BD, et al: MR of craniopharyngioma: Tumor delineation and characterization. AJNR 8:439–444, 1987.

54. Kaufman B: Perisellar lesions. In Taveras JM, Ferrucci JT (eds): Radiology: Diagnosis, Imaging, Intervention. Vol 3. Philadelphia, JB Lippincott Company, 1988, pp 1–11.

55. Kucharczyk W, Peck WW, Kelly WM, et al: Rathke cleft cysts: CT, MR imaging, and pathologic features. Radiology 165:491–495, 1987.

56. Graif M, Pennock JM: MR imaging of histiocytosis X in the central nervous system. AJNR 7:21–23, 1986.

57. Sartor K, Karnaze MG, Winthrop JD, et al: MR imaging in infra-, para- and retrosellar mass lesions. Neuroradiology 29:19–29, 1987.

58. Atlas SW, Grossman RI, Goldberg HI, et al: Partially thrombosed giant intracranial aneurysms: Correlation of MR and pathologic findings. Radiology 162:111–114, 1987.

59. Wiener SN, Pearlstein AE, Eiber A: MR imaging of arachnoid cysts. J Comput Assist Tomogr 11:236–241, 1987.

60. Steffey DJ, De Filipp GJ, Spera T, Gabrielsen TO: MR imaging of primary epidermoid tumors. J Comput Assist Tomogr 12:438–440, 1988.

61. Yuh WTC, Barloon TJ, Jacoby CG, et al: MR of fourth ventricular epidermoid tumors. AJNR 9:794–798, 1988.

62. Vion-Dury J, Vincentelli F, Jiddane M, et al: MR imaging of epidermoid cysts. Neuroradiology 29:333–338, 1987.

63. Gentry LR, Jacoby CG, Turski PA, et al: Cerebellopontine angle-petromastoid lesions: Comparative study of diagnosis with MR imaging and CT. Radiology 162:513–520, 1987.

64. MacKay IM, Bydder GM, Young IR: MR imaging of central nervous system tumors that do not display increase in T1 or T2. J Comput Assist Tomogr 9:1055–1061, 1985.

65. Hahn FJ, Ong E, McComb RD, et al: MR imaging of ruptured intracranial dermoid. J Comput Assist Tomogr 10:888–889, 1986.

66. Roosen N, Gahlen D, Stork W, et al: Magnetic resonance imaging of colloid cysts of the third ventricle. Neuroradiology 29:10–14, 1987.

67. Scotti G, Scialfa G, Colombo N, et al: MR in the diagnosis of colloid cysts of the third ventricle. AJNR 8:370–372, 1987.

68. Donaldson JO, Simon RH: Radiodense ions within a third ventricle colloid cyst. Arch Neurol 37:246, 1980.

69. Kingsley DPE, Brooks GB, Leving AW-L, Johnson MA: Acoustic neuromas: Evaluation by magnetic resonance imaging. AJNR 6:1–5, 1985.

70. Curati WL, Graif M, Kingsley DPE, et al: MRI in acoustic neuroma: A review of 35 patients. Neuroradiology 28:208–214, 1986.

71. Mikhael MA, Ciric IS, Wolff AP: MR diagnosis of acoustic neuromas. J Comput Assist Tomogr 11:232–235, 1987.

72. Press GA, Hesselink JR: MR imaging of cerebellopontine angle and internal auditory canal lesions at 1.5 T. AJNR 9:241–252, 1988.

73. Curati WL, Graif M, Kingsley DPE, et al: Acoustic neuromas: Gadolinium-DTPA enhancement in MR imaging. Radiology 158:447–451, 1986.

74. Daniels DL, Millen SJ, Meyer GA, et al: MR detection of tumor in the internal auditory canal. AJNR 8:249–252, 1987.

75. Mikhael MA, Ciric IS, Wolff AP: Differentiation of cerebellopontine angle neuromas and meningiomas with MR imaging. J Comput Assist Tomogr 9:852–856, 1985.

76. Daniels DL, Pech P, Pojunas KW, et al: Trigeminal nerve: Anatomic correlation with MR imaging. Radiology 159:577–583, 1986.

77. Daniels DL, Schenck JF, Foster T, et al: Magnetic resonance imaging of the jugular foramen. AJNR 6:699–703, 1986.

78. Bonstelle CT, Kaufman B, Benson JE, et al: Magnetic resonance imaging in the evaluation of the brainstem. Radiology 150:705–712, 1984.

79. Hueffle MG, Han JS, Kaufman B, Benson JE: MR imaging of brain stem gliomas. J Comput Assist Tomogr 9:263–267, 1985.

80. Lee BCP, Kneeland JB, Walker RW, et al: MR imaging of brainstem tumors. AJNR 6:159–163, 1985.

81. Peterman SB, Steiner RE, Bydder GM, et al: Nuclear magnetic resonance imaging (NMR), (MRI), of brain stem tumors. Neuroradiology 27:202–207, 1985.

82. Oot RF, Davis KR: Intra-axial posterior fossa neoplasms. *In* Taveras JM, Ferrucci JT (eds): Radiology: Diagnosis, Imaging, Intervention. Vol 3. Philadelphia, JB Lippincott Company, 1988, pp 1–9.

83. Randell CP, Collins AG, Young IR, et al: Nuclear magnetic resonance imaging of posterior fossa tumors. AJNR 4:1027–1034, 1983.

84. Zimmerman RA, Bilaniuk LT: Applications of magnetic resonance imaging in disease of the pediatric central nervous system. Magn Reson Imaging 4:11–24, 1986.

85. Barnes PD, Lester PD, Yamanashi WS, et al: Magnetic resonance imaging in childhood intracranial masses. Magn Reson Imaging 4:41–50, 1986.

86. Sze G, Uichanco LS, Brant-Zawadzki MN, et al: Chordomas: MR imaging. Radiology 166:187–192, 1988.

87. Oot RF, Melville G, New PFJ, et al: The role of MR and CT in evaluating clival chordomas and chondrosarcomas. AJNR 9:715–724, 1988.

88. Olsen WL, Dillon WP, Kelly WM, et al: MR imaging of paragangliomas. AJNR 7:1039–1042, 1986.

89. Daniels DL, Czervionke LF, Pech P, et al: Gradient recalled echo MR imaging of the jugular foramen. AJNR 9:675–678, 1988.

16

BRAIN: Spontaneous Hemorrhage

HEINRICH P. MATTLE, GERALD V. O'REILLY, ROBERT R. EDELMAN, and KEITH A. JOHNSON

MR APPEARANCE AND EVOLUTION OF BRAIN HEMORRHAGE

MAGNETIC STATES OF MATTER

THE EFFECTS OF PARAMAGNETIC SUBSTANCES ON SIGNAL INTENSITY

T₂ Shortening
T₁ Shortening

EVOLUTION OF SIGNAL INTENSITY CHANGES ON MR IMAGES

Very Acute Hematoma
Acute Hematoma
Subacute Hematoma
Chronic Hematoma

USE OF GRADIENT-ECHO PULSE SEQUENCES TO IMPROVE CHARACTERIZATION OF HEMATOMAS

Diffusion Causes Signal Loss on Spin-Echo Images
Static Magnetic Field Inhomogeneities Cause Signal Loss on Gradient-Echo Images
Boundary Effect

EFFECT OF OXYGENATION ON THE APPEARANCE OF HEMORRHAGE

EXTRACEREBRAL HEMORRHAGE

DIFFERENTIAL DIAGNOSIS OF HEMORRHAGE ON MR IMAGES

Fat Versus Hemorrhage
Proteinaceous Fluid Versus Hemorrhage
Flow Voids Versus Hemorrhage
Melanin Versus Hemorrhage
Calcification Versus Hemorrhage

GENERAL COMMENTS ON SPONTANEOUS BRAIN HEMORRHAGE

PATHOGENESIS OF BRAIN HEMORRHAGE

TIME COURSE OF BLEEDING

ETIOLOGY, LOCATION, AND FREQUENCY

CLINICAL PRESENTATION

ETIOLOGY OF HEMORRHAGE BY LOCATION AND ASSOCIATED BRAIN ABNORMALITIES

HYPERTENSIVE (DEEP) HEMORRHAGE

Putaminal Hemorrhage
Caudate Hemorrhage
Thalamic Hemorrhage
Brain Stem Hemorrhage
Cerebellar Hemorrhage

LOBAR HEMORRHAGE

Hemorrhage from Aneurysms
Vascular Malformations
Amyloid Angiopathy
Subcortical "Slit" Hemorrhage
Bleeding Diathesis
Drug Use and Abuse
Hemorrhage Associated with Tumor
Hemorrhagic Infarction
Miscellaneous Rare Types of Hemorrhage

PRIMARY INTRAVENTRICULAR HEMORRHAGE

PITUITARY HEMORRHAGE

INTRACEREBRAL HEMORRHAGE OF UNDETERMINED CAUSE

FACTORS INFLUENCING OUTCOME OF INTRACEREBRAL HEMORRHAGE AND THERAPEUTIC IMPLICATIONS

Spontaneous brain hemorrhage is defined as bleeding into the brain substance by any cause that is of nontraumatic origin. There are many causes of such hemorrhage, but by far the most common is uncontrolled chronic systemic arterial hypertension. Until the advent of computed tomography (CT) in 1972, the diagnosis of spontaneous brain hemorrhage could only be inferred from the angiographic findings of an avascular intracranial mass in a patient with a sudden stroke syndrome. Unless a ruptured aneurysm or arteriovenous malformation was also visualized on angiography, a conclusive antemortem diagnosis of brain hemorrhage was always questionable. Such an avascular mass could also have been

483

the result of an infarction, tumor, or abscess. Since its inception, CT so revolutionized the diagnosis of intracranial disease that it became, and still is, the primary diagnostic tool in the evaluation of a patient presenting with an acute stroke. For the first time, CT made it possible to distinguish between an ischemic and a hemorrhagic event in the brain by a noninvasive means.

However, CT does have significant limitations in its diagnostic capabilities. Small petechial hemorrhages in the brain stem, some hemorrhagic infarctions, and many chronic hematomas may escape detection by CT. This is partly due to low contrast resolution and bone artifacts, which often result in poor definition of posterior fossa structures, and also to partial volume effects, which tend to lessen sensitivity for the presence of small quantities of blood within an acute infarct. Another issue is that on CT scans, a brain hematoma gradually evolves over several weeks from high density, through an isodense phase, to low density. This change in scan appearance is due to an alteration in tissue density rather than actual resorption of the hematoma. As a consequence, after some months the CT findings of a brain hemorrhage are often indistinguishable from an old infarction, even though pathologically there is still evidence of a hematoma in the brain. Finally, CT or even angiography may, in some cases, fail to provide a specific diagnosis of the cause of the original hemorrhage, such as a vascular malformation or tumor.

While CT, despite these limitations, remains the diagnostic procedure most useful in the emergency management of an acute stroke patient, MR imaging may prove to be the ultimate method of refining the diagnosis. Pragmatically, many patients who have suffered a brain hemorrhage are not clinically suitable to undergo MR in the acute phase, due to restlessness or the need for life support equipment. Therefore, once the hemorrhagic nature of a lesion is identified by CT, MR can be used later to increase diagnostic information by more accurately defining the extent of the lesion, assessing the age of its hemorrhagic component, and detecting the presence of any underlying lesion. However, the various MR patterns of brain hemorrhage will need careful evaluation if correct deductions are to be made, as the evolution of hemorrhage is one of the more complex and controversial aspects of MR imaging. For instance, the impact of petechial hemorrhages detected within infarctions by MR imaging, but not CT, on the therapeutic application of anticoagulants remains to be determined.

MR APPEARANCE AND EVOLUTION OF BRAIN HEMORRHAGE

Intracranial hemorrhage has been studied extensively by MR imaging.[1–23b] The biochemical and physiochemical details of hemorrhage are reviewed in depth in Chapter 8. This section will review the basic concepts involved in interpreting the appearance of brain hemorrhage on MR images.

The complex manifestations of hemorrhage on MR images relate to the formation of a series of substances with potent magnetic properties, which result from the breakdown of oxyhemoglobin. These substances include deoxyhemoglobin, methemoglobin, ferritin, and hemosiderin. As a result of the magnetic properties of these hemoglobin breakdown products, intracerebral hemorrhage has a variety of appearances on MR images which depend on several factors: (1) pulse sequence; (2) field strength; (3) age of hemorrhage; and (4) state of oxygenation of the hemorrhage, which relates to its location.

MAGNETIC STATES OF MATTER

Matter can exist in several different magnetic states. These states are described in terms of their "magnetic susceptibility," which represents the degree to which the presence of a substance tends to attract or repel magnetic lines of force (Fig. 16–1). The magnetic susceptibility of a substance is predominantly determined by the configuration of the orbital electrons (see Chapter 8). Because of their smaller mass, these electrons have magnetic moments more than a thousand times greater than those of protons. The categories of magnetic susceptibility relevant to interpreting the appearance of hemorrhage on MR images include diamagnetism, paramagnetism, and superparamagnetism.

Most substances, including oxyhemoglobin, are diamagnetic. The orbital electrons in diamagnetic substances are paired, which reduces the effect of their magnetic moments. The paired electrons weakly

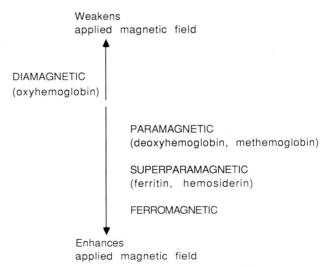

FIGURE 16–1. Magnetic susceptibility of hemoglobin breakdown products.

oppose an applied magnetic field, but to such a minimal extent that the magnetic properties of these electrons have a negligible effect on the appearance of the image. On the other hand, paramagnetic substances, which include all of the above-mentioned hemoglobin breakdown products, have a profound effect on signal intensity. Paramagnetic substances contain unpaired orbital electrons; in the case of hemoglobin breakdown products, the unpaired electrons are localized to iron atoms.

THE EFFECTS OF PARAMAGNETIC SUBSTANCES ON SIGNAL INTENSITY

The effects of a paramagnetic substance on signal intensity depend on several factors, including the concentration of the paramagnetic substance and the degree to which water molecules have access to it. Depending on the situation, paramagnetic hemoglobin breakdown products can predominantly induce either T_2 shortening, resulting in signal loss, or T_1 shortening, resulting in signal enhancement.

T_2 Shortening

Because paramagnetic molecules have a sizeable magnetic moment, their concentration within a restricted region produces a disturbance in the local magnetic field. The disturbance in magnetic field homogeneity produced by the concentration of these paramagnetic substances is analogous to the effect of placing an iron bar within the bore of the MR magnet. Examples of paramagnetic substances associated with this phenomenon include intracellular deoxyhemoglobin and intracellular methemoglobin.

Water molecules diffusing past these concentrated paramagnetic centers experience an inhomogeneous field, with resultant rapid dephasing (T_2 shortening) and signal loss (Fig. 16–2). This signal loss is seen on T_2-weighted images because T_2-weighted acquisitions use a long echo time (TE). As the TE is increased, there is more time available for the water molecules to diffuse through the inhomogeneous magnetic field, causing further dephasing and greater signal loss.

Ferritin and hemosiderin are categorized as superparamagnetic (see Chapters 7 and 8). Because of their very large magnetic moment, these superparamagnetic substances produce marked signal loss in smaller concentrations than intracellular deoxyhemoglobin and methemoglobin.

The superparamagnetic iron-containing cores of ferritin and hemosiderin are largely excluded from contact with water molecules. The same is true for deoxyhemoglobin, because the region of the globin molecule containing paramagnetic iron is hydrophobic and repels water molecules. However, T_1 relaxation processes depend on close interaction between water molecules and the paramagnetic center; these interactions decrease with the sixth power of the

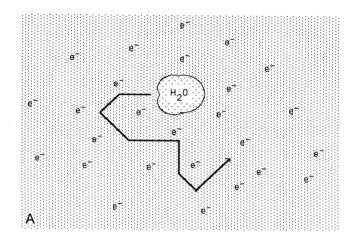

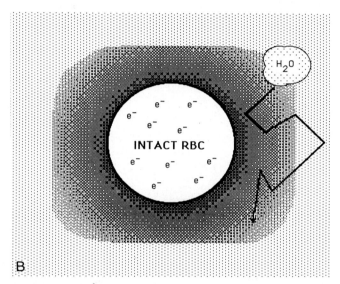

FIGURE 16–2. *A,* When water molecules diffuse through normal brain matter, they experience a homogeneous magnetic field. *B,* When paramagnetic or superparamagnetic substances such as hemoglobin breakdown products concentrate locally after hemorrhage, the homogeneity of the magnetic field in the brain is disturbed. The ensuing local magnetic field inhomogeneity increases dephasing and signal loss when water molecules diffuse past these substances. The signal loss is most pronounced on T_2-weighted images because of the long echo time (RBC = red blood cell.)

distance between molecules. As a result, these substances produce only minimal changes in T_1 relaxation.

T_1 Shortening

Paramagnetic molecules, which are distributed freely in solution, produce quite different alterations in signal intensity from those just discussed. Extracellular methemoglobin is an example of such a substance. Following erythrocyte lysis, methemoglobin is released into the extracellular space, where it distributes uniformly in solution and in reduced concentration. The magnetic moments of these unpaired electrons enhance the applied field. If water

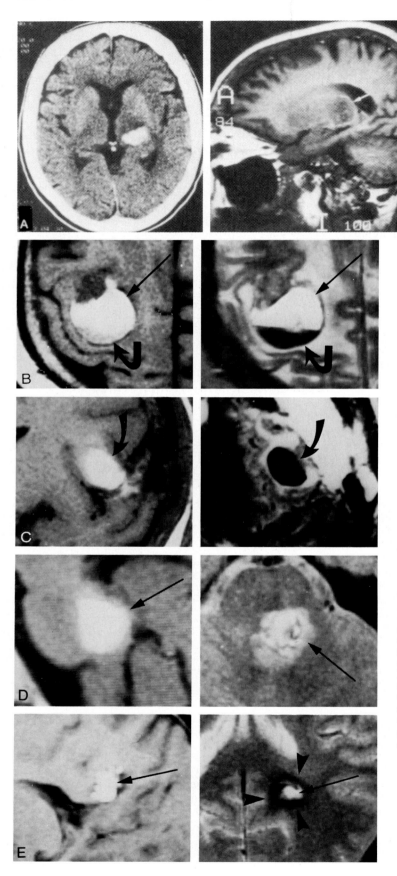

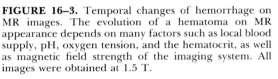

FIGURE 16–3. Temporal changes of hemorrhage on MR images. The evolution of a hematoma on MR appearance depends on many factors such as local blood supply, pH, oxygen tension, and the hematocrit, as well as magnetic field strength of the imaging system. All images were obtained at 1.5 T.

A, Acute hypertensive left thalamic hemorrhage. Left, Unenhanced CT within 12 hours of hemorrhage. Middle, T_1-weighted spin-echo image within 24 hours. Right, T_2-weighted spin-echo image. Note slight hypointensity of hemorrhage on T_1-weighted image and marked hypointensity on T_2-weighted image with surrounding bright edema *(arrow)*. (From Gomori JM, Grossman RI, Goldberg HI, et al: Intracranial hematomas: Imaging by high-field MR. Radiology 157:87–93, 1985; with permission.)

B, Subacute right parietal hemorrhage shows bright signal on T_1-weighted image *(left)* due to extracellular methemoglobin formation. Fluid-fluid level is seen with high intensity in supernatant *(straight arrow)* and decreased signal intensity in clot *(curved arrow)*. Signal loss is most pronounced on T_2-weighted image *(right)*. *C,* Subacute left parietal hemorrhage at later stage than *(B)* shows complete filling in of bright signal on T_1-weighted image *(left)*, uniform hypointensity on T_2-weighted image *(right)* due to intracellular deoxyhemoglobin and methemoglobin, and perihemorrhage edema *(arrow)*. *D,* Late subacute pontine hemorrhage shows bright signal throughout lesion on both T_1-weighted *(left)* and T_2-weighted *(right)* images. *E,* Chronic left occipital hemorrhage shows bright signal *(straight arrows)* on T_1-weighted *(left)* and T_2-weighted *(right)* images. Dark rim *(arrowheads)* is seen on T_2-weighted image representing superparamagnetic ferritin and hemosiderin.

molecules, through random diffusional processes, come within proximity of these paramagnetic centers, they experience fluctuating magnetic fields from the unpaired electrons. These fluctuating magnetic fields promote T_1 relaxation in nearby water molecules (dipole-dipole interaction). Although T_2 relaxation is also promoted by dipole-dipole interactions, the dominant effect in T_1-weighted images is usually an increase in signal, resulting from the T_1 shortening.

Because the methemoglobin molecules go into the extracellular space in a relatively uniform distribution and in reduced concentration, they no longer produce a significant degree of magnetic field inhomogeneity. As a result, in contrast to intracellular methemoglobin, the predominant effect of extracellular methemoglobin is to increase the signal from the hematoma.

EVOLUTION OF SIGNAL INTENSITY CHANGES ON MR IMAGES

The MR appearance of an intracerebral hematoma follows a well-defined, though somewhat variable, course. The evolution of the signal intensity changes is largely related to the paramagnetic effects described above. Table 16–1 summarizes the physical and magnetic properties of hemoglobin breakdown products. However, it is important to note that the appearance of the hemorrhage is strongly dependent on the field strength of the magnet and on the type of pulse sequence used (spin echo or gradient echo). Also, the time course shown below is only a rough approximation and varies depending on the size of the hemorrhage and other factors. We will first consider the appearance of a hematoma on spin-echo images obtained on a high field (1.5 tesla) system (Figs. 16–3 and 16–4 and Table 16–2).

Very Acute Hematoma (< 3 hours)

Immediately following an intracerebral bleed, there is a liquefied mass within the brain substance. This mass contains oxyhemoglobin but as yet no paramagnetic substances. As a result, the mass appears like any other proteinaceous fluid collection,

that is, dark to slightly hyperintense on T_1-weighted images and intermediate to bright signal on T_2-weighted images.

Acute Hematoma (3 hours to 3 days)

Over a period of several hours to several days, reduction in the oxygen tension within the hematoma results in the formation of intracellular deoxyhemoglobin and methemoglobin within intact red blood cells. Because of their distribution, these paramagnetic substances produce T_2 shortening, so that the hematoma appears dark (Fig. 16–3A). The loss of signal is roughly proportional to the square of the magnetic field strength and is most pronounced on images acquired with a long TE (e.g., 90 msec).

As in CT, fluid-fluid levels can be seen in MR images of hematoma. The lower compartment initially contains sedimented red blood cells and appears dark on T_2-weighted images due to the effects of intracellular paramagnetic substances and clot. The upper compartment contains fluid-rich plasma and appears bright on T_2-weighted images.

In addition to the region of signal loss associated with the hematoma, there is usually a thin rim of increased signal seen on T_2-weighted images surrounding the hematoma, which represents edema.

Subacute Hematoma (3 days to 3 weeks)

Over a period of several days to weeks, there is lysis of red blood cells. Redistribution of methemoglobin into the extracellular space changes the effect of this paramagnetic substance on signal intensity. Now the predominant effect is one of T_1 shortening (Fig. 16–3B–D). This results in signal enhancement, seen on T_1-weighted images and also to a lesser extent on T_2-weighted images, which begins in the rim of the hematoma and extends inward over time.

There are several reasons why the signal enhancement is seen on T_2-weighted images:

1. Because of the erythrocyte lysis, T_2 shortening disappears.
2. Osmotic effects draw fluid into the hematoma.
3. The repetition times (TR) in general use for T_2-weighted images (e.g., 2000 to 2500 msec) are not

TABLE 16–1. SUMMARY OF PHYSICAL AND MAGNETIC PROPERTIES OF HEMOGLOBIN BREAKDOWN PRODUCTS

Molecule	Iron Form	No. Unpaired Electrons	Distribution	ΔT_1	ΔT_2
Oxy-Hgb	Ferrous	1	Intact RBCs	—	—
Deoxy-Hgb	Ferrous	4	Intact RBCs	—	↓↓
			Lysed RBCs	—	—
Met-Hgb	Ferric	5	Intact RBCs	↓	↓↓
			Lysed RBCs	↓↓	↓
Ferritin	Ferric	~10,000 (insoluble)	Intracellular	—	↓↓
Hemosiderin	Ferric	~10,000 (insoluble)	Intracellular	—	↓↓

$\Delta T_1, \Delta T_2$ = change produced by molecule in T_1 and T_2 relaxation times.

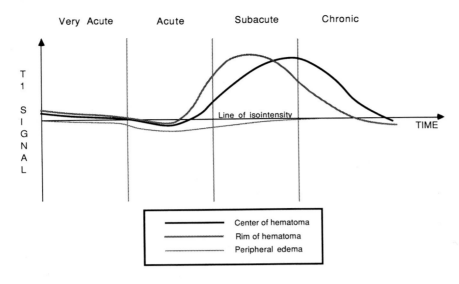

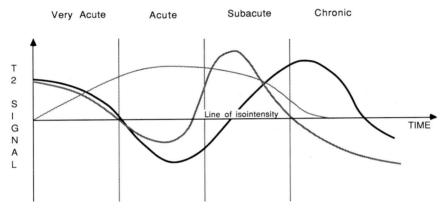

FIGURE 16–4. Graph showing evolution of signal intensity of cerebral hematoma on MRI.

sufficiently long to completely eliminate T_1-contrast effects in the image.

As a result of the combination of these effects, the hematoma becomes bright on T_2-weighted images.

Edema, of vasogenic type due to leakage of proteinaceous fluid into the intercellular space of the brain tissue, is now visible surrounding the hematoma. This fluid spreads along the fiber tracts giving the edema an appearance as though fingers ("edema fingers") are reaching into the normal brain tissue.

TABLE 16–2. TIME COURSE OF HEMORRHAGE SIGNAL INTENSITY COMPARED WITH BRAIN IN SPIN-ECHO MR IMAGES

Stage	T_1-Weighted Image	T_2-Weighted Image
0–3 hrs (very acute)	Intermediate*	Intermediate to bright
3 hrs–3 days (acute)	Intermediate to dark	Dark
3 days–3 wks (subacute)	Bright rim	Dark center, bright rim, later bright center
3 wks–3 mos + (chronic)	Bright or dark	Dark rim or completely dark

*Intermediate signal = signal similar to brain tissue.

Sometimes, dark areas persist in the hematoma even after one would have expected erythrocyte lysis to be complete. To some extent, this may represent persistent hyperconcentration of paramagnetic substances such as methemoglobin in portions of the hematoma. However, physical alterations in the structure of the hematoma, such as clot retraction, likely produce significant signal changes as well. It has been demonstrated that the increased hematocrit in retracted blood clots contributes to T_2 shortening, independent from any paramagnetic effect.[24] This effect can be demonstrated on images from both high and low field systems (for an example of this, see Fig. 16–20).

Chronic Hematoma (3 weeks to 3 months +)

Over a variable period of time, phagocytic cells invade the hemorrhage, beginning at the outer rim and working inward. These phagocytes metabolize the hemoglobin breakdown products and store the iron in the form of particulate ferritin and hemosiderin. In this form, iron is superparamagnetic and produces T_2 shortening. The T_2 shortening produces signal loss in the rim of the hematoma, most pronounced on T_2-weighted images but seen to a lesser extent on T_1-weighted images (Fig. 16–3E). Signal loss may be seen in old hematomas for many years due to persistent hemosiderin deposition.

USE OF GRADIENT-ECHO PULSE SEQUENCES TO IMPROVE CHARACTERIZATION OF HEMATOMAS

Magnetic susceptibility effects are field strength dependent (see Chapter 8). As a result, T_2 shortening is much less pronounced on lower field systems and, in many cases, may be unobservable on low field images obtained using spin-echo pulse sequences. To some extent, the problem can be overcome by increasing the TE. Diffusion-related effects, such as T_2 shortening, rapidly increase as the TE is lengthened. However, the interpretation of images obtained with a long TE (e.g., > 100 msec) may be hampered by a reduction of the signal-to-noise (S/N) ratio.

This problem may be overcome using gradient-echo pulse sequences. Gradient-echo pulse sequences differ from spin-echo sequences in that they lack the 180-degree radiofrequency (RF) refocusing pulse. Acute hematomas will appear dark on gradient-echo images, even when obtained on a low field system. On a high field system, gradient-echo acquisitions improve the sensitivity for the detection of acute, as well as old, hemorrhage[5] (Fig. 16–5). However, the mechanism that causes a hematoma to appear dark on gradient-echo images is different from that proposed for spin-echo images. As we shall now review, spin-echo images are primarily sensitive to the effects of *diffusion*, whereas gradient-echo images are primarily sensitive to the effects of *static magnetic field inhomogeneities*.

Diffusion Causes Signal Loss on Spin-Echo Images

Diffusion is a rapid, random motion of molecules. Such diffusional motion through an inhomogeneous magnetic field produces phase shifts, which will vary among water molecules within the same voxel. Because the phase shifts are different, there is signal loss. Furthermore, because of their random motion, the diffusing water molecules experience different amounts of dephasing before and after a 180-degree RF refocusing pulse used in the spin-echo pulse sequence. As a result, the signal loss produced by diffusion-related dephasing is irreversible, unlike that produced by static magnetic field inhomogeneities.

The signal loss produced by diffusion increases as the TE is lengthened and is pronounced on spin-echo images acquired with a long TE. However, gradient-echo images are acquired with a much shorter TE than in spin-echo imaging. Because the TE is short, diffusion effects are reduced on gradient-echo images and have a lesser role in producing signal loss.

Static Magnetic Field Inhomogeneities Cause Signal Loss on Gradient-Echo Images

Unlike spin-echo images, gradient-echo images are directly sensitive to the effects of static magnetic field inhomogeneities produced by paramagnetic hemoglobin breakdown products. Because of local magnetic field inhomogeneities, water molecules at different positions within a voxel experience different magnetic field strengths, independent of diffusional processes (Fig. 16–6). These static field inhomogeneities result in some spins precessing faster than others. The end result is that the hemoglobin breakdown products, which represent the main source of local field inhomogeneity, produce dephasing and signal loss from surrounding water molecules. Gradient-echo images, acquired without RF refocusing, are highly sensitive to these effects. However, the dephasing effects of static magnetic field inhomogeneities, unlike diffusion, are constant over time and are eliminated by the RF refocusing on a spin-echo image.

Boundary Effect

A related point is that the dark rim surrounding a hematoma on T_2-weighted gradient-echo images does not always represent deposition of hemoglobin breakdown products such as ferritin and hemosiderin. Signal loss can be encountered at the boundary between two regions having differing magnetic susceptibilities, even if no paramagnetic substances are located there. For example, one commonly sees this effect on cranial images, where there is signal loss at the surface of the brain adjacent to the paranasal sinuses (Fig. 16–7). This loss of signal is produced by the local field inhomogeneity between a region of higher (brain) and lower (air-containing sinus) magnetic susceptibility. A similar effect is produced at the border between a hematoma (higher susceptibility) and brain (lower susceptibility).

EFFECT OF OXYGENATION ON THE APPEARANCE OF HEMORRHAGE

Signal loss in an acute hematoma is dependent on the formation of deoxyhemoglobin. Deoxyhemoglobin will only form when the intracellular oxygen tension is reduced. Because of the high oxygen tension of cerebrospinal fluid (CSF), an acute hemorrhage into the subarachnoid space and ventricular system will not usually demonstrate paramagnetic-induced T_2 shortening (Fig. 16–8). A hemorrhagic cortical infarction may also show a lesser degree of T_2 shortening and signal loss on T_2-weighted images, because of the increase in oxygen tension due to "luxury perfusion."[25]

Although acute subarachnoid and intraventricular hemorrhages can be difficult to detect by MR, such

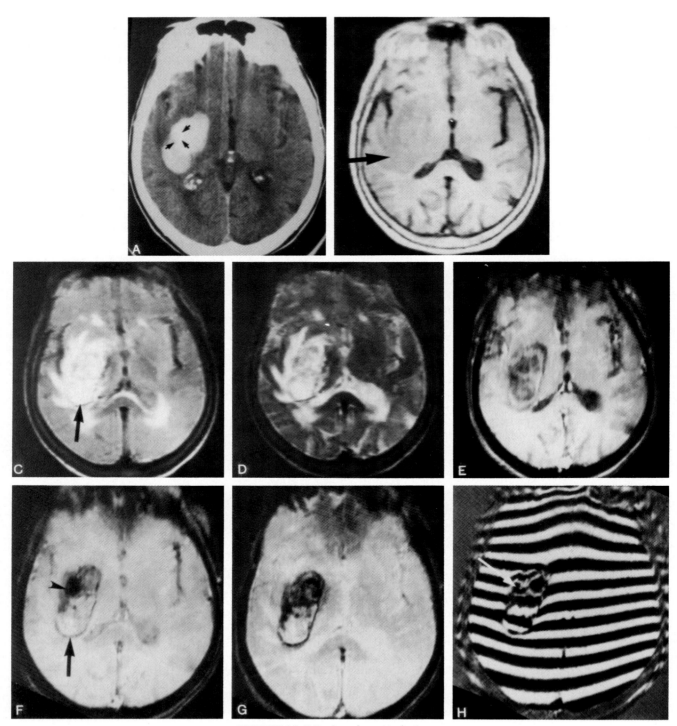

FIGURE 16–5 *See legend on opposite page*

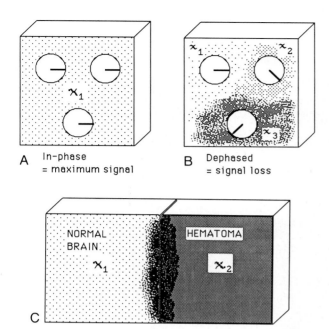

FIGURE 16–6. Illustration of signal loss due to intravoxel and intervoxel variations in magnetic susceptibility. *A*, In a voxel with uniform magnetic susceptibility (χ_1), the magnetic field is homogeneous and spins precess in phase. *B*, Within a voxel, variations in magnetic susceptibility (χ_1, χ_2, χ_3) due to paramagnetic hemoglobin breakdown products cause some spins to precess faster than others, leading to dephasing and signal loss. Signal loss is most pronounced on gradient-echo images. *C*, Field inhomogeneity at the boundary between two voxels having different magnetic susceptibilities (χ_1, χ_2) results in signal loss. This explains the dark rim seen at the border between an acute hematoma (higher magnetic susceptibility) and the surrounding brain (lower magnetic susceptibility).

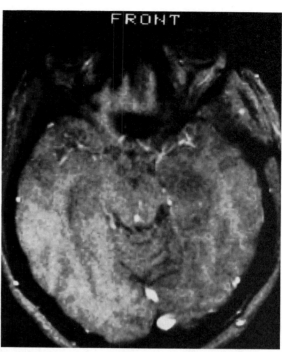

FIGURE 16–7. Axial FLASH MR image at 1.5 T. Area of signal loss in front of the circle of Willis is not due to hemorrhage, but instead represents a magnetic susceptibility effect where the brain is adjoining the air-containing sphenoid sinus.

hemorrhages may occasionally be seen as a region of increased signal intensity in the CSF on spin-echo images (Fig. 16–8). This signal increase, representing T_1 shortening, is probably a nonspecific effect of increased protein content. In the latter stages, subarachnoid and intraventricular hemorrhages may demonstrate regions of increased signal due to the formation of extracellular methemoglobin.

EXTRACEREBRAL HEMORRHAGE

An extracerebral hematoma results from such entities as subdural and epidural bleeding, aneurysmal rupture into the subarachnoid space, venous thrombosis, arterial dissection, and musculoskeletal hemorrhage. It shows an MR pattern of evolution similar to that of an intracerebral hematoma[14] but with one exception. Macrophages, which ingest iron in an hematoma, can transport iron from an extracerebral hematoma more readily than the phagocytic cells within the brain. This probably relates to the absence of a blood-brain barrier. Pituitary hematomas behave

FIGURE 16–5. Acute right putaminal hemorrhage in a patient with history of hypertension. The MR was performed 15 hours after the ictus on a 0.6-T system. *A*, CT scan done shortly before MR examination shows hyperdense hemorrhage with a more focal region of hyperdensity *(arrows)* of higher attenuation (9H) than rest of hemorrhage. *B*, T_1-weighted spin-echo image shows nonspecific lesion *(arrow)* isointense with gray matter. *C*, T_2-weighted spin-echo image (TR 2000 msec, TE 60 msec) shows hyperintense lesion. There is suggestion of a low-density halo *(arrow)*. Mild central hypointense area is similar in intensity to white matter. Outside the low density halo there is hyperintense signal suggesting vasogenic edema spreading along white fiber tracts. Findings suggest hemorrhage. *D*, A more T_2-weighted spin-echo image (TR 2000 msec, TE 120 msec) shows similar findings to *B*. *E*, T_1-weighted gradient-echo image (TR 100 msec, TE 16 msec) shows hypointensity within lesion, in contrast to *A*. *F*, Moderately T_2-weighted gradient-echo image (TR 100 msec, TR 30 msec) shows a definite low-intensity halo *(arrow)*; also seen is a focal area of marked hypointensity *(arrowhead)* which corresponds to area of increased density on CT in *A*. *G*, A more T_2-weighted gradient-echo image (TR 100 msec, TR 50 msec) shows pronounced hypointense halo as well as a markedly hypointense area that is much lower in intensity than white matter. Diagnosis of hemorrhage is unequivocal. *H*, Phase-sensitive zebra-stripe reconstruction (see Chapter 4) shows marked phase shifts in halo due to magnetic susceptibility gradient at junction of hemorrhage and brain. Also note focally increased phase shift *(arrow)* in the region of focal hypointensity seen in *E*. (From Edelman RR, Johnson K, Buxton R, et al: MR of hemorrhage: A new approach. AJNR 7:751–756, 1986; © by American Society of Neuroradiology.)

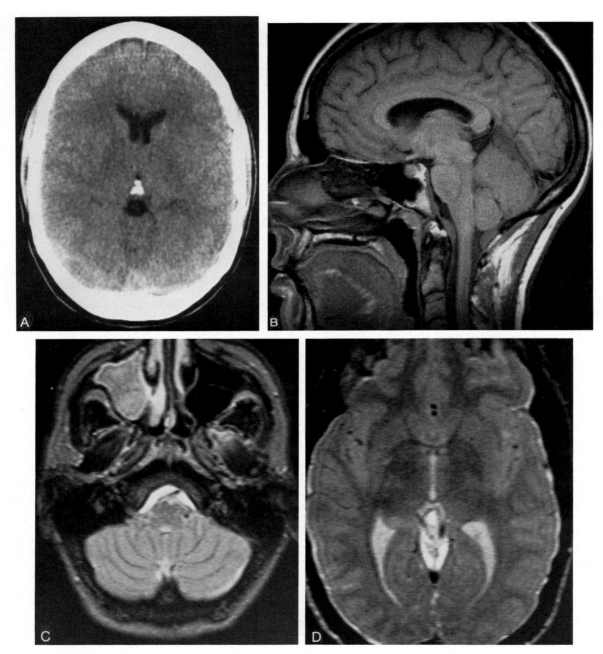

FIGURE 16–8. 38-year-old woman who suffered a subarachnoid hemorrhage (SAH) 10 days previously. Since subarachnoid blood is dispersed and removed from the cerebrospinal fluid within the first days after subarachnoid hemorrhage, the SAH was no longer seen on CT. Although SAH is usually difficult to perceive on MR images, in this case it was clearly demonstrated.

A, Normal CT scan. In the displayed CT slice no blood was visible in the quadrigeminal plate or superior cerebellar cisterns. *B*, Parasagittal T_1-weighted spin-echo MR image (TR = 720 msec, TE = 26 msec, 1.0 T) demonstrating a subarachnoid blood clot, isointense to brain, anterior to the brain stem, in the inferior and superior cerebellar cisterns and in the quadrigeminal plate cistern. *C*, Axial T_2-weighted spin-echo MR image (TR = 2500 msec, TE = 80 msec) demonstrates clot with markedly hyperintense signal anterior to the brain stem. *D*, Axial T_2-weighted spin-echo MR image (TR = 2500 msec, TE = 80 msec) showing blood as hyperintense signal in the superior cerebellar cisterns.

like extracerebral hematomas, since the pituitary gland is not separated from the general circulation by a blood-brain barrier. As a result, the peripheral rim of signal loss, due to storage of iron in the form of ferritin and hemosiderin, is sometimes thin or absent (e.g., see Fig. 16–26).

DIFFERENTIAL DIAGNOSIS OF HEMORRHAGE ON MR IMAGES

Fat, proteinaceous solutions, subacute hemorrhage, metastatic melanoma, and occasionally calcified basal ganglia can all appear bright on T_1-weighted images. Flow voids, melanin, calcification, and acute hemorrhage can all appear dark on T_2-weighted images. This can lead to considerable diagnostic confusion. Strategies for making this differentiation include the following.

Fat Versus Hemorrhage

Signal Intensity Comparisons

Compare the signal intensity of the tissue in question to nearby fat (e.g., subcutaneous fat in the scalp). If the tissue represents fat, then both regions should have a similar signal intensity on all pulse sequences. Because fat has a moderate T_2 relaxation time, it darkens uniformly as the TE is increased. On images obtained with a TE of 80 to 90 msec, fat appears moderately dark. Unlike fat, at least some portions of a subacute hematoma appear bright on T_2-weighted images, depending on the hematoma's state of evolution. Although portions of a subacute hematoma may appear dark on a high field system, the signal intensity is nearly always inhomogeneous. Furthermore, when imaged with a long TE, these portions of the hematoma will usually appear darker than scalp fat.

Comparisons between the signal intensities of different tissues can be somewhat difficult when imaging with a surface coil, as in spine imaging. Signal from tissues near the surface coil will appear artifactually enhanced when compared with deeper tissues, due to the fall off of sensitivity with depth. In this situation, a comparison should be made between tissues that are approximately at the same depth from the coil.

Chemical Shift-Selective Saturation

Where available, chemical shift-selective saturation (CHESS) pulses can be used to suppress fat signal (see Chapter 10). These pulses will not alter or suppress the signal from hemorrhage.

Boundary Effect

On spin-echo images, look for low signal at borders between the tissue in question and that of normal surrounding tissue. If the low signal is present only on one side of the lesion, it represents chemical shift artifact, and the lesion is probably fat. If the low signal, to some degree, is circumferential, it most likely represents magnetic susceptibility artifact from hemorrhage. (Gradient-echo images, such as FLASH or GRASS, can be misleading. Chemical shift artifacts can surround fatty lesions on gradient-echo images if the TE happens to produce a phase-contrast image [see Chapter 5]).

Proteinaceous Fluid Versus Hemorrhage

Infrequently, a lesion containing highly proteinaceous fluid (e.g., a follicular thyroid cyst) can produce very high signal intensity on T_1-weighted images, mimicking a subacute hematoma. However, the high signal in such a hematoma usually begins as a thin rim that evolves toward the center of the lesion. A lesion containing proteinaceous fluid tends to be more uniform in appearance. Furthermore, unlike a subacute hematoma, it does not usually have higher-than-normal magnetic susceptibility, and therefore, would not show signal loss at its interface with normal tissue.

Flow Voids Versus Hemorrhage

Blood vessels can also produce signal voids, but these can be evaluated using flow-compensated gradient-echo pulse sequences, which produce increased signal from flowing blood (see Chapter 4).

Melanin Versus Hemorrhage

Within melanin, stable free radicals have been detected which are paramagnetic and decrease both T_1 and T_2 relaxation times.[26, 27] This effect may make some melanomas appear brighter than the surrounding brain on T_1-weighted images and darker on T_2-weighted images. These signal characteristics are similar to those of an acute intracerebral hematoma containing intracellular deoxyhemoglobin and intracellular methemoglobin. However, the issue is confused by the high incidence of hemorrhage in melanoma metastases,[26, 27] so that the effects of hemorrhage may dominate those of the free radicals. This would explain why even an amelanotic melanoma may demonstrate the signal intensity changes characteristic of hemorrhage. Usually additional MR signs of a tumor are present which allow differentiation of a melanotic metastasis from a primary brain hemorrhage. The differentiation may be further aided by the administration of a contrast agent such as gadolinium-DTPA.

Calcification Versus Hemorrhage

Calcification produces local variations in magnetic susceptibility. These susceptibility variations may result in a signal void, indistinguishable from a subacute

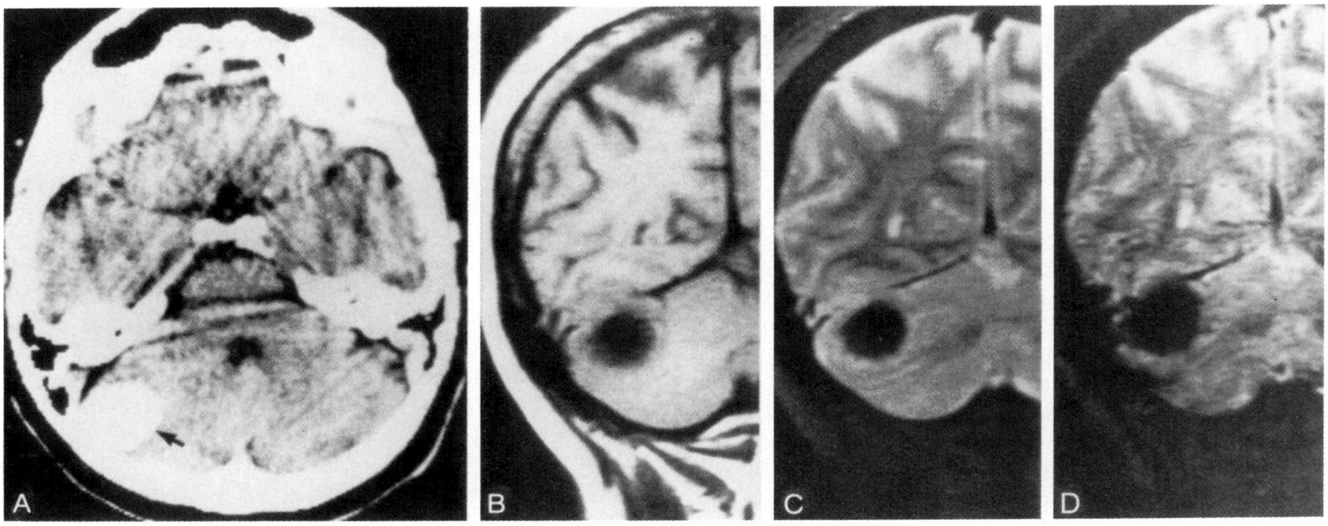

FIGURE 16–9. **Densely calcified posterior fossa meningioma.** *A*, On CT scan, lesion *(arrow)* appears hyperdense. *B*, Coronal spin-echo MR image (TR = 600 msec, TE = 20 msec, 1.5 T). *C*, Coronal spin-echo MR image (TR = 2500 msec, TE = 80 msec). *D*, Coronal GRASS image (TR = 750 msec, TE = 50 msec, flip angle = 10°).

Lesion is hypointense throughout most of the area of calcification on both spin-echo MR images. Note that hypointensity is more profound and extensive on gradient-echo image, due to decreased mobile proton density and magnetic susceptibility differences between the lesion and adjacent brain (From Atlas SW, Grossman RI, Hackney DB, et al: Calcified intracranial lesions: Detection with gradient-echo acquisition rapid MR imaging. AJR 150:1383–1389, 1988; © by American Roentgen Ray Society.)

hematoma (Fig. 16–9). In an old hematoma, regions of signal loss may persist on T_2-weighted images for months or years after the methemoglobin has been absorbed and T_1 signal enhancement has disappeared. In this situation, CT may be necessary to differentiate calcification from a hematoma.

Unlike a hematoma, calcification is not usually associated with high signal on MR images. One exception is the infrequent observation of bright signal within the basal ganglia on T_1-weighted images, raising the question of subacute hemorrhage (Fig. 16–10). This appearance has been reported in association with calcification without hemorrhage. Presumably, these calcifications are hydrated. It has been suggested that the slower motion of water molecules within the hydration layer results in T_1 shortening and, therefore, increased signal (diamagnetic effect). On T_2-weighted images, these regions may appear dark, presumably representing the susceptibility effect of calcium. This diagnosis is most likely when the bright signal regions are symmetric and have no mass effect (Fig. 16–10), and when there is no evidence of bright signal on T_2-weighted images.[29]

GENERAL COMMENTS ON SPONTANEOUS BRAIN HEMORRHAGE

PATHOGENESIS OF BRAIN HEMORRHAGE

Traditional teaching has emphasized that nearly all spontaneous brain hemorrhages are caused by chronic hypertensive damage to penetrating and subcortical arteries and arterioles. A mechanism that can provoke bleeding in these patients is an acute increase in blood flow and/or pressure leading to vessel rupture. However, even in situations without prior hypertension, acute increases in blood flow and/or pressure can produce hemorrhage.[30] Examples are (1) acute increases in blood flow after removal or improvement of focal arterial obstructions, and (2) reperfusion of ischemic or injured tissue. In the former situation, for example, in migraine[31] or after carotid endarterectomy,[32] bleeding occurs at the site of normal arterioles and capillaries. In the latter situation (e.g., reperfusion following embolic infarction), bleeding takes place in vessels and brain tissues that have suffered ischemic damage. Further mechanisms of brain hemorrhage include rupture of vascular malformations and aneurysms, bleeding from abnormally fragile arteries (e.g., arteritis or amyloid angiopathy), hemorrhage with bleeding diathesis, head trauma, and bleeding into preexisting lesions such as primary or metastatic tumors or granulomas.

TIME COURSE OF BLEEDING

The period of active bleeding in spontaneous brain hemorrhage is commonly believed to last a fraction of an hour, which generally implies that the active bleeding has ceased by the time the patient arrives at a hospital.[33] The mechanism of later clinical deterioration is less certain. Rebleeding is rare. In a study with chromium-labeled red blood cells injected at the

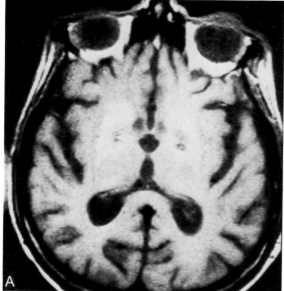

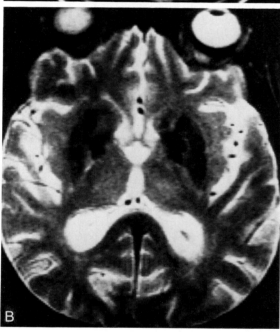

FIGURE 16–10. In this 50-year-old man, CT (not shown) showed extensive basal ganglia calcification. *A*, The axial T$_1$-weighted image (TR = 700 msec, TE = 18 msec, 1.5 T) demonstrates bright signal surrounding an area of signal loss bilaterally in the basal ganglia. The signal loss is in the globus pallidus. *B*, On the T$_2$-weighted image (TR = 2500 msec, TE 90 msec) there is signal loss in the putamen and even more marked in the globus pallidus. The symmetry of the lesions helps to differentiate them from a hematoma in the subacute stage. The appearance has been on the basis of T$_1$ and T$_2$ shortening due to dipole-dipole interactions between water and calcium.[29] The role of iron, if any, in producing this appearance is uncertain.

time of admission for hypertensive hemorrhage, it was found that patients who died had virtually no evidence of labeling in the original hemorrhage, whereas the Duret hemorrhages in the midbrain, which reflected the postadmission fatal cerebral her-

niation, were easily labeled.[34] Only occasionally CT or MRI scan will show enlargement of the hematoma after admission. The chief mechanism for subsequent worsening is the development of edema and ischemic necrosis around the lesion.[35]

ETIOLOGY, LOCATION, AND FREQUENCY

Spontaneous brain hemorrhage patients tend to be on average a decade younger than ischemic stroke patients. Hemorrhage accounts for around 10 to 13 per cent of all strokes.[36–38] The frequency of underlying causes varies with age. In children, vascular malformations, aneurysms, trauma, and hematologic disorders such as thrombocytopenia, leukemia, and hemophilia account for the majority of cases. Frequency and causes of brain hemorrhage in young adults are listed in Table 16–3; the etiologies of intracerebral hemorrhage in adults are summarized in Table 16–4.

Arterial hypertension is the presumed cause in 70 to 90 per cent of nontraumatic brain hemorrhage cases,[36] though the precise frequency depends on whether one examines autopsy specimens, clinical cases, or CT/MRI series. Distribution figures for a study of 100 unselected patients with brain hemorrhage are shown in Table 16–5. When etiology is correlated with the site of brain hemorrhage, hypertensive arteriopathy is the major cause of lenticulocapsular, cerebellar, brain stem, and thalamic hemorrhages. In lobar hemorrhages the etiologies are much more diverse. They comprise anticoagulant-related hemorrhages, rupture of aneurysms and vascular malformations, intratumoral bleedings, cerebral amyloid angiopathy, angiitis, and drug abuse.

CLINICAL PRESENTATION

Spontaneous brain hemorrhage occurs characteristically during physical exertion, and onset during

TABLE 16–3. CAUSES AND FREQUENCY OF SPONTANEOUS INTRACEREBRAL HEMORRHAGES IN THE YOUNG

Clinical Diagnosis	No.	(%) of Patients
Ruptured arteriovenous malformation	21	(29.1)
Arterial hypertension	11	(15.3)
Ruptured saccular aneurysm	7	(9.7)
Sympathomimetic drug abuse	5	(6.9)
Tumor	3	(4.2)
Acute alcohol intoxication	2	(2.8)
Preeclampsia/eclampsia	2	(2.8)
Superior sagittal sinus thrombosis	1	(1.4)
Systemic lupus erythematosus	1	(1.4)
Moyamoya	1	(1.4)
Cryoglobulinemia	1	(1.4)
Undetermined	17	(23.6)
Total	72	(100.0)

Adapted from Toffel GJ, Biller J, Adams HP: Nontraumatic intracerebral hemorrhage in young adults. Arch Neurol 44:483–485, 1987.

TABLE 16–4. CAUSES OF INTRACEREBRAL HEMORRHAGE

Hemorrhage from chronic hypertension
Hemorrhage from aneurysms
Bleeding from vascular malformations
   arteriovenous malformation
   cavernous angioma
   capillary telangiectasia
   venous angioma
Abnormally fragile arteries
   amyloid angiopathy
   arteritis
Bleeding diathesis
   warfarin, heparin
   thrombocytopenia
   hemophilia
   leukemia
   fibrinolysis
Drug abuse
Venous and sinus thrombosis
Infective endocarditis, septic emboli
Head trauma (into contusion site, tear of lenticulostriate arteries)
Bleeding into preexisting lesions such as:
   primary and metastatic tumors
   granulomas
Hemorrhagic stroke, hemorrhage into infarcts
Miscellaneous rare causes:
   migraine
   medical conditions with acute hypertension such as eclampsia,
      pheochromocytoma, glomerulonephritis
   vasopressor drugs
   after carotid endarterectomy
   upon exertion
   severe dental pain; painful urologic examination
   exposure to cold weather
   fat embolism to the brain
   supratentorial hemorrhage after posterior fossa surgery
   after occlusion of arteriovenous fistula

sleep is rare.[41] In 78 per cent there is a focal neurologic deficit[38] depending on the site of the hemorrhage and the disruption of brain tissue. Severe headaches occur in about 40 per cent of patients with brain hemorrhage,[37, 38] as opposed to 5 to 15 per cent in patients with infarction,[38] and seizures occur in 9 per cent.[38] Vomiting is present in 29 per cent, consciousness decreases in 50 to 57 per cent,[37] and coma supervenes in 21 per cent.[38] The latter symptoms correlate with either intraventricular extension of the

TABLE 16–5. DISTRIBUTION BY SITE OF 100 UNSELECTED PATIENTS WITH SPONTANEOUS BRAIN HEMORRHAGE

Type	Number of Cases
Putaminal	34
Lobar	24
Thalamic	20
Cerebellar	7
Pontine	6
Caudate	5
Putaminothalamic	4

From Kase CS, Mohr JP: Supratentorial intracerebral hemorrhage. *In* Barnett HJM, Mohr JP, Stein BM, Yatsu FM (eds): Stroke. Pathophysiology, Diagnosis, and Management. New York, Churchill-Livingstone, 1986, pp 525–548; with permission.

hemorrhage or increased intracranial pressure due to large hematoma size and transtentorial herniation.

There is almost always associated arterial hypertension.[36, 38] In many instances it occurs as a reflex to maintain adequate cerebral perfusion and does not necessarily signify a history of hypertension. Physical signs indicative of previous hypertension include left ventricular hypertrophy and hypertensive retinopathy. Subhyaloid hemorrhages in the ocular fundi are virtually diagnostic of subarachnoid hemorrhage and will occur in spontaneous brain hemorrhage only exceptionally.

ETIOLOGY OF HEMORRHAGE BY LOCATION AND ASSOCIATED BRAIN ABNORMALITIES

Although identification of a hematoma is extremely important, it is the underlying cause of the hemorrhage that is critical to patient management. The identification of the cause of a hemorrhage by MR may preclude the need for invasive diagnostic procedures. In the following sections we will review the clinical symptoms and signs and the significance of the location and MR appearance of various types of spontaneous brain hemorrhage. It should be recognized, however, that not all brain hematomas have an appearance on MR or CT images which renders a specific diagnosis.

HYPERTENSIVE (DEEP) HEMORRHAGE

More than a century ago, Charcot and Bouchard drew attention to "miliary aneurysms" from brains of hypertensive hemorrhage patients.[42] Fisher considered them a last link in a pathogenetic chain.[41] Hypertension causes degenerative changes in penetrating arteries in the form of lipid-rich hyaline subintimal material, called *lipohyalinosis*. The lipohyalinosis disrupts muscle and elastic elements and allows bulging of arterial walls. This process can interrupt blood flow and lead to lacunar infarcts. Alternatively, this process can result in hemorrhage at the site of aneurysmal outpouchings. Once the hemorrhage has started, secondary arterial ruptures at the periphery of the enlarging hematoma follow in avalanche fashion.

By anatomic site of penetrating arteries, hypertensive hemorrhages are located either in the basal ganglia, internal capsule, thalamus, pons, or deep in the cerebellum. Furthermore, small cortical perforators can lead to subcortical "slit" hemorrhages oriented parallel to the overlying cortex.

Hypertensive hemorrhages almost never are multiple. Multiple hemorrhages are much more likely due to bleeding diathesis, metastatic tumors, or cerebral amyloid angiopathy. Angiography has little role in the evaluation of this disorder.[43]

Putaminal Hemorrhage

Figure 16–5 shows a hypertensive putaminal hemorrhage. Most commonly it arises from a lateral branch of the striate arteries, and if sufficiently large it can extend to adjacent structures. The clinical spectrum reflects the size and the pattern of extension of the hemorrhage. All patients exhibit some form of a motor deficit, in addition to which a sensory disorder and eventually a hemianopsia will ensue due to involvement of the optic tract.

Caudate Hemorrhage

The sources of caudate hemorrhages are typically deep penetrating branches of the anterior and middle cerebral arteries.[44] The caudate also receives its blood supply from ependymal arteries. These vessels

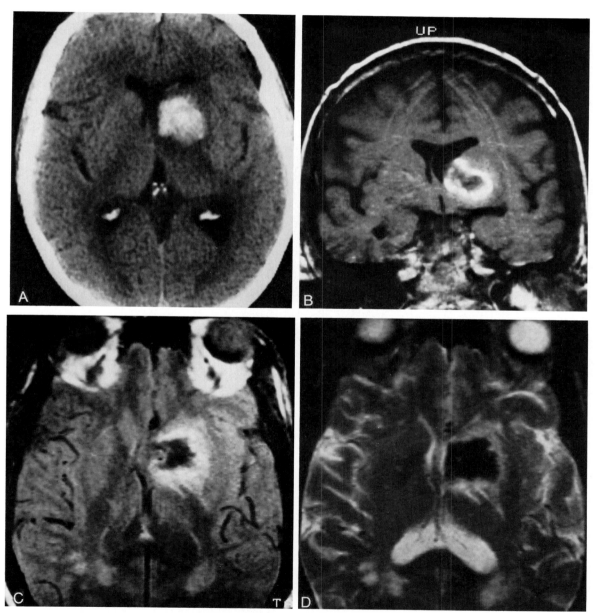

FIGURE 16–11. 57-year-old man with a history of hypertension. *A*, The CT shows an acute hemorrhage in the typical location of hypertensive bleeds. *B–D*, High field MRI performed three days after the bleeding episode shows involvement of the head of the caudate nucleus, anterior limb of the internal capsule, and lentiform nucleus. On the coronal T_1-weighted image *(B)*, a bright rim (extracellular methemoglobin) surrounds a dark center. The axial proton density–weighted image *(C)* shows a bright rim (extracellular methemoglobin and edema) and a dark center (intracellular methemoglobin and deoxyhemoglobin). The T_2-weighted image *(D)* shows more extensive signal loss due to the prolonged echo time and correspondingly greater sensitivity to dephasing effects from concentrated paramagnetic substances. The thin rim with increased signal intensity probably represents edema.

are not usually affected by hypertensive vasculopathy but, nonetheless, can be a source of bleeding due to the occasional vascular malformation. Hemorrhages occur in the head of the caudate nucleus, and extension into adjacent structures and the lateral ventricle is a common feature[45] (Fig. 16–11).

The clinical picture resembles that of subarachnoid hemorrhage: abrupt onset with headache, vomiting, and temporary behavioral abnormalities. In approximately half the cases, additional clinical features include gaze and contralateral hemiparesis.[45] The outcome in caudate hemorrhage is usually benign. Hydrocephalus can complicate the caudate hemorrhage. The hydrocephalus tends to disappear as the hemorrhage resolves, and ventriculoperitoneal shunting is required in most instances only temporarily.[45]

Thalamic Hemorrhage

In the majority of cases, thalamic hemorrhages are due to hypertensive arteriopathy (Fig. 16–12, see also Fig. 16–3A). The clinical presentation reflects again the size and extension of the hematoma.[46, 47] The patients present with a hemisensory syndrome associated with a motor deficit. Usually there is loss of all the sensory modalities over the contralateral limbs, face, and trunk. From a clinical point of view, these findings and the distribution of motor and sensory symptoms do not help to unequivocally differentiate thalamic from putaminal hemorrhage.

Thalamic hematomas have a high rate of intraventricular extension. This or the hemorrhage itself may cause hydrocephalus, requiring emergency ventric-

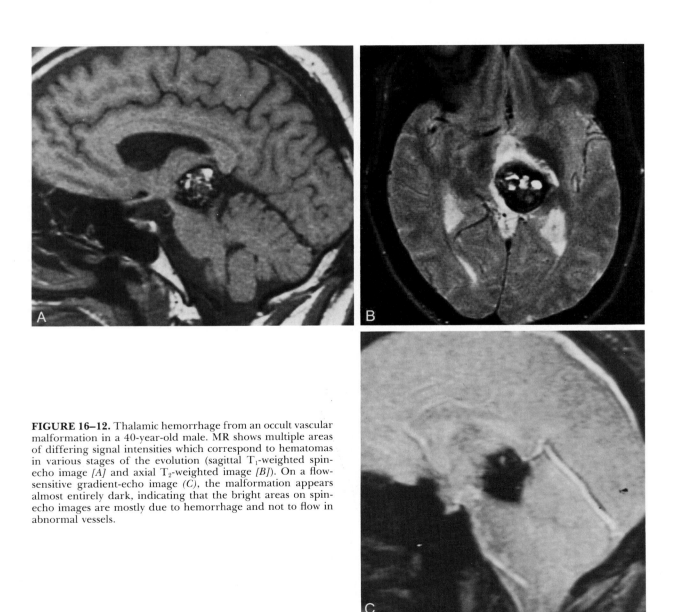

FIGURE 16–12. Thalamic hemorrhage from an occult vascular malformation in a 40-year-old male. MR shows multiple areas of differing signal intensities which correspond to hematomas in various stages of the evolution (sagittal T$_1$-weighted spin-echo image [A] and axial T$_2$-weighted image [B]). On a flow-sensitive gradient-echo image (C), the malformation appears almost entirely dark, indicating that the bright areas on spin-echo images are mostly due to hemorrhage and not to flow in abnormal vessels.

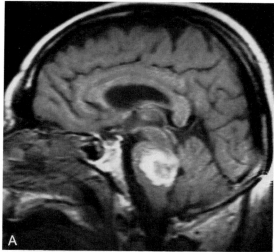

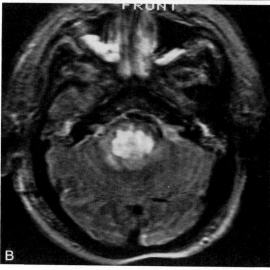

FIGURE 16–13. Pontine hemorrhage. 57-year-old man with history of hypertension who developed tetraparesis associated with ataxia, bilateral horizontal gaze palsy, and decrease of consciousness. The MR, obtained a few days after the onset of symptoms, shows subacute hemorrhage extending bilaterally into the pontine tegmentum. In the periphery of the hematoma there is hyperintense signal on both T_1-weighted *(A)* and T_2-weighted *(B)* spin-echo images, while the center is still isointense to adjacent brain tissue.

ular drainage. The outcome of hematomas larger than 3 cm in diameter is bleak.

Brain Stem Hemorrhage

Figure 16–13 shows a brain stem hemorrhage. Most brain stem hemorrhages occur in the pons, which is another classic location for hypertensive hemorrhage. Occasionally, these hemorrhages are due to arteriovenous malformations and other causes. CT and MRI permit hemorrhages to be confidently distinguished from ischemic brain stem lesions.[9, 48] Hypertensive brain stem hemorrhages present within minutes, whereas the clinical signs of hemorrhages due to leakage from arteriovenous malformations evolve gradually over two or more days.[49]

Pontine hemorrhages have been categorized according to location.[50–52] They result from rupture of perforating or long circumferential arteries. At onset of a massive pontine hemorrhage, roughly one third of the patients complain of severe occipital headache,[51] and vomiting or motor phenomena giving a false impression of seizures may ensue. Focal pontine signs evolve within a few minutes, including quadriplegia, abnormal muscle tone, ophthalmoplegia, pinpoint pupils, and irregular respiration.[53] Massive pontine hemorrhage is almost always fatal. When the patient survives, a so-called locked-in syndrome may ensue.

Unilateral hemorrhages limited to the pontine tegmentum demonstrate ipsilateral gaze palsy.[52] Bilateral tegmental hemorrhages cause ophthalmoplegia.[54] Hemorrhages limited to one side of the basis pontis produce contralateral limb weakness. Small pontine hemorrhages usually have a favorable outcome.

Hematomas in the mesencephalon[55–58] (Fig. 16–14) and *medulla oblongata*[59] are rare.[60] Their clinical presentation depends on location.[61, 62] Vascular malformations are a more common etiology than hypertension.

Cerebellar Hemorrhage

The leading cause of cerebellar hemorrhage is hypertension followed by anticoagulant-related hemorrhage;[63, 64] coagulopathies, aneurysms, vascular malformations (e.g., see Fig. 16–17), and cerebral emboli represent other rare causes. Cerebellar hemorrhages commonly arise in the region of the dentate nuclei and seldom in the vermis.[65, 66]

The hemorrhage acts as an acute posterior fossa mass and compresses the brain stem, often leading to necrosis of the tegmentum and acute hydrocephalus[67] (Fig. 16–15). The most constant initial symptoms are occipital headache, dizziness, and inability to stand or walk.[63, 64] A triad of limb ataxia, ipsilateral gaze palsy, and peripheral facial palsy is characteristic.[63] Involvement of the vermis results in severe truncal ataxia. Cerebellar hemorrhage is commonly misdiagnosed as brain stem stroke, labyrinthine disturbance, and subarachnoid hemorrhage (SAH).

Since clinical findings cannot reliably distinguish between extrinsic compression and intrinsic lesions of the brain stem, CT and MRI play an important role in their diagnosis. Aside from location and extent of the hemorrhage, these imaging modalities will show obliteration and displacement of the fourth ventricle, hydrocephalus, effacement of the basal cisterns, and blood in the ventricular system. In medically unstable patients, CT is the imaging modality of choice.

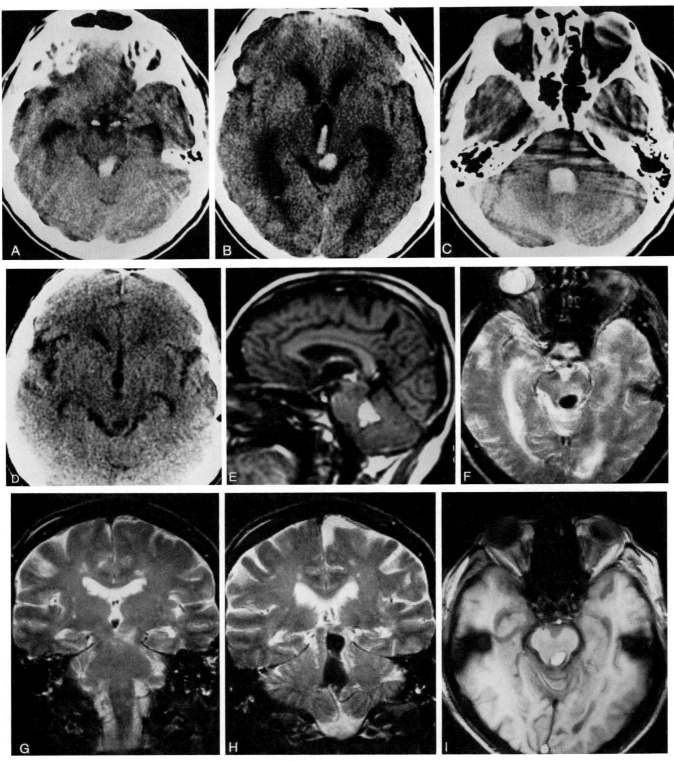

FIGURE 16–14 *See legend on opposite page.*

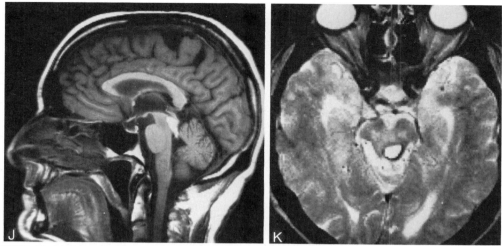

FIGURE 16–14. 64-year-old man with midbrain hemorrhage of unknown etiology. On CT a mesencephalic hematoma around the aqueduct *(A)* with breakthrough into the third *(B)* and fourth ventricle *(C)* is seen. Four weeks later CT demonstrates hypodensity at the site of the original hematoma *(D)*. Four days after the ictus, the sagittal T₁-weighted spin-echo (SE) MR image demonstrates bright blood in the posterior part of the third ventricle and in the fourth ventricle *(E)*. The axial T₂-weighted MR images show dark blood in the mesencephalic tegmentum *(F)*, in the third ventricle *(G)*, and in the fourth ventricle *(H)*. Three weeks later, on the axial and sagittal T₁-weighted SE images, blood in the midbrain, appearing bright, is still present *(I* and *J)* but is no longer seen in the ventricles *(J)*. On the T₂-weighted SE image, blood now appears bright, due to red cell lysis and increased water content as a consequence of osmotic effects *(K)*.

LOBAR HEMORRHAGE

Lobar hemorrhage is defined as a hemorrhage in the cerebral hemisphere, outside the basal ganglia

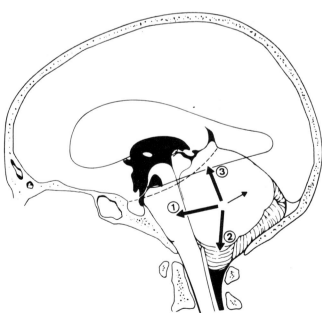

FIGURE 16–15. Illustration showing possible mass effects from a posterior fossa hemorrhage. The hemorrhage may compress the brain stem (1), leading to necrosis of the tegmentum, and cause cerebellar tonsillar herniation (2) and/or superior cerebellar tentorial herniation (3). Hydrocephalus may ensue due to compromise of CSF outflow. (Courtesy of U. Ebeling, University of Bern, Switzerland.)

and thalamus (Fig. 16–16). Less than 25 per cent of spontaneous brain hemorrhages are lobar in site, and hypertensive subcortical bleeding accounts for approximately one third of these.[37, 68] Apart from hypertension, the causes of lobar hemorrhage include the rupture of an aneurysm or vascular malformation; bleeding from abnormally fragile arteries (e.g., amyloid angiopathy, arteritis);[69] hemorrhage due to a bleeding diathesis, anticoagulant therapy, or drug abuse; bleeding into a preexisting lesion such as a primary or metastatic tumor; and bleeding associated with endocarditis[70] (see Table 16–4). Very rarely, these entities bleed in deep structures, where hypertensive hematomas are usually found, resulting in diagnostic confusion.

The etiology of lobar hemorrhage also varies with age. In the elderly, the most common cause is chronic hypertension, and only occasionally is amyloid angiopathy the etiology. Berry aneurysm rupture producing an intracerebral hematoma is more often seen in middle-aged adults (see Table 16–4). The leading causes of brain hemorrhage in young adulthood are ruptured vascular malformations and hypertension (see Table 16–3). In children, vascular malformations and hematologic disorders such as leukemia or thrombocytopenia account for the majority of cases. The clinical presentation depends on the location of the hematoma.[71]

Hemorrhage from Aneurysms

It is estimated that there are more than 28,000 cases of aneurysmal SAH in North America each year.[72] Of these, about 60 per cent of patients will

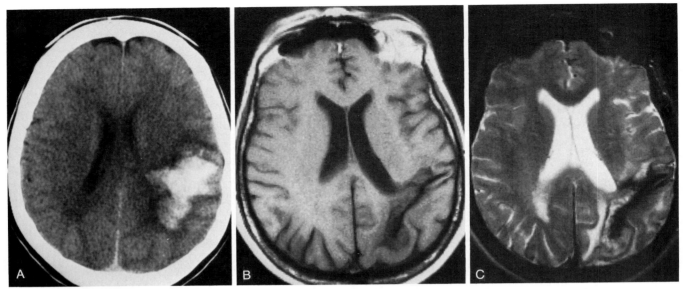

FIGURE 16–16. 64-year-old woman with a left parietal lobar hemorrhage. *A*, CT scan of the acute hemorrhage. *B*, High field MR scan performed 10 months later. The axial T_1-weighted spin-echo image demonstrates enlargement of the posterior horn of the left lateral ventricle and adjacent to it a long subcortical low intensity stripe. *C*, On the T_2-weighted spin-echo image (TR = 2800 msec, TE = 90 msec), the area of the previous hemorrhage is predominantly hypointense. The signal loss is due to old hemoglobin breakdown products such as ferritin and hemosiderin. These substances are superparamagnetic and produce T_2 shortening.

also suffer an associated brain hemorrhage because the ruptured aneurysm had embedded itself in the adjacent brain parenchyma.[73] The subarachnoid location of a ruptured aneurysm will determine the site of origin of a hematoma, most of which are found in the frontal and temporal lobes. The finding of a hematoma in the precallosal or septal area is characteristic of a ruptured anterior communicating artery aneurysm. An anterior temporal lobe hematoma, in conjunction with an SAH, is typical of a ruptured middle cerebral artery aneurysm (see Chapter 17).[74]

Vascular Malformations

Vascular malformations of the brain are categorized as arteriovenous malformations (AVMs), cavernous angiomas, capillary telangiectasias, and venous malformations (Figs. 16–17 and 16–18, see also Fig. 16–12). AVMs are more commonly located in the cerebral hemispheres, whereas capillary telangiectasias are most often found in the diencephalon, brain stem, and cerebellum.[75] An AVM contains a tangle of congenitally malformed vascular channels buried in the brain, known as a nidus. Within the nidus there are direct arteriovenous communications that permit marked increase in regional blood flow through the lesion. The feeding arteries have lost the capability of autoregulation, and the draining veins are usually dilated because of increased blood flow. Because an AVM is often in continuity with the ventricles or cerebral surface, a rupture of the nidus can produce parenchymatous as well as subarachnoid

and intraventricular hemorrhage. A cavernous angioma and a capillary telangiectasia are low-flow malformations of the arterioles and capillaries, respectively, without enlarged feeding arteries or draining veins; a venous angioma is a cluster of deep medullary veins draining abnormally, in a centripetal fashion, to a venous nidus.

MR is an extremely sensitive imaging modality for the detection of a vascular malformation and is capable of demonstrating the precise anatomic relationship of its feeding arteries, nidus, and draining veins.[1, 76–79] On spin-echo sequences signal loss in an AVM is due to either hemorrhage, rapidly flowing blood, or calcification. On gradient-echo images blood vessels with flowing blood have a bright signal because of flow-related enhancement, whereas hemosiderin and calcification are seen as a signal void (see Fig. 16–12). However, so-called bright blood gradient-echo techniques (see Chapter 4) may underestimate the true extent of the vascularity of an AVM, since rapid and turbulent flow can result in nonrecoverable signal loss within the AVM. Calcification within an AVM is best evaluated by CT. It should be noted that the presence of hemosiderin in an AVM does not necessarily indicate previous clinical episodes of bleeding, because on histology hemosiderin-laden macrophages are often found in the walls of an uncomplicated AVM (Fig. 16–18). Gradient-echo imaging may also be useful for demonstrating residual flow in an AVM after a recent hemorrhage, where the compressive effects of the hematoma on the AVM make contrast CT difficult to interpret.[76]

MR is superior to CT in detecting so-called occult

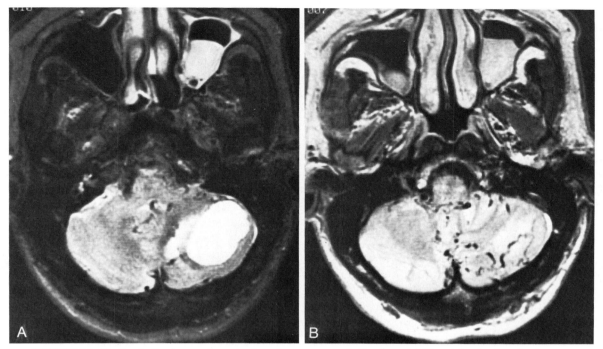

FIGURE 16–17. Cerebellar hemorrhage in the subacute stage. *A,* On the axial T$_2$-weighted spin-echo image the hemorrhage appears bright. *B,* The proton density–weighted spin-echo image of an adjacent slice shows multiple flow voids, consistent with an arteriovenous malformation.

or cryptic vascular malformations in the brain, which are defined as vascular malformations not demonstrated by angiography[77, 81, 82] (Fig. 16–18). Occult vascular malformations (OVM) are usually low-flow vascular lesions that have a propensity to bleed. Histologically, they include capillary telangiectasia, cavernous angioma, venous angioma, and rarely some true AVMs. On CT, all of these vascular lesions may contain punctate calcification. Furthermore, they may all show mild or no enhancement and exhibit minimal or no mass effect on adjacent structures. There is seldom any associated surrounding edema. On CT the differential diagnosis of such a lesion includes a calcified glioma, granuloma, hamartoma, or old hemorrhage.

On MR an OVM has a characteristic appearance. It consists of a circumscribed region of low signal intensity, most prominent on T$_2$-weighted images, representing hemosiderin deposition, which is on the periphery of the lesion (Fig. 16–18). Within the hemosiderin rim are multiple areas of higher but differing signal intensities which correspond to hematomas in various stages of evolution. Often scattered within the areas of hemorrhage are further foci of decreased signal caused by calcification and more hemosiderin. Simple hematomas associated with trauma, surgery, hypertension, or tumors have a single cavity. Hemorrhagic contusions and infarctions may have multiple collections but are of the same age and have other associated parenchymal findings. The diagnostic feature of an OVM on MR is the recognition of a lesion-containing hemorrhage

in various stages of evolution, indicative of recurrent bleeding. In a series of 63 vascular malformations of the brain stem, Abe and colleagues found that clinical data, in conjunction with the MR findings, were helpful in determining the true nature of such lesions.[49] However, a word of caution: although the MR appearance was initially thought to be diagnostic for an OVM, a recent report has shown a number of hemorrhagic neoplasms with similar MR features.[80] Further details of MR and vascular malformations are given in Chapter 17.

Amyloid Angiopathy

It is estimated that amyloid angiopathy accounts for 2 to 10 per cent of all brain hemorrhages.[83, 84] Amyloid deposition in small and medium-sized cerebral vessels without systemic amyloidosis has been found in 18 per cent of men and 28 per cent of women at autopsy.[85] Its frequency increases with age and there is an association with Alzheimer-type changes such as neuritic plaques and neurofibrillary tangles, but there is no correlation with hypertension or atherosclerosis. The frontal lobes are more frequently affected than the parietal, occipital, or temporal lobes.[85] Vessel walls, weakened and made brittle by amyloid deposition, may undergo spontaneous or traumatic rupture or develop miliary aneurysms with subsequent hemorrhage.[86] Lobar hemorrhages due to amyloid angiopathy commonly affect the elderly and are usually located in the cortex or subcortical

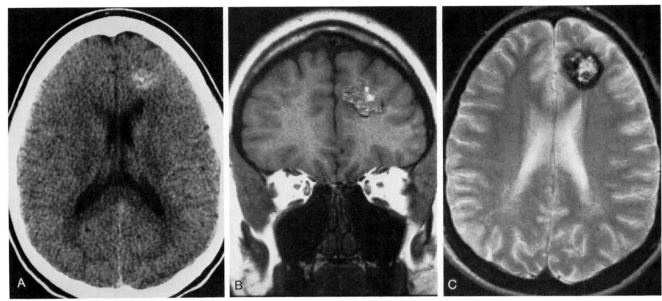

FIGURE 16–18. Occult vascular malformation in a 22-year-old woman, who suffered from seizures for many years. *A*, CT scan shows irregular hyperdensity in the left frontal lobe most likely representing calcification within a vascular malformation but indistinguishable from a calcified low-grade glioma. *B*, On the coronal T_1-weighted spin-echo image, small areas of bright signal are seen due to either flow-related enhancement within abnormal vessels or extracellular methemoglobin from small subclinical hemorrhages. *C*, T_2-weighted spin-echo image shows a hypointense ring around the vascular malformation. The presence of this ring is considered to be the result of chronic hemosiderin deposition developing from previous subclinical bleeds and also the consequence of a magnetic susceptibility effect because of subtle differences in the local magnetic fields between vascular malformation and surrounding brain. A hypointense ring rarely occurs around low-grade gliomas.

white matter. Sometimes there is associated subarachnoid, subdural, or intraventricular hemorrhage.[86] An additional feature is a tendency to produce recurrent hemorrhages over periods of months or years[84] (Fig. 16–19). In about one third of patients a progressive dementia of the Alzheimer type is present. Although confirmation of the diagnosis of amyloid angiopathy needs a surgical or autopsy specimen, it is suggested by the MR findings of two or more lobar hematomas of varying age in an elderly patient. Unfortunately, there is no therapeutic measure to prevent progression of the disease.

Subcortical "Slit" Hemorrhage

Cole and Yates described cortical penetrators as an additional site for aneurysm formation in hypertensive patients.[87] These can bleed and give rise to small hematomas at the junction between cortical gray and underlying white matter. The appearance of these hematomas is lens- or slit-shaped. When slit hemorrhages are seen, but there is no evidence or history of hypertension, other etiologies of lobar hemorrhage must be sought.

Bleeding Diathesis

Hemorrhagic disorders that occur with anticoagulants (Coumadin, heparin), thrombocytopenia, leukemia, liver disease, hemophilia, fibrinolysis,[88] and other rare diseases predispose to intracranial hemorrhage. Coumadin, widely used as an oral anticoagulant for the prevention of arterial and venous thrombosis and embolism, increases the risk of brain hemorrhage between 8- and 11-fold.[89] Anticoagulation-related brain hemorrhages represent the most serious side effect of anticoagulant treatment and generally have a dismal prognosis. Compared with hypertensive hemorrhage, an apparent difference in topographic distribution has been noted. Anticoagulation-related brain hemorrhages show a predilection for the cerebral lobes and the cerebellum (Fig. 16–20). The onset of clinical signs tends to be slower than with hypertensive hemorrhage.[90] Neither CT nor MRI shows any special features with this hemorrhage type. The diagnosis relies on history and laboratory findings.

Drug Use and Abuse

A number of "street drugs" such as heroin,[91] methamphetamine, amphetamine, pseudoephedrine,[92, 93] pentazocine and tripelenamine,[94] phenylpropanolamine,[95] and cocaine especially in the form of "crack"[96] have been implicated to cause brain hemorrhage. Transiently elevated blood pressure and/or angiographic changes suggestive of vasculitis have been implicated as etiologic factors.[92, 97] Generally cerebrovascular complications of these drugs present

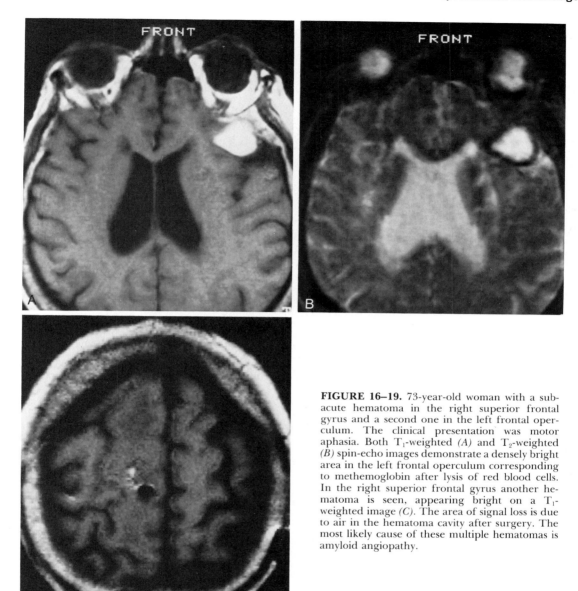

FIGURE 16–19. 73-year-old woman with a subacute hematoma in the right superior frontal gyrus and a second one in the left frontal operculum. The clinical presentation was motor aphasia. Both T_1-weighted *(A)* and T_2-weighted *(B)* spin-echo images demonstrate a densely bright area in the left frontal operculum corresponding to methemoglobin after lysis of red blood cells. In the right superior frontal gyrus another hematoma is seen, appearing bright on a T_1-weighted image *(C)*. The area of signal loss is due to air in the hematoma cavity after surgery. The most likely cause of these multiple hematomas is amyloid angiopathy.

as ischemic stroke but occasionally as brain hemorrhage closely following their use. The majority of the hematomas are located in the subcortical hemispheral white matter, and occasionally multiple hemorrhages occur simultaneously. Except for antithrombotics and antiplatelets, medically used drugs hardly ever cause brain hemorrhage as an unwanted side effect. One rare example is brain hemorrhage associated with L-asparaginase.[98]

Hemorrhage Associated with Tumor

Bleeding into preexisting brain tumors accounts for 10 per cent of all brain hemorrhages.[99] The clinical manifestation is either an acute new focal neurologic deficit or worsening of a pre-existing deficit, often associated with decreased level of consciousness. Only 1 to 2 per cent of primary or metastatic tumors present as a hemorrhage.[99] Of primary brain tumors that bleed, glioblastoma multiforme, oligodendroglioma, and ependymoma are the most common types. Metastases most prone to bleed are those of melanoma, choriocarcinoma, and bronchogenic, renal cell, and thyroid carcinoma.[100] Primary brain tumors are usually deeply seated and therefore produce deep bleeds, whereas metastases and their hemorrhages are more often subcortical or cortical in location.[101] The pathogenesis of tumoral

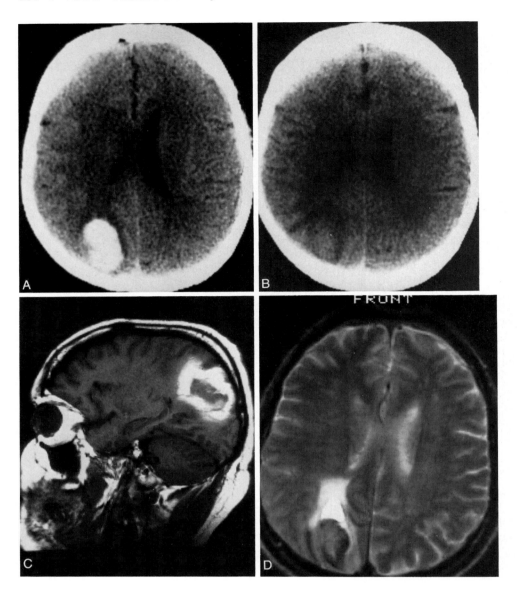

FIGURE 16–20. 51-year-old normotensive man who suffered a right parietooccipital subcortical hemorrhage due to anticoagulation. *A,* Acute clot appears hyperdense on CT scan. *B,* A follow-up CT scan 6 weeks later shows the resolving hematoma demarcated by a hypodense rim. The center is isodense with normal brain parenchyma. *C,* High field T_1-weighted spin-echo image obtained 10 days after the first CT scan demonstrates T_1 shortening in the periphery of the hematoma. *D,* On the T_2-weighted SE image there is retracted blood clot and supernatant plasma. The fluid-rich plasma is bright, while the clot appears darker.

hemorrhage is probably dependent on the degree of malignancy as well as on the rate of growth and vascularity of the tumor.

In general, the diagnosis of tumor as the underlying cause of a brain hemorrhage is difficult, since the hematoma may obliterate evidence of the neoplasm. However, Atlas and colleagues[16] and Destian and coworkers[3] have reported MR findings on spin-echo images which appear to be specific for tumoral hemorrhage (Fig. 16–21). They compared the signal intensity patterns of simple intracerebral hematomas with those hematomas due to an underlying neoplasm. Their findings may be summarized as follows.

1. Signal intensity patterns are generally more heterogeneous with neoplasia than with simple hematomas. In contrast to the orderly evolution of signal intensity changes in simple hematomas, multiple stages of hematoma evolution are often present simultaneously in a tumor.

2. Evolution of a tumoral bleed is slower than that of a simple hematoma.

3. Presence of a well-defined, complete hemosiderin rim found around simple hematomas is reduced or absent in tumoral bleeds. However, in later stages tumoral bleeds may also demonstrate a hemosiderin ring, though usually incomplete or attenuated.

4. Areas of abnormal signal intensity typical of tumor tissue suggest underlying neoplasia. This abnormal signal is usually hypointense or isointense relative to cortex on T_1-weighted spin-echo images and hyperintense on T_2-weighted images.

5. Tumoral bleed is suggested by the presence of edema that persists in the subacute and chronic stages, unlike transient perihematoma edema seen in acute simple hematomas. Figure 16–21 illustrates these findings.

6. Unlike simple hematomas, in which high signal intensity on T_1-weighted images originates in the rim

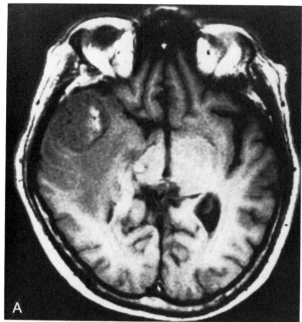

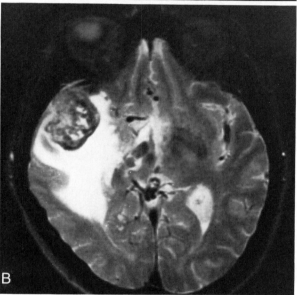

FIGURE 16–21. 70-year-old male with lung carcinoma. The T_1-weighted (A) and T_2-weighted (B) spin-echo images demonstrate hemorrhage into a temporal lobe metastasis. The diagnosis is suggested by the more heterogeneous signal intensity pattern than is encountered in simple hematomas, the presence of marked edema, and an ill-defined hemosiderin ring around the lesion. Unlike in a simple hematoma, where methemoglobin formation starts at the periphery, the bright signal resulting from methemoglobin is seen centrally on the T_1-weighted image.

of the lesion, increased signal (due to paramagnetic methemoglobin formation) may originate centrally within some tumoral bleeds. The reason for this discrepancy may relate to the oxygen tension.[102] In a simple hematoma, the oxygen tension may be so low centrally as to inhibit the oxidation of deoxyhemoglobin to methemoglobin. This delays the develop-

ment of central high signal intensity on T_1-weighted images. On the other hand, there is evidence that the oxygen tension in the central portions of neoplasms is greater than in simple hematomas (though lower than in normal tissues). In tumoral bleeds, enough oxygen may be present in the central region to support methemoglobin formation.

Aside from these features, the simplest means to differentiate tumor from nontumor bleeds is to administer an MR contrast agent such as gadolinium-DTPA.

In many cases, it is possible to differentiate hemorrhagic neoplasm from hematoma on the basis of the MR appearance. However, in some instances the diagnosis is only suspected by the finding of systemic malignancy, or by biopsy of the hematoma cavity following its surgical evacuation.

Hemorrhagic Infarction

Hemorrhagic infarction (HI) occurs in about 20 per cent of all infarcts, and the hemorrhage almost always originates in the cortex[25] (Fig. 16–22) or from deep perforators (Fig. 16–23). There are four conditions that predispose ischemic brain tissue to hemorrhage,[25, 103] and all are due to the phenomenon of reperfusion: (1) when an arterial embolus lyses and moves distally (Fig. 16–24); (2) when collaterals supply ischemic brain tissue; (3) when hypotension is followed by restoration of normal blood pressure; and (4) when temporal lobe herniation transiently occludes a posterior cerebral artery. The first two conditions predispose watershed zones to hemorrhagic infarction. Other causes of hemorrhagic infarction include hypertension, anticoagulation, fat embolism, and venous infarction.[104, 105] In fat embolism, multiple petechial hemorrhages in the cerebral white matter are a common finding, and occasionally larger hemorrhagic infarctions are seen in this entity.[106] Cerebral venous or sinus thrombosis may cause hemorrhagic infarction or frank hemorrhage[107] (Fig. 16–25). Contrast-enhanced CT can make the diagnosis of complete sagittal sinus thrombosis ("delta sign") but is insensitive to partial sinus thrombosis as well as cortical venous occlusion.[108] MR imaging, particularly in conjunction with flow imaging techniques, may prove superior to CT in this disorder.[109, 110]

In autopsy studies, some infarcts are devoid of blood and therefore pallid (pale infarction), others show mild congestion especially at their margins, and still others show extensive extravasation of blood from many small vessels in the infarcted tissue (red or hemorrhagic infarction). While many infarcts are of the same type, either pale or hemorrhagic, others are mixed.

Hemorrhagic infarction remained an autopsy diagnosis until the advent of CT. Because of the paramagnetic properties of blood and its degradation products, MR is even more sensitive than CT in the detection of hemorrhagic infarction. The MR ap-

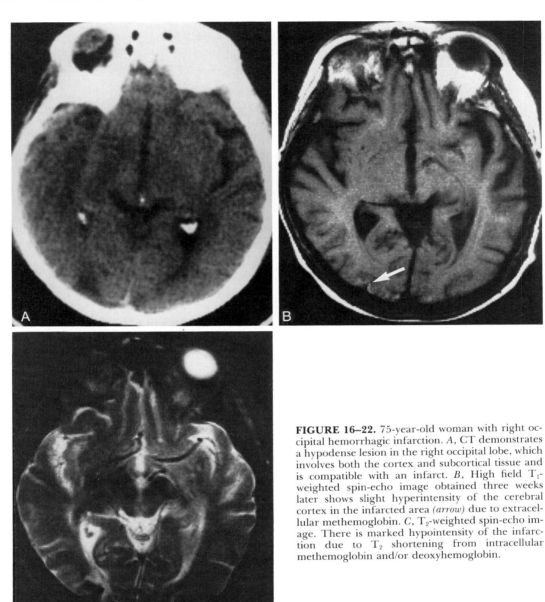

FIGURE 16–22. 75-year-old woman with right occipital hemorrhagic infarction. *A*, CT demonstrates a hypodense lesion in the right occipital lobe, which involves both the cortex and subcortical tissue and is compatible with an infarct. *B*, High field T_1-weighted spin-echo image obtained three weeks later shows slight hyperintensity of the cerebral cortex in the infarcted area *(arrow)* due to extracellular methemoglobin. *C*, T_2-weighted spin-echo image. There is marked hypointensity of the infarction due to T_2 shortening from intracellular methemoglobin and/or deoxyhemoglobin.

pearances are those of subcortical edema due to the ischemia, added to which are the various stages of a hemorrhage, as described earlier. However, there is one important difference. Hecht-Leavitt and coworkers[25] observed that in the acute stage of hemorrhagic infarction there was less low intensity on T_2-weighted images than in intraparenchymal hemorrhage. They believe this to be the result of a higher local pO_2 in hemorrhagic infarction because of early vascular recanalization and luxury perfusion (Fig. 16–24*B*). (See Chapter 17 for additional information on cerebral ischemia and infarction.)

Miscellaneous Rare Types of Hemorrhage

In addition to the mentioned brain hemorrhages, miscellaneous other rare types have been reported, some of them associated with acute rise in arterial pressure: medical conditions with acute hypertension such as eclampsia, pheochromocytoma, and glomerulonephritis; following carotid endarterectomy;[32] after surgical correction of congenital heart defects;[111] upon exertion and exposure to cold weather;[112] after administration of vasopressor drugs;

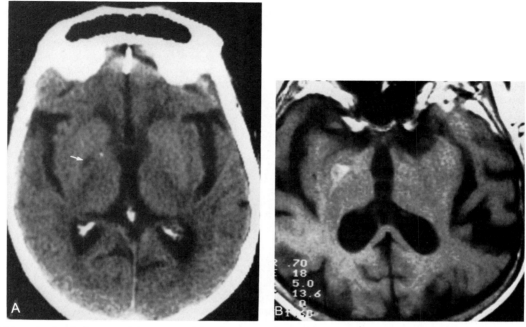

FIGURE 16–23. 74-year-old woman with a hemorrhagic lacunar infarct in the right internal capsule. *A,* The CT scan shows a small hypodense lesion *(arrow)* anterolateral to the thalamus representing a lacunar infarction. Medial to it is a small punctate calcification. There is moderate brain atrophy. *B,* High field T₁-weighted spin-echo image obtained at a slightly different angle than the CT scan demonstrates a triangular hyperintensity, consistent with extracellular methemoglobin, corresponding to the CT hypodensity. The hemorrhagic component in the infarction could not be seen on CT.

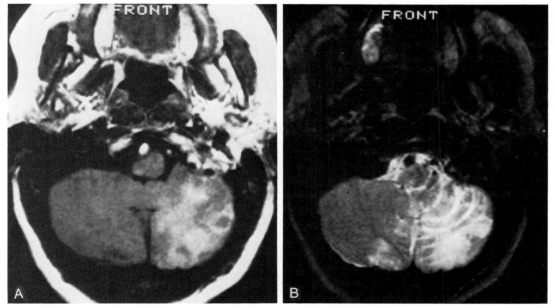

FIGURE 16–24. 69-year-old woman with an embolic hemorrhagic cerebellar infarction in the PICA territories. Inhomogeneous signal involving the left and, to a lesser extent, the right cerebellar hemisphere. *A,* On the T₁-weighted image, bright areas representing hemorrhage are interspersed with normal-appearing tissue. This appearance is atypical for most simple hematomas and occurs because of the inhomogeneous distribution of hemorrhage within the infarct. *B,* On the T₂-weighted image the entire infarction appears bright and the hemorrhagic components are poorly distinguished. The cerebellar folia are well seen indicating no mass effect of the infarct.

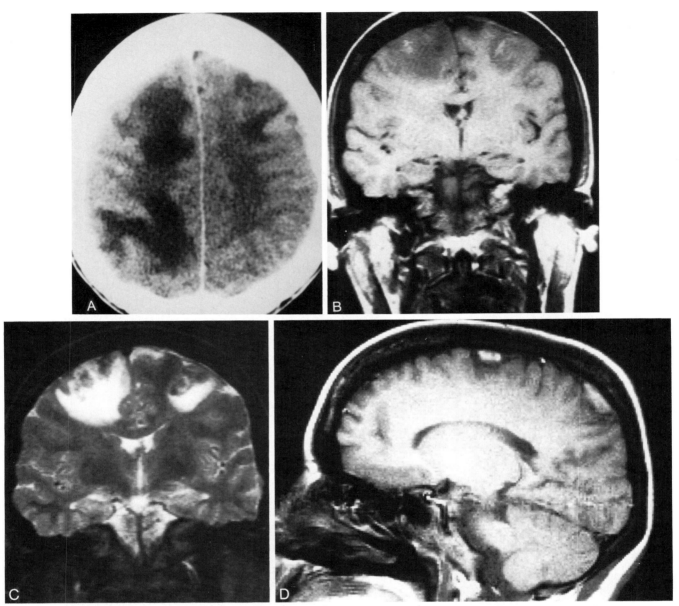

FIGURE 16–25. 32-year-old 34-week pregnant woman who suffered bilateral cortical venous thrombosis resulting in venous infarction. *A,* The CT scan shows hypodense areas in the high convexity slices suggesting bilateral infarction. High field T_1-weighted *(B)* and T_2-weighted *(C)* images show intermixed bright and dark signal adjoining the superior sagittal sinus. Although the appearances could represent hemorrhagic metastases, the distribution is suggestive of sagittal sinus thrombosis. The MR venogram (see Fig. 4–77) showed the superior sagittal sinus was partially thrombosed with obliteration of the feeding cortical veins. *D,* One month later, a T_1-weighted image shows subacute hemorrhage within the infarct, which is surrounded by edema.

and following sympathetic stimulation with severe dental pain[113] or painful urologic examination. Furthermore, supratentorial brain hemorrhage has complicated posterior fossa surgery.[114, 115] All these hemorrhages are preferentially located in the cerebral lobes. Brain stem and thalamic hemorrhage combined with SAH have followed balloon occlusion of an extracranial vertebral arteriovenous fistula.[116]

PRIMARY INTRAVENTRICULAR HEMORRHAGE

Intraventricular hemorrhages (IVH) can be separated into two groups: (1) IVHs without clinical or neuroradiologic evidence of a lesion in the adjacent brain parenchyma, and (2) IVHs resulting from erosion of the ventricular wall by a juxtaventricular lesion or rupture of a hemorrhage into the ventricles as outlined above[117, 118] (for an example, see Fig. 16–14). The first group is commonly referred to as primary IVH and is rare. Primary IVH has been described with aneurysms, vascular malformations, and tumors within the choroid plexus or involving the anterior choroidal or lenticulostriate vessels,[117, 119] but in many cases the cause is never detected. Primary IVH is also a common complication in premature infants.[120] The presenting features include headache, confusion, altered sensorium to a variable extent, and minimal or absent focal neurologic signs. Clinical distinction between SAH and primary IVH is impossible. The diagnosis is made by CT or MRI. Occasionally, on CT and/or MRI, a localized clot in the ventricles instead of diffusely spreading blood is seen simulating tumor. However, tumor can easily be ruled out on a follow-up scan. Altered sensorium as an initial presentation is associated with a grave prognosis, while in uncomplicated primary IVH the outcome is rather favorable.[118] When neurologic deterioration appears to be secondary to acute hydrocephalus, temporary ventriculostomy is indicated.

PITUITARY HEMORRHAGE

Degenerative changes such as small cysts or areas of hemorrhage occur as a gross or microscopic feature of nearly 28 per cent of pituitary adenomas[121] (Fig. 16–26). They are far more frequent than the catastrophic entities of pituitary apoplexy (see Fig. 15–16) or hemorrhage into a normal pituitary gland (Sheehan's syndrome). The frequency of small intra-tumoral bleeds in pituitary adenomas has been attracting recent attention, as MR imaging has made hemorrhagic foci within the adenomas easier to detect. However, decreased signal due to the paramagnetic field effects of hemosiderin is much less common in intratumoral hemorrhage in pituitary adenomas. This is probably because these extracerebral tumors lack a blood-brain barrier, so that there is less accumulation of hemosiderin-laden macrophages. There is evidence that pituitary adenomas treated with bromocriptine are at greater risk for intratumoral hemorrhage, which is often asymptomatic.[122]

INTRACEREBRAL HEMORRHAGE OF UNDETERMINED CAUSE

In a certain group of patients, the clinical and radiologic work-up will not be able to detect the reason for the hemorrhage. In patients in whom hypertension or amyloid angiopathy is not the likely cause of an hemorrhage, angiography is needed to help decide whether there is an anatomic explanation such as a vascular malformation or tumor causing the hemorrhage. If the initial angiogram is negative, in many institutions the study is repeated in 2 to 3 months when pressure from the hematoma has subsided.[35] If no abnormality is seen at that time, a CT or MRI scan 4 to 6 months later is suggested to be certain not to overlook an underlying pathology. Once the sensitivity of MRI is established for detecting these lesions in the acute and later stages, it should further reduce the need for angiography.

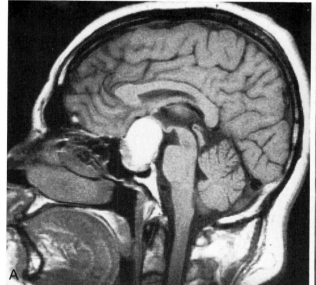 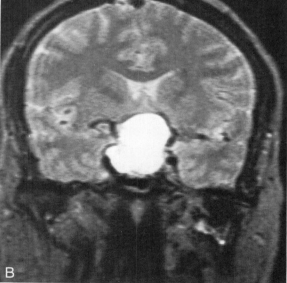

FIGURE 16–26. 40-year-old man with surgically proven hemorrhage into chromophobe pituitary adenoma. The sagittal T_1-weighted image (A) as well as the coronal T_2-weighted image (B) show bright signal consistent with extracellular methemoglobin. Note the absence of a dark rim around the hematoma, which is usually present around intracerebral hematomas. This is considered a consequence of an absent blood-brain barrier in the pituitary enabling iron-laden macrophages to mobilize away from the hematoma.

FACTORS INFLUENCING OUTCOME OF INTRACEREBRAL HEMORRHAGE AND THERAPEUTIC IMPLICATIONS

Alertness is bound to integrity of the reticular activating system. A unilateral mass can jeopardize its function either by displacing the brain stem laterally[123] or by impaction of portions of the medial temporal lobe between the tentorial edge and the adjacent brain stem causing compression and damage of the midbrain.[124] The oculomotor nerve is compressed as well. This process is called *transtentorial herniation*. Bilateral cerebral masses may compress the low diencephalon in the tentorial opening without shifting it horizontally. This is termed central or central descending transtentorial herniation. Pupillary enlargement and/or altered level of consciousness are considered the surest clinical signs of transtentorial herniation.

On CT scans, effacement of the tentorial cisterns, horizontal shift and depression of the pineal body, and contralateral hydrocephalus are the findings in tentorial herniations with a unilateral mass. In central herniation there is obliteration of the basal subarachnoid cisterns associated with downward shift of the pineal calcium.[125] In MRI the displacement and torquing of the brain stem can be appreciated directly.

Negative prognostic signs in patients with intracerebral hemorrhage include initial stupor or coma, significant midline shift on angiogram[126] or CT,[127, 128] large hemorrhage size, and intraventricular extension of blood. Patients with large temporal or temporoparietal hematomas appear to be at greater risk for brain stem compression than those with hematomas in other locations.[129] Of patients who survive the hemorrhage, only one quarter show persistent severe neurologic deficits at one year.[130]

Medical treatment is of critical importance. Blood pressure must be maintained within acceptable limits. Increased intracranial pressure can rarely be managed by medical means alone, and medical measures usually have to be followed by surgical evacuation of the hematoma. It is generally agreed that in patients with large lobar and putaminal hematomas and decreasing levels of consciousness, surgical evacuation of the hematoma can be lifesaving. In cerebellar hematomas a worsening sensorium is a distinct indication for surgery.[35] The clinical course of cerebellar hemorrhage is unpredictable.[63, 66] Rapid deterioration to coma and death can occur without warning. Hematomas with a diameter of 3 cm or less on CT usually have a favorable outcome with medical treatment.[131, 132] However, these patients need careful monitoring in the intensive care unit of an adequately equipped center for at least 48 hours. With larger lesions immediate surgical removal should be considered, since the morbidity of surgical intervention is low and the chance of rapid and irreversible deterioration considerable.[133] When a patient is in deep coma, removal of the hematoma can still result in good recovery, especially if the interval between decrease of consciousness and surgery is short. Ventricular drainage may be necessary to treat persisting hydrocephalus after evacuation of the hematoma. Ventricular drainage alone does not relieve pressure on the brain stem and bears the danger of superior cerebellar tentorial herniation.[134]

If there is loss of pupillary reaction and brain stem function, then surgery offers little chance for clinical improvement. There is also little to be gained by surgery in patients with thalamic and pontine hemorrhage. When hydrocephalus develops in thalamic hemorrhage, emergency ventricular drainage may be necessary as an isolated measure or in conjunction with surgical evacuation of the clot.

In suspected amyloid angiopathy, surgery should be avoided and delayed as long as possible, since the vessels are very fragile and surgical evacuation is often attended by uncontrollable hemorrhage and postoperative recurrent bleeding.[135] Hematomas due to aneurysms, arteriovenous malformations, and tumors are treated essentially in the same way as other forms of spontaneous brain hemorrhage. In patients who require surgical removal of the hematoma, efforts should be made to repair the aneurysm or arteriovenous malformation at the same operation to prevent postoperative bleeding.[35] When a tumor is suspected, the wall of the hematoma cavity should be biopsied for microscopic examination. The role of stereotactic techniques to remove hematomas needs to be studied further, and also the place of surgery in the neurologically stable patient is not yet established. Currently it is not proved that hematoma evacuation in a neurologically stable patient would improve the outcome and, therefore, is usually not done.

Other therapeutic measures are useful in certain conditions. In anticoagulant-related hemorrhage, administration of vitamin K and clotting factors or fresh frozen plasma may help to stem bleeding.[136] Thrombocytopenic patients may benefit from platelet transfusion,[137] and hemophiliacs from infusion of appropriate clotting factors.[138]

REFERENCES

1. Smith HJ, Strother CM, Kikuchi Y, et al: MR imaging in the management of supratentorial intracranial AVMs. AJNR 9:225–235, 1988.
2. Gomori JM, Grossman RI, Hackney DB, et al: Variable appearances of subacute intracranial hematomas on high-field spin-echo MR. AJNR 8:1019–1026, 1988.
3. Destian S, Sze G, Krol G, Zimmerman RD, Deck MDF: MR imaging of hemorrhagic intracranial neoplasms. AJNR 9:1115–1122, 1988.
4. Di Chiro G, Brooks RA, Girton ME, et al: Sequential MR studies of intracerebral hematomas in monkeys. AJNR 7:193–199, 1986.
5. Edelman RR, Johnson K, Buxton R, et al: MR of hemorrhage: A new approach. AJNR 7:751–756, 1986.

6. Grossman RI, Gomori JM, Goldberg HI, et al: MR of hemorrhagic conditions. Acta Radiol Suppl 369:56–58, 1986.

7. Tanaka T, Sakai T, Uemura K, et al: MR imaging as predictor of delayed posttraumatic cerebral hemorrhage. J Neurosurg 69:203–209, 1988.

8. Zimmerman RD, Heier LA, Snow RB, et al: Acute intracranial hemorrhage: Intensity changes on sequential MR scans. AJNR 9:47–57, 1988.

9. Komiyama M, Baba M, Hakuba A, et al: MR imaging of brainstem hemorrhage. AJNR 9:261–268, 1988.

10. Jenkins A, Hadley DM, Teasdale GM, et al: Magnetic resonance imaging of acute subarachnoid hemorrhage. J Neurosurg 68:731–736, 1988.

11. Satoh S, Kadoya S: Magnetic resonance imaging of subarachnoid hemorrhage. Neuroradiology 30:361–366, 1988.

12. Nose T, Enomoto T, Hyodo A, et al: Intracerebral hematoma developing during MR examination. J Comput Assist Tomogr 11:184, 1987.

13. Hosoda K, Tamaki N, Masuruma M, et al: Magnetic resonance images of chronic subdural hematomas. J Neurosurg 67:677–683, 1987.

14. Grossman RI, Gomori JM, Goldberg HI, et al: MR imaging of hemorrhagic conditions of the head and neck. RadioGraphics 8:441–454, 1988.

15. Hackney DB, Atlas SW, Grossman RI, et al: Subacute intracranial hemorrhage: Contribution of spin density to appearance on spin-echo images. Radiology 165:199–202, 1987.

16. Atlas SW, Grossman RI, Gomori JM, et al: Hemorrhagic intracranial malignant neoplasms: Spin-echo MR imaging. Radiology 164:71–77, 1987.

17. Winkler ML, Olsen WL, Mills TC, Kaufman L: Hemorrhagic and nonhemorrhagic brain lesions: Evaluation with 0.35-T fast MR imaging. Radiology 165:203–207, 1987.

18. Atlas SW, Mark AS, Grossman RI, Gomori JM: Intracranial hemorrhage: Gradient-echo MR imaging at 1.5 T. Radiology 168:803–807, 1988.

19. Bradley WG Jr: MRI of hemorrhage and iron in the brain. *In* Stark DD, Bradley WG Jr (eds): Magnetic Resonance Imaging. St. Louis, CV Mosby Company, 1988, pp 359–374.

20. Norman D: Vascular disease: Hemorrhage. *In* Brant-Zawadzki M, Norman D (eds): Magnetic Resonance Imaging of the Central Nervous System. New York, Raven Press, 1987, pp 209–220.

21. Gomori JM, Grossman RI: Mechanisms responsible for MR appearance and evolution of intracranial hemorrhage. RadioGraphics 8:427–440, 1988.

22. Barkovich AJ, Atlas SW: Magnetic resonance imaging of intracranial hemorrhage. Radiol Clin North Am 26:801–820, 1988.

23. Schlesinger SD: MRI of intracranial hematomas and closed head trauma. *In* Pomeranz SJ (ed): Craniospinal Magnetic Resonance Imaging. Philadelphia, WB Saunders Company, 1989, pp 399–435.

23a. Hayman LA, McArdle CB, Tabes KH, et al: MR imaging of hyperacute intracranial hemorrhage in the cat. AJNR 10:681–686, 1989.

23b. Brooks RA, DiChiro G, Patronas N: MR imaging of cerebral hematomas at different field strengths: Theory and applications. J Comput Assist Tomogr 13:194–206, 1989.

24. Hayman LA, Ford JJ, Taber KH, et al: T2 effect of hemoglobin concentration: Assessment with in vitro MR spectroscopy. Radiology 168:489–491, 1988.

25. Hecht-Leavitt C, Gomori JM, Grossman RI, et al: High-field MRI of hemorrhagic cortical infarction. AJNR 7:581–585, 1986.

26. Woodruff WW, Djang WT, McLendon RE, et al: Intracerebral malignant melanoma: High-field-strength MR imaging. Radiology 165:209–213, 1987.

27. Gomori JM, Grossman RI, Shields JA, et al: Choroidal melanomas: Correlation of NMR spectroscopy and MR imaging. Radiology 158:443–445, 1986.

28. Atlas SW, Grossman RI, Hackney DB, et al: Calcified intracranial lesions: Detection with gradient-echo-acquisition rapid MR imaging. AJR 150:1383–1389, 1988.

29. Dell LA, Brown MS, Orrison WW, et al: Physiologic intracranial calcification with hyperintensity on MR imaging: Case report and experimental model. AJNR 9:1145–1148, 1988.

30. Caplan L: Intracerebral hemorrhage revisited (editorial). Neurology 38:624–627, 1988.

31. Cole A, Aube M: Late-onset migraine with intracerebral hemorrhage: A recognizable syndrome. Neurology 37(Suppl 1):238, 1987.

32. Pomposelli FB, Lamparello PJ, Riles TS, et al: Intracranial hemorrhage after carotid endarterectomy. J Vasc Surg 7:248–255, 1988.

33. Ojemann RG, Mohr JP: Hypertensive brain hemorrhage. Clin Neurosurg 23:220–244, 1976.

34. Herbstein DS, Schaumburg HH: Hypertensive intracerebral hematoma. An investigation of the initial hemorrhage and rebleeding using chromium Cr51-labeled erythrocytes. Arch Neurol 30:412–414, 1974.

35. Ojemann RG, Heros RC: Spontaneous brain hemorrhage. Stroke 14:468–475, 1983.

36. Mohr JP, Caplan LR, Melski JW, et al: The Harvard Cooperative Stroke Registry: A prospective registry. Neurology 28:754–762, 1978.

37. Bogousslavsky J, Van Melle G, Regli F: The Lausanne Stroke registry: Analysis of 1,000 consecutive patients with first stroke. Stroke 19:1083–1092, 1988.

38. Foulkes MA, Wolf PA, Price TR, et al: The Stroke Data Bank: Design, methods, and baseline characteristics. Stroke 19:547–554, 1988.

39. Toffel GJ, Biller J, Adams HP: Nontraumatic intracerebral hemorrhage in young adults. Arch Neurol 44:483–485, 1987.

40. Gross CR, Kase CS, Mohr JP, et al: Stroke in south Alabama: Incidence and diagnostic features—A population based study. Stroke 15:249–255, 1984.

41. Fisher CM: Pathological observations in hypertensive cerebral hemorrhage. J Neuropathol Exp Neurol 30:536–550, 1971.

42. Charcot JM, Bouchard C: Nouvelles recherches sur la pathogénie de l'hémorrhagie cérébrale. Arch Physiol Norm Pathol 1:110–127, 643–665, 725–734, 1868.

43. Loes DJ, Smoker WRK, Biller J, Cornell SH: Nontraumatic lobar intracerebral hemorrhage: CT/angiographic correlation. AJNR 8:1027–1030, 1987.

44. Huber P Krayenbühl/Yasargil. Zerebrale Angiographie für Klinik und Praxis. Stuttgart, Thieme Publishers, 1979.

45. Stein RW, Kase CS, Hier DB, et al: Caudate hemorrhage. Neurology 34:1549–1554, 1984.

46. Kase CS, Mohr JP: Supratentorial intracerebral hemorrhage. *In* Barnett HJM, Mohr JP, Stein BM, Yatsu FM (eds): Stroke—Pathophysiology, Diagnosis, Management. New York, Churchill Livingstone, 1986, pp 525–547.

47. Weisberg LA: Thalamic hemorrhage: Clinical-CT correlations. Neurology 36:1382–1386, 1986.

48. Huang CY, Woo E, Yu YL, Chan FL: Lacunar syndromes due to brainstem infarct and haemorrhage. J Neurol Neurosurg Psychiat 51:509–515, 1988.

49. Abe M, Kjellberg RN, Adams RD: Clinical presentations of vascular malformations of the brain stem: Comparison of angiographically positive and negative types. J Neurol Neurosurg Psychiat 52:167–175, 1989.

50. Kase CS, Maulsby GO, Mohr JP: Partial pontine hematomas. Neurology 30:652–655, 1980.

51. Silverstein A: Primary pontine hemorrhage. *In* Vinken PJ, Bruyn GW (eds): Handbook of Clinical Neurology. Vol 12, Vascular Diseases of the Nervous System, Part II. Amsterdam, North Holland Publishing Co., 1972, pp 37–53.

52. Caplan LR, Goodwin JA: Lateral tegmental brainstem hemorrhages. Neurology 32:252–260, 1982.

53. Fisher CM: Some neuro-ophthalmological observations. J Neurol Neurosurg Psychiat 30:383–392, 1967.

54. Henn V, Lang W, Hepp K, Reisine H: Experimental gaze

palsies in monkeys and their relation to human pathology. Brain 107:619–636, 1984.

55. Sand JJ, Biller J, Corbett JJ, et al: Partial dorsal mesencephalic hemorrhages: Report of three cases. Neurology 36:529–533, 1986.

56. Weisberg LA: Mesencephalic hemorrhages: Clinical and computed tomographic correlations. Neurology 36:713–716, 1986.

57. Stern LZ, Bernick C: Spontaneous, isolated mesencephalic hemorrhage (letter). Neurology 36:1627, 1986.

58. Mangiardi JR, Epstein FJ: Brainstem haematomas: Review of the literature and presentation of five new cases. J Neurol Neurosurg Psychiat 51:966–976, 1988.

59. Biller J, Gentry LR, Adams HP Jr, Morris DC: Spontaneous hemorrhage in the medulla oblongata: Clinical MR correlations. J Comput Assist Tomogr 10:303–306, 1986.

60. Kase CS, Caplan LR: Hemorrhage affecting the brain stem and cerebellum. *In* Barnett HJM, Mohr JP, Stein BM, Yatsu FM (eds): Stroke—Pathophysiology, Diagnosis, Management. New York, Churchill Livingstone, 1986, pp 621–641.

61. Mumenthaler M: Neurologie. 8. Erweiterte Auflage. Stuttgart, Thieme Publishers, 1986.

62. Caplan LR, Stein RW: Stroke: A Clinical Approach. Boston, Butterworth Publishers, 1986.

63. Ott KH, Kase CS, Ojemann RG, Mohr JP: Cerebellar hemorrhage: Diagnosis and treatment. Arch Neurol 31:160–167, 1974.

64. Dunne JW, Chakera T, Kermode S: Cerebellar haemorrhage—diagnosis and treatment: A study of 75 consecutive cases. Q J Med 64:739–754, 1987.

65. McKissock W, Richardson A, Walsh L: Spontaneous cerebellar haemorrhage. Brain 83:1–9, 1960.

66. Fisher CM, Picard EH, Polak A, et al: Acute hypertensive cerebellar hemorrhage: Diagnosis and surgical treatment. J Nerv Ment Dis 140:38–57, 1965.

67. Ebeling U, Huber P: Der akute raumfordernde Prozess in der hinteren Schädelgrube. Klinik und computertomographischer Befund. Schweiz Med Wochenschr 116:1394–1401, 1986.

68. Kase CS, Williams PJ, Wyatt DA, Mohr JP: Lobar intracerebral hematomas: Clinical and CT analysis of 22 cases. Neurology 32:1146–1450, 1982.

69. Hilt DC, Buchholz D, Krumholz A, et al: Herpes zoster ophthalmicus and delayed contralateral hemiparesis caused by cerebral angiitis. Diagnosis and management approaches. Ann Neurol 14:543–553, 1983.

70. Hart RG, Kagan-Hallet K, Joerns SE: Mechanisms of intracranial hemorrhage in infective endocarditis. Stroke 18:1048–1056, 1987.

71. Ropper AH, Davis KR: Lobar cerebral hemorrhages: Acute clinical syndromes in 26 cases. Ann Neurol 8:141–147, 1980.

72. Ausman JI, Diaz FG, Malik GM, et al: Current management of cerebral aneurysms: Is it based on facts or myths? Surg Neurol 24:625–635, 1985.

73. Jellinger K: Pathology and aetiology of intracranial aneurysms. *In* Pia HW, Langmaid C, Zierski J (eds): Cerebral Aneurysms. Advances in Diagnosis and Therapy. Berlin, Springer Verlag, 1979, pp 5–41.

74. Hayvard RD, O'Reilly GV: Intracranial haemorrhage. Accuracy of computerized transverse axial scanning in predicting the underlying aetiology. Lancet 1:1–4, 1976.

75. Mohr JP, Nichols FC, Tatemichi TK, Stein BM: Vascular malformations of the brain: Clinical considerations. *In* Barnett HJM, Mohr JP, Stein BM, Yatsu FM (eds): Stroke—Pathophysiology, Diagnosis, Management. New York, Churchill Livingstone, 1986, pp 679–705.

76. Needell WM, Maravilla KR: MR flow imaging in vascular malformations using gradient recalled acquisition. AJNR 9:637–642, 1988.

77. Rigamonti D, Drayer BP, Johnson PC, et al: The MRI appearance of cavernous malformations (angiomas). J Neurosurg 67:518–524, 1987.

78. Rigamonti D, Spetzler RF, Drayer BP, et al: Appearance of

venous malformations on magnetic resonance imaging. J Neurosurg 69:535–539, 1988.

79. Farmer JP, Cosgrove GR, Villemure JG, et al: Intracerebral cavernous angiomas. Neurology 38:1699–1704, 1988.

80. Sze G, Krol G, Olsen WL, et al: Hemorrhagic neoplasms: MR mimics of occult vascular malformations. AJNR 8:795–802, 1987.

81. Gomori JM, Grossman RI, Goldberg HI, et al: Occult cerebral vascular malformations: High-field MR imaging. Radiology 158:707–713, 1986.

82. Ogilvy CS, Heros RC, Ojeman RG, New PF: Angiographically occult arteriovenous malformations. J Neurosurg 69:350–355, 1988.

83. Jellinger K: Cerebrovascular amyloidosis with cerebral haemorrhage. J Neurol 214:195–206, 1977.

84. Vinters HV: Cerebral amyloid angiopathy: A critical review. Stroke 18:311–324, 1987.

85. Masuda J, Tanaka K, Ueda K, Omae T: Autopsy study of incidence and distribution of cerebral amyloid angiopathy in Hisayama, Japan. Stroke 19:205–210, 1988.

86. Cosgrove CR, Leblanc R, Meagher-Villemure K, Ethier R: Cerebral amyloid angiopathy. Neurology 35:625–631, 1985.

87. Cole FM, Yates P: Intracerebral microaneurysms and small cerebrovascular lesions. Brain 90:759–768, 1967.

88. Carlson SE, Aldrich MS, Greenberg HS, Topol EJ: Intracerebral hemorrhage complicating intravenous tissue plasminogen activator treatment. Arch Neurol 45:1070–1073, 1988.

89. Wintzen AR, de Jonge H, Loeliger EA, Bots GTAM: The risk of intracerebral hemorrhage during oral anticoagulant treatment: A population study. Ann Neurol 16:553–558, 1984.

90. Kase CS, Robinson RK, Stein RW, et al: Anticoagulant-related intracerebral hemorrhage. Neurology 35:943–948, 1985.

91. Brust JCM, Richter RW: Stroke associated with addiction to heroin. J Neurol Neurosurg Psychiat 39:194–199, 1976.

92. Rumbaugh CL, Bergeron RT, Fang HC, McCormick R: Cerebral angiographic changes in the drug abuse patient. Radiology 101:335–344, 1971.

93. Delaney P, Estes M: Intracranial hemorrhage with amphetamine use. Neurology 30:1125–1130, 1980.

94. Caplan LR, Thomas C, Banks G: Central nervous system complications of addiction to "T's and Blues." Neurology 32:623–628, 1982.

95. Fallis RJ, Fisher M: Cerebral vasculitis and hemorrhage associated with phenylpropanolamine. Neurology 35:405–407, 1985.

96. Levine SR, Welch KMA: Cocaine and stroke. Stroke 19:779–783, 1987.

97. Kase CS: Intracerebral hemorrhage: Non-hypertensive causes. Stroke 17:590–595, 1986.

98. Feinberg WM, Swenson MS: Cerebrovascular complications of L-asparaginase therapy. Neurology 38:127–133, 1988.

99. Scott M: Spontaneous intracerebral hematoma caused by cerebral neoplasms. Report of eight verified cases. J Neurosurg 42:338–342, 1975.

100. Mandybur TI: Intracranial hemorrhage caused by metastatic tumors. Neurology 27:650–655, 1977.

101. Zimmerman RA, Bilaniuk LT: Computed tomography of acute intratumoral hemorrhage. Radiology 135:355–359, 1980.

102. Gatenby RA, Coia LR, Richter MP, et al: Oxygen tension in human tumors: In vivo mapping using CT-guided probes. Radiology 156:211–214, 1985.

103. Fisher CM, Adams RD: Observations on brain metabolism with special reference to the mechanism of hemorrhagic infarction. J Neuropathol Exp Neurol 10:92–93, 1951.

104. Ott BR, Zamani A, Kleefield J, Funkenstein HH: The clinical spectrum of hemorrhagic infarction. Stroke 17:630–637, 1986.

105. Lodder J, Krijne-Kubat B, Broekman J: Cerebral hemorrhagic infarction at autopsy: Cardiac embolic cause and

the relationship to the cause of death. Stroke 17:626–629, 1986.

106. McCarthy M, Norenberg MD: Pontine hemorrhagic infarction in nontraumatic fat embolism. Neurology 38:1645–1647, 1988.

107. Bousser MG, Chiras J, Sauron B, et al: Cerebral venous thrombosis—A review of 38 cases. Stroke 16:199–213, 1985; and Erratum Stroke 16:738, 1985.

108. Buonanno FS, Moody DM, Ball MR, Laster DW: Computed cranial tomographic findings in cerebral sinovenous occlusion. J Comput Assist Tomogr 2:281–290, 1978.

109. Sze G, Simmons B, Krol G, et al: Dural sinus thrombosis: Verification with spin-echo techniques. AJNR 9:679–686, 1988.

110. Edelman RR, Wentz KU, Mattle H, et al: Projection arteriography and venography in the body and head: Initial clinical results using magnetic resonance. Radiology 172:351–357, 1989.

111. Humphreys RP, Hoffman HJ, Mustard WT, Trusler GA: Cerebral hemorrhage after heart surgery. J Neurosurg 43:671–675, 1975.

112. Caplan LR, Neely S, Gorelick PB: Cold-related intracerebral hemorrhage. Arch Neurol 41:227, 1984.

113. Barbas N, Caplan L, Baquis G, et al: Dental chair intracerebral hemorrhage. Neurology 37:511–512, 1987.

114. Seiler RW, Zurbrügg HR: Supratentorial intracerebral hemorrhage after posterior fossa operation. Neurosurgery 18:472–474, 1986.

115. Haines S, Maroom J, Janetta P: Supratentorial intracerebral hemorrhage following posterior fossa surgery. J Neurosurg 49:881–886, 1978.

116. Kondoh T, Tamaki N, Takeda N, et al: Fatal intracranial hemorrhage after balloon occlusion of an extracranial vertebral arteriovenous fistula. J Neurosurg 69:945–948, 1988.

117. Gates PC, Barnett HJM, Vinters HV, et al: Primary intraventricular hemorrhage in adults. Stroke 17:872–877, 1986.

118. Verma A, Maheshwari MC, Bhargava S: Spontaneous intraventricular haemorrhage. J Neurol 234:233–236, 1987.

119. Darby DG, Donnan GA, Saling MA, et al: Primary intraventricular hemorrhage: Clinical and neuropsychological findings in a prospective stroke series. Neurology 38:68–75, 1988.

120. Volpe JJ: Neonatal intraventricular hemorrhage. N Engl J Med 304:886–891, 1981.

121. Kraus JF: Neoplastic diseases of the human hypophysis. Arch Pathol 39:343–349, 1945.

122. Yousem DM, Arrington JA, Zinreich SJ, et al: Pituitary adenomas: Possible role of bromocriptine in intratumoral hemorrhage. Radiology 170:239–243, 1989.

123. Ropper AH: Lateral displacement of the brain and level of consciousness in patients with an acute hemispheral mass. N Engl J Med 314:953–958, 1986.

124. Plum F, Posner JB: The Diagnosis of Stupor and Coma. 3rd ed. Philadelphia, FA Davis Company, 1980.

125. Hahn F, Gurney J: CT signs of central descending transtentorial herniation. AJNR 6:844–845, 1985.

126. McKissock W, Richardson A, Tyler J: Primary intracerebral haemorrhage. A controlled trial of surgical and conservative treatment in 180 unselected cases. Lancet 2:221–226, 1961.

127. Portenoy RK, Lipton RB, Berger AR, et al: Intracerebral haemorrhage: A model for the prediction of outcome. J Neurol Neurosurg Psychiat 50:976–979, 1987.

128. Tuhrim S, Dambrosia JM, Price TR, et al: Prediction of intracerebral hemorrhage survival. Ann Neurol 24:258–263, 1988.

129. Andrews BT, Chiles BW, Olsen WL, Pitts LH: The effect of intracerebral hematoma location on the risk of brainstem compression and on clinical outcome. J Neurosurg 69:518–522, 1988.

130. Fieschi C, Carolei A, Fiorelli M, et al: Changing prognosis of primary intracerebral hemorrhage: Results of a clinical and computed tomographic follow-up study of 104 patients. Stroke 19:192–195, 1988.

131. Little JR, Tubman DE, Ethier R: Cerebellar hemorrhage in adults. J Neurosurg 48:575–579, 1978.

132. Heiman TD, Satya-Murti S: Benign cerebellar hemorrhages. Ann Neurol 3:366–368, 1978.

133. Crowell RG, Ojemann RG: Spontaneous brain hemorrhage: Surgical considerations. In Barnett HJM, Mohr JP, Stein BM, Yatsu FM (eds): Stroke—Pathophysiology, Diagnosis, Management. New York, Churchill Livingstone, 1986, pp 1191–1206.

134. Cuneo RA, Caronna JJ, Pitts L, et al: Upward transtentorial herniation: Seven cases and a literature review. Arch Neurol 36:618–623, 1979.

135. Tyler KL, Poletti CE, Heros RC: Cerebral amyloid angiopathy with multiple intracerebral hemorrhages. Neurosurgery 57:286–289, 1982.

136. Mattle H, Kohler S, Huber P, et al: Anticoagulation-related intracranial extracerebral haemorrhage. J Neurol Neurosurg Psychiat 52:829–837, 1989.

137. Woerner FJ, Abildgaard CF, French BN: Intracranial hemorrhage in children with idiopathic thrombocytopenic purpura. Pediatrics 67:453–460, 1981.

138. Yoshida M, Hayashi T, Kuramoto S, et al: Traumatic intracranial hematomas in hemophiliac children. Surg Neurol 12:115–118, 1979.

17

BRAIN: Vascular Diseases

RICHARD J. HICKS, JOHN R. HESSELINK, GARY L. WISMER,
and KENNETH R. DAVIS

OCCLUSIVE CEREBROVASCULAR
DISEASE
   INFARCTION
   ARTERIAL OCCLUSION
   ARTERIAL DISSECTION
   VENOUS OCCLUSION
   ARTERITIS
   MIGRAINE
VASCULAR MALFORMATIONS
   ARTERIOVENOUS MALFORMATION
   CAVERNOUS ANGIOMA

CAPILLARY TELANGIECTASIA
VENOUS MALFORMATION
ANEURYSMS
   CONGENITAL BERRY ANEURYSMS
   SUBARACHNOID HEMORRHAGE
   COMPLICATIONS OF HEMORRHAGE
   GIANT ANEURYSMS
   OTHER TYPES OF ANEURYSMS
   POSTSURGICAL ASSESSMENT
FUTURE OF VASCULAR IMAGING

The utility of MR in vascular processes such as cerebral infarction, vessel thrombosis, vascular malformation, and giant aneurysm stems mainly from the sensitivity of MR to flow, subacute and chronic hemorrhage, and differences in water content and structure. The dynamic MR appearance of hemorrhage is described in detail in Chapter 16. The imaging of flow is also discussed more completely elsewhere in this text (Chapter 4) but is briefly mentioned here as it relates to neuroimaging of vascular lesions. Rapidly flowing blood undergoes high-velocity signal loss because the excited protons leave the section prior to signal generation.[1, 2] In slower flowing vessels, flow-related enhancement can be noted owing to the introduction of fully magnetized protons into the imaging plane. Relatively slow flow parallel to the imaging plane may undergo enhancement because of even-echo rephasing, exhibiting brighter signal on the even echoes of a symmetric echo train. The imaging of blood flow becomes even more complex with multislice acquisitions and oblique flow, so that even-echo rephasing is not often noted clinically in vascular malformations.[3] Vessels perpendicular to the imaging plane often exhibit flow-related enhancement in the end slices of an imaging stack if the flow is directed from outside into the imaging volume. A method of adjusting slice thickness and repetition time (TR) in single-slice acquisitions for flow-related enhancement of specific velocities using time-of-flight effects has been reported.[4] This method has been used with some success in demonstrating flow patterns within lesions. Out-of-plane flow enhancement can be augmented by gradient-echo (GRE) imaging using a short TR, and with a short enough TR this technique can be used for in-plane flow as well.

OCCLUSIVE CEREBROVASCULAR DISEASE

INFARCTION

Stroke is the third most common cause of death in the United States. Embolic strokes characteristically begin suddenly, with the deficit quickly reaching its peak, while thrombotic strokes may have a slower or more stuttering onset over hours or days. Thrombotic strokes are more likely to have prodromal transient ischemic attacks (TIAs). The most important risk factors are diabetes and hypertension, with valvular disease and atrial fibrillation being additional risk factors for embolic disease. Infarctions will involve one or more discrete vascular territories (most often the middle, anterior, and posterior cerebral arteries) with clinical findings referable to the involved portion of the brain. A low-flow state, such as severe hypotension, may result in "watershed" infarctions at the borders of adjacent vascular territories. Hemorrhagic infarction is most frequently secondary to an embolus that subsequently dissolves, with reconstitution of flow into vessels with damaged endothelium. Lacunar infarcts occur most often in the setting of hypertension and are due to occlusion of small penetrating branches originating from the proximal major cerebral arteries. They typically involve the basal ganglia, internal capsule, thalamus, and brain stem. Lacunar strokes often produce characteristic clinical syndromes such as pure motor hemiparesis, pure hemisensory syndrome, ataxic hemiparesis, and dysarthria–clumsy hand syndrome.[5]

MR is well suited for imaging brain infarcts owing to its exquisite sensitivity to edema. Experimentally, MR has yielded abnormal findings as soon as 2 to 4 hours after vessel occlusion, at a time when CT has shown no abnormality[6, 7] (Fig. 17–1). Experimental evidence has suggested that the lengthening of T_1 and T_2 may be greatest in very early ischemia before breakdown of the blood-brain barrier (BBB) allows protein leakage into edematous tissue. The exact structure of water within ischemic tissue, rather than water content alone, may also be a significant mechanism in the relaxation time and signal intensity changes in early stroke.[8] The difficulty of imaging

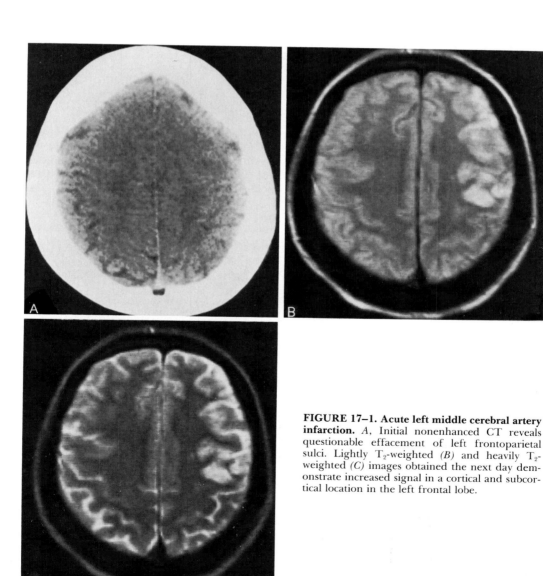

FIGURE 17–1. Acute left middle cerebral artery infarction. *A,* Initial nonenhanced CT reveals questionable effacement of left frontoparietal sulci. Lightly T_2-weighted *(B)* and heavily T_2-weighted *(C)* images obtained the next day demonstrate increased signal in a cortical and subcortical location in the left frontal lobe.

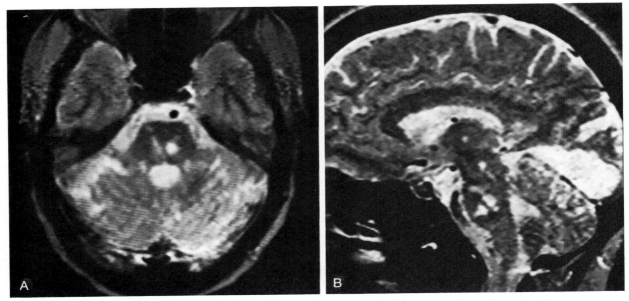

FIGURE 17–2. Brain stem and left occipital infarctions in a 42-year-old patient with multiple cranial nerve palsies. Left vertebral artery occlusion was demonstrated angiographically. Heavily T$_2$-weighted axial *(A)* and sagittal *(B)* images demonstrate multiple foci of increased signal in the pons, midbrain, and middle cerebellar peduncles, with a larger area of signal abnormality in the occipital lobe. A normal flow void is noted in the basilar artery.

acute hemorrhage is an important factor limiting the role of MR in the evaluation of acute infarction. In the subacute stage, MR may be more sensitive than CT for parenchymal hemorrhages.[9, 10] Salgado and colleagues,[11] in a study of 60 patients, found more abnormalities with MR, but MR missed cortical infarcts seen with enhanced CT, and MR was unable to distinguish between subacute and chronic hemorrhagic infarcts. MR does have an advantage over CT for imaging midbrain, pontine, and medullary infarctions, and it can also help assess patency of the major arteries[12] (Figs. 17–2 and 17–3). Others have noted that the multiplicity of lesions identified with non–contrast-enhanced MR in patients with pontine infarctions, sometimes bilateral and in multiple vascular territories, may limit the correlation with neurologic deficits.[13] In these cases, follow-up contrast-enhanced MR scans 2 to 3 weeks after the acute event may reveal enhancement of the more recent infarct.

The classic pattern of cerebral infarction is a wedge-shaped abnormality that involves both the cortex and a variable amount of the subcortical tissue, in either a major vascular territory or a watershed area. The amount of vascular territory affected depends on the adequacy or insufficiency of the leptomeningeal collateral circulation. Acute infarcts are associated with both cytotoxic and vasogenic edema. They are hyperintense on T$_2$-weighted and proton density–weighted images and hypointense on T$_1$-weighted images (Figs. 17–4 and 17–5). Hemorrhage into infarcts often represents oozing of blood from

damaged capillaries rather than frank hematoma formation. This type of hemorrhage is seen on MR as a cortical ribbon of low or high signal, depending on the stage of hemorrhage and pulse sequence selection[14] (Figs. 17–6 and 17–7).

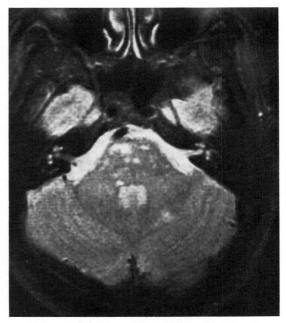

FIGURE 17–3. Brain stem infarction. Multiple small pontine infarctions are noted on this T$_2$-weighted image.

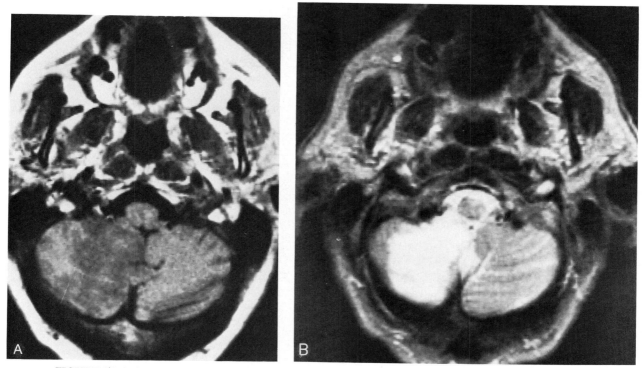

FIGURE 17–4. Acute cerebellar infarct. T_1-weighted (A) and T_2-weighted (B) images show areas of prolonged T_1 and T_2 in the right inferior cerebellar hemisphere, with slight mass effect on the inferior cerebellar peduncle. The infarct involves the territory of the posterior inferior cerebellar artery.

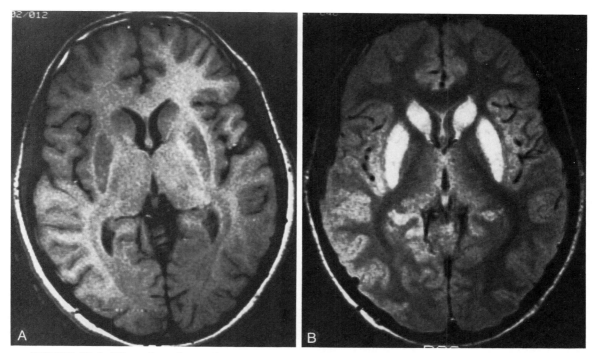

FIGURE 17–5. Bilateral caudate and putamen infarctions after severe hypotension. A, T_1-weighted image reveals decreased signal predominantly in the putamen bilaterally. B, T_2-weighted image illustrates strikingly increased signal in the head of the caudate nucleus and putamen bilaterally. The pattern is similar to that seen from severe hypoxia due to near-drowning and carbon monoxide poisoning.

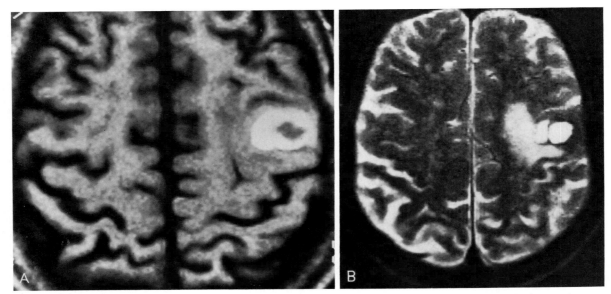

FIGURE 17–6. Hemorrhagic infarct. *A*, T_1-weighted image 10 days after onset of expressive aphasia reveals hemorrhage in the left precentral gyrus, shown as increased signal caused by the presence of methemoglobin. *B*, T_2-weighted image demonstrates an area of increased signal surrounded by hypointensity from early hemosiderin deposition. Edema is seen medially as a less well marginated area of increased signal.

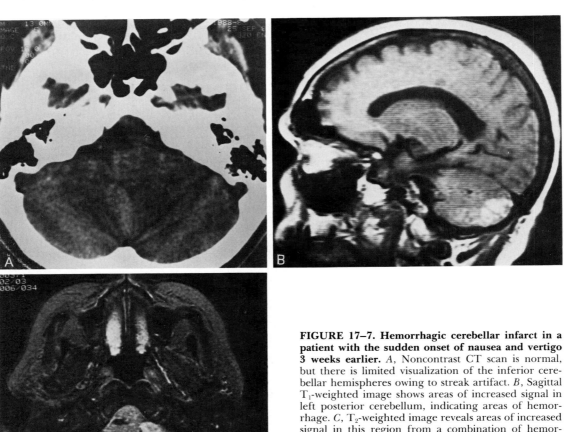

FIGURE 17–7. Hemorrhagic cerebellar infarct in a patient with the sudden onset of nausea and vertigo 3 weeks earlier. *A*, Noncontrast CT scan is normal, but there is limited visualization of the inferior cerebellar hemispheres owing to streak artifact. *B*, Sagittal T_1-weighted image shows areas of increased signal in left posterior cerebellum, indicating areas of hemorrhage. *C*, T_2-weighted image reveals areas of increased signal in this region from a combination of hemorrhage and edema. No hemosiderin deposition is present.

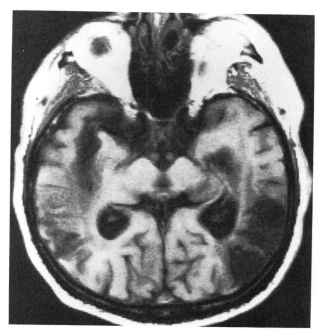

FIGURE 17–8. Chronic left temporal infarction. Left posterior temporal encephalomalacia is shown as an area of low signal with mild, asymmetric dilatation of the lateral ventricular trigone.

Old infarcts may have a more complex signal pattern. In addition to hemorrhagic components, evolution of infarcts results in areas of microcystic and macrocystic encephalomalacia and gliosis. Microcystic encephalomalacia and gliosis follow the signal intensity pattern described previously for acute infarcts. Macrocystic encephalomalacia follows the signal intensity of cerebrospinal fluid (CSF) and is discriminated best on proton density–weighted scans as areas slightly hypointense to brain (Fig. 17–8).

Several studies have shown a decided advantage of MR over CT for imaging lacunes.[15–17] In one study of 22 patients with presumed lacunar TIAs or stroke, CT revealed only 28 per cent of the lesions demonstrated by MR.[15] Lacunes are most often slitlike or ovoid lesions and are hyperintense relative to parenchyma on long TR sequences, with T_2-weighted sequences being the most sensitive. Lacunes may exhibit central cavitation and assume the signal characteristics of CSF. This is seen best on proton density–weighted images (long TR, short echo time [TE]), on which the liquid center is isointense or slightly hypointense to brain and is surrounded by a thin rim of high signal, representing edema or gliosis (Fig. 17–9).

Dilated Virchow-Robin spaces are commonly seen in the same group of patients at risk for lacunar infarctions. While these may mimic lacunes at first glance, they can often be differentiated because dilated Virchow-Robin spaces are isointense to CSF, round or linear, and usually smaller than lacunes (Fig. 17–10). These dilated perivascular spaces, which have also been termed *état criblé*, are most often seen in the anterior perforated substance, putamen, and internal capsule, (see Chapter 18).[18]

In studies of enhancement of infarcts with gadolinium–diethylene triamine pentaacetate (DTPA), also called gadopentetate dimeglumine (Magnevist, Berlex Laboratories, Wayne, NJ), nonenhanced T_2-weighted images have been as sensitive as enhanced T_1-weighted images, but nonenhanced images have not been as specific.[19, 20] Breakdown of the BBB is depicted similarly to enhanced CT but is more conspicuous on enhanced MR. At this point, the role of contrast enhancement in assessing strokes is limited in MR, as it is with CT. Nevertheless, enhanced scans assist with differential diagnosis, to distinguish infarct from a neoplastic or infectious process. Infarcts characteristically exhibit a serpiginous cortical pattern of enhancement (Fig. 17–11). In addition, the disruption of the BBB is only temporary in infarcts, occurring usually between 2 and 6 weeks. Finally, the increased conspicuity of BBB breakdown with gadolinium-enhanced MR may be of importance in the pathophysiologic investigation of cerebral infarction and may provide a means of assessing early therapy.

ARTERIAL OCCLUSION

Since the major cerebral arteries are visualized on spin-echo (SE) MR scans as areas of flow void, they should be scrutinized on the images to assess their patency. Although MR cannot identify calcified arteriosclerotic plaques as well as CT, the presence of a flow void or lack thereof gives information about flow through the vessel. If any intraluminal signal is present, a flow abnormality should be suspected, but interpretation of the aberrant flow can be difficult. High signal might indicate thrombosis with intraluminal subacute clot (methemoglobin), but it could also result from slow flow and flow enhancement. Signal isointense to brain could also result from slow flow or a complete occlusion with old fibrosed clot (Fig. 17–12). GRE images may clarify the situation because only vessels with flow will be hyperintense. The combination of GRE and SE images may help distinguish complete occlusion from a tight stenosis with slow flow. It remains to be determined how accurate GRE and other fast-scan techniques can be for detecting residual flow distal to a critical stenosis. At this point, angiography is still the definitive procedure for imaging vascular anatomy.

MR can image the extracranial vessels as well as the intracranial circulation. Of primary interest in stroke patients are the carotid, vertebral, and basilar arteries, which deliver blood to the brain parenchyma. Stenosis or occlusion of these major arteries is most often due to atherosclerosis but also result from embolus, dissection, trauma, surgery, neoplastic involvement, or arteritis.

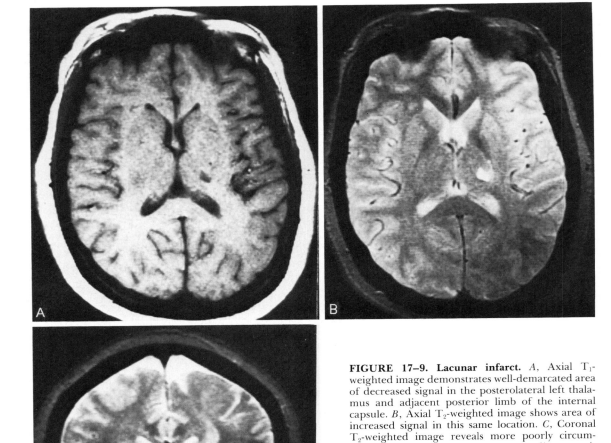

FIGURE 17–9. Lacunar infarct. *A,* Axial T_1-weighted image demonstrates well-demarcated area of decreased signal in the posterolateral left thalamus and adjacent posterior limb of the internal capsule. *B,* Axial T_2-weighted image shows area of increased signal in this same location. *C,* Coronal T_2-weighted image reveals more poorly circumscribed area of increased signal extending superiorly from the internal capsule into the corona radiata, consistent with an additional area of infarction, with resultant gliosis rather than encephalomalacia.

ARTERIAL DISSECTION

Arterial dissection often occurs spontaneously but has also been associated with fibromuscular dysplasia and trauma. Patients may present with neck pain, Horner's syndrome, and infarcts related to emboli or arterial occlusion. The internal carotid arteries are more often involved, but the vertebral arteries can also be affected. The false lumen is typically filled with clot, and the angiogram demonstrates a long segment of narrowing, usually terminating at the skull base. Complete occlusion is not uncommon.

MR has been successfully used to show areas of high signal intensity surrounding a constricted flow void on both T_1- and T_2-weighted images, best depicted in the axial plane.[21] The residual lumen is often placed eccentrically to one side of the high-signal region (Fig. 17–13). Acute dissections may be difficult to identify owing to decreased conspicuity

of hypointense acute hemorrhage on T_2-weighted images adjacent to low-signal fat and flow void. MR is a noninvasive way to follow the evolution of a dissection, such as progression from a stenosis to complete occlusion or pseudoaneurysm formation. On the other hand, an occluded vessel may recanalize and reestablish flow.

VENOUS OCCLUSION

Venous thrombosis is an uncommon but likely underdiagnosed condition, most often manifesting with headaches and papilledema. Focal deficits, seizures, and coma are evident in approximately 25 per cent of patients, usually in more advanced cases. Infectious etiologies are less common than in the preantibiotic era. In a study of 34 patients with cerebral venous thrombosis, 4 cases were related to

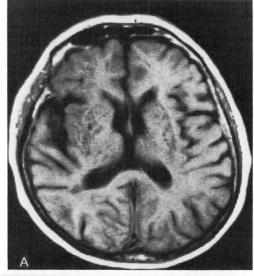

FIGURE 17–10. Dilated Virchow-Robin spaces. T_1-weighted (A) and heavily T_2-weighted (B) images best demonstrate the multiple punctate foci of signal abnormality in the putamen and external capsule bilaterally. These foci are isointense with CSF. C, A lightly T_2-weighted or spin-density image causes most of these areas to be obscured owing to the relative isointensity of CSF and brain on this sequence. A larger ovoid left external capsule lesion is hyperintense, consistent with a lacunar infarct.

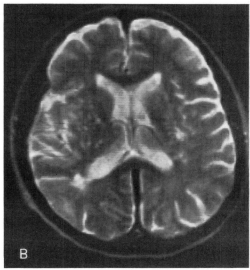

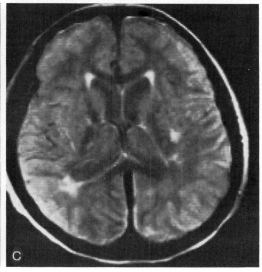

infections, 5 were due to local causes, 19 were related to "general causes" (Behçet's disease, puerperium, oral contraceptives, remote tumors), and 10 were idiopathic.[22] The most frequently occluded dural sinuses are the superior sagittal sinus and lateral (transverse) sinus, often with associated cortical vein thrombosis. This condition is considered to have a high incidence of venous infarction, hemorrhage, and death, but in this series hemorrhage was noted in only 3 of 25 cases and 4 patients died. Findings on CT (such as the "dense triangle" and "delta sign") can be suggestive, but diagnosis usually required angiography prior to the advent of MR.

There has been considerable interest in using MR to diagnose cerebral venous thrombosis noninvasively. The findings of replacing the normal flow void of the involved sinus with high signal on both the T_1- and T_2-weighted images has been noted[23, 24] (Figs. 17–14 and 17–15). The frequent appearance of flow-related enhancement has been a confounding factor.

The use of gradient recalled acquisitions may help, because the patent sinus more consistently exhibits flow-related enhancement and the clot darkens from magnetic susceptibility effects. The use of a nonselective 180-degree refocusing pulse to eliminate flow-related enhancement has recently been reported, and this may help further in this condition.[25] The MR diagnosis of cavernous sinus thrombosis has also been reported, with the findings of short T_1 and long T_2 in the cavernous sinus and superior ophthalmic vein.[26]

ARTERITIS

Vasculitis or arteritis comprises a broad group of diseases that feature inflammatory changes in blood vessels. The presenting neurologic symptoms are most often related to vascular compromise from an arteritis. Infectious arteritides are due to meningo-

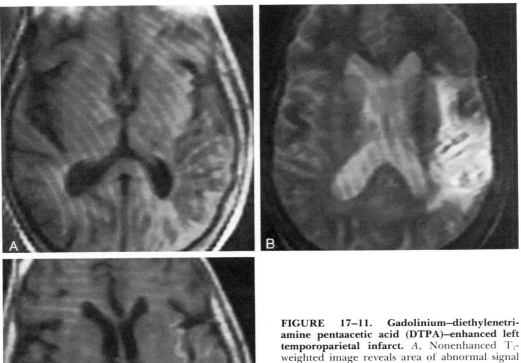

FIGURE 17–11. Gadolinium–diethylenetriamine pentaacetic acid (DTPA)–enhanced left temporoparietal infarct. *A,* Nonenhanced T₁-weighted image reveals area of abnormal signal intensity in the posterior temporal and parietal lobes on the left. *B,* T₂-weighted image shows additional involvement of the insular cortex. *C,* Gd-DTPA–enhanced T₁-weighted image demonstrates cortical ribbon of enhancement in both regions.

vascular syphilis, tuberculous meningitis, fungal meningitis, and subacute forms of bacterial meningitis, usually involving the vessels at the base of the brain. Necrotizing angiitis includes polyarteritis nodosa, giant cell arteritis, and Wegener's granulomatosis. Systemic lupus erythematosus can be classified under collagen vascular arteritis. The common noninfectious arteritides may involve the extracranial vessels, distinguishing them from the infectious group.[27] Systemic lupus erythematosus is particularly prone to affect the central nervous system and may cause seizures, cognitive impairment, alterations in the level of consciousness, and cranial nerve deficits.

MR has shown more brain parenchymal abnormalities than CT in this condition, with several different patterns of signal aberration.[28, 29] Cerebral infarctions (mostly involving white matter) and nonspecific focal lesions in the white matter and gray matter have been noted (Fig. 17–16). Miller and associates[30] proposed that vasculitis can be distinguished from multiple sclerosis by the milder periventricular changes in vasculitis and the association

of vasculitis with discrete hemispheric lesions or infarcts. Given the spectrum of signal abnormalities in multiple sclerosis, the utility of these differentiating features remains to be proved (see Chapter 18).

MIGRAINE

Migraine is a familial disorder characterized by severe, recurrent, usually unilateral, throbbing headaches. They begin in adolescence or early adult life and become less frequent during later years. Although many forms of migraine have been reported and considerable variability exists among patients, three major clinical syndromes are recognized. Classic migraine headaches are preceded by visual disturbances (aura), whereas common migraine occurs without the visual symptoms. Both forms respond to ergotamine. Complicated migraine is associated with neurologic deficits, such as confusion, drowsiness, dizziness, aphasia, and numbness and tingling or weakness in an extremity. The neurologic symptoms

FIGURE 17–12. Occluded right internal carotid artery. *A*, Coronal T₁-weighted image demonstrates replacement of the normal flow voids within the cavernous and supraclinoid portions of the right internal carotid artery with intermediate signal intensity (*arrows*). The lack of definite hyperintensity suggests a more chronic occlusion. *B*, Axial proton density–weighted image shows mild hyperintensity of cavernous carotid artery thrombus on the right (*arrow*). *C*, Axial proton density–weighted image seen more inferiorly reveals lack of a flow void within the horizontal portion of the right internal carotid artery (*arrows*).

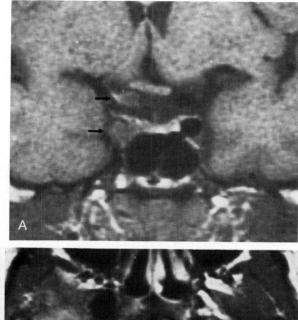

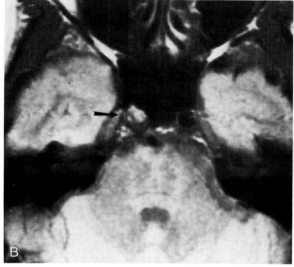

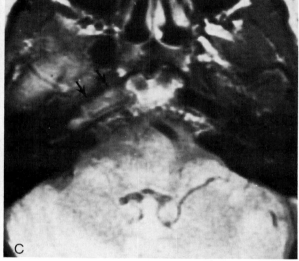

usually resolve after 5 to 15 minutes, but the headaches, nausea, and vomiting associated with all forms of migraine may last from a few hours to a few days.[31, 32]

Although the pathophysiology of migraine is not entirely understood, a vascular etiology is generally accepted. Initial vasoconstriction of the extracranial and intracranial arteries leads to cerebral ischemia, which is clinically manifested by the aura and neurologic deficits. A second phase of reactive vasodilatation and hyperemia is responsible for the subsequent throbbing headaches. One theory proposes that the vascular events are induced by release of vasoactive amines, such as norepinephrine, epinephrine, serotonin, and histamine. Inherent vascular hypersensitivity to these substances and abnormalities of the autonomic nervous system in patients with migraine may contribute to the problem.[31]

In a review by Soges and associates[32] of 24 patients with migraine, MR demonstrated parenchymal brain abnormalities in 41 per cent of patients with classic or common migraine and in 57 per cent with complicated migraine. The MR abnormalities consisted mainly of focal, discrete hyperintensities within the subcortical white matter (Fig. 17–17). Some patients in the complicated migraine group also had cortical lesions resembling infarcts that correlated with neurologic symptoms. The white matter lesions of migraine are similar to those seen in multiple sclerosis and deep white matter ischemia, and differentiation often requires correlation with the clinical picture.

VASCULAR MALFORMATIONS

Vascular malformations are developmental anomalies but are dynamic and may progress with time. Approximately 10 per cent of patients with subarachnoid hemorrhage or intracerebral hematoma have an underlying vascular malformation, most often presenting between the ages of 10 and 40 years.

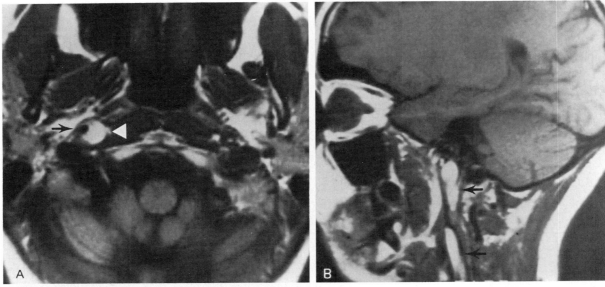

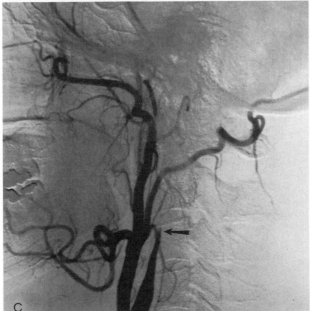

FIGURE 17–13. Internal carotid artery dissection. *A,* Axial T$_1$-weighted image shows hemorrhage of high signal intensity about the right internal carotid artery just below the skull base. The subintimal clot *(arrowhead)* is positioned eccentrically at the medial aspect of the flow void of the residual lumen *(arrow)*. *B,* Sagittal T$_1$-weighted image reveals high-signal hemorrhage *(arrows)* along the course of the internal carotid artery in the neck. *C,* Lateral view of right common carotid angiogram illustrates typical long, tapered occlusion of carotid artery dissection *(arrow)*.

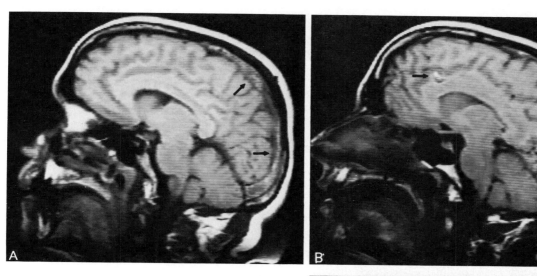

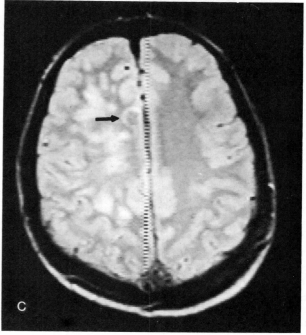

FIGURE 17–14. Superior sagittal sinus (SSS) thrombosis with hemorrhagic infarct. *A*, Sagittal T$_1$-weighted image shows mottled, slightly hyperintense signal in the posterior aspect of the SSS *(arrows)*. *B*, Parasagittal T$_1$-weighted image demonstrates small area of high-signal hemorrhage in the right cingulate gyrus *(arrow)*. *C*, Axial lightly T$_2$-weighted image reveals additional areas of high signal in the subcortical white matter and centrum semiovale consistent with ischemia and edema. The acute hemorrhage *(arrow)* is isointense on this sequence. A flow void is present in the SSS anteriorly, but mottled signal persists posteriorly. There was no filling of the posterior SSS at angiography (not illustrated).

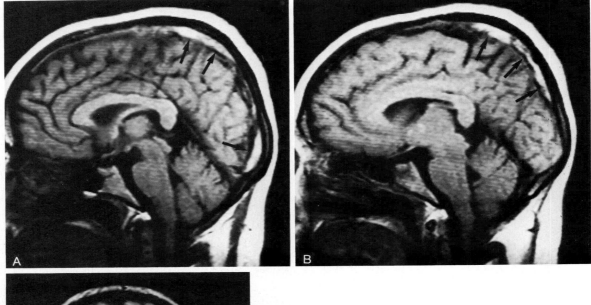

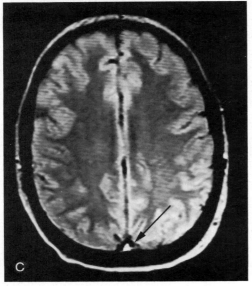

FIGURE 17–15. SSS thrombosis. *A* and *B*, Sagittal T₁-weighted images demonstrate increased signal within the SSS extending from the vertex to the torcular *(arrows)*. *C*, Axial T₂-weighted image reveals high signal intensity centrally within the posterior portion of the SSS *(arrow)*. The surrounding signal void may represent patent collateral veins about the SSS.

Patients may also present with seizures, stroke (secondary to a steal phenomenon), and headaches. Pathologically, vascular malformations are categorized as arteriovenous malformations, cavernous angiomas, capillary telangiectasias, and venous malformations. When these malformations are small or partially or completely thrombosed, the flow within them is too reduced to permit angiographic identification, and they are referred to as cryptic or occult malformations.

ARTERIOVENOUS MALFORMATION

Arteriovenous malformations (AVMs) are the most common vascular malformation. These consist of the classic tangle of dilated arteries and veins, usually with rapid arteriovenous shunting. Close to 50 per cent of patients will present with hemorrhage, and by the age of 40 years, 40 per cent of AVMs will have bled.[33] The hemorrhage is usually more benign than that due to a ruptured aneurysm. Ninety-five per cent of AVMs are in the supratentorial compartment, in either a lobar or a deep location, and 10 per cent are in the infratentorial region. One should suspect AVM as the cause of an intracerebral hemorrhage if the hemorrhage is lobar and away from the territories of the anterior communicating and middle cerebral arteries and also as the cause of deep hemorrhages in younger, normotensive patients. AVMs can thrombose either spontaneously or as a result of compression by the hematoma. Dural arterial supply is more commonly found with infratentorial AVMs, although it is important to remember that any AVMs adjacent to a dural surface can receive dural contributions.

Patients with an intracranial AVM are more likely to have a coexisting intracranial aneurysm, often on

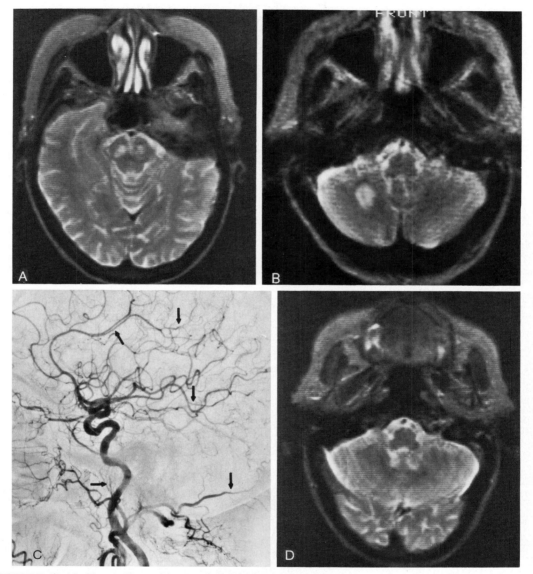

FIGURE 17–16. Giant cell arteritis. *A* and *B*, Initial axial T$_2$-weighted images demonstrate high signal areas in the cerebral peduncles bilaterally and deep right cerebellar hemisphere, suggesting multiple small infarcts. *C*, Lateral common carotid angiogram reveals multiple sites of narrowing in both internal and external carotid artery branches *(arrows)*. *D*, Axial T$_2$-weighted image 2 weeks later shows resolution of the right cerebellar lesion, consistent with reversal of ischemia.

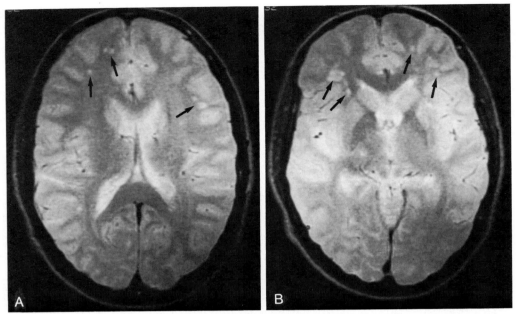

FIGURE 17–17. Migraine headaches with associated white matter lesions. *A* and *B*, Axial T_2-weighted images reveal multiple small lesions *(arrows)* in the subcortical white matter, primarily involving the frontal lobes.

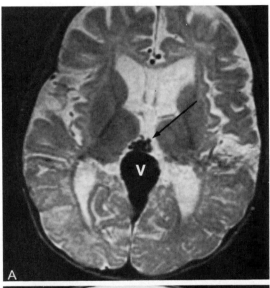

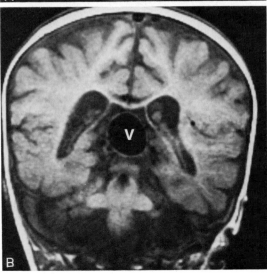

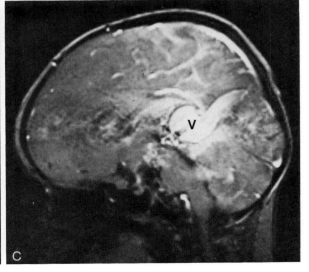

FIGURE 17–18. Vein of Galen vascular malformation in a 5-month-old male infant. *A*, Axial T_2-weighted image reveals small tangle of flow voids *(arrow)* representing feeding arterial vessels immediately anterior to the dilated vein of Galen (V). The brain is diffusely atrophic. *B*, Coronal T_1-weighted image provides a cross-sectional image of the dilated draining vein (V). *C*, GRE image produces flow-related enhancement and results in high signal intensity within the draining veins (V). Apparent drainage seen superiorly suggests straight sinus occlusion, possibly from high-flow angiopathy. Inhomogeneous signal anterior to the vein of Galen is related to artifact in the phase-encoding direction from pulsatile flow.

a feeding vessel. A vein of Galen malformation, mislabeled as aneurysm in the past, consists of a fistulous communication, most often between a dilated posterior cerebral artery and the vein of Galen or basal vein of Rosenthal (Fig. 17–18). In Wyburn-Mason syndrome, AVMs involve the midbrain and ipsilateral retina, with an ipsilateral facial nevus.

The MR appearance of AVMs consists of evidence of flow (usually voids or paradoxical enhancement) and hemorrhage (Figs. 17–19 to 17–21). Flow voids are most commonly produced by the vascular components of AVMs, also demonstrated by angiography and contrast-enhanced CT. In a comparative study of these three modalities in 15 patients,[34] MR was superior to CT and angiography for defining the exact relationship of the nidus, feeding arteries, and draining veins to the surrounding brain parenchyma. MR was also useful in evaluating the exact extent of nidus obliteration after embolization, detecting associated parenchymal abnormalities and subacute hem-

orrhage (see Fig. 16–17). Because of the difficulty in distinguishing between calcification, flow voids, and hemosiderin, MR had less sensitivity for old hemorrhage in the setting of AVMs undergoing embolization. The use of GRE imaging partially solves the problem by producing flow-related enhancement, so that remaining voids will represent hemosiderin or calcification.

Angiography is still needed for demonstrating the exact details of the distal distribution of feeding vessels and is the only technique, aside from positron-emission tomography (PET) scanning, capable of evaluating for steal phenomena. Dural AVMs may be difficult to identify with both CT (enhanced vessels obscured by high-attenuation calvarium) and MR (signal voids obscured by low-signal calvarium and dura); however, any enlarged arteries or veins traversing the subarachnoid space can be seen on T_2-weighted images. Again, GRE imaging should be of help in increasing the conspicuity of these lesions.

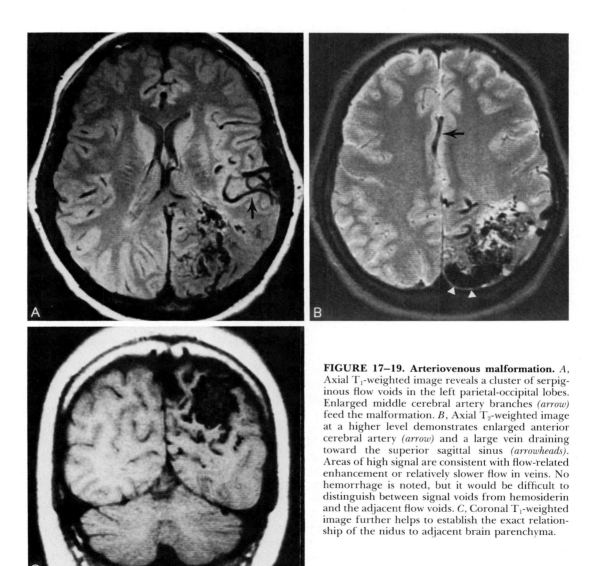

FIGURE 17–19. Arteriovenous malformation. *A*, Axial T_1-weighted image reveals a cluster of serpiginous flow voids in the left parietal-occipital lobes. Enlarged middle cerebral artery branches *(arrow)* feed the malformation. *B*, Axial T_2-weighted image at a higher level demonstrates enlarged anterior cerebral artery *(arrow)* and a large vein draining toward the superior sagittal sinus *(arrowheads)*. Areas of high signal are consistent with flow-related enhancement or relatively slower flow in veins. No hemorrhage is noted, but it would be difficult to distinguish between signal voids from hemosiderin and the adjacent flow voids. *C*, Coronal T_1-weighted image further helps to establish the exact relationship of the nidus to adjacent brain parenchyma.

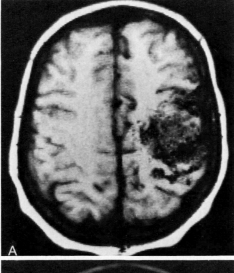

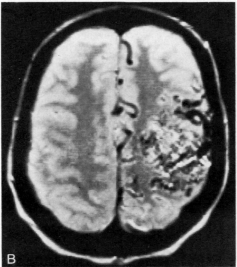

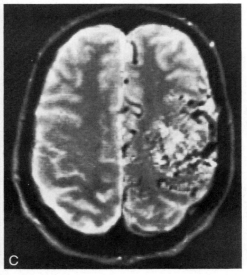

FIGURE 17–20. Frontoparietal arteriovenous malformation. *A,* T_1-weighted image shows multiple flow voids in the large arteriovenous malformation. Lightly T_2-weighted *(B)* and heavily T_2-weighted *(C)* images reveal a progressive increase in signal intensity in portions of the lesion, primarily because of slower flow within these vessels.

It is in the diagnosis of angiographically occult malformations that MR has come to be the most important imaging modality.[3, 35–38] Usually, flow effects are not seen, but the evidence of prior hemorrhage is the helpful sign (Fig. 17–22). The problem with many studies to date has been the difficulty of obtaining histologic proof, as most lesions are not surgically treated. Although lesions manifested by punctate foci of enhancement and calcification will be missed by noncontrast MR (2 of 15 lesions in one series),[36] others report that hemosiderin and ferritin deposition is more common than calcification and cite the detection of only 24 lesions by CT compared with 46 lesions by MR. A comparison of high field (1.5 T) and low field (0.12 T and 0.35 T) MR by Gomori and coworkers[37] revealed that high fields were superior for the detection of occult vascular malformations. Low field and midfield systems can partially compensate for this deficiency by utilizing GRE techniques that are more sensitive to magnetic susceptibility effects. In many cases, hemosiderin can be distinguished from calcification by comparing proton density, T_2-weighted, and GRE images, because the hemosiderin ring becomes progressively thicker and more pronounced on those images. Gd-DTPA enhancement increases the sensitivity of MR for occult malformations.

CAVERNOUS ANGIOMA

Cavernous angiomas consist of dilated vascular spaces without interspersed neural tissue and are often subcortical in location. They may be visualized on CT by means of calcification or enhancement and are usually occult on angiography. Approximately one third of cavernous angiomas manifest with seizures, and another one third manifest with hemorrhage.[39] These lesions have not been specifically investigated, but it is anticipated that the increased sensitivity of MR for detecting the cryptic AVMs would translate to improved detection of cavernous angiomas as well (Fig. 17–23).

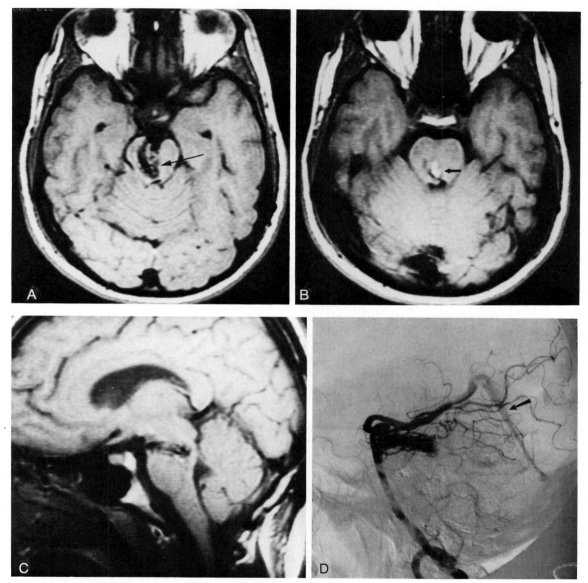

FIGURE 17–21. Midbrain arteriovenous malformation. *A,* Axial T₁-weighted image reveals serpiginous flow voids *(arrow)* in the midbrain, extending posteriorly from the flow void of the basilar artery. *B,* Axial T₁-weighted image demonstrates small area of increased signal consistent with hemorrhage *(arrow)*. Sagittal T₁-weighted image *(C)* correlates well with lateral view of vertebral angiogram *(D)*. Large vessels extend into the midbrain from the distal basilar artery and proximal posterior cerebral artery, with early filling of the straight sinus *(arrow)*.

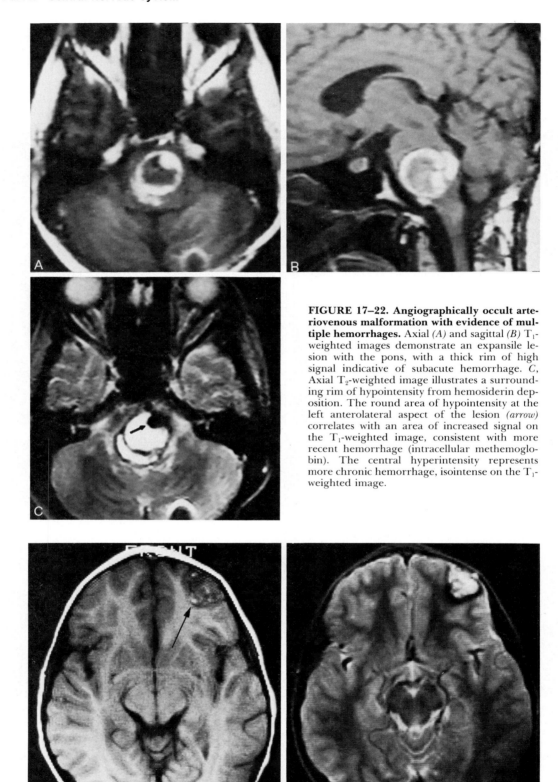

FIGURE 17–22. Angiographically occult arteriovenous malformation with evidence of multiple hemorrhages. Axial *(A)* and sagittal *(B)* T$_1$-weighted images demonstrate an expansile lesion with the pons, with a thick rim of high signal indicative of subacute hemorrhage. *C,* Axial T$_2$-weighted image illustrates a surrounding rim of hypointensity from hemosiderin deposition. The round area of hypointensity at the left anterolateral aspect of the lesion *(arrow)* correlates with an area of increased signal on the T$_1$-weighted image, consistent with more recent hemorrhage (intracellular methemoglobin). The central hyperintensity represents more chronic hemorrhage, isointense on the T$_1$-weighted image.

FIGURE 17–23. Cavernous angioma in a 12-year-old patient with a chronic seizure disorder and a calcified lesion on CT. *A,* Axial T$_1$-weighted image reveals inhomogeneous left frontal lesion *(arrow),* with a few small areas of increased signal representing hemorrhage. *B,* Axial T$_2$-weighted image demonstrates more high signal within the lesion and a thick hemosiderin rim.

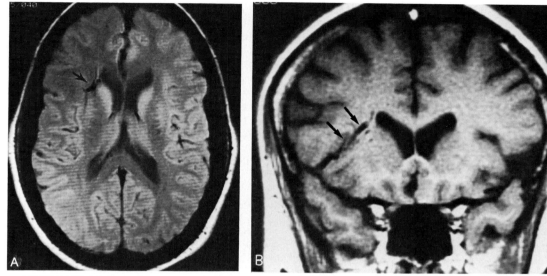

FIGURE 17–24. Frontal venous angioma. *A*, Spin-density image reveals the body of the venous angioma as a small stellate cluster of flow voids adjacent to the frontal horn of the right lateral ventricle *(arrow)*. *B*, Coronal T$_1$-weighted image demonstrates typical straight course of the draining vein *(arrows)*, perpendicular to the cortical surface.

CAPILLARY TELANGIECTASIA

Capillary telangiectasias are composed of dilated capillaries with interposed neural parenchyma. These are primarily found incidentally in the pons at autopsy and rarely become symptomatic. They are also occult radiographically.

VENOUS MALFORMATION

Venous malformations solely involve the venous system and are almost all venous angiomas. Classi-

cally, venous angiomas have a radiating or spokelike pattern of tributaries (medullary veins) draining into a single enlarged vein that courses perpendicular to the surface of the brain to enter a major vein or dural sinus. The exact origin of venous angiomas is controversial, but it is thought that they represent an abnormal prominence of collateral venous drainage in response to underdevelopment of the normal venous pathways. Rupture of venous angiomas is uncommon, but for unknown reasons, posterior fossa lesions are more prone to hemorrhage.

Venous angiomas have been imaged with MR[40, 41] by visualization of an enlarged draining vein (Figs.

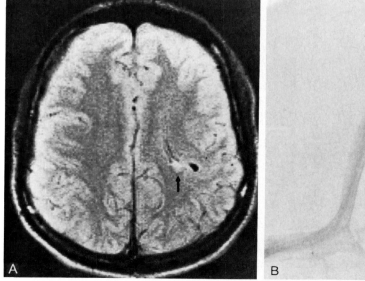
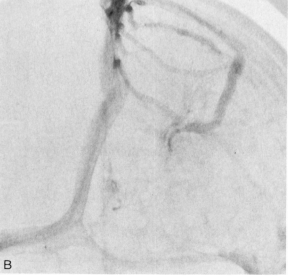

FIGURE 17–25. Parietal venous angioma. *A*, Axial T$_2$-weighted image reveals increased signal within the body of the venous angioma *(arrow)*, with a prominent draining vein seen laterally. *B*, Anteroposterior (AP) angiogram shows typical radiating pattern of tributary veins entering the draining vein.

17–24 to 17–26). Four of seven patients were also noted to have increased signal in the body of the angioma. Evidence of hemorrhage is usually lacking. It is unclear whether MR has any unique advantage in imaging these lesions, except in the posterior fossa, owing to the lack of artifact, or possibly in detecting an associated cryptic malformation.

ANEURYSMS

Ruptured aneurysms account for 72 per cent of all spontaneous subarachnoid hemorrhages. The remaining cases are secondary to bleeding AVMs (10 per cent) or are associated with primary intracerebral hemorrhage (12 per cent); in 6 per cent, no etiology is found. Types of aneurysms include congenital berry, arteriosclerotic, traumatic, mycotic, and neoplastic aneurysms. Most aneurysms manifest with sudden onset of severe headache secondary to rupture; others produce specific neurologic symptoms from mass effect, and some are found incidentally at angiography. Imaging studies are important to document the subarachnoid hemorrhage, to localize the site, to determine the type of aneurysm involved, and to evaluate the complicating factors, such as cerebral hematoma, ventricular rupture, hydrocephalus, cerebral infarction, impending uncal herniation, and rebleed.

CONGENITAL BERRY ANEURYSMS

Most intracranial aneurysms are saccular or berry aneurysms. There is controversy about their exact

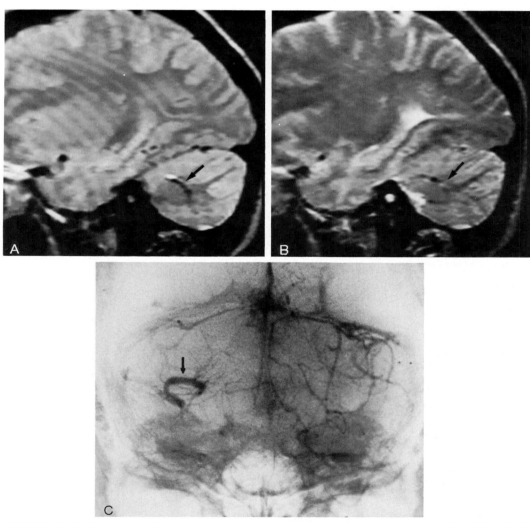

FIGURE 17–26. Right cerebellar venous angioma. *A*, Sagittal lightly T$_2$-weighted image (TR 2000, TE 60) reveals a flow void *(arrow)* in the right cerebellar hemisphere. *B*, Sagittal heavily T$_2$-weighted image (TR 2000, TE 120), the second echo of a symmetric sequence, reveals an area of even-echo rephasing in the draining vein *(arrow)*. *C*, AP vertebral angiogram shows vein draining laterally into the transverse sinus *(arrow)*.

etiology, but they probably result from developmental or acquired defects in the media and elastica. With time, an outpouching develops and grows into an aneurysm. The process is particularly apt to occur at sites of vessel branching. The internal carotid system is involved in 85 to 90 per cent of aneurysms, most often at the sites of the anterior communicating, posterior communicating, and middle cerebral arteries. Other less common sites include the cavernous portion of the internal carotid artery, the bifurcation of the basilar artery, and the origins of the three cerebellar arteries from the vertebrobasilar system.

Aneurysms may be multiple in 15 to 20 per cent of cases. Berry aneurysms frequently measure 1 cm or less in size, but they can attain larger sizes.[42]

Data about the risk of aneurysm rupture are difficult to obtain because many aneurysms remain asymptomatic and undetected throughout life. Autopsy studies have shown the incidence of congenital aneurysms in the general population to be between 1 and 2 per cent, but most of these are tiny outpouchings at bifurcations that are of no consequence clinically. Perhaps most relevant is the fact that if a patient has an unruptured aneurysm noted by CT

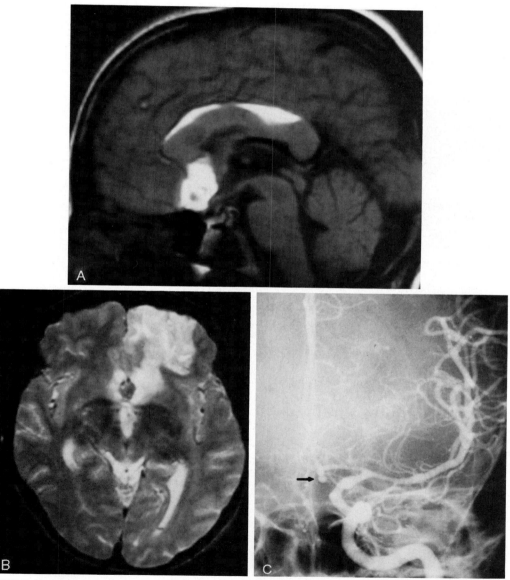

FIGURE 17–27. Anterior communicating artery aneurysm and subarachnoid hemorrhage. *A*, Sagittal T_1-weighted image demonstrates extensive high-signal subarachnoid blood in the suprasellar and pericallosal cisterns. *B*, Axial T_2-weighted image reveals high signal in the left frontal lobe consistent with ischemia from vessel spasm. *C*, AP left internal carotid angiogram shows the anterior communicating artery aneurysm *(arrow)* and areas of spasm in the anterior and middle cerebral arteries proximally. (Courtesy of Anthony Stauffer, Mission Community Hospital, Mission Viejo, CA.)

or angiography, the risk of bleeding is about 1 to 2 per cent per year. Saccular aneurysms are usually asymptomatic prior to rupture, at which time they produce subarachnoid hemorrhage and manifest with headache and variable alterations in the level of consciousness. Rarely, an aneurysm, usually arising from the cavernous portion of the internal carotid artery, can bleed into the subdural space, resulting in a subdural hematoma. The prognosis of patients with ruptured aneurysms is tempered by delayed complications (discussed further on) and by their propensity to rebleed, most frequently in the first 8 weeks but continuing to occur at the rate of 3 to 4 per cent per year for the first 10 years.[42]

Aneurysms generally produce a flow void on MR, but it is quite difficult on routine studies to distinguish the smaller ones from normal vessels (Figs. 17–27 to 17–29). Bondi and colleagues[43] studied 17 patients with 19 aneurysms using MR. Although all

aneurysms were identified, they noted that the findings were ambiguous in three of the smaller ones. Most of the aneurysms in this series were intermediate to giant in size. MR angiography, using three-dimensional (3D) acquisition techniques for thin sections and high resolution, combined with short TE GRE imaging for flow-related enhancement, is a promising technique that may make identification of these lesions more reliable. MR has been useful in at least one case of multiple aneurysms by revealing focal subacute hemorrhage about the bleeding aneurysm.[44]

SUBARACHNOID HEMORRHAGE

The ability of MR to detect subarachnoid hemorrhage has been very limited, with the exception of focal clots in the subarachnoid space[45, 46] (Figs. 17–

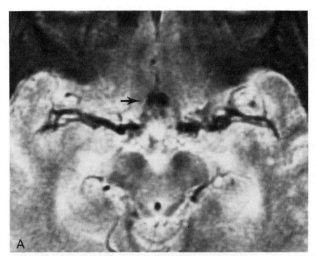

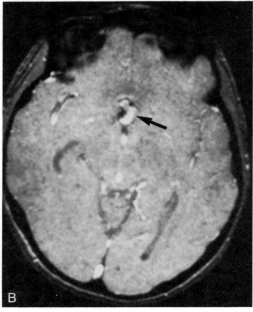

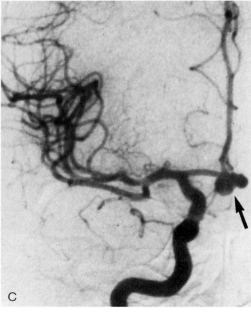

FIGURE 17–28. Anterior communicating artery aneurysm. A, Axial T$_2$-weighted image reveals lobular flow void *(arrow)* in the region of the anterior communicating artery. B, Axial GRE image (GRASS, flip angle 10, TR 150, TE 15) demonstrates flow-related enhancement within the aneurysm *(arrow)*. C, AP internal carotid angiogram illustrates lobulated anterior communicating artery aneurysm *(arrow)*.

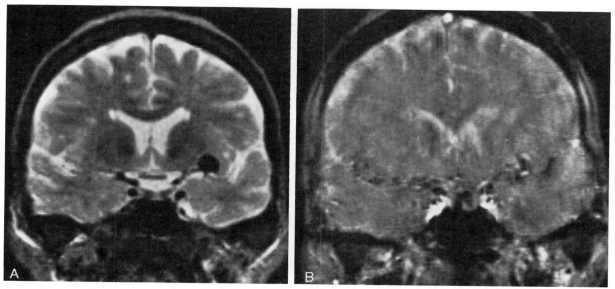

FIGURE 17–29. Large left middle cerebral artery aneurysm discovered incidentally on MR examination done for a parietal tumor. *A,* Coronal T$_2$-weighted image demonstrates a round flow void extending superiorly from the left middle cerebral artery bifurcation. *B,* GRE image (FISP, flip angle 20, TR 20, TE 10) reveals incomplete filling of the aneurysm by intermediate to high signal intensity, precluding the possibility that the signal void represented calcification.

27, 17–30, and 17–31; also see Fig. 16–8). Unless some novel pulse sequences are designed to improve detection of subarachnoid blood, CT will remain the front-line imaging technique in patients with suspected aneurysm rupture. Nevertheless, if subarachnoid clots are detected by MR, the distribution of the blood within the cisterns may suggest the location of the aneurysm. An anterior communicating aneurysm is suggested by blood in the cisterna lamina terminalis, anterior pericallosal cistern, and interhemi-

spheric fissure. There may be extension of blood into the septum pellucidum and lateral ventricle, as well as hematoma in the inferomedial frontal lobe. Localizing posterior communicating artery aneurysms is more difficult because the blood is usually diffuse within the cisterns. Intracerebral hematoma or ventricular rupture is unusual with posterior communicating aneurysms. Rupture of a middle cerebral aneurysm is characterized by blood in the sylvian fissure and a hematoma in the temporal lobe that

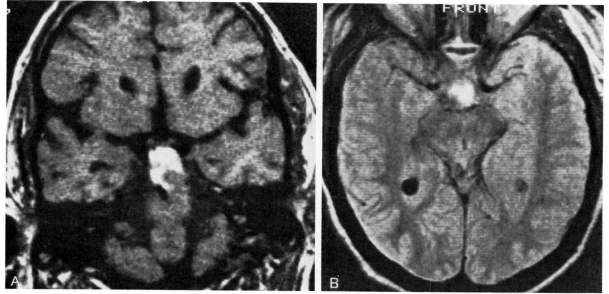

FIGURE 17–30. Subarachnoid hemorrhage. Coronal T$_1$-weighted *(A)* and axial T$_2$-weighted *(B)* images demonstrate a clot of high signal intensity in the prepontine cistern. (Signal void in the deep right parietal region represents the calcified glomus of the choroid plexus.)

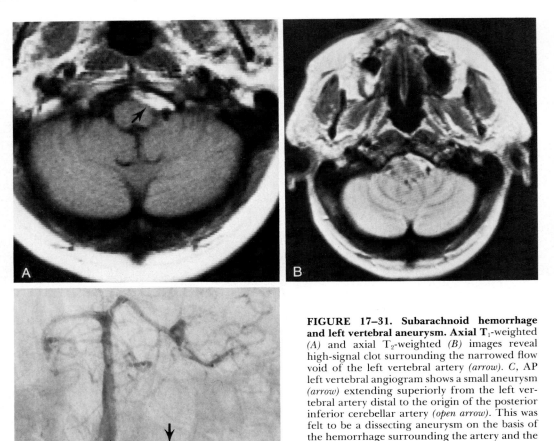

FIGURE 17–31. Subarachnoid hemorrhage and left vertebral aneurysm. Axial T_1-weighted (A) and axial T_2-weighted (B) images reveal high-signal clot surrounding the narrowed flow void of the left vertebral artery (arrow). C, AP left vertebral angiogram shows a small aneurysm (arrow) extending superiorly from the left vertebral artery distal to the origin of the posterior inferior cerebellar artery (open arrow). This was felt to be a dissecting aneurysm on the basis of the hemorrhage surrounding the artery and the unusual location of the aneurysm, but an aneurysm without evidence of dissection was found at surgery.

may also extend into the adjacent temporal horn. Posterior fossa aneurysms often do not have good localizing findings.

With regard to cerebral hematomas associated with aneurysms, anterior communicating artery aneurysms rupture into the inferomedial frontal lobe, middle cerebral aneurysms into the temporal lobe, and pericallosal aneurysms into the corpus callosum. Intracerebral hemorrhage is uncommon with the other aneurysms.

A fascinating picture of chronic subarachnoid hemorrhage is imaged only by MR. As a result of multiple small bleeds, some of which may even be subclinical, hemosiderin and ferritin are deposited within the meninges. The magnetic susceptibility effect of the hemosiderin produces low signal intensity that lines the cisternal spaces on T_2-weighted images (Fig. 17–32). The effect is more pronounced with GRE acquisitions. Zimmerman and associates[47] reported seven adult patients with bilateral progressive hearing loss. All other imaging studies were normal. T_2-weighted MR scans disclosed extensive hypointense "pial siderosis" outlining the posterior fossa subarachnoid space. They postulated meningeal-based cryptic AVMs as the likely source of the hemorrhages.

COMPLICATIONS OF HEMORRHAGE

The initial subarachnoid hemorrhage from aneurysm rupture often has devastating clinical consequences. Any associated intracerebral hematoma destroys brain parenchyma. Another major cause of morbidity and mortality is the cerebral vasospasm and infarction that occur later. The vasospasm develops after 72 hours and is maximal between 7 and 17 days. If the vasospasm is severe, cerebral ischemia and infarction may ensue.[42]

Hydrocephalus can be acute or delayed and may require shunting. The acute form is usually associated with ventricular hemorrhage and obstruction at the outlet foramina.

Transtentorial herniation can occur from the mass

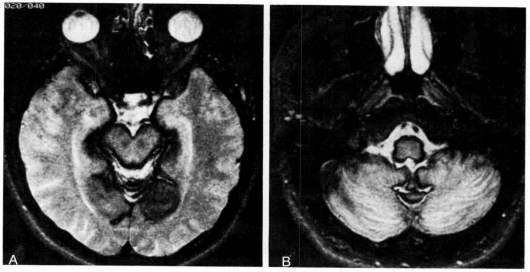

FIGURE 17–32. Pial siderosis. *A* and *B*, Axial T$_2$-weighted images demonstrate extensive hypointensity along the pial surfaces in the posterior fossa caused by hemosiderin deposition, presumably from multiple episodes of subarachnoid hemorrhage. (Courtesy of Peter McCreight, Scripps Memorial Hospital, La Jolla, CA.)

effect associated with cerebral hematoma, hydrocephalus, or infarction and brain edema. Herniation is suggested on MR by compression of the basal cisterns, displacement of the temporal lobe medially into the suprasellar cisterns, and shift of the midbrain to the opposite side. Coronal scans are best for demonstrating the inferior displacement of the uncus through the tentorial notch.

GIANT ANEURYSMS

Giant aneurysms, defined as those larger than 2.5 cm in diameter, have been studied more frequently with MR.[43, 48–50] Most giant aneurysms are located on the internal carotid artery but may also be seen on the basilar, anterior cerebral, and middle cerebral arteries. Giant aneurysms may be atherosclerotic in origin, and a few are mycotic, classically related to subacute bacterial endocarditis. Giant aneurysms slowly expand by accretion of clot within their lumen or organization of surface bleeding from small leaks. Spontaneous rupture is uncommon, and the aneurysms more often manifest with neurologic findings related to the compression of cranial nerves within the cavernous sinus or basal cisterns. Less frequently, they may produce emboli related to the clot and turbulent flow within the aneurysm lumen.

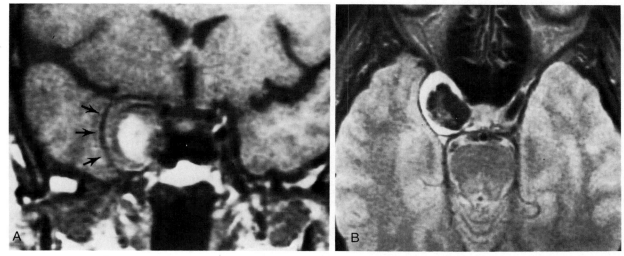

FIGURE 17–33. Giant internal carotid artery aneurysm. *A*, Coronal T$_1$-weighted image shows central hyperintensity and peripheral intermediate signal within a giant aneurysm of the cavernous portion of the right internal carotid artery *(arrows)*. *B*, Axial T$_2$-weighted image demonstrates reversal of the relative signal intensities. The findings are consistent with older thrombus peripherally and more acute thrombus centrally, or, less likely, flow-related enhancement in the residual lumen seen on the shorter TR T$_1$-weighted sequence.

The appearance on MR is usually distinctive, with the finding of a flow void surrounded by thrombus. The clot may be laminated, with layering of signal intensities representing different stages of clot evolution[48] (Figs. 17–33 and 17–34). Flow patterns are complex, and at times it is difficult to define the cause of intraluminal signal.[43] Intraluminal signal emanating from nonthrombosed stationary blood was reported by Olsen and associates[51] to be of intermediate signal intensity on T_1-weighted images and hyperintense on T_2-weighted images. Tsuruda and coworkers[49] reported the benefit of cine-MR using low flip angle GRE imaging for evaluation of large (1.0 to 2.5 cm) and giant aneurysms. This technique produces fairly consistent flow-related enhancement within the lumen, as opposed to routine SE imaging, which often displays mixed signal from flow void,

flow-related enhancement, and even-echo rephasing. Cine-MR can image pulsatile mass effects dynamically and may improve visualization of the aneurysm neck. MR has also been used to follow aneurysms after occlusion with detachable balloons.[48, 50] The progression of thrombus can be clearly imaged and may obviate follow-up angiography.

OTHER ANEURYSMS

Arteriosclerotic aneurysms usually have a fusiform shape and do not have a defined neck. They occur in an older age group and are associated with hypertension, arteriosclerotic disease, and generalized ectasia of the major intracranial arteries. The intracranial carotid and basilar arteries are the common sites

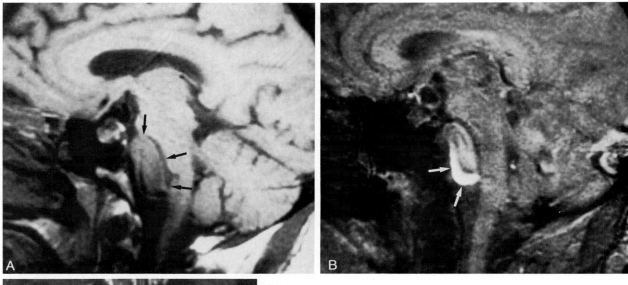

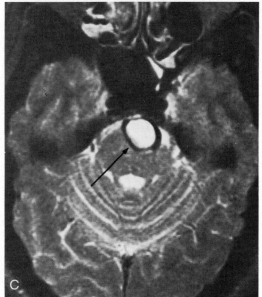

FIGURE 17–34. Fusiform giant basilar artery aneurysm. *A,* Sagittal T_1-weighted image demonstrates a mass *(arrows)* ventral to the brain stem that indents the pons. The mass is slightly hypointense compared with brain. The linear low signal intensity seen anteriorly within the mass suggests a patent lumen. *B,* On a GRE image (GE 33/13, flip angle 30 degrees), the high signal *(arrows)* observed anteriorly confirms a patent lumen within the aneurysm. *C,* Axial heavily T_2-weighted image reveals peripheral hypointensity from hemosiderin deposition *(arrow).* The central hyperintensity represents old thrombus.

of aneurysm formation. By the time of presentation, many arteriosclerotic aneurysms have enlarged to the point of entering the category of giant aneurysms. Symptoms are most often related to mass effect or to ischemia from occlusion of small penetrating arteries that supply the brain stem, internal capsule, or basal ganglia. Since the parent artery is incorporated into the aneurysm, surgical treatment is complex and hazardous.[42]

Traumatic, mycotic, and neoplastic aneurysms are relatively rare and occur in smaller distal arteries, away from the circle of Willis. These aneurysms are also small and below the resolution of MR, but MR can detect the associated parenchymal abnormalities, such as brain contusion, abscess, or tumor. Penetrating trauma, such as a gunshot injury, is usually necessary to result in a traumatic aneurysm. As mentioned previously, mycotic aneurysms usually occur in the setting of subacute bacterial endocarditis.[42]

POSTSURGICAL ASSESSMENT

Several studies have described the use of MR in patients with intracranial aneurysm clips.[52–54] Obviously, precise knowledge of the type and composition of the aneurysm clip used is required to ensure that it is nonferromagnetic or so weakly ferromagnetic that no appreciable torque will be applied. The clips caused metallic artifact, but this was less of a hindrance than with CT, and satisfactory examination of the brain was accomplished with MR in most cases. In giant aneurysms, evaluation of residual flow was possible, but in smaller aneurysms, artifact obscured the region of the aneurysm itself. MR demonstrated lesions related to the surgery better than CT; many of these lesions were small brain stem infarcts.[54]

FUTURE OF VASCULAR IMAGING

Perhaps in vascular disease more than in any other category of central nervous system disease, there is enormous potential for further advances in MR technology. Progress continues to be made with vascular imaging (see Chapter 4). With the use of GRE techniques, cine-MR, thick-slice, and projectional methods, the images of carotid bifurcations are approaching clinical usefulness (Fig. 17–35).[55, 56] Further studies are necessary to determine the accuracy of these methods compared with ultrasound and arteriography. There is hope that refinements of flow imaging will permit screening of the circle of Willis and other major intracranial vessels. Potential also exists for measuring cerebral blood flow and perfusion using ultrafast imaging systems in conjunction with gadolinium or some other paramagnetic agent.

Considerable experimental work has been done investigating cerebral metabolism with MR spectros-

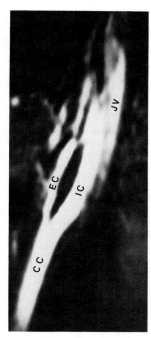

FIGURE 17–35. Cine-MR of carotid bifurcation. CC = common carotid artery; IC = internal carotid artery; EC = external carotid artery; JV = internal jugular vein.

copy. Measurements of phosphorus-31 metabolites can give information about the viability of ischemic brain tissue and the chance for recovery after reperfusion. Such methods can also be used to assess the effects of various therapies on cerebral ischemic disease (see Chapter 9). Studies are being designed to bring these spectroscopic techniques into the clinical arena to assist in the diagnosis and therapy of stroke and cerebrovascular disease.

REFERENCES

1. Bradley WG, Waluch V: Blood flow—magnetic resonance imaging. Radiology 154:443–450, 1985.
2. Mills CM, Brant-Zawadzki M, Crooks LE, et al: Nuclear magnetic resonance: Principles of blood flow imaging. AJNR 4:1161–1166, 1983.
3. Kucharczyk W, Lemme-Pleghos L, Uske A, et al: Intracranial vascular malformations: MR and CT findings. Radiology 156:383–389, 1985.
4. Kucharczyk W, Kelly WM, Davis DO, et al: Intracranial lesions: Flow-related enhancement on MR images using time-of-flight effects. Radiology 161:767–772, 1986.
5. Fisher CM: Lacunar strokes and infarcts: A review. Neurology 32:871–876, 1982.
6. Brant-Zawadzki M, Pereira B, Weinstein P, et al: MR imaging of acute experimental ischemia in cats. AJNR 7:7–11, 1986.
7. Unger EC, Gado MH, Fulling KF, Littlefield JL: Acute cerebral infarction in monkeys: An experimental study using MR imaging. Radiology 162:789–795, 1987.
8. Unger E, Littlefield L, Gado M: Water content and water structure in CT and MR signal changes: Possible influence in detection of early stroke. AJNR 9:687–691, 1988.
9. Hecht-Leavitt C, Gomori JM, Grossman RI, et al: High-field MRI of hemorrhagic cortical infarction. AJNR 7:581–585, 1986.

10. Brant-Zawadzki M, Weinstein P, Bartkowski H, Moseley M: MR imaging and spectroscopy in clinical and experimental cerebral ischemia: A review. AJNR 8:39–48, 1987.

11. Salgado M, Weinstein M, Furlan AJ, et al: Proton magnetic resonance imaging in ischemic cerebral vascular disease. Ann Neurol 20:502–507, 1986.

12. Fox AJ, Bogousslavsky J, Carey L, et al: Magnetic resonance imaging of small medullary infarctions. AJNR 7:229–233, 1986.

13. Biller J, Adams HP Jr, Dunn V, et al: Dichotomy between clinical findings and MR abnormalities in pontine infarction. J Comput Assist Tomogr 10:379–385, 1986.

14. Hesselink JR, Healy ME, Dunn WM, et al: Magnetic resonance imaging of hemorrhagic cerebral infarction. Acta Radiol [Suppl] 369:46–48, 1986.

15. Brown JJ, Hesselink JR, Rothruck JF: MR and CT of lacunar infarcts. AJNR 9:477–482, 1988.

16. Dewitt LD: Clinical use of magnetic resonance imaging in stroke. Stroke 17:328–331, 1985.

17. Biller J, Graff-Radford NR, Smoker WRK, et al: MR imaging in lacunar hemiballismus. J Comput Assist Tomogr 10:793–797, 1986.

18. Braffman BH, Zimmerman RA, Tojanowski JQ, et al: Pathologic correlation with gross and histopathology. 1.Lacunar infarction and Virchow-Robin spaces. AJNR 9:621–628, 1988.

19. NcNamara MT, Brant-Zawadzki M, Berry I, et al: Acute cerebral ischemia: MR enhancement using Gd-DTPA. Radiology 158:701–705, 1986.

20. Virapongse C, Mancuso A, Quisling R: Human brain infarcts: Gd-DTPA–enhanced MR imaging. Radiology 161:785–794, 1986.

21. Goldberg HI, Grossman RI, Gomori JM, et al: Cervical internal carotid artery dissecting hemorrhage: Diagnosis using MR. Radiology 158:157–161, 1986.

22. Bousser M-G, Chiras J, Bories J, Castaigne P: Cerebral venous thrombosis—a review of 38 cases. Stroke 16:191–213, 1985.

23. Macchi PJ, Grossman RI, Goldberg HI, et al: High field MR imaging of cerebral venous thrombosis. J Comput Assist Tomogr 10:10–15, 1986.

24. McMurdo SK, Brant-Zawadzki M, Bradley WG, et al: Dural venous thrombosis: Study using intermediate field strength MR imaging. Radiology 161:83–86, 1986.

25. Sze G, Simmons B, Krol G, et al: Dural sinus thrombosis: Verification with spin-echo techniques. AJNR 9:679–686, 1988.

26. Savino PJ, Grossman RI, Schatz DJ, et al: High-field magnetic resonance imaging in the diagnosis of cavernous sinus thrombosis. Arch Neurol 43:1081–1082, 1986.

27. Ferris EJ, Levine HL: Cerebral arteritis: Classification. Radiology 109:327–341, 1973.

28. Vermess M, Bernstein SM, Bydder GM, et al: Nuclear magnetic resonance (NMR) imaging of the brain in systemic lupus erythematosus. J Comput Assist Tomogr 7:461–467, 1983.

29. Aisen AM, Gabrielsen TO, McCune WJ: MR imaging of systemic lupus erythematosus involving the brain. AJNR 6:197–201, 1985.

30. Miller DH, Ormerod IEC, Gibson A, et al: MR brain scanning in patients with vasculitis: Differentiation from multiple sclerosis. Neuroradiology 29:226–231, 1987.

31. Adams RD, Victor M: Principles of Neurology. 2nd ed. New York, McGraw-Hill Book Company, 1981, pp 121–126.

32. Soges LJ, Cacayorin ED, Petro GR, Ramachandran TS: Migraine: Evaluation by MR. AJNR 9:425–429, 1988.

33. Wilkins RH: Natural history of intracranial vascular malformations: A review. Neurosurgery 16:421–430, 1985.

34. Smith HJ, Strother CM, Kikuchi Y, et al: MR imaging of supratentorial intracranial AVMs. AJNR 9:225–235, 1988.

35. New PFJ, Ojemann RG, Davis KR, et al: MR and CT of occult vascular malformations of the brain. AJNR 7:771–779, 1986.

36. Lemme-Pleghos L, Kucharczyk W, Brant-Zawadzki M, et al: MR imaging of angiographically occult vascular malformations. AJNR 7:217–222, 1986.

37. Gomori JM, Grossman RI, Goldberg HI, et al: Occult cerebral vascular malformations: High-field MR imaging. Radiology 158:707–713, 1986.

38. Griffin C, DeLaPaz R, Enzmann D: Magnetic resonance appearance of slow flow vascular malformations of the brainstem. Neuroradiology 29:506–511, 1987.

39. Simard JM, Garcia-Bengochea F, Ballinger WE, et al: Cavernous angioma: A review of 126 collected and 12 new clinical cases. Neurosurgery 18:162–172, 1986.

40. Augustyn GT, Scott JA, Olson E, et al: Cerebral venous angiomas: MR imaging. Radiology 156:391–395, 1985.

41. Cammarata C, Han JS, Haaga JR, et al: Cerebral venous angiomas imaged by MR. Radiology 155:639–643, 1985.

42. Fox JL: Intracranial aneurysms. Vol I. New York, Springer-Verlag, 1983, pp 1–603.

43. Bondi A, Scialfi G, Scotti G: Intracranial aneurysms: MR imaging. Neuroradiology 30:214–218, 1988.

44. Hackney DB, Lesnick JE, Zimmerman RA, et al: MR Identification of bleeding site in subarachnoid hemorrhage with multiple intracranial aneurysms. J Comput Assist Tomogr 10:878–880, 1986.

45. Bradley WG, Schmidt PG: Effect of methemoglobin formation on the MR appearance of subarachnoid hemorrhage. Radiology 156:99–103, 1985.

46. Chakeres DW, Bryan RN: Acute subarachnoid hemorrhage: In vitro comparison of magnetic resonance and computed tomography. AJNR 7:223–228, 1986.

47. Zimmerman RA, Hesselink JR, Bilaniuk LT, et al: Bilateral pial siderosis and hearing loss: Syndrome with negative CT and positive high-field MR imaging findings. Presented at the 74th Scientific Assembly and Annual Meeting, Radiological Society of North America, Chicago, November 27–December 2, 1988.

48. Atlas SW, Grossman RI, Goldberg HI, et al: Partially thrombosed giant intracranial aneurysms: Correlation of MR and pathologic findings. Radiology 162:111–114, 1987.

49. Tsuruda JS, Halbach W, Higashida RT, et al: MR evaluation of large intracranial aneurysms using cine low flip angle gradient-refocused MR imaging. AJNR 9:415–424, 1988.

50. Kwan ES, Wolpert SM, Scott RM, Runge V: MR evaluation of neurovascular lesions after endovascular occlusion with detachable balloons. AJNR 9:523–532, 1988.

51. Olsen WL, Kucharczyk W, Keyes WD, et al: Magnetic resonance characterization of non-flowing intravascular blood. Acta Radiol [Suppl] 369:63–66, 1986.

52. Becker RL, Norfray JF, Teitelbaum GP, et al: MR imaging in patients with intracranial aneurysm clips. AJNR 9:885–889, 1988.

53. Holtas S, Olsson M, Romner B, et al: Comparison of MR imaging and CT in patients with intracranial aneurysm clips. AJNR 9:891–897, 1988.

54. Brothers MF, Fox AJ, Lee DH, et al: MR of postoperative cerebral aneurysm. Presented at the 26th Annual Meeting, American Society of Neuroradiology, Chicago, May 15–20, 1988.

55. Wagle WA, Cousins JP, Dumoulin CL, Souza SP: Magnetic resonance angiography of the cervical and intracranial vasculature. Presented at the eighth annual meeting and exhibition of the Society of Magnetic Resonance in Medicine, Amsterdam, The Netherlands, August 12–18, 1989.

56. Nitz WR, Mawad ME, Wendt RE: Magnetic resonance angiography of the cerebral circulation. Presented at the eighth annual meeting and exhibition of the Society of Magnetic Resonance in Medicine, Amsterdam, The Netherlands, August 12–18, 1989.

18

BRAIN: Periventricular White Matter Abnormalities

JOHN R. HESSELINK and RICHARD J. HICKS

VIRCHOW-ROBIN SPACES
AGING AND WHITE MATTER ISCHEMIA
MULTIPLE SCLEROSIS
LEUKOENCEPHALOPATHY, LEUKODYSTROPHY, AND

LEUKOENCEPHALITIS
RADIATION INJURY
HYDROCEPHALUS AND CEREBROSPINAL FLUID FLOW
DIFFERENTIAL DIAGNOSIS

As a result of the high sensitivity of T_2-weighted spin-echo (SE) pulse sequences, MR images frequently reveal high-signal foci within the periventricular white matter. Estimates of the incidence of these hyperintensities in the brains of healthy, elderly persons have ranged from 10 per cent[1] to 30 per cent.[2] Gerard and Weisberg[1] found periventricular lesions in only 10 per cent of patients older than 60 years unless cerebrovascular symptoms or risk factors were present; if both were present, the incidence increased to 84 per cent.

The presence of these hyperintensities limits the sensitivity of MR for white matter disease. They are often normal variants or related to deep white matter ischemia, but they can be mistaken for, or can obscure, more serious pathology. Differential diagnosis includes Virchow-Robin perivascular spaces, *état criblé*, subcortical arteriosclerotic encephalopathy, infarction, multiple sclerosis, vasculitis, other white matter diseases, and transependymal cerebrospinal fluid (CSF) flow. Distinguishing among these etiologies is important for appropriate therapeutic planning. Their MR appearances are very similar. The

diagnostic groups are reviewed in the following sections, followed by a discussion of differential features.

VIRCHOW-ROBIN SPACES

When nutrient vessels penetrate the brain substance, the pia mater is carried along with the vessel for a variable distance. The small subarachnoid space that follows the pia is called the Virchow-Robin space. These perivascular CSF spaces appear as punctate areas of high signal on T_2-weighted images. They are commonly seen within the superficial white matter on higher axial sections through the cerebral hemispheres, where nutrient arteries for the deep white matter enter the brain (Fig. 18–1). The bright spots are usually no more than 1 or 2 mm. Another common location is in the lower basal ganglia at the level of the anterior commissure, where the lenticulostriate arteries enter the anterior perforated substance (Fig. 18–2). They are often clustered around the lateral aspects of the anterior commissure. If

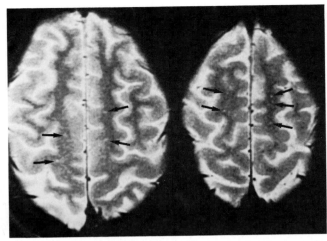

FIGURE 18–1. Normal Virchow-Robin spaces. Axial scans (spin echo [SE] 3000/80) through the vertex show multiple punctate hyperintense foci *(arrows)* within the white matter, representing normal perivascular CSF spaces.

small high-signal foci are observed in these areas, they should be dismissed as normal structures, unless corroborative evidence of disease is found on other brain sections.

AGING AND WHITE MATTER ISCHEMIA

As the brain ages, structural, chemical, and metabolic changes occur that are reflected on the MR images. Most important for MR interpretation are the changes related to deep white matter ischemia. The deep white matter of the cerebral hemispheres receives its blood supply from long, small-caliber arteries and arterioles that penetrate the cerebral cortex and traverse the superficial white matter fiber tracts. The white matter does not have as generous a blood supply as the gray matter and is more susceptible to ischemia. As the nutrient arteries become narrowed by arteriosclerosis and lipohyaline deposits within the vessel walls, the white matter becomes ischemic on a chronic basis.

Pathologically, one of the first changes in the aging brain is an increase in the perivascular fluid spaces, predominantly at the arteriolar level of the vascular tree. As the brain loses volume, it retracts away from the vessels and extracellular fluid fills the space. On postmortem studies, these perivascular fluid spaces appear like a network of tunnels within the brain substance. These changes have been termed *état criblé* (sievelike) by Durand-Fardel.[3] Similarly, shrinkage of the brain substance results in dilatation of the Virchow-Robin spaces. Differentiation between these

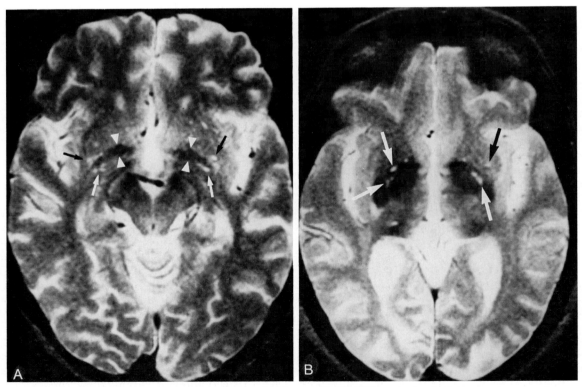

FIGURE 18–2. Normal Virchow-Robin spaces. *A,* Axial scan (SE 3000/80) at the level of the anterior commissure *(arrowheads)* reveals small high-signal foci *(arrows)* clustered about the lateral aspects of the commissure. *B,* On a slightly higher section (SE 3000/80), additional hyperintensities *(arrows)* are seen, all representing Virchow-Robin spaces surrounding penetrating lenticulostriate arteries.

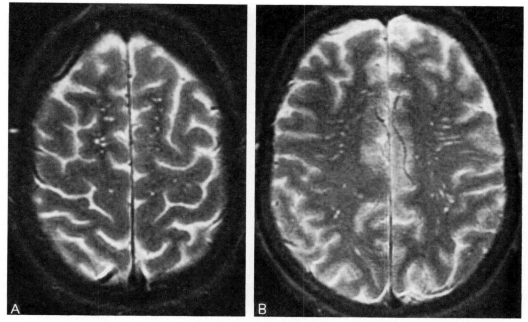

FIGURE 18–3. Abnormally dilated perivascular spaces. *A,* An axial scan (SE 3000/80) through the vertex shows many round hyperintensities within the white matter that are more prominent than normally seen. *B,* On a lower section, the hyperintensities have a more linear character, as if following the course of vessels.

two entities would depend on whether or not the perivascular fluid is enclosed by pial membrane. On T_2-weighted images, the dilated perivascular spaces appear as punctate hyperintense foci if cut in cross-section or may have a linear, vessel-like configuration if sectioned longitudinally (Fig. 18–3). On proton density–weighted and T_1-weighted scans, the fluid spaces should follow the signal characteristics of CSF or water.

With continued progressive ischemia, additional histologic changes are observed, including atrophy of axons and myelin and tortuous, sclerotic, and thickened vessels.[2] Maintenance of the myelin becomes deficient, resulting in "myelin pallor" on microscopic sections. Mild gliosis and increased interstitial fluid accompany the changes in the myelin.[4] This process has been called atrophic perivascular demyelination,[2] perivascular atrophy,[5] leuko-araiosis,[6] incomplete infarction,[7] deep white matter infarction,[8] microangiopathic leukoencephalopathy,[9] Binswanger's disease, and subcortical arteriosclerotic encephalopathy (SAE).[10, 11] None of these terms are very satisfying because they do not accurately reflect all the observed histologic changes, and they seem to overstate their clinical significance.

Necrosis is not seen until severe ischemia leads to frank infarction of brain tissue. In the larger white matter lesions, Marshall and colleagues[8] demonstrated central areas of necrosis, axonal loss, and demyelination characteristic of true infarction. The central infarct is surrounded by a large peripheral zone of astrocytic reaction. The peripheral zone of "isomorphic gliosis" also exhibits high signal on T_2-

weighted images and makes the lesion appear much larger than the actual size of the infarct. Their findings give support to the idea that the white matter hyperintensities represent a spectrum of pathologic changes associated with the vascular abnormalities.

As mentioned previously, the observed changes are secondary to chronic ischemia of the deep white matter and are found more often in patients with ischemic cerebrovascular disease, hypertension, and aging. A combination of arteriolar disease and episodic brain hypoperfusion probably leads to the histopathologic changes. Hypoperfusion can be caused by episodes of hypotension, hypoxia secondary to cardiac or carotid artery disease, hypertension, and/or aging.[9]

There is no general agreement about what terminology most correctly describes the periventricular hyperintensities seen on T_2-weighted MR images. It seems clear that the varied histologic changes are depicted on MR images as nonspecific foci of high signal that, at present, cannot be distinguished. Therefore, more nonspecific terms might be appropriate, such as *deep white matter ischemia* or *white matter hyperintensities of aging.*

The most common locations for the hyperintensities are the periventricular white matter, optic radiations, basal ganglia, centrum semiovale, and brain stem, in decreasing order of frequency.[4] The lesions are high signal on T_2-weighted and proton density–weighted images and have well-defined but irregular margins (Fig. 18–4) (also see Fig. 18–14A). They are mildly hypointense on T_1-weighted images, but the contrast between the lesions and the normal brain is

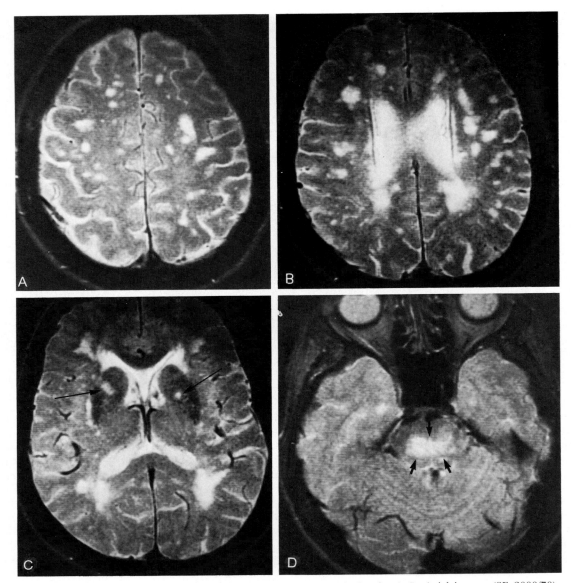

FIGURE 18–4. A 65-year-old woman with deep white matter ischemia. *A–D,* Axial images (SE 2000/70) demonstrate multiple hyperintense foci throughout the white matter of the brain. The hyperintensities are of various shapes and sizes. Some are discrete and well defined; others are irregular with indistinct margins. Lesions in the internal capsule and basal ganglia *(long arrows)* cannot be distinguished from lacunar infarcts. The pons is also involved *(short arrows).*

much less than on T_2-weighted images. The white matter changes are not associated with breakdown of the blood-brain barrier (BBB) and do not enhance. The process tends to be multifocal, but as the lesions enlarge, a more confluent pattern may develop.[12] As mentioned, lesions are often found in the internal capsule and putamen, common locations for lacunar infarcts (Fig. 18–5) (also see "Differential Diagnosis" further on), and the brain stem can be involved. In fact, if patchy foci are seen within the brain stem without symptomatology and with associated changes of periventricular white matter ischemia, very likely the brain stem foci represent changes of chronic

ischemia as well. The subcortical U-fibers receive their blood supply from shorter cortical arteries and generally are not involved by the process. Similarly, the corpus callosum is usually spared because it is supplied by the nearby pericallosal arteries.

There is also considerable debate about the significance of the white matter hyperintensities. In general, correlation between these findings and neurologic function is poor. A patient may have many high-signal foci within the white matter and be functioning perfectly normally. Nonetheless, they are not necessarily a normal part of aging because many elderly patients do not have them. Careful neuropsy-

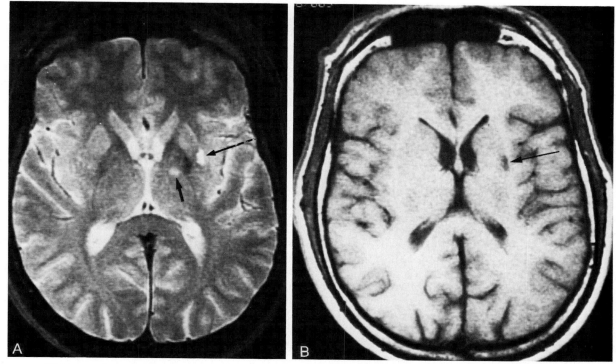

FIGURE 18–5. Lacunar infarcts. *A,* A T$_2$-weighted image (SE 2000/70) reveals two high-signal foci, one in the putamen *(long arrow)* and another in the region of the internal capsule *(short arrow)*. *B,* On a T$_1$-weighted scan (SE 600/20), the putaminal infarct *(arrow)* is hypointense owing to cystic necrosis. The other lesion is isointense, with signal characteristics identical with those of deep white matter ischemia. The clinical picture suggested a second infarct. (*A* from Brown JJ, Hesselink JR, Rothrock JF: MR and CT imaging of lacunar infarcts. AJNR 9:477–482, 1988; © by American Society of Neuroradiology.)

chologic studies have revealed that patients who have more of these lesions perform less well on neuropsychologic tests and are more likely to have cognitive deficits.[13] Steingart and colleagues[14] also noted a correlation with abnormalities of gait, limb power, plantar response, and the rooting and palmomental reflexes. They concluded that the observed white matter abnormalities may play a role in the development of intellectual impairment in the elderly. Drayer[9] suggested calling the process "normal aging" when a patient has the hyperintensities and "successful aging" when no lesions are present.

T$_2$-weighted images, having high sensitivity for increased water content of the brain, detect the changes of deep white matter ischemia much earlier than CT. They may be found as early as the mid or late forties, and then it becomes a clinical problem to decide what further tests, if any, are necessary to rule out, beyond a reasonable doubt, other significant pathology. An additional problem is how to relate the scan findings to the patient without causing undue alarm. Perhaps we must accept that the brain degenerates with aging just like other organ systems. Everyone develops degenerative changes in the joints with aging, some more than others. Probably, a similar phenomenon occurs in the brain. Fortunately, the brain has a large reserve, so that minor structural changes do not significantly alter function.

MULTIPLE SCLEROSIS

Multiple sclerosis (MS) is a chronic inflammatory disease of myelin that features a relapsing and remitting course with evidence of disseminated lesions in the central nervous system white matter. It is found predominantly in the northern climates of Canada, the United States, and Europe. The incidence of MS is 30 to 80 individuals per 100,000 population, and it is more prevalent in women than men (1.7:1.0). More than 250,000 Americans are afflicted, and MS is the most common disabling neurologic disease of young adults. More than two thirds of patients are between 20 and 40 years old.[15]

The clinical course is characterized by acute, transient attacks of focal neurologic dysfunction. The presenting symptom is usually weakness and/or numbness in one or more extremities or visual loss secondary to optic neuritis. Repeated attacks result in permanent white matter damage and chronic disability.[15]

The diagnosis of MS is usually established by a combination of history, physical examination, laboratory tests, and imaging findings. The McAlpine criteria for diagnosis are based on a group of clinical findings.[16] The most definitive laboratory evidence is oligoclonal bands in the CSF demonstrated by protein electrophoresis. The MR findings are discussed further on.

The etiology of MS is uncertain, but the most popular view is that an initial viral infection is followed sometime later by an autoimmune reaction that attacks the myelin. On histologic examination, acute MS plaques show partial or complete destruction and loss of myelin with sparing of axon cylinders. They occur in a perivenular distribution and are associated with a neuroglial reaction and infiltration of mononuclear cells and lymphocytes. Active demyelination is accompanied by transient breakdown of the BBB. Chronic lesions show predominantly gliosis. MS plaques are distributed throughout the white matter of the optic nerves, chiasm, and tracts, the cerebrum, the brain stem, the cerebellum, and the spinal cord.[15]

The sensitivity of MR imaging has been reported as 67 per cent in definite or probable multiple sclerosis[17] and as 76 per cent[18] to 85 per cent[19] in definite multiple sclerosis. These rates compare with published sensitivity figures for CT ranging from 25 per cent (routine enhanced CT)[19] to 60 per cent (double-dose enhanced CT).[18] In general, contrast-enhanced CT performs as well as plain MR in detecting acute plaques that are associated with breakdown of the BBB and enhance, but MR is far superior for evaluating patients with chronic progressive MS. Reports indicate that MR is more helpful than evoked potentials or CSF findings[20] for diagnosing MS, and in patients with isolated cord symptoms, MR of the brain was more sensitive than the

laboratory tests.[21] Detection of spinal cord plaques remains problematic because the images are often degraded by swallowing artifacts and by respiratory and cardiac motion. The lesions of optic neuritis are not reliably imaged.

MS plaques are seen best with T_2-weighted SE pulse sequences (long repetition time [TR] and long echo time [TE]), except for lesions closely apposed to an ependymal surface, where they may be obscured by the high-signal CSF. These lesions are depicted better by proton density–weighted scans (long TR and short TE) because the high-signal plaques are contrasted against the lower signal CSF (Fig. 18–6). In general, T_1-weighted images are less sensitive. MS plaques are hyperintense on T_2-weighted and proton density–weighted images (Fig. 18–7) and hypointense on T_1-weighted scans. They are usually discrete foci with well-defined margins and have a homogeneous texture without evidence of cystic or necrotic components. Hemorrhage is not a feature of MS lesions. Edema and mass effect are also uncommon.

The MS plaques are found in a periventricular distribution, particularly along the lateral aspects of the atria (Fig. 18–6B) and occipital horns. The corpus callosum (Fig. 18–7A), corona radiata, internal capsule, and centrum semiovale (Fig. 18–6A) are also commonly involved. When more than a few lesions are present, symmetric involvement of the cerebral hemispheres seems to be the rule. Any structures that contain myelin can harbor MS plaques, including the brain stem, spinal cord, subcortical U-fibers (Fig.

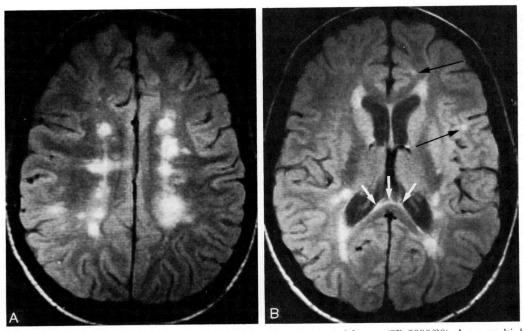

FIGURE 18–6. A 22-year-old woman with multiple sclerosis. *A,* Axial scan (SE 3000/20) shows multiple plaques within the centrum semiovale bilaterally. *B,* On a proton density–weighted image (SE 3000/20), MS plaques are clustered about the lateral atria. Two additional plaques *(black arrows)* are present in the subcortical U-fibers. A long, arcing plaque *(white arrows)* involves the inner fibers of the splenium of the corpus callosum.

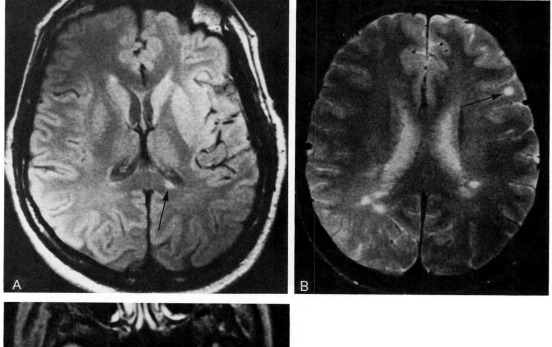

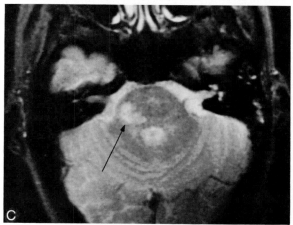

FIGURE 18–7. Multiple sclerosis. *A*, Proton density–weighted image (SE 3000/20) reveals a solitary plaque *(arrow)* in the splenium. *B*, A T_2-weighted scan (SE 3000/70) demonstrates a cortical plaque *(arrow)*, as well as other plaques in the white matter posterior to the ventricles. *C*, A section (SE 3000/70) through the pons shows a plaque *(arrow)* at the fifth nerve root entry zone.

18–6*B*), and even within the gray matter of the cerebral cortex (Fig. 18–7*B*) and basal ganglia. A distinctive site in the brain stem is the ventrolateral aspect of the pons at the fifth nerve root entry zone (Fig. 18–7*C*).

Lesions of the corpus callosum have been a special focus of study. On axial sections, plaques in the corpus callosum above the lateral ventricles have a characteristic horizontal orientation. In a review of 40 patients by Simon and colleagues,[22] 30 per cent had focal plaques in the corpus callosum. Over half also had long, inner callosal-subcallosal lesions that they describe as "arcing" transversely through the corpus callosum and crossing the midline (Fig. 18–6*B*). The lesions were between 1 and 8 mm thick and were most often seen on axial sections through the genu and splenium.

Brain atrophy can be a prominent part of long-standing, chronic MS. Ventricular dilatation and sulcal enlargement are the most obvious changes. Atrophy of the corpus callosum is also present in 40 per cent of patients and is seen best on T_1-weighted sagittal images. The atrophy progresses from the ependymal surface toward the outer fibers of the corpus callosum. When Simon and associates[22] compared their 40 MS patients with a control group, the corpus callosum measured 6.0 mm (range, 5.0 to 7.2 mm) in the normal group and only 4.3 mm (range, 3.0 to 5.4 mm) in the MS patients.

Nonenhanced MR cannot accurately reveal lesion activity, as plaques almost always remain evident after they disappear on CT.[17] The clinical correlation of signs and symptoms with supratentorial lesions is poor because most of the lesions seen on MR are old and inactive. Since up to 83 per cent of patients with brain stem and cerebellar plaques exhibit acute neurologic deficits, the correlation is better with posterior fossa lesions.[17, 19] In MS patients with internuclear ophthalmoplegia, MR has detected corresponding midbrain plaques even though CT findings were normal.[23, 24] A system of grading disease severity by MR has been found to correlate with clinical rating scales.[25]

Since acute MS plaques are associated with transient breakdown of the BBB, gadolinium-diethylene-triamine pentaacetate (Gd-DTPA) will produce enhancement (increased signal intensity) of these lesions on T_1-weighted images (Fig. 18–8). Enhancement will be observed for up to 8 weeks following acute demyelination. Thus, Gd-enhanced MR can be used to assess lesion activity just like contrast-enhanced CT. Either nodular or ringlike enhancement may be seen early after contrast injection, but the central areas tend to fill in and become more homogeneous on delayed scans. Immediate postcontrast scans are most sensitive for detecting MS, and delayed scanning is not necessary. In a study by Grossman and associates,[26] Gd-enhanced MR detected more enhancing lesions than "high-iodine" CT, and the lesions found correlated better with clinically active disease and recent deficits. Contrast-enhanced MR can be used to follow the progression of disease and to assess the response to therapy. Occasionally, large MS plaques may produce mass effect and simulate a tumor. Lack of enhancement or the enhancement pattern may help characterize these unusual plaques.

In patients with advanced disease, Drayer and associates[27] noted decreased signal intensity (T_2 shortening) in the putamen and thalamus on T_2-weighted images. They postulate that the effect is likely due to abnormal accumulation of iron or other trace metals.

In summary, MR is without question the diagnostic imaging procedure of choice in patients with clinically suspected MS. Moreover, it can be conclusively stated that CT is inadequate. MR is so exquisitely sensitive for detecting MS that the absence of plaques on an MR scan makes the diagnosis of active MS involving the brain extremely unlikely. Finally, the interpretation of MR studies is aided by the usual occurrence of MS in a younger group of patients than that associated with the more benign periventricular hyperintensities of aging. When an atypical presentation of MS is being considered in an older patient, the nonspecificity of white matter lesions becomes very troublesome. This problem is discussed later under "Differential Diagnosis."

LEUKOENCEPHALOPATHY, LEUKODYSTROPHY, AND LEUKOENCEPHALITIS

These groups include a long list of diseases that affect the cerebral white matter. The terminologies are confusing, and the methods of categorization are complex. Separate discussion of all these diseases is beyond the scope of this text, and the reader is referred to any neurology textbook for a more complete review. Only the more common entities are discussed below.

Progressive multifocal leukoencephalopathy (PML) is a demyelinating disease that results from reactivation of latent papovavirus in an immunocompromised individual. In the past, most cases occurred in patients with Hodgkin's disease, in those with chronic lymphocytic leukemia, or in those treated with steroids or immunosuppressive drugs. More recently, an increasing number of cases of PML are occurring with acquired immunodeficiency syndrome (AIDS). In addition to demyelination, histologic examination reveals deformed oligodendrocytes and reactive astrocytes. There is no effective therapy, and death ensues within a few months.[15]

The white matter lesions of PML are patchy and round or oval at first but then become confluent and large. The process is often distinctly asymmetric and initially involves the peripheral white matter, following the contours of the gray-white matter interface to give outer scalloped margins (Fig. 18–9). It is not primarily a periventricular process, but as the disease progresses, the deeper white matter is also affected (see Fig. 19–31). The prolonged T_1 and T_2 relaxation times reflect the loss of myelin and increased water. Mass effect and contrast enhancement are rarely seen.[28]

The *leukodystrophies* include *adrenoleukodystrophy, Krabbe's globoid cell* and *metachromatic leukodystrophy,* as well as other less well known entities. They have in common a genetic origin and involve the peripheral nerves as well as the central nervous system. Each is caused by a specific inherited biochemical defect in the metabolism of myelin proteolipids that results in abnormal accumulation of a metabolite in brain tissue. Progressive visual failure, mental deterioration, and spastic paralysis develop early in life.[15]

The leukodystrophies are characterized by symmetric, massive destruction of the white matter. Adrenoleukodystrophy primarily involves the parietooccipital and temporooccipital lobes but extends forward as the disease progresses. Sites of active demyelination along the advancing edges may be associated with BBB disruption and enhance with contrast. Unlike the focal plaquelike character of MS, adrenoleukodystrophy tends to be contiguous within fiber tracts and often is confluent within the larger white matter bundles of the centrum semiovale (see Fig. 19–40).[29]

Acute disseminated encephalomyelitis (ADEM) is a demyelinating disease that is thought to be of autoimmune origin. It usually occurs within 2 weeks after one of the childhood viral infections, such as measles or chickenpox, or following vaccination against rabies or smallpox. The clinical picture is one of abrupt onset with a monophasic course, to distinguish it from MS and most other white matter diseases. Lesions are found in the brain stem, cerebrum, and cerebellum and as a rule are asymmetric and few in number. Since it is a myelinoclastic process, lesions usually correlate with discrete clinical symptoms.[30] Acute hemorrhagic leukoencephalitis is a more fulminant variant of ADEM (see Figs. 19–25 and 19–26).

Another disease process that is being encountered with increasing frequency in the AIDS population is a *subacute white matter encephalitis,* secondary to either

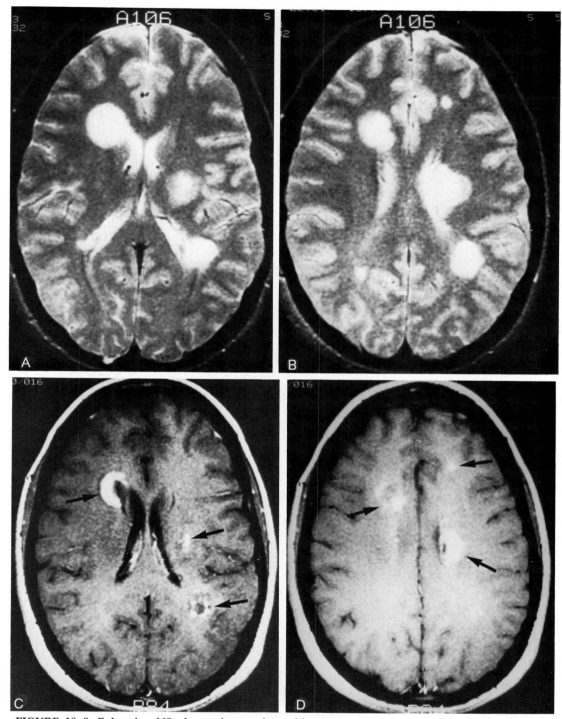

FIGURE 18–8. Enhancing MS plaques in a patient with acute presentation. *A* and *B*, T_2-weighted (SE 3000/80) images show multiple plaques in the periventricular white matter. *C* and *D*, On contrast-enhanced scans (SE 600/20, Gd-DTPA), many of the plaques enhance *(arrows)*, indicating that they are active lesions. (Courtesy of Dean Berthoty, Sunrise Diagnostic Center, Las Vegas, NV.)

human immunodeficiency virus (HIV) or cytomegalovirus (CMV) (see Chapter 19). The two viruses often coexist in brain specimens taken from AIDS patients. The MR picture is one of bilateral, diffuse, patchy to confluent areas of increased signal intensity with poorly defined margins involving the white matter of the cerebrum, cerebellum, and brain stem (see Fig. 19–32).[31] The MR appearance is distinct from that of PML, and the clinical setting readily separates it from other white matter abnormalities.

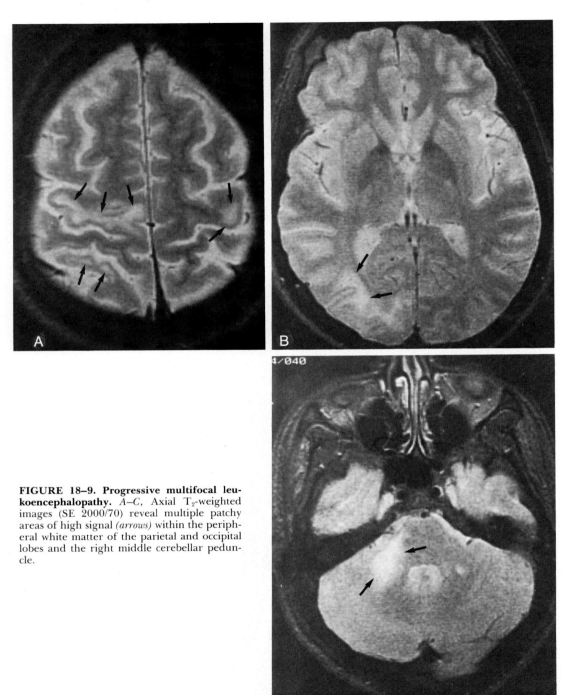

FIGURE 18–9. Progressive multifocal leukoencephalopathy. *A–C,* Axial T₂-weighted images (SE 2000/70) reveal multiple patchy areas of high signal *(arrows)* within the peripheral white matter of the parietal and occipital lobes and the right middle cerebellar peduncle.

RADIATION INJURY

Radiation to the brain produces acute and delayed changes. The acute changes occur during the course of irradiation and represent mild vasogenic edema secondary to an acute inflammatory response of the capillary endothelium. The endothelium is the most radiosensitive tissue in the brain. These changes resolve after therapy and are not observed on imaging studies. After a few weeks to a few months, focal demyelination is seen histologically, associated with proliferation of the glial elements and mononuclear cells. This condition can progress to irreversible damage to the capillary endothelium, perivascular inflammation, breakdown of the BBB, diffuse vasogenic edema of the cerebral white matter, necrotic foci, vacuolation, and petechial hemorrhage. Endothelial hyperplasia also occurs, resulting in reduced cerebral blood flow. The pathologic changes of radiation necrosis continue to evolve for a number of years after the initial radiation. The location and amount of brain injury are related to the radiation dose, fractionation methods, and the portals used.[32]

The effects of radiation injury to the brain are first detected on imaging studies about 6 to 8 months following the initial therapy. The possibility that MR visualizes radiation lesions earlier than CT has been raised but not fully explored. MR detects more lesions than CT, and the abnormalities appear more extensive on MR than on CT.[33, 34] The characteristic pattern of radiation injury is symmetric, high-signal foci on T_2-weighted images in the periventricular white matter (Fig. 18–10). The changes parallel those seen in ischemia, but the lesions are more prevalent and a confluent pattern usually develops.[35] As the process extends outward to involve the peripheral arcuate fibers of the white matter, the margins become scalloped (Fig. 18–11), a helpful feature in the differential diagnosis.[36] With time, atrophy becomes a part of the picture, as shown by enlargement of the ventricles and cortical sulci. There is relative sparing of the posterior fossa, basal ganglia, and internal capsules, but in more severe cases these structures are also involved. Deposition of hemosiderin in the basal ganglia has been reported.[37]

As observed histologically, imaging findings may continue to progress for 2 or more years after radiation therapy. With high-dose therapy, radiation ne-

crosis may lead to profound edema and focal mass effect and contrast enhancement with Gd-DTPA. Especially in these cases, distinguishing radiation change from recurrent tumor can be extremely difficult, if not impossible. Frequently, biopsy is required to clarify the issue.[35]

Enhancement of radiation lesions depends on the degree of BBB breakdown. With mild injury to the BBB, only vasogenic edema may be observed. More severe injuries result in leakage of the macromolecules of contrast agents across the BBB into the interstitial space to produce enhancement of the area. In an experimental study of radiation injury, Hecht-Leavitt and colleagues[37] noted that the nonenhancing lesions showed only edema and demyelination, while the enhancing lesions demonstrated histologic changes of necrosis with inflammatory infiltrates.

HYDROCEPHALUS AND CEREBROSPINAL FLUID FLOW

Hydrocephalus means an increased amount of CSF within the cranial cavity, usually associated with dilatation of the ventricles. Hydrocephalus has been subdivided into (1) noncommunicating hydrocephalus (obstruction within the ventricular system); (2) communicating hydrocephalus (obstruction around the basal cisterns or over the cerebral convexities); (3) normal-pressure hydrocephalus (no elevation of CSF pressure); and (4) hydrocephalus ex vacuo (in-

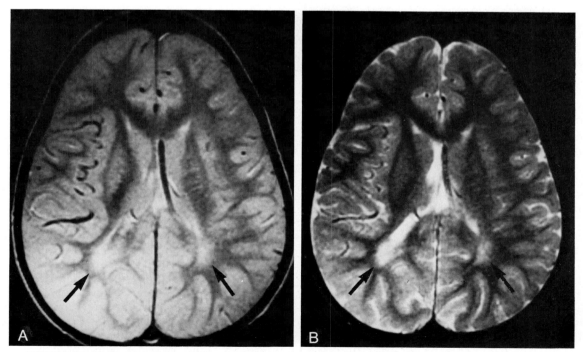

FIGURE 18–10. Early radiation injury 8 months after radiotherapy for a posterior fossa tumor. *A* and *B*, Axial scans (SE 3000/30,80) show focal areas of high signal *(arrows)* within the forceps major bilaterally. A shunt catheter is present in the left lateral ventricle.

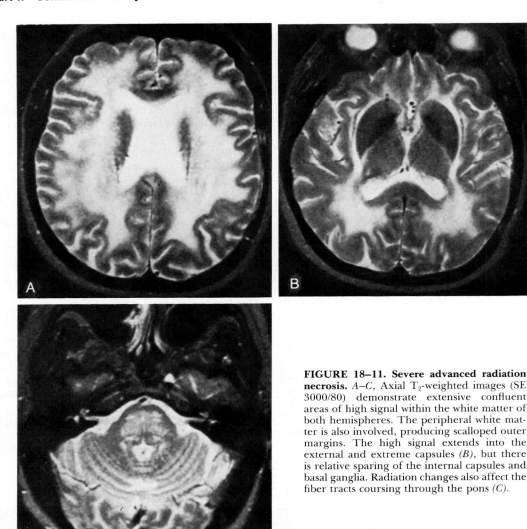

FIGURE 18–11. Severe advanced radiation necrosis. *A–C*, Axial T₂-weighted images (SE 3000/80) demonstrate extensive confluent areas of high signal within the white matter of both hemispheres. The peripheral white matter is also involved, producing scalloped outer margins. The high signal extends into the external and extreme capsules *(B)*, but there is relative sparing of the internal capsules and basal ganglia. Radiation changes also affect the fiber tracts coursing through the pons *(C)*.

creased CSF secondary to brain atrophy). The term hydrocephalus ex vacuo is not used much anymore and has been replaced with "atrophy" or simply "volume loss," which more correctly describes the pathologic process.

A basic knowledge of CSF physiology is important for understanding the concepts of hydrocephalus and the problems associated with imaging and diagnosis. Normally, the total CSF volume measures between 90 and 150 ml, and it is renewed four to five times daily. Most of the CSF is produced by the choroid plexus within the ventricles, but some is also contributed by the blood vessels in the subependymal regions and pia. The CSF flows from the lateral ventricles into the third and fourth ventricles, exits through the foramina of Magendie and Luschka, and diffuses into the basal cisterns and up over the cerebral convexities. Absorption occurs through the arachnoid villi that project into the large meningeal

veins and dural sinuses. The larger arachnoid villi, called pacchionian granulations, are found in a parasagittal location along the superior sagittal sinus and sometimes along the transverse sinuses.[15]

Hydrocephalus can result from obstruction anywhere along the path of CSF flow, from the lateral ventricle to the parasagittal cisterns. The term "noncommunicating hydrocephalus" is really a misnomer because some communication always exists. Complete obstruction is incompatible with life.

Clinically, obstructive hydrocephalus manifests with an enlarging head (in patients under 5 years old), headache, and papilledema. With time, a frontal lobe disorder evolves, consisting of inattentiveness, distractibility, and inability to carry out complex mental functions. Continued pressure leads to a progressive gait disorder and sphincteric incontinence.[15]

Normal-pressure hydrocephalus (NPH) is characterized by the classic triad of ataxia, dementia, and incontinence. The onset is more insidious than that of acute obstructive hydrocephalus. It occurs predominantly in the elderly and is easily confused with other causes of dementia, both clinically and on imaging studies. The etiology often is never established. Most cases are likely due to a mild but chronic meningeal inflammation secondary to a subclinical subarachnoid hemorrhage or infection or from an asymptomatic fibrosing meningitis of unknown etiology. CSF absorption is only mildly compromised, and as the ventricles dilate, CSF formation equilibrates with absorption, and pressure approaches normal. Nevertheless, the low pressure in enlarged ventricles still exerts significant pressure against the periventricular white matter and, over time, induces degeneration of those fiber tracts.[15]

The MR diagnosis of hydrocephalus is fraught with uncertainties. The major diagnostic dilemma is distinguishing hydrocephalus from brain atrophy in the older patient with sufficient certainty to direct appropriate therapy. Nonetheless, there are a number of imaging criteria that can help in differential diagnosis. Some of these signs have been taken directly from earlier imaging techniques, such as pneumoencephalography and CT; other findings have been learned more recently from MR investigations.

The common denominator of hydrocephalus is enlargement of the ventricular system out of proportion to the cortical sulci (Figs. 18–12 and 18–13). Although sometimes brain atrophy may be primarily central, the general rule is dilatation of both the ventricles and the sulci (Fig. 18–14). Conversely, communicating hydrocephalus may show enlargement of the sulci, although it is not often a prominent feature. With acute obstructive hydrocephalus, the temporal horns, in particular, are dilated. Moreover, the portions of the frontal horns anterior to the

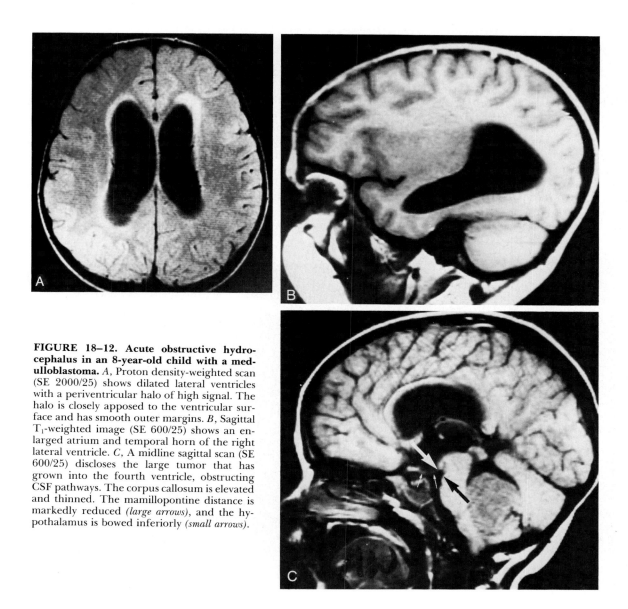

FIGURE 18–12. Acute obstructive hydrocephalus in an 8-year-old child with a medulloblastoma. A, Proton density-weighted scan (SE 2000/25) shows dilated lateral ventricles with a periventricular halo of high signal. The halo is closely apposed to the ventricular surface and has smooth outer margins. B, Sagittal T_1-weighted image (SE 600/25) shows an enlarged atrium and temporal horn of the right lateral ventricle. C, A midline sagittal scan (SE 600/25) discloses the large tumor that has grown into the fourth ventricle, obstructing CSF pathways. The corpus callosum is elevated and thinned. The mamillopontine distance is markedly reduced (large arrows), and the hypothalamus is bowed inferiorly (small arrows).

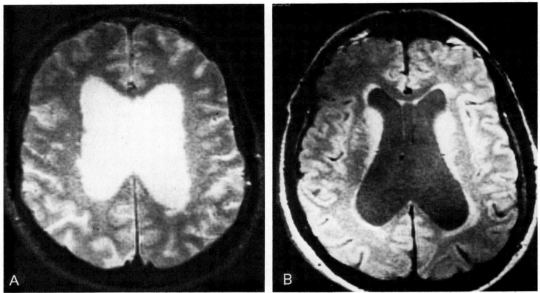

FIGURE 18–13. Normal-pressure hydrocephalus. *A* and *B*, On T_2-weighted and proton density–weighted scans (SE 2000/25,70), the lateral ventricles are enlarged out of proportion to the cortical sulci. A periventricular halo of high signal is also present.

caudate nuclei usually have a rounded or ballooned configuration on axial scans. Dilatation of the fourth ventricle is evidence for a communicating hydrocephalus, but it is not a reliable sign because obstruction at the foramina of Luschka or Magendie gives a similar appearance. On the other hand, the presence of a small fourth ventricle, with dilated lateral and third ventricles, indicates a problem at the level of the aqueduct. Dilatation of the lateral ventricles with a normal third ventricle suggests an obstructing le-

sion at the foramen of Monro, such as a colloid cyst (see Fig. 15–25).

Expansion of the inferior recesses of the third ventricle is an attribute of all forms of hydrocephalus and helps distinguish hydrocephalus from the atrophic or normal brain. In patients with hydrocephalus, El Gammal and associates[38] noted a reduction in the mamillopontine distance caused by dilatation of the anteroinferior third ventricle and inferior bowing and displacement of the hypothala-

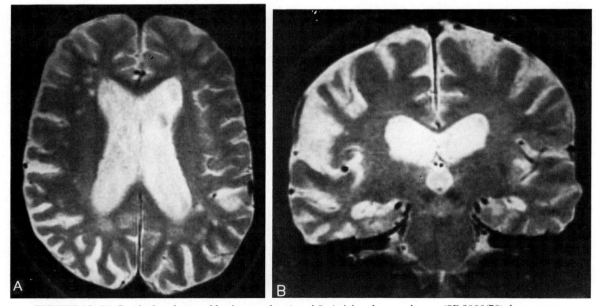

FIGURE 18–14. Cortical and central brain atrophy. *A* and *B*, Axial and coronal scans (SE 3000/70) demonstrate dilatation of both the ventricles and the cortical sulci, indicating generalized brain volume loss. Multiple hyperintensities within the white matter are consistent with changes of deep white matter ischemia.

mus (see Fig. 18–12C). The distance is measured from the anterior base of the mamillary body to the top of the pons parallel to the anterior aspect of the mesencephalon. The average mamillopontine distance was 7.5 mm for the hydrocephalic group, compared with 11.5 mm and 12.0 mm for the normal and atrophic groups, respectively. A measurement below 10 mm was considered strong evidence for hydrocephalus. They also noted depression of the posterior fornix in patients with hydrocephalus.

The corpus callosum often provides clues for the correct diagnosis. On the sagittal view, uniform thinning (below 6 mm) and smooth elevation of the corpus callosum are evidence for hydrocephalus (see Fig. 18–12C).[38]

The phenomenon of transependymal CSF flow has been looked at exhaustively to differentiate atrophy from hydrocephalus, particularly NPH. It has not been a reliable sign on CT scans, and it has proved to be equally perplexing on MR. Upon reviewing 365 consecutive MR scans, Zimmerman and coworkers[12] detected mild periventricular hyperintensity in most patients (93.5 per cent), including patients with no evidence of intracranial pathology. They concluded that mild periventricular hyperintensity is a nonspecific sign and does not indicate either demyelinating disease or hydrocephalus.

A common finding on axial T_2-weighted images is a cap of high signal around the frontal horns of the lateral ventricles (Fig. 18–15). Histologic studies of this subependymal area by Sze and associates[39] revealed a loose network of axons with low myelin content. They also noted a patchy loss of the ependyma in the frontal horns. Unfortunately, this porous ependyma has been given the name "ependymitis granularis," which sounds more like a disease than a histologic observation. Another factor to explain the MR finding is laboratory evidence that water normally passes from periventricular vessels into the interstitial space and is resorbed across the ependymal lining into the lateral ventricles.[40] Moreover, the interstitial fluid tends to converge at the dorsolateral angle of the frontal horns. In any case, the cap of high signal about the frontal horns is a normal finding and should not be mistaken for pathology. The centripetal flow of interstitial fluid in the periventricular regions could also partially explain the presence of mild periventricular hyperintensity in normal patients.

More extensive periventricular hyperintensity suggests a pathologic process but is also nonspecific. In hydrocephalus, the peripheral margins of the halo tend to be smooth and more or less of even thickness (see Figs. 18–12A and 18–13B). If irregular, the margins are blunted and do not extend very far out into the white matter. With MS and white matter ischemia, the margins are more sharply angulated and may extend out to the corticomedullary junction.[12]

The pulsatile nature of CSF flow provides an opportunity to exploit the dynamic capabilities of MR. The appearance of a flow void in regions of rapid CSF flow and pulsation has been imaged at field strengths ranging from 0.35 to 1.5 T.[41] This flow void has been attributed to velocity, turbulence, and out-of-phase pulsatile flow.[42] Citrin and associates[43] applied cardiac gating to CSF imaging and revealed more prominent hypointensity in the aqueduct and foramen of Magendie during the systolic arterial pulse wave. They related this finding to transmission of the arterial pulse wave into the thin-walled cerebral venous system and ultimately the brain and CSF. Normal CSF flow voids are seen best on T_2-weighted images at areas of maximal narrowing and flow. CSF flow voids have been identified in normal patients in the aqueduct of Sylvius (67 per cent) (Fig. 18–16A), the caudal fourth ventricle (32 per cent), and, less frequently, the third ventricle (4 per cent).[42, 44]

In studies of patients with ventriculomegaly and hydrocephalus, the presence of a flow void was more useful than its absence, as its absence indicated possible obstruction but did not directly indicate the level of obstruction. Absence of a flow void in the aqueduct was noted in 13 patients with obstruction or stenosis of the aqueduct but also in 1 patient with a colloid cyst. Moreover, if the scan series does not encompass the entire ventricular system, flow enhancement may be observed on the end slices of the series (Fig. 18–16B). Flow voids are more pronounced in patients with larger ventricles, but they cannot be used to differentiate patients with atrophy from those with extraventricular obstructive hydrocephalus.[41, 44] In a comparison of chronic NPH, acute communicating hydrocephalus, and atrophy, CSF

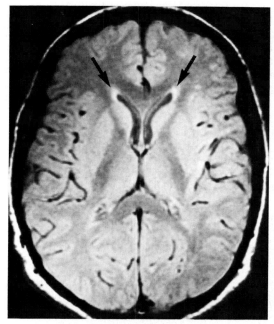

FIGURE 18–15. Normal frontal CSF caps. On a proton density–weighted image (SE 3000/20), hyperintensity (arrows) surrounds the tips of the frontal horns of both lateral ventricles, representing normal accumulation of fluid in the area.

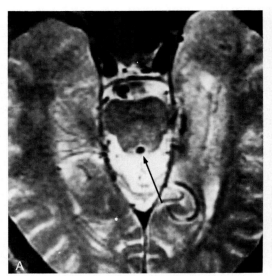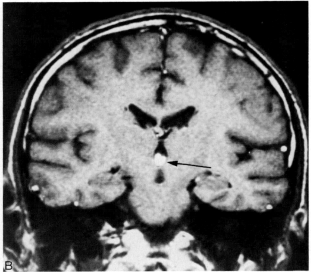

FIGURE 18–16. Normal CSF flow phenomena. *A,* Axial T_2-weighted scan (SE 3000/80) reveals a flow void within the aqueduct of Sylvius *(arrow). B,* The end slice of a coronal T_1-weighted sequence (SE 600/20) demonstrates flow enhancement within the third ventricle *(arrow).*

flow voids were most pronounced with chronic NPH, possibly correlating with a reduced ventricular compliance. The flow voids were less prominent in acute communicating hydrocephalus and were seen least often with atrophy.[45] A rapid method of mapping and quantifying pulsatile CSF flow using subtraction of image pairs derived from gradient-echo (GRE) pulses has been reported by Edelman and coworkers.[46] Perhaps this technique will prove to be of more help in differentiating between ventriculomegalic states.

The signal intensity on T_2-weighted images has been noted to be higher in intraventricular CSF than in extraventricular CSF. The signal is also higher in arachnoid cysts, in intraventricular cysts, and in association with spinal block.[47, 48] Although it has been postulated that this higher signal may be due to subtle differences in protein (15 to 30 mg/dl), in vitro studies have revealed a low sensitivity of MR to small changes in protein concentration.[49] More likely, the higher intensity is due to nonpulsatile flow and the lack of signal loss from spin dephasing.[47] CSF pulsations can also complicate image interpretation by causing signal loss and artifacts that can simulate space-occupying lesions within the ventricular system.

MR has been helpful in identifying the cause for noncommunicating hydrocephalus owing to its greater sensitivity for lesion detection, its capability of direct sagittal imaging of the aqueduct and fourth ventricle, and the ability to visualize intraventricular lesions without the use of intraventricular contrast. In particular, small midbrain lesions about the aqueduct are much more evident with MR than with CT.[23, 24, 50] Extraventricular hydrocephalus due to basilar meningitis, on either an inflammatory or a carcinomatous basis, is not reliably imaged with plain MR, but after intravenous injection of Gd-DTPA, the characteristic cisternal enhancement pattern may be displayed on T_1-weighted images (see Chapter 19).

DIFFERENTIAL DIAGNOSIS

Since the periventricular hyperintensities have common histologic features, such as increased interstitial water, demyelination, and gliosis, it should not be surprising that their MR appearance can be quite similar. Nevertheless, differential clues are often present on the images. The normal Virchow-Robin spaces should not be a problem. They are round, are no more than 1 or 2 mm in size, and are seen on the higher axial sections through the cerebral hemispheres and on lower sections through the basal ganglia at the level of the anterior commissure.

The major problem is distinguishing MS from the chronic changes of deep white matter ischemia and aging. MS is a disease of young adults, while the changes of ischemia are seen predominantly in patients over 60 years old, but overlap of the age groups does occur. MS plaques tend to be closely apposed to the atria and occipital horns of the lateral ventricles. The corpus callosum is frequently involved, and plaques can be found in the subcortical U-fibers and even the cortical gray matter. The plaques in the corpus callosum often have a characteristic horizontal orientation. Lesions at the fifth nerve root entry zone and in the spinal cord are further evidence for MS.

White matter ischemia usually spares the corpus callosum and the subcortical U-fibers. There is often a history of hypertension, stroke, and cardiovascular disease. A multifocal process with little or no neurologic dysfunction also suggests the diagnosis.

Many of the other white matter diseases have

special features. PML occurs in an immunocompromised host and involves the peripheral white matter in a patchy and asymmetric fashion. The leukodystrophies occur in children and exhibit a symmetric, diffuse, and confluent pattern of involvement. The white matter encephalitides have an acute clinical course and a history of a recent viral infection, vaccination, or AIDS.

Vasculitic disorders, such as systemic lupus erythematosus (SLE) and Behçet's disease, can also result in multifocal periventricular hyperintensities. Moreover, these diseases occur in young adults and can produce a neurologic picture similar to that of MS. Associated systemic features are important diagnostic clues for vasculitis, and the brain images usually reveal cortical infarcts in addition to the periventricular lesions (see Chapter 17).[51, 52]

Migraine is another neurologic problem associated with periventricular abnormalities. In a study by Soges and colleagues,[53] periventricular hyperintensities were found in 41 per cent of patients with classic or common migraine and in 57 per cent of patients with complicated migraine. The white matter lesions resemble those of MS and deep white matter ischemia, but the classic pattern of headaches usually identifies these patients (see Chapter 17).

Transependymal CSF flow usually appears as a smooth halo of relatively even thickness and has the associated findings of lateral ventricles that are enlarged out of proportion to the cortical sulci, dilated inferior recesses of the third ventricle, and smooth elevation and even thinning of the corpus callosum. In general, radiation necrosis exhibits a confluent pattern of high signal intensity within the periventricular white matter, with scalloped margins that extend out to involve the subcortical U-fibers.

The proton density–weighted image is often helpful to differentiate significant disease from the more benign processes. Virchow-Robin spaces, *état criblé* without gliosis, brain cysts, and ventricular diverticula are all isointense on the proton density–weighted image. The other entities show increased signal. Unfortunately, the changes of deep white matter ischemia are also of higher signal than the brain and CSF. Cystic or necrotic components of lacunar infarcts may be isointense on proton density–weighted images, but they have an associated peripheral zone of increased signal (see Chapter 17).[54]

Enhancement is a very helpful feature. Acute MS plaques, subacute infarcts, radiation necrosis, and adrenoleukodystrophy are associated with breakdown of the BBB and enhance with Gd-DTPA. Enhancement patterns provide additional diagnostic clues. The CSF spaces and chronic changes of white matter ischemia and aging will not enhance.

Mirowitz and colleagues[55] noted hyperintense foci in the posterior limb of the internal capsule on T_2-weighted images in 56 per cent of patients imaged at 1.5 tesla. The foci were low signal on T_1-weighted images and were round or oval, homogeneous, well-defined, and symmetrical. Correlative anatomic studies showed these hyperintense foci to represent the parietopontine tract, containing axons that were less heavily myelinated compared with the surrounding fibers of the internal capsule.

All of the above features are helpful in evaluating periventricular white matter abnormalities. Sometimes, a definitive diagnosis cannot be made from the images alone, and a list of differential diagnoses must be considered and correlated with clinical information.

REFERENCES

1. Gerard G, Weisberg LA: Magnetic resonance imaging in adult white matter disorders and hydrocephalus. Semin Neurol 6:17–23, 1986.
2. Kirkpatrick JB, Hayman LA: White-matter lesions in MR imaging of clinically healthy brains of elderly subjects: Possible pathologic basis. Radiology 162:509–511, 1987.
3. Durand-Fardel M: Traité du Ramollissement du Cerveau. Paris, Bailliere, 1843.
4. Awad IA, Johnson PC, Spetzler RF, et al: Incidental subcortical lesions identified on magnetic resonance imaging in the elderly. II. Postmortem pathological correlations. Stroke 17:1090–1097, 1986.
5. Challa VR, Moody DM: White-matter lesions in MR imaging of elderly subjects. Radiology 164:874–878, 1987.
6. Hachinski VC, Potter P, Merskey H, et al: Leuko-araiosis. Arch Neurol 44:21–23, 1987.
7. Brun A, Englund E: A white matter disorder in dementia of the Alzheimer type: A pathoanatomical study. Ann Neurol 19:253–262, 1986.
8. Marshall VG, Bradley WG, Marshall CE, et al: Deep white matter infarction: Correlation of MR imaging and histopathologic findings. Radiology 167:517–522, 1988.
9. Drayer BP: Imaging of the aging brain. Part I. Normal findings. Radiology 166:785–796, 1988.
10. Olszewski J: Subcortical arteriosclerotic encephalopathy. World Neurol 3:359–375, 1962.
11. Burger PC, Burch JG, Kunze U: Subcortical arteriosclerotic encephalopathy (Binswanger's disease): A vascular etiology of dementia. Stroke 7:626–631, 1976.
12. Zimmerman RD, Fleming CA, Lee BCP, et al: Periventricular hyperintensity as seen by magnetic resonance: Prevalence and significance. AJNR 7:13–20, 1986.
13. Brant-Zawadzki M, Fein G, Van Dyke C, et al: MR imaging of the aging brain: Patchy white-matter lesions and dementia. AJNR 6:675–682, 1985.
14. Steingart A, Hachinski VC, Lau C, et al: Cognitive and neurologic findings in subjects with diffuse white matter lucencies on computed tomographic scan (leuko-araiosis). Arch Neurol 44:32–35, 1987.
15. Adams RD, Victor M: Principles of Neurology. 2nd ed. New York, McGraw-Hill Book Company, 1981, pp 524–702.
16. McAlpine D, Compston MD: Some aspects of the natural history of disseminated sclerosis. Q J Med 21:135, 1952.
17. Jacobs L, Kinkel PR, Kinkel WR: Impact of nuclear magnetic resonance imaging on the assessment of multiple sclerosis patients. Semin Neurol 6:24–32, 1986.
18. Jackson JA, Leake DR, Schneiders NJ, et al: Magnetic resonance imaging in multiple sclerosis: Results in 32 cases. AJNR 6:171–176, 1985.
19. Sheldon JJ, Siddharthan R, Tobias J, et al: MR imaging of multiple sclerosis: Comparison with clinical and CT examinations in 74 patients. AJNR 6:683–690, 1985.
20. Gebarski SS, Gabrielsen TO, Gilman S, et al: The initial diagnosis of multiple sclerosis: Clinical impact of magnetic resonance imaging. Ann Neurol 17:469–474, 1985.
21. Edwards MK, Farlow MR, Stevens JC: Cranial MR in spinal cord MS: Diagnosing patients with isolated cord symptoms. AJNR 7:1003–1006, 1986.

22. Simon JH, Holtas SL, Schiffer RB, et al: Corpus callosum and subcallosal-periventricular lesions in multiple sclerosis: Detection with MR. Radiology 160:363–367, 1986.

23. Bogousslavsky J, Fox AJ, Corey LS, et al: Correlates of brainstem oculomotor disorders in multiple sclerosis: Magnetic resonance imaging. Arch Neurol 43:460–463, 1986.

24. Atlas SW, Grossman RI, Savino PJ, et al: Internuclear ophthalmoplegia: MR-anatomic correlation. AJNR 8:243–247, 1987.

25. Edwards MK, Farlow MR, Stevens JC: Multiple sclerosis: MRI and clinical correlation. AJNR 7:595–598, 1986.

26. Grossman RI, Gonzalez-Scarano F, Atlas SW, et al: Multiple sclerosis: Gadolinium enhancement in MR imaging. Radiology 161:721–725, 1986.

27. Drayer B, Burger P, Hurwitz B, et al: Reduced signal intensity on MR images of thalamus and putamen in multiple sclerosis: Increased iron content? AJNR 8:413–419, 1987.

28. Guilleux MH, Steiner RE, Young IR: MR imaging in progressive multifocal leukoencephalopathy. AJNR 7:1033–1035, 1986.

29. Kumar AJ, Rosenbaum AE, Naidu S, et al: Adrenoleukodystrophy: Correlating MR imaging with CT. Radiology 165:497–504, 1987.

30. Atlas SW, Grossman RI, Goldberg HI, et al: MR diagnosis of acute disseminated encephalomyelitis. J Comput Assist Tomogr 10:798–801, 1986.

31. Post MJD, Tate LG, Quencer RM, et al: CT, MR and pathology in HIV encephalitis and meningitis. AJNR 9:469–476, 1988.

32. Lampert PW, Davis RL: Delayed effects of radiation on the human CNS—"early" and "late" delayed reactions. Neurology 14:912–917, 1964.

33. Dooms GC, Hecht S, Brant-Zawadzki M, et al: Brain radiation lesions—MR imaging. Radiology 158:149–155, 1986.

34. Frytak S, Earnest F, O'Neill BP, et al: Magnetic resonance imaging for neurotoxicity in long-term survivors of carcinoma. Mayo Clin Proc 60:803–812, 1985.

35. Tsuruda JS, Kortman KE, Bradley WG, et al: Radiation effects on cerebral white matter: MR evaluation. AJNR 8:431–437, 1987.

36. Curnes JT, Laster DW, Ball MR, et al: Magnetic resonance imaging of radiation injury to the brain. AJNR 7:389–394, 1986.

37. Hecht-Leavitt C, Grossman RI, Curran WJ, et al: MR of brain radiation injury: Experimental studies in cats. AJNR 8:427–430, 1987.

38. El Gammal T, Allen MB, Brooks BS, et al: MR evaluation of hydrocephalus. AJNR 8:591–597, 1987.

39. Sze G, De Armond SJ, Brant-Zawadzki MB, et al: Foci of MRI signal (pseudo lesions) anterior to the frontal horns: Histologic correlations of a normal finding. AJNR 7:381–387, 1986.

40. Cserr HF, Ostrach LH: Bulk flow of interstitial fluid after intracranial injection of Blue Dextran 2000. Exp Neurol 45:50–60, 1974.

41. Sherman JL, Citrin CM, Gangarosa RE, Bowen BJ: The MR appearance of CSF flow in patients with ventriculomegaly. AJNR 7:1025–1032, 1986.

42. Sherman JL, Citrin CM: Magnetic resonance demonstration of normal CSF flow. AJNR 7:3–6, 1986.

43. Citrin CM, Sherman JL, Gangarosa RE, Scanlon D: Physiology of the CSF flow-void sign: Modification by cardiac gating. AJNR 7:1021–1024, 1986.

44. Sherman JL, Citrin CM, Bowen BJ, Gangarosa RE: MR demonstration of altered CSF flow by obstructive lesions. AJNR 7:571–579, 1986.

45. Bradley WG, Kortman KE, Burgoyne B: Flowing cerebrospinal fluid in normal and hydrocephalic states: Appearance on MR images. Radiology 159:611–616, 1986.

46. Edelman RR, Wedeen VJ, Davis KR, et al: Multiphasic MR imaging: A new method for direct imaging of pulsatile CSF flow. Radiology 161:779–783, 1986.

47. Enzmann DR, Rubin JR, DeLaPaz R, Wright A: Cerebrospinal fluid pulsation: Benefits and pitfalls in MR imaging. Radiology 161:773–778, 1986.

48. Brant-Zawadzki M, Kelly W, Kjos B, et al: Magnetic resonance imaging and characterization of normal and abnormal intracranial cerebrospinal fluid (CSF) spaces. Neuroradiology 27:3–8, 1985.

49. Hackney DB, Grossman RI, Zimmerman RA, et al: Low sensitivity of clinical MR to small changes in the concentration of nonparamagnetic protein. AJNR 8:1003–1008, 1987.

50. Sherman JL, Citrin CM, Barkovich AJ, Bowen BJ: MR imaging of the mesencephalic tectum: Normal and pathologic variations. AJNR 8:59–64, 1987.

51. Aisen AM, Gabrielsen TO, McCune WJ: MR imaging of systemic lupus erythematosus involving the brain. AJNR 6:197–201, 1985.

52. Miller DH, Ormerod IEC, Gibson A, et al: MR brain scanning in patients with vasculitis: Differentiation from multiple sclerosis. Neuroradiology 29:226–231, 1987.

53. Soges LJ, Cacayorin ED, Petro GR, Ramachandran TS: Migraine: Evaluation by MR. AJNR 9:425–429, 1988.

54. Brown JJ, Hesselink JR, Rothrock JF: MR and CT imaging of lacunar infarcts. AJNR 9:477–482, 1988.

55. Mirowitz S, Sartor K, Gado M, Torack R: Focal signal–intensity variations in the posterior internal capsule: Normal MR findings and distinction from pathologic findings. Radiology 172:535–539, 1989.

19

BRAIN: Trauma, Inflammation, and Degenerative and Metabolic Disorders

RICHARD J. HICKS, JOHN R. HESSELINK, GARY L. WISMER, and KENNETH R. DAVIS

TRAUMA
    EXTRACEREBRAL HEMORRHAGE
    CONTUSIONS
    SHEAR INJURIES
    THE ROLE OF MR
INFLAMMATION
    ABSCESS
    Bacterial
    Fungal
    Cysticercosis
    MENINGITIS
    Bacterial
    Tuberculosis
    Sarcoidosis
    Neurosyphilis
    ENCEPHALITIS
    Herpes Simplex
    Acute Disseminated Encephalomyelitis

AIDS-RELATED INFECTIONS
    Toxoplasmosis
    Cryptococcosis
    Progressive Multifocal Leukoencephalopathy
      (PML)
    Human Immunodeficiency
      Virus/Cytomegalovirus Encephalitis
DEGENERATIVE DISEASES
    PARKINSONISM
    ALZHEIMER'S DISEASE
    PICK'S DISEASE
    HUNTINGTON'S CHOREA
METABOLIC DISORDERS
    CENTRAL PONTINE MYELINOLYSIS
    LEIGH'S DISEASE
    WILSON'S DISEASE
    HALLERVORDEN-SPATZ DISEASE
    ADRENOLEUKODYSTROPHY

TRAUMA

Patients with head trauma constitute a large percentage of the cases referred for neuroimaging. Initially, the role of MR in these patients was considered limited owing to the time required for the examination, difficulty in using life support and monitoring equipment within the scanning room, and problems in imaging acute hemorrhage. Although some of these problems still remain, MR has come to be used more frequently in these patients, particularly in the subacute period.

The most common head injuries result from blunt or nonpenetrating trauma. These frequently induce a temporary or longer loss of consciousness, and the brain may suffer gross damage despite the lack of a skull fracture or penetrating injury. Skull fractures may indicate the presence of significant trauma, but the absence or presence of a skull fracture cannot be used to predict the presence or severity of intracranial injury.

Cerebral concussion is a clinical diagnosis in which there is reversible paralysis of nervous function, occurring immediately at the time of injury.[1] The brain is subject to shearing stresses caused by rotational forces encountered in both acceleration and deceleration injuries. These motions result in injuries typically involving the inferior frontal and anterior and inferior temporal lobes, where the brain comes into contact with bony protuberances. Pathologically, many concussive episodes are unassociated with any abnormalities, but in other, more severe, cases bruises, lacerations, hemorrhages, localized swellings, and herniation of tissue may be found. Delayed bleeding into contusions has been seen with CT in a small percentage of patients.[2]

EXTRACEREBRAL HEMORRHAGE

Extraaxial collections (epidural and subdural hematomas) differ clinically from concussion in that a lucid interval may be present. Acute epidural hematomas are often associated with skull fractures and lacerations of the dural vessels, most often meningeal arteries and veins but occasionally a dural sinus. Two thirds of epidural hematomas are in the temporoparietal region, and they usually have a biconvex or

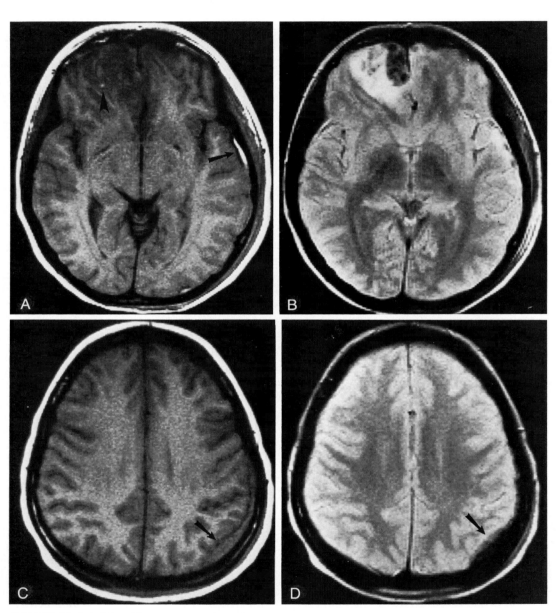

FIGURE 19–1. Subdural hematoma, epidural hematoma, and hemorrhagic contusion 3 days after injury. *A,* T_1-weighted image shows high-signal left temporal subdural hematoma *(arrow)* and small focus of hemorrhage in the right frontal lobe *(arrowhead).* *B,* Proton density image demonstrates the low signal of deoxyhemoglobin in the acute right frontal hemorrhage, with edema seen laterally. Increased signal is also noted in a bland left temporal contusion, adjacent to the site of the subdural hematoma, which is not well seen with this sequence. *C,* T_1-weighted image reveals isointense left parietal extraaxial collection with convex margins *(arrow).* *D,* Proton density image illustrates the low signal of acute hemorrhage in this epidural hematoma.

lentiform configuration. Epidural hematomas are limited by the firmer attachment of the dura at the suture margins, but they may cross the midline, especially with superior sagittal sinus lacerations, and they can also bridge the supratentorial and infratentorial compartments with tears along the torcular and transverse sinuses.

Subdural hematomas, both acute and chronic, are most often caused by bleeding from torn bridging dural veins. A lucid interval is seen less commonly with acute subdural than with epidural hematomas. Subdural hematomas are less frequently associated with skull fractures but more often associated with parenchymal brain damage. The subdural space is a more freely communicating space, and the hematomas form a crescent-shaped layer over the brain surface. Subdural hematomas readily cross suture lines but do not cross the midline. Instead, they extend along the dura of the falx into the interhemispheric fissure and onto the tentorium, which epidural hematomas cannot do. Both epidural and subdural hemorrhages occur within the confined space of the bony calvarium and compress the adjacent brain, often requiring emergency evacuation.

Chronic subdural hematomas are usually related to a slower venous bleed without accompanying cerebral parenchymal injury. A thick, vascular dural membrane forms that can be a source for repeated episodes of hemorrhage. These collections are more often biconvex, rather than the crescentic shape of acute subdural hematomas. The injury leading to a chronic subdural hematoma can be relatively minor and may have occurred weeks before presentation. Patients often present with disturbances of mentation and conciousness rather than focal or lateralizing signs. An iatrogenic cause is overshunting or too rapid decompression of chronic hydrocephalus.

Subdural hygromas or effusions consist of collections of cerebrospinal fluid (CSF) in the subdural spaces, presumably resulting from a traumatic arachnoid tear, or they may also develop after ventricular shunting. They may accumulate slowly during the first few days following head trauma, especially in the pediatric population.

Multiple studies have demonstrated improved visualization of extraaxial hemorrhage with MR compared with CT, largely related to the high conspicuity of hyperintense subacute hemorrhage (methemoglobin) on T_1-weighted images and the multiplanar capabilities of MR[3, 4, 5–7] (Figs. 19–1 to 19–4). Coronal images are very helpful for identifying subtemporal collections and hemorrhage adjacent to the tentorium cerebelli. MR has been helpful in distinguishing chronic subdural hematomas (usually hyperintense on T_2-weighted images with variable hyperintensity on T_1-weighted images, depending on age) (Figs. 19–5 and 19–6) from subdural hygromas (isointense with CSF on all sequences) (Fig. 19–7). Chronic subdural hematomas are often isointense with gray matter on T_1-weighted images, probably owing to dilution and partial resorption or breakdown of free methemoglo-

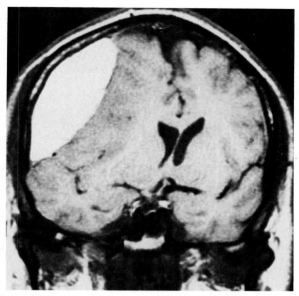

FIGURE 19–2. Subdural hematoma. The broad-based, high-signal extraaxial collection has a convex, rather than concave, medial surface in this instance. Cingulate herniation is well demonstrated, and deformity of the suprasellar cistern suggests descending transtentorial herniation.

bin. High T_1 signal within what otherwise appears to be a chronic subdural hematoma suggests rebleeding. Hemosiderin is rarely seen in subdural hematomas without repeated episodes of bleeding,[8] because of either low macrophage activity or removal of hemosiderin that has formed. The presence of membranous strands coursing through an extraaxial collection is additional evidence for a chronic subdural hematoma. The thick subdural membranes will also enhance following contrast infusion.

As mentioned previously, acute hemorrhages are more difficult to evaluate with MR because they can be isointense to the brain. Many physical and chemical changes are happening rapidly and concurrently in acute hematomas, making the MR appearance variable and interpretation difficult. The specific causes of the observed MR signal are likely multifactorial. The reader is referred to Chapters 8 and 16.

The utility of MR in imaging subarachnoid blood has generally been limited, with only large clots in the subarachnoid space being evident.[3, 5] One study noted better visualization of these subarachnoid clots as hyperintensity on T_2-weighted images, with the T_1-weighted images being negative.[3] The low sensitivity of MR for detecting subarachnoid hemorrhage may in part reflect differences in methemoglobin formation between blood in the subarachnoid space and intraparenchymal hemorrhage and the faster resorption of blood from the subarachnoid space.

CONTUSIONS

Damage to the brain parenchyma is a common component of head trauma. The type, location, and

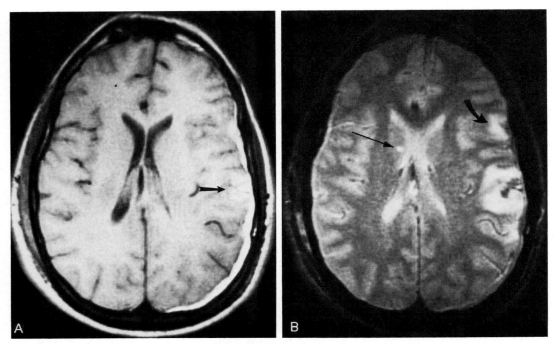

FIGURE 19–3. Subdural hematoma and hemorrhagic contusion. *A*, T₁-weighted image reveals high-signal left temporoparietal collection. An area of high signal is also present within the left temporal lobe *(arrow)*. *B*, The extraaxial collection is subacute and isointense with parenchyma on this T₂-weighted sequence. The temporal lobe contusion demonstrates low-signal acute hemorrhage with high-signal edema peripherally. The difference in the signal intensity of parenchymal and extraaxial hemorrhages is not uncommon. Another contusion is present in the left frontal lobe *(curved arrow)*, as well as a focal shear injury in the left caudate nucleus *(long arrow)*.

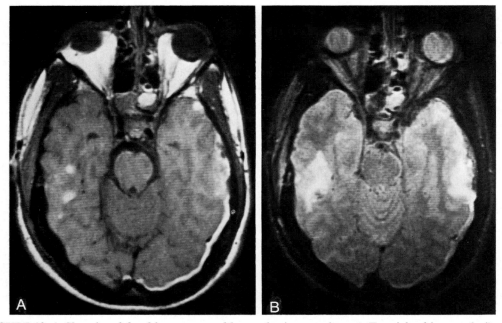

FIGURE 19–4. Chronic subdural hematoma and hemorrhagic contusions. *A*, T₁-weighted image of a 7-year-old child with learning disabilities 6 months after head trauma reveals high-signal left temporoparietal subdural hematoma and several foci of increased signal in the temporal lobes bilaterally. *B*, T₂-weighted image shows mild hyperintensity of subdural hematoma and areas of presumed gliosis and microcystic encephalomalacia about the parenchymal hemorrhages.

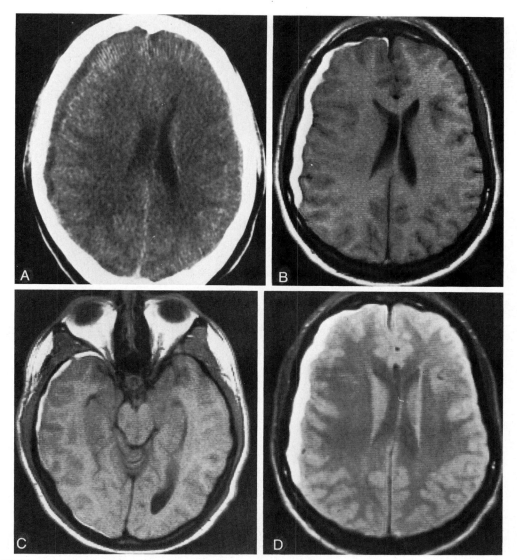

FIGURE 19–5. Subdural hematoma imaged 2 weeks after injury. *A,* CT reveals an extraaxial collection of slightly greater than CSF attenuation, accompanied by midline shift. *B* and *C,* Axial T$_1$-weighted images demonstrate high-signal hemorrhage with extension seen inferiorly along the temporal lobe. *D,* Proton density image shows high signal persisting in the subdural hematoma.

degree of brain injury are determined to a large extent by the physical properties of the skull and brain. The skull is very hard and rigid and protects the brain from direct injury. However, the inner table of the skull has roughened edges and ridges of bone along the floor of the anterior cranial fossa, sphenoid wings, and petrous ridges that can contuse the brain surface during the compressive forces of trauma.[9]

Injury of the brain parenchyma sets in motion a series of events. Tissue disruption and cell injury are associated with release of vasoactive substances and other by-products. Subsequent increase in vascular permeability to serum proteins results in a progressive increase in interstitial fluid. Over a period of several days, the edema fluid spreads within the white matter, producing mass effect on adjacent structures and possible further damage. More serious injuries may be associated with vascular disruption and hemorrhage into contusions.[9–11]

Cortical contusions are usually multiple, measuring approximately 2 to 4 cm, and 30 to 50 per cent of lesions are hemorrhagic. Approximately 50 to 75 per cent of cortical contusions involve the frontal and temporal lobes, particularly the lateral surfaces of both lobes and the inferior surface of the frontal lobes.[3, 12] Although less common, the occipital and parietal lobes can also be involved by contusions.

Varying signal intensity patterns are seen on MR, depending on the age and amount of hemorrhage present. In several studies, MR has had a decided advantage over CT in the imaging of bland contu-

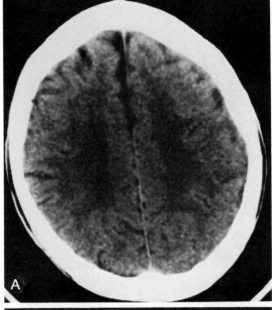

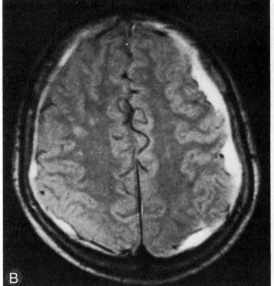

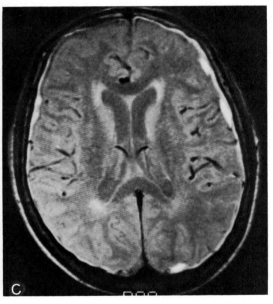

FIGURE 19–6. Chronic subdural hematoma. *A,* CT of a 77-year-old man reveals changes of diffuse atrophy, with prominent CSF spaces over the frontal lobes. *B* and *C,* Proton density images reveal extensive but thin bilateral subdural hematomas.

sions and has been roughly equivalent to CT in imaging hemorrhagic contusions[3–5, 12] (Fig. 19–8). Overall, MR has shown approximately 90 per cent of all cortical contusions imaged by either modality.

In general, T_2-weighted images are best for evaluating brain contusions. T_1-weighted images are helpful in looking for any associated hemorrhage. Nonhemorrhagic contusions are hyperintense on T_2-weighted scans and hypointense on T_1-weighted scans owing to brain edema and increased water content in the lesions. The brain edema increases during the first few days, producing mass effect on adjacent brain structures. With time, the edema subsides and the dead tissues are removed, resulting in areas of encephalomalacia and compensatory focal dilatation of adjacent ventricles and sulci.[12]

The MR appearance of hemorrhagic contusions is more dynamic, changing over time as the internal chemistry of the hematoma changes. In fact, the signal intensities on T_1- and T_2-weighted images often provide clues about the approximate age of hemorrhagic contusions (see Chapter 16). The central hypointensity of acute hemorrhagic contusions on T_2-weighted images is often highlighted by the surrounding edema. After a few days, methemoglobin forms and gives a mottled pattern of high signal on T_1-weighted images resulting from the multifocal nature of hemorrhage into cortical contusions (Figs. 19–9 to 19–12).

The brain stem is also subject to injury from head trauma. Although it is protected from direct injury by its location, acceleration-deceleration forces asso-

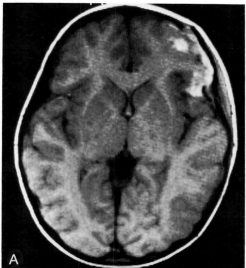

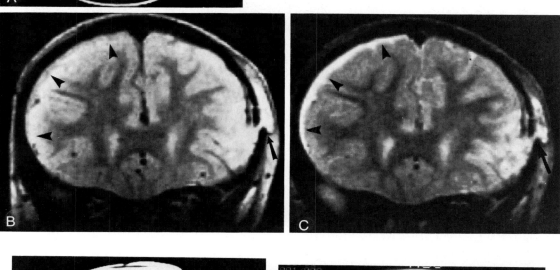

FIGURE 19–7. Subdural hygroma, hemorrhagic contusion, and skull fracture 1 week after trauma. *A,* Axial T₁-weighted image demonstrates high-signal hemorrhage in the left frontal lobe with a possible small subdural hematoma. *B,* Coronal proton density image reveals an isointense right frontal subdural collection *(arrowheads).* A skull fracture *(arrow)* is present on the left. *C,* Coronal T₂-weighted image illustrates edema in the left frontal lobe. A right frontal extraaxial collection *(arrowheads)* is isointense with CSF, consistent with a subdural hygroma. A left posterior frontal skull fracture *(arrow)* is well shown, with high signal extending through the defect into the subgaleal tissues. If this defect is due to a dural tear, it can result in the formation of a leptomeningeal cyst.

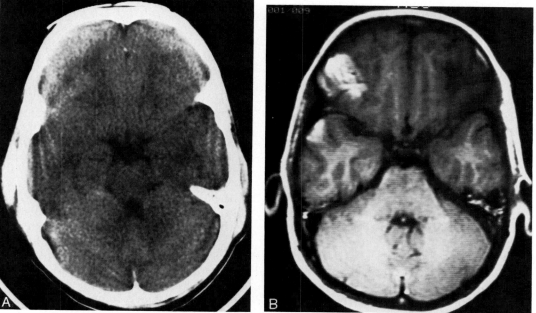

FIGURE 19–8. Hemorrhagic contusions. *A,* Two days after injury, CT scan is normal. *B,* T₁-weighted image 10 days after injury reveals high-signal hemorrhage in the right inferior frontal and temporal lobes. This may represent delayed hemorrhage into contusions or may indicate a false-negative CT scan. (From Hesselink JR, Dowd CF, Healy ME, et al: MR imaging of brain contusions: A comparative study with CT. AJNR 9:269–278, 1988; © by American Society of Neuroradiology.)

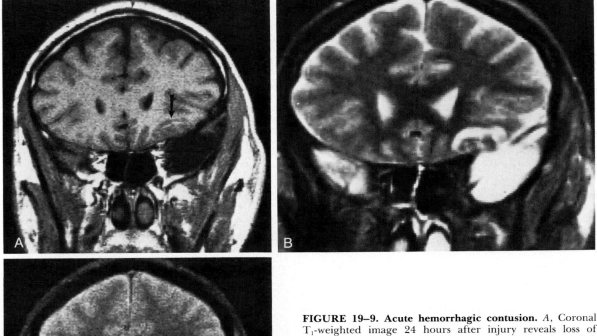

FIGURE 19–9. Acute hemorrhagic contusion. *A,* Coronal T_1-weighted image 24 hours after injury reveals loss of normal gray-white matter differentiation in the inferior left frontal lobe, with a thin rim of increased signal seen superiorly *(arrow).* A left temporal arachnoid cyst is isointense with CSF. *B,* Coronal T_2-weighted image demonstrates isointense acute hemorrhage with surrounding edema. *C,* Coronal gradient-echo (GRE) image (FISP with flip angle of 20 degrees, repetition time [TR] 300 msec, echo time [TE] 22 msec) reveals drop-out of signal from acute hemorrhage because of the greater sensitivity of GRE sequences to magnetic susceptibility effects.

ciated with impact to the head may produce displacement and twisting of the brain stem. These forces can result in tearing of penetrating arteries or veins and in compression of the brain stem against the sharp edges of the tentorium or surfaces of the clivus and petrous bones[9, 13] (Fig. 19–13).

SHEAR INJURIES

Severe head injuries are often associated with rotational forces that produce shear stresses on the brain parenchyma. The brain itself has very little rigidity and is extremely noncompressible. Brain volume can be decreased only by exerting great pressure. On the other hand, the brain is soft and malleable. Relatively little effort is required to distort the shape of the brain. The parenchyma is of relatively uniform density, except for differences between the CSF of the ventricles and surrounding brain tissue. Slight differences in density also exist between gray and white matter.[9]

When the skull is rapidly rotated, it carries along the superficial brain parenchyma, but the deeper structures lag behind, causing axial stretching and separation and disruption of nerve fiber tracts. Shear stresses are most marked at junctions between tissues of differing densities.[9, 13] As a result, shear injuries commonly occur at gray and white matter junctions, but they are also found in the deeper white matter of the corpus callosum, centrum semiovale, brain stem (mostly the midbrain and rostral pons), and cerebellum.[14] Lesions in the basal ganglionic regions are usually found along the borders between the ganglia and the internal or external capsules—in other words, the deep gray and white matter junctions of the cerebral hemispheres. Thalamic and basal ganglia injuries are hemorrhagic in slightly more than 50 per cent of cases[2, 12] (Fig. 19–14). On the other hand, shear injuries of the corpus callosum and centrum semiovale are more often nonhemorrhagic[3, 4] (Fig. 19–15).

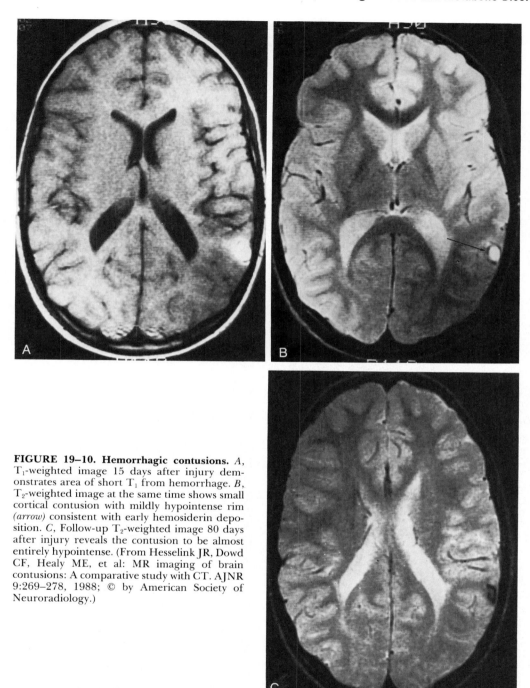

FIGURE 19–10. Hemorrhagic contusions. *A,* T_1-weighted image 15 days after injury demonstrates area of short T_1 from hemorrhage. *B,* T_2-weighted image at the same time shows small cortical contusion with mildly hypointense rim *(arrow)* consistent with early hemosiderin deposition. *C,* Follow-up T_2-weighted image 80 days after injury reveals the contusion to be almost entirely hypointense. (From Hesselink JR, Dowd CF, Healy ME, et al: MR imaging of brain contusions: A comparative study with CT. AJNR 9:269–278, 1988; © by American Society of Neuroradiology.)

Attempts to correlate CT findings with acute and chronic sequelae of closed head trauma have been discouraging, largely because of the insensitivity of CT to many cerebral injuries. Chief among these, poorly seen by CT and well seen by MR, are the diffuse axonal injuries or white matter shear injuries. These injuries constitute the most frequent findings on MR in head trauma, accounting for 40 per cent of all lesions in one study of 40 patients.[2] Shear injuries are most often multiple, ovoid, and parallel

to white matter fiber bundles. They are hyperintense on T_2-weighted scans and hypointense on T_1-weighted scans, unless hemorrhagic components are present, in which case more complex patterns are observed. During transition phases of hematoma evolution, combinations of methemoglobin, hemosiderin rings, and peripheral edema can result in layers of differing signal intensity and a targetlike appearance.

The axial plane is the primary plane of imaging

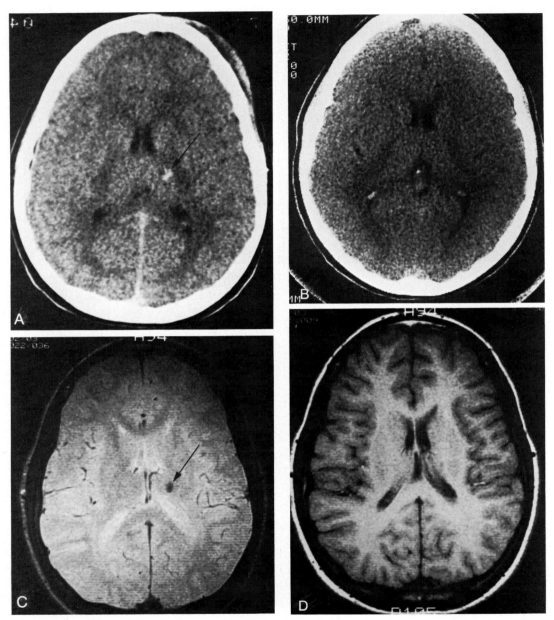

FIGURE 19–11. Hemorrhagic thalamic contusion. *A,* CT scan 1 day after trauma reveals hemorrhage in the left thalamus *(arrow).* *B,* Follow-up CT 6 months later is normal. *C,* T_2-weighted image 2 years after injury demonstrates low signal at the site of hemorrhage *(arrow),* presumably from hemosiderin deposition. *D,* T_1-weighted image reveals relative isointensity of the old hemorrhage. (From Hesselink JR, Dowd CF, Healy ME, et al: MR imaging of brain contusions: A comparative study with CT. AJNR 9:269–278, 1988; © by American Society of Neuroradiology.)

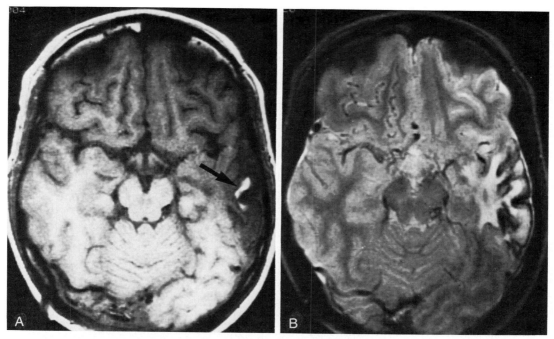

FIGURE 19–12. Hemorrhagic infarct as a complication of head trauma. *A*, T$_1$-weighted image reveals a small area of high signal within the left temporal lobe *(arrow)*, with larger areas of low signal present in the temporal lobe laterally. *B*, T$_2$-weighted image demonstrates serpiginous low signal in the cortex caused by hemosiderin deposition from chronic hemorrhage into the infarct.

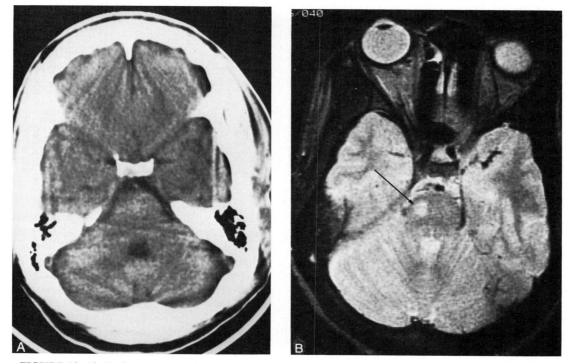

FIGURE 19–13. Brain stem contusion. *A*, CT scan reveals no abnormality of the brain stem. *B*, T$_2$-weighted image demonstrates high signal in the pons *(arrow)* from a bland contusion. (From Hesselink JR, Dowd CF, Healy ME, et al: MR imaging of brain contusions: A comparative study with CT. AJNR 9:269–278, 1988; © by American Society of Neuroradiology.)

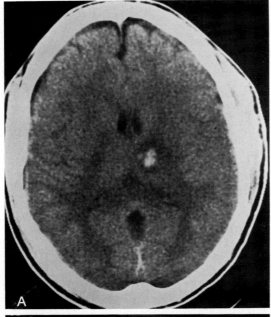

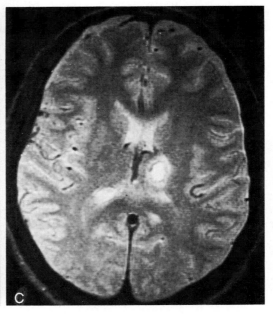

FIGURE 19–14. Hemorrhagic thalamic contusion. *A,* CT scan 2 days after injury reveals hemorrhage in the left thalamus. *B,* T_1-weighted image 13 days after injury shows high-signal methemoglobin from subacute hemorrhage. *C,* T_2-weighted image reveals high signal centrally with a low-signal rim from hemosiderin deposition, surrounded by higher signal edema. (From Hesselink JR, Dowd CF, Healy ME, et al: MR imaging of brain contusions: A comparative study with CT. AJNR 9:269–278, 1988; © by American Society of Neuroradiology.)

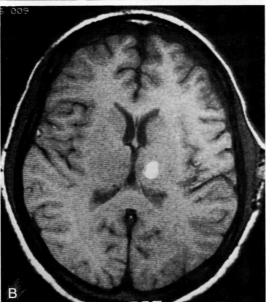

for both cortical contusions and shear injuries, but supplemental coronal views are helpful to assess injuries to the body of the corpus callosum and the inferior frontal and temporal lobes. Fast scan techniques or gradient-echo (GRE) images have lower resolution but are useful in uncooperative patients. Contrast enhancement has little role in the evaluation of brain contusions.

THE ROLE OF MR

There are indications that the added information provided by MR in many traumatic conditions is clinically useful. MR defines the exact extent of large collections and the presence of small collections better than CT, but to date very rarely has the surgical management of the patient been altered by this information. However, the medical management and prognosis of the patient have often been altered significantly by the additional information provided by MR.[4, 6] Diffuse axonal injuries have been associated with impaired consciousness and poor prognosis.[2, 5] Exact correlation of MR with clinical status has been variable. In a study of 20 patients with mild and moderate closed head injuries, lesions documented by MR correlated more closely with deficits on neuropsychologic testing than did lesions noted

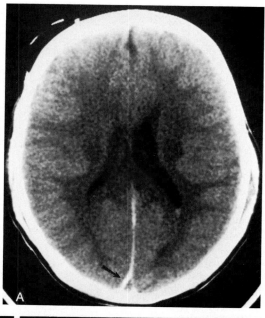

FIGURE 19–15. Shear injury of the corpus callosum, bilateral subdural hygromas, and small subdural hematoma. *A*, CT scan illustrates blood along the posterior falx *(arrow)*. No abnormality of the corpus callosum is identifiable. *B*, Proton density image demonstrates high-signal contusion in the splenium of the corpus callosum *(arrow)* and small right occipital subdural hematoma. Isointense subdural collections are present over the frontal lobes bilaterally, consistent with subdural hygromas *(arrowheads)*. *C*, T$_2$-weighted image demonstrates similar findings. (From Hesselink JR, Dowd CF, Healy ME, et al: MR imaging of brain contusions: A comparative study with CT. AJNR 9:269–278, 1988; © by American Society of Neuroradiology.)

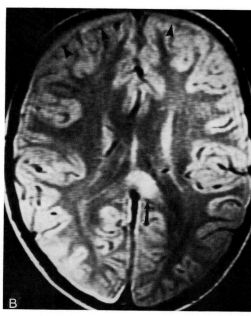

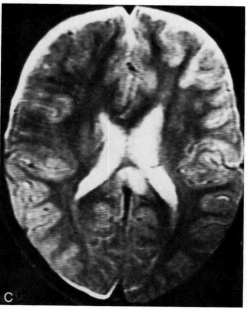

on CT.[15] Kelly and colleagues[6] studied 100 patients with head trauma, and in the 24 patients with post-traumatic syndrome (a constellation of complaints including headache, vertigo, memory loss, attention deficits, and emotional instability), all had normal findings on CT and MR.

Overall, most investigators feel that MR is superior to CT for imaging head trauma in all cases except acute (less than 48 to 72 hours) moderate to severe head trauma. In these cases, the ease and rapidity of obtaining a CT scan and its high sensitivity for acute hemorrhage make it the preferred imaging modality. The role of MR in symptomatic patients after minimal head trauma remains uncertain, given the high percentage of normal studies in these cases. MR is especially indicated in patients whose signs and symptoms are disproportionately greater than expected on the basis of CT findings.

INFLAMMATION

Inflammatory diseases of the brain include abscess, meningitis, encephalitis, and vasculitis. The brain is protected from invading infectious agents by the calvarium, dura, and blood-brain barrier. Moreover, the cerebral tissue itself is relatively resistant to infection. A common precursor to infection is infarction of tissue by arterial occlusion or venous thrombosis, leading to the formation of a culture medium composed of dead tissue.[1] Most pyogenic infections are hematogenous and related to septicemia and endocarditis. Direct extension from an infected paranasal sinus or middle ear or mastoid is less common than in the preantibiotic era.

Fungal infections are much less common than bacterial infections but are taking on more importance in patients with acquired immunodeficiency syndrome (AIDS) and those immunocompromised by way of chemotherapy, neoplasia, or immunosuppressive therapy for organ transplantation. Fungal infections may cause meningitis and meningoencephalitis, intracranial thrombophlebitis, brain abscesses, and mycotic aneurysms. The most common infections are cryptococcosis, coccidioidomycosis, mucormycosis, aspergillosis, and candidiasis.

The most important viral infections of the central nervous system (CNS) from an imaging point of view are aseptic meningitis, encephalitis, and progressive multifocal leukoencephalopathy (PML). Herpes simplex is responsible for a fulminant viral encephalitis, and both the human immunodeficiency virus (HIV) and cytomegalovirus (CMV) produce a white matter encephalitis associated with the AIDS epidemic.

ABSCESS

Bacterial

Brain abscesses may be related to infections of the paranasal sinuses, mastoids, and middle ears, as well as hematogenous seeding, but in 20 per cent of cases a source is not discovered. Very rarely an abscess is

secondary to meningitis. In children, more than 60 per cent of cerebral abscesses are associated with congenital heart disease and right-to-left shunts. Presenting symptoms of a cerebral abscess include headache, drowsiness, confusion, seizures, and focal neurologic deficits. Fever and leukocytosis are common during the invasive phase of a cerebral abscess but may resolve as the abscess becomes encapsulated. Organisms most frequently cultured from brain abscesses in otherwise immunocompetent individuals are staphylococci and streptococci.

When the brain is inoculated with a pathogen, a local cerebritis develops. Pathologically, an area of cerebritis consists of vascular congestion, petechial hemorrhage, and brain edema. The infection goes through a stage of cerebral softening, followed by liquefaction and central cavitation. With time, the central necrotic areas become confluent and are encapsulated after 1 to 2 weeks. Edema, a prominent feature of cerebral abscess, may actually subside after the capsule forms.

In the cerebritis stage, MR reveals high signal intensity on T_2-weighted images, both centrally from inflammation and peripherally from edema. Areas of low signal are variably imaged on T_1-weighted scans. As the progression to abscess ensues, there is further prolongation of T_1 and T_2 centrally. The capsule becomes highlighted as a relatively isointense structure containing and surrounded by low signal on T_1-weighted images and high signal on T_2-weighted images[16–18] (Figs. 19–16 and 19–17). Mottled areas of enhancement are seen on MR enhanced with gadolinium–diethylene triamine pentaacetic acid (Gd-DTPA) during the cerebritis stage, with an enhancing rim developing as the abscess matures

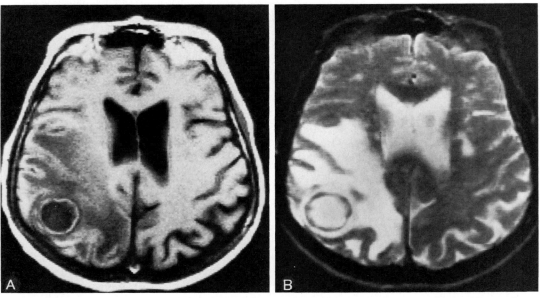

FIGURE 19–16. *Nocardia* **abscess in a patient taking steroids on a chronic basis.** *A*, T_1-weighted image shows central hypointense necrosis with isointense capsule surrounded by low-signal edema. *B*, T_2-weighted image reveals hypointense capsule highlighted by increased signal centrally and peripherally.

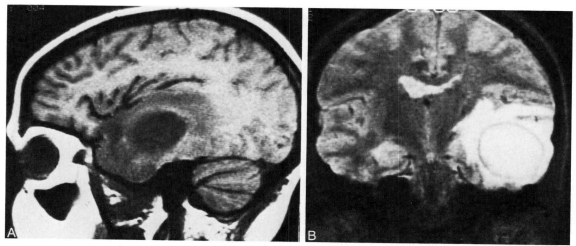

FIGURE 19–17. Left temporal lobe abscess. *A*, Sagittal T_1-weighted image demonstrates low-signal lesion with surrounding edema; a discrete capsule is not seen. *B*, Coronal T_2-weighted image reveals a well-defined capsule.

(Fig. 19–18). The enhancing rim may appear late in the cerebritis stage, prior to actual central necrosis.[18, 19] In some instances, the central area of necrosis has also enhanced on delayed scans, but not as commonly as is seen in necrotic tumors.

CT and MR have contributed significantly to decrease the mortality and morbidity of cerebral abscesses. First, they afford earlier diagnosis and therapy. Second, one can monitor the response to medical therapy, to determine if the therapy is effective or whether surgical drainage is necessary. Possible indications for surgery include an enlarging abscess, demonstration of a mature capsule, and proximity to a ventricle. Finally, it is possible to localize the abscess cavity accurately for surgery or CT- or MR-guided needle aspiration.

Fungal

Infection with fungal organisms can start as a meningitis or cerebral abscess, or the organisms can invade directly from an extracranial compartment. As mentioned previously, fungal infections are primarily found in immunocompromised hosts. In immunocompetent patients, fungal abscesses tend to evolve more slowly than bacterial abscesses, but that is not the case in patients with deficient immunity. In general, there are no specific MR imaging features to distinguish the infecting agent.

Coccidioidomycosis is endemic to the central valley regions of California and desert areas of the southwestern United States. Infection occurs by inhalation of dust from soil usually heavily infected with arthrospores. Primary coccidioidomycosis, a pulmonary infection, is followed by dissemination in only about 0.2 per cent of immunocompetent patients. CNS involvement most often is a meningitis, but cerebral abscess and granuloma formation can also occur (Fig. 19–19).

Mucormycosis is seen most often in patients with poorly controlled diabetes. It starts as a necrotizing vasculitis of the nose and sinuses and spreads by direct invasion of adjacent facial compartments. Extension into the intracranial cavity occurs through the cribriform plate, superior orbital fissure, and basal foramina or indirectly via involvement of vascular structures. Once within the intracranial cavity, it produces a purulent meningitis, cerebral infarction from arterial occlusion, and acute cerebritis resulting from direct invasion of the olfactory tracts and inferior frontal and temporal lobes. Cranial nerve involvement and cavernous sinus thrombosis are common.

The MR findings reflect the observed pathologic changes. Regions of meningeal and cerebral inflammation are hyperintense on T_2-weighted and proton density–weighted MR images. Infarction and edema account for additional high-signal parenchymal abnormalities. Gadolinium-enhanced T_1-weighted scans show enhancement of the basal meningeal inflammation, as well as the adjacent cerebral involvement. Coronal scans are especially helpful to display the relationships of the meningeal process to the brain and adjacent extracranial compartments.[20]

Aspergillosis is an aggressive opportunistic fungal infection. The organism gains entrance with inhalation of infected grains or dusts and results in primarily a pulmonary infection. Pathologic changes include a combination of suppuration and granulomas. Dissemination to the CNS may start as a basal meningitis, but the organism readily invades vascular structures and extends into the brain parenchyma.

Cysticercosis

Neurocysticercosis is the most frequently encountered parasitic infestation of the CNS. Originally

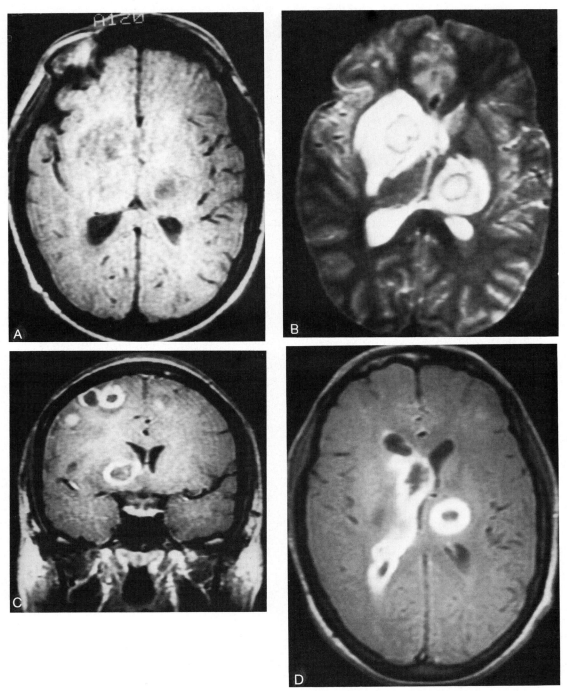

FIGURE 19–18. *Streptococcus* **abscess progressing to ependymitis.** *A*, Axial T_1-weighted image reveals areas of low signal adjacent to the frontal horn of the right lateral ventricle and in the left thalamus. *B*, Axial T_2-weighted image demonstrates capsules, heterogeneous central necrosis, and peripheral edema. *C*, Coronal T_1-weighted image with Gd-DTPA enhancement illustrates multiple enhancing rims and several homogeneous areas of enhancement consistent with cerebritis. *D*, Axial T_1-weighted image with Gd-DTPA enhancement 1 week later reveals extensive ependymal enhancement on the right from ependymitis. (Courtesy of Mark Healy, Mission Community Hospital, Mission Viejo, CA.)

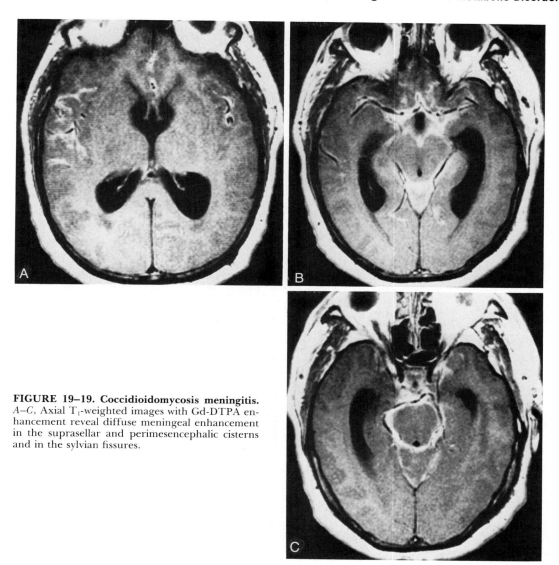

FIGURE 19–19. Coccidioidomycosis meningitis.
A–C, Axial T_1-weighted images with Gd-DTPA enhancement reveal diffuse meningeal enhancement in the suprasellar and perimesencephalic cisterns and in the sylvian fissures.

endemic in underdeveloped countries—predominantly Latin America, Africa, Asia, and some portions of eastern Europe—it is becoming increasingly frequent in North America in immigrant populations.[21, 22] Humans become accidental hosts for the larval stage of *Taenia solium*, the pork tapeworm, by ingesting contaminated material. The eggs hatch in the stomach, and larvae burrow through the gut wall and become distributed by the circulatory system. There is a predilection for involvement of the brain. Patients most often present with seizures, elevated intracranial pressure, focal neurologic abnormalities, and altered mental status. Asymptomatic infections are common.

Four forms of neurocysticercosis are described: meningeal, parenchymal, ventricular, and mixed. In all locations, death of the larva provokes a more intense inflammatory response and, in the case of an intraventricular lesion, may lead to ependymitis. Parenchymal lesions consist of small cysts, large cysts, and calcified lesions (Fig. 19–20). Small (approxi-

mately 1.5 cm in diameter) cysts may have a central area of relatively shorter T_1 (isointense or hyperintense to cortex) and are uniformly hyperintense on T_2-weighted images. Large (4 to 7 cm) cysts are usually multiloculated, are adjacent to the subarachnoid space, and may contain a mural nodule. The presence of a mural nodule or a T_2-hypointense rim in encapsulated lesions may correlate with larval death. Visualization of calcified lesions has been variable with MR; overall, there is an advantage for CT in this regard.[23, 24] Sometimes, calcified lesions are surrounded by edema, making them more conspicuous on MR. Basal cistern lesions can be difficult to identify but have been visualized as areas of intermediate signal intensity on T_1-weighted images. Intraventricular cysticercosis results in deformable and mobile cysts that may cause intermittent hydrocephalus. Rhee and associates[25] noted three of four lesions to be hypointense relative to CSF on heavily T_2-weighted images. Occasionally, they may appear relatively hyperintense to CSF on proton density se-

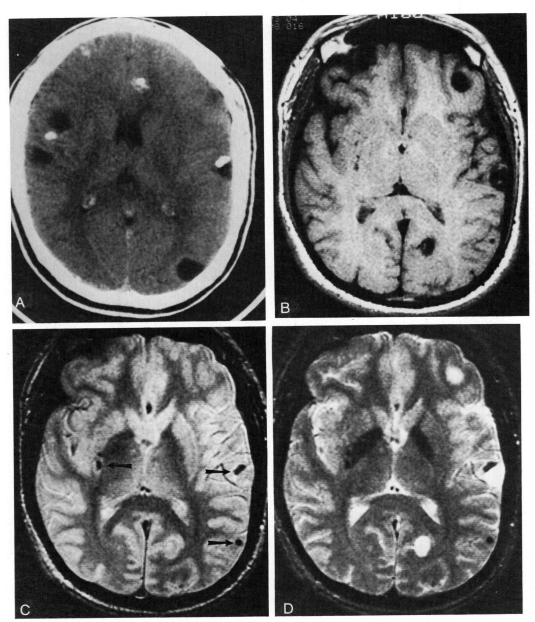

FIGURE 19–20. Parenchymal cysticercosis. *A,* CT scan demonstrates multiple parenchymal cysts, several of which are partially calcified. *B,* T₁-weighted image reveals areas of low signal in the left frontal, temporal, and occipital lobes. Calcifications are difficult to identify. *C,* Proton density image shows areas of calcification as low signal *(arrows)*. The cysts are isointense. *D,* T₂-weighted image reveals high signal within the parenchymal cysts.

quences. MR has the potential to replace ventriculography in the study of patients with intraventricular cysticercosis (Fig. 19–21).

MENINGITIS

Bacterial

Bacterial meningitis is an infection of the pia and arachnoid and adjacent CSF. The outer arachnoid serves as a barrier to the spread of infection, but involvement of the subdural space can occur, resulting in a subdural empyema. This complication is more common in children than adults. The most common organisms involved are *Haemophilus influenzae*, *Neisseria meningitidis*, and *Diplococcus pneumoniae*. Patients present with fever, headache, seizures, altered consciousness, and neck stiffness. The overall mortality ranges from 5 to 15 per cent for *H. influenzae* and meningococcal meningitis to as high as 30 per cent for pneumococcal meningitis. In addition,

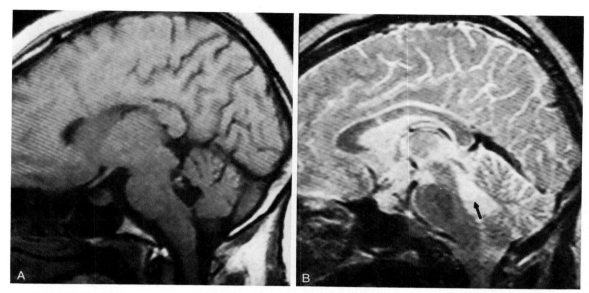

FIGURE 19–21. Intraventricular cysticercosis. *A*, Sagittal T_1-weighted image shows the fourth ventricle to be enlarged, with abnormal increased signal within it superiorly. The patient had previously been shunted for hydrocephalus. *B*, T_2-weighted image reveals mildly hyperintense cyst in the fourth ventricle *(arrow)*.

persistent neurologic deficits are found in 10 per cent of children after *H. influenzae* meningitis and in 30 per cent of patients with pneumococcal meningitis.[1]

The ability of nonenhanced MR to image meningitis is extremely limited, and the majority of patients appear to have normal findings or mild hydrocephalus. In severe cases, the basal cisterns may be completely obliterated, with high signal intensity replacing the normal CSF signal on proton density images. Intermediate signal intensity may be seen in the basal cisterns on T_1-weighted images in these cases.[16] Infection within the ventricles, caused by either direct extension from a shunt or abscess or progression of meningitis, may lead to ependymitis, resulting in hyperintensity outlining the ventricles on T_2-weighted images and enhancement of the ependyma on T_1-weighted images with Gd-DTPA (see Fig. 19–19). Subdural empyemas are better seen with MR than with CT, and the signal characteristics of the exudate in subdural empyema (higher signal than CSF) help to differentiate it from benign extraaxial collections.[26]

As mentioned previously, the meningeal inflammation may produce a basal arachnoiditis with obstruction of CSF pathways and communicating hydrocephalus. If there is an associated ventriculitis, a noncommunicating hydrocephalus can develop. Adhesions and loculated CSF collections can occur in the basal cisterns. Moreover, cerebral infarction can result from congestion in leptomeningeal vessels, cortical vein thrombosis, or vasculitis. If left untreated, a meningitis may evolve into a cerebritis and cerebral abscess.

Thrombophlebitis of the dural sinuses can occur as a complication of meningitis or direct spread of adjacent infection. The lateral and sigmoid sinuses in particular may be affected by infections in the middle ear and mastoid. The clinical and imaging features of dural sinus thrombosis are discussed in Chapter 17.

Tuberculosis

Tuberculous meningitis remains an important discrete entity, becoming more common as an infectious agent in AIDS patients. As a rule, the evolution is less rapid than in pyogenic infections. Vasculitis and cerebral infarction, caused by inflammatory changes in the basal cisterns, are more prevalent. The MR features of tuberculous meningitis are similar to those of bacterial meningitis, but the chronic inflammation induces thick granulation tissue that produces a more striking enhancement pattern. Actual intracranial tuberculomas are rare in the United States. Mature tuberculomas are T_2 hypointense. Central necrosis in some lesions results in a T_2-bright core with a rim of low signal intensity.[27]

Sarcoidosis

Sarcoidosis is a granulomatous disease of unknown etiology. In approximately 5 per cent of cases, the CNS is involved as a granulomatous infiltration of the meninges and underlying parenchyma, most notably at the base of the brain. It may also affect cranial or peripheral nerves as isolated disease. Cranial nerve palsies, chronic meningitis, and hypothalamic-pituitary dysfunction are frequent manifestations.[28]

Experience with MR in intracranial sarcoidosis has been relatively limited.[29, 30] MR is well suited to imaging focal pituitary and hypothalamic lesions and the white matter lesions that have been noted in these patients. The basal cisterns may enhance in patients with meningeal sarcoidosis, but a nodular pattern

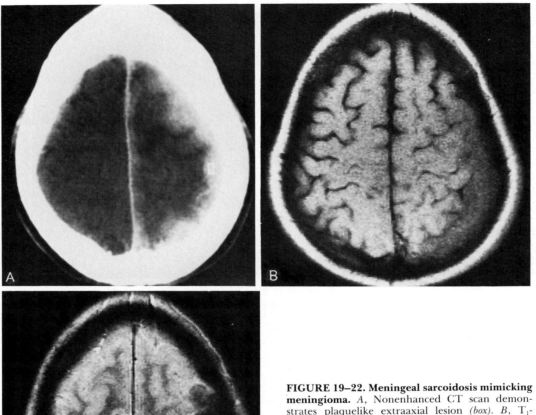

FIGURE 19–22. Meningeal sarcoidosis mimicking meningioma. *A*, Nonenhanced CT scan demonstrates plaquelike extraaxial lesion *(box)*. *B*, T_1-weighted image reveals lesion to be mildly hypointense. *C*, T_2-weighted image demonstrates marked hypointensity of the lesion. Sarcoidosis was found at surgery. (MR images courtesy of Paul Markarian, M.D., Mercy Hospital, Springfield, MA.)

usually distinguishes it from the infectious varieties. A particularly interesting form of meningeal sarcoid results in thick meningeal plaques, often over the convexities. These may mimic meningiomas in that they remain isointense or hypointense relative to cortex on T_2-weighted as well as T_1-weighted images (Fig. 19–22).

Neurosyphilis

The most important feature of neurosyphilis is its meningeal involvement, presenting early as meningitis and meningovascular syphilis and later as tabes dorsalis and meningomyelitis. Meningovascular syphilis consists of inflammatory reaction in the walls of subarachnoid vessels and their accompanying Virchow-Robin spaces. This reaction leads to wall thick-

ening, vessel narrowing, and occlusion. Angiography demonstrates areas of narrowing in the large and medium-sized vessels at the base of the brain. These vascular changes cannot be reliably imaged by MR at this point. However, MR clearly displays the multiple small areas of ischemia or infarction, suggesting the diagnosis of vasculitis.[31]

ENCEPHALITIS

Acute encephalitis of the nonherpetic type manifests with signs and symptoms similar to those of meningitis, but with the added features of any combination of convulsions, delirium, altered consciousness, aphasia, hemiparesis, ataxia, ocular palsies, and facial weakness. The major causative agents are arthropod-borne arboviruses (eastern and western equine encephalitis, St. Louis encephalitis, California virus encephalitis). Eastern equine encephalitis is the most serious but fortunately also the least frequent of the arbovirus infections.

Brain stem encephalitis is a reversible syndrome, usually presenting with midbrain signs, especially ophthalmoplegia, and followed by rostrocaudal progression. Most patients have a preceding respiratory illness. CT findings are most often normal, but MR may show lesions with increased T_2 signal in the brain stem.[32] Occasionally, there may be frank enlargement of the midbrain and pons.

Herpes Simplex

Herpes simplex is the most common and gravest form of acute encephalitis, with a 30 to 70 per cent fatality rate and an equally high morbidity rate. It is almost always caused by type 1 virus, except in neonates, in whom type 2 predominates. Symptoms may reflect the propensity to involve the inferomedial frontal and temporal lobes—hallucinations, seizures, personality changes, and aphasia. For medical therapy to be effective, it must be instituted within 5 days of the onset of the illness. Since the medical therapy produces its own morbidity, brain biopsy is usually performed before starting therapy. Therefore, early detection by imaging studies is critical.

MR has demonstrated positive findings in viral encephalitis as soon as 2 days after symptoms, more quickly and definitively than CT. Early involvement of the limbic system and temporal lobes is characteristic of herpes simplex encephalitis. The cortical abnormalities are first noted as ill-defined areas of high signal on T_2-weighted scans, usually beginning unilaterally but progressing to become bilateral[16, 26] (Figs. 19–23 and 19–24). Edema, mass effect, and gyral enhancement may also be present. Since MR is more sensitive than CT for detecting these early changes of encephalitis, it is hoped that it will improve the prognosis of this devastating disease.

Acute Disseminated Encephalomyelitis

Acute disseminated encephalomyelitis is an acute demyelinating disease thought to represent an immune-mediated complication of infection, rather than a direct viral infection of the CNS. It is also known as postinfectious encephalitis. The clinical presentation is one of confusion, seizures, headaches, and fevers. Ataxia may occur. Spinal cord involvement may lead to paraplegia or quadriplegia. The most common viral diseases implicated are measles, rubella, smallpox, and chickenpox. It is occasionally seen after vaccination or nondescript respiratory infections.

MR demonstrates lesions in the cerebrum, cerebellum, and brain stem, often while CT is normal or nondiagnostic. The lesions may be patchy and may involve the deep and subcortical white matter. Clinical findings have correlated with the location of lesions shown by MR, and progressive resolution has occurred concurrently with clinical improvement[33, 34] (Figs. 19–25 and 19–26).

AIDS-RELATED INFECTIONS

AIDS results in neurologic symptoms in approximately one third of patients.[35, 36] The most commonly reported CNS complications include opportunistic fungal, viral, and protozoan infections and lymphoma. Recently, direct infection of the CNS with HIV has been reported.[37, 38] In one of the largest reviews of the neurologic manifestations of AIDS,[39] of a total of 315 patients with CNS complications,

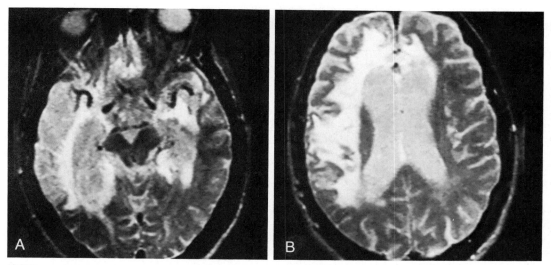

FIGURE 19–23. Herpes simplex encephalitis. *A* and *B*, T_2-weighted images demonstrate increased signal in virtually the entire right temporal lobe and medial portion of the left temporal lobe. The involvement of the right frontal lobe spares portions of the cortex.

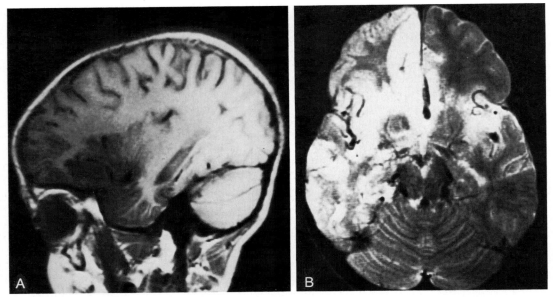

FIGURE 19–24. Herpes simplex encephalitis. *A*, Sagittal T_1-weighted image reveals abnormal signal in the left temporal lobe and operculum. *B*, Axial T_2-weighted image shows asymmetric involvement, with more extensive signal abnormality in the right temporal and frontal lobes.

viral syndromes were seen in 94 patients. These consisted of subacute encephalitis (54), atypical septic meningitis (21), herpes simplex encephalitis (9), PML (6), viral myelitis (3), and varicella-zoster encephalitis (1). Nonviral infections included those caused by *Toxoplasma gondii* (103), *Cryptococcus neoformans* (41), *Candida albicans* (6), mycobacteria (6), *Treponema pallidum* (2), and *Mycobacterium tuberculosis, Aspergillus,* and *Escherichia coli* (1 each). Neoplasms included primary CNS lymphoma (15), systemic lymphoma with CNS involvement (12), and metastatic Kaposi's sarcoma (3). Cranial and peripheral nerve complications were seen in 51 patients. Many of these neuropathies, as well as the cases of subacute encephalitis and atypical septic meningitis, may have been due to direct infection with HIV.

Toxoplasmosis

Toxoplasma gondii, a protozoan, is the most common opportunistic infection in AIDS patients, accounting for between 13.4 per cent[40] and 33 per cent[39] of all CNS complications. Haitian AIDS patients appear to be particularly susceptible to this infection. The characteristic MR appearance is multiple ring-enhancing lesions located at the corticomedullary junction, but the basal ganglia and white matter are also frequently involved. The amount of peripheral edema is variable. Earlier in the evolution of the abscesses, the nodule may exhibit more homogeneous enhancement with little mass effect or edema (Figs. 19–27 to 19–29). In general, fungal abscesses evolve more slowly than bacterial ones, but in immunocompromised individuals, the fungal lesions can be quite aggressive.[41, 42] Dual infections are common in AIDS

patients. In such cases, invariably one of the pathogens is *Toxoplasma gondii.*[39] Toxoplasmosis may also coexist with lymphoma. Another confounding fact is that the inflammatory reaction to toxoplasmosis may mimic lymphoma on biopsy or CSF cytology.[43]

Cryptococcosis

Cryptococcosis is the most common CNS fungal infection in AIDS, occurring in 8.7 to 13 per cent of patients.[39, 40] *Cryptococcus neoformans* has a peculiar propensity to affect individuals with deficiencies in cell-mediated immunity, and it usually produces a meningitis. CSF antibody titers are not always reliable for diagnosis because the immune response in AIDS patients is so variable. Imaging studies may be negative or may show only mild ventricular dilatation. Since cerebral atrophy is common in AIDS patients, distinguishing central atrophy from hydrocephalus is not always easy, and sometimes follow-up studies or correlation with the clinical picture is necessary. Meningeal enhancement is not often present unless a chronic inflammation has developed. A chronic relapsing infection can result in cryptococcal brain abscesses (Fig. 19–30).

Progressive Multifocal Leukoencephalopathy (PML)

PML is a disorder characterized by widespread foci of demyelination caused by reactivation of a latent papovavirus. Most cases occur in immunocompromised hosts secondary to neoplasia, chemotherapy, and, increasingly, AIDS. The lesions are initially round or oval, becoming larger and more confluent

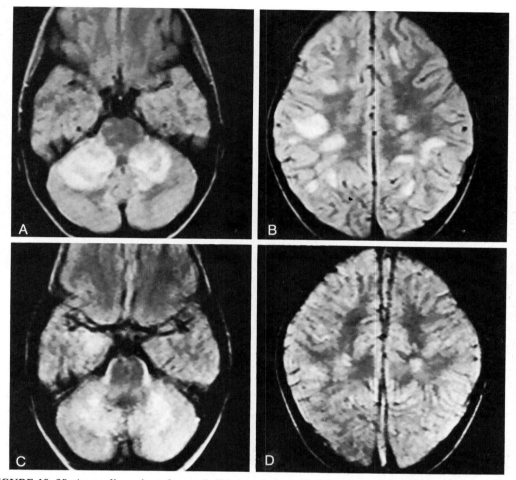

FIGURE 19–25. Acute disseminated encephalitis in a 4-year-old child who presented with cerebellar signs after an upper respiratory infection. *A,* T$_2$-weighted image reveals abnormal signal in the middle cerebellar peduncles and adjacent cerebellar hemispheres. *B,* T$_2$-weighted image illustrates subcortical white matter abnormalities in both cerebral hemispheres. *C* and *D,* T$_2$-weighted images 2 months later reveal marked improvement, correlating with the patient's clinical condition.

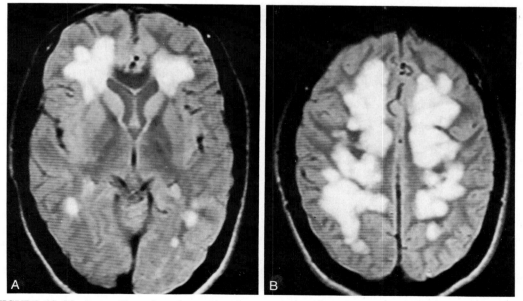

FIGURE 19–26. Acute disseminated encephalitis. *A* and *B,* Proton density images demonstrate multiple confluent lesions in the periventricular white matter and centrum semiovale.

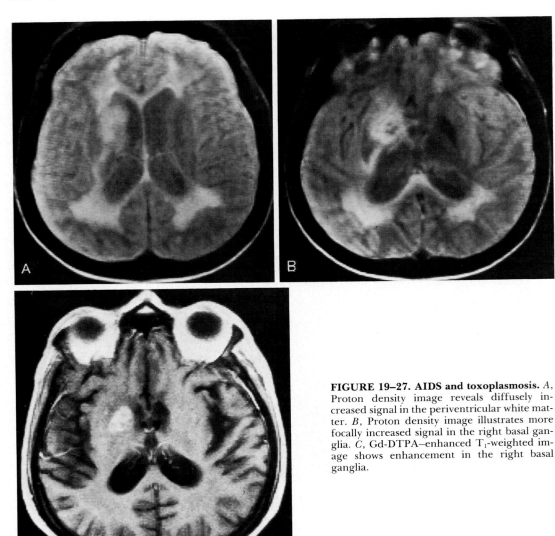

FIGURE 19–27. AIDS and toxoplasmosis. *A*, Proton density image reveals diffusely increased signal in the periventricular white matter. *B*, Proton density image illustrates more focally increased signal in the right basal ganglia. *C*, Gd-DTPA–enhanced T_1-weighted image shows enhancement in the right basal ganglia.

with time.[44] Subcortical white matter may be the first area of involvement, with later spread to the deeper white matter. The pattern is often asymmetric (Fig. 19–31). The MR appearance reflects the long T_1 and long T_2 of the lesions, typically without mass effect (see Fig. 18–9). The high T_2 signal is related to both demyelination and edema. These lesions do not usually enhance on CT, and preliminary experience with MR suggests that most do not enhance with Gd-DTPA.

Human Immunodeficiency Virus/Cytomegalovirus Encephalitis

More recently, interest has centered on a subacute encephalitis involving the white matter because of its association with HIV infection of the brain[45] and

correlation with a primary AIDS dementia complex.[46, 47] Subacute encephalitis is seen in up to 30 per cent of patients with AIDS, and CMV may be the causal agent in some cases. Levy and associates[39] reported that 54 (17 per cent) of 315 patients in their clinical series had subacute encephalitis. In another series,[40] 31.4 per cent had microglial nodular encephalitis suggesting HIV, and CMV was found in only 14.4 per cent of those cases. The two viruses often coexist in brain specimens taken from AIDS patients.

In a study of 21 patients with HIV encephalitis,[48] both CT and MR were found to be relatively insensitive to the early stages of involvement, manifested pathologically by widespread microscopic microglial nodules with multinucleated giant cells. The secondary changes of atrophy were well seen by both modalities in the majority of patients, while parenchymal lesions consistent with demyelination were noted in

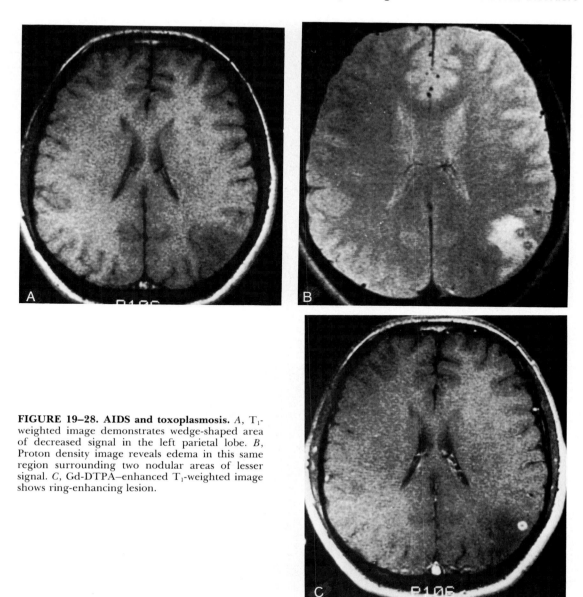

FIGURE 19–28. AIDS and toxoplasmosis. *A*, T_1-weighted image demonstrates wedge-shaped area of decreased signal in the left parietal lobe. *B*, Proton density image reveals edema in this same region surrounding two nodular areas of lesser signal. *C*, Gd-DTPA–enhanced T_1-weighted image shows ring-enhancing lesion.

three of seven patients studied by MR. In this same study, CT was superior to nonenhanced MR for the detection of one case of HIV encephalitis.

Correlative radiologic-pathologic studies in our laboratory also revealed that MR has difficulty in detecting microglial nodules, unless they occur in clusters. The problem in detecting microglial nodules is probably due to their small size (50 to 100 μm). The in-plane resolution of MR images is about 0.7 mm (700 μm), and the 5-mm-thick sections are subject to partial volume effects from adjacent normal brain parenchyma. This finding is supported by the fact that the microglial nodules (with associated infarction or necrosis) detected by MR in our series were large clusters of microglial nodules, greater than 3 mm.

As is evident from the preceding discussion, CNS

pathology in AIDS is quite varied. MR is assuming an increasingly important role in the diagnostic work-up of these patients. T_2-weighted images are most sensitive for detecting the brain abnormalities. MR is especially better than CT for assessing white matter diseases and other abnormalities with an intact blood-brain barrier.[49] Contrast enhancement is helpful for differentiating lesions from surrounding edema, discriminating between lesions in close proximity, judging lesion activity, and defining small cortical lesions with minimal edema.

The problem in interpreting MR images in AIDS patients has been the lack of specificity of the findings, the frequent coexistence of different pathologies, and the relatively infrequent pathologic proof. Jarvik and associates[50] describe four patterns of signal abnormality with corresponding pathology. The best

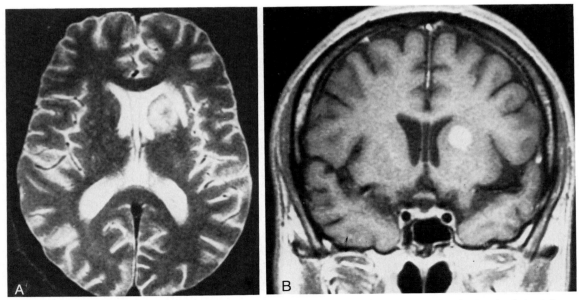

FIGURE 19–29. Toxoplasmosis. *A*, T₂-weighted image reveals high-signal edema in the head of the left caudate nucleus and adjacent external capsule. *B*, Coronal Gd-DTPA–enhanced image shows enhancement of central area, with slight mass effect on the adjacent ventricle. Incidentally noted is a cavum septi pellucidi.

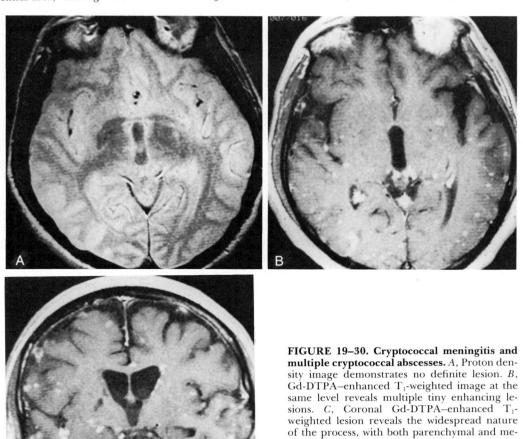

FIGURE 19–30. Cryptococcal meningitis and multiple cryptococcal abscesses. *A*, Proton density image demonstrates no definite lesion. *B*, Gd-DTPA–enhanced T₁-weighted image at the same level reveals multiple tiny enhancing lesions. *C*, Coronal Gd-DTPA–enhanced T₁-weighted lesion reveals the widespread nature of the process, with both parenchymal and meningeal enhancement.

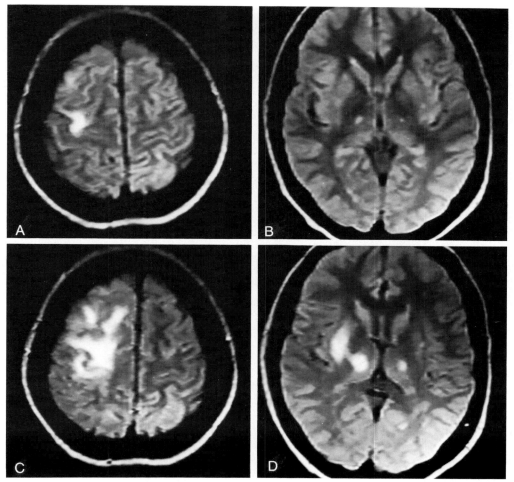

FIGURE 19–31. Progressive multifocal leukoencephalopathy. *A* and *B*, Proton density images reveal lesions in the right frontal subcortical white matter and posterolateral thalamus bilaterally. *C* and *D*, Proton density images 2 months later demonstrate progression of the previously noted lesions and a new area of signal abnormality in the right putamen. No mass effect is present.

correlation was that between a pattern of multiple, small, discrete foci of high signal intensity and toxoplasmosis and PML. Toxoplasmosis lesions tended to be heterogeneous with discrete margins, and PML lesions were homogeneous with indistinct margins. In addition, PML involves the subcortical white matter and only rarely enhances. Another differentiating feature is the lack of mass effect with PML. Lymphoma can mimic toxoplasmosis in AIDS patients. Less common infections, such as aspergillosis and tuberculosis, are occasionally encountered. Other patterns described had more limited pathologic proof. Large, bilateral, patchy to confluent lesions in white matter were seen with encephalitis from CMV and HIV (Fig. 19–32). Solitary lesions with high T_2 signal were due to nonviral opportunistic infections. The final pattern of atrophy was associated with chronic HIV infections, as described earlier. With further experience with Gd-DTPA in these patients,

additional differentiating features should be forthcoming.

Olsen and coworkers[51] found white matter abnormalities in 31 per cent of the AIDS patients that they studied. Clinical findings and course were used to determine the exact etiology in most instances, as pathologic material was available in a minority of cases. They reported patterns of signal abnormality and clinical correlations similar to those described previously. Diffuse, widespread involvement correlated with AIDS dementia complex. Rarely, punctate or patchy lesions were noted with AIDS dementia complex. Focal white matter lesions were noted in all six patients with PML, two patients with lymphoma, and one patient with toxoplasmosis. Focal white matter lesions were not seen with AIDS dementia complex. Clinical features may also be a differentiating feature in that only 2 of 33 patients with AIDS dementia complex had focal neurologic findings.

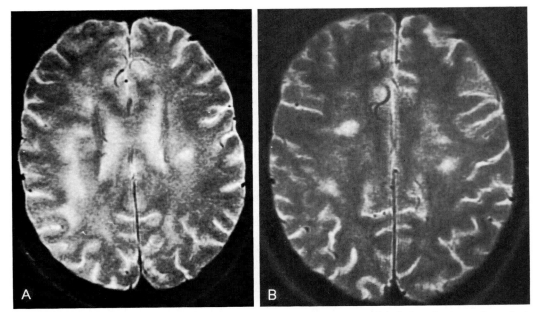

FIGURE 19–32. HIV encephalitis. *A,* T$_2$-weighted image demonstrates multiple lesions in the periventricular white matter, becoming confluent in the right hemisphere. *B,* A higher image reveals more focal abnormalities in the centrum semiovale.

DEGENERATIVE DISEASES

Imaging of degenerative disorders with CT has generally been disappointing, and attempts have been made to apply MR to this area with hopes of demonstrating more specific findings. The key to the MR imaging of many of these disorders may rest in understanding the normal and pathologic distribution of iron in the brain. Iron is visualized as areas of hypointensity on T$_2$-weighted and GRE images caused by local field inhomogeneity and magnetic susceptibility effects. Drayer and colleagues[52] noted decreased signal in the globus pallidus, reticular substantia nigra, red nucleus, and dentate nucleus (Fig. 19–33). These areas correlated closely with sites of preferential accumulation of ferric iron on Perls' stains in normal brains post mortem. This iron deposition becomes greater with increasing age, with iron stains first becoming positive at 6 months in the globus pallidum and at 3 to 7 years in the dentate

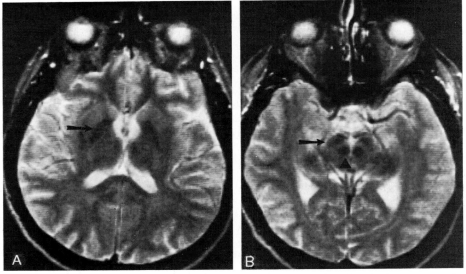

FIGURE 19–33. Normal iron deposition in a 36-year-old man. *A,* T$_2$-weighted image demonstrates decreased T$_2$ signal in the globus pallidus *(arrow). B,* T$_2$-weighted image reveals decreased signal from iron deposition in the reticular portion of the substantia nigra *(arrow)* and red nucleus *(arrowhead).*

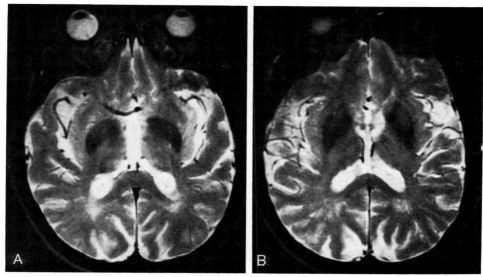

FIGURE 19–34. Normal iron deposition in an 80-year-old man. *A* and *B*, T$_2$-weighted images show profound hypointensity in both the globus pallidus and the putamen bilaterally.

nucleus. With advanced age (approximately the ninth decade), there may be enough iron deposition in the putamen to render it as hypointense as the globus pallidus (Fig. 19–34).

Iron may play a role in neurotransmitter metabolism, and several degenerative disorders have been reported to be associated with increased iron deposition in the brain. This has been described in Hallervorden-Spatz disease, Huntington's chorea, Parkinson's disease and multisystem atrophy variants, Alzheimer's disease, and multiple sclerosis.[53]

PARKINSONISM

Parkinson's disease begins most frequently in persons between 40 and 70 years of age. The characteristic features include slowness of movement, poverty of facial expression, flexed posture, immobility, and static tremor. Pathologically, there is a loss of pigmented cells in the pars compacta of the substantia nigra. Parkinson plus syndromes include patients with more severe symptoms and lesser responses to drug therapy. These syndromes include striatonigral degeneration, Shy-Drager orthostatic hypotension (multiple system atrophy), olivopontocerebellar atrophy, and progressive supranuclear palsy[54–56] (Fig. 19–35).

Generalized atrophy with prominent sulci and arachnoid spaces is a common finding in these patients, and the only finding identified with CT in most cases. MR has revealed areas of hypointensity, which appear to correlate with sites of iron deposition. Findings that have been described include hypointensity of the putamen, a return to normal signal intensity rather than the usual low signal intensity of the dorsolateral aspect of the substantia nigra, and narrowing of the band of relatively increased signal

between the hypointense red nucleus and the pars reticulata of the substantia nigra. This last finding corresponds anatomically with the pars compacta of the substantia nigra. Varying levels of significance have been reported for these findings in different studies, with the putaminal hypointensity being least significant and the narrowing of the pars compacta appearing to be the most significant.[57–59]

Initial studies suggested that the putaminal changes were more frequent in Parkinson plus syndromes, but this has not been found to be the case in a more recent study by Rutledge and associates.[58]

In progressive supranuclear palsy, atrophy of the

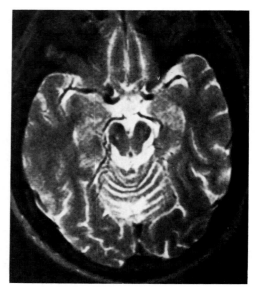

FIGURE 19–35. Progressive supranuclear palsy. Axial T$_2$-weighted scan discloses atrophy of the midbrain, with prominence of the perimesencephalic cisterns.

midbrain is present. Tissue loss involving the medulla, pons, brachium pontis, and cerebellum is noted in olivopontocerebellar atrophy.

ALZHEIMER'S DISEASE

Alzheimer's disease (including senile and presenile forms) is the most common and important of the degenerative diseases of the brain. Most affected patients are in their fifties or sixties. The incidence of moderate to severe dementia over the age of 60 has been estimated to be approximately 5 per cent, and 60 per cent of these cases are the result of Alzheimer's disease.[60] Disorders of memory are first noted, with language disturbances and visuospatial disorientation following. CT reveals enlargement of the ventricular system and cortical sulci, but this is usually not significantly different from that in age-matched controls. The real utility of CT in Alzheimer's disease lies in the exclusion of other treatable disorders. MR reveals the same atrophic changes but can better image focal enlargement of the temporal horns of the lateral ventricles, correlating with hippocampal atrophy (Fig. 19–36). This atrophy is best seen in the coronal plane. Areas of increased T_2 signal were identified in 5 of 12 patients with Alzheimer's disease by Fazekas and associates.[60] In that particular study, there was no difference in the frequency of periventricular and deep white matter T_2-hyperintense lesions between controls and patients with Alzheimer's disease. A more extensive smooth halo of periventricular hyperintensity was noted in 50 per cent of patients with Alzheimer's disease compared with controls. Although there are few specific findings in Alzheimer's disease, the absence of white matter abnormality, hydrocephalus, mass lesion, or metabolic disorder in a demented patient strongly indicates Alzheimer's or Parkinson's disease.

PICK'S DISEASE

Pick's disease has symptoms largely indistinguishable from those of Alzheimer's disease, although focal disturbances may be more common in Pick's disease. There is striking atrophy of both gray and white matter, typically involving the inferior frontal and temporal lobes.[1]

HUNTINGTON'S CHOREA

Huntington's chorea is characterized by a dominant inheritance of dementia and choreoathetosis. It most often manifests in the fourth and fifth decades.[1] Atrophy of the head of the caudate nucleus and putamen bilaterally and moderate frontotemporal atrophy produce findings identifiable with both CT and MR[61] (Fig. 19–37). The ease of coronal imaging with MR and the greater gray-white matter contrast result in some advantages over CT in diagnosing this condition, but there are no specific MR signal abnormalities in Huntington's chorea.

METABOLIC DISORDERS

CENTRAL PONTINE MYELINOLYSIS

Central pontine myelinolysis is a disorder characterized pathologically by dissolution of the myelin sheaths of fibers within the central aspect of the basis pontis. In extreme cases, there may be extension to the pontine tegmentum, midbrain, thalamus, internal capsule, and cerebral cortex.[1] Many patients are asymptomatic, and at the other extreme are patients whose symptoms are masked by coma. Most patients with clinically diagnosed cases present with spastic quadriparesis, pseudobulbar palsy, and acute changes

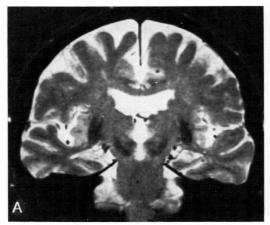
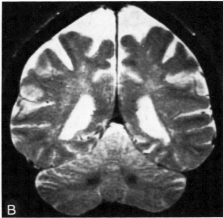

FIGURE 19–36. Alzheimer's disease. *A* and *B*, Coronal images show moderate to severe cortical atrophy. The lateral and third ventricles are also dilated, indicating central atrophy as well. The temporal horns are not enlarged, but the hippocampal structures are small.

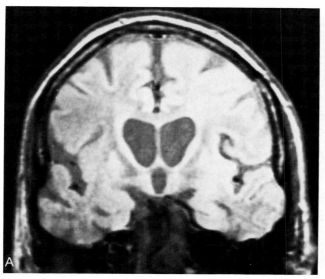
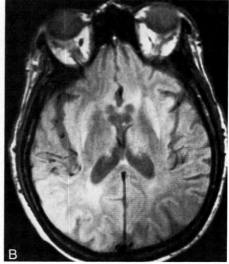

FIGURE 19–37. Huntington's disease. *A*, A coronal proton density–weighted scan demonstrates atrophy of the caudate nuclei, associated with dilatation of the frontal horns of the lateral ventricles. *B*, On an axial scan, the putamen is also small and atrophic bilaterally.

in mental status, with possible progression to altered levels of consciousness and death. Survival is possible, with varying residual neurologic deficits. Although initial reports were largely confined to chronic alcoholics, central pontine myelinolysis has also been seen in patients with electrolyte disturbances, particularly hyponatremia, which has been rapidly corrected.

Use of MR has increased the number of patients with central pontine myelinolysis and abnormal imaging studies. In a study by Miller and colleagues[62] of 13 patients with central pontine myelinolysis (5 diagnosed clinically, 8 diagnosed at autopsy), only 1 of 9 CT examinations were abnormal, while 10 of 11 patients had abnormal MR studies. The lesions on MR were best seen as areas of hypointensity on inversion recovery (IR) images and hyperintensity on T_2-weighted images in the central pons, with sparing of the pontine tegmentum and ventrolateral pons. All lesions had an oval shape on sagittal images, a batwing configuration on coronal images, and various shapes on the axial images (Fig. 19–38). Associated lesions were noted in three patients in the periventricular white matter, basal ganglia, and corticomedullary junction. In looking for possible mimicking lesions in other groups of patients, a pontine lesion was noted in 5 per cent of patients with supratentorial white matter disease. This combination of prominent supratentorial disease with pontine lesions was not noted in patients with central pontine myelinolysis, and this may be a differentiating feature. Follow-up scans at 6 months and 1 year revealed little or no change despite clinical recovery. Pathologically involved areas correlate with the areas of MR signal abnormality.[62, 63]

LEIGH'S DISEASE

Leigh's disease (subacute necrotizing encephalomyelopathy) is a familial disorder with autosomal recessive inheritance. Onset is usually in the first year of life in more than half of cases, but occasionally it can first manifest in adulthood.[1] Presenting signs and symptoms range from hypotonia, seizures, and myoclonic jerks in the first year of life to ataxia, dysarthria, and nystagmus in the second year. Death, most often from respiratory failure, usually occurs before 3 years of age. The exact biochemical defect remains unknown but may involve pyruvate metabolism. Bilaterally symmetric foci of necrosis and spongiform degeneration are noted pathologically. CT has revealed symmetric areas of decreased attenuation in the basal ganglia, brain stem, and cerebellum. MR has shown these same lesions as areas of increased T_2 signal (Fig. 19–39) and has also shown involvement of the tectum, tegmentum, and medullary olive in instances when CT has revealed normal findings in these areas.[64, 65]

WILSON'S DISEASE

Wilson's disease (hepatolenticular degeneration) is an autosomal recessive disorder of copper metabolism. Onset of symptoms is usually during the second or third decade. The classic syndrome is dysphagia, slowness and rigidity of movements, dysarthria, and tremor. Pathologic changes primarily involve the lentiform nuclei and range from frank cavitation to softening and atrophy. MR has demonstrated abnor-

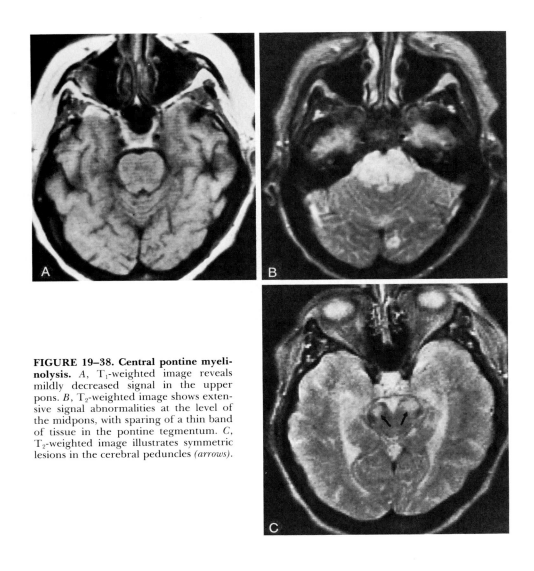

FIGURE 19–38. Central pontine myelinolysis. *A*, T$_1$-weighted image reveals mildly decreased signal in the upper pons. *B*, T$_2$-weighted image shows extensive signal abnormalities at the level of the midpons, with sparing of a thin band of tissue in the pontine tegmentum. *C*, T$_2$-weighted image illustrates symmetric lesions in the cerebral peduncles *(arrows)*.

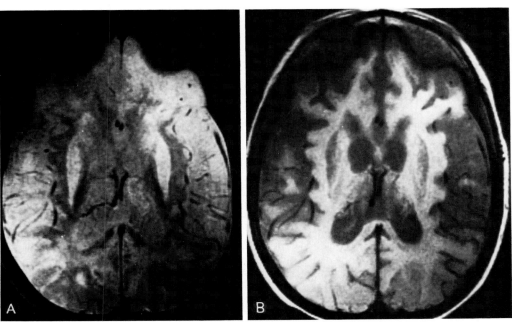

FIGURE 19–39. Leigh's disease. *A*, Axial T$_2$-weighted scan reveals high-signal abnormalities within the basal ganglia bilaterally. *B*, On a T$_1$-weighted scan, the lesions are distinctly hypointense and heterogeneous, consistent with necrosis of brain tissue. Also note the profound cortical atrophy.

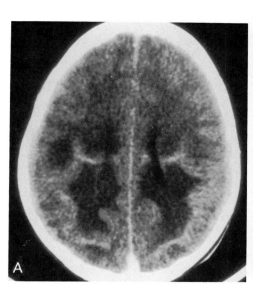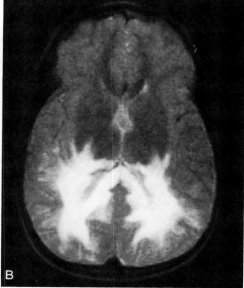

FIGURE 19–40. Adrenoleukodystrophy. *A,* CT scan of a young child demonstrates bilateral hypodense areas within the white matter of the occipital and posterior parietal lobes. The involvement is relatively symmetric and confluent. *B,* A T₂-weighted MR scan in the same child shows hyperintensity in the same areas of the posterior cerebral white matter. The posterior temporal lobe is also involved, and the abnormality extends into the splenium of the corpus callosum.

mally increased T_2 signal in the putamen and caudate most commonly but also in the thalamus, dentate nuclei, midbrain, and subcortical white matter. Generalized atrophy and ventricular dilatation are seen as well.[66, 67] In a study of 22 patients by Starosta-Rubinstein and associates,[67] lesions in the putamen and caudate correlated well with clinical findings.

HALLERVORDEN-SPATZ DISEASE

Hallervorden-Spatz disease is a progressive movement disorder in which there is abnormal iron deposition in the globus pallidus, reticular zone of the substantia nigra, and red nucleus.[68] It is inherited as an autosomal recessive trait. Onset is in late childhood or early adolescence, with both corticospinal and pyramidal motor findings. MR has revealed decreased T_2 signal in the lentiform nuclei and perilentiform white matter, related to this excess iron deposition. Areas of increased signal in the periventricular white matter have been noted, and these may correlate with disordered myelination. Disproportionate atrophy of the brain stem and cerebellum is also seen.[68, 69]

ADRENOLEUKODYSTROPHY

Adrenoleukodystrophy is a metabolic encephalopathy affecting boys between the ages of 4 and 8 years in the classic form. The neurologic findings of behavioral problems, intellectual impairment, and long

tract signs can appear before or after adrenal gland insufficiency. Several forms have been described, some of which can manifest later in life. Degeneration of myelin, often asymmetric, occurs in various parts of the cerebrum, brain stem, optic nerves, and sometimes spinal cord.[1] The typical CT findings are large, symmetric, low-density lesions with peripheral enhancement involving the occipital, posterior parietal, and temporal lobes (Fig. 19–40). Atypical CT findings include frontal lobe involvement, unilateral involvement, calcifications, and mass effect.[70] A comparison of CT with MR in six patients demonstrated the advantages of MR for subcortical white matter lesions and improved depiction of involvement of the auditory and visual pathways[70] (also see Chapter 18).

REFERENCES

1. Adams RD, Victor M: Principles of Neurology. 3rd ed. New York, McGraw-Hill Book Company, 1985, p 644.
2. Gentry LR, Godersky JC, Thompson B: MR imaging of head trauma: Review of the distribution and radiopathologic features of traumatic lesions. AJNR 9:101–110, 1988.
3. Gentry LR, Godersky JC, Thompson B, Dunn VD: Prospective comparative study of intermediate-field MR and CT in the evaluation of closed head trauma. AJNR 9:91–100, 1988.
4. Zimmerman RA, Bilaniuk LT, Hackney DB, et al: Head injury: Early results of comparing CT and high-field MR. AJNR 7:757–764, 1986.
5. Snow RB, Zimmerman RD, Gandy SE, Deck MDF: Comparison of magnetic resonance imaging and computed tomography in the evaluation of head injury. Neuroradiology 18:45–52, 1986.
6. Kelly AB, Zimmerman RD, Snow RB, et al: Head trauma:

Comparison of MR and CT—experience in 100 patients. AJNR 9:699–708, 1988.

7. Hans JS, Kaufman B, Alfidi RJ, et al: Head trauma evaluated by magnetic resonance and computed tomography: A comparison. Radiology 150:71–77, 1984.

8. Fobben ES, Grossman RI, Hackney DB, et al: The MR appearance of subdural hematomas and hygromas. Presented at the Twenty-sixth Annual Meeting of the American Society of Neuroradiology, Chicago, May 15–20, 1988.

9. Holbourn AHS: Mechanisms of head injuries. Lancet 2:438–441, 1943.

10. Tornheim RA: Traumatic edema in head injury. *In* Becker DP, Povlishock JT (eds): Central Nervous System Trauma: Status Report. Bethesda, MD, National Institute of Neurological and Communicative Diseases and Stroke, 1985, pp 431–442.

11. Jennett B, Teasdale G: Dynamic Pathology in Management of Head Injuries. Philadelphia, FA Davis, 1981, pp 45–75.

12. Hesselink JR, Dowd CF, Healy ME, et al: MR imaging of brain contusions: A comparative study with CT. AJNR 9:269–278, 1988.

13. Adams JH, Mitchell DE, Graham DI, Doyle D: Diffuse brain damage of immediate impact type: Its relationship to primary brainstem damage in head injury. Brain 100:489–502, 1977.

14. Peerless SJ, Rewcastle NB: Shear injuries of the brain. Can Med Assoc J 96:577–582, 1966.

15. Levin HS, Amparo E, Eisenberg HM, et al: Magnetic resonance imaging and computerized tomography in relation to the neurobehavioral sequelae of mild and moderate head injuries. J Neurosurg 66:706–713, 1987.

16. Davidson HD, Steiner RM: Magnetic resonance imaging in infections of the central nervous system. AJNR 6:499–504, 1985.

17. Brant-Zawadzki M: NMR imaging of experimental brain abscess: Comparison with CT. AJNR 4:250–253, 1983.

18. Runge VM, Clanton JA, Price AC, et al: Evaluation of contrast enhanced MR imaging in a brain-abscess model. AJNR 6:139–149, 1985.

19. Grossman RI, Joseph PM, Wolf G, et al: Experimental intracranial septic infarction: Magnetic resonance imaging. Radiology 155:649–653, 1985.

20. Press GA, Weindling SM, Hesselink JR, et al: Rhinocerebral mucormycosis: MR manifestations. J Comput Assist Tomogr 12:744–749, 1988.

21. Colli BO, Martelli N, Assiriti JA, et al: Results of surgical treatment of neurocysticercosis in 69 cases. J Neurosurg 18:419–427, 1986.

22. Leblanc R, Knowles KF, Melanson D, et al: Neurocysticercosis: Surgical and medical management with praziquantel. Neurosurgery 18:419–427, 1986.

23. Lotz J, Albert B, Bowen R: Neurocysticercosis: Correlative pathomorphology and MR imaging. Neuroradiology 30:35–41, 1988.

24. Suss RA, Maravilla KR, Thompson J: MR imaging of intracranial cysticercosis: Comparison with CT and anatomopathologic features. AJNR 7:235–242, 1986.

25. Rhee RS, Kumasaki DY, Sarwar M, et al: MR imaging of intraventricular cysticercosis. J Comput Assist Tomogr 11:598–601, 1988.

26. Schroth G, Kretzschmar K, Gawehn J, Voigt K: Advantage of magnetic resonance imaging in the diagnosis of cerebral infections. Neuroradiology 29:120–126, 1987.

27. Gupta RK, Jena A, Sharma A, et al: MR imaging of intracranial tuberculomas. J Comput Assist Tomogr 12:280–285, 1988.

28. Ho SU, Berenberg RA, Kim KS, et al: Sarcoid encephalopathy with diffuse infiltration and focal hydrocephalus shown by sequential CT. Neurology 29:1161–1165, 1979.

29. Ketonen L, Oksanen V, Kuulialu I: Preliminary experience of magnetic resonance imaging in neurosarcoidosis. Neuroradiology 29:127–129, 1987.

30. Sherman JL, Hayes WS, Stern BJ, et al: MR evaluation of intracranial sarcoidosis: Comparison with CT. Presented at the Twenty-Fifth Annual Meeting of the American Society of Neuroradiology, New York, May 10–15, 1987.

31. Holland BA, Perrett LV, Mills CM: Meningovascular syphilis: CT and MR findings. Radiology 158:439–442, 1986.

32. Furman JM, Brownstone PK, Baloh RW: Atypical brainstem encephalitis: Magnetic resonance imaging and oculographic findings. Neurology 35:438–440, 1985.

33. Dunn V, Bale JF, Zimmerman RA, et al: MRI in children with postinfectious disseminated encephalomyelitis. Magn Reson Imaging 4:25–32, 1986.

34. Atlas SW, Grossman RI, Goldberg HI, et al: MR diagnosis of acute disseminated encephalomyelitis. J Comput Assist Tomogr 10:798–801, 1986.

35. Levy RM, Rosenbloom S, Perrett LV: Neuroradiologic findings in AIDS: A review of 200 cases. AJNR 7:833–839, 1986.

36. Belman AL, Ultmann MH, Horovpian D: Neurologic complications in infants and children with acquired immunodeficiency syndrome. Ann Neurol 18:560–566, 1985.

37. Resnick L, DiMarzo-Veronese F, Schupbach J, et al: Intrablood-brain-barrier synthesis of HTLV-III–specific IgG in patients with neurologic symptoms associated with AIDS or AIDS-related complex. N Engl J Med 313:1498–1504, 1985.

38. Ho DD, Rota TR, Schooley RT, et al: Isolation of HTLV-III from cerebrospinal fluid and neural tissues of patients with neurologic syndromes from acquired immunodeficiency syndrome. N Engl J Med 313:1493–1497, 1985.

39. Levy RM, Bredesen DE, Rosenbloom ML: Neurologic manifestations of the acquired immunodeficiency syndrome (AIDS): Experience at UCSF and review of the literature. J Neurosurg 62:475–495, 1985.

40. Anders KH, Guerra WF, Tomiyasu U, et al: The neuropathology of AIDS: UCLA experience and review. Am J Pathol 124:537–557, 1986.

41. Kelly WM, Brant-Zawadzki M: Acquired immunodeficiency syndrome: Neuroradiologic findings. Radiology 149:485–491, 1983.

42. Elkins CM, Leon E, Grenell SL, Leeds NE: Intracranial lesions in the acquired immunodeficiency syndrome: Radiological (computed tomographic) features. JAMA 253:393–396, 1985.

43. Whalen MA, Kricheff II, Handler M, et al: Acquired immunodeficiency syndrome: Computed tomographic manifestations. Radiology 149:477–484, 1983.

44. Guilleux M-H, Steiner RE, Young IR: MR imaging in progressive multifocal leukoencephalopathy. AJNR 7:1033–1035, 1986.

45. Wiley CA, Schrier RD, Nelson JA, et al: Cellular localization of human immunodeficiency virus infection within the brains of acquired immune deficiency syndrome patients. Proc Natl Acad Sci USA 83:7089–7093, 1986.

46. Holland JC, Tross S: The psychosocial and neuropsychiatric sequelae of the acquired immunodeficiency syndrome and related disorders. Ann Intern Med 103:760–764, 1985.

47. Navia BA, Jordan BD, Price RW: The AIDS dementia complex: I. Clinical features. Ann Neurol 19:517–524, 1986.

48. Post JMD, Tate LG, Quencer RM, et al: CT, MR, and pathology in HIV encephalitis and meningitis. AJNR 9:469–476, 1988.

49. Post JMD, Sheldon JJ, Hensley GT, et al: Central nervous system disease in acquired immunodeficiency syndrome: Prospective correlation using CT, MR imaging and pathologic studies. Radiology 158:141–148, 1986.

50. Jarvik JG, Hesselink JR, Kennedy C, et al: Acquired immunodeficiency syndrome: Magnetic resonance patterns of brain involvement with pathological correlation. Arch Neurol 45:731–736, 1988.

51. Olsen WL, Longo FM, Mills CM, Norman D: White matter disease in AIDS: Findings at MR imaging. Radiology 169:445–448, 1988.

52. Drayer B, Burger P, Darwin R, et al: Magnetic resonance imaging of brain iron. AJNR 7:373–380, 1986.

53. Drayer BP: Imaging of the aging brain. Part 1. Normal findings. Radiology 166:785–796, 1988.

54. Drayer BP: Imaging of the aging brain. Part 2. Pathologic conditions. Radiology 166:797–806, 1988.
55. Drayer BP, Olanow W, Burger P, et al: Parkinson Plus Syndrome: Diagnosis using high-field MR imaging of brain iron. Radiology 159:493–498, 1986.
56. Pastakia B, Polinsky R, DiChiro G, et al: Multiple system atrophy (Shy-Drager syndrome): MR imaging. Radiology 159:499–502, 1986.
57. Duguid JR, DeLaPaz R, DeGroot J: Magnetic resonance imaging of the midbrain in Parkinson's disease. Ann Neurol 20:744–747, 1986.
58. Rutledge JN, Hilal SK, Silver AJ, et al: Study of movement disorders and brain iron by MR. AJNR 8:397–411, 1988.
59. Braffman BH, Grossman RI, Goldberg HI, et al: MR imaging of Parkinson disease with spin-echo and gradient-echo techniques. AJNR 9:1093–1099, 1988.
60. Fazekas F, Chawluk JB, Alavi A, et al: MR signal abnormalities at 1.5 T in Alzheimer's dementia and normal aging. AJNR 8:421–426, 1987.
61. Simmons J, Pastakia B, Chase TN, Shults CW: Magnetic resonance imaging in Huntington disease. AJNR 7:25–28, 1986.
62. Miller GM, Baker HC Jr, Okazaki H, Whisnant JP: Central pontine myelinolysis and its imitators: MR findings. Radiology 168:795–802, 1988.
63. Thompson AJ, Brown MM, Swash M, et al: Autopsy validation of MRI in central pontine myelinolysis. Neuroradiology 30:175–177, 1988.
64. Geyer CA, Sartor KJ, Preasky AJ, et al: Leigh disease (subacute necrotizing encephalomyelopathy): CT and MR findings in five cases. J Comput Assist Tomogr 12:40–44, 1988.
65. Davis PC, Hoffman JC, Braun IF, et al: MR of Leigh's disease (subacute necrotizing encephalomyelopathy). AJNR 8:71–75, 1987.
66. Aisen AM, Martel W, Gabrielsen TO, et al: Wilson disease of the brain: MR imaging. Radiology 157:137–141, 1985.
67. Starosta-Rubinstein S, Young AB, Kluin K, et al: Clinical assessment of 31 patients with Wilson's disease: Correlation with structural changes on magnetic resonance imaging. Arch Neurol 44:365–370, 1987.
68. Littrup PJ, Gebarski SS: MR imaging of Hallervorden-Spatz disease. J Comput Assist Tomogr 9:491–493, 1985.
69. Tanfani G, Mascalchi M, Dal Pozzo GC, et al: MR imaging in a case of Hallervorden-Spatz disease. J Comput Assist Tomogr 11:1057–1058, 1987.
70. Kumar AJ, Rosenbaum AE, Naidu S, et al: Adrenoleukodystrophy: Correlating MR imaging with CT. Radiology 165:497–504, 1987.

20

THE ORBIT

STEVEN E. HARMS

ORBITAL ANATOMY
TECHNICAL CONSIDERATIONS
    RADIOFREQUENCY COIL
    PULSE SEQUENCES
    TIMING PARAMETERS AND TIP ANGLES
    ACQUISITION METHODS

PATHOLOGY
    OCULAR LESIONS
    INTRACONAL LESIONS
    OPTIC NERVE AND SHEATH LESIONS
    EXTRAOCULAR MUSCLE LESIONS
    EXTRACONAL LESIONS

A variety of clinical presentations of ophthalmic disease require further evaluation by an imaging method. Some of these problems include decreased vision, double vision, orbital deformity, orbital mass, periorbital mass, intracranial mass, exophthalmos, ptosis, localized inflammation, and trauma. Until recently, plain radiographs, ultrasound, and x-ray CT were the imaging modalities most commonly used.

The resolution and contrast available on CT revolutionized the imaging evaluation of orbital lesions. The primary advantage of CT is the ability to localize the lesion. As far as characterizing orbital lesions, CT differential diagnoses are commonly defined according to the anatomic location. These anatomic categories are (1) ocular, (2) intraconal, (3) optic nerve or sheath, (4) extraocular muscle, and (5) extraconal.

The high soft tissue contrast available on MR imaging,[1-9] combined with newer high-resolution techniques,[10-16] provides superior anatomic detail of many orbital structures. In addition, since MR signals are a more sensitive probe of the molecular environment, differences in signals can vary, with the tissue pathology providing even more diagnostic information than can be gained by anatomy alone.[9, 10, 14, 16] Multiple imaging planes are directly available by MR. Artifacts secondary to high-density dental materials within the mouth, noted frequently on coronal CT scans, are not a problem on MR. The radiation exposure to the lens on a CT examination[17] can be eliminated by using MR. These advantages are rapidly making MR a major diagnostic tool for evaluating orbital lesions.

ORBITAL ANATOMY

The optic globe is divided into two compartments: the anterior chamber, filled with aqueous humor, and the posterior chamber, filled with vitreous humor. These compartments are separated by the lens apparatus. On MR images, the vitreous and aqueous humors have signal intensities similar to that of cerebrospinal fluid (CSF) owing to the high fluid content (Figs. 20–1 and 20–2). The signal is low on T_1-weighted images, moderately low on proton density (N[H]) images, isointense on cross-over images, and relatively high on T_2-weighted images compared with brain.

The globe is a multilayered structure composed of an inner retina and an outer sclera, with choroid between the two. Two layers can be seen on T_1- and N(H)-weighted images. The choroid and retina are higher in signal than is the vitreous or sclera on T_1- and N(H)-weighted images. The sclera has low signal on all images.

The optic nerve is divided into four segments: intraocular, intraorbital, intracanalicular, and intracranial. The intraorbital and intracranial portions are well seen by CT because of adequate contrast with surrounding structures. The intraocular portion is

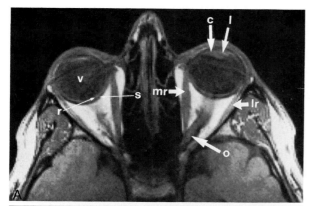

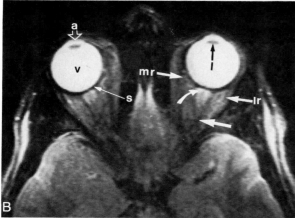

FIGURE 20–1. Two-dimensional (2D) multislice images. A T_1-weighted (spin echo [SE] 500/30) image *(A)* obtained with a 2D multislice technique using 5-mm slices and 1-mm gaps. The orbital fat has the highest signal, and the vitreous has the lowest signal. Optic nerve and muscle are intermediate in signal. A T_2-weighted (SE 2000/120) image *(B)* demonstrates the highest signal from the vitreous. The orbital fat has moderate signal on this heavily T_2-weighted image. Fluid within the dural sheath *(curved arrow)* around the optic nerve has high signal and can easily be separated from surrounding fat on T_2-weighted images. The lens has moderate signal on the T_1-weighted image and low signal on the T_2-weighted images. The aqueous humor (a), ciliary body (c), lens (l), lateral rectus (lr), medial rectus (mr), optic nerve (o), retina and choroid (r), sclera (s), and vitreous (v) are labeled. Normally, some fluid can be seen within the dural sheath *(curved arrow)* on the T_2-weighted images.

only about 1 mm in length and is poorly seen by CT. High-resolution, thin-slice MR is capable of producing quality images of this anatomy. The demonstration of the intracanalicular portion is frequently limited on CT by the surrounding high-density bone of the optic canal.[18] Bone does not produce artifact on MR. The optic nerve is similar to brain in signal intensity. The signal of the nerve is moderately high on T_1-weighted images, moderately high on N(H)-weighted images, isointense on cross-over images, and moderately low on T_2-weighted images compared with CSF or vitreous.

The extraocular muscles are well visualized on T_1- and N(H)-weighted images as moderate signal intensity surrounded by high-signal fat. Muscle has a very short T_2 and rapidly loses signal relative to surround-

ing tissue with T_2 weighting (long repetition time [TR], long echo time [TE] images).

Orbital fat has a short T_1 and a moderate T_2. The very short T_1 results in a high signal intensity on T_1-weighted images. It often becomes necessary to reduce the relative signal of orbital fat to unmask tumors that are surrounded by fat. This signal reduction is achieved with more heavily T_2-weighted images.

Flow within vessels usually results in a signal void in high contrast with surrounding structures. The ophthalmic artery arises from the internal carotid artery and passes through the optic canal within the dural sheath inferolateral to the optic nerve. Shortly after entering the orbit, the ophthalmic artery courses over the nerve in 85 per cent of cases. The superior ophthalmic vein courses from its origin in the nasal aspect of the orbit in a posterolateral direction deep to the superior rectus muscle through the superior orbital fissure. The inferior ophthalmic vein follows the inferior rectus muscle and passes through the inferior orbital tissue. Flow-related enhancement can produce high signal within vessels, particularly on partial saturation images. Slower flow within veins is sometimes enhanced on even echoes owing to even-echo rephasing.

The anterior soft tissues of the orbit are separated from the rest of the orbit by a thin connective tissue membrane called the orbital septum. The orbital septum extends from the bony periosteum to the tarsal plates of the eyelids. The septum divides the orbit into the anterior preseptal space and the posterior retrobulbar space. The septum acts as a major barrier to the spread of inflammatory processes of the preseptal space from the rest of the orbit.[19] The septum is seen as a moderate- to low-signal structure on T_1-weighted images.

Cortical bone has low signal on all MR images because of a low proton density and a short T_2. Bone is visualized as a signal void surrounded by the higher signal soft tissue. Even the mucoperiosteum of the paranasal sinuses provides enough signal to separate bone from air within the sinuses.

The normal lacrimal gland is an almond-sized, well-defined structure located anteriorly in the superolateral portion of the orbit. The normal lacrimal gland has moderate signal on all images.

TECHNICAL CONSIDERATIONS

The technique choices for MR examinations are divided into the following major categories: (1) radiofrequency (RF) coil, (2) pulse sequences, (3) timing parameters and tip angles, and (4) acquisition method.[20–24]

The selection of a particular magnetic field strength for orbital imaging is not critical. High-quality images have been produced at fields of 0.15 to 1.5 T. The lower field strength systems have the

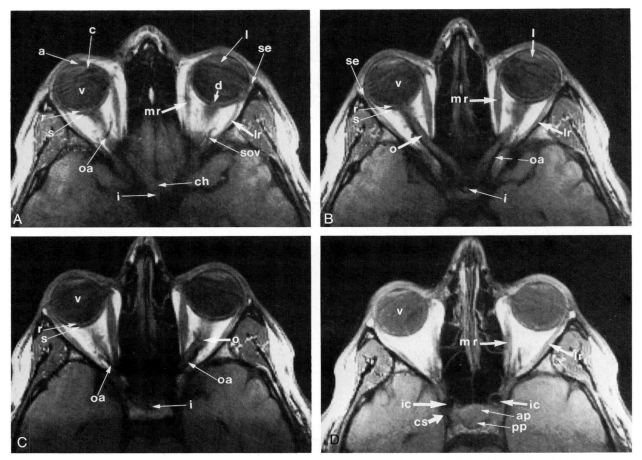

FIGURE 20–2. Three-dimensional (3D) images. Adjacent T_1-weighted (SE 300/26) 3D images through the optic nerve *(A–D)* demonstrate sharper anatomic detail than do the 2D multislice images in Figure 20–1 owing to a much thinner slice thickness (1.6 mm) and no gaps between slices. The imaging times for both 2D and 3D examinations were virtually the same. A multiecho 3D examination using echo times (TEs) of 40 *(E)*, 80 *(F)*, 120 *(G)*, and 160 *(H)* msec demonstrates proton density weighting *(E)*, with increasing T_2 weighting on progressing echoes. These slices are 3.2 mm thick. Note the high signal-to-noise (S/N) on even the very long TE 160 msec *(H)* image because of the inherently improved S/N of 3D imaging. The aqueous humor (a), optic chiasm (ch), ciliary body (c), cavernous sinus (cs), lens (l), infundibulum (i), internal carotid artery (ic), optic nerve (o), retina (r), sclera (s), medial rectus (mr), lateral rectus (lr), orbital septum (se), ophthalmic artery (oa), superior ophthalmic vein (sov), anterior lobe pituitary (ap), and posterior lobe pituitary (pp) are labeled.

advantages of generally shorter tissue T_1 values, allowing for faster TRs without saturation, and improvement in the signal-to-noise ratio (S/N) with surface coils. The higher field strength systems generally have an overall improvement in S/N, but the images are degraded by chemical shift artifacts.

RADIOFREQUENCY COIL

The major advancement in MR technology allowing the production of high-quality orbital imaging has been the introduction of surface coils.[10–15] The improvement in the S/N can be used to produce higher resolution and thinner slices without "data starvation." Initially, small, circular surface coils were used to obtain images of a single orbit.[11, 12] More

recently, specialized orbit coils have been used to obtain images of both orbits simultaneously at the expense of some S/N.[10, 14] The orbit coil approach is useful in orbital imaging because the imaging of the opposite orbit and deep structures near the chiasm is often necessary for a complete orbital examination. Improved designs are expected in the future.

PULSE SEQUENCES

Several pulse sequences are available on current commercial instruments: (1) single spin echo (SE), (2) multiple SE, (3) inversion recovery (IR), and (4) gradient echo (GRE).

The SE sequence is the workhorse of almost all commercial systems. The ability of this technique for

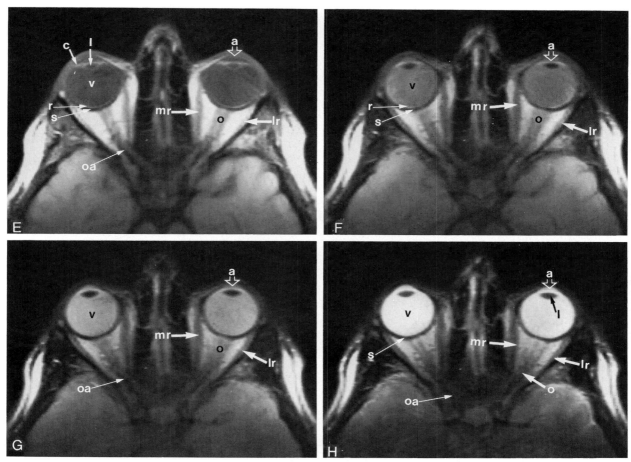

FIGURE 20–2 *Continued*

producing T_1 weighting is limited by T_1 and T_2 values of the tissues in question. Most normal orbital tissues, such as fat, muscle, and fibrous tissue, have relatively short T_2 values.[20] A significant amount of signal is lost owing to T_2 effects if the TE is long. T_2 weighting is efficiently done by an SE sequence. Multiple echo sequences can be employed for producing images of increasing T_2 weighting on progressive echoes.

The IR sequence produces images with more T_1 weighting than conventional SE sequences. Some workers indicate that short T_1 inversion recovery (STIR) images may be useful for contrast reversal in brain and orbital imaging.[25] At present, it appears that the SE sequence produces adequate T_1 weighting for orbital imaging. IR will, in general, have a longer imaging time than a comparable T_1-weighted SE sequence. The relative difference in time is probably the greatest contributor to the lack of popularity of this sequence. As more modern systems emerge with a higher inherent S/N, single or fractional excitation methods make the time penalty for IR much less than on previous instruments. The major benefit of STIR is the suppression of fat signal within the orbit. Fat signal can be suppressed in other ways, such as chemical shift imaging, chemical shift selective imaging, fat saturation pulses, and bidirectional slice

excitation. These other methods can be implemented with conventional SE sequences.

Newer GRE pulse sequences that have recently emerged on commercial imagers include FLASH, GRASS, FISP, and FAST.[26–29] These sequences utilize a narrow tip angle RF pulse and a gradient-refocused echo.[26] Since less RF power is used, the recovery time is reduced, resulting in an overall more efficient acquisition. Gradient echoes can be used to reduce the TE for decreasing signal loss due to T_2 effect. At present, these sequences have limited application in the orbit because of signal loss from magnetic susceptibility effects. Stimulated echo sequences (STEAM) and steady-state sequences (SSFP, CE-FAST, CE-SSFP) are expected to emerge in the future for specialized imaging tasks.[28, 29] These techniques are addressed in depth in Chapter 5.

TIMING PARAMETERS AND TIP ANGLES

Timing parameters and tip angles are used to vary tissue contrast based upon the inherent T_1, T_2, and N(H) of the tissue (Figs. 20–1 and 20–2). With the exception of the vitreous and aqueous humors, most of the orbital contents, such as fat, muscle, and fibrous tissue, have relatively short T_2 values. A short TE is helpful in reducing signal loss caused by the short T_2 of the normal tissues. The T_1 values for muscle, connective tissue, and fat are moderate to short.

When planning an imaging sequence to produce good anatomic images efficiently, T_1 weighting seems most appropriate, considering the relative T_1 values of the tissues. An SE sequence with as short a TE and TR as possible provides excellent anatomic detail with a very short acquisition time.

T_2-weighted images are useful in characterizing lesions or in more precisely defining the extent of some disease that may be poorly seen on the T_1-weighted images. Since orbital fat has a very short T_1 and a moderate T_2, heavily T_2-weighted images are often necessary to separate high-signal fat due to short T_1 from a disease process. At 0.6 T, a TR 2000, TE 120 image has adequate T_2 weighting to enhance vitreous, aqueous, and most lesions compared with orbital fat. If a shorter TE is desired, then a longer TR could be used to achieve a similar goal. If a shorter TR is desired, then the TE would need to be lengthened to produce similar contrast.

Proton density–weighted images are useful for producing good anatomic images and for characterizing some orbital tumors. Compared with T_1-weighted images, N(H) weighting is generally more time consuming and achieves less contrast. More slices are available with N(H)-weighted, two-dimensional (2D), multislice acquisitions, since a longer TR is used. On some instruments with long duty cycles, it may be necessary to acquire N(H)-weighted images instead of T_1-weighted images to generate an adequate number of slices.

A cross-over image or balanced T_1-T_2 image refers to an image of decreased contrast at or near the isointensity point of two tissues on SE signal intensity plots. At 0.6 T, the cross-over image for brain and CSF lies between TE 60 and TE 90 at a TR of 2000. Cross-over images are useful for characterizing certain orbital lesions but have poor anatomic detail.

If a long TR multiecho sequence is used, the images will be primarily N(H) weighted on the initial echo and can progress through the cross-over or isointense images to the more heavily T_2-weighted images on the later echoes. When a short TR multiecho sequence is used, the short TE image will be more T_1 weighted, and each additional image will be more T_2 weighted. Cross-over images are still obtained with a short TR, but N(H) weighting is reduced.

The relative T_1 or T_2^* weighting of a GRE sequence is varied by the use of tip angles. Tip-angle adjustment can be used in addition to or instead of the usual TE and TR timing parameter adjustments. A usual tip for the initial RF pulse of an SE sequence is 90 degrees. T_1-weighted GRE sequences are impaired by higher signal generated at the slice edges than at the center, resulting in a double slice effect. A wide tip angle and a short TR produce a T_1-

weighted GRE sequence. As the tip angle is reduced, the sequence becomes more proton density weighted. Lengthening the TE produces more T_2^* weighting. Because of motion sensitivity and magnetic susceptibility artifacts, GRE techniques have been difficult to apply in the orbit.

ACQUISITION METHODS

Most MR systems currently use 2D single-slice and 2D multislice acquisition methods (Fig. 20–1). The 2D single slice is very useful for surface coil localization and angulation measurements. The 2D multislice SE is at present the standard acquisition technique of most commercial imagers. It is an efficient method for acquiring a set of long TR, relatively short TE (proton density–weighted), and long TE (T_2-weighted) images.

When T_1-weighted images are desired, the shorter TR severely limits the number of available slices per SE scan, particularly on machines with long duty cycles. For orbital imaging, in which only a small number of slices are necessary, the reduced number of slices with a heavily T_1-weighted SE sequence is not usually a significant problem.

The ability to produce thin slices by 2D methods is limited by the narrowest bandwidth of the slice-selection pulse and the strength of the slice-selection gradients. Since no RF slice excitation is perfectly square, the excitation of the slice is uneven, and some tissue outside the slice is excited. Gaps are usually produced between slices to reduce saturation of signals from adjacent slices. The difficulty in achieving thin, contiguous sections by 2D multislice acquisitions is the greatest limitation of this method for orbital imaging.

Three-dimensional (3D) acquisition methods (Fig. 20–2) are emerging as an effective way for producing very thin slices of the orbit without gaps between slices[30] and is currently our choice for orbital imaging. A slab of tissue is selected by a slice-selection pulse, and the slab is further divided into slices by additional phase encoding in the slice-selection direction. Since each slice is not individually selected by a selective excitation, the width of the slice is not limited by the RF bandwidth or the gradient strength. The signal contribution from the central 3D slices does not fall off toward the edge, as in 2D methods. Because of the more even tip angle within the slice, the S/N is improved. Since each slice is not individually selected by a selective excitation, as in 2D methods, no gap is necessary between slices. Since a narrow-bandwidth RF pulse is not needed for the excitation, the bandwidth can be widened for shorter TE studies. A long TR is not necessary for exciting additional slices, as in 2D multislice methods. A short TR (T_1-weighted) study does not limit the number of slices. The 3D approach is an effective way of improving the S/N, since the S/N of a 3D acquisition improves with the square root of the number of slices. Fast scan sequences, such as FLASH, more efficiently utilize the 3D method for signal averaging than 2D multislice, since the repetition rate is not limited by a long recovery time.[26]

The imaging time of 3D acquisitions greatly increases with TR. Therefore, long TR sequences are not efficiently obtained by this method. T_2-weighted studies can be obtained at a shorter TR, but the TE would need to be increased to produce similar contrast compared with 2D data. T_2^*-weighted fast scan images are not restrictive, since a longer TR is not critical.

The 3D multislab method employs the use of a selective excitation for defining separate slabs of tissue in a manner similar to 2D multislice. These slabs are further divided into slices with phase-encoding gradients like conventional 3D acquisitions. This method combines some of the attributes of both techniques.[31, 32]

PATHOLOGY

The excellent anatomic definition of the orbit seen on MR imaging provides the foundation for the anatomic categorization of orbital disease. The MR behavior of tissues can be further used to develop improved differential diagnoses based upon both anatomic and MR signal intensity patterns.

OCULAR LESIONS

Ocular lesions can be categorized clinically into two groups: those occurring in childhood and those occurring in adulthood. The MR image intensities of ocular lesions are summarized in Table 20–1.

Retinoblastoma is the most common intraocular tumor in children.[34] The average age at the time of diagnosis is 18 months.[35] Up to 30 per cent of cases are bilateral.[34, 36, 37] Correct staging of this lesion is important, since tumors confined to the globe have

TABLE 20–1. OCULAR LESIONS OF CHILDHOOD AND ADULTHOOD

Lesion	T_1	T_2
Childhood		
Retinoblastoma	High	Low
Coats' disease	High	High
PHPV	High	High
Hemorrhage	High	High
Toxocara canis endophthalmitis	High	High
Posterior scleritis	Low	Low
Adulthood		
Melanoma	High	Low
Metastases	Moderate	Low-Moderate
Hemorrhage	High	High
Phthisis bulbi	Low	Low

a cure rate approaching 90 per cent. When tumors extend beyond the globe, the cure rate drops to below 20 per cent.[38, 39] Retinoblastomas are treated by radiation, enucleation, or both, depending upon the stage of the disease. Accurate staging is, therefore, very important in treatment planning.

Evaluation of retinoblastomas for early extension through the globe or into the optic nerve is difficult by CT.[40] Typically, retinoblastomas have high signal on T_1- and N(H)-weighted images. Highly T_2-weighted images demonstrate lower signal tumor compared with vitreous (Fig. 20–3). A high-signal subretinal effusion is typically seen adjacent to the tumor mass on T_1, T_2, N(H), and cross-over images. The fact that sclera has low signal because of a short T_2 is important for determining the extension of tumor through the sclera. The optic nerve should be evaluated for focal masses, thickening, or abnormal signal to indicate spread of disease along the nerve. Calcifications seen commonly by CT are not usually well demonstrated by MR.[9, 10, 14] Calcifications, however, are not diagnostic of retinoblastoma.

Though rare, other conditions can occur at about the same time of life as retinoblastoma and can present diagnostic problems. These lesions include Coats' disease, persistent hyperplastic primary vitreous (PHPV), *Toxocara canis* endophthalmitis, retrolental fibroplasia, and Norrie's disease (retinal dysplasia).

Coats' disease is a retinal anomaly characterized by telangiectasias of the retina with a lipoproteinaceous exudate in the retina and subretinal space (Fig. 20–4). Coats' disease could be confused clinically and by most imaging methods with a necrotic retinoblastoma.[41] The distinction is important, since Coats' disease can be treated by laser and the vision preserved. On MR, the lesion of Coats' disease has homogeneous high signal on both T_1- and T_2-weighted images.[9, 10]

PHPV usually manifests at birth or infancy as a unilaterally small globe. The disorder is a congenital persistence and hyperplasia of the embryonic hyaloid vascular system.[42] On MR, a small globe filled with high-signal hemorrhage on both T_1- and T_2-weighted images is seen (Fig. 20–5). Fluid levels can be present.[14, 43]

Posterior scleritis[44] and phthisis bulbi are chronic inflammatory processes that have thickened low-signal sclera on both T_1- and T_2-weighted images.

Hemorrhage (Fig. 20–6) in the extracellular methemoglobin phase usually has inhomogeneous high signal on both T_1- and T_2-weighted images.[9, 14] Chronic hemorrhage has low signal on T_2-weighted images resulting from the magnetic susceptibility effects of hemosiderin and iron salts. Hyperacute hemorrhage can have lower signal on T_1-weighted images.

Toxocara canis endophthalmitis has high signal on both T_1- and T_2-weighted images. The larval granulomas can be seen as high signal within the lower signal inflamed sclera on T_1-weighted images.[9]

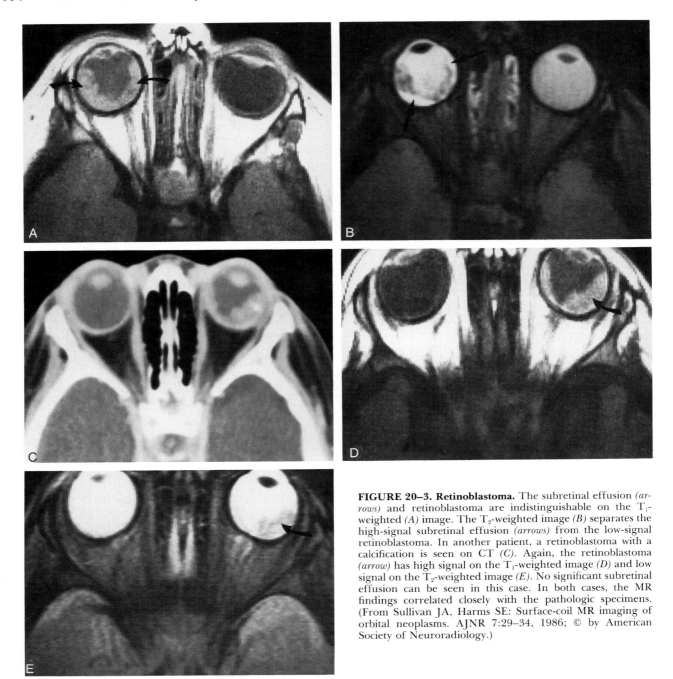

FIGURE 20–3. Retinoblastoma. The subretinal effusion *(arrows)* and retinoblastoma are indistinguishable on the T_1-weighted *(A)* image. The T_2-weighted image *(B)* separates the high-signal subretinal effusion *(arrows)* from the low-signal retinoblastoma. In another patient, a retinoblastoma with a calcification is seen on CT *(C)*. Again, the retinoblastoma *(arrow)* has high signal on the T_1-weighted image *(D)* and low signal on the T_2-weighted image *(E)*. No significant subretinal effusion can be seen in this case. In both cases, the MR findings correlated closely with the pathologic specimens. (From Sullivan JA, Harms SE: Surface-coil MR imaging of orbital neoplasms. AJNR 7:29–34, 1986; © by American Society of Neuroradiology.)

Choroidal melanoma (Fig. 20–7) is the most common malignancy of the globe and is most frequently encountered in those between the ages of 50 and 70.[35, 36] Melanomas have high signal on the T_1-weighted images and low signal on the T_2-weighted images.[9, 12, 16] An associated subretinal effusion, exhibiting high signal on both T_1- and T_2-weighted images, is common.[10, 14, 45, 46] Primary melanoma of the globe is usually treated by enucleation.[35]

The primary differential diagnosis for melanoma is choroidal metastasis. Metastatic breast and lung carcinomas are most common, followed by gastroin-testinal and genitourinary tumors.[47] In 50 per cent of cases involving ocular metastases, the primary tumor is undiagnosed at the time of presentation.[48] The distinction between melanoma and choroidal metastasis is important, since metastatic disease is not typically treated by enucleation. Carcinomas usually have moderate signal on T_1-weighted images and higher signal on T_2-weighted images. Melanoma usually has high signal on T_1-weighted images and low signal on T_2-weighted images. Metastases can often be distinguished from melanoma on the basis of their MR appearance.[49–51] Hemorrhage, having very high

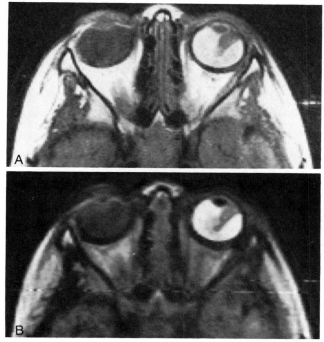

FIGURE 20–4. Coats' disease. The high-signal subretinal exudate is seen on the T_1-weighted *(A)* and T_2-weighted *(B)* images. The lipoproteinaceous exudate is demonstrated by ophthalmoscopy. (From Sullivan JA, Harms SE: Characterization of orbital lesions by surface coil MR imaging. RadioGraphics 7:9–28, 1987; with permission.)

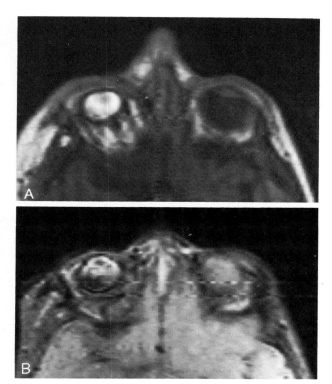

FIGURE 20–5. Persistent hyperplastic primary vitreous (PHPV). Mixed high signal is seen within the small globe on both the T_1-weighted *(A)* and the T_2-weighted *(B)* images. (From Sullivan JA, Harms SE: Characterization of orbital lesions by surface coil MR imaging. RadioGraphics 7:9–28, 1987; with permission.)

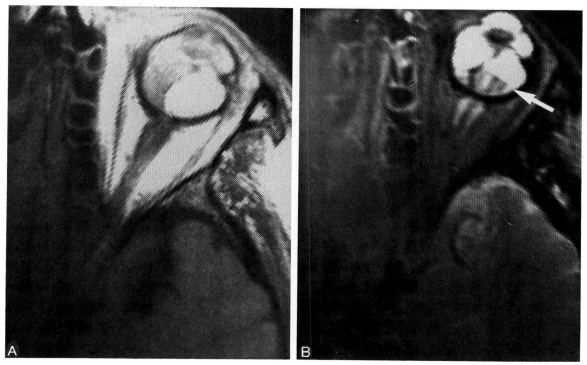

FIGURE 20–6. Hemorrhage. High signal is seen on both the T_1-weighted *(A)* and the T_2-weighted *(B)* images. Note the fluid level *(arrow)*.

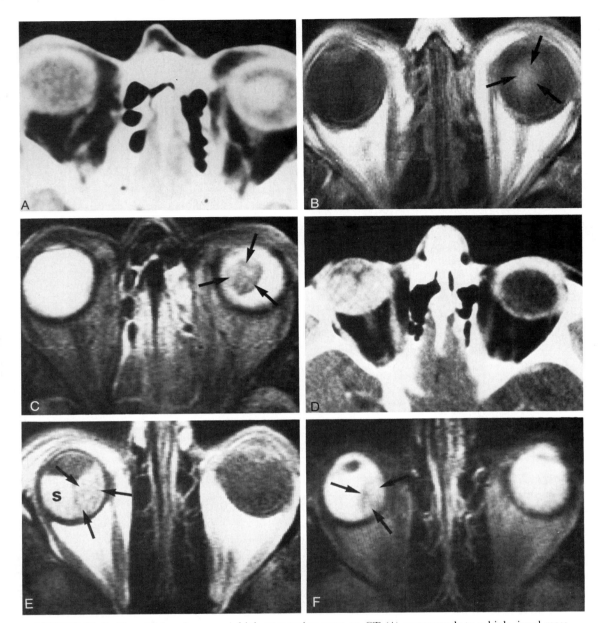

FIGURE 20–7. Choroidal melanoma. A high-attenuation mass on CT *(A)* corresponds to a high-signal mass *(arrows)* on the T₁-weighted image *(B)* and a low-signal mass *(arrows)* on the T₂-weighted image *(C).* When a large subretinal exudate is present, the CT scan *(D)* overestimates the size of the mass. MR correctly differentiates the mass *(arrows)* as an area of slightly lower signal than the subretinal effusion (S) on the T₁-weighted image *(E)* and much lower signal than the subretinal effusion (S) on the T₂-weighted image *(F).* (From Sullivan JA, Harms SE: Surface-coil MR imaging of orbital neoplasms. AJNR 7:29–34, 1986; © by American Society of Neuroradiology.)

signal on all images, is easily distinguished from most ocular masses in this age group.[10, 14]

INTRACONAL LESIONS

The MR image intensities in a variety of intraconal lesions are summarized in Table 20–2.

Cavernous hemangioma is the most common benign orbital neoplasm.[52–54] These lesions typically

TABLE 20–2. INTRACONAL LESIONS

Lesion	T_1	T_2
Vascular lesions	Low	Low
Pseudotumor	Low	Low
Hemangioma	Low	High
Lymphoma	Low	High
Most sarcoma, carcinoma	Low	High
Hemorrhage (subacute)	High	High
Lipoma	High	Low

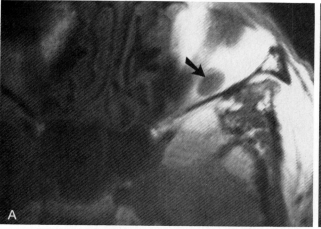

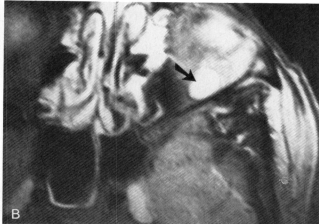

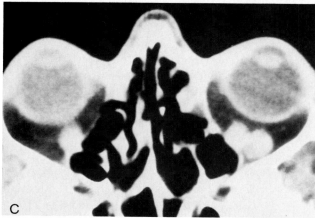

FIGURE 20–8. Cavernous hemangioma. A well-defined intraconal mass with low signal *(arrow)* on the T_1-weighted *(A)* and high signal *(arrow)* on the T_2-weighted *(B)* images is typical of a cavernous hemangioma. These findings correlate with the homogeneous enhancing mass shown on the contrast CT *(C)*. (From Sullivan JA, Harms SE: Surface-coil MR imaging of orbital neoplasms. AJNR 7:29–34, 1986; © by American Society of Neuroradiology.)

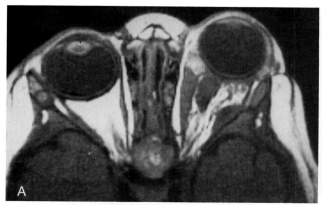

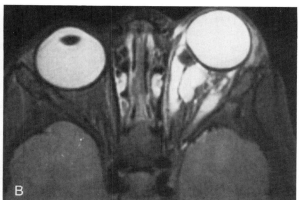

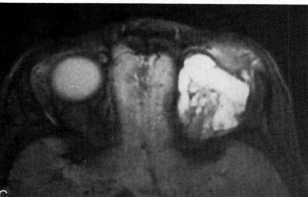

FIGURE 20–9. Lymphangioma. Proton density–weighted *(A)* and T_2-weighted *(B and C)* axial scans show a heterogeneous mass within the left orbit of a 9-month-old child. The mass involves both the intraconal and the extraconal compartments. Multiple cystic components are hypointense to fat on proton density–weighted images and hyperintense to fat on T_2-weighted images. The globe is markedly proptotic.

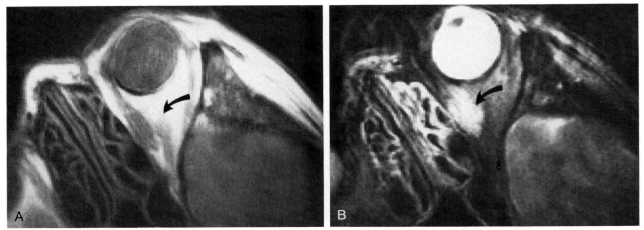

FIGURE 20–10. Lymphoma. An ill-defined enlargement of the medial rectus is produced in this case of lymphoma. Lymphoma *(arrow)* typically is low signal on T_1-weighted *(A)* and high signal on T_2-weighted *(B)* images. (From Sullivan JA, Harms SE: Surface-coil MR imaging of orbital neoplasms. AJNR 7:29–34, 1986; © by American Society of Neuroradiology.)

occur in the intraconal region, lateral to the optic nerve.[54] The lesions are usually well-defined ovoid masses with low signal on T_1-weighted images and high signal on T_2-weighted images (Fig. 20–8). Calcifications commonly occur but are rarely seen on MR.[10, 14, 55, 56] Lymphangiomas are usually extraconal but often involve both compartments. They occur in children and have a heterogeneous texture with cystic components (Fig. 20–9). These lesions are important because of their tendency to hemorrhage, resulting in acute proptosis. The presence of hemorrhage on MR may also help distinguish lymphangioma from cavernous hemangioma.

Lymphomas (Fig. 20–10) can have well-defined margins and a signal intensity pattern similar to that of hemangioma.[10, 14, 55, 56] Ill-defined margins and the invasion of surrounding structures are important differentiating features of lymphoma (Fig. 20–10).

Lymphomas are usually homogeneous. Sarcomas and carcinomas are typically inhomogeneous.

Orbital pseudotumor is a nonspecific inflammation of orbital tissues. It tends to be unilateral and accounts for 25 per cent of all cases of unilateral exophthalmos. This condition can be remitting or chronic and progressive. It may regress spontaneously or respond to steroids. It involves predominantly the tissues immediately behind the globe. An infiltrative process, it often involves both the extraconal and the intraconal spaces.

Orbital pseudotumor can have an appearance similar to that of a number of lesions. The MR signal characteristics are, however, quite unusual (Fig. 20–11). These chronic inflammatory lesions, having low signal on both T_1- and T_2-weighted images, can be distinguished from most other lesions on the basis of MR signals.[10, 14, 57]

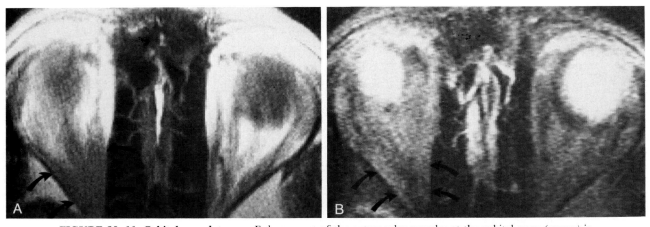

FIGURE 20–11. Orbital pseudotumor. Enlargement of the extraocular muscles at the orbital apex *(arrows)* is typical of orbital pseudotumor. This mass has low signal on T_1-weighted *(A)* and T_2-weighted *(B)* images. Lymphoma is less likely, since there is no T_2 enhancement.

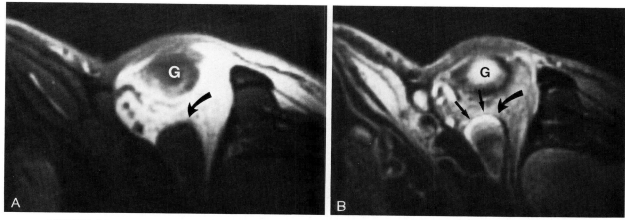

FIGURE 20–12. Orbital varix. T_1-weighted *(A)* and T_2-weighted *(B)* scans show a mass *(curved arrow)* within the orbital apex. A small portion of the globe (G) is sectioned anteriorly. The mass is low signal on the T_1-weighted image but exhibits heterogeneous signal intensity on the T_2-weighted image related to turbulent flow within the patent lumen of the varix. Some flow enhancement *(small arrows)* is present in the dome of the mass.

Vascular lesions of the orbit include orbital varix, arteriovenous malformation, and carotid-cavernous fistula. High flow usually results in signal void on all images owing to a wash-out effect. Flow enhancement can be seen on partial saturation 2D examinations. An orbital varix could conceivably have even-echo rephasing, resulting in increased signal on even echoes owing to slow flow, or high intensity on T_2-weighted images because of the long T_2 of venous blood (Fig. 20–12). The varices appear as fusiform or globular masses, often near the orbital apex. By increasing venous pressure with a Valsalva maneuver, the varix may enlarge, confirming the diagnosis. Carotid-cavernous fistula frequently shows a dilated superior ophthalmic vein and proptosis.[53]

OPTIC NERVE AND SHEATH LESIONS

The MR appearance of a variety of lesions associated with the optic nerve and sheath is summarized in Table 20–3.

Optic gliomas usually manifest in children between 2 and 6 years of age, and 90 per cent of them are apparent by age 20.[36, 48] There is a strong association with neurofibromatosis. A homogeneous fusiform enlargement of the optic nerve is a common anatomic picture (Fig. 20–13). MR aids in the staging of this lesion, since the homogeneous high signal on T_2-weighted images can demonstrate the extent of tu-

mor without evidence of nerve enlargement[10, 14] (Fig. 20–14). Optic gliomas can extend posteriorly through the optic canal to involve the optic chiasm. From there, they can involve either the opposite optic nerve or the optic tracts.

Meningiomas (Fig. 20–15) can arise from the nerve sheath or can extend from a primary intracranial meningioma along the optic nerve sheath. Meningiomas most often affect women (80 per cent) in the third, fourth, and fifth decades of life.[58] Meningiomas are usually poorly seen by MR, since the lesions are nearly isointense with the optic nerve. If a mass can be defined, very few lesions have this appearance, and the diagnosis can easily be made by MR (Fig. 20–15). In most cases, however, meningiomas will be better diagnosed and followed with a contrast CT.[10] With the advent of MR contrast agents, the advantage of CT in the evaluation of meningiomas is eliminated. The superiority of MR in the evaluation of the orbital apex and optic canal makes contrast-enhanced MR the favored imaging method over CT for the evaluation of nerve sheath meningiomas.[59]

Optic neuritis, pseudotumor, endocrine ophthalmopathy, and papilledema have been associated with an enlarged optic nerve sheath. Optic neuritis from a demyelinating disease such as multiple sclerosis can be seen as a high-signal plaque on T_2-weighted images without evidence of sheath enlargement. Changes from radiation therapy have homogeneous high signal on T_2-weighted images.

TABLE 20–3. OPTIC NERVE AND SHEATH LESIONS

Lesion	T_1	T_2	Cross-over	N(H)
Meningioma	Low-isointense	Low-isointense	Isointense	Isointense
Glioma	Low	High	High	High
Radiation change	Isointense	High	High	High
Optic neuritis	Isointense	High	High	High

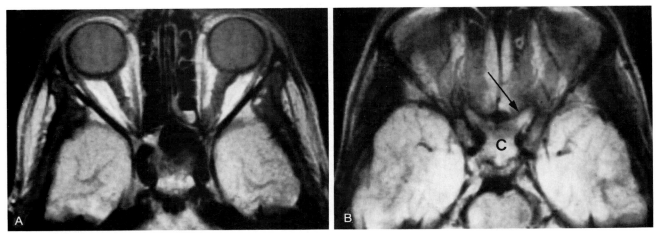

FIGURE 20–13. Optic glioma. A proton density–weighted scan *(A)* through the midorbits discloses fusiform enlargement of the left optic nerve. On a higher section, the proximal portion of the nerve *(long arrow)* is also enlarged as it enters the optic chiasm (C).

EXTRAOCULAR MUSCLE LESIONS
(Table 20–4)

Endocrine ophthalmopathy, a process of unknown etiology, is the most common cause of enlargement of the extraocular muscles and the most common cause of bilateral proptosis.[60] Endocrine ophthalmopathy typically occurs in patients with Graves' disease, but extraocular muscle changes have been seen in euthyroid patients as well.[61] Seventy per cent of cases are bilateral and symmetric. There is a 4 to 1 female preponderance. The histopathologic picture of the muscles is similar to that of orbital pseudotumor.[14] The MR signal characteristics are also indistinguish-

able from those of orbital pseudotumor (Fig. 20–16). The inferior and medial recti are most commonly involved. The greatest mass is often in the midportion of the muscle, with sparing of the spinal portion of the muscle. Pseudotumor, on the other hand, ordinarily involves the apical portion of the muscle.[61]

Rhabdomyosarcoma and lymphoma (Fig. 20–10) typically have high signal on T_2-weighted images, which distinguishes them from endocrine ophthalmopathy and pseudotumor. Rhabdomyosarcoma is the most common primary orbital malignancy in children.[62] It is a very aggressive tumor and often shows extensive destruction on MR scans. Both rhabdomyosarcoma and lymphoma can be homogeneous

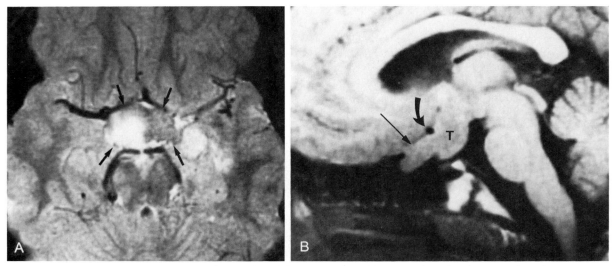

FIGURE 20–14. Optic glioma. A 7-year-old child with visual problems was found to have a chiasmal mass *(arrows)* on an axial T_2-weighted image *(A)*. The mass fills much of the suprasellar cisterns and has a heterogeneous internal texture. On a T_1-weighted sagittal image, the tumor (T) in the chiasm has extended forward into the left optic nerve *(arrow)*. The A1 segment of the anterior cerebral artery *(curved arrow)* is positioned between the mass and the adjacent frontal lobe.

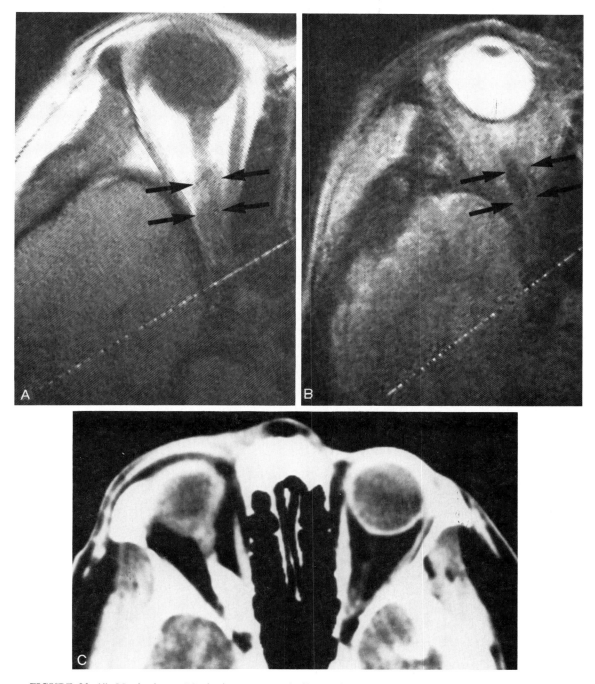

FIGURE 20–15. Meningioma. Meningiomas are typically nearly isointense with the optic nerve on all MR images. The T₁-weighted *(A)* and T₂-weighted *(B)* images show a focal area that is slightly lower in signal than optic nerve *(arrows)*. The CT scan *(C)* demonstrates this calcified meningioma better than MR.

TABLE 20–4. EXTRAOCULAR MUSCLE LESIONS

Lesion	T$_1$	T$_2$
Endocrine ophthalmopathy	Low	Low
Pseudotumor	Low	Low
Brown's syndrome	Low	Low
Rhabdomyosarcoma	Low	High
Lymphoma	Low	High

in signal intensity and can demonstrate infiltration and invasion of adjacent structures.

Brown's syndrome (Fig. 20–17) is a focal enlargement of the superior oblique muscle, limiting nasal upward gaze.[63] The scar has signal characteristics similar to those of muscle, with moderately low signal on T$_1$-weighted images and low signal on T$_2$-weighted images.

EXTRACONAL LESIONS

The typical MR signal intensity patterns for a variety of extraconal lesions are shown in Table 20–5.

Many extraconal tumors arise from the lacrimal

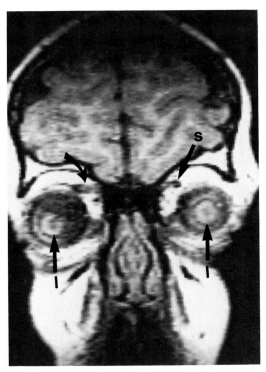

FIGURE 20–17. Brown's syndrome. Focal enlargement of the superior oblique muscle *(curved arrow)* is shown compared with the normal superior oblique muscle (s) on these 0.8-mm-thick slices obtained with a selective 3D technique. Note the inferolateral deviation of the lens (l) on the affected side compared with the opposite unaffected eye.

gland in the superolateral aspect of the orbit. Fifty per cent of primary lacrimal gland masses are of epithelial origin,[64, 65] equally divided between benign mixed adenomas and carcinomas, most frequently adenoid cystic carcinomas (Fig. 20–18). The remaining 50 per cent of lacrimal gland masses include lymphoid lesions, such as dacryoadenitis and pseudotumors. Most carcinomas are poorly circumscribed, inhomogeneous lesions of low signal on T$_1$-weighted images and high signal on T$_2$-weighted images. Demonstration of invasion of surrounding structures is a sign of malignancy.

Dermoid cysts are congenital lesions arising from epithelial rests, typically presenting as painless, discrete masses. Anatomically, the lesions are well-circumscribed masses, often displacing, but not infiltrating, adjacent structures.[36, 64, 65] Characteristic fat-fluid levels are often seen on MR (Fig. 20–19), even in the absence of a fluid level or fat attenuation on CT. The presence of fat excludes most other orbital neoplasms. The dependent fluid excludes lipoma.[10, 14] Another common appearance for dermoid tumors is homogeneous high signal on both T$_1$- and T$_2$-weighted images.

Epidermoid tumors have low signal on T$_1$-weighted images and high signal on T$_2$-weighted images like most other tumors (Fig. 20–20). These tumors can be differentiated from other neoplasms by the lack of T$_2$ enhancement on N(H) or cross-over images.[14]

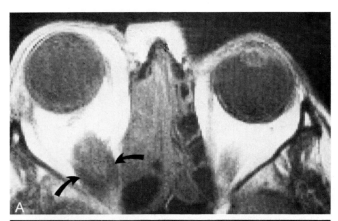

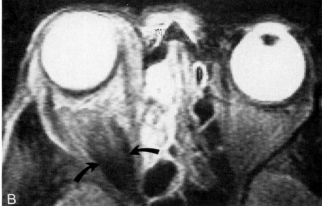

FIGURE 20–16. Endocrine ophthalmopathy. Enlargement of the midportion of the inferior rectus *(arrows)* is seen. This mass has low signal on both T$_1$-weighted *(A)* and T$_2$-weighted *(B)* images.

TABLE 20–5. EXTRACONAL LESIONS

Lesion	T₁	T₂	N(H)	Cross-over
Carcinoma	Low	High	High	High
Lymphoma	Low	High	High	High
Hemangioma	Low	High	High	High
Epidermoid	Low	High	Moderate	Isointense
Encephalocele	Low	High	Moderate-low	Isointense
Lipoma	High	Moderate	High	High
Dermoid	High-moderate	Moderate-high	High-moderate	Isointense
Osteoma	Low	Low	Low	Low
Fibrous dysplasia	Low	Low	Low	Low
Tolosa-Hunt syndrome	Low	Low	Low	Low
Hemorrhage (subacute)	High	High	High	High
Mucocele	High	High	High	High

Encephaloceles are homogeneous, well-defined lesions having nearly CSF intensity on T_1, T_2, N(H), and cross-over images. Mucoceles (Fig. 20–21) typically have high signal on N(H)- and T_2-weighted images.[14]

Orbital cellulitis is an acute bacterial infection that most often represents extension of an infection from the paranasal sinuses or eyelid. The orbits are pre-disposed to infections because, first, they are surrounded by the paranasal sinuses, which are commonly infected. Second, the thin lamina papyracea offers little resistance to an aggressive process in the ethmoid sinuses. Finally, the veins of the face do not have valves and thus serve as another pathway for extension of inflammation into the orbit.

Preseptal cellulitis appears as an area of increased

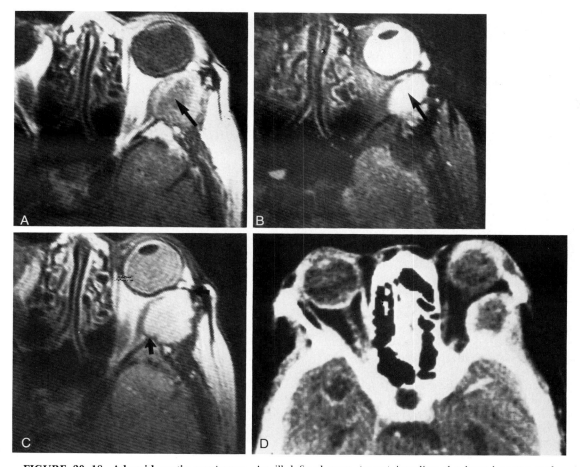

FIGURE 20–18. Adenoid cystic carcinoma. An ill-defined mass *(arrow)* invading the lateral rectus and breaking through the lateral wall of the orbit is shown on the T_1-weighted *(A)*, T_2-weighted, *(B)*, and N(H)-weighted *(C)* images. The central necrosis is most evident on the T_2-weighted image. The orbital anatomy is much better demonstrated on the MR than on the contrast-enhanced CT scan *(D)*. (From Sullivan JA, Harms SE: Surface-coil MR imaging of orbital neoplasms. AJNR 7:29–34, 1986; © by American Society of Neuroradiology.)

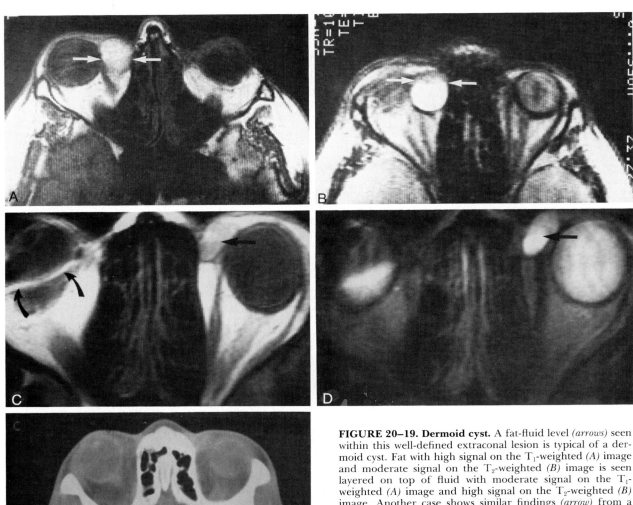

FIGURE 20–19. Dermoid cyst. A fat-fluid level *(arrows)* seen within this well-defined extraconal lesion is typical of a dermoid cyst. Fat with high signal on the T_1-weighted *(A)* image and moderate signal on the T_2-weighted *(B)* image is seen layered on top of fluid with moderate signal on the T_1-weighted *(A)* image and high signal on the T_2-weighted *(B)* image. Another case shows similar findings *(arrow)* from a smaller lesion on the T_1-weighted *(C)* and T_2-weighted *(D)* images. A subtle and nonspecific mass is seen on the corresponding CT scan *(E)*. The artifact in the right orbit *(C)* *(curved arrows)* is due to cosmetics. (From Sullivan JA, Harms SE: Surface-coil MR imaging of orbital neoplasms. AJNR 7:29–34, 1986; © by American Society of Neuroradiology.)

signal on T_2-weighted images (Fig. 20–22), with swelling of the anterior orbital tissues and obliteration of the fat planes. The fibrous orbital septum offers some resistance to extension of the infection into the posterior compartment of the orbit. Often, the first sign of involvement of the orbit is slight edema of the orbital fat. This is followed by development of more discrete abnormalities as the infectious process progresses. In most cases, the cellulitis is confined to the extraconal space, but if left untreated, it can enter the muscle cone and intraconal space.

Orbital cellulitis can lead to orbital abscess formation (Fig. 20–23). Extension of an ethmoiditis into the orbit usually begins as a subperiosteal abscess. This abscess can be identified on MR scan as a thin layer of low or high signal immediately lateral to the lamina papyracea.

Tolosa-Hunt syndrome is a lesion pathologically similar to orbital pseudotumor that involves the cavernous sinus and superior orbital fissure, producing painful ophthalmoplegia.[66] The lesion has a signal intensity similar to that of orbital pseudotumor on MR (Fig. 20–24). Clinically, a response to steroids is said to be diagnostic, but similar responses have been seen with other orbital lesions.[67] The MR findings could provide useful clinical information for patients with suspected Tolosa-Hunt syndrome.

Skin lesions, such as basal cell carcinoma (Fig. 20–25), frequently involve the eyelid. Basal cell carcinoma has low signal on T_1-weighted images and high signal on T_2-weighted images.[10, 14] Some squamous cell carcinomas do not enhance with T_2 weighting.

Obstruction or inflammation of the nasolacrimal sac can lead to dilatation of the sac (dacryocystitis),

Text continued on page 620

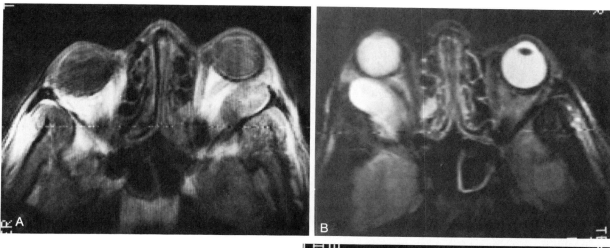

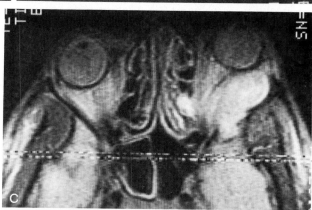

FIGURE 20–20. Epidermoid. Epidermoid tumors have low signal on T_1-weighted *(A)* images and high signal on T_2-weighted *(B)* images. These tumors can be distinguished from most other orbital tumors by their lack of enhancement on cross-over *(C)* and N(H)-weighted images. (From Sullivan JA, Harms SE: Characterization of orbital lesions by surface coil MR imaging. RadioGraphics 7:9–28, 1987; with permission.)

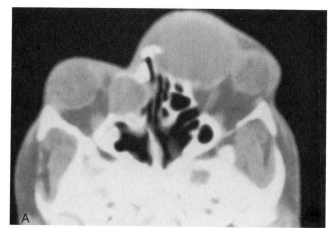

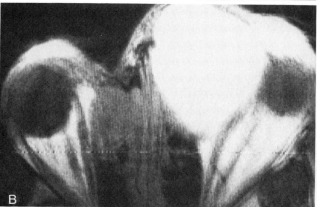

FIGURE 20–21. Mucocele. This mucocele could not be distinguished from an encephalocele by CT *(A)*. On MR, mucoceles have homogeneous high signal on both T_1-weighted *(B)* and T_2-weighted *(C)* images. Encephaloceles tend to follow CSF in signal intensity. (From Sullivan JA, Harms SE: Characterization of orbital lesions by surface coil MR imaging. RadioGraphics 7:9–28, 1987; with permission.)

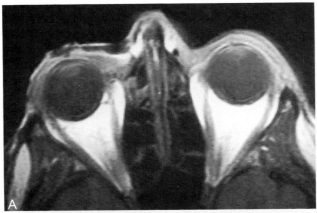

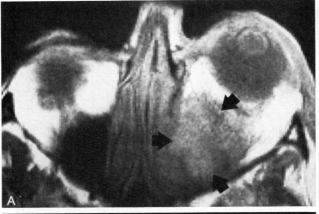

FIGURE 20–22. Cellulitis. The cellulitis is confined to the preseptal space by the orbital septum. Cellulitis has low signal on the T_1-weighted (A) and high signal on the T_2-weighted (B) images. The ulcer is secondary to a treated basal cell carcinoma.

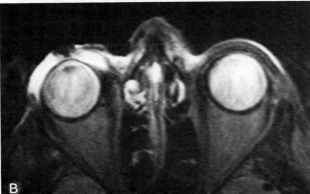

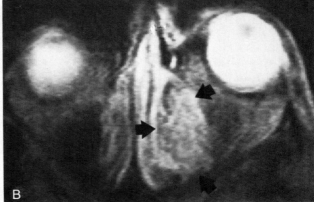

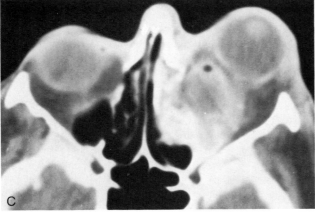

FIGURE 20–23. Abscess. Abscess has low signal (arrows) on T_1-weighted (A) and high signal (arrows) on T_2-weighted (B) images. A comparative CT scan (C) with gas in the abscess is shown.

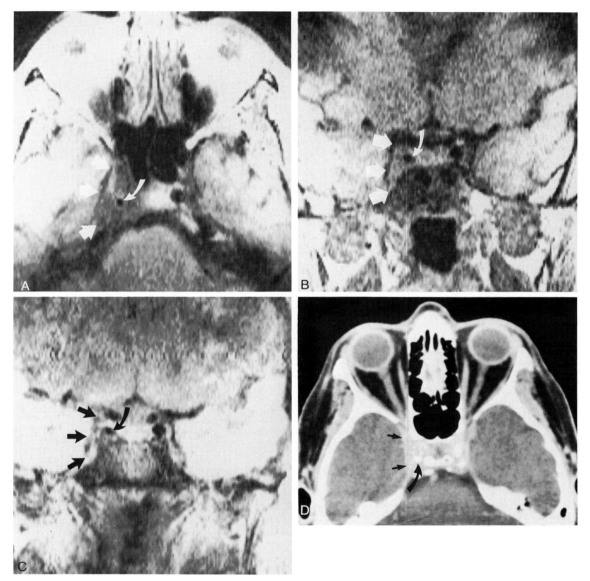

FIGURE 20–24. Tolosa-Hunt syndrome. The Tolosa-Hunt syndrome is seen as a low-signal mass *(arrows)* in the region of the cavernous sinus on the transverse T_1-weighted *(A)*, coronal T_1-weighted *(B)*, and transverse T_2-weighted *(C)* images. The narrowed internal carotid artery *(curved arrow)* is seen. A contrast-enhanced CT scan *(D)* shows a subtle mass *(arrows)* and a narrowed internal carotid artery *(curved arrow)*.

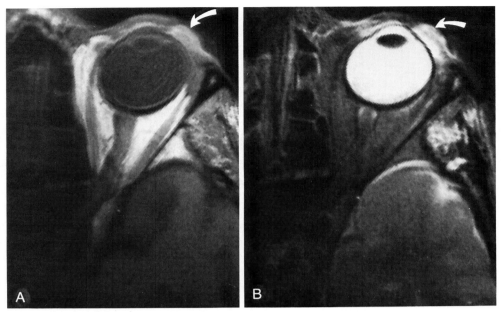

FIGURE 20–25. Basal cell carcinoma. The mass of basal cell carcinoma *(arrow)* has low signal on the T₁-weighted *(A)* and high signal on the T₂-weighted *(B)* images.

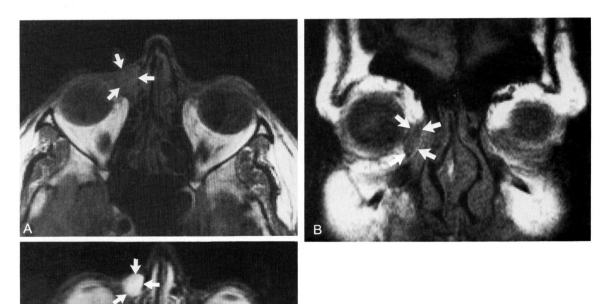

FIGURE 20–26. Dacryocystitis. A well-defined, homogeneous, enlarged nasolacrimal sac *(arrows)* is evidence of dacryocystitis. The sac is filled with fluid having low signal on the transverse *(A)* and coronal *(B)* T₁-weighted images and high signal on the T₂-weighted *(C)* image.

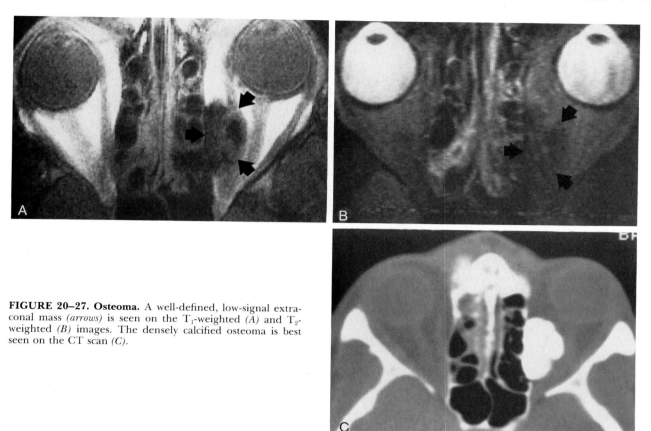

FIGURE 20–27. Osteoma. A well-defined, low-signal extraconal mass *(arrows)* is seen on the T_1-weighted *(A)* and T_2-weighted *(B)* images. The densely calcified osteoma is best seen on the CT scan *(C)*.

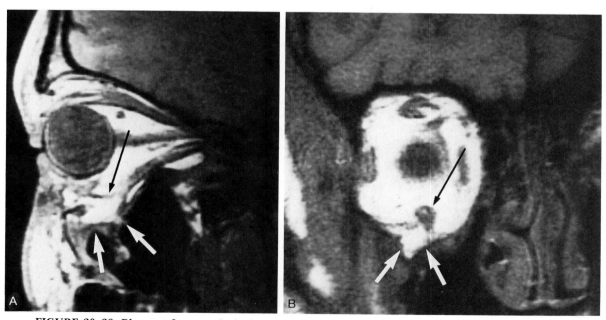

FIGURE 20–28. Blow-out fracture. Sagittal *(A)* and coronal *(B)* T_1-weighted scans demonstrate a blow-out fracture of the right orbit with depression of the orbital floor *(arrows)* into the superior maxillary sinus. The inferior rectus muscle *(long arrow)* is clearly identified and is not entrapped by the floor fracture.

as shown in Figure 20–26.[68] A well-defined, homogeneous, long T_1 and T_2 fluid intensity extraconal mass in the inferomedial orbit is typical of dacryocystitis.

Bone lesions can involve the orbit. Fibrous dysplasia frequently involves the superior lateral orbit. Osteomas (Fig. 20–27) are common, particularly in patients with Gardner's syndrome.[14] Other possible lesions include osteosarcoma, giant cell tumor, and metastatic disease. Osteomas have low signal on all images. Fibrous dysplasia also has low signal on all images but is not quite as low in signal as a densely calcified osteoma. Osteogenic osteosarcoma is more aggressive in appearance, with mixed high and low signal on T_2-weighted images. Although CT is the primary imaging modality for evaluating orbital fractures, the multiplanar capability of MR and high soft tissue contrast are helpful to assess possible muscle entrapment with blow-out fractures (Fig. 20–28).

REFERENCES

1. Li KC, Poon PY, Hinton P, et al: MR imaging of orbital tumors with CT and ultrasound correlations. J Comput Assist Tomogr 8:1039–1047, 1984.
2. Hawkes RC, Holland GN, Moore WS, et al: NMR imaging in the evaluation of orbital tumors. AJNR 4:254–256, 1983.
3. Jan JS, Benson JE, Bonstelle CT, et al: Magnetic resonance imaging of the orbit: A preliminary experience. Radiology 150:755–759, 1984.
4. Sobel DF, Kelly W, Kjos BO, et al: MR imaging of orbital and ocular disease. AJNR 6:259–264, 1985.
5. Edward JH, Hyman RA, Vacirca SJ, et al: 0.6 T magnetic resonance imaging of the orbit. AJNR 6:253–258, 1985.
6. Sobel DF, Mills C, Char D, et al: NMR of the normal and pathologic eye and orbit. AJNR 5:345–350, 1984.
7. Moseley I, Brant-Zawadzki M, Mills C: Nuclear magnetic resonance imaging of the orbit. Br J Ophthalmol 67:333–342, 1983.
8. Char DH, Sobel D, Kelly WM, et al: Magnetic resonance scanning in orbital tumor diagnosis. Ophthalmology 92:1305–1310, 1985.
9. Haik BG, Louis LS, Smith ME, et al: Magnetic resonance imaging in the evaluation of leukocoria. Ophthalmology 92:1143–1152, 1985.
10. Sullivan JA, Harms SE: Surface coil MR imaging of orbital neoplasms. AJNR 7:29–34, 1986.
11. Schenck JF, Foster TH, Henkes JL, et al: High-field surface-coil MR imaging of localized anatomy. AJNR 6:181–186, 1985.
13. Harms SE, Wilk RM, Wolford LM, et al: The temporomandibular joint: Magnetic resonance imaging using surface coils. Radiology 157:133–136, 1985.
14. Sullivan JA, Harms SE: Characterization of orbital lesions by surface coil MR imaging. RadioGraphics 7:9–28, 1987.
15. Bilaniuk LT, Schenck JF, Zimmerman RA, et al: Ocular and orbital lesions: Surface coil MR imaging. Radiology 156:669–674, 1985.
16. Gomori JM, Grossman RI, Shields JA, et al: Choroidal melanomas: Correlation of NMR spectroscopy and MR imaging. Radiology 158:443–445, 1986.
17. Rosenkranz G, Tellkamp H, Köhler K, et al: Radiation exposure to the lens during CT of the orbital area. Digitale Bilddiagn 5:66–69, 1985.
18. Unsold R, Newton T, Hoyt WF: CT examination technique of the optic nerve. J Comput Assist Tomogr 4:560–563, 1980.
19. Alker GJ, Banna M, Rudin S, et al: Computed tomography of the orbit. CRC Crit Rev Diagn Imaging 15:27–93, 1981.
20. Harms SE, Kramer DM: Fundamentals of magnetic resonance imaging. CRC Crit Rev Diagn Imaging 25:79–111, 1985.
21. Kramer DM: Basic principles of magnetic resonance imaging. Radiol Clin North Am 22:765–778, 1984.
22. Harms SE, Morgan TJ, Yamanashi WS, et al: Principles of nuclear magnetic resonance imaging. RadioGraphics 4:26–43, 1984.
23. Harms SE, Siemers PT, Hildebrand P, Plum G: Multiple spin-echo magnetic resonance imaging of the brain. Radio-Graphics 6:117–134, 1980.
24. Rosen BR, Brady TJ: Principles of nuclear magnetic resonance for medical applications. Semin Nucl Med 13:308–318, 1984.
25. Bydder GM, Young IR: MR imaging: Clinical use of the inversion recovery sequence. J Comput Assist Tomogr 9:659–675, 1985.
26. Frahm J, Hasse A, Matthari W: Rapid three-dimensional MR imaging using the FLASH technique. J Comput Assist Tomogr 10:363–368, 1986.
27. Hasse A, Frahm J, Matthaei W, Hanicke KD: Rapid images and NMR movies. *In* Program of the Society of Magnetic Resonance in Medicine, 1985, pp 980–981.
28. Frahm J, Merboldt KD, Hanicke W, Haase A: Stimulated echo imaging. J Magn Reson 64:81–93, 1985.
29. Haase A, Frahm J: NMR imaging of spin-lattice relaxation using stimulated echoes. J Magn Reson 65:481–490, 1985.
30. Harms SE, Muschler G: Three dimensional MR imaging of the knee using surface coils. J Comput Assist Tomogr 10:733–777, 1986.
31. Harms SE, Kramer DM: Clinical use of the 3D multislab acquisition method for imaging neurologic disorders. *In* Program of the Society of Magnetic Resonance in Medicine, 1986, pp 641–642.
32. Haacke EM, Bearden FH, Clayton JR, Linga NR: Reduction of MR imaging time by the hybrid fast-scan technique. Radiology 158:521–529, 1986.
33. Mansfield P: Multi-planar image formation using NMR spin echoes. J Phys [C] 10:55–58, 1977.
34. Danziger A, Price HI: CT findings in retinoblastoma. JAMA 133:783, 1979.
35. Reese AB: Tumors of the Eye. New York, Harper and Row, 1976.
36. Jacobs L, Wiesberg LA, Kinkel WR: Computerized Tomography of the Orbit and Sella Turcica. New York, Raven Press, 1980.
37. Zimmerman RA, Bilaniuk LT: Computed tomography of the evaluation of patients with bilateral retinoblastomas. J Comput Tomogr 3:251–257, 1979.
38. Brown DH: The clinicopathology of retinoblastomas. Am J Ophthalmol 61:508, 1966.
39. Harris GJ, Williams AL, Reeser FH: Intra-ocular evaluation by computed tomography. Int Ophthalmol Clin 22:197–217, 1982.
40. Reese AB, Ellsworth RM: The evaluation and current concept of retinoblastoma therapy. Trans Am Acad Ophthalmol Otolaryngol 67:164, 1963.
41. Sherman JL, McLean IW, Brallier DR: Coats' disease, CT-pathologic correlation in two cases. Radiology 146:77–78, 1983.
42. Mafee MF, Goldberg MF, Valvassori GE, Capek V: Computed tomography in the evaluation of patients with persistent hyperplastic primary vitreous (PHPV). Radiology 145:713–717, 1982.
43. Mafee MF, Goldberg MF: Persistent hyperplastic primary vitreous (PHPV): Role of computed tomography and magnetic resonance. Radiol Clin North Am 25:683–692, 1987.
44. Armstrong EA, Smith TH, Harms SE: Brawny scleritis of the eye: Correlation of CT and MRI anatomy. Presented at European Society of Paediatric Radiology, Glasgow, 1985.
45. Peyman GA, Mafee MF: Uveal melanoma and similar lesions: The role of magnetic resonance imaging. Radiol Clin North Am 25:471–486, 1987.

46. Mafee MF, Peyman GA: Retinal and choroidal detachments: Role of magnetic resonance imaging and computed tomography. Radiol Clin North Am 25:509–528, 1987.
47. Hesselink JR, Davis KR, Weber AL, et al: Radiological evaluation of orbital metastases with emphasis on computed tomography. Radiology 137:363, 1980.
48. Jones ES, Jakobiec FA: Diseases of the Orbit. Hagerstown, MD, Harper and Row, 1979.
49. Gomori JM, Grossman RI, Shields JA, et al: Choroidal melanomas: Correlation of NMR spectroscopy and ME imaging. Radiology 158:443–445, 1986.
50. Mafee MF, Peyman GHA, Grissland JE, et al: Malignant uveal melanoma simulating lesions: MR imaging evaluation. Radiology 160:773–780, 1986.
51. Peyster RG, Augsburger JJ, Shields JA, et al: Intraocular tumors: Evaluation with MR imaging. Radiology 168:773–779, 1988.
52. Forbes GS, Sheedy PF II, Waller RR: Orbital tumors evaluated by computed tomography. Radiology 136:101, 1980.
53. Lloyd GAS: CT scanning in the diagnosis of orbital disease. J Comput Tomogr 3:227, 1979.
54. Davis KR, Hesselink JR, Dallow RL, Grove AS Jr: CT and ultrasound diagnosis of cavernous hemangioma and lymphangioma of the orbit. J Comput Tomogr 4:98–104, 1980.
55. Bilaniuk LT, Atlas SW, Zimmerman RA: Magnetic resonance imaging of the orbit. Radiol Clin North Am 25:509–528, 1987.
56. Mafee MF, Putterman A, Valvassori GE, et al: Orbital space occupying lesions: Role of magnetic resonance imaging and computed tomography—a review of 145 cases. Radiol Clin North Am 25:529–560, 1987.
57. Atlas SW, Grossman RI, Savino PJ, et al: Surface-coil MR of orbital pseudotumor. AJNR 8:141–146, 1987.
58. Wright JE: Primary optic nerve meningiomas: Clinical presentation and management. Trans Am Acad Ophthalmol Otolaryngol 83:617–624, 1977.
59. Daniels DL, Yu S, Pech P, Haughton VM: Computed tomography and magnetic resonance imaging of the orbital apex. Radiol Clin North Am 25:803–818, 1987.
60. Rothfus WE, Curtin HD: Extraocular muscle enlargement: A CT review. Radiology 150:409–415, 1984.
61. Alper MG: Endocrine orbital disease. In Arger PH (ed): Orbit Roentgenology. New York, Wiley, 1977.
62. Vade A, Armstrong D: Orbital rhabdomyosarcoma in childhood. Radiol Clin North Am 25:701–714, 1987.
63. Goldhammer Y, Smith JL: Acquired intermittent Brown's syndrome. Neurology 24:666, 1974.
64. Hesselink JR, Davis KR, Dallow RL, et al: Computed tomography of masses in the lacrimal gland region. Radiology 137:363, 1980.
65. Stewart WB, Krobel GB, Wright JE: Lacrimal gland and fossa lesions: Approach to diagnosis and management. Ophthalmology 86:886, 1979.
66. Glaser JS: Neuro-ophthalmology. Hagerstown, MD, Harper and Row, 1978.
67. Thomas JE, Yoss RF: The parasellar syndrome: Problems in determining etiology. Mayo Clin Proc 45:617, 1970.
68. Russell EJ, Czervionke L, Huckman M, et al: CT of the inferomedial orbit and the lacrimal drainage apparatus: Normal and pathologic anatomy. AJNR 6:759–766, 1985.

21

HEAD AND NECK

BARBARA L. CARTER, P. KOENIGSBERG, MARK S. BANKOFF,
and VAL M. RUNGE

INDICATIONS

TECHNIQUE

TEMPORAL BONE AND POSTERIOR
FOSSA

NASOPHARYNX, INFRATEMPORAL
FOSSA, AND PARAPHARYNGEAL
SPACE

PARANASAL SINUSES AND NASAL
CAVITY

SALIVARY GLANDS

OROPHARYNX, LARYNX, AND NECK

ORAL CAVITY AND MANDIBLE

LARYNX

NECK

TEMPOROMANDIBULAR JOINT

In the past, the radiographic evaluation of the ear, nose, and throat (ENT) has been limited to plain films, fluoroscopy, pleuridirectional tomography, and CT, with heavy emphasis recently on CT.[1] CT has been extremely useful in evaluating the head and neck region in areas that are difficult to visualize directly or palpate, such as the nasopharynx, infratemporal fossa, and parapharyngeal space. In other areas, CT has shown the deep extent of disease previously unsuspected by visual inspection, and it has altered the evaluation and management of patients dramatically since its advent. In recent years, MR imaging has gained acceptance in the study of ENT cases,[2] and early data indicate that it not only is beneficial but also will probably become the imaging modality of choice for many patients, depending on availability and cost.[3–6] MR has many potential advantages over CT because of its finer soft tissue detail and its capability of identifying fluid-containing structures and abnormal soft tissue lesions without the use of intravenous iodinated contrast material.[7] By obtaining direct sagittal and coronal images, one can determine the total extent of a tumor in a plane that is better for the surgeon and radiation oncologist, who are attempting to plan the most appropriate treatment. MR is also used in assessing the response of a tumor to treatment and in detecting recurrent disease.

INDICATIONS

MR is now the imaging modality of choice in the posterior fossa for identifying acoustic neuromas within the cerebellopontine angle and internal auditory canal and for differentiating between an acoustic neuroma and other mass lesions in the area, such as epidermoid tumors.[8–11] MR has the advantage of depicting centrally placed lesions, such as an infarct or small tumor in the vicinity of the nuclei of cranial nerves V to XII when patients present with signs and symptoms that could be due to a lesion anywhere along the course of these and the other cranial nerves. This new imaging modality is also evolving as the procedure of choice in evaluating patients suspected of having tumors of the temporal bone, skull base, nasopharynx, and infratemporal fossa.[12, 13] Note should be made that CT may be needed to supplement the MR image for detailed analysis of involvement of cortical bone and the dense otic capsule containing the cochlea, vestibule, and semicircular canals. CT is still the procedure of choice for evaluating the minute detail of the middle ear with its ossicular chain in the case of congenital anomalies, trauma, and localized infection.

In other ENT areas, MR is also evolving as being equal to or superior to CT in patients suspected of having a tumor. This improvement is particularly apparent in the nasopharynx and infratemporal fossa but is also evident in the nasal cavity, paranasal sinuses, oropharynx, hypopharynx, larynx, salivary glands, and neck. For example, tumors of the nasal cavity, such as the esthesioneuroblastoma, have the potential for intracranial extension, requiring careful evaluation of the area immediately above and below the cribriform plate. Malignant lesions of the paranasal sinuses often involve the orbit, infratemporal fossa, and pterygopalatine space, requiring the best detail possible of the soft tissue structures in the area. Bone marrow involvement by tumor and infection is discernible by MR but difficult to detect by CT unless there is cortical bone destruction or reactive sclerosis. In other regions, MR is at least equal to CT in the evaluation of patients with tumors of the salivary glands, parapharyngeal space, oropharynx, larynx, and neck, including the thyroid and parathyroid glands. Exquisite soft tissue detail is needed for determining the total extent of disease and for identifying metastatic nodes. Finally, temporomandibular joint abnormalities are a common problem, particularly among young females. These have been studied progressively over the past few years with pleuridirectional tomography, arthrography, CT, and now MR.[14] The last technique has the advantage of superior soft tissue detail for visualizing the anterior and posterior bands and the intermediate zone of the meniscus, and it is therefore becoming the procedure of choice for assessing temporomandibular joint (TMJ) dysfunction.[15–18]

TECHNIQUE

All portions of the head and neck area should be studied with T_1-weighted images (short repetition time [TR], short echo time [TE] sequences) to obtain the best soft tissue detail possible. These images are usually acquired in the axial plane and are supplemented by coronal images through the area of interest. Thin (≤ 3 mm) slices are needed for the detailed analysis of small areas, such as the internal auditory canal and skull base. Thicker slices (8 mm) permit review of larger areas of the neck for identification of metastatic nodes. An intermediate slice thickness (5 mm) may be used in other areas, such as the larynx and sinuses.

T_2-weighted images (long TR, long TE sequences) through the area of interest can permit better differentiation of the abnormality in question. The newest fast scan techniques, such as FLASH and FISP, may offer additional information. These sequences demonstrate some flow sensitivity, permit the acquisition of breath-hold images, and may eventually provide—with three-dimensional (3D) volume acquisition—improved detail on thin, 1-mm, adjacent sections.

The actual pulse sequence for T_1- and T_2-weighted images varies with the strength of the magnet. For the Siemens 1-T magnet (Siemens, Iselin, NJ), 256 × 256 data acquisition is used, with a spin-echo (SE) technique using a TR of 0.6 second and a TE of 17 msec for mild T_1-weighted images. Sequential images separated by 1-mm spacing are obtained. Four acquisitions are used for thin (3 mm) sections to improve signal-to-noise ratio (S/N), and two are used for the thicker sections. For the T_2 sequence, a TR of 3.0 seconds is used with a TE of 45/90 msec, using either a 256 × 256 matrix or a 256 × 128 true rectangular pixel. Gradient moment nulling with a two-axis first-order correction is used to compensate for motion on T_2-weighted images.

A head coil is used for the temporal bone, skull base, nasopharynx, paranasal sinuses, and oral pharynx. A surface coil or other specially designed receiver coil should be used for assessment of the TMJ, neck, larynx, thyroid, and parathyroid glands and for finer detail of the temporal bone.[19] Paramagnetic contrast agents such as gadolinium–diethylene triamine pentaacetic acid (Gd-DTPA) are now approved for use in intracranial lesions[8] and are being evaluated for other areas, such as the upper aerodigestive tract.

TEMPORAL BONE AND POSTERIOR FOSSA

MR has become the imaging procedure of choice for the evaluation of the posterior fossa, including possible tumors of the temporal bone. By using a paramagnetic contrast agent such as Gd-DTPA, MR is even more sensitive for detecting a tumor or an infectious process. The superior soft tissue detail and lack of bone hardening artifact permit visualization of the region of the nuclei in the pons[20] and of the peripheral course of the cranial nerves[12] throughout the basilar cisterns, the cerebellopontine angle, the internal auditory canal, the jugular fossa, and the hypoglossal canal to the neck (Fig. 21–1). These features largely negate the need for intravenous iodinated contrast enhancement and for air cisternography.[21, 22]

The dorsal and ventral nuclei of the cochlear nerve produce an eminence, the acoustic tubercle adjacent to the inferior cerebellar peduncle in the caudal portion of the pons.[20] The nuclei of the vestibular nerve are located more posteromedially, near the floor of the fourth ventricle. The cochlear nerve, passing through the anteroinferior portion of the internal auditory canal, ends in the spiral ganglion within the modiolus of the cochlea; the vestibular nerves, in the posterior portion of the internal auditory canal, end in the vestibular ganglion and supply the semicircular canals (Fig. 21–1). The facial nerve, originating medial to the vestibular and cochlear nerves, travels in the anterosuperior portion of the internal auditory canal, entering the facial nerve canal. It courses anterolaterally to the geniculate

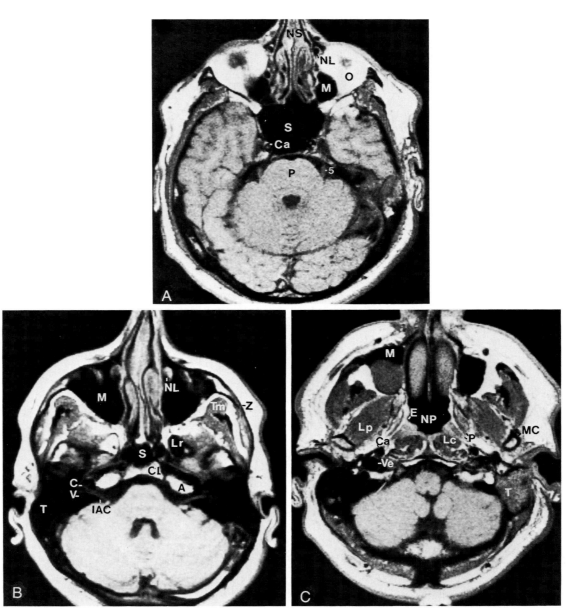

FIGURE 21–1. Normal temporal bone and posterior fossa. T_1-weighted axial images (TR 0.8/TE 17). *A*, A view through the pons (P) and sphenoid sinus (S) that shows the fifth cranial nerve (5), the internal carotid artery (Ca), the nasal septum (NS), the nasolacrimal duct (NL), infraorbital fat (O), and the apex of the maxillary sinus (M). *B*, A view slightly caudad through the internal auditory canal (IAC) containing the seventh and eighth cranial nerves. This leads to the inner ear with the cochlea (C) and vestibule (V), with limited visualization of the semicircular canals. The temporal bone (T) containing pneumatized mastoid air cells and the maxillary sinus are air containing and thus have no signal. The nasolacrimal duct (NL) is along the medial wall of the maxillary sinus. The temporalis muscle (Tm) is deep to the zygoma (Z). Marrow within the clivus (Cl) and petrous apex (A) has a strong signal, whereas the sphenoid sinus (S), with the left lateral recess (Lr), is aerated. *C*, A view further caudad through the medulla and cerebellar tonsils. The internal jugular vein (Ve) and internal carotid (Ca) have a low signal. The longus capitis muscle (Lc) forms the posterior wall of the nasopharynx (NP), and the tensor and levator palatini muscles (P) arise inferior to the eustachian tube (E). The lateral pterygoid muscle (Lp) passes from the pterygoid plate to the mandibular condyle (MC) and condylar neck. A retention cyst is present in the right maxillary sinus (M). The left temporal bone (T) is altered by previous mastoidectomy.

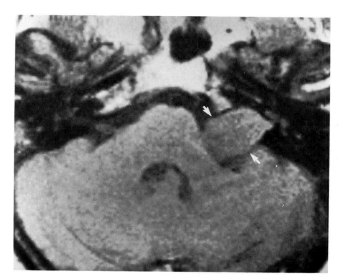

FIGURE 21–2. **Large left acoustic neuroma** *(arrows).* Axial T$_1$-weighted image (TR 0.8/TE 17). Note enlargement of the left cerebellopontine (CP) angle cistern and slight displacement of the fourth ventricle by the large tumor.

ganglion area, and then the canal takes a hairpin turn posteriorly, passing above the oval window and below the lateral semicircular canal. It then turns vertically to exit through the stylomastoid foramen. The facial nerve then enters the parotid gland and divides into five to seven branches. Cranial nerves IX, X, and XI originate in the medulla medial to the jugular fossa, where they exit via the pars nervosa to the carotid sheath. Cranial nerve XII arises from an elongated nucleus in the hypoglossal triangle of the floor of the fourth ventricle. The fibers, passing ventrally through the medulla, emerge as a linear series of 10 to 15 rootlets through the anterolateral sulcus between the pyramid and olive, receiving fibers

from other areas, all of which unite as the hypoglossal nerve, passing through the hypoglossal canal to enter the carotid sheath deep to the internal jugular vein.

Acoustic neuromas account for approximately 80 per cent of tumors in the cerebellopontine angle, and the majority of these tumors extend into the internal auditory canal (Fig. 21–2). MR is needed to identify the small intracanalicular tumors (Fig. 21–3) originating from the vestibular nerve.[23, 24] These patients may present with tinnitus or vertigo, or both, prior to any hearing loss. Any attempt to preserve hearing would require early detection of these schwannomas.[10] MR is the screening procedure of choice for the early detection of small acoustic neuromas. Even further sensitivity is attained with the use of Gd-DTPA[8] (see Fig. 15–26). Other tumor masses to be considered in the cerebellopontine angle area are meningiomas (see Fig. 15–10), epidermoid tumors (Fig. 21–4), aneurysms, cysts (Fig. 21–5), and metastatic lesions. According to Mawhinney,[22] 40 per cent of the neurilemmoma group have a markedly prolonged T$_1$, whereas meningiomas tend to have a somewhat shorter T$_1$, similar to the T$_1$ of brain. Epidermoid tumors often have an irregular outline and moderate heterogeneity (see Fig. 21–4).[25] Both high and low signals on T$_1$-weighted images have been reported, the majority with low signals. The same authors found a high signal in the cerebellopontine angle to mitigate against the diagnosis of meningioma. The axial scan is good for showing mass effect and extension into the internal auditory canal. The coronal plane is useful to supplement the axial plane for showing the total extent of tumor and the relationship of the mass to the tentorium (see also Chapter 15).

Schwannomas may occur anywhere along the course of the cranial nerves and should be considered the most likely cause of a tumor along the course of

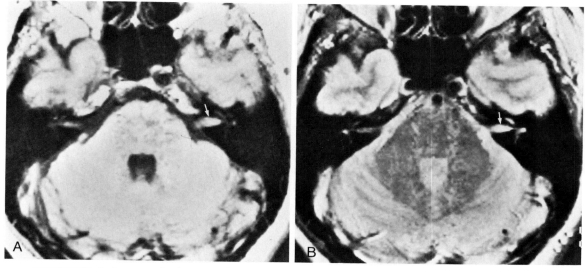

FIGURE 21–3. **Intracanalicular acoustic neuroma.** Axial images. *A,* T$_1$-weighted image (TR 0.65/TE 20). *B,* T$_2$-weighted image (TR 3.00/TE 45). A small acoustic neuroma is contained within the canal *(arrow).*

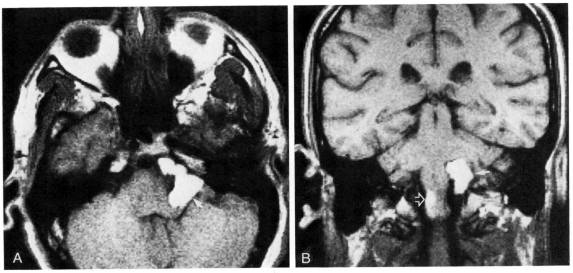

FIGURE 21–4. Epidermoid tumor. T_1-weighted image (TR 0.7/TE 17). Axial *(A)* and coronal *(B)* images. A large, irregular, bright lesion is present in the left CP angle *(closed arrow)*, and a small lesion *(open arrow)* is seen in the right. At surgery, a ruptured epidermoid tumor was found, with soft, yellow mucoid material surrounding the cranial nerves.

the facial nerve within the temporal bone, as described previously. A schwannoma or a paraganglioma may manifest as tumor mass in the region of the jugular fossa and hypoglossal nerve canal. When arising within the tympanic cavity from Jacobson's or Arnold's nerve, the paraganglioma[26] is known as a glomus tympanicum (Fig. 21–6), whereas in the jugular fossa, it has been referred to as a glomus jugulare (Fig. 21–7). These tumors are usually benign but are often locally invasive (see Fig. 15–35) and will recur if not completely excised. Three per cent of paragangliomas may be seen in more than one area,[27] partic-

ularly when seen in patients with familial tendencies (26 per cent). Both temporal bones, the carotid bifurcation, and the course of the vagus nerve into the chest are areas that should be examined when there is a familial history of paraganglioma. Although rare, paragangliomas may be malignant (Fig. 21–7) and metastasize to nodes and other areas in the body. Schwannomas (Figs. 21–8 and 21–9) are usually more sharply defined, but they, too, can extend into the posterior fossa and inferiorly below the skull and into the neck (Fig. 21–9). The coronal plane is preferable for identifying the total extent of tumor,

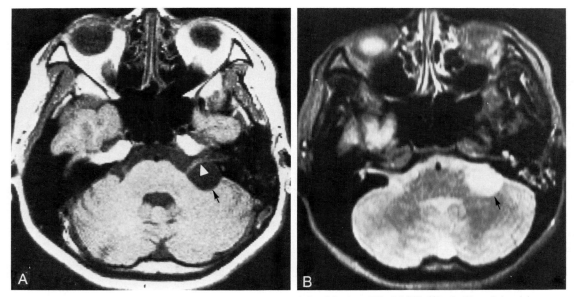

FIGURE 21–5. Arachnoid cyst. Axial images. *A*, T_1-weighted image (TR 0.6/TE 17). *B*, T_2-weighted image (TR 3.0/TE 70). A fluid-containing structure *(arrow)* is displacing the seventh and eighth cranial nerves *(arrowhead)* anteriorly.

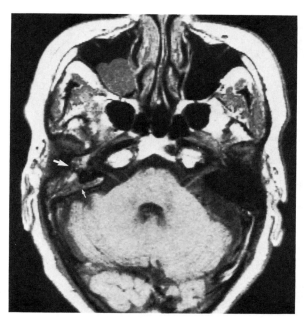

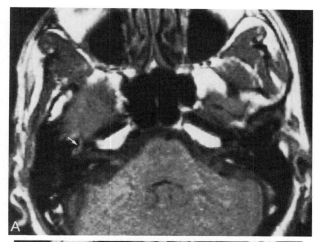

FIGURE 21–6. Glomus tympanicum. Axial image, T_1-weighted (TR 0.8/TE 17). The tumor is extending throughout the tympanic cavity and mastoid air cells *(arrows)*, but not into the jugular fossa or below the skull base. Note excellent visualization of the seventh and eighth cranial nerves and the retention cyst in the right maxillary sinus.

and this is best accomplished with MR. CT has the advantage of better detail of compact bone and is needed at present for careful analysis of the more invasive types of tumors of the temporal bone. The

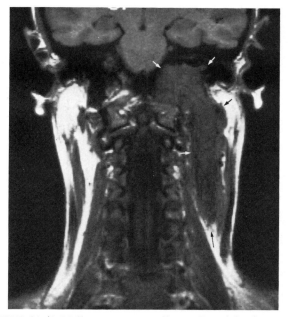

FIGURE 21–7. Malignant paraganglioma. T_1-weighted coronal image (TR 0.6/TE 17). Tumor is extending from the jugular fossa down to the neck within the internal jugular vein *(arrows)*. The serpiginous appearance is attributed to variations in flow. This tumor barely projects into the tympanic cavity and extends to the posterior fossa (not shown). It later metastasized to bones and liver.

FIGURE 21–8. Schwannoma, seventh cranial nerve. Axial plane, *A* cephalad to *B*. T_1-weighted images (TR 0.6/TE 17). A tumor of the seventh cranial nerve extends posteriorly from the geniculate ganglion area *(closed arrow)* through the horizontal portion of the facial nerve canal, as seen in *A*, and down through the vertical portion of the canal *(open arrow)*, as seen in *B*.

CT scan is preferable for evaluating destruction of such fine structures as the tegmen tympani, the floor of the hypotympanum, and portions of the otic capsule and even for determining minimal invasion of the tympanic cavity. This destruction of the temporal bone is particularly evident in patients with a carcinoma or sarcoma of the area. CT remains the procedure of choice for the evaluation of trauma, cholesteatoma, and mastoiditis because of the importance of defining minute detail of the ossicular chain, the tegmen, and the various recesses of the tympanic cavity. As surface-coil images of the temporal bone become more available or with other technologic advances, MR may become equal to or surpass CT in some of these areas (Fig. 21–10). Extensive infection that is apt to extend outside the temporal bone, as with malignant external otitis, is more within the realm of MR for an evaluation of the adjacent soft tissue structures and the bone marrow (Fig. 21–11). Similarly, systemic diseases such as Wegener's granulomatosis, sarcoidosis, and histiocytosis are probably

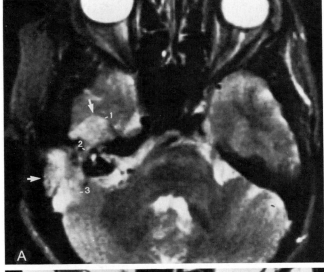

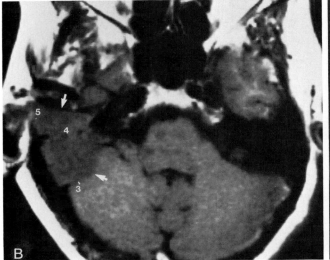

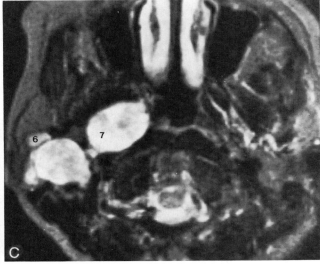

FIGURE 21–9. Huge schwannoma. Axial images. *A* and *C*, T$_2$-weighted images (TR 30/TE 90). *B*, T$_1$-weighted image (TR 0.65/TE 20). *A* is cephalad to *B*, which is cephalad to *C*. Note the large tumor *(arrows)* extending from the facial nerve canal anteriorly to the middle cranial fossa (1) and back through the horizontal portion of the facial nerve canal (2) to the posterior cranial fossa (3). *B* shows the tumor in the region of the vertical portion of the facial nerve canal (4) extending into the posterior cranial fossa (3) and external auditory canal (5). *C* shows tumor in the parotid gland (6) extending anteromedially deep to the parotid gland and to the parapharyngeal space (7). (Case referred from ENT Department, Boston City Hospital, Boston, MA.)

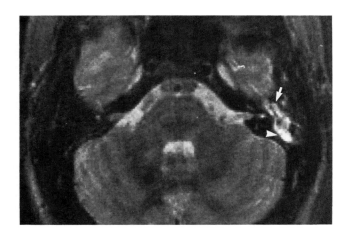

FIGURE 21–10. Cholesteatoma, left tympanic cavity. T$_2$-weighted axial image (TR 3.0/TE 90). Enlargement of the epitympanum *(arrow)* and mastoid antrum *(arrowhead)* is a result of bone destruction by the cholesteatoma.

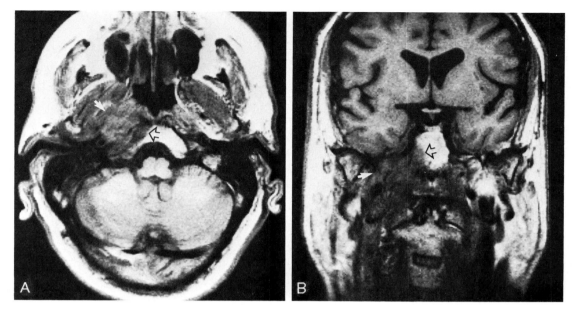

FIGURE 21–11. Malignant external otitis media with osteomyelitis, skull base. *A,* Axial image. *B,* Coronal image. T_1-weighted images (TR 0.8/TE 17). A large mass *(closed arrow)* is present in the right side of the nasopharynx encroaching on the parapharyngeal space. Decreased signal *(open arrow)* in the clivus indicates bone marrow involvement by the proven inflammatory mass. The right external otitis had responded to antibiotics prior to the MR imaging study.

better candidates for MR because of adjacent soft tissue involvement. MR has additional advantages over CT in the posterior fossa, with its superior detail of the brain stem. Small infarcts or tumors in this area may simulate a more peripheral lesion. Other considerations for the advantages and disadvantages of MR versus CT are listed in Table 21–1. Stapes prostheses are a potential contraindication for MR, but studies to date[28] have not shown any evidence of motion of the prosthesis by the magnetic field.

NASOPHARYNX, INFRATEMPORAL FOSSA, AND PARAPHARYNGEAL SPACE

The *nasopharynx* (Figs. 21–12 to 21–17), located immediately below the sphenoid sinus and clivus, is enclosed by the superior pharyngeal constrictor muscle with the pharyngobasilar fascia, the salpingopharyngeus muscles adjacent to the torus tubarius of the eustachian tube, the tensor and levator palatini

TABLE 21–1. ADVANTAGES AND DISADVANTAGES OF MR AND CT

MR Advantages	CT Advantages	MR Disadvantages	CT Disadvantages
No radiation	Superior bone detail	Contraindications	Bone hardening artifact
Superior detail of soft tissues and brain stem	Availability	Aneurysm clip	Dental filling artifact
Multiple pulse sequences—	Lower cost to patient	Pacemaker	Allergy to iodinated contrast material
T_1, T_2, and so on	Biopsy for suspected tumor	Cochlear implant	Radiation exposure
No bone hardening artifact	Drainage of abscess cavities	Pregnancy	
Dental artifacts localized		Higher cost	
Multiplanar capability		Motion artifact:	
No iodinated contrast		Respiration	
Intrinsic sensitivity to blood flow		Vessel pulsation	
		Cerebrospinal fluid pulsation	
		Prolonged scanning time	
		Absence of signal from dense cortical bone and calcium	
		Critically ill patients with life support mechanisms more difficult	
		Claustrophobia more severe than with CT	

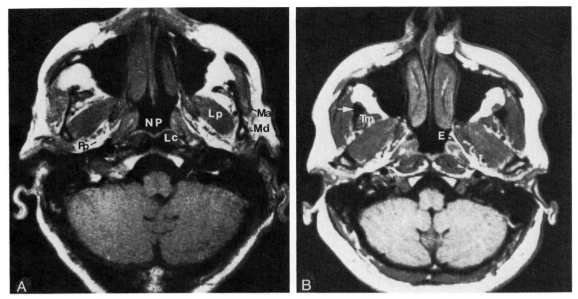

FIGURE 21–12. Normal nasopharynx, infratemporal fossa, and parapharyngeal space. T_1-weighted image, axial plane (TR 0.8/TE 17). *A,* The mucosa of the nasopharynx (NP) has a higher signal than does the longus capitis muscle (Lc). The parapharyngeal space (Pp) is a fat plane between the muscles of the nasopharynx and the lateral pterygoid muscle (Lp). The masseter muscle (Ma) is lateral to the mandible (Md). *B,* The opening of the eustachian tube (E) is clearly seen. The temporalis muscle (Tm) is inserting on the coronoid process *(arrow)* of the mandible.

muscles, and the stylopharyngeus muscle.[29, 30] The *infratemporal fossa,* located below the middle cranial fossa, contains the inferior portion of the temporalis muscle and the lateral pterygoid muscle. It is limited laterally by the mandible, anteriorly by the maxillary sinus and pterygoid plates, and posteriorly by the deep portion of the parotid gland. The *parapharyngeal*

space[31] is a fat plane between the infratemporal fossa and pharynx. It is an inverted triangle extending from the skull base posteromedial to the lateral pterygoid muscle and extends caudad to the level of the submandibular and masticator spaces. Anatomically, the internal jugular vein, carotid artery, and cranial nerves within the carotid sheath are consid-

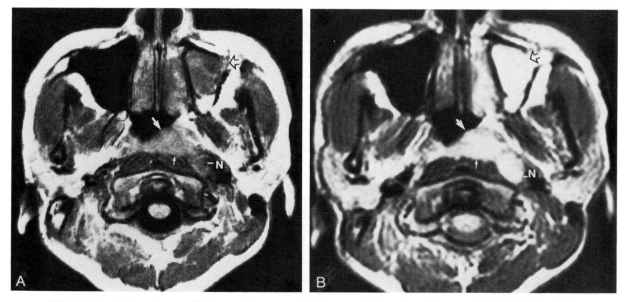

FIGURE 21–13. Carcinoma of left nasopharynx. Axial images. *A,* T_1-weighted image (TR 0.7/TE 17). *B,* T_2-weighted image (TR 2.5/TE 30). Carcinoma of nasopharynx *(closed arrows)* with metastasis to the node of Rouviere (N). Both lesions have intermediate signal on the T_1-weighted image *(A)* and increased signal on the T_2-weighted image *(B).* The left maxillary sinusitis *(open arrow)* has similar signal characteristics.

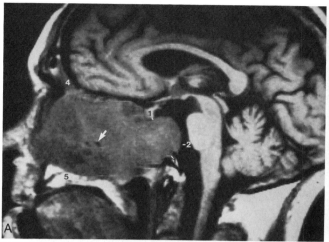
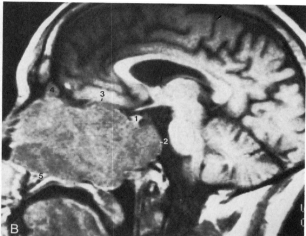
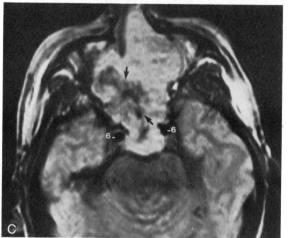

FIGURE 21–14. Chordoma. *A*, Sagittal T₁-weighted image (TR 0.65/TE 20). *B*, Sagittal T₁-weighted image after gadolinium (TR 0.65/TE 20). *C*, Axial scan, T₂-weighted image (TR 3.0/TE 25). A huge tumor occupying the entire nasal cavity and nasopharynx extends back through the clivus (1) to the pontine cistern (2). It extends superiorly through the roof of the ethmoid air cells to the floor of the anterior cranial fossa (3) and anterosuperiorly to the frontal sinus (4). Inferiorly, it is encroaching on the hard palate (5). The irregular low signals noted within the lesion are due to calcifications *(arrows)*. Note how the tumor is partially encompassing the carotid arteries (6).

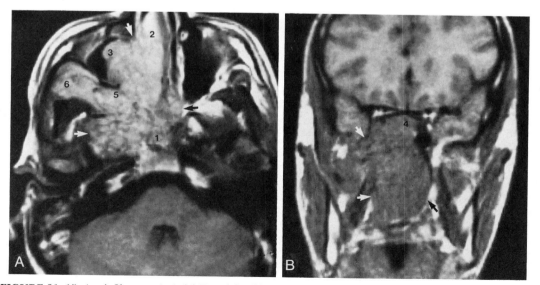

FIGURE 21–15. Angiofibroma. *A*, Axial T₁-weighted image after gadolinium (TR 0.65/TE 19). *B*, Coronal T₁-weighted image before gadolinium (TR 0.65/TE 19). A huge angiofibroma *(arrows)* is extending from the nasopharynx (1) to the nasal cavity (2), maxillary sinus (3), and sphenoid sinus (4) and out through the pterygopalatine fossa (5) to the infratemporal fossa (6). The patient presented with nasal stuffiness.

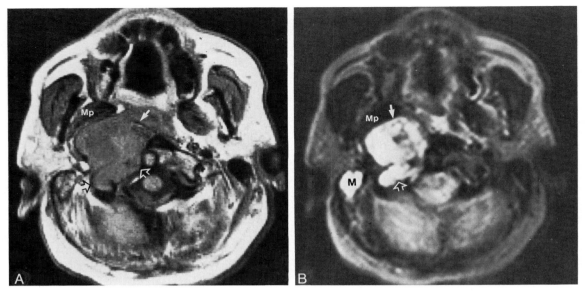

FIGURE 21–16. Benign schwannoma, C1 nerve root. Axial images. *A*, Proton density–weighted image (TR 1.5/TE 17). *B*, T₂-weighted image (TR 3.0/TE 100). This large mass *(closed arrow)* encroaching on the right parapharyngeal space and medial pterygoid muscle (Mp) is destroying the lateral mass of C1 *(open arrows)*. The internal carotid artery, jugular vein, and vertebral artery are displaced posterolaterally. Retained fluid in the right mastoid tip (M) is due to obstruction of the eustachian tube.

ered to be in the posterior compartment of the parapharyngeal space. This neurovascular bundle is located posteromedial to the styloid process and the deep portion of the parotid gland.

Squamous cell carcinoma is the most common malignant tumor seen in the nasopharynx (Fig. 21–13). It tends to be locally invasive and may erode through the skull base into the intracranial cavity.[27, 32, 33] Metastatic nodes in the neck are commonly seen and may be the first sign and symptom of tumor in the area. Other malignant tumors to be considered in the nasopharynx are lymphoepithelioma or poorly differentiated carcinoma, adenocarcinoma, sarcoma, lymphoma, chordoma, and metastatic carcinoma. Rhabdomyosarcoma is more often seen in young children. Chordomas arising from the skull base (Fig. 21–14) (also see Fig. 15–34) are often observed in the region of the sphenooccipital synchondrosis. They tend to recur locally. The chondroid chordoma with an abundant cartilaginous component tends to have a better prognosis with a longer survival rate.[27]

Benign tumors do occur in the nasopharynx but are less common. Angiofibroma (Fig. 21–15), a vascular tumor seen in male teenagers, may arise from

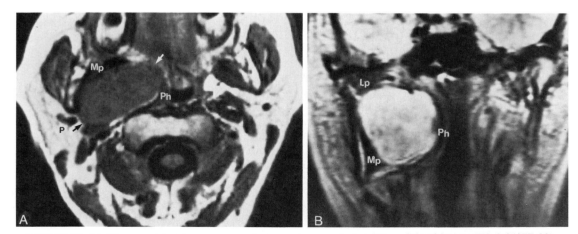

FIGURE 21–17. Pleomorphic adenoma, parapharyngeal space. *A*, Axial T₁-weighted image (TR 0.65/TE 20). *B*, Coronal T₂-weighted image (TR 3.00/TE 45). A mass in the parapharyngeal space *(arrows)* is deep to and separate from the parotid gland (P). It is displacing the lateral pterygoid muscle superiorly (Lp) and the medial pterygoid muscle laterally and anteriorly (Mp). It is also displacing the pharyngeal muscle (Ph) medially and thus encroaching slightly on the airway.

the nasopharynx or nasal cavity.[34] These tend to be locally aggressive and may extend laterally into the pterygopalatine fossa and superiorly to the sphenoid and ethmoid sinuses. Other unusual benign tumors seen within or adjacent to the nasopharynx include Tornwaldt's cyst, hemangiomas, lymphangioma, lipoma, and chondroma. Occasionally, a meningioma or chromophobe adenoma may extend caudad to the nasopharynx.

Tumors of the *parapharyngeal space* include the paraganglioma and schwannoma in the posterior compartment and tumors of salivary gland origin in the anterior compartment. Other masses seen in the area are lipomas, branchial cleft cysts, dermoids, teratomas, and enlarged nodes.

The paraganglioma (also known as chemodectoma and glomus tumor) originates from the neural crest cells. The tumors may arise from the carotid body at the carotid bifurcation or from the nodose ganglia of the vagus nerve in the neck and superior mediastinum. Schwannomas and neurofibromas may arise from cranial nerves IX to XII in the posterior compartment of the parapharyngeal space or in the more peripheral branches (Fig. 21–16), as in the infratemporal fossa. Aneurysms of the carotid artery have been reported in the neck and nasopharynx following trauma. Hemangiomas may also occur in this area.[35]

Tumors of minor salivary gland origin may be benign, such as the pleomorphic adenoma or mixed tumor, but tumors of minor salivary gland origin have a higher incidence of malignancy (especially the adenoid cystic carcinoma) than those arising from the major salivary gland.[1, 27] An attempt should be made to distinguish between tumors of the deep portion of the parotid gland and tumors of minor salivary gland origin in the parapharyngeal space (Fig. 21–17). The identification of a fat plane between the tumor and the deep portion of the parotid gland makes this distinction possible.

MR is superior to CT in the evaluation of these tumors because of its exceptional soft tissue detail and its ease of imaging in the coronal and sagittal as well as the axial planes.[36] The T_1-weighted image is used to obtain anatomic detail of the area. T_2-weighted images are valuable for better defining a tumor-bearing area, normal muscle, and vessels. The paraganglioma has been described as having a typical serpiginous appearance because of the marked vascularity in the tumor with varying rates of blood flow.[26] Metastatic nodes to the neck often have a heterogeneous high signal intensity on the T_2-weighted image (Fig. 21–13), but this does not necessarily differentiate an enlarged homogeneous inflammatory node from a metastatic node. Biopsy of the primary tumor and of the enlarged node is still necessary to establish the correct diagnosis. It has been stated that MR is more sensitive than CT in the detection of recurrent tumor and in the differentiation between postradiation fibrosis and residual tumor, but this remains to be proved. Paramagnetic contrast agents such as Gd-DTPA may enhance the detection of the primary tumor and the recurrent tumor and may improve the detection of tumor in the presence of postoperative and postradiation fibrosis.

PARANASAL SINUSES AND NASAL CAVITY

The paranasal sinuses and nasal cavity are air-containing structures with an absent signal on MR because of the lack of hydrogen protons (Figs. 21–1 and 21–18). The mucous membrane of this area becomes edematous with a minimal degree of inflammatory disease, whether it be on an allergic or inflammatory basis. This edema alters the signal characteristics, resulting in a long T_1 or low signal with the T_1-weighted image and a long T_2 or high signal with the T_2-weighted image (Fig. 21–19). A large proportion of patients having an MR study of the head will have evidence of some degree of sinusitis as an incidental and often asymptomatic finding. Retention cysts are commonly seen in the sinuses, especially in the maxillary sinus (see Fig. 21–6). Edematous turbinates are also a common finding.

Most patients needing medical attention for sinusitis are adequately studied with plain film examination. Patients requiring additional studies for a suspected complication of sinusitis may need tomography. Pleuridirectional tomography has been supplanted by CT. MR is now beginning to replace CT in this and other areas of the head and neck.[34, 37] Even though MR is limited in the depiction of bone detail, particularly for the thin, bony septa and thin walls seen in the paranasal sinuses, it is superior for assessing bone marrow changes in the skull, zygoma, palate, and mandible. MR is the superior modality for the identification of an abscess in the orbit or in the intracranial cavity and for the detection of cavernous sinus thrombosis. CT may be required for identifying minute bone changes, but MR has definite advantages for identifying complications of sinusitis.

Obstruction of the ostium of a sinus, with continued production of mucus, results in expansion of the sinus with remolding of its walls and in encroachment on adjacent structures. This development of a mucocele (Fig. 21–20) may occur as a result of chronic inflammatory disease, trauma, or tumor. If the mucocele becomes secondarily infected, it is known as a pyocele. Mucoceles occur most commonly in the frontal sinuses but are also seen in the ethmoid, sphenoid, and rarely the maxillary sinuses. The enlargement can be seen with either CT or MR. The latter has the advantage of clearly showing the fluid content with the T_2-weighted image and of displaying the sinus in a coronal plane as well as an axial plane. The coronal plane is important for demonstrating relationships to adjacent structures, such as the contents of the orbit and the cavernous sinus.

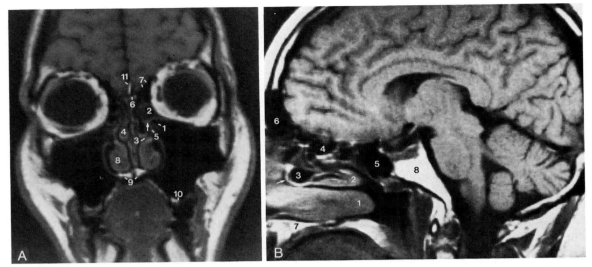

FIGURE 21–18. Normal sinuses. *A,* Coronal T$_1$-weighted image (TR 0.65/TE 20). The ostium of the maxillary sinus (1) opens to an infundibulum, which leads to the hiatus semilunaris *(arrow)* under the ethmoidal bulla (2). Air flows from the hiatus to the middle meatus (3), which is bordered by the middle turbinate (4) and the uncinate process (5). The middle turbinate has a vertical attachment to the cribriform plate (6). Also note the roof of the ethmoid air cells (7), the inferior turbinate (8), the hard palate (9), and the floor of the maxillary sinus (10). The crista galli (11) has a bright signal because of marrow fat. Incidentally, note that the left middle turbinate is pneumatized, a phenomenon that is often seen, this turbinate being part of the ethmoid bone. *B,* Sagittal T$_1$-weighted image (TR 0.65/TE 20). The inferior (1) and middle turbinates (2) are clearly seen. An air pocket at the anterior edge of the middle turbinate (3) is the bulla ethmoidalis, identifying the region of the hiatus semilunaris *(arrow)* opening to the middle meatus, under the middle turbinate. The ethmoid air cells (4) and sphenoid sinus (5) are clearly seen, as is the frontal sinus (6). Also note the high signal in the fat of the marrow of the palate (7) and clivus (8).

Tumors of the paranasal sinuses are most often squamous cell in origin, and they usually occur in the maxillary sinus (Fig. 21–21). Adenocarcinoma has a much lower incidence than squamous cell carcinoma, but it is seen in wood workers and cabinet makers because of their inhalation of wood dust.

Other types of malignant tumors to be considered in this area are esthesioneuroblastoma (olfactory neuroblastoma), occurring most often in the upper nasal cavity. About 11 per cent of patients with this tumor may have intracranial extension. These tumors tend to invade and destroy and to recur if inadequately

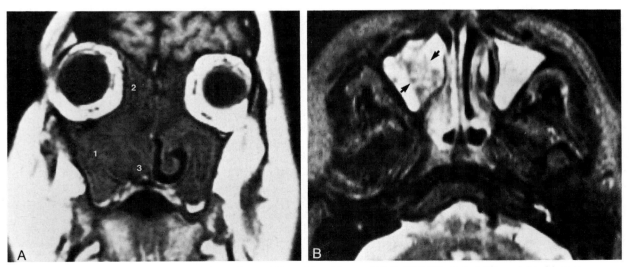

FIGURE 21–19. Chronic sinusitis. *A,* Coronal T$_1$-weighted image (TR 0.6/TE 17). *B,* Axial T$_2$-weighted image (TR 3.0/TE 90). These show diffuse opacification of the paranasal sinuses by acute and chronic inflammatory disease. The maxillary sinuses (1) and ethmoid sinuses (2) are completely opacified, as is the right nasal cavity (3). The bright signal on the T$_2$-weighted image in *B* is attributed to acute edematous changes in the soft tissues. More chronic inflammatory disease is manifest as a mixed lower signal *(arrows).*

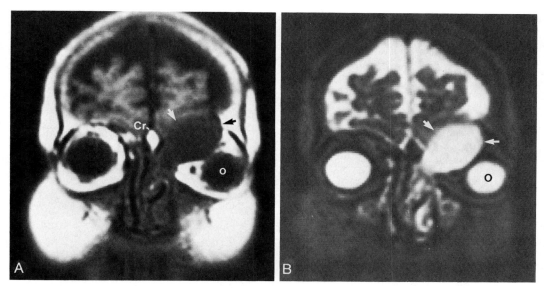

FIGURE 21–20. Mucocele, left supraorbital ethmoid sinus. Coronal images. *A,* T$_1$-weighted image (TR 0.8/TE 17). *B,* T$_2$-weighted image (TR 2.5/TE 80). The expanded supraorbital sinus *(arrows)* is displacing the globe (O) inferiorly and laterally. Note fat within the crista galli (Cr). (From Carter BL: Part II: Paranasal sinuses, nasal cavity, pterygoid fossa, nasopharynx, and infratemporal fossa. *In* Valvassori GE, Hanafee W, Carter BL et al [eds]: ENT Diagnostic Imaging. Stuttgart, Georg Thieme Verlag, 1988.)

excised. Malignant melanoma, extramedullary plasmacytoma, lymphoma, adenoid cystic carcinoma, and sarcomas are other malignant lesions to be considered in the differential diagnosis (Fig. 21–22). Of the metastatic tumors occurring in the paranasal sinuses, the kidney is the most common primary lesion, but lung and breast tumors are also possible sources.[27]

Differentiation between chronic inflammatory disease and tumor requires biopsy. Bone destruction is usually evident in the presence of tumor, and this is easier to appreciate on the CT scan. Bone marrow involvement of the palate may not be accompanied by destruction; however, MR is the best modality for an evaluation of the marrow (Fig. 21–22). The multiple pulse sequences used with MR make it easier to differentiate between solid tumor mass and inflammatory reaction. A strong signal with a long T$_2$ is to be expected in the presence of acute inflammatory

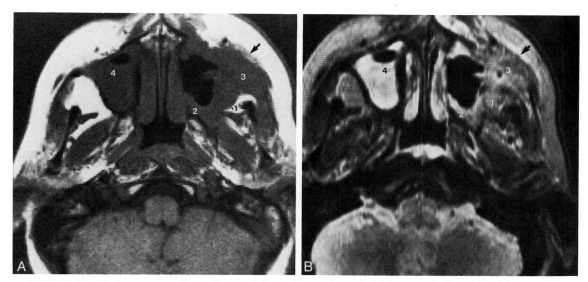

FIGURE 21–21. Squamous cell carcinoma, left maxillary sinus. Axial images. *A,* T$_1$-weighted image (TR 0.6/TE 17). *B,* T$_2$-weighted image (TR 3.0/TE 45). Destruction of the posterolateral wall of the maxillary sinus is due to the carcinoma, which is extending posterolaterally to the infratemporal fossa (1) and posteriorly to the pterygopalatine fossa (2) and laterally through the zygoma (3) to encroach on the subcutaneous fascia *(arrow)*. Sinusitis of the right maxillary sinus (4) is also evident with an air-fluid level.

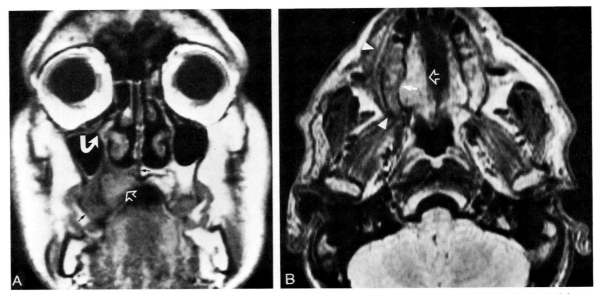

FIGURE 21–22. Adenoid cystic carcinoma, palate. *A*, Coronal T₁-weighted image (TR 0.6/TE 17). *B*, Axial T₂-weighted image (TR 2.5/TE 35). Carcinoma of the hard palate *(closed arrows)* and superior alveolar ridge is also involving the soft tissues *(open arrow)* of the palate and the mucous membrane of the right maxillary sinus *(curved arrow)* and extends posterolateral to the buccinator muscle *(arrowheads)* and back to the pterygoid plate and pterygopalatine fossa.

disease. Tumor may obstruct the ostium to the sinus, resulting in soft tissue changes within the sinus caused by tumor (low signal on T₂) or retained fluid (bright signal on T₂).

Differentiation between tumor and retained fluid is much more evident with MR, particularly with the T₂-weighted image. Tumor has a lower and more varied signal, whereas edema or fluid has a brighter and more homogeneous signal. It should be noted, however, that chronic inflammatory disease may also give a low mixed signal. The presence of bone destruction implies malignancy. Biopsy is necessary for the final distinction. The minute detail needed for planning radical surgery and radiotherapy re-

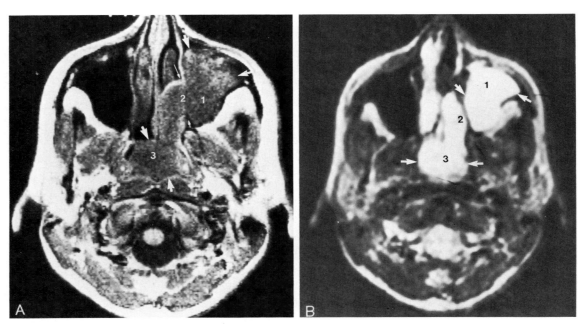

FIGURE 21–23. Antrochoanal polyp. Axial images. *A*, T₁-weighted image (TR 0.8/TE 17). *B*, T₂-weighted image (TR 2.5/TE 70). The polyp *(arrows)* extends from the left maxillary sinus (1) through the ostium to the nasal cavity (2) and nasopharynx (3). The high signal on the T₂-weighted image *(B)* clearly shows the extent of the polyp.

quires thin-section images with both CT and MR in the coronal and axial planes. Extension into the lacrimal sac area, infraorbital nerve canal, orbit, pterygopalatine fossa, infratemporal fossa, and cavernous sinus must be determined as accurately as possible. This can be accomplished with either modality, but MR has several advantages.[38] Dental artifacts are less of a problem, coronal images are easier to obtain, and intravenous contrast is not needed. Baseline studies should be obtained with either modality after surgery and radiotherapy and used as a baseline for the detection of early recurrent disease.

Benign tumors can usually be adequately studied by CT, but they can be imaged equally well with MR. The fluid content of the cystic lesion is readily apparent with its long T_2. A true polyp has characteristics different from those of a retention cyst. This observation is exemplified by the antrochoanal polyp (Fig. 21–23), in which the heterogeneity can be seen owing to fibrous tissue, blood vessels, and mucous glands. Other benign growths in the area to be considered are the inverting papilloma; schwannoma; neurofibroma; nasal glioma; osteoma; odontogenic cysts (Fig. 21–24), and tumors; and nonodontogenic cysts, such as the globulomaxillary (Fig. 21–25), nasoalveolar, nasopalatine, and fissural cysts. Calcifications within the tumor and dense bone are better studied by CT. Cystic lesions are more readily identified by MR because of the long T_2.

Congenital abnormalities with possible intracranial extension are better shown with MR because of the greater anatomic detail of the intracranial structures.[39] Nasodermoid lesions may communicate through the nasal septum and foramen cecum to the region of the falx or may communicate directly through the nasion. Encephaloceles occasionally pre-

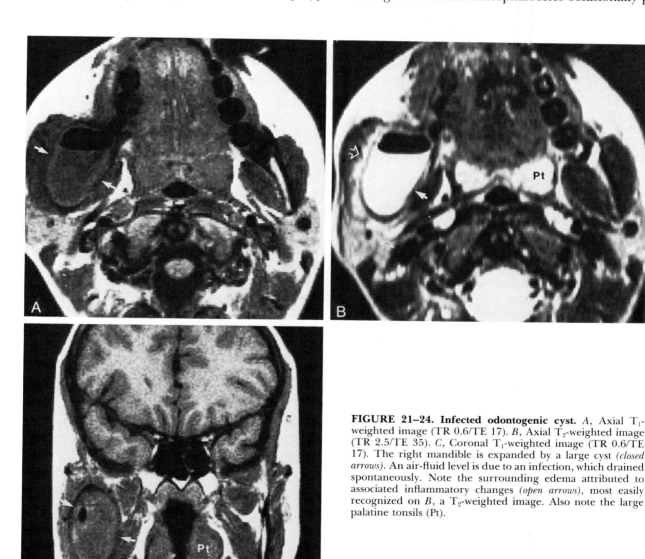

FIGURE 21–24. Infected odontogenic cyst. *A*, Axial T_1-weighted image (TR 0.6/TE 17). *B*, Axial T_2-weighted image (TR 2.5/TE 35). *C*, Coronal T_1-weighted image (TR 0.6/TE 17). The right mandible is expanded by a large cyst *(closed arrows)*. An air-fluid level is due to an infection, which drained spontaneously. Note the surrounding edema attributed to associated inflammatory changes *(open arrows)*, most easily recognized on *B*, a T_2-weighted image. Also note the large palatine tonsils (Pt).

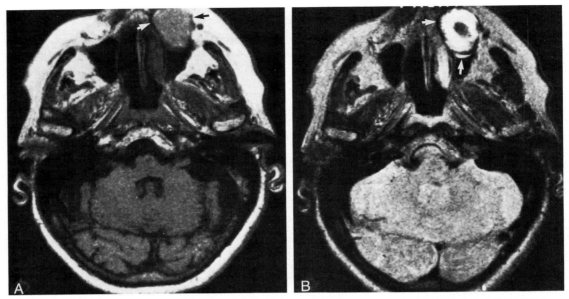

FIGURE 21–25. Left maxillary nonodontogenic cyst. Axial images. *A*, T$_1$-weighted image (TR 0.8/TE 17). *B*, T$_2$-weighted image (TR 2.0/TE 70). Inflammatory debris with acute and chronic changes and cholesterol clefts were found within the cyst *(arrows)*. A T$_2$-weighted image *(B)* shows the cyst to best advantage with a central core of tissue and calcification.

sent as mass lesions in the nasal cavity through a defect in the cribriform plate or roof of the ethmoid air cell.

SALIVARY GLANDS

The major salivary glands—the parotid, submandibular, and sublingual glands—are clearly seen on MR (Fig. 21–26). The parotid and submandibular glands are readily apparent on CT, but the sublingual glands are more difficult to visualize. The parotid often has a higher fat content than the submandibular gland and thus a shorter T$_1$, with a bright signal on T$_1$-weighted images.[40] MR has been reported to show the facial nerve within the parotid gland by obtaining axial images inclined slightly caudad.[2, 41] MR or CT may be used to identify a mass and to determine its position relative to the known course of the facial nerve lateral to the retromandibular vein. MR has the advantage of obtaining better detail with dense parotid glands, which have an attenuation similar to that of muscle on CT.[42, 43] With the dense gland, it is more difficult to identify a tumor with CT. The T$_2$-weighted image of MR shows to best advantage the tumor with a longer T$_2$ in general and thus a higher signal than the parenchyma of the gland (Figs. 21–27 and 21–28). A tumor in the deep portion of the parotid gland (i.e., deep to the facial nerve) requires careful dissection to protect the facial nerve, and this relationship should be identified prior to surgery (Fig. 21–29). Tumors of the deep portion of the parotid gland, medial to the mandible, may encroach on the parapharyngeal space. This type of

mass should be differentiated from a tumor arising from the parapharyngeal space (see Fig. 21–17) because of the different surgical approach used for complete excision.

Numerous (750 to 1000) minor salivary glands are found in the submucosa of the upper aerodigestive tract, including the lips, the cheeks, the hard and soft palates, the tonsillar pillars, and the base and lateral edges of the tongue,[1] but ectopic glands may be found scattered throughout the neck and within the submucosa of the trachea. Pleomorphic adenomas are the most common benign tumors of the salivary glands and are seen most often in the parotid gland but can occur in any of the major or minor salivary glands.[27] A Warthin's tumor or adenolymphoma is less common (about 8 per cent of all parotid tumors), as are other adenomas, oncocytomas, and hemangiomas (Figs. 21–29 and 21–30). All benign tumors are sharply defined and usually have a long T$_1$ (low signal) and long T$_2$ (high signal). Unfortunately, the CT and MR characteristics of a mass lesion are not diagnostic of a benign tumor. A malignant lesion may have a similar appearance (Fig. 21–31). A biopsy is needed for the identification of the type of tumor. When the malignant tumor is invasive, such as a squamous cell carcinoma, it can be identified as malignant by its morphologic appearance (Fig. 21–32). The various types of malignancy involving the salivary glands include malignant mixed tumor, mucoepidermoid carcinoma, adenoid cystic carcinoma, adenocarcinoma, squamous cell carcinoma, lymphoma (Fig. 21–33), metastatic tumor, and others. The minor salivary glands do have a higher incidence of malignancy (adenoid cystic carcinoma) than the major salivary glands.[27]

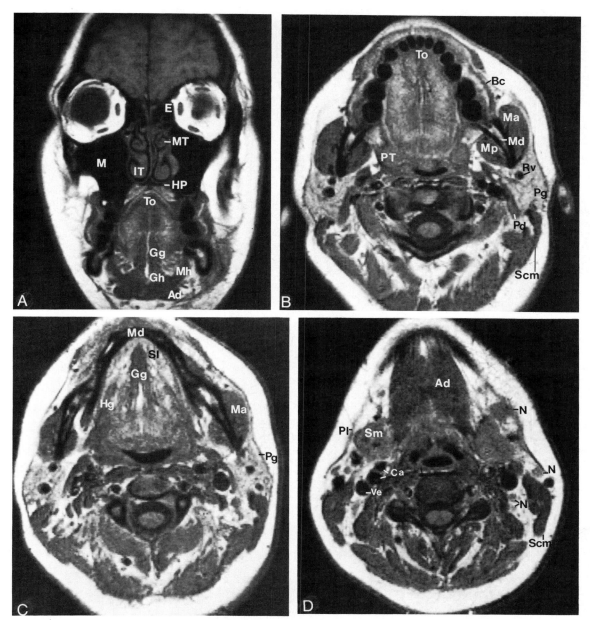

FIGURE 21–26. Normal oropharynx and salivary glands. *A,* Coronal image. *B–D,* Axial images. *B* is cephalad to *C,* which is cephalad to *D.* T₁-weighted images (TR 0.8/TE 17). *A* is through the oropharynx, maxillary sinuses, and nasal cavity. The intrinsic muscles of the tongue (To) can be seen separate from the extrinsic muscles: genioglossus (Gg); and the suprahyoid group, the geniohyoid (Gh), mylohyoid (Mh), and anterior belly of the digastric (Ad). Note also the hard palate (HP), the inferior turbinate (IT), and the middle turbinate (MT). The maxillary sinus (M) and ethmoid air cells (E) are air containing and without signal. *B* shows the intrinsic muscles of the tongue (To); the palatine tonsils (PT); the medial pterygoid muscle (Mp); the masseter muscle (Ma); the mandible (Md), which contains marrow; and the parotid gland (Pg), which contains the retromandibular vein (Rv). The posterior belly of the digastric (Pd) is deep to the parotid gland, and the sternocleidomastoid muscle (Scm) is behind the parotid gland. The buccinator muscle (Bc) is lateral to the mandibular teeth. *C* is further caudad through the extrinsic muscles of the tongue, showing the mandible (Md), the genioglossus muscle (Gg), the hyoglossus muscle (Hg), the sublingual glands (Sl), the masseter muscle (Ma), and the tail or inferior portion of the parotid gland (Pg). *D* is a section through the submandibular gland (Sm), just above the hyoid bone at the level of the anterior belly of the digastric (Ad). The platysma muscle (Pl) is located superficially. The sternocleidomastoid muscle (Scm) is overlying the internal jugular vein (Ve) and the carotid artery (Ca). Lymph nodes (N) are present around the submandibular gland, superficial and deep to the sternocleidomastoid muscle.

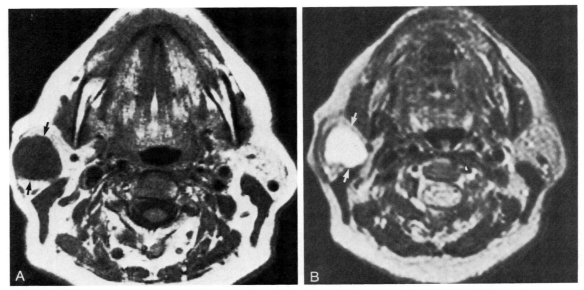

FIGURE 21–27. Pleomorphic adenoma. Axial images. *A*, T$_1$-weighted image (TR 0.8/TE 17). *B*, T$_2$-weighted image (TR 3.0/TE 70). A fairly characteristic low signal is present with a T$_1$-weighted image, and a high signal is seen with a T$_2$-weighted image *(arrows)*.

Inflammatory disease of the major salivary glands may be identified by either modality, particularly when there is a question of an abscess. Sialography remains the procedure of choice for the assessment of ductal stricture, ductal dilatation, and sialadenitis, as with Sjögren's syndrome. Abnormalities of the gland (Fig. 21–34) and gross dilatation of the duct can be seen on MR. Plain film studies are used primarily for the identification of opaque calculi, which occur most often in Wharton's duct of the submandibular gland (Fig. 21–35). The ranula, a

cystlike fluid collection due to obstruction of a sublingual gland, is usually diagnosed by clinical examination but may be an incidental finding on the MR study (Fig. 21–36).

OROPHARYNX, LARYNX, AND NECK

The normal anatomy of this area is illustrated in Figures 21–26 and 21–37. The tongue[44, 45] is com-

Text continued on page 645

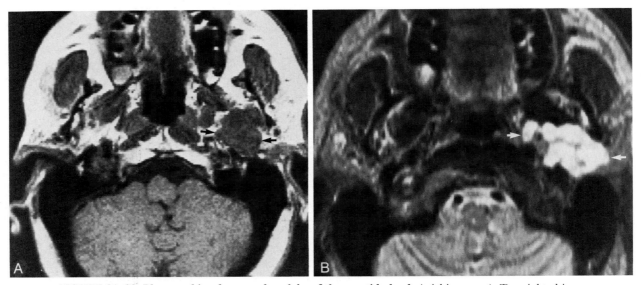

FIGURE 21–28. Pleomorphic adenoma, deep lobe of the parotid gland. Axial images. *A*, T$_1$-weighted image (TR 0.6/TE 17). *B*, T$_2$-weighted image (TR 3.0/TE 70). A multilobulated mass *(arrows)* is present in the deep portion of the parotid gland, deep to the facial nerve and to the retromandibular vein. It is multilobulated, with a somewhat mixed signal—low on the T$_1$-weighted image, bright on the T$_2$-weighted image—as seen in *B*.

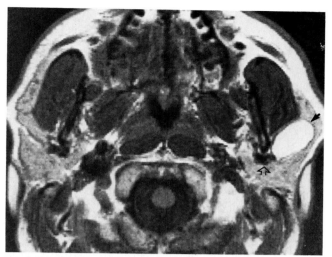

FIGURE 21–29. Lipoma, parotid gland. T_1-weighted axial image (TR 0.6/TE 17). This sharply defined fat-containing tumor *(closed arrow)* was found to be deep to the facial nerve and thus is technically within the deep portion of the parotid gland, although it is superficial to the retromandibular vessels *(open arrow)*.

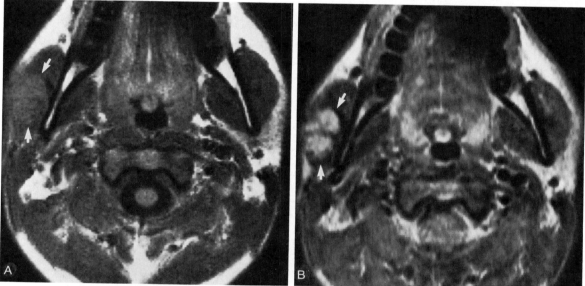

FIGURE 21–30. Hemangioma, masseter muscle. Axial images. *A,* T_1-weighted image (TR 0.6/TE 17). *B,* T_2-weighted image (TR 2.5/TE 35). A mass *(arrows)* was felt by physical examination to be within the parotid gland but proved to be anterior to the parotid, within the masseter muscle. The signal is slightly brighter than muscle on T_1 *(A)* and much brighter on T_2 *(B)*.

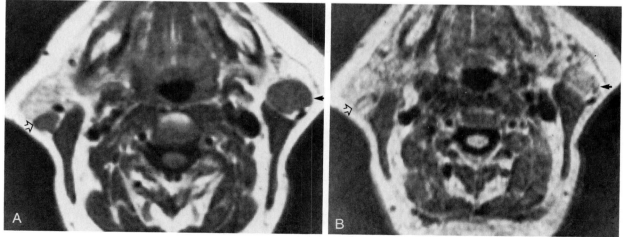

FIGURE 21–31. Mucoepidermoid carcinoma, left parotid gland. Axial images. *A,* T_1-weighted image (TR 0.6/TE 17). *B,* T_2-weighted image (TR 3.0/TE 45). These show a sharply defined *(closed arrow)* tumor that looks benign but in fact was found to be malignant. It has a low signal in *A* but is isointense with the parotid in *B.* A sharply defined tumor *(open arrow)* is also present in the right parotid gland.

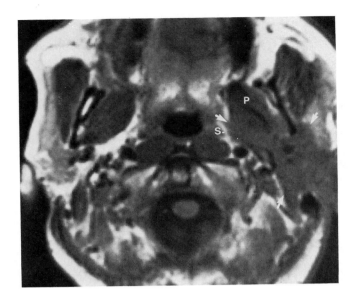

FIGURE 21–32. Recurrent adenocarcinoma of the parotid gland. T₁-weighted axial image (TR 0.6/TE 17). A diffusely infiltrating mass *(arrows)* is extending from the superficial portion of the parotid gland to the deep portion and encroaching on the parapharyngeal space (S) and medial pterygoid muscle (P).

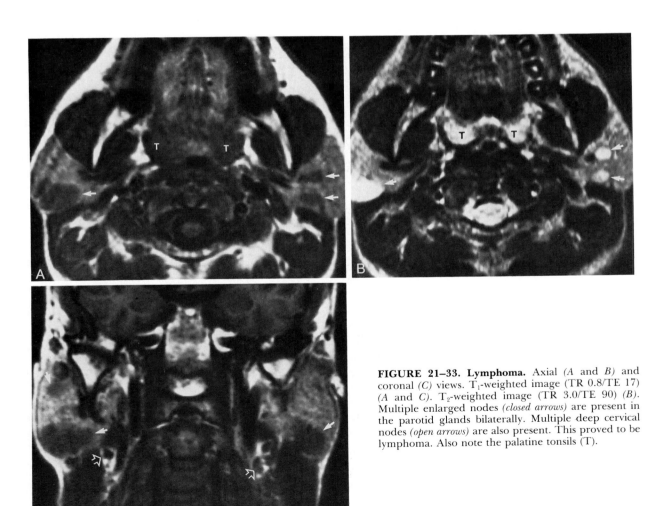

FIGURE 21–33. Lymphoma. Axial *(A and B)* and coronal *(C)* views. T₁-weighted image (TR 0.8/TE 17) *(A and C).* T₂-weighted image (TR 3.0/TE 90) *(B).* Multiple enlarged nodes *(closed arrows)* are present in the parotid glands bilaterally. Multiple deep cervical nodes *(open arrows)* are also present. This proved to be lymphoma. Also note the palatine tonsils (T).

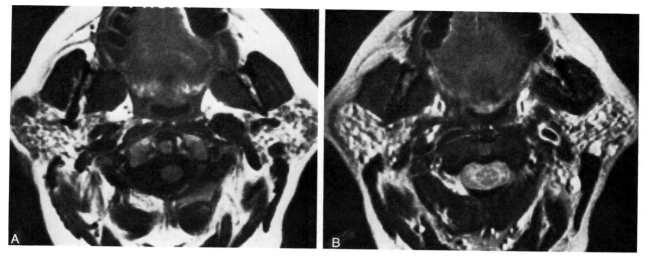

FIGURE 21–34. Sjögren's syndrome. Axial images. *A*, T_1-weighted image (TR 0.75/TE 17). *B*, T_2-weighted image (TR 3.0/TE 45). Bilateral sialadenitis with lymphoproliferative disease involving the salivary glands has resulted in a mixed signal bilaterally. Distention of the small peripheral ducts within the gland is due to lymphocytic infiltration.

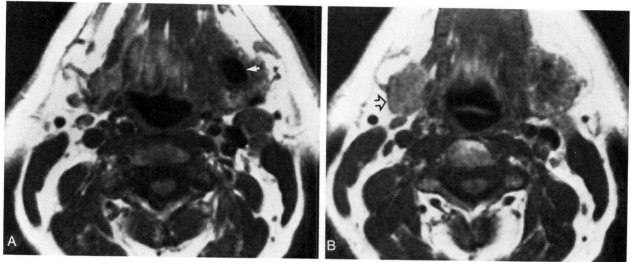

FIGURE 21–35. Chronic inflammatory changes in the submandibular gland secondary to obstruction. T_1-weighted axial images (TR 0.65/TE 20). *A* is cephalad to *B*. A stone *(closed arrow)* with a very low signal is present in the hilum of the gland. This was causing chronic obstruction and a chronic inflammatory reaction of the gland, which is enlarged. Note the normal-appearing right submandibular gland *(open arrow)*.

FIGURE 21–36. Ranula. T_2-weighted axial image (TR 3.0/TE 45). An obstructed sublingual gland *(arrow)* is evident as a fluid-containing cyst in the floor of the mouth. This is lateral to the genioglossus muscle (1) and above the mylohyoid muscle. Also note the palatine tonsils (2) and deep cervical nodes (3), which have a brighter signal on T_2-weighted images, particularly with any degree of inflammatory change.

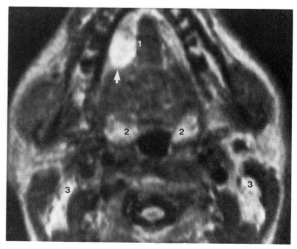

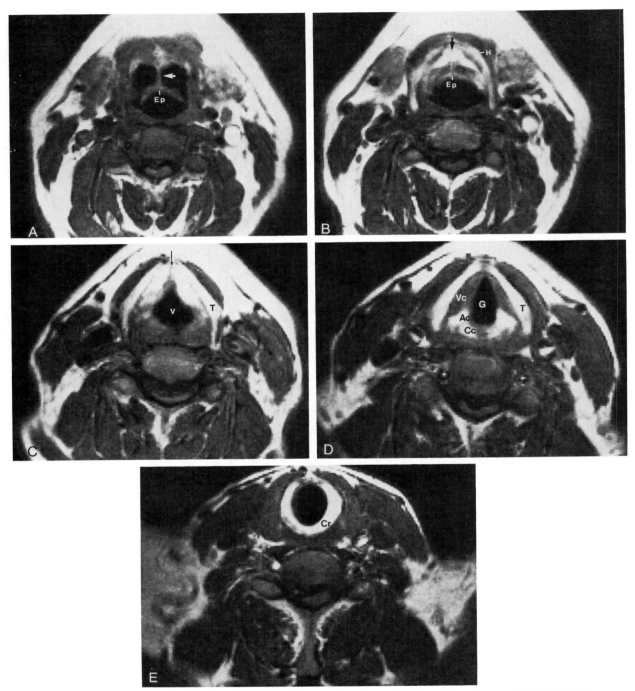

FIGURE 21–37. Normal larynx. Axial images, *A* cephalad to *E* caudad. T$_1$-weighted images (TR 0.8/TE 17). *A* is through the tip of the epiglottis (Ep), showing the glossoepiglottic fold *(arrow)* anteriorly. *B* is slightly caudad through the hyoid bone (H) showing the preepiglottic fat *(arrow)*. *C* is further caudad through the thyroid cartilage (T), showing fat *(arrow)* in the preepiglottic space and the vestibule (V) to the larynx. *D* is further caudad through the vocal cords (Vc), arytenoid cartilage (Ac), and cricoid cartilage (Cc). Also note the thyroid cartilage (T) and the glottis (G). The cartilage is bright because of fat in the marrow. *E* is through the cricoid ring (Cr) in the subglottic area.

posed of intrinsic muscles and supported by extrinsic muscles (genioglossus, hyoglossus, and styloglossus muscles) and the suprahyoid muscles (mylohyoid, geniohyoid, and digastric muscles). The palatine tonsils (see Fig. 21–26) are bounded by the anterior and posterior pillars, which in turn are continuous with the soft palate located posterior to the hard palate. The lingual tonsil is located at the posterior aspect of the tongue, with the adenoids in the nasopharynx completing Waldeyer's ring. The hypopharynx contains the valleculae at the base of the tongue, the suprahyoid portion of the epiglottis, and the piriform sinuses and leads to the larynx anteriorly and into the cervical esophagus posteriorly. The vestibule to the larynx contained by the aryepiglottic folds from top of the epiglottis to the arytenoids extends to the glottis, located between the true cords.[46–48] The supraglottic portion of the larynx contains the epiglottis, the aryepiglottic folds, the arytenoids, the false cords, and the ventricles. The true glottis lies between the true cords and the anterior commissure, whereas the subglottis is the area caudad to the true cords to the lower limit of the larynx. The laryngeal skeleton consists of the hyoid bone, epiglottis, thyroid cartilage, arytenoid cartilages, and cricoid cartilage. No signal is emitted from the compact portion of the hyoid bone or from the calcification of the cartilaginous skeleton. However, these structures often contain a fatty marrow, which does emit a strong signal on the T_1-weighted image.

The epiglottis is a curved, leaflike structure that tapers inferiorly to a point, the petiole, where it is attached to the thyroid lamina via the thyroepiglottic ligament (Fig. 21–37). Fat is normally present in the preepiglottic space down to this ligament. The thyroid cartilage consists of two laminae, which fuse anteriorly at the laryngeal prominence. The superior thyroid notch between these laminae lying above the glottis should not be confused with cartilaginous destruction. The superior cornua of the thyroid cartilage attach posteriorly to the hyoid bone via the thyrohyoid ligaments, whereas the inferior cornua articulate posteriorly with the cricoid cartilage at the cricothyroid joint. Calcification and ossification of the thyroid cartilage are quite variable but are usually symmetric between the two sides. The arytenoid cartilages, with the vocal process attaching to the vocalis muscles, articulate with the cricoid cartilage at the cricothyroid joint. The arytenoid cartilages adduct and rotate toward the midline during phonation and with breath holding. The cricoid cartilage, a signet ring–shaped structure, forms the base of the larynx and defines the subglottic space to the first tracheal ring.

Physical examination with direct visualization and palpation usually identifies the presence of most tumors in these areas. Additional study with CT or MR is needed for determining the total extent of local disease (Figs. 21–38 to 21–40), degree of bone destruction, cartilaginous invasion, and proximity to and involvement of large vessels in the area and for identifying metastatic adenopathy.[45, 46, 49] Congenital malformation, infections, trauma, and miscellaneous diseases are usually adequately studied by plain films and fluoroscopic procedures, but additional imaging with CT or MR is occasionally needed for the identification of a cyst (see Fig. 21–44), a benign lesion such as hemangioma (see Fig. 21–30), or an abscess.

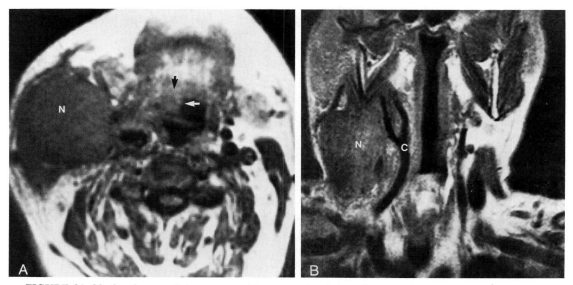

FIGURE 21–38. Carcinoma of the tongue with metastatic adenopathy. T_1-weighted image (TR 0.8/TE 17). *A,* Axial. *B,* Coronal. The primary tumor *(arrows)* of the base of the tongue encroaching on the vallecula is relatively small. Metastatic nodes to the neck (N) are very large and are displacing the carotid artery (C) medially. Note the advantage of the coronal image for showing the total extent of metastasis.

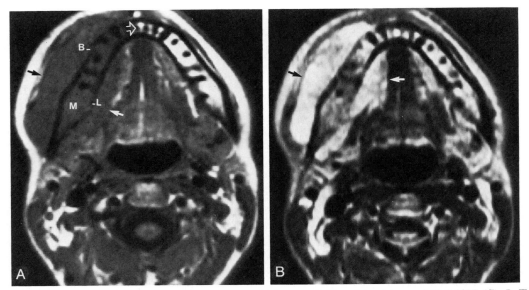

FIGURE 21–39. Osteosarcoma of the mandible. Axial images. *A,* T$_1$-weighted image (TR 0.8/TE 17). *B,* T$_2$-weighted image (TR 3.0/TE 45). The tumor *(closed arrows)* is infiltrating the marrow of the body of the mandible (M). It extends to the midline *(open arrow)* and back to the angle of the mandible. It is also extending through the buccal (B) cortex to the subcutaneous area and through the lingual (L) cortex to the floor of the mouth.

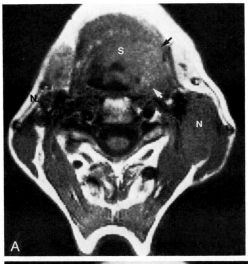

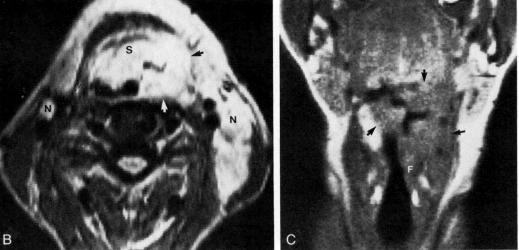

FIGURE 21–40. Large supraglottic carcinoma with cervical node metastases. Axial *(A)* and coronal *(C)* T$_1$-weighted images (TR 0.6/TE 17). *B,* Axial T$_2$-weighted image (TR 3.0/TE 45). A large tumor *(arrows)* of the epiglottis and pharyngoepiglottic fold is extending anteriorly to the preepiglottic space (S) and across the midline to the right. This also extends inferiorly to the level of the false cords (F). Note metastasis to the cervical nodes (N) bilaterally.

ORAL CAVITY AND MANDIBLE

The most common malignant tumor of the oral cavity is squamous cell carcinoma of the tongue, floor of mouth (see Fig. 21–38), peritonsillar area, and hypopharynx.[49] This type of tumor tends to have a low signal with the T_1- and T_2-weighted image and is therefore a little more difficult to identify than other types of tumors. Paramagnetic contrast agents such as Gd-DTPA are expected to improve the sensitivity of MR in the early identification of this lesion. Other malignant tumors to be considered are those of salivary gland origin, such as the adenoid cystic carcinoma, adenocarcinoma, sarcoma, and lymphoma, which require biopsy for diagnosis. These same tumors may affect the mandible and maxilla (Fig. 21–39). Benign tumors of the mandible and maxilla are odontogenic in origin; examples include the ameloblastoma, odontoma, and the odontogenic cysts, such as the dentigerous, radicular, and primordial cysts. The nonodontogenic tumors include osteoma, giant cell reparative granuloma, granular cell myoblastoma, aneurysmal bone cyst, and ossifying fibroma.

Plain film studies are usually adequate for assessing benign tumors. CT or MR or both are needed for determining the total extent of a malignant lesion. MR has the advantage of demonstrating marrow involvement. Dental artifacts degrade the image more with CT than with MR.

LARYNX

Tumors of the larynx are usually categorized according to their location in the supraglottic, glottic, and subglottic areas (Fig. 21–40). When extending throughout the larynx, these are known as transglottic tumors. CT or MR is indicated for evaluating the total extent of these tumors deep to the mucosa and for identifying any destruction of the laryngeal cartilage and extension of tumor beyond the confines of the larynx.[47, 50, 51] These modalities are also used for identifying metastatic nodes to the neck in staging the disease and in following the patient's response to therapy and for the discovery of any recurrent disease.

The shorter scan time of CT permits imaging with different maneuvers that demonstrate cord mobility and distensibility of the hypopharynx and laryngeal ventricle. MR has the advantage of displaying the larynx in a coronal plane, which permits better visualization of the laryngeal ventricle and subglottic area. Relatively narrow slices (4 mm or less) should be used when evaluating the larynx, whether by CT or MR. There are certain pitfalls and limitations with both CT and MR when evaluating cartilaginous invasion by tumor, particularly with the irregular pattern of calcification and ossification seen. Only moderately advanced or far-advanced neoplastic involvement can be diagnosed with confidence. The paralaryngeal space lateral to the cords may contain a thin line of fat, which should be symmetric.[47] Asymmetry of this fat line is highly suggestive of tumor invasion of the paralaryngeal space. Invasion of the endolarynx may be seen with tumors arising from the piriform sinus. Such tumors tend to be more aggressive than laryngeal tumors, and they have a higher incidence of cartilaginous invasion and metastatic adenopathy.

NECK

Three different compartments involving the entire length of the neck include visceral, neurovascular, and retropharyngeal space. The visceral compartment, containing the larynx, hypopharynx, and esophagus (discussed previously), also contains the thyroid and parathyroid glands.[52, 53] Nuclear medicine and ultrasound studies have been and still are the imaging modalities of choice for most patients with an abnormality of the thyroid and parathyroid glands. These structures can also be visualized by both CT and MR, particularly when enlarged (Fig. 21–41).[54–58] These two modalities are used for assess-

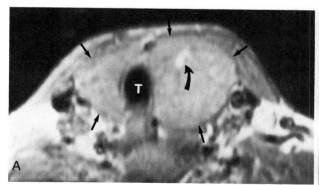
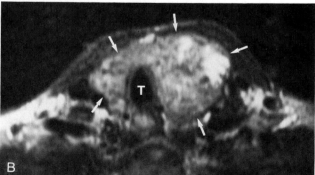

FIGURE 21–41. Multinodular goiter. *A* and *B*, Axial proton density–weighted and T_2-weighted images (TR 3.0/TE 20,70). The thyroid gland *(arrows)* is markedly enlarged, particularly the left lobe, and surrounds the trachea (T). The gland has a heterogeneous texture, and a few foci of hemorrhage *(curved arrow)* are present. (Courtesy of Robert M. Mattrey, University of California, San Diego, CA.)

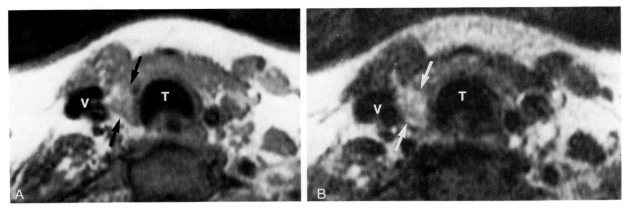

FIGURE 21–42. Parathyroid adenoma. *A* and *B*, Axial proton density–weighted and T_2-weighted scans (TR 3.0/TE 20,65). A 1-cm hyperintense mass *(arrows)* lies immediately medial to the neurovascular sheath (V) on the right. The mass is along the posterior margin of the deep lobe of the right thyroid gland (T), but no cleavage plane can be identified. Location and appearance are consistent with a parathyroid adenoma. (Courtesy of Robert M. Mattrey, University of California, San Diego, CA.)

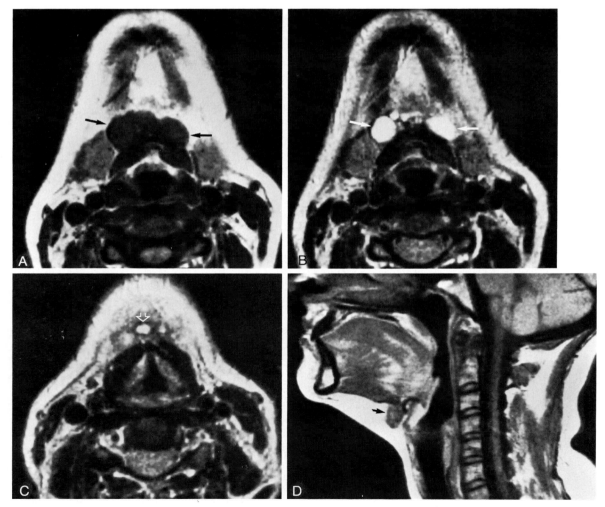

FIGURE 21–43. Thyroglossal duct cyst. *A*, Axial T_1-weighted image (TR 0.5/TE 40). *B* and *C*, Axial T_2-weighted images (TR 1.5/TE 80). *D*, Sagittal T_1-weighted image (TR 0.5/TE 30). An atypical bilobed cyst extends from the prehyoid area *(closed arrows)* down to a small tract *(open arrow)*, anterior to the thyroid cartilage. This proved to be a thyroglossal duct cyst containing a small colloid-producing cancer.

ing extension of tumor into the mediastinum directly or by metastases and for trying to identify ectopic parathyroid tumors in the mediastinum. Although a specialized surface coil is preferable for studying structures in the neck, the body coil is needed when attempting to determine extension into or involvement of the mediastinum. T_2-weighted images have been used for showing parathyroid adenomas (Fig. 21–42) and thyroid and parathyroid cysts.[59, 60] The few shown to date have had a long T_2, with increased signal on the T_2-weighted image.

The other two compartments of the neck are the neurovascular compartment, containing the carotid artery, internal jugular vein, vagus nerve, and lymph nodes, and the retropharyngeal space, containing the prevertebral space and prevertebral muscles. Benign tumors occurring in these compartments include paragangliomas, schwannomas, and neurofibromas.[61, 62]

Cystic structures in the neck are generally a result of congenital anomalies. The thyroglossal duct cyst located anteriorly in the midline may be found anywhere from the base of the tongue to the thyroid isthmus (Fig. 21–43). Branchial cleft cysts arising primarily from the second branchial cleft occur most commonly at the anterior border of the sternocleidomastoid muscle, posterior to the submandibular gland,[63] but they may be seen in the parotid gland and in the parapharyngeal area (Fig. 21–44). Cystic hygromas arising from lymphoid tissue may be seen in the posterior triangle of the neck or in the anterior triangle. Other cysts in the neck[64] have been reported, such as cervical thymic tissue, plunging ranula, and so forth.[65]

Enlarged lymph nodes are most commonly due to metastatic carcinoma or to lymphoma but are also seen in diffuse inflammatory disease, in cat scratch disease, in tuberculosis, and in patients with acquired immunodeficiency syndrome (AIDS)–related lymphadenopathy. Other benign lesions to be considered are lipoma, hemangioma,[16] lymphangioma, and other vascular diseases (Fig. 21–45). An aneurysm of the carotid artery occurring after trauma (Fig. 21–46) may also manifest as a mass in the neck.[66] An abscess in the neck is often secondary to dental caries, trauma, or a surgical procedure involving the mandible. An abscess cavity is to be differentiated from an infected branchial cleft cyst.[63]

CT has been used to good advantage in studying all of these abnormalities of the neck, but it requires the use of intravenous contrast enhancement. MR again has the advantage of showing these abnormalities in the coronal plane as well as the axial plane and in identifying the abnormality without the use of intravenous contrast. T_2-weighted images often show the abnormality to best advantage, although the T_1-weighted or proton density image has the capability of showing the best anatomic detail. The T_2-weighted image identifies the abnormality but is not specific enough for differentiating among be-

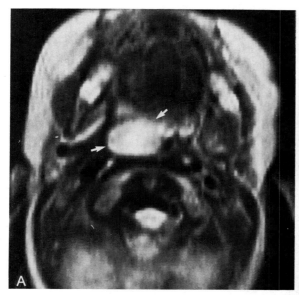
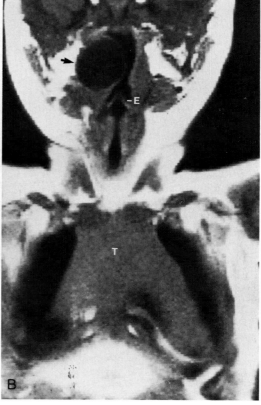

FIGURE 21–44. Pharyngeal cyst. *A*, Axial T_2-weighted image (TR 3.0/TE 45). *B*, Coronal T_1-weighted image (TR 0.6/TE 17). These show a large cyst *(arrows)* on the right side of the pharynx encroaching on the airway. This is cephalad to the epiglottis (E). Incidentally, note the prominent thymus (T).

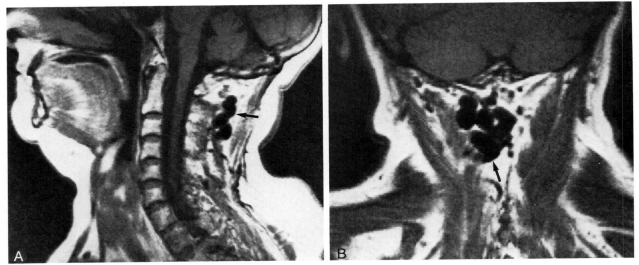

FIGURE 21–45. Vascular malformation of the neck. T_1-weighted images (TR 0.6/TE 17). *A*, Sagittal. *B*, Coronal. Enlarged tortuous vessels *(arrows)* are being supplied by the vertebral arteries.

nign, malignant, and inflammatory disease. MR spectroscopy and newly developed pulse sequences may shed further light on this differential diagnosis in the head and neck area.[7, 10]

TEMPOROMANDIBULAR JOINT

Patients with derangement of the TMJ (see Chapter 38) may present with a number of different complaints, ranging from headache, facial pain, and neck tenderness to the more classic symptoms of clicking, grinding, and joint pain. Clinical examination may be limited in those patients unable to open their mouths because of pain. Radiographic examination has progressed from plain films and tomography to arthrography, CT, and recently MR.[14, 15, 67] MR has the advantage of showing the meniscus itself in a normal position or displaced anteriorly in an abnormal fashion.[68] A surface coil is positioned over the joint, and images are obtained with both the open and closed mouth position. T_1-weighted images show to best advantage the anatomic detail of the area. Coronal T_1-weighted images are used to supplement the sagittal plane for the identification of mediolat-

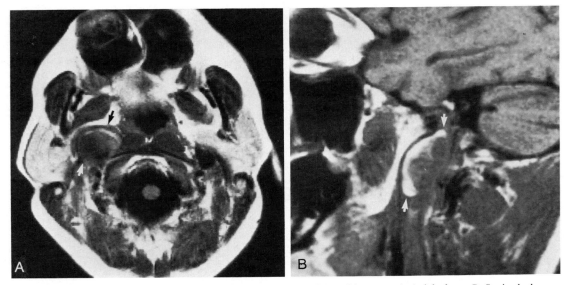

FIGURE 21–46. Traumatic aneurysm *(arrows)*, **right internal carotid artery.** *A*, Axial plane. *B*, Sagittal plane. T_1-weighted images (TR 0.8/TE 17). The high signal in the periphery is attributed to clot, and the somewhat irregular low signal in the rest of the aneurysm is attributed to turbulent flow. This aneurysm is encroaching on the right parapharyngeal space and deep portion of the parotid gland.

eral disk displacements. Dynamic studies with fast imaging techniques permit an evaluation of one complete cycle of opening and closing.

Derangement of the TMJ usually follows trauma, often an automobile accident. CT has the advantage of showing bone detail, but MR is better suited for evaluating the meniscus. These patients may have degenerative disease of the TMJ, narrowing of the joint space, or an anteriorly positioned meniscus when the mouth is closed. The last can be corrected to some extent with a specially designed bite device to position the mandibular condyle slightly more anteriorly within the condylar fossa. An anterior meniscus in the open and closed position or a "closed lock" is indicative of a more advanced derangement of the joint. Pain is due to stretching of the nerve fibers in the posterior attachment of the meniscus as it is stretched and torn with the anterior displacement.

ACKNOWLEDGMENTS: Sincere appreciation is extended to Nancy Williams for typing the manuscript and to S. M. Wolpert, M.D., Chief of Neuroradiology, for the use of cases 45 and 46.

REFERENCES

1. Colman MT, Hanafee WH: Diagnostic imaging of the head and neck. *In* Cummings CW, Fredrickson JM, Hacker LA (eds): Otolaryngology Head and Neck Surgery. St Louis, CV Mosby, 1986.
2. Mancuso AA, Hanafee WN (eds): Computed Tomography and Magnetic Resonance Imaging of the Head and Neck. 2nd ed. Baltimore, The Williams & Wilkins Company, 1985.
3. Baker SR, Latack JT: Magnetic resonance imaging of the head and neck. Otolaryngol Head Neck Surg 95:82–89, 1986.
4. Bilaniuk LT, Schenck JF, Zimmerman RA, et al: Ocular and orbital lesions: Surface coil MR imaging. Radiology 156:669–674, 1985.
5. Dietrich RB, Lufkin RB, Kangarloo H, et al: Head and neck MR imaging in the pediatric patient. Radiology 159:769–776, 1986.
6. Mafee MF, Rasouli F, Spigos DG, et al: Magnetic resonance imaging in the diagnosis of nonsquamous tumors of the head and neck. Otolaryngol Clin North Am 19:523–536, 1986.
7. Daniels DL, Pech P, Mark L, et al: Magnetic resonance imaging of the cavernous sinus. AJR 144:1009–1014, 1985.
8. Curati WL, Graif M, Kingsley DPE, et al: Acoustic neuromas: Gd-DTPA enhancement in MR imaging. Radiology 158:447–451, 1986.
9. Daniels DL, Herfkins R, Koehler PR, et al: Magnetic resonance imaging of the internal auditory canal. Radiology 151:105–108, 1984.
10. Daniels DL, Millen SJ, Meyer GA, et al: MR detection of tumor in the internal auditory canal. AJR 148:1219–1222, 1987.
11. Daniels DL, Schenck JF, Foster T, et al: Surface-coil magnetic resonance imaging of the internal auditory canal. AJR 145:469–472, 1985.
12. Daniels DL, Pech P, Pojunas KW, et al: Trigeminal nerve: Anatomic correlation with MR imaging. Radiology 159:577–583, 1986.
13. Han JS, Huss RG, Benson JE, et al: MR imaging of the skull base. J Comput Assist Tomogr 8:944–952, 1984.
14. Harms SE, Wilk RM: MRI of the temporomandibular joint. RadioGraphics 7:521–542, 1987.
15. Harms SE, Wilk RM, Wolford LM, et al: The temporomandibular joint: Magnetic resonance imaging using surface coils. Radiology 157:133–136, 1985.
16. Itoh K, Nishimura K, Togashi K, et al: MR imaging of cavernous hemangioma of the face and neck. J Comput Assist Tomogr 10:831–835, 1986.
17. Roberts D, Schenck J, Joseph P, et al: Temporomandibular joint: Magnetic resonance imaging. Radiology 155:829–830, 1985.
18. Westesson P, Katzberg RW, Tallents RH, et al: Temporomandibular joint: Comparison of MR images with cryosectional anatomy. Radiology 164:59–64, 1987.
19. Koening H, Lenz M, Sauter R: Temporal bone region: High-resolution MR imaging using surface coils. Radiology 159:191–194, 1986.
20. Flannigan BD, Bradley WG, Mazziotta JC, et al: Magnetic resonance imaging of the brain stem: Normal structure and basic functional anatomy. Radiology 154:375–383, 1985.
21. Gentry LR, Jacoby CG, Turski PA, et al: Cerebellopontine angle–petromastoid mass lesions: Comparative study of diagnosis with MR imaging and CT. Radiology 162:513–520, 1987.
22. Mawhinney RR, Buckley JH, Worthington BS: Magnetic resonance imaging of the cerebellopontine angle. Br J Radiol 59:961–969, 1986.
23. Mikhael MA, Ciric IS, Wolff AP: MR diagnosis of acoustic neuromas. J Comput Assist Tomogr 11:232–235, 1987.
24. Press GA, Hesselink JR: MR imaging of cerebellopontine angle and internal auditory canal lesions at 1.5 T. AJR 150:1371–1381, 1988.
25. Latack JT, Kartush JM, Kemink JL, et al: Epidermoidomas of the cerebellopontine angle and temporal bone: CT and MR aspects. Radiology 157:361–366, 1985.
26. Olsen WL, Dillon WP, Kelly WM, et al: MR imaging of paragangliomas. AJR 148:201–204, 1987.
27. Batsakis JG: Tumors of the Head and Neck: Clinical and Pathological Considerations. Baltimore, The Williams & Wilkins Company, 1979, pp 369–379.
28. Applebaum EL, Valvassori GE: Effects of magnetic resonance imaging fields on stapedectomy prostheses. Arch Otolaryngol 111:820–821, 1985.
29. Carter BL: Upper aerodigestive tract and neck. *In* Haaga JR, Alfidi R (eds): Computed Tomography of the Whole Body. 2nd ed. St. Louis, CV Mosby, 1988, pp 445–488.
30. Dillon WP, Mills CM, Kjos B, et al: Magnetic resonance imaging of the nasopharynx. Radiology 152:731–738, 1984.
31. Lloyd GAS, Phelps PD: The demonstration of tumours of the parapharyngeal space by magnetic resonance imaging. Br J Radiol 59:675–683, 1986.
32. Teresi LM, Lufkin RB, Vinuela F, et al: MR imaging of the nasopharynx and floor of the middle cranial fossa. Part I. Normal anatomy. Radiology 164:811–816, 1987.
33. Teresi LM, Lufkin RB, Vinuela F, et al: MR imaging of the nasopharynx and floor of the middle cranial fossa. Part II. Malignant tumors. Radiology 164:817–821, 1987.
34. Carter BL: Part II. Paranasal sinuses, nasal cavity, pterygoid fossa, nasopharynx, and infratemporal fossa. *In* Valvassori GE, Hanafee W, Carter BL, et al (eds): ENT Diagnostic Imaging. Stuttgart, Georg Thieme Verlag, 1988, pp 174–250.
35. Levine E, Wetzel LH, Neff JR: MR imaging and CT of extrahepatic cavernous hemangiomas. AJR 147:1299–1304, 1986.
36. Teresi LM, Lufkin RB, Wortham DG, et al: Parotid masses: MR imaging. Radiology 163:405–409, 1987.
37. Lloyd GAS, Lund VJ, Phelps PD, et al: Magnetic resonance imaging in the evaluation of nose and paranasal sinus disease. Br J Radiol 60:957–968, 1987.
38. Belkin B, Papageorge M, Bankoff M, et al: A comparative study of magnetic resonance imaging versus computed tomography for evaluation of maxillary and mandibular tumors. J Oral Maxillofac Surg 48:1039–1047, 1988.

39. Lusk RP, Lee PC: Magnetic resonance imaging of congenital midline nasal masses. Otolaryngol Head Neck Surg 95:303–306, 1986.

40. Rice DH, Becker T: Magnetic resonance imaging of the salivary glands: A comparison with computed tomographic scanning. Arch Otolaryngol Head Neck Surg 113:78–80, 1987.

41. Teresi LM, Kolin E, Lufkin RB, et al: MR imaging of the intraparotid facial nerve: Normal anatomy and pathology. AJR 148:995–1000, 1987.

42. Casselman JW, Mancuso AA: Major salivary gland masses: Comparison of MR imaging and CT. Radiology 165:183–189, 1987.

43. Mandelblatt SM, Braun IF, Davis PC, et al: Parotid masses: MR imaging. Radiology 163:411–414, 1987.

44. Lufkin RB, Larsson SG, Hanafee WN: Work in progress: NMR anatomy of the larynx and tongue base. Radiology 148:173–175, 1983.

45. Unger JM: The oral cavity and tongue: Magnetic resonance imaging. Radiology 155:151–153, 1985.

46. Lufkin RB, Hanafee WN: Application of surface coils to MR anatomy of the larynx. AJNR 6:491–497, 1985.

47. Lufkin RB, Hanafee WN, Wortham D, et al: Larynx and hypopharynx: MR imaging with surface coils. Radiology 158:747–754, 1986.

48. McArdle CB, Bailey BJ, Amparo EG: Surface coil magnetic resonance imaging of the normal larynx. Arch Otolaryngol Head Neck Surg 112:616–622, 1986.

49. Lufkin RB, Wortham DG, Dietrich RB, et al: Tongue and oropharynx: Findings on MR imaging. Radiology 161:69–75, 1986.

50. Hoover LA, Wortham DG, Lufkin RB, et al: Magnetic resonance imaging of the larynx and tongue base: Clinical applications. Otolaryngol Head Neck Surg 97:245–250, 1987.

51. Wortham DG, Hoover LA, Lufkin RB, et al: Magnetic resonance imaging of the larynx: A correlation with histologic sections. Otolaryngol Head Neck Surg 94:123–133, 1986.

52. Kier R, Herfkens RJ, Blinder RA, et al: MRI with surface coils for parathyroid tumors: Preliminary investigation. AJR 147:497–500, 1986.

53. Kneeland JB, Krubsack AJ, Lawson TL, et al: Enlarged parathyroid glands: High-resolution local coil MR imaging. Radiology 162:143–146, 1987.

54. Charkes ND, Maurer AH, Siegel JA, et al: MR imaging in thyroid disorders: Correlation of signal intensity with Graves disease activity. Radiology 164:491–494, 1987.

55. Gefter WB, Spritzer CE, Eisenberg B, et al: Thyroid imaging with high-field strength surface-coil MR. Radiology 164:483–490, 1987.

56. Higgins CB, McNamara MT, Fisher MR, et al: MR imaging of the thyroid. AJR 147:1255–1261, 1986.

57. Stark DD, Moss AA, Gamsu G, et al: Magnetic resonance imaging of the neck. Part 1. Normal anatomy. Radiology 150:447–454, 1984.

58. Stark DD, Moss AA, Gamsu G, et al: Magnetic resonance imaging of the neck. Part 2. Pathologic findings. Radiology 150:455–461, 1984.

59. Noma S, Nishimura K, Togashi K, et al: Thyroid gland: MR imaging. Radiology 164:495–499, 1987.

60. Spritzer CE, Gefter WB, Hamilton R, et al: Abnormal parathyroid glands: High-resolution MR imaging. Radiology 162:487–491, 1987.

61. Glazer HS, Niemeyer JH, Balfe DM, et al: Neck neoplasms: MR imaging. Part I. Initial evaluation. Radiology 160:343–348, 1986.

62. Glazer HS, Niemeyer JH, Balfe DM, et al: Neck neoplasms: MR imaging. Part II. Posttreatment evaluation. Radiology 160:349–354, 1986.

63. Kreipke DL, Lingeman RE: Cross-sectional imaging (CT, NMR) of branchial cysts: Report of three cases. J Comput Assist Tomogr 8:114–116, 1984.

64. Som PM, Sacher M, Lanzieri CF, et al: Parenchymal cysts of the lower neck. Radiology 157:399–406, 1985.

65. Charnoff SK, Carter BL: Plunging ranula: CT diagnosis. Radiology 158:467, 1986.

66. Goldberg HI, Grossman RI, Gomori JM, et al: Cervical internal carotid artery dissecting hemorrhage: Diagnosis using MR. Radiology 158:157–161, 1986.

67. Burnett KR, Davis CL, Read J: Dynamic display of the temporomandibular joint meniscus by using "fast-scan" MR imaging. AJR 149:959–962, 1987.

68. Katzberg RW, Bessette RW, Tallents RH, et al: Normal and abnormal temporomandibular joint: MR imaging with surface coil. Radiology 158:183–189, 1986.

22

THE BRACHIAL PLEXUS

RENÉE FITZMORRIS GLASS

TECHNICAL CONSIDERATIONS

ANATOMY

PATHOLOGY
POSTTRAUMATIC
NONTRAUMATIC

Pain and numbness in the shoulder and arm are the presenting symptoms of a number of significant entities, including lesions of the brachial plexus. The physician must exclude disorders of the shoulder, cervical spine, peripheral nerves, and vascular supply to arrive at the correct diagnosis. Not only can these processes mimic a plexopathy, but also the symptomatology of primary brachial plexus lesions is variable, depending on the nature of the lesion and the exact anatomic location. Both the physical examination and electromyography are of limited utility in this area, and so the need for an imaging tool arises. Prior to the advent of MRI, the radiologist had plain film techniques, myelography, and CT as the principal means of investigation. The limitation of myelography is readily apparent, since it evaluates the structures within and adjacent to the thecal sac: cervical cord, dura, and nerve roots. With respect to the brachial plexus, myelography is most useful in a posttraumatic situation to detect nerve root avulsion from the spinal cord, but it cannot assess more peripheral abnormalities.[1] The development of CT brought a marked improvement, because of its good contrast discrimination and spatial resolution. Unfortunately, in this particular region, several difficulties cause lesion conspicuity to be diminished. The shoulder artifact, resulting from beam hardening from the scapula and humeral head, is the most important of these. Difficulties in interpretation can also arise from poorly timed intravenous contrast injection, resulting in suboptimal vascular enhancement. Finally, the axial plane of section can be suboptimal for evaluating the oblique course of the plexus.[2-10] With the development of MRI, a significant new technique is available. Many problems exist in imaging the body with MR due to vascular flow and respiratory and cardiac motion, but these are not usually significant in the evaluation of the brachial plexus. The multiplanar capability of MRI, and the excellent soft tissue contrast it affords, allow detailed images of the brachial plexus to be created.

TECHNICAL CONSIDERATIONS

As experience with MR imaging grows, so does the variety of techniques applied to imaging any given area of anatomy. The radiologist has an extensive list of parameters from which to choose in attempting to optimize lesion conspicuity, including type of coil, pulsing sequences, plane of section, and so on, while trying to minimize the multitude of artifacts inherent in MR imaging. The literature is replete with examples utilizing various combinations, many of which prove to be impractical in day to day imaging.

There are two goals in imaging the brachial plexus. Of primary interest is the ability to demonstrate precisely the anatomic features of this complex region, and multiplanar imaging is helpful in this regard. The second is to generate a diagnosis or differential diagnosis. Although tissue characterization is not perfect with MR imaging, the information can be useful in narrowing the list of possibilities and helping direct patient care. To meet these goals, the plexus is optimally examined in at least two planes, and images with both T_1 and T_2 weighting are obtained. Gradient-echo (GRE) sequences suffer from decreased signal-to-noise ratio (S/N) and spatial resolution and are primarily useful for screening or

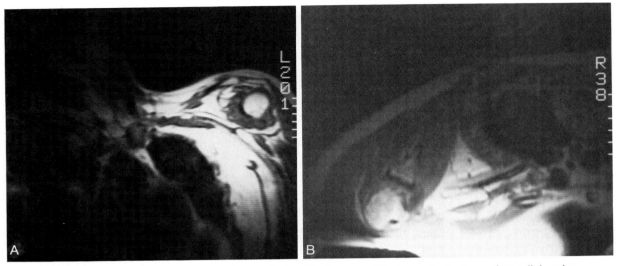

FIGURE 22–1. Example of surface-coil degradation. Excellent detail is obtained with the surface coil, but the high signal from subcutaneous fat and the rapid drop-off in signal with increasing distance from the coil compromise image quality. *A*, Coronal image, TR 500/TE 20, 1 excitation, 5-mm slice. *B*, Axial image, TR 2000/TE 20, 2 excitations, 5-mm slice.

localizer sequences, although as software improves, these may become more diagnostic.

The next question to be considered is the type of coil to be used to gather data. Some authors have advocated the use of surface coils,[11–13] because of the superiority of S/N in this design. The trade-off is the marked degradation in image quality with increasing distance from the coil. Limiting the images to those obtained with the surface coil may significantly compromise the area effectively scanned (Figs. 22–1 and 22–6). Since it is often clinically difficult to localize a neurologic deficit to a specific anatomic junction, the capability of imaging a large area must be preserved. The body coil can satisfy this requirement, especially with the use of the off-center field-of-view (FOV). Using this feature, an acceptably small FOV can be obtained, without sacrificing homogeneity of signal (Fig. 22–2). In the most complex cases, it may be useful to use the surface coil in a slightly more creative way. With most MR systems, the body coil is able to demonstrate the brachial plexus well, but it is very unsatisfactory in evaluating the spinal canal and neural foramina. In patients with an unrevealing or confusing neurologic examination, it may be advantageous to position the patient with a surface coil beneath the posterior neck, so that a screening image of the cervical spine can be obtained.[14] If this study is normal, then the plexus can be evaluated without repositioning the patient. In this way, high S/N and high-resolution images of the cervical spine are obtained, and yet the plexus can be evaluated without signal drop-off. In addition, the posterior position of the surface coil prevents the coil edge artifact from being in a significant area of anatomy when the plexus is imaged.

The plane of section is another area of debate. In general, coronal and axial planes are able to delineate pathology exquisitely. Some authors advocate the sagittal plane,[15] but if this is used exclusively, the ability to compare with the asymptomatic side is lost. In general, it is preferable to begin with a coronal T_1-weighted sequence, using an FOV large enough to image both right and left superior sulci and to avoid significant wraparound (aliasing). Selection of the FOV is dependent on the patient's size, varying from 32 to 38 cm. In most cases of neoplastic involvement of the plexus, this sequence will depict the mass rather clearly outlined by the normal fat of the supraclavicular fossa. This sequence is also necessary to position accurately the off-center axial images, obtained with a T_2-weighted pulse sequence. The anatomic landmarks that are important to consider include the midline, to demonstrate the proximal aspect of the great vessels and the origins of the nerve roots, and the axillary recess. The optimal FOV will again depend on the patient's size, usually ranging from 28 to 34 cm, and can be accurately predicted from the coronal views if necessary. A double echo is gathered on the T_2 sequence to obtain images of intermediate and heavy T_2 weighting. Occasionally, depending on the setting, a sagittal sequence may provide more information than the axial, such as the extent of invasion of a known Pancoast tumor.[2]

In areas such as the brachial plexus, where respiratory motion can be a limitation, reordering of the phase-encoding steps can also be helpful in reducing the ghosts seen from the periodic chest motion of respiration. Since only a reordering of data acquisition is involved in these sequences, there is no time penalty associated with them. These sequences have various acronyms according to the manufacturer, such as ROPE (*r*espiratory *o*rdering of *p*hase *e*ncoding) (Picker International, Highland Heights, OH)

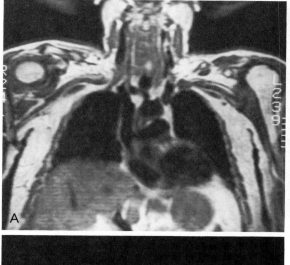

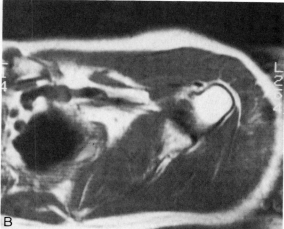

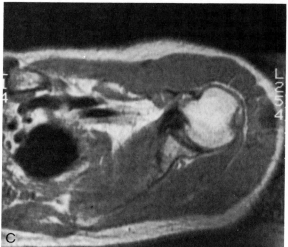

FIGURE 22–2. Surface coil with off-center FOV. With use of the body coil both to transmit and to receive signal, as well as the off-center FOV, images both have detailed resolution and do not suffer from signal drop-off. *A*, Coronal image, TR 800/TE 20, 4 excitations, 5-mm slice. *B*, Axial image, TR 800/TE 20, 4 excitations, 10-mm slice. *C*, Axial image, TR 2500/TE 20, 128 matrix, 2 excitations, 5-mm slice.

and EXORCIST (General Electric Company, Milwaukee, WI). Usually, images will be of diagnostic quality without using these sequences. Although some authors use gating routinely, it does have significant time penalties, and diagnostic information can be obtained without it. The images shown here do not use cardiac gating. When blood flow is important to document, such as in a possible superior vena cava syndrome, GRE techniques can be utilized. Although spatial resolution will be limited, as mentioned previously, the presence of flow can be determined, which can thereby obviate either nuclear medicine flow studies or angiography.

Since T_1-weighted images have higher S/N compared with that of T_2-weighted images, the coronal sequences can be obtained with a 5-mm slice thickness. The T_2 sequences, however, are better when a 10-mm slice thickness is used. In the body, where respiration, flowing blood, and slight motion by the patient all combine to degrade image quality, the 128 matrix is usually superior to the 256 matrix. With this matrix size, two to four excitations are recommended. As more variation is allowed in matrix size by the equipment manufacturers, other matrix sizes may be preferred and may alter the number of excitations needed.

ANATOMY[16, 17]

The brachial plexus is formed by the union of the ventral primary divisions of C5 through C8 and the first dorsal nerve, with some inconstant contributions from the fourth cervical and second dorsal nerves. The arrangement of the nerves within the plexus is subject to considerable variation, but most commonly, the fifth and sixth cervical nerve roots unite to form the upper trunk, the seventh cervical nerve forms the middle trunk, and the eighth and first dorsal nerves form the lower trunk. The roots and trunks can be identified as they exit the intervertebral foramina and course anterolaterally to pass between the anterior and middle scalenus muscles. In axial plane of section, therefore, the scalenus muscles form essential landmarks that should always be identified.

The anterior scalenus arises from the transverse

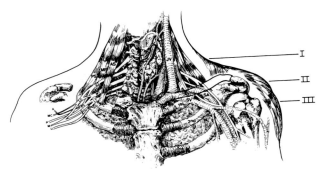

FIGURE 22–3. Coronal anatomy. AS = anterior scalene muscle; 5R–1R = fifth cervical nerve root to the first thoracic nerve root; JV = internal jugular vein; MS = middle scalene muscle; PS = posterior scalene muscle; SA = subclavian artery; SV = subclavian vein; 1st = first rib; 2nd = second rib. (Courtesy of H. R. Harnsberger, M.D.)

processes of the third, fourth, fifth, and sixth cervical vertebrae and inserts on the first rib. The middle scalenus, a bulkier and longer muscle, arises from the posterior aspect of the transverse processes of the lower six cervical vertebrae and has a broad insertion along the first rib. A posterior scalenus muscle does exist but is not often discrete from the middle scalenus. It arises from the transverse processes of C5 through C7 and inserts onto the second rib. The insertion of the anterior and middle scaleni is separated by a groove on the first rib in which the subclavian artery and the brachial plexus travel. The subclavian vein travels anteriorly to the anterior scalene, beneath the clavicle and the subclavian muscle.

At this point, the trunks of the proximal brachial plexus intermingle, forming the divisions first, then the cords, and finally the individual nerves. The details of this complex anatomy are rarely clinically significant and vary from individual to individual.

The importance at this level of the plexus is that these nerves surround the axillary artery at its second part (posterior to the pectoralis minor muscle). The cords are named for their position relative to the axillary artery, that is, posterior, medial, or lateral. By the level of the third portion of the axillary artery, distal to the pectoralis muscle, the plexus has divided into its terminal branches, which still surround the artery (Figs. 22–3 and 22–4).

Although the vessels and the scalenus muscles form the major anatomic landmarks, several other anatomic features should be noted. Other muscles that should be recognized include the serratus anterior, the pectoralis minor, and the small subclavius and omohyoid muscles. Both the serratus anterior and the pectoralis minor are familiar structures, since they are usually well seen on CT.[9] The serratus anterior muscle arises from the eight upper ribs and inserts onto the ventral aspect of the scapula. The pectoralis minor arises from the third through fifth ribs and inserts onto the coracoid process. The subclavius parallels the clavicle, originating from the first rib and costal cartilages and inserting into the undersurface of the clavicle. The smallest muscle, since it is perhaps the least familiar, gives rise to the most confusion. This is the omohyoid muscle. It has two bellies, which are united by a central tendon. The superior belly is one of the strap muscles, originating from the hyoid bone and extending inferiorly to the central tendon. The inferior belly then extends from the central tendon to the superior border of the scapula, just medial to the coracoid process. Another common anatomic feature is the anterior scalenus lymph node chain, part of the deep cervical chain, which is seen in normal volunteers.[18]

The signal characteristics of the normal structures are constant and can be helpful in accurately assessing this region. Muscle tissue is of an intermediate

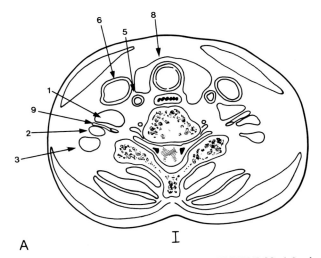

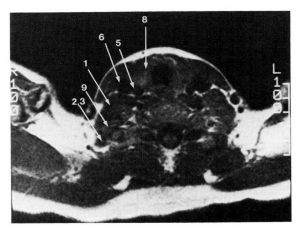

FIGURE 22–4 *See legend on opposite page*

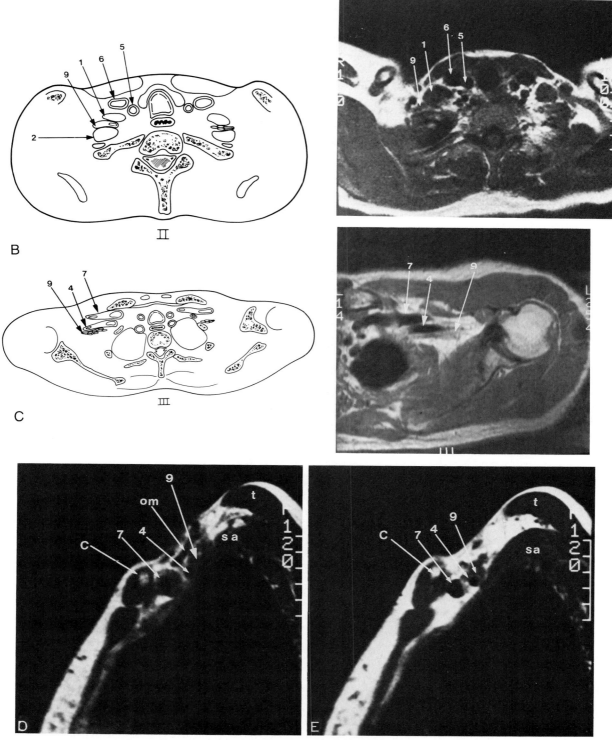

FIGURE 22–4. Axial schematics in three sections with corresponding axial MR images. Levels I to III refer to those diagrammed in Figure 22–3. *A*, The level of the thyroid bed. Proximal nerve roots that have already exited the neural foramina lie between the two scalene muscles. On the diagram, more distal nerve roots still lie in their foramina. *B*, The level of the cervicothoracic junction, just superior to the pulmonary apex. The brachial plexus now lies between the scalene muscles. *C*, The level of the apex of the axillary recess, where the brachial plexus lies posterior to the subclavian artery and vein. *D*, Sagittal plane, axillary recess. *E*, Sagittal plane, medial to *D*. 1 = Anterior scalene muscle; 2 = middle scalene muscle; 3 = posterior scalene muscle; 4 = subclavian artery; 5 = carotid artery; 6 = internal jugular vein; 7 = subclavian vein; 8 = thyroid gland; 9 = brachial plexus; C = clavicle; om = omohyoid muscle; sa = serratus anterior muscle; t = trapezius muscle.

signal intensity on all pulse sequences, and the structures of the plexus are similar or slightly less intense. The vessels are more variable, with the usual artifacts of flow commonly associated with imaging vascular structures. Usually, on at least one of the obtained pulse sequences, a homogeneous loss of signal intensity will be present throughout the vascular lumen. If signal is seen on all sequences, then the possibility of thrombus should be considered and further imaging directed toward this diagnosis. Lymph nodes and neoplasm are most often of low signal on T_1 and higher signal on T_2. Size remains an important criterion for distinguishing benign from malignant lymphadenopathy. Neoplasia, while typically following this general appearance, may be complicated by radiation, necrosis, and hemorrhage (see "Pathology").

PATHOLOGY

POSTTRAUMATIC

In discussions of brachial plexopathies, it is common to divide the population of patients into traumatic and nontraumatic subsets. The posttrauma patient most often has a documented clinical history of significant injury. The brachial plexopathy seen in this setting may be from diverse causes. Nerve root avulsions, with or without an associated pseudomeningocele, clavicular or rib fractures and dislocations, posttraumatic neuromas, and hematomas are all found. A subgroup of this population includes those patients with a plexopathy following anesthesia or axillary arteriography. Depending on the mechanism of injury in this latter group, hematoma, nerve ische-

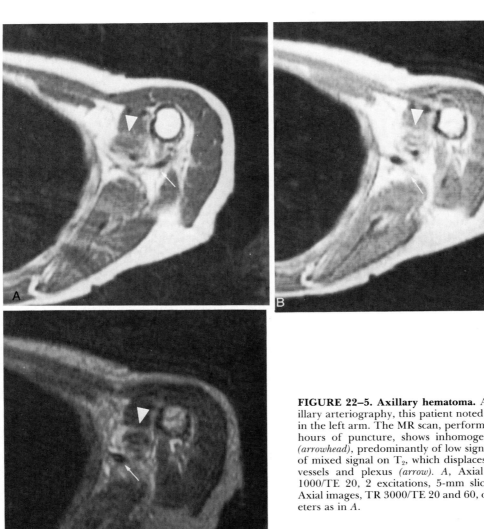

FIGURE 22–5. Axillary hematoma. After left axillary arteriography, this patient noted paresthesias in the left arm. The MR scan, performed within 48 hours of puncture, shows inhomogeneous tissue *(arrowhead)*, predominantly of low signal on T_1 and of mixed signal on T_2, which displaces the axillary vessels and plexus *(arrow)*. *A*, Axial image, TR 1000/TE 20, 2 excitations, 5-mm slice. *B* and *C*, Axial images, TR 3000/TE 20 and 60, other parameters as in *A*.

mia, and possibly nerve section may be the etiology of the symptoms.[19-23]

The appearance of hematoma on MR imaging has been fairly well described.[24-29] Depending on the age of the hematoma, the degree of encapsulation from the surrounding tissues, and the field strength used, the signal characteristics will vary (see Chapters 8 and 16). Most often, both acute hematoma and acute intraparenchymal hemorrhage will be of low signal intensity on T_1-weighted images because of the presence of deoxyhemoglobin. The appearance in the acute stage on T_2 weighting is most dependent on field strength. At higher field strengths, the T_2 shortening by the magnetically susceptible deoxyhemoglobin in intact red blood cells becomes apparent as a region of low intensity. This shortening is apparent in hematomas, in which the central core is slower to oxidize to methemoglobin than is the outer core. Hemorrhage and hematoma will often be visualized in the subacute and chronic phases. The definition of these phases is not precise, but "subacute" generally refers to 2 days to several weeks after the initial hemorrhage, whereas "chronic" refers to several weeks to months after the initial event. At the cellular level, these terms describe the gradual oxidation of deoxyhemoglobin to methemoglobin. Methemoglobin results in shortening of T_1 (high intensity on T_1-weighted images) and lengthening of T_2 (high intensity on T_2-weighted images). As the macrophages are attracted to the hematoma rim and convert the heme iron into hemosiderin, the paramagnetic hemosiderin produces a low-intensity margin on T_2-weighted images. This effect is field strength dependent and thus most evident at the higher field strengths. GRE techniques, owing to their sensitivity to magnetic susceptibility effects, are especially sensitive to the presence of hemosiderin (Figs. 22–5 and 22–8).

The nerve root avulsions and pseudomeningoceles are uniform in appearance, generally following the signal characteristics of cerebrospinal fluid (CSF), and are typical in location, associated with the ipsilateral neural foramina. The actual discontinuity of the nerve root is more difficult to demonstrate than the CSF collection (Fig. 22–6). Several cases are cited in the literature that show increased signal within the nerves on T_2 weighting, and this has been interpreted as consistent with edema[13] (Fig. 22–7).

NONTRAUMATIC

The second large group of patients comprises those with no significant history of trauma. Frequently, their presentation is vague or atypical. Symptoms may include pain or numbness in the neck or shoulder, paresthesias, and upper extremity weakness.[30] With this complaint, such diverse causes as cervical spondylitis, rotator cuff tears, peripheral nerve entrapment syndromes,[31, 32] and thoracic outlet syndromes,[33] as well as lesions of the brachial plexus, need to be considered.[30] The physical examination may be unrevealing, since palpation of the region is difficult owing to the deep location of the neural elements. Electromyography can also be misleading or incomplete and does not distinguish between a mass lesion and other causes of plexopathy.[34-36] Therefore, this group of patients will often be referred for an imaging study. Unlike the posttrauma patients, in whom there is some rationale for including myelography, abnormalities in this group will be best approached with MR imaging. The differential diagnosis in a brachial plexopathy includes secondary malignancies in patients with known primary tumors,

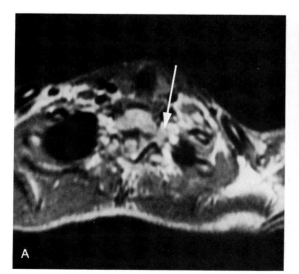
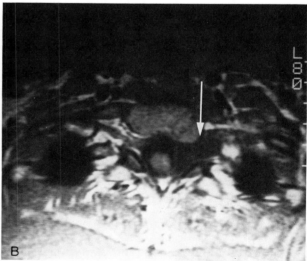

FIGURE 22–6. Nerve avulsion. Typical posttraumatic pseudomeningocele *(arrow)*, with the same signal characteristics as that of CSF. *A*, Axial image, body coil, TR 2500/TE 20, 128 matrix, 2 excitations, 5-mm slice. *B*, Axial image, surface coil, TR 1000/TE 20, 128 matrix, 4 excitations, 3-mm slice.

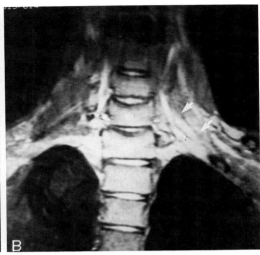

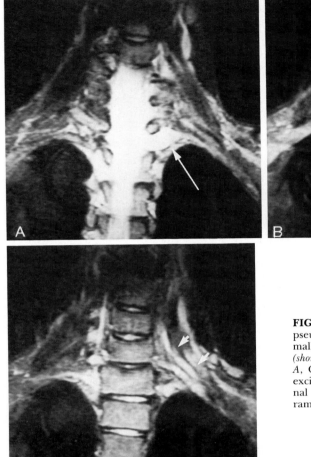

FIGURE 22–7. Nerve edema. Posttraumatic pseudomeningocele *(long arrow, A)* and abnormally increased signal in nonavulsed nerve roots *(short arrows, B* and *C)* on T_2-weighted images. *A,* Oblique coronal image, TR 2000/TE 70, 2 excitations, 5-mm slice. *B* and *C,* Oblique coronal images, TR 2000/TE 30 and 70, other parameters as in *A.*

primary neoplasia of the plexus, radiation injury, and idiopathic plexopathy. On occasion, MR imaging will be useful in elucidating an abnormality suggested on CT, such as vascular ectasia.

The most common etiology of plexopathy is involvement by a metastatic lesion.[37] Malignancies that ordinarily involve this region include lymphomas, sarcomas, and carcinomas from lung, breast, kidney, and the head and neck. When these lesions form masses, the diagnosis is straightforward (Fig. 22–8). Of more difficulty is the infiltrative involvement, which may have a normal appearance on MR imaging[12] (Fig. 22–9). Metastatic lesions may involve the plexus in one of two ways, either by hematogenous spread, including both the masses and the infiltrative types, or by direct extension, most commonly the Pancoast type of lung cancer. In these cases, it is important to demonstrate the relationship of the tumor to the pulmonary apex, and either the coronal or the sagittal image can do this reliably. An important limitation to keep in mind in evaluating these images is how the respiratory motion can de-

grade the image, making the pulmonary component obscure (Fig. 22–10). The bulky masses will characteristically be of low to intermediate signal on T_1 weighting and will be relatively hyperintense on T_2 weighting. These lesions are often inhomogeneous, especially as they increase in size, owing to areas of hemorrhage and necrosis (Fig. 22–11).

A subset of this group is composed of patients who not only have a known primary tumor but also have received radiation therapy to the superior sulcus.[37–39] Radiation injury can occur with doses above 6000 rads but has been reported with pathologic confirmation at doses as low as 4800 rads. In one study, the interval between radiation therapy and the onset of plexopathy was from 18 months to 10 years.[3] Initial reports in the literature suggested that radiation fibrosis might be reliably distinguished from recurrent tumor on MR imaging, based on signal characteristics.[40] Since the pathologic appearance of irradiated tissue changes over time, with repair and involution, the MR appearance should be expected to be variable over time as well. In the final stages of

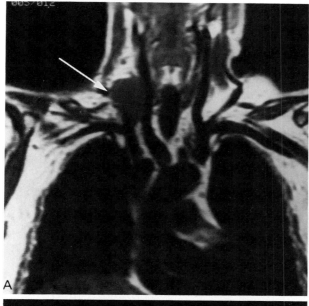

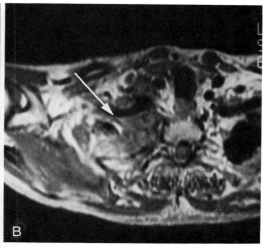

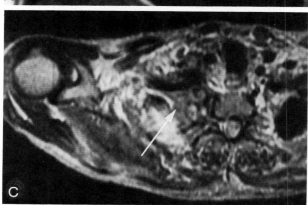

FIGURE 22–8. Bulky metastatic mass. Metastatic adenocarcinoma forming a bulky soft tissue mass *(arrow)* adjacent to the right common carotid artery and surrounding the internal jugular vein. This tumor is less bright on T_2 *(C)* than is often seen with metastases. *A,* Coronal image, TR 600/TE 20, 4 excitations, 5-mm slice. *B* and *C,* Axial images, TR 2500/TE 20 and 60, 2 excitations, other parameters as in *A.*

repair, when fibrotic tissue has completely replaced edema and inflammatory cells, the MR images would be expected to show low signal characteristics on all sequences. However, the early and intermediate stages following radiation therapy may contain areas of high signal on T_2 weighting. MR imaging will be unable to distinguish between edema and necrosis, and recurrent or residual tumor, in these cases. Complicating this issue is the unpredictability of the time required for fibrotic repair in a field of radiation in any given patient[41] (Fig. 22–12).

Although less commonly seen than the metastatic lesions, primary tumors of the plexus do occur.[42] These are most likely to be neurofibromas, 10 per cent of which are malignant, and schwannomas (neurilemmomas). The signal characteristics of these lesions are not reliably distinct from those of the malignant lesions and require a tissue diagnosis (Fig. 22–13).

Miscellaneous causes of brachial plexopathy should be mentioned. Among these are a variety of anatomic impingements that can be symptomatic and have been loosely grouped under the heading of thoracic outlet syndromes.[31–33] Included in this list are the scalenus anticus and cervical rib syndromes, the scalenus medius bands, and the costoclavicular syndrome. Since these syndromes are most often positional, and the anatomic abnormality subtle, it may be difficult to identify these prospectively. Knowledge of the patient's history and a physical examination suggesting an intermittent neuropathy and abnormalities of arterial or venous flow (or both) are essential. Posttraumatic injuries, especially of the clavicle, are often included in the thoracic outlet syndromes. Granulation tissue from an old clavicular fracture or a clavicular nonunion may compromise the plexus and subclavian vessels (Figs. 22–14 and 22–15).

A final significant cause of brachial plexopathy has been variously described in the literature by such terms as paralytic brachial neuritis, acute shoulder neuritis, acute brachial radiculitis, and so on.[35, 43] Perhaps idiopathic brachial plexus neuropathy provides a satisfactory description, since this disorder has been associated with multiple causes. Currently, it is thought that this neuropathy may be a manifes-

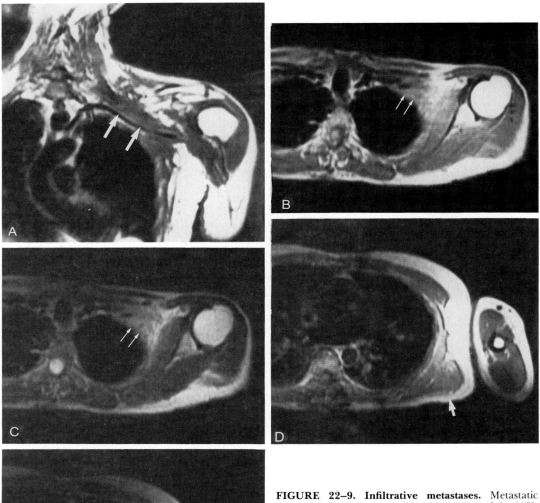

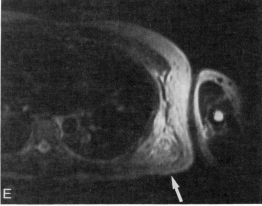

FIGURE 22–9. Infiltrative metastases. Metastatic breast adenocarcinoma in a male patient, of the infiltrative type *(arrows)*. Multiple pulmonary nodules are also evident. Note the extension along the posterior chest wall, which displays typical signal characteristics. The tumor in the superior sulcus is more isointense on all sequences. *A*, Coronal image, TR 800/TE20, 4 excitations, 5-mm slice. *B* and *C*, Axial images, TR 3000/TE 20 and 70, 10-mm slice, 2 excitations. *D* and *E*, Axial images, other parameters as in *B* and *C*.

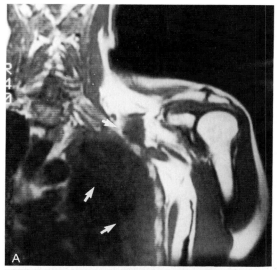

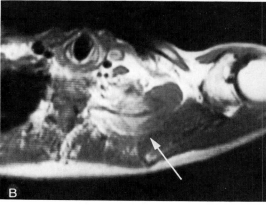

FIGURE 22–10. Pancoast-type tumor. In this tumor, the respiratory motion causes significant image degradation and decreases conspicuity of the bulky lung mass and pleural fluid. The supraclavicular and apical components are well seen. On axial images, the tumor mass *(arrows)* is of high intensity with T_2 weighting. *A,* Coronal image, TR 600/TE 20, 128 matrix, 4 excitations, 5-mm slice. *B* and *C,* Axial images, TR 2500/TE 20 and 70, 10-mm slice, 2 excitations.

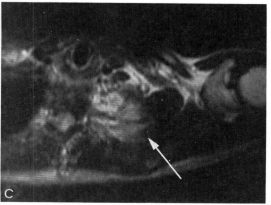

tation of an infectious disorder or the result of a hypersensitivity reaction. Well-documented cases exist of the onset of the plexopathy after administration of sera or vaccines. It has also been seen in patients with primary malignancies, when no involvement of

the plexus could be demonstrated, and on follow-up, gradual resolution of these symptoms occurred.[34] Thus, this entity should be kept in mind when evaluating the cancer patient with shoulder and arm pain.

FIGURE 22–11. Tumor with heme. Tumor in the left pulmonary apex *(arrow)* extends into the supraclavicular fossa and contains areas of bright signal on T_1, likely representing intratumoral hemorrhage. TR 600/TE 20, 4 excitations, 10-mm slice.

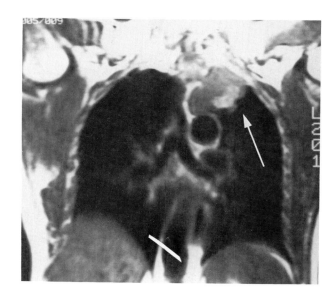

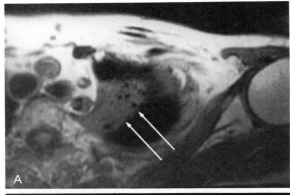

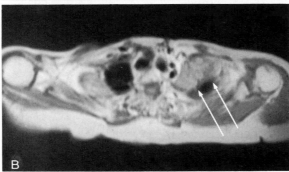

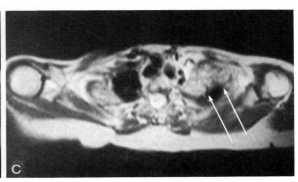

FIGURE 22–12. High-signal radiation fibrosis, after 18 years. Eighteen years prior to the MR scan, the patient had a mastectomy and radiation therapy, with chronic secondary lymphedema. No clinical evidence of recurrent tumor was present at the time of imaging or in 1 year of subsequent clinical follow-up. The radiation fibrosis *(arrows)* in this patient is unusual in its bright signal on T_2 weighting. *A,* Axial image, TR 800/TE 20, 4 excitations, 5-mm slice. *B* and *C,* Axial images, TR 2000/TE 20 and 70, 2 excitations, 10-mm slice.

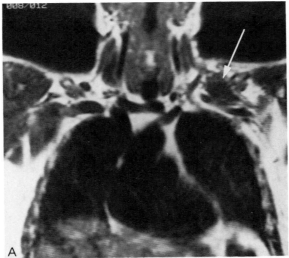

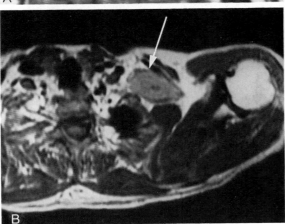

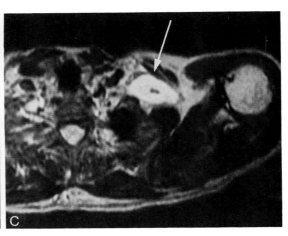

FIGURE 22–13. Schwannoma. This well-encapsulated mass *(arrow)* was demonstrated to be a benign schwannoma at surgery. This pattern of signal characteristics can be seen in both benign and neoplastic tumors and is nonspecific. *A,* Coronal image, TR 600/TE 20, 4 excitations, 5-mm slice. *B* and *C,* Axial images, TR 2500/TE 20 and 70, 2 excitations, other parameters as in *A.*

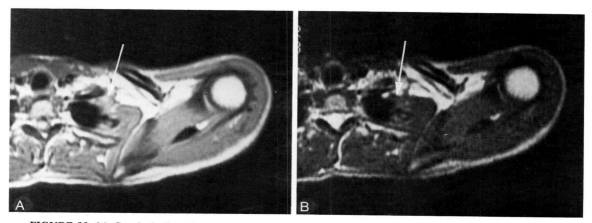

FIGURE 22–14. Cervical rib with extra soft tissue. By comparison with plain films and careful examination of the multiple slices, it was demonstrated that the extra soft tissue *(arrow)* at the left pulmonary apex was related to a cervical rib. *A* and *B*, Axial images, TR 2000/TE 20 and 70, 4 excitations, 5-mm slice.

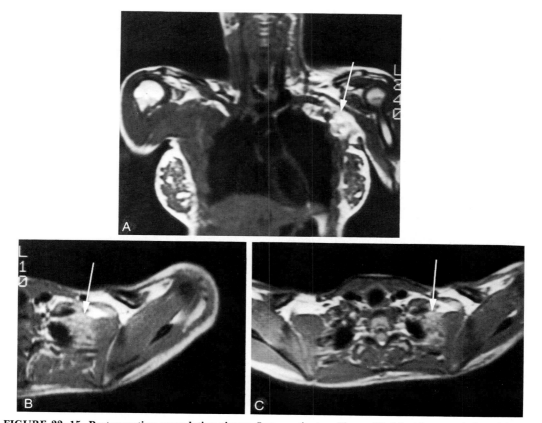

FIGURE 22–15. Postoperative granulation tissue. Same patient as Figure 22–14. After surgical excision of the cervical rib, symptoms gradually recurred over a period of days to weeks. Repeat examination demonstrates extensive tissue *(arrow)*, presumably granulation tissue and hemorrhage, surrounding the brachial plexus and subclavian and axillary vessels. The asymmetry with the contralateral apex is seen in *C. A*, Coronal image, TR 800/TE 20, 4 excitations, 5-mm slice. *B* and *C*, Axial images, TR 3000/TE 20, 2 excitations, other parameters as in *A*.

REFERENCES

1. Armington WG, Harnsberger HR, Osborn AG, Seay AR: Radiographic evaluation of brachial plexopathy. AJNR 8:361–367, 1987.
2. Heelan RT, Demas BE, Caraveli JF, et al: Superior sulcus tumors: CT and MR imaging. Radiology 170:637–641, 1989.
3. Cascino TL, Kori S, Krol G, Foley KM: CT of the brachial plexus in patients with cancer. Neurology 33:1553–1557, 1983.
4. Gebarski KS, Glazer GM, Gebarski SS: Brachial plexus: Anatomic, radiologic, and pathologic correlation using computed tomography. J Comput Assist Tomogr 6:1058–1063, 1982.
5. Powers SK, Norman D, Edwards MSB: Computerized tomography of peripheral nerve lesions. J Neurosurg 59:131–136, 1983.
6. Stewart JD, Schmidt B, Wee R: Computed tomography in the evaluation of plexopathies and proximal neuropathies. Can J Neurol Sci 10:244–247, 1983.
7. Takasagi JE, Godwin JD, Halvorsen RE, et al: Computed tomographic evaluation of lesions in the thoracic apex. Invest Radiol 33:1553–1557, 1985.
8. Usselman JA, Vint VC, Waltz TA: CT demonstration of a brachial plexus neuroma. AJNR 1:346–347, 1980.
9. Vock P, Owens A: Computed tomography of the normal and pathologic thoracic inlet. Eur J Radiol 2:187–193, 1982.
10. Webb WR, Jeffrey RB, Godwin JD: Thoracic computed tomography in superior sulcus tumors. J Comput Assist Tomogr 5:361–365, 1981.
11. Castagno AA, Shuman WP: MR imaging in clinically suspected brachial plexus tumor. AJR 149:1219–1222, 1987.
12. Kneeland JB, Kellman GM, Middleton WD, et al: Diagnosis of diseases of the supraclavicular region by use of MR imaging. AJR 148:1149–1151, 1987.
13. Rapoport S, Blair DN, McCarthy SM, et al: Brachial plexus: Correlation of MR imaging with CT and pathologic findings. Radiology 167:161–165, 1988.
14. Flannigan BD, Lufkin RB, McGlade C, et al: MR imaging of the cervical spine: Neurovascular anatomy. AJR 248:785–790, 1987.
15. Blair DN, Rapoport S, Sostman HO, Blair OC: Normal brachial plexus: MR imaging. Radiology 165:763–767, 1987.
16. Anderson JE: Grant's Atlas of Anatomy. 7th ed. Baltimore, The Williams & Wilkins Company, 1978.
17. Hollinshead WH, Rosse C: Textbook of Anatomy. Philadelphia, Harper and Row, 1985, pp 182–190.
18. Kellman GM, Kneeland JB, Middleton WD, et al: MR imaging of the supraclavicular region: Normal anatomy. AJR 148:77–82, 1987.
19. Jackson L, Keats AS: Mechanisms of brachial plexus palsy following anesthesia. Anesthesiology 26:190–194, 1965.
20. Lyon BB, Hansen BA, Mygind T: Peripheral nerve injury as a complication of axillary arteriography. Acta Neurol Scand 51:29–36, 1975.
21. Molnar W, Paul DJ: Complications of axillary arteriotomies: An analysis of 1,762 consecutive studies. Radiology 104:269–276, 1972.
22. O'Keefe DM: Brachial plexus injury following axillary arteriography. J Neurosurg 53:853–857, 1980.
23. Orkin FK, Cooperman LH: Complications of Anesthesia. Philadelphia, JB Lippincott, 1983, pp 648–654.
24. Bradley WG Jr, Schmidt PG: Effect of methemoglobin formation on the MR appearance of subarachnoid hemorrhage. Radiology 156:99–103, 1985.
25. Cohen MD, McGuire W, Cory DA, Smith JA: MR appearance of blood and blood products: An in vitro study. AJR 146:1293–1297, 1986.
26. Edelman RR, Johnson K, Buxton R, et al: MR of hemorrhage: A new approach. AJNR 7:751–756, 1986.
27. Gomori J, Grossman RI, Goldberg HI, et al: Intracranial hematomas: Imaging by high-field MR. Radiology 157:87–93, 1985.
28. Swensen SJ, Keller PL, Berquist TH, et al: Magnetic resonance imaging of hemorrhage. AJR 145:921–927, 1985.
29. Unger EC, Glazer HS, Lee JKT, Ling D: MRI of extracranial hematomas: Preliminary observations. AJR 146:403–407, 1986.
30. Adams RD, Victor M (eds): Principles of Neurology. New York, McGraw-Hill, 1981, pp 917–922.
31. Hare WSC, Rogers WJ: The scalenus medius band and the seventh cervical transverse process. Diagn Imag 50:263–268, 1981.
32. McCormick CC, Gubbay SS, Lekias JS: Upward dislocation of the first rib: A rare cause of nerve entrapment, producing brachialgia. Br J Radiol 54:140–142, 1981.
33. Lord JW, Rosati LM: Thoracic outlet syndromes. Ciba Clin Symp 23:1–32, 1971.
34. Kori S, Foley K, Posner J: Brachial plexus lesions in patients with cancer: 100 cases. Neurology 31:45–50, 1981.
35. Pezzimenti JF, Bruckner HW, DeConti RC: Paralytic brachial neuritis in Hodgkin's disease. Cancer 31:626–629, 1973.
36. Synek VM, Cowan JC: Somatosensory evoked potentials in patients with metastatic involvement of the brachial plexus. Electromyogr Clin Neurophysiol 23:545–551, 1983.
37. Posner JB: Neurological complications of systemic cancer. Med Clin North Am 63:783–800, 1979.
38. Lederman RJ, Wilbourn AJ: Brachial plexopathy: Recurrent cancer or radiation? Neurology 34:1331–1335, 1984.
39. Thomas JE, Colby MY: Radiation-induced or metastatic-brachial plexopathy? JAMA 222:1392–1395, 1971.
40. Glazer HS, Lee JKT, Levitt RG, et al: Radiation fibrosis: Differentiation from recurrent tumor by MR imaging. Work in progress. Radiology 156:721–726, 1985.
41. Match RM: Radiation-induced brachial plexus paralysis. Arch Surg 110:384–386, 1975.
42. Dart LH, MacCarty CS, Love JG, Dockerty MB: Neoplasms of the brachial plexus. Minn Med 53:959–964, 1970.
43. Tsairis P, Dyck P, Mulder D: Natural history of brachial plexus neuropathy. Arch Neurol 27:109–117, 1972.

23

MR IMAGING OF THE CERVICAL AND THORACIC SPINE

GREGORY M. SHOUKIMAS and JOHN R. HESSELINK

EXAMINATION TECHNIQUE
GENERAL CONSIDERATIONS
PULSE SEQUENCES
ALGORITHMS
ANATOMY

SPINAL CORD DISEASE (INTRAMEDULLARY)
TUMORS
SYRINGOHYDROMYELIA
INFLAMMATORY/DEGENERATIVE
ISCHEMIA/INFARCTION
VASCULAR MALFORMATIONS
DEGENERATIVE SPINAL DISEASE (EXTRADURAL)
INTERVERTEBRAL DISK DISEASE
SPONDYLOSIS

SPINAL STENOSIS
POSTOPERATIVE (See Chapter 24)
VERTEBRAL AND PARAVERTEBRAL ABNORMALITIES (EXTRADURAL)
METASTATIC DISEASE
PRIMARY BONE LESIONS
BONE MARROW DISEASE
PARASPINAL TUMORS
INFECTION
INTRADURAL EXTRAMEDULLARY DISEASE
NERVE SHEATH TUMORS
MENINGIOMA
METASTATIC DISEASE
TRAUMA
CRANIOVERTEBRAL ABNORMALITIES

Cross-sectional imaging of the spine and spinal cord has contributed substantially to the detection, characterization, and, in many cases, histopathologic identification of a number of diseases of the spine and spinal cord. The distinct advantages of direct axial and computer-reformatted multiplanar imaging of the spine using computed x-ray tomography have been reviewed.[1] Despite the advantages achieved by computed x-ray tomography, intrathecal contrast administration is required in a large number of cervical and thoracic examinations to visualize pathologic conditions of neural, bony, and ligamentous structures.

Although newer nonionic and low-osmolality con-

trast agents are less toxic,[2, 3] their administration is not entirely without danger, and some centers require hospitalization, thereby increasing the cost of the examination beyond that of a magnetic resonance (MR) study. Furthermore, in a setting where clinical localization of a lesion(s) is difficult, axial imaging with CT of the entire spine may be indicated but is clearly not practical.

MR has several advantages over CT and is effectively challenging CT for supremacy in the diagnosis of diseases of the spine. A major benefit of MR is the ability to directly image the spinal cord. The MR images not only show the external contours of the cord but also reveal differences in signal intensity in diseased portions. Moreover, since different signal intensities are obtained from the cortical bone, epidural fat, cerebrospinal fluid (CSF), and spinal cord, MR is well-suited for imaging extradural, subarachnoid, and intramedullary abnormalities within the spinal canal.[4]

EXAMINATION TECHNIQUE

An understanding of the basic principles of MR imaging is essential to achieve the appropriate tissue contrast (T_1- or T_2-weighting), spatial resolution, an adequate number of images, and the optimal imaging plane and signal-to-noise ratios (S/N) required for diagnosing spinal disorders. S/N is influenced by most of the imaging parameters, as well as the selection of receiver coil (body coil versus a variety of surface coils). These considerations are reviewed in detail Chapters 1 and 2.

GENERAL CONSIDERATIONS

MR imaging has the capacity to produce images that are well suited for diagnosis of spine and spinal cord disorders. Direct sagittal, coronal, axial, and oblique imaging can be performed without repositioning the patient. Since data are obtained directly in the desired plane of imaging, no computer reformatting artifact is generated. Surface coils are used to enhance the magnetic coupling of the receiver coil to the body, thereby improving spatial resolution to the extent that MR images achieve spatial resolution comparable to that of high-resolution CT scanners. Currently, high-resolution MR images have a spatial resolving power of approximately 0.5 mm.

Tissue contrast is determined by operator selection of pulse parameters and can be manipulated to achieve T_1- or T_2-weighted images. On many MR units, selection of the TR and TE is essentially infinite, whereas on others a limited menu of pulse sequences is available. Despite these differences, the capacity to obtain a range of variable T_1- and T_2-weighted sequences appropriate for most clinical situations is essentially unaffected. The decision to apply a particular pulse sequence should be based primarily on the clinical problem and the likelihood of finding intra-versus extradural disease.

Although conventional T_1- and T_2-weighted studies are routinely performed with standard spin-echo sequences, the demand for greater patient throughput, the desire to reduce CSF flow artifacts, and the hope that quantification of physiologic parameters such as blood and cerebrospinal fluid flow can be achieved have led to the development of "fast scan" pulse sequences. These techniques have been given a number of acronyms, including FISP, FLASH, and GRASS. They are discussed in more detail in Chapter 5. Briefly, they employ a variable initial flip angle that may be smaller than the conventional 90-degree angle used in spin-echo techniques. Also, rather than using a 180-degree refocusing pulse, gradient reversal is employed to maximize signal refocusing. With gradient-echo techniques, T_1- and T_2-weighted images can be obtained in a considerably shorter amount of time than required with spin-echo techniques. These methods also reduce flow and pulsation artifacts that may obscure image detail.

When spin-echo techniques are required, cardiac gating decreases flow artifacts. With this technique, the patient's heart rate (R-R interval) or a multiple thereof determines the TR. Because data are acquired at precisely the same time during the cardiac cycle, artifacts generated by cardiac pulsation are reduced. Flow compensation techniques or gradient motion rephasing methods are also effective in reducing CSF flow artifacts. Switching the phase and frequency encoding axes to orient the phase axis along the long axis of the spine reduces swallowing, cardiac, respiratory, and CSF pulsation artifacts (Fig. 23–1), but it also increases chemical shift artifact

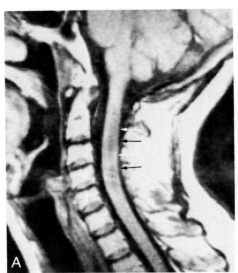 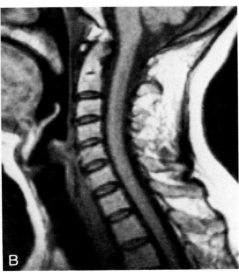

FIGURE 23–1. Phase artifact simulating intraparenchymal lesion. *A,* SE 500/40 sagittal 5-mm image. Phase-encoding axis is in the horizontal (x) direction, which generates artifact through the spinal cord from mandible and tongue motion *(arrows).* In this situation, failure to recognize the artifactual nature of the finding might lead to the erroneous diagnosis of a cord lesion in this patient with a cervical myelopathy. T_2-weighted images showed a similar phase artifact. *B,* SE 500/40 sagittal 5-mm image. Changing the phase-encoding axis to the vertical direction eliminates phase-encoding artifact across the spinal cord, yielding a normal diagnostic study.

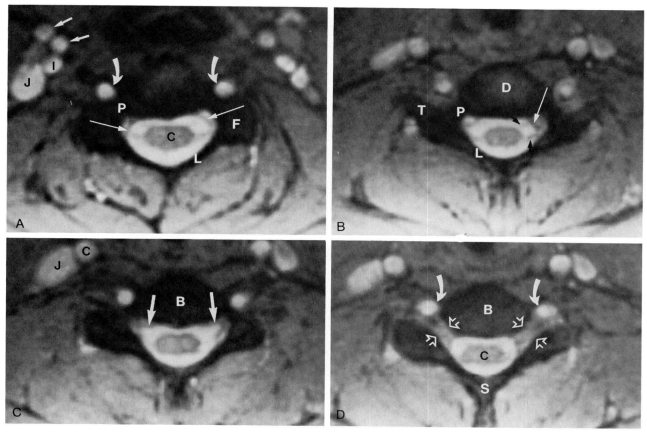

FIGURE 23–3. Normal axial anatomy, gradient-echo scans (GRE 25/13, flip angle = 8 degrees). *A,* Level of pedicle. The intermediate-signal spinal cord (C) is surrounded by hyperintense CSF. Long arrows = Dura of thecal sac; P = pedicle; F = facet/lateral mass; L = lamina; curved arrows = vertebral arteries; J = jugular vein; I = internal carotid artery; short arrows = branches of external carotid artery. *B,* Level of intervertebral disk. The high signal of the disk (D) is confined to the central portion. P = Pedicle; T = transverse process; L = lamina; short arrows = anterior and posterior rootlets; long arrow = dura. *C,* Level of root sleeves. The root sleeves *(arrows)* are budding off the thecal sac and beginning to enter the neural foramina. B = Vertebral body; C = common carotid artery; J = jugular vein. *D,* Level of neural foramina. The tissues in the neural foramina *(open arrows)* are of intermediate signal and contrast with the hypointense bordering bone and the hyperintense thecal sac medially. B = Vertebral body; C = cord; S = spinous process; curved arrows = vertebral arteries.

because its long axis parallels the sagittal plane. In patients with severe scoliosis, coronal scans may incorporate a longer segment of the cord in the imaging plane if the kyphosis or lordosis is not too extreme. Axial or angled axial (oblique) images may be necessary to further characterize the degree of cord compression, to document a suspected lesion seen on long-axis views, and to determine the lateral extent of an intraspinal process.

Assessment of cervical *radiculopathy* has been a challenge for MR because of the small amount of epidural fat, the difficulty in resolving the anatomy of the smaller neural foramina, and the problem of obtaining thin sections with adequate S/N. Despite its limitations, MR capabilities exceed those of plain myelography and approach the accuracy of CT with myelography (CTM).[11] MR is an effective screening technique for cervical radiculopathy; CTM can be reserved for selected cases in which the MR is equiv-

ocal or negative in patients with strong clinical findings.

Both T_1-weighted and gradient-echo images are required in the sagittal plane to evaluate the causes of radicular symptoms. The gradient-echo images give the best contrast between osteophytes and hyperintense thecal sac. Disk fragments are also usually well seen, but on occasion the disk is nearly isointense to the CSF. In these cases, the anatomy may be displayed better on the T_1-weighted images. The T_1-weighted image is also important for screening the cord.

Since the cervical neural foramina are oriented in an oblique plane, they are not adequately imaged in the sagittal plane. Therefore, additional views in the axial plane are necessary to assess foraminal disease. With our present technology, gradient-echo scans seem to give the best anatomic detail in the axial plane. Effacement of the hyperintense thecal sac

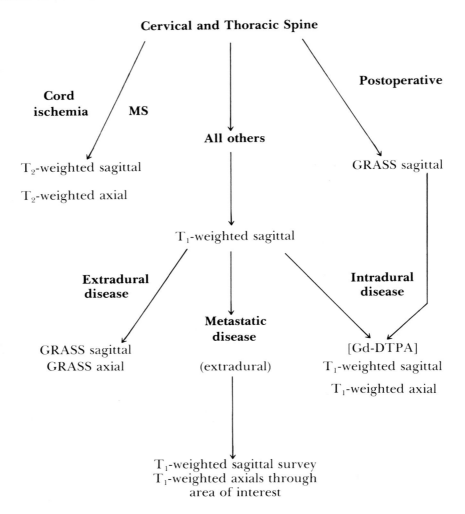

Cervical and Thoracic Spine

Cord ischemia   **MS**

All others

Postoperative

T₁-weighted sagittal
T_2-weighted sagittal
T_2-weighted axial

GRASS sagittal

T_1-weighted sagittal

Extradural disease

Intradural disease

GRASS sagittal
GRASS axial

Metastatic disease

(extradural)

[Gd-DTPA]
T_1-weighted sagittal

T_1-weighted axial

T_1-weighted sagittal survey
T_1-weighted axials through
area of interest

identifies any abnormality within the spinal canal, and the tissues within the foramina provide sufficient signal to display encroachment upon the foramina. In the postoperative patient, Gd-DTPA is valuable, as it enhances epidural scar and allows distinction from recurrent disc herniation to be made.

Owing to more compact anatomy in the cervical region, sections should be as thin as possible to avoid volume-averaging effects. At high field strength, 3-mm sections may be employed, whereas at intermediate field strengths, 4- to 5-mm sections are used to maintain S/N. Using gradient-echo imaging with thin sections should minimize the number of cases requiring additional imaging studies for lesion confirmation and presurgical planning.

From the foregoing discussion, an algorithm (see above) can be devised, taking into account the clinical findings and pertinent history.

ANATOMY

Much of the cervical and thoracic spinal anatomy is displayed best with a T_1-weighted pulse sequence (TR = 600 msec; TE = 20 msec). With this sequence, the cord has a higher signal than the surrounding CSF (Figs. 23–2A and 23–4). CSF (water signal) has a very long T_1 relaxation time and thus emits very little signal when a short TR and TE are employed. The normal cord has smooth ventral and dorsal margins, and it follows the normal lordotic and kyphotic curves of the spine. Its anteroposterior diameter is relatively constant, except for mild cervical and distal thoracic enlargements.

A common artifact on sagittal MR scans of the spine acquired with lower matrix sizes (256 × 128) is a thin line down the center of the cord. The line is of low signal intensity on T_1-weighted scans and high signal intensity on gradient-echo and T_2-weighted scans. At first, it was thought that the line might represent the central canal, and in some cases it was misinterpreted as a syrinx. Further studies identified the line as a "Gibbs" or "truncation" artifact due to undersampling of data (see Chapter 3). The artifact is markedly reduced by using matrix sizes of 256 × 256 or larger.

Ligamentous structures, dura, and cortical bone also exhibit low signal intensity on T_1-weighted images, and differentiation of these structures from one

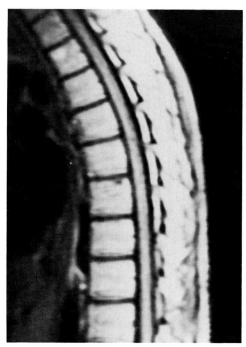

FIGURE 23–4. Normal mid-sagittal view of thoracic spine, T_1-weighted scan (SE 600/20). The thoracic cord is outlined by the low-signal CSF. The vertebral bodies are hyperintense, and the intervertebral disks are of intermediate signal intensity. The disks are partially obscured by chemical shift artifact.

another or from CSF may not be possible. The cervical spinal canal does not contain much epidural fat, but Gd-DTPA may enhance the retrovertebral plexus to separate the posterior longitudinal ligament from the anterior dura. The intervertebral disk is contrasted against the hypointense vertebral end plates above and below and the ligaments anteriorly and posteriorly (Fig. 23–2A and B).

Bone marrow normally has a high fat content unless it is pathologically involved, and the very short T_1 of fat renders the marrow hyperintense on T_1-weighted images (Fig. 23–4). Paravertebral musculature has an intermediate T_1 and thus has signal characteristics intermediate between normal marrow and CSF. When interpreting signal characteristics on images obtained with a surface coil, one must keep in mind that the signal intensity progressively decreases as the anatomy gets farther away from the coil.

On gradient-echo images, anything with high water content or flow is hyperintense (see Fig. 23–3). CSF, jugular veins, and carotid and vertebral arteries have high signal intensity. Intervertebral disks, neural structures, and muscles are of intermediate signal intensity. Bone, marrow, and fat are hypointense. The soft tissues within the neural foramina are highlighted against the dark cortical bone.[12] The cord is clearly seen surrounded by the hyperintense CSF, and on good-quality scans the anterior and posterior rootlets can be identified traversing the subarachnoid

space. Also, on higher-matrix scans the gray and white matter of the spinal cord can be recognized.[13]

SPINAL CORD DISEASE (INTRAMEDULLARY)

MR has added a new dimension to spinal cord imaging, as it is the only technique that can reliably image the internal architecture of the cord. As a result, solid and cystic portions of intramedullary lesions can be identified, and the longitudinal extent can be defined more accurately than was possible before. The addition of Gd-DTPA has further enhanced the ability of MR to localize tumor nidus, to differentiate benign and reactive processes from neoplastic lesions, and to determine the activity of lesions.[14]

TUMORS

Primary cord neoplasms consist predominantly of *ependymoma* (60 per cent) (Fig. 23–5) and *astrocytoma* (25 per cent) (Fig. 23–6), with the statistics varying according to location in the spine. Astrocytoma is slightly more common in the cervical region, the two are about equal in the thoracic area, and ependymoma predominates at the level of the conus medullaris and below. These gliomas exhibit more benign behavior than their intracranial counterparts. *Oligodendroglioma* and *hemangioblastoma* (Fig. 23–7) are less common cord neoplasms, and rarely *teratoma, dermoid* (Fig. 23–8), and *lipoma* have been identified.[15] Except for lipoma, no distinct MR morphology has been described that consistently enables precise histologic identification without biopsy. Evidence of hypervascularity suggests hemangioblastoma. Hematogenous *metastases* from breast or lung carcinoma and melanoma may produce an appearance similar to that of primary intramedullary neoplasms (Fig. 23–9), although metastases may involve several segments of the cord and subarachnoid spread of tumor is common.[16] Regardless of the etiology, the MR appearance of these neoplasms varies widely, making a specific diagnosis difficult in most cases.

On T_1-weighted images expansion of the cord is the hallmark of intramedullary neoplasm (Fig. 23–5A and B). On T_2-weighted images, the expanded segment of cord demonstrates T_2 prolongation (Fig. 23–6) that may be limited to the segment of abnormal appearing cord on T_1-weighted images. Areas of increased T_2 in the other nonexpanded segments represent microinfiltration of tumor or tumor-associated edema. Conventional MR techniques cannot reliably make this distinction. Gd-DTPA enhances areas of blood-brain barrier breakdown to help detect, characterize, and define the extent of intramedullary neoplasms (Figs. 23–5 and 23–7).[17, 18]

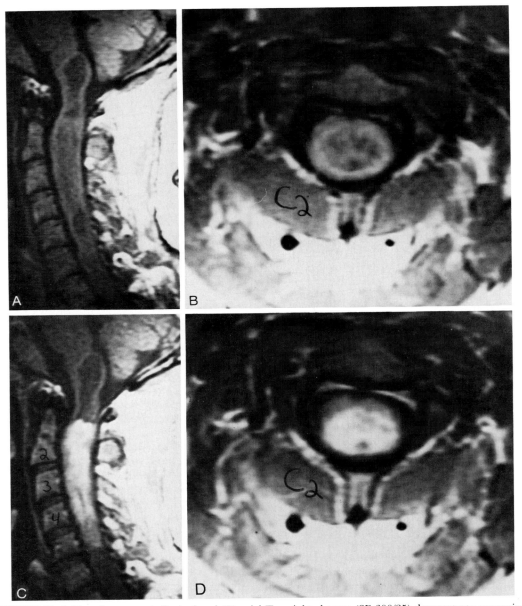

FIGURE 23–5. Ependymoma. *A*, Sagittal and *(B)* axial T_1-weighted scans (SE 600/25) demonstrate expansion of the upper cervical cord. The mass is heterogeneous, and an apparent cystic component superiorly extends above the foramen magnum. *C* and *D*, Contrast-enhanced scans (SE 600/25, Gd-DTPA) reveal enhancement of the central portion of the mass extending from C1 down to C5. The perimeter of the cyst superiorly also enhances slightly.

Focal areas of either increased or decreased T_1 may be present within the expanded parenchyma owing to the presence of cysts or necrotic cavities. The concentration of protein and the presence of hemorrhage determine the degree of T_1 shortening or lengthening (Fig. 23–7). Cavities containing high concentrations of protein have a shorter T_1 than does CSF. Focal areas of subacute hemorrhage, depending on the time the scan is performed after hemorrhage, have a shortened T_1 owing to the paramagnetic effect of methemoglobin. T_2 lengthening may also be seen

in these circumstances. Intraoperative ultrasonography has been shown to be of value for definition of cystic and necrotic components of cord tumors.[19]

Defining cyst cavities as either primary, as in syringohydromyelia, or a result of an intramedullary tumor is sometimes difficult, although several features have been described that may facilitate this distinction.[20] Fluid isointense to CSF, smooth distinct internal margins, and thinned adjacent parenchyma without evidence of T_2 prolongation within the parenchyma are signs of a primary cavity. Even cavities

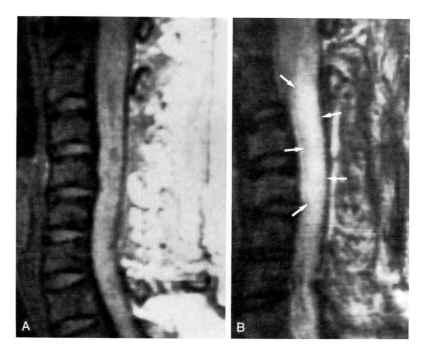

FIGURE 23–6. Astrocytoma. *A*, Sagittal T₁-weighted scan (SE 600/25). Patient has had a previous laminectomy extending from C3 to C6. The entire cervical cord is enlarged and has a heterogeneous internal texture. *B*, A T₂-weighted image (SE 2000/70) shows an area of high signal intensity *(arrows)* in the cord from C3 to C5. Margins of the lesion are indistinct and blend in with the normal cord tissue. Findings are consistent with an intramedullary tumor.

of this description can be associated with an intramedullary or extramedullary neoplasm at a level distant from the cavity.[21] For this reason, examination of the entire spinal cord may be indicated when cavitation occurs in the absence of a Chiari malformation or history of previous trauma.

Tumor cavities, on the other hand, often have a slightly shorter T₁, perhaps secondary to a higher protein concentration and the presence of necrotic debris. On T₂-weighted images, the fluid may have signal characteristics that do not parallel CSF but show greater signal compared to CSF. The internal margins may be irregular, and the contiguous cord parenchyma may be irregularly thickened (Fig. 23–5). The signal of adjacent parenchyma is frequently increased on T₂-weighted images owing to the presence of tumor cells, edema, or both. According to Williams et al,[22] when multifactorial analysis is applied, the distinction between tumor and nonneoplastic cavities approaches a specificity of 88 per cent

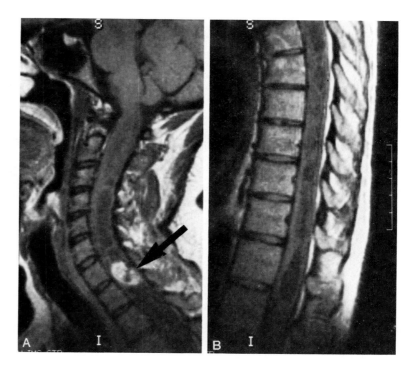

FIGURE 23–7. Hemangioblastoma. Sagittal enhanced scans (SE 500/40, Gd-DTPA) disclose cystic enlargement of the entire cord extending from the foramen magnum down to the conus. A 2 × 1 cm tumor nodule *(arrow)* enhances at the cervicothoracic junction. The central nonenhancing area likely represents the vascular pedicle of the hemangioblastoma. The heterogeneous appearance of the cystic component is probably due to flow effects and cyst loculations with varying protein concentrations.

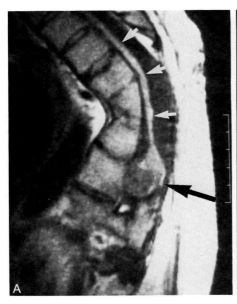
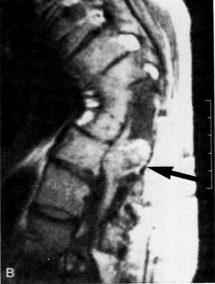

FIGURE 23–8. Recurrent intraspinal dermoid. Sagittal images (SE 500/40) demonstrate a mass (black arrow) with mixed signal intensities. The high-signal areas posteriorly correspond to fat, and the other soft-tissue elements are of intermediate signal intensity. The spinal cord is markedly atrophic (white arrows). The mass is contiguous with the cord, and the cord is draped anteriorly over the mass. At surgery the dermoid tumor was found to have invaded the cord but was predominantly exophytic.

for simple cysts and 60 per cent for tumor-associated cavities. Other authors have suggested that the absence of signal within an intramedullary cavity on flow-sensitive pulse sequences may also be a good indicator of a simple, nonneoplastic cavity.[23]

Although the sagittal plane is best for screening the cord, the images are more susceptible to partial volume effects that can make interpretation difficult. Axial images eliminate some of the volume-averaging artifacts and help define cord lesions identified on the sagittal scans. Furthermore, axial images may help differentiate a contiguous extramedullary mass causing cord flattening from a true intramedullary process.

Despite the profound improvement achieved by MR in the evaluation of cord neoplasms, there may

still be a role for angiography in a subgroup of patients with von Hippel–Lindau disease with suspected hemangioblastoma or vascular malformations of the cord. Conventional MR spin-echo sequences and even some of the newer MR angiographic techniques have not achieved the resolution or specificity required to define the vascularity of these lesions.[24]

MR is a noninvasive means of evaluating cord morphology for evidence of recurrent or residual tumor, for change in previously identified cavities, and for response to therapy. Unfortunately, because T_2-weighted images are rather nonspecific with respect to causes of T_2 prolongation, the distinction between gliosis, tumor, edema, and radiation-induced necrosis may not be possible. Gadolinium is particularly helpful in postoperative cases (Fig. 23–

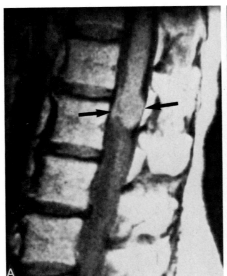
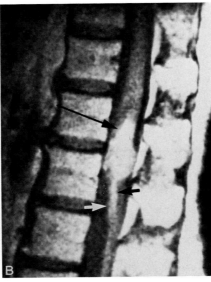

FIGURE 23–9. Intramedullary metastasis to the conus from breast carcinoma. A, Noncontrast scan (SE 500/40) reveals nodular expansion (arrows) of the conus. The mass is isointense to the cord. B, Contrast-enhanced scan (SE 500/40, Gd-DTPA) demonstrates enhancement of the nodule as well as the conus (long arrow) above the nodule and the proximal cauda equina (short arrows), indicating infiltration of the contiguous neural structures. A head MR showed an additional cerebral metastasis (not shown). At surgery, an intramedullary metastasis with exophytic growth was found.

8), because cord tumors invariably enhance as discrete solid lesions. In general, distinguishing postoperative changes from residual or recurrent tumor is easier for cord tumors than for intraaxial brain lesions. In questionable cases, follow-up studies may be necessary.

SYRINGOHYDROMYELIA

Prior to the advent of MR, the diagnosis of intramedullary cavities was based on not only the presence of cord expansion but also the entrance of contrast media into the cavity after a delay of 4 to 6 hours. On delayed CTM, contrast uptake occurs in about 80 to 90 per cent of cases.[25] Because contrast uptake in the cord can be seen in a number of other processes, such as tumor or inflammation, confusion in diagnosis often occurred. Direct evaluation of the cord with MR and of the entire spinal neuraxis with surface coils provides more sensitive and specific evaluation of syringohydromyelia.

In the largest series by Sherman et al,[26] four separate groups of patients were identified based on the appearance of the cavities and any associated anomaly or relevant history. Approximately 41 per cent had syringomyelia associated with tonsillar ectopia (Chiari I malformation) (Fig. 23–10), 28 per cent had posttraumatic syrinx, 15 per cent were associated with neoplasm, and 15 per cent were idiopathic. When the cavities were analyzed for specific characteristics, a few observations were made. At least one third of patients with nonneoplastic cavities had associated high signal intensity in the cord contiguous to the cavity or in the parenchyma distal or proximal to the cavity. This high signal intensity in a simple syrinx is speculated to represent

gliosis, edema, demyelination, or microcystic malformation.[27, 28] The presence of edema is supported by the return of the hyperintense parenchyma to normal signal intensity following myelotomy and shunt decompression of the cyst.[29]

As discussed above in the section on intramedullary neoplasms, the cerebrospinal fluid flow void signal (CFVS) most likely represents a combination of phase-shift and time-of-flight phenomena and may be a reliable indicator of nonneoplastic parenchymal cavities, approaching a sensitivity of 80 per cent.[30] In cavities less than 3 mm in diameter, however, the CFVS is unreliable, as these small channels may not demonstrate signal void. In the majority of cases, however, the diagnosis of a simple (primary) syrinx can be made based on thinning of the parenchyma adjacent to the expanded cavity (Fig. 23–11). The internal margins are smooth but may be interrupted by septations that can be continuous or incomplete. The latter results in a haustrated appearance of the cord (Fig. 23–10).

Again, Gd-DTPA markedly increases the certainty of distinguishing a primary syrinx from a cystic neoplasm. If a cavity is noted within the cord on screening T_1-weighted sagittal scans, rather than struggling with T_2-weighted images, Gd-DTPA should be given and the T_1-weighted scans repeated in sagittal and axial planes. If no enhancing nodule is seen, a cord neoplasm is unlikely.

Examination of the entire spinal cord with T_1-weighted sagittal images is mandatory. In regions where a cavity is suspected but somewhat equivocal in the sagittal projection, axial T_1-weighted scans should be done. Failure to examine the entire spinal neuraxis may result in missing cavities that are separated from the primary or larger cavity. Long segments of normal-appearing cord may intervene between a cervical cavity and one located in the conus

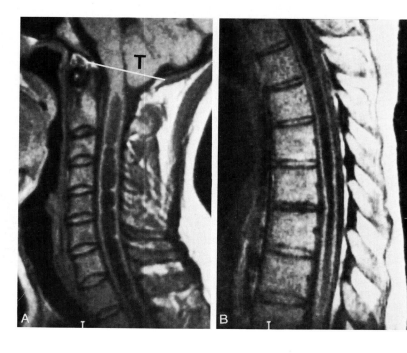

FIGURE 23–10. Syringohydromyelia with Chiari I malformation. Sagittal T_1-weighted images (SE 500/40) show an intramedullary cystic cavity extending from the cervicomedullary junction down to the level of the conus. In the cervical region the syrinx has a haustrated appearance. The cerebellar tonsil (T) is positioned below the foramen magnum (line).

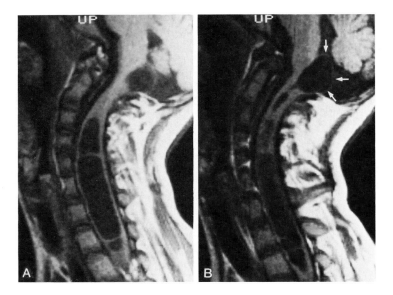

FIGURE 23–11. Syringohydromyelia with cyst of the central canal. SE 550/21 sagittal images demonstrate multiloculated, cystic expansion of the cervical spinal cord. Note that the cord parenchyma is thinned adjacent to the cavity, and, despite the septations, the margins are smooth and regular. There is focal cystic expansion of the central canal at the obex *(B)* with the cyst *(arrows)* bulging into the cisterna magna. The spinal canal is also enlarged and the vertebral bodies are eroded and remodeled, indicating the longstanding nature of the abnormality.

medullaris.[31] Failure to recognize an additional cavity could result in inappropriate or incomplete shunting and subsequent failure of the patient to improve clinically.

INFLAMMATORY/DEGENERATIVE

In patients with suspected *multiple sclerosis,* isolated symptoms related to the spinal cord are seen approximately 15 to 20 per cent of the time. Symptoms consist of progressive or intermittent spastic para- or quadriparesis. The finding of high signal foci in the brain in patients with demyelinating disease improves the diagnostic specificity in patients with isolated spinal cord symptoms, since approximately 60 per cent of these patients have a positive brain MR as well (Fig. 23–12)[32] (see Chapter 18). While autopsy studies of MS patients have consistently demonstrated extensive spinal cord disease,[33] the sensitivity of MR for detection of cord plaques is not as good as for brain lesions. This lower sensitivity is likely

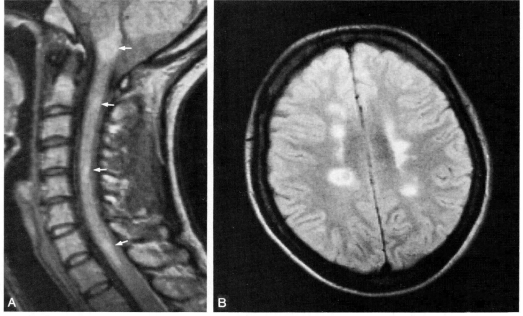

FIGURE 23–12. Multiple sclerosis. *A,* T$_2$-weighted sagittal image (SE 2000/40) reveals multiple hyperintense foci in the cervical spinal cord and the lower medulla *(arrows),* compatible with a diagnosis of demyelinating disease. *B,* Axial brain image (SE 3000/40) shows multiple high-signal foci in the centrum semiovale characteristic of multiple sclerosis plaques.

related to the lower S/N of the T_2-weighted spin-echo images of the spine and to image degradation from CSF pulsations, respiration, peristalsis, and gross body motion. For the same reasons, the detection rate is higher in the cervical cord than in the thoracic region.[34]

Demyelinating disease in the spinal cord may be unifocal or multifocal and may involve long or short segments of the cord (Fig. 23–12). In a number of patients, focal, mild cord expansion is associated with a demyelinating lesion. In rare cases a slit-like cavity associated with an area of increased T_2 has been seen in patients with suspected MS. At intermediate field strength, a T_1 sequence with a TE of 40 msec may reveal subtle areas of increased signal in cord plaques. This is due to the relatively long TE of 40 msec and the contribution of T_2 effects. Of note, unlike the brain, where MS plaques may be hypointense with T_1 sequences, plaques in the spinal cord do not exhibit low signal.

Detection of high-signal lesions in the cord is often hindered by flow artifacts that commonly accompany examinations of both the cervical and thoracic spine. Flow artifacts can be reduced by using flow compensation techniques such as MAST or FRODO or by using cardiac gating. However, these techniques do not eliminate all the artifacts, and the diagnosis of spinal cord MS remains a challenge. Initial expectations that the problem would be overcome with partial flip or gradient-echo studies have not yet been realized. Gradient-echo images have their own artifacts and the overall S/N is less.

The role of Gd-DTPA has not been clarified. Acute MS plaques are associated with transient breakdown of the blood-brain barrier and do enhance.[35] Enhancing plaques are quite obvious on T_1-weighted images. The question remains whether or not contrast enhancement is essential or cost effective for screening the spinal cord for MS. It cannot replace the T_2-weighted spin-echo sequence, which demonstrates nonenhancing plaques. Doing both significantly increases scanning time. At this point, Gd-DTPA is probably useful for the more challenging cases, in which the diagnosis of MS is not certain, brain lesions are absent or are not characteristic of MS, and the patient has perplexing symptoms referable to the spinal cord. Also, enhancement features of MS plaques can be used to judge the effects of therapy.

High-signal foci seen in the cord are somewhat nonspecific and can be seen in myelitis from other inflammatory causes (i.e., *sarcoid, Wegener's granulomatosis*), in posttraumatic myelomalacia, and in association with arteriovenous malformation. The history and course of the illness are often helpful in differential diagnosis. The diagnosis of arteriovenous malformations can be very difficult, but the finding of abnormal vessels in the subarachnoid or epidural space provides a clue. Lastly, high signal may be seen focally in the cord in areas of spondylotic compression on T_2 images (see Fig. 23–19). This is presumed

to be secondary to inflammation, gliosis, or edema and should be readily apparent because of the associated extradural compression.

There are many *degenerative diseases* of the spinal cord that remain to be investigated, and it is hoped that MR will provide insights into these diseases. *Amyotrophic lateral sclerosis* (ALS) is characterized by degeneration of anterior horn cells, bulbar motor nuclei, and corticospinal and corticobulbar pathways. The disease presents in middle-aged adults and has a uniformly dismal prognosis, with death occurring within 5 years of onset. Preliminary studies of ALS with MR have revealed atrophy of the ventral aspects of the spinal cord with sparing of the dorsal columns.[36] Cord swelling without abnormal signal changes in the cord parenchyma has been noted in *acute transverse myelitis*.[37] A case report of Devic's disease, another demyelinating disorder, disclosed cord swelling acutely, followed by progressive cord atrophy on later scans.[38]

ISCHEMIA/INFARCTION

The spinal cord is susceptible to ischemia and infarction because its collateral circulation is relatively poor. The cord receives its direct blood supply from a single anterior spinal artery and two smaller posterior spinal arteries. The anterior spinal artery supplies the anterior two thirds of the cord parenchyma, including the anterior horns and corticospinal tracts. Branches from the vertebral arteries supply the cervical cord, a supreme intercostal artery supplies the upper thoracic cord, and the artery of Adamkiewicz is the predominant source for the lower thoracic cord and conus medullaris.

There are many causes of spinal cord ischemia that can lead to paraplegia or quadriplegia, depending on the level of cord damage. Probably the most common cause is related to extrinsic compression, with trauma being high on the list. Any lesion that compresses the cord can produce focal ischemia or a more generalized ischemic syndrome by obstructing flow through the anterior spinal artery. Cord infarction can result from ligation of intercostal arteries at the time of paraspinal surgery for tumor or thoracic disks, and it is a recognized complication of coarctation repair (Fig. 23–13). Paraplegia rarely results from diagnostic angiography. Another cause of cord ischemia is spinal arteriovenous malformation, either due to vascular steal phenomenon or as a complication of surgery or embolization therapy.

MR gives us the first opportunity to study cord ischemia and infarction because no other technique can reliably detect the subtle changes. Needless to say, our experience with imaging this entity is limited. The findings on MR include focal edema and cord swelling, reflected on the images as areas of high signal intensity on T_2-weighted scans (Fig. 23–13). As in the brain, if the abnormality follows a vascular distribution, involving the anterior two thirds of the

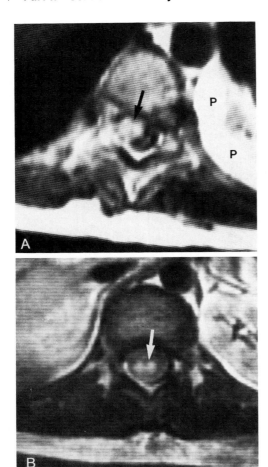

FIGURE 23–13. Hemorrhagic infarction of the thoracic spinal cord. Patient became paraplegic immediately following surgical repair of a coarctation of the aorta. *A,* Axial T_1-weighted scan (SE 600/25) obtained 1 week after surgery reveals high signal intensity *(arrow)* within the cord on the right, consistent with subacute hemorrhage (methemoglobin). The high signal intensity in the posterior left chest (P) represents hemorrhagic pleural fluid secondary to the recent thoracotomy. *B,* Axial T_2-weighted scan (SE 2000/70) at the level of the conus shows high-signal edema *(arrow)* within the cord.

cord, for example, a vascular etiology is more likely. With time, the infarct evolves to leave an area of myelomalacia and cord atrophy. Spinal angiography remains the definitive method for identifying the arterial supply to the cord.

VASCULAR MALFORMATIONS

Because of the inability to reliably image flow using currently available MR techniques, the sensitivity of MR in the detection of arteriovenous malformations (AVMs) remains questionable. However, reports in the literature demonstrate utility of this technique in assessing spinal AVMs, and some cases have shown specific advantages of MR over myelography, delayed intrathecal contrast CT, and even arteriography.[39]

Using T_1- and T_2-weighted pulse sequences, variable appearances have been reported. Large vessels in the cord or on the pial surface may give the cord a scalloped appearance. Focal parenchymal low or high signal from flow-related enhancement or signal void may be seen within these vessels. These flow phenomena may take the form of either punctate or curvilinear structures (Fig. 23–14). Some investigators have also identified inhomogeneous areas of high and low signal, which they speculate represent thrombosed or ligated vessels in a vascular malformation that has been partially resected.[40] Focal areas of low signal on T_2 images can result from the deposition of hemosiderin-laden macrophages. Modic et al[41] reported three cases in which high signal intensity was seen in the spinal cord distal to an AVM. The abnormal signal was theorized to represent edema or possibly the effects of chronic vascular insufficiency from a steal syndrome, with high signal representing the effects of chronic ischemia (i.e., gliosis and demyelination).

In cavernous hemangioma of the spinal cord, focal cord enlargement has been identified as a diagnostic feature of these lesions.[42] Although the MR charac-

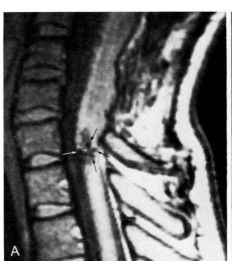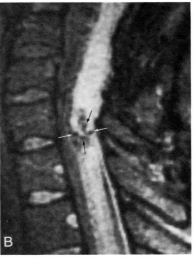

FIGURE 23–14. Intramedullary arteriovenous (AV) malformation. Patient has had previous laminectomy and cordotomy for removal of an intramedullary hematoma. T_1-weighted (SE 600/20) *(A)* and T_2-weighted (SE 2000/70) *(B)* scans demonstrate multiple punctate areas of low signal intensity *(arrows)* within the cord, representing vessels of an AV malformation. The cord above is markedly distorted by previous hemorrhage and surgery.

teristics of spinal vascular malformations are varied, they are usually highly suggestive of the diagnosis. MR is especially effective for evaluating the intramedullary malformations.[43] Confusion in diagnosis can arise in cases in which hypervascularity in an intramedullary neoplasm can simulate the appearance of a vascular malformation. Even diagnostic spinal angiography may not clarify the diagnostic dilemma in all cases, and ultimately surgical exploration and biopsy may be required. Newer techniques using three-dimensional flow imaging may substantially increase the diagnostic sepecificity of MR in AVM. Their use at this time is experimental, and the utility of these techniques in the spine is unproven.

DEGENERATIVE SPINAL DISEASE (EXTRADURAL)

As discussed in the technique section, examinations of the cervical and thoracic spine should employ both sagittal and axial scans. A sagittal T_1 study shows the margins of the spinal cord with respect to other structures within the spinal canal. Subtle scalloping of the cord may be present owing to encroachment posteriorly by ligamentum flavum hypertrophy or anteriorly by disk or spondylosis. Because disk, ligament, and bone have low or absent signal on T_1-weighted images, it may not be possible to differentiate these structures from one another.[11] In addition, low-signal CSF on T_1 images can silhouette a low-signal epidural lesion such as disk or osteophyte. The increased contrast between the CSF-containing thecal sac and adjacent structures on gradient-echo images improves visualization of extradural lesions that impinge on the thecal sac.[44] T_1-weighted axial images frequently enable identification of lateralizing disk and osteophyte, but gradient-echo scans often improve lesion conspicuity.

INTERVERTEBRAL DISK DISEASE

Disk degeneration is accompanied by loss of water content and therefore signal intensity on MR images. The traditional findings of decrease in disk height and presence of calcification and gas assist in diagnosing this condition. In the cervical spine, chronic disk degeneration is commonly associated with spondylotic changes.

Loss of disk signal is not a necessary prerequisite for disk herniation. On T_1 images a herniated disk generally has the same signal characteristics as the parent disk and is seen as an extrusion of disk material into the spinal canal (Fig. 23–15).[45] Herniated disks can be midline or lateral, and it is important to clearly identify the location of the disk fragment for surgical planning (Fig. 23–16).[46]

It is not always possible to determine whether a herniated disk is subligamentous or has dissected through the posterior longitudinal ligament. Since the ligament is thicker and stronger in the midline, central disks are more likely than lateral ones to be subligamentous. The sagittal view is often best for determining the relationship of the disk to the ligament (Fig. 23–17). Once a disk fragment has extended into the epidural space, it can migrate more easily away from the interspace.[47]

High signal above and below a herniated disk is frequently seen and most likely represents flow enhancement in engorged epidural veins containing slowly flowing blood (Fig. 23–18). On parasagittal scans, flow enhancement in these veins may be the only indicator of an epidural abnormality when a central component is absent. It is important to differentiate this common phenomenon from sequestration of disk material. Sequestered disk fragments can have a higher signal than the parent disk on both T_1- and T_2-weighted scans, especially on the first echo of a T_2-weighted multiecho sequence employing a long TR. Usually the distinction is made on the basis of size and eccentric relationship to the disk space, occurring either rostral or caudal to the interspace. On axial scans the imaging plane is orthogonal to the veins and often results in loss of the high signal seen in the veins on the sagittal images. High signal persists in sequestered disk material regardless of the plane of imaging.

At intermediate field strengths, T_1 or proton-density imaging (long TR/short TE) is routinely used to assess the spinal canal and neural foramina. Midline extradural lesions can be identified on sagittal views by cord effacement, but when eccentric they may be seen better on the axial views (Fig. 23–19). High signal in the neural foramina may also be diminished owing to either displacement of epidural veins or foraminal fat. At higher field strength, gradient-echo imaging provides excellent tissue-contrast resolution. Sensitivity for detection of extradural disease appears to be high regardless of field strength.

When either herniated disks or osteophytes impinge on the spinal cord, cord injury can result, which points out the importance of prompt, accurate diagnosis and definitive therapy. As with any contusion, cord edema and swelling develop, which may be seen as focal high signal intensity on T_2-weighted scans (Fig. 23–20). There may also be disruption of the blood-brain barrier and enhancement may be observed with Gd-DTPA.

SPONDYLOSIS

Spondylosis can take the form of marginal endplate osteophytes, uncovertebral process hypertrophy, or facet joint disease. When marginal osteophytes form along the vertebral end plates, the posterior longitudinal ligament is pushed posteriorly. Since the outer fibers of the disk anulus are attached to the posterior longitudinal ligament, the disk is also pulled posteriorly, resulting in a disk sandwich with

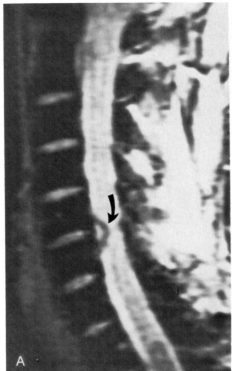

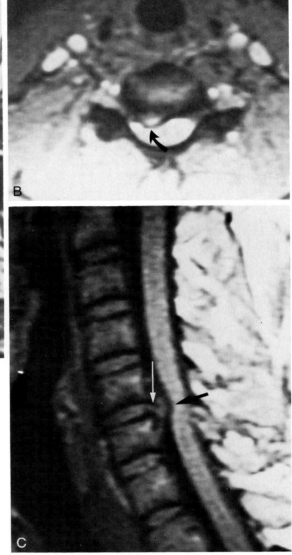

FIGURE 23–15. Herniated disk in a 28-year-old man with a right C6 radiculopathy and a myelopathy. Sagittal *(A)* and axial *(B)* GRASS images (GRE 25/13, flip angle = 8 degrees) demonstrate a herniated disk *(curved arrow)* at the level of C5-C6, lateralized to the right side and effacing the hyperintense CSF-containing thecal sac. The bright signal in the middle is the fragment of hydrated disk, and the border of low signal represents a combination of the dura, remnants of the posterior longitudinal ligament, and possibly some hemorrhage. *C,* A sagittal T₁-weighted image (SE 600/25) shows marked indentation *(black arrow)* of the ventral surface of the cord. The disk fragment has maintained a thin attachment *(white arrow)* to the parent intervertebral disk.

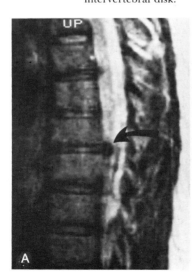

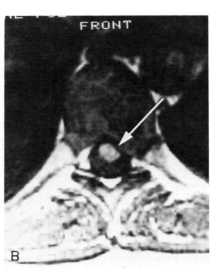

FIGURE 23–16. Herniated thoracic disk. *A,* A sagittal T₂-weighted scan (SE 2300/80) discloses a herniated disk *(curved arrow)* at the level of T9-T10. *B,* On a T₁-weighted axial image (SE 580/26), the disk lateralizes to the left side and indents the ventrolateral aspect of the cord *(arrow).*

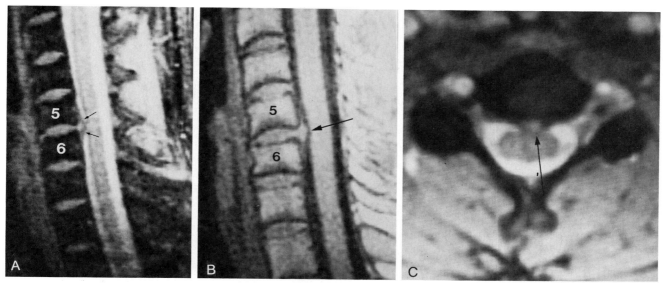

FIGURE 23–17. Subligamentous disk herniation. *A*, Gradient-echo scan (GRE 25/13, flip angle = 4 degrees). A small disk fragment has herniated posteriorly at C5-C6 and effaces the ventral thecal sac. The posterior longitudinal ligament *(arrows)* has been pulled off the adjacent vertebral bodies. *B*, T$_1$-weighted scan (SE 600/20). The disk fragment is contiguous with the C5-C6 interspace and indents the ventral cord slightly *(arrow)*. *C*, Axial gradient-echo scan confirms a small central herniated disk *(arrow)*.

the disk in the middle and the end-plate osteophytes above and below (Figs. 23–21 and 23–22). The disk sandwich accounts for the exaggerated projection of the intervertebral disk behind the vertebral body on the sagittal view.

Osteophytes are hypointense on all pulse sequences. Identification of central osteophytes re-

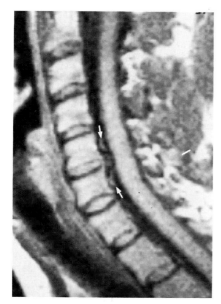

FIGURE 23–18. Disk herniation with engorged venous plexus. SE 500/40 sagittal 5-mm image. At C5-C6, disk material has extruded posteriorly and impinges on the ventral aspect of the spinal cord. Above and below the herniated disk are crescentic regions of high signal intensity *(arrows)* representing engorged epidural veins.

quires gradient-echo or T$_2$-weighted images to achieve good contrast between the osteophytes and the hyperintense CSF within the thecal sac. On T$_1$-weighted scans, osteophytes may be silhouetted by the low-signal CSF (Fig. 23–21). Posterior ridging osteophytes produce broad ventral impressions on the thecal sac (Fig. 23–22). If large, the posterior bony ridges can cause repeated trauma to the cord with neck motion, eventually resulting in cord deformity, atrophy, and a myelopathy. Acute cord contusion in spinal stenosis may have even more devastating consequences with quadriplegia.

Evaluation of the neural foramina is the ultimate challenge for MR. The anatomy is small, the signal intensity from foraminal tissues is only moderate, and the bright CSF of the thecal sac is not available to help assess encroachment by spondylotic disease. Osteophytes develop at the uncovertebral joints and the facet joints and project into the lateral spinal canal and foramina (Fig. 23–23). Symptoms are caused by impingement of nerve roots as they exit the foramina.

Accurate assessment of mild foraminal narrowing requires high-quality images and is aided by careful patient positioning so that both foramina are sectioned together on the axial images. MR performs better in cases of moderate to severe foraminal disease (Fig. 23–24).[46] Oblique images obtained perpendicular to the plane of the exiting nerve roots may improve the diagnosis of foraminal encroachment,[48, 49] but this technique requires two additional acquisitions to visualize the left and right neural foramina.

At this point, CT still has higher resolution for measuring foraminal narrowing by spondylotic disease, and we do not hesitate to recommend CTM if

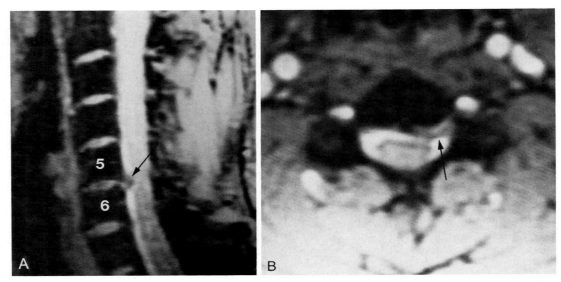

FIGURE 23–19. Herniated cervical disk. Sagittal *(A)* and axial *(B)* gradient-echo images (GRE 25/13, flip angle = 4, 8 degrees). Disk material *(arrow)* has herniated posteriorly into the spinal canal at C5-C6. The disk lateralizes to the left and extends into the neural foramen. It effaces the thecal sac and slightly distorts the cord. The disk space at C5-C6 is also narrowed.

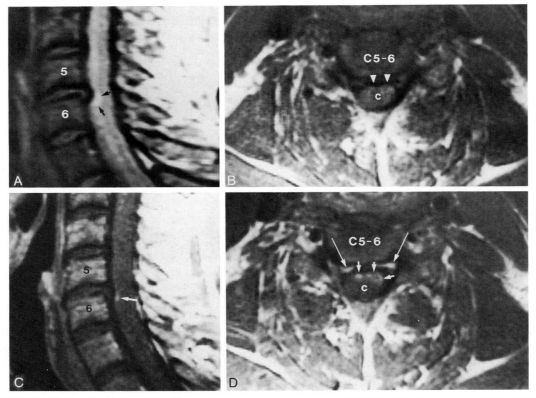

FIGURE 23–20. Herniated disk with cord injury. Noncontrast sagittal (SE 2000/80) *(A)* and axial (SE 600/20) *(B)* views. On the T_2-weighted scan, the disk at C5-C6 projects posteriorly into the canal to compress the cord. The high signal *(arrows)* in the cord represents either edema or gliosis. The abnormal disk is difficult to see on the axial scan, but it extends back to the edge of the arrowheads. The cord (c) appears normal. *C* and *D*, Contrast-enhanced scans (SE 600/20, Gd-DTPA) reveal enhancement *(short arrows)* of the anterior cord adjacent to the herniated disk. Cord contusion can result from disk or osteophytes that impinge on the cord (c). Note enhancement of some epidural veins *(long arrows)*. (Courtesy of Dean Berthoty, Sunrise Diagnostic Center, Las Vegas, Nevada.)

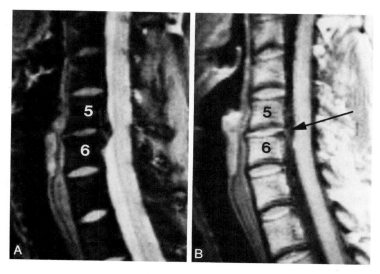

FIGURE 23–21. Spondylosis. *A,* A gradient-echo scan (GRE 300/22, flip angle = 6 degrees) reveals a large osteophyte at the C5-C6 level, projecting posteriorly into the spinal canal. The osteophyte effaces the thecal sac and lies against the cord but does not compress it. Also noted is disk space narrowing at the same level. *B,* On a T₁-weighted scan (SE 710/26), the osteophyte is silhouetted by the low-signal CSF. The disk projects posteriorly *(arrow)* beyond the apparent posterior margin of the vertebral bodies.

the MR scan is equivocal or negative in a patient who clearly has radicular symptoms. Nonetheless, MR is a reasonable screening method because it can detect moderate to severe foraminal stenosis, the grades of disease that merit surgical consideration.[11] Volume acquisition methods with oblique image reconstruction and improvements in surface coil design with higher S/N may make MR more competitive for evaluating patients with cervical radiculopathy.

Although thoracic disk herniation is a well-recognized entity,[45] a thoracic radiculopathy secondary to spondylosis is uncommon. The rib cage stablizes the thoracic spine so that degenerative changes of the joints do not develop readily. A radicular syndrome at the thoracic level is more likely due to a neurofibroma or some other paraspinal neoplastic process.

SPINAL STENOSIS

When bulging disks, spondylosis, and ligamentum flavum hypertrophy progress to constrict the spinal canal and cord, spinal stenosis develops. These changes are depicted on sagittal gradient-echo or T₂-weighted images as hourglass narrowing of the thecal sac, usually involving multiple levels in the mid- and lower cervical region (Fig. 23–25). On T₁-weighted scans, canal stenosis results in scalloping of the normally smooth dorsal and ventral margins of the cord. As learned from myelography, the degree of canal stenosis and cord scalloping shown on the images is greater when the neck is in a hyperextended position. Repositioning the patient for neutral or hyperflexed views may define more accurately the true cord

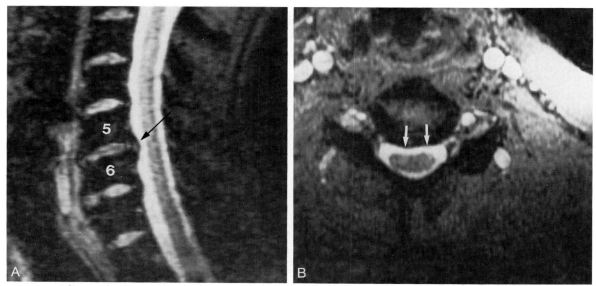

FIGURE 23–22. Spondylosis with posterior ridging. *A,* Gradient-echo scan (GRE 25/13, flip angle = 4 degrees) demonstrates degenerative disk disease at C5-C6 and posterior osteophytes *(arrow)* projecting into the spinal canal. The disk is sandwiched between the adjacent osteophytes. *B,* On an axial scan at the same level, a ridge of bone *(arrows)* effaces the ventral thecal sac. Even though the osteophytes do not touch the cord, the cord is flattened owing to long-standing canal narrowing at that level. The neural foramina are widely patent.

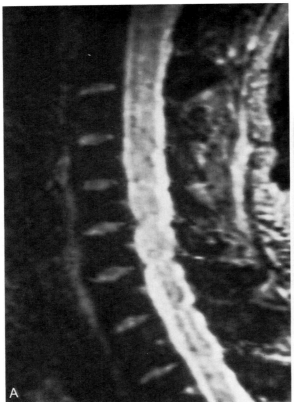

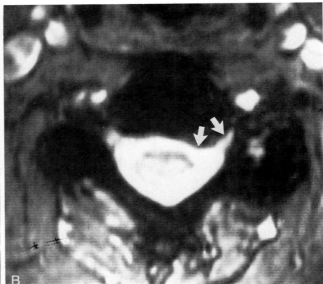

FIGURE 23–23. Spondylosis with foraminal narrowing. *A,* A sagittal GRASS image (GRE 25/13, flip angle = 8 degrees) shows posterior ridging osteophytes at several levels. *B,* On an axial GRASS image, the osteophyte *(arrows)* at C5-C6 lateralizes to the left side, effaces the thecal sac, and compromises the left neural foramen.

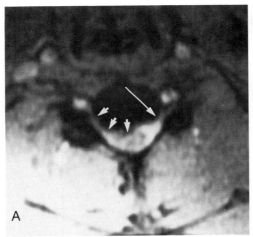

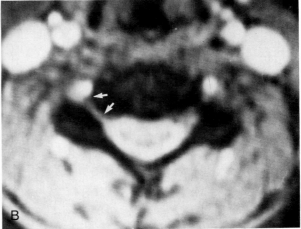

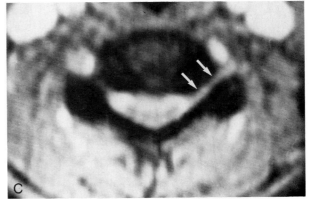

FIGURE 23–24. Examples of foraminal stenosis, axial gradient-echo images (GRE 25/13, flip angle = 8 degrees). *A,* A large osteophyte *(short arrows)* projects into the right ventrolateral canal, effacing the thecal sac and touching the cord. It also causes severe stenosis of the right neural foramen. There is also moderate narrowing of the left neural foramen by an osteophyte *(long arrow).* The marked hypointensity distinguishes osteophytes from herniated disk material. *B,* A prominent osteophyte *(arrows)* arising from the right joint of Luschka produces severe compromise of the neural foramen. *C,* There is moderate to severe narrowing of the left neural foramen *(arrows)* by spondylosis.

FIGURE 23–25. Spinal stenosis. *A*, T_2-weighted scan (SE 2000/70) demonstrates the characteristic hourglass configuration of the thecal sac with spinal stenosis. There is anterior subluxation of C4 on C5. Disk degeneration is associated with disk space narrowing at C4-C5, C5-C6, and C6-C7, as well as posterior osteophytes at all these levels and at C3-C4. Hypertrophy of the ligamentum flavum *(arrows)* is present at C2-C3, C3-C4, and C4-C5. The degree of spinal stenosis is most severe at C4-C5. *B*, A lateral plain film confirms the severe degenerative changes of the lower cervical spine and the subluxation at C4-C5.

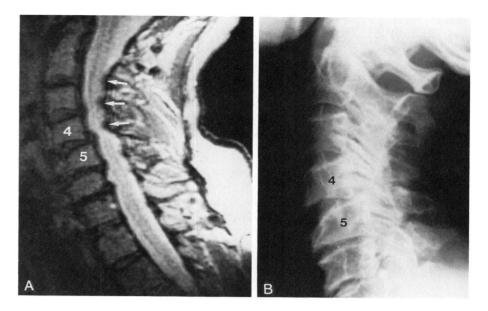

compression (Fig. 23–26). Nonetheless, the hyperextended view illustrates what happens to the cord when the patient assumes that position. The spinal cord is more susceptible to traumatic injury in patients with a compromised spinal canal.

In patients with myelopathy secondary to spondylosis and spinal stenosis, defining the extent of anterior, lateral, and posterior impingement is necessary to plan the surgical approach. It is also important to correlate the degree of cord compression with the patient's clinical presentation and neurologic examination. Although cord effacement may be present in many patients, Teresi et al[50] have shown that a myelopathic syndrome may not become apparent until there is at least a 30 per cent reduction in cross-sectional area of the spinal cord at the affected level. Although some patients may become symptomatic with less compression, in their study no patients with less than a 16 per cent reduction in cord cross-sectional area developed symptoms.

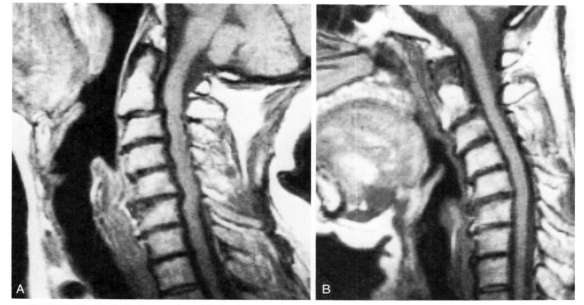

FIGURE 23–26. Spinal stenosis, with flexion-extension views. *A*, SE 500/40 sagittal 5-mm section. With the neck in a hyperextended position, the cord has a markedly scalloped appearance, suggesting cord compression due to multilevel marginal osteophytes. Also, there is mild anterior subluxation of C2 on C3. *B*, SE 500/40 sagittal 5-mm section. Repositioning the neck into a hyperflexed position changes the appearance of the cord dramatically, with reduction of the apparent spinal stenosis. The mild subluxation of C2 on C3 remains unchanged. Changes in neck position account for much of the discrepancy between myelography (usually performed in the hyperextended position) and postmyelographic CT or MR (performed in a neutral position).

VERTEBRAL AND PARAVERTEBRAL ABNORMALITIES (EXTRADURAL)

METASTATIC DISEASE

The spine is a common site for metastatic disease. The more common primary tumors to metastasize to the spine are lung and breast carcinoma, followed by prostatic carcinoma and lymphoma. Any malignancy has the potential to metastasize to bone. In patients with a known malignancy, a skeletal survey is a routine part of the metastatic work-up, and this is effectively done with a radionuclide bone scan. On the other hand, an acute or insidious onset of a myelopathy mandates immediate evaluation with an imaging study that can identify an epidural mass compressing the spinal cord or cauda equina. Since a myelopathy is often progressive and the duration of cord compression determines the potential for recovery, an expeditious examination of the entire spinal neuraxis is of paramount importance so that therapy can be instituted without delay.

Historically, such an examination was first achieved by air-contrast myelography and later improved upon with the introduction of oil-based radiopaque contrast media. Subsequently, water-soluble media were introduced that permitted computed tomography with intrathecal contrast (CTM) to be performed. Despite the benefits of these techniques, certain disadvantages may be encountered when the lumbar puncture is unsuccessful or a technically inadequate study is produced in a distressed and neurologically disabled patient. Furthermore, myelographic examination via the lumbar route may be limited to the identification of a single large obstructing lesion in the caudal portion of the spinal canal. This may be supplemented by CT, but it is inefficient for screening large distances of the spinal neuraxis. If complete obstruction to the flow of contrast is encountered, the addition of contrast from the C1-C2 route may be necessary to define the rostral margin of the blocking lesion. If two obstructing lesions are encountered, one rostral and the other caudal, the intervening regions of the spinal canal may fail to opacify. This decreases the capability of myelography and CTM to identify additional lesions in this location.[51, 52]

Using the body coil for localization purposes and a series of overlapping surface coil studies in the sagittal plane, the entire spinal neuraxis can be thoroughly studied with MR. Areas suspected of harboring a mass lesion can be studied with supplemental axial images. Specifically, the technique consists of obtaining a body coil sagittal image set using a short TR/TE with 64 or 128 y-gradients and 1/2 or 1 excitation. This can be done in less than 2 minutes and provides information for localization of thoracic levels, which can be difficult to define on the surface coil study. The surface coil is employed to provide high S/N images with spatial resolution that permits

morphologic characterization of the entire spine and spinal neuraxis. Using an overlapping series of 5-mm-thick sagittal images with a short TR and short TE (SE 500–600/20–30), the anatomy of the osseous spine, ligaments, spinal cord, cauda equina, and individual nerve roots can be identified (see anatomy section). T_2-weighted studies are not routinely employed but may have some utility in defining the paravertebral extent of tumor that can appear isointense with muscle on T_1-weighted images. Gd-DTPA has been used in the assessment of patients with acute myelopathy, and the preliminary results suggest that it does not have a role. In fact, Gd-DTPA may mask metastases by increasing the signal of osseous metastases so that they appear isointense to normal marrow on T_1 images.[53]

Using the T_1-weighted study, the medullary cavity should have a relatively homogeneous high-signal appearance owing to the presence of marrow fat. Metastases, primary osseous neoplasms, and some hematopoietic or metabolic disorders result in replacement of the high-signal fat by lower-signal substrates such as neoplastic tissue, fibrosis, or abnormally increased extracellular fluid (Fig. 23–27). The pattern of replacement may be characteristic, but the clinical history is often equally important. Varying degrees of decreased signal in the marrow cavity from osseous metastases can be seen on T_1 images, depending on the amount of blastic reaction (Fig. 23–28).[54] Not infrequently, MR detects osseous metastases when the plain films are normal and the CT scan demonstrates only very subtle changes in the trabecular pattern. Nuclear medicine studies may also be normal, especially in multiple myeloma and lymphoma.

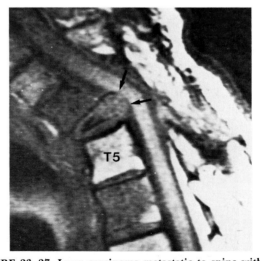

FIGURE 23–27. Lung carcinoma metastatic to spine with cord compression. A sagittal T_1-weighted image (SE 600/25) reveals a kyphotic deformity of the upper thoracic spine. Multiple metastases have replaced the normal high-signal marrow with intermediate-signal tumor tissue. T5 and T7 have relatively normal marrow signal. T4 has collapsed, and tumor tissue *(arrows)* has extruded posteriorly into the spinal canal, compressing the cord.

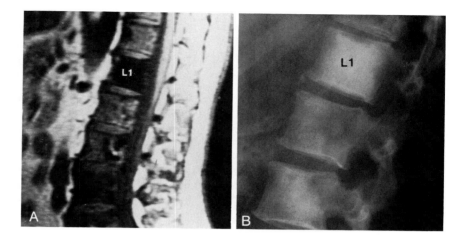

FIGURE 23–28. Prostatic carcinoma metastatic to spine. *A*, A sagittal T₁-weighted scan (SE 600/20) discloses multiple abnormal areas of low signal in the thoracic and lumbar spine. The L1 vertebral body is markedly hypointense. *B*, A plain radiograph reveals sclerotic metastases with markedly increased density of L1. The signal intensity on MR depends on the ratio of sclerotic bone reaction to soft-tissue tumor component.

The low signal is accounted for by replacement of marrow fat by tumor and its associated edema or desmoplastic reaction. In older patients with osteoporosis and vertebral compression deformities, difficulty may arise in trying to distinguish this entity from neoplasm, but the marrow in osteoporosis maintains its fat component (see section on bone marrow disease). Multiple vertebral bodies may show compression deformities with the typical end-plate depression of osteoporosis. Correlation with the plain films can be very helpful. When areas of low signal are seen in vertebrae of normal height, suspicion of metastases should arise. An exception to this rule is the solitary bone island that can be easily clarified with plain films or CT. In general, high-signal foci on T₁ images are indicative of more benign processes such as fat islands, hemangiomas, or (less likely) hemorrhagic infarction.

Except in unusual circumstances, epidural metastatic disease occurs in association with osseous metastases. Osseous disease by itself, while important to identify, is frequently observed clinically but not treated. It is, however, of paramount importance to identify any soft-tissue masses, particularly epidural components that are likely to manifest with neurologic sequelae (Figs. 23–29, 23–30). Once a soft-tissue mass is identified, additional features require characterization, including definition of the caudal-rostral and paravertebral extent, identification of any additional soft-tissue involvement, and quantification of the degree of cord, cauda equina, and root compression.[55] Finally, the MR findings should always be correlated with the patient's clinical symptoms.

Historically, the definition of obstruction to contrast flow has changed relative to the myelographic technique available. With Pantopaque, a lower-grade obstruction is more likely to block contrast flow than with a less viscous, water-soluble contrast agent. With the application of CT, contrast may be detected cephalad to a "block" that was not seen by plain film myelographic technique. Also, it is well known that a small lesion may cause significant neurologic dysfunction if it is located in a position that results in

occlusion of radiculomedullary vessels. A larger, less strategically located, slower growing mass may be relatively asymptomatic. Overall, a "myelographic block" is rather nonspecific. More important is the visualization and definition of the epidural mass, and this can be done rapidly, effectively, and noninvasively with MR.

Epidural neoplasm on T₁ images is usually slightly lower in signal than spinal cord (Fig. 23–27). Effacement of the margins of the cord results in scalloping of the ventral or dorsal surface when the mass is

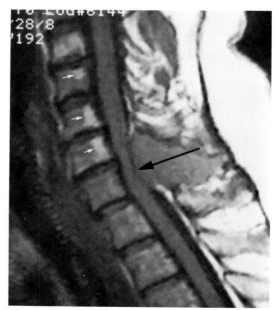

FIGURE 23–29. Thyroid carcinoma metastases with myelopathy. SE 400/28 sagittal image. Metastasis to the spinous process of C7 has produced posterior impingement on the cord *(black arrow)*, resulting in a myelopathy. Surgical decompression in this case could be achieved through a posterior approach rather than the more difficult anterior approach. Characterization of the causative lesion with respect to anterior, lateral, or posterior location is necessary to plan surgical therapy. Note the high-signal foci in segments of vertebral bodies *(small white arrows)*, representing fatty replacement of the marrow from previous radiation therapy.

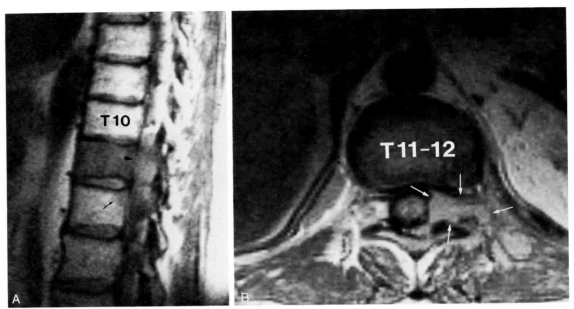

FIGURE 23–30. Non-Hodgkin's lymphoma, metastatic to spine. *A,* SE 500/40 parasagittal image. Tumor has replaced much of the normal marrow of the T11 vertebral body. The tumor has broken through the cortex posteriorly *(arrowhead)* to displace the high-signal epidural fat. Note that the posterosuperior portion of T12 has decreased signal consistent with tumor involvement *(small arrow)*. *B,* SE 1000/40 axial scan through the T11-T12 foramen. Tumor *(arrows)* has infiltrated the epidural space on the left, compressing the left side of the thecal sac and filling the left neural foramen.

located anteriorly or posteriorly. When an epidural mass compresses and flattens the cord, it often produces pseudoexpansion of the cord in one plane. This appearance should not be confused with an intramedullary lesion that enlarges the cord in both dimensions. When severe cord compression is present, a persistent rim of low signal may surround the cord despite complete obstruction to CSF flow on myelography. This is best seen on axial T_1 images and represents the investing dural membranes of the spinal cord.

From the surgical perspective, whether the compression is predominantly anterior or posterior in origin determines the surgical approach and nature of the decompressive procedure. In cases of anterior compression by a solitary metastasis, transabdominal or thoracic decompression followed by stabilization and fusion may be indicated, whereas, with posterior or lateral compression, a less complicated posterior decompressive laminectomy is all that is required. Clearly, detection of multiple lesions may alter the therapeutic approach and dissuade one from the surgical approach. With regard to radiation therapy, each lesion requires characterization of its caudal-rostral and paravertebral extent to determine portal dimensions. In most cases, treatment can be instituted without further radiographic evaluation. Biopsy may be required if the primary neoplasm is unknown. Despite the excellent tissue contrast resolution afforded by MR between neoplasm and normal tissue, the technique is not yet capable of distinguishing different tumor types. Potentially, MR spectroscopy

may be the ultimate complement to this already powerful technique.

PRIMARY BONE LESIONS

Detection of *vertebral hemangiomas* by CT and plain films has been limited to those relatively large lesions that demonstrate a coarse, vertically striated trabecular pattern. While hemangiomas of the spine are usually incidental findings and of little clinical significance, occasionally they expand and break through the cortex to cause a myelopathic or radiculopathic syndrome. In those cases, embolization and surgical extirpation may be required to relieve compression.

As in other compressive lesions in the spinal canal, MR is particularly well-suited for demonstrating areas of cord and root involvement. The trabecular pattern characteristic on plain films and CT may also be seen on MR. On short TR/TE sequences, the trabeculae maintain a low signal intensity, but the high signal of the intervening matrix usually predominates and tends to obscure the bony trabeculae (Fig. 23–31). Pathologic and chemical shift studies have shown that the matrix of a hemangioma is composed mostly of adipose tissue. On long TR/TE sequences, high signal in the hemangioma is also seen, owing to the presence of angiomatous tissue. Contrary to their appearance in the vertebral body, extraosseous components of hemangiomas have an intermediate T_1 and a relatively long T_2. The longer T_1 is explained by the absence of fat in the extraosseous compo-

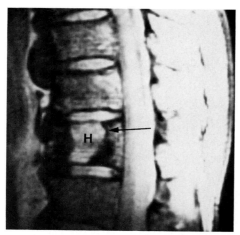

FIGURE 23–31. Vertebral hemangioma. Sagittal image (SE 2000/25) discloses a high-signal lesion (H) within a lower thoracic vertebral body. The lesion is well-defined, and a discrete cortical margin is evident posteriorly *(arrow)*. Vertebral hemangiomas are often hyperintense on both T_1- and T_2-weighted scans owing to a combination of adipose and angiomatous tissue.

nent.[56] In many otherwise normal spines, small hyperintense foci are found in the vertebral body marrow on short TR/TE sequences. Postmortem studies of these foci have revealed small hemangiomas or intraosseous islands of fat.[57] Distinction between *fat islands* and hemangiomas should be possible on T_2 images, because the hemangioma maintains the high signal but the fat becomes progressively lower in signal on longer TE sequences.

There are a host of other *primary bone tumors* that can occur in the spine, but they are relatively uncommon. Many of them have characteristic plain film findings, but sectional imaging studies are required to assess soft-tissue components. Investigations to date have shown MR to be superior to plain CT and equal to CTM for defining bone involvement, spinal canal invasion, paraspinal soft-tissue extension, and vascular involvement. CT is better for showing subtle cortical bone erosion and calcified tumor matrix.[58]

Most bone tumors have prolonged T_1 and T_2 relaxation times. Even lesions that appear relatively dense on CT may have sufficient soft-tissue matrix to render them hyperintense on T_2-weighted images (see also Chapter 40). Dense calcification and reactive bone are hypointense, but much of the calcification within the tumor matrix is invisible to MR. The presence of hemorrhage or fat alters the signal characteristics.[59]

As with conventional imaging studies, location, character of bone destruction, amount of blastic response, and soft-tissue component are clues to tumor histology. Grossly lytic lesions with large soft-tissue masses are likely malignant, such as *osteosarcoma* or *chondrosarcoma*. *Osteoblastoma* (Fig. 23–32) and *aneurysmal bone cyst* exhibit expansile features with surrounding reactive bone, indicating more slowly growing benign lesions. Although MR is less sensitive than CT for detecting bone, reactive sclerosis can usually be seen as a band of low signal.[60] The MR appearance of aneurysmal bone cyst can be quite specific, with a thick hypointense rim and multiple cysts with internal septations and fluid-fluid levels. The fluid levels result from sedimented red blood cells and serum, and the cyst contents have varying signal intensities owing to hemorrhage of different ages.[61]

In *eosinophilic granuloma*, the soft-tissue matrix is of intermediate signal on T_1-weighted images and hyperintense on T_2-weighted scans (Fig. 23–33). If vertebral collapse occurs, the soft tissue may extrude posteriorly into the spinal canal.[62]

BONE MARROW DISEASE

The vertebral body is composed of three tissues: bone, hematopoietic (red) marrow, and fatty (yellow) marrow. With aging, the bone becomes demineralized and the ratio of hematopoietic to fatty marrow changes. MR studies of patients of varying ages have revealed that the T_1 relaxation time of bone marrow progressively decreases with age. The T_1 shortening is due to replacement of hematopoietic marrow by fatty marrow. At birth the vertebral marrow consists entirely of hematopoietic tissue. The fatty component increases to about 15 per cent by age 10, 35 per cent by age 25, and 60 per cent by age 80.[63]

As a result of increased marrow fat, the T_2 relaxation time also decreases with age except in women over 50. The greater loss of bone mineral in postmenopausal women is postulated as the cause of the variation. The bone mineral content remains relatively constant until age 45. After that age, osteoporosis gradually develops, and the loss of bone mineral is more rapid and significant in women. By age 75, bone mineral content has decreased by 40 per cent in men and 55 per cent in women. Bone mineral affects the T_2 relaxation time of marrow. Magnetic susceptibility effects reduce the apparent T_2 of protons at bone-tissue interfaces, making those protons invisible to MR. With osteoporosis (loss of bone mineral), the protons are "unmasked," resulting in an increase in spin density and T_2 relaxation time.[64]

There are many diseases that affect the bone marrow, including metastatic disease (see section above), tumors of blood cell origin, blood dyscrasias and anemias, and radiation therapy. In normal marrow there are two populations of protons (water and fat protons), and the two populations are more or less balanced. Any disease process that upsets that balance affects the MR signal.[63] In the adult, the active red marrow of the body is found mostly in the axial skeleton. Primary and secondary marrow malignancies preferentially infiltrate areas of active hematopoiesis, so the spine and pelvis are commonly affected.[65] Replacement of the normal marrow by abnormal soft tissues results in increased marrow

FIGURE 23–32. Osteoblastoma. *A* and *B*, Long TR sagittal scans (SE 2000/30,70) reveal a large mass (M) arising from the posterior elements of the upper thoracic spine. The mass is well-defined and has a heterogeneous internal texture. It has expanded into the posterior epidural space, compressing the thecal sac and spinal cord. *C* and *D*, On T$_1$-weighted sagittal and axial images (SE 800/20), the mass (M) has destroyed much of the posterior elements on the left. It also involves the left pedicle and the posterior lateral aspect of the adjacent vertebral body *(arrowheads)*. The tumor has also extended into the paraspinal soft tissues on the left *(black arrows)*. The spinal cord *(long arrow)* is markedly flattened by the epidural component. (Courtesy of Dean Berthoty, Sunrise Diagnostic Center, Las Vegas, Nevada.)

cellularity, a greater number of water protons, and prolongation of T$_1$ and T$_2$.

Plasmacytoma and *multiple myeloma* are neoplasms of plasma cells that commonly involve the spine. Plasmacytoma is a solitary lesion that destroys a vertebra and frequently breaks through the cortex to produce a soft-tissue mass. Multiple myeloma causes widespread skeletal destruction and is associated with anemia, hypercalcemia, renal impairment, and in-

creased susceptibility to infections. Both lesions are osteolytic and often lead to vertebral collapse. If the soft-tissue components enter the epidural space, cord compression and a myelopathy may result. Signal characteristics can be identical to metastatic disease; however, multiple myeloma usually exhibits more diffuse involvement of the bone marrow (Fig. 23–34).[66]

Prolongation of T$_1$ of the marrow has been noted

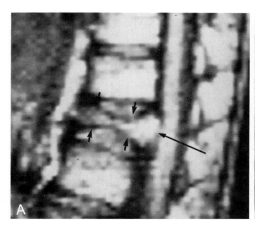
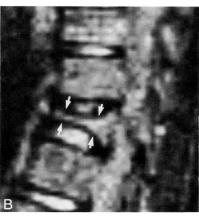

FIGURE 23–33. Eosinophilic granuloma. *A,* T$_1$-weighted (SE 500/40) and *B,* T$_2$-weighted (SE 2000/40) images demonstrate compression (vertebra plana) *(short arrows)* of the T11 vertebral body. Soft tissue *(long arrow)* also projects posteriorly into the ventral epidural space. The intervertebral disks are not involved. (Courtesy of David Sobel, Scripps Clinic, La Jolla, California.)

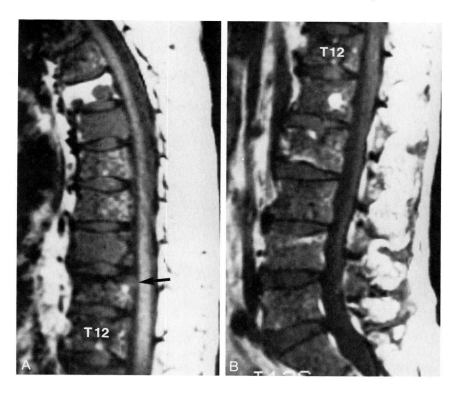

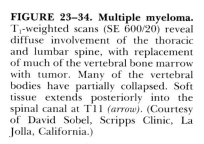

FIGURE 23–34. Multiple myeloma. T_1-weighted scans (SE 600/20) reveal diffuse involvement of the thoracic and lumbar spine, with replacement of much of the vertebral bone marrow with tumor. Many of the vertebral bodies have partially collapsed. Soft tissue extends posteriorly into the spinal canal at T11 *(arrow)*. (Courtesy of David Sobel, Scripps Clinic, La Jolla, California.)

in children with *acute lymphocytic leukemia* (ALL).[67] The T_1 lengthening and low signal on T_1-weighted images are most pronounced in newly diagnosed ALL, moderately prolonged with ALL in relapse, and within normal range in ALL in remission. Detection of marrow infiltration is more difficult in young children because the marrow is already very cellular and has a relatively long T_1.

Polycythemia vera also results in increased marrow cellularity and decreased signal on T_1-weighted scans. Close correlation has been demonstrated between the estimated T_1 relaxation time and the cellularity of the marrow on histology.[68] *Lymphoma* produces focal nodules of tumor in the marrow to distinguish it from the more diffuse myeloproliferative disorders (see Fig. 23–30).

Other studies indicate that MR may have merit for evaluating response of marrow diseases to chemotherapy.[69] Following therapy, the signal characteristics of the marrow slowly return to normal over a period of months.

Disease processes that reduce marrow cellularity or destroy the hematopoietic tissue have the reverse effect on MR signal characteristics. The water protons decrease and the fat protons increase, shortening T_1 and T_2 relaxation times. This effect is observed with the anemias and following radiation and chemotherapy.

Aplastic anemia results in diffuse loss of marrow cellularity. Relaxation measurements show shortening of T_1 due to increased fat, but the effect is difficult to see on spin-echo T_1-weighted images. However, the change in the marrow is apparent with

chemical-shift imaging methods.[65] *Myelofibrosis* produces a similar effect, but the marrow involvement is more patchy.

Changes occurring in the spine within the portals of the *radiation* field have been described.[70] During the months following irradiation, fatty degeneration of the bone marrow occurs, resulting in profound shortening of T_1 (see Fig. 23–29). In some patients, we have found a return of the marrow signal to normal. This may result from repopulation of the marrow by hematopoietic elements or possibly the occurrence of mixed fibrosis and fat. Also, if discrete low-signal foci are present within the fatty marrow, regrowth of tumor should be considered. Fatty replacement of marrow can also occur adjacent to areas of degenerative spinal disease, but its focal nature is usually characteristic.[71]

PARASPINAL TUMORS

Neuroblastomas are tumors of the sympathetic nervous system that occur in children. Two thirds originate in the adrenal medulla and the remainder in the paravertebral sympathetic plexus. A prominent soft-tissue mass is often found at the time of presentation. Of major concern is the potential of these tumors to extend through the adjacent neural foramina to enter the epidural space and compress the cord. MR can accurately assess both the paraspinal and intraspinal components so that myelography is no longer necessary in these patients (Fig. 23–35). On T_2-weighted images neuroblastoma is hyperin-

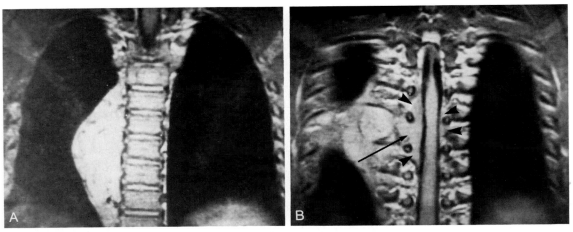

FIGURE 23–35. Thoracic neuroblastoma. *A,* A coronal scan (SE 600/25) through the posterior chest discloses a large right paraspinal mass. The mass is well-defined and slightly heterogeneous. *B,* On a section more posterior, the tumor has extended through a neural foramen *(arrow)* to involve the epidural space *(arrowheads).*

tense relative to the adjacent tissues in the mediastinum and epidural space. Proton density–weighted scans give good contrast between epidural tumor and the thecal sac.[72] Neuroblastoma also has the potential to spread to the bone marrow.

Another common tumor of the paravertebral region is *lymphoma.* It usually starts in the paraaortic lymph nodes and extends from there to involve adjacent structures (Fig. 23–36). Like other paraspinal tumors or infections, lymphomas have ready access to the epidural space via the neural foramina.

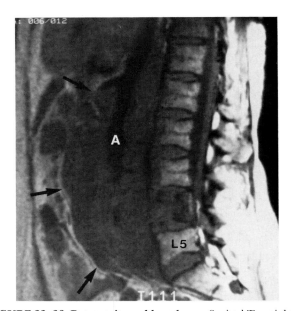

FIGURE 23–36. Retroperitoneal lymphoma. Sagittal T_1-weighted image (SE 600/20) demonstrates a large retroperitoneal mass *(arrows).* The aorta (A) is encased by the tumor and displaced anteriorly. The L4 vertebral body is largely destroyed, and the anterior portions of L2 and L3 are also involved. (Courtesy of David Sobel, Scripps Clinic, La Jolla, California.)

Osseous involvement is also possible. MR is gaining in importance for staging of lymphomas.

INFECTION

The early diagnosis of spinal *diskitis* and *osteomyelitis* has important implications with respect to reducing the morbidity associated with these infections. Instituting prompt antibiotic therapy is the goal in order to avoid the necessity for surgical decompression after epidural abscess has ensued. Early diskitis and osteomyelitis have a typical appearance on T_1- and T_2-weighted images (Fig. 23–37). On short TR/TE sequences, the earliest signs of infection include loss of signal in both the disk space and the end-plate marrow of the contiguous vertebral bodies. There is also disruption of the low signal end-plate band separating the marrow cavity from the nucleus pulposus of the disk. Narrowing of the disk space also occurs in the early stages. On long TR/TE images, there is an increase in signal in the disk and in the contiguous vertebral body marrow cavities that may appear more extensive than the changes seen on the T_1-weighted studies.

While these signal alterations are also seen in the marrow of patients with primary or metastatic neoplastic disease, as a rule tumor does not breach the end plate. Moreover, although extensive involvement of the marrow cavity may be present with neoplasia, including vertebral destruction and collapse, the disk space often remains intact or is only minimally affected.

In infectious vertebral osteomyelitis, changes in the disk and proximal marrow cavity are likely a result of pyogenic infection with organisms, white cells, and edema. More distal marrow changes are probably due to the associated edema. By applying chemical-shift techniques, the increase in marrow water con-

FIGURE 23–37. *Staphylococcus aureus* **diskitis/osteomyelitis.** *A*, SE 400/28 scan shows early changes of diskitis and osteomyelitis, with low signal in the vertebral bodies of L1 and L2. There is thinning and disruption of the normal low-signal band of the cortical bone of the vertebral end plates *(arrow)*. No epidural abscess is seen, but there is slight expansion of the superior posterior margin of L2 *(arrowhead)*. *B*, SE 2000/60. High signal is present in the inferior aspect of L1 and superior aspect of L2, consistent with inflammatory changes with edema. Inhomogeneity of the disk material signal is noted with discontinuity of the end plate *(arrow)*. *C*, SE 400/28 image obtained 6 weeks after antibiotic therapy. There is decrease in the disk space height and persistent abnormal signal in the vertebral bodies. The better-defined hypointense line at the inferior margin *(arrows)* probably represents reactive bony sclerosis as part of the healing process. *D*, SE 2000/120. Corresponding T_2-weighted image demonstrates high signal in the vertebral bodies, with loss of signal and height in the disk space. Changes in the disk space are likely to persist, but the vertebral bodies may return to normal with continued therapy. High signal most likely reflects residual edema or debris from previous infection.

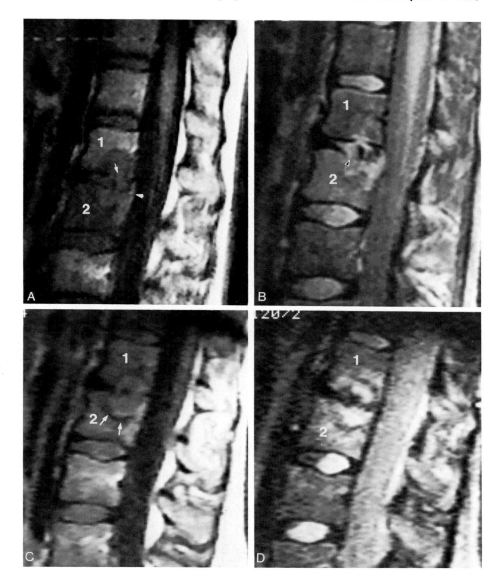

tent secondary to edema and the infectious process itself may be appreciated more readily.[73] After institution of appropriate antibiotic therapy, the changes described above may reverse almost entirely. The return of normal marrow signal is more complete if treatment commences early after the onset of disease. If disk space destruction occurs to any significant degree, the disk height and signal likely remain abnormal despite resolution of the infection.

Based on the morphologic features of vertebral diskitis and osteomyelitis, Modic et al[74] was able to demonstrate a 96 per cent sensitivity, a 93 per cent specificity, and a 94 per cent accuracy of MR in 37 patients with this disease. These statistics demonstrate a significant improvement of MR over more conventional plain film radiography, nuclear medicine, and computed tomography.

When early diskitis and osteomyelitis go undetected and untreated, *epidural* or *paravertebral abscess*

may develop, requiring surgical drainage. Failure to intervene promptly can result in severe and permanent neurologic sequelae due to epidural compression and meningitis. Most frequently, untreated vertebral osteomyelitis results in a paravertebral soft-tissue abscess.[75] Epidural abscess can also result from septicemia or a pelvic infection or can follow spine surgery (Fig. 23–38).

As discussed above, changes in the bone and disk space enable distinction between abscess and neoplasm in most cases. Because of the ability to obtain direct sagittal and axial images, MR is equipped better to define the extent of epidural abscess for planning surgical therapy and for follow-up during the resolution phase. The ability to define the relationship between epidural abscess and contiguous neural structures with CT is only truly achieved after the introduction of intrathecal contrast agents. If the thecal sac puncture is inadvertently done at the

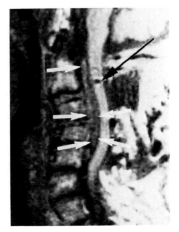

FIGURE 23–38. Postoperative epidural abscess. A few weeks after surgery at C3-C4, the patient developed neck pain and a myelopathy. SE 580/12 sagittal 4-mm slice. A large soft-tissue mass is located ventral to the spinal cord from C2 to C4-C5 *(white arrows)*. The cord is displaced posteriorly into a large laminectomy defect. When the patient worsened following surgery, a C1-C2 puncture was attempted for myelography. Low signal in the cord at C2 represents inadvertent needle placement in the cord with either air or hemorrhage present *(black arrow)*.

infection site, the risk of meningitis is increased. MR avoids this potential complication.

INTRADURAL EXTRAMEDULLARY DISEASE

Reliable distinction between intra- and extradural masses that closely appose the dura can be difficult. Some of the features learned from myelography can be applied to the MR images. For instance, when an intraspinal mass lies in the epidural space and compresses the thecal sac, an extradural "cap sign" may be present as a result of the epidural fat remaining interposed between the margins of tumor and the dura. Intradural lesions expanding the thecal sac have not demonstrated this phenomenon. Moreover, extradural masses compress both the thecal sac and the cord, narrowing the subarachnoid space on both sides of the cord. An intradural extramedullary mass displaces the cord to the opposite side and widens the subarachnoid space on the side of the mass, leaving a cap of CSF above and below. As discussed in the section on spinal cord disease, intramedullary lesions expand both the cord and the thecal sac. When a mass becomes large enough to obliterate all three compartments, localization becomes much more difficult.

Analysis of large series of patients with intraspinal neoplasms has demonstrated a slightly higher incidence of nerve sheath tumors (35 per cent) than of meningiomas (25 per cent).[15] Distinction between the two groups of neoplasms is based on the signal characteristics, location within the spinal canal, presence of bone erosion, and growth patterns.

NERVE SHEATH TUMORS

Nerve sheath tumors include both neurofibroma and neurilemoma (schwannoma). They originate from Schwann cells of the myelin sheath that invest the nerve roots as they exit the spinal column. Neurilemomas are usually solitary lesions and do not incorporate the nerve root. Neurofibromas are associated with neurofibromatosis and are generally multiple, and the nerve fibers become entangled within the tumor, making resection difficult without sacrificing the nerve.[15] The nerve sheath tumors can be intradural, extradural, or both, giving them a dumbbell appearance.

Bone erosion with scalloping of the vertebral body margins or widening of the neural foramen with erosion of the pedicles is the hallmark of nerve sheath tumors (Fig. 23–39). Even in the absence of bone

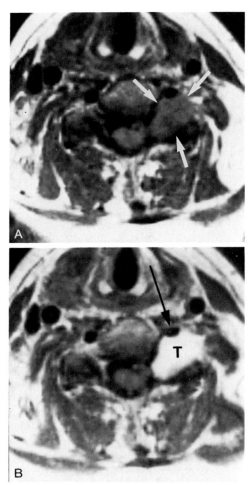

FIGURE 23–39. Neurofibroma. *A,* Noncontrast axial scan (SE 500/40) shows a soft-tissue mass *(arrows)* in the left C6-C7 neural foramen. The mass erodes the adjacent vertebral body and facets to enlarge the foramen. *B,* Enhanced scan (SE 500/40, Gd-DTPA) reveals homogeneous uptake by the tumor (T). The tumor is entirely extradural. The soft tissue at the left anterolateral margin of the cord does not enhance and may represent compressed nerve roots or venous plexus. The vertebral artery *(arrow)* is displaced anteriorly.

erosion, extension of a soft-tissue mass through the neural foramen with a dumbbell configuration is quite characteristic.[76] Although CT provides better bone detail, MR can easily detect changes in contours of the vertebral bodies and pedicles associated with an intraspinal mass.

The signal characteristics of nerve sheath tumors are somewhat different from those of meningiomas. Nerve sheath tumors typically have a T_1 that is slightly longer than or equal to that of the spinal cord. Lengthening of TR and TE with increased T_2-weighting results in brightening of the tumor (Fig. 23–39). T_2-weighted images give good contrast between the hyperintense schwannoma, medium-intensity paravertebral muscles, and hypointense fat.[77] With larger intraspinal lesions, cord compression can occur, producing a myelopathy, and, in these cases, separation of tumor and cord can be difficult (Fig. 23–40). Axial and sagittal images demonstrating deviation of the cord at levels above or below the lesion are clues to an extramedullary mass, but an exophytic cord tumor can produce a similar appearance. With extradural lesions, a low signal rim may separate the thecal sac from the tumor. This low-signal rim most likely represents the dura, since it seems to persist despite severe cord compression.

Neurofibromas and neurilemomas enhance brightly and uniformly with Gd-DTPA (Fig. 23–40). Enhancement is most helpful for intradural lesions—for detection of the smaller ones and definition of the larger ones. Gadolinium is less helpful for extradural lesions because the enhancing tumor becomes isointense to the surrounding fat.

Although less common, other mass lesions can enlarge a neural foramen or produce vertebral erosions, simulating a primary neoplasm. Differential diagnosis includes a list of cystic lesions, such as large arachnoid diverticula (see Fig. 24–14), synovial cysts, or lateral meningoceles (see below). Marked scalloping of the vertebral bodies is also associated with dural ectasia, a feature of neurofibromatosis. The fluid nature of these lesions should be readily apparent by examining signal intensities and enhancement features.[78] In rare cases, subarachnoid seeding of a root sleeve by metastases can result in foraminal expansion.

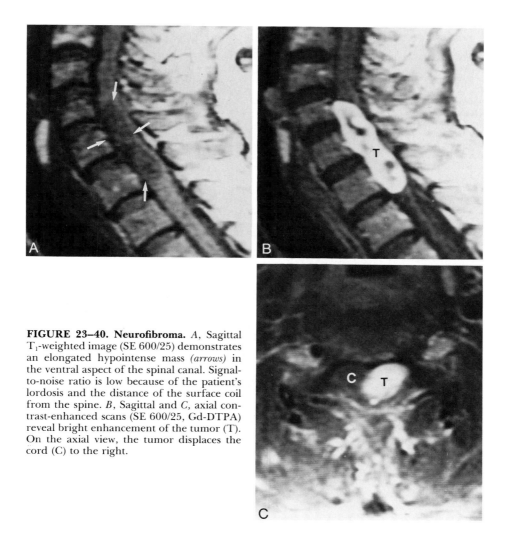

FIGURE 23–40. Neurofibroma. A, Sagittal T_1-weighted image (SE 600/25) demonstrates an elongated hypointense mass (arrows) in the ventral aspect of the spinal canal. Signal-to-noise ratio is low because of the patient's lordosis and the distance of the surface coil from the spine. B, Sagittal and C, axial contrast-enhanced scans (SE 600/25, Gd-DTPA) reveal bright enhancement of the tumor (T). On the axial view, the tumor displaces the cord (C) to the right.

MENINGIOMA

Meningiomas arise from the meninges surrounding the spinal cord and are found primarily in the intradural extramedullary compartment. They are much more common in females and become symptomatic from cord compression during middle age or later. Over 80 per cent occur in the thoracic region; another common site is the craniovertebral junction.

Meningiomas have many of the same imaging features of a subarachnoid-based mass as described for nerve sheath tumors. They often have similar signal characteristics on T_1-weighted images, but, as in the head, meningiomas tend to maintain signal intensity similar to that of the grey matter of the cord on T_2-weighted images.[79] Pathologically, calcification is common in meningioma and rare in neurofibroma, but the insensitivity of MR to calcification makes this diagnostic criterion of little value in MR interpretation. Meningiomas have been shown in early investigational trials to enhance rapidly and densely (Fig. 23–41), whereas neuromas take up the contrast more slowly.[17]

METASTATIC DISEASE

The ability to examine the spinal cord and cauda equina directly without injection of intrathecal contrast agents gives MR an advantage for examining patients with suspected intradural metastases. Drop metastases generally originate from either primary or less commonly metastatic disease of the brain with subsequent seeding into the subarachnoid space. Because of either the dynamics of cerebrospinal fluid flow or gravitation, neoplastic cells implant on the spinal arachnoid or pia, resulting in a variety of appearances attributable to intradural metastases. Intradural metastases may also occur from direct spread of extradural tumor or from lymphatic or hematogenous dissemination. Primary brain neoplasms that may lead to drop metastases include medulloblastoma, ependymoma, germinoma, choroid plexus carcinoma, teratoma, glioblastoma, and pineoblastoma. Secondary neoplasms metastatic to brain with a predilection for drop metastases include lymphoma, melanoma, and breast, lung, and renal cell carcinoma.

Using a short TR/TE sequence, several appearances of intradural tumor seeding have been noted. Most common are focal nodular masses that may vary substantially in size, ranging from only a few millimeters to greater than 1 cm (Figs. 23–42 and 23–43). They are frequently spread throughout the subarachnoid space, including laterally in the recesses and root sleeves.[80] On occasion with longstanding disease, erosion of the bony margins of the lateral recesses has also been observed, and the appearance can resemble multiple neurofibromata. Signal characteristics may not distinguish the two entities because T_1 and T_2 values similar to those of neurofibroma have been reported. Obviously, a history of preexisting primary malignancy is important information. Detection of an occult lesion in the brain may clarify the situation.

A second appearance that has been seen with intradural metastases is diffuse coating of the spinal cord with tumor, resulting in either smooth or nodular pseudoexpansion of the cord. This appearance may actually simulate an intramedullary lesion on routine noncontrast MR.[81] The third expression of

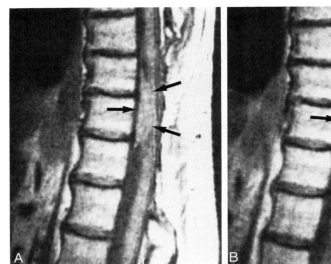
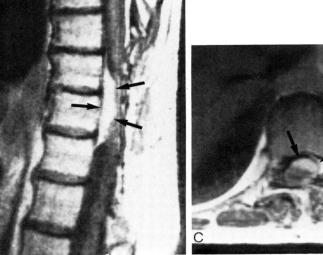

FIGURE 23–41. Recurrent thoracic meningioma. *A*, Plain MR scan (SE 500/40) shows a mass *(arrows)*, isointense to the cord, in the ventral spinal canal, displacing the cord posteriorly. The patient has had a previous laminectomy in the area. Following contrast injection, sagittal *(B)* and axial *(C)* scans (SE 500/40, Gd-DTPA) disclose a hyperintense dural-based mass *(arrows)* within the thecal sac, typical of meningioma. Spinal meningiomas can also have a more globular shape.

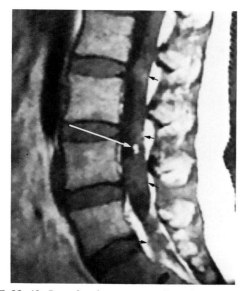

FIGURE 23–42. Intradural metastases from breast carcinoma. SE 310/20 sagittal unenhanced image shows multiple nodular lesions *(small arrows)* of varying sizes in the subarachnoid space. These lesions are indistinguishable from multiple neurofibromas. Note a small focus of high signal *(long arrow)* in the spinal canal at L4, corresponding to a droplet of Pantopaque.

intradural metastatic disease is a homogeneous increase in signal within the subarachnoid space. This effect is seen predominantly in the lumbar region and is probably due to a combination of increased protein content within the CSF, malignant cells, and damping of CSF pulsations.

Gd-DTPA should be used in all cases of suspected intradural or "drop" metastases. It significantly increases the sensitivity for detection of the smaller nodules and readily distinguishes the pseudoexpansion described above from an intramedullary process.[82]

TRAUMA

The role of MR in spinal trauma has not been entirely defined. At present, most diagnostic algorithms for the work-up of acute injuries maintain plain films and CT as the primary imaging modalities. Plain films effectively assess spinal alignment, major fractures, and degree of instability. CT is used to detect nondisplaced fractures of the vertebral arch, migration of fragments into the spinal canal, and

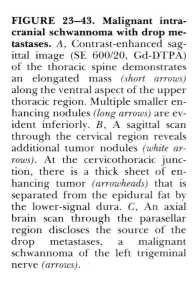

FIGURE 23–43. Malignant intracranial schwannoma with drop metastases. *A,* Contrast-enhanced sagittal image (SE 600/20, Gd-DTPA) of the thoracic spine demonstrates an elongated mass *(short arrows)* along the ventral aspect of the upper thoracic region. Multiple smaller enhancing nodules *(long arrows)* are evident inferiorly. *B,* A sagittal scan through the cervical region reveals additional tumor nodules *(white arrows).* At the cervicothoracic junction, there is a thick sheet of enhancing tumor *(arrowheads)* that is separated from the epidural fat by the lower-signal dura. *C,* An axial brain scan through the parasellar region discloses the source of the drop metastases, a malignant schwannoma of the left trigeminal nerve *(arrows).*

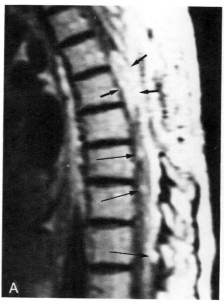

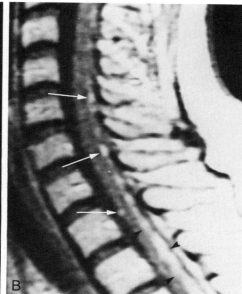

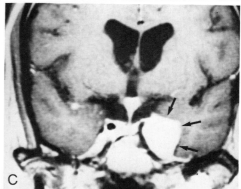

associated herniated disks. MR has not made many inroads into the arena of acute spinal trauma because the examination takes longer, the images lack bone detail, and much of the life-support equipment and many of the stabilizing devices are not MR compatible. Nonetheless, evidence is accumulating in the literature that MR can be done rapidly and safely in an emergency setting and that the information obtained may have important implications for therapy.[83]

The immediate goals of therapy depend on the patient's clinical condition. If the deficit is complete and fixed with no motor or sensory function below the level of injury, the primary goal is to stabilize the spine to facilitate rehabilitation. On the other hand, if the deficit is incomplete, emergent diagnosis of any compressive lesion of the cord must be made so that surgical decompression can be done without delay.

Assuming that the technical problems of scanning times and MR compatibility of support equipment are solved, what are the capabilities of MR for evaluating the acutely traumatized patient? With multiplanar imaging, MR can certainly detect any malalignment of the spine and major fractures of the vertebral elements. Flexion/extension views can be obtained readily with sagittal imaging to assess stability, and the exquisite contrast resolution of MR may reveal information about ligamentous injury.

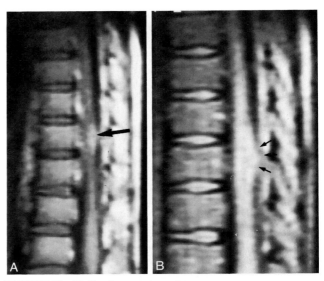

FIGURE 23–45. **Cord contusion with parenchymal hemorrhage.** *A,* SE 500/32 sagittal slice. Focal area of high signal intensity *(arrow)* with expansion in the dorsal aspect of the cord is consistent with cord hemorrhage. No epidural hematoma is evident. *B,* SE 2000/60 sagittal slice. This T_2-weighted image again shows focal cord expansion with a nodular area posteriorly *(arrows)*. These findings were confirmed by CT/myelography, and the nodular area probably represents a small subpial hematoma.

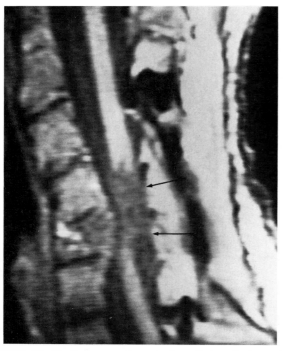

FIGURE 23–44. **Severe cord contusion.** Patient had previous anterior fusion of a cervical spine fracture and a posterior decompressive laminectomy. A sagittal T_1-weighted scan (SE 600/20) shows a severe cord contusion *(arrows)* at the levels of C4 and C5. The damaged cord is hypointense and has irregular, poorly defined margins. (From Hesselink JR: Spine imaging: History, achievements, remaining frontiers. AJR 150:1223–1229, 1988; © by American Roentgen Ray Society.)

Admittedly, MR cannot match CT for defining fractures of the pedicles, facets, and laminae.

Again, of primary importance is the evaluation of the status of the cord, and it is here that MR outperforms any other imaging modality. First, MR can detect fragments of bone within the canal that might be compressing the cord because the fragments invariably contain some marrow. Moreover, epidural hematomas requiring evacuation are easily seen by MR but often elude detection by CT unless intrathecal contrast is given. MR is also better for demonstrating associated disk herniation.[84]

Cord injuries can have a variable appearance. Severe injuries may reveal marked disruption of cord structure or even complete transection (Fig. 23–44). Milder contusions show high-signal areas within the cord on T_2-weighted images, representing edema and perhaps cord swelling.[85, 86] The signal characteristics of hemorrhagic components depend on the age of the hemorrhage, the field strength of the magnet, and the pulse sequence used (Fig. 23–45) (see Chapters 8 and 16). McArdle et al[87] reported that the presence of an intramedullary hematoma indicates a poorer prognosis for recovery than if the contusion is nonhemorrhagic. Much of the MR information on acute cord injuries is relatively new, and the clinical and therapeutic implications are still uncertain.

MR has already assumed a role in the evaluation of cord injuries during the subacute and chronic stages. After the patient has stabilized medically, the MR examination can be performed to assess the degree of cord damage, myelomalacia, atrophy, scarring, and fibrosis. More important, in the setting of

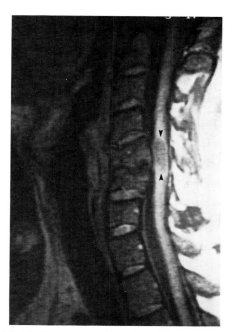

FIGURE 23–46. Post-traumatic syrinx. The trauma occurred a few months earlier. The patient returns with progressing neurologic symptoms. Proton-density weighted scan (SE 2000/70) reveals the residua of the anterior spinal fractures, with marked deformity of the C5 and C6 vertebral bodies. Bone projects posteriorly to produce mild compromise of the spinal canal. The cord is widened at that level and contains a cystic cavity *(arrowheads)*. The cavity is hypointense and has well-defined margins, consistent with a post-traumatic syrinx. The high-signal areas within the cord above and below the syrinx represent either residual edema or gliosis.

new or progressive signs of neurologic dysfunction, MR can facilitate the diagnosis of delayed complications, such as disk herniation, arachnoid cyst, and posttraumatic cord syrinx.[88] The syrinx or intramedullary cyst (Fig. 23–46) first forms at the site of injury but can extend some distance beyond and become quite large. MR readily distinguishes between syrinx and other posttraumatic changes. Myelomalacia and gliosis are focal processes with poorly defined margins and are associated with cord atrophy. A syrinx has well-defined margins and frequently expands the cord. Both are hyperintense on T_2-weighted scans; however, on proton density–weighted images gliosis is hyperintense to cord tissue, but the fluid-containing syrinx is usually hypointense. Dynamic studies of cyst pulsation have disclosed that those with prominent pulsation and fluid motion are more likely to expand and cause progressive symptoms. Fluid motion can be measured with gradient-echo scans or cine-MR. Results of these studies may have important clinical implications for shunting of posttraumatic syringomyelia.[89]

CRANIOVERTEBRAL ABNORMALITIES

Most congenital anomalies of the spine occur in either the upper cervical or lower thoracic and lum-

bar regions. They are found as isolated entities or in combination with one another, such as in Chiari malformation type II with an associated tethered cord and myelomeningocele (see Chapter 24). The age of clinical presentation ranges from birth to adulthood depending on the type and severity of the malformation. MR using short TR/TE sequences in the sagittal plane has been particularly valuable in the assessment of these patients, yielding information regarding the position of the cerebellar tonsils and inferior vermis and the presence of hydro- or syringomyelia, low occipital or cervical meningocele, and, rarely, a cervical diastematomyelia. With the widespread use of MR, it appears that the detection of Chiari I malformation (Fig. 23–47) has increased substantially because of the ability to see clearly the cervicomedullary junction on T_1 sagittal images.[90, 91] The correlation between Chiari I malformation and symptomatology requires scrutiny, as low-lying tonsils may be considered an incidental and clinically unimportant finding. Vertebral anomalies, such as Klippel-Feil deformity, may be present with a Chiari I malformation and are also readily visible on MR sagittal images, although plain films and CT may be of more value in characterizing the subtle osseous changes that may occur (see Chapter 14).

Abnormalities or deformities at the craniovertebral junction can develop from trauma or from neoplastic, degenerative, and inflammatory diseases.[92] T_1-weighted sagittal images give an exquisite display of the anatomy of this area, clearly showing the relationships of bone and soft tissue to the spinal cord.

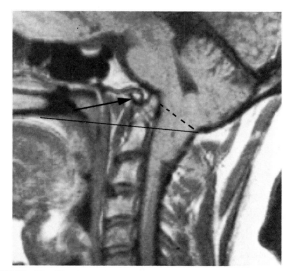

FIGURE 23–47. Chiari I malformation with platybasia and basilar invagination. SE 500/40 sagittal 5-mm image. The cerebellar tonsils are positioned inferiorly below the plane of the foramen magnum *(dashed line)*. Chamberlain's line *(solid line)* from the hard palate to the opisthion passes through the mid-dens, consistent with basilar invagination. The anterior arch of C1 *(arrow)* is fused to the occiput, and the lower clivus is elevated to an abnormally horizontal position. The dens behind the anterior arch of C1 lies against the brain stem, and the brain stem is kinked at the pontomedullary junction. No syringohydromyelia was found.

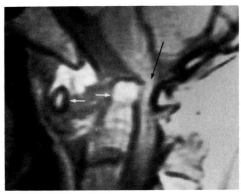

FIGURE 23–48. Psoriatic arthritis with C1-C2 subluxation. Sagittal T$_1$-weighted scan (SE 600/20) reveals markedly increased distance between the anterior arch of C1 and the odontoid *(white arrows)*. The soft tissue in between is inflammatory granulation tissue. The upper cervical cord *(black arrow)* is severely compressed between the odontoid and the posterior arch of C1. (From Hesselink JR: Spine imaging: History, achievements, remaining frontiers. AJR 150:1223–1229, 1988; © by American Roentgen Ray Society.)

Rheumatoid and psoriatic arthritis (Fig. 23–48) produce inflammatory changes in synovial joints. Exuberant inflammatory tissue or pannus erodes articular surfaces and weakens supporting ligaments, which can lead to subluxation and cord compression.[93, 94]

REFERENCES

1. Rothman SLG, Glenn WV (eds): Multiplanar CT of the Spine. Baltimore, University Park Press, 1985.
2. Caille JM, Gioux M, Arne P, Paty J: Neurotoxicity of nonionic iodinated water soluble contrast media in myelography: Experimental study. AJNR 4:1185–1189, 1983.
3. Ratcliff G, Sandler S, Latchaw R: Cognitive and affective changes after myelography: A comparison of metrizamide and iohexol. AJNR 6:683–687, 1986.
4. Haughton VM: MR imaging of the spine. Radiology 166:297–301, 1988.
5. Enzmann DR, Griffin C, Rubin JB: Potential false-negative MR images of the thoracic spine in disk disease with switching of phase- and frequency-encoding gradients. Radiology 165:635–637, 1987.
6. Enzmann DR, Rubin JB: Cervical spine: MR imaging with a partial flip angle, gradient-refocused pulse sequence. Part 1. General considerations and disk disease. Radiology 166:467–472, 1988.
7. Hesselink JR: Spine imaging: History, achievements, remaining frontiers. AJR 150:1223–1229, 1988.
8. Modic MT, Weinstein MA, Pavlicek W, et al: Magnetic resonance imaging of the cervical spine: Technical and clinical observations. AJR 141:1129–1136, 1983.
9. Modic MT, Hardy RW, Weinstein MA, et al: Nuclear magnetic resonance of the spine: Clinical potential and limitations. Neurosurgery 15:583–592, 1984.
10. Stimac GK, Porter BA, Olson DO, et al: Gadolinium-DTPA–enhanced MR imaging of spinal neoplasms: Preliminary investigation and comparison with unenhanced spin-echo and STIR sequences. AJNR 9:839–846, 1988.
11. Modic MT, Masaryk TJ, Mulopulos GP, et al: Cervical radiculopathy: Prospective evaluation with surface coil MR imaging, CT with metrizamide and metrizamide myelography. Radiology 161:753–760, 1986.
12. Czervionke LF, Daniels DL, Ho PSP, et al: Cervical neural

13. Czervionke LF, Daniels DL, Ho PSP, et al: The MR appearance of gray and white matter in the cervical spinal cord. AJNR 9:557–582, 1988.
14. Sze G, Krol G, Zimmerman RD, Deck MDF: Intramedullary disease of the spine: Diagnosis using gadolinium-DTPA–enhanced MR imaging. AJNR 9:847–858, 1988.
15. Russell DS, Rubenstein LJ: Pathology of Tumours of the Nervous System. 4th ed. Baltimore, Williams & Wilkins Company, 1977.
16. Post MJD, Quencer RM, Green BA, et al: Intramedullary spinal cord metastases, mainly of nonneurogenic origin. AJNR 8:339–346, 1987.
17. Bydder GM, Brown J, Niendorf HP, Young IR: Enhancement of cervical intraspinal tumors in MR imaging with intravenous gadolinium-DTPA. J Comput Assist Tomogr 9(5):847–851, 1985.
18. Valk J: Gd-DTPA in MR of spinal lesions. AJNR 9:345–350, 1988.
19. Enzmann DR, Murphy IK, Silverberg GD, et al: Spinal cord tumor imaging with CT and MR. AJNR 6:95–99, 1985.
20. Rubin JM, Aisen AM, DiPietro MA: Ambiguities in MR imaging of tumoral cysts in the spinal cord. J Comput Assist Tomogr 10:395–398, 1986.
21. Goy AMC, Pinto RS, Raghavendra BN, et al: Intramedullary spinal cord tumors: MR Imaging, with emphasis on associated cysts. Radiology 161:381–386, 1986.
22. Williams AL, Haughton VM, Pojunas KW, et al: Differentiation of intramedullary neoplasms and cysts by MR. AJNR 8:527–532, 1987.
23. Sherman JL, Citrin CM, Gangarosa RE, Bowen BJ: The MR appearance of CSF pulsations in the spinal canal. AJNR 7:879–884, 1986.
24. Rebner M, Gebarski SS: Magnetic resonance imaging of spinal-cord hemangioblastoma. AJNR 6:287–289, 1985.
25. Aubin ML, Vigneaud J, Jardin C, Bar D: Computed tomography in 75 clinical cases of syringomyelia. AJNR 2:199–204, 1981.
26. Sherman JL, Barkovich AJ, Citrin CM: The MR appearance of syringomyelia: New observations. AJNR 7:985–995, 1986.
27. Yeates A, Brant-Zawadzki M, Norman D, et al: Nuclear magnetic resonance imaging of syringomyelia. AJNR 4:234–237, 1983.
28. Lee BCP, Zimmerman RD, Manning JJ, Deck MDF: MR imaging of syringomyelia and hydromyelia. AJNR 6:221–228, 1985.
29. Barkovich AJ, Sherman JL, Citrin CM, Wippold FJ II: MR of postoperative syringomyelia. AJNR 8:319–327, 1987.
30. Enzmann DR, O'Donohue J, Rubin JB, et al: CSF pulsations within nonneoplastic spinal cord cysts. AJNR 8:517–525, 1987.
31. Samuelsson L, Bergstom K, Thuomas K-A, et al: MR imaging of syringohydromyelia and Chiari malformations in myelomeningocele patients with scoliosis. AJNR 8:539–546, 1987.
32. Edwards MK, Farlow MR, Stevens JC: Cranial MR in spinal cord MS: Diagnosing patients with isolated cord symptoms. AJNR 7:1003–1005, 1986.
33. Ikuta F, Zimmerman HM: Distribution of plaques in seventy autopsy cases of multiple sclerosis in the United States. Neurology 26(suppl):26–28, 1976.
34. Maravilla KR, Weinreb JC, Suss R, Nunnally RL: Magnetic resonance demonstration of multiple sclerosis plaques in the cervical spinal cord. AJR 144:381–385, 1985.
35. Grossman RI, Gonzalez-Scarano F, Atlas SW, et al: Multiple sclerosis: Gadolinium enhancement in MR imaging. Radiology 161:721–725, 1986.
36. Sherman JL, Drachman DB, Citrin CM: MR evaluation of amyotrophic lateral sclerosis (ALS). Presented at the annual meeting of the American Society of Neuroradiology, New York City, May, 1987.
37. Merine D, Wang H, Kumar AJ, et al: CT myelography and

MR imaging of acute transverse myelitis. J Comput Assist Tomogr 11:606–608, 1988.

38. Tashiro K, Ito K, Maruo Y, et al: MR imaging of the spinal cord in Devic disease. J Comput Assist Tomogr 11:516–517, 1987.
39. Minami S, Sagoh T, Nishimura K, et al: Spinal arteriovenous malformation: MR imaging. Radiology 169:109–115, 1988.
40. DiChiro G, Doppman JL, Dwyer AJ, et al: Tumors and arteriovenous malformations of the spinal cord: Assessment using MR. Radiology 156:689–697, 1985.
41. Masaryk TJ, Ross JS, Modic MT, et al: Radiculomeningeal vascular malformations of the spine: MR imaging. Radiology 164:845–849, 1987.
42. Fontaine S, Melanson D, Cosgrove R, Bertrand G: Cavernous hemangiomas of the spinal cord: MR imaging. Radiology 16:839–841, 1988.
43. Dormont D, Gelbert F, Assouline E, et al: MR imaging of spinal cord arteriovenous malformations at 0.5 T: Study of 34 cases. AJNR 9:833–838, 1988.
44. Hedberg MC, Drayer BP, Flom RA, et al: Gradient echo (GRASS) MR imaging in cervical radiculopathy. AJNR 9:145–151, 1988.
45. Ross JS, Perez-Reyes N, Masaryk TJ, et al: Thoracic disk herniation: MR imaging. Radiology 165:511–515, 1987.
46. Brown BM, Schwartz RH, Frank E, Blank NK: Preoperative evaluation of cervical radiculopathy and myelopathy by surface-coil MR imaging. AJNR 9:859–866, 1988.
47. Karnaze MG, Gado MH, Sartor KJ, Hodges FJ III. Comparison of MR and CT myelography in imaging the cervical and thoracic spine. AJR 150:397–403, 1988.
48. Daniels DL, Hyde JS, Kneeland JB, et al: The cervical nerves and foramina: Local-coil MR imaging. AJNR 7:129–133, 1986.
49. Modic MT, Masaryk TJ, Ross JS, et al: Cervical radiculopathy: Value of oblique MR imaging. Radiology 163:227, 1987.
50. Teresi LM, Lufkin RB, Reicher MA, et al: Asymptomatic degenerative disk disease and spondylosis of the cervical spine: MR imaging. Radiology 164:83–88, 1987.
51. Fink IJ, Garra BS, Zabell A, Doppman JL: Computed tomography with metrizamide myelography to define the extent of spinal canal block due to tumor. J Comput Assist Tomogr 8(6):1072–1075, 1984.
52. Wang AM, Lewis ML, Rumbaugh CL, et al: Spinal cord or nerve root compression in patients with malignant disease: CT evaluation. J Comput Assist Tomogr 8(3):420–428, 1984.
53. Sze G: Gadolinium-DTPA in spinal disease. Radiol Clin North Am 26:1009–1024, 1988.
54. Colman LK, Porter BA, Redmond J III, et al: Early diagnosis of spinal metastases by CT and MR studies. J Comput Assist Tomogr 12:423–426, 1988.
55. Smoker WRK, Godersky JC, Knutzon RK, et al: The role of MR imaging in evaluating metastatic spinal disease. AJNR 8:901–908, 1987.
56. Ross JS, Masaryk TJ, Modic MT, et al: Vertebral hemangiomas: MR imaging. Radiology 165:165–169, 1987.
57. Hajek PC, Baker LL, Goobar JE, et al: Focal fat deposition in axial bone marrow: MR characteristics. Radiology 162:245–249, 1987.
58. Beltran J, Noto AM, Chakeres DW, Christoforidis AJ: Tumors of the osseous spine: Staging with MR imaging versus CT. Radiology 162:565–569, 1987.
59. Zimmer WD, Berquist TH, McLeod RA, et al: Bone tumors: Magnetic resonance imaging versus computed tomography. 155:709–718, 1985.
60. Aisen AM, Martel W, Braunstein EM, et al: MRI and CT evaluation of primary bone and soft-tissue tumors. AJR 146:749–756, 1986.
61. Beltran J, Simon DC, Levy M, et al: Aneurysmal bone cysts: MR imaging at 1.5 T. Radiology 158:689–690, 1986.
62. Haggstrom JA, Brown JC, Marsh PW: Eosinophilic granuloma of the spine: MR demonstration. J Comput Assist Tomogr 12:344–345, 1988.
63. McKinstry CS, Steiner RE, Young AT, et al: Bone marrow in leukemia and aplastic anemia: MR imaging before, during, and after treatment. Radiology 162:701–707, 1987.
64. Dooms GC, Fisher MR, Hricak H, et al: Bone marrow imaging: Magnetic resonance studies related to age and sex. Radiology 155:429–432, 1985.
65. Porter BA, Shields AF, Olson DO: Magnetic resonance imaging of bone marrow disorders. Radiol Clin North Am 24:269–279, 1986.
66. McKissock W, Bloom WH, Chynn KY: Spinal cord compression caused by plasma-cell tumors. J Neurosurg 18:68–73, 1961.
67. Moore SG, Gooding CA, Brasch RC, et al: Bone marrow in children with acute lymphocytic leukemia: MR relaxation times. Radiology 160:237–240, 1986.
68. Nyman R, Rehn S, Glimelius B, et al: Magnetic resonance imaging in diffuse malignant bone marrow diseases. Acta Radiol [Diagn] 28:199–205, 1987.
69. Cohen MD, Klatte EC, Baehner R, et al: Magnetic resonance imaging of bone marrow disease in children. Radiology 151:715–718, 1984.
70. Ramsey RG, Sacharias CE: MR imaging of the spine after radiation therapy: Easily recognizable effects. AJNR 6:247–252, 1985.
71. de Roos A, Kressel H, Spritzer C, et al: MR imaging of marrow changes adjacent to end plates in degenerative lumbar disk disease. AJR 149:531, 1987.
72. Siegel MJ, Jamroz GA, Glazer HS, et al: MR imaging of intraspinal extension of neuroblastoma. J Comput Assist Tomogr 10:593–595, 1986.
73. Bertino RE, Porter BA, Stimac GK, Tepper SJ: Imaging spinal osteomyelitis and epidural abscess with short TI inversion recovery (STIR). AJNR 9:563–564, 1988.
74. Modic MT, Feiglin DH, Piraino DW, et al: Vertebral osteomyelitis: Assessment using MR. Radiology 157:157–166, 1985.
75. Van Lom KJ, Kellerhouse LE, Pathria MN, et al: Infection versus tumor in the spine: Criteria for distinction with CT. Radiology 166:851–855, 1988.
76. Zimmermann RA, Bilaniuk LT: Imaging of tumors of the spinal canal and cord. Radiol Clin North Am 26:965–1007, 1988.
77. Burk DL, Brunberg JA, Kanal E, et al: Spinal and paraspinal neurofibromatosis: Surface coil MR imaging at 1.5 T. Radiology 162:797–801, 1987.
78. Geremia GK, Russell EJ, Clasen RA: MR imaging characteristics of a neurenteric cyst. AJNR 9:978–980, 1988.
79. Scotti G, Scialfa N, Colombo N, Landoni L: MR imaging of intradural extramedullary tumors of the cervical spine. J Comput Assist Tomogr 9:1037–1041, 1985.
80. Barloon TJ, Yuh WTC, Yang CJC, Schultz DH: Spinal subarachnoid tumor seeding from intracranial metastases: MR findings. J Comput Assist Tomogr 11:242–244, 1987.
81. Berns DH, Blaser S, Ross JS, et al: MR imaging with Gd-DTPA in leptomeningeal spread of lymphoma. J Comput Assist Tomogr 12:499–500, 1988.
82. Sze G, Abranson A, Krol G, et al: Gadolinium-DTPA in the evaluation of intradural extramedullary spinal disease. AJNR 9:153–163, 1988.
83. Mirvis SE, Giesler FH, Jelinek JJ, et al: Acute cervical spine trauma: Evaluation with 1.5 T MR imaging. Radiology 166:807–816, 1988.
84. Kulkarni MV, McArdle CB, Kopanicky D, et al: Acute spinal cord injury: MR imaging at 1.5 T. Radiology 164:837–843, 1987.
85. Chakeres DW, Flickinger F, Bresnahan JC, et al: MR imaging of acute spinal cord trauma. AJNR 8:5–10, 1987.
86. Hackney DB, Asato R, Joseph P, et al: Hemorrhage and edema in acute spinal cord compression: Demonstration by MR imaging. Radiology 161:387–390, 1986.
87. McArdle CB, Crofford MJ, Mirfakhraee M, et al: Surface coil MR of spinal trauma: Preliminary experience. AJNR 7:885–893, 1986.

88. Quencer RM, Sheldon JJ, Post MJD, et al: MRI of the chronically injured cervical spinal cord. AJNR 7:457–464, 1986.

89. Quencer RM: The injured spinal cord: Evaluation with magnetic resonance and intraoperative sonography. Radiol Clin North Am 26:1025–1045, 1988.

90. Ahmed OA, Sartor K, Geyer CA, Gado MH: Position of cerebellar tonsils in the normal population and in patients with Chiari malformation: A quantitative approach with MR imaging. J Comput Assist Tomogr 9:1033–1036, 1985.

91. Barkovich AJ, Wippold FJ, Sherman JL, Citrin CM: Significance of cerebellar tonsillar position on MR. AJNR 7:795–799, 1986.

92. Sze G, Brant-Zawadzki MN, Wilson CR, et al: Pseudotumor of the craniovertebral junction associated with chronic subluxation: MR imaging studies. Radiology 161:391–394, 1986.

93. Bundschuh C, Modic MT, Kearney F, et al: Rheumatoid arthritis of the cervical spine: Surface-coil MR imaging. AJNR 9:565–571, 1988.

94. Pettersson H, Larsson EM, Holtas S, et al: MR imaging of the cervical spine in rheumatoid arthritis. AJNR 9:573–577, 1988.

24

MR IMAGING OF THE LUMBAR SPINE

JOHN R. HESSELINK and GREGORY M. SHOUKIMAS

EXAMINATION TECHNIQUE
   GENERAL CONSIDERATIONS
   PULSE SEQUENCES
   ALGORITHMS
ANATOMY
DEGENERATIVE SPINAL DISEASE
(EXTRADURAL)
   INTERVERTEBRAL DISK DISEASE
   SPONDYLOSIS
   SPINAL STENOSIS
POSTOPERATIVE SPINE
VERTEBRAL AND PARAVERTEBRAL
ABNORMALITIES (EXTRADURAL)
(see Chapter 23)

SACRAL LESIONS
   CHORDOMA
   TERATOMA
   PAGET'S DISEASE

INTRADURAL EXTRAMEDULLARY
DISEASE
   ARACHNOIDITIS
   PANTOPAQUE
   TUMORS (see Chapter 23)

SPINAL DYSRAPHISM

Magnetic resonance (MR) has many noteworthy features for imaging the lumbar spine. It is entirely noninvasive. So far as we know, there are no adverse effects from MR imaging. The spine and neural elements can be imaged without the injection of intravenous or intrathecal contrast agents. Images can be obtained in any plane. Owing to the strong magnetic fields employed, MR imaging should not be performed on patients with cardiac pacemakers, intraocular metallic foreign bodies, or intracranial aneurysm clips. Also, it is not recommended during the first trimester of pregnancy.

Although cortical bone gives essentially no MR signal, the hypointense bone is contrasted against the higher signal of the adjacent soft tissues. In addition, the marrow within the vertebral bodies and posterior elements of the spine contains blood and fat, both of which produce an MR signal. As a result, any disease process that distorts the architecture of the marrow can be detected. The MR images provide much better contrast resolution than does CT. In addition, major vascular structures, such as the aorta and vena cava, are imaged because of the phenomenon of signal void from flowing blood. The application of surface coils has further improved the spatial and contrast resolution of MR images of the spine.

EXAMINATION TECHNIQUE

GENERAL CONSIDERATIONS

The requirements for MR imaging of the lumbar spine are a little different than for the cervical and thoracic spine. The cord does not normally extend down into the lumbar region. The anatomy is larger and does not require such thin sections. In general, the images are better because there are fewer artifacts from CSF pulsations, and cardiac and respiratory motion have little effect in the lumbar region.

In the vast majority of cases, interest can be focused on the lower lumbar levels because most patients have radicular symptoms related to disk disease or degenerative joint disease. Nevertheless, in examination of the lumbar spine, one of the sagittal views should include the conus medullaris to exclude a higher lesion that could be responsible for radicular-type symptoms. As in the upper levels, surface coils are preferable for lumbar scans, the specific type depending on the MR system being used. A thorough evaluation of the lumbar spine requires imaging in both the sagittal and axial planes. (See Chapter 23 for a more detailed description of spinal examination techniques.)

PULSE SEQUENCES

The same pulse sequences are available for the lumbar spine as for the cervical: T_1- and T_2-weighted spin-echo and gradient-echo methods. The basic scan parameters include a 256 × 256 or 256 × 128 matrix and two to four excitations (four to six for GRASS), depending on the specific pulse sequence. A 5-mm slice thickness with a 1-mm interslice gap is used for all sequences and imaging planes. One of the sagittal sequences should use a 24-cm field of view to include the conus; additional scans can use an 18- to 20-cm field of view to get better spatial resolution. The axial scans are prescribed from a sagittal view, with angled sets of scans parallel to each interspace (Fig. 24–1). When the scans are angled to each interspace, they overlap posteriorly and locally degrade the images. That does not interfere with interpretation unless the overlapped areas extend forward into the spinal canal. A 16- to 20-cm field of view is used for the axial scans.

The T_1-weighted scan is obtained with a TR of 500 to 800 msec and a TE of 20 to 30 msec. As for the cervical spine, the hyperintense bone marrow, epidural fat, and paraspinal fat contrast nicely with the hypointense cortical bone and CSF and the intermediate-signal neural structures and paravertebral muscles (Fig. 24–2A and B). T_1-weighted sequences are also used in conjunction with gadolinium (Gd)-DTPA enhancement.

The T_2-weighted pulse sequence is slightly different than for the upper spinal levels (TR = 1800 to 2500 msec; TE = 30 to 40/60 to 80 msec). Flow compensation is used routinely, and symmetric echoes capture more signal with even-echo rephasing. The first echo images have higher signal-to-noise ratio (S/N) and show the soft tissues better (Figs. 24–2C and 24–3). The high-signal CSF on the second echo is best for visualizing the nerve roots within the thecal sac and for evaluating extradural compressions of the thecal sac (Fig. 24–4).

Pulse parameters for gradient-echo scans (GRASS, FLASH, FISP) include a TE of 12 to 30 msec and a TR ranging from 25 to 50 msec for a single slice and 300 to 500 msec for multislice acquisitions. A flip angle of 6 to 25 degrees results in a good myelographic effect (see Fig. 24–2D).

ALGORITHMS

Based on the clinical presentation, algorithms can be designed for MR imaging of the lumbar spine (See Appendix I, MRI Scan Protocols). In general, the algorithms are rather straightforward because the large category of spinal cord diseases is not a consideration. Most protocols start with gradient-echo and T_1-weighted sagittal scans. This combination assures adequate evaluation of the bony structures, disks, and epidural and subarachnoid space. An alternative is to replace the above two sequences with a T_2-weighted spin-echo scan. This dual-echo sequence gives similar information in about the same amount of time. Since the neural foramina in the lumbar spine are oriented 90 degrees to the sagittal plane, the scans should extend far enough laterally to include the foramina.

In the nonoperated back, the T_2-weighted sequence seems to give the most information in the axial plane, and the TR is sufficiently long to cover all the interspaces of interest with one acquisition. In the postoperative back, a gradient-echo sagittal scan is followed by Gd-DTPA injection and T_1-weighted scans in both sagittal and axial planes.

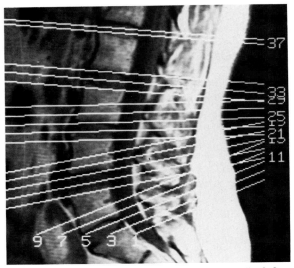

FIGURE 24–1. Technique. Axial scans are prescribed from a sagittal view, angling the sections parallel to each interspace.

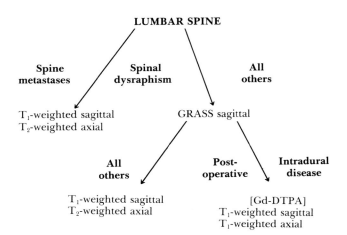

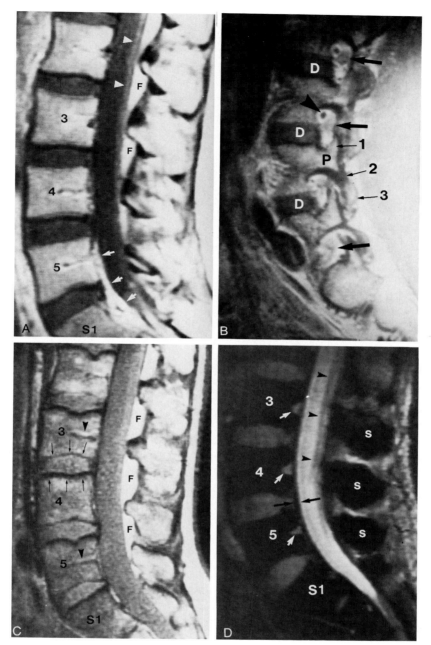

FIGURE 24–2. Normal sagittal anatomy. *A*, Midsagittal T_1-weighted scan (SE 600/20). The CSF is hypointense, the bone marrow and fat (F) are hyperintense, and the disks are of intermediate signal. Cortical bone remains black. Patient has a generous amount of ventral epidural fat *(arrows)* behind L5 and S1. The neural elements *(arrowheads)* are clustered posteriorly within the thecal sac. *B*, Parasagittal T_1-weighted scan (SE 600/20). The nerve roots *(large arrows)* are positioned in the upper part of the neural foramina, surrounded by high-signal fat. The hypointense dot anterosuperior to the root is a radicular vein *(arrowhead)* that connects the retrovertebral plexus with the paravertebral plexus of veins. The intervertebral disks (D) border the inferior aspects of the foramina. Posterior elements include the pedicle (P), superior facet (1), pars interarticularis (2), and inferior facet (3). *C*, Proton density–weighted scan (SE 2000/25). Tissues are more isointense, except for epidural fat (F), which is bright. Tissues closer to the coil (more posterior) are of higher signal than tissues farther away (anterior). CSF is of slightly lower signal intensity than the intervertebral disks. The superior end plate of L4 appears thicker and darker than the inferior end plate of L3 owing to chemical shift artifact *(arrows)* in the frequency-encoding direction. The parallel bright and dark lines of the basivertebral veins *(arrowheads)* are due to chemical shift and flow displacement artifact. *D*, Gradient-echo scan (GRE 25/13, flip angle = 6) produces a myelographic effect. Anything with high water content or flow appears bright. Normal disks have enough water to make them hyperintense. The basivertebral veins *(white arrows)* are bright because of flow. Vertebral bodies (L3-S1) and spinous processes (S), including cortical bone and marrow, are hypointense. Nerve roots *(arrowheads)* are clustered posteriorly. Hypointense line *(black arrows)* at the posterior interspace represents a combination of dura, posterior longitudinal ligament, and outer fibers of the anulus.

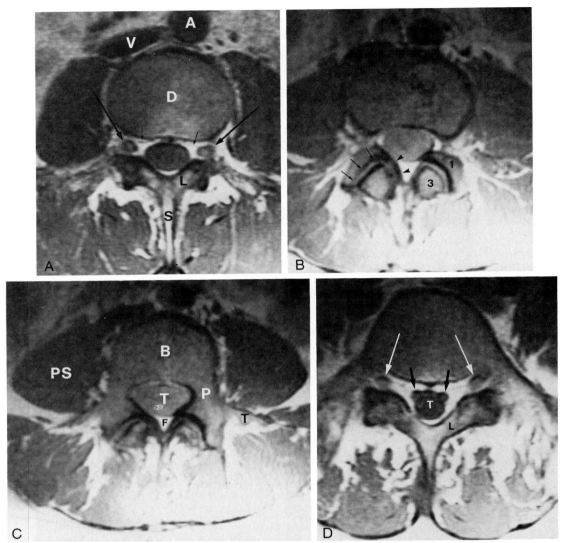

FIGURE 24–3. Normal axial anatomy, proton density–weighted scans (SE 1800/30). *A*, Level of disk and neural foramina, L4-L5. The L4 nerve roots *(long arrows)* are surrounded by epidural fat in the neural foramina. The hypointense beaded linear structures *(short arrows)* are epidural veins. A = Aorta; V = inferior vena cava; D = disk; L = lamina; S = spinous process. *B*, Level of facet joints, L4-L5. 1 = Superior facet of L5; 3 = inferior facet of L4; arrows = facet joint; arrowheads = ligamentum flavum. *C*, Level of pedicles, L5. B = Vertebral body; P = pedicle; white T = thecal sac; F = epidural fat; PS = psoas muscle; black T = transverse process. *D*, Level of neural foramina, L5-S1. The L5 nerve roots *(white arrows)* are exiting through their foramina. The S1 nerve roots *(black arrows)* are budding off the thecal sac (T). The spinal canal has a generous amount of high-signal epidural fat. L = Lamina.

ANATOMY

In imaging patients with back pain, the primary anatomic areas of interest are the intervertebral disks, spinal canal, neural foramina, and facet joints. The intervertebral disk consists of the nucleus pulposus surrounded by the anulus fibrosus. Both the anulus and the nucleus are composed of collagen and proteoglycans (chondroitin-6-sulfate, keratan sulfate, hyaluronic acid, and chondroitin-4-sulfate). The nucleus contains relatively more proteoglycans to give it a looser gelatinous texture. It blends in with the surrounding anulus without clear anatomic demarcation. The anulus has more collagen, and the collagen becomes progressively more compact and tougher at the periphery. The outer anulus is attached to the adjacent vertebral bodies at the site of the fused epiphyseal ring by Sharpey fibers and to the anterior and posterior longitudinal ligaments. Normal disks are well hydrated, the nucleus containing 80 to 85 per cent water and the anulus about 80 per cent.[1] Together with the cartilaginous end plates of the adjacent vertebral bodies, the intervertebral disk forms a disk complex that gives structural integ-

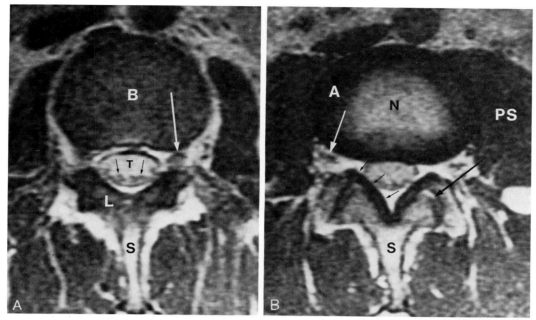

FIGURE 24–4. Normal axial anatomy, T₂-weighted scans (SE 1800/60), L4-L5. *A,* Level of neural foramina and inferior vertebral body. B = Vertebral body; L = lamina; S = spinous process; T = thecal sac. The nerve roots *(small arrows)* are clustered in the posterior thecal sac (T). The left L4 nerve root *(long white arrow)* lies within the neural foramen. *B,* Level of intervertebral disk and inferior neural foramina. The L4 nerve root *(white arrow)* has exited the foramen and is positioned along the posterolateral aspect of the disk space. A = Anulus fibrosus/vertebral end plate complex; N = nucleus pulposus; PS = psoas muscle; S = spinous process. The facet joint *(long black arrow)* is bounded by the superior facet of L5 laterally and the inferior facet of L4 medially. The ligamentum flavum *(short arrows)* is hypointense. Note the relatively high signal of the epidural fat on this lightly T₂-weighted image.

rity to the interspace and cushions the mechanical forces applied to the spine.

Normally, the disk has a concave margin posteriorly and is symmetric. The anulus is hypointense on all pulse sequences; the nucleus is of intermediate signal on T₁-weighted images (see Fig. 24–2A) and hyperintense on gradient-echo (see Fig. 24–2D) and T₂-weighted scans (Fig. 24–4B). On axial views the high signal of the nucleus is confined to the central portion of the disk.

The dural sac extends from C1 to the sacrum and is highlighted by epidural fat and connective tissues (see Fig. 24–2A). Fat is invariably present in the posterior part of the spinal canal, with smaller amounts ventrally but increasing on more caudal sections. On T₂ images the spinal nerves of the cauda equina are outlined by the high-signal CSF and are usually clustered posteriorly in the thecal sac (Fig. 24–4). On progressively more caudal axial images, the nerves march forward in pairs (anterior and posterior rootlets) on either side on their way to their respective root sleeves. When the nerves leave the root sheath at the medial aspects of the neural foramina, they are enveloped by the epidural fat. At this point, they become more visible on proton-density and T₁-weighted images. The nerves exit through their respective foramina below the pedicle of the corresponding vertebrae (see Figs. 24–2B and 24–3A and D). The nerve root ganglion is located at the lateral aspect of the foramen.

Recognition of spinal veins as normal structure on MR scans is important. The retrovertebral plexus lies on the dorsal surface of the vertebral body beneath the posterior longitudinal ligament. The basivertebral vein (see Fig. 24–2C and D) within the vertebral body drains into the retrovertebral plexus. Radicular veins course through the neural foramina (see Fig. 24–2B), connecting the retrovertebral plexus with the paravertebral venous plexus.

The posterior longitudinal ligament is adherent to the posterior surfaces of the vertebral end plates and intervertebral disks and cannot be separated from the dura, anulus, or bony cortex on MR scans (see Fig. 24–2D). The ligamentum flavum can be identified as a structure of intermediate signal intensity between the laminae (see Figs. 24–3B and 24–4B).[2] The intermediate-signal cartilage of the facet joints is lined on either side by hypointense cortical bone (see Fig. 24–3B).

DEGENERATIVE SPINAL DISEASE (EXTRADURAL)

INTERVERTEBRAL DISK DISEASE

Degenerative disk disease is a major cause of chronic disability in the adult working population and a common reason for referral to an MR imaging center. The normal disk was described above in the anatomy section. With aging, certain biochemical and structural changes occur in the intervertebral disks. There is an increase in the ratio of keratan sulfate to chondroitin sulfate, and the proteoglycans lose their close association with the disk collagen. The disk also loses its water-binding capacity and the water content decreases down to 70 per cent. The vertebral end plates also becomes thinner and more hyalinized.[3] This degree of disk degeneration is considered a normal part of aging.

With more advanced degeneration, dense disorganized fibrous tissue replaces the normal fibrocartilaginous structure of the nucleus pulposus, leaving no distinction between the nucleus and anulus fibrosus. Also, fissures develop in the cartilaginous end plates, and regenerating chondrocytes and granulation tissue form in the area. In an anatomic and MR study of cadaveric spines, Yu et al[4] found three types of anular tears in degenerated disks. Concentric tears had fluid-filled spaces between adjacent lamellae, radial tears represented rupture through all layers of the anulus, and transverse tears were ruptures of Sharpey's fibers at the periphery of the anulus. MR demonstrated only the radial and transverse tears. They also noted that disks with anular tears were of lower signal intensity and had slightly reduced height compared to normal disks, suggesting that anular tears may be partly responsible for the degenerative process.[5] In a separate report,[6] the same group disclosed that complete radial tears were commonly associated with prominently bulging disks. Therefore, a degenerated bulging disk does not necessarily imply that the anulus is intact.

The terminology for describing abnormal disks can be quite confusing and includes a long list, such as "degeneration," "bulge," "protrusion," "herniation," "prolapse," "extrusion," "sequestration," and "free fragment." Part of the reason for the confusion has been the subtlety and in some cases the inaccuracy of the distinguishing features on conventional imaging studies. With its higher contrast resolution, MR promises to clarify disk abnormalities. "Disk degeneration" refers to the biochemical and structural changes described above, but the term is also used to refer to disk disease as a whole. A bulging disk enlarges circumferentially in a symmetric fashion; subtle anular tears may be present (see above) but there is no major disruption of the anulus. Some use "protrusion" and "bulge" interchangeably; we prefer to use the term "protrusion" for a bulging disk that is eccentric to one side, indicating that the nucleus pulposus is beginning to dissect through the anular fibers and thin the anulus. Perhaps protrusions or eccentric bulges occur at sites of radial tears and are potential sites for future herniation.

"Herniated disk" implies rupture of the anulus with extrusion of nucleus pulposus through the defect. The extruded portion remains connected to the parent disk. The term "disk prolapse" has been used to describe a herniated disk covered by a few remaining anular fibers.[7] Perhaps a disk prolapse could also be called a severe protrusion. This is not meant to be facetious, because with the increased resolution of MR, these terms may come to have specific meaning and clinical utility. A sequestered disk is a free fragment of disk material that is no longer attached to the parent disk. Free fragments can migrate above or below the disk space.

Regardless of the terminology, what is most important is the precise relationship between the disk

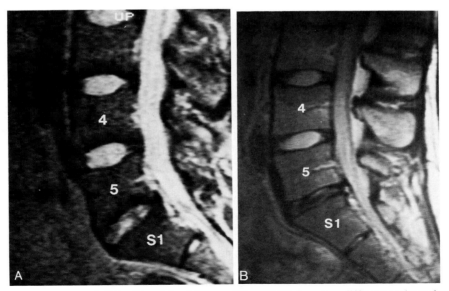

FIGURE 24–5. Degenerated disks. T_2-weighted images (SE 1500/70) from two different patients demonstrate degenerated disks at L5-S1. The disks are relatively hypointense owing to decrease in water content. Degeneration of the disk fibrocartilage and loss of structural integrity result in compression of the disk and decrease in height of the interspace. The disks also bulge slightly posteriorly into the spinal canal. The disks at L3-L4 and L4-L5 are normally hydrated, and the high signal is confined to the central part of the disk.

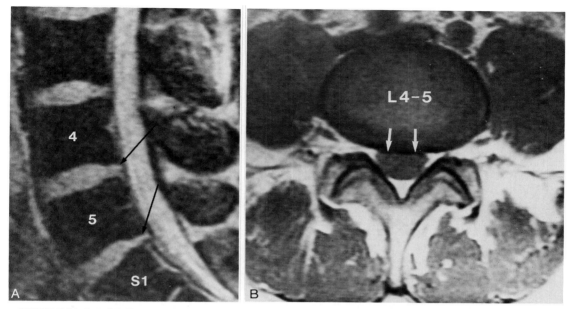

FIGURE 24–6. Mild disk bulge. *A,* Gradient-echo sagittal scan (GRE 33/13, flip angle = 8 degrees). The disks have retained their water content, but the high signal extends more posteriorly *(arrows)* than normal. (Compare with Fig. 24–5, levels L3-L4 and L4-L5.) *B,* Axial proton-density scan (SE 1800/30) confirms a mild central bulging disk *(arrows)* at L4-L5, slightly effacing the ventral thecal sac.

margin and the contiguous neural structures. Clearly, there is a wide range of clinical symptomatology from patient to patient which may not be related so much to the size or shape of an abnormal disk as to the relationship of the disk to the nerve roots.

Degeneration of an intervertebral disk results in a rounded, symmetric bulging of the disk beyond the margins of the vertebral body. MR can detect early disk degeneration because, as the disks lose water, the MR signal decreases on gradient-echo and T_2-weighted images (Fig. 24–5).[8] On T_1-weighted images, the bulging disk may be outlined posteriorly by a low-signal rim delineating the slightly higher-signal disk. This rim of low signal corresponds to the intact anulus and the posterior longitudinal ligament. A bulging disk encroaches on the ventral spinal canal and inferior portion of the foramina but does not displace the nerve roots (Figs. 24–6 and 24–7). The combination of sagittal and axial views provides excellent visualization of the relationships of the disk to the spinal canal and neural foramina.

On the sagittal view, dissection of a degenerated nucleus through fibers of the anulus is clearly depicted (Fig. 24–8). Defects in the anulus with disk extending posteriorly are indicative of herniation. In the sagittal plane, a herniated disk has an hourglass appearance along the posterior disk margin, which could be described as a "squeezed toothpaste" effect

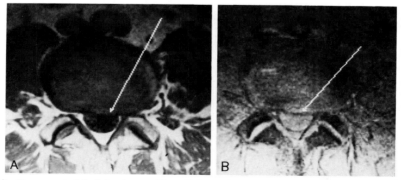

FIGURE 24–7. Degenerated bulging/protruding disk. *A,* SE 650/21 axial 4-mm image. L4-L5 disk bulge *(arrow)* is eccentric to the left and minimally effaces the left ventral thecal sac. The eccentricity could put the abnormality in the category of disk protrusion. *B,* Axial 5-mm gradient-echo image (GRE 100/13, flip angle = 15 degrees) at the same level as *A.* Distinction between the disk and the thecal sac is better secondary to the myelographic effect created by this sequence. The high signal of the nucleus pulposus extends farther out toward the periphery than in a normal disk. (Compare with Fig. 24–4*B.*) The low-signal rim around the disk is the anulus fibrosus and around the thecal sac is the dura.

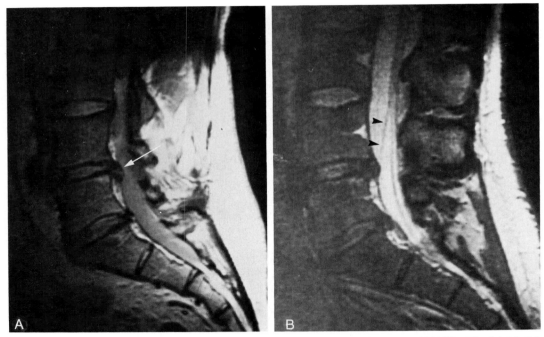

FIGURE 24–8. Herniated intervertebral disk. *A,* Proton density–weighted scan (SE 2000/25). The L4-L5 disk has dissected through the posterior anulus and herniated into the ventral spinal canal *(arrow). B,* On a T$_2$-weighted image (SE 2000/70), the abnormal disk is noted to lie against the L5 nerve root *(arrowheads).* The L5-S1 disk is also degenerated and protruding posteriorly.

(Fig. 24–9). Axial scans show either asymmetry of the posterior disk margin or a soft-tissue mass displacing the adjacent nerve root.[9] Disk fragments are found most often in the ventral-lateral aspect of the canal because the tough posterior longitudinal ligament resists posterior extension near the midline. The neural foramina are visualized on parasagittal images of the lumbar spine, and disk herniation can be detected by obliteration of foraminal fat. Nevertheless, axial images are required for a complete examination of the epidural space around the disk (Fig. 24–10).

A herniated or bulging disk usually impinges on the nerve root as it courses inferiorly toward the foramen at the next lower level. For example, an L4-L5 herniated disk impinges on the L5 root (see Fig. 24–8). The L4 root is likely to be unaffected unless there is lateral and cephalad migration of a free fragment into the neural foramen. Free fragments, or sequestrations, can migrate some distance cephalad or rostral to the disk space (Fig. 24–11), and it is important to alert the surgeon to their precise location. Sequestered disks may have either high or low signal on T$_1$- and T$_2$-weighted images (Fig. 24–12).[7] We have seen a number of cases of extruded fragments that were hyperintense on spin-density images.

Just as with CT, axial MR has the advantage of being able to visualize lateral disk herniations.[10] This type of disk compresses the nerve root within the foramen or just beyond its lateral margin distal to the nerve root sheath (Fig. 24–13) and therefore is often missed on the myelogram. Lateral disks may not be evident on the midsagittal image, and parasagittal views display confusing anatomic relationships of the disk to nearby structures.

Other lesions that can be found in a neural foramen include neurofibromas, synovial cysts, arachnoid diverticula (Fig. 24–14), and soft-tissue extension of neoplasms of the spine and paraspinal regions (see Chapter 23). Although differentiation of these lesions from a sequestered disk may be difficult, it is often possible to distinguish them on the basis of signal characteristics, anatomic location, and clinical history.

A number of conditions can mimic herniated disks. The most common problem is postoperative scarring in patients with recurrent or persistent back pain (see below). Other entities include epidural abscess, epidural tumor, spinal stenosis (see appropriate sections), and conjoint nerve roots. The conjoint root is an anomaly in which two root sleeves, usually L5 and S1, leave the thecal sac together (Fig. 24–15). On axial images it appears as a mass in the ventral-lateral aspect of the spinal canal. The mass is usually located at the midportion of the vertebral body, and on more inferior axial images the nerve root is positioned anteriorly, an important clue for conjoint root. A herniated disk displaces the root posteriorly. Another clue is enlargement of the lateral recess at the same level, indicating the longstanding nature of the abnormality. In doubtful situations, a myelogram readily clarifies the condition.

The determination of clinically significant disk disease is an important radiologic and clinical decision because the possible consequences of back surgery

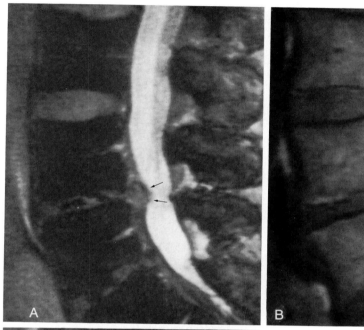

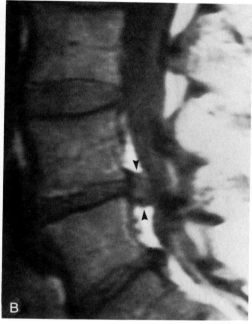

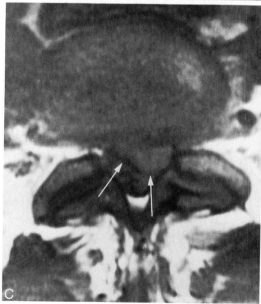

FIGURE 24–9. Herniated intervertebral disk. *A*, Gradient-echo MR scan (GRE 33/13, flip angle = 8 degrees) discloses a herniated disk *(arrows)* at the level of L4-L5, producing a ventral extradural impression on the thecal sac. The intervertebral disks at both L4-L5 and L5-S1 are degenerated, with decreased signal intensity and disk height. The markedly hypointense areas within the disks represent either calcification or air. *B*, On a T₁-weighted image (SE 600/20), the disk fragment *(arrowheads)* is outlined by the hyperintense epidural fat. The disk at L5-S1 also bulges posteriorly into the spinal canal. This bulging disk is difficult to see on the gradient-echo image *(A)* because the degenerated disk is isointense to the epidural fat and does not efface the thecal sac. *C*, An axial scan (SE 600/20) confirms the large herniated disk *(arrows)* located in the left anterolateral aspect of the spinal canal, compressing the thecal sac and nerve roots. (From Hesselink JR: Spine imaging: History, achievements, remaining frontiers. AJR 150:1223–1229, 1988.)

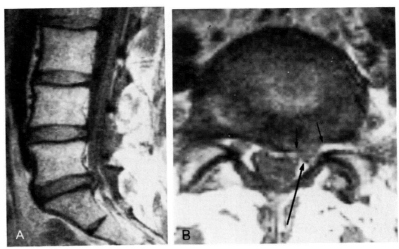

FIGURE 24–10. Herniated/extruded disk. *A,* SE 500/40 sagittal 5-mm image. A bulging disk is noted at L5-S1, indenting the ventral aspect of the thecal sac. *B,* SE 1000/40 axial 5-mm image. In addition to the bulging disk, an extruded fragment *(long arrow)* is present in the left lateral recess and impinges on the left S1 nerve root. Note the defect in the anulus *(small arrows)* and the asymmetry of the epidural fat in the ventral lateral spinal canal.

are not insignificant. Identification of displacement of a spinal nerve root or severe effacement of the thecal sac, especially ventrolaterally, that correlates with radicular pain or a muscle weakness pattern supports the operative approach to therapy when conservative medical therapy has failed.[11] At times, direct visualization of the nerve root can be difficult. Asymmetry of the epidural fat with displacement of fat out of the ventrolateral canal or neural foramen is an important sign for disk herniation.[12] When there is a generalized paucity of epidural fat, producing an MR "myelogram" with gradient-echo or T_2-weighted images may be beneficial. Using this technique, it is frequently easier to identify the interface between the disk and thecal sac. As with CT, MR is also helpful in those patients with a wide epidural space at the level of L5-S1. Prominent epidural fat results in increased distance between the disk space and the ventral margin of the thecal sac and therefore an insensitive myelogram.

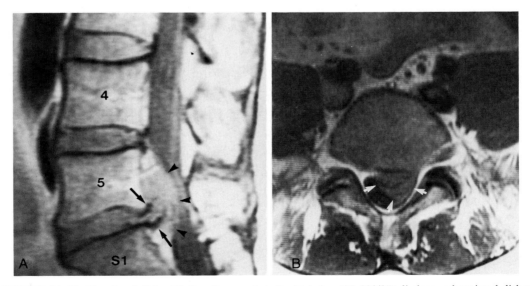

FIGURE 24–11. Herniated disk with free fragment. *A,* Sagittal view (SE 600/25) discloses a herniated disk at L5-S1 with a large free fragment *(arrowheads)* that has migrated superiorly. The ragged-appearing hypointensities *(arrows)* are remnants of the anulus and posterior longitudinal ligament. *B,* Axial view (SE 1800/30) shows the large fragment *(arrows)* of disk in the ventrolateral spinal canal.

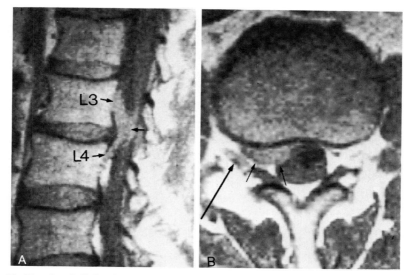

FIGURE 24–12. Herniated disk with sequestration. *A,* SE 500/40 sagittal image. At L3-L4, there is a large fragment of disk *(arrows)* in the ventral epidural space that is separated from its parent disk. This free fragment (sequestration) has migrated superiorly along the posterior margin of the L3 vertebral body. The signal characteristics of the fragment are similar to those of disk material. Note that the contiguous disc space is slightly narrowed. *B,* SE 500/40 axial image. The sequestered disk *(small arrows)* identified on the sagittal images extends posteriorly to efface the ventrolateral aspect of the thecal sac and laterally into the neural foramen to displace the L3 nerve root and ganglion posteriorly *(long arrow).* Typically, extruded fragments maintain signal characteristics similar to those of normal nucleus pulposus.

SPONDYLOSIS

Some degree of spondylosis is invariably associated with degenerative disk disease. Decrease in height of the intervertebral disk places more stress on the facet joints, leading to degenerative joint disease. Moreover, with the loss of structural strength at the disk level, exaggerated motion occurs at the facet joints, accelerating the degenerative changes and placing stress upon the posterior supporting ligaments as well.

Not all back pain or sciatica is due to herniated disks. Since the facet joints are innervated by branches of the posterior root ganglion, *facet joint disease* can produce radicular pain. The first change noted in the facet joints is bony sclerosis, which

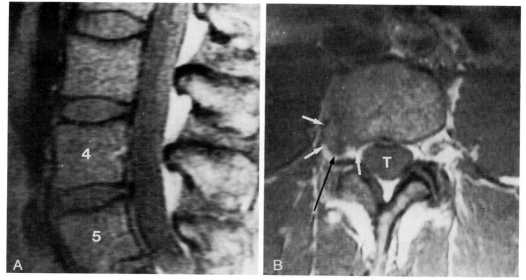

FIGURE 24–13. Lateral herniated disk. *A,* Midsagittal scan (SE 600/25) shows only mild degeneration and bulging of the disk at L4-L5. *B,* Axial view (SE 1800/30) reveals a large lateral herniated disk *(white arrows).* The right L4 nerve root *(black arrow)* is displaced posteriorly. The normal left root is surrounded by epidural fat. The thecal sac (T) is not deformed.

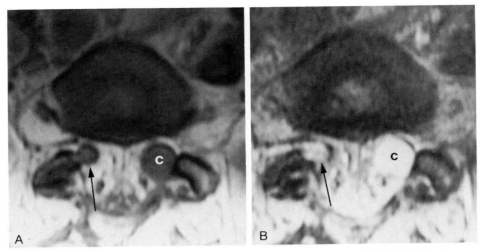

FIGURE 24–14. Tarlov's cyst. Proton-density *(A)*, and T$_2$-weighted *(B)* scans (SE 1800/30,60) demonstrate a round cystic mass (C) in the left ventrolateral spinal canal. On the T$_2$-weighted scan, it becomes hyperintense and follows the signal intensity of the opposite root sleeve *(arrow)*. Findings are consistent with a Tarlov's cyst or a root sleeve diverticulum.

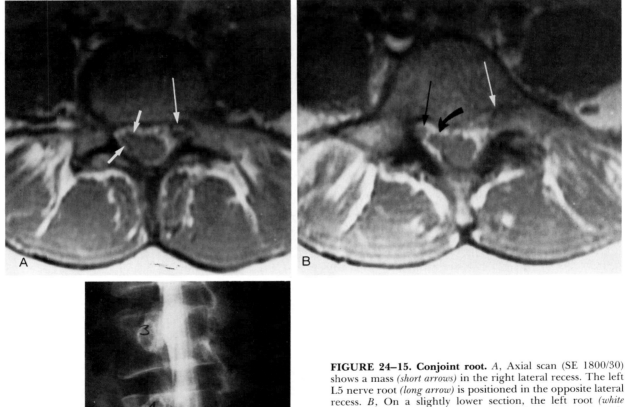

FIGURE 24–15. Conjoint root. *A*, Axial scan (SE 1800/30) shows a mass *(short arrows)* in the right lateral recess. The left L5 nerve root *(long arrow)* is positioned in the opposite lateral recess. *B*, On a slightly lower section, the left root *(white arrow)* is in the foramen. The right L5 nerve root *(straight black arrow)* has separated from the "mass," leaving the S1 root *(curved arrow)* within the epidural space. *C*, A lumbar myelogram confirms that the L5 and S1 nerve roots *(arrows)* exit the thecal sac together.

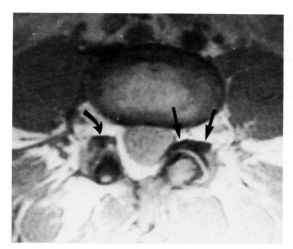

FIGURE 24–16. Facet joint disease. The left superior facet *(arrows)* is sclerotic and hypertrophied. Degenerative changes of the right facet joint *(curved arrow)* are also present, with some sclerosis, facet hypertrophy, and irregularity of the joint space.

appears black on the MR images (Fig. 24–16). These changes are associated with narrowing and irregularity of the articular surfaces, followed by bony hypertrophy of the facets (Fig. 24–17). Facet joint hypertrophy, along with osteophyte formation along the posterior lateral margins of the vertebral body, can encroach upon the lateral recesses of the spinal canal and the neural foramina.[13] Compression of the existing nerve roots results in a radicular pain syndrome called the *lateral recess syndrome.*

When the operative approach to treatment is considered, the distinction between hypertrophic bone formation and herniated disk is important. The dis-

tinction can usually be made by MR on a morphologic basis, but it becomes more difficult when the disk is severely degenerated and desiccated, making it more isointense to bone. The dense sclerotic bone of an osteophytic spur is markedly hypointense on MR. With larger ones, a component of marrow extends into the osteophyte (Fig. 24–18). Osteophytes encroaching on neural foramina are contrasted nicely by foraminal fat on T_1-weighted scans. Visualization of those that project into the spinal canal depends on the amount of fat that is present in the ventral epidural space. If no fat is there to provide contrast, the marrow component of the osteophyte is still seen, but the cap of bone may be silhouetted by adjacent low-signal CSF within the thecal sac. In those cases, T_2-weighted or gradient-echo images display the abnormal anatomy better. Other low-signal abnormalities, such as calcification or air in a bulging degenerated disk, can have a similar appearance, but usually the combination of sagittal and axial scans differentiates these lesions.

SPINAL STENOSIS

Spinal stenosis is due to congenitally short pedicles or may be acquired as a result of combined facet hypertrophy, degenerated bulging disk, and hypertrophy of the ligamentum flavum. Spondylolisthesis and surgical fusion are other causes of spinal stenosis.

Spinal stenosis is graphically displayed in the sagittal plane by gradient-echo pulse sequences (Fig. 24–19). The hyperintense thecal sac is effaced anteriorly by the bulging disk and osteophytes and posteriorly by the ligamentum flavum, resulting in an hourglass configuration. Acquired spinal stenosis is usually associated with moderate to severe multilevel disk degeneration, consisting of loss of normal signal, disk space narrowing, and calcification and air within the disks. The calcification and air cannot be identified with certainty on MR. On axial views the constricted canal often has a triangular or trefoil shape due to encroachment on the ventral-lateral aspect of the canal by hypertrophied facets.[13]

Owing to normal variations in spinal canal size, radiographic studies may suggest spinal stenosis when clinically patients are free from symptoms of this disease. This is more likely to occur with CT because the inherent contrast of plain CT does not permit accurate assessment of the degree of cauda equina crowding in the spinal canal. Myelography, on the other hand, demonstrates obstruction to contrast flow or constriction with an hourglass appearance of the thecal sac in severe cases of spinal stenosis. The CSF(contrast):nerve root ratio is markedly decreased. MR can also demonstrate "crowding" or clumping of nerve roots on axial and sagittal images. With T_1-weighting, a focal increase in signal can be seen in the thecal sac where the cauda equina roots pass through the stenotic canal. Similarly, the roots within the thecal sac are outlined by high-signal CSF

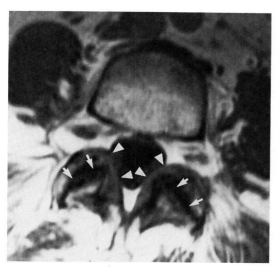

FIGURE 24–17. Severe facet joint disease. A T_1-weighted scan (SE 600/25) demonstrates severe degenerative disease of the facet joints bilaterally. The joint spaces *(arrows)* are markedly narrowed and irregular, and the articular surfaces are sclerotic. The ligamentum flavum *(arrowheads)* is also hypertrophied on both sides.

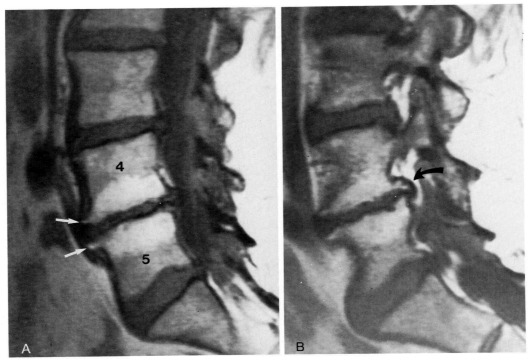

FIGURE 24–18. Spondylosis with foraminal stenosis. Patient has had previous laminectomies and diskectomies at L4-L5. *A*, T_1-weighted scan (SE 600/25) demonstrates severe degenerative changes at L4-L5, with marked disk space narrowing and irregularity of the vertebral end plates. Prominent osteophytes *(arrows)* are present anteriorly. The bands of bright signal in the adjacent vertebral bodies represent fatty replacement of bone marrow. *B*, On a parasagittal section (SE 600/25), a large osteophyte *(curved arrow)* projects into the inferior aspect of the left L4-L5 neural foramen. Note that the marrow extends into the base of the osteophyte.

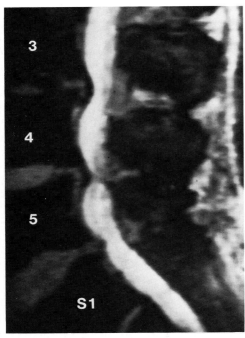

FIGURE 24–19. Spinal stenosis. Sagittal gradient-echo image (GRE 33/13, flip angle = 15 degrees) demonstrates constriction of the spinal canal at multiple levels owing to bulging, degenerated disks. Hypertrophy of the ligamentum flavum contributes to a severe stenosis at L4-L5.

on T_2-weighted and gradient-echo images. When approaching a stenotic area on successive sections, the nerve roots become crowded together and the amount of CSF becomes progressively diminished.

Spondylolisthesis refers to forward displacement of one vertebra over another, usually of the fifth lumbar over the body of the sacrum, or of the fourth lumbar over the fifth. It is often associated with a spondylolysis, a developmental defect, or fracture of the pars interarticularis (Fig. 24–20). The pars defect is demonstrated best in the sagittal plane and is easier to see if the bone has a generous component of marrow or if soft tissue is interposed between the bone fragments.[14] A spondylisthesis results in elongation of the spinal canal in its anteroposterior dimension because the vertebral body moves forward, leaving the posterior elements behind. Spondylolisthesis is graded according to how far the vertebral body moves forward on the one below (grade 1 = 25 per cent; grade 2 = 50 per cent; grade 3 = 75 per cent).

A degenerative spondylolisthesis develops when there are severe degenerative changes and excess motion of the facet joints. Subluxation at the facet joints allows forward or posterior movement of one vertebra over another. A degenerative spondylolisthesis narrows the spinal canal and is more likely to compromise the neural foramina.

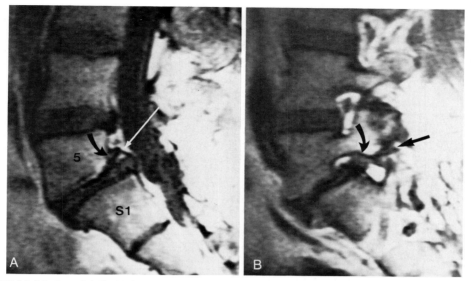

FIGURE 24–20. Spondylolisthesis with spondylolysis. *A,* A sagittal scan (SE 600/20) shows anterior subluxation of L5 on S1 (grade 1 spondylolisthesis). The intervertebral disk has maintained its relationship to S1, and the posterior longitudinal ligament *(white arrow)* has been torn off the posterior body of L5. There is erosion of the posteroinferior aspect of L5 *(curved arrow)*, with formation of an osteophyte. *B,* A parasagittal scan reveals discontinuity (spondylolysis) of the pars interarticularis *(straight arrow)*. The L5 nerve root *(curved arrow)* is compressed with the neural foramen.

POSTOPERATIVE SPINE

The decision to perform surgery on patients with lumbar pain syndromes in the absence of objective neurologic deficit(s) must be weighed carefully against the potential for postoperative failed back syndrome with its attendant chronic pain and limited functional recovery. Reportedly, failed back syndrome occurs in 10 to 40 per cent of postoperative patients. Explanations for this include recurrent disk herniation, epidural scar formation, lateral recess or neural foraminal stenosis, and arachnoiditis.[15] More commonly, the radiologist is asked to evaluate patients with recurrent back pain sometime following surgery, and the primary differential diagnosis is between recurrent disk herniation and epidural scarring. Myelography and noncontrast CT are very difficult to interpret in this group of patients. CT with intravenous contrast has been reported to be 74 to 87 per cent accurate for distinguishing recurrent disk herniation from epidural scar.[16] However, unless rigorous bolus injection techniques are used, the results are often less satisfactory. In our experience, referring clinicians have limited faith in the ability of these techniques to distinguish scar from recurrent disk herniation.

In the early postoperative period, interpretation of the MR images is extremely difficult. The presence of fat graft, hematoma (Fig. 24–21), gas, and inflammation (see Fig. 23–38) complicates the observed signal intensities.[17] Moreover, recurrent disk and epidural scar exhibit similar topographical and signal characteristics (hypo- or isointense to disk on T₁-weighted images and hyperintense to disk on T₂-weighted images).

After about 1 month, the acute postoperative changes resolve, making it easier to distinguish scar from disk. As before surgery, recurrent disk is often in continuity with the parent disk (Fig. 24–22). Dis-

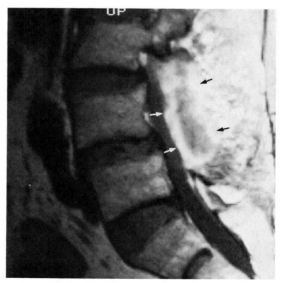

FIGURE 24–21. Postoperative epidural hematoma. Patient had a recent laminectomy at L4 and L5. A sagittal section (SE 550/21) reveals a retrothecal mass that has a rim of high signal *(arrows)* and a central region of intermediate signal. The high-signal rim on this T₁-weighted image is due to the paramagnetic effect of methemoglobin in the hematoma. Note the degenerated L4-L5 disk and slight anterior subluxation of L4 on L5.

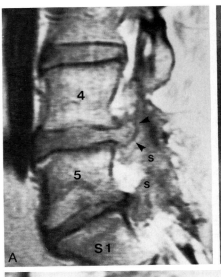

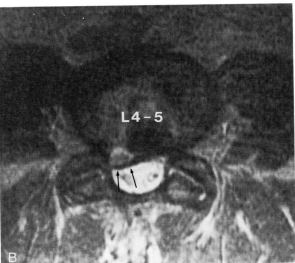

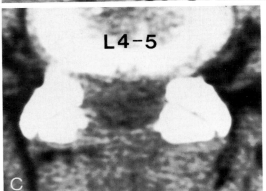

FIGURE 24–22. Recurrent herniated disk. Patient had previous laminectomies and disk excisions at L4-L5 and L5-S1. *A*, Sagittal MR scan (SE 2000/25) reveals a fragment of disk material *(arrowheads)* herniated posteriorly from the L4-L5 interspace. Intermediate signal scar tissue *(small s's)* is present at both operated levels. A thin black line separates the disk from the scar. *B*, On a T₂-weighted axial image (SE 2000/70), the extruded disk *(arrows)* compresses the right ventrolateral thecal sac and the proximal L5 root sleeve. (From Hesselink JR: Spine imaging: History, achievements, remaining frontiers. AJR 150:1223–1229, 1988.) *C*, On a corresponding CT scan, the disk cannot be distinguished from epidural scar.

continuity in the anulus fibrosus is not entirely reliable because it can result from the surgical incision as well as from disk rupture. Unless the disk material has become separated as a free fragment or sequestration, it remains similar in signal characteristics to the parent disk on both T₁- and T₂-weighted images (Fig. 24–23). In general, herniated disks are relatively well-defined and, in some cases, have a hypointense rim.[18] The hypointense perimeter probably represents a combination of remnants of the anulus and posterior longitudinal ligament, dura, and focal hemorrhage at the time of surgery. The observation that the dark rim becomes thicker and more obvious on T₂-weighted images is suggestive of hemosiderin or chronic hemorrhage.

On the other hand, epidural scar has poorly defined margins and is either isointense or hypointense on short TR/TE sequences compared to the adjacent disk (see Fig. 24–22).[19] With more T₂-weighting, scar generally increases in signal, but to a lesser degree many months or years after surgery. In addition, if the soft-tissue abnormality can be followed posteriorly along the lateral margin of the spinal canal to the region of the laminectomy, it is probably scar (Fig. 24–24). Retraction of the thecal sac to the side of the soft tissue is another sign favoring postoperative scar.

Gd-DTPA should be used routinely in the postoperative back because it is a valuable aid for differentiating the various postoperative tissues. Epidural scar enhances to a much greater degree on MR than on contrast-enhanced CT. The enhancing scar clearly identifies nerve roots trapped within the scar (Fig. 24–25) and outlines any retained or recurrent disk fragments. A disk fragment induces a local inflammatory reaction, and vascular granulation tissue often forms about its perimeter. As a result, the perimeter of a herniated disk may enhance with Gd-DTPA, but the central part will not, thus distinguishing it from epidural scar (Fig. 24–26).

SACRAL LESIONS

CHORDOMA

Chordomas are relatively rare skeletal neoplasms that arise from notochordal remnants in the skull and spine. About one half of chordomas occur in the sacrum, another 35 per cent in the clivus, and the remainder in the vertebrae. They are slow-growing tumors but locally aggressive and invasive. They are

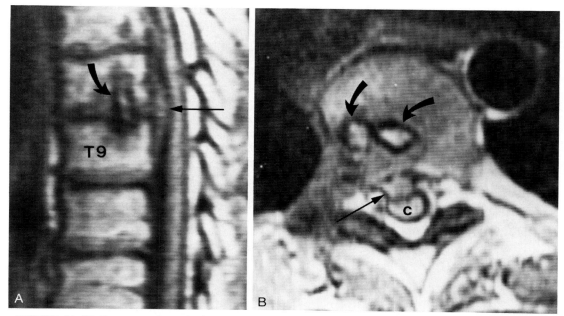

FIGURE 24–23. Recurrent thoracic disk. Patient has had previous disk excision and anterior fusion at T8-T9. *A,* Sagittal and *B,* axial scans (SE 600/20) show recurrent disk herniation *(long arrow)* at T8-T9. The disk fragment compresses the thecal sac and ventrolateral aspect of the cord (c). Two bone fragments *(curved arrows)* have been surgically placed to aid fusion at that interspace.

predominantly lytic and commonly break through the bony cortex to extend into the presacral and pelvic regions. Calcifications and bone remnants are often scattered within the soft-tissue mass. The sacral nerve roots are generally entangled within the mass.[20]

Sagittal MR images are particularly good for displaying the destroyed areas of the sacrum and the relationship of the tumor to the pelvic viscera anteriorly and the gluteal muscles posteriorly.[21] Chordomas are slightly hypointense on T_1-weighted images and hyperintense on T_2-weighted images (Fig. 24–27). They often have a heterogeneous internal texture owing to calcification, necrosis, and gelatinous mucoid collections.[22, 23]

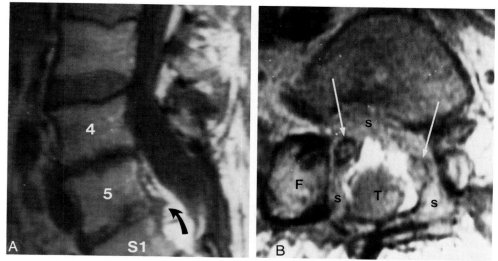

FIGURE 24–24. Postoperative epidural scar. Patient has had laminectomy and multiple disk excisions at L4-L5 and L5-S1. *A,* Sagittal view (SE 600/20) shows disk space narrowing and degenerative changes at both operated levels. Some soft-tissue intensity *(curved arrow)* is present posteriorly at L5-S1. *B,* Axial scan (SE 1800/35) at L5-S1. F = Lateral fusion bone; T = thecal sac; s = epidural scar. There is extensive scarring in the epidural space. Some high-signal epidural fat is positioned between the thecal sac and the scar. The S1 nerve roots *(arrows)* are embedded within the scar tissue. No disk material is identified.

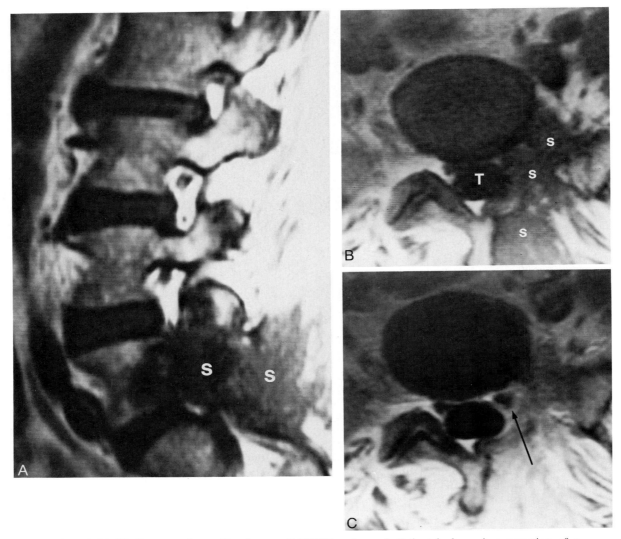

FIGURE 24–25. Postoperative epidural scar, Gd-DTPA enhanced. Patient had previous resection of a neurofibroma. *A* and *B*, Plain T₁-weighted scans (SE 600/20) show extensive scar tissue (s's) along the lateral aspect of L5. The posterior scar tissue is of higher signal intensity because it is closer to the surface coil. The CSF-containing thecal sac (T) is hypointense. *C*, Following contrast injection (SE 600/20, Gd-DTPA) the scar tissue enhances to distinguish it from disk. The S1 nerve root sleeve *(arrow)* is embedded within the scar.

TERATOMA

Teratomas are multipotential tumors that contain tissues of all three germ layers, such as skin, hair, and teeth of ectodermal origin; cartilage, connective tissue, and fat of mesodermal origin; and intestinal epithelium and glandular tissue of endodermal origin. The sacrococcygeal region is a favorite site in infancy and childhood. Teratomas cause marked destruction of the sacrum and can grow into quite large masses, filling the pelvic cavity. Malignant transformation into carcinomas and sarcomas is common.[24]

Their varied histology is reflected in their distinctly heterogeneous appearance on MR. The solid soft-tissue parts are of intermediate signal, dental elements are hypointense, and cystic areas are hyperintense on T₂-weighted images, and the fatty components are hyperintense on T₁-weighted scans.

PAGET'S DISEASE

Paget's disease, or osteitis deformans, is an acquired disorder of unknown etiology. Normal bone is destroyed and replaced by poorly mineralized osteoid matrix. The new defective bone is associated with a large soft-tissue component that contains a great deal of fibrous tissue. The bones most often involved are the pelvis, skull, femur, and spine,

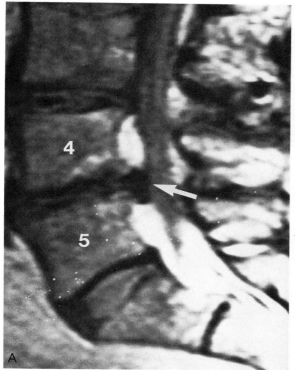

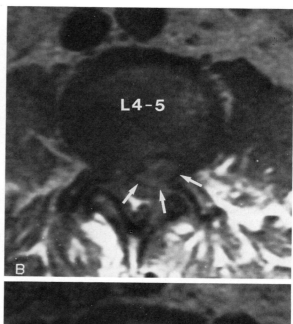

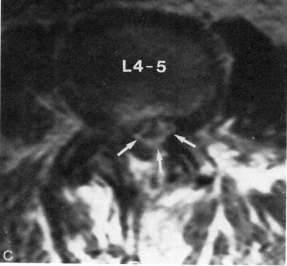

FIGURE 24–26. Recurrent herniated disk, Gd-DTPA enhanced. Patient had previous left laminectomy and disk excision at L4-L5. *A*, A sagittal scan (SE 600/20) demonstrates degenerated disks at L3-L4 and L4-L5, associated with disk space narrowing. Low signal within the disks represents air or calcification. A hypointense mass *(arrow)* projects posteriorly from the L4-L5 interspace. *B*, Noncontrast axial scan (SE 600/20) reveals a poorly defined mass *(arrows)* in the left ventrolateral spinal canal at L4-L5. *C*, Axial scan (SE 600/20, Gd-DTPA). Following contrast injection, the perimeter of the mass *(arrows)* enhances, but the central portion does not, consistent with a herniated disk. Note enhancement of the scar tissue at the laminectomy site posteriorly.

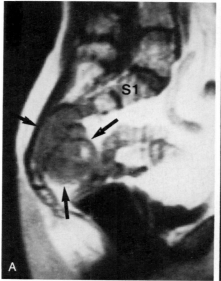

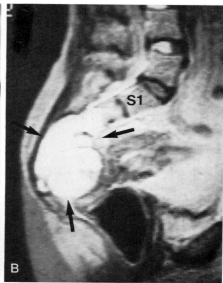

FIGURE 24–27. Sacral chordoma. *A*, T$_1$-weighted (SE 500/30) and *B*, T$_2$-weighted (SE 1500/60) images demonstrate a destructive lesion *(arrows)* involving the mid-sacral segments. A soft-tissue mass extends into the pelvic cavity. The tumor is hypointense on the T$_1$ image and hyperintense on the T$_2$ image.

followed by other long bones and the mandible. The pagetoid bone is structurally weak, and vertebral compression fractures are common.[25]

Paget's disease results in enlarged, expanded bone that has a heterogeneous texture. The soft-tissue matrix accounts for the intermediate signal intensity on T_1-weighted images and hyperintensity on T_2-weighted images. The mineralized components, underestimated by MR, become more prominent in later stages of the disease.

Many other diseases of the bone and marrow can also involve the sacrum and coccyx. Metastatic disease, primary bone tumors, and bone marrow diseases are discussed in Chapter 23 in the section on vertebral and paravertebral abnormalities. Moreover, neoplasia of the pelvic organs can secondarily involve the sacrum. Many of the spinal dysraphic states affect the sacrum (see section on spinal dysraphism).

INTRADURAL EXTRAMEDULLARY DISEASE

ARACHNOIDITIS

One of the complications occurring after surgery, meningitis, subarachnoid hemorrhage, and Pantopaque myelography is the development of arachnoiditis. Unfortunately, this condition can result in a debilitating pain syndrome that has no effective treatment. In many patients with low back and extremity pain, morphologic evidence of extradural root compression is absent, and in a small number of these patients, the cause is arachnoiditis. This condition results from adhesion of nerve roots and the occasional formation of loculated cavities within the thecal sac that may expand and cause mechanical compression of contiguous neural structures. Water-soluble contrast myelography with CT is very sensitive for the detection of this phenomenon because of the excellent spatial and tissue-contrast resolution achieved with contrast and radiographic technique. As both spatial and tissue-contrast resolution of MR improve with better surface coil design, the diagnosis of arachnoiditis can be made noninvasively but not easily. Morphologic signs of arachnoiditis include clumping of the nerve roots within the thecal sac with the creation of an intradural pseudomass (Fig. 24–28). Adhesion of individual nerve roots to the inner margins of the arachnoid mater gives the appearance of an empty thecal sac.[26] The intradural cysts can be difficult to detect if their contents have signal characteristics similar to those of CSF. If their protein content is increased, T_1 shortening results in increased signal on T_1-weighted images. Damping of CSF pulsations may become apparent on gradient-echo or T_2-weighted sequences. No study performed to date has shown, however, that MR is more sensitive than myelography and CTM in the diagnosis of arachnoiditis. Fortunately, since Pantopaque has

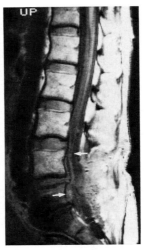

FIGURE 24–28. Arachnoiditis, postoperative lumbar spine. SE 650/12 sagittal 4-mm slice. Intradural nerve roots of the cauda equina have a serpiginous course within the thecal sac and, in some regions, appear clumped *(arrows)*. While not specific, these changes suggest arachnoiditis. No cystic loculations are evident. Note degenerative changes at L4-L5 and L5-S1.

been replaced by nonionic, water-soluble agents for myelography, arachnoiditis has become much less common.

PANTOPAQUE

Residual Pantopaque continues to be found in patients who previously had myelography with this agent. On both CT and plain films, its detection poses no real problem. However, to the unwary, residual Pantopaque may look like other pathology on MR. Pantopaque has a short T_1 and short T_2 (Fig. 24–29)[27] and may have identical signal characteristics to an intraspinal lipoma or hemorrhage (intracellular methemoglobin). Droplets of Pantopaque are usually spherical and sharply marginated. Nevertheless, reported cases and our own experience have demonstrated that while the differentiation between Pantopaque and an intraspinal lesion should be straightforward, this is not always the case. When doubt exists, plain films should be obtained.

SPINAL DYSRAPHISM

A tethered spinal cord is associated with a large number of the dorsal dysraphic states, including myelomeningocele, lipomyeloschisis (dorsal dysraphism with lipoma), myelocystocele, dorsal dermal sinus, and caudal regression. Identifying the tethered cord is paramount (Fig. 24–30). Although this can be accomplished with myelography and CTM, the risk of puncturing the tethered cord or injecting contrast into a loculated fluid collection is avoided

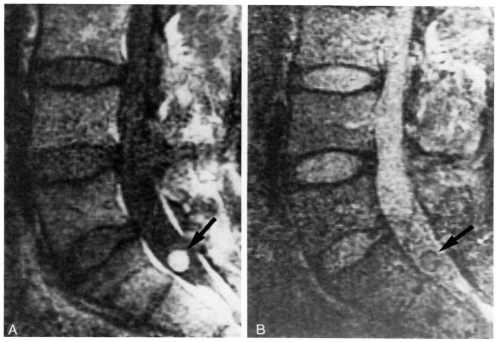

FIGURE 24–29. Pantopaque. *A*, T_1-weighted (SE 600/25) and *B*, T_2-weighted (SE 1800/60) scans disclose a globule of Pantopaque *(arrow)* in the caudal thecal sac. Pantopaque is a fatty oil and follows the signal intensity of fat (hyperintense on T_1- and hypointense on T_2-weighted images).

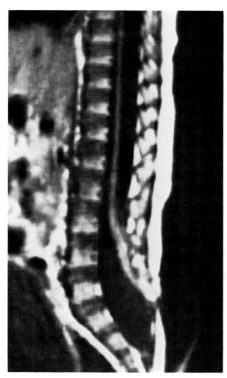

FIGURE 24–30. Spinal dysraphism with tethered cord. On a sagittal scan (SE 600/25), the cord continues down into the lumbar region and is tethered posteriorly at the lumbosacral junction. The lower canal is widened and the posterior bony elements are deficient.

with MR, which provides all the necessary information in the vast majority of cases. A thickened filum may be difficult to distinguish on MR, especially when the conus terminates at a normal level. Thickening of the filum can be simulated by normally clumped ventral and dorsal roots situated in the posterior aspect of the thecal sac.

Subsequent to identification of a tethered cord, the etiology must be determined. Intraspinal lipoma is seen as a high-signal lesion on short TR/TE sequences and may have both intramedullary and extramedullary components (Fig. 24–31). The mass may be confined to an intraspinal intradural location (Fig. 24–32), or it may extend into a dysraphic abnormality (lipomyelomeningocele). In dorsal dermal sinus, the tethered cord may extend into the sinus, and the tract itself can be traced to its exit zone at the skin surface. A number of other features associated with tethered cord require definition, such as the location of the neural placode, fibrovascular tethering band(s), ventral and dorsal roots, dorsal root entry zones, any nerve roots crossing in an aberrant fashion, and associated hydrosyringomyelia.[28] Some features can be inferred, as in lipomyeloschisis, by the location of the "kinked" dorsal surface of the cord (fibrovascular band) and the more caudal location of the neural placode. It has been noted that a flattened neural placode may be inseparable from the thecal sac. Additionally, it may be difficult to determine whether a low-lying placode in a dorsal meningocele is actually tethered or simply positioned in the me-

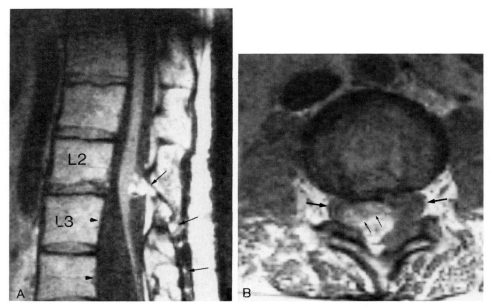

FIGURE 24–31. Tethered cord with lipomyeloschisis. *A*, SE 500/40 sagittal image. Tethered cord with a thickened filum is identified. The conus terminates at L3. There is a multilobulated lipoma intimately associated with the spinal cord, with small lobules of fat extending dorsally and inferiorly into an endodermal sinus tract *(arrows)* that communicates with the skin surface (not shown). Dural ectasia is also demonstrated with slight scalloping of lower vertebral bodies *(arrowheads)*. *B*, SE 500/40 axial image. There appears to be a broad site of attachment of the spinal cord to the lipoma *(small arrows)*. The position of coursing roots is not clearly defined owing to the technique's limits of resolution. As in *A*, note the dural ectasia with expansion of the root sleeves *(large arrows)*.

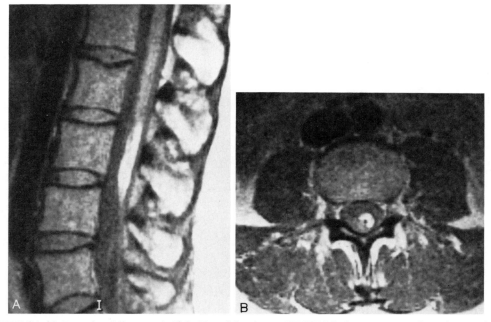

FIGURE 24–32. Intradural lipoma. *A*, Plain T_1-weighted scan (SE 500/40) demonstrates a hyperintense lesion in the intradural space contiguous with the conus. There was no history of previous Pantopaque myelogram or acute event to suggest hemorrhage. Patient had two previous CT scans at L4-S1 for low back pain and right leg radicular syndrome. *B*, On an axial scan (SE 1500/40), the high-signal lipoma is located on the left anterior surface of the cord. Focal low signal in the center of the lesion most likely represents the filum terminale.

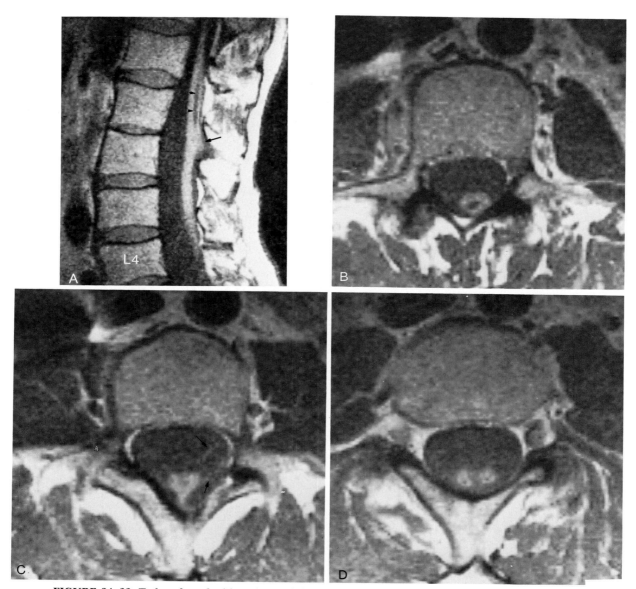

FIGURE 24–33. Tethered cord with syrinx and diastematomyelia. *A*, SE 500/40 sagittal image. The conus terminates at L4, consistent with tethering. There is a band of tissue similar in signal to cord parenchyma that extends dorsally at L1-L2 *(arrow)*, but no definite association with a lipoma or meningocele is seen. Immediately rostral to the site of tethering, there is a low-signal zone within the cord parenchyma, suggesting an associated syrinx cavity *(arrowheads)*. *B–D*, SE 500/40 axial images from L1 to L3. The most rostral image *(B)* demonstrates a clearly defined low-signal syrinx cavity within the cord. At the point of tethering *(C)*, the cord has an irregular configuration, with a "tail" of tissue extending into the retrothecal region. The thecal sac is expanded (dural ectasia) with minimal scalloping of the posterior margin of L2. Small dorsal and central roots *(arrows)* are seen coursing toward the neural foramina. In *D*, the cord is split into two distinct structures.

ningocele as a result of tethering more cephalic by the fibrovascular band.[29] At the present time, spatial resolution of state-of-the-art MR does not permit clear visualization of individual nerve roots, and the roots may not be adequately assessed by this technique. When surgical planning requires this information, further study with intrathecal contrast CT may be needed.

In the thoracic spine diastematomyelia and diplomyelia (true split cord) have been identified and may simulate the appearance of a hydromyelia on sagittal images. Further evaluation with axial images defines the true nature of the abnormality by characterizing the two round or ovoid components of the split cord (Fig. 24–33).[30] On short TR/TE images, the osseous spur, unless it contains marrow, or a fibrous septum may be difficult to distinguish from a CSF cleft that may be present between the two elements of separated spinal cord. Gradient-echo or long TR/TE sequences that produce a myelographic effect often clarify the situation because a dark spur or septum is contrasted against the bright CSF.[31] In some cases, differentiation between these two structures may require further evaluation with plain CT. Diastematomyelia or diplomyelia is frequently associated with a tethered cord.

REFERENCES

1. Coventry MB: Anatomy of the intervertebral disk. Clin Orthop 67:9–15, 1969.
2. Ho PSP, Yu S, Sether LA, et al: Ligamentum flavum: Appearance on sagittal and coronal MR images. Radiology 168:469–472, 1988.
3. Modic MT, Masaryk TJ, Ross JS, Carter JR: Imaging of degenerative disk disease. Radiology 168:177–186, 1988.
4. Yu S, Haughton VM, Sether LA, Wagner M: Anulus fibrosus in bulging intervertebral disks. Radiology 169:761–763, 1988.
5. Yu S, Haughton VM, Ho PSP, et al: Progressive and regressive changes in the nucleus pulposus. Part II. The adult. Radiology 169:93–97, 1988.
6. Yu S, Sether LA, Ho PSP, et al: Tears of the anulus fibrosus: Correlation between MR and pathologic findings in cadavers. AJNR 9:367–370, 1988.
7. Masaryk TJ, Ross JS, Modic MT, et al: High-resolution MR imaging of sequestered lumbar intervertebral disks. AJNR 9:351–358, 1988.
8. Hesselink JR: Spine imaging: History, achievements, remaining frontiers. AJR 150:1223–1229, 1988.
9. Lee SH, Coleman PE, Hahn FJ: Magnetic resonance imaging of degenerative disk disease of the spine. Radiol Clin North Am 26:949–964, 1988.
10. Osborn AG, Hood RS, Sherry RG, et al: CT/MR spectrum of far lateral and anterior lumbosacral disk herniations. AJNR 9:775–778, 1988.
11. Modic MT, Hardy RW, Weinstein MA, et al: Nuclear magnetic resonance of the spine: Clinical potential and limitations. Neurosurgery 15:583–592, 1984.
12. Edelman RR, Shoukimas GM, Stark DD, et al: High resolution surface-coil imaging of lumbar disk disease. AJNR 6:479–485, 1985.
13. Grenier N, Kressel HY, Schiebler ML, et al: Normal and degenerative posterior spinal structures: MR imaging. Radiology 165:517–525, 1987.
14. Johnson DW, Farnum GN, Latchaw RE, Erba SM: MR imaging of the pars interarticularis. AJNR 9:1215–1220, 1988.
15. Burton CV, Kirkaldy-Willis WH, Yong-Hing K, Heithoff KB: Causes of failure of surgery on the lumbar spine. Clin Orthop 157:191–199, 1981.
16. Firvoznia H, Kricheff II, Rafii M, et al: Lumbar spine after surgery: Examination with intravenous contrast enhanced CT. Radiology 163:221–226, 1987.
17. Ross JS, Masaryk TJ, Modic MT, et al: Lumbar spine: Postoperative assessment with surface-coil MR imaging. Radiology 164:851–860, 1987.
18. Hochhauser L, Kieffer SA, Cacayorin ED, et al: Recurrent postdiskectomy low back pain: MR-surgical correlation. AJNR 9:769–774, 1988.
19. Bundschuh CV, Modic MT, Ross JS, et al: Epidural fibrosis and recurrent disk herniation in the lumbar spine: MR imaging assessment. AJNR 9:169–178, 1988.
20. Rich TA, Schiller A, Suit HD, Mankin HJ: Clinical and pathologic review of 48 cases of chordoma. Cancer 56:182–187, 1985.
21. Petterson H, Hudson T, Hamlin D, et al: Magnetic resonance imaging of sacrococcygeal tumors. Acta Radiol [Diagn] 26:161–165, 1985.
22. Yuh WTC, Flickinger FW, Barloon TJ, Montgomery WJ: MR imaging of unusual chordomas. J Comput Assist Tomogr 12:30–35, 1988.
23. Rosenthal DI, Scott JA, Mankin HJ, et al: Sacrococcygeal chordoma: Magnetic resonance imaging and computed tomography. AJR 145:143–147, 1985.
24. Russell DS, Rubinstein LJ: Pathology of Tumours of the Nervous System. 4th ed. Baltimore, Williams & Wilkins Company, 1977.
25. Robbins SL: Pathology. 3rd ed. Philadelphia, WB Saunders Company, 1967.
26. Ross JS, Masaryk TJ, Modic MR, et al: MR imaging of lumbar arachnoiditis. AJNR 8:885–892, 1987.
27. Mamourian AC, Briggs RW: Appearance of Pantopaque on MR images. Radiology 158:457–460, 1986.
28. Naidich TP, McLone DG, Mutluer S: A new understanding of dorsal dysraphism with lipoma (lipomyeloschisis): Radiologic evaluation and surgical correction. AJR 140:1065–1078, 1983.
29. Davis PC, Hoffman JC, Ball TI, et al: Spinal abnormalities in pediatric patients: MR imaging findings compared with clinical, myelographic and surgical findings. Radiology 166:679–685, 1988.
30. Altman NR, Altman DH: MR imaging of spinal dysraphism. AJNR 8:533–538, 1987.
31. Han JS, Benson JE, Kaufman B, et al: Demonstration of diastematomyelia and associated abnormalities with MR imaging. AJNR 6:215–219, 1985.

PART III

CHEST AND ABDOMEN

25

MR IMAGING OF THE THORAX

THERESA C. McLOUD and MARK W. RAGOZZINO

TECHNIQUES
NORMAL ANATOMY
THE MEDIASTINUM
    MEDIASTINAL MASSES
    THYMUS
    TRACHEA

THE STAGING OF BRONCHOGENIC
CARCINOMA
THE HILUM
THE LUNG

The chest is well suited for magnetic resonance imaging because of the inherent contrast among lung, fat, muscle, and flowing blood. In addition, MR offers the advantage of visualization of the lungs, mediastinum, and major vessels in several planes without the use of contrast material. MR has already proven to be a valuable technique in the evaluation of the mediastinum[1–4] and hila[2, 5–7] and in the staging of bronchogenic carcinoma.[5, 8–10] This chapter illustrates the strengths as well as some of the weaknesses of this technique.

TECHNIQUES

Chest imaging is routinely performed using a spin-echo technique. In general, short (250 to 500 msec) TR values and short TE values (14 to 30 msec) are employed. Although standard spin-echo pulse sequences that use a moderately short repetition time (TR) and moderately short echo time (TE) are widely used (500/30), degradation of image quality produced by cardiac and respiratory motion is frequently noted with these pulse sequences. For this reason we have implemented very short TR/TE pulse sequences that, in conjunction with extensive signal averaging, minimize both cardiac and respiratory motion artifacts and provide high T_1 contrast.[11, 12] The use of a short TR permits multiple signal averages to be obtained in a relatively short acquisition period; the short TE permits high T_1 contrast and minimizes within-view phase shifts and resultant ghost artifacts. T_2-weighted images with long TR intervals (1500 to 2000 msec) and long TE values (60 to 120 msec) are not used routinely in the chest. Such images suffer from further quality degradation due both to respiratory motion and to ghosting artifacts from pulsatile flow in the heart and great vessels. However, T_2-weighted images may be useful in certain instances, particularly in determining tissue characteristics of certain lesions in the chest, such as mediastinal cysts and hematomas, and in highlighting tissue plane separation between pathologic processes and normal structures. MR features of normal anatomy and pathologic processes described in this chapter are those noted on T_1-weighted images unless otherwise designated.

Initial imaging of the chest is done using the body coil with multislice acquisition. The time required to perform the examination varies with the pulse sequences and the number of phase-encoding steps used. Generally, 128 phase-encoding steps are adequate and provide a spatial resolution of approximately 3 mm. By employing the short TR and TE values mentioned above, the acquisition time ranges from 4 to 6 minutes, and 10 to 12 slices can be obtained. T_2-weighted images with correspondingly longer TR and TE pulse sequences may require an imaging time varying from 8 to 12 minutes.

In general, transaxial imaging is performed. However, the ideal imaging plane is perpendicular to the

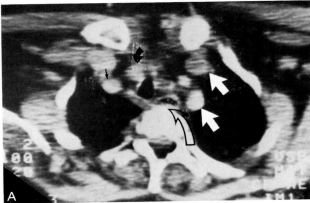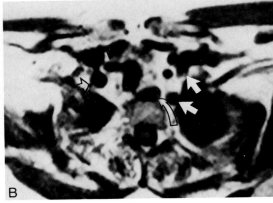

FIGURE 25–1. CT (A) and MR (B) scans at the level of the thoracic inlet. Right subclavian artery (*A, small black arrow*). Left subclavian artery (posterior) and left subclavian vein (anterior) (*large arrows*). Innominate artery (*closed curved arrow*). Esophagus (*B, open curved arrow*).

tissue interface of interest. In many patients, sagittal or coronal imaging may be preferred. Sagittal and coronal images are particularly useful in the evaluation of structures that lie in the coronal plane, such as the trachea, major airways, and great vessels, and in examining such regions as the aorticopulmonary window and lung apices.[13–16]

Because of the length of time required to obtain the images, patients are instructed to breathe quietly during the examination. If the respiratory rate is rapid, scan quality is poor. Generally patients are supine, with their arms positioned at their sides.

Gating image acquisition to the ECG can significantly increase the resolution of the heart, mediastinum, great vessels, pulmonary hila, and paracardiac mediastinal masses by reducing flow artifact.[1, 17–19] However, ECG gating is often not necessary if very short TR and TE pulse sequences are employed. There are a number of disadvantages to cardiac gating: (1) it does not reduce respiratory motion; (2) the TR must be matched to the patient's R-R interval, which alters tissue contrast; and (3) gating increases the set-up time for the study. However, ECG gating is recommended in patients with vascular lesions or those with inferior mediastinal (paracardiac masses) or lung masses abutting the heart.

Respiratory gating of image acquisition can also be used to reduce motion artifact. However, clinical experience with this technique is limited.[1, 20, 21] Respiratory gating is associated with markedly increased scan time. Other techniques that reduce respiratory motion artifacts, such as STIR pulse sequence and dynamic reordering of the phase-encoded gradient steps (ROPE, COPE, and EXORCIST), have been described.[21, 22]

NORMAL ANATOMY

The thorax can be conveniently divided into three components: the chest wall, the lungs, and the me-

diastinum. The MR characteristics of components of these structures determine their appearance on MR imaging. Fat, which is characterized by short T_1 and medium T_2 values, has high signal intensity on T_1-weighted images and moderate intensity on T_2-weighted images. Muscle has long T_1 and short T_2 values and has low signal intensity on T_1- and T_2-weighted images. Cortical bone, ligaments, tendons, fascia, and the lungs generate little signal on either T_1 or T_2 sequences.

In normal subjects, most mediastinal structures that can be identified by computed tomography (CT) are visible on transaxial MR. The lumens of mediastinal vessels generally show low signal intensity and are identified by their sharp contrast with high-intensity mediastinal fat. The aortic arch and its large vessels, the brachiocephalic veins, the subclavian

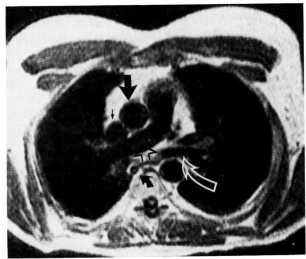

FIGURE 25–2. MR scan at the level of the bifurcation of the pulmonary artery. Superior vena cava (*small closed arrow*). Ascending aorta (*large closed arrow*). Right pulmonary artery (*open arrow*). Azygos vein (*closed curved arrow*). Left main bronchus (*open curved arrow*).

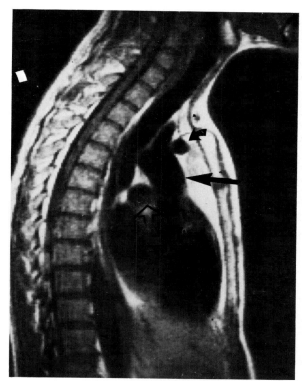

FIGURE 25-3. Sagittal scan at midline. The trachea is well visualized. Ascending aorta (*large black arrow*). Right pulmonary artery (*open arrow*). Left innominate vein (*curved black arrow*).

veins, and the vena cava are always identified (Fig. 25-1). The azygos vein and arch are visible in most patients. The main pulmonary artery, left and right pulmonary arteries, right interlobar pulmonary artery, right truncus anterior, and descending left pulmonary artery are all usually well seen, as are the large pulmonary veins[1, 6, 24] (Figs. 25-2 and 25-3).

The normal pulmonary hilum consists primarily of bronchi and the pulmonary arteries and veins. The main bronchi and the bronchus intermedius are almost always visible on MR scanning, but they cannot be differentiated from vessels except by location because of their low signal intensity[1] (see Fig. 25-2).

Other structures in the mediastinum which can consistently be identified on MR scanning include normal-sized mediastinal lymph nodes, the thymus gland, and the esophagus. They are intermediate in signal intensity, being less intense than fat and more intense than air-filled lung or mediastinal vessels.

THE MEDIASTINUM

The mediastinum is ideally suited to MR imaging because of the inherent contrast between the bright signal intensity of mediastinal fat and the signal void produced by flowing blood within the heart and mediastinal vessels. The goal of most imaging procedures in the mediastinum is threefold: (1) to iden-

tify mediastinal lesions and determine their extent; (2) to characterize the tissue components of such lesions, particularly with regard to fat and calcium content, blood and fluid (cysts, hematomas, and lipomas); and (3) to differentiate enlarged nodes from vessels in patients with bronchogenic carcinoma and lymphoma. Finally, determination of the relationship of mediastinal lesions to adjacent structures is important in surgical planning. The relative merits of MR imaging and CT scanning of the chest are discussed in relationship to all of these issues. Vascular lesions such as aneurysms and dissections are discussed elsewhere in the text.

MEDIASTINAL MASSES

MR facilitates the identification of lesions within the mediastinum. Tumor demonstrates lower intensity than fat.[1, 24-26] Although the spatial resolution of MR is less than that of CT scanning, its superior contrast resolution allows for the detection of infiltrating tumor in the mediastinum which may not be visible on CT (Fig. 25-4). Contrast between mediastinal vessels and tumor permits evaluation without the use of contrast material, although care must be taken to avoid confusing paradoxical enhancement with soft-tissue masses. Another advantage of MR relative to CT is that it allows direct imaging in the sagittal and coronal planes without degradation of spatial resolution.[13-15] Imaging in multiple planes reduces the chance of misinterpretation as a result of volume averaging, a common problem with axial imaging alone.

With regard to benign mediastinal lesions, MR may provide definitive diagnoses in specific instances. For example, benign fatty masses occur frequently in the mediastinum. Examples of such lesions include diffuse widening of the mediastinum due to lipomatosis secondary to exogenous obesity, Cushing's disease, and the administration of steroids; focal masses such as benign lipomas; prominent pericardial fat pads; and omental herniations through the esophageal hiatus. Although such entities are easily diagnosed by CT scanning because of their low attenuation coefficients, MR provides equivalent diagnostic information because of the bright signal intensity of fatty masses on T_1-weighted images. Cysts containing high concentrations of mucin or protein, such as bronchogenic cysts, have short T1 values and often appear bright on both T1- and T2-weighted images (Fig. 25-5). On the other hand, cystic masses containing serous fluid, such as simple thymic or pericardial cysts, typically have long T_1 and T_2 values.[25, 26] On T_1-weighted images, simple cysts appear as lesions of low signal intensity comparable to that of cerebrospinal fluid. However, when scans are performed with long TR and TE values (T$_2$-weighted images), there is a significant relative increase relative in signal because of the long T_2 value of water (Fig. 25-6).

Localized hematomas are unusual in the mediastinum. Following major trauma diffuse bleeding is a

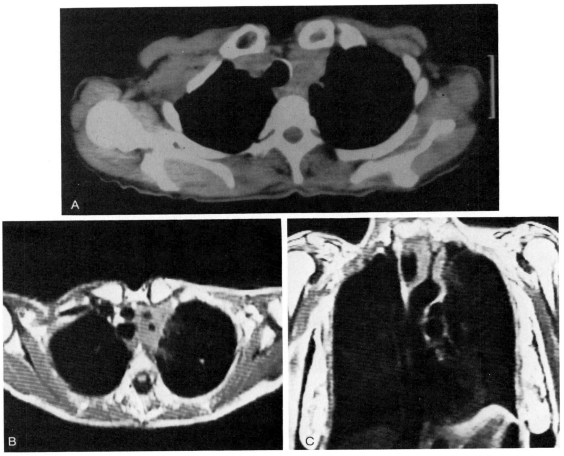

FIGURE 25–4. Middle-aged woman with chest pain and weight loss. *A,* CT scan performed without contrast fails to delineate a definite mass, although there is loss of mediastinal fat planes. *B,* Axial and *(C)* coronal T_1-weighted MR scans show a medium signal intensity tumor surrounding and encasing the left carotid and left subclavian arteries. An ill-defined border is identified extending into the left lung. The diagnosis is bronchogenic carcinoma arising in the left upper lobe and directly invading the mediastinum.

more common event, usually secondary to rupture of the aorta or the great vessels. Such injuries are managed surgically on an emergent basis. However, occasionally localized hematomas can be identified in the mediastinum, and they may present as isolated mediastinal masses. The MR characteristics of hematomas in either the subacute or early chronic stage have been well described. They characteristically appear as areas of bright signal intensity on T_1-weighted images. Such signal characteristics are attributed to

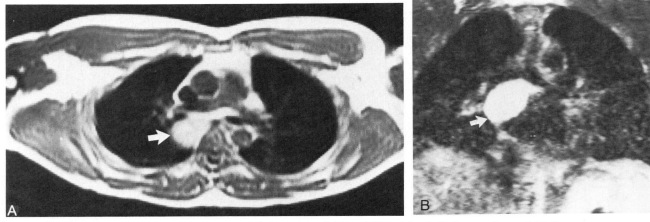

FIGURE 25–5. Bronchogenic cyst. Both T_1-weighted *(A)* and T_2-weighted *(B)* images show a high-intensity mass *(arrow).*

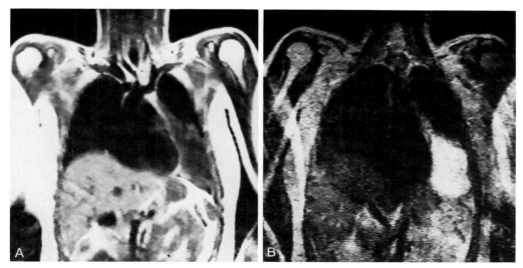

FIGURE 25–6. Thymic cyst. *A,* T_1-weighted image shows a low signal intensity mass in the inferior anterior mediastinum. *B,* T_2-weighted image (second echo—120 msec) shows a marked increase in signal intensity characteristic of a cyst.

the presence of methemoglobin (Fig. 25–7). In addition, a thin low-intensity rim may be identified at the periphery of the mass owing to hemosiderin-laden macrophages, though less commonly than in intracerebral hematomas.

Goiters can be readily diagnosed on CT scanning. CT characteristics include heterogeneous areas of attenuation, calcification, continuity of the lesion with the thyroid in the neck, and intense opacification following the administration of contrast material.[28, 29] Similarly, goiters exhibit characteristic features on MR imaging.[30] Both cystic and solid areas can be identified in most cases. On T_2-weighted images, colloid cysts appear as high signal intensity areas that are brighter than subcutaneous fat. Areas of hemorrhage may produce bright signal intensity on both T_1- and T_2-weighted images[26] (Fig. 25–8). Although calcification may not be detected on MR imaging, in some cases large deposits of calcification produce highly visible areas of signal void. In addition, sagittal and coronal MR images often provide better visualization of both the extent of the intrathoracic component and its contiguity with the thyroid in the neck, information that may be crucial in planning the surgical approach.

The ability to identify mediastinal lymph nodes in order to determine if they are enlarged and to distinguish them from vessels is an important function of any imaging technique in the mediastinum. T_1-weighted MR images permit the visualization of normal-size nodes (less than 1 cm) and most mediastinal nodes that are borderline in size or enlarged. MR is therefore equivalent to CT in the detection of mediastinal adenopathy.[1] However, the poorer spatial resolution of MR may result in blurring of the edges of individual discrete nodes that are in close proximity, suggesting that they are a single larger mass.[8] MR, however, does have the advantage of ready differentiation of normal and enlarged nodes from mediastinal vessels. Although such a distinction can be readily accomplished by CT scanning with contrast, MR offers an advantage in patients in whom contrast represents a hazard (Fig. 25–9).

Calcification within a mediastinal mass or lymph node usually cannot be recognized on MR.[26, 31] This represents a drawback for MR, since calcium may be an important discriminator in the mediastinum between benign and malignant lymph node enlargement. In addition, the detection of calcium may be helpful in the evaluation of other mass lesions, such as aortic aneurysms and goiters.

Generally speaking, benign mediastinal lesions cannot be differentiated from malignant tumors except for the situations mentioned in the preceding paragraphs. T_1 and T_2 values do not appear to differ significantly.[24, 26, 32] Preliminary evidence suggests that tumors that recur following therapy may be distinguished from post-therapy fibrosis on T_2-weighted images, since tumors may appear relatively bright and fibrosis relatively dark.[33] Unfortunately, this distinction may not be accurate in the months immediately following therapy, since actively growing or inflamed fibrotic tissue may mimic neoplasm.

Mediastinal Hodgkin's lymphoma commonly has a heterogeneous appearance on T_2-weighted MR images. After treatment, the appearance may change significantly. In one study, mass/fat signal intensity ratios of inactive lymphomas (0.3) were much lower than active lymphomas (0.9) in T_2-weighted images.[33a] The results of this study suggest that persistent high signal intensity on T_2-weighted images, or an increase in signal intensity over time, is suspect

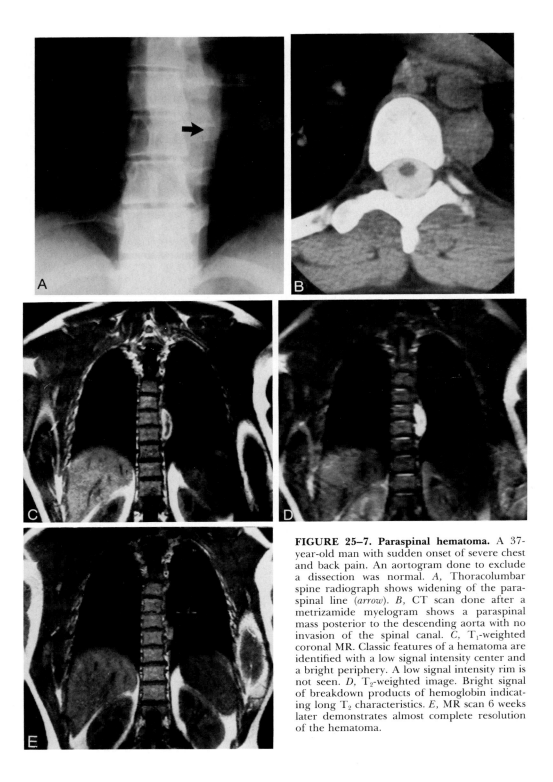

FIGURE 25–7. Paraspinal hematoma. A 37-year-old man with sudden onset of severe chest and back pain. An aortogram done to exclude a dissection was normal. *A,* Thoracolumbar spine radiograph shows widening of the paraspinal line *(arrow)*. *B,* CT scan done after a metrizamide myelogram shows a paraspinal mass posterior to the descending aorta with no invasion of the spinal canal. *C,* T_1-weighted coronal MR. Classic features of a hematoma are identified with a low signal intensity center and a bright periphery. A low signal intensity rim is not seen. *D,* T_2-weighted image. Bright signal of breakdown products of hemoglobin indicating long T_2 characteristics. *E,* MR scan 6 weeks later demonstrates almost complete resolution of the hematoma.

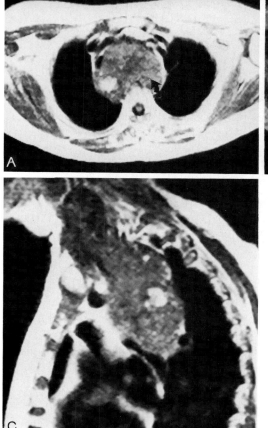

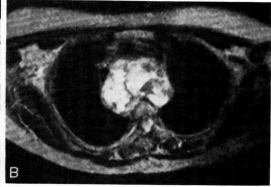

FIGURE 25–8. Large intrathoracic goiter. *A*, T_1-weighted image. The mass is composed of mostly low signal intensity circular structures (*arrow*). There is one bright area identified. *B*, T_2-weighted image. Marked increase in signal intensity of most of the goiter. The areas of long T_1 and T_2 relaxation times represent colloid cysts. The area of bright signal intensity in both *A* and *B* is an area of hemorrhage. *C*, Sagittal scan demonstrates extension into the neck above and the subcarinal area below.

for recurrent tumor. Another study has suggested that MRI obtained pretreatment can be used to predict the size of residual masses posttreatment.[33b] Dark regions of the tumor, possibly representing fibrosis, were found to persist posttreatment, whereas brighter regions, presumably representing active tumor, disappeared.

With regard to the relationship of mediastinal masses to other structures, MR offers some unique advantages. In general, the relationship between a mediastinal mass and adjacent vessels and the presence of vascular compression or obstruction are better demonstrated with MR than with contrast-enhanced CT.[1, 6, 24] In addition, coronal and sagittal imaging of structures that are oriented in the longitudinal plane, such as the trachea, superior vena cava, and aorta, permit better resolution of the edges of such structures than transaxial imaging. Therefore, the interface between such normal structures in the mediastinum and mediastinal tumors can be better appreciated. The diaphragm, which is often difficult to detect on axial CT images, is clearly identified as an area of low signal intensity on MR sagittal and coronal images when a tumor or other pathologic process abuts it. This is a result of the inherent contrast between muscle and adjacent tumor (Fig. 25–10).

THYMUS

A recent study by de Greer et al[34] indicates that MR scanning may be superior to CT in the evaluation of the normal thymus. The thymus generally appeared thicker and more easily identifiable on MR images in patients over the age of 20. This observation was due mainly to the fact that the thymus could be distinguished from fat on MR images because of differences in proton density. MR appeared to be better than CT in distinguishing between a thymus partially replaced by fat and mediastinal fat.

TRACHEA

The trachea is another organ that is ideally suited to MR imaging. We had the opportunity to study five normal volunteers and 20 patients with a variety of tracheal lesions, including tracheal stenosis and primary and secondary neoplasms of the trachea.[35] The trachea is best imaged with a spin-echo technique using short TR and TE pulsing sequences and multiplanar imaging. A surface coil can be employed for studies of the cervical trachea. MR images of the trachea provide excellent spatial resolution and anatomic detail of the larynx, the entire trachea, and the carina and main bronchi.

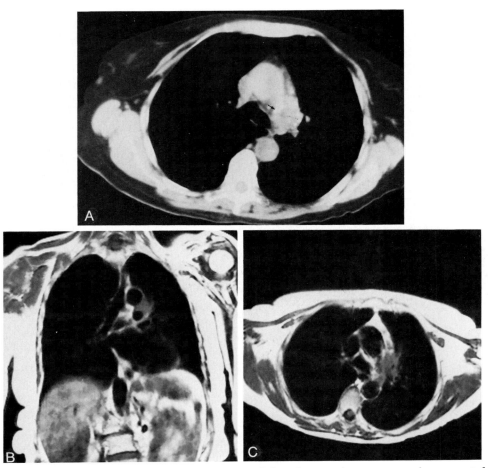

FIGURE 25–9. Lymphadenopathy versus aneurysm. Subaortic mass in a woman who presented with hoarseness. *A,* CT scan done without contrast shows an AP window mass with a small partial rim of calcium, raising the possibility of an aneurysm (*arrow*). The patient refused contrast because of a previous reaction. MR scan in (*B*) coronal and (*C*) axial planes shows a definite soft-tissue mass in the area consistent with lymphadenopathy. The diagnosis is bronchogenic carcinoma with mediastinal metastases.

CT scanning does provide a major advance in tracheal imaging. Axial projections permit ready determination of cross-sectional area and therefore the degree of tracheal obstruction; CT clearly shows the relationship of the trachea to major mediastinal vessels and, in the case of tumors, identifies intraluminal lesions, extraluminal extension, and associated adenopathy.[36, 37] However, CT lacks some of the advantages of imaging in the coronal and sagittal planes, particularly the ability to determine accurately the length of tracheal lesions and their extent relative to the carina and main bronchi. Such a determination is an essential component of preoperative evaluation. Modern anesthetic and surgical techniques have made extensive tracheal resections possible; however, lesions of inordinate length may not allow adequate mobilization for reanastomosis of the airway.[38]

MR appears to be an ideal method for imaging the trachea because it demonstrates the airway, mediastinal vessels, and other structures simultaneously in at least three different planes. Among the tracheal lesions that we studied, MR was highly accurate in estimation of both the length and degree of tracheal occlusion. In the evaluation of tracheal stenosis, however, MR does not appear to offer any particular advantage over conventional radiography. However, MR offers definite advantages in the evaluation of patients with primary and secondary tracheal neoplasms. In primary tumors, direct invasion of tumor into the mediastinum occurs in 30 to 40 per cent of patients. Although CT is a fairly accurate method of delineating mediastinal invasion by such neoplasms, our experience suggests that MR may be superior to CT in this regard (Fig. 25–11). The advantage of MR may be related to several factors, including multiplanar imaging and better contrast between soft tissue and mediastinal fat. The latter permits thin fat planes, such as that between the trachea and the esophagus, to be visualized more easily and also aids in the distinction between bulky intramural tumor, which displaces mediastinal fat, and tumor invasion. In regard to secondary invasion of the trachea by

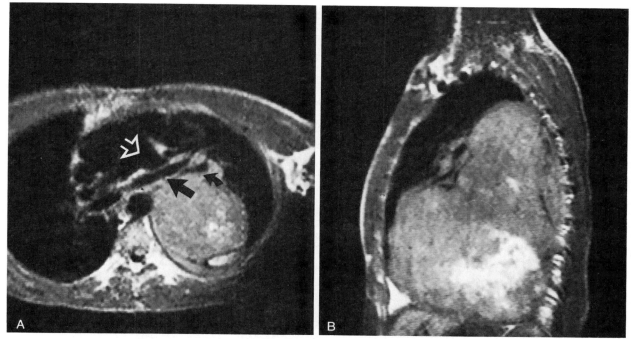

FIGURE 25–10. Metastatic Ewing's sarcoma to left chest. A 25-year-old patient with isolated metastasis to left hemithorax being evaluated for possible left pneumonectomy. *A*, Axial MR shows that the main pulmonary artery is not invaded, allowing an adequate resection margin (*open arrow*). Tumor is seen displacing the left main bronchus anteriorly (*black arrow*) and encasing the descending branch of the left pulmonary artery (*curved black arrow*). Note the small hematoma posteriorly which occurred secondary to a needle biopsy. *B*, Sagittal MR scan shows the diaphragm as a curvilinear structure of low signal intensity. The tumor does not extend into the abdominal cavity.

other tumors, our study suggests that direct invasion of the tracheal wall is identified more consistently with MR scanning than with CT.

THE STAGING OF BRONCHOGENIC CARCINOMA

Initial experience suggests that evaluation of the mediastinum with MR is approximately equal to that of CT with regard to the staging of bronchogenic carcinoma.[5, 7–10] These data, however, are somewhat limited. Webb et al[8] reported a series of 33 patients in which they compared staging done with MR with staging done with CT and surgery. They found that CT and MR provided comparable information regarding the presence and size of mediastinal nodes. MR better discriminated mediastinal nodes from vascular structures than did noncontrast CT. However, in 2 of their 11 patients with multiple mediastinal lymph nodes that were normal in size at CT examination and surgery, MR suggested a confluent abnormal mass, probably because of poorer spatial resolution (Fig. 25–12). Musset et al[10] studied 44 patients with bronchogenic carcinoma prospectively by both computed tomography and magnetic resonance imaging. Both T_1- and T_2-weighted sequences and coronal and sagittal images were performed. They found no statistically significant differences between the two imaging methods in the evaluation

of either tumor extent or nodal involvement. Their experience was similar to that of other investigators who reported that calculation of the relaxation times T_1 and T_2 are not useful in differentiating benign from malignant adenopathy.

MR, however, may be useful in the assessment of lesions that directly invade the chest wall and mediastinum (Fig. 25–13). In a recent report, Haggar et al[39] reported that MR imaging was useful in the evaluation of chest wall invasion by carcinoma of the lung. They studied 19 patients, 13 of whom underwent surgery. MR findings indicative of chest wall invasion included a high signal focus within the chest wall and/or chest wall thickening on T_2-weighted images. TR values at 2500 msec and TE values at 50 to 100 msec were employed. Contrast differences between normal and invaded chest wall could be appreciated on these T_2-weighted images, and coronal and sagittal imaging facilitated identification of tumor contiguity with extrathoracic structures.

Superior sulcus carcinomas are defined as bronchogenic carcinomas occurring at the extreme apex of the lung. Such tumors may be considered resectable and are usually managed with radiation therapy followed by surgery with chest wall resection if there is no evidence of mediastinal or distant metastases. However, accurate assessment of the local extent of disease is an important aspect in the staging of these lesions. We have found MR to be useful in determin-

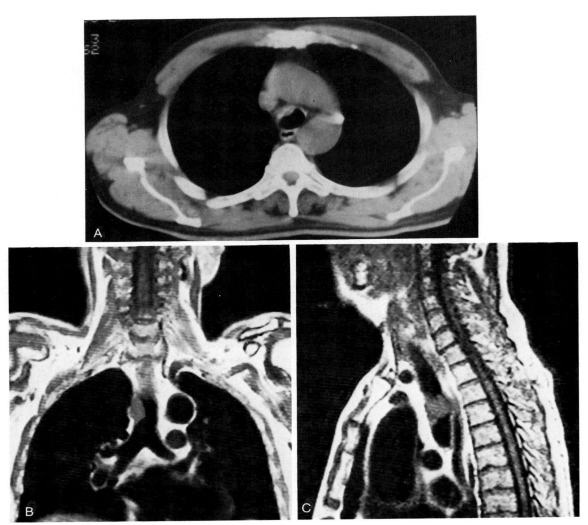

FIGURE 25–11. Adenoid cystic carcinoma of the trachea. *A*, CT scan. There is a mass arising from the anterolateral wall of the trachea. A well-defined fat plane can be identified between the mass and adjacent mediastinal structures. *B*, Coronal MR scan shows direct invasion of mediastinal fat and extension to the pleura of the right lung. *C*, Sagittal scan. The tumor extends through the posterior tracheal wall to invade the esophagus. Findings confirmed at surgery.

ing certain parameters of unresectability, such as invasion of the vertebral body and involvement of the subclavian artery and brachial plexus (Fig. 25–14). Sagittal and coronal images are particularly useful in imaging such lesions. T_2-weighted images help to differentiate apical tumor from surrounding muscle and to define the extent of the tumor in the base of the neck.

THE HILUM

The normal pulmonary hilum consists primarily of bronchi and the pulmonary arteries and veins. CT has become the method of choice for the evaluation of the hilum. An adequate CT study requires a large bolus of contrast and dynamic imaging. This allows differentiation between abnormal soft tissue and vascular structures. MR is ideally suited for evaluation of the hilum. Although, for the most part, MR images of the normal hilum show only the walls of the bronchi and hilar vessels, Webb and colleagues[7] have recently described collections of soft tissue representing both fat and normal-sized nodes which may be confused with a mass or lymphadenopathy.[1, 7] These occur in three specific locations: on the right at the level of the bifurcation of the right pulmonary artery and at the origin of the right middle lobe bronchus and on the left at the level of the left upper lobe bronchus. Normal-sized lymph nodes in the range of 3 to 5 mm can also be identified.[1, 7]

Indications for MR include (1) evaluation of the enlarged hilum; (2) differentiation of an enlarged hilum due to prominent vessels from a hilar soft tissue mass; and (3) detection of hilar adenopathy in

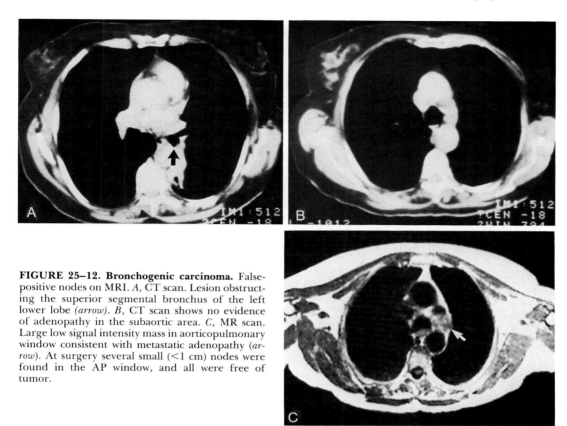

FIGURE 25–12. Bronchogenic carcinoma. False-positive nodes on MRI. *A,* CT scan. Lesion obstructing the superior segmental bronchus of the left lower lobe *(arrow). B,* CT scan shows no evidence of adenopathy in the subaortic area. *C,* MR scan. Large low signal intensity mass in aorticopulmonary window consistent with metastatic adenopathy *(arrow).* At surgery several small (<1 cm) nodes were found in the AP window, and all were free of tumor.

the staging of bronchogenic carcinoma and lymphoma. MR studies of the hilum are best performed with cardiac gating and a T_1-weighted sequence. In a study of hilar masses and lymphadenopathy, Webb et al[7] reported that MR allowed a confident diagnosis of a hilar mass in each case and clearly showed the relationship of the mass to normal vessels and large bronchi[7, 24] (Fig. 25–15). When compared to CT scans performed following the injection of a contrast bolus, MR largely confirmed the CT findings but made the diagnosis of hilar mass much easier and better showed the relationship of the mass to vessels at multiple levels. MR is clearly superior to CT in defining a hilar mass lesion when a bolus injection of contrast is suboptimal, when no contrast is given, or when the mass is small.[1, 6, 40]

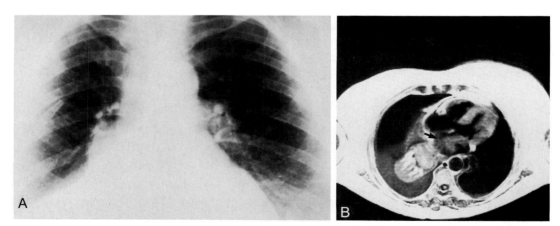

FIGURE 25–13. Bronchogenic carcinoma invading the left atrium. *A,* Standard radiograph in a patient with bronchoscopically proven large cell carcinoma arising in the right intermediate bronchus. There is collapse of the right middle and lower lobes. *B,* During radiation therapy the patient developed a cardiac murmur. Cardiac gated MR scan shows that the tumor has directly invaded and is filling the lumen of the left atrium *(arrow).*

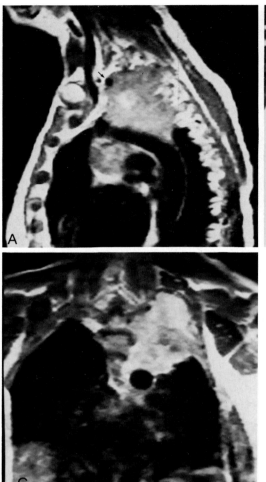

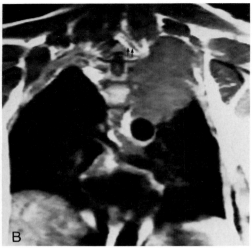

FIGURE 25–14. Superior sulcus carcinoma. *A,* Sagittal image shows the superior extent of the tumor. It extends to but does not invade the subclavian artery *(arrow)*. Enlarged subaortic nodes are also identified. *B,* T_1- and *(C)* T_2-weighted coronal images. On the T_2-weighted image the bright signal intensity of tumor allows ready differentiation from surrounding low signal intensity muscle. Branches of the brachial plexus can also be identified *(double arrow).*

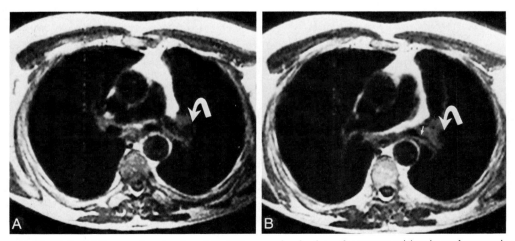

FIGURE 25–15. Left hilar carcinoma. *A* and *B,* MR scans clearly show the tumor arising in and narrowing the superior segmental bronchus of the left lower lobe *(B, small arrow)* and surrounding the left pulmonary artery and displacing it laterally *(curved arrow).*

With regard to the staging of bronchogenic carcinoma, Glazer et al[5] surveyed 19 patients with bronchogenic carcinoma who also had surgery. Nine of these were proven to have hilar lymph node metastases, whereas five others had enlarged (10 mm or greater) lymph nodes that were not involved by tumor. In all of these 14, MR was interpreted as showing node enlargement. The results of MR were closely comparable to those found on CT examinations of these patients. It appears that MR must be considered at least as sensitive as CT in detecting hilar lymph node enlargement.

In the assessment of the major airways, MR does offer the advantage of imaging in sagittal and coronal planes. This avoids the problem of partial volume averaging which occurs with axial imaging of the airways. However, both CT and conventional tomography provide better spatial resolution, and evidence so far suggests that these imaging modalities provide more accurate evaluation of the major bronchi in the hilar areas.

THE LUNG

Unfortunately, the lung is not well suited to MR imaging. On spin-echo images in normal subjects, little signal is obtained from the lung parenchyma. This is due to two factors: the very low proton density of air and the long T_1 of lung, which is similar to that of muscle. Areas of consolidation and masses can usually be identified, but the degree to which they can be differentiated has yet to be fully established. However, MR has been found to be less sensitive than CT in the detection of small nodules. This is primarily the result of the better spatial resolution of CT and respiratory motion during the MR study.[41] In addition, the morphologic characteristics of larger nodules are not as well defined on MR as on CT.

Several studies have been devoted to the evaluation

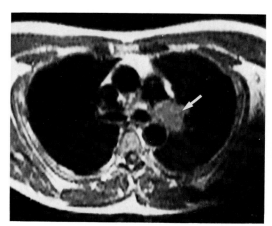

FIGURE 25–16. Metastatic renal cell carcinoma. MR scan shows low signal intensity tumor embolus (*arrow*) in the left pulmonary artery.

of pulmonary emboli using MR scanning. Because blood flowing in central pulmonary arteries produces no signal in normal patients, pulmonary emboli within central vessels can be recognized on ECG-gated or ungated studies. Emboli usually produce an intense signal that is readily detectable.[1] Pulmonary emboli have been detected in humans using MR,[42–44] but such emboli are usually large and central in location (Fig. 25–16). Experimental studies in dogs[45] have shown that more than 60 per cent of emboli are detectable on MR scanning. However, it does not appear that MR will replace other studies in the evaluation of pulmonary embolism.

In summary, MR appears to be particularly useful in the evaluation of the mediastinum and the hilum. Although MR has several advantages over CT, namely the facts that contrast material is not necessary and that multiple planar imaging can be done, it is not apparent at this time that MR offers such distinct advantages that it will replace CT in the evaluation of the thorax.

REFERENCES

1. Webb WR: Magnetic resonance imaging of the thorax: Review of uses and comparison with computed tomography. Proceedings of Categorical Course in Chest Radiology, American Roentgen Ray Society, 1986, p 59.
2. Webb WR: Magnetic resonance imaging of the mediastinum, hila, and lungs. J Thorac Imag 1:65, 1985.
3. von Schulthess GK, McMurdo K, Tscholakoff D, et al: Mediastinal masses: MR imaging. Radiology 158:289, 1986.
4. Epstein DM, Kressel H, Gefter W, et al: MR imaging of the mediastinum: A retrospective comparison with computed tomography. J Comput Assist Tomogr 8:670, 1984.
5. Glazer GM, Gross BH, Aisen AM, et al: Imaging of the pulmonary hilum: A prospective comparative study in patients with lung cancer. AJR 145:245, 1985.
6. Cohen AM, Creviston S, LiPuma JP, et al: Nuclear magnetic resonance of the mediastinum and hila: Early impressions of its efficacy. AJR 141:1163, 1983.
7. Webb WR, Gamsu G, Stark D, et al: Magnetic resonance imaging of the normal and abnormal pulmonary hila. Radiology 152:89, 1984.
8. Webb WR, Jensen BG, Sollitto R, et al: Bronchogenic carcinoma: Staging with MR compared with staging with CT and surgery. Radiology 156:117, 1985.
9. Poon PY, Bronskill MJ, Henkelman RM, et al: Mediastinal lymph node metastases with bronchogenic carcinoma: Detection with MR imaging and CT. Radiology 162:651, 1987.
10. Musset D, Grenier P, Carette M, et al: Primary lung cancer staging: Prospective comparative study of MR imaging with CT. Radiology 160:607, 1986.
11. Stark DD, Wittenberg J, Edelman RR, et al: Detection of hepatic metastases: Analysis of pulse sequence performance in MR imaging. Radiology 159:365, 1986.
12. Stark DD, Hendrick RE, Hahn PF, Ferrucci JT Jr: Motion artifact reduction with fast spin-echo imaging. Radiology 164:183–191, 1987.
13. Webb WR, Gamsu G, Crooks LE, et al: Multisection sagittal and coronal magnetic resonance of the mediastinum and hila. Work in progress. Radiology 150:475, 1984.
14. Webb WR, Jensen BG, Gamsu G, et al: Coronal magnetic resonance imaging of the chest: Normal and abnormal. Radiology 153:729, 1984.
15. O'Donovan PB, Ross JS, Sivak ED, et al: Magnetic resonance imaging of the thorax: The advantages of coronal and sagittal planes. AJR 143:1183, 1984.

16. Batra P, Brown K, Stechel RJ, et al: MR imaging of the thorax: A comparison of axial, coronal, and sagittal imaging planes. J Comput Assist Tomogr 12:75, 1988.

17. Lanzer P, Botvinck EH, Schiller NB, et al: Cardiac imaging using gated magnetic resonance. Radiology 150:121, 1984.

18. Lieberman JM, Alfidi RJ, Nelson AD, et al: Gated magnetic resonance imaging of the normal and diseased heart. Radiology 152:465, 1984.

19. Amparo EG, Higgins CB, Farmer D, et al: Gated MRI of cardiac and paracardiac masses: Initial experience. AJR 143:1151, 1984.

20. Runge VM, Clanton JA, Partain CL, et al: Respiratory gating in magnetic resonance imaging at 0.5 tesla. Radiology 151:521, 1984.

21. Eliman RL, McNamara MT, Pollack M, et al: Magnetic resonance imaging with respiratory gating: Techniques and advantages. AJR 143:1175, 1984.

22. Bailes DR, Gilderdale DJ, Bydder GM, et al: Respiratory ordered phase-encoding (ROPE): A method of reducing respiratory motion artifacts in MR imaging. J Comput Assist Tomogr 9:835, 1985.

23. Bydder GM, Young IR: MRI: Clinical use of the inversion recovery sequence. J Comput Assist Tomogr 9:659, 1985.

24. Gamsu G, Webb WR, Sheldon P, et al: Nuclear magnetic resonance imaging of the thorax. Radiology 147:473, 1983.

25. Webb WR, Gamsu G, Stark DD, et al: Evaluation of magnetic resonance sequences in imaging mediastinal tumors. AJR 143:723–777, 1984.

26. Gamsu G, Stark DD, Webb WR, et al: Magnetic resonance imaging of benign mediastinal masses. Radiology 151:709, 1984.

27. Hahn PF, Stark DD, Vici LG, Ferrucci JT: Duodenal hematoma: The rim sign in MR imaging. Radiology 159:379, 1985.

28. Bashist B, Ellis K, Gold PR: Computed tomography of intrathoracic goiters. AJR 140:455, 1983.

29. Glazer GM, Axel L, Moss AA: CT diagnosis of mediastinal thyroid. AJR 138:495, 1982.

30. Higgins CB, McNamara MT, Fisher MR, et al: Imaging of the thyroid. AJR 147:1255, 1986.

31. Higgins CB, Stark DD, McNamara M, et al: Multiplane magnetic resonance imaging of the heart and major vessels. Studies in normal volunteers. AJR 142:661, 1984.

32. Ross JS, O'Donovan PB, Novoa R, et al: Magnetic resonance of the chest: Initial experience with imaging and in vivo T_1 and T_2 calculations. Radiology 152:95, 1984.

33. Glazer HS, Lee JHT, Levitt RG, et al: Radiation fibrosis: Differentiation from recurrent tumor by MR imaging. Radiology 156:721–726, 1985.

33a. Zerhoun EA, Fishman EK, Jones R, et al: MRI of "sterilized" lymphoma (abstr.) Radiology 161(P):207, 1986.

33b. Nyman RS, Rehn SM, Glimelins BLG, et al: Residual mediastinal masses in Hodgkin disease: Prediction of size with MRI. Radiology 170:435–440, 1989.

34. de Greer G, Webb WR, Gamsu G: Normal thymus: Assessment with MR and CT. Radiology 158:313, 1986.

35. Laissy JP, Rebibo G, Iba Zizen MT, et al: MRI in the preoperative assessment of tracheal compression. Case report. Eur J Radiol 7:281–287, 1987.

36. Gamsu G, Webb WR: Computed tomography of the trachea: Normal and abnormal. AJR 139:321, 1982.

37. Spizarny DL, Shepard JO, McLoud TC, et al: CT of adenoid cystic carcinoma of the trachea. AJR 146:1129, 1986.

38. Grillo HC: Tracheal tumors: Surgical management. Ann Thorac Surg 26:112, 1978.

39. Haggar AM, Pearlberg JL, Froelich JW, et al: Chest-wall invasion by carcinoma of the lung: Detection by MR imaging. AJR 148:1075, 1987.

40. Cohen AM, Creviston S, Li Puma JP, et al: NMR evaluation of hilar and mediastinal lymphadenopathy. Radiology 148:737, 1983.

41. Muller NL, Gamsu G, Webb WR: Pulmonary nodules: Detection using magnetic resonance and computed tomography. Radiology 155:687, 1985.

42. Moore EH, Gamsu G, Webb WR, et al: Pulmonary embolus: Detection and follow-up using magnetic resonance. Radiology 153:471, 1984.

43. Thickman D, Kressel HY, Axel L: Demonstration of pulmonary embolism by magnetic resonance imaging. AJR 142:921, 1984.

44. White RD, Winkler ML, Higgins CB: MR imaging of pulmonary arterial hypertension and pulmonary emboli. AJR 149:15, 1987.

45. Gamsu G, Hirji M, Moore EH, et al: Experimental pulmonary emboli detected using magnetic resonance. Radiology 153:467, 1984.

26

FRONTIERS IN CARDIAC MAGNETIC RESONANCE

HOWARD L. KANTOR

ULTRAFAST CARDIAC IMAGING

EVALUATION OF CARDIAC PERFUSION

IMAGING OF CORONARY BYPASS GRAFTS AND NATIVE CORONARY ARTERIES

  CORONARY BYPASS GRAFTS

  CORONARY ARTERIES

SPECTROSCOPY

  PHOSPHORUS SPECTROSCOPY

  Myocardial Ischemia
  Segmental Ischemia
  Transmural Metabolite Distribution in Ischemia

Phasic Alteration in Myocardial Metabolites Workload
Myocardial Protection
Cardiac Transplantation

CARBON-13 SPECTROSCOPY

PROTON SPECTROSCOPY

Lactate

SODIUM AND POTASSIUM

HUMAN SPECTROSCOPY

Cardiac Application
Skeletal Muscle Investigation in Congestive Heart Failure

ULTRAFAST CARDIAC IMAGING

One general goal of MR imaging techniques is to increase the speed of the examination, both to enhance cost effectiveness and to reduce patient discomfort. For MR studies of the heart, however, the need to minimize the duration of image acquisition is even greater, given that cardiac anatomy in a prolonged study may be obscured even if gating is performed (owing to irregularities in the heart rhythm) and because cardiac anatomy and physiology change throughout the heart cycle. Although motion reduction algorithms and intelligent gating systems can reduce the effect of motion, an instantaneous technique that produces a snapshot of the heart would be an invaluable imaging modality.

An MR imaging technique that meets these needs is called echo-planar imaging (EPI).[1-5] As previously discussed in Chapter 5, EPI represents a significant departure from standard two-dimensional Fourier transform (2DFT) imaging methods in which one phase-encoding step is applied after each radiofrequency (RF) excitation. With 2DFT methods, only one projection is acquired with each repetition time (TR) interval, so that the image acquisition time is relatively lengthy. Moreover, for cardiac imaging the need to synchronize data acquisition to the cardiac cycle precludes using very short TR. To overcome these limitations, the EPI method acquires all the projections needed to create an image after a single RF excitation. This is accomplished by rapidly oscillating the frequency-encoding gradient during the envelope of a spin-echo signal. First, a spin echo is produced by application of a 90-degree and a 180-degree RF pulse, with the echo peaking at the echo time (TE), as in a standard spin-echo pulse sequence. However, rather than apply a single phase-encoding gradient and a constant frequency-encoding gradient, the frequency-encoding gradient is rapidly oscillated during the build-up and decay of the spin echo. A series of gradient echoes are thereby produced, each of which is separately phase-encoded by

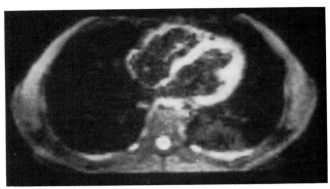

FIGURE 26–1. Transaxial echo-planar image of the thorax of a normal volunteer obtained on a 2.0 tesla imager (Advanced NMR Systems, Inc., Woburn, MA). Note the high signal intensity of cerebrospinal fluid within the spinal canal and of a small amount of posteriorly layering pleural fluid. (TE = 30 msec, TR = infinite).

application of a very brief phase-encoding gradient pulse. After the data are appropriately filtered and resorted, the image is reconstructed.

Echo-planar images are somewhat different in appearance from conventional 2DFT images. First, because all data are acquired after a single RF pulse, the TR is nearly infinite. As a result, the images are free from T_1 weighting and can be strongly T_2 weighted, with the degree of T_2 weighting depending on the TE. Tissues with long T_2 relaxation times, such as cerebrospinal fluid or simple cysts, appear brightest, as shown in the axial image in Figure 26–1[6] obtained in a transaxial section. (Currently, EPI systems generally use only one oscillating gradient [x-gradient] and allow acquisitions only in the axial plane. However, this limitation is temporary and will be overcome in future implementations of these systems.) Second, although the read-out time for each gradient echo is extremely short (submillisecond), resulting in a large signal bandwidth (see Chapter 10), the total read-out time for the whole series of

gradient echoes is relatively long. This results in severe chemical shift artifact as well as sensitivity to magnetic susceptibility effects. Chemical artifact is avoided with chemical shift-selective RF pulses that result in water-only or fat-only images. Finally, it is not currently feasible to apply the extra gradient pulses needed for flow compensation within the short time interval for EPI image acquisition. As a result, flowing blood may appear dark or have mixed signal intensity because of flow-related dephasing (see Chapter 4).

Recent reports have suggested an enormous clinical potential for EPI.[7–16] For the instant heart studies shown in this chapter, a prototype 2.0-T EPI-dedicated system was used, although 1.5-T whole-body systems capable of both standard and EPI imaging are becoming commercially available. Special hardware is required, such as powerful gradient amplifiers, sinusoidally resonating gradients capable of submillisecond rise and fall times, and wide bandwidth receivers. These requirements differ from conventional 2DFT imaging, which typically uses trapezoidal gradients with more modest peak amplitudes and smaller signal bandwidths. Patient set-up is similar to that for a standard MR examination. Although the image acquisition time is very short (e.g., 20 to 30 msec for a 128 × 64 or 128 × 128 acquisition matrix), ECG leads are still applied to permit sorting of images according to the phase of the cardiac cycle. In addition to the EPI images, which currently have limited multiplanar capability and limited spatial resolution, we usually acquire at least one standard set of gated spin-echo images for optimal anatomic definition.

Although clinical studies using EPI are all preliminary, there are several areas in which potentially useful applications have been shown. For instance, using chemical shift-selective pulses, one can unambiguously determine the lipid composition of a lesion, even if it is moving in an irregular manner. Figure 26–2A shows a water-only EPI image from a patient

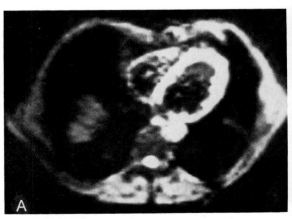
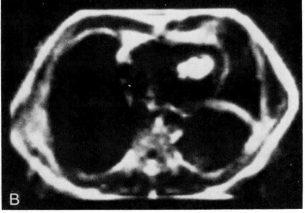

FIGURE 26–2. A, Chemical shift selective echo-planar water image of a patient known to have a left ventricular mass by echocardiography. No mass is seen. B, Chemical shift selective echo-planar fat image of the same patient. Note the bright mass in the left ventricular apex which appears to partially penetrate the apex. The mass is a lipoma.

reported to have an intracardiac mass by echocardiography. An EPI image also was performed with a fat-selective pulse (Fig. 26–2B). This shows an apical intracardiac lipoma, as well as the superficial adipose tissue.

Echo-planar imaging is especially well suited for pediatric imaging, given the need for careful evaluation of complex congenital anomalies in uncooperative patients and a need to limit exposure to ionizing radiation. Two studies[7, 8] have shown the efficacy of EPI in pediatric imaging. Even when patients are in atrial fibrillation or are demonstrating other cardiac irregularities, good image quality can be obtained.

In addition to spin-echo EPI images, it is possible to obtain gradient-echo EPI images. The acquisition method is similar to that for spin-echo EPI, except that the series of separately phase-encoded gradient echos are acquired under the envelope of a gradient-echo signal produced by a single alpha RF pulse. Gradient-echo EPI images are predominantly proton density and T_2^* weighted. Such images show a very bright blood pool signal except, analogous to conventional MR imaging, when there is intravoxel phase dispersion (e.g., due to turbulence). EPI can show low intensity jets from turbulent flow through an incompetent valve, as shown in Figure 26–3. Note that the images are free of respiratory motion artifact, although the patient did not suspend breathing. This is because the image acquisition times are short relative to the period of respiratory motion.

A series of gradient-echo EPI images can be obtained spanning one or a few cardiac cycles and can be played back in a closed loop to produce a cineangiogram-like study. This method is capable of displaying wall motion abnormalities and permits rapid calculation of ejection fractions and cardiac chamber volumes.

A particularly intriguing capability of EPI is that it can show transient phenomena, some of which could not be detected by standard MR imaging routines. We have investigated the transient response of myocardial signal to the lanthanide contrast agents gadolinium-DTPA (Gd-DTPA) and dysprosium-DTPA (Dy-DTPA).[17] Following intravascular administration, these agents distribute into the intravascular and interstitial spaces (see Chapters 7 and 8). In cardiac studies using standard spin-echo methods, Gd-DTPA has been reported to have a transient effect on T_1, with only a minor effect on T_2 in the standard doses (<0.2 mmol/kg).[18] However, using spin-echo EPI, a very different effect from bolus administration of Gd-DTPA was observed in a canine model. Instead of the expected rise in signal intensity, there was a loss of signal intensity (T_2 effect) (Fig. 26–4). The plot in Figure 26–5 shows the time course of signal changes in 50 images taken every 1.5 seconds, as part of an 80 data image set. The Gd-DTPA bolus had a maximal effect lasting approximately 15 seconds, occurring within 10 to 15 seconds after the injection. The experiment was repeated after an injection of dipyridamole to produce coronary vasodilation and increase coronary blood flow, demonstrating an even more profound signal reduction with an earlier time-to-peak effect. A similar effect is produced by Dy-DTPA. The loss of signal is caused by a marked shortening in the T_2 relaxation time of the myocardium. The T_2 shortening is due to diffusion of water molecules through an inhomogeneous magnetic field produced by high concentrations of the paramagnetic agents.

In order to investigate a clinically relevant problem, that of coronary stenosis detection, we applied a balloon occluder to the left anterior descending (LAD) coronary of a dog[19] and observed the signal

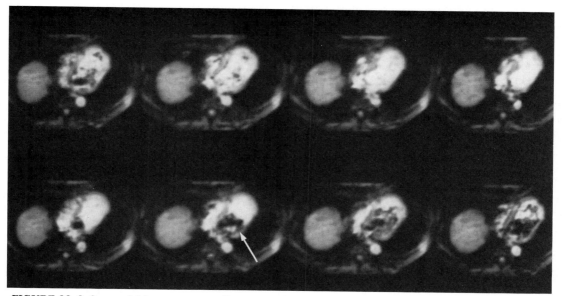

FIGURE 26–3. Sequential instant scan gradient-echo images of a patient with aortic regurgitation. All the images can be acquired within a single heart beat. The dark region in the left ventricle (arrow) corresponds to a jet from the aorta.

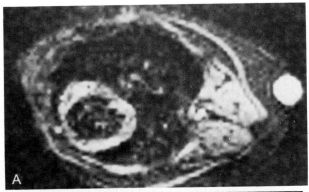

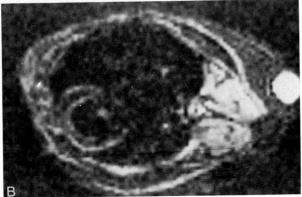

FIGURE 26–4. *A,* Echo-planar image obtained from a dog in the control state. *B,* Image obtained after injection of Gd-DTPA into the jugular vein, demonstrating marked signal reduction due to T₂ shortening (magnetic susceptibility effect).

intensity change after Dy-DTPA injection. The study was done in four parts: (1) after applying the deflated balloon occluder to the LAD, (2) after inflation of the occluder to reduce the distal LAD pressure by 20 to 40 mm, (3) after administration of dipyridamole while the occluder was inflated, and (4) after deflation of the occluder and with a second, smaller injection of dipyridamole. As shown in Figure 26–6, the baseline data set shows a significant difference between the LAD zone and a myocardial region supplied by another coronary artery (remote zone). This is likely an artifact from the surgical preparation, which re-

sulted in increased flow to the zone supplied by the manipulated coronary artery. Application of the occluder to produce a stenosis blunted the Dy-DTPA effect in the LAD zone. Administration of dipyridamole to increase blood flow enhanced the contrast between the normally perfused remote zone and the region of reduced perfusion (LAD zone). Finally, removal of the stenosis did not appear to change the Dy-DTPA effect in the remote region but did significantly increase the contrast effect in the LAD zone. These data suggest that contrast-enhanced EPI imaging may prove useful in detecting significant coronary stenoses. This study would not be possible with conventional MR methods, which do not permit adequate temporal resolution.

Recently, another method for producing first-pass perfusion studies of the heart has been described.[20] This method, which is a variant of an inversion recovery (IR) technique, differs from EPI in that it produces T₁-weighted rather than T₂-weighted images. As a result, administration of Gd-DTPA predominantly causes an increase, rather than a decrease, in myocardial signal. The method (Fig. 26–7) employs an initial 180-degree RF pulse to invert the spins. Next, an inversion delay (TI) is allowed to elapse, during which differences in longitudinal magnetization (i.e., T₁ contrast) evolve depending on the T₁ relaxation times of the various tissues (see Chapter 1). Finally, a very rapid gradient-echo acquisition using an ultrashort TR (e.g., 4 msec) and an ultrashort TE (e.g., 2 msec) is performed. The total time for data acquisition (32 phase-encoding steps) is on the order of 100 msec, which is short relative to the T₁ relaxation time of myocardium. The use of a small field-of-view partly compensates for the loss of resolution from the small acquisition matrix.

By selecting an appropriate TI (e.g., 400 msec at 1.5 T) the signal from myocardium is eliminated. After administration of Gd-DTPA as a bolus injection (0.05 to 0.1 mmol/kg over 5 to 10 sec) into a peripheral vein, ultrafast inversion recovery images are acquired every 2 to 3 seconds for up to 2 minutes. The application of each 180-degree RF pulse is synchronized to the ECG to ensure that each cardiac image is acquired at the same point of the cardiac

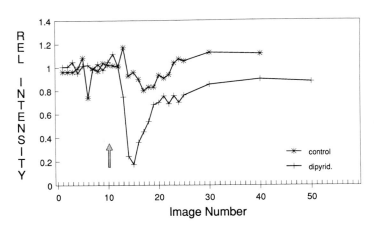

FIGURE 26–5. Plot of relative signal intensity versus image number, with approximately 1.5 seconds between each echo-planar image acquisition. The Gd-DTPA was injected into the jugular vein at the time of the tenth image *(arrow)*. The contrast agent produced a signal reduction in the initial study, which is more pronounced after treatment with dipyridamole.

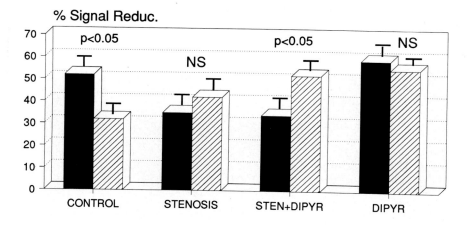

FIGURE 26–6. A plot of signal reduction on echo-planar images as a result of Dy-DTPA intravenous injection. Black area = LAD zone; shaded area = remote zone. The administration of dipyridamole increased tissue contrast between the stenotic region and normally perfused myocardium.

cycle. In a study of healthy human subjects, bolus administration of Gd-DTPA produced an approximate threefold signal enhancement of perfused myocardium (Fig. 26–8). The time course of the enhancement was relatively slow, with a gradual increase in myocardial signal occurring over approximately 20 seconds after contrast agent administration, followed by a gradual decrease in signal due to contrast agent wash-out which occurred over tens of seconds. The prolonged wash-out can be attributed to the prolonged wash-in and to the interstitial distribution of gadolinium-DTPA. The prolonged wash-in, due to spreading of the peripherally injected bolus in the arm veins, represents a problem in human subjects with respect to quantitating wash-out curves (see further on). A portion of the original bolus may still be arriving at the heart as long as 20 seconds after the original intravenous injection and thereby overlaps the second-pass recirculation of the contrast agent.

The ultrafast inversion recovery method has also been applied to the study of abnormal perfusion in the ischemic heart. In a perfused rat heart model, administration of Gd-DTPA with ultrafast inversion recovery imaging produced marked signal enhance-

ment of perfused myocardium, whereas an infarct that had been induced by occluding a coronary artery showed no enhancement (Fig. 26–9).

EVALUATION OF CARDIAC PERFUSION

Gd-DTPA has been proved safe and efficacious for studies in the central nervous system. Clinical application to human studies of ischemic heart disease is also feasible, and such studies are currently underway. However, interpretation of the results of these studies will rely on knowledge gained from well-controlled animal studies as well as consideration of the basic principles of indicator dilution studies of organ perfusion (i.e., tissue blood flow), which we will now review.

For studying tissue perfusion, the Stewart-Hamilton equation states that after injection of a bolus of contrast agent into the blood, the tissue blood flow (F) can be determined as:

$$F = m/[\int_0^\infty c(t)dt]$$

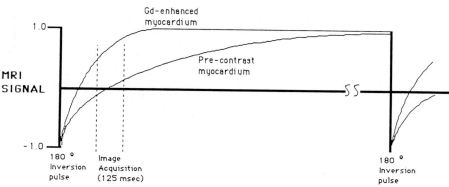

FIGURE 26–7. Diagram of acquisition method for ultrafast inversion recovery imaging. The spins are inverted by a 180-degree pulse at the R wave. Four hundred msec later, an image is acquired over a period of 125 msec.

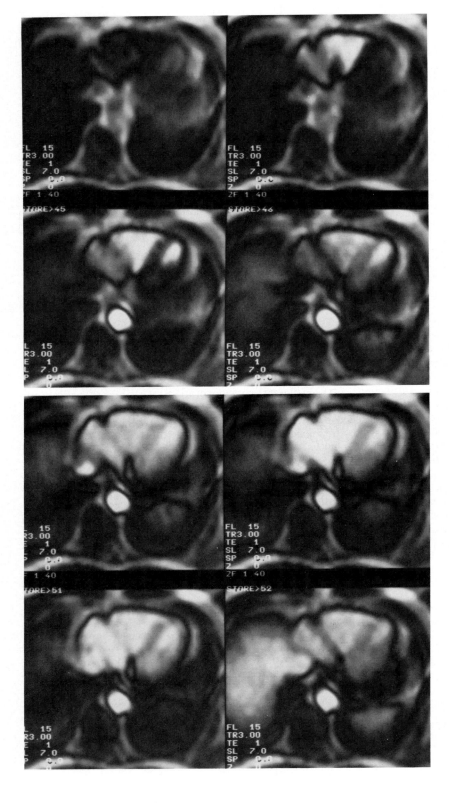

FIGURE 26–8. First-pass cardiac perfusion study of a healthy human subject using the instant inversion recovery sequence with bolus administration of Gd-DTPA. There is marked enhancement of the left ventricular myocardium. Note the dark lines around the right atrial and ventricular cavities when the contrast agent first appears, representing a boundary effect between regions of differing magnetic susceptibility.

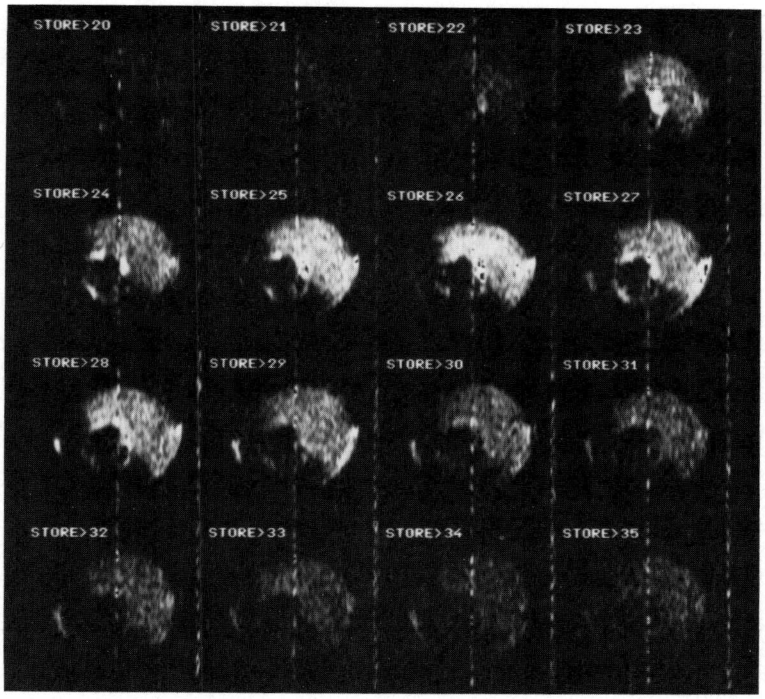

FIGURE 26–9. Ultrafast inversion recovery images acquired at 5-second intervals following administration of Gd-DTPA in a perfused rat heart model. The left coronary artery was occluded. Note the marked enhancement of the perfused myocardium (upper right segment of heart) and absence of signal change in the nonperfused region (lower left segment).

where m = mass of contrast agent injected, and c(t) = instantaneous concentration of the contrast agent in the tissue. Since the actual mass of contrast agent delivered to the tissue is unknown, other methods may be more practical for MR quantification of perfusion. For instance, one can attempt to measure the mean transit time of the contrast agent, which is related to the shape of the time-concentration curve of the contrast agent (arterial input function). For a nondiffusible (purely intravascular) contrast agent, this method provides a flow per unit vascular volume. In order to compute flow per unit tissue volume, the fraction of tissue that is vascular must be known.[21–23]

There are major practical difficulties in applying these approaches to MR contrast studies. For example, the relationship between signal intensity and concentration of contrast agent is not precisely known. The fractional vascular volume of the tissue is another unknown.

Still another issue is the distribution of contrast agent between tissue and blood. Gd-DTPA can cross the endothelial barrier and distributes between the interstitial and intravascular spaces. Changes in myocardial signal intensity following administration of Gd-DTPA therefore depend on tissue perfusion but also on the volume of the interstitial space into which the contrast agent distributes. For instance, reperfused infarcts may show increased contrast enhancement relative to normal regions because of edema and a resulting increase in the extracellular space, without necessarily indicating whether blood flow is increased.[24, 25] Quantitative measurement of perfusion therefore requires a knowledge of the partition coefficient of the contrast agent between the intra- and extravascular space.

In this regard, superparamagnetic iron oxide (e.g., ferrites) may have an advantage. It is a particulate agent that cannot cross through the capillary wall and therefore remains within the intravascular space. Because this agent is superparamagnetic (see Chapter 8), it is also potent, so that very small doses will cause a marked reduction in myocardial signal intensity. We have recently investigated the myocardial effects of a prototype superparamagnetic agent[26] (AMI-25, Advanced Magnetics Inc., Cambridge, MA). Our results showed that with as low a dose as 36 micromoles of iron per kilogram of body weight and conventional spin-echo pulse sequences, we were able to detect an approximate 40 per cent signal reduction, which was homogeneous throughout the myocardium. The signal drop results partly from diffusion, as determined from CPMG experiments, and partly from relaxivity effects unrelated to diffusion.

Although precise quantitation of cardiac perfusion may prove elusive, even qualitative evaluation of contrast agent studies is likely to provide useful clinical information about myocardial ischemia. Rapid contrast-enhanced studies of the heart using ultrafast scanning methods, perhaps in conjunction with stress-inducing maneuvers such as exercise or dipyridamole administration, have the potential for improving the accuracy with which ischemic heart disease is evaluated. Even without ultrafast scanning techniques, perfusion deficits have been shown in the setting of acute and subacute myocardial infarction. Several investigators have studied the usefulness of contrast-enhanced MR with Gd-DTPA and standard spin-echo methods.[27–29] These studies have suggested that contrast administration improves detection of myocardial infarcts in both the acute and subacute stages. In acute occlusive infarcts, there is generally reduced enhancement of the infarct relative to normal myocardium due to reduced delivery of contrast agent to the infarcted region. In subacute infarcts, the situation is more complex because of edema and collateral circulation. As mentioned above, this may result in increased enhancement of the infarct relative to myocardium.

IMAGING OF CORONARY BYPASS GRAFTS AND NATIVE CORONARY ARTERIES

CORONARY BYPASS GRAFTS

Coronary bypass graft surgery is a common surgical procedure, with more than 200,000 performed annually in the United States.[30] Because bypass graft closure is a late complication, requiring accurate diagnosis and appropriate clinical investigation to improve patency, a noninvasive method of accurate diagnosis is needed. To this end, several investigators have employed MRI to examine bypass graft patency.[31–33]

White and colleagues[34] examined 27 patients with 72 grafts using spin-echo imaging and found a predictive accuracy of 78 per cent. Rubinstein and coworkers[35] in a slightly smaller group detected a sensitivity of 92 per cent and a specificity of 85 per cent, with a similar result obtained by Jenkins and colleagues.[36] Frija and associates,[37] also using spin-echo imaging, detected 38 out of 39 patent normal grafts. They had much greater difficulty in identifying diseased grafts because of inability to view the entire bypass graft. White and coworkers[38] reported the use of a gradient-echo (bright blood) sequence and found a sensitivity for graft patency of 93 per cent, with a specificity of 86 per cent, and an overall predictive accuracy of 89 per cent.

We have been examining bypass graft patency with a combination of spin-echo and gradient-echo methods. Instead of using the standard imaging planes (i.e., axial, coronal, sagittal), axes are defined with respect to the patient's cardiac anatomy, guided by the surgeon's operative report. This requires an understanding of the typical location of the grafts (Fig. 26–10). This is especially important with sequential grafts, for which patency in all segments must be determined. Figure 26–11 shows an image in the plane of the pulmonary outflow tract, chosen to examine grafts to the diagonal and circumflex coronaries. In this orientation the grafts are likely to be running through the plane, minimizing partial volume effects. If graft patency is still a question, a gradient-echo sequence is performed, with the results displayed in Figure 26–12. Note that the high signal grafts are easily identified. Another imaging plane would be chosen to detect an LAD graft. Preliminary results of 96 proximal graft anastomoses reveal that

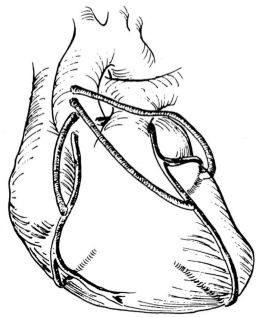

FIGURE 26–10. Schematic diagram showing the predominantly superficial locations of coronary bypass grafts. These grafts are well suited for surface coil imaging. (From Moncada R, Salinas M, Churchill R, et al: Patency of saphenous aortocoronary-bypass grafts demonstrated by computed tomography. N Engl J Med 303:5–13, 1980; with permission of the New England Journal of Medicine.)

of 74 patent proximal anastomoses by x-ray cineangiography, 72 were detected by MRI (Holmvang et al, in preparation).

There are several potential pitfalls in evaluating bypass graft patency. Artifactual signal voids from

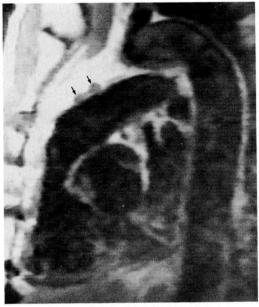

FIGURE 26–11. Spin-echo image of the heart oriented to demonstrate the coronary bypass grafts (arrows) crossing the pulmonary outflow tract.

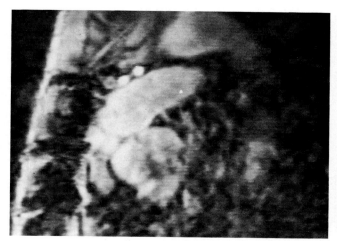

FIGURE 26–12. Gradient-echo image of the patient in Figure 26–11. Note the bright signal from the bypass grafts to the diagonal and circumflex coronary arteries. (From Boucher CA, Kantor HL, Okada RD, Strauss HW: Radionuclide imaging and magnetic resonance imaging. *In* Eagle KA, et al (eds): The Practice of Cardiology. Boston, Little, Brown, 1989; with permission.)

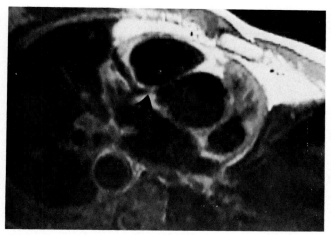

FIGURE 26–13. A spin-echo image demonstrating the left coronary artery at its origin. The arrow indicates a region of apparent stenosis (see text). (From Holmvang G: Noninvasive imaging of the coronary arteries. *In* Miller D (ed): Clinical Cardiac Imaging. New York, McGraw-Hill Book Co., 1988; with permission.)

sternal wires may obscure portions of the graft; however, in our experience this is an infrequent occurrence. On gated spin-echo images, the signal intensity within the graft, as well as the position of the graft, may vary over the cardiac cycle, making identification of contiguous regions difficult. The small size of internal mammary grafts is near the limit of spatial resolution of the MR images, and clips are often placed at multiple sites along these grafts, producing signal voids. Use of surface coils to image the bypass grafts, which are mostly superficial in location, can improve signal-to-noise ratio (S/N) and thereby permit higher spatial resolution to be obtained than with body coils. Finally, proper interpretation of the MR images requires a solid knowledge of the usual anatomic configurations of different types of grafts.

Identifying graft patency will have some clinical utility; however, a more significant impact would be anticipated if projection angiograms showing the entire length of the graft could be obtained or if flow down the graft could be measured. To date, this goal has not been obtained. Measurement of graft flow using phase imaging or time-of-flight techniques might also prove useful. However, this work is still at a very preliminary stage.

CORONARY ARTERIES

Imaging of the coronary arteries is among the most difficult tasks facing MRI technology. The coronary arteries are moving with each cardiac cycle as well as with respiration. Normal flow velocities in the coronary arteries approach 1 meter per second, which can produce signal loss from flow-related dephasing. The native arteries range in size from 1 to 5 mm. In addition, coronary flow is phasic, with peak

flow during early diastole, which limits the available time window for coronary imaging. Despite all these difficulties, coronary arteries are often quite well visualized by MRI. Figure 26–13 shows the LAD coming off the aorta, and Figure 26–14 shows the full extent of the left coronary system, with branching into the circumflex and LAD coronaries. The major problem, even with these images which demonstrate the coronaries, is the inability to discern diseased from normal regions. In Figure 26–13, there appears to be a left main coronary artery stenosis, but in fact the appearance is a result of the vessel leaving the plane of the image (Fig. 26–15). Partial volume averaging is also a limitation, particularly with spin-echo techniques, and calcified plaques may increase the signal void and overestimate the region of flow.

It is clear from these bypass graft studies that an alternative adjunct to spin-echo imaging may im-

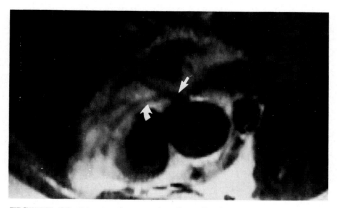

FIGURE 26–14. An image showing the branching of the left coronary system *(arrows)*. Despite the finding of an 80 per cent LAD stenosis during cardiac catheterization, the artery appears normal. (From Holmvang G: Noninvasive imaging of the coronary arteries. *In* Miller D (ed): Clinical Cardiac Imaging. New York, McGraw-Hill Book Co., 1988; with permission.)

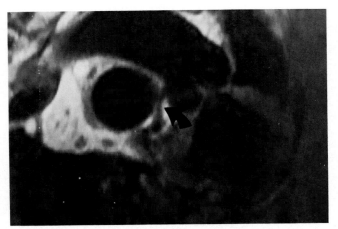

FIGURE 26–15. An orthogonal image of the patient in Figure 26–13, in which the left coronary curves up toward the pulmonary artery. This curvature resulted in the apparent stenosis on the axial image.

prove the accuracy of MR. One approach being pursued uses a preinversion pulse followed by projective imaging, alternated with a standard projective sequence without preinversion. Image subtraction then reveals only the vessels filled by blood from the preinverted region. The problem with this method is that for coronary imaging in a projective format, blood pool from the ventricle must not be excited. Therefore, the inversion should only be applied to the aortic root and in a region suitably close to the coronary ostia to reduce mixing and allow complete filling of the coronaries. Nishimura and colleagues[39] have devised a method for applying inversion pulses to a limited three-dimensional (3D) volume without affecting tissues outside the volume. This method employs a modulation of the gradients as well as the RF pulses. To date, however, no convincing image of the coronary arteries has been produced. Initial results using a STEAM sequence to selectively tag blood in the aortic root and image inflow into the proximal coronary arteries have shown promise in a perfused rat heart model (D. Burstein, personal communication, 1989), but the method has not yet been applied in humans. Another approach is to acquire a series of contiguous 2D gradient-echo cine images spanning the proximal arteries and postprocess them into a projection angiogram using a maximal intensity projection method, but again the results are too preliminary for adequate evaluation.

An additional challenge is posed by flow turbulence, especially around stenotic lesions, which will cause signal loss. This may cause overestimation of the severity of the lesion or make one appear where none exists. The most clear-cut method to reduce the signal loss from turbulence, beyond just using flow compensation, is to use ultrashort TE (see Chapter 4). Nonetheless, in severe stenoses some degree of signal loss will persist. Also, use of very short TE necessarily limits spatial resolution, given finite peak gradient amplitudes and rise times. Use of 3D meth-

ods to reduce the voxel size and thereby overcome flow-related dephasing has proven effective for studies of the cerebrovascular circulation, but application to the coronary arteries is problematic due to respiratory and cardiac motion. It is possible that the limitations imposed by motion could be resolved using EPI methods. However, the requisite spatial resolution is far beyond that currently available with ultrafast scanning methods. For at least the immediate future, perfusion imaging with contrast agents is likely to have greater clinical potential than anatomic imaging for the noninvasive detection of coronary artery stenosis.

SPECTROSCOPY

The heart is an especially appropriate organ to be studied by MR spectroscopy (MRS) because of the great magnitude of cardiovascular-related illness in this country and the potential applicability of MRS for examination of the most prevalent cardiac disease process, myocardial ischemia.

PHOSPHORUS SPECTROSCOPY

Initial in vitro studies of cells and tissues centered around the evaluation of bioenergetics. ^{31}P MRS is a valuable tool in this endeavor because a typical spectrum has resonances from ATP, phosphocreatine (PCr), inorganic orthophosphate (Pi), as well as phosphomonoesters, phosphodiesters, and small contributions from ADP and NAD. Early studies showed that PCr and ATP are 100 per cent MRS observable, making these investigations even more appropriate. It had also been shown that MRS metabolite measurements in tissues could be obtained within reasonable acquisition times (i.e., <1 hour). Studies done in yeast[40, 41] and cell suspensions[42–46] were extended to intact organs such as skeletal muscle,[47–51] brain,[52–58] liver,[59–67] and kidney.[68–70] Cardiac studies were initially performed by Gadian and coworkers.[71] These investigators demonstrated that the phosphates of ATP and phosphocreatine as well as resonances from inorganic orthophosphate and sugar phosphates could be demonstrated. They examined the metabolic changes in an excised rat heart that had been rapidly cooled to zero degrees centigrade. With gradual warming to 30 degrees, an acidic shift of the inorganic orthophosphate peak was noted as well as degradation of the high energy phosphorylated metabolites. These studies were extended to the observation of hearts under more steady-state conditions using an in vitro retrograde perfusion apparatus.[72] With this preparation, examinations could be performed over an approximate three-hour period with maintenance of baseline metabolites and with a left ventricular balloon in place allowing measurement of ventricular function throughout the experiment. Using this model, several aspects of myocardial metabolism and physiology have been examined: (1) the investigation of myocardial ischemia and the correlation of high energy metabolites with persistent functional impairment related to transient ischemia (stunned myocardium), (2) the variation of phosphorus metabolites throughout the cardiac cycle, (3) the effect of workload on myocardial metabolites and the control of myocardial respiration, and (4) the assessment of myocardial protection. With improved probe design and the advent of horizontal bore magnets capable of accepting whole animals and humans, these studies were extended to in vivo examinations, with the goal of understanding cardiac physiology in health and disease.

Myocardial Ischemia

It was quite well known before in vivo MRS experiments were performed that severe ischemia caused a loss of high energy phosphates.[73, 74] Cellular and nonperfused skeletal muscle preparations[50, 75–77] demonstrated a similar gradual reduction in PCr and ATP, with increasing Pi. Jacobus and colleagues[78] and Garlick and associates[79] extended this work to the perfused beating heart model, showing similar results. Additionally there is an acidic shift of the Pi peak as a result of the byproducts of anaerobic metabolism (predominantly lactic acid).

Several groups have examined the effect of transient ischemia on the recovery of high energy phosphates and/or myocardial systolic function.[80–89] There is a rapid reduction in PCr and an increase in Pi with ischemia, as well as an acidic shift and a drop in function. With a modest duration of complete ischemia (12 to 14 minutes) or a less severe flow reduction, the ATP does not significantly change, and almost complete recovery of function is achieved. Clarke and Willis[83] performed graded perfusion studies and suggested that under ischemic conditions, cytosolic metabolite levels may limit contractile function, but that under high flow conditions, other factors may govern function (Fig. 26–16). During the recovery period, PCr increases rapidly and usually overshoots the control concentration, Pi returns to normal, and almost complete recovery of function is achieved. With a greater duration of total ischemia (more than 20 minutes), the ATP falls and may not fully recover, and ATP concentration correlates with reduced functional recovery.[88, 90] Although this association during reperfusion has been supported by some investigators with analytical techniques,[91–93] its causal relationship is counter to data from other laboratories[94–98] and requires further study.

Segmental Ischemia

More recently, interest has centered on the study of models of myocardial ischemia that correspond more closely to the classic clinical problem—in vivo

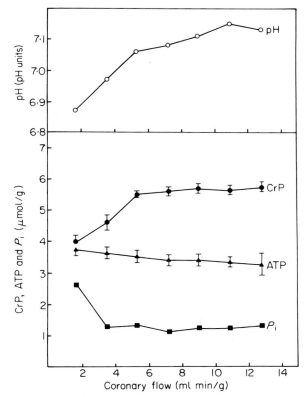

FIGURE 26–16. Relationship among PCr, ATP, and Pi, in the isovolumic rat heart, with variation in coronary flow. (From Clarke K, Willis RJ: Energy metabolism and contractile function in rat hearts during graded, isovolumentric perfusion using ^{31}P nuclear magnetic resonance spectroscopy. J Mol Cell Cardiol 19:1153–1160, 1987; with permission.)

segmental partial or complete myocardial ischemia in the setting of a persistent or reversible flow disturbance.[99–102] The first studies of segmental ischemia were done be Hollis and colleagues[103] in a rat model. They found that after LAD ligation, two Pi peaks became visible, consistent with the low and normal pH regions corresponding to the normal and ischemic myocardium. Guth and colleagues[99] induced anterior wall myocardial ischemia by occluding the LAD coronary artery and obtained ^{31}P spectra from a 2.5-cm surface coil placed over the region supplied by the LAD. Using the relative localizing capability of the surface coil, which preferentially collects signal within one diameter away from the surface coil, it was shown that PCr decreased to 46 per cent after 17 minutes of LAD occlusion, and ATP fell to approximately 75 per cent of control. After 22 minutes of reperfusion the PCr had returned to baseline while the ATP remained depressed. There was a correlation between postreperfusion fractional ATP content and fractional recovery of contractile function. A similar study was done by Schaefer and coworkers,[104] in which they examined the effect of graded myocardial ischemia, with relative flow assessed by microspheres. A flow reduction of 50 per cent or less was associated with a significant fall in PCr, and relative

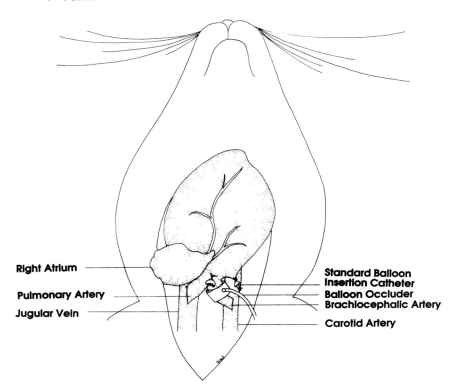

FIGURE 26–17. Model of the heterotopic rat heart transplant. (From Rozenman Y, Kantor HL: Heterotopic transplanted rat heart: A model for in vivo determination of phosphorus metabolites during ischemia and perfusion. Magn Reson Med 1989 [in press].)

Right Atrium

Pulmonary Artery

Jugular Vein

Standard Balloon Insertion Catheter

Balloon Occluder

Brachiocephalic Artery

Carotid Artery

flow was found most highly correlated with PCr/Pi. In contrast to the study of Guth and associates, there was no significant reduction in ATP up to a relative flow of 0.2. This is most consistent with data obtained on a rat transplant model of global myocardial ische-

RF Coil

Coaxial Cable

Balloon Occluder

Femoral Artery Catheter

Femoral Vein Catheter

FIGURE 26–18. Position of the rat in the NMR probe with the surface coil transceiver in place. (From Rozenman Y, Kantor HL: Heterotopic transplanted rat heart: A model for in vivo determination of phosphorus metabolites during ischemia and perfusion. Magn Reson Med 1989 [in press].)

mia.[105] In this study an isogenic heterotopic heart transplantation procedure is performed 2 to 5 days before MRS examination (Figs. 26–17 and 26–18). A balloon occluder is positioned around the trans-

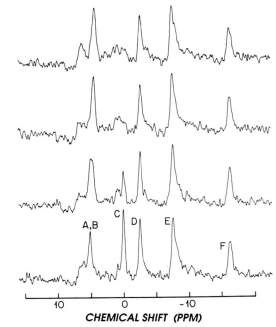

A,B   C   D   E

F

10   0   -10

CHEMICAL SHIFT (PPM)

FIGURE 26–19. NMR spectra from the transplanted heart during a control period (bottom) and sequentially during global ischemia. The peak assignments are: A,B = 2,3 DPG and Pi; C = PCr; D = gamma phosphate of ATP; E = alpha phosphate of ATP and NAD; F = beta phosphate of ATP. (From Rozenman Y, Kantor HL: Heterotopic transplanted rat heart: A model for in vivo determination of phosphorus metabolites during ischemia and perfusion. Magn Reson Med 1989 [in press].)

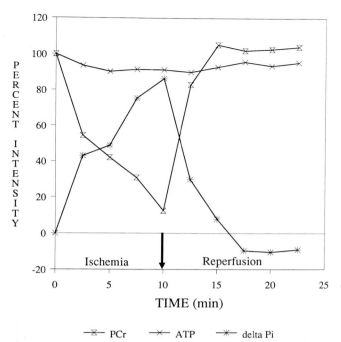

FIGURE 26–20. Time course of metabolite concentrations during ischemia and reperfusion. (From Rozenman Y, Kantor HL: Heterotopic transplanted rat heart: A model for in vivo determination of phosphorus metabolites during ischemia and perfusion. Magn Reson Med 1989 [in press].)

planted brachiocephalic artery, allowing occlusion of the retrograde flow while in the magnet. An intraventricular standard allows quantitation of the spectrum, adjustment of the pulse duration for reproducible B_1, and an isovolumetric working state. The results revealed no significant change in ATP, even at peak ischemia when PCr was 13 per cent of the control concentration (Figs. 26–19 and 26–20). This result, and the data of Schaefer and colleagues, are consistent with the suggested near equilibrium of the creatine kinase reaction.[106] Using the normal measured concentrations of the creatine kinase reactants,[107] it can be calculated that for a 10 per cent residual concentration of PCr, the ATP would fall by

only 7 per cent, which is within the experimental error of our measurement. The likely explanation for the results of Guth and associates is that regions of more severe ischemia or infarction contributed to their spectra. This assessment is consistent with the excellent coronary collateral blood flow in the dog, which is not present in the pig, allowing for a more homogeneous ischemic region in the pig.

Transmural Metabolite Distribution in Ischemia

Myocardial blood flow during states of increased workload (such as aortic stenosis) and during myocardial ischemia[108–114] result in an inhomogeneous transmural distribution of blood flow. During a period of acute occlusion, myocardial necrosis in both canines and humans begins in the subendocardium, consistent with this blood flow distribution.[115–118] Two groups have begun examining this phenomenon and its effect on high energy phosphate content. Gober and coworkers[119] examined porcine myocardial ischemia using an epicardial surface coil, and the Fourier series window technique (FSW).[120, 121] This method of spectral localization takes advantage of the spatial inhomogeneity afforded by a surface coil.[122, 123] Rather than collecting an entire B_1 imaging data set in this technique, only data that significantly contribute to locations of interest are obtained (Figs. 26–21 and 26–22). With this method in a porcine model, they were able to demonstrate an increased Pi peak in the subendocardium during reduced coronary perfusion (Fig. 26–23), which was not evident in the subepicardium. This effect was associated with a reduced relative perfusion to the subendocardium as compared with the subepicardium (Fig. 26–24). Robitaille and associates[124, 125] used an alternative method that employs adiabatic pulses to achieve uniform slice selection in a defined region using an ISIS technique, generating a localized region of interest. An FSW experiment is then performed on this region, producing spectra localized to slices that do not have wings of mixed spatial selection, such as those encountered in standard FSW experiments.

Using this technique, the canine myocardium was

FIGURE 26–21. Diagram of a surface coil B_1 contours on a plane phantom showing desired location of signal acquisition, which is used in modelling and pulse sequence optimization. Representative regions are: Epi, subepicardium; Endo, subendocardium; Cavity, ventricular chamber. HMPT is a standard sample of hexamethylphosphorus triamide. (From Gober J, Schaefer S, Camacho SA, et al: Epicardial and endocardial localized ^{31}P magnetic resonance spectroscopy: Evidence for metabolic heterogeneity during regional ischemia. Magn Reson Med [in press].)

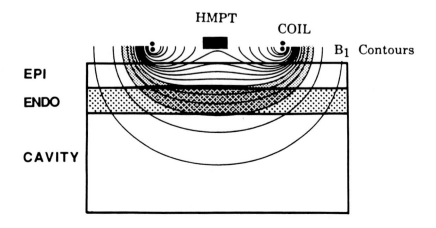

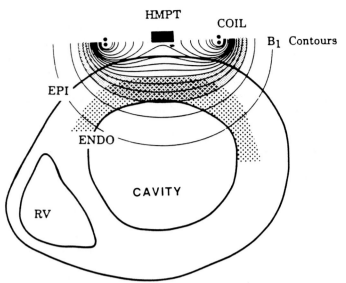

FIGURE 26–22. A diagram of the coil positioned on a heart. (From Gober J, Schaefer S, Camacho SA, et al: Epicardial and endocardial localized ^{31}P magnetic resonance spectroscopy: Evidence for metabolic heterogeneity during regional ischemia. Magn Reson Med [in press].)

examined in systole after coronary flow reduction. With a 20 per cent reduction in coronary flow there was an increase in Pi that was homogeneous across the myocardial thickness. However, when a 75 per cent flow reduction was implemented, Pi increased in a more subendocardial layer. In an even deeper slice the peaks from 2,3 diphosphoglycerate (2,3 DPG) of blood become apparent. These data demonstrate the feasibility of MR spectroscopic measurement of the transmural heterogeneity of myocardial perfusion, which should improve the overall sensitiv-

ity of MRS for detecting significant myocardial ischemia.

The study by Robitaille and coworkers[125] also discussed a problem that is unique to cardiac spectroscopic applications. Because the heart is in motion, data acquired with B_0 gradient localization must be gated in order to ensure reproducible positioning. The position can be determined for both systole and diastole, but it must be understood that wall thickness will vary during the cardiac cycle. A spectrum obtained with a B_1 gradient FSW method from the inner half of the myocardium in diastole will not represent the inner half of the myocardium during systole. More importantly, during ischemia when myocardial akinesis (absence of motion) or dyskinesis (paradoxical motion) may be observed, the resultant spectral localization may be even more unpredictable. Conclusions regarding spectra obtained from different phases of the cardiac cycle must therefore be reached after considering changes in myocardial thickness.

Phasic Alteration in Myocardial Metabolites

In 1980 Fossel and colleagues[126] demonstrated in a Langendorff perfused rat heart with glucose as its metabolic substrate that PCr and ATP levels are reduced during systole and that Pi is increased. Additionally they found that a cycling of sugar phosphates increased during systole and decreased during diastole. This experiment was ideally suited to the capability of MRS for performing very rapid measurements gated to the heart rate. Collection of the free induction decay can be done with short acquisition times (<50 msec), thus indeed reflecting the state of the myocardium during a very short interval

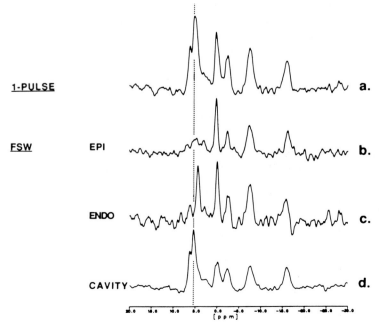

FIGURE 26–23. Spectra of an ischemic pig heart acquired with a standard one-pulse sequence compared with those obtained with the Fourier series window (FSW) method, localized to the three myocardial regions. (From Gober J, Schaefer S, Camacho SA, et al: Epicardial and endocardial localized ^{31}P magnetic resonance spectroscopy: Evidence for metabolic heterogeneity during regional ischemia. Magn Reson Med [in press].)

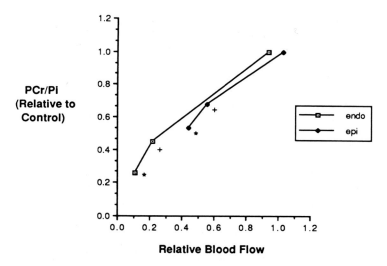

FIGURE 26–24. Myocardial PCr/Pi as a function of relative blood flow. (From Gober J, Schaefer S, Camacho SA, et al: Epicardial and endocardial localized ^{31}P magnetic resonance spectroscopy: Evidence for metabolic heterogeneity during regional ischemia. Magn Reson Med [in press].)

of systole or diastole. Despite this interesting result and some agreement with freeze clamping studies in glucose perfused hearts, data collected by other investigators did not corroborate the results; however, these experiments were done in different model systems. In vivo studies using an implanted coil and other in vivo studies using a catheter coil[127] showed no cyclic changes of high energy phosphates. As noted in Figure 26–25 the spectrum collected from four phases of the cardiac cycle in this canine model did not significantly change. More recently, an examination of myocardial metabolites using one-dimensional spatial selectivity with a B_1 imaging technique demonstrated that in the baseline state of normal perfusion there was no change in myocardial metabolites throughout the cardiac cycle. However, in the setting of ischemia one could see subendocardial changes during portions of the cardiac cycle. Robataille and associates[125] suggested that these variations with ischemia reflect a change in heart wall thickness in ischemic regions, with wall thinning producing an apparent change in metabolite concentration, ATP, and PCr content. This cyclic variation of high energy phosphates requires further investigation for corroboration.

Workload

Glucose perfused rat heart studies have demonstrated a reduction in steady-state high energy metabolites with increasing workload.[128, 129] This has been shown by several groups and has been related to creatine kinase flux changes. The increase in creatine kinase flux was associated with a calculated increase in ADP assuming a near equilibrium condition for creatine kinase. These data suggest that myocardial oxygen consumption is very strongly coupled with ADP concentrations through the creatine

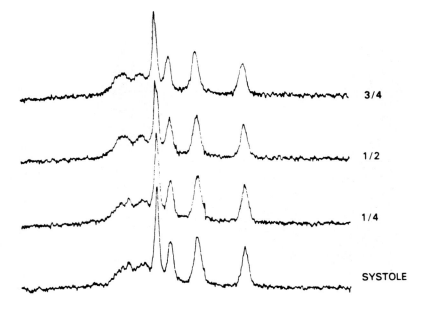

FIGURE 26–25. Gated ^{31}P magnetic resonance spectra of the canine heart obtained with a catheter coil, for each of four phases of the cardiac cycle. (From Kantor HL, et al: Am J Physiol 251:H171–H175, 1986; with permission.)

kinase reaction. A similar result was seen in an in vivo rat heart model, which revealed an approximate 2½-fold increase in creatine kinase flux with an increase in workload. This was found despite the fact that high energy phosphate content did not substantially change; this result does not generally agree with the perfused heart data. Several other investigators have sought to study this phenomenon and have found both a species variability as well as a substrate variability of the effective workload on phosphorus metabolites. Balaban and coworkers[130] studied this same problem in canine hearts using a catheter coil (Fig. 26–26). They examined five dogs without the need for thoracotomy by inserting an MRS receiver coil transvenously or transarterially into the right or left ventricle, respectively. After insertion of right atrial pacing leads, animals were paced to heart rates ranging from 60 to 180 per minute, with no significant effect on high energy phosphate metabolites detectable (Fig. 26–27). It has been proposed that the disparity in results may reflect the differing substrates in these experiments. Glucose perfused hearts may be more susceptible to high energy phosphate changes with increased workload than blood perfused hearts, in which fatty acids are the primary energy source, suggesting a different rate limiting step in metabolism for the two substrates. More recently, it has been shown that in vivo creatine kinase fluxes measured in pigs do not significantly change with changes in workload,[131] once again supporting the hypothesis that in vivo heart preparations do not behave like the glucose perfused rat heart.

Myocardial Protection

In this era of heart surgery with cardiopulmonary bypass, myocardial protection has been a paramount issue. In fact, the technique of cardiopulmonary bypass was developed in order to allow the surgeon to operate on an incised heart while perfusing the

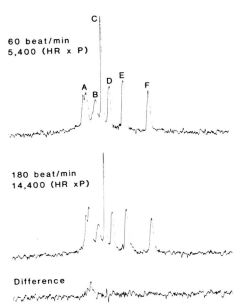

FIGURE 26–27. Canine heart ^{31}P spectra obtained at two different pacing rates. The peak assignments are: A = 2,3 DPG and Pi; B = phosphodiesters; C = PCr; D = gamma phosphate of ATP; E = alpha phosphate of ATP and NAD; and F = beta phosphate of ATP. The difference of the two spectra is shown in c. (From Balaban RS, Kantor HL, Katz LA, Briggs RW: Relation between work and phosphate metabolites in the in vivo paced mammalian heart. Science 232:1121–1123, 1986; with permission.)

other organs. However, in order to maintain a bloodless field while bypassing the coronaries, it is necessary to cross-clamp the aorta, thereby causing the heart to become ischemic. Although some surgeons prefer to cannulate the coronaries and perfuse them separately, cardiac preservation during this period of ischemia is of utmost importance.

Hollis and colleagues[132] investigated the effect of normothermic potassium chloride (KCl) arrest on perfused rabbit hearts after 40 minutes of global ischemia. They demonstrated that the KCl arrested heart retains most of its ATP and upon reperfusion returns to full function, while the control heart only retains a portion of its ATP and produces 70 per cent of its systolic function. This effect is associated with a pH of 7.0 in the treated hearts and with a more acidic pH of 6.1 in the control hearts. To further simulate the clinical situation, Flaherty and coworkers[133] compared the protective effects of hypothermia versus KCl arrest and hypothermia. The KCl perfused hypothermic hearts had a greater postischemic ATP recovery as well as a greater recovery of left ventricular function than the control hypothermic hearts (Fig. 26–28). In addition, as seen in the previous study, the addition of KCl was associated with less acidic change in pH. Further studies have examined the effects of lower temperatures,[134] perfusate containing fluorocarbon,[135] nifedipine plus hypothermia,[136] propranolol,[137] verapamil,[138] prostaglandin (PGBx),[139] and adenosine deaminase inhibitors.[140]

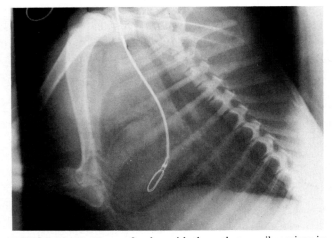

FIGURE 26–26. X-ray of a dog with the catheter coil receiver in the right ventricle.

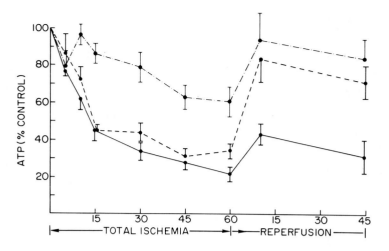

FIGURE 26–28. The time course of myocardial ATP during ischemia and reperfusion. Hypothermia *(solid line)*, single dose of hyperkalemic cardioplegia *(dashed line)*, three doses of hyperkalemic cardioplegia at 20-minute intervals *(dash-dot line)*. (From Flaherty JT, Weisfeldt M, Bulkley BH, et al: Mechanisms of ischemic myocardial cell damage assessed by phosphorus-31 nuclear magnetic resonance. Circulation 65:561, 1982; with permission.)

Cardiac Transplantation

With the greater application of immunosuppressive therapy, cardiac transplantation has become more successful, and the need to follow the course and early treatment of rejection has grown. Most of the investigations of transplant rejection have centered around the measurement of T_1 and T_2. Animal studies in rats and dogs indicated that relaxation times were prolonged with rejection.[141–143] Wisenberg and associates[144] studied 25 patients after recent cardiac transplantation. They found that within the first 25 days after surgery all patients had prolonged relaxation times. However, later imaging showed a significant increase in T_1 and T_2 only in patients with biopsy-proven rejection. A more recent study[145] examined T_2 relaxation in five normal subjects and nine transplant patients. T_2 values in patients with biopsy-proven rejection were significantly elevated. In another study using a rat model, administration of Gd-DTPA produced a marked increase in enhancement on T_1-weighted images in animals with transplant rejection.[146] Phosphorus MRS studies have indicated that reductions in high energy phosphates occur with cardiac rejection, and reversal of rejection is associated with an improvement in these metabolites.[147, 148]

CARBON-13 SPECTROSCOPY

Because of the low sensitivity and low natural abundance of carbon-13, ^{13}C MRS has not been applied to in vivo cardiac spectroscopic applications as often as ^{31}P and ^{1}H. However, because of the large chemical shift spectrum for ^{13}C, the presence of carbon in virtually all metabolic substrates, and the utility of ^{13}C as a tracer to measure cellular exchange rates and fluxes, ^{13}C MRS has been utilized extensively for the examination of cellular applications.[149–156] The first in vivo investigation was performed by Alger and colleagues.[157] They examined metabolism in the rat liver of 1-^{13}C-glucose into glycogen and also obtained spectra from the rat head, abdomen, and hind limb.

The first cardiac ^{13}C MRS study, performed by Neurohr and coworkers,[158] showed that spectra could be obtained in 6 minutes. They were able to demonstrate the build-up of labeled glycogen in the heart after a ^{13}C-glucose infusion and the degradation of glycogen within 6 minutes of anoxia associated with generation of ^{13}C-labeled lactate. Additionally, after infusion of 2-^{13}C-acetate, they demonstrated the appearance of C4, C2, and C3 resonances of glutamine and glutamate, consistent with the scrambling of the label through tricarboxylic acid cycle (TCA cycle) intermediates. A follow-up study by the same group[159] confirmed that virtually all of the carbons in glycogen contribute to the MR signal, suggesting the great utility of this method for quantitative examination of glycogen depletion, as would be anticipated in severe ischemia.

Of great interest to several investigators was a determination of the substrate utilization in intermediary metabolism and of the factors that alter this utilization. Chance and associates[160] perfused rat hearts with 5 mM glucose and either 5 mM acetate or 1 mM pyruvate, then replaced the latter two substrates with ^{13}C-labeled pyruvate or acetate. The results showed that TCA flux was greater for pyruvate than acetate for comparable levels of oxygen consumption and indicated the utility of ^{13}C MRS and mathematical modeling for examining in vivo metabolic flux. Malloy and Sherry and coworkers[161–163] utilized mathematical modeling with ^{13}C spectra from beating hearts as well as extracts to determine substrate preference and fractional enrichment. They first showed that lactate is preferred over glucose by the guinea pig heart in the presence of insulin.[164] Then a mathematical model was developed for determining the fractional enrichment of various molecules when supplied with ^{13}C-labeled pyruvate, propionate, or acetate. The method involves examining the multiplet structure of glutamate (Fig. 26–29). Illustrated is the C3 resonance of glutamate, which may be a singlet if no neighboring carbons are

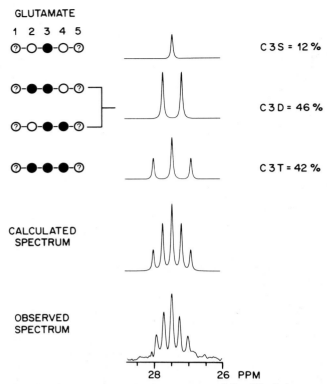

FIGURE 26–29. The multiplet structure of the C3 of glutamate with the fractional contribution to the calculated spectrum below. See text for full description. (From Malloy CR, Sherry AD, Jeffrey FM: Evaluation of carbon flux and substrate selection through alternate pathways involving the citric acid cycle of the heart by ^{13}C NMR spectroscopy. J Biol Chem 263:6964–6971, 1988; with permission.)

enriched, a doublet if either the C2 or C4 are also enriched (it is a coincidence that the coupling constants are very similar for these two positions), or a quintet if C2, C3, and C4 are enriched with [13]C. Similar multiplet structure calculations can be made for the C2 and C4 resonances, allowing calculation of the percentage of enrichment at each site. These data allow calculation of the fractional enrichment of the acetyl-CoA pool, which forms citrate in the TCA cycle, and determination of TCA intermediate sources, which are unrelated to acetyl-CoA supply, the anaplerotic pathways. These pathways include pyruvate carboxylation, as well as protein degradation, to form TCA intermediate skeletons. Results showed that about 15 per cent of oxidative flux was through an anaplerotic pathway when hearts were perfused with pyruvate, and that coperfusion with acetate did not significantly alter this measurement.

Another group of investigators sought to examine the effect of anoxia or ischemia on the concentration of enriched metabolites.[165, 166] They perfused guinea pig hearts with 3-^{13}C-pyruvate and found the label under normoxic conditions in alanine glutamate and aspartate. However, during anoxia the glutamate and aspartate labels decreased and appeared in succinate, indicating that anaerobic metabolism of glutamate

and aspartate, which occurs in skeletal muscle, is also present in the guinea pig perfused heart. These investigators then examined the effect of glucose-insulin-potassium (GIK) infusion on metabolism during global ischemia in a perfused guinea pig heart preparation.[166] This experiment is unique in that simultaneous interleaved ^{31}P and ^{13}C spectra were acquired using two MRS consoles interfaced to the MRS probe. Typical spectra are shown in Figure 26–30. The results revealed that GIK did not significantly reduce acidosis, high energy phosphate depletion, or lactate accumulation; however, glycogenolysis was diminished by the GIK.

PROTON SPECTROSCOPY

The ^{1}H MRS spectrum contains information about a large number of metabolites that are important in evaluating disease processes. One of the first proton spectra of a beating heart was obtained by Ugurbil and associates[167] examining the perfused heart preparation. The water signal was reduced (see further on) by applying a saturating pulse train to the water resonance in a spin-echo sequence. They found that resonances from carnitine, creatine and phosphocreatine, taurine, and lactate could be observed, and they detected an increase in the lactate signal in the presence of ischemia. This report indicated the great potential of ^{1}H spectroscopy, especially for detecting lactate, a sensitive indicator of myocardial ischemia.

Lactate

The human myocardium cannot function normally under anaerobic conditions, which activate glycolysis. Lactate, a product of glycolysis, is useful in defining the onset of anaerobic metabolism and is considered a sensitive indicator of the imbalance between oxygen supply and demand.[168–170] The application of ^{1}H spectroscopic methods for in vivo lactate determination requires suppression of the broad water peak, which reduces dynamic range of the digitized data and obscures the baseline of the lactate signal, making quantitation difficult. Because lactate is indistinguishable on the basis of chemical shift from the lipid methylene peak in biologic samples, it is also imperative to eliminate this lipid peak from the ^{1}H spectrum. Several methods must therefore be combined to accomplish these goals.

The most common water suppression technique currently used in biologic MRS is a selective excitation method.[171, 172] This method consists of the formation of a shaped radiofrequency profile in the frequency domain by the application of a binomial sequence of pulses (the Fourier transform of which forms a $\sin^n$ function). The pulses in a sample 4-pulse binomial sequence, with alternating phase and relative amplitudes 1-3-3-1, produces a $\sin^3$ frequency profile. By adjusting the spacing between pulses to equal the inverse of twice the chemical shift difference between

FIGURE 26–30. ^{13}C *(A)* and ^{31}P *(B)* spectra of an isolated perfused guinea pig heart. Note the decrease in glycogen (glyc C1) and the increase in lactate (lac C3) and alanine (ala C3) during ischemia. The ^{31}P spectra show a loss of PCr and increase in Pi. (From Hoekenga DE, Brainard JR, Hudson JY: Rates of glycolysis and glycogenolysis during ischemia in glucose-insulin-potassium–treated perfused hearts: A ^{13}C, ^{31}P nuclear magnetic resonance study. Circ Res 62:1065–1074, 1988; with permission.)

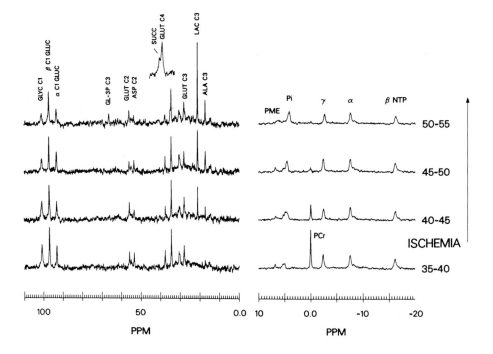

the peak desired and that suppressed, a region of the spectrum distant from the water resonance can be observed. Other functions (e.g., sech) or nonanalytical sequences are also capable of a high degree of frequency selection.

Using a long spin-echo sequence, lipid signal can be diminished by taking advantage of the longer T_2 of lactate compared with that of fat. Another approach uses the coherence transferred from the coupled protons of lactate. When a frequency-selective pulse train is applied to the CH proton resonance, there is a 180-degree phase modulation of the CH_3 lactate signal. By subtracting the two spectra, with and without this phase modulating pulse, only lactate remains visible (with a small residual water peak). This method has been used successfully in examining the brain[173–176] and the perfused heart in a modified form.[177] The difficulty with this method is that in order to use it with surface coil–associated B_1 inhomogeneity, multiple pulses are necessary[178–181] to allow for phase cycling of the receiver and transmitter. An alternative approach, which represents another method of displaying the coherence between spins, displays the effects of the multiple or zero quantum transitions of a multispin system.[182–187] In this technique, the multiple quantum coherences, which are not directly observable, are established and allowed to evolve before being converted back to a single quantum effect in order to be detected. This requires at least a three-pulse sequence and eliminates water, which has no strongly coupled protons, but detects lactate.

An alternative approach that does not require intricate phase cycling or subtraction of spectra has been suggested by Meyer,[188] based on an earlier investigation,[189] in which repetitive pulses are applied

in a time short with respect to T_1 to produce a steady-state magnetization with an echo that peaks at the time of the next pulse (a negative or rising echo). This negative echo has a T_1, T_2, diffusion, and pulse angle dependence, with a broad excitation profile. Keller[190] used this sequence to examine the effect of ischemia on a perfused heart. He determined that a peak corresponding to the lactate methyl chemical shift increased appropriately during ischemia, and in the presence of iodoacetate—an inhibitor of glycolysis—this rise was blunted. This was convincing evidence that lactate concentration was being measured.

We have recently applied this method to the surface coil MRS evaluation of myocardial lactate production in vivo using the heterotopic isogenic transplanted heart model in the neck.[191] As seen in Figure 26–31, during occlusion of the blood supply to the transplanted heart, lactate accumulation is detected with an excellent S/N ratio and a temporal resolution of 1 minute. We were able to show that if diffusion is not neglected, shorter repetition times will improve S/N, and calculations suggest that lipid suppression will still be effective.

SODIUM AND POTASSIUM

Given that muscular contraction is intimately related to transmembrane potential, the capability of measuring transmembrane distributions of cations is certain to play a major role in our understanding of cardiac function in health and disease. Two problems exist in examining potassium and sodium concentrations: (1) identifying the relative compartments of these cations when one compartment contains a much lower concentration of ion than the other, and (2)

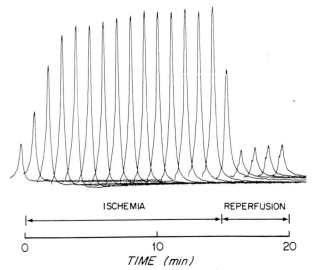

ISCHEMIA   REPERFUSION

0   10   20

TIME (min)

FIGURE 26–31. Time course of lactate production over 15 minutes of occlusion and 5 minutes of reperfusion. (From Rozenman Y, Kantor HL: Heterotropic transplanted rat heart: A model for in vivo determination of phosphorus metabolites during ischemia and perfusion. Magn Reson Med 1989 [in press].)

the difficulty of examining a nucleus with spin greater than ½ (both sodium and potassium are spin 3/2 nuclei) (see Chapter 9). The latter problem is related to the nonzero nuclear quadrupole moment of such nuclei, causing interaction with electric fields and thereby substantially increasing resonance linewidths. Very broad resonance components may not in fact be observable, producing an MRS-invisible component.

The identification of intra- and extracellular compartments is performed with shift or relaxation agents, which produce their effects over short distances. Two common shift reagents, Dy(TTHA)[192] and Dy(PPP),[193] have been used to study the myocardium. Pike and colleagues[194] examined perfused beating rat hearts, demonstrating that the addition of ouabain or the presence of low potassium medium showed influx of extracellular sodium. They suggested that the sodium and potassium visibility are less than 20 per cent. Burstein and Fossel[195] also examined changes in intracellular sodium with ouabain, in addition to rapid pacing, noting a 4.6-fold and a 40 per cent increase in intracellular sodium with the respective stimuli. They have also examined the T_2 relaxation of intracellular sodium, finding biexponential behavior. This suggested two distinct compartments of sodium in the cell, or that quadrupolar effects alter the T_2 (though this would predict a relative amplitude for the two components of 60:40, which was not observed). The answer likely lies in a combination of the two explanations. Similar studies of the intracellular potassium[196] also demonstrate two T_2 components, again attesting to intracellular heterogeneity.

HUMAN SPECTROSCOPY

Cardiac Application

Human applications of cardiac MRS spectroscopy have been more difficult than those for other organ systems, such as the brain, because of the deep location of the heart, making for low S/N (because surface coils cannot be applied in close proximity), and because of the constant motion of the heart, which complicates accurate spectral localization. The motion problem can be partially resolved with gating signal acquisition to the ECG; however, the asynchrony of cardiac and respiratory motion produces further difficulties.

The first human in vivo cardiac spectroscopy investigation was done by Whitman and coworkers.[197] They examined ^{31}P MRS spectra from an 8-month-old girl with a congenital cardiomyopathy and demonstrated an increased PCr/Pi and a reduced PCr/ATP compared with a control 18-month-old child (Fig. 26–32). They were able to demonstrate that intravenous glucose or oral carbohydrate loading reduced PCr/Pi and increased PCr/ATP to approximately the control levels. This result suggested a defect in oxidative metabolism, which could be compensated by an increase in anaerobic metabolism. This examination was possible because of the thin chest wall of both children examined, permitting the assumption that a surface coil on the chest principally obtained signal from the heart.

In order to apply this method to the adult population, a method of localization was necessary to both eliminate signal from skeletal muscle and permit evaluation of regional myocardial abnormalities, such as would appear in coronary artery disease. The first method which was employed involved using the B_0 gradient to select a disk of myocardium from the sensitive volume of a surface coil (DRESS technique).[198] Bottomley[199] used this method to obtain spectra from a normal volunteer, and the PCr/ATP ratios measured were consistent with deeper spectra coming predominantly from the heart. Bottomley and colleagues then examined four patients for 5 to 9 days after acute anterior myocardial infarction. They found two of the four had abnormally low PCr/Pi ratios. This same technique was also used to examine five volunteers[200] for systolic and diastolic ^{31}P spectra; no significant difference was found.

Blackledge and associates,[201] using the rotating-frame MRS technique (B_1 imaging), examined six volunteers to determine normal metabolite ratios. This method permits visualization of spectra acquired from several layers of the myocardium and thus allows evaluation of skeletal muscle contamination (which yields a high PCr/ATP) and blood contribution (containing a large amount of 2,3 DPG). As shown in Figure 26–33, the deepest spectrum has substantial 2,3 DPG while the most superficial layer has a high PCr/ATP. A plot of PCr/ATP reveals that the ratio levels off at about 1.6, consistent with open

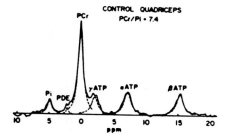

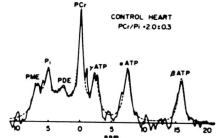

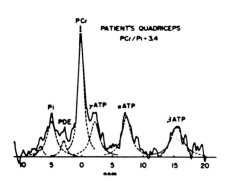

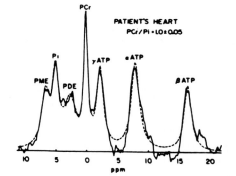

FIGURE 26–32. [31]P spectra obtained at 1.9 tesla in a healthy control subject and in an eight-month-old girl with congenital cardiomyopathy. Note the increased Pi and reduced PCr/ATP in the patient. (From Whitman GJR, Chance B, Bode H, et al: Diagnosis and therapeutic evaluation of a pediatric case of cardiomyopathy using phosphorus-31 nuclear magnetic resonance spectroscopy. J Am Coll Cardiol 5:745, 1985; with permission.)

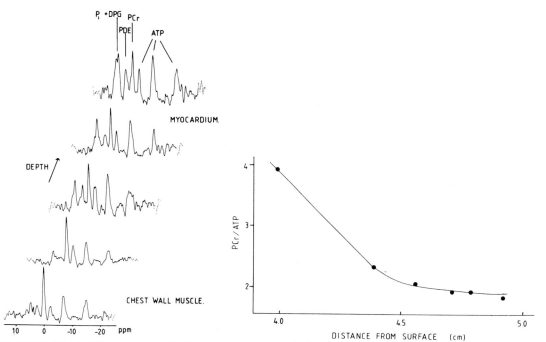

FIGURE 26–33. [31]P spectra acquired using the rotating frame method in a healthy subject. Note the increase in 2,3 DPG with deeper spectra, representing signal from blood in the ventricular chambers, and the gradual reduction of PCr/ATP with a plateau at approximately 1.6. (From Blackledge MJ, Rajagopalan B, Oberhaensli RD, et al: Quantitative studies of human cardiac metabolism by ^{31}P rotating-frame NMR. Proc Natl Acad Sci USA 84:4283–4287, 1987; with permission.)

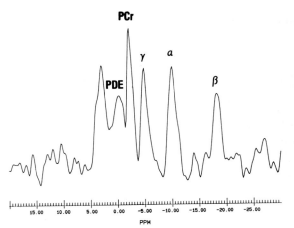
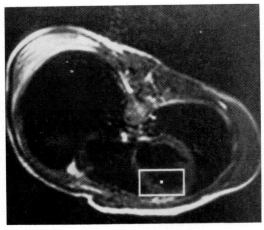

FIGURE 26–34. [31]P spectrum of the human heart obtained with an ISIS technique in 40 minutes. On the right is a ^{1}H MR image of the patient with the region of ^{31}P spectral acquisition. (From Matson GB, Twieg DB, Karczmar GS, et al: Application of image-guided surface coil P-31 MR spectroscopy to human liver, heart, and kidney. Radiology 169:541–547, 1988; with permission.)

chest measurements in animals.[202] This same group has examined spectra from patients with hypertrophic cardiomyopathy,[203] and when compared to normals at rest they were unable to discriminate among the subjects. More recently, normal subjects undergoing lower extremity exercise have been examined,[204] revealing no significant change in PCr/ATP despite an almost threefold increase in oxygen consumption. This study paves the way for similar examinations of patients with ischemic heart disease.

An alternative localizing method is being used by two groups to localize spectral acquisition.[205, 206] The ISIS method[207] permits 3D localization with frequency-selective inverting pulses (see Chapter 9). Each group has obtained good quality cardiac ^{31}P spectra (Fig. 26–34).

The final human spectroscopy method to be discussed is full 3D chemical shift imaging (CSI).[208] In this method the chemical shift is encoded in one of the axes, and a representative image seen in Figure 26–35 has both spectral and spatial information displayed.[209] Clinical application of this method to cardiac patients has yet to be attempted.

Other nuclei have also been examined in humans.

[1]H spectroscopy can be used to observe resonances other than water and fat. Barany and colleagues[210] were able to obtain water-suppressed ^{1}H spectra (Fig. 26–36), with the dominant peak derived from PCr-creatine at 3.02 ppm.

A potential major improvement in human spectroscopy is on the horizon. With the limited availability of 4.0-T large bore magnets for human examination, spectroscopy for clinical applications should take a major leap forward. It has been demonstrated[211–213] that the theoretically predicted increased S/N at higher fields is achieved, with a significant improvement in spectral resolution. This should vastly improve the capability of performing spectroscopy studies, especially for the more insensitive nuclei.

Skeletal Muscle Investigation in Congestive Heart Failure

The role of skeletal muscle metabolic alterations to fatigue in congestive heart failure has been an area of great research and clinical interest, noting the high prevalence of heart disease and the desire to

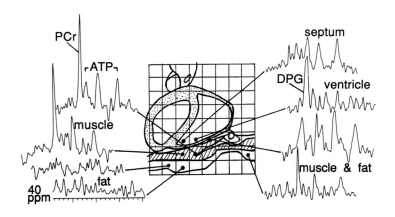

FIGURE 26–35. [31]P 3D CSI obtained at 1.5 tesla. (From Bottomley PA: Human *in vivo* NMR spectroscopy in diagnostic medicine: Clinical tool or research probe? Radiology 170:1–15, 1989; with permission.)

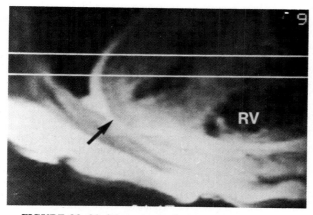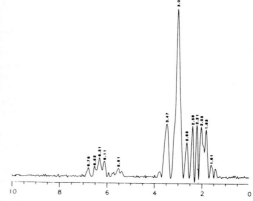

FIGURE 26–36. ¹H spectrum from a human heart obtained with a modified DRESS technique, with the image and image-selected spectrum slice shown at the left. (From Barany M, Langer BG, Glick RP, et al: *In vivo* H-1 spectroscopy in humans at 1.5 T. Radiology 167:839–844, 1988; with permission.)

ameliorate a major accompanying symptom. There have been many investigations into the alterations of ³¹P MRS–detected high energy phosphorylated metabolites.[214–216] Similar investigations have been extended to the study of exercising muscle in congestive heart failure.[217–222] Results showed that excessive loss of PCr and more severe acidosis occur in patients with congestive heart failure when compared with controls. There was, however, no relationship between plethysmographically determined blood flow and any clinical or metabolic variables. These data suggest that congestive heart failure is associated with increased muscle glycolysis and reduced efficiency, thereby partially accounting for patient fatigue.

REFERENCES

1. Mansfield P: Multi-planar image formation using NMR spin echoes. J Phys C. Solid State Physics 10:L55–58, 1977.
2. Mansfield P, Pykett IL: Biological and medical imaging by NMR. J Magn Reson 29:355–373, 1978.
3. Mansfield P, Morris PG: NMR Imaging in Biomedicine. New York, Academic Press, 1982.
4. Mansfield P, Grannell PK: NMR diffraction in solids? J Phys C Solid State Physics 6:L422–426, 1973.
5. Mansfield P, Grannell PK: Diffraction and microscopy in solids and liquids by NMR. Phys Rev 12:3618–3634, 1975.
6. Holmwang G, Drucker EA, Rzedzian RR, et al: Ultra-fast cardiac NMR imaging (abstr). Circulation (Suppl II) 78:590, 1988.
7. Chrispin A, Small P, Rutter N, et al: Transectional echo planar imaging of the heart in cyanotic congenital heart disease. Pediatr Radiol 16(4):293–297, 1986.
8. Chrispin A, Small P, Rutter N, et al: Echo planar imaging of normal and abnormal connections of the heart and great arteries. Pediatr Radiol 16(4):289–292, 1986.
9. Stehling MJ, Howseman AM, Ordidge RJ, et al: Whole-body echo-planar MR imaging at 0.5 T. Radiology 170:257–263, 1989.
10. Howseman AM, Stehling MK, Chapman B, et al: Improvements in snap-shot nuclear magnetic resonance imaging. Br J Radiol 61(729):822–828, 1988.
11. Ordidge RJ, Coxon R, Howseman A, et al: Snapshot head imaging at 0.5 T using the echo planar technique. Magn Reson Med 8(1)110–115, 1988.
12. Pykett IL, Rzedzian RR: Instant images of the body by magnetic resonance. Magn Reson Med 5(6):563–571, 1987.
13. Doyle M, Mansfield P: Chemical shift imaging: A hybrid approach. Magn Reson Med 5(3):255–261, 1987.
14. Chapman B, Turner R, Ordidge RJ, et al: Real-time movie imaging from a single cardiac cycle by NMR. Magn Res Med 5:246–254, 1987.
15. Chapman B, Turner R, Ordidge RJ, et al: Real-time movie imaging from a single cardiac cycle by NMR. Magn Reson Med 5(3):246–254, 1987.
16. Rzedzian RR, Pykett IL: Instant images of the human heart using a new, whole-body MR imaging system. AJR 149(2):245–250, 1987.
17. Kantor HL, Rzedzian RR, Buxton R, et al: Transient effects of Gd-DTPA and Dy-DTPA on myocardial MR image intensity using ultra-high speed MR imaging. Magn Res Med (submitted).
18. Johnston DL, Liu P, Lauffer RB, et al: Use of gadolinium-DTPA as a myocardial perfusion agent: Potential applications and limitations for MRI. J Nucl Med 28:871–877, 1987.
19. Kantor HL, Rzedzian RR, Berliner E, et al: Detection of coronary stenoses by ultra-fast NMR: The utility of dysprosium-DTPA. Circulation (submitted).
20. Atkinson DJ, Burstein D, Edelman RR: Evaluation of first-pass cardiac perfusion by instant magnetic resonance imaging: Radiology (in press).
21. Zierler KL: Equations for measuring blood flow by external monitoring of radioisotopes. Circ Res 16:309–321, 1965.
22. Zierler KL: Theory of the use of arteriovenous concentration differences for measuring metabolism in steady and non-steady states. Circ Res 40:2111–2125, 1961.
23. Axel L: Cerebral blood flow determination by rapid-sequence computed tomography. Radiology 137:679–686, 1980.
24. Saeed M, Wagner S, Wendland MF, et al: Occlusive and reperfused myocardial infarcts: Differentiation with Mn-DPDP-enhanced MR imaging. Radiology 172:59–64, 1989.
25. Peshock RM, Malloy CR, Buja A, et al: MR imaging of acute myocardial infarction: Gadolinium-DTPA pentaacetic acid as a marker of reperfusion. Circulation 74:1434–1440, 1986.
26. Rozenman Y, Zou X, Kantor HL: Cardiovascular MRI with iron oxide particles: The utility of a superparamagnetic contrast agent and the role of diffusion in signal loss. Radiology (in press).
27. Rehr RB, Peshock RM, Malloy CR, et al: Improved in vivo MR imaging of acute myocardial infarction after intravenous paramagnetic contrast agent administration. Am J Cardiol 57:864–868, 1986.
28. McNamara MT, Tscholakoff D, Revel D, et al: Differentiation of reversible and irreversible myocardial injury by MR imaging with and without gadolinium-DTPA. Radiology 158:765–769, 1986.
29. Wesbey GE, Higgins CB, McNamara MT, et al: Effect of

gadolinium-DTPA on the magnetic relaxation times of normal and infarcted myocardium. Radiology 153:165–169, 1984.

30. Hurst JW (ed): Clinical Essays on the Heart. Vol 2. New York, McGraw-Hill Book Co., 1984.

31. Jenkins JPR, Isherwood I, Love HG, et al: Coronary artery bypass graft patency as assessed by magnetic resonance imaging (MRI) (abstr). Soc Magn Reson Med 2:390, 1986.

32. Holmvang G: Noninvasive imaging of the coronary arteries. *In* Miller D (ed): Clinical Cardiac Imaging. New York, McGraw-Hill Book Co., 1988.

33. Gnomes AS, Lois JF, Drinkwater DC, Corday SR: Coronary artery bypass grafts: Visualization with MR imaging. Radiology 162:715, 1987.

34. White RD, Caputo GR, Mark AS, et al: Coronary artery bypass graft patency: Noninvasive evaluation with MR imaging. Radiology 164(3):681–686, 1987.

35. Rubinstein RI, Askenase AD, Thickman D, et al: Magnetic resonance imaging to evaluate patency of aortocoronary bypass grafts. Circulation 76(4):786–791, 1987.

36. Jenkins JP, Love HG, Foster CJ, et al: Detection of coronary artery bypass graft patency as assessed by magnetic resonance imaging. Br J Radiol 61(721):241, 1988.

37. Frija G, Schouman-Claeys E, Lacombe P, et al: A study of coronary artery bypass graft patency using MR imaging. J Comput Assist Tomogr 12(2):226–231, 1989.

38. White RD, Pflugfelder PW, Lipton MJ, Higgins CB: Coronary artery bypass grafts: Evaluation of patency with cine MR imaging. AJR 150(6):1271–1274, 1988.

39. Nishimura DG, Macovski A, Jackson JI, et al: Magnetic resonance angiography by selective inversion recovery using a compact gradient echo sequence. Magn Reson Med 8:96–103, 1988.

40. Alger JR, den Hollander JA, Shulman RG: In vivo phosphorus-31 nuclear magnetic resonance saturation transfer studies of adenosinetriphosphatase kinetics in *Saccharomyces cervisiae*. Biochemistry 21:2957–2963, 1982.

41. Campbell SL, Jones KA, Shulman RG: In vivo ^{31}P nuclear magnetic resonance saturation transfer measurements of phosphate exchange reactions in the yeast *Saccharomyces cervesiae*. FEBS Lett 193:189–193, 1985.

42. Balaban RS: The application of nuclear magnetic resonance to the study of cellular physiology. Am J Physiol 246 (Cell Physiol 15):C10–C19, 1984.

43. Ugurbil K, Shulman RG, Brown TR: High resolution ^{31}P and ^{13}C NMR studies of *Escherichia Coli* cells in vivo. *In* Shulman RG (ed): Biological Applications with Magnetic Resonance. New York, Academic Press, 1979, pp 537–589.

44. Evans FE: ^{31}P nuclear magnetic resonance studies on relaxation parameters and line broadening of intracellular metabolites of HeLa cells. Arch Biochem Biophys 193:63–75, 1979.

45. Shulman RG, Brown TR, Ugurbil K, et al: Cellular applications of ^{31}P and ^{13}C NMR. Science 205:160–168, 1979.

46. Burt CT, Moore RR, Roberts MF, Brady TJ: The fluorinated anesthetic halothane as a potential NMR biologic probe. Biochim Biophys Acta 805:375–381, 1984.

47. Chance B, Eleff S, Leigh JS, et al: Mitochondrial regulation of phosphocreatine/inorganic phosphate ratios in exercising human muscle: A gated ^{31}P NMR study. Proc Natl Acad Sci USA 78:6714–6718, 1981.

48. Dawson MJ, Gadian DG, Wilkie DR: Muscular fatigue investigated by phosphorus nuclear magnetic resonance. Nature 274:861–866, 1978.

49. Dawson MJ, Gadian DG, Wilkie DR: Mechanical relaxation rate and metabolism studied in fatiguing muscle by phosphorus nuclear magnetic resonance. J Physiol 299:465–484, 1980.

50. Hoult DI, Busby SJW, Gadian DG, et al: Observation of tissue metabolites using ^{31}P nuclear magnetic resonance. Nature 252:285–287, 1974.

51. Kushmerick MJ, Meyer RA: Chemical changes in rat leg muscle by phosphorus nuclear magnetic resonance. Am J Physiol 248:C542–C549, 1985.

52. Hope PL, Cady EB, Tofts PS, et al: Cerebral energy metabolism studied with phosphorus NMR spectroscopy in normal and birth-asphyxiated infants. Lancet 2:366–369, 1984.

53. Peeling J, Wong D, Sutherland GR: Nuclear magnetic resonance study of regional metabolism after forebrain ischemia in rats. Stroke 20:633–640, 1989.

54. Azzopardi D, Wyatt JS, Cady EB, et al: Prognosis of newborn infants with hypoxic-ischemic brain injury assessed by phosphorus magnetic resonance spectroscopy. Pediatr Res 25:445–451, 1989.

55. Behar KL: Nuclear magnetic resonance of the brain: Evaluation of ^1H, ^{31}P, and ^{13}C spectra in normal and pathological states *in vivo*. PhD Thesis, Yale University, 1985.

56. Behar KL, den Hollander JA, Petroff OAC, et al: Effect of hypoglycemic encephalopathy upon amino acids, high energy phosphates and pH; in the rat brain in vivo: Detection by sequential ^{1}Hand ^{31}P NMR spectroscopy. Neurochemistry 44:1045–1055, 1985.

57. Prichard JW, Alger JR, Behar KL, et al: Cerebral metabolic studies in vivo by ^{31}P NMR. Proc Natl Acad Sci USA 80:2748–2751, 1983.

58. Petroff OAC, Prichard JW, Behar KL, et al: In vivo phosphorus nuclear magnetic resonance spectroscopy in status epilepticus Ann Neurol 16:169–177, 1984.

59. Thoma WJ, Ugurbil K: Rapid ^{31}P NMR test of liver function. Magn Reson Med 8:220–223, 1988.

60. Oberhaensli RD, Galloway GJ, Taylor DJ, et al: Assessment of human liver metabolism by phosphorus-31 magnetic resonance spectroscopy. Br J Radiol 59:695, 1986.

61. Grivegnee AR, Segebarth C, Luyten PR, Den Hollander JA: P31 MR spectroscopy of the human liver: Assessment of fructose metabolism (abstr). Radiology 165:67, 1987.

62. Vock P, Cotting J, Labebeck R, et al: Effect of intravenous fructose on the P31 spectrum of the liver: Dose response curve in normal volunteers (abstr). Radiology 165:346, 1987.

63. Thoma WJ, Henderson LM, Ugurbil K: Removal of the broad resonance in P31 NMR spectra of intact tissues. J Magn Reson 61:141–144, 1985.

64. Thoma WJ, Ugurbil K: Saturation-transfer studies of ATP-Pi exchange in isolated perfused rat liver. Biochim Biophys Acta 893:225, 1987.

65. Tanaka A, Chance B, Quistorff B: A possible role of inorganic phosphate as a regulator of oxidative phosphorylation in combined urea synthesis and gluconeogenesis in perfused rat liver. A phosphorus magnetic resonance spectroscopy study. J Biol Chem 264:10034–10040, 1989.

66. Vine W, Thoma WJ, Ugurbil K: Biochemical differences between Ringer's lactate and Collins' solution in hepatic preservation: Detection by ^{31}P magnetic resonance spectroscopy. Transplant Proc Feb. 21(1 pt. 2) 1338–1339, 1989.

67. Jue T, Rothman DL, Tavitian BA, Shulman RG: Natural abundance ^{13}C NMR study of glycogen repletion in human liver and muscle. Proc Natl Acad Sci USA 86:1439–1442, 1989.

68. Herman HV, Elliott WC, Gorlin R: An electrocardiographic, anatomic, and metabolic study of zonal myocardial ischemia in coronary heart disease. Circulation 35:834, 1987.

69. Ackerman JJ, Lowry M, Radda GK, et al: The role of intrarenal pH in regulation of ammoniagenesis: [31P] NMR studies of the isolated perfused rat kidney. J Physiol 319:65–79, 1981.

70. Freeman D, Bartlett S, Radda GK, Ross BD: Energetics of sodium transport in the kidney saturation transfer 31P-NMR. Biochim Biophys Acta 762:325–336, 1983.

71. Gadian DG, Hoult DI, Radda GK, et al: Phosphorus nuclear magnetic resonance studies on normoxic and ischemic cardiac tissue. Proc Natl Acad Sci USA 73:4446–4448, 1976.

72. de Leiris J, Harding DP, Pestre S: The isolated perfused rat heart: A model for studying myocardial hypoxia or ischaemia. Basic Res Cardiol 79:313–321, 1984.

73. Jennings RB, Reiner KA, Hill ML, et al. Total ischemia in dog hearts in vitro. Circ Res 49:892, 1981.

74. DeBoer LWV, Ingwall JS, Kloner RA, Braunwald E: Prolonged derangements of canine myocardial purine metabolism after a brief coronary artery occlusion not associated with anatomic evidence of necrosis. Proc Natl Acad Sci USA 77:5471–5475, 1980.

75. Burt CT, Glonek T, Barany M: Analysis of phosphate metabolites, the intracellular pH, and the state of adenosine triphosphate in intact muscle by phosphorus nuclear magnetic resonance. J Biol Chem 251:2584–2591, 1976.

76. Salhaney JM, Yamane T, Shulman RG, Ogawa S: High resolution 31P nuclear magnetic resonance studies of intact yeast cells. Proc Natl Acad Sci USA 72:4966–4970, 1975.

77. Burt CT, Glonek T, Barany M: Analysis of living tissue by phosphorus-31 magnetic resonance. Science 195:145–149, 1977.

78. Jacobus WE, Taylor G, Hollis DP, Nunnally RL: Phosphorus nuclear magnetic resonance of perfused working rat hearts. Nature 265:756–758, 1977.

79. Garlick PB, Radda GK, Seeley PJ, Chance B: Phosphorus NMR studies on perfused heart. Biochem Biophys Res Commun 74:1256–1262, 1977.

80. Bailey IA, Seymour A: The effects of reperfusion on the 31P NMR spectrum of ischaemic rat hearts. Biochem Soc Trans 9:234–236, 1981.

81. Grove TH, Ackerman JJH, Radda GK, Bore PJ: Analysis of rat heart in vivo by phosphorus nuclear magnetic resonance. Proc Natl Acad Sci USA 77:299–302, 1980.

82. Hollis DP, Nunnally RL, Taylor GJ, et al: Phosphorus nuclear magnetic resonance studies of heart physiology. J Magn Reson 29:319–330, 1978.

83. Clarke K, Willis RJ: Energy metabolism and contractile function in rat hearts during graded, isovolumic perfusion using 31P nuclear magnetic resonance spectroscopy. J Mol Cell Cardiol 19:1153–1160, 1987.

84. Whitman G, Kieval R, Wetstein L, et al: The relationship between global myocardial ischemia, left ventricular function, myocardial redox state, and high energy phosphate profile. J Surg Res 35:332–339, 1983.

85. Camacho SA, Lanzer P, Toy BJ, et al: In vivo alterations of high energy phosphates and intracellular pH during reversible regional ischemia: A 31P magnetic resonance spectroscopy study. Am Heart J 116:701–708, 1988.

86. Brooks WM, Willis RJ: 31P nuclear magnetic resonance study of the recovery characteristics of high energy phosphate compounds and intracellular pH after global ischemia in the perfused guinea pig heart. J Mol Cell Cardiol 15:495–502, 1983.

87. Flaherty JT, Weisfeldt ML, Bulkley BH, et al: Mechanisms of ischemic myocardial cell damage assessed by phosphorus-31 nuclear magnetic resonance. Circulation 65:561–571, 1982.

88. Kupriyanov VV, Steinschneider AY, Ruuge EK, et al: Regulation of energy reaction velocity through the creatine kinase reaction in vitro and in perfused rat heart. 31P-NMR studies. Biochim Biophys Acta 805:319–331, 1984.

89. Balaban RS: The application of nuclear magnetic resonance to the study of cellular physiology. Am J Physiol 246:C10–C19, 1984.

90. Whitman GJR, Kieval RS, Brown J, et al: Optimal hypothermic preservation of arrested myocardium in isolated perfused rabbit hearts: A 31P NMR study. Surgery 105:100–108, 1989.

91. Braunwald E, Kloner RA: The stunned myocardium: Prolonged post-ischemic ventricular dysfunction. Circulation 68:170–182, 1983.

92. Reimer KA, Hill ML, Jennings RB: Prolonged depletion of ATP and of the adenine nucleotide pool due to delayed resynthesis of adenine nucleotides following reversible myocardial ischemic injury in dogs. J Mol Cell Cardiol 13:229–239, 1981.

93. Swain JL, Sabina RL, McHale PA, et al: Prolonged myocardial nucleotide depletion after brief ischemia in the open-chest dog. Am J Physiol 242:H818–H826, 1982.

94. Ellis SG, Wynne J, Braunwald E, et al: Response of reper-

fusion-salvaged, stunned myocardium to inotropic stimulation. Am Heart J 107:13–19, 1984.

95. Becker LC, Levine JH, DiPaula AF, et al: Reversal of dysfunction in post-ischemic stunned myocardium by epinephrine and postextrasystolic potentiation. J Am Coll Cardiol 7:580–589, 1986.

96. Przyklenk K, Kloner RA: Superoxide dismutase plus catalase improve contractile function in the canine model of the "stunned myocardium." Circ Res 58:148–156, 1986.

97. Hoffmeister HM, Mauser M, Schaper W: Effect of adenosine and AICAR on ATP content and regional contractile function in reperfused canine myocardium. Basic Res Cardiol 80:445–458, 1985.

98. Taegtmeyer H, Roberts AFC, Raine AEG: Energy metabolism in reperfused heart muscle: metabolic correlates to return of function. J Am Coll Cardiol 6:864–870, 1985.

99. Guth BG, Martin JF, Heusch G, Ross J Jr: Regional myocardial blood flow, function and metabolism using phosphorus-31 nuclear magnetic resonance spectroscopy during ischemia and reperfusion in dogs. J Am Coll Cardiol 10:673–681, 1987.

100. Stein PD, Goldstein S, Sabbah HN, et al: In vivo evaluation of intracellular pH and high-energy phosphate metabolites during regional myocardial ischemia in cats using 31P nuclear magnetic resonance. Magn Reson Med 3:262–269, 1986.

101. Sievers RE, Schmiedl U, Wolfe CL, et al: A model of acute regional myocardial ischemia and reperfusion in the rat. Magn Reson Med 10:172–181, 1989.

102. Kavanaugh KM, Aisen AM, Fechner KP, et al: Regional metabolism during coronary occlusion, reperfusion, and reocclusion using phosphorus31 nuclear magnetic resonance spectroscopy in the intact rabbit. Am Heart J 117:53–59, 1989.

103. Hollis DP, Nunnally RL, Jacobus WE, Taylor GJ: Detection of regional ischemia in perfused beating hearts by phosphorus nuclear magnetic resonance. Biochem Biophys Res Commun 75:1086–1091, 1977.

104. Schaefer S, Camacho SA, Gober J, et al: Response of myocardial metabolites to graded regional ischemia: 31P NMR spectroscopy of porcine myocardium in vivo. Circ Res 64:968–976, 1989.

105. Rozenman Y, Kantor HL: Heterotopic transplanted rat heart: A model for in vivo determination of phosphorus metabolites during ischemia and reperfusion. Magn Reson Med 1989 (in press).

106. Matthews PM, Bland JL, Gadian DG, Radda GK: The steady-state rate of ATP synthesis in the perfused rat heart measured by 31P NMR saturation transfer. Biochem Biophys Res Comm 103:1052–1059, 1981.

107. Bittl JA, Delayre J, Ingwall JS: Rate equation for creatine kinase predicts the in vivo reaction velocity: 31P NMR surface coil studies in brain, heart, and skeletal muscle of the living rat. Biochemistry 26:6083, 1987.

108. Vinten-Johansen J, Rosenkranz ER, Buckberg GD, et al: Metabolic and histochemical benefits of regional blood cardioplegic reperfusion without cardiopulmonary bypass. J Thorac Cardiovasc Surg 92:535, 1986.

109. Hoffman JI: Transmural myocardial perfusion. Prog Cardiovasc Dis 29:429, 1987.

110. Rivas F, Cobb FR, Bache RJ, Greenfield JC: Relationship between blood flow to ischemic regions and extent of myocardial infarction. Serial measurement of blood flow to ischemic regions in dogs. Circ Res 38:439–447, 1976.

111. Forman R, Kirk ES, Downey JM, Sonnenblick EH: Nitroglycerin and heterogeneity of myocardial blood flow. Reduced subendocardial blood flow and ventricular contractile force. J Clin Invest 52:905, 1973.

112. Griggs DM Jr, Nakamura Y: Effects of coronary constriction on myocardial distribution of iodoantipyrine-I131. Am J Physiol 215:1082, 1968.

113. Buckberg GD, Fixler DE, Archie JP, Hoffman JIE: Experimental subendocardial ischemia in dogs with normal coronary arteries. Circ Res 30:67, 1972.

114. Rouleau J, Boerboom LE, Surjadhana A, Hoffman JIE: The role of autoregulation and tissue diastolic pressures in the transmural distribution of left ventricular blood flow in anesthetized dogs. Circ Res 45:804, 1979.

115. Reimer KA, Lowe JE, Rasmussen MM, Jennings RB: The wavefront phenomenon of ischemic cell death. I. Myocardial infarct size vs. duration of coronary occlusion in dogs. Circulation 56:786, 1977.

116. Reimer KA, Jennings RB: The "wavefront phenomenon" of myocardial ischemic cell death. II. Transmural progression of necrosis within the framework of ischemic bed size (myocardium at risk) and collateral flow. Lab Invest 40:633, 1979.

117. Schaper W, Frenzel H, Hort W, Winkler B: Experimental coronary artery occlusion. II. Spatial and temporal evolution of infarcts in the dog heart. Basic Res Cardiol 74:233, 1979.

118. Forman R, Cho S, Factor SM, Kirk ES: Acute myocardial infarct extension into a previously preserved subendocardial region at risk in dogs and patients. Circulation 67:117, 1983.

119. Gober J, Schaefer S, Camacho SA, et al: Epicardial and endocardial localized ^{31}P magnetic resonance spectroscopy: Evidence for metabolic heterogeneity during regional ischemia. Magn Reson Med (in press).

120. Garwood M, Schleich, Ross BD, et al: A modified rotating frame experiment based on Fourier Series Window Function. J Magn Reson 65:239, 1985.

121. Metz KR, Briggs RW: Spatial localization of NMR spectra using Fourier series analysis. J Magn Reson 64:172, 1985.

122. Ackerman JJH, Grove TH, Wong GG, et al: Mapping of metabolites in whole animals by ^{31}P NMR using surface coils. Nature 283:167, 1980.

123. Evelhoch JL, Crowley MG, Ackerman JJH: Signal-to-noise optimization and observed volume localization with circular surface coils. J Magn Reson 56:110–124, 1984.

124. Robitaille P, Merkle H, Sublett E, et al: Spectroscopic imaging and spatial localization using adiabatic pulses and applications to detect transmural metabolite distribution in the canine heart. Magn Reson Med 10:14–37, 1989.

125. Robitaille P, Lew B, Merkle H, et al: Transmural metabolite distribution in regional myocardial ischemia as studied with ^{31}P NMR. Magn Reson Med 10:108–118, 1989.

126. Fossel ET, Morgan HE, Ingwall JS: Measurement of changes in high-energy phosphates in the cardiac cycle by using gated P-31 NMR. Proc Natl Acad Sci USA 77:3654, 1980.

127. Kantor HL, Briggs RW, Balaban RS: *In vivo* ^{31}P nuclear magnetic resonance measurements in canine heart using a catheter-coil. Circ Res 55:261–266, 1984.

128. Ingwall JS: Phosphorus nuclear magnetic resonance spectroscopy of cardiac and skeletal muscles. Am J Physiol 242:H729, 1982.

129. Bittl JA, Ingwall JS: Reaction rates of creatine kinase and ATP synthesis in the isolated rat heart. A P-31 magnetization transfer study. J Biol Chem 260:3512, 1985.

130. Balaban RS, Kantor HL, Katz LA, Jacobus RW: Relation between work and phosphate metabolites in the in vivo paced mammalian heart. Science 232:1121–1123, 1986.

131. Martin JF, Guth BD, Griffey RH, Hoekenga DE: Myocardial creatine kinase exchange rates and ^{31}P NMR relaxation rates in intact pigs. Magn Reson Med 11:64–72, 1989.

132. Hollis DP, Nunnally RL, Taylor GJ, et al: Phosphorus nuclear magnetic resonance studies of heart physiology. J Magn Reson 29:319–330, 1978.

133. Flaherty JT, Weisfeldt M, Bulkley BH, et al: Mechanisms of ischemic myocardial cell damage assessed by phosphorus-31 nuclear magnetic resonance. Circulation 65:561, 1982.

134. Bathe-Smith EC, Bendall JR: Rigor mortis and adenosine triphosphate. J Physiol 106:177, 1947.

135. Bernard M, Menasche P, Canioni P, et al: Enhanced cardioplegic protection by a fluorcarbon-oxygenated reperfusate: A phosphorus-31 nuclear magnetic resonance study. J Surg Res 39:216, 1985.

136. Bernard M, Menasche P, Fontanarava E, et al: Effect of nifedipine in hypothermic cardioplegia. A phosphorus-31 nuclear magnetic resonance study. Clin Chim Acta 152:43, 1985.

137. Nakazawa M, Katano Y, Imai S, et al: Effects of 1- and d-propranolol on the ischemic myocardial metabolism of the isolated guinea pig heart as studied by ^{31}P NMR. J Cardiovasc Pharmacol 4:700, 1982.

138. Nunally RL, Bottomley PA: Assessment of pharmacological treatment of myocardial infarction of phosphorus-31 NMR with surface coils. Science 211:177, 1981.

139. Pieper GM, Wu ST, Salhany JM: A polymeric prostaglandin (PGBx) attenuates adenine nucleotide loss during global ischemia and improves myocardial function during reperfusion. J Mol Cell Cardiol 17:775–783, 1985.

140. Dhasmana JP, Digerness SB, Geckle JM, et al: Effects of adenosine deaminase inhibitors on the heart's functional and biochemical recovery from ischemia: A study utilizing the isolated rat heart adapted to ^{31}P nuclear magnetic resonance. J Cardiovasc Pharmacol 5:1040, 1983.

141. Eugene M, Lechat P, Hadjiisky P, et al: NMR and proton relaxation times in experimental heterotopic heart transplantation. J Heart Transplant 5:39, 1986.

142. Sasaguri S, LaRaia PJ, Fabri BM, et al: Early detection of cardiac allograft detection with proton NMR. Circulation 72:231, 1985.

143. Tscholakoff D, Aherne T, Yee ES, et al: Cardiac transplantation in dogs: Evaluation with MR. Radiology 157:697, 1985.

144. Wisenberg G, Pflugfelder PW, Kostuk WJ, et al: Diagnostic applicability of MR imaging in assessing human cardiac allograft rejection. Am J Cardiol 60:130–136, 1987.

145. Lund G, Morin RL, Olivari MT, Ring WS: Serial myocardial T2 relaxation time measurements in normal subjects and heart transplant recipients. J Heart Transplant 7:274–279, 1988.

146. Konstam MA, Aronovitz MJ, Runge VM, et al: MR imaging with Gd-DTPA for detecting cardiac transplant rejection in rats. Circulation 78:1187–1194, 1988.

147. Fraser CD, Chacko VP, Jacobus WE, et al: Metabolic changes preceding functional and morphologic indices of rejection in heterotopic cardiac allografts. A 31P MR study. Transplantation 46:346–351, 1988.

148. Haug CE, Shapiro JI, Chan L, Weil R: P-31 NMR spectroscopy evaluation of heterotopic cardiac allograft rejection in the rat. Transplantation 44:175–178, 1987.

149. Shulman RG, Brown TR, Ugurbil K, et al: Cellular applications of ^{31}P and ^{13}C nuclear magnetic resonance. Science 205:160, 1979.

150. Cohen SM, Ogawa S, Shulman RG: ^{13}C NMR studies of gluconeogenesis in rat liver cells. Utilization of labeled glycerol by cells from euthyroid and hyperthyroid rats. Proc Natl Acad Sci USA 76:1603, 1979.

151. Cohen SM, Shulman RG, McLaughlin AC: Effects of ethanol on alanine metabolism in perfused mouse liver studied by ^{13}C NMR. Proc Natl Acad Sci USA 76:4808, 1979.

152. den Hollander JA, Brown TR, Ugurbil K, et al: ^{13}C nuclear magnetic resonance studies of anaerobic glycolysis in suspensions of yeast cells. Proc Natl Acad Sci USA 76:6096, 1979.

153. Cohen SM, Glynn P, Shulman RG: ^{13}C NMR study of gluconeogenesis from labeled alanine in hepatocytes from euthyroid and hyperthyroid rats. Proc Natl Acad Sci USA 78:60, 1981.

154. den Hollander JA, Behar KL, Shulman RG: ^{13}C NMR study of transamination during acetate utilization by *Saccharomyces cerevisiae*. Proc Natl Acad Sci USA 78:2693, 1981.

155. Scott AI, Baxter RL: Applications of ^{13}C NMR to metabolic studies. Annu Rev Biophys Bioeng 10:151, 1981.

156. Alger JR, Sillerud LO, Behar KL, et al: *In vivo* carbon-13 nuclear magnetic resonance studies of mammals. Science 214:660, 1981.

157. Alger JR, Rothman DL, Shulman RG: Natural abundance C-13 NMR measurement of hepatic glycogen in the living rabbit. J Magn Reson 56:334, 1984.

158. Neurohr KJ, Barrett EJ, Schulman RG: *In vivo* carbon-13

nuclear magnetic resonance studies of heart metabolism. Proc Natl Acad Sci USA 80:1603, 1983.

159. Neurohr KJ, Gollin G, Neurohr JM, et al: Carbon-13 nuclear magnetic resonance studies of my myocardial glycogen metabolism in live guinea pigs. Biochemistry 23:5029–5035, 1984.

160. Chance EM, Seeholzer SH, Kobayashi K, Williamson JR: Mathematical analysis of isotope labeling in the citric acid cycle with applications to ^{13}C NMR studies in perfused rat hearts. J Biol Chem 258:13785–13794, 1983.

161. Malloy CR, Sherry AD, Jeffrey FM: Carbon flux through citric acid cycle pathways in perfused heart by ^{13}C NMR spectroscopy. FEBS Lett 212:58–62, 1987.

162. Malloy CR, Sherry AD, Jeffrey FM: Evaluation of carbon flux and substrate selection through alternate pathways involving the citric acid cycle of the heart by ^{13}C NMR spectroscopy. J Biol Chem 263:6964–6971, 1988.

163. Sherry AD, Malloy CR, Roby RE, et al: Propionate metabolism in the rat heart by ^{13}C NMR spectroscopy. Biochem J 254:593–598, 1988.

164. Sherry AD, Nunnally RL, Peshock RM: Metabolic studies of pyruvate- and lactate-perfused guinea pig hearts by ^{13}C NMR. Determination of substrate preference by glutamate isotopomer distribution. J Biol Chem 260:9272–9279, 1985.

165. Brainard JR, Hoekenga DA, Hutson JY: Metabolic consequences of anoxia in the isolated, perfused guinea pig heart: Anaerobic metabolism of endogenous amino acids. Magn Reson Med 3:673–684, 1986.

166. Hoekenga DE, Brainard JR, Hudson JY: Rates of glycolysis and glycogenolysis during ischemia in glucose-insulin-potassium–treated perfused hearts: A ^{13}C, ^{31}P nuclear magnetic resonance study. Circ Res 62:1065–1074, 1988.

167. Ugurbil K, Petein M, Maidan R, et al: High resolution proton NMR studies of perfused rat hearts. FEBS Lett 167:73–78, 1984.

168. Herman HV, Elliott WC, Gorlin R: An electrocardiographic, anatomic, and metabolic study of zonal myocardial ischemia in coronary heart disease. Circulation 35:834, 1987.

169. Gerz EW, Wisneski JA, Neese R, et al: Myocardial lactate metabolism: Evidence of lactate release during net chemical extraction in man. Circulation 63:1273, 1981.

170. Peuhkurinen KJ, Takala TES, Nuutinen EM, Hassinen IE: Tricarboxylic acid cycle metabolites during ischemia in isolated perfused rat heart. Am J Physiol 244:H281, 1983.

171. Hore PJ: A new method of water suppression in the proton NMR spectra of aqueous solutions. J Magn Reson 54:539, 1983.

172. Hore PJ: Solvent suppression in Fourier transform nuclear magnetic resonance. J Magn Reson 55:283, 1983.

173. Hetherington HP, Avison MJ, Shulman RG: ^{1}H homonuclear editing of rat brain using semiselective pulses. Proc Natl Acad Sci USA 82:3115–3118, 1985.

174. Rothman DL, Behar KL, Hetherington HP, Shulman RG: ^{1}H double resonance difference spectroscopy of the rat brain in vivo. Proc Natl Acad Sci USA 81:6330, 1984.

175. Rothman DL, Behar KL, Hetherington HP, et al: ^{1}H observe ^{13}C decouple measurements of lactate and glutamate in the rat brain in vivo. Proc Natl Acad Sci USA 82:1633, 1985.

176. Williams SR, Proctor E, Allen K, et al: Quantitative estimation in lactate in the brain by ^{1}H NMR. Magn Reson Med 7:425–431, 1988.

177. Richards TL, Terrier F, Sievers RE, et al: Lactate accumulation in ischemic and anoxic-isolated rat hearts assessed by H-1 spectroscopy. Invest Radiol 22:638–641, 1987.

178. Bedall MR: Elimination of high-flux signals near surface coils and field gradient sample localization using depth pulses. J Magn Reson 59:406–429, 1984.

179. Hetherington HP, Avison MJ, Shulman RG: ^{1}H homonuclear editing of the rat brain using semi-selective pulses. Proc Natl Acad Sci USA 82:3115, 1985.

180. Hetherington HP, Rothman DL: Phase cycling of refocusing pulses to eliminate dispersive refocusing magnetization. J Magn Reson 65:348, 1985.

181. Hetherington HP, Wishart D, Fitzpatrick SM, et al: The application of composite pulses to surface coil NMR. J Magn Reson 66:313, 1986.

182. Dumoulin CL: The application of multiple-quantum techniques for the suppression of water signals in ^{1}H NMR spectra. J Magn Reson 64:38–46, 1985.

183. Sotak CH, Freeman DM: A method for volume-localized lactate editing using zero-quantum coherence created in a stimulated-echo pulse sequence. J Magn Reson 77:382–388, 1988.

184. Sotak CH, Freeman DM, Hurd RE: The unequivocal determination of in vivo lactic acid using two-dimensional double-quantum coherence-transfer spectroscopy. J Magn Reson 78:355–361, 1988.

185. Dumoulin CL, Williams EA: Suppression of uncoupled spins by single-quantum homonuclear polarization transfer. J Magn Reson 66:86–92, 1986.

186. McKinnon GD, Boesiger P: Communication: A one-shot lactate-editing sequence for localized whole-body spectroscopy. Magn Reson Med 8:355–361, 1988.

187. Knuttel A, Rommel E, Clausen M, Kimmich R: Integrated volume-selective/spectral editing ^{1}H NMR and postdetection signal processing for the sensitive determination of lactate. Magn Reson Med 8:70–79, 1988.

188. Meyer RA: Echo acquisition during frequency-selective pulse trains for proton spectroscopy of metabolites in vivo. Magn Reson Med 4:297–301, 1987.

189. Kaiser R, Bartholdi E, Ernst RR: Diffusion and field-gradient effects in NMR fourier spectroscopy. J Chem Phys 69:2966–2979, 1974.

190. Keller AM, Sorce DJ, Sciacca RR, et al: Very rapid lactate measurement in ischemic perfused hearts using ^{1}H MRS continuous negative echo acquisition during steady-state frequency selective excitation. Magn Reson Med 7:65–78, 1988.

191. Rozenman Y, Kantor HL: A method for rapid in vivo cardiac lactate determination using MR spectroscopy with a surface coil. Magn Reson Med (in press).

192. Gupta RK, Gupta P, Moore RD: NMR studies of intracellular metal ions in intact cells and tissues. Annu Rev Biophys Bioeng 13:221–246, 1984.

193. Springer CS Jr, Pike MM, Balschi JA, et al: Use of shift reagents for nuclear magnetic resonance studies of the kinetics of ion transfer in cells and perfused hearts. Circulation 72:89–93, 1985.

194. Pike MM, Frazer JC, Dedrick DF, et al: 23Na and 39K nuclear magnetic resonance studies of perfused rat hearts. Discrimation of intra- and extracellular ions using a shift reagent. Biophys J 48(1):159–173, 1985.

195. Burstein D, Fossel ET: Nuclear magnetic resonance studies of intracellular ions in perfused frog heart. Am J Physiol 252:1138–1146, 1987.

196. Burstein D, Litt HI, Fossel ET: NMR characteristics of "visible" intracellular myocardial potassium in perfused rat hearts. Magn Reson Med 1:66–78, 1989.

197. Whitman GJR, Chance B, Bode H, et al: Diagnosis and therapeutic evaluation of a pediatric case of cardiomyopathy using phosphorus-31 nuclear magnetic resonance spectroscopy. J Am Coll Cardiol 5:745, 1985.

198. Bottomley PA, Foster TH, Darrow J: Depth-resolved surface-coil spectroscopy (DRESS) for in vivo H-1, P-31, and C-13 NMR. J Magn Reson 59:338, 1984.

199. Bottomley PA: Noninvasive study of high-energy phosphate metabolism in human heart by depth-resolved ^{31}P NMR spectroscopy. Science 229:769–772, 1985.

200. Grist TM, Kneeland JB, Rilling WR, et al: Gated cardiac MR imaging and P-31 MR spectroscopy in humans at 1.5 T. Radiology 170:357–361, 1989.

201. Blackledge MJ, Rajagopalan B, Oberhaensli RD, et al: Quantitative studies of human cardiac metabolism by ^{31}P rotating-frame NMR. Proc Natl Acad Sci USA 84:4283–4287, 1987.

202. Kantor HL, Briggs RW, Balaban RS: In vivo ^{31}P nuclear magnetic resonance measurements in canine heart using a catheter-coil. Circ Res 55:261–266, 1984.

203. Rajagopalan B, Blackledge MJ, McKenna WJ, et al: Measurement of phosphocreatine to ATP ratio in normal and diseased human heart by ^{31}P magnetic resonance spectroscopy using rotating frame-depth selection technique. Ann NY Acad Sci 508:321–332, 1987.

204. Conway MA, Bristow JD, Blackledge MJ, et al: Cardiac metabolism during exercise measured by magnetic resonance spectroscopy. Lancet 2:692, 1988.

205. Matson GB, Twieg DB, Karczmar GS, et al: Application of image-guided surface coil P-31 MR spectroscopy to human liver, heart, and kidney. Radiology 169:541–547, 1988.

206. Luyten PR, Groen JP, Vermeulen JWAH, den Hollander JA: Experimental approaches to image localized human ^{31}P NMR spectroscopy. Magn Reson Med 11:1–21, 1989.

207. Ordidge RY, Connelly A, Lohman JAB: Image-selected *in vivo* spectroscopy (ISIS): A new technique for spatially selective NMR spectroscopy. J Magn Reson 66:283–294, 1986.

208. Brown TR, Kincaid BM, Ugurbil K: NMR chemical shift imaging in three dimensions. Proc Natl Acad Sci USA 79:3523–3526, 1982.

209. Bottomley PA: Human *in vivo* NMR spectroscopy in diagnostic medicine: Clinical tool or research probe? Radiology 170:1–15, 1989.

210. Barany M, Langer BG, Glick RP, et al: *In vivo* H-1 spectroscopy in humans at 1.5 T. Radiology 167:839–844, 1988.

211. Barfuss H, Fischer H, Hentschel D, et al: Whole-body MR imaging and spectroscopy with a 4-T system. Radiology 169:811–816, 1988.

212. Ortendahl DA: Whole-body MR imaging and spectroscopy at 4 T: Where do we go from here? Radiology 169:864–865, 1988.

213. Hardy CJ, Bottomley PA, Roemer PB, Redington RW: Rapid ^{31}P spectroscopy on a 4-T whole-body system. Magn Reson Med 8:104–109, 1988.

214. Chance B, Leigh JS Jr, Clark BJ, et al: Control of oxidative metabolism and oxygen delivery in human skeletal muscle: A steady-state analysis of the work/energy cost transfer function. Proc Natl Acad Sci USA 82:8384–8388, 1985.

215. Arnold DL, Taylor DJ, Radda GK: Investigation of human mitochondrial myopathies by phosphorus magnetic resonance spectroscopy. Ann Neurol 18:189–196, 1985.

216. Meyer RA, Kushmerick MJ, Brown TR: Application of ^{31}P NMR spectroscopy to the study of striated 3d muscle metabolism. Am J Physiol 242:C1–C11, 1982.

217. Massie B, Conway M, Yonge R, et al: Skeletal muscle metabolism in patients with congestive heart failure: Relation to clinical severity and blood flow. Circulation 76:1009–1019, 1987.

218. Massie BM, Conway M, Rajagopalan B, et al: Skeletal muscle metabolism during exercise under ischemic conditions in congestive heart failure. Circulation 78:320–326, 1988.

219. Massie BM, Conway M, Yonge R, et al: ^{31}P nuclear magnetic resonance evidence of abnormal skeletal muscle metabolism in patients with congestive heart failure. Am J Cardiol 60:309–315, 1987.

220. Wilson JR, Fink L, Maris J, et al: Evaluation of energy metabolism in skeletal muscle of patients with heart failure with gated phosphorus-31 nuclear magnetic resonance. Circulation 71:57–62, 1985.

221. Wiener DH, Fink LI, Maris J, et al: Abnormal skeletal muscle bioenergetics during exercise in patients with heart failure: Role of reduced muscle flow. Circulation 73:1127–1136, 1986.

222. Rajagopalan B, Conway MA, Massie B, Radda GK: Alterations of skeletal muscle metabolism in humans studied by phosphorus 31 magnetic resonance spectroscopy in congestive heart failure. Am J Cardiol 62:53E–57E, 1988.

27

EXAMINATION OF THE ADULT HEART AND GREAT VESSELS

R. DINSMORE

IMAGING TECHNIQUE

SELECTION OF IMAGE PLANES

TECHNIQUE FOR MR OF THE THORACIC AORTA

ACQUIRED DISEASES OF THE AORTA

    AORTIC ANEURYSMS

    DISSECTING HEMATOMA

CONGENITAL HEART DISEASE

    SPECIFIC ANOMALIES

    Coarctation of the Aorta
    Atrial Septal Defect
    Anomalies of Systemic Veins
    Interventricular Septal Defects
    Systemic-Pulmonary Surgical Shunts
    Transposition Complexes
    Congenital Aortic Stenosis
    Right Ventricular Outflow Obstruction

PULMONARY HYPERTENSION

LEFT VENTRICULAR DIMENSIONS AND FUNCTION

    Regional Left Ventricular Function
    Left Ventricular Dimensions
    Global Left Ventricular Function

PERICARDIAL AND MYOCARDIAL DISEASES

    Normal Pericardium
    Pericardial Effusion
    Constrictive Pericarditis and Restrictive Cardiomyopathy
    Dilated or Congestive Cardiomyopathy
    Hypertrophic Cardiomyopathy
    Pericardial Cysts
    Cardiac Tumors and Thrombus
    Intracardiac Thrombus
    Lipomatous Hypertrophy of the Interatrial Septum

CORONARY ARTERY DISEASE

The clinical value of MR imaging of the heart and great vessels may be divided into four areas: (1) display of anatomy and gross pathology, (2) evaluation of cardiac dimensions and mechanical function, (3) study of blood flow, and (4) characterization of normal and abnormal tissues. The usefulness of MR for anatomic and pathologic display is well established, particularly for evaluation of the diseases of the aorta and pericardium, congenital heart disease, and cardiac tumors. MR provides images of uniformly high quality throughout a large field, including cardiac chambers, major vessels, and other thoracic structures without need for contrast medium. In this respect, MR is unique among imaging methods, whether invasive or noninvasive. MR images are tomographic, eliminating overlap of structures, and may be obtained in any desired image plane so that anatomy can be optimally displayed.

MR studies of cardiac function are at an earlier stage, but initial work suggests that this is one of the most promising applications. MR has some important advantages over other methods in this area. The flexibility of image plane selection is an asset for obtaining measurements and functional information, since it allows examinations to be rigorously standardized. Because of the absence of biologic effect, MR studies can be repeated as often as desired. Since it does not require radiopaque contrast medium, the examination itself does not affect function. Electrocardiographic (ECG) synchronization allows static image acquisition at any point in the cardiac cycle, and newly developed methods now provide motion display.

The potential ability of MR for tissue characterization has had very promising but still limited applications in the heart. It has been used primarily in the study of acute myocardial infarction but has also been useful in pericardial disease and in the identification and evaluation of the extent of tumor spread. Blood flow imaging using MR cineangiography will be considered in Chapters 28 and 29.

IMAGING TECHNIQUE

Because of cardiac motion, ECG synchronization is required for MR studies of the heart and is desirable for the aorta, particularly the thoracic portion. A telemetry system with nonmagnetic wires and three standard electrodes on the extremities is used for ECG synchronization. For most studies oriented to anatomic display of the heart and great vessels, spin-echo (SE) pulse sequences with echo delay (echo time [TE]) equal to or less than 30 msec and repetition time (TR) related to the ECG R-R interval are used. Images are acquired in a matrix of 128 vertical (interpolated to 256) × 256 horizontal picture elements. Multiple echoes may be obtained for tissue discrimination. For example, a TE 30/60 sequence is useful in the evaluation of acute myocardial infarct. This will be further discussed under "Coronary Artery Disease."

SELECTION OF IMAGE PLANES

For most studies of the heart, image planes should be oriented to intrinsic cardiac axes rather than to the conventional transverse, sagittal, or coronal axes through the thorax, which are normally used for noncardiac studies.[1] Image planes through precisely defined cardiac axes provide an optimal anatomic display and are necessary for precise measurements and function evaluation. They also allow for standardized technique, which is not possible with thorax-oriented image planes, since the position of the heart in the thorax varies widely from patient to patient and, in some instances, from examination to examination in the same patient. In addition, studies of the left ventricular myocardium for thickness or signal intensity should be done with image planes perpendicular to the left ventricular wall to avoid errors caused by the partial volume phenomenon when the image plane is oblique to the myocardium[2] (Figs. 27–1 and 27–2).

At the Massachusetts General Hospital, three standardized axial image planes are used for cardiac studies, all oriented to the long axis through the left ventricle, that is, the axis between the aortic valve and the apex (Fig. 27–3).[1] These three image planes are a *short-axis series* perpendicular to the long axis (Fig. 27–4) and *two long-axis planes.* One is approximately *parallel to the septum* (Fig. 27–5), and the other, rotated 90 degrees on the long axis, is approximately *perpendicular to the septum* (Fig. 27–6). The aortic valve and apex are used as anatomic landmarks for the reference axis because each is relatively small and

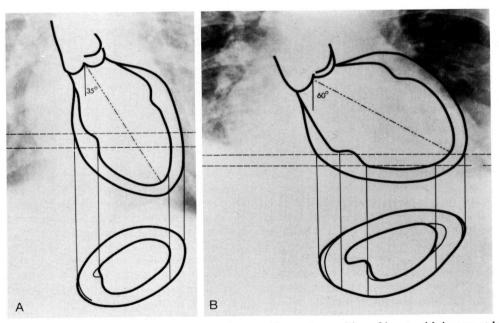

FIGURE 27–1. Variation in projected transverse image with varying position of heart, with images at level of posterior papillary muscles. *A,* Relatively vertical heart. *B,* Nearly average position. Note falsely increased thickness of projected myocardial wall. (From Dinsmore RE, Wismer GL, Miller SW, et al: Magnetic resonance imaging of the heart using image planes oriented to cardiac axes: Experience with 100 cases. AJR 145:1177–1183, 1985; © by American Roentgen Ray Society.)

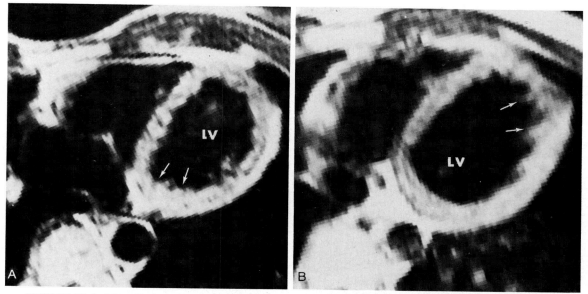

FIGURE 27–2. Diastolic MR image in plane transverse to thorax in two normal subjects. Apparent relative increase in left ventricular myocardial thickness (*arrows*) posteriorly in *A* and in anterolateral area in *B*. LV = left ventricle. (From Kaul S, Wismer GL, Brady TJ, et al: Measurement of normal left heart dimensions using optimally oriented MR images. AJR 146:75–79, 1986; © by American Roentgen Ray Society.)

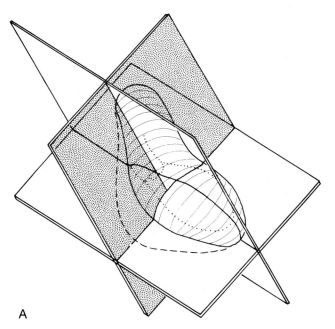

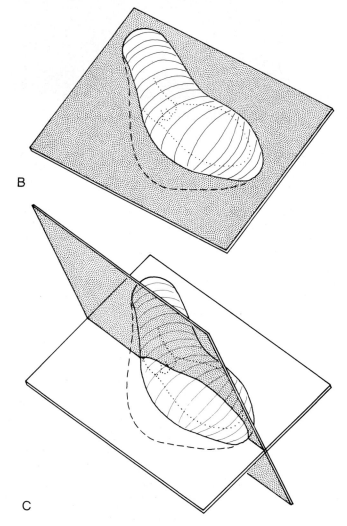

FIGURE 27–3. Three-dimensional (3D) diagrams of heart, with right side rotated 30 degrees anteriorly. *A,* Plane (*shaded area*) of image through short axis of left ventricle. *B,* Plane (*shaded area*) of image through long axis of left ventricle parallel to interventricular septum. *C,* Plane (*shaded area*) of image through long axis of left ventricle perpendicular to septum. (From Dinsmore RE, Wismer GL, Levine RA, et al: Magnetic resonance imaging of the heart: Positioning and gradient angle selection for optimal imaging planes. AJR 143:1135–1142, 1984; © by American Roentgen Ray Society.)

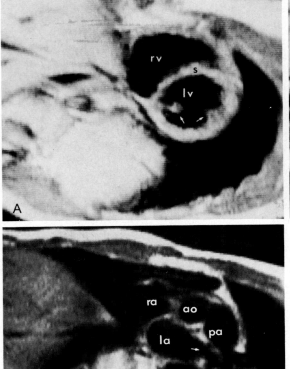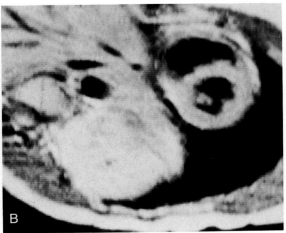

FIGURE 27–4. MR images of plane through short axis of left ventricle at level of papillary muscles (*arrows*). *A*, End-diastole. *B*, End-systole. *C*, Through base showing aorta (ao), pulmonary artery (pa), both atria (ra, la), and pulmonary vein (*arrow*). lv = left ventricle; rv = right ventricle; s = interventricular septum. (From Dinsmore RE, Wismer GL, Levine RA, et al: Magnetic resonance imaging of the heart: Positioning and gradient angle selection for optimal imaging planes. AJR 143:1135–1142, 1984; © by American Roentgen Ray Society.)

distinctive and because a line through these points is nearest to a true long axis. A set of multislice images through each of these planes provides an essentially complete anatomic display; however, images in all three planes are not routinely obtained in all patients. Because of the anatomic relationship of the interventricular and interatrial septa and the atrioventricular valves with the long axis of the left ventricle, these image planes are useful for a wide range of cardiac conditions, in addition to specific studies of the left ventricle, as will be described later in this chapter. Possible exceptions include studies of the pericardium, the pulmonary veins, the left atrium, and the main pulmonary artery and bifurcation, which, because of their orientation, are well shown on images transaxial to the thorax.

After determining which image planes are appropriate for a given examination, the next step is to locate these planes through the patient as expeditiously as possible to avoid prolonging the examination. Our method is to begin with an initial multislice series done with a 30-degree rotation from the coronal plane to achieve the equivalent of rotating the patient's right shoulder 30 degrees anteriorly[1] (Fig.

FIGURE 27–5. *A–C*, MR images. *A*, Through long axis of left ventricle, parallel to septum. Aortic valve and apex (*arrows*). Also note right atrium (ra), venae cavae, and parts of pulmonary arteries. Image plane is shown as straight line in *D*. *B*, Plane similar to that in *A* but more posterior. Also shown are the left atrium (la), pulmonary veins (v), mitral valve (*arrow*), left ventricle (lv), and anterior (a) and posterior (p) papillary muscles. Image plane is shown as straight line in *E*. *C*, Plane more anterior than in *A*. Note right ventricle (rv), right atrium (ra), main pulmonary artery (mpa) and its right branch, and closed pulmonic valve (*arrow*). Image plane is shown as straight line in *F*. *D–F*, Sixty-degree left anterior oblique radiographs showing relations of cardiac chambers and image planes (*straight lines*) equivalent to MR images through long axis of left ventricle (LV) parallel to septum. AO = aorta; RV = right ventricle; RA = right atrium; SVC = superior vena cava; MPA = main pulmonary artery; RPA and LPA = right and left pulmonary arteries, respectively; IVC = inferior vena cava. (From Dinsmore RE, Wismer GL, Levine RA, et al: Magnetic resonance imaging of the heart: Positioning and gradient angle selection for optimal imaging planes. AJR 143:1135–1142, 1984; © by American Roentgen Ray Society.)

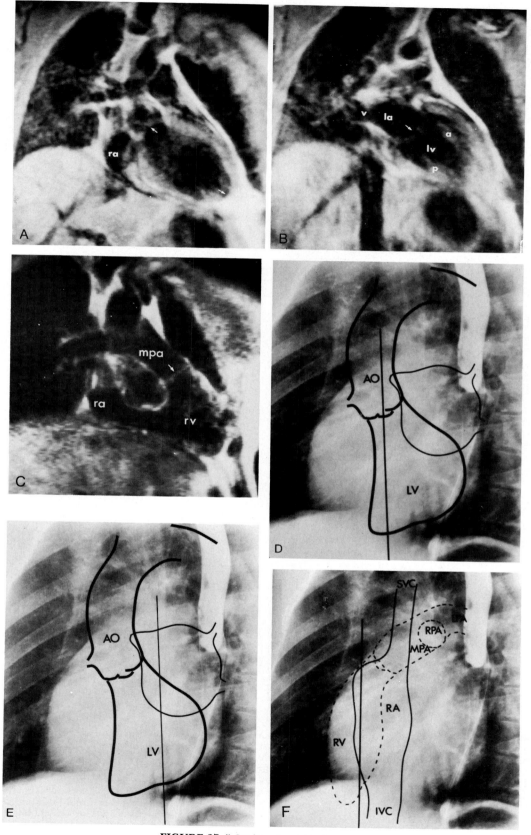

FIGURE 27–5 *See legend on opposite page*

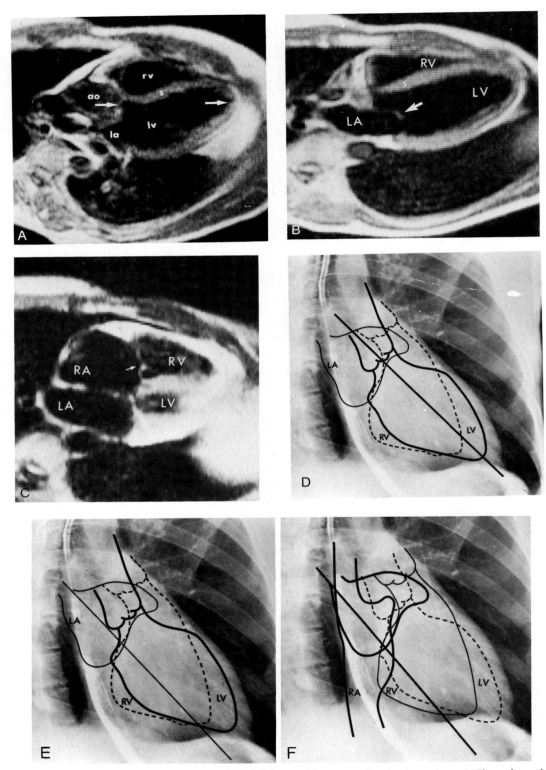

FIGURE 27–6. MR image through long axis of left ventricle, perpendicular to septum. *A,* Plane through aortic valve and apex (*arrows*). Image was acquired at end-diastole, hence the increased signal intensity in aortic root and sinuses (ao) in comparison with that in cardiac chambers. Image plane is similar to that shown as straight line in *D. B,* Plane offset to right, through anterior (*arrow*) and posterior leaflets of mitral valve. Image plane is similar to that shown as straight line in *E. C,* Plane further offset to right, similar to that shown as straight line in *F.* Display of both atria, interatrial septum, and anterior and septal (*arrow*) leaflets of tricuspid valve. *D–F,* Thirty-degree right anterior oblique radiographs showing relations of cardiac chambers and image planes (*straight lines*) equivalent to MR images through long axis of left ventricle, perpendicular to septum. RV and LV = right and left ventricles, respectively; S = interventricular septum; LA = left atrium; RA = right atrium. (From Dinsmore RE, Wismer GL, Levine RA, et al: Magnetic resonance imaging of the heart: Positioning and gradient angle selection for optimal imaging planes. AJR 143:1135–1142, 1984; © by American Roentgen Ray Society.)

27–7*A*). (Alternatively, this examination could also be done by rotating the patient and using the magnet's coordinate axes for a coronal image series [Fig. 27–7*B*].) A 30-degree rotation was selected because, based on experience with quantitative ventriculographic studies,[3, 4] and, subsequently, MR,[1, 25] this rotation consistently produces long-axis images through the aortic valve–apex axis. It also results in long-axis images that are approximately parallel (or, rotated 90 degrees, perpendicular) to the septum. Direct measurement of a septal angle can be done;[5] however, it is questionable whether this is of practical value, since the septum has a spiral configuration, changing with the cardiac cycle and affected by such conditions as regional ischemia and right ventricular pressure or volume overload. The initial series of images through the left ventricle is analogous to a 30-degree right anterior oblique left ventriculogram (see Fig. 27–5*A* and *B*), and images more anteriorly offset through the right ventricle and right atrium are also similar to a right anterior oblique angiogram (Fig. 27–5*C*). The information needed to locate the basic image planes can be determined on this examination. The aortic valve and left ventricular apex are located, and the angle between this axis and the

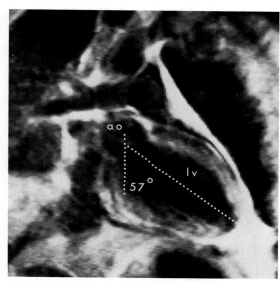

FIGURE 27–8. MR image in plane through long axis of left ventricle (lv) parallel to interventricular septum, at level through aortic valve and left ventricular apex. Method for measurement of the angle of this axis with the long axis of the body is illustrated. ao = aortic root. (From Dinsmore RE, Wismer GL, Miller SW, et al: Magnetic resonance imaging of the heart using image planes oriented to cardiac axes: Experience with 100 cases. AJR 145:1177–1183, 1985; © by American Roentgen Ray Society.)

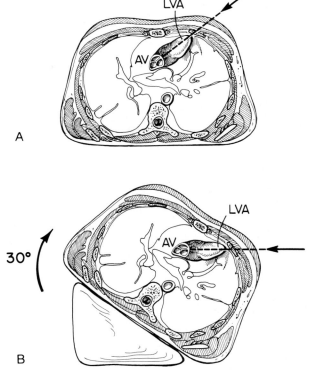

FIGURE 27–7. Transverse section through thorax as viewed from below. Position of line drawn through aortic valve (AV) and left ventricular apex (LVA) with patient supine (*A*) and with right shoulder rotated 30 degrees anteriad (*B*). (From Dinsmore RE, Wismer GL, Levine RA, et al: Magnetic resonance imaging of the heart: Positioning and gradient angle selection for optimal imaging planes. AJR 143:1135–1142, 1984; © by American Roentgen Ray Society.)

z-axis is measured (Fig. 27–8). This angle, describing a rotation on the newly defined y-axis, then allows one to obtain an image series through the long axis of the left ventricle perpendicular to the septum (see Fig. 27–7). A further 90-degree rotation on the same axis defines the plane through the short axis of the left ventricle (see Fig. 27–4).

TECHNIQUE FOR MR OF THE THORACIC AORTA

Our technique for image plane selection in examination of the aorta is as follows. An initial TE 30/60-msec short-axis multislice series is done using a transaxial image plane, that is, a plane transverse to the thorax. Next a TE 30-msec long-axis series is done by the following method.[6] From a transverse image slice at or immediately below the arch, a line is projected through the center of the ascending and descending aorta (Fig. 27–9*A*). The angle between this line and the vertical is measured. Then a multislice series of images is obtained with the measured rotation on the magnetic z-axis, off the sagittal plane. This results in a long-axis aortic view showing the entire sweep of the aortic arch (Fig. 27–9*B*). If the aorta is not tortuous, the entire thoracic aorta may be shown on one image slice. As an alternative to rotation of the magnet's coordinate axis, the patient can be rotated (right shoulder raised) the same number of degrees, and images can be obtained with the magnet's coordinate axes for a sagittal series.

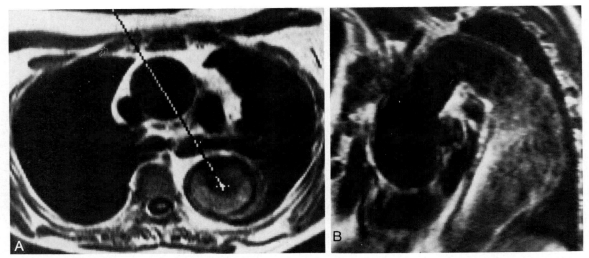

FIGURE 27–9. A 64-year-old man with fusiform aneurysm of ascending aorta and of distal arch and descending aorta. Short-axis (*A*) and long-axis (*B*) MR images with 30-msec TEs. Line drawn through ascending and descending parts of aorta in *A* is 28 degrees from vertical, indicating degree of rotation either in patient or of magnetic gradient angle to achieve long-axis image in *B*. (From Dinsmore RE, Wismer GL, Miller SW, et al: Magnetic resonance imaging of the heart using image planes oriented to cardiac axes: Experience with 100 cases. AJR 145:1177–1183, 1985; © by American Roentgen Ray Society.)

ACQUIRED DISEASES OF THE AORTA

MR is particularly well suited to aortic studies. Image plane flexibility and large field-of-view (FOV) of uniformly high quality give MR imaging important advantages over CT and two-dimensional (2D) echo-cardiography, respectively. The accuracy of MR in depicting the whole of the thoracic aorta has been demonstrated by the correlation of aortic diameters at multiple levels from sinuses of Valsalva to descending aorta obtained from MR with measurements from echocardiography, CT, and aortography (Fig. 27–10).[6]

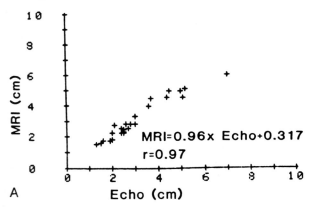

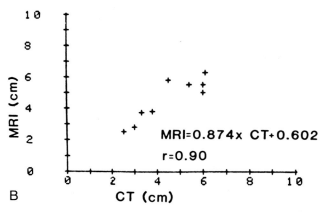

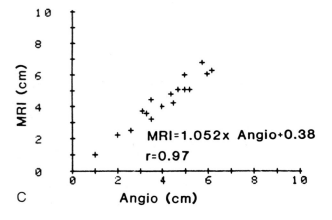

FIGURE 27–10. Comparison of measurements of aorta by MRI with those from other imaging methods. Measurements of aorta at multiple levels by MRI are compared in *A* with echocardiography (Y [MRI measurements] = 0.96 × [echo measurements] + 0.32, r = 0.97), in *B* with CT (Y [MRI measurements] = 0.87 × [CT measurements] + 0.6, r = 0.90), and in *C* with aortography (Y [MRI measurements] = 1.05 × [angio measurements] + 0.38, r = 0.97). (From Dinsmore RE, Liberthson RR, Wismer GL, et al: Magnetic resonance imaging of thoracic aortic aneurysms: Comparison with other imaging methods. AJR 146:309–314, 1986; © by American Roentgen Ray Society.)

AORTIC ANEURYSMS

A number of authors have described the use of MR in evaluation of aortic aneurysms.[6–10] Measurement of maximal aneurysm diameter by MR imaging corresponds closely to measurements from aortography, CT, and 2D echocardiography in a variety of types of aneurysms (Fig. 27–11).[6, 9] MR appears to be sensitive in detection of aneurysms; in our initial series of 15 patients, 20 aneurysms were detected by MR imaging compared with 19 detected by other imaging techniques.[6] A small saccular atherosclerotic aneurysm that was missed on transaxial CT images was well shown on a long-axis MR image, attesting to the advantage of image plane flexibility (Fig. 27–12). There has been excellent agreement between MR and other imaging techniques regarding aneurysm morphology and extent.[6, 9]

Atherosclerotic aneurysms of the thoracic aorta most commonly involve the distal arch and upper descending aorta. Chest pain, which is the most frequent symptom, suggests expansion and possible impending rupture. These aneurysms may also produce symptoms by compressing adjacent structures, such as the tracheal bronchial tree or the esophagus, or, less commonly, the great systemic veins or pulmonary arteries. Thus, an important advantage of MR over other methods of aortic imaging is the excellent demonstration of each of these structures on routine aortic studies. Typical saccular aneurysms of the descending thoracic aorta caused by atherosclerosis are shown in Figure 27–12 and 27–13*A*. In a study of abdominal aortic aneurysms, it was shown that MR imaging may give a better evaluation of aneurysm diameter than aortography.[7] This report cited a case in which marked thickening of the aneurysmal wall by thrombus resulted in only slight dilation of the lumen, with the result that aortography under-

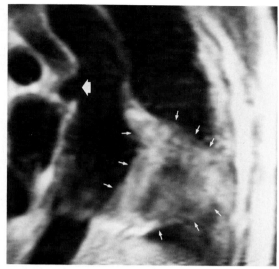

FIGURE 27–12. Detail of an MR image of descending thoracic aorta, in long axis, of 84-year-old man with two saccular aneurysms. Large arrow indicates small aneurysm that was not detected by CT. Arrows outline area of bright signal due to thrombus in large aneurysm. (From Dinsmore RE, Liberthson RR, Wismer GL, et al: Magnetic resonance imaging of thoracic aortic aneurysms: Comparison with other imaging methods. AJR 146:309–314, 1986; © by American Roentgen Ray Society.)

estimated the aneurysm diameter. However, MR imaging clearly defined the lumen and the thickened wall.

Difficulties sometimes arise, however, in distinguishing MR signal originating in thrombus from that due to turbulent or slowly flowing blood in an aneurysm. This distinction can sometimes be made by comparing images obtained in diastole with those obtained in systole.[11] Another method involves obtaining an examination with a first and second echo (TE approximately 30 and 60 msec).[7] The second-echo image tends to show an increase in the signal intensity of slowly flowing blood and a decrease in the signal intensity of thrombus. However, exceptions have been described,[12] probably because signal intensity is affected by a number of factors in addition to the velocity of moving blood. A method for distinguishing thrombus from slowly flowing blood that is independent of signal intensity using a first-order phase-shift technique for display of flow is illustrated in Figure 27–13.[13] Although clinical experience with this method is small, it promises to be highly accurate.[13, 14] Spatial presaturation, using additional radiofrequency (RF) pulses, is useful for reducing flow signal. It is particularly effective for imaging of flow perpendicular to the plane of section but is less effective for flow within the plane of section and for slow flow (see Chapter 4).

The status of MR in evaluation of *Takayasu's arteritis* is not yet clear. Amparo and colleagues[7] described concentric thickening of the aortic wall of the involved part of the abdominal aorta and of brachiocephalic branches, of medium signal intensity. How-

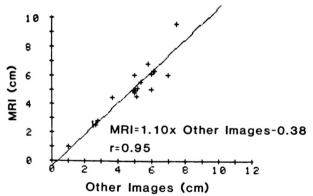

MRI=1.10x Other Images-0.38
r=0.95

FIGURE 27–11. Comparison of measurements of maximal aneurysm diameter by MR imaging with maximal diameters obtained with other imaging techniques. Relation is described by the regression equation: Y (MRI diameters) = 1.1 × (diameters, other imaging techniques) − 0.38, r = 0.95). (From Dinsmore RE, Liberthson RR, Wismer GL, et al: Magnetic resonance imaging of thoracic aortic aneurysms: Comparison with other imaging methods. AJR 146:309–314, 1986; © by American Roentgen Ray Society.)

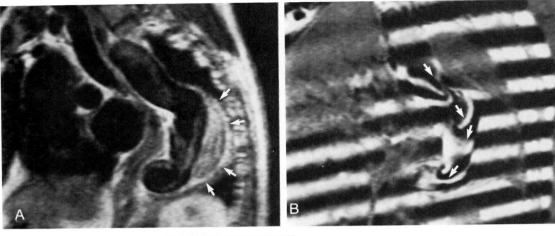

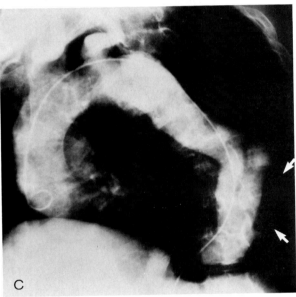

FIGURE 27–13. *A,* MR image in long axis, showing detail of descending thoracic aortic aneurysm in systole. Note intraluminal signal throughout aorta, though it is most intense in periphery of aneurysm (*arrows*). *B,* Phase-shift image in diastole, showing no deflection of phase stripes in periphery of aneurysm, and antegrade deflection in a central channel, indicating flowing blood (*arrows*). *C,* Thoracic aortogram confirming presence of peripheral thrombus (*arrows*) and central open channel. (From Dinsmore RE, Wedeen V, Rosen B, et al: Phase-offset technique to distinguish slow blood flow and thrombus on MR images. AJR 148:634, 1987; © by American Roentgen Ray Society.)

ever, Miller and associates[15] found a significant number of false-positive and false-negative examinations in display of the details of Takayasu's lesions in comparison to aortography. We have seen a patient with *giant cell aortitis* and a fusiform thoracic aneurysm who showed thickening at the margins of the aneurysm primarily involving the nonaneurysmal portion of the aorta[6] (Fig. 27–14).

Aneurysms due to *cystic medial necrosis,* commonly a manifestation of the *Marfan syndrome,* are fusiform and usually limited to the proximal aorta, typically with maximal dilation of the aortic sinuses. This combination of features results in a characteristic appearance on long-axis examinations, as shown in Figure 27–15. These aneurysms are potentially life threatening because of the frequent complications of dissecting hematoma or left ventricular failure due to aortic regurgitation. Aortic regurgitation is initially a result of dilation of the aortic valve ring but may be exacerbated by disruption of the valve by dissecting hematoma. Surgical intervention before these

complications develop now offers the possibility of improved prognosis for these patients but is, at present, technically feasible only when the aorta reaches a diameter of 6 cm or more.[59] Thus, noninvasive serial examination of asymptomatic patients has become important. MR now appears to be the method of choice for this evaluation.[60]

DISSECTING HEMATOMA

The diagnosis of *dissecting hematoma* is usually first suggested clinically by development of acute, severe, "tearing" chest pain and such physical signs as changing pulse deficits and development of new signs of aortic regurgitation. Although these findings may be highly characteristic, diagnostic imaging is necessary not only to confirm the diagnosis but also to show the location and extent of involvement of the aorta and the presence of complications such as compression or occlusion of branches of the aorta, since these

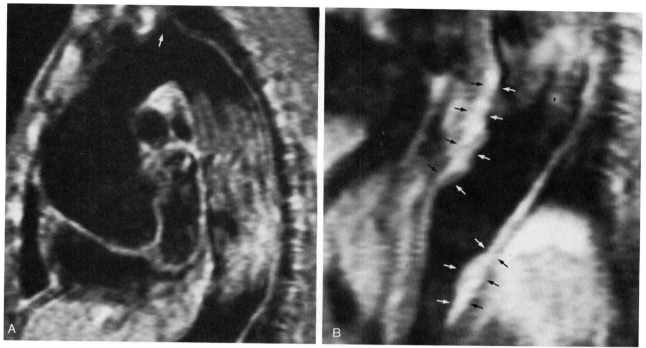

FIGURE 27–14. MR images of 28-year-old man with giant cell aortitis and fusiform aneurysm involving ascending and descending thoracic aorta. *A*, Thoracic aorta in long axis. Arrow indicates occluded left subclavian artery. *B*, Thoracoabdominal aorta in long axis. Arrows indicate thickened aortic wall. Note that thickening extends into nonaneurysmal part of aorta. (From Dinsmore RE, Liberthson RR, Wismer GL, et al: Magnetic resonance imaging of thoracic aortic aneurysms: Comparison with other imaging methods. AJR 146:309–314, 1986; © by American Roentgen Ray Society.)

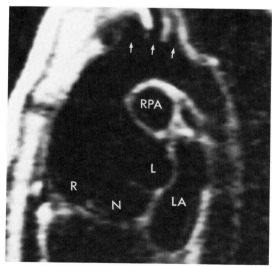

FIGURE 27–15. MR image of aorta, in long axis, of 29-year-old woman with the Marfan syndrome. Note origins of brachiocephalic branches (*arrows*) and normal thickness of aortic wall in comparison with patient in Figure 27–16. RPA = right pulmonary artery; LA = left atrium; L, R, N = left, right, and noncoronary sinuses of Valsalva, respectively. (From Dinsmore RE, Liberthson RR, Wismer GL, et al: Magnetic resonance imaging of thoracic aortic aneurysms: Comparison with other imaging methods. AJR 146:309–314, 1986; © by American Roentgen Ray Society.)

factors influence the choice of therapy. *Type A dissections* involve the ascending aorta, are frequently associated with aortic incompetence or compromised coronary blood flow, and are usually considered an indication for surgery. *Type B dissections* involve the descending thoracic aorta distal to the left subclavian artery and may be treated either medically or surgically. MR has been shown to be highly sensitive and specific for the diagnosis of aortic dissection.[61] MR imaging has been very successful in demonstration of the diagnosis and extent of dissection and in confirming or excluding involvement of major aortic branches, including the brachiocephalic, celiac, and superior mesenteric and renal arteries.[11, 16, 17] A disadvantage is the difficulty of studying an acutely ill patient with life support systems in a relatively inaccessible position within a powerful magnet. For this reason, the method is currently most promising for the relatively stable patient and for follow-up studies after surgery or medical treatment.

The diagnosis of dissection by MR is established by demonstration of true and false channels, separated by a thin, membranous structure (the intima and a portion of the media) (Figs. 27–16 and 27–17). In some instances, flow is rapid in both channels, resulting in absence of signal (flow void) on either side of the partition. Particularly in diastole, slower

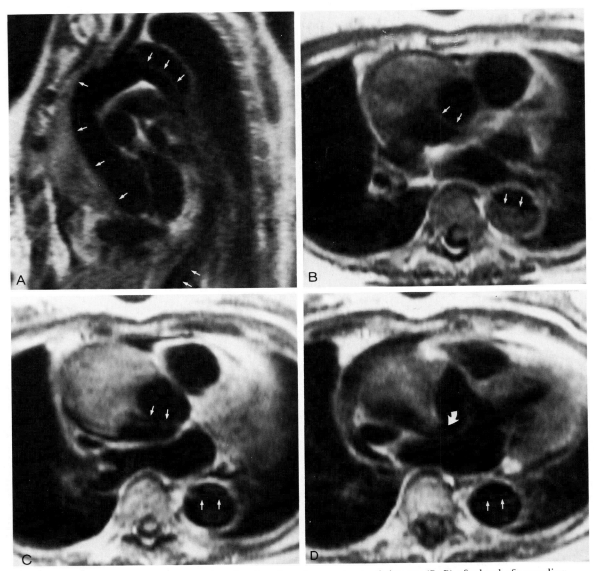

FIGURE 27–16. Long-axis image (*A*) and series of contiguous short-axis images (*B–D*) of a level of ascending aorta in a patient with dissecting hematoma. Arrows indicate partition between aortic lumen and false channel. *D,* Curved arrow indicates communication between true and false channels at intimal tear. (From Dinsmore RE, Wedeen VJ, Miller SW, et al: MRI of dissection of the aorta: Recognition of the intimal tear and differential flow velocities. AJR 146:1286–1288, 1986; © by American Roentgen Ray Society.)

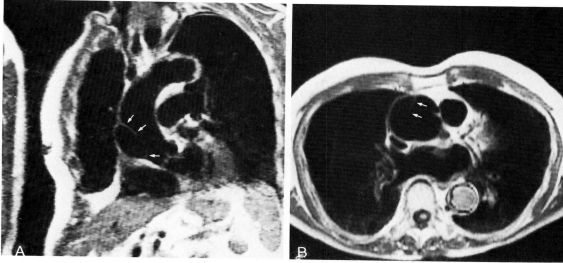

FIGURE 27–17. Long-axis image (*A*) and short-axis image (*B*) of the aorta of a patient with a local dissecting hematoma of the ascending aorta above the sinuses of Valsalva. The arrows indicate the intimal flap. Note the communication (intimal tear) between the true and false channels.

flow in the false channel may give rise to signal also with a characteristic appearance (Figs. 27–18 and 27–19), usually including flattening of the contour of the true lumen. The intimal flip is often best shown by cine techniques (Fig. 27–20). The long-axis image plane is particularly useful in evaluation of dissection, since it shows the arch in continuity. Display of the two separate channels may be enhanced by use of the phase-shift technique for display of different rates of flow and to exclude thrombus in the false channel.[17] Another potentially important advantage of MR imaging over CT in evaluation of dissection is that it is possible to identify precisely the site of the intimal tear (Figs. 27–16*B–D* and 27–17).[17] This information is frequently useful if surgical treatment is contemplated.

Early experience suggests that MR will make a particularly important contribution to management of the patient after either medical or surgical treatment.[62] The aortic graft and the presence of any residual false channel are readily shown (Fig. 27–21). Phase display and spatial presaturation techniques may be especially useful for this evaluation. Complications, such as late aneurysmal dilation of the false channel or infection, as shown in Figure 27–22, are well demonstrated by this method.

CONGENITAL HEART DISEASE

Two-dimensional echocardiography is the principal noninvasive method for imaging studies of congenital heart disease in infants and small children, though MR is assuming an increasing role (see Chapter 29). However, after early childhood, echocardiography has increasing technical problems related to availability of the echo window, limiting the quality and extent of examination possible in many patients. It is in these cases that MR appears to have its strongest potential role for demonstrating congenital heart disease. Congenital abnormalities of cardiac

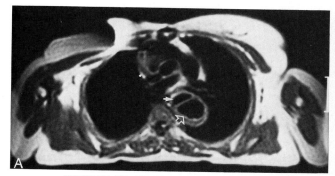
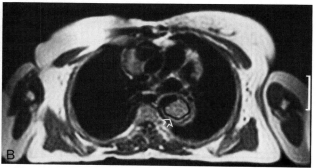

FIGURE 27–18. Dissection of the descending thoracic aorta, showing the effect of slow flow on signal intensity in the false lumen. *A*, The true (*closed arrow*) and false (*open arrow*) lumens are shown during systole. *B*, During diastole, signal intensity in the false lumen is increased, consistent with slow flow (*arrow*). (Courtesy of Drs. Tom Hedrick and Donald Johnston, The Methodist Hospital, Houston, TX.)

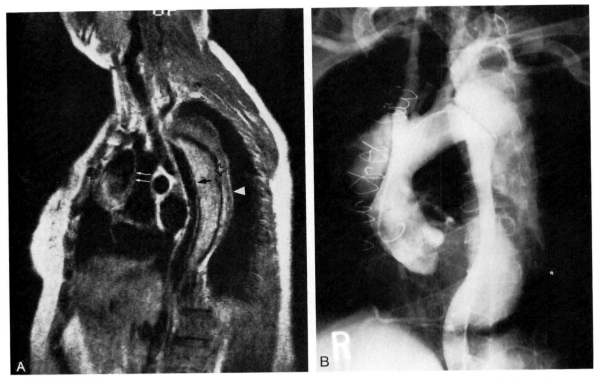

FIGURE 27–19. Type A dissection of the aorta. *A,* Long-axis view showing the true lumen of the descending aorta with flow void *(closed arrow),* signal in the false channel *(open arrow),* and thrombus *(arrowhead).* The false channel of the ascending aorta is indicated by double arrows. *B,* Aortogram showing true and false channels. (Courtesy of Drs. Thomas Hedrick and Donald Johnston, The Methodist Hospital, Houston, TX.)

valves may be evaluated using cine MR imaging techniques; nonetheless, echocardiography is, at the present time, the method of choice when satisfactory studies can be obtained.

SPECIFIC ANOMALIES

COARCTATION OF THE AORTA.[18, 19] A routine aortic examination in the short and long axes provides an excellent demonstration of the lesions associated with coarctation. The examination readily shows such details as the length and severity of coarctation, the size of the ascending aorta and arch, the relationship of the origins of brachiocephalic branches to the narrowed segment, the presence of poststenotic dilation, and the size of the descending aorta (Fig. 27–23). Although the sensitivity of MR for evaluation of collateral vessels, information that is important for planning surgery, has not yet been established, it is likely to be high with use of cine MR imaging. MR

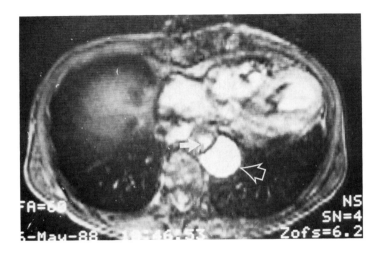

FIGURE 27–20. Axial cine image in a patient with a type B dissection. The dark intimal flap between the true lumen *(closed arrow)* and false lumen *(open arrow)* is well seen. (Courtesy of H. Kantor, M.D.)

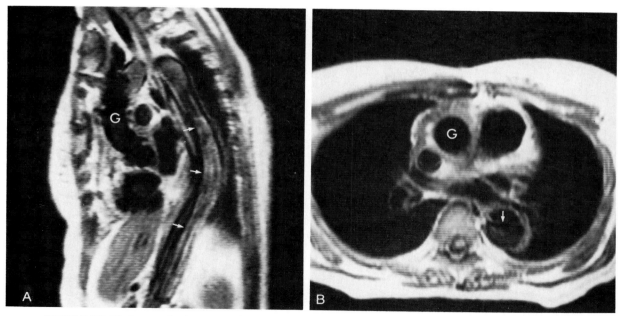

FIGURE 27–21. Long-axis view (*A*) and short-axis view (*B*) of the aorta 1 week after composite graft of the ascending aorta for dissecting hematoma. Note persistence of two channels in the descending aorta (*arrows*). The preoperative examination of this patient is shown in Figure 27–16. G = ascending aortic graft.

imaging appears to be particularly useful for follow-up studies after surgical repair of coarctation[20] (Fig. 27–24).

ATRIAL SEPTAL DEFECT. MR images provide exquisite detail of the interatrial septum, unmatched by other imaging techniques, whether invasive or noninvasive. In our experience, a combination of multiple short- and long-axis (perpendicular to the septum) images provides excellent detail of the septum and its relationship to other structures, including mitral and tricuspid valves, the cavae, and the pulmonary veins (Fig. 27–25).[21] The long-axis view is

especially useful in determining the type of defect, since the locations of primum, secundum, and sinus venosus defects are best displayed in this image plane, which shows the length of the septum from superior to inferior, as well as the atrioventricular valves (Figs. 27–25 to 27–27). Initial experience has shown good correlation between the estimated size of the defect measured on the long-axis images perpendicular to the septum and the size measured at surgery.[21]

MR imaging appears to be very sensitive in the detection of interatrial septal defects; Diethelm and coworkers[22] found a sensitivity of 97 per cent in 30

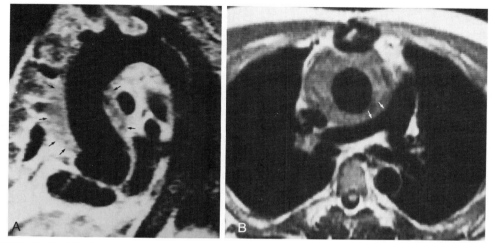

FIGURE 27–22. MR image of a 38-year-old man 8 months following graft replacement of the ascending aorta for fusiform aneurysm resulting from cystic medial necrosis. *A*, Long-axis image. The ascending aortic graft is surrounded by an abscess of medium signal intensity (*arrows*). *B*, Short-axis image at the level of the pulmonary artery. The abscess surrounding the aortic graft slightly compresses the pulmonary artery (*arrows*). The abscess was later drained surgically.

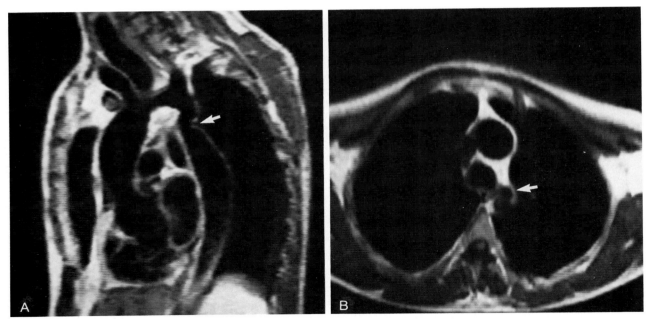

FIGURE 27–23. Long-axis view (*A*) and short-axis view (*B*) of the aorta of a patient with congenital coarctation of the aortic isthmus (*arrow*).

patients with proven atrial defects. In a review of MR imaging of 33 subjects without congenital heart disease, we found three apparent defects (9 per cent) in the interatrial septum.[21] In each instance, these false defects were shown on only one of multiple images. Diethelm and coworkers[22] found a similar false-positive rate, with a specificity of 90 per cent in their series. This instance of false-positive cases is considerably lower than the rate, as high as 50 per cent, that has been reported with 2D echocardiography.[23] Even with improving MR image quality, a small proportion of false-positive diagnoses by MR imaging may continue to occur because of normal thinning of the septum in the fossa ovalis region (Figs. 27–6C and 27–26B). Errors can probably be minimized by requiring that the demonstration of defects be reproducible on at least two acquisitions[21] and that they have sharp, thick margins rather than gradual tapering of the edges, which may be more characteristic of a thin fossa ovalis or signal dropout.[22]

Pulmonary veins are well demonstrated by MR on images through the long and short axes of the heart or on transaxial images. Diethelm and coworkers[22] found, in a study of transaxial MR in 64 patients, demonstration of at least two pulmonary veins in 98 per cent, at least three veins in 94 percent, and four veins in 86 per cent. This sensitivity is greater than that described in the detection of pulmonary veins by 2D echocardiography.[24] The demonstration on MR imaging of partial and total anomalous venous drainage has been described[18, 25] (Fig. 27–28). Although experience is still limited, it appears likely that MR imaging will be the best noninvasive method for delineating anomalies of pulmonary venous drainage, because of its characteristics of good resolution throughout the imaging field.

ANOMALIES OF SYSTEMIC VEINS. Anomalies of large systemic veins, such as persistent left superior vena cava, are readily diagnosed by MR imaging.[21, 26] Figure 27–29 shows an anomalous left superior vena cava with drainage into the coronary sinus, which is typically dilated.

INTERVENTRICULAR SEPTAL DEFECTS. MR has been found to be sensitive in the detection of interventricular septal defects.[27] In our experience, the long-axis view perpendicular to the septum is particularly useful for demonstration of the defect and its precise location within the septum and in relation to the atrioventricular and semilunar valves (Fig. 27–30).[25] However, defects may be accurately diagnosed and localized by transaxial images.[27]

SYSTEMIC-PULMONARY SURGICAL SHUNTS. Jacobstein and colleagues[28] described the successful MR demonstration of patency of palliative shunts (Figs. 27–31 to 27–33). Katz and associates[20] found MR imaging to be in complete agreement with angiography, CT, or surgery in 17 cases with patent shunts and 6 with occluded shunts. However, MR was less sensitive in the detection of stenoses in nonoccluded shunts (8, or 66.7 per cent) in this series.

TRANSPOSITION COMPLEXES. The anatomy and relationships of the great vessels are well shown by MR, since the full extent of the vessels and the branching patterns are well displayed (Figs. 27–34 and 27–35). Visceral atrial situs is readily determined by MR, with its large FOV. Guit and associates[29] used coronal images to display central bronchial anatomy and positions of the inferior vena cava, abdominal aorta, liver, and stomach. Atrial anatomy is well demon-

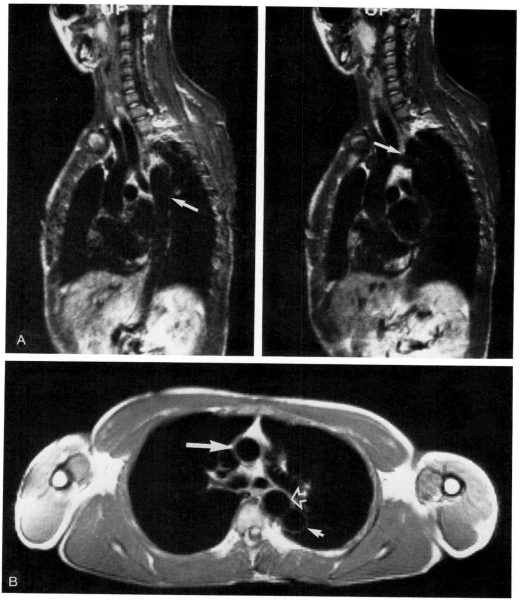

Figure 27–24. Coarctation repair with placement of a bypass graft. *A,* Sagittal images at two levels through the region of the coarctation. The graft is seen joining the descending aorta (*arrow*) (*left*) and the arch above the coarctation (*arrow*) (*right*). The transverse image (*B*) shows the ascending aorta (*closed arrow*), the descending aorta (*open arrow*), and the adjacent graft (*arrowhead*). (Courtesy of Drs. Tom Hedrick and Donald Johnston, The Methodist Hospital, Houston, TX.)

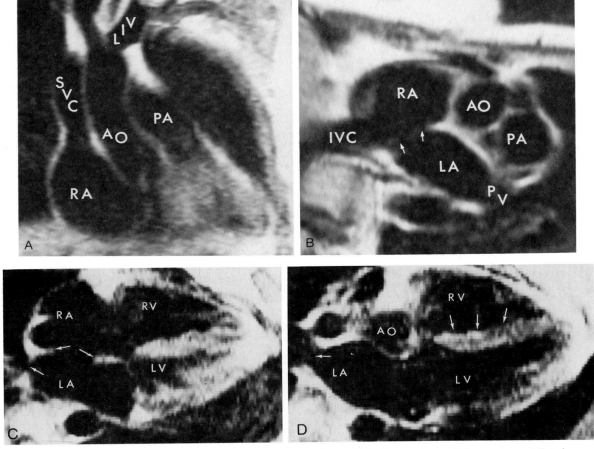

FIGURE 27–25. **Secundum interatrial septal defect.** *A,* Through the long axis parallel to septum. Dilated right atrium (RA) and pulmonary artery (PA) with normally draining superior vena cava (SVC). *B,* Through the short axis. Interatrial septal defect (*arrows*), inferior vena cava (IVC), and left pulmonary vein (PV), which enters left atrium (LA), are seen. *C,* Through long axis perpendicular to septum at level of interatrial septum. Defect in secundum position (*arrows*). Pulmonary vein (*single arrow*) drains normally into left atrium (LA). *D,* Through long axis perpendicular to septum at level of aortic root (AO) in diastole. Dilated right ventricle (RV), concavity of interventricular septum on right ventricular side (*arrows*), and pulmonary vein, which enters left atrium (LA), (*arrow*), are seen. LIV = left innominate vein; LV = left ventricle. (From Dinsmore RE, Wismer GL, Guyer D, et al: Magnetic resonance imaging of the interatrial septum and atrial septal defects. AJR 145:697–703; © by American Roentgen Ray Society.)

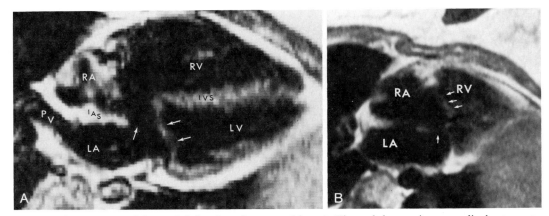

FIGURE 27–26. **Interatrial septal defect in primum position.** *A,* Through long axis perpendicular to septa. Note relation to interatrial defect (*single arrow*), to anterior leaflet of mitral valve (*double arrows*), and to interventricular septum (IVS). *B,* Parallel image with rightward offset, showing atria and interatrial septum (IAS). Tricuspid valve (*triple arrows*) and primum interatrial defect (*single arrow*) are seen, as well as an apparent defect in fossa ovalis area. Unusual degree of thinning of septum in this region was found at surgery. RA = right atrium; RV = right ventricle; LA = left atrium; LV = left ventricle; PV = pulmonary vein. (From Dinsmore RE, Wismer GL, Guyer D, et al: Magnetic resonance imaging of the interatrial septum and atrial septal defects. AJR 145:697–703; © by American Roentgen Ray Society.)

FIGURE 27–27. Sinus venosus atrial septal defect. A long-axis image perpendicular to the interatrial septum shows the defect (*arrow*) superiorly, in the sinus venosus portion of the septum. RA = right atrium; LA = left atrium; RV = right ventricle.

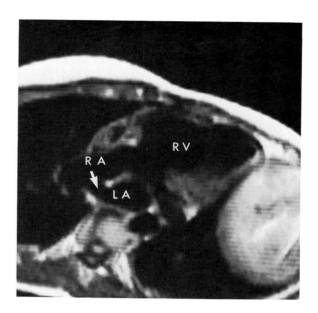

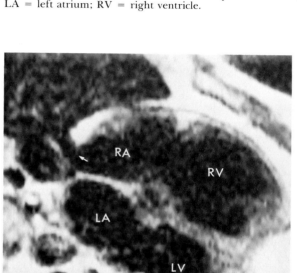

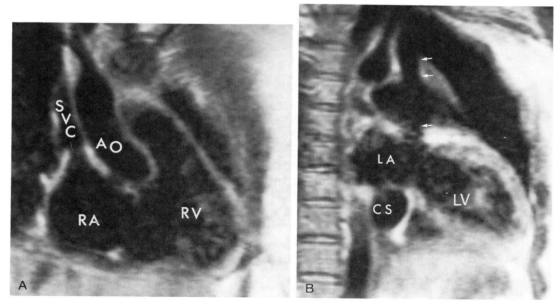

FIGURE 27–28. A 64-year-old man with partial anomalous pulmonary venous return from right lung to right atrium (RA), with intact interatrial septum, confirmed at cardiac catheterization and pulmonary angiography. Long-axis image perpendicular to septa shows dilated right-sided chambers, intact interatrial septum, and anomalous pulmonary vein (*arrow*) entering right atrium. RV = right ventricle; LA = left atrium; LV = left ventricle. (From Dinsmore RE, Wismer GL, Miller SW, et al: Magnetic resonance imaging of the heart using image planes oriented to cardiac axes: Experience with 100 cases. AJR 145:1177–1183, 1985; © by American Roentgen Ray Society.)

FIGURE 27–29. Persistent left superior vena cava (SVC) draining into coronary sinus (CS). *A*, Through long axis parallel to septum at right ventricular level. Dilated right ventricle (RV) and right atrium (RA) and a small superior vena cava (SVC) can be seen. *B*, Through long axis parallel to septum at left atrial (LA) and left ventricular (LV) levels. Persistent left superior vena cava (*arrows*) and dilated coronary sinus (CS) can be noted. AO = aorta. (From Dinsmore RE, Wismer GL, Guyer D, et al: Magnetic resonance imaging of the interatrial septum and atrial septal defects. AJR 145:697–703, 1985; © by American Roentgen Ray Society.)

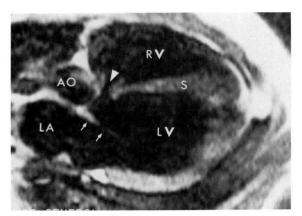

FIGURE 27–30. A 25-year-old man with interventricular septal defect (*arrowhead*) high in membranous septum, confirmed at catheterization and surgery. MR image through long axis of left ventricle (LV) perpendicular to interventricular septum (S). Diameter of defect was estimated at 7 mm by MR imaging and was found to be 8 mm at surgery. Anterior leaflet of mitral valve (*arrows*). RV = right ventricle; AO = aortic root; LA = left atrium. (From Dinsmore RE, Wismer GL, Miller SW, et al: Magnetic resonance imaging of the heart using image planes oriented to cardiac axes: Experience with 100 cases. AJR 145:1177–1183, 1985; © by American Roentgen Ray Society.)

strated on transaxial cardiac images. Ventricular morphology, including trabecular pattern, relationship of atrial ventricular and semilunar valves, and the presence of an infundibulum, is well observed on axial cardiac views.

CONGENITAL AORTIC STENOSIS. MR has not been useful in the evaluation of the aortic valve leaflets themselves, although this may change as motion techniques develop further. However, MR imaging has been shown to be useful in the diagnosis of subvalvular and supravalvular aortic stenosis (Fig. 27–36).[30, 31] At the same time, left ventricular wall thickness and contractile function can be demonstrated.

RIGHT VENTRICULAR OUTFLOW OBSTRUCTION. As in the case of the aortic valve, MR has not yet been useful in demonstration of isolated pulmonic valve stenosis. However, right ventricular infundibular stenosis in patients with *tetralogy of Fallot* and *pulmonary branch stenosis* are well shown by MR (Fig. 27–37). Flexibility of image plane selection is particularly useful in such cases. For example, the image plane can be aligned with the right ventricular infundibulum for optimal display of the obstruction in tetralogy of Fallot. Similarly, images through the long axis perpendicular to the septum show the position of the interventricular septal defect and of the overriding aorta. Surgical pulmonary bands are readily demonstrated.

PULMONARY HYPERTENSION

Patients with pulmonary arterial hypertension have been shown to have increased right ventricular wall thickness demonstrable by MR, as well as persisting MR signal in the pulmonary artery throughout the cardiac cycle.[32] The persisting signal is due to slow pulmonary blood flow in these patients. Although these observations must be considered to be in a preliminary stage, this information is potentially very useful as an adjunct to the disordered anatomy of patients with congenital heart disease.

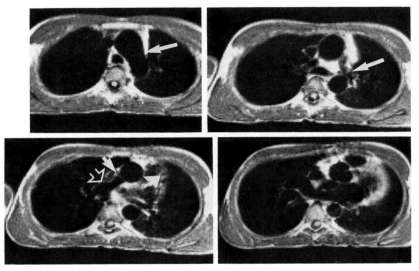

FIGURE 27–31. Tricuspid atresia and Waterson shunt. The upper left image shows the aortic arch (*arrow*). A markedly stenosed left pulmonary artery (*arrow*) is present at a lower level (*right upper*). The lower left image shows the shunt (*closed arrow*) joining the ascending aorta (*arrowhead*) to the stenosed right pulmonary artery (*open arrow*).

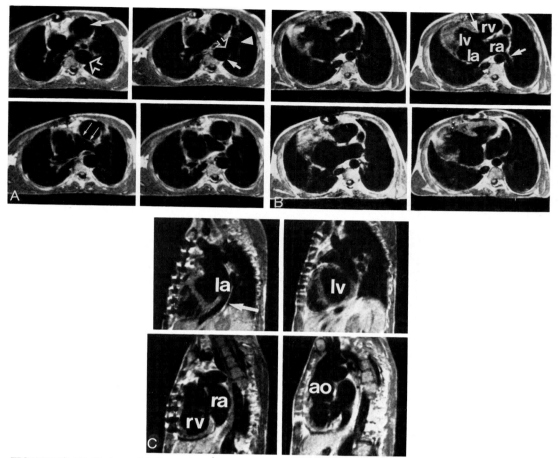

FIGURE 27–32. Patient with Potts shunt for pulmonic valve stenosis. Dextrocardia, ventricular septal defect, and atrial septal defect were also present. *A,* The ascending (*closed arrow*) and descending (*open arrow*) aorta are visualized in the most superior image (*upper left*). In the upper right image, the distal left pulmonary artery (*arrowhead*) is shown connected with the descending aorta (*closed arrow*) via the Potts shunt (*open arrow*). The proximal left pulmonary artery is also visualized (*small arrows*). *B,* These images were obtained at a lower thoracic level. Dextrocardia is apparent. The left ventricle (lv), right ventricle (rv), left atrium (la), and right atrium (ra) are seen. The right upper image shows the ventricular septal defect (*long arrow*). A pulmonary vein is seen entering the right atrium (*short arrow*). The lower images were obtained more inferiorly. *C,* Sagittal plane images of the same patient. The left atrium (la) is seen, with a hepatic vein entering inferiorly (*arrow*). The left ventricle (lv) is noted in the right upper image. In moving from right to left, the right ventricle (rv) becomes visible (*left lower image*). A dilated aorta (ao) is demonstrated in the right lower image.

FIGURE 27–33. Rastelli repair of pulmonary atresia and ventricular septal defect. The upper left image shows the aortic arch (*arrow*). The left pulmonary artery is visualized in the upper right image (*arrow*). The conduit (*open arrow*) to the small right pulmonary artery is shown in the lower right image (*closed arrow*). (Courtesy of Drs. Tom Hedrick and Donald Johnston, The Methodist Hospital, Houston, TX.)

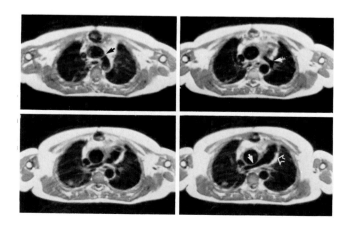

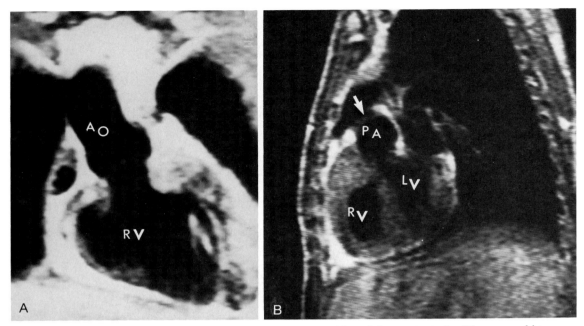

FIGURE 27–34. MR images of a 16-year-old boy with transposition of the great arteries. There was a history of pulmonary artery banding and subsequent Senning repair, including closure of a ventricular septal defect (VSD). *A,* An image plane parallel to the septum. *B,* An image plane perpendicular to the septum. The aorta is shown to arise from the right ventricle in *A* and the pulmonary artery from the left ventricle in *B*. AO = ascending aorta; PA = main pulmonary artery; RV = right ventricle; LV = left ventricle; arrow indicates the pulmonary band. (From Dinsmore RE: The use of MRI in congenital heart disease. *In* Osbakken M [ed]: NMR Techniques in the Study of Cardiovascular Structure and Function. Mt. Kisco, NY, Futura Publishing Co., 1988, pp 123–136.)

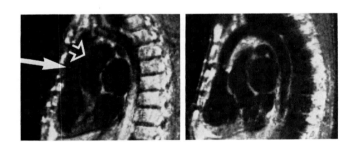

←
FIGURE 27–35. Corrected transposition shown at two levels (left image is to the right side of the thorax). The aorta lies anterior (*closed arrow*) to the pulmonary artery (*open arrow*).

FIGURE 27–36. MR image of the left ventricle of a 32-year-old man in a plane perpendicular to the long axis of the septum, showing focal subaortic stenosis by a congenital bar (*arrow*). (From Dinsmore RE: The use of MRI in congenital heart disease. *In* Osbakken M [ed]: NMR Techniques in the Study of Cardiovascular Structure and Function. Mt. Kisco, NY, Futura Publishing Co., 1988, pp 123–136.)

→

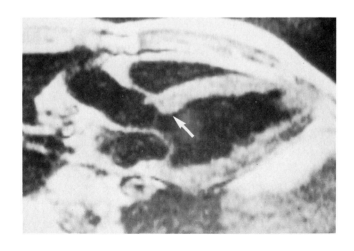

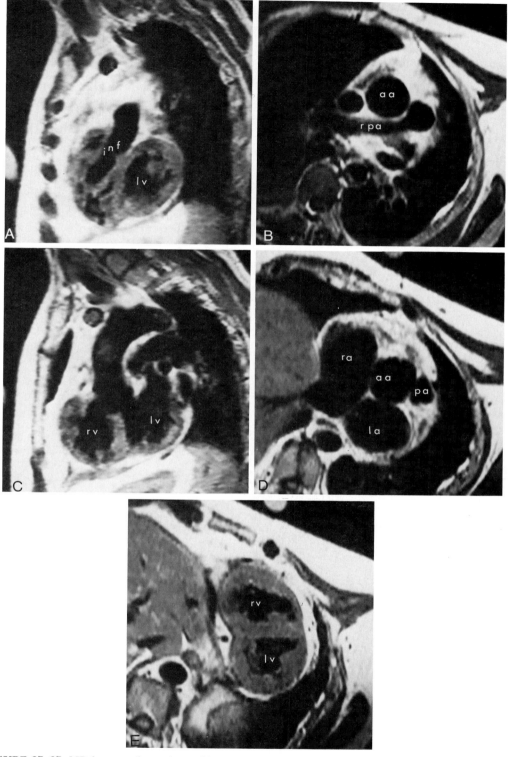

FIGURE 27–37. MR images of a patient with tetralogy of Fallot. *A*, A plane through the long axis of the right ventricular outflow tract showing mild tubular infundibular narrowing. *B*, Transaxial images through the pulmonary trunk and through a diffusely narrowed right pulmonary artery. *C*, A plane through the long axis of the ascending aorta showing overriding, interventricular septal defect, and right ventricular hypertrophy. *D*, Short-axis image at the base showing relative size of aorta and pulmonary arteries. *E*, Short-axis image at ventricular level showing the markedly hypertrophied right ventricle. rv = right ventricle; inf = infundibulum; lv = left ventricle; pa = pulmonary trunk; rpa = right pulmonary artery; aa = ascending aorta. (From Dinsmore RE: The use of MRI in congenital heart disease. *In* Osbakken M [ed]: NMR Techniques in the Study of Cardiovascular Structure and Function. Mt. Kisco, NY, Futura Publishing Co., 1988, pp 123–136.)

LEFT VENTRICULAR DIMENSIONS AND FUNCTION

The use of MR to measure the heart and study its function is in its infancy. Nonetheless, the evidence available suggests that MR may well become the best and most accurate method for measurement of the heart. Since it is completely noninvasive, the examination itself has no effect on function and can be repeated as frequently as needed. The flexibility of image plane selection available, along with the uniformly high image quality throughout the image plane, makes it possible to obtain measurements through precisely defined anatomic landmarks on standardized examinations.

Although conventional transaxial images have been used for cardiac measurements in normal volunteers, it is difficult to validate these measurements, since the image plane is different from that used by other techniques. Furthermore, such examinations cannot be standardized. The transaxial image plane is oblique to intrinsic cardiac axes, with a degree of obliquity that varies from patient to patient. In a group of 100 cases, we found that the angle between the long axis of the left ventricle and the long axis of the body varies from 33 degrees to 76 degrees, with a mean of 57 degrees ± 9 degrees (see Fig. 27–1).[25] The transaxial plane is oblique through much of the myocardial wall, particularly in the inferior area, making measurements unreliable (see Figs. 27–1 and 27–2). Precise identification of left ventricular segmental anatomy is difficult with image planes oriented to the chest.

For function studies, we use images oriented to an axis between the aortic valve and left ventricular apex, that is, through the long axis of the left ventricle. A complete examination of the left ventricle in our laboratory consists of a series of short-axis images, perpendicular to the long axis, and two long-axis series (see Figs. 27–4 to 27–6).[1] One long-axis series is approximately parallel to the interventricular septum, and the other is perpendicular to the septum.

REGIONAL LEFT VENTRICULAR FUNCTION. The study of regional function depends upon precise and reproducible display of segmental anatomy. A technique for left ventricular segmental anatomic display is illustrated in Figure 27–38.[25] The left ventricle is divided along its long axis (apex–aortic valve) into three short-axis sections. The basal and middle sections are further divided into four quadrants, each giving a total of nine segments. The system is compatible with standard angiographic and echocardiographic segmental nomenclature systems. Figure 27–39 illustrates the use of MR imaging in the study of regional wall motion abnormality.

LEFT VENTRICULAR DIMENSIONS. Normal dimensions from MR imaging are shown in Table 27–1.[2]

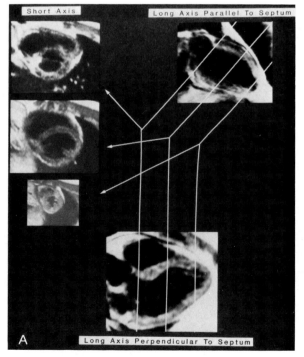
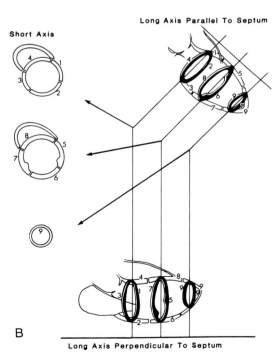

FIGURE 27–38. Composite illustration of images in three standard planes oriented to axis through aortic valve and left ventricular apex. *A,* MR images. *B,* Diagram of images showing nine left ventricular wall segments: (1) anterobasal, (2) posterior, (3) posterobasal, (4) basal septal, (5) anterolateral, (6) posterolateral, (7) diaphragmatic, (8) apical septal, and (9) apical. (From Dinsmore RE, Wismer GL, Miller SW, et al: Magnetic resonance imaging of the heart using image planes oriented to cardiac axes: Experience with 100 cases. AJR 145:1177–1183, 1985; © by American Roentgen Ray Society.)

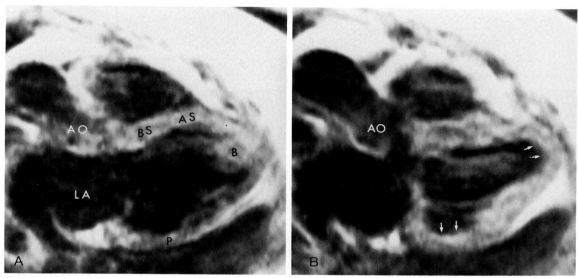

FIGURE 27–39. A 64-year-old woman with severe three-vessel coronary artery disease. MR images in plane through long axis of left ventricle. *A,* Diastolic image. Thinning of posterior segment (P) and increased blood pool signal (B) in apical area. *B,* Systolic image. Akinesia and absence of systolic thickening (*arrows*) of posterior and apical segments. AO = aortic root; LA = left atrium; BS = basal septal segment; AS = apical septum. (From Dinsmore RE, Wismer GL, Miller SW, et al: Magnetic resonance imaging of the heart using image planes oriented to cardiac axes: Experience with 100 cases. AJR 145:1177–1183, 1985; © by American Roentgen Ray Society.)

These measurements were taken from long- and short-axis images in normal volunteers (Fig. 27–40), with comparison with 2D echocardiograms in comparable positions. There was no significant difference between the individual measurements made by the two methods in left ventricular cavity dimension, thickness of interventricular septum and posterior wall, and left atrial cavity dimension.

GLOBAL LEFT VENTRICULAR FUNCTION. Studies of *global left ventricular function* (ejection fraction) have been done with two approaches. The first and simpler method uses a single image through the long axis in systole and diastole, with calculation of the ejection fraction by the area-length method (Fig. 27–41). This method has shown a good correlation with ejection fraction calculated from left ventriculograms in patients with coronary artery disease, with a relatively low interobserver variability.[33, 34] The other method

TABLE 27–1. NORMAL LEFT VENTRICULAR DIMENSIONS

Dimension: Location	Diastole	Systole
Left ventricular cavity diameter (mm):		
Chordal level	46.4 ± 5.5	33.6 ± 3.8
Papillary muscle level	43.4 ± 4.4	29.9 ± 4.8
Septum thickness (mm):		
Chordal level	10.3 ± 0.5	15.5 ± 1.4
Papillary muscle level	10.4 ± 1.8	15.6 ± 2.5
Posterior wall thickness (mm):		
Chordal level	10.2 ± 0.5	15.7 ± 1.0
Papillary muscle level	10.3 ± 1.2	15.4 ± 1.4
Left atrial diameter (mm):		
Anteroposterior	25.6 ± 4.2	

From Kaul S, Wismer GL, Brady TJ, et al: Measurement of normal left heart dimensions using optimally oriented MR images. AJR 146:75–79, 1986; © by American Roentgen Ray Society.

uses multiple short-axis image slices in systole and diastole, from aortic valve to apex, with calculation of ventricular volumes and ejection fraction by the use of Simpson's rule.[35] This method is technically more complex but has the prospect of ultimately being the more accurate method. It provides a more complete examination of the left ventricle than is obtained by left ventriculography. Another advantage is that it eliminates the geometric assumption, inherent in the area-length method, that the left ventricle is an ellipsoid of revolution. Since this is an important source of error, particularly in patients with coronary artery disease whose ventricles do not contract symmetrically, the advantage of this approach is significant. To obtain the systolic and diastolic image series rapidly, a short TE can be used, allowing the acquisition of a multislice cluster of images during isovolumic diastole and another during isovolumic systole. Initial results with the use of this method have been promising.[35] New techniques for more rapid acquisition of MR images using gradient-echo cineangiography (see Chapter 28) can be expected to accelerate the development of MR cardiac function studies.[36–38]

PERICARDIAL AND MYOCARDIAL DISEASES

NORMAL PERICARDIUM. The normal pericardium appears on MR images as a 1- to 3-mm curved line of low signal intensity around the heart. It is defined internally by the adjacent myocardium, of medium signal intensity, or epicardial fat, of high intensity, and is defined externally by the high-intensity peri-

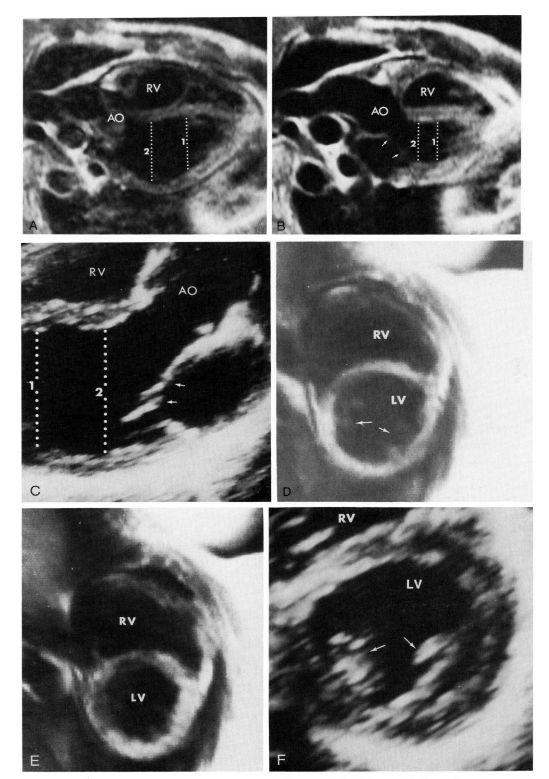

FIGURE 27–40. Diastolic (*A*) and systolic (*B*) long-axis images of the left ventricle in a plane through the aortic valve and apex, perpendicular to the septum. *C,* Parasternal long-axis two-dimensional (2D) echo, diastole. Left ventricular diameters were measured at mid papillary muscle level (1) and chordal level (2). Diastolic (*D*) and systolic (*E*) short-axis MR image of left ventricle at mid papillary muscle level. *F,* Parasternal short-axis 2D echo at mid papillary muscle level in diastole. AO = aortic sinuses; RV = right ventricle; double arrows = mitral valve plane; single arrows in *D* = papillary muscles. (From Kaul S, Wismer GL, Brady TJ, et al: Measurement of normal left heart dimensions using optimally oriented MR images. AJR 146:75–79, 1986; © by American Roentgen Ray Society.)

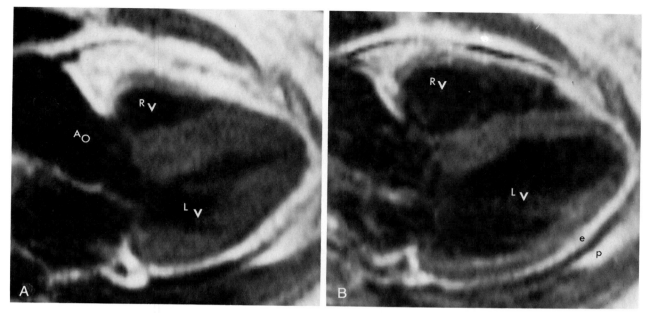

FIGURE 27–41. Long-axis MR image, perpendicular to the septum, of the left ventricle. *A,* End-systole. *B,* End-diastole. These images were used to calculate left ventricular ejection fraction by the area-length method. Note, in *B,* the normal pericardium shown as a curved line of low signal intensity between the high-intensity epicardial (e) and pericardial (p) fat stripes. LV = left ventricle; RV = right ventricle; AO = aorta. (From Stratemeier EJ, Thompson R, Brady TJ, et al: Ejection fraction determination by MR imaging: Comparison with left ventricular angiography. Radiology 158:775–777, 1986; with permission.)

cardial fat. The low-intensity stripe probably includes both layers of the pericardium and the small amount of fluid normally present. Since the visceral pericardium normally consists of a single cell layer, it is the thicker parietal pericardium, of low signal intensity fibrous tissue, that probably contributes more to the normal pericardial stripe.[63] The anterior pericardium may appear artifactually thickened, owing to motion-related signal loss (Fig. 27–42).

PERICARDIAL EFFUSION. The principal method for diagnosis of pericardial effusion is echocardiography. The examination can be done rapidly and at the bedside or in the hospital emergency ward. Extensive experience has shown it to be both sensitive and specific for detection of pericardial effusion. However, loculated pericardial effusion may be missed by

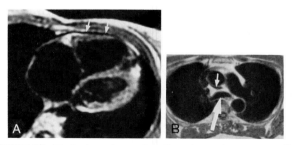

FIGURE 27–42. *A,* Anterior pericardium (*arrows*) appears artifactually thick owing to motion. *B,* More superiorly, superior pericardial recess (*short arrow*) is noted posterior to ascending aorta. Long arrow = carina.

echocardiography, and in some cases satisfactory study cannot be done. Thus, MR is useful if echocardiography is unsuccessful or the results equivocal, or if loculated fluid is suspected in, for example, a patient in the postoperative period. Echocardiography has not been successful in quantitation of pericardial fluid, probably because of nonuniform distribution of fluid. MR appears to have the potential for greater accuracy, but this remains to be investigated. In the presence of pericardial effusion, the width of the pericardial stripe is increased. Nonhemorrhagic effusion (Fig. 27–43) tends to have a low signal intensity. Effusions due to uremia, trauma, or tuberculosis may show regions of high signal intensity[39, 40] (Fig. 27–44).

CONSTRICTIVE PERICARDITIS AND RESTRICTIVE CARDIOMYOPATHY. In contrast to pericardial effusion, the accuracy of echocardiography in diagnosis of constrictive pericarditis has been poor. At present, most cases of constrictive pericarditis are a late result of viral pericarditis, and, unlike tuberculous pericarditis, the pericardium is seldom calcified. Even with the combination of echocardiography and catheterization studies, the clinical distinction between constrictive pericarditis and restrictive cardiomyopathy can be difficult. In both, heart size is normal or only mildly increased, and systolic ventricular function is normal or only mildly depressed. At catheterization, both have elevated right-sided and left-sided diastolic filling pressures. In the case of constrictive pericardial disease, this is due to the constraint on diastolic filling by inflexible pericardial scar, and in those with re-

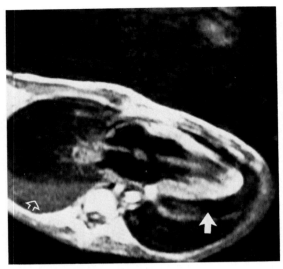

FIGURE 27–43. Long-axis view of the heart perpendicular to the septum, showing a large pericardial effusion with low signal intensity (*arrow*). The effect of gravity is seen in the posterior location of both the pericardial and the right pleural effusion (*open arrow*). (From Miller SW, Brady TJ, Dinsmore RE, et al: Cardiac magnetic resonance imaging: The Massachusetts General Hospital Experience. Radiol Clin North Am 23:745–764, 1985; with permission.)

strictive myocardial disease, the heart muscle itself has decreased compliance and is usually uniformly thickened. The most common cause of restrictive cardiomyopathy in the United States is amyloid heart disease; a less frequent cause is endomyocardial disease. Although studies of sensitivity and specificity are yet to be done, it now appears that MR may be

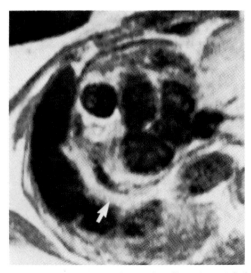

FIGURE 27–44. Pericarditis. The pericardium (*arrow*) behind the left atrioventricular sulcus is thick. The pericardial fluid has increased signal intensity with an irregular distribution, probably representing fibrous stranding. (From Miller SW, Brady TJ, Dinsmore RE, et al: Cardiac magnetic resonance imaging: The Massachusetts General Hospital Experience. Radiol Clin North Am 23:745–764, 1985; with permission.)

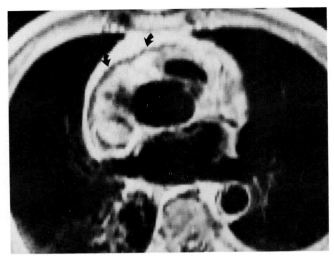

FIGURE 27–45. Transaxial image at the level of the aortic valve in a 60-year-old patient with constrictive pericarditis, showing thickened, irregularly defined pericardial stripe of medium signal intensity.

able to distinguish between the two conditions reliably. Patients with constrictive disease have been shown to have thickened pericardium, usually of medium signal intensity (Fig. 27–45).[40] When calcification is present, it shows a low signal intensity but, unlike pericardial fluid, has an irregular border. It tends to occupy the atrioventricular grooves (Fig. 27–46), in contrast to pericardial fluid, which typically lies predominately adjacent to the cardiac chambers, particularly the left ventricle and right atrium. Patients with restrictive cardiomyopathy due to amyloid show uniformly increased myocardial thickness and normal left ventricular size and constriction. They commonly have pericardial effusions, which are usually small and have low signal intensity (Fig. 27–47). The demonstration of pericardial thickening in a patient with physiologic changes of constrictive versus restrictive heart disease is clinically important, since the former is treated by surgical stripping of the pericardium and the latter is treated medically.

DILATED OR CONGESTIVE CARDIOMYOPATHY. This condition is characterized by left ventricular dilation and depression of systolic function, with normal to slightly increased myocardial thickness. Similar changes appear in the right ventricle, although they may be less severe. Dilated cardiomyopathies are most commonly idiopathic, though less frequently specific causes, such as alcoholic cardiomyopathy or myocarditis, can be identified. MR is an excellent method for evaluation of chamber size and thickness, systolic function, and the presence of functional mitral regurgitation, a frequent complication. However, it is not possible to assess the severity of left ventricular failure or to exclude underlying coronary artery disease by MR at present.

HYPERTROPHIC CARDIOMYOPATHY. This condition is associated with marked hypertrophy of the left ventricle and sometimes also the right ventricle. The hypertrophy is occasionally concentric but more typ-

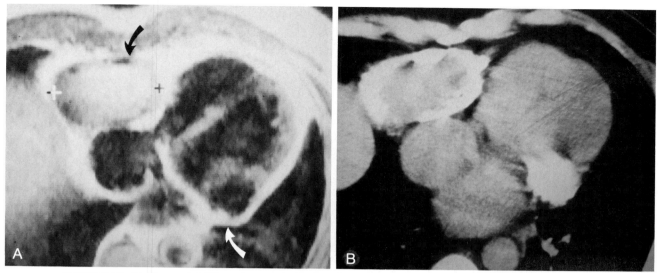

FIGURE 27–46. Transaxial MR at the ventricular level (*A*) and CT scan at similar level (*B*) in a 65-year-old man with tuberculous constrictive pericarditis. Note fibrous and calcific masses in the anterior (*black arrow*) and posterior (*white arrow*) atrioventricular grooves. Calcification is shown as irregularly defined absence of signal on the MR image.

ically disproportionately affects the septum (Fig. 27–48) or, in some patients, the apex (Fig. 27–49). A majority have obstruction to left ventricular outflow at some point in the course of the disease. This obstruction is associated with systolic anterior motion of the anterior leaflet of the mitral valve, bringing it into close proximity or contact with the interventricular septum, a phenomenon that is now generally considered to be the cause of obstruction.

Because of its high resolution and flexibility of image plane selection, MR is an excellent method for characterization of the hypertrophic pattern in patients with hypertrophic cardiomyopathy.[45] With cine

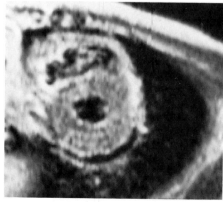

FIGURE 27–47. Amyloid heart disease. A short-axis image using spin-echo (SE) sequence (TE = 60 msec) delineated the concentric hypertrophy of both the right and the left ventricles. There is a slight inhomogeneous appearance to the myocardium. A small pericardial effusion is layered posteriorly. (From Miller SW, Brady TJ, Dinsmore RE, et al: Cardiac magnetic resonance imaging: The Massachusetts General Hospital Experience. Radiol Clin North Am 23:745–764, 1985; with permission.)

MR imaging, it is now possible to demonstrate systolic anterior motion as well, though sensitivity of MR for this purpose is not known.

PERICARDIAL CYSTS. These cysts have demonstrated a low signal intensity, increasing on second-echo images, and are surrounded by a line of low intensity presumably due to the parietal pericardium[40] (Fig. 27–50). The demonstration of typical features is diagnostic and should not require further studies or intervention.

CARDIAC TUMORS AND THROMBUS. As a rapidly growing literature attests, MR has become an important method for evaluation of cardiac masses.[41–44, 64–66] Echocardiography has been the principal non-invasive method for evaluation of cardiac tumors and thrombus. Since at present most cases studied by MR have been previously investigated by echocardiography, the sensitivity and specificity of MR in the detection of cardiac masses are not known. Since echocardiography is widely available and less expensive than MR, it is the appropriate screening method at the present time. In some cases, a high-quality echo is diagnostic, and no further studies need to be done. Examples include the typical left atrial myxoma, with a mobile mass attached to the fossa ovalis (Fig. 27–51); left atrial thrombus with a sessile mass in a patient with mitral stenosis; or left ventricular thrombus in an aneurysm. In other instances, MR is indicated following the initial echo study. Examples include the following:

1. The echocardiogram is technically unsatisfactory (Fig. 27–52).

2. The echocardiogram is satisfactory but shows atypical features in an otherwise diagnostic study (e.g., unusual site of attachment of suspected myxoma [Fig. 27–53]), or the study is not diagnostic

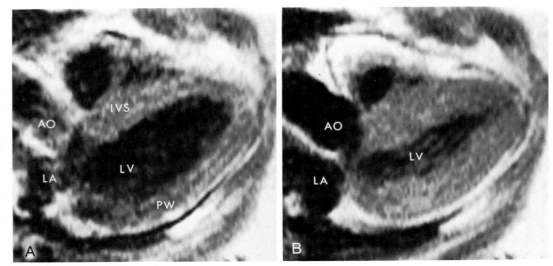

FIGURE 27–48. A 66-year-old man with idiopathic hypertrophic subaortic stenosis. MR images through long axis of left ventricle (LV) in plane perpendicular to septum. *A,* Diastole. Asymmetric hypertrophy. Upper septal thickness was 27 mm; posterior wall (PW) was 15 mm. Measurements from 2D echocardiography were 24 and 14 mm, respectively. *B,* Systole. Marked systolic thickening and small end-systolic cavity with exaggerated reduction in short-axis diameter, which are findings characteristic of hypertrophic cardiomyopathy. AO = aortic root; LA = left atrium; IVS = interventricular septum. (From Dinsmore RE, Wismer GL, Miller SW, et al: Magnetic resonance imaging of the heart using planes oriented to cardiac axes: Experience with 100 cases. AJR 145:1177–1183, 1985; © by American Roentgen Ray Society.)

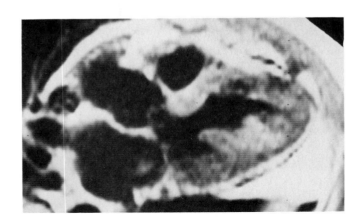

FIGURE 27–49. A 44-year-old man with the apical form of hypertrophic cardiomyopathy. Note marked, lobulated thickening of the myocardium near the apex.

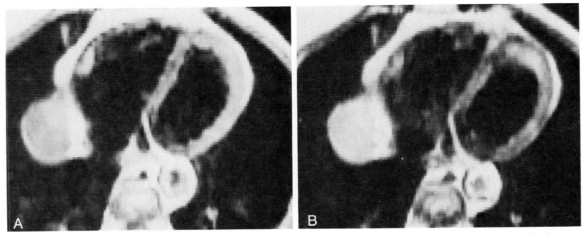

FIGURE 27–50. Transaxial MR of a pericardial cyst. *A,* First-echo (TE = 30 msec) image. *B,* Second-echo (TE = 60 msec) image. The well-encapsulated cyst shows a relative increase in signal intensity on the second-echo image.

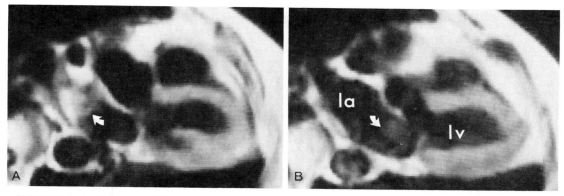

FIGURE 27–51. Long-axis MR image, perpendicular to the septum, of a 70-year-old woman with left atrial myxoma. *A*, Systole showing the myxoma (*arrow*), which was attached by a stalk to the fossa ovalis, in the posterior part of the left atrium. *B*, Diastole showing the tumor adjacent to the mitral valve. la = left atrium; lv = left ventricle.

of tumor type or extent. In these cases, MR may be helpful because of its superior resolution.

3. Suspected invasive tumors (e.g., with echo demonstration of an intracardiac mass and pericardial fluid or mass) are not adequately defined by echocardiography. Their extent is usually well shown by MR, since the signal intensity of invasive tumors is usually distinguishable from that of normal myocardium, though similar (Fig. 27–54).

4. Tumors arising in adjacent organs, such as the lung, esophagus, or liver, and invading the heart are better shown by MR because of its wide FOV (Figs. 27–55 and 27–56).

INTRACARDIAC THROMBUS. The intracardiac thrombus usually shows an increase in signal intensity compared with normal myocardium on a first-echo (TE, 28 msec) image, with further increase in contrast on the second image (TE, 56 msec).[67] However, exceptions with lower signal intensity have also been described[68] (Fig. 27–57). In some instances, thrombus may be difficult to distinguish from blood pool signal.

This distinction is aided by showing reproducibility of the signal on successive images, characteristic changes with double-echo sequences, or persistence on cine MR imaging loops.

LIPOMATOUS HYPERTROPHY OF THE INTERATRIAL SEPTUM. This condition is characterized pathologically by infiltration of adipose tissue between cardiac muscle fibers. In contrast to cardiac lipomas, lipomatous hypertrophy is an unencapsulated, infiltrative process. It is frequently seen in overweight patients and is often associated with atrial fibrillation. It is usually detected by echocardiography, often as an incidental finding. However, the tissue characteristics cannot be determined by this method. MR provides a specific diagnosis with accurate display of the extent of involvement and of characteristic signal intensity for fatty tissue (Fig. 27–58). Chemical shift techniques show a mixture of fat and water.[69] In contrast, intracardiac lipomas may be shown to consist entirely of lipid cells. These benign tumors are encapsulated and contain mature fat cells (Fig. 27–59).

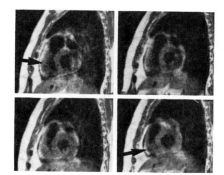

FIGURE 27–52. Regional right ventricular hypertrophy mistaken for a mass on 2D echocardiography. The upper left image is the most rightward image, with thickening along most of the anterior free wall of the right ventricle (*arrow*). The lower right image shows regional hypertrophy at the apex of the right ventricle (*arrow*). (Courtesy of Drs. Tom Hedrick and Donald Johnston, The Methodist Hospital, Houston, TX.)

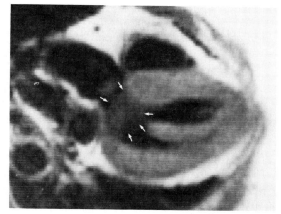

FIGURE 27–53. Long axis perpendicular to the interventricular septum in a 70-year-old woman with a myxoma in the left ventricular outflow tract (*arrows*). The tumor is attached to the interventricular septum.

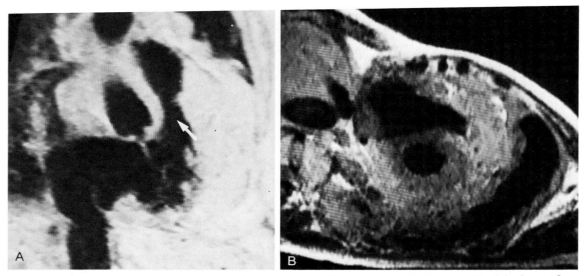

FIGURE 27–54. Long-axis MR image parallel to the septum (*A*) and short axis MR image (*B*) of the heart of a patient with lymphoma. Note extensive invasion of the walls of the heart, with compression of the right ventricular tract (*arrow*).

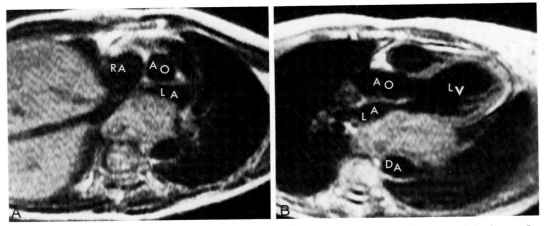

FIGURE 27–55. Short-axis (*A*) and long-axis (*B*) (perpendicular to the septum) MR images of the heart of a patient, showing extension into the heart of a carcinoma of the esophagus. The tumor occupies most of the left atrial cavity. RA = right atrium; AO = ascending aorta; LV = left ventricle; DA = descending aorta; LA = left atrial cavity.

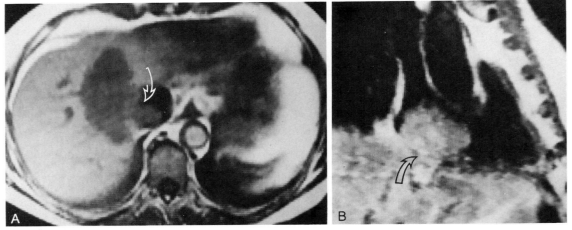

FIGURE 27–56. Biliary carcinoma arising in the liver and extending through the hepatic vein to the right atrium. *A*, Transaxial image showing the tumor in the liver invading its hepatic vein (*arrow*). *B*, Coronal view showing the mass in the right atrium. The patient was referred for MR imaging after echocardiography showed a mass of uncertain origin in the right atrium.

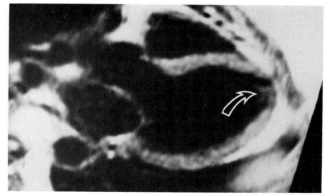

FIGURE 27–57. Long-axis MR image perpendicular to the septum in a patient with an apical myocardial infarction and apical left ventricular thrombus (*arrow*). Note thinning of the myocardium at the apex adjacent to the thrombus.

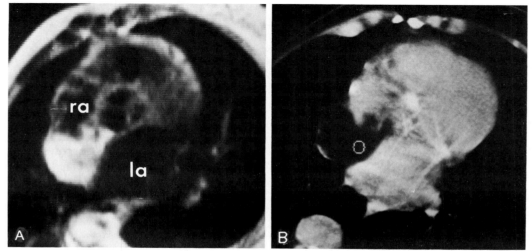

FIGURE 27–58. **Lipomatous hypertrophy of the interatrial septum in a middle-aged woman.** *A*, Transverse MR image at the level of the aortic valve and atria showing lobulated thickening of the interatrial septum with high signal intensity. *B*, CT scan at a similar level showing a lobulated fat lucency but lacking detail of intracardiac structures. ra = right atrium; la = left atrium.

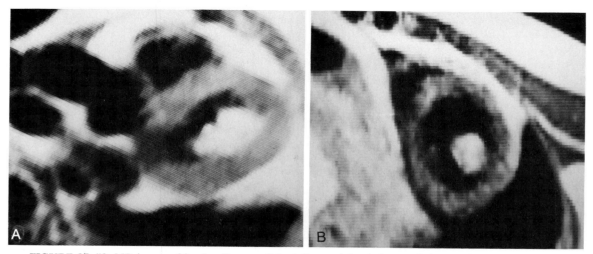

FIGURE 27–59. **MR image of benign lipoma of the left ventricle.** *A*, Long-axis image plane perpendicular to the septum. *B*, Short-axis image showing a well-defined mass of high signal intensity near the apex.

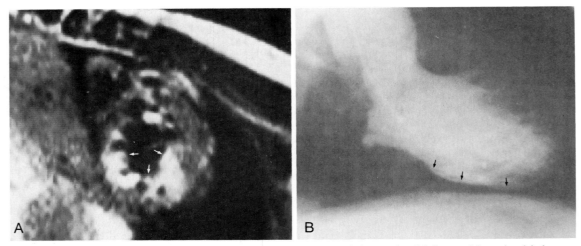

FIGURE 27–60. *A,* SE image (TE = 60 msec) through plane of short axis of left ventricle at level below papillary muscles. Area of increased signal (*arrows*) in diaphragmatic left ventricular segment (segment 7, Figure 27–38), extending into posterolateral segment (segment 6). Small area of bright signal adjacent to septum originates in blood pool. *B,* Right anterior oblique left ventriculogram in systole. Area of akinesia (*arrows*) in diaphragmatic segment. (From Dinsmore RE, Wismer GL, Miller SW, et al: Magnetic resonance imaging of the heart using image planes oriented to cardiac axes: Experience with 100 cases. AJR 145:1177–1183, 1985; © by American Roentgen Ray Society.)

CORONARY ARTERY DISEASE

Although myocardial ischemia without infarction does not appear to be detectable by MR imaging at the present time, patients studied within the first few weeks after acute myocardial infarction show an increase in signal intensity in the region of infarction (Fig. 27–60).[46] This increase in intensity is associated with an increase in T_1[47, 48] and T_2[46] relaxation times. The changes are presumably related to the edema that occurs with acute infarction. The increase in signal intensity may be associated with regional wall thinning.[49] The location of the increased signal intensity on transaxial images has demonstrated good correlation with ECG localization,[50] and, on short-axis images of the left ventricle, with angiographic location.[51, 52] The use of a series of contiguous short-axis images through the left ventricle has been shown to allow calculation of total infarct volume, with good correlation with the length of the severely hypokinetic segment on ventriculography, in patients with acute myocardial infarction.[53] Care must be taken

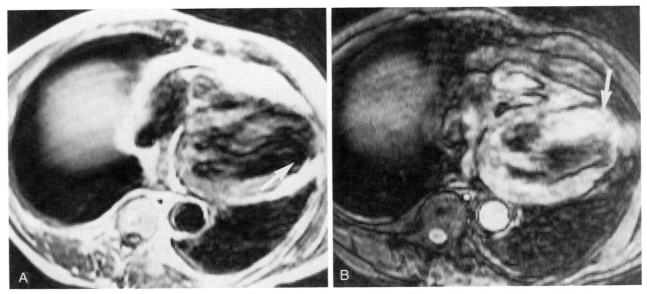

FIGURE 27–61. True LV aneurysm. Note thinning of myocardium at LV apex (*arrow*) on SE image (*A*) and blood stasis (*arrow*) in cine-FLASH image (*B*).

not to confuse signal from slowly flowing blood adjoining the hypokinetic segment with high signal from infarcted myocardium.

Old myocardial infarcts usually show thinning and decrease in signal intensity to less than that of normal myocardium, consistent with the development of fibrous scar, although signal intensity in some cases is similar to that of normal myocardium.[54] Areas of old infarction consistently show systolic thinning, which can be correlated with left ventriculographic findings on axial images, in contrast with normal thickness of adjacent myocardium[55] (see Fig. 27–39). Aneurysms associated with old infarcts are well shown (Fig. 27–61).

Portions of the proximal right and left coronary arteries are often demonstrated on transaxial or short-axis images of the heart. Demonstration can be enhanced by the use of surface coils[56] (Fig. 27–62); however, these studies are of limited clinical usefulness at the present time. Coronary artery bypass grafts are technically easier to evaluate than coronary arteries because of their straighter course and usually larger diameter. Gomes and associates[57] studied 20 patients with 64 grafts, using a body coil and SE pulse sequence (TE, 28 msec) in transaxial, coronal, and coronal-oblique sections, and detected 84 per cent of patent grafts on prospective studies. Holmvang and colleagues[58] studied patients with 37 grafts and detected all 29 patent grafts using a surface coil in most cases. In addition, multiple angled views were used for optimal definition. Patent grafts are shown as areas of low signal intensity, which are circular if on end (Fig. 27–63) or tubular if in long longitudinal sections. The ultimate sensitivity and specificity of the method, as well as the possibility of estimation of flow volume in patent grafts, await further investigation. However, flow imaging methods and perfusion imaging methods using magnetic

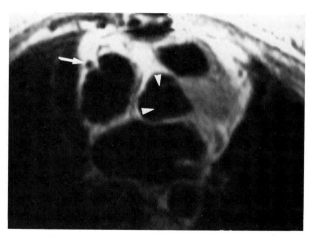

FIGURE 27–63. Axial surface-coil image of a patient with a right coronary artery bypass graft, at the level of the aortic valve (*arrowheads*). The graft is shown adjacent to the right atrium in cross-section (*arrow*). (Courtesy of Dr. Robert Edelman, Beth Israel Hospital, Boston, MA.)

susceptibility agents (Chapter 26) offer great promise for assessment of coronary artery disease and may have a major clinical impact in the future.

REFERENCES

1. Dinsmore RE, Wismer GL, Levine RA, et al: Magnetic resonance imaging of the heart: Positioning and gradient angle selection for optimal imaging planes. AJR 143:1135–1142, 1984.
2. Kaul S, Wismer GL, Brady TJ, et al: Measurement of normal left heart dimensions using optimally oriented MR images. AJR 146:75–79, 1986.
3. Newman WM, Spronll RF: Principles of Interactive Computer Graphics. 2nd ed. New York, McGraw-Hill, 1979.
4. Greene DG, Carlisle R, Grant C, Bunnell IL, et al: Estimation of left ventricular volume by one-plane cineangiography. Circulation 35:61, 1967.
5. Feiglin DM, George CR, MacIntyre WJ, et al: Gated cardiac magnetic resonance structural imaging: Optimization by electronic axial rotation. Radiology 154:129, 1985.
6. Dinsmore RE, Liberthson RR, Wismer GL, et al: Magnetic resonance imaging of thoracic aortic aneurysms: Comparison with other imaging methods. AJR 146:309–314, 1986.
7. Amparo EG, Higgins CB, Moddick W, et al: Magnetic resonance imaging of aortic disease: Preliminary results. AJR 143:1203–1209, 1984.
8. Evancho AM, Osbakken M, Weidner W, et al: Comparison of NMR imaging and aortography for preoperative evaluation of abdominal aortic aneurysm. Magn Reson Med 2:41–55, 1985.
9. Schaeffer S, Peshock RM, Mallory CR, et al: Nuclear magnetic resonance imaging in Marfan's syndrome. J Am Coll Cardiol 9:70–74, 1987.
10. Zeitler E, Kaiser W, Schuiere G, et al: Magnetic resonance imaging of aneurysms and thrombi. Cardiovasc Intervent Radiol 8:321–328, 1986.
11. Geisinger MA, Risius B, O'Donnell JA, et al: Thoracic aortic dissections: Magnetic resonance imaging. Radiology 155:407–412, 1985.
12. Glazer HS, Gutierrez FR, Levitt RG, et al: The thoracic aorta studied by MR imaging. Radiology 157:149, 1985.
13. Dinsmore RE, Wedeen V, Rosen B, et al: Phase-offset technique to distinguish slow blood flow and thrombus on MR images. AJR 148:634, 1987.
14. White EM, Edelman RR, Wedeen VJ, Brady TJ, et al: Intra-

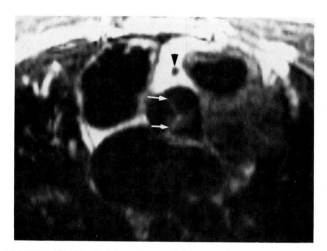

FIGURE 27–62. Axial surface-coil image, of 3.2-mm thickness, through the heart of a normal volunteer at the level of the aortic valve (*white arrows*). The right coronary artery (*black arrowhead*) is shown in cross-section as an area of low signal intensity (Courtesy of Dr. Robert Edelman, Beth Israel Hospital, Boston, MA.)

vascular signal in MR imaging: Use of phase display for differentiation of blood-flow signal from intraluminal disease. Radiology 161:245–249, 1986.

15. Miller DL, Reinig JW, Volkman DJ, et al: Vascular imaging with MRI: Inadequacy in Takayasu's arteritis compared with angiography. AJR 146:949–954, 1986.

16. Amparo EG, Higgins CB, Hricak H, Sollito R, et al: Aortic dissection: Magnetic resonance imaging. Radiology 155:399–406, 1985.

17. Dinsmore RE, Wedeen VJ, Miller SW, et al: MRI of dissection of the aorta: Recognition of the intimal tear and differential flow velocities. AJR 146:1286–1288, 1986.

18. Didier D, Higgins CB, Fisher MR, et al: Congenital heart disease: Gated MR imaging in 72 patients. Radiology 158:227, 1986.

19. Fletcher BD, Jacobstein MD: MRI of congenital abnormalities of the great arteries. AJR 146:941–948, 1986.

20. Katz ME, Glazer MS, Siegel MJ, et al: Mediastinal vessels: Postoperative evaluation with MR imaging. Radiology 161:647–651, 1986.

21. Dinsmore RE, Wismer GL, Guyer D, et al: Magnetic resonance imaging of the interatrial septum and atrial septal defects. AJR 145:697–703, 1985.

22. Diethelm L, Dery R, Lipton MJ, Higgins CB, et al: Atrial-level shunts: Sensitivity and specificity of MR in diagnosis. Radiology 162:181–186, 1987.

23. Shapiro JN, et al: Single and two-dimensional echocardiographic features of left intra-atrial septum in normal subjects and patients with an atrial septal defect. Am J Cardiol 43:816–819, 1979.

24. Bansal RC, Jajik AJ, Seward JB, Offord KP, et al: Feasibility of detailed two-dimensional echocardiographic examination in adults: Prospective study in 200 patients. Mayo Clin Proc 55:291–308, 1980.

25. Dinsmore RE, Wismer GL, Miller SW, et al: Magnetic resonance imaging of the heart using image planes oriented to cardiac axes: Experience with 100 cases. AJR 145:1177–1183, 1985.

26. Fisher MR, Hricak H, Higgins CB, et al: Magnetic resonance imaging of developmental venous anomalies. AJR 145:705, 1985.

27. Didier D, Higgins CB: Identification and localization of ventricular septal defect by gated magnetic resonance imaging. Am J Cardiol 57:1363–1368, 1986.

28. Jacobstein MD, Fletcher BD, Nelson AD, et al: Magnetic resonance imaging: Evaluation of palliative systemic-pulmonary shunt. Circulation 70:650, 1984.

29. Guit GL, Bluemm R, Rohmer J, et al: Levotransposition of the aorta: Identification of segmental cardiac anatomy using MR imaging. Radiology 161:673–679, 1986.

30. Miller SW, Brady TJ, Dinsmore RE, et al: Cardiac magnetic resonance imaging: The Massachusetts General Hospital Experience. Radiol Clin North Am 23:745–764, 1985.

31. Boxer RA, Fishman MC, LaCorte MA, et al: Diagnosis and postoperative evaluation of supravalvular aortic stenosis by magnetic resonance imaging. Am J Cardiol 58:367–368, 1986.

32. Bouchard A, Higgins CB, Byrd BF, et al: Magnetic resonance imaging in pulmonary arterial hypertension. Am J Cardiol 56:938–942, 1985.

33. Stratemeier EJ, Thompson R, Brady TJ, et al: Ejection fraction determination by MR imaging: Comparison with left ventricular angiography. Radiology 158:775–777, 1986.

34. Buckwalter KA, Aisen AM, Dilworth LR, et al: Gated cardiac MRI: Ejection fraction determination using the right anterior oblique view. AJR 147:33–37, 1986.

35. Edelman RR, Thompson R, Kantor H, et al: Cardiac function: Evalution with fast-echo MR imaging. Radiology 162:611–615, 1987.

36. Utz JA, Herfkens RJ, Heinsimer JA, et al: Cine MR determination of left ventricular ejection fraction. AJR 148:839, 1987.

37. Rzedzian RR, Pykett IL: Instant images of the human heart using a new, whole body MR imaging system. AJR 149:245–250, 1987.

38. Drucker EA, et al: Preliminary evaluation of a new high-speed MR imaging system for the assessment of cardiac function in normal volunteers. Book of Abstracts. Soc Magn Reson Med 1:17, 1987.

39. Stark DD, Higgins CB, Lanzer P, et al: Magnetic resonance imaging of the pericardium: Normal and pathologic findings. Radiology 150:469, 1984.

40. Sechtum U, Tscholakoff D, Higgins CB, et al: MRI of the abnormal pericardium. AJR 147:245, 1986.

41. Conces DJ, Vix VA, Klatte EC, et al: Gated MR imaging of left atrial myxomas. Radiology 156:445–447, 1985.

42. Boxer RA, La Corte MA, Singh S, et al: Diagnosis of cardiac tumors in infants by magnetic resonance imaging. Am J Cardiol 56:831–832, 1985.

43. Go RT, O'Donnell JK, Underwood DA, et al: Comparison of gated cardiac MRI and 2D echocardiography of intracardiac neoplasms. AJR 145:21–25, 1985.

44. Amparo EG, Higgins CB, Farmer D, et al: Gated MRI of cardiac and paracardiac masses: Initial experience. AJR 143:1151–1156, 1984.

45. Thompson RC, et al: MRI along the true left ventricular axes in hypertrophic heart disease: Accurate characterization of cardiac hypertrophy. Circulation 72:122, 1985.

46. McNamara MT, Higgins CB, Schechtmann N, et al: Detection and characterization of acute myocardial infarction in man with use of gated magnetic resonance. Circulation 71:717, 1985.

47. Been M, Smith MA, Ridgeway JP, et al: Characterisation of acute myocardial infarction by gated magnetic resonance imaging. Lancet 1:348, 1985.

48. Been M, Smith MA, Ridgway JP, et al: Serial changes in the T1 relaxation parameter after myocardial infarction in man. Br Heart J 59:1–8, 1988.

49. Filipchuk NG, Peshock RM, Malloy CR, et al: Detection and localization of recent myocardial infarction by magnetic resonance imaging. Am J Cardiol 58:214, 1986.

50. Fisher MR, McNamara MT, Higgins CB, et al: Acute myocardial infarction: MR evaluation in 29 patients. AJR 148:247, 1987.

51. Johnston DL, Thompson RC, Lin P, et al: Magnetic resonance imaging during acute myocardial infarction. Am J Cardiol 57:1059, 1986.

52. Dinsmore RE, et al: Characterization of myocardial signal intensity by MRI in proven normal and infarcted myocardial segments. Radiology 157:147, 1985.

53. Johns J, et al: Measurement of myocardial infarct volume by MRI. J Am Coll Cardiol 7:197A, 1986.

54. McNamara MT, Higgins CB, et al: Magnetic resonance imaging of chronic myocardial infarcts in man. AJR 146:315, 1986.

55. Akins EW, Hill JA, Sievers RW, Conti CR, et al: Assessment of left ventricular wall thickness in healed myocardial infarction by magnetic resonance imaging. Am J Cardiol 59:24, 1987.

56. Rubenstein RI, Askenase AD, Thickman D, et al: MRI to evaluate patency of aortocoronary bypass grafts. Circulation 76:786–791, 1987.

57. Gomes AS, Lois JF, Drinkwater DC, Corday SR, et al: Coronary artery bypass grafts: Visualization with MR imaging. Radiology 162:175, 1987.

58. Holmvang G, et al: Coronary artery bypass graft patency by MRI. Circulation 44:42, 1986.

59. Gott VL: Surgical treatment of aneurysms of the ascending aorta in the Marfan syndrome. N Engl J Med 315:1070, 1986.

60. Soulen R, Fishman EK, Pyeritz RE, et al: Marfan syndrome evaluation with MRI versus CT. Radiology 165:697, 1987.

61. Kersting-Summerhoff BA, Higgins CB, White RD, et al: Aortic dissection: Sensitivity and specificity of MRI. Radiology 166:651, 1988.

62. White RD, Ullyot DJ, Higgins CB, et al: MRI of the aorta after surgery before aortic dissection. AJR 150:87, 1988.

63. Sechtum U, Tscholakoff D, Higgins CB, et al: MRI of the normal pericardium. AJR 147:239, 1986.

64. Freedberg RS, Kronzon I, Rumoncik WM, Liebeskind D, et al: The contribution of MRI to the evaluation of intracardiac tumors diagnosed by echocardiography. Circulation 77:96, 1988.

65. Winkler M, Higgins CB, et al: Suspected intracardiac masses: Evaluation with MRI. Radiology 165:117, 1987.

66. Gomes AS, Lois JF, Child JS, et al: Cardiac tumors and thrombus: Evaluation with MRI. AJR 149:895, 1987.

67. Dooms GC, et al: MRI of cardiac thrombi. J Comput Assist Tomogr 10:415, 1986.

68. Gomes AS, Lois JF, Child JS, et al: Cardiac tumors and thrombus: Evaluation with MRI. AJR 149:895, 1987.

69. Levine RA, Weyman AE, Dinsmore RE, et al: Noninvasive tissue characterization: Diagnosis of lipomatous hypertrophy of the atrial septum by NMR imaging. J Am Coll Cardiol 7:688, 1986.

28

CINE MR IMAGING OF THE HEART

IAIN A. SIMPSON, ROB NEWMAN, JOEL F. MARTIN, and KYUNG J. CHUNG

PHYSICAL PRINCIPLES OF CINE MR IMAGING

THE IMAGING METHOD

Fast Scan Pulse Sequence
Continuous Sampling Throughout the Cardiac Cycle
Retrospective Sorting and Reconstruction

LIGHTENING ARTIFACT

ELECTROCARDIOGRAM

PHYSIOLOGIC GATING

CINE MR IMAGE INTERPRETATION

METHODS OF EXAMINATION

IMAGING COILS

PREPARING THE PATIENT

POSITIONING THE PATIENT

IMAGING PLANES

Long-Axis Imaging
Short-Axis View
Other Oblique Views

PRACTICAL ASPECTS OF CINE MR IMAGING

ASSESSMENT OF SPECIFIC CARDIAC ABNORMALITIES

LEFT VENTRICULAR FUNCTION

RIGHT VENTRICULAR FUNCTION

MYOCARDIAL INFARCTION

VALVE REGURGITATION

MISCELLANEOUS LESIONS

PROBLEMS AND PITFALLS

FUTURE APSECTS OF CINE MR IMAGING

CONCLUSION

As we have seen in Chapter 27, conventional electrocardiographic (ECG) gated MR imaging can provide superb definition of cardiac anatomy. However, because of the inherent nature of this spin-echo (SE) technique, with its relatively long repetition time (TR), it does not allow a dynamic appreciation of cardiac function or visualization of intracardiac blood flow. Clearly, this is a major limitation of conventional ECG-gated MR imaging, since visualization of blood flow and ventricular wall motion may be of considerable importance for the functional assessment of many cardiac disorders. Precise detail of cardiac anatomy is particularly important for the assessment of congenital heart disease, but even here, as in almost all adult cardiac lesions, it is the related flow distubances and their hemodynamic consequences that often determine prognosis and the need for and timing of surgical intervention.

Thus, noninvasive techniques, such as two-dimensional (2D) echocardiography, cardiac Doppler ultrasound, color Doppler flow mapping, and nuclear cardiology, which yield functional hemodynamic information, have gained much acceptance as diagnostic techniques for the evaluation of many cardiac lesions and have proved to be extremely valuable for the assessment of patients with a wide range of cardiac disorders. However, ultrasound techniques are somewhat limited by the problems of ultrasound window and penetration, which pertains particularly to the investigation of patients in the postoperative period and those with significant respiratory disease. Although radionuclide angiography can overcome some of these problems, it has only very limited spatial resolution and, in addition to requiring the injection of radioactive isotopes, does not provide adequate structural information.

Although valuable information can be gained from these conventional noninvasive techniques, even when used in combination they do not always allow a complete diagnostic profile to be obtained without the need for cardiac catheterization and angiography. This is particularly true for the structural and functional assessment of complex cardiac lesions or those associated with multisystem disorders. There is a continuing need, therefore, for a repeatable noninvasive technique, such as cine MR imaging, which combines the highest possible resolution imaging of dynamic structural information combined with visualization and quantitative assessment of associated intracardiac and extracardiac blood flow.

This chapter deals with cine MR imaging as it relates to adult cardiology; it describes the basic principles of cine MR imaging, as well as the particular examination methods commonly employed with this technique. It should also provide an insight into the value and potential application of cine MR imaging in a wide variety of adult cardiac disorders and serves to illustrate how it can enhance understanding of the pathophysiology of many of these lesions, in addition to improving our diagnostic capabilities.

It should be emphasized at this point that cine MR imaging, as a new imaging technique, is in a developmental stage even in relation to the more established conventional ECG-gated imaging. As a result, it is a rapidly expanding and developing technology, and much of the information displayed by cine MR imaging is still not fully understood. Considerable research is required before the true clinical value of cine MR imaging is entirely established, and this research is only now beginning. Advances in image quality and temporal resolution, acquisition and reconstruction time, and pulse sequences, as well as the future possibility of real-time cine MR imaging (see Chapter 26), can only help expand the emerging applications of what is already becoming recognized as a very exciting technology for the investigation of cardiac disease.

PHYSICAL PRINCIPLES OF CINE MR IMAGING

THE IMAGING METHOD

There are substantial differences between a conventional SE cardiac gated sequences and the cine MR scan (Fig. 28–1). Cine has the following:

1. A short TR, gradient-echo (GRE) (fast scan) sequence.

2. Continuous execution of the pulse sequence throughout the cardiac cycle.

3. Retrospective sorting and reconstruction of the MR data (for optimal implementation of the method; an alternative, less effective method is prospective gating, discussed further on).

The result is a time-efficient scan sequence producing "bright blood," with high temporal resolution images evenly spaced throughout the R-R interval.

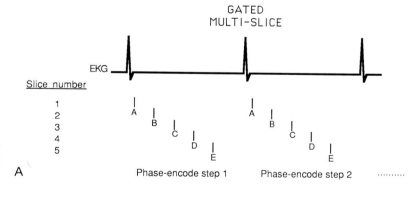

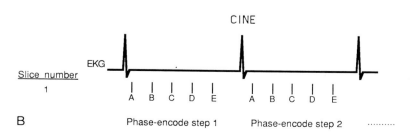

FIGURE 28–1. Comparison between cardiac imaging methods. *A*, Conventional SE imaging. Different slices (1–5) are acquired at different phases (*A–E*) of the cardiac cycle. *B*, Single-slice cine MR imaging. One slice is acquired at multiple phases (*A–E*) in the cardiac cycle. Alternatively, two to four slices can be acquired, with a proportional reduction in the number of phases sampled.

Fast Scan Pulse Sequence

To generate an MR signal with conventional spin echoes in cardiac or other imaging applications, spins must be present within a slice for both the slice-selective 90-degree and the slice-selective 180-degree radiofrequency (RF) pulses (see Chapter 4). This condition is fulfilled by the spins of the myocardium, but not by those of the moving blood in the cardiac chambers. Thus, while there is a signal from the myocardium, rapid blood flow provides no signal (a flow void).

In the cine scan sequence, a very different process is at work. The T_1/T_2 of the heart muscle at 1.5 T is approximately 800/40 msec, respectively, and the T_1/T_2 of blood is approximately 1000/300 msec, respectively. For a short TR, fast scan sequences are generally T_1 or proton density weighted (see Chapter 5). If we were to ignore flow for a moment, this would leave little T_1 contrast between the myocardium and the blood within the heart when using cine or other fast scan techniques. Because of the short TR of the pulse sequence and the long T_1 of the tissues, both would be relatively saturated, thus returning a low signal. However, there are two phenomena that result in increased contrast: (1) the presence of rapidly flowing blood and (2) the short echo time (TE) (relative to spin echo) of a fast scan.

1. Because the heart muscle is relatively stationary in the slice being imaged, it is continuously being reexcited by the rapid RF pulses, and its spins never fully recover between successive excitations (partial saturation). Thus it returns little signal. However, blood moving into the selected slice has not been exposed to any of the previous RF pulses (is not saturated) and can return a very strong signal.

2. The second contrast mechanism of cine fast scan is caused by the fact that no 180-degree RF refocusing pulse is used in the cine pulse sequence. Nine to 17 msec after the initial RF pulse, the signal is recovered via a gradient echo. This rapid refocus-ing and read-out are completed before the spins in the blood have moved very far from their initial location.

Through both of these mechanisms, the blood appears much brighter than the myocardium in cine images. The cine pulse sequence also has the option for flow motion compensation (first-order gradient moment rephasing), which serves to improve the refocusing of the moving spins of blood, further increasing their signal intensity.

T_1 weighting in fast scan images is controlled primarily through the flip angle of the pulse sequence and the selection of TR relative to the T_1 of the tissue being imaged. The shortest possible TR should be used in cine to provide the maximal temporal resolution over the cardiac cycle.

T_2 weighting of the scan is controlled by the TE selected. However, there is the same motivation as before to keep the scan sequence as short as possible to provide the maximal number of samples possible during the cardiac cycle. In addition, a short TE results in a minimum of signal loss from turbulent or accelerated flow or from susceptibility artifacts. In general, a fast scan sequence having short TR and TE with a moderate flip angle is generally used.

Continuous Sampling Throughout the Cardiac Cycle

Unlike conventional SE imaging, the retrospectively gated cine pulse sequence is not synchronized with the cardiac cycle but is continuously sampling data at regularly spaced intervals (typically every 66 msec for a two-slice scan) throughout the entire cardiac cycle (Fig. 28–2). The view (phase-encoding gradient) is held constant over a single R-R interval and is incremented only when a valid cardiac trigger is detected. Thus, a 128 matrix × 2 NEX (number of excitations) scan will take 256 heartbeats to complete. As each echo data point is stored, the elapsed time from the last R-wave trigger is included. One

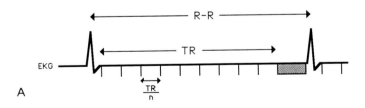

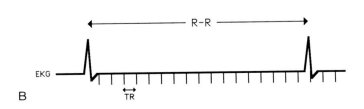

FIGURE 28–2. Comparison between ECG gating methods. *A,* Prospective gating uses R wave as trigger for start of each series of data acquisitions. Extra time left over at end of each R-R interval (*shaded area*) may produce a "lightening" artifact for the first slice after the R wave. *B,* Retrospective gating. Data are acquired independently from the ECG, and the data are sorted and interpolated in conjunction with the stored ECG tracing after the acquisition is completed.

result of this technique is that for each individual R-R interval the first data sample point will occur at different delay times (0 to 65 msec) from the QRS trigger point. The second result of this asynchronous sampling is that as the patient's R-R interval changes over the period of the scan, more or less samples will be taken in each R-R interval. The sorting method used before the cine reconstruction takes both of these factors into consideration.

Retrospective Sorting and Reconstruction

The optimal method for reconstruction of cine images is retrospective: The operator prescribes the scan parameters; data are collected based on the patient's cardiac activity; and after the completion of the scan, the operator chooses how many time phase images of the cardiac cycle are desired.

The sorting and interpolation of the echo data are completed in four steps. After the completion of a scan, in a single continuous file there will be data for 1 to 32 slice locations, with as many data points as fit in the R-R interval for each heartbeat.

1. The data are sorted by slice location, producing N files, where N is the number of physical slice locations prescribed in the scan.

2. On each of the slice files, the R-R interval for each individual cardiac cycle is divided into M equal intervals, M being the number of phases selected by the operator. For a scan with an average heart rate of 60 beats per minute and 16 phases selected, there will be 64 msec between calculated points.

3. Echo data are calculated for each of the M phases over the [NEX × matrix size, typically 256] heartbeats by interpolating data from the two closest actual data points that were collected during the scan. Interpolation is used to ensure that all images have the same effective TR, even if the R-R interval varies over the course of the acquisition (i.e., an arrhythmia). For instance, while 17 actual echo data points may have been taken in one R-R interval, and 15 in another, 16 interpolated points can be calculated for each interval. As a practical matter, as the number of reconstructed phases is increased beyond the actual number of data samples taken during each R-R interval, image quality will decrease.

4. All of the data for the first phase over all 256 heartbeats of the scan are collected and processed by a normal two-dimensional Fourier transform (2DFT) reconstruction. A similar process is used for each of the succeeding (M − 1) temporal locations throughout the cardiac cycle. The result is an array of (N physical locations) by (M temporal phases) images.

LIGHTENING ARTIFACT

High signal intensity in cine images is usually due to rapid blood flow. However, in certain types of cine acquisitions, the first image may have a higher signal intensity than the other images, unrelated to flow.[38] The origin of this "lightening" artifact depends on whether a prospective or retrospective method was used to acquire the data.

PROSPECTIVE ACQUISITION. In this method, a series of data acquisitions are initiated by each R wave (Fig. 28–2A). The slices are acquired over the user-selected interval TR (which should be <90 per cent of the R-R interval to account for normal variations in the heart rate), and the time interval between slices is (TR/n), where n = number of slices. After the data for all n slices have been acquired, some time elapses before the next R wave. This time interval (RR-TR) may be longer than the time interval (TR/n) between slices. As a result, the first slice after each R wave experiences more T_1 relaxation and produces a stronger signal than the other slices.

There are two ways to minimize this artifact: (1) the first slice may be discarded, which will not significantly reduce the temporal resolution if a large number of slices were acquired; (2) the signal intensity of the first image may be normalized to equal that of the other images. This is accomplished by first determining a signal intensity ratio of background tissues (such as fat) in the first image and another image and then reducing the signal intensities in the first image by this factor.

RETROSPECTIVE ACQUISITION. This method is generally preferred to prospective gating for cardiac imaging and is the method now used for all of our studies, because it is less sensitive to arrhythmias. Retrospective gating also permits reordering of the phase-encoding steps according to the respiratory phase, to correct for ghost artifacts due to respiratory motion. However, it requires much more data processing than does prospective gating. As discussed earlier, data are acquired at constant short intervals of TR, independent of the R wave (Fig. 28–2B). Therefore, all slices experience the same amount of T_1 relaxation and should appear equally bright.

In fact, a lightening artifact can also be seen with retrospective acquisitions. At each R wave, the phase-encoding gradient is incremented to acquire a new projection, and the RF phase is alternated. The sudden change in RF phase disturbs the steady-state precession of the transverse magnetization and results in increased signal in the first slice after the R wave. This artifact can be eliminated by changing the order of the phase-encoding steps and alternating the RF phase only once during the acquisition, as illustrated in Figure 28–3. Now the sudden change in signal occurs only at a single phase-encoding step, rather than at every step.

Finally, one should note that flow is not the only type of motion that produces increased signal on cine acquisitions. Over the course of the cardiac cycle, the heart undergoes complex motions, such as shortening along its long axis from apex to base and torsion around the long axis. As a result, different portions of the heart may move into and out of the

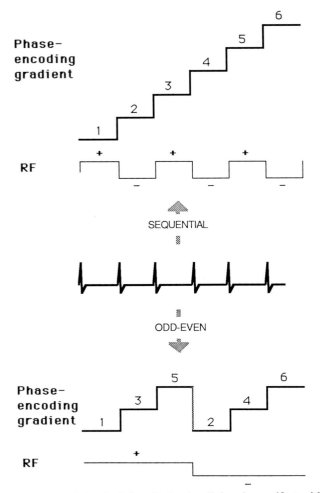

FIGURE 28–3. Method for eliminating lightening artifact with retrospective gating. *Top,* Routine, sequential acquisition of phase-encoding steps, with alternation of RF phase after each R wave, results in disruption of the steady state, producing the lightening artifact. *Bottom,* By using odd-even acquisition of phase-encoding steps, only a single transition is required, thereby eliminating the lightening artifact.

imaging plane. This may result in artifactual enhancement of myocardial signal, similar to flow-related enhancement.

ELECTROCARDIOGRAM

Location and placement of the ECG leads constitute the most sensitive part of the cine scan process. It is very important to note that there is no one best lead configuration for all patients. The electrical patterns of the heart detected on the surface of the body are affected by four factors: (1) the electrical patterns of the heart (which may be altered by cardiac damage or disease); (2) the physical orientation of the heart; (3) surrounding pulmonary conditions, such as pleural effusion or emphysema; and (4) signals generated by rapid blood flow in the magnetic

field of the scanner. Whereas the first three factors are general, the fourth is unique to MR. Research has shown that the neuromuscular electrical patterns of the heart itself are not altered by the magnetic field; however, once the patient is moved into the magnet, the effect of the flowing blood within the magnetic field can cause the T wave to appear inverted or elevated. This flow signal phenomenon is induced only by the charged particles (hemoglobin) moving within a magnetic field and disappears once the patient is removed from the magnet.[1-3]

PHYSIOLOGIC GATING

Recently, another method has been proposed for gating that eliminates the need for ECG electrodes. In this method, called "physiologic gating," data are acquired continuously, as in retrospective ECG gating.[41] The GRE pulse sequence is modified to produce two echoes. This first echo is flow compensated and phase encoded normally and is used to produce the cine images. The second echo (which has also been called a "navigator" or "monitor" echo) is *not* phase encoded. As a result, it represents a projection of all signal intensities along the phase-encoding direction. Furthermore, it is not flow compensated. Therefore, in organs with substantial blood pools, such as the heart, the signal intensity of the navigator echo will vary with changes in flow velocity over the cardiac cycle. The precise signal pattern will depend on the region being sampled; for instance, the aorta has flow dynamics different from those of the left ventricle. In general, during slower diastolic flow, the navigator echo will have a large signal intensity, whereas during fast systolic flow it will be reduced in intensity. The peak signal generally occurs during late diastole, near the R wave.

By using this peak signal like an R wave, the acquired data can be retrospectively sorted to produce a cineangiogram. Respiration also produces a subtle, lower frequency variation in signal intensity of the navigator echo. This information can be used to reorder the phase-encoding steps to minimize artifacts, without the need for mechanical monitoring of respiration. To date, physiologic gating has not proved as reliable as ECG gating for cine imaging, but this may change with further technical development.

CINE MR IMAGE INTERPRETATION

The fast scan technique used for cine[4-6] employs a low flip angle GRE sequence. The TR for cine is much shorter than that for standard SE sequences. A series of cine MR images can therefore be acquired during each cardiac cycle, allowing a dynamic appreciation of cardiac motion with excellent temporal resolution. Data acquired over a series of cardiac cycles can then be reconstructed into a dynamic cine loop format with as many as 32 frames per cardiac cycle. By selecting multiple slice locations, it is possible to visualize dynamic structural and flow information over the entire left ventricle using one cine MR imaging acquisition. It is therefore possible to make an accurate assessment of global and regional left ventricular function. Note that with the cine technique, blood is seen as a high-intensity signal compared with the surrounding myocardium rather than as the absence of signal, which is associated with conventional ECG-gated imaging. This is a result of the spins within the myocardium and other stationary structures within the slice being continuously reexcited, producing partial saturation and a decrease in signal intensity. In comparison, flowing blood is unsaturated prior to entering the slice and will return a very high-intensity signal as it continues to flow, and this enhances the contrast between flowing blood and myocardium. The optimal flow contrast is obtained with a flip angle near 30 degrees. Substantially smaller or larger flip angles produce worsened flow contrast and/or image quality (Fig. 28–4).

While this contrast principle is true for laminar flow, the presence of hydrodynamic turbulence and acceleration will cause considerable loss of signal intensity, so that laminar flow and turbulence are also easily distinguished. This finding is demonstrated in the in vitro model seen in Figure 28–5.

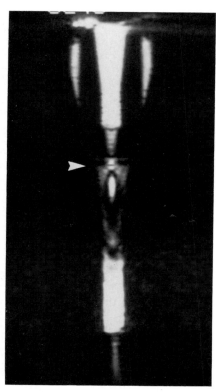

FIGURE 28–5. In vitro flow model of valve stenosis with flow from top to bottom, with the position of obstruction indicated by an arrowhead. Note that the laminar flow seen proximally is associated with a uniformly high intensity signal. Distal to the obstruction, there is a high-velocity jet with a laminar central core of high signal intensity surrounded by a turbulent zone with loss of signal. Downstream there is relaminarization of flow, with a resultant increase in signal intensity to its original value.

This is an important observation, since most cardiac lesions of clinical significance are associated with turbulent flow, which will be readily apparent and easily distinguished from normal flow in cine MR imaging. In clinical examinations, cine MR imaging displays loss of flow signal intensity proximal to obstructive (Fig. 28–6) and regurgitant lesions (Fig. 28–7) in a flow zone that would be expected to be hydrodynamically laminar. It is now well recognized from color Doppler flow map studies that acceleration of flow occurs proximal to obstructive and regurgitant lesions.[7, 8] Since spatial acceleration causes a range of velocities and accelerations to be present within each voxel, significant signal loss occurs on cine MR imaging in volumes of laminar accelerating flow. The identification of this region by cine MR imaging may be of some clinical value, allowing identification of the origin of regurgitant lesions. It may also be predictive of the severity of obstructive lesions,[9] with the length of the zone of proximal acceleration, as identified by the zone of proximal signal loss, increasing at higher pressure gradients across valvular or arterial obstructions. Signal intensity patterns on cine cardiac images are summarized in Table 28–1.

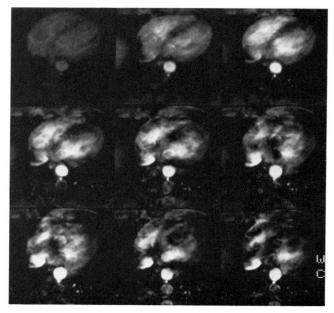

FIGURE 28–4. Effect of flip angle on axial cine images (TR = 30 msec). Flip angles increase from 10 degrees (*upper left*) to 90 degrees (*lower right*). At very small flip angles (e.g., 10 degrees), contrast between ventricular cavity and myocardium is small. At large flip angles, ghost artifacts and image quality worsen. (Courtesy of R. Edelman, M.D.)

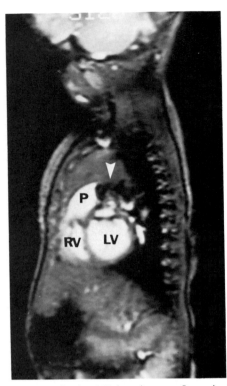

FIGURE 28–6. Systolic cine MR imaging stop frame in the sagittal view in a patient with a pulmonary artery (P) band. Note that proximal to the band in the right ventricular outflow tract (*arrowhead*) there is a zone of signal loss, in a laminar zone of spatial flow acceleration. LV = left ventricle; RV = right ventricle.

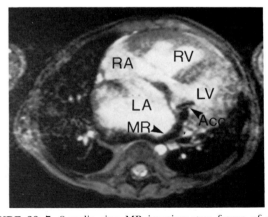

FIGURE 28–7. Systolic cine MR imaging stop frame of mitral regurgitation in the axial view. The plane of the mitral valve is indicated by arrowheads. Notice that there is signal loss in the left atrium associated with the turbulent jet of mitral insufficiency, but there is also some signal loss proximal to the regurgitant orifice on the left ventricular side of the valve. Again, this is a zone of laminar spatially accelerating flow (Acc). Note that this view is quite similar to a four-chamber view, as imaged by echocardiography, with the right ventricle (RV), right atrium (RA), left ventricle (LV), and left atrium (LA) visualized as well as the tricuspid and mitral valves.

TABLE 28–1. SUMMARY OF SIGNAL INTENSITIES IN MR CINEANGIOGRAMS

1. *Normal heart:* Blood pool appears homogeneously bright; myocardium appears dark. Transient low signal may be seen near the opening mitral and tricuspid valves during early diastole and during closure of these valves.
2. *Ischemic heart disease:* Stationary blood in akinetic segments has moderate or low signal intensity without change over the cardiac cycle.
3. *Valvular regurgitation:* Dark jet, due to turbulent dephasing, originates from the abnormal valve. Size of jet provides qualitative assessment of the severity of regurgitation.
4. *Valvular stenosis:* Dark jet, due to turbulent dephasing, originates from the abnormal valve. Size of jet depends on shape of stenotic lesion as well as severity of stenosis.
5. *Paracardiac/intracardiac masses, intracardiac thrombus:* Low or moderate signal intensity that does not change over the cardiac cycle.
6. *Pericardium:* Free pericardial fluid appears bright. Fibrosis or calcium appears dark.
7. *Central pulmonary emboli[40]:* Low or moderate signal intensity that does not change over the cardiac cycle.
8. *Implants:* Sternal wires, bypass clips, and cardiac valve prostheses produce signal voids of varying size.

METHODS OF EXAMINATION

Much of the methodology used for performing cardiac cine MR imaging is common either to MR in general or to the ECG-gated technique. However, to obtain high-quality cine MR images, our experience would suggest that a number of aspects of the examination technique are particularly important. These relate mainly to the use of different imaging coils, positioning of the patient and appropriate instruction prior to study, attention to ECG gating, and utilization of a variety of individually specified imaging planes.

IMAGING COILS

In general, the higher signal-to-noise (S/N) provided by surface coils or extremity coils for MR imaging allows smaller fields-of-view (FOVs) and higher spatial resolution imaging; this also pertains to cardiac cine MR imaging. In adults, it is standard procedure to use the main body coil of the magnet but for infants and young children a head coil should always be used whenever possible. Children up to the age of 5 years can almost always fit adequately within the head coil. In addition, in our experience, it is also possible to use, in newborn infants, the extremity coil normally used for imaging knees. When children are unable to fit into the head coil, then a 5-inch surface coil can be applied to the anterior chest by lying the patient supine on top of the coil, but the signal strength falls off quite quickly from the anterior chest surface, and deeper structures may not be imaged adequately, precipitating the need for using the main body coil. However, even in adults, surface coils may be of value if particularly high-resolution imaging of the anterior right ventricular surface of the heart or anterior pericardium is required. The application of these imaging coils is discussed more fully in Chapter 29.

PREPARING THE PATIENT

The most important aspect of patient preparation that relates specifically to cardiac imaging is obtaining a satisfactory ECG for gating purposes. Since cine MR imaging averages data over many cardiac cycles, problems encountered in triggering from the ECG will cause significant image degradation. To obtain consistently good ECG triggering, our experience would suggest that adult ECG electrodes be used even in infants and children and that the skin be vigorously cleansed with alcohol wipes to ensure good electrical contact. Unlike the practice with standard monitoring, we would recommend that all four electrodes be placed adjacent to each other on the patient's back just to the left of the spine (see also Chapter 2). This practice will almost always provide an adequate ECG signal and avoids problems with progressively decreasing R-wave amplitude during the scan. It is important to check that a high-quality ECG signal is present and that the gating software of the system is triggering on each R wave without T-wave interference. This checking should be done prior to placing the patient in the magnet and also after the patient is positioned within the magnet, as the magnetic field can occasionally cause alteration in the signal.

A second important consideration for the ECG leads is the placement of the ECG cables (see Chapter 2). The cables should be braided together to minimize the area between the leads and should be placed away from the patient's skin. This practice will reduce pickup induced by the magnetic field gradients and the likelihood of a false R-wave trigger. More important, burns to the patient are possible if a large loop of ECG lead is placed against the patient's skin.

Because cine MR imaging relies on averaged information obtained over many cardiac cycles (usually 256 for 128-matrix imaging with 2 excitations), significant variation in the R-R interval will also cause image degradation. Therefore, difficulties will be encountered with cine MR imaging of patients with significant arrhythmias, particularly atrial fibrillation with a variable ventricular response, or of patients with frequent supraventricular or ventricular ectopic activity. Our experience would suggest that it is not usually possible to obtain high-quality imaging in these patients. Ultrafast imaging methods (see Chapter 26) are needed for these patients.

POSITIONING THE PATIENT

The patient can be placed in the magnet either feet first or head first, and which method is used is immaterial (as mentioned earlier, the T-wave appearance depends on the magnetic field direction and, therefore, on the orientation of the patient) as long as the appropriate position is entered in the data entry so that the images are properly labeled. This procedure may appear somewhat obvious, but it is extremely important, since untold confusion can arise when attempting to prescribe oblique images if the image labels have been reversed. The patient should not be touching the sides of the magnet and should be warned to remain absolutely still during each individual scan. Cine MR imaging is particularly susceptible to motion artifacts, and the patient should be warned of this prior to study. For the same reason, they should be told to breathe normally but not excessively. The noise level of the gradient-echo pulse sequence used for cine imaging is also much higher than that with conventional imaging, and many patients require ear plugs as a result.

IMAGING PLANES

For cine MR imaging, all clinical magnets have the facility for imaging in the three orthogonal planes: sagittal, axial (Fig. 28–8), and coronal (Fig. 28–9). These three imaging planes can be quite useful in many cardiac conditions. They are often adequate when merely looking for anatomic definition using conventional ECG-gated MR imaging, in which case the operator can build up a three-dimensional (3D) picture of the anatomy in his or her mind. However, the heart does not conform to these standard orthogonal planes, and imaging in these planes alone may limit the diagnostic capabilities of cine MR imaging. The implementation of software that allows manipulation of the magnetic field gradients can provide oblique images in any desired plane of the heart by rotation around any one or a combination of the three standard orthogonal axes. Oblique imaging is an integral part of any cine MR imaging examination, since it allows imaging of the true axes of the heart and can also be tailored to the individual needs of the patient being studied.

Long-Axis Imaging

The plane of the long axis of the heart is from the right shoulder to the cardiac apex and is a standard imaging plane for echocardiographic examination. For MR imaging in the same view, it is best first to perform a conventional ECG-gated localizing scan in the standard coronal plane. By then prescribing cine MR imaging in an oblique plane that intersects the aortic valve and the cardiac apex on the coronal images, a long-axis view of the heart can be obtained (Fig. 28–10). Some MR imaging systems will allow a graphic prescription to be performed directly from the coronal images, with a line superimposed at an operator-determined angle to achieve the long-axis view. Alternately, the exact 3D coordinates of the

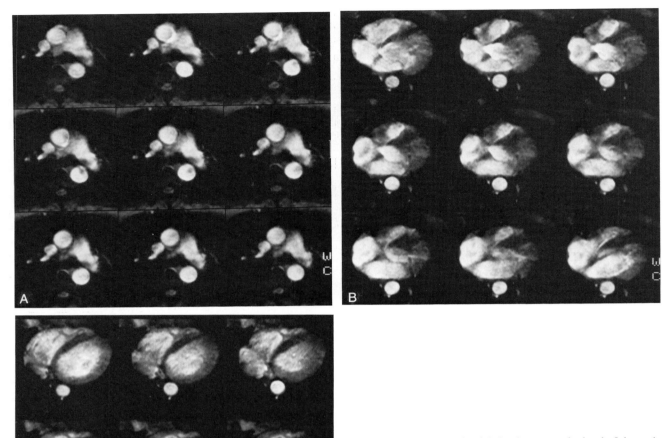

FIGURE 28–8. Standard axial cine images at the level of the main pulmonary artery (*A*), aortic root (*B*), and midventricles (*C*). Note the variation in displayed anatomy over the cardiac cycle, due to the complex rotational and translational motions of the heart.

start and end locations can be input to achieve effectively the same imaging plane and the appropriate number of slice locations.

Short-Axis View

It is also possible to obtain sequential short-axis images of the left ventricle (Fig. 28–11), allowing accurate assessment of left ventricular function. An apparent short-axis view can be obtained by simply prescribing multiple slice locations in an anteroposterior direction at 90 degrees to the line between the right shoulder and apex. However, this is not a true short-axis image, since the apex is situated more

anteriorly than the base of the heart and the rotations required to achieve a true short-axis image are more complicated. A true short-axis image can be obtained in one of two ways. Either a graphic prescription can be performed from the long-axis view, as described above, subsequently obtaining sequentially slices perpendicular to a line between the aortic valve and apex, or the exact 3D coordinates of the aortic valve and apex can be input and scanning can be performed in a plane perpendicular to these points. Either of these methods will produce sequential true short-axis slices of the left ventricle, from which the most accurate estimation of left ventricular function and left ventricular volumes can be obtained.

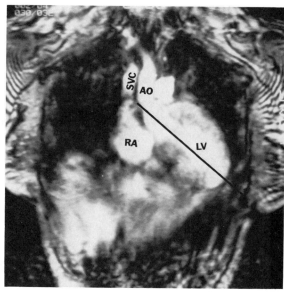

FIGURE 28–9. Standard orthogonal coronal view of cine MR imaging stop frame. Note that the left ventricular (LV) cavity is well demonstrated, as well as the left ventricular outflow tract and ascending aorta (AO). The superior vena cava (SVC) and right atrium (RA) are also well imaged in this view. From this coronal image, it is possible to prescribe an oblique image along the line between the aortic valve and apex as shown, from which a long-axis view of the heart will be obtained.

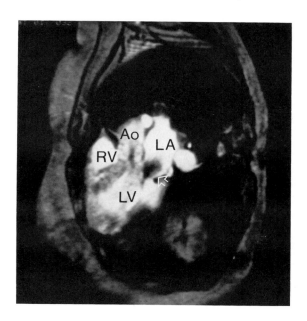

FIGURE 28–10. Long-axis view of the heart as prescribed from a coronal image (see Fig. 28–6). Accurate estimates of global and regional left ventricular function can easily be made from this view, with the left ventricle (LV) being well visualized along its major axis. Mitral regurgitation is also seen as a zone of signal loss in the left atrium (LA) on this early systolic frame (*arrow*). Note that the image appears quite similar to the standard long-axis view as imaged by two-dimensional (2D) echocardiography. AO = aorta; RV = right ventricle.

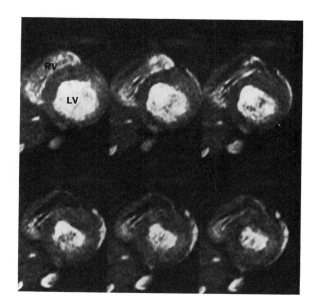

FIGURE 28–11. Short-axis view of the heart as prescribed directly from the long-axis view (see Fig. 28–7). Six representative time frames are shown from end-diastole (*top left*) to end-systole (*bottom right*). LV = left ventricle; RV = right ventricle.

Other Oblique Views

With a little practice, it is possible to use the standard orthogonal planes as a basis for imaging in any desired plane of the heart or great vessels. For example, to perform cine MR imaging in the true plane of the aorta, a conventional ECG-gated scan is first performed in the standard axial view. This scan allows imaging of both the ascending and the descending portions of the aorta in cross-section. A graphic prescription that transects these two structures will allow cine MR images to visualize the whole of the aorta (Fig. 28–12) and thereby enhance the ability to diagnose such abnormalities as coarctation of the aorta, as shown in Figure 28–13. In our experience,[10] we have found that the facility for multiplanar oblique imaging is absolutely essential for cardiac imaging and provides considerably more diagnostic information than using the standard orthogonal planes alone.

PRACTICAL ASPECTS OF CINE MR IMAGING

There are several imaging parameters that are fairly standard for cine MR imaging in adults. First, it is necessary to image using the standard body coil. Second, for standard cine imaging, a flip angle of 30 degrees is usual, with a slice thickness of 10 mm. Third, cine MR imaging should always be preceded by conventional ECG-gated imaging. Conventional ECG-gated MR imaging is an important adjunct to cine MR imaging not only as a technique that enhances resolution of structural detail but also as a

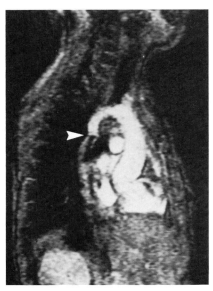

FIGURE 28–13. Cine MR imaging in the long axis of the aorta. Note that the ascending aorta, aortic arch, and descending aorta are well visualized. There is a narrowed region in the proximal descending aorta that is consistent with a discrete coarctation of the aorta (*arrowhead*). This is further confirmed by the presence of a dark jet of turbulent high-velocity flow seen at and distal to the coarctation site. (From Simpson IA, Chung KJ, Glass RF, et al: Cine MRI for evaluation of anatomy and flow relations in infants and children with coarctation of the aorta. Circulation 78:142–148, 1988; by permission of the American Heart Association, Inc.)

method of choosing the appropriate slice locations for subsequent cine imaging. Finally, we have tended not to use any interslice spacing for either ECG-gated or cine MR imaging to avoid missing any important anatomic or flow-related information. In clinical terms, this does not usually cause any noticeable image degradation, especially in cine mode.

In patients with labored breathing or significant variation in heart rate, particularly those with atrial fibrillation, the quality of cine MR images is much reduced. As a result, we have tended not to image these individuals, as it is unusual to obtain images of sufficient quality for diagnostic purposes.

The temporal resolution of cine MR imaging is directly related to the TR used, which can be lower than 12 msec for a single slice location. However, increasing the number of slice locations reduces temporal resolution, so that if two slice locations are chosen, then the TR doubles and, as a result, temporal resolution is halved. Similarly, with three slice locations, the number of images obtained per cardiac cycle is a third of that obtained from just one slice location. For most adults, with heart rates less than 100 beats per minute, good temporal resolution of at least 16 image frames per cardiac cycle can be obtained using two slice locations per cine acquisition sequence. The acquisition time for a single cine scan is not normally much different from a conventional gated imaging sequence, usually 2 to 3 minutes, dependent on heart rate; but whereas the gated

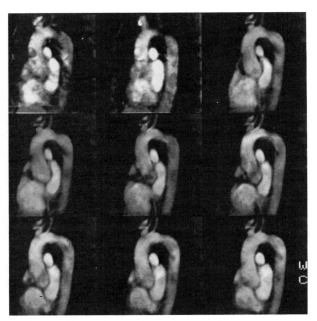

FIGURE 28–12. Long axis cine images of a normal aorta.

images are available immediately following the end of data acquisition, the cine data require lengthier reconstruction. This reconstruction may take a further 5 minutes or more for each cine acquisition. The extra time required for cine reconstruction, in combination with the fact that each cine acquisition consists of only four slice locations covering as little as 4 cm at a time, means that it is important to know the exact scan locations prior to commencing the cine scan sequence. These locations can easily be obtained by first performing a much less time-consuming ECG-gated imaging sequence, which allows as many as 20 different slice locations, from which the most appropriate can be chosen for subsequent cine MR imaging.

In attempting a comprehensive assessment of the structure and function of the heart by cine MR imaging, it is recommended that ECG-gated localizing scans first be performed in all three standard orthogonal planes. The long- and short-axis views can be prescribed from the coronal images, as described above. Sagittal views provide the location for cine MR imaging used to assess right ventricular function, and the axial view usually provides an excellent four-chamber equivalent view (see Fig. 28–7). For a complete cardiac assessment in an individual patient, cine MR imaging should be performed at two slice locations in each of the long-axis view, the axial four-chamber view, and the sagittal view at the locations of the left and right ventricular cavities. This practice requires three separate cine acquisitions of around 2 to 3 minutes each, which can be reconstructed at the end of the examination to minimize the patient's time within the magnet. If a detailed assessment of left ventricular function and regional wall motion is required, then multiple short-axis views of the heart can be obtained using a single sequence that performs several acquisitions at different locations to maintain temporal resolution. Six different slice locations (three acquisitions) are usually necessary to cover the entire left ventricle. A complete cardiac assessment, as described above, will usually require the patient to be in the magnet for no more than 1 hour and 30 minutes and will allow an accurate assessment of all aspects of cardiac structure and function. The examination can easily be tailored to each individual if it is necessary to investigate only specific cardiac lesions, and, indeed, in many instances, the patient's time within the magnet may be only 30 to 45 minutes.

ASSESSMENT OF SPECIFIC CARDIAC ABNORMALITIES

Cine MR imaging is a very versatile diagnostic tool, and the value of the technique in a wide range of cardiac abnormalities is only now beginning to be realized. The combination of structural and functional information makes it ideal for the investigation of congenital heart disease, as detailed in Chapter 29, but it also has considerable application to adult cardiology. The following description of the use of cine MR imaging in a variety of cardiac disorders reflects the initial clinical experience with the technique, but it is likely to be some time before the full range of possible applications are explored and its true clinical value is fully appreciated.

LEFT VENTRICULAR FUNCTION

The excellent temporal resolution of dynamic cine MR imaging, combined with the high image resolution of this inherently volumetric technique, probably now makes cine MR imaging the noninvasive technique of choice for the assessment of global and regional left ventricular function.[11]

Since 16 or even 32 dynamic images throughout the cardiac cycle can be obtained, it is possible to determine end-systolic and end-diastolic frames with considerable accuracy. It has already been demonstrated that cine MR imaging can be used to measure left ventricular stroke volume and ejection fraction and to make accurate assessments of left ventricular volume and cardiac output.[12–15] Probably the most accurate method of assessing these parameters of left ventricular function by cine MR imaging is using contiguous short-axis sections that encompass the entire left ventricle. Cine MR imaging has also been shown to assess accurately regional left ventricular wall motion abnormalities in animals[16] and in patients with coronary artery disease.[17]

Volumetric assessment of the left ventricle using cine MR imaging is considerably more accurate than other imaging techniques, since, unlike cardiac ultrasound, each slice is inherently volumetric (usually 1 cm per slice for adults) and the image resolution obtained is far superior to radionuclide techniques. The technique is successful in a higher proportion of patients than is ultrasound for providing high-resolution images of the entire myocardial contour, and the planar imaging technique of cine MR imaging allows much more precise definition of regional wall motion. It is probably a more accurate technique for the assessment of global and regional left ventricular function even than cine angiography, which, unlike cine MR imaging is limited by superimposition of regional information.

RIGHT VENTRICULAR FUNCTION

The geometric shape of the right ventricle makes it difficult to assess function accurately using any imaging technique. However, our experience with infants and children would suggest that cine MR imaging is able to assess right ventricular function quite accurately compared with right ventricular ejection fraction measured by angiography,[18, 19] almost certainly because of the 3D volumetric nature of the angiographic technique. Right ventricular function evaluation is generally best achieved from the standard sagittal view, which provides a dynamic volumetric assessment of the right ventricle, with accurate estimates of right ventricular ejection fraction being obtained from the end-systolic and end-diastolic images. This view also allows excellent visualization of the right ventricular outflow tract, where dynamic outflow obstruction and pulmonary regurgitation can easily be assessed. The axial four-chamber equivalent view can also be useful for visualizing right ventricular function and is particularly valuable for assessing abnormalities of right ventricular inflow.

MYOCARDIAL INFARCTION

Cine MR imaging has considerable potential for the evaluation of patients with myocardial infarction, but, again, there is limited information available at present. This is due, in part at least, to the difficulties in imaging acutely ill patients, compounded by the fact that in many instances the MR facilities are somewhat remote from the coronary care units. However, there are some data to suggest that in acute myocardial infarction cine MR imaging can provide a sensitive noninvasive method for characterizing both functional and anatomic changes. The area of infarction is associated with decreased signal intensity on tissue characterization and with regional wall motion abnormality,[20] which not only can prove valuable for determining the presence and site of infarction but also may prove to be of help in the accurate, noninvasive sizing of infarcts clinically. The reported sensitivity and specificity of cine MR imaging in acute myocardial infarction with respect to the assessment of regional wall motion abnormalities compare favorably with those of 2D echocardiography and with thallium-201 scintigraphy of perfusion defects.[21] In chronic infarctions, there may be wall thinning and abnormal wall motion (Fig. 28–14).

VALVE REGURGITATION

In recent years, there has been considerable interest in assessing the severity of valve regurgitation, since this can often be quite difficult clinically. Doppler ultrasound, particularly color Doppler flow mapping, has added a new dimension to the evaluation of valve regurgitation, and this has been shown to provide a semiquantitative estimate of severity.[22–26] However, it is apparent from in vitro studies that the flow velocity information displayed by color Doppler flow mapping in valve regurgitation is considerably more complex than initially thought and is related to many factors other than merely the volume of regurgitation.[27]

Little information is currently available regarding the role of cine MR imaging in quantifying valve regurgitation, but there is no doubt that the turbulent

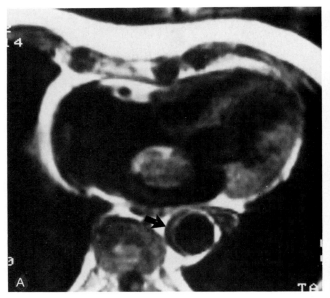
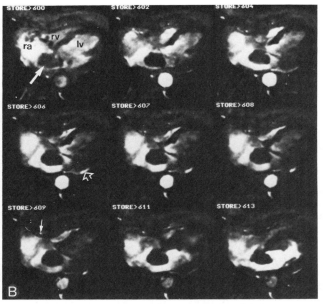

FIGURE 28–14. Patient with apical and septal infarctions and suspected left atrial myxoma. *A,* Gated SE image obtained with flow presaturation shows thinning of left ventricular septum and apex, as well as mass in left atrium, which is attached to the interatrial septum. Note incidentally "pseudodissection" (*arrow*) of descending aorta, representing chemical shift artifact. *B,* Cine images demonstrate marked hypokinesis of the left ventricular apex and septum. Mass (*large arrow*) appears dark, in contrast to bright signal from flowing blood. Also note the rather complex signal pattern in the descending aorta, which is a normal finding. Small arrow = right coronary artery; open arrow = normal amount of fluid in dependent portion of pericardium.

spray area caused by valve regurgitation can easily be identified by cine MR imaging (Figs. 28–15 and 28–16). However, although the imaging algorithms of color Doppler flow mapping and cine MR imaging are quite different, it is essentially the same turbulent spray area that is imaged by both techniques. It is somewhat naive, therefore, to expect that the distribution of the turbulent regurgitant jet spray will in itself be able to provide an accurate quantitative assessment of valve regurgitation, as has been suggested for both mitral[28, 29] and aortic[30, 31] regurgitation, since it has not been possible to demonstrate this with color Doppler flow mapping. To date, only very limited in vitro data exist to substantiate the effects of hemodynamic variables on the display of flow information in valve regurgitation by cine MR imaging,[32] and much more work is required in this area before the role of cine MR imaging for the qualitative and quantitative assessment of valve regurgitation is established.

One major limitation of the cine technique for the evaluation of valve regurgitation is that despite being volumetric to some extent, as a planar technique, cine MR imaging cannot rapidly alter the exact imaging plane, as can color Doppler flow mapping. The direction of regurgitant jets can be quite unpredictable, and it is impossible to ensure that cine MR imaging is consistently imaging the maximal jet distribution. However, cine MR imaging can certainly identify the presence of valve regurgitation, and the origin of the regurgitant jet may be seen from the flow void caused by the zone of spatial acceleration seen proximal to the regurgitant orifice (see Fig. 28–7). This feature may prove to be of particular value

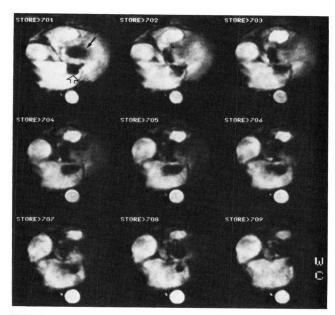

FIGURE 28–16. Axial cine MR imaging showing dark jets from moderate mitral (*open arrow*) and aortic (*closed arrow*) regurgitation. Note incidentally the increased myocardial signal in the first (*upper left*) image. This represents a lightening artifact caused by the use of prospective gating.

in the assessment of prosthetic valve regurgitation, in which the site of origin may be of some importance and in which color Doppler flow mapping may be difficult to perform.[33]

MISCELLANEOUS LESIONS

The clinical applications of cine MR imaging are undoubtedly wide ranging, but because of the very recent introduction of the technique, they have yet to be fully established. The assessment of intracardiac tumors and pericardial lesions (Figs. 28–14 and 28–17) is likely to remain the realm of conventional ECG-gated imaging, in which high-resolution anatomic detail at a single phase of the cardiac cycle is more important and T_2-weighted imaging can more readily differentiate tissue characteristics. However, even in this case cine MR imaging may provide valuable additional information by visualizing the dynamic characteristics of these lesions, particularly the motion of intracardiac masses, which can facilitate assessment of their intracardiac attachments. Cine MR imaging may prove superior to conventional ECG-gated imaging in the detection of intracardiac thrombus, which causes a signal void on cine MR imaging. The differentiation of thrombus from stagnant blood flow can, at times, be difficult using ECG-gated imaging. Although sluggish, swirling, or slowly moving blood often produces some signal loss on cine MR imaging and, in many circumstances, it can be difficult to distinguish this from freshly formed thrombus, once again the dynamic aspects of cine imaging are of particular value in making this dis-

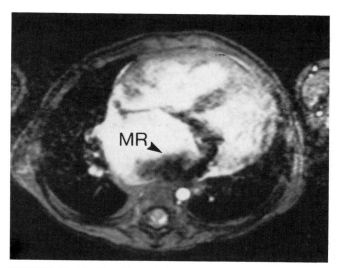

FIGURE 28–15. Cine MR imaging in the axial view in a patient with significant mitral regurgitation (MR). In this systolic stop frame, a swirling dark jet (*arrowhead*) of turbulent, high-velocity regurgitant flow is seen to originate proximal to the posterior mitral valve leaflet and extend into the left atrium and swirl around the posterior left atrial wall. An identical appearance of the regurgitant jet was seen on color Doppler flow mapping.

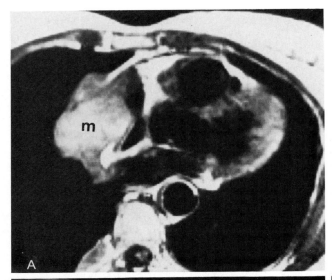

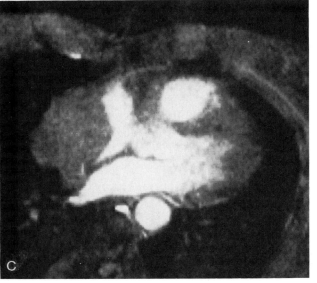

FIGURE 28–17. Pericardial mesothelioma (m) compressing the right atrium. *A.* Gated SE image with flow presaturation. *B,* Systolic cine MR image. *C,* Diastolic cine MR image.

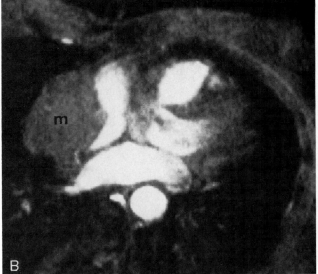

tinction. The presence of thrombus is usually associated with a signal void that persists throughout the cardiac cycle (Fig. 28–18) whereas a sluggish or stagnant blood flow is characterized by its intermittent appearance.

The flow-enhanced signal on cine MR imaging can be quite useful in clinical situations in which it is important to demonstrate flow to assess the patency of blood vessels. This practice is most readily applied to coronary artery bypass grafts, in which the loss of signal intensity is indicative of lack of flow caused by a blocked graft.[34] Cine MR imaging has yet to be successfully applied to the reliable evaluation of native coronary artery disease, and because of the tortuosity of the coronary vessels, it is likely that this will require some combination of cine imaging, 3D reconstruction, and flow sensitization, which itself is at an early stage of development,[35] to provide a reliable quantitative assessment of coronary artery blood flow.

Cine MR imaging is certainly valuable for the noninvasive assessment of cardiomyopathies. In congestive cardiomyopathy, systolic left and right ventricular function can be easily and accurately studied, as has been described previously, and diastolic compliance problems may be identified in patients with restrictive cardiomyopathies. In hypertrophic cardiomyopathy, the distribution and full extent of the ventricular hypertrophy can be seen on long-axis (Figs. 28–19 and 28–20) views, the systolic and diastolic function can be assessed, and any intraventricular obstruction can be identified. The presence of intracavitary obstruction is usually apparent from the turbulent flow void visualized within the ventricular outflow tract, with its origin usually seen at the point of systolic anterior motion of the mitral valve.

It is likely that as cine MR imaging becomes more widely available and its use in clinical practice expands, the clinical value of this technology for as-

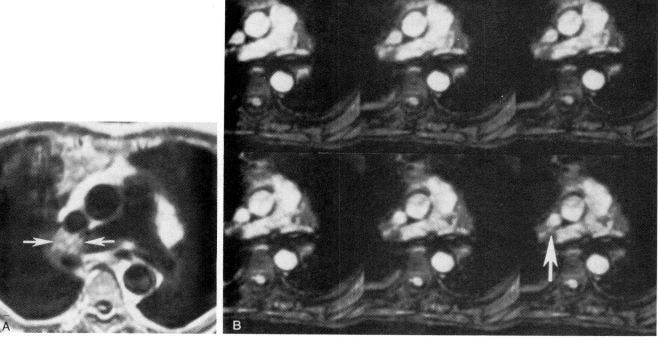

FIGURE 28–18. Central pulmonary embolus. *A,* SE images show filling defect (*arrows*) with intermediate signal intensity in the right pulmonary artery. It is difficult to be certain this does not represent flow signal. *B,* Cine MR images show persistence of abnormal signal without significant change over the cardiac cycle. (From Posteraro RH, Sostman HD, Spritzer CE, Herfkens RJ: Cine–gradient-refocused MRI of central pulmonary emboli. AJR 152:465–468, 1989; © by American Roentgen Ray Society.)

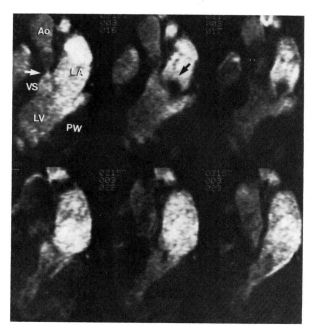

FIGURE 28–19. Long-axis cine MR image in a patient with hypertrophic cardiomyopathy at various time intervals throughout the cardiac cycle. Note the extensive left ventricular (LV) hypertrophy associated with the slitlike ventricular cavity at peak systole (*white arrow*). There is also an early systolic signal void (*black arrow*) in the left atrium (LA) immediately behind the mitral valve, indicating some degree of mitral regurgitation. AO = aorta; PW = posterior wall; VS = ventricular septum.

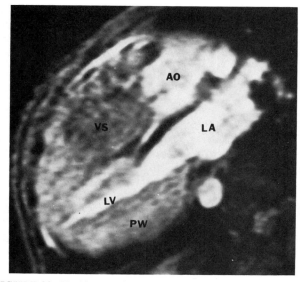

FIGURE 28–20. Cine MR image of hypertrophic cardiomyopathy in the long-axis view. Again note the extensive myocardial hypertrophy with a small left ventricular (LV) cavity during systole. AO = aorta; LA = left atrium; PW = posterior wall; VS = ventricular septum.

sessing a wide range of cardiologic conditions will become increasingly apparent.

PROBLEMS AND PITFALLS

There are a number of problems and pitfalls associated with the general usage of MR imaging, and these have been discussed throughout this text. However, there are also certain potential problems that pertain to adult cardiology and to cine MR imaging in particular, which should be borne in mind. The first major problem encountered with the MR imaging of patients with cardiac disorders is that it is necessary for the patient to lie flat, as the bore of the magnet is quite small. Patients often have to lie flat for a considerable time, and this can be difficult in those with severely compromised left ventricular function or severe valvular heart disease, and there is a real danger of precipitating pulmonary edema in these patients. If only very specific diagnostic information is required in these patients, it may be possible to perform a very limited study, concentrating on one specific aspect of cardiac anatomy and flow. Similarly, the magnet is not the ideal environment for those patients who are critically ill, particularly those requiring intensive monitoring and those who may be subject to life-threatening arrhythmias. It should be remembered that the presence of arrhythmias, even if they do not cause hemodynamic upset, is still a problem, since these may cause significant deterioration in the image quality.

It is also worth reemphasizing at this point that patients with active cardiac pacemakers (temporary as well as permanent) or those who still have a pacemaker lead in situ, even though nonfunctioning, cannot be allowed into the magnet, as an electrical discharge via the pacing electrode may occur and will cause considerable pacemaker damage and may in itself be life threatening. This is one of the very few absolute contraindications to MR imaging, but it is clearly important to establish the presence of a possible pacemaker prior to considering any patient for MR imaging.

The presence of metallic vascular clips or any metal implantation, such as prosthetic valves, is not in itself a contraindication to MR imaging, and good imaging of the surrounding structures can be obtained by conventional ECG-gated imaging. However, the gradient recalled pulse sequence of cine MR imaging is highly susceptible to these extraneous materials, which can cause large artifactual signal voids on the cine MR images (Fig. 28–21). It is unusual to confuse these with any abnormality of cardiovascular flow, since the artifactual signal voids are quite large and do not vary during the cardiac cycle and will often be seen to extend outside the vascular structures. Sternal wires are invariably present after sternotomy; but the signal voids caused by these rarely interfere with imaging of the heart, and at worst the signal

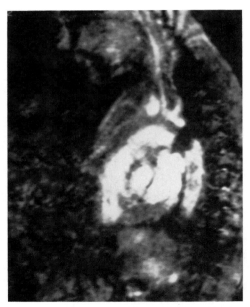

FIGURE 28–21. Cine MR image in an oblique view in a patient studied following repair of a coarctation of the aorta. A large image void is seen in the proximal descending aorta in the region of the coarctation repair. This void is associated with the presence of vascular clips and note that it extends outside the vascular structures, unlike the turbulent jet seen with coarctation of the aorta in Figure 28–13.

void will encroach only onto the anterior right ventricular surface. Vascular clips in other areas are much more problematic. Radiopaque vascular markers are often inserted at the time of cardiac surgery to identify the origin of coronary artery bypass grafts in case subsequent coronary angiography is required, and vascular clips are often used for the repair of vascular lesions, such as coarctation of the aorta. Their presence causes considerable image voids on cine MR imaging at and surrounding the main region of interest, and this makes it impossible to comment on either the structural detail of the lesion or the associated flow abnormalities. This is of some concern because of our clinical experience with cine MR imaging in assessing abnormalities of the great vessels, in which high-resolution imaging by cardiac ultrasound is often difficult. We believe that cine MR imaging is now the technique of choice for the investigation of these patients and can often obviate subsequent or repeated angiography. As a result, it has become the policy of the cardiac surgeons in our institution to use vascular clips only when they are thought to be essential at the time of surgery.

FUTURE ASPECTS OF CINE MR IMAGING

The fundamental aspects of cine MR imaging are now well established, but it is a rapidly developing technology and many of the current problems are likely to be overcome. In addition, advances will occur in the acquisition of data, in their reconstruction, and in the nature of the display of the considerable information available from cine MR imaging. It is likely that better magnets, gradients, pulse sequences, and reconstruction techniques will provide even more information in cine imaging. Real-time cine MR imaging is also being developed, and this will add a new dimension to cine MR imaging and overcome many of the problems caused by significant heart rate variation or arrhythmias in some patients.

Although inherently volumetric, cine MR imaging is essentially still a planar imaging technique and is therefore limited to some extent by its inability to display 3D information spatially. Three-dimensional reconstruction of cine MR images is in its infancy but promises much for the assessment of complex structural abnormalities and the associated, often complex, flow relationships.

The development of different pulse sequences will allow cine MR imaging to provide information on actual flow velocities, and these velocity-encoding sequences will not only measure velocities that are angle independent but also provide accurate spatial velocity information and hence accurate velocity profiles.[36] It will therefore be possible to measure absolute flow in the aorta and pulmonary artery and hence left and right ventricular outputs, in addition to being able to measure flow in coronary artery bypass grafts and potentially in native coronary vessels.[37] This velocity information can be directionally color coded and displayed simultaneously with structural MR imaging information, providing a spatial appreciation of both anatomy and flow similar to that obtained by color Doppler flow mapping.

In at least one aspect, MR cineangiography can provide important functional information not available from either ultrasound or angiography. During systole, the heart normally contracts along its long axis (apex to base). This motion is well shown by MR cineangiography, ultrasound, and angiography. However, the heart also undergoes complex twisting

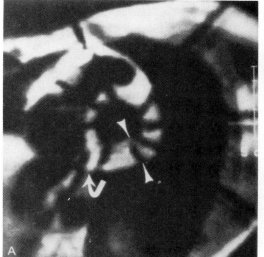
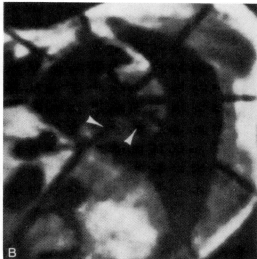
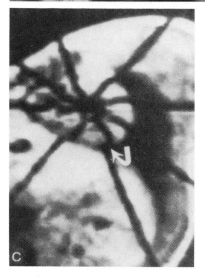

FIGURE 28–22. Conventional cine MR images are insensitive to twisting motion. More sensitive evaluation is obtained by tagging segments of the myocardium with preinversion pulses, which then appear dark, and then imaging over the cardiac cycle to follow their motion. Three slices obtained at early systole—base (*A*), middle (*B*), and apex (*C*)—are shown, displaying global counterclockwise rotation of the heart. There is twisting of some intramyocardial tag lines, especially in the inferior and left lateral wall (*arrowheads*), representing different degrees of twisting between subendocardial and subepicardial regions. Tag motion is most pronounced in the inferior wall tags (*curved arrow*). (From Zerhouni EA, Parish DM, Rogers WJ, et al: Human heart: Tagging with MR imaging—a method for noninvasive assessment of myocardial motion. Radiology 169:59–63, 1988; with permission.)

motions. These motions will not be well shown by ultrasound or angiography. For instance, an ischemic, hypokinetic segment of the heart may appear to move normally, because the abnormal segment is passively displaced by the motion of other, normal segments. Subtle wall motion abnormalities can be detected more precisely by tagging segments of the myocardium with RF presaturation or preinversion pulses and then following the motion of these tags over the cardiac cycle[39, 39a] (Fig. 28–22). With use of this method, absence of the normal twisting motion and abnormal myocardial compliance in ischemic heart disease can be demonstrated much more reliably than by other imaging techniques.

CONCLUSION

Cine MR imaging is an exciting development in the field of noninvasive cardiac imaging. The dynamic spatial appreciation of high-resolution structural information, combined with a dynamic display of cardiac blood flow that is not limited by the problems of ultrasound penetration, makes this technique both unique and extremely valuable. The exact role that cine MR imaging will play in adult cardiology continues to expand and develop and has yet to be fully established. Much critical research is required with the cine MR imaging technology already available, in addition to the developing technology, before the exact sensitivity, specificity, and diagnostic capabilities of the technique can be fully appreciated.

The similarity in the display of cine MR images to those obtained at angiography should serve to illustrate the considerable potential of this technique, but it is worth remembering that as a planar rather than a projection-type technique, considerable expertise is required both in choosing the appropriate imaging planes for individual patients and in interpreting the cine MR images obtained. In our experience, it is quite helpful to have both the radiologist and the cardiologist actively involved not only in the interpretation of cardiac cine MR imaging but also in its prescription of scan technique to tailor the examination most precisely to each patient.

Conventional ECG-gated MR imaging and cine MR imaging are clearly complementary techniques, and although cine MR imaging provides considerably more information on cardiac flow and function, conventional ECG-gated imaging yields generally better structural detail and information on tissue characterization and is currently always required in conjunction with cine MR imaging to choose the most appropriate slice locations for cine imaging.

On the basis of our clinical experience with cine MR imaging and the initial research that is only now becoming available, it is clear that cine MR imaging is a considerable advance in the field of cardiac imaging and will play an increasingly valuable diagnostic and management role in the future of adult cardiology.

REFERENCES

1. Glover G, Pelc N: A rapid gated cine MRI technique. *In* Kressel H (ed): The Magnetic Resonance Annual. New York, Raven Press, 1988, pp 299–333.
2. James TL, Margulis AL: Biomedical Magnetic Resonance. Radiology Research and Education Foundation, San Francisco, 1984, pp 421–441.
3. Saunders RD, Smith H: Safety aspects of NMR clinical imaging. Br Med Bull 40:148–154, 1984.
4. Fram J, Haase A, Mathaei D: Rapid three-dimensional MR imaging using the FLASH technique. J Comput Assist Tomogr 10:363–368, 1986.
5. Wehrli FW: Introduction to Fast-Scan Magnetic Resonance. Milwaukee, WI, General Electric, 1986.
6. Haase A, Mathaei D, Hanicke W: FLASH imaging: Rapid NMR imaging using low-flip angle pulses. J Magn Res 67:258–266, 1986.
7. Simpson IA, Valdes-Cruz LM, Yoganathan AP, et al: Spatial velocity distribution and acceleration in serial subvalve tunnel and valvular obstructions: An in vitro study using Doppler color flow mapping. J Am Coll Cardiol 13:241–248, 1989.
8. Simpson IA, Sahn DJ, Valdes-Cruz LM, et al: Color Doppler flow mapping in coarctation of the aorta: New observations and improved evaluation using color flow diameter and proximal acceleration as predictors of severity. Circulation 77:736–744, 1988.
9. Simpson IA, Chung KJ, Powell JB, et al: Cine magnetic resonance imaging for the evaluation of pulmonary artery banding in infants and children. J Am Coll Cardiol 11:248A, 1988.
10. Simpson IA, Chung KJ, Glass RF, et al: Cine magnetic resonance imaging for evaluation of anatomy and flow relations in infants and children with coarctation of the aorta. Circulation 78:142–148, 1988.
11. Sechtem U, Pflugfelder PW, White RD, et al: Cine MR imaging: Potential for evaluation of cardiovascular function. AJR 148:239–246, 1987.
12. Utz JA, Herfkens RJ, Heinsimer JA, et al: Cine MR determination of left ventricular ejection fraction. AJR 148:839–843, 1987.
13. Sechtem U, Pflugfelder PW, Gould RG, et al: Measurement of right and left ventricular volumes in healthy individuals with cine MR imaging. Radiology 163:667–670, 1987.
14. Pflugfelder PW, Sechtem U, Gould RR, et al: Concordance of right and left ventricualr stroke volume measurements in normal subjects by cine MRI. J Am Coll Cardiol 9:46A, 1987.
15. Meese RB, Spritzer CE, Negro-Vilar R, et al: A new technique for quantification of left and right ventricular stroke volumes utilizing rapid dynamic magnetic resonance imaging. J Am Coll Cardiol 11:156A, 1988.
16. Askenase A, Chen G, Thompson W, et al: Oblique cine magnetic resonance blood flow imaging to assess changes in wall motion. Circulation 76[Suppl IV]:IV–29, 1987.
17. Holmvang F, Edelman R, Pearlman JD, et al: Left ventricular wall motion analysis by cine NMR. J Am Coll Cardiol 11:156A, 1988.
18. Chung KJ, Simpson IA, Sahn DJ, et al: Cine magnetic resonance imaging in congenital heart disease. Dynam Cardiovasc Imaging 1:133–138, 1987.
19. Chung KJ, Simpson IA, Newman R, et al: Cine magnetic resonance imaging for evaluation of congenital heart disease: Role of pediatric cardiology compared with echocardiography and angiography. J Pediatr 113:1028–1035, 1988.
20. Meese RB, Herfkens RJ, Negro-Vilar R, et al: Rapid dynamic magnetic resonance images of the heart in evaluation of acute myocardial infarction. Circulation 76[Suppl IV]:IV–31, 1987.
21. Rokey R, O'Neill P, Nitz W, et al: Left ventricular wall motion assessment by cine nuclear magnetic resonance imaging: Comparison with two-dimensional echocardiography and

thallium-201 tomography. J Am Coll Cardiol 11:156A, 1988.

22. Miyatake K, Okamoto M, Kinoshita N, et al: Clinical applications of a new type of real-time two-dimensional Doppler flow imaging system. Am J Cardiol 54:857–868, 1984.

23. Omoto R, Yokote Y, Takamoto S, et al: The development of real-time two-dimensional Doppler echocardiography and its clinical significance in acquired valvular diseases. Jpn Heart J 25:325–340, 1984.

24. Miyatake K, Izumi S, Okamoto M, et al: Semiquantitative grading of severity of mitral regurgitation by real-time two-dimensional Doppler flow imaging technique. J Am Coll Cardiol 7:82–88, 1986.

25. Helmcke F, Nanda NC, Hsuin MC, et al: Color Doppler assessment of mitral regurgitation with orthogonal planes. Circulation 75:175–183, 1987.

26. Otsuji Y, Tei C, Kisanuki A, et al: Color Doppler echocardiographic assessment of the change in the mitral regurgitation volume. Am Heart J 114:349–354, 1987.

27. Simpson IA, Valdes-Cruz LM, Sahn DJ, et al: Color Doppler flow mapping of simulated in vitro regurgitant jets: Evaluation of the effects of orifice size and hemodynamic variables. J Am Coll Cardiol 13:1195–1207, 1989.

28. Aurigemma G, Reicheck N, Schieblar M, et al: Evaluation of mitral regurgitation by cardiac cine magnetic resonance imaging. Circulation 76[Suppl IV]:IV–31, 1987.

29. Aurigemma G, Reicheck N, Axel L, et al: Cardiac cine magnetic resonance imaging: Detection of mitral and aortic regurgitation. J Am Coll Cardiol 9:159A, 1987.

30. Pflugfelder PW, Landzberg JS, Cassidy MM, et al: Comparison of cine magnetic resonance imaging with Doppler-echocardiography for the evaluation of aortic regurgitation. AJR 152:729–735, 1989.

31. Aurigemma G, Reicheck N, Schiebler M, et al: Evaluation of aortic regurgitation by cine magnetic resonance imaging. J Am Coll Cardiol 11:155A, 1988.

32. Cook SL, Maurer G, Berman DS, et al: Effect of flow rate and orifice size on flow jets visualized by fast NMR imaging: A phantom study. J Am Coll Cardiol 11:156A, 1988.

33. Sprecher DL, Adamick R, Adams D, Kisslo J: In vitro color flow, pulsed and continuous wave Doppler ultrasound masking of flow by prosthetic valves. J Am Coll Cardiol 9:1306–1310, 1987.

34. Aurigemma G, Reicheck N, Schiebler M, et al: Noninvasive determination of coronary bypass graft patency using cine magnetic resonance imaging. Circulation 76[Suppl IV]:IV–29, 1987.

35. Weinberg PM, Chin AJ, Axel L, et al: Three dimensional motion pictures of the beating heart with congenital heart defects from in vivo magnetic resonance images. J Am Coll Cardiol 11:247A, 1988.

36. Klipstein RH, Firmin DN, Underwood SR, et al: Blood flow patterns in the human aorta studied by magnetic resonance. Br Heart J 58:316–323, 1987.

37. Underwood SR, Firmin DN, Klipstein RH, et al: MR velocity mapping: Clinical application of a new technique. Br Heart J 57:404–412, 1987.

38. Glover GH, Pelc NJ: A rapid gated cine MRI technique. In Kressel HY (ed): Magnetic Resonance Annual. New York, Raven Press, 1988, pp 209–333.

39. Zerhouni EA, Parish DM, Rogers WJ, et al: Human heart: Tagging with MR imaging—a method for noninvasive assessment of myocardial motion. Radiology 169:59–63, 1988.

39a. Axel L, Dougherty L: Heart wall motion: Improved method of spatial modulation of magnetization for MR imaging. Radiology 172:349–350, 1989.

40. Posteraro RH, Sostman HD, Spritzer CE, Herfkens RJ: Cine-gradient-refocused MRI of central pulmonary emboli. AJR 152:465–468, 1989.

41. Spraggins TA, Owens SF, Margosian PM: Retrospective cardiac gating requiring no physiological monitoring. Presented as a work in progress abstract at the 7th Annual Meeting of the Society of Magnetic Resonance in Medicine, San Francisco, August 20–26, 1988.

29

CINE MR IMAGING OF CONGENITAL HEART DISEASE

KYUNG J. CHUNG and IAIN A. SIMPSON

TECHNIQUE AND METHOD OF
EXAMINATION
CLINICAL APPLICATIONS IN
CONGENITAL HEART DISEASE
RIGHT HEART LESIONS
Tetralogy of Fallot
Hypoplastic Right Heart Syndrome
Transposition of the Great Arteries

DISEASES OF THE GREAT ARTERIES
AND VEINS
Coarctation of the Aorta
Pulmonary Artery Banding for Ventricular
Septal Defect or Single Ventricle

LEFT HEART AND SHUNT LESIONS

DISCUSSION

ECG-gated conventional spin-echo magnetic resonance imaging has been widely used to assess cardiac anatomy and function.[1-7] Clinical investigators have reported their experiences with this new technique for evaluation of congenital heart disease.[8-15] Recently, rapid MRI techniques (cine MRI) using low flip angles, gradient-refocused echoes, and short repetition times have provided dynamic visualization of blood flow. This new cine MRI technique allows us to appreciate the complex anatomic and flow relationships of congenital cardiac defects as moving rather than stationary images.[16-22]

It is well recognized that two-dimensional echocardiography can assess anatomic and functional aspects of congenital heart disease. However, adequate imaging of the right ventricle and pulmonary arteries, especially after median sternotomy for open heart surgery, is not always feasible, and therefore cardiac catheterization and angiography have been used to assess these areas.

Magnetic resonance imaging is a noninvasive technique that is not limited by the problems of acoustic penetration required by ultrasound examination, and it provides excellent visualization of structural and functional details of congenital heart lesions. We used this technique for evaluation of infants and children with various congenital cardiac defects and discuss our preliminary experience with the applicability and efficacy of this new diagnostic modality.

TECHNIQUE AND METHOD OF EXAMINATION

The physical principles of cine MRI were discussed in the previous chapter. Briefly, we perform cine MRI using 30-degree flip angle excitation pulses and a short repetition time that allow steady-state MR acquisition with good signal-to-noise ratios. Gradient-recalled echoes are used for rephasing of spins and to allow short echo times. The gradient reversal is a nonslice-selective refocusing technique. Spins excited by initial 30-degree pulses are refocused even if flow carries them out of the imaging slice, and therefore flowing blood is bright on cine MRI rather than low signal intensity shown on standard spin-echo images. The bright signal provides sharp contrast between the myocardium and flowing blood (Fig. 29–1). Up to 32 time frames per each R-R interval are available per image slice, depending on the patient's heart rate. A 5- or 10-mm slice thickness is used for the cine mode. No gap or a 1-mm gap is used with a 5-mm slice thickness, but a 1 to 2 mm interslice gap is used with a 10-mm slice thickness to avoid cross-talk.

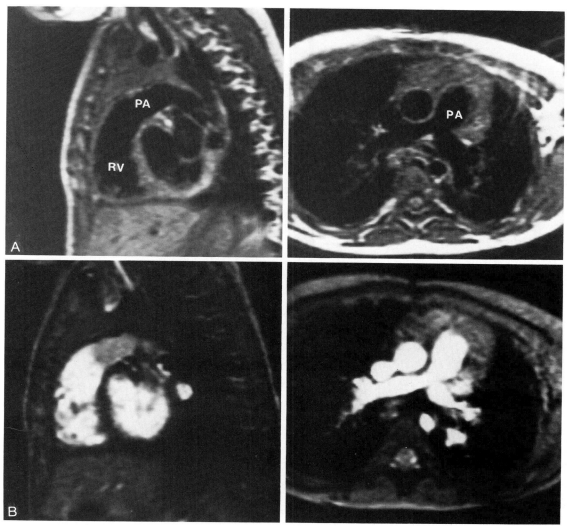

FIGURE 29–1. Conventional ECG-gated and cine MRI in sagittal and axial planes. Flowing blood through the right ventricle (RV) and the pulmonary artery (PA) is dark in ECG-gated images *(A)*, whereas it is bright on cine mode *(B)*.

Images are obtained using two excitations and an acquisition matrix of 128 × 258. Cine MRI images are reconstructed with Fourier transform methods and are displayed continuously in dynamic form throughout the cardiac cycle for analysis. Observation of the changes of anatomic configuration and blood flow signal intensity throughout the cardiac cycle are facilitated with this method. The anatomy of the cardiac chambers, myocardium, cardiac valves, and great vessels can be appreciated. Specific anatomic details are then analyzed more closely using stop frame images.

Our cine MRI is performed with a commercially available system operating at a field strength of 1.5 tesla. For children weighing less than 20 kilograms, a 16 or 24 cm cylindrical coil (knee or head) is used. These small coils not only provide excellent images of the heart and great vessels without interfering with ECG gating, but also give a safety feature by reducing potential movement of the babies during

the procedure. Older children are placed in a regular body coil. At present, the smallest field-of-view for the cine MRI on our system is 24 cm. ECG-gated spin-echo imaging is initially performed in a multi-slice mode to select the optimal slice location for cine MRI. To select the optimal imaging planes for various cardiac structures, several tomographic planes are used. Coronal, axial, and sagittal planes are used for initial localization. Then, an oblique angle software program is manipulated to obtain the optimal angle for specific areas of interest without changing the patient's position. A variety of views are acquired depending on which features are most important for diagnosis. For the vena caval system, right atrium, and right ventricle, coronal views are usually sufficient. For the ventricular outflow tract and for the main and branch pulmonary arteries, sagittal, axial, and sitting-up views display the anatomy nicely. The sitting-up views are particularly important in patients with complex pulmonary artery anomalies. For abnormalities of the aorta, such as coarctation of the great arteries, and for the great artery relationships in transposition of the great arteries, the sagittal or left anterior oblique equivalent views are chosen to image in the true planes of these structures. For the systemic and pulmonary venous returns, axial and coronal views are utilized. In postoperative cases with systemic-to-pulmonary artery shunts and Fontan operations, coronal or sagittal views are preferred.

There are two important technical factors when attempting to obtain high-quality images. Any patient movement during scanning can cause significant image degradation; therefore, it is extremely important that young children be sedated appropriately, and older children should be instructed about the importance of staying still during image acquisition. Any child who is under five years of age or who is uncooperative should be sedated with chloral hydrate (80 to 100 mg/kg) orally, approximately 30 minutes prior to the procedure. This medication works in 95 per cent of cases, but occasionally a small dose of Versed (0.05 mg/kg) intravenously may be necessary to initiate proper sedation, even after a full dose of chloral hydrate. At our MR institute, this sedation protocol has provided excellent sedation in all patients without respiratory or circulatory compromise. Another important technical part to obtain high-quality images is proper ECG gating. It is imperative to obtain clean ECG recordings with tall R waves without T-wave interference. Although not often a major problem, significant heart rate variation due to arrhythmia can be a potential difficulty with this technique, and it has been our experience that high-resolution images cannot be achieved in patients with significant arrhythmia. Another potential problem that pertains particularly to patients with complex cardiac surgery is that vascular clips produce signal voids. Similar signal voids have been seen in patients with sternal wires, and these artifacts also interfere with cine MR images of the right ventricle.

CLINICAL APPLICATIONS IN CONGENITAL HEART DEFECTS

RIGHT HEART LESIONS

Anatomic and functional assessments of the right ventricle and the pulmonary arteries are extremely important for managing cardiac defects. Serial cardiac catheterization and angiography have been the gold standard for pre- and postoperative management of pediatric patients with congenital heart disease. Echocardiography can provide useful information in assessing the right ventricle and pulmonary arteries, especially the pressure gradient across the pulmonic valve with the Doppler method. However, difficulties often arise in imaging these areas, especially the branch pulmonary arteries in older children

and in postoperative patients due to the scarring process from median sternotomy. MR imaging can provide accurate and complete imaging of the right heart anatomy and flow relationships in patients with cardiac defects because it allows multiplanar imaging of the heart and great vessels.

In our studies, image quality was excellent in 81 per cent of the cases, providing complete documentation of diagnostic features. The images provided substantial diagnostic information in another 14 per cent and was nondiagnostic in only 5 per cent. This technique was most useful for evaluating areas of the right ventricle (95 per cent), great arteries (95 per cent), vena caval system (94 per cent), and pulmonary venous systems (91 per cent). Poor quality images were due mainly to patient motion, variation of heart rate, mistriggering of the ECG-gating circuit due to T-wave interference, and flow artifact produced by turbulent high velocity flow in the cine mode. Usually, clearly defined anatomy or function of the cardiac valves was not adequately accessible, though their motions during the cardiac cycle were easily appreciated. Flow voids documenting tricuspid and pulmonary insufficiency were obtained, however, in a patient in whom valvular regurgitation was present.

The anatomy and the blood flow patterns of the right atrium, right ventricle, and pulmonary artery were studied utilizing specific imaging planes to obtain maximum information. For abnormality of the right atrium and right ventricle, coronal, sagittal, and axial views were used. The right ventricular outflow tract and main and branch pulmonary arteries were well visualized on sagittal and axial views, but these areas were better appreciated with sitting-up views, and this particular view provided superb visualization of the pulmonary annulus, main pulmonary, and bifurcation of the pulmonary arteries.

We compared the results of MR imaging in these patients with data obtained by echocardiography and conventional cineangiography. By utilizing multiple MRI views, the right side of the heart was clearly visualized, documenting anatomy similar to the views obtained by cineangiography. MRI was far superior than echocardiography, especially in older children after surgical repair, for defining the anatomy of the right ventricle and pulmonary arteries. Spectral and color Doppler echocardiography provided valuable information with regard to the right ventricular pressure and the pressure gradient across the stenotic areas, but MRI provided more useful information regarding right ventricular function and anatomy of the pulmonary arteries.

Tetralogy of Fallot

Tetralogy of Fallot is the most common cyanotic congenital heart disease. It consists of a large ventricular septal defect, valvular and infundibular pulmonary stenosis with varying degrees of hypoplastic pulmonary annulus and arteries, aortic overriding, and right ventricular hypertrophy (Fig. 29–2). The hemodynamic changes in patients with tetralogy of Fallot are very similar. They all have systemic right ventricular pressure and aortic desaturation due to right-to-left shunting through the ventricular septal defect. On the other hand, the anatomy of the right ventricular outflow tract and pulmonary arteries is variable in each patient, and approximately 15 per cent of patients have the left anterior descending coronary artery arising from the right coronary artery, precluding extensive right ventricular outflow tract reconstruction. For these reasons angiocardiography is performed preoperatively in all patients with tetralogy of Fallot. Preoperatively, the status of the entire right ventricle and pulmonary artery can be accurately assessed by ECG-gated MRI using axial, sagittal, and angled axial views (Fig. 29–3). However, these areas cannot be assessed adequately with cine MRI, because the turbulent flow through the obstructive area creates significant signal loss in the areas of the right ventricular outflow tract and the pulmonary artery. Although MRI can provide accurate functional and anatomic data in this lesion, preoperative angiography is necessary to study the coronary artery anatomy. As of yet, MRI cannot provide essential information about the distributions of the coronary arteries.

On the other hand, the combination of ECG-gated and cine MRI can completely evaluate these patients postoperatively. Important findings in tetralogy of Fallot after surgery are the anatomic status of the right ventricular outflow tract and pulmonary artery, the degree of pulmonary insufficiency, right ventricular function, and residual ventricular septal defect. MRI provides excellent visualization of the right ventricle and pulmonary artery (Fig. 29–4), and cine MRI can detect any pulmonary valve insufficiency

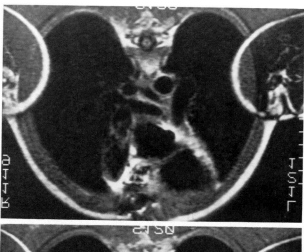

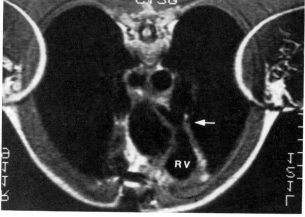

FIGURE 29–3. Tetralogy of Fallot. Sitting-up views of right ventricle (RV) and pulmonary artery obtained by ECG-gated MRI show entire RV, narrow RV outflow tract (arrow), and main pulmonary artery in lower panel and its branches in upper panel.

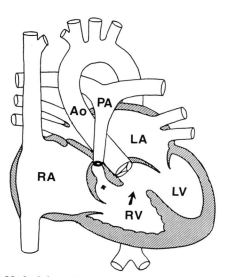

FIGURE 29–2. Schematic drawing of tetralogy of Fallot shows narrow right ventricular (RV) outflow tract (small arrow), ventricular septal defect (large arrow), overriding of the aorta (Ao), and RV hypertrophy. LA = left atrium, RA = right atrium.

(Fig. 29–5) and can assess right ventricular function (Fig. 29–6) in these patients after surgery. Spectral and color flow Doppler echocardiography can assess the residual ventricular septal defect and residual gradient across the right ventricular outflow area, whereas MRI can provide information about the anatomy and the function of the right heart. Thus, the combination of echocardiography and MRI, both noninvasive techniques, can give a complete assessment of these patients in the postoperative state.

Hypoplastic Right Heart Syndrome

The syndrome of hypoplastic right heart includes a small, underdeveloped right ventricle, pulmonary atresia with intact ventricular septum, and/or tricuspid atresia (Fig. 29–7). Since the right ventricle is invariably small in this lesion, the sizing of the true right ventricular chamber and the pulmonary artery preoperatively, and monitoring the growth of the right ventricle and patency of the pulmonary valve after the surgery are the main concerns. In patients with pulmonary atresia with intact ventricular sep-

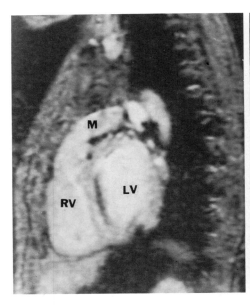 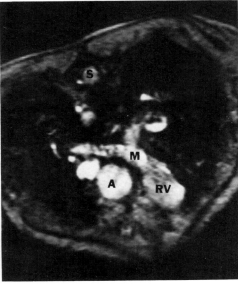

FIGURE 29–4. Sagittal *(left)* and angled axial *(right)* views in a child after surgical repair of tetralogy of Fallot show wide right ventricular (RV) outflow tract as well as main (M), right, and left pulmonary arteries. A = aorta, LV = left ventricle, S = spine.

tum, the right ventricular chamber size and the wall thickness and anatomy of the pulmonary artery are accurately measured preoperatively with MRI (Fig. 29–8). After pulmonary valvotomy, the growth of the right ventricle and the flow pattern through the pulmonic valve are also easily assessed (Fig. 29–9), and the right ventricular function data correlate well with those obtained by cardiac catheterization and angiocardiography (Fig. 29–10). In children after Fontan operation for tricuspid atresia, which is an anastomosis between the right atrium and the main pulmonary artery (Fig. 29–11), blood flow through the conduit between the right atrium and the pulmonary artery can be seen (Fig. 29–12). With further development of the cine MRI technique, allowing more quantitative flow analysis, precise functional and anatomic assessments of the results of the Fontan procedure can be expected.

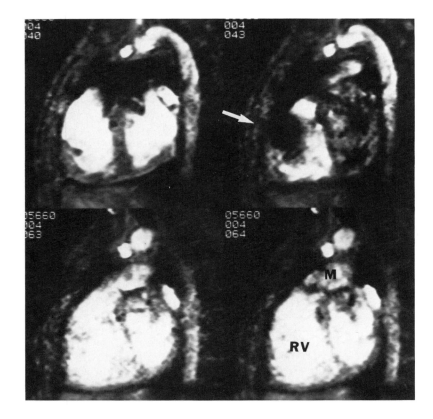

FIGURE 29–5. Four selected cine MR images are shown from a child after surgical repair of tetralogy of Fallot. Early diastolic image shows area of low signal intensity *(arrow)* extending from main pulmonary artery (M) to right ventricle (RV) due to pulmonary regurgitation.

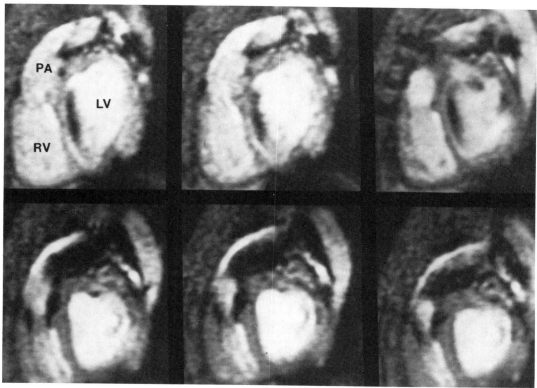

FIGURE 29–6. These cine MRI images were obtained from a one-year-old child after surgical repair of tetralogy of Fallot. Six selected images are shown from diastole *(top, left)* to systole *(bottom, right)*. The imaging sequence from diastole to systole is visible, and the ejection fraction can be obtained by measuring systolic and diastolic volumes. LV = left ventricle, PA = pulmonary artery, RV = right ventricle.

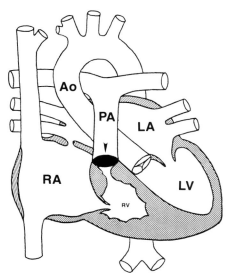

FIGURE 29–7. Schematic drawing of hypoplastic right heart syndrome. This syndrome consists of a small, underdeveloped right ventricular (RV) chamber, atretic pulmonary valve *(arrow)*, and intact ventricular septum. Tricuspid valve can be hypoplastic or atretic, but the pulmonary arteries (PA) are usually normal. Ao = aorta, LA = left atrium, LV = left ventricle, RA = right atrium. (From Chung KJ, Simpson IA, Newman R, et al: Cine MRI for evaluation of congenital heart disease: Role in pediatric cardiology compared with echocardiography and angiography. J Pediatr 113:1028–1035, 1988.)

Transposition of the Great Arteries

Systemic or pulmonary venous pathway obstruction is the most common anatomic complication of the intra atrial baffle procedure by either Mustard or Senning method for d-transposition of the great arteries (Fig. 29–13). Functional impairment such as tricuspid insufficiency and right ventricular or systemic ventricular dysfunction have been other problems after this procedure, because the right ventricle and the tricuspid valve are not structured for systemic load. Systemic and pulmonary venous pathways have been extensively evaluated by two-dimensional and Doppler echocardiography, radionuclide imaging, and digital subtraction angiography. All these techniques have drawbacks. Cine MRI has a great advantage over these modalities since it can provide information regarding vena caval (Fig. 29–14) and pulmonary venous entry anatomy after surgical repair in these children. Also, right ventricular ejection fraction can be measured (Fig. 29–15) with an accuracy that is extremely close to angiographic values. In patients with tricuspid valve insufficiency, signal loss beneath the valve is well appreciated. A recent advance in surgical technique for this lesion is an arterial switch operation using the Jatene procedure. The most common complication from this procedure

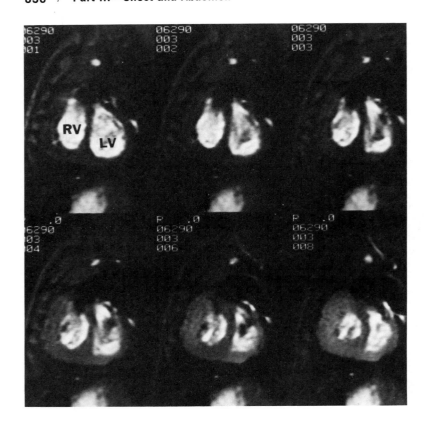

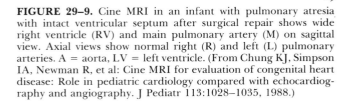

← **FIGURE 29–8.** Six selected cine images from a baby with pulmonary atresia with intact ventricular septum show a small right ventricular (RV) chamber, with no flow through the RV outflow tract. Also note marked hypertrophy of the RV wall.

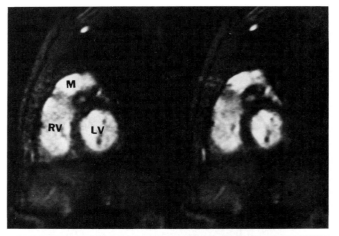

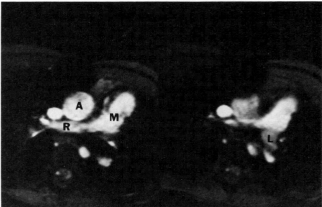

→

FIGURE 29–9. Cine MRI in an infant with pulmonary atresia with intact ventricular septum after surgical repair shows wide right ventricle (RV) and main pulmonary artery (M) on sagittal view. Axial views show normal right (R) and left (L) pulmonary arteries. A = aorta, LV = left ventricle. (From Chung KJ, Simpson IA, Newman R, et al: Cine MRI for evaluation of congenital heart disease: Role in pediatric cardiology compared with echocardiography and angiography. J Pediatr 113:1028–1035, 1988.)

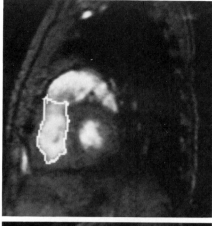

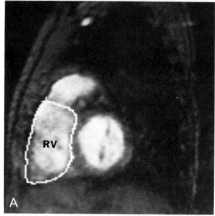

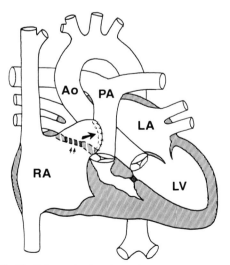

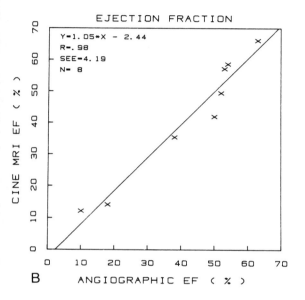

FIGURE 29–10. Right ventricular (RV) area ejection fraction (EF) is measured by planimetry of systolic *(top)* and diastolic *(bottom)* areas *(A)*, and the value correlates well with the EF obtained by angiography *(B)*.

is coronary arterial obstruction causing myocardial infarction. Using a paramagnetic agent with ultrafast MRI techniques (see Chapter 26), it may eventually prove feasible to detect early changes in the myocardium in these patients after arterial switch operation.

FIGURE 29–11. Schematic drawing of Fontan procedure shows anastomosis *(single arrow)* between right atrium (RA) and the pulmonary artery (PA). The atrial septal defect is closed *(double arrows)*. Ao = aorta, LA = left atrium, LV = left ventricle, RA = right atrium.

DISEASES OF THE GREAT ARTERIES AND VEINS

The anatomic and functional status of the great arteries and veins is extremely well defined by cine MRI, which has proved to be far superior to any other noninvasive technique currently available.

Coarctation of the Aorta

It is well recognized that two-dimensional echocardiography can diagnose and estimate the severity of coarctation of the aorta. Adequate imaging of the coarctation site is usually possible in neonates, but difficulties can arise in patients after surgery due to scarring and in older children because the distance between the ultrasound transducer and the descending aorta is greater, resulting in poorer image resolution. Doppler ultrasound has further enhanced the noninvasive assessment of these patients and has produced favorable results in predicting the pressure gradient across the coarctation. However, the pressure gradient measured across a coarctation may not necessarily reflect the degree of obstruction, since it is dependent on a number of other factors, including the length and shape of the obstruction, the amount of flow through the coarctation, and the presence and extent of collateral blood flow. As a result,

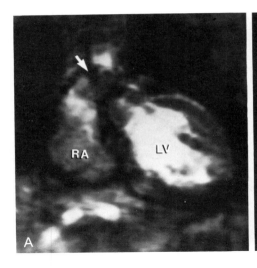 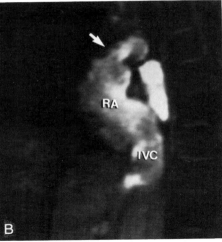

FIGURE 29–12. Coronal *(A)* and sagittal *(B)* views from a child after Fontan operation. There is slight narrowing *(arrow)* at the junction of right atrium (RA) and pulmonary artery anastomosis. IVC = inferior vena cava, LV = left ventricle.

although Doppler ultrasound can measure the pressure gradient from the peak velocity, it may not always accurately reflect the severity of coarctation, since coarctations are sometimes long segments with tortuous obstruction. In addition, confusion can arise in newborn infants with a restrictive right-to-left shunting ductus arteriosus, because this lesion can produce a flow-velocity pattern in the descending aorta that mimics coarctation.

Conventional ECG-gated MRI provides excellent visualization of structural detail in coarctation of the aorta (Fig. 29–16), but it does not give dynamic information about flow through the narrowed area and collateral circulation. On the other hand, cine MRI yields both anatomic and functional information

about coarctation of the aorta. Cine MRI performed in the sagittal or rotated sagittal plane (equivalent to left anterior oblique view) with slice locations chosen from previous localizing gated scan (Fig. 29–17) displays excellent definition of the severity of the coarctation, as well as the anatomic status of the aorta proximal and distal to the coarctation, and the status of the collateral vessels (Fig. 29–18). The anatomic severity of coarctation assessed by cine MRI was similar to that obtained by conventional angiography in our study (Fig. 29–19), but flow velocity observation added information about physiology and severity. Diastolic lucent jets from high velocity flow across

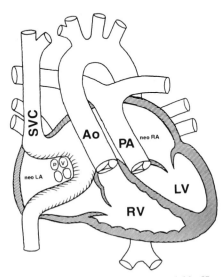

FIGURE 29–13. Schematic drawing of intraatrial baffle procedure for transposition of the great arteries. Note that the systemic venous (SVC) return is directed to the left ventricle (LV) through the neo right atrium (RA) and further to the pulmonary artery (PA). The pulmonary venous return (PV) is directed to the right ventricle (RV) through the neo left atrium (LA) and further to the aorta (Ao).

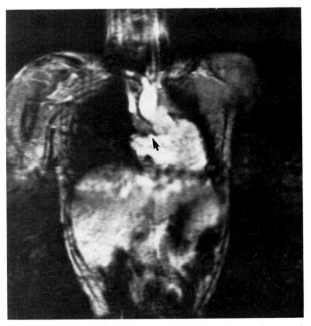

FIGURE 29–14. Cine MRI in a child after Mustard operation. Coronal image demonstrates narrowing at the junction of the superior vena cava and the right atrium *(arrow)*. A dark area is seen just above the obstruction, presumably due to turbulent flow associated with obstruction.

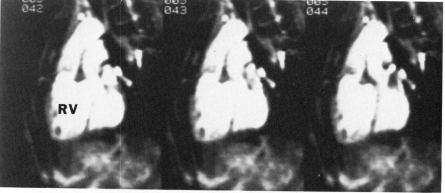

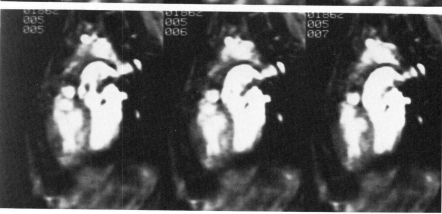

FIGURE 29–15. Sagittal cine images in a six-year-old child after intraatrial baffle procedure (Mustard operation) for transposition of the great arteries. Top, diastolic frames. Frame 42 *(top left)* is end-diastole. Bottom, systolic phases. Frame 7 *(bottom right)* is late systole. Right ventricular (RV) function can be assessed from these images. (From Chung KJ, Simpson IA, Glass RF, et al: Cine MRI in patients with transposition of the great arteries after surgical repair. Circulation 77:104–109, 1988; by permission of the American Heart Association, Inc.)

the coarctation were seen originating from the coarctation site. The lucent jets were always associated with high diastolic flow velocities. The maximum length of the lucent jets imaged on cine MRI correlated well with the coarctation severity measured by angiography and at surgery (Fig. 29–20). However, no lucent jets were identified with mild coarctation or in patients who had significant collaterals.

The capability of oblique plane imaging is essential for accurate assessment of aortic coarctation by MRI, since the sagittal view yields adequate information in less than 50 per cent of cases. In patients with severe coarctation, the anatomy of the aorta can be consid-

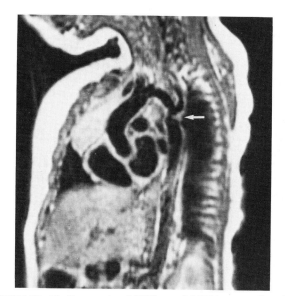

FIGURE 29–16. Conventional ECG-gated MRI in rotated sagittal view in an infant with severe coarctation of the aorta *(arrow)*. Note discrete narrowing at the site of coarctation.

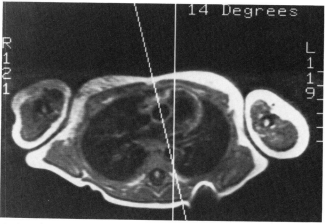

FIGURE 29–17. Axial view of ECG-gated MRI. It shows angle of rotation *(dotted line)* required to allow subsequent imaging in the plane of the aorta, with the line transecting the ascending and descending portions of the aorta in cross-section. (From Simpson IA, Chung KJ, Glass RF, et al: Cine MRI for evaluation of anatomy and flow relationships in infants and children with coarctation of the aorta. Circulation 78:142–148, 1988; by permission of the American Heart Association, Inc.)

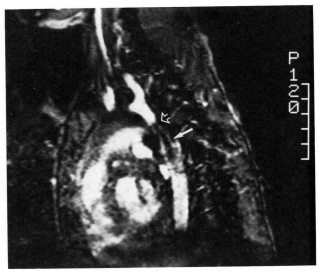

FIGURE 29–18. Stop frame of a cine MRI sequence from a child with coarctation of the aorta shows discrete narrowing *(open arrow)* in the descending thoracic aorta just distal to the subclavian artery take-off, and the lucent high velocity jet *(white arrow)* originating from the coarctation site and extending distally into the descending aorta. (From Simpson IA, Chung KJ, Glass RF, et al: Cine MRI for evaluation of anatomy and flow relationships in infants and children with coarctation of the aorta. Circulation 78:142–148, 1988; by permission of the American Heart Association, Inc.)

erably distorted, and the versatility of oblique imaging is necessary. The signal void produced by the vascular clips often used at the surgical repair site is an important consideration. Recently, vascular clips have been avoided or replaced by nonmetallic clips, if necessary, thus eliminating the possibility of false signal loss.

The high resolution real-time imaging and dynamic spatial and temporal velocity information now

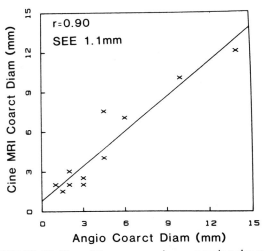

FIGURE 29–19. Plot of linear regression comparing the smallest flow diameter at the coarctation site on cine MRI with the diameter measured at angiography. (From Simpson IA, Chung KJ, Glass RF, et al: Cine MRI for evaluation of anatomy and flow relationships in infants and children with coarctation of the aorta. Circulation 78:142–148, 1988; by permission of the American Heart Association, Inc.)

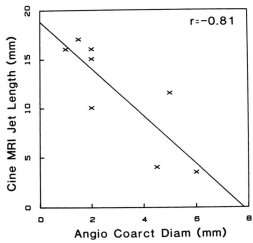

FIGURE 29–20. Graph of linear regression comparison of the maximum jet length of the lucent high velocity jets on cine MRI with the severity of coarctation of the aorta at angiography. (From Simpson IA, Chung KJ, Glass RF, et al: Cine MRI for evaluation of anatomy and flow relationships in infants and children with coarctation of the aorta. Circulation 78:142–148, 1988; by permission of the American Heart Association, Inc.)

provided by echocardiography make it unlikely that MRI will replace ultrasound as the primary noninvasive method for assessment of coarctation of the aorta in newborn infants and neonates. MRI will be used for patients in whom further information with respect to anatomic detail and flow relationships is required after echocardiographic examination to confirm the echo findings, and in cases in which the echocardiogram gives incomplete information. It has a more important role in older infants and children and in serial follow-up of patients after surgical repair of coarctation, because echocardiographic examination can be quite difficult in these patients.

Pulmonary Artery Banding for Ventricular Septal Defect or Single Ventricle

Pulmonary artery banding is a common palliative surgical procedure for young infants with large or multiple ventricular septal defects or single ventricle with complex cardiac anatomy. The subsequent clinical course of these patients and their ultimate surgical options are determined by the band providing adequate protection of pulmonary vasculature from the development of pulmonary vascular disease, and by the patient's ability to grow in the absence of ongoing congestive heart failure. Problems related to the postoperative results of pulmonary artery banding usually are associated with loosening of the band and/or its migration and displacement toward the branch pulmonary arteries or pulmonary valve. The slippage or displacement can cause preferential obstruction with distortion of one branch pulmonary artery and unobstructed flow in the other or valvular dysfunction. Therefore, noninvasive evaluation of the pulmonary artery band is very important. Accurate evaluation of the status of a pulmonary artery band must be made on a serial basis with respect to its anatomy or position.

Cine MRI provides accurate, high-resolution anatomic definition of the pulmonary artery and pulmonary artery bands in young infants as well as valuable information about flow dynamics proximal and distal to the band (Fig. 29–21). As a planar technique, cine MRI assesses the narrowest diameter of the band probably better than angiography. Whereas similar high-resolution detail of the position and anatomy of the band can be obtained using conventional ECG-gated MRI (Fig. 29–22), the cine technique gives additional functional information by imaging flow through and distal to the band. The pressure gradient between the right ventricle and the main pulmonary artery measured at the cardiac catheterization has correlated well with the narrowest flow diameter across the band on cine MRI (Fig. 29–23). Accurate estimation of the pressure gradient across the band can be obtained using continuous wave Doppler. The combination of cine MRI and Doppler echocardiogram offers an excellent alternative to cardiac catheterization and angiography for establishing the status of the pulmonary artery band,

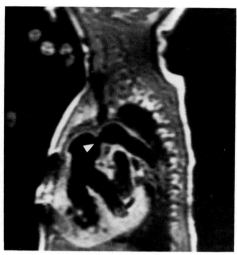

FIGURE 29–22. ECG-gated MRI in sagittal view in an infant after pulmonary artery (PA) banding shows discrete narrowing *(arrowhead)* at the site of banding.

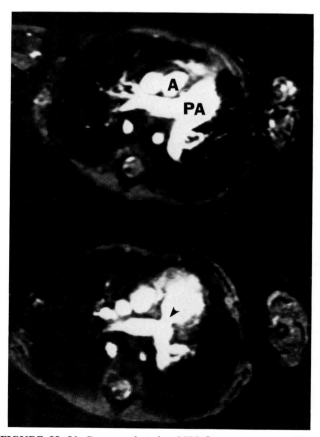

FIGURE 29–21. Preoperative cine MRI from a neonate with a large ventricular septal defect and congestive heart failure shows large pulmonary artery (PA) on axial view *(top)*. Cine MRI obtained from the same baby 3 months after PA banding shows a discrete narrowing *(arrow)* at the midportion of the main PA due to previous banding *(bottom)*. A = aorta.

and also serves as an aid to appropriate patient management without need for invasive investigation.

Other abnormalities of the aorta and systemic or pulmonary venous system were evaluated, and cine MRI provided useful information, especially for the pulmonary venous return (Fig. 29–24).

LEFT HEART AND SHUNT LESIONS

Magnetic resonance imaging does provide some useful information of left heart lesions, such as hypertrophic cardiomyopathy, dilated cardiomyopathy, and discrete subaortic stenosis. It is of very limited value for assessing the severity of valvular aortic stenosis due to signal loss during the systolic phase of the cardiac cycle. Extensive work has been done to assess the regurgitant volumes in patients with mitral and aortic regurgitation. So far, cine MRI has been able to provide quantitative information of valvular regurgitation comparable to that obtained by color Doppler echocardiography, but the precise quantitative data are not available at the present time. In patients with ventricular or atrial septal defects, and in those with patent ductus arteriosus, cine MRI does not add much more information to that obtained from two-dimensional and Doppler echocardiography. However, the precise anatomy of the pulmonary arteries by cine MRI can effectively rule out any pathology, and that added information may obviate an invasive procedure (Fig. 29–25).

DISCUSSION

Cine MRI alone can provide accurate and complete imaging of anatomy and flow relationships in patients

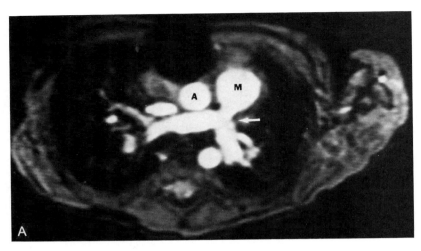

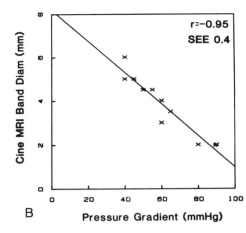

FIGURE 29–23. Linear regression analysis comparing the diameter of the pulmonary artery band *(arrow)* on cine MRI *(A)* to the pressure gradient across the band *(B)*. The narrowest flow diameter across the band on cine MRI correlated well with the pressure gradient between the right ventricle and pulmonary artery.

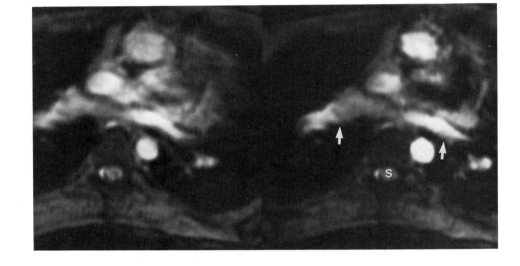

FIGURE 29–24. Axial views show normal right and left pulmonary venous return. The arrows point to pulmonary veins. S = spine.

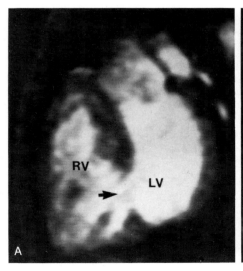

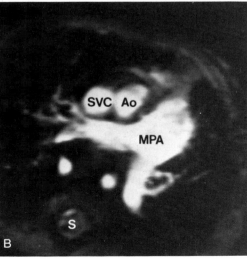

FIGURE 29–25. A, A stop frame of cine MRI in the sagittal view shows a large ventricular septal defect *(arrow)*. B, An axial view demonstrates enlarged main (MPA) and branch pulmonary arteries due to increased left-to-right shunt through a large ventricular septal defect. AO = aorta; LV = left ventricle, RV = right ventricle, SVC = superior vena cava.

with congenital cardiac defects, since it allows multiplanar imaging of the heart and great vessels. Cine MRI uses a new pulse sequence with small flip angle and gradient-refocused echoes.[23-25] Unlike its appearance on conventional ECG-gated MRI, flowing blood has bright signal compared with that of myocardium on cine MRI. Because the myocardium is relatively stationary in the slice being imaged, it is continuously reexcited by the rapid radiofrequency pulses, its spins never fully recover between successive excitations, and, therefore, the myocardium stays saturated and returns little signal. Because of its rapid flowing motion, the blood, however, is not saturated and returns a very bright signal. Through this mechanism, laminar blood flow appears much brighter than the myocardium in cine mode and yields excellent contrast between the two.

Abnormalities of the heart and great vessels have been studied by two-dimensional and Doppler echocardiography, radionuclide imaging, and digital subtraction angiography.[26-32] All of these techniques have drawbacks. Echocardiography has excellent spatial resolution for identifying anatomic detail, but its tomographic nature and limited depth resolution restrict its value in visualizing extracardiac structures, particularly when they are distant from the transducer. Also, imaging with two-dimensional echocardiography may be limited in patients after median sternotomy for surgical repair because of its scarring process. However, Doppler echocardiography provides estimates of hemodynamic data in a quantitative form not yet available with cine MRI. Radionuclide imaging is a sensitive detector of physiologic data, but it gives suboptimal spatial orientation and anatomic detail, and it also requires injection of radioactive isotopes. Digital subtraction angiography provides efficient use of x-rays and excellent quality images, but its invasive nature and the amount of radiation required are disadvantages in small children. Cine MRI, the newest imaging technique, can now provide not only accurate anatomy of cardiac structures but also functional, noninvasive assessment of the cardiac chambers and walls and flow relationships.[16-21] The major advantage of cine MRI over other noninvasive methods is that it has no limitation of imaging planes, nor are technical difficulties encountered due to a small cardiac window or previous chest surgery. Also, unlike the cine CT technique, it requires no injection of contrast media and does not involve radiation. The quality of the images we obtained was further enhanced by studying the younger patients either in the head or knee coil.

We are able to obtain good-quality images with cine MRI for anatomic and functional analysis of cardiac chambers and great vessels in 95 per cent of the patients with congenital heart disease before and after surgical repair. The anatomy of right ventricular outflow tract and pulmonary arteries is comparable to that in the images obtained by cineangiography and is far superior to echocardiography. The status of great artery relationships is accurately assessed, but echocardiography also is diagnostic in this regard. Structures outside the cardiac chambers, such as the vena cava and pulmonary venous systems are evaluated better by cine MRI than by echocardiography. The high-resolution real-time imaging and dynamic spatial and temporal velocity information now provided by two-dimensional and color flow Doppler mapping make it unlikely that cine MRI will have a significant clinical impact on the assessment of intracardiac lesions, such as atrial and ventricular septal defects. However, difficulties can arise with ultrasound imaging after surgical repair and in older children, especially in imaging extracardiac structures and venous and arterial anatomy. The site and the severity of coarctation of the aorta can be readily evaluated with cine MRI, and this technique is extremely useful for both pre- and postoperative states.

Cine MRI is in its early stage of development and still has several drawbacks. Cine MRI provides superb anatomic detail, but assessing cardiac function may be limited because images are not acquired in real-time, and their acquisition is somewhat time consuming. The information is compiled from cumulative data from 128 cardiac cycles, but it simulates real-time cardiac imaging like radionuclide angiography, and functional analysis comparable to angiography can be achieved.

In conclusion, our preliminary experience suggests that cine MRI can provide anatomic and functional information equivalent to cineangiography. It produces dynamic, high-resolution, and flow-enhanced images that are inherently volumetric in any desired plane through the heart and great vessels. It is particularly applicable to small children, since it is entirely noninvasive and uses no radiation yet provides sufficient data for patient management. Cine MRI carries a clean safety record so far.[33] Its only drawback at the present time is that it cannot estimate pressures and resistances, knowledge of which may be necessary for proper management in certain patients with complex cardiac lesions. Cine MRI, however, will not replace echocardiography, which is well-

TABLE 29–1. COMPARISON OF MRI AND ECHOCARDIOGRAPHY: RELATIVE STRENGTHS AND ADVANTAGES

	MRI	Echocardiogram
Anatomic	Great arteries and veins, right heart lesions, post-operative	VSD, ASD, PDA, left heart lesions
Functional	Volumetric: ideal, impractical now	Global, practical
Valvular regurgitation	Qualitative	Qualitative
Valvular stenosis	Not useful	Quantitative
Pericardium	Effusion, mass constrictive pericarditis	Effusion
Miscellaneous	Spectroscopy: future potential, expensive	Bedside examination, economical

established and an important part of a diagnostic sequence for assessing congenital heart disease (Table 29–1). With the complementary information from echocardiography and cine MRI, we are now close to providing a comprehensive noninvasive assessment of congenital heart disease. Certainly, serial angiography for evaluating chamber growth and postoperative function is no longer required. We believe the combined use of echocardiography and cine MRI will play an increasingly important role in pediatric cardiology.

REFERENCES

1. Higgins CB: Overview of MR of the heart. AJR 146:907–918, 1986.
2. Byrd BF, Schiller NB, Botvinick EH, Higgins CB: Normal cardiac dimensions by magnetic resonance imaging. Am J Cardiol 55:1440–1442, 1985.
3. Markiewicz W, Sechtem U, Higgins CB: Evaluation of the right ventricle by magnetic resonance imaging. Am Heart J 113:8–15, 1987.
4. Buckwater KA, Aisen AM, Dilworth LR, et al: Gated cardiac MRI: Ejection fraction determination by using the right anterior oblique view. AJR 147:33–37, 1986.
5. Stratemeier EJ, Thompson R, Brady TJ, et al: Ejection fraction determination by MR imaging: Comparison with left ventricular angiography. Radiology 158:775–777, 1986.
6. Kaul S, Wismer GL, Brady TJ, et al: Measurement of normal left heart dimensions using optimally oriented MR images. AJR 146:75–79, 1986.
7. Fisher MR, vonSchulthess GK, Higgins CB: Multiphase cardiac magnetic resonance imaging: Normal regional left ventricular wall thickening. AJR 145:27–30, 1985.
8. Higgins CB, Byrd BF, Farmer DW, et al: Magnetic resonance imaging in patients with congenital heart disease. Circulation 70:851–860, 1984.
9. Didier D, Higgins CB, Fisher MR, et al: Congenital heart disease: Gated MR imaging in 72 patients. Radiology 158:227–235, 1986.
10. Fletcher BD, Jacobstein MD, Nelson AD, et al: Gated magnetic resonance imaging of congenital cardiac malformations. Radiology 150:137–140, 1984.
11. Boxer RA, Singh S, LaCorte MA, et al: Cardiac magnetic resonance imaging in children with congenital heart disease. J Pediatrics 109:460–464, 1986.
12. Jacobstein MD, Fletcher BD, Nelson AD, et al: Magnetic resonance imaging: Evaluation of palliative systemic-pulmonary artery shunt. Circulation 70:650–656, 1984.
13. Kersting-Sommerhoff BA, Sechtem UP, et al: MR imaging of congenital anomalies of the aortic arch. AJR 143:1192–1194, 1984.
14. Bank ER, Aisen AM, Rocchini AP, Hernandez RJ: Coarctation of the aorta in children undergoing angioplasty: Pretreatment and posttreatment MR imaging. Radiology 162:235–240, 1987.
15. Amparo EG, Higgins CB, Shafton EP: Demonstration of coarctation of the aorta by magnetic resonance imaging. AJR 143:1192–1194, 1984.
16. Chung KJ, Simpson IA, Glass RF, et al: Cine magnetic resonance imaging in patients with transposition of the great arteries after surgical repair. Circulation 77:104–109, 1988.
17. Simpson IA, Chung KJ, Glass RF, et al: Cine magnetic resonance imaging for evaluation of anatomy and flow relationships in infants and children with coarctation of the aorta. Circulation 78:142–148, 1988.
18. Sechtem U, Pflugfelder P, Cassidy MC, et al: Ventricular septal defect: Visualization of shunt flow and determination of shunt size by cine MR imaging. AJR 149:689–692, 1987.
19. Sechtem U, Pflugfelder P, White RD, et al: Cine MR imaging: Potential for the evaluation of cardiovascular function. AJR 148:239–246, 1987.
20. Utz JA, Herfkens RJ, Heinsimer JA, et al: Cine MR determination of left ventricular ejection fraction. AJR 148:839–843, 1987.
21. Sechtem U, Pflugfelder PW, Gould RG, et al: Measurement of right and left ventricular volumes in healthy individuals with cine MR imaging. Radiology 163:697–670, 1987.
22. Chung KJ, Simpson IA, Newman R, et al: Cine magnetic resonance imaging for evaluation of congenital heart disease: Role in pediatric cardiology compared with echocardiography and angiography. J Pediatrics 113:1028–1035, 1988.
23. Fralm J, Haase A, Mathaei D: Rapid three-dimensional MR imaging using the FLASH technique. J Comput Assist Tomogr 10:363–368, 1986.
24. Wehrli FW: Introduction to fast-scan magnetic resonance. General Electric, 1986, Milwaukee, Wisconsin.
25. Haase A, Mathaei D, Hanicke W: FLASH imaging: Rapid NMR imaging using low-flip angle pulses. J Magn Reson 67:258–266, 1986.
26. Silverman NA, Snider R, Colo J, et al: Superior vena caval obstruction after Mustard operation: Detection by two-dimensional contrast echocardiography. Circulation 64:392–396, 1981.
27. Chin AJ, Sanders SP, Williams RG, et al: Two-dimensional echocardiographic assessment of caval and pulmonary venous pathways after the Senning operation. Am J Cardiol 52:118–126, 1983.
28. Keane JF, Williams R, Treves S, et al: Assessment of the postoperative patient by non-invasive techniques. Prog Cardiovasc Dis 18:57–74, 1975.
29. Hurwitz RA, Papaincolaon N, Treves S, et al: Radionuclide angiography in evaluation of patients after repair of transposition of the great arteries. Am J Cardiol 49:761–765, 1982.
30. Torso SD, Kelly MJ, Kalff V, Venables AW: Radionuclide assessment of ventricular contraction at rest and during exercise following the Fontan procedure for either tricuspid atresia or single ventricle. Am J Cardiol 55:1127–1132, 1985.
31. Hagler DJ, Seward JB, Tajik AJ, Ritter DJ: Functional assessment of the Fontan operation: Combined M-mode, two-dimensional and Doppler echocardiographic studies. J Am Coll Cardiol 4:756–764, 1984.
32. Chung KJ, Hesselink JR, Chernoff HL, et al: Digital subtraction angiography in patients with transposition of the great arteries after Senning repair. J Am Coll Cardiol 5:113–117, 1985.
33. Shellock FG: Biological effects of MRI: A clean safety record so far. Diag Imag 9:96–101, 1987.

30

MR IMAGING OF THE UPPER ABDOMEN AND ADRENAL GLANDS

ROBERT MATTREY, MICHAEL TRAMBERT, and ROBERT R. EDELMAN

GENERAL APPROACH TO IMAGING THE UPPER ABDOMEN

   OPTIMIZING SPATIAL AND CONTRAST RESOLUTION

   MOTION ARTIFACTS

   Respiratory Gating
   Phase Reordering
   Signal Averaging
   Surface Coil Imaging
   Breath Holding

   BOWEL MOTION AND SIGNAL

   OUR IMAGING APPROACH FOR THE UPPER ABDOMEN

LIVER

   INTRODUCTION

   GENERAL INDICATIONS

   IMAGING STRATEGIES

   Pulsing Sequence
   Imaging Planes

   NORMAL ANATOMY

   LIVER PATHOLOGY

   Malignant Masses
   Benign Masses
   Hemorrhage
   Infiltrative Disorders
   Inflammatory Disease
   Hepatic Vascular Disease

   ROLE OF MRI IN LESION DETECTION

BILIARY TREE

PANCREAS

   PULSE SEQUENCES

   ANATOMY

   FOCAL MASSES/INFLAMMATION

ADRENAL GLANDS

   PULSE SEQUENCES

   ANATOMY

   MASSES

   OUR APPROACH TO THE WORK-UP OF ADRENAL LESIONS

SPLEEN

CONCLUSION

Significant strides have been made toward a wider acceptance of magnetic resonance imaging of the upper abdomen. Whereas its ultimate role continues to be defined, its impact on liver, biliary tree, spleen, pancreas, and adrenal imaging has been impeded by several technical difficulties that have placed MRI second in line to CT or sonography. The latter well-established modalities are not only efficacious in assessing these structures but are also more accessible, less expensive, and have enjoyed wider acceptance among referring physicians.

This chapter is intended to highlight the present capabilities and limitations of MR imaging of the upper abdomen—the technically most challenging region to image—and to describe an imaging approach to minimize artifacts and maximize accuracy. It is also intended to present the reader with the normal MR appearance of organs in this region along with some commonly encountered pathologic conditions. It should be emphasized that advances in MRI on both technical and clinical fronts affect the field on a monthly basis, requiring reassessment of MRI's role in abdominal imaging. The advent of fast MRI and contrast media, for example, could eliminate some of MRI's limitations and add further capabilities. It is necessary, therefore, to keep an open mind when discussing the limitations of MRI, for such limitations may be temporary.

GENERAL APPROACH TO IMAGING THE UPPER ABDOMEN

The optimal pulsing sequences used to image each organ are discussed in their respective sections. Here, the approach to imaging the upper abdomen, which is aimed at minimizing artifacts and optimizing contrast, is highlighted. In this section, a short discussion on oral contrast agents is also presented.

OPTIMIZING SPATIAL AND CONTRAST RESOLUTION

Unless a surface coil is used, there is no hope for body MRI to compete with the spatial resolution of CT. However, the high contrast resolution afforded by MRI makes up for this deficit in most clinical settings.

Image quality is a balance of spatial and contrast resolution and acquisition time. An acquisition matrix of 256 × 256 is rarely used at our institution since, compared with 128 phase-encoding steps, the 256 phase-encoding steps decrease the signal-to-noise (S/N) ratio and double the acquisition time, precluding the use of multiple signal averages. Less signal averaging increases the conspicuity of motion-related ghost artifacts. Slice thickness of less than 10 mm is reserved for unusual circumstances in which high spatial resolution as well as contrast resolution are required. Thinning the slice by half decreases the signal by half without affecting imaging time. A field-of-view below 30 cm is rarely used, because of wrap-around. Also, a decrease from 35 to 30 cm, which produces slight improvement in spatial resolution (pixel width decreases from 1.4 to 1.2 mm), decreases the S/N ratio by 27 per cent.

To obtain T_2-weighted images with optimal contrast, it may be necessary to prescribe a wide interslice gap or to obtain the slices interleaved. This is because the 180-degree slice-select radiofrequency (RF) pulse of the spin-echo sequence is not a perfect square wave, thus radiating tissues outside the slice; this phenomenon is called cross-talk[1, 2] (see Chapter 2). The untimely excitation of these tissues shortens the effective repetition time (TR). A shorter TR decreases signal and increases T_1 weighting.[3] The effect of cross-talk on signal and contrast is shown in Figure 30–1. As can be seen, cross-talk affects tissues with long T_1 such as water, tumors, abscesses, and so forth. It occurs in all MR systems; however, the degree of cross-talk is specific to each system. Since the minimum interslice gap required to achieve maximum signal varies from system to system, the effect of interslice gap on signal should be determined as part of quality assurance.

When imaging a region of interest, the region must be located at isocenter or be centered within the imaging volume to ensure proper contrast resolution. Since RF power needed to achieve a 90-degree tip angle is optimized over the central slice, significant

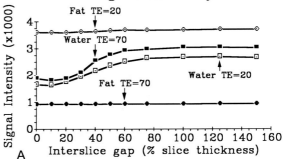

Effect of Interslice Gap on Signal Intensity

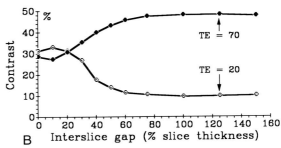

Effect of Interslice Gap on Fat/Water Contrast

FIGURE 30–1. The effect of interslice gap on signal and contrast was evaluated using two cylinders, one filled with water and the other with oil, placed in the magnet parallel to the static field and imaged transaxially (2000/20 and 70 msec) with 10-mm slice thickness using the body coil. Eleven series were obtained each with a different interslice gap (0 to 150 per cent slice thickness).

A, Fat and water signal, measured over the central slice, are shown as a function of interslice gap. While fat signal (material with short T_1) was unaffected by variations in the interslice gap, water signal (material with long T_1) increased by 50 per cent when the gap increased from 0 to 60 per cent slice thickness. *B,* Fat/water contrast calculated from *(A)* as the difference of fat and water signal divided by their sum and shown as a function of interslice gap. Note that since fat was unaffected, contrast decreased at TE = 20 (less T_1 weighting) and increased at TE = 70 (more T_2 weighting). (From Schwaighofer BW, Yu K, Mattrey RF: Diagnostic significance of interslice gap and imaging volume. AJR [in press].)

signal loss may occur as slices become further removed from the central slice owing to less optimal RF power.[3] RF power becomes suboptimal away from the central slice because of inhomogeneities in the RF and magnetic fields, and because the mix of tissues contained in the slice may differ (more or less air, and so forth). The effect of slice position on signal is shown in Figure 30–2. It can be observed that: (1) the fat and water signals decrease equally and gradually from the central slice outward in either direction; (2) there is 10 per cent signal loss by the twelfth centimeter and 30 per cent loss by the twentieth centimeter; (3) the effect is asymmetric when comparing the trailing and leading halves for an unknown reason. Therefore, on our system the maximum acceptable volume that can be scanned is 24 cm. This effect will be system-dependent. Whereas it

Percent Change in Signal From Isocenter

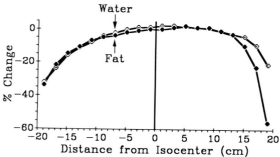

FIGURE 30–2. Effect of slice position on signal. Using the same phantom described in Figure 30–1, a transaxial series was obtained (2000/20 and 70) with 10-mm slice thickness, 100 per cent interslice gap, and an imaging volume of 40 cm (from −20 to +20 cm from isocenter). Fat and water signals measured on every slice are shown as a function of distance from isocenter. Note the asymmetric behavior over the leading and trailing halves. Also note that fat and water signals decrease equally (no effect on contrast) and remain within 10 per cent over the central 25-cm imaging volume. Signals on slices obtained beyond 12.5 cm from the central slice deteriorate significantly. (From Schwaighofer BW, Yu K, Mattrey RF: Diagnostic significance or interslice gap and imaging volume. AJR [in press].)

is tempting in abdominal imaging to cover as much distance as possible, top of liver to midpelvis for example, interpreting contrast on the first and last few slices should be done with caution (Fig. 30–3).

MOTION ARTIFACTS

Motion is a major problem in abdominal imaging because it produces blurring and ghost artifacts (see Chapter 3). These artifacts may dominate other noise sources[4] and, when severe, render the study nondiagnostic. Ghost artifacts occur in MR because of the use of two-dimensional Fourier methods for spatial localization, which propagates ghosts of moving structures in the phase-encoded direction due to the introduction of phase errors. Ghosting occurs with motion of any structure but becomes perceptible when structures have sufficient contrast with adjacent tissues, such as liver or bowel and fat. When projected over the liver, they may obscure liver texture or even produce focal abnormalities simulating masses (Fig. 30–4). Through several years of experience with reconstructed images we have learned to tone down conclusions when faced with images riddled with artifacts. While it may be easy to recognize motion when ghosts streak the image, motion on MRI can cause a more subtle effect that may go unnoticed, providing a false sense of security. This imperceptible artifact is produced in part by motion of low contrast structures which blurs the image and reduces the contrast-to-noise ratio. The other subtle effect of

motion is increased partial volume averaging. Since the sampling volume during data acquisition is occupied, for example, by a liver lesion part of the time and by the liver the other part, its resultant intensity is a weighted average of the two tissues. Therefore, small low contrast lesions that have diameter equal to or less than liver excursion during respiration may become obscured. To enhance the visibility of small lesions, their contrast with liver must be increased, as has been noted for example when the liver was made dark with ferrite particles.[5]

There are several approaches to minimize image degradation from motion, though none is particularly effective in uncooperative or dyspneic patients. Techniques to reduce motion artifacts are presented here in brief but are addressed in more detail in Chapter 3.

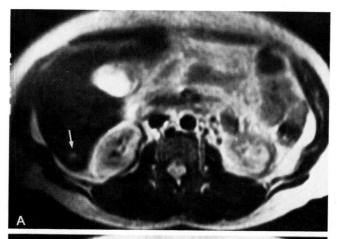

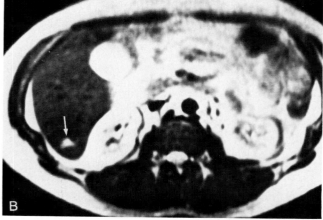

FIGURE 30–3. T₂-weighted images both obtained with identical parameters over a presumed hemangioma *(arrow)* and photographed with similar window and level. (TR = 2000, TE = 70, 256 × 128 matrix, 10-mm slice thickness, 50 per cent interslice gap, and 4 excitations). *A,* Slice position is at −11 cm from isocenter. Isocenter was located just caudal to sacral promontory. *B,* Slice position was at +8 cm from isocenter. Isocenter was located at midliver. Note increased contrast and sharpness when compared with *(A).* (From Schwaighofer BW, Yu K, Mattrey RF: Diagnostic significance or interslice gap and imaging volume. AJR [in press].)

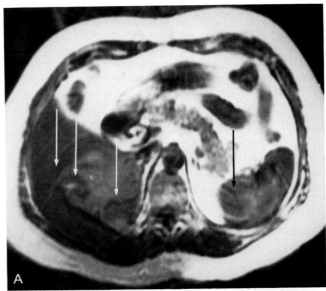

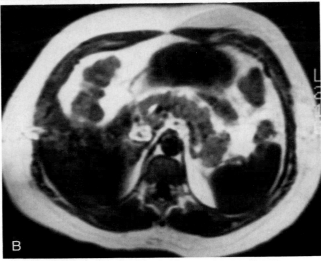

FIGURE 30–4. Ghosts from bowel can mimic lesions. *A*, Apparent liver and splenic lesions were produced by ghosts from bowel anterior to liver and spleen (phase-encoded direction is anteroposterior). Note that fat and bowel relationship anterior to liver was duplicated over liver. *B*, Lesions were eliminated when the phase-encode direction was oriented right/left.

Respiratory Gating

Degradation from respiratory motion can be eliminated by the use of true respiratory gating. This can be achieved by timing data acquisition to the respiratory cycle or by limiting data acquisition to one phase of respiration. Like cardiac gating, organs will be essentially "frozen" in a single position. However, unlike cardiac gating, the respiratory cycle is too long, resulting in up to four-fold increase in acquisition time.[6] Since this is not practical, respiratory gating can be used to eliminate deep breaths and sighs.

Phase Reordering

Ghosting is caused by a modulation in the phase direction produced by rhythmic or periodic motion. Therefore, if data collection in the phase direction is randomized relative to the respiratory cycle, periodicity is reduced.[7] Like respiratory gating methods, phase-reordering methods (e.g., ROPE, COPE, EXORCIST) require the use of a respiratory monitor but make efficient use of data, increasing acquisition time only slightly (typically <15 per cent). While phase reordering reduces ghost artifacts, it does not affect motion-induced blurring or partial volume averaging.

Signal Averaging

The intensity of ghost artifacts decreases with increased signal averages, resulting in marked improvement in image detail.[8] The use of eight or more excitations requires the use of a short TR to permit such acquisition to be completed within a reasonable time period (10 minutes or less).[9] However, gradient hardware limitations, pulse sequence design, or power deposition may preclude obtaining adequate numbers of slices to span the liver. Furthermore, since time constraints preclude the use of long TR, more than four excitations with 128 phase encodes cannot be used for T_2-weighted acquisitions.

Surface Coil Imaging

By having the patient lie on a flat surface coil, the dependent tissues "seen" by the limited field-of-view of the coil become relatively immobile. Since the mobile nondependent abdominal wall is in the far field, it reduces ghost artifacts. Surface coil imaging has been used to produce high resolution images of the liver (Fig. 30–5).[10] However, the limited field-of-view makes it impossible to screen the entire liver in a timely manner.

Breath Holding

Breath holding eliminates ghost artifacts, blurring, and motion-related partial volume averaging; however, slices must be imaged within 15 seconds. Methods have been described that permit MR images to be obtained in seconds and even milliseconds, rather than minutes, by the use of gradient-echo, rather than spin-echo, techniques.[11] These techniques are described in detail in Chapter 5. The impact of such techniques and the optimal sequences that increase lesion detection remain undetermined but hold great promise.

BOWEL MOTION AND SIGNAL

Respiration and peristalsis cause significant excursion of bowel loops. Since bowel is adjacent to fat,

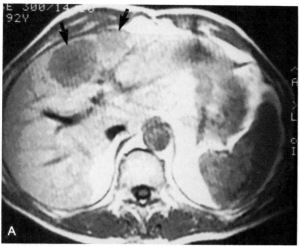

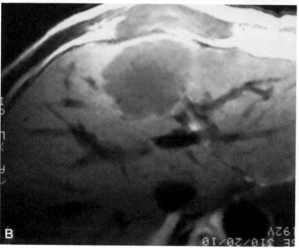

FIGURE 30–5. Spatial resolution can be markedly improved by using surface coil images. *A,* Short TR/short TE T_1-weighted body coil image at low field (pixel dimensions = 3.6 mm × 1.8 mm) demonstrates two superficial lesions *(arrows). B,* High resolution surface coil image (pixel dimensions = 0.9 mm × 0.9 mm), obtained with the same parameters but with the patient prone to restrain motion of the anterior abdominal wall, more sharply delineates the lesions as well as branching hepatic vessels.

ghosting from such interfaces, as well as blurring, can be observed. Peristaltic activity is effectively controlled with 1 mg glucagon (Fig. 30–6). Whereas its use is limited to select cases at some centers, it is routinely administered to all patients at our institution and others. Some administer glucagon intramuscularly, others subcutaneously. Since the long TR sequence is performed immediately following the T_1-weighted localizer, and since glucagon action, when given subcutaneously, begins in 4 to 6 minutes and lasts 20 minutes, its effect is maximized during the long acquisition time. Note, however, that glucagon is not totally benign. It is contraindicated in diabetic patients and can cause gastrointestinal and other symptoms in as many as 30 per cent of cases during the first few hours after administration.[12]

On all pulsing sequences, bowel loops can have an intensity similar to normal or abnormal tissues depending on their fluid and air content. Detailed evaluation of the bowel wall and lumen is precluded by peristaltic motion. However, with rapid MR imaging artifacts due to peristalsis are minimized, allowing a more clear delineation of bowel as air-containing structures than would be the case for longer conventional acquisitions. On rapid gradient-echo images, bowel loops appear as dark tubular structures with an outer dark ring, the latter representing a magnetic susceptibility boundary effect between air in the bowel lumen and the surrounding soft tissues (Fig. 30–7). However, magnetic susceptibility effects, which increase with increasing field strength, can also generate major artifacts that can limit interpretation of the image (Fig. 30–8). This problem is minimized by the use of thin slices and very short echo times (TEs) (e.g., 5 msec).

As with computed tomography, optimal MR visualization of normal and abnormal structures in the abdomen requires an effective oral contrast agent. Whereas oral contrast may not be necessary in many patients evaluated for liver or spleen pathology, left lobe lesions could be confused with stomach (Fig. 30–9), right lobe lesions with hepatic flexure, and spleen with stomach and small bowel, particularly in thin patients. Paramagnetic agents such as iron solutions (e.g., 500 cc dilute Geritol) or gadolinium–diethylene triamine pentaacetic acid (Gd-DTPA) increase the signal intensity from bowel.[13–15] Since their effect on signal intensity is dependent upon their concentration, bowel content affects their performance beyond the duodenum. The increase in bowel signal on both T_1- and T_2-weighted images may not only increase peristaltic ghost artifacts but may allow the confusion of bowel with fat or blood. We believe that darkening bowel on T_1- and particularly on T_2-weighted images would be more effective in highlighting abnormal regions, since the latter would become the only bright areas on the image. Gas, administered via effervescent tablets, only provides transitory contrast unless administered in conjunction with glucagon.[16] Gas administered in this fashion increases peristalsis and is less effective in the small bowel. The administration of magnetite destroys local magnetic field homogeneity, shortening T_2 and lowering signal from bowel.[17, 18] However, since it is given as a suspension, its effect is also dependent upon bowel content, making it less effective in the small bowel.[18]

We have described and tested the use of perfluorochemicals in animals and man.[19] Perfluorooctylbromide (PFOB), which is investigational at present, does not contain any hydrogen atoms and therefore appears as a signal void within bowel. It is heavier and immiscible with water, and therefore its effect is independent of bowel content (Fig. 30–10). Furthermore, PFOB has a fast transit through the bowel without added peristalses, owing to its low surface tension, thus requiring less volume and time to achieve distal bowel filling. Five hundred to 600 ml

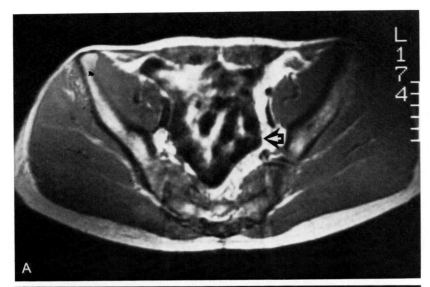

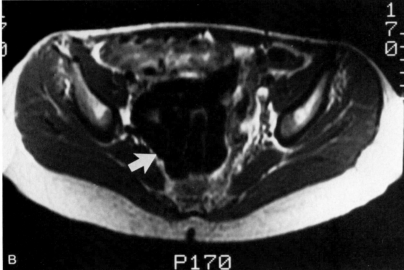

FIGURE 30–6. Effect of glucagon on image sharpness shown in two patients given perfluorooctylbromide (PFOB) orally, one without *(A)* and the other after 1 mg glucagon *(B)* given subcutaneously. *A,* Hydrogen density–weighted image (2000/20) obtained 30 minutes after ingesting 500 ml of PFOB. Note darkening of distal bowel *(arrow),* fuzzy bowel margins, and ghost artifacts anterior of abdominal wall *(small arrows). B,* Similar imaging parameters as *(A)* obtained in a different patient 30 minutes after ingesting 600 ml of PFOB. Note blacker signal in distal bowel *(arrow),* sharp bowel margin, and no ghosting anterior to abdominal wall because of absent bowel motion *(small arrows). (A* from Mattrey RF, Hajek PC, Gylys-Morin V, et al: Perfluorochemicals as gastrointestinal contrast agents for MR imaging: Preliminary studies in rats and humans. AJR 148:1259–1263, 1987; © by American Roentgen Ray Society.)

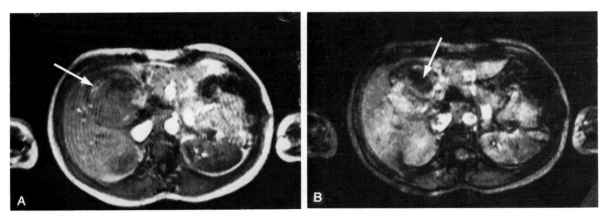

FIGURE 30–7. One-month-old hematoma secondary to liver biopsy. *A,* T₁-weighted gradient-echo image obtained with breath holding (TR/TE 100/11) shows some areas of hyperintensity *(arrow).* Note loss of signal in bowel in left upper quadrant secondary to magnetic susceptibility effect. *B,* T₂-weighted gradient-echo image obtained with breath holding (TR/TE 100/30) shows marked central hypointensity *(arrow)* due to magnetic susceptibility variations. At a longer echo delay (30 msec), the susceptibility effect at the air/tissue interface is more prominent, obscuring the bowel and left side abdominal muscles.

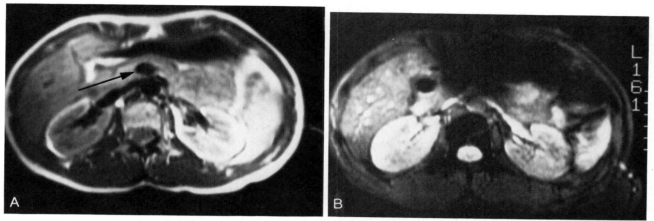

FIGURE 30–8. Magnetic susceptibility effect of gas/water interfaces. *A,* Hydrogen density–weighted image (2000/25) shows superior mesenteric vein *(arrow)* and pancreas posterior to gas-filled antrum. *B,* GRASS image, obtained with relative T_1-weighting, TR/TE of 34/12, and tip angle of 30 degrees at approximately the same level as *(A),* shows deterioration of the anatomy depicted in *(A)* secondary to the gas-filled antrum.

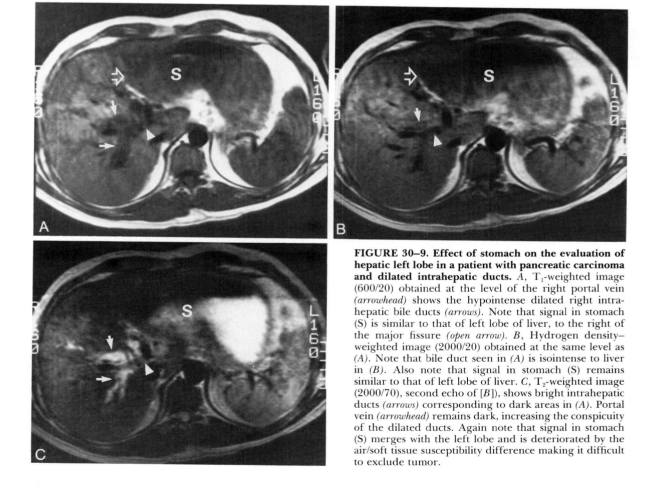

FIGURE 30–9. Effect of stomach on the evaluation of hepatic left lobe in a patient with pancreatic carcinoma and dilated intrahepatic ducts. *A,* T_1-weighted image (600/20) obtained at the level of the right portal vein *(arrowhead)* shows the hypointense dilated right intrahepatic bile ducts *(arrows).* Note that signal in stomach (S) is similar to that of left lobe of liver, to the right of the major fissure *(open arrow).* *B,* Hydrogen density–weighted image (2000/20) obtained at the same level as *(A).* Note that bile duct seen in *(A)* is isointense to liver in *(B).* Also note that signal in stomach (S) remains similar to that of left lobe of liver. *C,* T_2-weighted image (2000/70), second echo of [*B*]), shows bright intrahepatic ducts *(arrows)* corresponding to dark areas in *(A).* Portal vein *(arrowhead)* remains dark, increasing the conspicuity of the dilated ducts. Again note that signal in stomach (S) merges with the left lobe and is deteriorated by the air/soft tissue susceptibility difference making it difficult to exclude tumor.

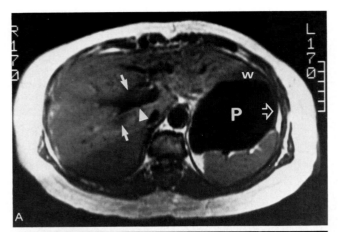

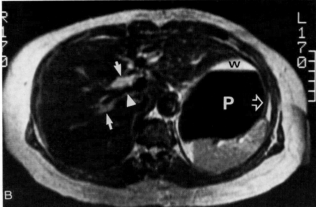

FIGURE 30–10. Effect of perfluorooctylbromide (PFOB) on imaging the left upper quadrant in a patient with pancreatic carcinoma and dilated intrahepatic bile ducts (not the same patient as in Fig. 30–9). *A*, Hydrogen density–weighted image (2000/20) obtained at the level of the right portal vein *(arrowhead)* and dilated bile duct *(arrows)*. Note that bile duct is slightly darker than liver. Also note that because PFOB (P) is heavier and immiscible with water (w), it assumes a dependent position and produces a PFOB/water level. Therefore, the degree of darkening achieved with PFOB is insensitive to bowel content. *B*, T_2-weighted image (2000/70, second echo of [*A*]) shows the increased signal of intrahepatic ducts *(arrows)*, while the portal vein remains dark *(arrowhead)*. Also note that the black signal of PFOB (P) and the bright signal of water in the stomach and the PFOB/water level aid in distinguishing stomach from left lobe of liver. Note that the gastric wall *(open arrow)* is seen only when contrasted against PFOB.

of PFOB reaches the colon within 30 minutes in most subjects. PFOB has undergone successful phase I and II testing and is presently in phase III trials.

OUR IMAGING APPROACH FOR THE UPPER ABDOMEN

It should be emphasized that there are significant differences in the approach to abdominal MR imaging. This approach is tempered by the equipment used and its field strength, local biases, and the patient population upon which techniques are tested.

The approach described below is what we have found most optimal at high field strength in our setting.

Our typical sequences utilize a 256 × 128 matrix, 10-mm slice thickness, and four acquisitions. On T_1-weighted short TR (usually 400 to 800 msec) sequences, we use either a 1- or 2-mm interslice gap. Although these gaps promote cross-talk, their effect is to increase T_1 weighting, which is acceptable, and decrease the S/N ratio, which is made up for by the four excitations.

On T_2-weighted images (TR = 2000), we utilize a 5-mm interslice gap to ensure a higher S/N ratio and T_2 contrast. The 128 matrix allows for four excitations, which decrease ghosting from motion. The T_2-weighted series requires 17.5 minutes of acquisition time. We have found that longer acquisition times decrease patient cooperation and increase motion artifacts. Although used at many sites, we do not use flow compensation techniques, which decrease motion-related signal loss and artifacts, because they increase signals from flowing blood. Since we seek bright areas on T_2-weighted images, vessels could potentially be confused with lesions. Similarly, we do not use even echoes (20/40, 35/70, and so forth), since the second echo also increases signals from flowing blood due to rephasing of moving protons (Fig. 30–11). Respiratory compensation is used in nearly all instances. We also use flow void (presaturation) techniques to eliminate signal from blood vessels.

All patients are given 1 mg glucagon subcutaneously just before they are advanced into the magnet. A 14-inch-wide strap, attached to the table, is tightly wrapped about the abdomen to minimize the excursion of the anterior abdominal wall. Bellows are placed about the lower chest to allow for phase reordering. If the study is to characterize a left lobe lesion, cardiac gating is used. Finally, arms are placed above the head, since wraparound artifacts from arms by the side of the patient can mimic liver lesions.

LIVER

INTRODUCTION

The liver, the chemical factory and detoxification center of the body, is one of the most complex organs. It has been endowed with a dual blood supply, which constitutes 30 per cent of its weight.[20] While its metabolic function predisposes the liver to storage diseases, injury, cirrhosis, and tumors, its abundant blood supply makes the liver a prime site for metastatic deposits. The high incidence of bowel malignancies with predilection to metastasize to liver, and the drastic change in management if such metastases are found, has made the liver the most important abdominal organ to study. The subdiaphragmatic location of the liver, its position under the ribs, and its significant excursion during respiration have made it one of the most challenging to image.

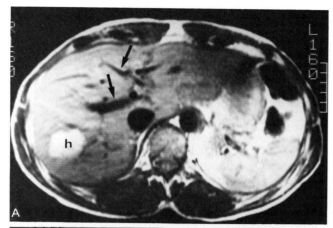

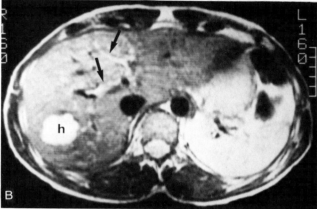

FIGURE 30–11. Effect of even-echo rephasing on portal vein signal. *A,* Hydrogen density–weighted image (2000/30) shows hyperintense hemangioma (h) and dark portal veins *(arrows). B,* Second echo after *(A)* at 2000/60 shows increased hemangioma (h) to liver contrast. However, portal veins are now filled with signal *(arrows).* Compare this image, the second echo of a 2000/30/60 sequence, with Figure 30–10B, also a second echo but obtained at 2000/20/70.

Nuclear medicine techniques rely upon Kupffer cell uptake of a tagged particle to detect space-occupying lesions, since the latter lack these phagocytes. While ideally it should be very accurate, radionuclide studies suffer from poor spatial resolution, intrahepatic vessels mimic defects, and lesions become hidden by surrounding parenchyma and respiratory motion, limiting the detection rate of liver lesions to 70 to 80 per cent.[21] The detection rate is somewhat improved when single photon emission tomography is used.[22]

Sonography is a powerful imaging modality capable of visualizing the liver in any plane and of differentiating vessels from lesions. It is the only modality unaffected by respiration; in fact, respiratory motion improves perception of lesions on real-time imaging. It is estimated that if the liver is well seen and imaged with proper transducers, better than 95 per cent of lesions are detected, as is suggested from intraoperative data.[23] However, in the clinical setting, sonography is limited by the thickness of the subcutaneous tissue and the proximity of ribs to liver, resulting in a detection rate of approximately 60 to 70 per cent.[24]

Detection of liver lesions by CT is restricted to the assessment of differences in mass density. CT without contrast detects 50 per cent of lesions.[25, 26] To take advantage of the difference in blood supply and vascularity, iodinated agents are utilized to assist CT in lesion detection. Because these agents quickly diffuse out of the vascular space,[20] they enhance the extracellular fluid that is similar for liver and neoplastic tissues. That this is true is evidenced by the poor detection rate when contrast is infused slowly.[25, 26] Very rapid infusion with dynamic CT,[27, 28] delayed scanning,[29] or, least practical for screening, CT-angiography[30–32] is needed to increase the detection rate of lesions greater than 1 cm to approximately 90 per cent.[30] Since CT scanning relies on suspension of respiratory motion for optimal image quality, and since full liver coverage requires multiple breath-holds, sampling errors can potentially miss lesions.

MR without intravenous contrast is more sensitive than dynamic CT for the detection of liver lesions.[26, 33] It possesses the imaging qualities of both CT and ultrasound, in that MRI can image the liver in any plane, it displays the vascular structures without the need for contrast media, and it provides a full field-of-view of the slice of interest unimpeded by bone or bowel gas. MRI has a higher detection rate because it differentiates liver from lesions by interrogating three parameters (T_1, T_2, and proton density) in lieu of only one (mass density). MRI, however, still has significant problems to overcome in imaging this complex organ. Data acquisition times are still too long relative to the periods of the respiratory cycle, bowel peristalsis, and circulatory events. Respiration moves the liver several centimeters, resulting in blurring of hepatic detail, masking lesions with low contrast with liver, and superimposing ghost artifacts that obscure the image. Pulsatile flow in vessels perpendicular to the plane of section (aorta and inferior vena cava on transverse images) projects vascular ghosts in the phase-encode direction over hepatic parenchyma. The intimate relationship of the stomach, duodenum, and hepatic flexure to the liver can demand discrimination provided only by a bowel contrast agent. Solid structures, such as small intrahepatic gallstones or hepatic calcifications, are difficult to detect on MRI, as is gas in the biliary system. Lastly, MRI is more costly when compared with other well-established imaging modalities.

All these limitations are being addressed by manufacturers and researchers, with solutions possible in the very near future. Acquisition times on the order of milliseconds are now possible. Acquisition gated to the cardiac cycle to eliminate pulsatile motion is already available. Oral and liver/spleen specific agents are in clinical trials. Reduction in examination time and improvements in efficiency may make MRI financially competitive with other modalities.

The array of MR accessible tissue characteristics, the multiplanar capability, the high detection rate without the need for contrast media, the possibility to image the entire liver with a single breath-hold, and the capabilities afforded by MR spectroscopy, offer the potential for making MR the method of choice for noninvasive investigation of liver disorders.

We consider MRI of the liver, when performed for the proper indications and with the appropriate techniques, to have become a valuable clinical tool. In the following sections, we will review liver imaging strategies and present the MR appearance of the normal and abnormal liver. This presentation should give the reader a clear perspective of the current role of MR relative to other imaging modalities, keeping in mind that this field is in its infancy.

GENERAL INDICATIONS

At our institution, MRI of the liver is performed to detect primary or metastatic neoplastic lesions, document patency of intrahepatic veins, define extent of disease for preoperative planning, differentiate hemangiomas from malignant neoplasm, and demonstrate vascular and portosystemic shunt patency. Given the high dependence of CT on contrast media for its efficacy, and given that MRI is comparable to contrast-aided CT, MRI should be the imaging modality of choice in any patient with a contraindication to contrast media.

IMAGING STRATEGIES

MR imaging techniques of the liver must be directed toward maximizing the contrast-to-noise ratio between liver and lesions and reducing motion artifacts. Methods to reduce motion artifacts were presented above.

Pulsing Sequence

In designing a pulse sequence to maximize contrast, relaxation properties of liver and lesions must be considered, as well as the magnetic field strength being used. The T_1 relaxation times of tissues converge with increasing field strength.[34] Since at low field, the T_1 difference between liver and tumor is greater than at high field, its ability to discriminate between liver and tumors is greater. However, when sufficient T_1 weighting is achieved at high fields by use of inversion recovery[35] or by use of very short TE times made possible with gradient-echo imaging (see Chapter 5), sufficient contrast can be achieved to demonstrate tumors. While T_2 relaxation is in general independent of field strength, it tends to be shorter for liver at high field, presumably due to its high metallic content affecting its magnetic susceptibility.[36] Since at high field the difference in T_1 of liver and tumor is smaller, liver T_2 is shorter, and the S/N ratio is greater, T_2-weighted sequences have

higher detection rates.[36] However, the contrast-to-noise ratio even at high field remains a limitation.[35] Given the different performance of liver imaging at different fields, the imaging strategies will be presented separately.

Imaging at Low Field

Since at low field strength the difference in T_1 between liver and lesions (approximately 40 per cent) is greater than the T_2 difference (approximately 20 per cent),[37] and since T_2 images are limited by low contrast-to-noise ratio, T_1-weighted pulse sequences provide better contrast. However, the short T_2 of the liver has an important consequence on T_1-weighted pulse sequences. Because tumors and other pathologic conditions have longer T_2 relaxation than liver, more signal is lost from liver for any given TE. Since tumors are darker than liver, contrast decreases with longer TE times. Thus, to maximize T_1 contrast, the shortest TE available must be used. As illustrated in Figure 30–12, a relatively short TE of 30 msec results in a substantial loss of tumor contrast compared with a TE of 18 msec. If TE less than 20 msec is not available on a particular system, an inversion recovery sequence should be used, since T_1 contrast with inversion recovery is less sensitive to the echo time.

For a given total acquisition time, shortening the TR to approximately 250 to 500 msec maximizes the contrast-to-noise ratio. Furthermore, the shorter TR permits more signal averaging for a given acquisition time, which reduces motion artifacts.[8] While the T_1-weighted sequence provides better detection of mass lesions,[26, 33] the T_2-weighted sequence is essential for tissue characterization.

At low field, since short TR must be used, a section thickness of 15 mm provides a voxel size small enough for adequate spatial resolution and large enough for sufficient contrast-to-noise ratio, as well as full coverage of the normal sized liver transaxially. Although most mass lesions will be detected at this slice thickness, thinner sections are needed for detecting small (<1 cm) lesions and for evaluating the pancreas and adrenal glands. With thin slices, two consecutive series through the liver may be required for complete coverage.

Imaging at High Field

At 1.0 T, the short inversion time inversion recovery (STIR) sequence maximizes contrast-to-noise ratio when compared with T_1- and T_2-weighted sequences.[38] However, its sensitivity and specificity remain unclear.

We have been disappointed with the sensitivity of T_1-weighted spin-echo sequences at high field because of a lesser T_1 difference between liver and lesions, and TEs of less than 18 msec are not available.[36] However, the significant difference in T_2 relaxation times of these two tissues, coupled with nearly similar T_1 relaxation, and the greater signal

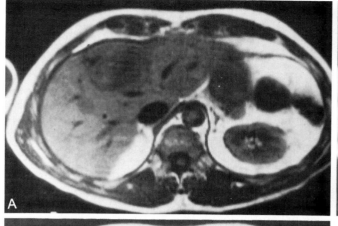

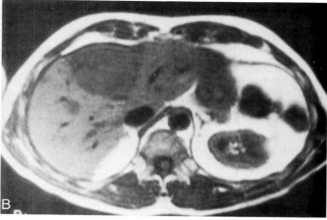

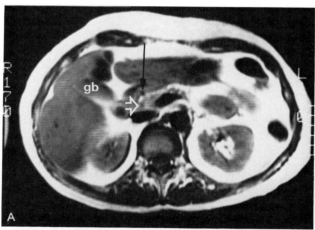

FIGURE 30–12. Effect of TR and TE on contrast between liver and metastatic lesions on spin-echo T₁-weighted images. *A,* Image obtained at 500/30 and 4 excitations shows only moderate liver-lesion contrast, because approximately half the signal from the liver (T_2 = 40 msec) is lost by the time the echo occurs. *B,* By shortening the TR and doubling the number of excitations (same acquisition time as [*A*]), T₁ contrast is improved. *C,* By shortening the TE as well as the TR, still better contrast is obtained. Note that the superficial lesion *(curved arrow)* was poorly visualized with the other sequences.

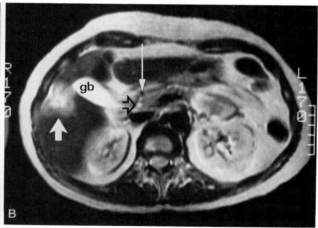

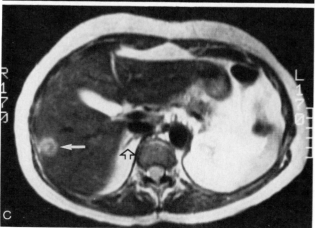

FIGURE 30–13. Appearance of metastases at high field strength. *A,* Hydrogen density image (2000/20) obtained at the level of the gallbladder (gb) and pancreatic head in a patient with colon carcinoma shows no evidence of disease. Note the darker appearance of the gastroduodenal artery (GDA) *(arrow)* compared with the common bile duct (CBD) *(open arrow)*. *B,* T₂-weighted image (2000/70, second echo of [*A*]) shows large intrahepatic metastasis with central high signal presumed to represent necrosis *(thick arrow)*. Also note the persistent dark signal in the GDA and the bright signal in the CBD. *C,* T₂-weighted image obtained 2.5 cm cephalad to (*B*) shows another lesion with different appearance *(arrow)*. Note outer bright rim of tumor surrounding a dark band around a bright center. Also note normal right adrenal *(open arrow)*, which is isointense with liver. Chemical shift artifact (bright line paralleling adrenal limb) is also seen. (Courtesy of Donald Widder, M.D.)

available at high field provide for high contrast-to-noise ratio on T₂-weighted images (Fig. 30–13). The inversion recovery sequence, which provides greater T₁ contrast than spin-echo sequence, was shown to be more sensitive than T₂-weighted images.[35] It was speculated that the 2000/600/20 (TR/TI/TE) inversion recovery sequence performed better than the spin-echo 2000/80 technique because of the lesser contrast-to-noise ratio achieved with the latter. Indeed, this study used only two excitations and a 33 per cent interslice gap, both of which can compromise T₂ contrast resolution. The inversion recovery sequence at high field was comparable to the T₁-weighted spin-echo technique at low field.[35]

Since multislice inversion recovery has not been available on our system, our standard imaging sequence for screening the liver has been a TR of 2 sec and asymmetric echoes obtained at 20 and 70 msec. The long TR provides ample slices to cover the liver and upper abdomen, and the asymmetric echoes maximize the chance for vessels to remain dark on T₂-weighted images. To decrease vascular signal further, we use flow presaturation, which delivers 90-degree RF pulses outside the imaging volume to decrease the influx of fully magnetized protons (see Chapter 4). To maximize the contrast-to-noise ratio, we utilize a matrix of 256 × 128, four excitations, and a slice thickness of 10 mm. To decrease the effect of cross-talk, we utilize a 50 per cent interslice gap. The 5-mm gap should not miss lesions, since the excursion of the liver during respiration is greater than 1 cm, and since lesions located in the 5-mm gap will enter the imaging voxel of the adjacent slices several times during the 17.5-minute acquisition.

In addition to the long TR sequence described above, we also use a T₁-weighted (TR = 600 and TE = 20 msec) sequence to provide tissue characterization and to allow the recognition of water (dark signal) (Fig. 30–14), tumor (darker or equal to liver) (Fig. 30–15), fat or old blood (brighter than liver) (Fig. 30–16).

Gradient-Echo Techniques

Recently, a gradient-echo approach to liver imaging was described (a variation on FLASH or GRASS) which permits multislice T₁-weighted or T₂-weighted images to be obtained in a single breath-holding interval.[4] This rapid imaging technique has been

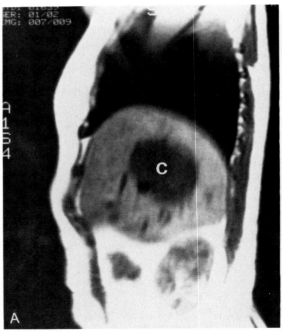

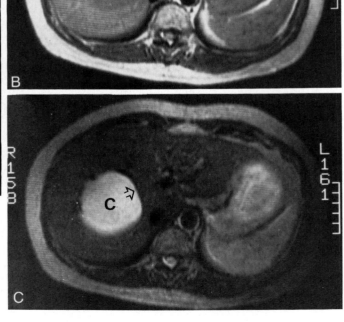

FIGURE 30–14. Appearance of uncomplicated intrahepatic cyst (C) at high field. *A*, T₁-weighted sagittal image (600/20) shows dark well-circumscribed lesion in the right lobe of liver. Note the sharp anterior and posterior margins and the fuzzy superior and inferior margins due to respiratory motion. *B*, Hydrogen density image (2000/20) shows marked decrease in contrast between cyst and liver. Note the well-defined dark margin *(open arrow)* and homogeneous internal signal. *C*, T₂-weighted image (2000/70, second echo of [*B*]) shows marked increase in signal relative to liver, well-defined dark margin *(open arrow)*, and homogeneous bright internal signal.

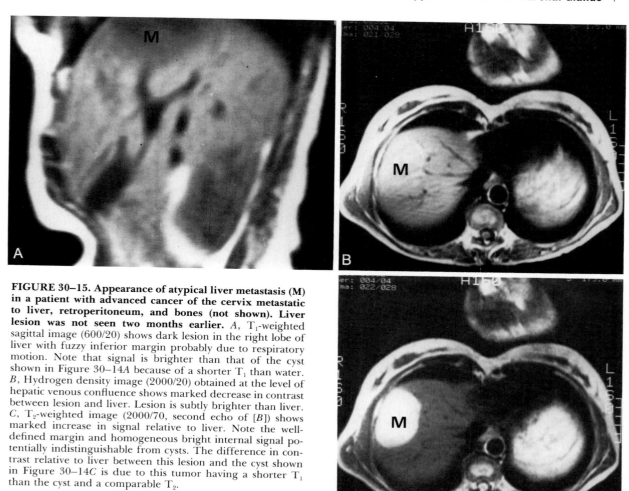

FIGURE 30–15. Appearance of atypical liver metastasis (M) in a patient with advanced cancer of the cervix metastatic to liver, retroperitoneum, and bones (not shown). Liver lesion was not seen two months earlier. *A*, T_1-weighted sagittal image (600/20) shows dark lesion in the right lobe of liver with fuzzy inferior margin probably due to respiratory motion. Note that signal is brighter than that of the cyst shown in Figure 30–14*A* because of a shorter T_1 than water. *B*, Hydrogen density image (2000/20) obtained at the level of hepatic venous confluence shows marked decrease in contrast between lesion and liver. Lesion is subtly brighter than liver. *C*, T_2-weighted image (2000/70, second echo of [*B*]) shows marked increase in signal relative to liver. Note the well-defined margin and homogeneous bright internal signal potentially indistinguishable from cysts. The difference in contrast relative to liver between this lesion and the cyst shown in Figure 30–14*C* is due to this tumor having a shorter T_1 than the cyst and a comparable T_2.

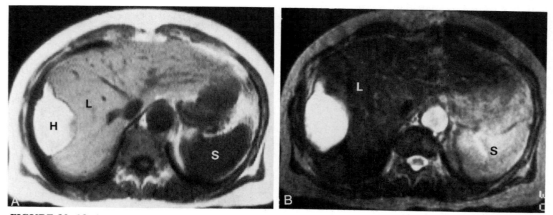

FIGURE 30–16. Appearance of subacute hematoma with FLASH at 1.5 tesla. *A*, T_1-weighted FLASH (TR = 100, TE = 5, and 80-degree flip angle) shows bright subcapsular hematoma (H). Note that liver (L) imaged at 1.5 T is markedly brighter than spleen (S). This degree of contrast is difficult to achieve with spin-echo techniques, since the minimum TE is greater than 18 msec. Also note absence of motion artifact. The entire liver was imaged in 18 sec during a single breath-hold. *B*, Lesion remains bright on T_2-weighted spin-echo image, consistent with old blood.

described in detail elsewhere. Briefly, T_1-weighted gradient-echo images are obtained using short TR (e.g., 100 msec), short TE (e.g., 5 msec), and large pulse angle (e.g., 75 degrees); the short TE minimizes T_2 contrast and the large pulse angle maximizes T_1 contrast. This technique uses a spoiler pulse applied after TE to eliminate the remaining transverse magnetization and stimulated echo artifact. This technique holds great promise since it provides greater T_1 contrast than is achieved with spin-echo techniques, and because the short TE decreases magnetic susceptibility related signal losses. Most advantageous is the ability to scan the liver with a single breath-hold, eliminating motion artifacts and motion-related signal losses (motion causes greater dephasing and hence shorter T_2) (Figs. 30–16 and 30–17). We await the widespread implementation of such a technique

to determine its impact on imaging the liver and upper abdomen.

T_2-weighted gradient-echo images are also obtained with short TR but with long TE (e.g., 40 msec) and small pulse angle (e.g., 15 degrees) in order to maximize T_2 contrast and minimize T_1 weighting. Because gradient-echo techniques do not use a 180-degree refocusing pulse, images obtained with long TE are T_2^* weighted. T_2^* weighting offers different fat/water phase-contrast properties and increased sensitivity to magnetic field inhomogeneity and susceptibility variations as compared with conventional T_2-weighted spin-echo images. The greater sensitivity to magnetic susceptibility effects can be useful for detecting subacute hemorrhage. However, gradient-echo techniques are still under development and have not replaced conventional spin-echo techniques at the present time.

At many institutions the spoiled gradient-echo technique and short TEs are not available. Standard gradient-echo sequences (e.g., GRASS), while fast, have not been useful in lesion detection due to a lesser contrast between liver and lesions. It is reserved to assess vascular anatomy and patency and to detect subacute hemorrhage (Fig. 30–18).

Imaging Planes

Liver imaging is performed in the axial plane, as with CT. This plane is most ideal for anatomic display of intrahepatic vessels and segmental anatomy. Other planes are used, usually with T_1 weighting, to evaluate the integrity of liver margins and to determine the anatomic origin of masses. The sagittal plane is well suited for the evaluation of liver margin with diaphragmatic dome and right kidney. Coronal or sagittal planes are also used to visualize the extrahepatic portal vein. However, to obtain the most optimal view of the portal vein, acquire either a sagittal series with the subject rotated 30 degrees right side up or, if available, an oblique sagittal plane graphically prescribed from a quick coronal localizer. Finally, to project ghost artifacts arising from pulsatile flow in the aorta and inferior vena cava away from the liver in the transaxial plane, the subject can be rotated 15 to 20 degrees left side up[39] or, if available, repeat the sequence but on the second series swap the frequency with the phase-encoded direction. Since ghosting occurs in the phase direction, ghosts will be projected once anteroposterior and once right-left, allowing the assessment of the entire liver free of artifact. The need for oblique positioning and the swapping of the phase-encoded direction has been essentially eliminated by the availability of the flow void (presaturation) technique.

NORMAL ANATOMY

Normal liver parenchyma is homogeneous on all pulsing sequences. On T_1-weighted images, the liver

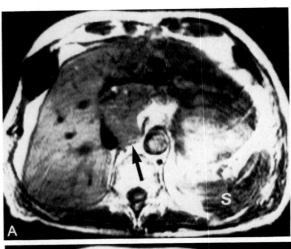
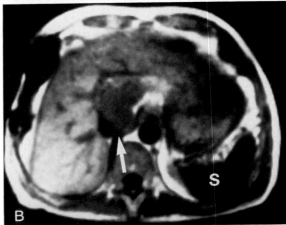

FIGURE 30–17. Appearance of malignant lesion with short TE FLASH. *A*, T_1-weighted spin-echo sequence (2000/20) at 1.5 T. Note the enlarged caudate *(arrow)*, which is minimally darker than liver, along with a small right lobe, consistent with alcoholic liver scarring. Also note that liver signal is nearly equal to that of spleen (S), which is compromised by ghost artifacts from respiratory motion. *B*, FLASH (TR = 100, TE = 5, and 80-degree flip angle) obtained during a single breath-hold in the same patient shows marked increase in contrast between liver and tumor, which fills the caudate lobe *(arrow)*, liver, and spleen (S). Note absence of respiratory motion artifacts.

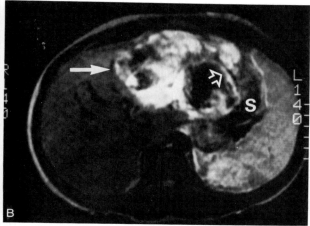

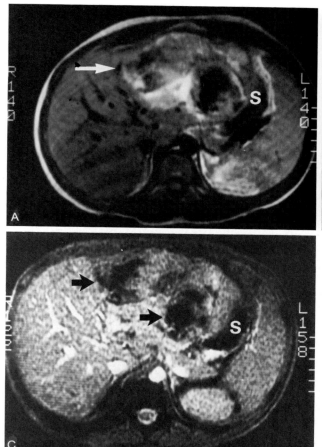

FIGURE 30–18. Hepatoblastoma in a 12-year-old with significant internal hemorrhage, characteristic of these lesions. *A,* Hydrogen density–weighted image (2000/20) shows a mixed intensity lesion *(arrow)* filling the left lobe of the liver. Regions of bright and dark signal are due to hemorrhage of different ages. Note that stomach (S) is indistinguishable from mass. *B,* T$_2$-weighted image (2000/70, second echo of [A]) shows the bright regions brighter and dark regions darker, consistent with old (bright) and new (dark) hemorrhage. Note that a white rim surrounds dark area *(open arrow)*, suggesting early methemoglobin formation at the periphery of the newer bleed. *C,* Gradient-echo image (29/20 at 8 degrees), which has more T$_2$ than T$_1$ contrast, shows area of new hemorrhage *(arrows)* as dark due to magnetic susceptibility effect caused by deoxyhemoglobin. Note that remainder of mass is isointense with liver.

has moderate signal intensity, similar to pancreas, brighter than kidneys, spleen, adrenals, muscle, and ascites, but substantially darker than subcutaneous fat. On T$_2$-weighted images, the liver, because of its short T$_2$, is as dark as muscle and adrenals, slightly darker than pancreas, and substantially darker than kidneys, normal spleen, and ascites. Due to the similarity of T$_1$ and T$_2$ relaxation times of normal spleen and tumors, the spleen could be used as an internal standard to ensure that the liver is imaged with proper T$_1$ weighting. Isointensity of the liver and spleen on a supposedly "T$_1$-weighted" image should be taken as evidence that the degree of T$_1$ weighting is suboptimal for detecting mass lesions. The spleen as an internal standard should be used with caution if it fails to increase in signal relative to fat on T$_2$-weighted sequences. The spleen, because of its reticuloendothelial function, can accumulate iron and other products that shorten its T$_2$ and darken its signal.

The hepatic venous system is well assessed by MR. Blood vessels appear dark on spin-echo images due to flow-related signal loss.[40] The confluence of the hepatic veins should always be demonstrable on good-quality images. Sharp visualization of segmental branches is a sign that image quality is sufficient to detect small lesions. On T$_2$-weighted images, the

slower flowing venous blood occasionally has high signal, particularly if symmetric echoes are used, due to even-echo rephasing. These branching bright lines should not be confused with bile ducts. The latter should not be seen if normal in size. The ligamentum venosum and ligamentum teres are of low intensity, but the fat-containing fissures in which they travel are bright.

The accurate localization of liver lesions is paramount to appropriate follow-up and to assess hepatic resectability. Segmental liver anatomy is highly ordered and best appreciated on axial images. All hepatic vessels obey the following rule: hepatic veins travel at the periphery of segments and lobes and portal veins travel in the center of segments and lobes. The three main hepatic veins meet with the inferior vena cava (IVC) as it is exiting the liver. The middle hepatic vein divides the liver into a right and left lobe. Each of these two lobes is then bisected by its respective hepatic vein into two segments—the anterior and posterior right segments, and the medial and lateral left segments. The main portal vein, traveling along the major fissure, center of liver, bifurcates to send the right and left portal veins in the center of their respective lobes. In turn, each portal vein bifurcates to send a branch along the center of each of the two segments of each lobe.

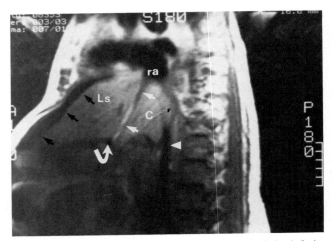

FIGURE 30–19. Sagittal 10-mm scan at the level of the inferior vena cava (IVC) *(arrowhead)* obtained with TR/TE of 800/20 shows the fat and ligament *(white arrows)* of ligamentum venosum, which in fetal life connected the main portal vein *(curved arrow)* and IVC as it entered the right atrium (ra). Note changes induced by alcohol: large caudate (c) and lateral segment (ls) of left lobe of liver, as well as ascites *(small black arrows)*, seen best in the anterior hepatic space.

In addition to the vascular branches outlining the internal geography, there are three superficial fissures. The major fissure, present along the inferior surface, bisects the liver in an oblique fashion into right and left lobes. This fissure contains the main portal vein, hepatic artery, common bile duct, and the neck of the gallbladder. The fissure of the ligamentum venosum is horizontal on transverse images but angles posteriorly as it proceeds cephalad (Fig. 30–19). It is the superior continuation of the major fissure, and it separates the caudate lobe from the lateral segment of the left lobe. In this fissure traveled the ductus venosus in fetal life carrying portal venous blood to the IVC. The third and last fissure is the fissure of the ligamentum teres, which travels at the base of the falciform ligament. It was the umbilical vein in fetal life which carried blood to the left portal vein. The falciform ligament, which is the fused leaves of the anterior peritoneal reflections, enters the anterior surface of the liver bisecting the left lobe into its two medial and lateral segments. The major fissure and the fissure of the ligamentum teres provide landmarks of hepatic segmental anatomy along its caudal end, and the hepatic veins and ligamentum venosum provide the landmarks at its cephalic end.

LIVER PATHOLOGY

Malignant Masses

Metastases

Metastases represent the most common malignancy of the liver. Because of their prolonged T_1 and T_2 relaxation times, most of these lesions appear darker than liver on T_1-weighted images and brighter than

liver on T_2-weighted images. Whereas the morphology of most lesions appears similar on T_1-weighted images, T_2 weighting may produce characteristics that allow recognition of metastases from other type of lesions (Figs. 30–20 and 30–21). Differentiation between metastases and benign lesions (cysts and hemangiomas) is possible since the former have T_2 relaxation times that are shorter than those of simple cysts and hemangiomas.[41] However, this differentiation is at times difficult (Figs. 30–15 and 30–22). MRI cannot differentiate between various cell types, since on T_2-weighted images most metastatic liver tumors have grossly similar signals. The intensity of these lesions on T_2-weighted images is similar to the intensity of the normal spleen but is less intense than cerebrospinal fluid (CSF) in the spinal canal. However, necrotic regions or areas of old hemorrhage within a tumor, as well as highly vascular metastases, may have signal on T_2 weighting overlapping those of hemangiomas and cysts.[42] One characteristic sign of malignancy is an intense ring surrounding a less intense core on T_2-weighted images (Fig. 30–21) or a target lesion (see Figs. 30–13C and 30–20B).

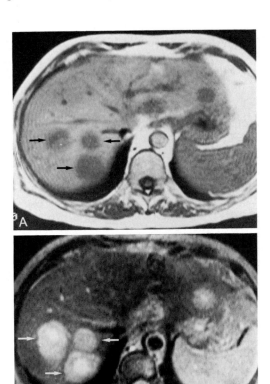

FIGURE 30–20. Metastasis from colon adenocarcinoma obtained at low field demonstrates the target sign, which is similar to that shown at high field (see Fig. 30–13C). *A,* On a T_1-weighted image, metastases appear homogeneous and darker than liver *(arrows). B,* On a T_2-weighted image, they assume a targetlike appearance, characteristic of malignant lesions. Note that they appear larger than on T_1 weighting *(A).* This may be due to necrosis, shown on T_1, in the center of a larger lesion, in which the periphery was not seen on T_1.

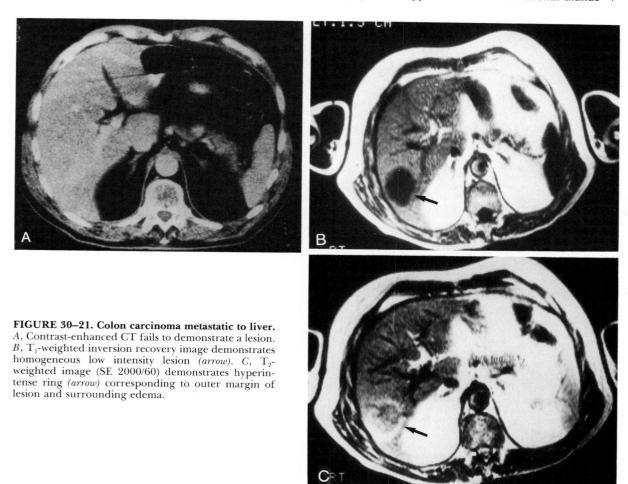

FIGURE 30–21. Colon carcinoma metastatic to liver. *A,* Contrast-enhanced CT fails to demonstrate a lesion. *B,* T₁-weighted inversion recovery image demonstrates homogeneous low intensity lesion *(arrow)*. *C,* T₂-weighted image (SE 2000/60) demonstrates hyperintense ring *(arrow)* corresponding to outer margin of lesion and surrounding edema.

It is possible, if even echoes or flow compensation are used, for vessels to become bright and therefore confused with mass lesions. If liver imaging is used with asymmetric echoes and with the flow void option to further decrease vascular signal, vessels in most instances will appear darker than liver. However, at low field, which may allow lesions to appear as dark as vessels on T₁-weighted images, care must be taken to avoid confusion, particularly in the central region of the liver where larger vessels may be seen in cross-section. Screening for small metastatic lesions may be difficult in the presence of dilated biliary ducts. Enlarged bile ducts are distinguished from vessels and lesions by their tortuous course, by their dark signal on T₁-weighted images, and by their brighter signal on T₂-weighted images (see Figs. 30–9, 30–10, and 30–23). While there may be overlap in signals at low field, at high field bile ducts and cysts are the intrahepatic structures consistently darker than liver on T₁-weighted spin-echo images (see Fig. 30–14). Thus, a bright region seen only on T₂-weighted images, particularly if bile ducts are seen in a different location on T₁-weighted images, would represent a focal lesion.

Hepatoma

Most primary liver tumors, such as hepatomas, are easily visualized by MR (Figs. 30–24 and 30–25).[43] Hepatomas are more common in Asia and Africa than in Western nations due to the high incidence of hepatic infections. In the United States, hepatomas are seen in patients with alcohol abuse, or hepatitis, or chemical injury. Hepatomas were described as having a dark rim seen on T₁-weighted images at low field.[41] This sign seen in 40 per cent of hepatomas[45] is not specific. It can be seen around other lesions and is therefore not helpful for differential diagnosis. It is thought, however, when hepatomas have a dark pseudocapsule, that these lesions are less aggressive and may be easily enucleated.[45] At high field, hepatomas on T₂-weighted images have a double capsular signal: an inner thin dark band, thought to be due to the tumor fibrous capsule, and an outer thin bright band, thought to be due to compressed vessels or new bile ducts.[45] A significant number of hepatomas (31 per cent) were hyperintense on T₁-weighted images.[45, 46] This is probably due to their high fat content.[47] Hepatomas have been the only solid neoplasms with bright signal on T₁-weighted sequences.

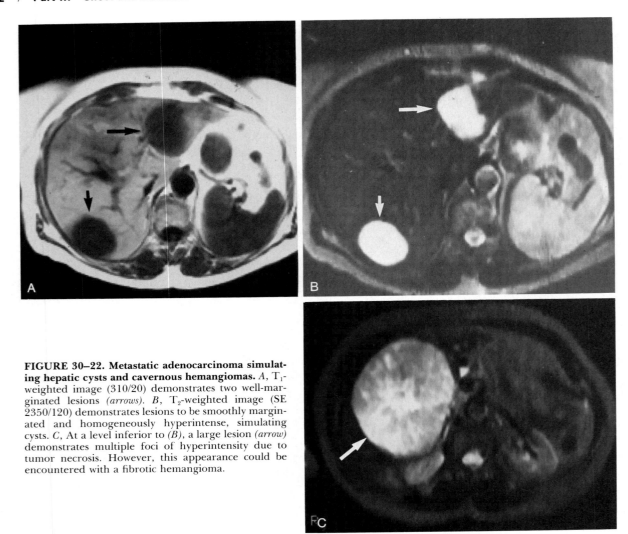

FIGURE 30–22. Metastatic adenocarcinoma simulating hepatic cysts and cavernous hemangiomas. *A*, T₁-weighted image (310/20) demonstrates two well-marginated lesions *(arrows)*. *B*, T₂-weighted image (SE 2350/120) demonstrates lesions to be smoothly marginated and homogeneously hyperintense, simulating cysts. *C*, At a level inferior to *(B)*, a large lesion *(arrow)* demonstrates multiple foci of hyperintensity due to tumor necrosis. However, this appearance could be encountered with a fibrotic hemangioma.

We have observed this in one of our few cases. While the tumor signal in these cases is inhomogeneous, it is uniformly bright. Since other solid liver lesions, except possibly focal nodular hyperplasia, rarely contain fat,[48] it is possible that this finding may be specific; however, more data would have to be accumulated for proof. Hepatic hamartomas may also contain fat. The MR appearance of these rare lesions has not been described. Given their appearance on CT,[48] it would be predicted that they would have a much brighter signal due to their pure fat content than the signal generated by a fat-containing hepatoma. Cysts, complicated by hemorrhage or high protein content, may be bright on T₁-weighted images. However, these cysts will be sharply demarcated and homogeneous in appearance and will be excessively bright on T₂-weighted images, potentially allowing their recognition.

MR sensitivity for the detection of hepatomas deteriorates when lesions become 2 cm or smaller. In one report 85 per cent of small lesions were detected,[45] while in another report only 33 per cent

were detected.[44] As previously discussed, respiratory motion is probably the cause for this insensitivity. We believe that MRI without the aid of contrast media and without breath holding will have difficulty in consistently visualizing lesions smaller than 2 to 3 cm.

In the differential diagnosis of hepatomas on MRI, the presence of daughter lesions, the thin single or double outer layer pseudocapsule, and vascular invasion add significantly to the specificity. The presence of a brighter lesion than liver on T₁-weighted images may add yet more specificity.

Other Malignant Lesions

Data on malignant lesions other than metastasis or hepatocellular carcinoma are scant and difficult to evaluate at present. For lymphomatous involvement of the liver, in a report in 1984 by Weinreb and colleagues done at low field, MR did very poorly in detecting lesions, thought to be due to the infiltrative nature of the disease.[49] In 1 of the 13 cases, a focal lesion seen on CT was also visible on MRI. In a more

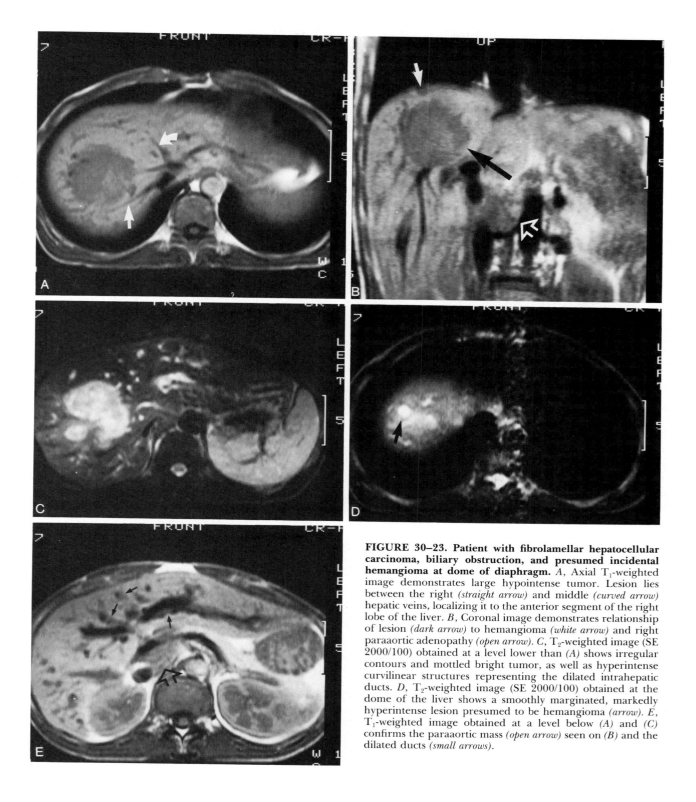

FIGURE 30–23. Patient with fibrolamellar hepatocellular carcinoma, biliary obstruction, and presumed incidental hemangioma at dome of diaphragm. *A,* Axial T_1-weighted image demonstrates large hypointense tumor. Lesion lies between the right *(straight arrow)* and middle *(curved arrow)* hepatic veins, localizing it to the anterior segment of the right lobe of the liver. *B,* Coronal image demonstrates relationship of lesion *(dark arrow)* to hemangioma *(white arrow)* and right paraaortic adenopathy *(open arrow). C,* T_2-weighted image (SE 2000/100) obtained at a level lower than *(A)* shows irregular contours and mottled bright tumor, as well as hyperintense curvilinear structures representing the dilated intrahepatic ducts. *D,* T_2-weighted image (SE 2000/100) obtained at the dome of the liver shows a smoothly marginated, markedly hyperintense lesion presumed to be hemangioma *(arrow). E,* T_1-weighted image obtained at a level below *(A)* and *(C)* confirms the paraaortic mass *(open arrow)* seen on *(B)* and the dilated ducts *(small arrows).*

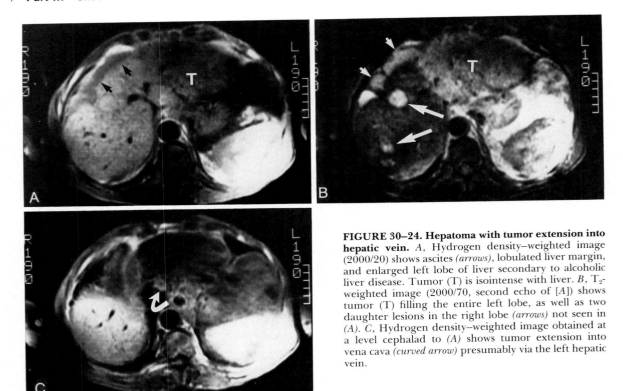

FIGURE 30–24. Hepatoma with tumor extension into hepatic vein. *A*, Hydrogen density–weighted image (2000/20) shows ascites *(arrows)*, lobulated liver margin, and enlarged left lobe of liver secondary to alcoholic liver disease. Tumor (T) is isointense with liver. *B*, T$_2$-weighted image (2000/70, second echo of [*A*]) shows tumor (T) filling the entire left lobe, as well as two daughter lesions in the right lobe *(arrows)* not seen in *(A)*. *C*, Hydrogen density–weighted image obtained at a level cephalad to *(A)* shows tumor extension into vena cava *(curved arrow)* presumably via the left hepatic vein.

recent study, MRI detected focal disease and missed the infiltrative type.[50] An example of a focal lymphomatous deposit is shown in Figure 30–26. No data, to the best of our knowledge, are available on leukemic involvement of the liver. Leukemic involvement can also be focal or infiltrative.[51] It is possible that MRI will have similarly disappointing results when leukemic infiltration is present.

Hepatoblastoma, the most frequent primary liver malignancy in infants, may have characteristic appearance on MRI. The lesion is typically multilobular and is characterized by multiple areas of intrinsic hemorrhage.[52] We have seen two children with this disease, both presenting similar appearances. The hemorrhage was easily seen on gradient-echo images (see Figs. 30–18 and 30–27).

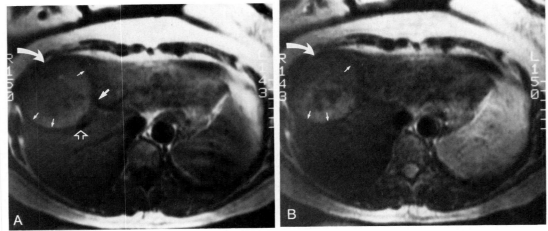

FIGURE 30–25. Hepatoma with shorter T$_1$ than liver. *A*, Axial hydrogen density–weighted image (2000/20) shows a well-circumscribed lesion *(curved arrow)* that deviates the middle hepatic vein anteriorly *(arrow)* and the right portal vein posteriorly *(open arrow)*, placing the lesion in the anterior half of the anterior segment of the right lobe. *B*, T$_2$-weighted image (2000/70), second echo of *(A)*, shows further increase in tumor signal relative to liver. Note that the lesion has a single layer capsule seen on hydrogen density *(A)* and T$_2$-weighted image *(B)* *(small arrows)*.

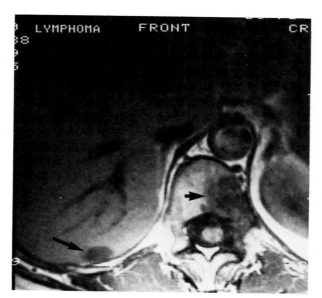

FIGURE 30–26. Mildly T_1-weighted (580/26) axial image obtained at 1.0 T using posterior circular surface coil shows a well-defined peripheral lymphomatous lesion in the liver *(arrow)* and bone lesion in vertebral body and pedicle *(short arrow)*.

Benign Masses

Cysts

Cysts are common incidental findings in the liver and may coexist with metastatic disease. Simple cysts are characterized by very long T_1 and T_2 relaxation times, similar to those of CSF. At low field strength, although they appear very dark on T_1-weighted images, simple cysts are best distinguished from malignant tumors on strongly T_2-weighted images and morphologically (e.g., SE 2000/120) (Fig. 30–28).[41] Cysts have similar appearance at high field as they do at low field, except that the contrast between cysts and liver is diminished on T_1-weighted images due to a lesser difference in T_1 relaxation contrast (compare Fig. 30–14 with Fig. 30–28). The most distinguishing feature is the well-defined smooth margin of a darker homogeneous signal than liver on T_1- or hydrogen density–weighted images where the S/N ratio is best, which becomes very bright and homogeneous on T_2 weighting, brighter than spleen or liver metastases, and as bright as CSF in the spinal canal. However, when complicated, small, or imaged with artifacts, cysts can become indistinguishable from tumors. In fact, in a patient at high risk for malignancy, ultrasound is considered the most specific imaging technique. Furthermore, when a lesion does not follow the classic appearance (smooth margin, homogeneous dark signal on T_1-weighted images, and homogeneous bright signal on T_2-weighted images), ultrasound confirmation of a cystic lesion is beneficial.

Hemangioma

Hemangiomas are the most common benign solid tumors of the liver. Their high prevalence, in nearly 10 per cent of the population, makes their differentiation from malignant disease of paramount importance, particularly in cancer patients. Radiology has struggled over the decades to provide this discrimination. At present, all noninvasive imaging studies fall short in their ability to make a definitive diagnosis to obviate a biopsy in a high-risk patient.

At the present time the highest specificity for hemangiomas larger than 2 to 3 cm is SPECT scanning following the administration of technetium-

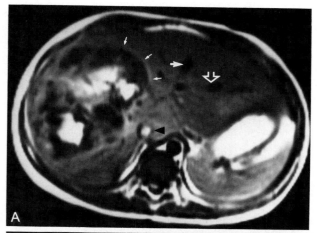

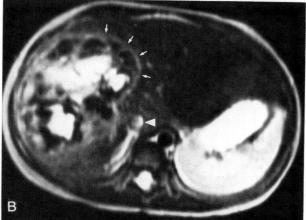

FIGURE 30–27. Hepatoblastoma in a 2-year-old, with partial caval thrombosis. *A,* Hydrogen density–weighted (2000/20) axial scan shows a large lesion filling the posterior segment of the right lobe. Note the very bright and very dark signals within this mass. Note the location of the mass relative to the middle hepatic vein *(small arrow)* and left hepatic vein *(open arrow)*. Note the bright signal within the vena cava *(arrowhead)*. *B,* T_2-weighted image (2000/70, second echo of [A]) shows that the regions that were bright on *(A)* remained bright and the dark areas remained dark. These are regions of hemorrhage within the mass, which is demarcated from liver by a bright rim *(small arrows)*, possibly representing early blood degradation. Note persistent bright signal within the cava consistent with clot most likely propagating from the nonvisualized right hepatic vein (clot seen better at other levels not shown).

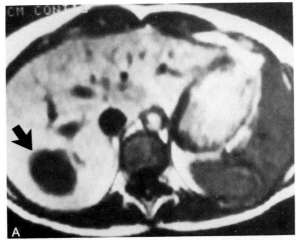

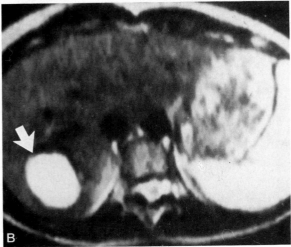

FIGURE 30–28. Hepatic cyst. *A,* Single well-marginated hepatic cyst is present in posterior segment of the right lobe of liver *(arrow).* It is markedly darker than liver and moderately darker than spleen on a T_1-weighted image obtained at low field strength. *B,* T_2-weighted image obtained at the same level as *(A)* shows the cyst to be smooth and well marginated with liver. Note it is as bright as CSF and spleen.

labeled RBC.[53] Classic hemangiomas have normal or diminished flow on the angiographic phase, followed by retention of the isotope on delayed scans relative to liver at 20 to 60 minutes.[53] Retention of the tracer on delayed scans, representing higher blood content than liver, was not seen in association with any other lesion in a recent report of a small series of 18 hemangiomas and 8 metastases.[53]

The typical appearance of hemangiomas on CT is low attentuation on the precontrast scans, peripheral fill-in of contrast following bolus injection, and delayed retention of contrast (lesion remains isodense or hyperdense with liver at 20 to 30 minutes).[54] This characteristic enhancement pattern is seen in 55 per cent of hemangiomas and in 1.5 per cent of metastases.[42, 54] Because of noncharacteristic hemangiomas, there is 14 per cent overlap in their appearance with metastases.[42]

Whereas there is a classic sonographic appearance for hemangiomas (small echogenic focus), there is significant overlap in the echo-texture of typical and atypical hemangiomas with metastasis, such that sonography offers little specificity in the high-risk patient. Findings on radioisotope, CT, and sonography, in combination with clinical data (high versus low-risk patient), increase specificity significantly. However, specificity is never 100 per cent. A patient at high risk for liver malignancy still requires needle biopsy for final diagnosis. Biopsy of hemangiomas is not entirely free of risk, and a conclusive diagnosis requires either a skilled cytologist to identify characteristic endothelial cells or multiple repeat biopsies that remain negative for malignancy.[55]

Because cavernous hemangiomas are essentially sacs of unclotted blood, they have long T_1 and T_2 relaxation times.[56, 57] Although the blood is flowing through dilated sinusoids, the velocity of flow is apparently too slow to significantly alter signal intensity. On T_2-weighted images, the signal intensity of cavernous hemangiomas is very bright, similar to CSF, and characteristically increases relative to liver with longer TEs (Fig. 30–29). Like all liver tumors, cavernous hemangiomas appear dark on heavily T_1-weighted images. However, on moderately T_1-weighted images, cavernous hemangiomas may appear nearly isointense with liver, whereas simple cysts will appear darker than liver because of their longer T_1. At high field strength, hemangiomas are typically isointense or darker than liver on T_1-weighted images, isointense or brighter than liver on hydrogen density images, and markedly brighter on T_2-weighted images (Fig. 30–29).

MR can differentiate cavernous hemangiomas from malignant tumors with an accuracy on the order of 90 per cent if several criteria are fulfilled: (1) smooth contours that are typically lobulated, (2) homogeneous on all pulse sequences, (3) high signal on T_2-weighted pulse sequences, and (4) continued increase of signal relative to liver with longer TEs (Fig. 30–29).[58] Relaxation parameter measurements, which are calculated from multiple images, may be less reliable than signal intensity ratios obtained from a single image due to the accumulation of inaccuracies caused by respiratory motion, variations in RF pulse angles, preamplifier gain, and so forth. Visual inspection should be relied upon in lieu of the cumbersome T_2 measurements by comparing lesion signal intensity to that of CSF on highly T_2-weighted images (SE TR = 2000 with TE = 120–180 at low field, TR 2000–2500 with TE 60–80 at high field).[59] At high field strength, given the similarity of T_1 relaxation of hemangiomas and liver and the markedly shorter T_2 of liver (nearly one third that of hemangioma[60]), TR/TE of 2000/80 is sufficiently T_2 weighted that further TEs, which add noise, are not necessary (Fig. 30–30). In a recent report, in which T_2 values of 97 hepatomas and 61 hemangiomas were measured, 80 msec was found to separate hemangiomas from hepatomas in 88 per cent of le-

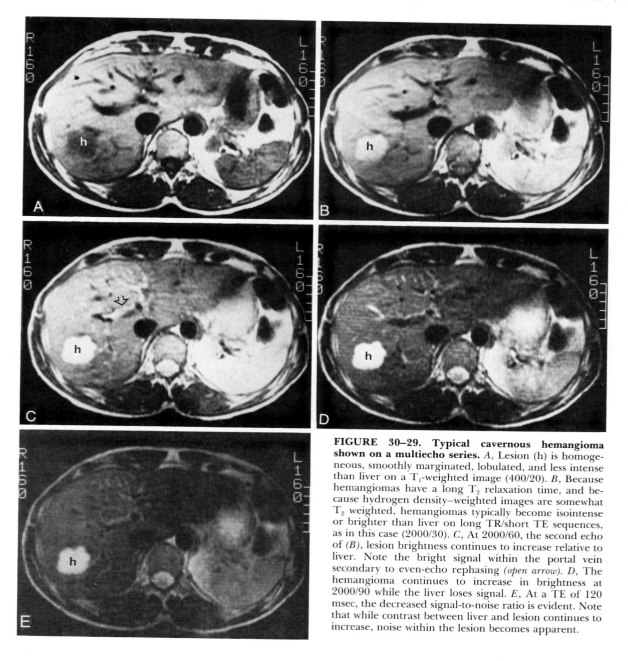

FIGURE 30–29. Typical cavernous hemangioma shown on a multiecho series. *A,* Lesion (h) is homogeneous, smoothly marginated, lobulated, and less intense than liver on a T₁-weighted image (400/20). *B,* Because hemangiomas have a long T₂ relaxation time, and because hydrogen density–weighted images are somewhat T₂ weighted, hemangiomas typically become isointense or brighter than liver on long TR/short TE sequences, as in this case (2000/30). *C,* At 2000/60, the second echo of *(B),* lesion brightness continues to increase relative to liver. Note the bright signal within the portal vein secondary to even-echo rephasing *(open arrow). D,* The hemangioma continues to increase in brightness at 2000/90 while the liver loses signal. *E,* At a TE of 120 msec, the decreased signal-to-noise ratio is evident. Note that while contrast between liver and lesion continues to increase, noise within the lesion becomes apparent.

sions.[60] The 12 per cent overlap was due to hemangiomas smaller than 2 cm in all but two lesions. Lesions smaller than 2 cm can be affected by partial volume averaging with the dark liver secondary to liver excursion during respiration and long imaging times. In another study hemangiomas could be differentiated prospectively from 97.5 per cent of hypovascular metastases but from only 61 per cent of hypervascular lesions.[61]

Preliminary experience with gadolinium-DTPA suggests that the enhancement patterns of cavernous hemangiomas are similar to those seen in contrast-enhanced CT with iodinated agents. Initially, there is peripheral rim enhancement with gradual filling

in and prolonged retention of contrast.[62a] As in CT, atypical enhancement patterns may be seen. The gradual enhancement observed in hemangiomas may be helpful in excluding a hypervascular metastasis. However, we have seen a few small (less than 2 cm) hemangiomas enhance immediately after contrast administration.

Unfortunately, MR evaluation for cavernous hemangioma does not offer a perfectly accurate result for several reasons. Not all hemangiomas have the classic characteristic appearance (Figs. 30–31 and 30–32). This may be due to partial thrombosis or fibrosis or to a yet unknown reason. More worrisome, a few metastases have been noted to be indistinguishable

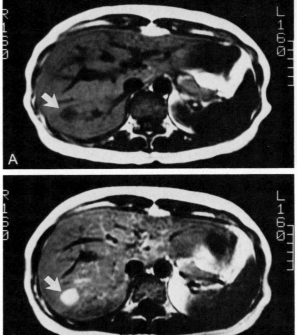

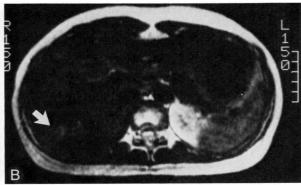

FIGURE 30–30. Typical hemangioma *(arrow)* that loses signal on long TE sequences. *A*, Hemangioma is darker than liver on a T_1-weighted (300/20) image obtained at 1.5 T. *B*, While lesion had characteristic appearance and signal increased on the first and second echoes (2000/30 and 60, not shown) relative to liver, it decreased slightly on the third echo (2000/90, not shown), and was hardly perceptible on the fourth echo (2000/120) because of increased noise. *C*, Same sequence as *(A)*, 300/20, acquired 5 minutes after 0.1 mmol/kg Gd-DTPA. Note the diffuse increase in lesion intensity, typical of hemangioma. (Courtesy of Dean P. Berthoty, M.D., Sunrise Hospital, Las Vegas, NV.)

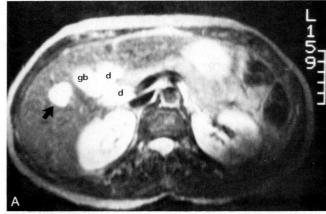

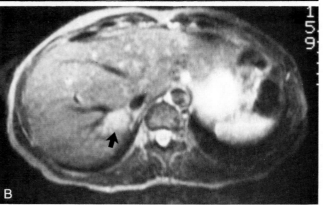

FIGURE 30–31. Mixed appearance of hemangioma. *A*, T_2-weighted image (2000/70) shows a biopsy-proven hemangioma in a patient with endometrial carcinoma. Note that the lesion *(arrow)* has typical characteristics: homogeneously bright, lobulated, and smoothly marginated. Note that its signal is comparable to gallbladder (gb), fluid-filled duodenum (d), and CSF. *B*, T_2-weighted image obtained within the same series as *(A)*, a few levels cephalad to *(A)*, shows a bubbly 3-cm lesion posterior to right hepatic vein *(arrow)*. Note poor margination with liver, darker signal than lesion in *(A)*, and the presence of central signals. This was also a hemangioma at biopsy.

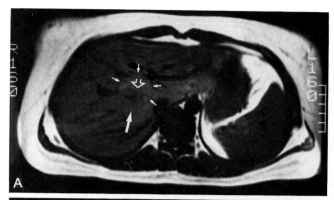

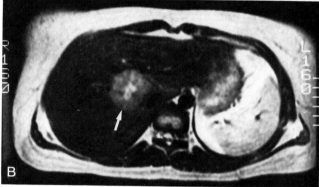

FIGURE 30–32. Atypical hemangioma. *A*, Mildly T_1-weighted image obtained at high field with TR/TE set at 1500/20. Note that lesion *(arrow)* is isointense with liver, has a faint capsule *(small arrows)*, and has central dark signal *(open arrow)*. *B*, Second echo of *(A)*, 1500/90 shows an inhomogeneous lesion with central high signal suggestive of malignancy with necrosis (compare with Fig. 30–22C). (Courtesy of Donald Widder, M.D.)

from cavernous hemangiomas, even on images obtained with prolonged TEs (Fig. 30–33).[61] Two of the many possible pathophysiologic mechanisms that are thought to produce atypical behavior of lesions are hypervascularity and necrosis. Given MRI's limited experience, the exact percentage of hemangiomas that do not have the classic appearance and the percentage of metastases with characteristics mimicking those of hemangiomas are not yet known. However, all 18 hemangiomas smaller than 4 cm had characteristic appearance, but only 1 of 6 lesions larger than 4 cm were typical.[61] Certainly, hemangiomas need not be homogeneously bright.[62]

From the data published to date it can be concluded that if lesions are smaller than 2 cm, there may be difficulty recognizing hemangiomas from malignant lesions;[60] if they are larger than 4 cm, they are mostly atypical in their appearance;[61] and if the patient is known to have a hypervascular primary, then MRI can err in 39 per cent of the cases.[61] These statistics are certainly discouraging and further suggest that in a high-risk patient, MRI, like the other imaging modalities, will not be sufficiently and consistently specific to obviate biopsy. However, with the added soft tissue contrast afforded by MRI, with the advent of MR contrast media, with added clinical

experience, and with the ability to evaluate the liver with sufficient speed to eliminate the effect of motion, we believe that MRI will eventually have a narrower gray zone than that of CT.

Despite these limitations, MR is still recommended for evaluating suspected cavernous hemangiomas in a subset of patients with small lesions and without known hypervascular tumors. Patients with large lesions (greater than 4 to 5 cm) benefit most from a blood pool SPECT study. In patients with multiple liver masses, MRI may identify the lesions more likely to be metastatic to increase the yield of biopsy. Of course, MR may not distinguish simple cysts from hemangiomas, but this failure is seldom of clinical significance, since in this setting sonography is very precise. Furthermore, with the availability of Gd-DTPA, MRI would easily differentiate the hypervascular hemangioma from the avascular cyst. At this time we believe that MRI adds yet another data point to the patient's work-up but does not offer a definitive diagnosis.

Other Benign Focal Lesions

The reported clinical experience with other benign liver masses is much smaller than for cysts and hemangiomas. Hepatic adenomas may be indistinguishable by MR criteria from malignant tumors (Fig. 30–34). Mattison and colleagues reported that focal nodular hyperplasia has similar signal intensity to liver on both T_1-weighted and T_2-weighted pulse sequences[63] (Fig. 30–35). This appearance is not surprising, since these tumors are composed of nodules of hepatocytes and Kupffer cells. These lesions may also demonstrate a central stellate pattern that is hypointense on T_1- and hyperintense on T_2-weighted images, consistent with the central scar. The bright signal on T_2-weighting may be due to the bile and vascular content of the central scar.[63] However, these authors also described a case of fibrolamellar hepatocellular carcinoma that was virtually indistinguishable from focal nodular hyperplasia. This suggests that additional clinical experience is needed.

Hemangioendotheliomas, present in neonates, are known for high arteriovenous shunts resulting in death in utero or in the neonatal period from high output cardiac failure. Palliative therapy after birth is usually sufficient. In large lesions, debulking may be necessary. MR characteristics of these lesions are not yet well characterized. In one case, the lesion was lobulated, well defined, and contained large vessels (Fig. 30–36). No other distinct features could be extracted.

Hemorrhage

The MR appearance of hemorrhage depends on several parameters, including the age of the lesion and magnetic field strength. These characteristics are presented in Chapter 8 and 16. At low and medium

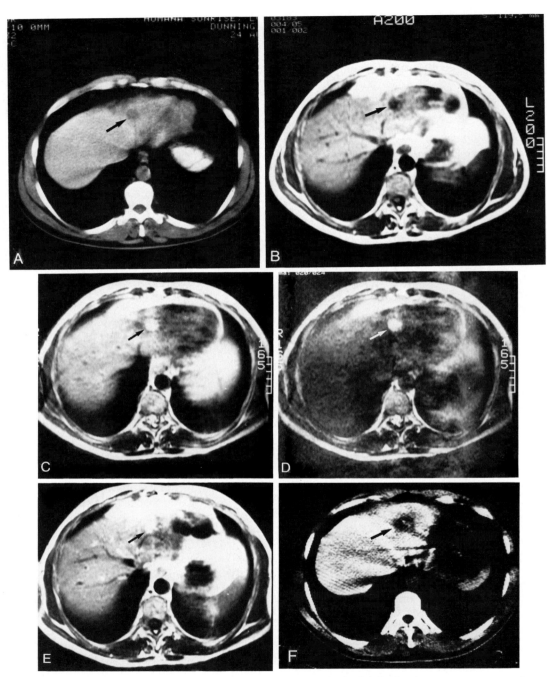

FIGURE 30–33. Atypical colon metastasis *(arrow).* *A,* CT scan obtained following intravenous contrast shows small hypodense lesion at the dome of the left lobe. *B,* T$_1$-weighted (300/20) scan shows lesion darker than liver. *C,* Second echo (2000/60) of a four-echo sequence (2000/30/60/90/120) shows bright lesion relative to liver. Lesion was brighter than liver at 2000/30 (not shown). *D,* Lesion becomes very bright on the fourth echo (2000/120). *E,* Lesion completely fills in by 20 minutes after 0.1mmol/kg Gd-DTPA, becoming isointense with fat anterior to liver. *F,* CT scan obtained as a follow-up 2 months later shows interval growth of colon metastasis. (Courtesy of Dean P. Berthoty, M.D., Sunrise Hospital, Las Vegas, NV.)

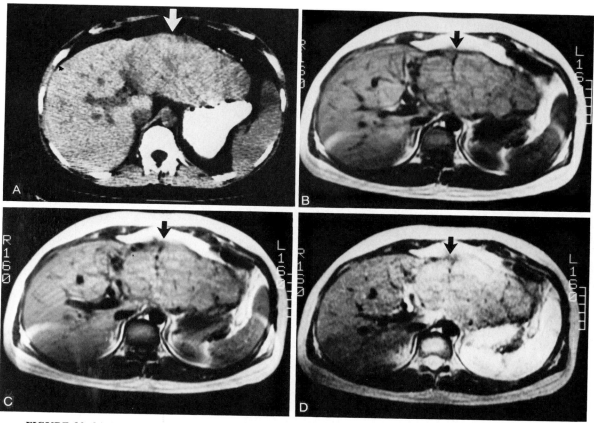

FIGURE 30–34. Hepatic adenoma. *A*, CT scan obtained without contrast shows enlarged lateral segment of left lobe *(arrow)* that is subtly less dense than remainder of liver. *B*, T_1-weighted image (600/20) obtained at nearly the same level as *(A)* shows the enlarged lateral segment that is isointense with remainder of liver but has a disarrayed architecture. *C*, A more hydrogen density–weighted image (1500/20) shows no significant difference from the T_1-weighted image *(B)*. *D*, More T_2 weighting (1500/80) shows lesion to be brighter than liver. These findings are not specific. They could also be seen with hepatomas or any other malignant process. (Courtesy of Donald Widder, M.D.)

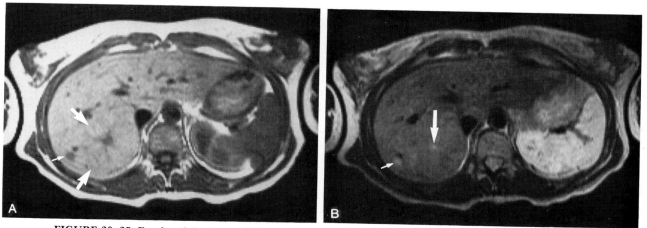

FIGURE 30–35. Focal nodular hyperplasia and cavernous hemangioma (surgically proven). *A*, T_1-weighted image shows poor contrast between lesion *(arrows)* and liver. Note radiating spokes of hypointensity secondary to fibrous septa, and incidental cavernous hemangioma *(small arrow)*. *B*, T_2-weighted image also shows poor liver/lesion contrast. Note the bright central "scar" *(arrow)* that was darker than liver on *(A)*. Also note that small cavernous hemangioma *(small arrow)* has lower signal intensity than expected, probably due to partial volume averaging.

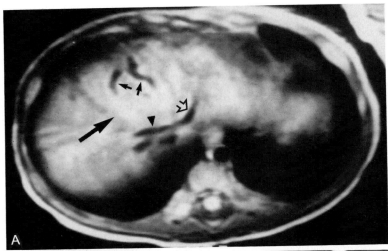

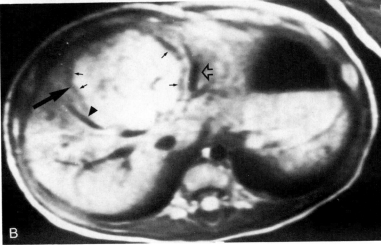

FIGURE 30–36. Hemangioendothelioma in a neonate. *A,* Transverse hydrogen density image (2000/20) shows the lesion *(arrow)* subtly brighter than liver. Note the splaying of the middle *(arrowhead)* and left hepatic *(open arrow)* veins by the mass, which locates it in the medial segment of the left lobe. Also note the two large vessels within the mass *(small arrows)*. *B,* T₂-weighted image obtained at a level just below *(A)* shows the lobulated, well-marginated, and bright lesion. Note the capsule about the lesion *(small arrows)* and the splayed hepatic veins shown here to a better advantage than on *(A)*.

field strengths, acute hematoma appears similar to other proteinaceous fluid collection, having a moderately long T_1 and T_2. At high fields, acute hematomas demonstrate central hypointensity on T_2-weighted images due to preferential T_2 shortening caused by deoxyhemoglobin.[64] These magnetic susceptibility effects are also well shown on lower field systems if gradient-echo techniques are used.[65] In contrast to acute hematomas, subacute (>72 hours old) hematomas have a short T_1 caused by methemoglobin (see Fig. 30–16). Subacute hematomas show regions of hyperintensity on T_1-weighted images, usually beginning at the rim and filling in over time (see Fig. 30–7).[66, 67] Some chronic hematomas develop a dark outer rim owing to hemosiderin deposition. Hemosiderin causes variations in magnetic susceptibility that result in predominant T_2 shortening. Intraparenchymal liver hemorrhages and hematomas are reabsorbed over a period of days to months, depending on their volume and whether or not they are mixed with bile. Note should be made that the presence of characteristic features of hem-

orrhage does not exclude the presence of an underlying malignancy (see Figs. 30–18, 30–27, and 30–37).

While the timing of events during the resolution of hematomas seems predictable in the CNS, it is less predictable in the body. No doubt hematomas undergo similar changes regardless of location. It is the time period spent in each stage which is dependent upon the surrounding environment. If the body has access to the extravasated blood, such as in the peritoneal space, red blood cells may be directly absorbed prior to their lysis and methemoglobin formation. If lysis occurs, it increases the osmotic pressure within the hematoma; water is absorbed, decreasing the concentration of methemoglobin. Furthermore, methemoglobin, which is water soluble, will be removed more efficiently from the space, further decreasing its concentration and effect. Unlike brain hemorrhages, hemorrhages in the body seldom show a low signal rim due to formation of hemosiderin, probably due to the easy access of hemosiderin-laden macrophages to lymphatic chan-

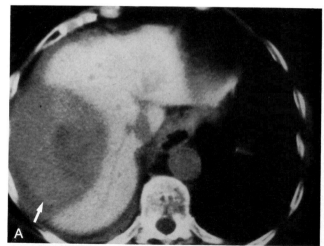

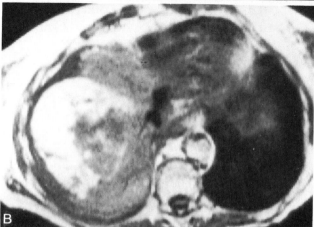

FIGURE 30–37. Metastatic leiomyosarcoma with hemorrhage. *A*, CT image shows slight hyperdensity of hemorrhage *(arrow)* in liver relative to blood in aorta. *B*, T_1-weighted image shows marked hyperintensity of the hemorrhage due to methemoglobin formation. Underlying tumor is not evident.

nels. If the body has limited access to the hematoma, such as hemorrhagic cysts of the ovaries, hematoceles, or hemorrhage in any closed space, the course seems to parallel that of the CNS.

Infiltrative Disorders

Fatty Infiltration

Despite a generally greater capacity for tissue characterization, conventional MR images demonstrate fatty infiltration poorly compared with CT (Fig. 30–38). Despite the short T_1 of fat, fatty infiltration in T_1-weighted images produces either no significant change or slight hyperintensity when compared with unaffected portions of the liver. The apparent lack of sensitivity to focal fat is because the focal fat is accompanied, in alcoholic hepatitis for example, with concomitant increase in water content. The shortening in T_1 from fat is therefore canceled by the lengthening of T_1 by water. However, this seeming

insensitivity to fat can be used to distinguish focal fatty infiltration from metastatic disease, a diagnosis that can be difficult to make with CT or ultrasound.

Although conventional pulse sequences display fatty infiltration poorly, phase-contrast pulse sequences are extremely sensitive to the presence of fat (Fig. 30–39).[68] These sequences are discussed in detail in Chapters 9 and 10. Briefly, phase-contrast sequences take advantage of the slight chemical shift between fat and water protons. Due to these differences, water protons resonate at approximately 3.5 parts-per-million (ppm) higher frequency than fat protons. On a conventional spin-echo pulse sequence where the 180-degree refocusing pulse is delivered at TE/2, fat and water protons are in phase at echo time and are therefore additive. If the 180-degree pulse is shifted from TE/2 by a precise amount, then the fat and water protons will be directly opposed at echo time, canceling each other out.[68] Therefore, each voxel containing water and fat will appear dark. Similar results can be achieved if a gradient-echo sequence is performed with an appropriate choice of TE for the given field strength. Phase-contrast effects can be helpful or detrimental. On T_1-weighted images, phase-contrast is undesirable because it lowers the signal intensity of the liver and reduces liver-to-lesion contrast (Fig. 30–40). However, on more T_2-weighted images, phase contrast decreases liver intensity further, making lesions more conspicuous (Fig. 30–39).[69, 70] We have not found the phase-contrast technique as consistently useful for the detection of mass lesions in the liver as speculated. It is mostly used to distinguish fatty infiltration from mass lesion.

Iron Deposition

Hemochromatosis is a disorder of excessive iron deposition which may be caused by excessive gut absorption of iron (primary form) or by increased red blood cell turnover rate (secondary form, for example, as caused by multiple transfusions). Hemochromatosis affects many organ systems, including liver, pancreas, spleen, heart, and skin. The effect of hemochromatosis is due to excessive deposition of hemosiderin which shortens T_2 with minimal effect on T_1. If T_2 is on the order of one half to one third TE, signal will be lost regardless of the TR used.[71, 72] Hepatic signal may be so minimal as to approach background noise levels (Fig. 30–41). Primary hemochromatosis, which spares the spleen, can be differentiated from the secondary form, which affects the spleen, by assessing splenic signal on T_2-weighted images.

The critical organ in hemochromatosis is the heart, since many of these patients die from iron-induced cardiomyopathy. Whereas MR can detect smaller quantities of iron than CT, attempts at quantifying iron concentration have been unsuccessful. Furthermore, it is not possible to distinguish iron in the reticuloendothelial system, which is relatively harm-

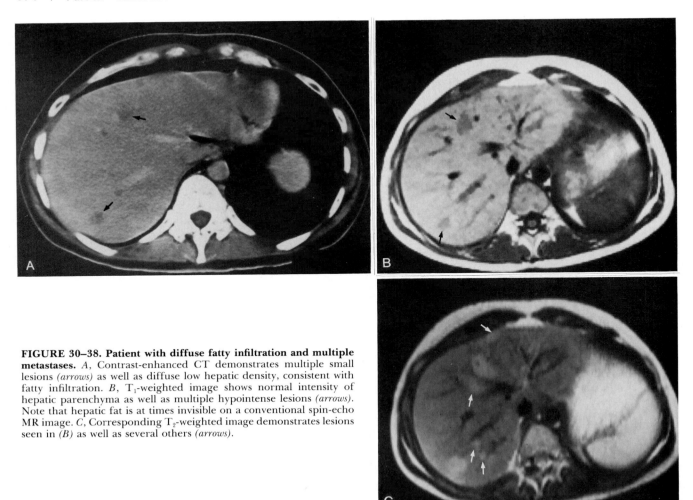

FIGURE 30–38. Patient with diffuse fatty infiltration and multiple metastases. *A*, Contrast-enhanced CT demonstrates multiple small lesions *(arrows)* as well as diffuse low hepatic density, consistent with fatty infiltration. *B*, T_1-weighted image shows normal intensity of hepatic parenchyma as well as multiple hypointense lesions *(arrows)*. Note that hepatic fat is at times invisible on a conventional spin-echo MR image. *C*, Corresponding T_2-weighted image demonstrates lesions seen in *(B)* as well as several others *(arrows)*.

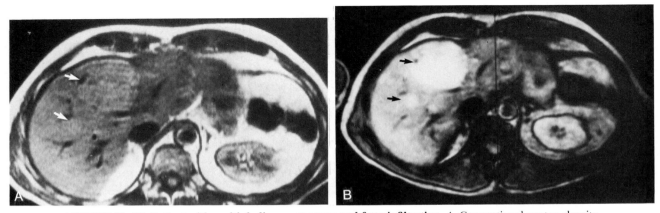

FIGURE 30–39. Patient with multiple liver metastases and fatty infiltration. *A*, Conventional proton density image (2000/30) shows poor contrast between liver and lesions *(arrows)*. *B*, Phase-contrast proton density image (2000/30) obtained using the Dixon technique shows much better liver-to-lesion contrast *(arrows)* due to the reduction in signal intensity from the fat-infiltrated liver. Also note the dark rim about the left kidney due to signal cancellation, since these dark voxels contain both fat and water.

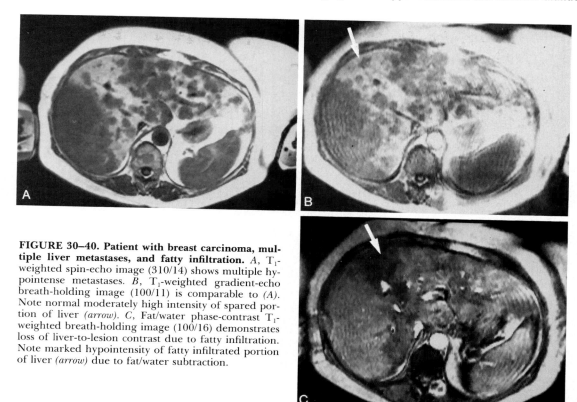

FIGURE 30–40. Patient with breast carcinoma, multiple liver metastases, and fatty infiltration. *A,* T_1-weighted spin-echo image (310/14) shows multiple hypointense metastases. *B,* T_1-weighted gradient-echo breath-holding image (100/11) is comparable to *(A)*. Note normal moderately high intensity of spared portion of liver *(arrow)*. *C,* Fat/water phase-contrast T_1-weighted breath-holding image (100/16) demonstrates loss of liver-to-lesion contrast due to fatty infiltration. Note marked hypointensity of fatty infiltrated portion of liver *(arrow)* due to fat/water subtraction.

less, from the more toxic hepatocyte accumulation. At the present time, while MR is more sensitive than CT, it has no clinical advantage over CT or other noninvasive methods[73] for the evaluation of hemochromatosis. However, given the effect of iron on liver signal, the detection of hepatomas—a consequence of this disease—is made easy.

Copper

Copper, which is deposited in the liver of patients with Wilson's disease, is also paramagnetic in its ionic form. However, cirrhosis develops in the advanced stages of the disease, which may in part account for the failure to observe consistent hepatic signal changes in these patients.[74] It is also possible that the conjugated copper, though paramagnetic, is hidden from mobile hydrogens.

Inflammatory Disease

MR has had very limited usefulness in the evaluation of hepatitis and cirrhosis. Inflammatory conditions of the liver cause a nonspecific increase in T_1 and T_2 relaxation times due to increased free water content.[75] Such an effect is detectable when the condition is focal, since there will be contrast between the normal and abnormal portions of the liver (Fig. 30–42). Chronic inflammation may lead to cirrhosis,

which is accompanied by a reduction in liver volume and changes in hepatic lobar morphology (see Figs. 30–17, 30–24, 30–43). Ascites, which frequently accompanies liver failure, is most commonly seen about the liver and is hypointense on T_1-weighted images and markedly hyperintense on T_2-weighted images (see Figs. 30–19, 30–24, and 30–43).

A report from Japan suggested that in cirrhosis, multiple small dark nodules can be seen studding the liver.[76] It is thought that these dark nodules on T_2-weighted images represent regenerating nodules characteristic of this disease. These dark nodules were seen in 9 of 25 patients (36 per cent). Of these 25 patients, 21 had cirrhosis on the basis of viral hepatitis. Although findings in alcoholic cirrhosis have not been fully described, we suspect that internal changes of the liver will be similar.

Hepatic abscesses have similar appearance to cysts on MRI. However, when complicated, they may assume different signals (Fig. 30–44).

Hepatic Vascular Disease

Because blood flow provides a form of endogenous vascular contrast, MR is well suited for evaluating vascular disorders of the liver as well as depicting normal and abnormal lobar morphology (Fig. 30–45). Patent vessels usually demonstrate a signal void within their lumen. However, at times increased intraluminal signal can be seen due to even-echo

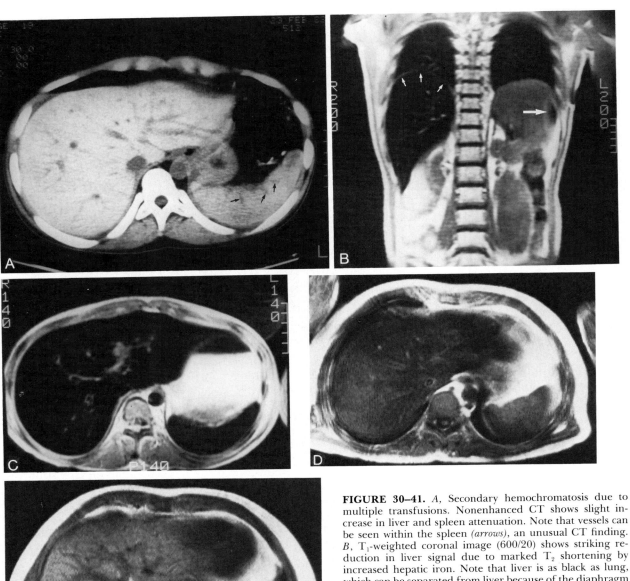

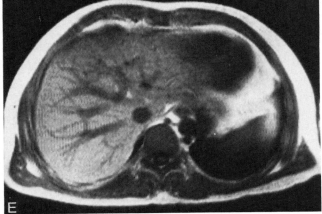

FIGURE 30–41. *A,* Secondary hemochromatosis due to multiple transfusions. Nonenhanced CT shows slight increase in liver and spleen attenuation. Note that vessels can be seen within the spleen *(arrows),* an unusual CT finding. *B,* T$_1$-weighted coronal image (600/20) shows striking reduction in liver signal due to marked T$_2$ shortening by increased hepatic iron. Note that liver is as black as lung, which can be separated from liver because of the diaphragm *(small arrows).* The dark tip of the spleen can be seen adjacent to stomach *(arrow). C,* Proton density image (2000/20) shows signal of liver and spleen to be equal to background. *D,* Different patient with primary hemochromatosis. Before therapy (serum ferritin = 721), the liver is dark in a T$_1$-weighted image. *E,* After six months of phlebotomy treatment (serum ferritin = 8), the liver has normal signal intensity.

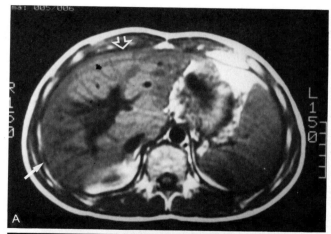

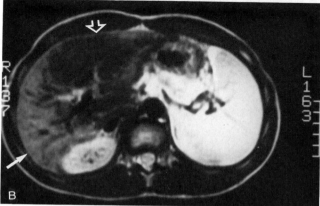

FIGURE 30–42. Acute focal CMV hepatitis in a child. *A,* T₁-weighted image (300/20) shows a dark right lobe *(arrow)*, as dark as spleen, and a brighter left lobe. Note the subtly dark subcapsular portion of the bright left lobe *(open arrow)*. *B,* T₂-weighted image (2000/70) looks like the negative image of *(A),* in that areas that were bright became dark, and areas that were dark became bright. The contrast between dark and bright, though reversed, is nearly equal. The dark areas in *(A)* are portions of the liver with increased water content which brighten on T₂ *(B).* The bright areas of the liver on *(A)* are the unaffected portions of the liver that darken normally on T₂ *(B).* The hydrogen density image (not shown) had similar appearance as the T₂-weighted image but with less striking contrast. (Courtesy of Dean P. Berthoty, M.D., Sunrise Hospital, Las Vegas, NV.)

rephasing (see Fig. 30–11) or slow flow in intrahepatic vessels (see Figs. 30–29*D* and 30–46) and particularly in portal veins when associated with portal hypertension. A positive statement of patency can be made with high confidence when a vessel is black. However, when vessels contain signal they may be patent or thrombosed. As a general rule for evaluating vessel patency with SE sequences, avoid using sequences that increase vascular signal, such as even echoes (e.g., 20/40, 25/50, or 30/60) or flow compensation techniques. Rather, use asymmetric echoes (e.g., 20/70) and sequences that promote flow void, such as the flow void option, thinner slices, and longer TEs. Of course care must be taken to maintain proper T₁ or T₂ weighting and S/N ratio. Since a thrombosed vessel contains stationary protons, it should show signal on any sequence and any plane.

Such a vessel could still be patent if it has stagnant blood or blood with extremely slow flow velocity.

Thrombosis of the hepatic veins (Budd-Chiari syndrome) can be equally evaluated by MR, contrast-enhanced CT, and duplex sonography. Failure to visualize the confluence of the hepatic veins and paucity or complete absence of their branches are reliable criteria for the diagnosis. However, care should be taken not to overcall this condition in cirrhotic livers, since compression of hepatic veins by fibrosis and increased intracapsular pressure could be mistaken for venous occlusion (see Fig. 30–43). The presence of comma-shaped venous collaterals in Budd-Chiari syndrome may be a useful distinguishing feature (Fig. 30–47).[77]

Portal hypertension can be accompanied by portal vein occlusion, venous collaterals, and splenomegaly (Fig. 30–48).[78] Varices appear as tortuous low intensity tubular structures (Fig. 30–48). When chronic splenic, superior mesenteric, and/or portal venous occlusion occurs, perivascular collaterals develop, called cavernous transformation (Fig. 30–49).[78] In patients with either spontaneous or surgical portal-venous shunting, shunt patency can be demonstrated by MRI as an intraluminal flow void at the level of the anastomosis (Fig. 30–50). Of course, color Doppler may be as sensitive and should be attempted first. Although the specificity of MRI for portal vein thrombosis was 100 per cent in a recent study of 15 patients with thrombosed portal veins,[79] the clinical utility of MR for this application will be enhanced by the implementation of methods for determining the velocity and direction of flow,[80] as is presently available with duplex sonography as well as MR angiographic techniques (see Chapter 4).

Intrahepatic portal vein occlusion can produce a triangular wedge-shaped region within the liver—the

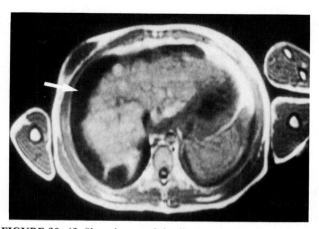

FIGURE 30–43. Shrunken, nodular liver and surrounding ascites *(arrow).* Note the loss of right lobe volume and increase in left lobe volume, characteristic of chronic alcoholic liver disease as in this patient with proven macronodular cirrhosis. Paucity of hepatic vessels can be due to compression from increased intracapsular pressure. Compression of hepatic veins may make it difficult to exclude Budd-Chiari syndrome.

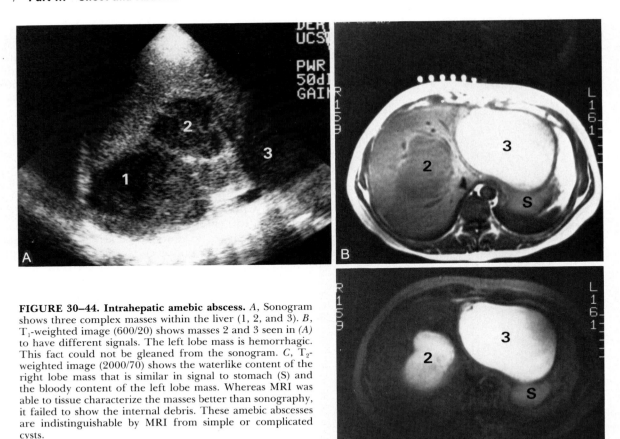

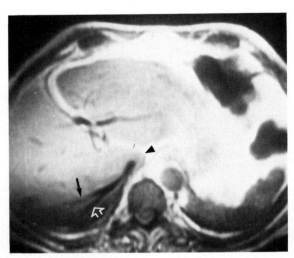

FIGURE 30–44. Intrahepatic amebic abscess. *A*, Sonogram shows three complex masses within the liver (1, 2, and 3). *B*, T_1-weighted image (600/20) shows masses 2 and 3 seen in *(A)* to have different signals. The left lobe mass is hemorrhagic. This fact could not be gleaned from the sonogram. *C*, T_2-weighted image (2000/70) shows the waterlike content of the right lobe mass that is similar in signal to stomach (S) and the bloody content of the left lobe mass. Whereas MRI was able to tissue characterize the masses better than sonography, it failed to show the internal debris. These amebic abscesses are indistinguishable by MRI from simple or complicated cysts.

FIGURE 30–45. Near total absence of the right lobe of the liver for unknown reason. Patient denied alcohol abuse. Furthermore, the caudate lobe *(arrowhead)* is also diminutive, which is unusual if right lobe volume loss was secondary to alcoholic liver disease. Note that the middle *(arrow)* and right *(open arrow)* hepatic veins are near each other because the anterior segment of the right lobe is minuscule. Also note that the right hepatic vein *(open arrow)* is near the posterior margin of the liver because the posterior segment of the right lobe is also minuscule.

apex of which is central and the base abutting the capsule—which is of high signal on T_2-weighted images.[81] It may possibly be due to infarction or edema. Hepatoma, in that series, was the most common reason for portal occlusion.[81]

ROLE OF MRI IN LESION DETECTION

CT is presently considered the imaging modality of choice as a screening test for the detection of liver masses and is the gold standard in some institutions.[32] CT has an estimated accuracy ranging from 50 to 96 per cent for liver metastases. Furthermore, CT can simultaneously assess the upper abdomen and offer the capacity for guided needle biopsy.[82–84] However, the high detection rate demands the use of rapid intravenous infusion of iodinated contrast medium in combination with advanced technology for dynamic scanning, arterial catheterization, and at times delayed scanning 4 hours later.

When optimized pulse sequences are used at low or high field,[26, 33, 35] MR was shown to be superior to CT in its sensitivity for liver lesion detection. However, others disagree.[32] Further investigation is therefore warranted. While reports suggest that high field

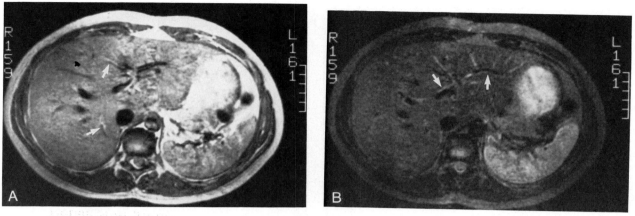

FIGURE 30–46. Branching white lines within the liver due to misregistration caused by a phase shift induced when protons flow within the imaging plane (flow-displacement artifact, see Chapter 4). *A*, Hydrogen density image (2000/20) shows normal liver with some vessels causing phase shift *(arrows)*. *B*, T$_2$-weighted image (2000/70) shows more branching white lines from phase shift mostly because the background is darker than in *(A)*. Note that the white lines *(arrows)* are superior to the right and inferior to left portal branches because blood flow is in opposite directions (see also Fig. 30–29*D*).

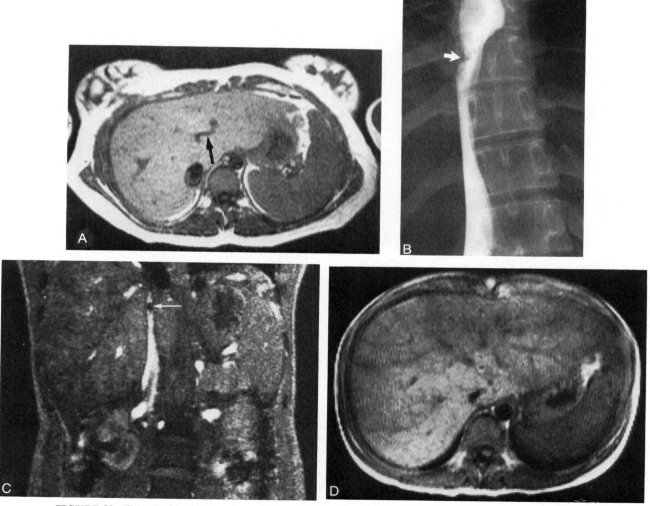

FIGURE 30–47. *A*, Budd-Chiari syndrome. Note absence of normal hepatic veins. Curvilinear collateral vessel *(arrow)* is characteristic of this disorder. *B*, Different patient with clot in inferior vena cava (IVC) and thrombosis of peripheral hepatic veins. Vena cavogram shows narrowing of IVC and clot *(arrow)*. *C*, Coronal flow-compensated breath-hold gradient-echo image (TR/TE/flip angle = 30 msec/10 msec/30°) shows clot *(arrow)* in IVC and abnormal paucity of small hepatic veins. *D*, Axial T$_1$-weighted image shows hepatomegaly and inhomogeneous liver texture.

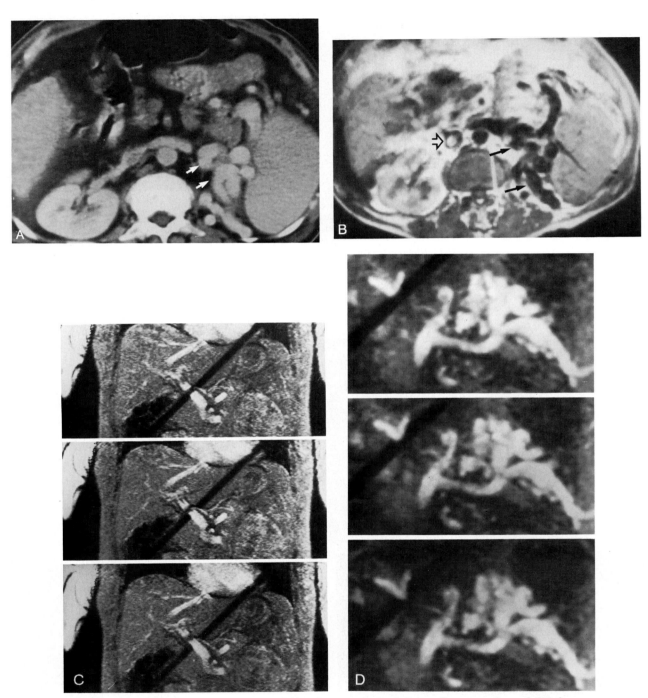

FIGURE 30–48. *A,* Portal hypertension, varices, splenomegaly, and ascites. Contrast-enhanced CT demonstrates dense tortuous vessels *(arrows)* near splenic hilum. *B,* MR readily demonstrates varices as low intensity structures *(arrows)* due to flow void. Note low intensity of ascites surrounding liver on this T$_1$-weighted image. Signal in vena cava *(open arrow)* is due to flow caused by incoming full magnetized protons from outside the imaging volume. *C,* MR angiograph techniques cn be useful for determining flow direction and patency of the portal vein. Breath-hold bolus track study in a healthy subject shows normal motion of a presaturated bolus of portal venous blood toward the liver. *D,* Different patient with alcoholic cirrhosis and portal hypertension. Note reversed direction of portal flow, and gastric varices. (From Edelman RR, Wentz K, Mattle M, et al: MR angiography and dynamic flow evaluation of the portal venous system. AJR 153:755–760, 1989.)

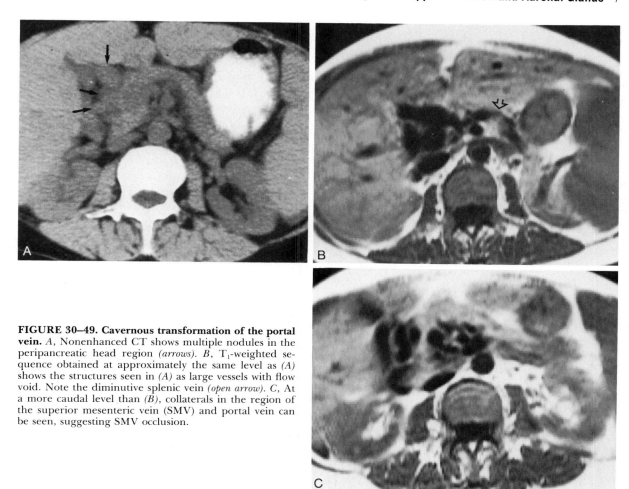

FIGURE 30–49. Cavernous transformation of the portal vein. *A,* Nonenhanced CT shows multiple nodules in the peripancreatic head region *(arrows). B,* T$_1$-weighted sequence obtained at approximately the same level as *(A)* shows the structures seen in *(A)* as large vessels with flow void. Note the diminutive splenic vein *(open arrow). C,* At a more caudal level than *(B),* collaterals in the region of the superior mesenteric vein (SMV) and portal vein can be seen, suggesting SMV occlusion.

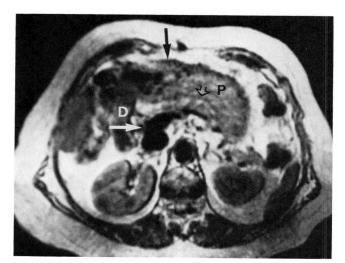

FIGURE 30–50. Patent portacaval shunt *(white arrow)* in a patient with acute pancreatitis. Note the phlegmon (P) in the lesser sac anterior to pancreas *(open arrow),* posterior to gastric antrum *(black arrow),* and left of duodenum (D). Signal within the phlegmon was indistinguishable from stomach on all pulsing sequences (not shown).

systems are more sensitive when using T$_2$-weighted sequences,[36] there is suggestion that heavily T$_1$-weighted sequences with inversion recovery at high field may be equally sensitive.[35] Since sonography and radionuclide imaging of the liver are known to be less accurate than CT, MR is emerging as potentially the most sensitive examination for patients with suspected hepatic metastases.[26] It is not clear what is the minimum size liver lesion consistently detectable by MRI. In one report MR sensitivity in detecting hepatomas was severely limited when lesions were less than 2 cm.[44]

Contrast agents have the potential to improve the performance of MR. In one study at mid-field (0.6 T), administration of ferrite, which eliminates the signal from normal liver parenchyma, produced a marked improvement in lesion detection.[5] However, no significant improvement was obtained on a high field system, when postcontrast scans were compared with T$_2$-weighted SE images.[81a] Additional studies will be needed to provide a more definitive assessment of the role of contrast agents in liver MRI.

Some studies have suggested that CT during arterial portography provides the best sensitivity for hepatic lesion detection.[84a, 84b] MR was much less sensitive than CT portography for detecting lesions smaller than 2 cm. However, the combination of CT-portography and MR may provide greater sensitivity than either method alone.[84b] Since CT-portography is not a routine screening procedure, this approach is reserved for patients who are candidates for hepatic resection.

The unavailability of oral and intravenous MR contrast media to distinguish bowel from normal and abnormal structures and to evaluate renal and vascularized tissues limits MRI's ability to fully assess the remainder of the upper abdomen.[84] While at present MRI may be the most sensitive imaging modality for liver lesion detection, it is reserved for patients in whom the discovery of a lesion missed by CT will significantly alter their management and for those patients with contraindication to iodinated contrast media.

The future of MRI is, however, different. Although not yet approved for body applications, Gd-DTPA is now available for clinical use. Gd-DTPA, like iodinated water soluble agents, is distributed in the extracellular fluid space. Since most imaging schemes require minutes to acquire, Gd-DTPA contrasts tissues with different extracellular fluid volumes. That mass lesions and liver have similar extracellular fluid volumes has been shown by the insensitivity of CT when iodinated agents are infused slowly. Areas of third space that equilibrate with the extracellular fluid slowly, such as the biliary tree, cysts, abscesses, and areas of necrosis, will be highlighted by Gd-DTPA.[85] Findings, described for enhanced CT scanning, are being shown feasible with Gd-DTPA–enhanced MRI.[86–88] We suspect that MRI with Gd-DTPA might suffer from similar inaccuracies as has been observed with CT following contrast administration (see Fig. 30–33). Gd-DTPA is, however, ideally suited for imaging kidneys, allowing MR for the first time to evaluate intrinsic renal masses. However, for the detection of intrinsic renal masses with Gd-DTPA, a word of caution is warranted. The time sequence of renal tissue enhancement versus renal tumor enhancement is not known for MRI. The so-called equilibrium image on CT obtained 3 minutes after contrast injection may by no means be an equilibrium image for MRI, in that the wash-out rate of Gd-DTPA from tumors is not known and MRI is more sensitive to small levels of Gd-DTPA than is CT for iodine levels. At 3 minutes after administration of Gd-DTPA, renal tumors may be isointense with kidneys. Oral MR contrast agents as well as ferrite particles are in phase III trials and may be approved by the time this text is published. The availability of oral contrast agents, Gd-DTPA, ferrite particles, and other yet investigational intravenous contrast media, along with significant technical advances allowing greater contrast with short

acquisition time, will require the reassessment of the role of MR in imaging the upper abdomen.

BILIARY TREE

Normal bile ducts are too small to be visualized, but when dilated they are seen as tortuous branching structures with low intensity on T_1-weighted images and with high intensity on T_2-weighted images (see Figs. 30–9, 30–10, and 30–23). It is important to see them adjacent to the portal veins on T_1-weighted sequences, since phase shift artifact from flow can

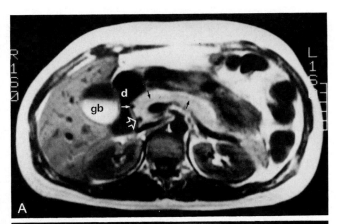

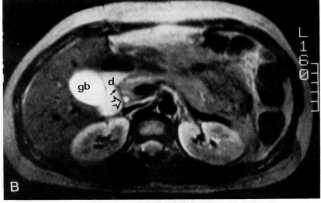

FIGURE 30–51. Normal gallbladder and pancreas in a fasting patient. *A*, T_1-weighted (600/20) image obtained at the level of the pancreas shows a fluid/fluid level in the gallbladder (gb). Upper layer is fresh, less concentrated bile, while lower layer is concentrated and denser in this fasting patient. Note that the bright signal of the pancreas (slightly brighter than liver and much brighter than water-filled duodenum [d] in this patient) allows the visualization of the normal intrapancreatic duct *(black small arrows)*, the gastroduodenal artery *(small white arrow)*, and distal common bile duct *(open arrow)*. *B*, On T_2 weighting (1500/80), the gallbladder (gb) becomes diffusely bright; the pancreas darkens but to a lesser degree than liver and is well demarcated from the bright fluid-filled duodenum (d); the normal pancreatic duct is no longer seen, probably due to decreased signal-to-noise ratio; the gastroduodenal artery is faintly seen *(small black arrow)*; and the distal common bile duct becomes intensely bright compared with the darkened pancreatic head *(open arrow)*. (Courtesy of Donald Widder, M.D.)

mimic their appearance on T_2-weighted images (see Figs. 30–29*D* and 30–46). The extrahepatic bile duct is easily seen when dilated. However, the normal distal common bile duct is frequently seen at the level of the pancreatic head where it is imaged in cross-section (see Figs. 30–13 and 30–51). Its signal intensity behavior is like that of water and that of the intrahepatic bile ducts. When dilated it can be traced from porta hepatis to pancreatic head. Pancreas is brighter than duct on T_1-weighted images and darker on T_2-weighted images (Figs. 30–13 and 30–51). On T_1-weighted images, the intrapancreatic duct is not typically seen when normal in size but at times can be visible (Fig. 30–51). When seen, it is darker than pancreas but becomes brighter than pancreas on T_2-weighted images. Like the measurements on CT, the common bile duct within the pancreatic head is a few millimeters in diameter, but a measurement of up to 1 cm can be normal.

The MR signal intensity within the gallbladder varies depending on the concentration of bile and therefore on the fasting status. In the normal gallbladder of fasting subjects, the concentrated bile appears hyperintense compared with liver on moderately T_1-weighted images (Fig. 30–51). However, fresh nonconcentrated bile in nonfasting patients is like that of the intrahepatic biliary tree and has signal behavior like that of water. In a spectroscopic analysis Demas and colleagues[89] found that the T_1 relaxation of bile was strictly related to the T_1 relaxation of water hydrogens and not to those contained in cholesterol, phospholipids, proteins, and bile salts. Bakan and Barnhart[90] studied the effects of bile constituents on T_1 shortening of water protons and found that of all the constituents, T_1 of bile related best with the concentration of bile salts, total proteins, and bile viscosity. Mixing of concentrated and fresh bile appears to be poor, since the more concentrated viscous

bile (bright bile) layers along the dependent portion of the gallbladder below the less concentrated bile (dark bile) (Fig. 30–51). Could the signal intensity of gallbladder contents help differentiate normal from abnormal gallbladders? In vitro T_1 and T_2 relaxation measurements reported by Loflin and coworkers[91] of bile collected from 6 patients who had normal gallbladders, and from 11 patients with acute and 41 patients with chronic cholecystitis during surgery, showed no significant difference between the groups. Their study, however, had a great deal of variability in the measurements requiring larger samples for statistical significance particularly between the normal and abnormal groups. In an in vivo study, McCarthy and colleagues[92] reported that the relationship of bile signal intensity was significantly related to health or disease. When bile was hyperintense relative to liver on a T_1-weighted image, it implied normalcy with 100 per cent specificity. However, when bile was isointense or hypointense relative to liver in a fasting patient on a T_1-weighted image, it implied disease in only 44 per cent of cases.[92] To truly assess the role of MRI in gallbladder disease, further work is needed to confirm these findings and prove efficacy.

Gallstones are solid structures. Like cortical bone, they have short T_2 relaxation times, appearing dark on all sequences. Therefore, gallstones appear as a signal void within the gallbladder contrasted against the white bile on T_2-weighted images[93] (Figs. 30–52 and 30–53). Some gallstones may demonstrate a high intensity nidus of yet uncertain etiology.[93] Unlike CT, MRI shows gallstones as regions of black signal void because of their solid nature rather than chemical composition, and unlike sonography shows all stones.

Whether of biliary, pancreatic, or metastatic origin, if associated with a dilated biliary tree, neoplastic tissue in the porta hepatis can be difficult to differ-

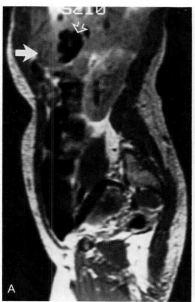 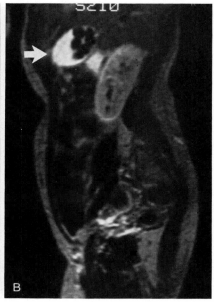

FIGURE 30–52. Gallstones either are black on all pulsing sequences or at times are black with central signal. *A*, Hydrogen density sagittal image (2000/20) shows gallbladder *(arrow)* with low signal bile and multiple black stones. Note subtle signal within some stones *(open arrow)*. *B*, Stones are highly contrasted to bright bile on a T_2-weighted image (2000/70).

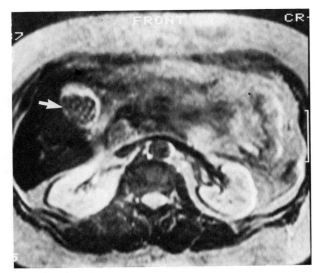

FIGURE 30–53. Gallstones *(arrow)* regardless of size and number can be easily seen on T_2-weighted images, as in this case, due to marked increase in contrast between black stones and white bile.

entiate from bile (Fig. 30–54) and at times from other normal structures in that region (Fig. 30–55). In this setting, Gd-DTPA and oral contrast can be of help since solid tissues will enhance while the biliary tree and bowel content will not, and the oral agent would outline the lumen of stomach and bowel (see Figs. 30–10 and 30–56). A retrospective study reported by Dooms and coworkers, utilizing a 0.35-T unit,[94] showed that MRI was capable of detecting 7 of 9 tumors. It is not clear from their report, however, whether MRI will be capable in detecting these lesions in prospect. In a case done at our institution at 1.5 T, it was difficult to delineate mass from the biliary tree (Fig. 30–54). The role of MRI in cholangiocarcinoma awaits further evaluation.

It has been well documented that the biliary tree is best assessed by ultrasound.[95] However, CT is better suited for the differential diagnosis of distal common bile duct obstruction.[96] The role of MRI in this setting is yet unclear. MRI can visualize the biliary tree and distal duct in any plane just like with sonography; it can visualize gallstones; it can recognize, particularly when aided with oral contrast, pancreas from duodenum; and it can evaluate the uncinate process of the pancreas on sagittal views, which may be easier to interpret than the transverse view. However, the future of MRI in the differential diagnosis of obstructive jaundice, while promising, awaits further investigation.

PANCREAS

At the present time, MR does not appear to have a significant role in the evaluation of pancreatic disorders.[97] Susceptibility to respiratory and bowel motion, confusion with surrounding bowel, inability

to demonstrate small calcifications, and somewhat inferior spatial resolution limit the role of MR vis-à-vis ultrasound and CT. However, in patients with known contrast hypersensitivity, MR can help differentiate vascular structures adjacent to the pancreas from parenchyma and tumor (see Figs. 30–13 and 30–51).

PULSE SEQUENCES

The pulse sequence considerations for pancreas and liver are the same, since the relaxation times of these two organs are somewhat similar. Anatomy is best demonstrated by T_1-weighted pulse sequences because of the excellent retroperitoneal fat/pancreas contrast (see Figs. 30–4, 30–13, and 30–51). We prefer the long TR/short TE sequence (hydrogen density) images, since these images have greater S/N ratio than T_1-weighted images. However, hydrogen density images have slightly less fat/tissue contrast. Administration of an oral contrast agent can improve the delineation of pancreas from stomach (Fig. 30–56). We use 1 mg glucagon subcutaneously on a routine basis to minimize blurring from bowel activity. We evaluate the pancreas on T_1-weighted sagittal images and on hydrogen density and T_2-weighted transaxial images. Slice thickness is usually 10 mm; however, on additional sequences, a 5-mm slice thickness is used to minimize partial volume. The sagittal plane demonstrates the uncinate process clearly (Fig. 30–57). A focal bulge suggests disease (Fig. 30–58). These localized bulges can be difficult to appreciate on transaxial images. We find the coronal plane of limited utility.

ANATOMY

The pancreatic morphology is variable in appearance. The gland may appear smooth or lobulated

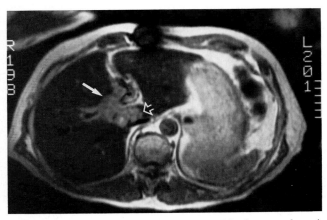

FIGURE 30–54. Cholangiocarcinoma *(arrow)* in the porta hepatis is invading the liver and causing biliary obstruction. It is indistinguishable from the dilated biliary tree that was easily depicted on a contrast-enhanced CT (not shown). Note invasion of the caudate lobe *(open arrow)*.

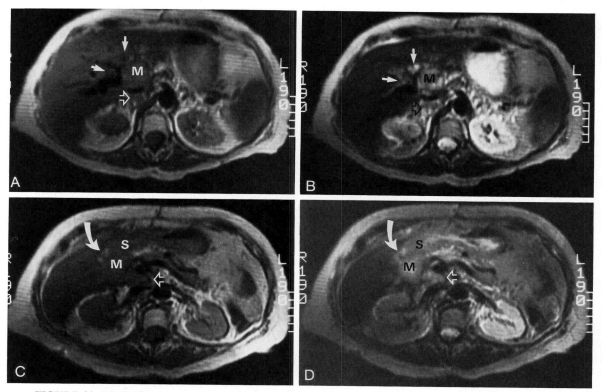

FIGURE 30–55. Gallbladder carcinoma in the porta hepatis. *A* and *B*, Hydrogen density (2000/20) *(A)* and T$_2$-weighted (2000/70) *(B)* images obtained at the level of the mass show the mass (M) with signals indistinguishable from dilated biliary tree *(small white arrows)*. Note the presence of retrocaval adenopathy *(open arrow)* with similar signal as primary lesion. *C* and *D*, Hydrogen density *(C)* and T$_2$-weighted *(D)* images, obtained within the same series as *(A)* and *(B)* but at a more caudal level, show the mass (M) with signals indistinguishable from gastric antrum (S) and pancreatic uncinate process *(open arrow)*. Note that gastric antrum could have been confused with left lobe involvement because the fat in the gastroduodenal ligament *(curved arrow)* could be mistaken for the ligamentum teres. Oral contrast would resolve this confusion. The darkened fat posterior to the right kidney and not to the left kidney is an artifact from shading. Note similar signal in subcutaneous fat.

FIGURE 30–56. Improved visualization of pancreatic head after ingestion of perfluorooctyl-bromide (PFOB). *A*, Axial hydrogen density image (2000/20) was obtained at the level of the pancreatic head. Note that the anterior margin of the pancreas appears nodular and indistinct. *B*, Repeat scan with identical parameters as in *(A)*, but after PFOB, shows smooth and clearly marginated pancreatic head secondary to the filling of the gastric antrum and duodenum. (From Mattrey RF, Hajek PC, Gylys-Morin V, et al: Perfluorochemicals as gastrointestinal contrast agents for MR imaging: Preliminary studies in rats and humans. AJR 148:1259–1263, 1987; © by American Roentgen Ray Society.)

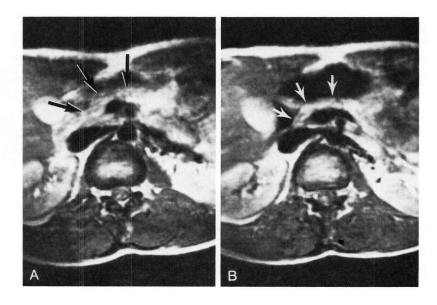

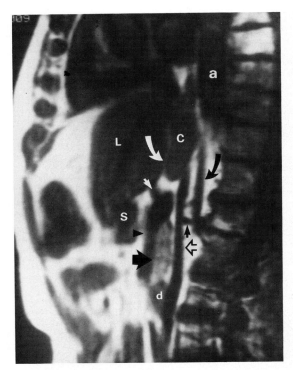

FIGURE 30–57. Normal uncinate process *(large black arrow)* is seen on a sagittal T$_1$-weighted scan (600/20) between the superior mesenteric vein *(arrowhead)* and inferior vena cava *(open arrow)*. Note on this plane the visualization of aorta (a), ligamentum venosum *(curved white arrow)* separating the caudate (C) from the lateral segment of left lobe (L), crux of diaphragm *(curved black arrow)*, hepatic artery *(small white arrow)*, stomach (s), right renal artery *(small black arrow)*, and third portion of duodenum (d).

(see Figs. 30–4 and 30–51) or may blend with surrounding tissues if replaced by fat. Pancreatic tissue is as bright or slightly darker than liver on T$_1$-weighted images and is slightly brighter than liver on T$_2$-weighted images. Pancreas has a short T$_2$, but not as short as that of liver. The normal pancreatic duct is too small to be routinely visualized on body coil images, but it has been demonstrated occasionally (Fig. 30–51) when high-resolution surface coils were used in thin subjects[98] or when the duct was dilated (Fig. 30–59). The common bile duct is, however, routinely seen on T$_2$-weighted images, particularly on the transaxial plane, since it has a much longer T$_2$ than that of pancreatic head and is seen in cross-section (see Figs. 30–13 and 30–51).

FOCAL MASSES/INFLAMMATION

Like liver tumors, pancreatic tumors appear hypointense compared with the normal parenchyma on T$_1$-weighted images, and at times hyperintense on T$_2$-weighted images.[97–99] Marked hyperintensity within a solid mass on highly T$_2$-weighted images suggests hypervascularity as in an islet cell tumor, tumor necrosis, and/or hemorrhage (Fig. 30–60). At

high field, based upon our limited experience, pancreatic cancer has had similar signals to normal pancreatic parenchyma. Final assessment of tumor signal behavior, however, requires further investigation.

Staging of pancreatic cancer may be more easily done with MRI, particularly in patients allergic to the iodinated contrast media. MRI offers greater ease in visualizing and evaluating the superior mesenteric and splenic arteries and veins for encasement and thrombosis (Figs. 30–59 and 30–61). Mesenteric fat is easily assessed for signal changes. Peripancreatic, celiac, and periportal nodes are more easily recognized adjacent to darkened vessels and liver (Fig. 30–61). While CT is very specific for nonresectability, its sensitivity is poor.[100] The sensitivity and specificity of MRI in this setting have not been defined but have great promise. These data are being accumulated presently through a national collaborative study supported by the National Institutes of Health (NIH).

MRI can demonstrate pancreatitis when it produces a phlegmonous mass (see Fig. 30–50) or when the inflammatory process infiltrates the peripancreatic tissues (Figs. 30–62 and 30–63). Although uncomplicated pseudocysts will demonstrate similar in-

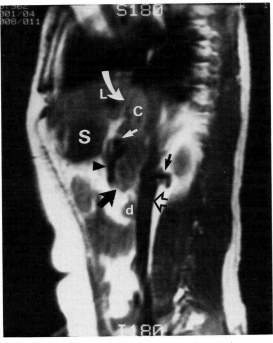

FIGURE 30–58. Pancreatic carcinoma in the uncinate process *(large black arrow)* is seen on a sagittal T$_1$-weighted scan (600/20) between the superior mesenteric vein (SMV) *(arrowhead)* and inferior vena cava *(open arrow)*. In contrast to the normal uncinate seen in Figure 30–57, note the mass effect on the SMV in this example. Also note that on this plane the ligamentum venosum *(curved white arrow)* separating the caudate (C) from the lateral segment of left lobe (L), hepatic artery *(small white arrow)*, stomach (S), right renal artery *(small black arrow)*, and third portion of duodenum (d) can be recognized.

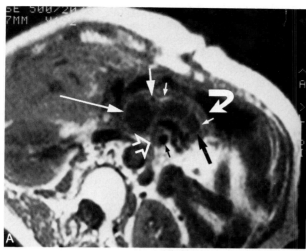

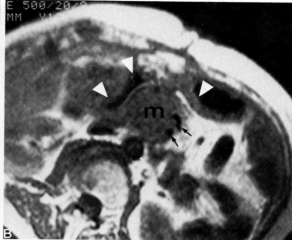

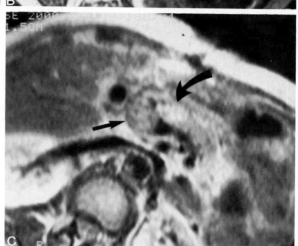

FIGURE 30–59. Pancreatic carcinoma with dilated pancreatic duct. *A*, T₁-weighted image shows dilated common bile duct *(long white arrow)* and pancreatic duct *(long black arrow)* within the brighter head and body of pancreas. Note that gastroduodenal artery *(short white arrow)* and narrow strip of fat *(small white arrows)* separate pancreas with atrophic body from posterior wall of stomach *(curved arrow)*. The black signal within the splenic vein defines the posterior margin of pancreas. Mass *(open arrow)*, better seen in *(B)*, extends posterior to superior mesenteric artery *(small black arrow)*. *B*, At slightly inferior level than *(A)*, T₁-weighted image shows large mass (m) separated from duodenum and posterior wall of stomach *(arrowheads)* by a thin strip of fat. Note that mass also encases superior mesenteric vessels *(small arrows)*. *C*, T₂-weighted image at a slightly higher level than *(A)* shows increased signal within the common bile duct *(arrow)* and pancreatic duct *(curved arrow)*. Note that the common bile duct is less intense than the pancreatic duct, most likely from sludge within it.

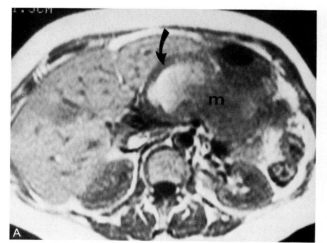

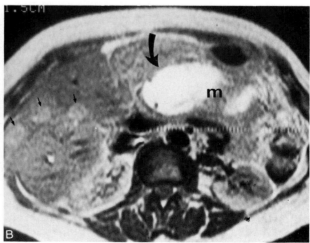

FIGURE 30–60. Hemorrhagic islet cell tumor. *A*, T₁-weighted image demonstrates mass (m) with hyperintense regions *(curved arrow)* due to subacute hemorrhage. *B*, T₂-weighted image shows persistence of hyperintense areas characteristic of old blood. Note faintly visualized liver metastases *(small arrows)*.

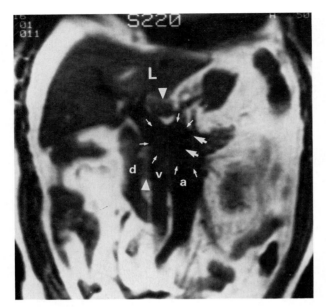

FIGURE 30–61. Pancreatic carcinoma *(small arrows)* is shown on this T₁-weighted (600/20) coronal scan obtained posterior to the level of the pancreas encasing the celiac axis and superior mesenteric artery *(white arrows)*. Note peripancreatic adenopathy *(arrowheads)* seen separate from duodenum (d), vena cava (v), aorta (a), and left lobe of liver (L).

tensity characteristics as CSF in the spinal canal, high protein content or infection can cause the relaxation times of these benign lesions to overlap with those of tumors. Furthermore, tumor infiltration of the pancreas may be difficult to distinguish from pancreatitis. Pancreatitis enlarges the gland, can produce infiltration of peripancreatic tissues and, when hemorrhagic, assumes signals of blood (Figs. 30–62 and 30–63).

The exact role of MRI in the assessment of the pancreas is still unclear. It certainly does not offer at present additional data not already gained from CT and sonography.[101] Its role in staging is also unclear. With more use of oral contrast and the availability of intravenous contrast, the ability of MRI to diagnose, stage, and differentiate pancreatic cancer from pancreatitis will have to be reassessed. With the increasing popularity of pancreatic tissue transplantation, MRI may serve a role in detecting rejection.[102]

ADRENAL GLANDS

The adrenal gland is a site for the development of a variety of primary and secondary tumors and, uncommonly, for inflammatory lesions. Because of its high spatial resolution, CT is an excellent modality to demonstrate small lesions. However, it has limited tissue characterization potential. Early results suggested that MR displays larger (> 2 cm) adrenal tumors as well as CT but with greater potential for lesion characterization.[103] In addition, because of the signal void in vessels and greater fat-to-adrenal contrast, MRI allows for easier recognition of the left

adrenal gland than does CT. Indeed, the left and right adrenal glands were seen on MRI in 99 per cent and 91 per cent of cases, respectively.[104]

There are three distinct settings in which adrenal lesions are encountered that require different diagnostic work-up. The first setting is in patients who have functioning adrenal lesions with symptoms or biochemical evidence of elevation of catecholamines, cortisone, or aldosterone. This group requires surgery. The goal of imaging is to identify the lesion for diagnosis and preoperative planning. In this setting, CT is the imaging modality of choice, given its ability to visualize the adrenal gland and its high spatial resolution.[104a] MRI could be helpful in finding

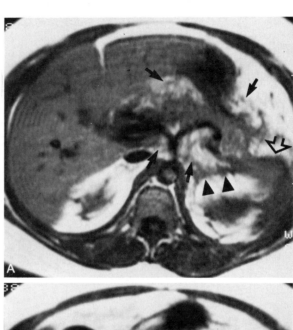

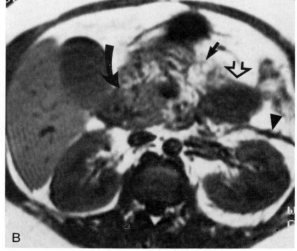

FIGURE 30–62. Acute pancreatitis with pseudocyst formation. *A*, T₁-weighted image obtained at the level of the pancreatic body shows infiltration of peripancreatic fat *(small arrows)*. Note thickening of left anterior perirenal space *(arrowheads)* and fluid near the tail of the pancreas *(open arrow)*. *B*, A few levels caudal to *(A)* within the same T₁-weighted series, there is enlargement of the pancreatic head *(curved arrow)*, infiltration of the peripancreatic fat *(small arrow)*, thickening of left anterior perirenal space *(arrowhead)*, and pseudocyst formation *(open arrow)*.

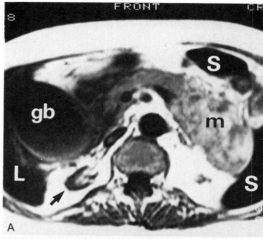

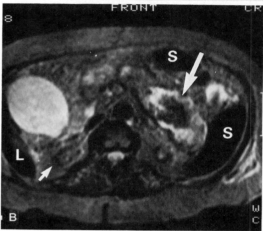

FIGURE 30–63. Hemorrhagic pancreatitis. *A*, T_1-weighted trans-axial image (600/14) obtained at the level of pancreatic body shows large, slightly hyperintense mass (m) in body and tail of pancreas. Note marked distention of gallbladder (gb). Also note dark liver (L) and spleen (S) secondary to hemochromatosis. *B*, T_2-weighted image (2340/100) obtained at approximately the same level as *(A)* shows darkening of pancreatic mass characteristic of subacute hemorrhage. Note the darkened liver (L) and spleen (S) as seen in *(A)*. Also note the small atrophic right kidney on both T_1- *(A)* and T_2-weighted images *(B) (arrow)*.

ectopic pheochromocytomas because these lesions are very bright on T_2-weighted images, can be found anywhere from the base of the skull to the perineum, and because coronal or sagittal scans can cover the entire region in two series.[105]

The second setting is in patients who are either normal or have known cancer, in whom a large incidental adrenal lesion is found during the course of upper abdominal imaging. It is accepted that the risk of malignancy increases in lesions larger than 5 cm. These lesions are surgical and do not require any further imaging. A biopsy to exclude metastasis may be of help in the cancer patient since metastases need not be resected.

The third setting is the topic of interest. This is when an incidental adrenal lesion less than 5 cm is found in normal or oncologic patients. These patients present a diagnostic dilemma frequently requiring

biopsy, since lesions could be malignant in the otherwise normal patient or could represent metastasis in patients with cancer. MRI could potentially be of help in this group of patients to decrease the frequency of adrenal biopsies. Since the solution to this problem remains investigational, we will present a summary of the collected knowledge on this topic as well as our approach to the problem.

PULSE SEQUENCES

Adrenal tissue appears dark on both T_1- and T_2-weighted images relative to the surrounding fat (see Figs. 30–22, 30–35, and 30–64). Its T_1 signal is intermediate, being equal to or slightly darker than liver and close to that of muscle. Its T_2 signal is dark, similar to that of muscle, equal to or slightly darker than liver. Given that fat is brightest on T_1-weighted sequences, this pulsing sequence is used for anatomic screening. If an abnormality is shown on the T_1-weighted image, then a T_2-weighted image is obtained for further tissue characterization. Our typical sequence includes a T_1-weighted coronal localizer (600/20) followed by a T_1-weighted transverse series with TR = 600, TE = 20, a 256 × 128 matrix, 10-mm thick every 12 mm, and four acquisitions. The third and last series is obtained in the transverse plane with TR = 2000, two TEs at 20 and 70 msec, a 256 × 128 matrix, 10-mm thick every 15 mm, and four acquisitions. If other planes are needed to localize large tumors, they are obtained with T_1 weighting (600/20).

Transverse images provide the best detail to assess the body and limbs of the adrenal gland for enlargement or the presence of mass lesions. When assessing abnormal glands, coronal images define the relationship between mass and kidney, whereas sagittal scans assess the relationship of mass to inferior vena cava.

It is tempting, given the size of the adrenal, to utilize a 5-mm slice thickness to improve spatial resolution and to stack the slices with minimal interslice gap in order not to miss small lesions. This added resolution might be accomplished at the expense of contrast resolution, defeating the purpose of the exam, since in most cases MRI is obtained as a secondary study for lesion characterization. If the lesion is small, 5-mm-thick slices may be necessary to minimize partial volume, which will affect T_2 contrast. When using 5-mm slices, ensure that the S/N ratio remains high by using a 256 × 128 matrix, a field-of-view not smaller than 34 cm, and four excitations. To search for small lesions for characterization, rather than decreasing the interslice gap, the lesion should be located with a T_1-weighted sequence, and then its T_2 contrast with liver or fat should be assessed on a properly T_2-weighted series obtained with appropriate interslice gap to minimize cross-talk and ensure maximal contrast (Fig. 30–65) (see above, "Optimizing Spatial and Contrast Resolution"). If stacked slices are needed, obtain them interleaved.

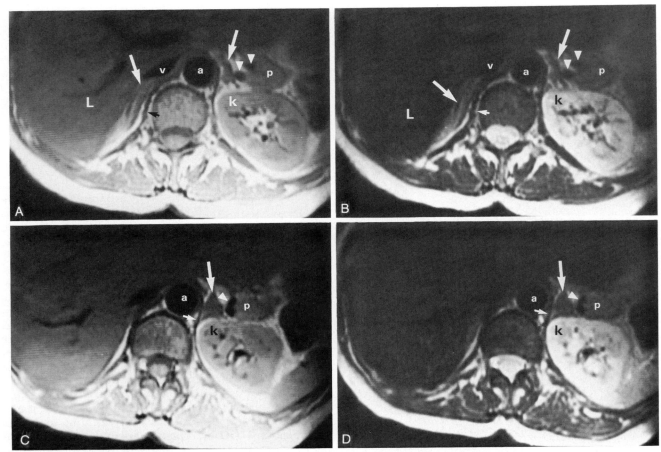

FIGURE 30–64. Normal adrenal gland and adrenal adenoma imaged with 5-inch circular surface coil centered at the L1 vertebral body. *A* and *B,* Hydrogen density (2000/20) *(A)* and T₂-weighted (2000/70) *(B)* images show both the right and left adrenal glands *(arrow).* Note that adrenals are darker than fat and are isointense with liver (L) and crus of diaphragm *(small arrow)* on both images. Note their relationship to the inferior vena cava (v), aorta (a), crus of diaphragm *(small arrow),* pancreas (p), kidney (k), and splenic vessels *(arrowheads).*

C and *D,* Hydrogen density *(C)* and T₂-weighted *(D)* images, obtained within the same series as *(A)* and *(B)* but at a more cephalic level, show a left adrenal lesion *(arrow)* that has similar signal characteristics as the normal adrenal (darker than fat on all sequences and as dark or darker than liver on all sequences). Again note the relationship of left adrenal lesion to the aorta (a), crus of diaphragm *(small arrow),* pancreas (p), kidney (k), and splenic vessels *(arrowhead).*

There is another technical detail needed to ensure the highest contrast-to-noise ratio. Since optimal power is only guaranteed at isocenter, which on transaxial images is the center of the imaging volume, adrenal lesions should be located in the center of the imaging volume and not on the edges (see "Optimizing Spatial and Contrast Resolution"). Including the adrenal glands on the same sequence that covers the lower chest or the remainder of the abdomen places the lesion at the edge of the imaging volume, decreasing the S/N ratio.[3] All one really needs is one high-quality T₂-weighted image obtained in the center of the lesion with minimum partial volume. Since that is not practical, ensure that the lesion is in the center of the imaging volume and select the optimal interslice gap.

High contrast and spatial resolution can be obtained with the use of surface coils. The commercially available 5-inch and license plate coils have been used in our institution for this purpose with mixed results. While they can provide excellent high resolution studies with less respiratory ghosting (Fig. 30–64), positioning is critical, and in obese patients, they can be ineffective. Anteriorly positioned glands in obese patients and malpositioning of the coil can place the adrenals at the fringes of the field-of-view, yielding worse contrast-to-noise ratio than can be achieved with the body coil.

ANATOMY

The adrenal glands have varied appearances. They are comprised of a body and two limbs, and the body is always located anteromedial to the limbs. Generally one limb is horizontal and the other vertical (Fig.

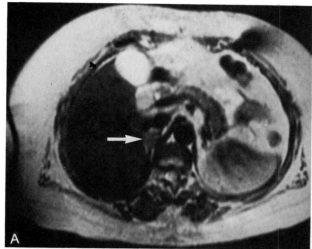

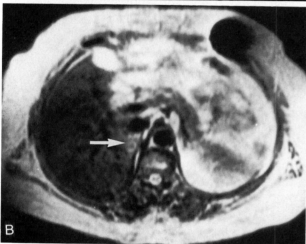

FIGURE 30–65. Effect of interslice gap on adrenal lesion tissue characterization is shown on two T$_2$-weighted images, both obtained with identical parameters over a presumed adrenal metastasis *(arrow)* and photographed with similar window and level. (TR = 3000, TE = 70, 256 × 128 matrix, 10mm slice thickness, and 2 excitations). *A,* Obtained with 20 per cent interslice gap. *B,* Obtained with 50 per cent interslice gap. Note that while lesion was darker than fat in *(A)* it became isointense with fat in *(B).* (From Schwaighofer BW, Yu K, Mattrey RF: Diagnostic significance of interslice gap and imaging volume. AJR [in press]; by permission of the American Roentgen Ray Society.)

30–66); however, more commonly on the right, both limbs can assume a vertical orientation (Fig. 30–64). The right adrenal gland is located superior to the upper pole of the kidney, posterior to the vena cava, medial to the liver, and lateral to the crus of the diaphragm. The left adrenal is typically located anteromedial to and at the level of the upper pole of the kidney, lateral to the crus, posterolateral to the aorta, and posteromedial to the splenic artery and vein and pancreas (Fig. 30–64). The location of the left adrenal gland relative to these landmarks is more variable than the location of the right adrenal to its landmarks. While the recognition of the left adrenal gland from the myriad of vessels in that location can at times be difficult on CT, the intermediate signal

of the adrenal is well contrasted with the white signal of fat and is easily recognized from the signal void of vessels and the dark signal of diaphragmatic crura on MRI. Due to the poor spatial resolution of MRI, we have not been able to reliably distinguish between adrenal cortex and medulla.

MASSES

Although simple adrenal cysts and myelolipomas have distinguishing density features on CT images, adrenal adenomas do not. Adrenal cysts and myelolipomas also have distinguishing features on MRI (Figs. 30–67 and 30–68). Adrenal adenomas, incidental findings on abdominal CT studies, tend to be distinguished by their small size (3 cm) but cannot be differentiated from carcinoma or metastasis by CT tissue characterization.[106] A recent report utilizing dynamic incremented CT during contrast administration suggested that CT can reliably distinguish benign from malignant lesions. When the investigators recognized a benign lesion they were correct 100 per cent of the time. However, when malignancy was suspected, they were correct 70 per cent of the time.[107] These data are comparable to those reported for MRI, with several reports describing near 30 per cent overlap between adenomas and metastatic disease.[108–110] However, the CT study was retrospective, with several limitations detailed by the authors that require further refinement and testing in a prospective manner, dampening the significance of their findings. It is also important to note that all reports investigating the tissue characterization potential of MRI were done at low field. It is not yet clear whether the specificity of high field units, with their added T$_2$ discrimination, will be comparable, better, or worse than low field units.

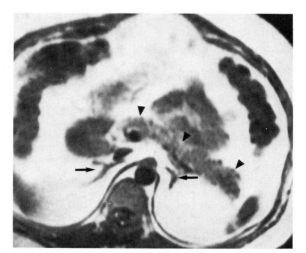

FIGURE 30–66. Normal adrenals *(arrows)* and pancreas *(arrowheads)* seen on a T$_1$-weighted image (600/20). Note the high contrast between adrenals and fat and the limbs of the adrenals, one being horizontal and the other vertical.

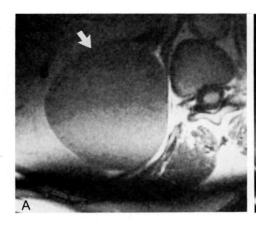
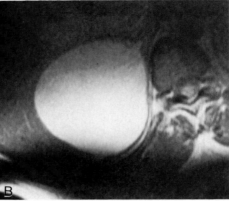

FIGURE 30–67. Simple adrenal cyst imaged with posteriorly positioned surface coil. *A*, Hydrogen density image shows large smooth mass involving the right adrenal gland *(arrow)*. Note the darker signal of mass when compared with surrounding liver. *B*, T₂-weighted image, second echo of *(A)*, shows the lesion markedly hyperintense relative to liver that is smooth and free of internal architecture, characteristic of cysts.

Reports suggested that adrenal hyperplasia and adenomas can be reliably differentiated from malignant tumors on the basis of the lesion-to-liver and/or lesion-to-fat signal intensity ratio. The failure of MR to identify calcification is an uncommon detriment since calcifications rarely occur in these tumors. Hyperplasia, as well as nonfunctioning adenomas, are nearly isointense or darker than liver on both T_1- and T_2-weighted images (see Fig. 30–64). Adrenal carcinoma (Fig. 30–69) and metastasis (Fig. 30–70) appear moderately hyperintense, and pheochromo-

cytomas (Fig. 30–71) and other functioning adenomas appear markedly hyperintense, compared with liver on T_2-weighted images.[111–113] The precise signal intensity ratio depends on the particular pulse sequence used, the magnetic field strength, the slice thickness, and the size of the lesion. Large lesions or thin slices will have less partial volume effect with fat or liver than smaller lesions or thicker slices. One study has suggested that T_2 relaxation times, rather than signal intensity ratios, provide the best characterization of adrenal lesions.[113a] Most adenomas had

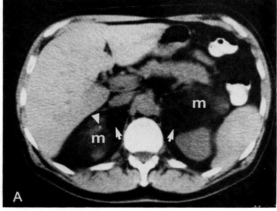
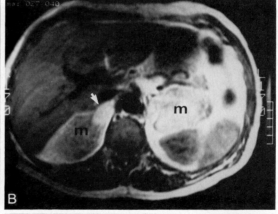
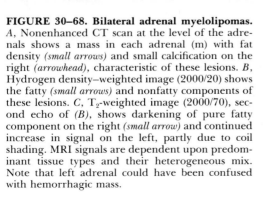
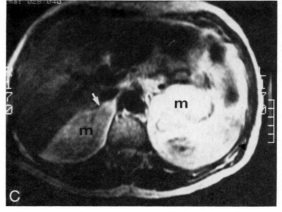

FIGURE 30–68. Bilateral adrenal myelolipomas. *A*, Nonenhanced CT scan at the level of the adrenals shows a mass in each adrenal (m) with fat density *(small arrows)* and small calcification on the right *(arrowhead)*, characteristic of these lesions. *B*, Hydrogen density–weighted image (2000/20) shows the fatty *(small arrows)* and nonfatty components of these lesions. *C*, T₂-weighted image (2000/70), second echo of *(B)*, shows darkening of pure fatty component on the right *(small arrow)* and continued increase in signal on the left, partly due to coil shading. MRI signals are dependent upon predominant tissue types and their heterogeneous mix. Note that left adrenal could have been confused with hemorrhagic mass.

T_2 values less than 60 msec, whereas nonadenomas had T_2 values greater than 61 msec.

Early clinical experience suggests that MR can obviate the need for biopsy in a subset of patients. The degree of overlap between adenomas and metastases is, however, significant (20 to 30 per cent).[108–110] To the time of this writing, the overlap has been when adenomas were bright. However, Glazer[105] reported three metastases that were dark on T_2-weighted images. The frequency of this occurrence and whether there was a reason for the dark signal, such as hemorrhage, are unknown. If metastases can assume a dark signal with significant frequency, then MRI would be of limited value.

Simple adrenal cysts, like cysts elsewhere, demonstrate marked hypointensity on T_1-weighted images and marked hyperintensity on highly T_2-weighted images (see Fig. 30–67). Subacute hemorrhage into a tumor, or fat in an adrenal myelolipoma, can be easily identified. Inflammatory lesions of the adrenals can be variable. In the literature, tuberculosis was bright on T_2-weighted images.[114] Histoplasmosis in one of our cases was dark (Fig. 30–72).

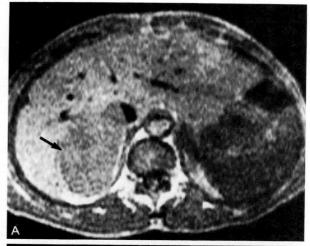
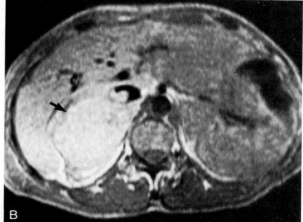

FIGURE 30–70. Metastases to adrenal glands generally have signals similar to those of liver metastases. *A*, On T_1-weighted image, lung carcinoma metastasis to right adrenal gland is hypointense compared with liver. Invasion of inferior vena cava by adrenal metastasis, as seen here, is infrequent. *B*, On a T_2-weighted image, obtained at nearly the same level as *(A)*, adrenal metastasis is mildly hyperintense relative to liver.

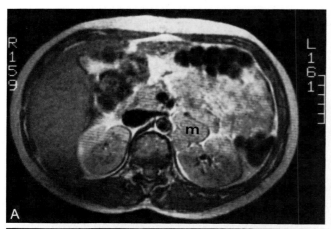
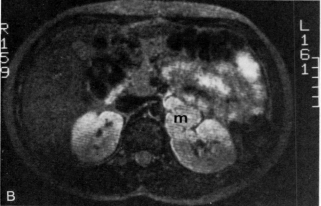

FIGURE 30–69. Primary adrenal adenocarcinoma (m) in a child. *A*, The large left adrenal mass is isointense with kidney, brighter than liver, and darker than fat on a hydrogen density–weighted image (2000/20). *B*, On a T_2-weighted image (2000/70), second echo of *(A)*, the lesion is isointense with kidney and brighter than liver and fat.

OUR APPROACH TO THE WORK-UP OF ADRENAL LESIONS

We influence the work-up of patients as discussed above. This approach is similar to that described by Bernardino.[115] We utilize a 1.5-T system and attempt to maximize contrast-to-noise as discussed above on a T_2-weighted image. We then subjectively compare the signal intensity of the lesion to that of liver, muscle, and fat. The liver-to-muscle contrast ensures that the liver is normal and can be used as a reference tissue. Otherwise, we use muscle as the reference tissue. It then depends whether the patient is known to have other malignancies.

In a patient with known malignancy, a lesion darker or as dark as liver is followed for one year. If the lesion is brighter than fat, we recommend biopsy. If it has intermediate signal, follow-up or biopsy is

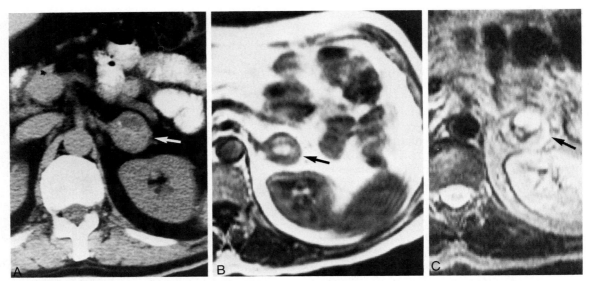

FIGURE 30–71. Pheochromocytoma involving left adrenal gland. *A*, CT scan shows an inhomogeneous left adrenal lesion *(arrow)*. *B*, T$_1$-weighted image shows the mass *(arrow)* to be darker than fat with high intensity region, presumably due to hemorrhage. *C*, T$_2$-weighted image demonstrates mass *(arrow)* to have similar signal intensity to fat in some areas and to be brighter in others.

recommended, depending on the degree of clinical suspicion or whether the lesion, if it is a metastasis, would significantly alter management.

In a patient not known to have an underlying malignancy, an incidental lesion darker or as dark as liver requires no further work-up. However, if the lesion is brighter than liver or as bright as fat, follow-up is recommended.

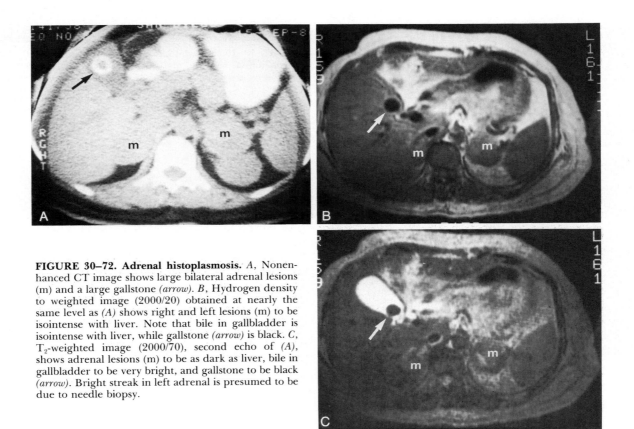

FIGURE 30–72. Adrenal histoplasmosis. *A*, Nonenhanced CT image shows large bilateral adrenal lesions (m) and a large gallstone *(arrow)*. *B*, Hydrogen density to weighted image (2000/20) obtained at nearly the same level as *(A)* shows right and left lesions (m) to be isointense with liver. Note that bile in gallbladder is isointense with liver, while gallstone *(arrow)* is black. *C*, T$_2$-weighted image (2000/70), second echo of *(A)*, shows adrenal lesions (m) to be as dark as liver, bile in gallbladder to be very bright, and gallstone to be black *(arrow)*. Bright streak in left adrenal is presumed to be due to needle biopsy.

SPLEEN

The spleen can be a site of metastatic disease, particularly in leukemia and lymphoma. Detection of splenic lesions is important. As with liver lesions, the discovery of metastasis alters patient management. Furthermore, in lymphoma, surgical resection done for staging could be obviated. If liver imaging for lesion detection is challenging, then splenic imaging is nearly impossible. The spleen is not only smaller than liver, more hidden by the rib cage, and moves with respiration, it displays pseudolesions on dynamic CT due to its inhomogeneous wash-in rate of contrast media.[116] To add to the difficulty in imaging the spleen, splenic MR relaxation parameters are similar to those of malignant lesions.[117] Focal masses and infiltrative neoplasms such as lymphoma generally display poor contrast with the normal spleen since both have long T_1 and T_2 times. However, when necrotic, cystic, or hemorrhagic, lesions can be well-demonstrated with sufficiently T_1- and T_2-weighted pulse sequences.[117] Dark siderotic nodules (Gamna-Gandy bodies) may be seen in patients with portal hypertension and should not be confused with neoplasm.[124]

A recent study evaluated several splenic lesion types in 22 patients at 1.5 T utilizing gradient-echo techniques and breath holding.[118] They reported a high lesion detection rate. All lesions appeared darker than spleen at a 30-degree flip angle. However, their MR sensitivity was comparable to CT and sonography, which are known to be poor.[119] Their experience is unique, very recent, and requires duplication and validation at other centers.

The development of specific reticuloendothelial system contrast agents, such as ferrite for MR, which is approaching phase III trials,[120, 121] or radiopaque particles for CT,[122, 123] will undoubtedly increase our sensitivity in detecting splenic lesions.

CONCLUSION

It should be clear from the above discussion that the role of MR in imaging the upper abdomen remains in constant flux. There are more unknown than known areas. The role of MRI relative to CT and sonography continues to be defined and then redefined when new technical or pharmacologic advances are introduced to the clinical setting.

We have presented the current role of MR imaging in this most challenging region of the body. The exact role remains unclear but, as can be seen, has advanced significantly since MRI was introduced in the early 1980s. There are maneuvers available to overcome most of the limitations of MRI. However, these ploys require additional sequences beyond the standard routine and the presence of an expert to guide the work-up. With the clinical demand placed on MRI for CNS and musculoskeletal imaging that

is technically straightforward, and with the as yet unsaturated market with MRI units, the complexity of abdominal imaging and its unclear role has hindered its advance. A set protocol of pulsing sequences (recipe approach), applicable to all patients in prospect, must be established. This protocol must minimize inaccuracies caused by artifacts and maximize the contrast-to-noise ratio between a region of interest and its surroundings, while maintaining adequate patient throughput to allow MRI to become a primary imaging modality in this difficult and complex region.

REFERENCES

1. Kneeland JB, Shimakawa A, Wehrli FW: Effect of intersection spacing on MR image contrast and study time. Radiology 158:819–822, 1986.
2. Kucharczyk W, Crawley AP, Kelly WM, Henkelman RM: Effect of multislice interference on image contrast in T2- and T1-weighted MR images. AJNR 9:443–451, 1988.
3. Schwaighofer BW, Yu K, Mattrey RF: Diagnostic significance of interslice gap and imaging volume. AJR (in press).
4. Edelman RR, Hahn PF, Buxton R, et al: Rapid MR imaging with suspended respiration: Clinical application in the liver. Radiology 161:125–131, 1986.
5. Stark DD, Weissleder R, Elizondo G, et al: Superparamagnetic iron oxide: Clinical application as a contrast agent for MR imaging of the liver. Radiology 168:297–301, 1988.
6. Ehman RL, McNamara MT, Pollack M, et al: MRI with respiratory gating: Techniques and advantages. AJR 143:1175–1182, 1984.
7. Bailes DR, Gilderdale DJ, Bydder GM, et al: Respiratory ordered phase-encoding (ROPE): A method for reducing respiratory motion artifacts in MR imaging. J Comput Assist Tomogr 9:835–838, 1985.
8. Axel L, Summers RM, Kressel HY, Charles C: Respiratory effects in two-dimensional Fourier transform MR imaging. Radiology 160:795–801, 1986.
9. Stark DD, Wittenberg J, Edelman RR, et al: Detection of hepatic metastasis by MRI: Analysis of pulse sequence performance. Radiology 159:365–370, 1986.
10. Edelman RR, McFarland E, Stark DD, et al: Surface coil MRI of abdominal viscera: Theory and initial clinical application. Radiology 157:425–432, 1985.
11. Frahm J, Haase A, Matthaei D: Rapid three-dimensional MR imaging using the FLASH technique. J Comput Assist Tomogr 10:363–368, 1986.
12. Miller RE, Chernish SM: On the use of glucagon-ancillary effects and other considerations. In Picazo J (ed): Glucagon in Gastroenterology and Hepatology. Lancaster, MTP Press, 1982, pp 55–67.
13. Wesbey GE, Brasch RC, Engelstad BL, et al: NMR contrast enhancement study of the gastrointestinal tract of rats and a human volunteer using nontoxic oral iron solutions. Radiology 149:175–180, 1983.
14. Runge VM, Stewart RG, Clanton JA, et al: Work in progress: Potential oral and intravenous paramagnetic NMR contrast agents. Radiology 147:789–791, 1983.
15. Laniado M, Kornmesser W, Hamm B, et al: MR imaging of the gastrointestinal tract: Value of Gd-DTPA. AJR 150:817–821, 1988.
16. Weinreb JC, Maravilla KR, Redman HC, Nunally R: Improved MR imaging of the upper abdomen with glucagon and gas. J Comput Assist Tomogr 8:835–838, 1984.
17. Renshaw PF, Owen CS, McLaughlin AC, et al: Ferromagnetic contrast agents: A new approach. Mag Res Med 3:217–225, 1986.
18. Widder DJ, Edelman RR, Greif WL, Monda L: Magnetite albumin suspension: A superparamagnetic oral MR contrast agent. AJR 149:839–843, 1987.

19. Mattrey RF, Hajek PC, Gylys-Morin V, et al: Perfluorochemicals as gastrointestinal contrast agents for MR imaging: Preliminary studies in rats and humans. AJR 148:1259–1263, 1987.

20. Dean PB, Kivisaari L, Kormano M: Contrast enhancement pharmacokinetics of six ionic and nonionic contrast media. Invest Radiol 18:368–374, 1983.

21. Alderson PO, Adams DF, McNeil BJ, et al: Computed tomography, ultrasound, and scintigraphy of the liver in patients with colon or breast carcinoma: A prospective comparison. Radiology 149:225–230, 1983.

22. Brendel AJ, Leccia F, Drouillard J, et al: Single photon emission computed tomography, planar scintigraphy, and transmission computed tomography: A comparison of accuracy in diagnosing focal hepatic disease. Radiology 153:527–532, 1984.

23. Machi J, Isomoto H, Yamashita Y, et al: Intraoperative ultrasonography in screening for liver metastases from colorectal cancer: Comparative accuracy with traditional procedures. Surgery 101:678–684, 1987.

24. Smith TJ, Kemeny MM, Sugarbaker PH, et al: A prospective study of hepatic imaging in the detection of metastatic disease. Ann Surg 195:486–491, 1982.

25. Sugarbaker PH, Vermess M, Doppman JL, et al: Improved detection of focal lesions with computerized tomographic examination of the liver using ethiodized oil emulsion (EOE-13) liver contrast. Cancer 54:1489–1495, 1984.

26. Reinig JW, Dwyer AJ, Miller DL, et al: Liver metastasis detection: Comparative sensitivities of MR imaging and CT scanning. Radiology 162:43–47, 1987.

27. Foley WD, Berland LL, Lawson TL, et al: Contrast enhancement technique for dynamic hepatic computed tomographic scanning. Radiology 147:797–803, 1983.

28. Alpern MB, Lawson TL, Foley WD, et al: Focal hepatic masses and fatty infiltration detected by enhanced dynamic CT. Radiology 158:45–49, 1986.

29. Bernardino ME, Erwin BC, Steinberg HV, et al: Delayed hepatic CT scanning: Increased confidence and improved detection of hepatic metastases. Radiology 159:71–74, 1986.

30. Miller DL, Simmons JT, Chang R, et al: Hepatic metastasis detection: Comparison of three CT contrast enhancement methods. Radiology 165:785–790, 1987.

31. Matsui O, Takashima T, Kadoya M, et al: Liver metastases from colorectal cancers: Detection with CT during arterial portography. Radiology 165:65–69, 1987.

32. Heiken JP, Weyman PJ, Lee JKT, et al: Detection of focal hepatic masses: Prospective evaluation with CT, delayed CT, CT during arterial portography, and MR imaging. Radiology 171:47–51, 1989.

33. Wittenberg J, Stark DD, Butch RJ, Ferrucci JT: Comparative accuracy of MRI and CT for liver metastases. Presented at the Fifth Annual Meeting of the Society of Magnetic Resonance in Medicine, August 19–22, 1986.

34. Bottomley PA, Hardy CJ, Argersinger RE: The field dependence of T1 contrast between normal and pathologic tissue: A review. In: Society of Magnetic Resonance in Medicine, Book of Abstracts. 2:407–408, 1986.

35. Reinig JW, Dwyer AJ, Miller DL, et al: Liver metastases: Detection with MR imaging at 0.5 and 1.5T. Radiology 170:149–153, 1989.

36. Foley WD, Kneeland BJ, Cates JD, et al: Contrast optimization for the detection of focal hepatic lesions by MR imaging at 1.5T. AJR 149:1155–1160, 1987.

37. Moss AA, Goldberg HI, Stark DD, et al: Hepatic tumors: MR and CT appearance. Radiology 150:141–147, 1984.

38. Paling MR, Abbitt PL, Mugler JP, Brookemann JR: Liver metastases: Optimization of MR imaging pulse sequences at 1.0T. Radiology 167:695–699, 1988.

39. Edelman RR, Stark DD, Saini S, et al: Oblique planes of section in MR imaging. Radiology 159:807–810, 1986.

40. Fisher MR, Wall SD, Hricak H, et al: Hepatic vascular anatomy on MRI. AJR 144:739–746, 1985.

41. Wittenberg J, Stark DD, Forman BH, et al: Differentiation of hepatic metastases from hepatic hemangiomas and cysts by using MR imaging. AJR 151:79–84, 1988.

42. Ferrucci JT, Freeny PC, Stark DD, et al: Advances in hepatobiliary radiology. Radiology 168:319–338, 1988.

43. Itai Y, Ohtomo K, Furui S, et al: MR imaging of hepatocellular carcinoma. J Comput Assist Tomogr 10:963–968, 1986.

44. Ebara M, Ohto M, Watanabe Y, et al: Diagnosis of small hepatocellular carcinoma: Correlation of MR imaging and tumor histologic study. Radiology 159:371–377, 1986.

45. Itoh K, Nishimura K, Togashi K: Hepatocellular carcinoma: MR imaging. Radiology 164:21–25, 1987.

46. Rummeny E, Weissleder R, Stark DD, et al: Primary liver tumors: Diagnosis by MR imaging. AJR 152:63–72, 1989.

47. Yoshikawa J, Matsui O, Takashima T, et al: Fatty metamorphosis in hepatocellular carcinoma: Radiologic features in 10 cases. AJR 151:717–720, 1988.

48. Roberts JL, Fishman EK, Hartman DS, et al: Lipomatous tumors of the liver: Evaluation with CT and US. Radiology 158:613–617, 1986.

49. Weinreb JC, Brateman L, Maravilla KR: Magnetic resonance imaging of hepatic lymphoma. AJR 143:1211–1214, 1984.

50. Weissleder R, Stark DD, Elizondo G, et al: MRI of hepatic lymphoma. Mag Res Imaging 6:675–681, 1988.

51. Heiberg E, Wolverson MK, Sundaram M, Shields JB: CT findings in leukemia. AJR 143:1317–1323, 1984.

52. Dachman AH, Pakter RL, Ros PR, et al: Hepatoblastoma: Radiologic pathologic correlation in 50 cases. Radiology 164:15–19, 1987.

53. Tumeh SS, Benson C, Nagel JS, et al: Cavernous hemangioma of the liver: Detection with single-photon emission computed tomography. Radiology 164:353–356, 1987.

54. Freeny PC, Marks WM: Hepatic hemangioma: Dynamic bolus CT. AJR 147:711–719, 1986.

55. Cronan JJ, Esparza AR, Dorfman GS, et al: Cavernous hemangioma of the liver: Role of percutaneous biopsy. Radiology 166:135–138, 1988.

56. Itai Y, Furui S, Araki T, et al: Computed tomography of cavernous hemangioma of the liver. Radiology 137:149–155, 1980.

57. Glazer GM, Aisen AM, Francis IR, et al: Hepatic cavernous hemangioma: MR imaging. Radiology 155:417–420, 1985.

58. Ferrucci JT: MR imaging of the liver. AJR 147:1103–1116, 1986.

59. Stark DD, Felder RC, Wittenberg J, et al: MRI of cavernous hemangioma of the liver. AJR 145:213–222, 1985.

60. Ohtomo K, Itai Y, Yoshikawa K, et al: Hepatocellular carcinoma and cavernous hemangioma: Differentiation with MR imaging. Efficacy of T2 values at 0.35 and 1.5T. Radiology 168:621–623, 1988.

61. Li KC, Glazer GM, Quint LE, et al: Distinction of hepatic cavernous hemangioma from hepatic metastases with MR imaging. Radiology 169:409–415, 1988.

62. Ros PR, Lubbers PR, Olmsted WW, Morillo G: Hemangioma of the liver: Heterogeneous appearance on T2-weighted images. AJR 149:1167–1170, 1987.

62a. Edelman RR, Siegel J, Singer A, et al: Dynamic MRI of the liver by using gadolinium-DTPA. AJR (in press).

63. Mattison GR, Glazer GM, Quint LE, et al: MR imaging of hepatic focal nodular hyperplasia: Characterization and distinction from primary malignant hepatic tumors. AJR 148:711–715, 1987.

64. Gomori J, Grossman RI, Goldberg HI, et al: Intracranial hematomas: Imaging by high-field MR. Radiology 157:87–93, 1985.

65. Edelman RR, Johnson K, Buxton RB, et al: MR imaging of hemorrhage: A new approach. AJNR 7:751–756, 1986.

66. Hahn PF, Stark DD, Vici L-G, Ferrucci JT Jr: Duodenal hematoma: The ring sign in MR imaging. Radiology 159:379–382, 1986.

67. Unger EC, Glazer HS, Lee JKT, et al: MRI of extracranial hematomas: Preliminary observations. AJR 146:403–407, 1986.

68. Dixon WT: Simple proton spectroscopic imaging. Radiology 153:189–194, 1984.

69. Lee JKT, Heiken JP, Dixon WT: Detection of hepatic metastases by proton spectroscopic imaging: Work in progress. Radiology 156:429–433, 1985.

70. Stark DD, Wittenberg J, Middleton MS, Ferrucci JT: Liver metastases: Detection by phase-contrast MR imaging. Radiology 158:327–332, 1986.

71. Brasch RC, Wesbey GE, Gooding CA, Koerper MA: MRI of transfusional hemosiderosis complicating thalassemia major. Radiology 150:767–771, 1984.

72. Stark DD, Moseley ME, Bacon BR, et al: MRI and spectroscopy of hepatic iron overload. Radiology 154:137–142, 1985.

73. Brittenham GM, Farrell DE, Harris JW, et al: Magnetic susceptibility measurement of human iron stores. N Engl J Med 307:1671–1675, 1982.

74. Lawler GA, Pennock JM, Steiner RE, et al: NMR imaging in Wilson disease. J Comput Assist Tomogr 7:1–8, 1983.

75. Stark DD, Bass NM, Moss AA, et al: NMR imaging of experimentally induced liver disease. Radiology 148:743–751, 1983.

76. Itai Y, Ohnishi S, Ohtomo K, et al: Regenerating nodules of liver cirrhosis: MR imaging. Radiology 165:419–423, 1987.

77. Stark DD, Hahn PF, Trey C, et al: MRI of the Budd-Chiari syndrome. AJR 146:1141–1148, 1986.

78. Bernardino ME, Steinberg HV, Pearson TC, et al: Shunts for portal hypertension: MR and angiography for determination of patency. Radiology 158:57–62, 1986.

79. Levy HM, Newhouse JH: MR imaging of portal vein thrombosis. AJR 151:283–286, 1988.

80. White EM, Edelman RR, Wedeen VJ, Brady TJ: Intravascular signal in MR imaging: Use of phase-display for differentiation of blood-flow signal from intraluminal disease. Radiology 161:245–249, 1986.

81. Itai Y, Ohtomo K, Kokubo T, et al: Segmental intensity differences in the liver on MR images: A sign of intrahepatic portal flow stoppage. Radiology 167:17–19, 1988.

81a. Marchal G, Mecke PV, Demaerel P, et al: Detection of liver metastases with superparamagnetic iron oxide in 15 patients: Results of MRI at 1.5 Tesla. AJR 152:771–775, 1989.

82. Snow JH Jr, Goldstein HM, Wallace S: Comparison of scintigraphy, sonography and computed tomography in the evaluation of hepatic neoplasms. AJR 132:915–918, 1979.

83. Scherer U, Rothe R, Eisenburg J, et al: Diagnostic accuracy of CT in circumscript liver disease. AJR 130:711–714, 1978.

84. Chezmar JL, Rumancik WM, Megibow AJ, et al: Liver and abdominal screening in patients with cancer: CT versus MR imaging. Radiology 168:43–47, 1988.

84a. Heiken JP, Weyman PJ, Lee JKT, et al: Detection of focal hepatic masses: Prospective evaluation with CT, delayed CT, CT during arterial portography, and MR imaging. Radiology 171:47–51, 1989.

84b. Nelson RC, Chezmar JL, Sugarbaker PM, Bernadino ME: Hepatic tumors: Comparisons of CT during arterial portography, delayed CT, and MRI for preoperative evaluation. Radiology 172:27–34, 1989.

85. Schmiedl U, Paajanen H, Arakawa M, et al: MR imaging of liver abscesses: Application of Gd-DTPA. Mag Res Imaging 6:9–16, 1988.

86. Mano I, Yoshida H, Nakabayashi K, et al: Fast spin echo imaging with suspended respiration: Gadolinium enhanced MR imaging of the liver. J Comput Assist Tomogr 11:73–80, 1987.

87. Ohtomo K, Itai Y, Yoshikawa K, et al: Hepatic tumors: Dynamic MR imaging. Radiology 163:27–31, 1987.

88. Hamm B, Wolf KJ, Felix R: Conventional and rapid MR imaging of the liver with Gd-DTPA. Radiology 164:313–320, 1987.

89. Demas BE, Hricak H, Moseley M, et al: Gallbladder bile: An experimental study in dogs using MR imaging and proton spectroscopy. Radiology 157:453–455, 1985.

90. Bakan DA, Barnhart JL: Determination of parameters effecting proton relaxation of hepatic and gallbladder biles in dogs. Hepatology 8:341–346, 1988.

91. Loflin TG, Simeone JF, Mueller PR, et al: Gallbladder bile in cholecystitis: In-vitro MR evaluation. Radiology 157:457–459, 1985.

92. McCarthy S, Hricak H, Cohen M, et al: Cholecystitis: Detection with MRI. Radiology 158:333–336, 1986.

93. Moon KL, Hricak H, Margulis AR, et al: NMR imaging characteristics of gallstones in vitro. Radiology 148:753–756, 1983.

94. Dooms GC, Kerlan RK, Hricak H, et al: Cholangiocarcinoma: Imaging by MR. Radiology 159:89–94, 1986.

95. Cooperberg PL, Gibney RG: Imaging of the gallbladder, 1987. Radiology 163:605–613, 1987.

96. Baron RL, Stanley RJ, Lee JKT, et al: A prospective comparison of biliary obstruction using computed tomography and ultrasonography. Radiology 145:91–98, 1982.

97. Tscholakoff D, Hricak H, Thoeni R, et al: MR imaging in the diagnosis of pancreatic disease. AJR 148:703–709, 1987.

98. Simeone JF, Edelman RR, Stark DD, et al: Surface coil MR imaging of abdominal viscera: The pancreas. Radiology 157:437–441, 1985.

99. Stark DD, Moss AA, Goldberg HI, et al: MR and CT of the normal and diseased pancreas: A comparative study. Radiology 150:153–162, 1984.

100. Freeny PC, Marks WM, Ryan JA, Traverso LW: Pancreatic ductal adenocarcinoma: Diagnosis and staging with dynamic CT. Radiology 166:125–133, 1988.

101. Steiner E, Stark DD, Hahn PF, et al: Imaging of pancreatic neoplasms: Comparison of MR and CT. AJR 152:487–491, 1989.

102. Yuh WTC, Hunsicker LG, Nghiem DD, et al: Pancreatic transplants: Evaluation with MR imaging. Radiology 170:171–177, 1989.

103. Shultz CL, Haaga JR, Fletcher BD, et al: MRI of the adrenal glands: A comparison with CT. AJR 143:1235–1240, 1984.

104. Chang A, Glazer HS, Lee JKT, et al: Adrenal gland: MR imaging. Radiology 163:123–128, 1987.

104a. Ikeda DM, Francis IR, Glazer GM, et al: The detection of adrenal tumors and hyperplasia in patients with primary aldosteronism: Comparison of scintigraphy, CT, and MR imaging. AJR 153:301–306, 1989.

105. Glazer GM: MR imaging of the liver, kidneys, and adrenal glands. Radiology 166:303–312, 1988.

106. Fishman EK, Deutch BM, Hartman DS, et al: Primary adrenocortical carcinoma: CT evaluation with clinical correlation. AJR 148:531–535, 1987.

107. Berland LL, Koslin DB, Kenney PJ, et al: Differentiation between small benign and malignant adrenal masses with dynamic incremental CT. AJR 151:95–101, 1988.

108. Doppman JL, Reinig JW, Dwyer AJ, et al: Differentiation of adrenal masses by magnetic resonance imaging. Surgery 102:1018–1026, 1987.

109. Reinig JW, Doppman JL, Dwyer AJ, Frank J: MRI of indeterminate adrenal masses. AJR 147:493–496, 1986.

110. Chezmar JL, Robbins SM, Nelson RC, et al: Adrenal masses: Characterization with T1-weighted MR imaging. Radiology 166:357–359, 1988.

111. Fink IJ, Reinig JW, Dwyer AJ, et al: MRI of pheochromocytomas. J Comput Assist Tomogr 9:454–458, 1985.

112. Reinig JW, Doppman JL, Dwyer AJ, et al: Adrenal masses differentiated by MR. Radiology 158:81–84, 1986.

113. Glazer GM, Woolsey EJ, Borrello J, et al: Adrenal tissue characterization using MRI. Radiology 158:73–79, 1986.

113a. Baker ME, Blinder R, Spritzer C, et al: MR evaluation of adrenal masses at 1.5 T. AJR 153:307–312, 1989.

114. Baker ME, Spritzer C, Blinder R, et al: Benign adrenal lesions mimicking malignancy on MR imaging: Report of two cases. Radiology 163:669–671, 1987.

115. Bernardino ME: Management of the asymptomatic patient with a unilateral adrenal mass. Radiology 166:121–123, 1988.

116. Glazer GM, Axel L, Goldberg HI, Moss AA: Dynamic CT of the normal spleen. AJR 137:343–346, 1981.

117. Hahn PF, Weissleder R, Stark DD, et al: MR imaging of focal splenic tumors. AJR 150:823–827, 1988.

118. Hess CF, Griebel J, Schmiedl U, et al: Focal lesions of the spleen: Preliminary results with fast MR imaging at 1.5T. J Comput Assist Tomogr 12:569–574, 1988.

119. Zornoza J, Ginaldi S: Computer tomography in hepatic lymphoma. Radiology 138:405–410, 1981.

120. Weissleder R, Hahn PF, Stark DD, et al: Superparamagnetic iron oxide. Enhanced detection of focal splenic tumors with MR imaging. Radiology 169:399–403, 1988.

121. Weissleder R, Elizondo G, Stark DD, et al: The diagnosis of splenic lymphoma by MR imaging: Value of superparamagnetic iron oxide. AJR 152:175–180, 1989.

122. Thomas JL, Bernardino ME, Vermess M, et al: EOE-13 in the detection of hepatosplenic lymphoma. Radiology 145:629–634, 1982.

123. Mattrey RF: Potential role of perfluorooctylbromide in the detection and characterization of liver lesions with CT. Radiology 170:18–20, 1989.

124. Minami M, Itai Y, Ohtomo K, et al: Siderotic nodules in the spleen: MR imaging of portal hypertension. Radiology 172:681–684, 1989.

31

MR IMAGING OF THE KIDNEY AND RETROPERITONEUM

NICHOLAS PAPANICOLAOU and RICHARD C. PFISTER

MR IMAGING OF THE KIDNEY

NORMAL ANATOMY

PATHOLOGY

Perinephric Space
Renal Hilum
Pyelocalyceal System
Kidney

CLINICAL APPLICATIONS

MR IMAGING OF THE RETROPERITONEUM

NORMAL ANATOMY

PATHOLOGY

Ureteral Dilatation
Retroperitoneal Fibrosis
Fluid Collection—Abscesses
Lymphadenopathy

MR IMAGING OF THE KIDNEY

The radiologic investigation of renal disease has rapidly expanded in recent years to include the use of cross-sectional imaging techniques and radionuclides in addition to intravenous urography and renal angiography. Magnetic resonance (MR) is the latest of the cross-sectional imaging modalities to emerge with the potential for adequate anatomic resolution, tissue-specific discrimination, and demonstration of blood flow. Some of the anticipated advantages of MR imaging of renal disorders have yet to materialize, whereas others are forthcoming, with improvements in hardware, software, and pulse sequence selection expected to continue. We discuss here the experience accumulated to date in evaluating the kidney by MR imaging and the relevant clinical applications of the modality as they are currently evolving.

NORMAL ANATOMY

MR imaging can define the normal anatomy of the kidney and perinephric space (Fig. 31–1).[1–7] The

presence of perinephric and renal hilar fat results in adequate separation of the kidney from adjacent structures. Since fat has short T_1 and moderate T_2 values, it displays high signal intensity on T_1-weighted

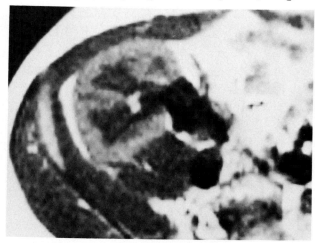

FIGURE 31–1. Normal renal anatomy by MR imaging in patient with kidney transplant. This SE 260/20 acquisition demonstrates the corticomedullary differentiation. Perinephric and pyelosinus fat are seen as high signal intensity areas. The renal vessels appear as signal-void tubular structures.

899

spin-echo (SE) images. The perinephric fascia may not always be visualized in normal individuals. When it is seen, it appears as a thin, low-intensity line. The renal hilar vessels are shown as low-intensity tubular structures, their low signal intensity caused by rapidly flowing blood. The renal capsule is not visible on MR images and should not be confused with the chemical shift artifact encountered along the periphery of the kidney at the interface between water-containing tissues and surrounding fat.[8]

The long T_1 of urine within the pyelocalyceal system results in low signal intensity on T_1-weighted images. This is nicely demonstrated in the presence of hydronephrosis (Fig. 31–2). Otherwise, the non-dilated collecting system usually is not distinguishable from the central pyelosinus fat. Short repetition time (TR) and echo delay time (TE) acquisitions are preferable for imaging the collecting system. With T_2-weighted images, the signal intensity of urine is greater than that of fat.

The separation between the renal cortex and medulla can be easily shown. The cortex emits higher signal intensity than the medulla in T_1-weighted images, and this difference becomes more apparent when the patient is well hydrated. The corticomedullary differentiation (CMD) is enhanced on short TR sequences but disappears when long TR and TE values are used.

Fat produces high signal intensity on some inversion recovery (IR) and gradient-echo techniques. The renal cortex appears homogeneous on all imaging techniques. On IR imaging (short TE and TR and inversion time set to optimize the T_1 contrast of the tissues imaged) the CMD may be seen better than on SE pulse sequences, but the overall anatomic detail may be degraded because of the resulting lower signal-to-noise ratio.[2, 3]

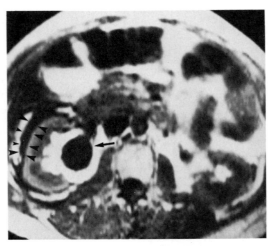

FIGURE 31–3. Perinephric urinoma in a 57-year-old man with right flank pain following extracorporeal lithotripsy for renal calculus. The SE 300/32 T_1-weighted image shows a very low signal intensity perinephric collection, consistent with urinoma *(arrowheads)*. The corticomedullary differentiation of the treated kidney is preserved. The dilated renal pelvis has a similar MR appearance *(arrow)*. (From Hahn PF, Saini S, Stark DS, et al: Intraabdominal hematoma: The concentric-ring in MR imaging. AJR 148:115–119, 1987; © by American Roentgen Ray Society.)

PATHOLOGY

Perinephric Space

A thickened perinephric fascia, as is the case with computed tomography (CT), usually represents inflammatory or neoplastic involvement.

Fluid collections in the perinephric space are readily demonstrable on MR images. It is often possible to distinguish blood from urine. Owing to the long T_1 value of urine, urinomas appear as low signal intensity collections on T_1-weighted pulse sequences (Fig. 31–3). On the other hand, the appearance of hematoma or hemorrhage is variable. Swensen and coworkers found that on T_1-weighted images acute hemorrhage displayed low signal intensity and therefore long T_1 values.[9] T_2-weighted images had a high signal intensity at low-medium field strengths, but low signal at 1.5 T. Hematomas are initially isointense with muscle or the renal medulla on T_1-weighted images and become more intense with time as the T_1 values decrease (Fig. 31–4).[10] Both abscesses and solid masses can simulate an early hematoma. These imaging features are in agreement with in vitro studies showing that acute hemorrhage and nonhemorrhagic fluid collections have overlapping distributions of relaxation parameters.[11] As early as 3 weeks after the bleeding, the hematoma may develop a thin, dark peripheral rim on all pulse sequences and a brighter inner ring best seen on T_1-weighted images.[10] These findings have been attributed to the paramagnetic effects of hemoglobin degradation to methemoglobin and hemosiderin digested by phagocytes surround-

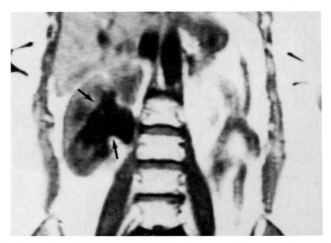

FIGURE 31–2. Hydronephrosis in a 60-year-old woman. Coronal SE 500/25 image demonstrates mild to moderate pyelocaliectasis of the right collecting system *(arrows)*.

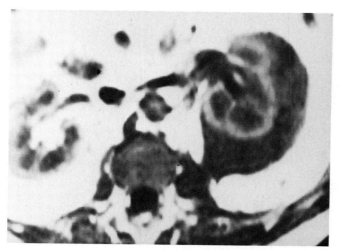

FIGURE 31–4. **Acute perirenal hematoma in a 66-year-old man several hours after extracorporeal lithotripsy for left renal calculus.** The SE 310/20 MR image shows a low to intermediate signal intensity left perirenal hematoma. The corticomedullary differentiation is preserved bilaterally. The fragmented calculus cannot be seen on MR imaging.

ing the hematoma.[12] The larger central area of the hematoma is brighter than muscle on all pulse sequences. This pattern tends to persist over time as the size of the blood collection decreases.

Mixed fluid collections result in considerable overlap and variability of relaxation parameters. Serial imaging demonstrating evolutionary changes within these collections may be helpful in improving the diagnostic yield of MR imaging.

Renal Hilum

The hilar vessels, the inferior vena cava, and the aorta can be easily seen on MR images. Currently, a significant clinical contribution of MR imaging is its ability to detect the presence of thrombus within the renal vein and the vena cava (Fig. 31–5). Hricak et al. were able to distinguish between thrombosis and sluggish blood flow on T_2-weighted images.[13]

The presence and direction of blood flow within veins and arteries can also be reliably documented by recently introduced imaging techniques.[14–16] Renal vein thrombi, if present in the main vein, are imaged with good reliability. Perihilar lymphadenopathy and parapelvic cysts have also been detected, the latter as low-intensity signal structures on T_1-weighted images owing to the presence of clear fluid within them.

Pyelocalyceal System

Hydronephrosis or a large extrarenal pelvis can be demonstrated by MR techniques owing to the low-intensity urine on T_1-weighted images (see Fig. 31–2). Renal parenchymal thinning can also be readily assessed. In experimentally induced hydronephrosis in the dog, the CMD was preserved early on but was lost in long-standing obstruction.[17] Similar findings were encountered in patients with hydronephrosis (see Fig. 31–2).[4, 7]

Detection of filling defects within the collecting system depends on their size, location, and nature. Soft-tissue calcifications are defined poorly or not at all by MR imaging. Densely calcified tissue generates a low-intensity signal because of its low density of mobile protons. Therefore, renal calculi, nephrocalcinosis, and tumoral calcinosis frequently escape diagnosis.

Limited spatial resolution, image degradation by motion artifacts, and chemical composition of a lesion are reasons for failure of MR to demonstrate filling defects. Differentiation between parapelvic cysts and renal sinus lipomatosis is easy because of the long T_1 of fluid and short T_1 of fat.

Kidney

Diffuse Parenchymal Disease (Medical Renal Disease)

A variety of diffuse renal parenchymal diseases have been imaged by MR. The finding most frequently encountered in medical renal disease is the loss of the normally observed CMD. In the normal kidney, both SE (short TR and TE) and IR techniques demonstrate the separation between cortex and medulla, whereas long TR and TE times on SE imaging usually result in its obliteration.

Leung et al. studied 12 patients with chronic glomerulonephritis utilizing IR (TR 1400/TE 400) technique and a variety of SE pulse sequences.[4] They also imaged patients with end-stage renal failure and others with significant renal artery stenosis. The CMD was not seen in any of the imaged kidneys. Hricak et al reported two cases of chronic glomerulonephritis in which the renal cortex was less intense than adjacent liver.[6] The renal cortex was more intense than the liver and the CMD was preserved on T_1-weighted images in a patient with glycogen storage disease.

Lande and coworkers found the intensity of the renal cortex decreased in 11 of 19 patients with sickle-cell nephropathy, a finding that was most evident on T_2-weighted images.[18] This was in part attributed to iron deposition in the cortex. However, six of their patients with thalassemia major and iron overload from repeated transfusions did not demonstrate the same feature. Therefore, they speculate that reduced cortical signal intensity may also reflect abnormal iron metabolism in the renal cortex of these patients. The renal medulla in the sicklers appeared similar to that of normal volunteers, both visually and quantitatively.[18]

In a case report of a patient with paroxysmal nocturnal hemoglobinuria, Mulopulos et al. described a reversal of the normally observed higher cortical intensity over that of the medulla on T_1-weighted images. Renal cortical intensity was very

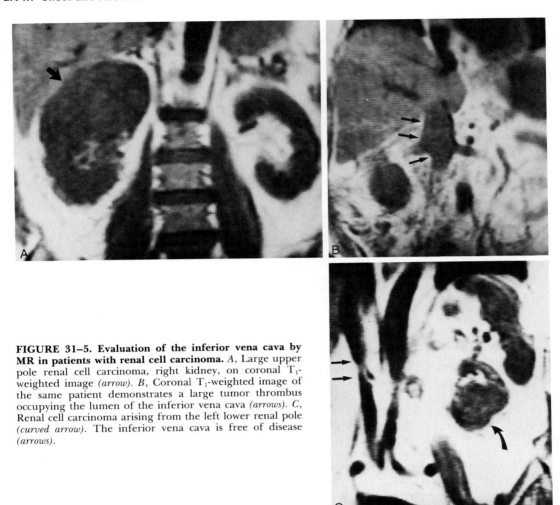

FIGURE 31–5. Evaluation of the inferior vena cava by MR in patients with renal cell carcinoma. *A,* Large upper pole renal cell carcinoma, right kidney, on coronal T_1-weighted image *(arrow). B,* Coronal T_1-weighted image of the same patient demonstrates a large tumor thrombus occupying the lumen of the inferior vena cava *(arrows). C,* Renal cell carcinoma arising from the left lower renal pole *(curved arrow).* The inferior vena cava is free of disease *(arrows).*

low on T_2-weighted images.[19] The findings were attributed to the paramagnetic effect of iron, which is deposited mostly in the renal cortex and causes shortening of its relaxation parameters.

Experimentally induced renal arterial and venous occlusion in animals was studied with MR imaging by Yuasa and Kundel and London and coworkers.[20, 21] Acute venous ligation resulted in renal enlargement and prompt cessation of urine formation. In acute arterial ligation, kidney size remained unchanged but excretory function was lost. Quantitative T_1 values were somewhat prolonged in both groups, but they also overlapped with normal relaxation times. In vivo and in vitro measurements of the relaxation times by Yuasa and Kundel revealed prolonged T_1 and T_2 in both venous and arterial ligation. Correlation with imaging in human patients is necessary before the clinical relevance of these observations can be established.

Renal Transplants

Currently, complications following renal transplantation are evaluated by renal sonography and radio-nuclide renography jointly, since neither modality can provide adequate anatomic and physiologic data simultaneously.

Experience with MR imaging of renal allografts has been limited.[3, 4, 22–24, 26] Hricak et al. imaged nine patients with normal renal transplants, all with morphologic features previously described for native normal kidneys (Fig. 31–6).[23]

Fluid collections around the transplant can be easily detected. Geisinger et al. described a hematoma with high signal intensity on both T_1- and T_2-weighted images and two lymphoceles of low intensity on T_1- but high intensity on T_2-weighted images.[22] Hricak et al. could not differentiate urinomas, seromas, and lymphoceles from each other, since all three types of collections demonstrated low signal intensity on T_1- and high signal intensity on T_2-weighted images (both T_1 and T_2 are long).[23] Hematomas and abscesses both had higher signal intensity T_1-weighted images than did the other three fluid types.

The distinction of acute graft rejection (GR) from acute tubular necrosis (ATN) is difficult on both clinical and imaging grounds. Rholl and coworkers used SE and IR techniques to image canine kidneys

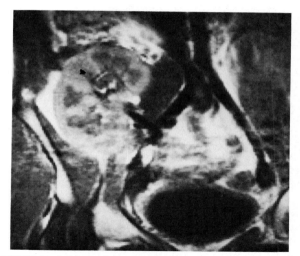

FIGURE 31–6. Normal renal transplant in the right lower quadrant. Coronal SE T_1-weighted image demonstrates normal renal anatomy.

with induced GR and ATN following transplantation.[25] Acute rejection resulted in obliteration, whereas ATN resulted in preservation of the CMD on T_1-weighted images. Hricak et al. documented normal MR allograft morphology in patients with ATN as well as cyclosporine-induced nephrotoxicity on T_1-weighted images.[23, 24] The preservation of the CMD in ATN has also been reported by LiPuma.[3] Leung et al. obtained similar results by imaging nontransplant patients with histologically proven ATN.[4] However, Winsett et al. have reported significant overlap in the corticomedullary intensity ratios obtained from patients with ATN, GR, and cyclo-

sporine toxicity, so that an accurate diagnosis could not be rendered by MR alone.[26]

Rejection has been associated with partial or complete loss of the CMD (Fig. 31–7).[22–26] The degree of CMD indistinction corresponds to the severity of the rejection. Acute rejection results in prolonged T_1 values, expressed as decreased signal intensity of the renal cortex and an indistinct CMD, whereas chronic rejection leads to complete effacement of the CMD.[22] In patients with chronic rejection, Geisinger et al. found a uniform signal intensity throughout the renal parenchyma on T_1-weighted images.[22] T_2-weighted images were noncontributory in differentiating between acute and chronic rejection. Additional MR features of acute rejection include renal transplant enlargement (swelling) and absence of renal hilar fat, the latter a sign of severe rejection.[24] Hricak et al. found MR imaging more accurate in diagnosing GR than either sonography or renal scintigraphy.[24] They encountered one patient with chronic rejection, in whom the graft had a mottled appearance and the CMD was obliterated. The renal sinus fat could not be identified either.

Focal Renal Masses

CYSTIC MASSES

Simple renal cysts appear on T_1-weighted images as homogeneous, low signal intensity structures without internal debris, whereas they display increased signal intensity on T_2-weighted images (Fig. 31–8).[1–5, 27–30] They are clearly separated from the adjacent renal parenchyma, and their contour is smooth. The wall of a simple cyst is not demonstrable by MR, but septations have been shown.

MR imaging may differentiate cysts from solid

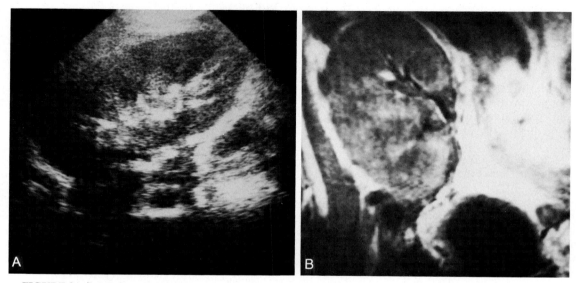

FIGURE 31–7. MR imaging of subacute renal transplant rejection four weeks following cadaveric transplant. *A,* Sagittal renal sonogram is normal except for slight parenchymal inhomogeneity. The central renal sinus is preserved, and no perinephric fluid collections are seen. *B,* Coronal T_1-weighted image of the transplant shows obliteration of the corticomedullary separation and disorganization of the central renal sinus, findings consistent with renal transplant rejection.

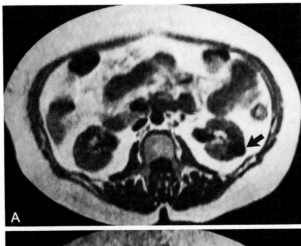

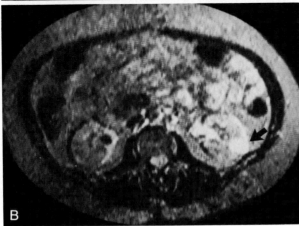

FIGURE 31–8. Simple renal cyst in patient with equivocal sonography and history of reaction to intravenous administration of contrast material. *A,* Transverse T$_1$-weighted image demonstrates a low signal intensity lesion in the lateral aspect of the left kidney *(arrow).* *B,* Transverse T$_2$-weighted image of the same patient shows the same lesion to be of high signal intensity, consistent with a fluid-containing cyst *(arrow).*

masses with an accuracy comparable to that of sonography and CT. In a study of 42 patients with complex and simple renal cysts, Marotti et al. concluded that when the fluid intensity by MR imaging was similar to that of normal urine, the cyst was benign regardless of its wall thickness or septal characteristics.[30] When the contents within a cystic mass did not have the MR characteristics of simple fluid, MR imaging was not helpful in characterizing that mass.

Hemorrhagic and infected cysts have relaxation times that differ from those of simple cysts.[2, 30, 31] Hemorrhagic cysts are of high intensity on SE and IR acquisitions because of their shorter T$_1$ values. Differences in intensity among multiple cysts reflect evolution of the hemorrhage, the cyst with the most recent bleeding appearing most intense. Infected cysts are of intermediate intensity between a simple and a hemorrhagic cyst.

The appearance of polycystic kidneys on MR images is a good example of the visual spectrum of cystic disease, with certain cysts containing clear fluid and others hemorrhagic (Fig. 31–9). The kidneys are enlarged and largely replaced by the cysts. The high-intensity layering seen within some cysts is attributed to iron-containing debris that has settled into the dependent part of the cyst.[31] Hilpert et al. examined nine patients with adult-type polycystic kidney disease by MR imaging, sonography, and CT.[31] They found that MR imaging differentiated between simple cysts, hemorrhagic cysts, and a large renal cell carcinoma. Hemorrhagic cysts were seen as homogeneous medium to high signal intensity structures, some of them containing high-intensity fluid-iron levels. The renal cell carcinoma appeared as a high-intensity lesion because of hemorrhage; however, no fluid-iron levels were found in the neoplasm.

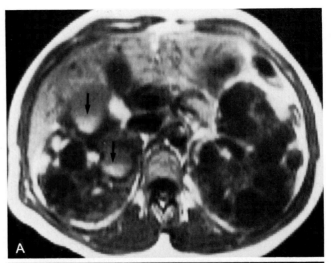

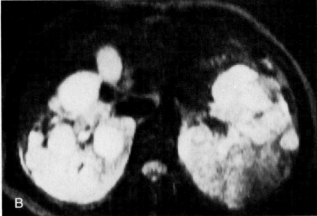

FIGURE 31–9. Adult-type polycystic kidney disease in a young woman with positive family history. *A,* Transverse SE 310/20 image shows bilaterally large kidneys containing mostly low signal intensity cysts. Higher signal intensity sediments probably represent hemorrhage *(arrows).* *B,* The SE 2350/180 image demonstrates the cysts to be of high signal intensity. (*A* from Papanicolaou N, Hahn PF, Edelman RE, et al: Magnetic resonance imaging of the kidney. Urol Radiol 8:139–150, 1986; with permission.)

SOLID RENAL MASSES

Solid masses may be easily distinguished from either simple cysts or normal parenchyma. Unfortunately, a tissue-specific discrimination that was hoped for has not yet materialized, and reliable differentiation between inflammatory and neoplastic masses has not been possible to date. Solid renal masses usually appear as heterogeneous structures that cause distortion of the renal contour and parenchyma relative to their size and location.[2–7, 27–29, 32–37] Their MR signal intensity varies extensively, depending upon tissue composition and pulse sequence acquisition.

Inflammatory renal masses have been imaged, although few in number (Fig. 31–10). Choyke and coworkers studied three such cases using partial-saturation T_1-weighted techniques and T_2-weighted SE sequences.[28] Two of the masses were well circumscribed, rather homogeneous, and of low signal intensity on T_1-weighted images, whereas the third was ill-defined and contained low- and high-intensity

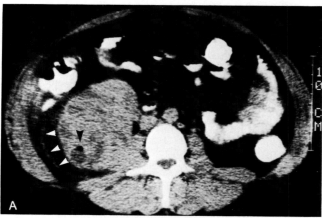

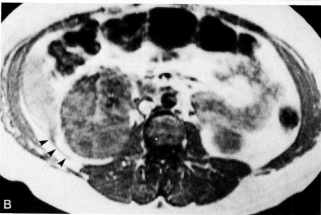

FIGURE 31–10. Diffuse pyelonephritis in a 45-year-old diabetic woman. Percutaneous needle biopsy of right kidney yielded pus and *Escherichia coli* bacteria, also cultured from the patient's urine and blood. *A*, Transverse CT scan demonstrates a right kidney of abnormal size (large) and appearance, with a small amount of air in the parenchyma *(black arrowhead)*. The perinephric fascia is thickened *(white arrowheads)*. *B*, Transverse SE 500/24 image at about the same level as the CT scan shows a diffusely abnormal right kidney, with some thickening of the perinephric fascia *(arrowheads)*.

areas. Hricak et al. described an abscess as an inhomogeneous, low-intensity solid mass on SE technique.[27] Hadley et al. and LiPuma reported cases of xanthogranulomatous pyelonephritis.[3, 32] The renal parenchyma had higher-than-normal intensity, and the purulent urine in the dilated collecting system was brighter than clear urine. Renal calculi, when present, could not be seen by MR imaging. The lipid-containing abnormal parenchyma was of different intensity from the adjacent retroperitoneal fat. Li-Puma also encountered two renal abscesses that appeared as inhomogeneous, low-intensity masses, indistinguishable from solid neoplasms.[3]

Renal cell carcinoma is the most extensively studied neoplasm, and its MR characteristics vary widely (see Fig. 31–5). A feature common to neoplasms on SE techniques is a relative prolongation of T_1 compared with normal parenchyma, assuming that areas of hemorrhage or necrosis are not included in the region of interest.[2–4, 27–29] T_2 values are usually similar to or higher than those of normal renal parenchyma. Clear cell–type carcinomas exhibited slightly higher intensity signal than normal cortex, whereas granular cell neoplasms showed low intensity on SE T_1-weighted imaging.[2]

Hemorrhage and necrosis are frequently encountered within the usually vascular renal cell carcinomas. Both processes have been shown to produce high signal intensity images. Kulkarni et al. reported long T_2 values in a case of necrotic tumor on a TR 1000/TE 60 SE pulse sequence.[29]

Experience with staging of renal cell carcinomas has yielded encouraging results. Hricak and coworkers correctly staged 26 of 27 tumors with MR imaging as compared with surgical staging.[13] MR imaging diagnosed the primary neoplasm in all patients, detected retroperitoneal lymphadenopathy and direct invasion of adjacent organs, and evaluated renal vein and caval patency for possible tumor thrombosis (Fig. 31–11A and B). Multiplanar image acquisition is an important advantage of MR imaging over other radiologic techniques; an additional advantage is the inherent ability of MR imaging to visualize vascular structures and their lumina without the need for intravascular contrast enhancement.

More recently, Hricak et al., in a larger series of patients with renal cell carcinoma, reported a somewhat decreased accuracy in the preoperative staging (82 per cent of the lesions detected). MR imaging was best in excluding vascular extension and tumor spread to adjacent structures but was not accurate in diagnosing bowel and mesentery involvement.[33] Of special interest was their finding that MR imaging missed five neoplasms smaller than 3 cm in diameter, prompting them to suggest that it should not be used as a screening modality for renal tumors. This observation was confirmed by other investigators, who were unable to detect tumors isointense with the renal parenchymal.[34] Application of dynamic imaging methods and gadolinium-DTPA (Chapter 7) will likely improve the accuracy of MRI (Fig. 31–11C and D).

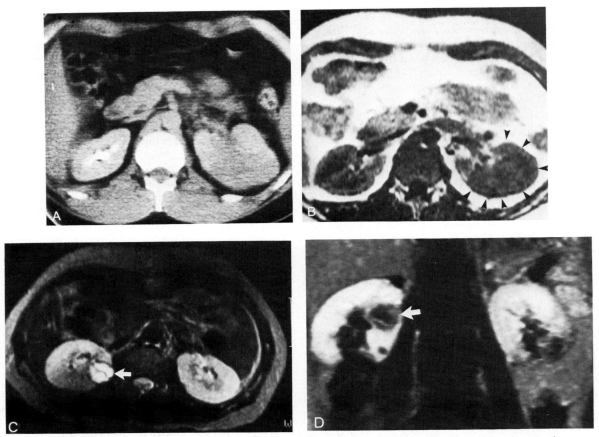

FIGURE 31–11. *A,* Infiltrating papillary renal cell carcinoma in a 35-year-old male with painless hematuria. Contrast-enhanced CT scan shows a normal right upper renal pole and a diffusely abnormal left upper kidney, with patchy perfusion and absent collecting system. *B,* The IR pulse sequence image shows the infiltrating process to occupy most of the left upper renal pole *(arrowheads).* The corticomedullary differentiation is obliterated, although it is better seen on the normal right kidney. *C,* Different patient with renal cell carcinoma, no invasion. T_2-weighted SE image (TRITE-2500 msc/90 msc) shows irregular, high intensity mass *(arrow).* *D,* Postgadolinium-DTPA T_1-weighted coronal gradient-echo image shows nonenhancing mass *(arrow).* Smaller mass inferiorly represents a cyst. (Courtesy of R. Edelman, M.D.) (*A* from Papanicolaou N, Hahn PF, Edelman RR, et al: Magnetic resonance imaging of the kidney. Urol Radiol 8:139–150, 1986; with permission.)

Three cases of papillary renal cell carcinoma have been reported to date.[7, 29, 35] One report showed a rather low-intensity lesion,[29] whereas the second described a high-intensity mass compared to normal tissue,[35] both with T_1-weighted SE techniques. A third case of papillary carcinoma was of lower signal intensity than that of normal tissue on T_1-weighted SE and IR pulse sequences (Fig. 31–11).[7] T_2-weighted SE images failed to demonstrate the process, indicating T_2 values similar to those of normal tissues.

The MR features of Wilms' tumor in 14 children were described.[36] Signal intensity was consistent with prolonged T_1 and T_2 relaxation times and quite variable, mainly because of coexisting necrosis and hemorrhage. Specific characteristics enabling differentiation of the tumor from other solid renal masses could not be found. Whereas local extension and spread of the disease into the liver and inferior vena cava were well documented, capsular invasion was missed in four cases. Of interest was the detection by both MR imaging and CT of enlarged retroperitoneal lymph nodes in five patients, with MR features similar to those of the primary neoplasm. Upon exploration, however, no tumor was found in the nodes.

Urothelial tumors may be impossible to detect unless they are of sufficient size or infiltrate the renal parenchyma. Leung et al. examined a urothelial neoplasm with IR and SE techniques.[4] On IR pulse sequences the lesion was isointense with the renal parenchyma. SE acquisitions showed a high signal intensity lesion. Papanicolaou et al. described a case of transitional cell carcinoma that presented as an infiltrating neoplasm, mostly homogeneous, of intermediate signal intensity and obliteration of the CMD on T_1-weighted SE technique.[7]

In two cases of renal lymphoma, the involved kidneys were grossly enlarged (Fig. 31–12).[7] The infiltrating process produced low-intensity, rather homogeneous masses on T_1-weighted SE technique. There was total loss of the CMD. Adjacent lymphadenopathy had a similar appearance. Three pediatric cases of leukemia and Burkitt's lymphoma re-

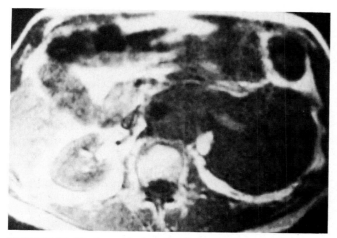

FIGURE 31–12. Systemic lymphoma involving the left kidney. Transverse SE 310/18 image demonstrates a low signal intensity, enlarged left kidney with retroperitoneal adenopathy surrounding the aorta.

ported by Dietrich and Kangarloo had similar MR features.[37] However, LiPuma reported a case of Burkitt's lymphoma, in which both kidneys contained areas of higher signal intensity on T_1-weighted SE technique, attributed to metastatic deposits.[3]

Metastatic disease to the kidneys from lung and breast primaries appears as low-intensity lesions on T_1-weighted SE and large flip angle gradient-echo techniques.[28, 29]

Angiomyolipoma of the kidney, a hamartoma with occasionally invasive character, has always been an interesting lesion to image radiologically (Fig. 31–13). It is highly echogenic by sonography and contains low attenuation areas on CT, both owing to its fat component. Its MR characteristics vary.[3, 4, 7, 27, 29] A common feature is its high signal intensity on T_1-weighted SE acquisitions, because of the short T_1 of fat. Likewise, T_2-weighted SE images show a moderate intensity lesion because of moderate T_2 values of fat. The neoplasm has been described as homogeneous and well-defined in some reports and heterogeneous and indistinguishable from the perinephric fat in others.

CLINICAL APPLICATIONS

The achievements of MR imaging are significant considering the short period of time the modality has been used in clinical practice. Experience with MR imaging of renal pathology is still limited. Early reports in the literature and subsequent larger series have attempted to define the yield and limitations of MR in a variety of disease entities. Normal renal anatomy can be demonstrated in multiple planes. Blood flow or lack thereof within large vessels can be documented in a noninvasive manner. Differentiation between cystic and solid renal lesions appears to

be reliable, and hemorrhage may be diagnosed and followed through its biochemical evolution. Preoperative staging of renal cell carcinoma has been relatively successful, although renal neoplasm screening has been problematic, and imaging of post-transplantation complications is promising.

Imaging and management of the indeterminate renal mass continue to generate controversy in clinical practice. When strict criteria are met, sonography and computed tomography are highly accurate in differentiating cystic from solid renal lesions (93 to 97 per cent).[38–40] The small percentage of indeterminate masses usually undergoes follow-up imaging, needle aspiration, or, depending on the clinical situation, exploration. Angiography often is noncontributory, since most of these masses are hypovascular or avascular. Marotti et al. imaged with MR a small number of patients with simple and complex renal

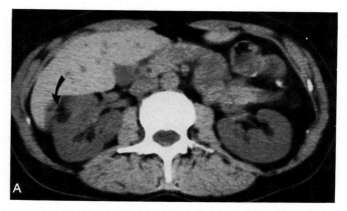

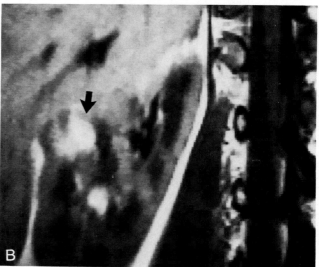

FIGURE 31–13. Angiomyolipoma of the right kidney in a 45-year-old woman with right flank pain. *A*, Plain CT scan through the kidneys shows a low-density lesion in the anterolateral aspect of the right kidney *(curved arrow)*. *B*, Coronal SE T_1-weighted image demonstrates the same lesion as a high signal intensity focus *(arrow)*. (*A* from Papanicolaou N, Hahn PF, Edelman RR, et al: Magnetic resonance imaging of the kidney. Urol Radiol 8:139–150, 1986; with permission.)

cysts.[30] They concluded that a cyst is benign, regardless of the thickness of its wall or septations, when the MR characteristics of its fluid are similar to those of urine. After studying nine patients with polycystic kidney disease, Hilpert et al. suggested that MR imaging may differentiate simple cysts from hemorrhagic cysts and neoplasms.[31] At the present time, both studies need to be confirmed by larger series of patients, before a definite indication for MR can emerge. Therefore, it is unlikely that MR will replace either sonography or CT in the near future in the investigation of an indeterminate renal mass or the screening for renal tumors; however, limited use in selected patients may be of help.

Preoperative staging of renal cell carcinoma is amenable to MR imaging and appears to be a useful clinical application at the present time. Extent of tumor, renal vein and caval thrombosis, and perihilar lymphadenopathy can all be diagnosed with accuracy.[13, 33] The proximal extent of the thrombus also can be demonstrated, obviating the need for cavography or CT with intravenous contrast enhancement. Multiplanar imaging capability makes MR imaging more advantageous than CT in the evaluation of local extent of and/or invasion by the neoplasm.

The role of MR imaging in the diagnosis of complications following transplantation is not yet well defined. The number of studies and patients currently is too small to allow useful applications to emerge. Most investigators agree that detection of graft rejection can be made safely, primarily on the basis of a swollen kidney with obliterated corticomedullary differentiation.[22-24] Acute tubular necrosis and cyclosporine-induced toxicity usually result in normal allograft images, so that neither process can be ruled out in the presence of a normal kidney; however, rejection would be unlikely. It appears that renal biopsy, sonography, and scintigraphy will continue to be performed in the work-up of patients with suspected post-transplantation complications, with MR imaging reserved for selected patients (high suspicion for graft rejection, biopsy contraindicated).

Current disadvantages of MR imaging include the lack of satisfactory tissue specificity in the differential diagnosis of solid renal masses and renal parenchymal diseases with a few exceptions, inability to demonstrate calcifications, image degradation because of motion artifacts, and prolonged scanning time. It is evident that many areas of the renal pathophysiology and anatomy are still waiting to be explored by MR, including in vivo spectroscopy, in a more systematic and quantitative fashion. In practical terms, renal MR imaging has not established itself yet as an indispensable, available, and time- and cost-effective diagnostic tool. If important physiologic applications of objective, quantitative data and development of useful pulse sequence techniques materialize, the clinical use of MR imaging will be enhanced, and what is now a promising technique will become an indispensable tool in the investigation of renal disease.

MR IMAGING OF THE RETROPERITONEUM

The high signal intensity of retroperitoneal fat on MR imaging contrasts nicely with the low signal intensity of vascular structures and the intermediate signal intensity of retroperitoneal and adjacent intraperitoneal solid organs. Physiologic motion (cardiac, respiratory, intestinal) usually causes limited degradation of the images of the retroperitoneum. Multiplanar MR scanning capability offers an advantage over CT in many clinical situations.

As with the kidney, clinical experience with MR imaging of the other retroperitoneal structures is limited. The adrenal glands, pancreas, and blood vessels have been discussed elsewhere. This section covers the ureters, lymphatic system, and retroperitoneal muscles, mainly the iliopsoas muscles.

NORMAL ANATOMY

The nondilated ureter and normal-size lymph nodes are difficult to demonstrate on MR imaging.[1, 2] Since the major retroperitoneal vessels, the aorta and the cava, are easily identified, they serve as landmarks for the localization of the ureters and lymph node chains. The ureter is more likely to be seen, because urine contrasts adequately with the high signal intensity of retroperitoneal fat on T_1-weighted images.

The iliopsoas muscles can be clearly outlined in normal individuals and are best seen in axial (transverse) and coronal planes using T_1-weighted pulse sequence.[3, 4] The signal intensity of muscle tissue is low on T_1-weighted images, because of its long T_1 and short T_2 relaxation times, as compared with the bright appearance of fat, which has a rather short T_1 relaxation time. High signal intensity bands within the muscles represent fat. The same bands may also be seen on computed tomography scans because of the different attenuation of the x-rays between muscle and fat.

The iliopsoas muscles usually are bilaterally symmetric in appearance, so an obvious asymmetry should be investigated further. Frequently, the cause of such asymmetry is malpositioning of the patient.

PATHOLOGY

Ureteral Dilatation

The dilated ureter is easily identified on axial and coronal T_1-weighted images. The coronal plane may be more suitable in the evaluation of the level and the cause of ureteral obstruction. On coronal images, long segments of the ureteral lumen can be seen on single images; therefore, the relation between the ureter and the obstructing lesion may be demonstrated to better advantage (Fig. 31–14). Displace-

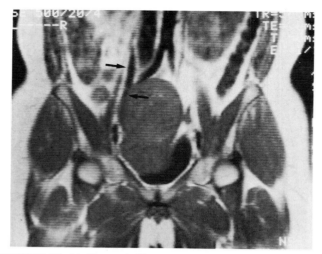

FIGURE 31–14. Ureteral dilatation secondary to large bladder neoplasm in a 35-year-old man. The mildly dilated right ureter is easily seen on SE T_1-weighted coronal MR image of the pelvis (arrows).

ment of the dilated ureter and the cause thereof are readily demonstrable on either axial or coronal images.

Retroperitoneal Fibrosis

The proliferation of fibrous tissue in the retroperitoneum often is confined to the prevertebral and paravertebral regions. The pathologic process may occur anywhere from the kidneys to the lower pelvis, and its extent and bulk vary. Clinical presentation frequently is nonspecific, as the fibrosis envelops various retroperitoneal structures, such as ureters, lymphatics, and blood vessels. Spread toward the porta hepatis and intraperitoneal bowel loops as well as rectum and uterus occurs infrequently.

Computed tomography can diagnose retroperitoneal fibrosis and assess its extent directly and definitively. Sonography also may occasionally be helpful. One study compared patients with benign and malignant retroperitoneal fibrosis.[41a] The signal intensity of the process was higher than that of the adjacent psoas muscle and considerably lower than that of retroperitoneal fat in T_1-weighted images (Fig. 31–15). More useful were T_2-weighted SE images, in which malignant processes generally showed high signal, similar to or slightly lower than fat, and a heterogeneous structure; whereas benign processes showed low signal, similar to muscle, and a homogeneous structure. However, further study is needed with larger numbers of patients. A potential unique contribution of MR imaging is its noninvasive assessment of the effect retroperitoneal fibrosis may have on blood flow through the aorta, cava, and iliac vessels. Changes in intraluminal arterial or venous signals have been seen and attributed to vascular constriction. Further studies, however, are necessary to confirm and explore the significance of alterations in blood flow.

Fluid Collections—Abscesses

Limited experience with MR imaging of retroperitoneal fluid collections and abscesses exists.[1, 3, 4, 6, 7] Transverse scans are preferable for demonstration of the retroperitoneal pathology. Sagittal images may be helpful if the process extends toward or into the spine.

It is generally accepted that MR imaging is quite sensitive in diagnosing abnormal fluid collections and inflammation in the retroperitoneum. Psoas abscesses usually were seen as areas of increased signal intensity compared to muscle tissue on both T_1- and T_2-weighted images.[3, 4] Elsewhere, abscesses presented as low or intermediate signal intensity collections, either homogeneous or heterogeneous, on short TR images, with increased intensity on longer TR images.[6, 7] Pancreatic phlegmon, exudative pancreatitis, and a chronic hematoma had similar appearance on T_1- and T_2-weighted images.[6] Post–lymph node dissection lymphoceles appear as well-defined, low signal intensity (lower than muscle) structures on T_1-weighted images and become quite bright on T_2-weighted images (Fig. 31–16). Measurements of T_1 and T_2 relaxation times allowed Dooms et al. to distinguish lymphoceles from lymph node masses.[41] Both parameters were much longer for lymphoceles than for abnormal lymph nodes.

Differentiation between abscesses, neoplasms, and complex fluid collections often is problematic with MR imaging. Therefore, most investigators agree that needle aspiration or biopsy is necessary for specific diagnosis.

Lymphadenopathy

Enlarged retroperitoneal lymph nodes can be identified on MR imaging (Fig. 31–17).[41, 42, 44, 48, 49] The

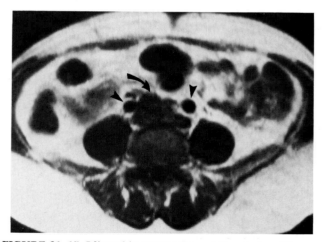

FIGURE 31–15. Idiopathic retroperitoneal fibrosis in a 65-year-old man who presented with mild hypertension and bilateral hydronephrosis. SE T_1-weighted transverse MR image demonstrates a low signal intensity retroperitoneal mass surrounding the large vessels, which are indistinct (curved arrow). Both ureters are dilated (arrowheads).

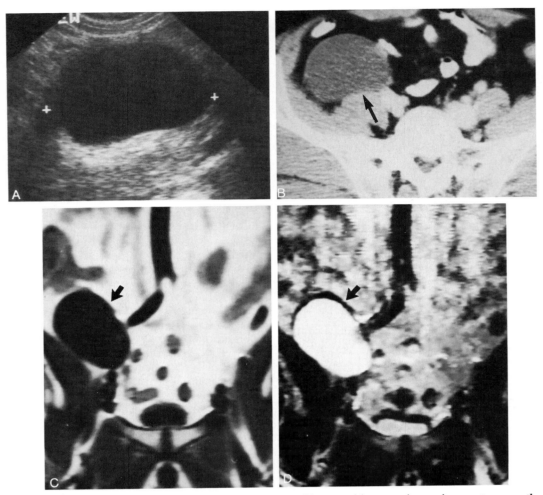

FIGURE 31–16. Postoperative lymphocele in a 52-year-old man with prostatic carcinoma, two months following lymph node dissection. *A*, Transverse sonogram of the pelvis shows a well-defined echolucent structure, with enhancement of the sound beam posteriorly, consistent with fluid collection. *B*, Axial plain CT scan of the pelvis shows well-circumscribed low-density collection anterior to the right psoas muscle and lateral to the iliac vessels *(arrow)*. *C*, SE T_1-weighted coronal MR image of the pelvis demonstrates low signal intensity collection in the right lower quadrant *(arrow)*. *D*, The same collection, seen on SE T_2-weighted coronal image, appears to be of very high signal intensity *(arrow)*. This change in signal intensity is highly suggestive of a fluid collection.

exact accuracy of MR detection as a function of lymph node size cannot be assessed; however, nodes as small as 7 or 8 mm have been seen.[41, 48] Transverse imaging is by far the best imaging plane. MR imaging offers the added advantage over computed tomography that the aorta and cava can be outlined clearly on routine imaging. With T_1-weighted imaging, nodes appear of relatively low intensity. Lee et al. found that the best pulse sequence for lymph node imaging is an SE sequence with TR 900/TE 30 or TR500/TE 30.[44] The former provided images of excellent contrast between lymph nodes and surrounding fat, whereas the latter had a slightly better contrast but also a noisier image. Contrast between nodes and adjacent muscle was better when the TR was longer. Dooms et al. found that optimal demonstration of lymphadenopathy required two pulse sequences, one with long TR and TE and one with

short TR.[41] They agreed with Lee et al. that the best contrast between abnormal nodes and fat was obtained with TR of 500 msec. With T_2-weighted imaging, nodes appear relatively bright and may be difficult to distinguish from fat.

It is generally agreed that CT with intravenous contrast enhancement and MR imaging are comparable in the detection of retroperitoneal lymphadenopathy. Both modalities detect abnormal nodes on the basis of size increases rather than tissue characteristics. CT has somewhat better spatial resolution and requires shorter scanning time. CT is also most suitable for guidance of percutaneous needle biopsy of suspicious nodes. Metallic clips create significant artifacts in CT-generated images, but they have little effect on MR images. MR imaging has superior tissue contrast resolution, an advantage over CT that allows for easier separation of adjacent structures such as

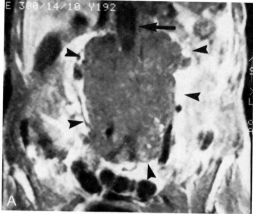

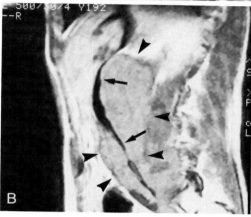

FIGURE 31–17. Massive retroperitoneal lymphadenopathy in a 70-year-old man with metastatic prostatic carcinoma. *A,* Coronal SE T$_1$-weighted MR image of the abdomen shows a large medium signal intensity retroperitoneal mass *(arrowheads),* surrounding the aorta *(arrow). B,* Sagittal SE T$_1$-weighted MR image shows the large mass of lymph nodes *(arrowheads)* displacing and deforming the inferior vena cava *(arrows).*

muscle, vessels, and bowel loops. The use of oral contrast material is of paramount importance to CT scanning and a similar agent, appropriate for MR imaging, will improve MR diagnostic accuracy.

For practical purposes, until MR imaging can provide tissue-specific information that will permit characterization of the disease process involving lymph nodes, CT will remain the screening diagnostic procedure of choice for patients in whom retroperitoneal lymphadenopathy is a concern.

REFERENCES

Kidney

1. Newhouse JH: Urinary tract imaging by nuclear magnetic resonance. Urol Radiol 4:171–175, 1982.
2. Hricak H, Newhouse JH: MR imaging of the kidney. Radiol Clin North Am 22:287–296, 1984.
3. LiPuma JP: Magnetic resonance imaging of the kidney. Radiol Clin North Am 22:925–941, 1984.
4. Leung AWL, Bydder GM, Steiner RE, et al: Magnetic resonance imaging of the kidneys. AJR 143:1215–1227, 1984.
5. Williams RD, Hricak H: Magnetic resonance imaging in urology. J Urol 132:641–649, 1984.
6. Hricak H, Crooks L, Sheldon P, Kaufman L: Nuclear magnetic resonance imaging of the kidney. Radiology 146:425–432, 1983.
7. Papanicolaou N, Hahn PF, Edelman RR, et al: Magnetic resonance imaging of the kidney. Urol Radiol 8:139–150, 1986.
8. Babcock EE, Brateman L, Weinreb JC, et al: Edge artifacts in MR images: Chemical shift effect. J Comput Assist Tomogr 9:252–257, 1985.
9. Swensen SJ, Keller PL, Berquist TH, et al: Magnetic resonance imaging of hemorrhage. AJR 145:921–927, 1985.
10. Hahn PF, Saini S, Stark DS, et al: Intraabdominal hematoma: The concentric-ring in MR imaging. AJR 148:115–119, 1987.
11. Brown JJ, vanSonnenberg E, Gerber KH, et al: Magnetic resonance relaxation times of percutaneously obtained normal and abnormal body fluids. Radiology 154:727–731, 1985.
12. Bradley WG Jr, Schmid PG: Effect of methemogloblin formation on the MR appearance of subarachnoid hemorrhage. Radiology 156:99–103, 1985.
13. Hricak H, Demas BE, Williams RD, et al: Magnetic resonance imaging in the diagnosis and staging of renal and perirenal neoplasms. Radiology 154:709–715, 1985.
14. Wedeen VJ, Rosen BR, Chesler D, Brady TJ: MR velocity imaging by phase display. J Comput Assist Tomogr 9:530–536, 1985.
15. Axel L: Blood flow effects in magnetic resonance imaging. AJR 143:1157–1166, 1984.
16. Wehrli FW, Shimakawa A, MacFall JR, et al: MR imaging of venous and arterial flow by selective saturation-recovery spin echo (SSRSE) method. J Comput Assist Tomogr 9:537–545, 1985.
17. Thickman D, Kundel H, Brery D: Magnetic resonance evaluation of hydronephrosis in the dog. Radiology 152:113–116, 1984.
18. Lande IM, Glazer GM, Sarnaik S, et al: Sickle-cell nephropathy: MR imaging. Radiology 158:379–383, 1986.
19. Mulopulos GP, Turner DA, Schwartz MM, et al: MRI of the kidneys in paroxysmal nocturnal hemoglobinuria. AJR 146:51–52, 1986.
20. Yuasa Y, Kundel HL: Magnetic resonance imaging following unilateral occlusion of the renal circulation in rabbits. Radiology 154:151–156, 1985.
21. London DA, Davis PL, Williams RD, et al: Nuclear magnetic imaging of induced renal lesions. Radiology 148:167–172, 1983.
22. Geisinger MA, Risius B, Jordan ML, et al: Magnetic resonance imaging of renal transplants. AJR 143:1229–1234, 1984.
23. Hricak H, Terrier F, Demas BE: Renal allografts: Evaluation by MR imaging. Radiology 159:435–441, 1986.
24. Hricak H, Terrier F, Marotti M, et al: Post-transplant renal rejection: Comparison of quantitative scintigraphy, US and MR imaging. Radiology 162:685–688, 1987.
25. Rholl KS, Lee JKT, Ling D, et al: Acute renal rejection versus acute tubular necrosis in a canine model: MR evaluation. Radiology 160:113–117, 1986.
26. Winsett MZ, Amparo EG, Fawcett HD, et al: Renal transplant dysfunction: MR evaluation. AJR 150:319–323, 1988.
27. Hricak H, Williams RD, Moon KL Jr, et al: Nuclear magnetic resonance imaging of the kidney: Renal masses. Radiology 147:765–772, 1983.
28. Choyke PL, Kressel HY, Pollack HM, et al: Focal renal masses: Magnetic resonance imaging. Radiology 152:471–477, 1984.
29. Kulkarni MV, Shaff MI, Sandler MP, et al: Evaluation of renal masses by MR imaging. J Comput Assist Tomogr 8:861–865, 1984.
30. Marotti M, Hricak H, Fritzsche P, et al: Complex and simple renal cysts: Comparative evaluation with MR imaging. Radiology 162:679–684, 1987.
31. Hilpert PL, Friedman AC, Radecki PD, et al: MRI of hemorrhagic renal cysts in polycystic kidney disease. AJR 146:1167–1172, 1986.
32. Hadley MDM, Nichols DM, Smith FW: Nuclear magnetic resonance tomographic imaging in xanthogranulomatous pyelonephritis. J Urol 127:301–303, 1982.

33. Hricak H, Thoeni RF, Carroll PR, et al: Detection and staging of renal neoplasms: A reassessment of MR imaging. Radiology 166:643–649, 1988.

34. Glazer GM: MR imaging of the liver, kidneys, and adrenal glands. Radiology 166:303–312, 1988.

35. Herman SD, Friedman AC, Siegelbaum M, et al: Magnetic resonance imaging of papillary renal cell carcinoma. Urol Radiol 7:168–171, 1985.

36. Belt TG, Cohen MD, Smith JA, et al: MRI of Wilms' tumor: Promise as the primary imaging method. AJR 146:955–961, 1986.

37. Dietrich RB, Kangarloo H: Kidneys in infants and children: Evaluation with MR. Radiology 159:215–221, 1986.

38. Pollack HM, Banner MP, Arger PH, et al: The accuracy of gray-scale renal ultrasonography in differentiating cystic neoplasms from benign cysts. Radiology 143:741–745, 1982.

39. McClennan BL, Stanley RJ, Melson GL, et al: CT of renal cyst: Is cyst aspiration necessary? AJR 133:671–675, 1979.

40. Balfe DM, McClennan BL, Stanley RJ, et al: Evaluation of renal masses considered indeterminate on computed tomography. Radiology 142:421–428, 1982.

Retroperitoneum

41. Dooms GC, Hricak H, Crooks LE, Higgins CB: Magnetic resonance imaging of the lymph nodes: Comparison with CT. Radiology 153:719–728, 1984.

41a. Arrive L, Hricak H, Tavares NJ, Miller TR: Malignant versus nonmalignant retroperitoneal fibrosis: Differentiation with MR imaging. Radiology 172:139–143, 1989.

42. Lawson TL, Foley WD, Thorsen MK, et al: Magnetic resonance imaging of discrete and conglomerate lymph node masses. Radiographics 5:971–984, 1985.

43. Weinreb JC, Cohen JM, Maravilla KR: Iliopsoas muscles: MR study of normal anatomy and disease. Radiology 156:435–440, 1985.

44. Lee JKT, Glazer HS: Psoas muscle disorders: MR imaging. Radiology 160:683–687, 1986.

45. Hricak H, Higgins CB, Williams RD: Nuclear magnetic resonance imaging in retroperitoneal fibrosis. AJR 141:35–38, 1983.

46. Cohen JM, Weinreb JC, Maravilla KR: Fluid collections in the intraperitoneal and extraperitoneal spaces: Comparison of MR and CT. Radiology 155:705–708, 1985.

47. Wall SD, Fisher MR, Amparo EG, et al: Magnetic resonance imaging in the evaluation of abscesses. AJR 144:1217–1221, 1985.

48. Lee JKT, Heiken JP, Ling D, et al: Magnetic resonance imaging of abdominal and pelvic lymphadenopathy. Radiology 153:719–728, 1984.

49. Dooms GC, Hricak H, Moseley ME, et al: Characterization of lymphadenopathy by magnetic resonance relaxation times: Preliminary results. Radiology 155:691–697, 1985.

PART IV

PELVIS

32

MR IMAGING OF THE PELVIS

EVE K. COHEN and HERBERT Y. KRESSEL

TECHNIQUE
MALE PELVIS
   NORMAL ANATOMIC FEATURES
   PATHOLOGIC CHANGE
   Prostate
   Bladder
   Testes
   Rectum and Colon

FEMALE PELVIS
   NORMAL ANATOMY
   PATHOLOGIC CHANGE
   Leiomyoma
   Endometrial Carcinoma
   Cervical Carcinoma
   Adnexa
   Endometriosis
   Recurrence and Postoperative Appearances

Since its inception, MR imaging has had wide application in the pelvis. This has been due in part to the relative paucity of motion-related artifacts, with resultant improvement in image quality (particularly when compared to the upper abdomen) and in parenchymal detail for genitourinary organs in the male and female pelvis, as well as the obvious benefits in understanding the relationship of disease processes to adjacent structures through the use of multiplanar imaging. In this chapter we will review a technical approach to acquiring pelvic images, describe the normal anatomic features of the pelvis, and review significant areas of MR imaging applications in a variety of disease processes.

TECHNIQUE

The relative lack of respiratory motion artifacts in the pelvis does tend to simplify the overall approach to pelvic imaging. In general, respiratory gating, motion compensation algorithms, and the use of highly signal averaged techniques for imaging are not required. While each examination is somewhat tailored to the specific clinical problem presented, a number of general features are worth noting.

Air insufflation in the rectum provides an easy method of obtaining good air contrast with the colon and of separating the rectum and sigmoid from other structures of the pelvis. The patient should be examined in the prone position to facilitate rectosigmoid air accumulation and to provide contrast between the rectal vault and adjacent structures. The prone position has the additional advantage of reducing patient claustrophobia and decreasing motion artifacts due to respiration. The use of 1 mg of glucagon intramuscularly just prior to the onset of the examination helps reduce intestinal peristalsis and preserve distention of the colon following air insufflation. Preparation of the bladder is useful as well. In contrast to preparation for an ultrasound examination, in which full bladder distention is critical, in MR imaging the benefits of bladder distention in delineation of bowel loops and bladder wall may be somewhat mitigated by the relative increase in gross patient motion and discomfort during the study if the bladder is overdistended. As a result, we prefer a partially distended bladder at the beginning of the examination. The use of a vaginal tampon in female patients facilitates localization of the vagina and determination of its relation to other pelvic organs such as the uterus. This is particularly useful in evaluating patients with cervical or vulvar carcinoma.

A general approach to imaging the pelvis has been to obtain both short TR/TE (TR 600, TE 20 msec) images in at least one plane and long TR/TE images in the same plane to categorize the T_1 and T_2 relaxation properties of suspected abnormalities. In general, axial imaging remains the primary plane of data

TABLE 32–1. PARAMETERS IN MR IMAGING OF THE PELVIS

Organ	Plane	Sequence (SE TR/TE)
Vagina	axial	600/20; 2500/40, 80
	sagittal	2500/40, 80
	(coronal)	2500/40, 80
Uterus, cervix	axial	600/20; 2500/40, 80
	sagittal	2500/40, 80
	(coronal)	
Adnexa	axial	600/200; 2500/40, 80
	coronal	(2500/40, 80); 600/20
	(sagittal)	
Prostate	axial	2500/40, 80; 600/20
	sagittal	2500/40, 80
	coronal	2500/40, 80
Seminal vesicles	axial	2500/40, 80
Bladder	axial	600/20; 2500/40, 80
	sagittal	2500/40, 80
Rectum	axial	600/20; 2500/40, 80
	sagittal	2500/40, 80

Parentheses = as clinically indicated.

acquisition, although frequently these images are supplemented with coronal or sagittal images. In the female, the adnexa, ovaries, and broad ligament and their relationship to the uterine fundus and pelvic floor are best visualized in the coronal plane. Axial images facilitate visualization of the cervix, ovaries, vagina, and pelvic side wall structures. In the male pelvis, coronal images define the relationships of the prostate gland to the levator ani muscles. Axial images provide a ready means for identifying zonal anatomy of the prostate gland and the seminal vesicles in addition to lymph nodes, muscles, and bony structures of pelvic side walls. The sagittal acquisitions are particularly useful in identifying the relationships of pathologic processes to portions of bladder and rectum in both male and female patients (Table 32–1). Sagittal acquisitions are also helpful in displaying uterine, cervical, and vaginal relationships and the anteroposterior extent of lesions in these structures. Although imaging is generally performed with the body coil, significant improvements in spatial resolution can be achieved by using external or intrarectal surface coils.[1a]

MALE PELVIS

NORMAL ANATOMIC FEATURES

The prostate, seminal vesicles, testes, and vasa deferens are well demonstrated on MR images (Fig. 32–1). As in the rest of the pelvis, contrast with surrounding fat is optimized on the short TR/TE images, but intraparenchymal detail is best delineated on the long TR/TE images.

The zonal architecture of the prostate as described by McNeal[1, 2] can be delineated on MR images.[3, 4] The transitional, central, and peripheral zones of the gland may be demonstrated. The central and transitional zones appear as areas of relative signal decrease in the prostate, whereas the peripheral zone, particularly in males older than 30, is demonstrated as an area of high signal intensity on long TR/TE images. In addition, the periprostatic venous plexus in both its anterior and posterolateral components may be demonstrated (Fig. 32–2).

The seminal vesicles are of intermediate intensity on short TR/TE images and are demonstrated as high signal on the long TR/TE images (Fig. 32–1). Asymmetry in the signal intensity of the seminal vesicles, or lack of increase in signal in the long TR/TE images, implies pathology.[5–7] The inner aspect of the bladder wall is not easily separated from its fluid content on short TR/TE sequence but is outlined by the high signal of the fluid on long TR/TE. However, the outer serosal margins are best delineated on short TR/TE, using the high-signal perivesicle fat as contrast. Occasionally, a chemical shift artifact[8] may distort the appearance of the thickness of the bladder wall in the frequency-encoded direction. In cases with equivocal findings, rescanning the patient in a different plane or switching the directions of the frequency- and phase-encoding gradients is useful in excluding chemical shift artifact as the cause of the apparent distortion in wall thickness. The normal corpus cavernosum and corpora spongiosum are readily identified on the long TR/TE sequences as the corporal parenchyma demonstrate high signal intensity, presumably owing to the static blood pool (see Fig. 32–1A and B).

The normal testicular anatomy is best demonstrated with surface coils. The testes are of relatively high signal and homogeneous on long TR/TE pulse sequences. The epididymis and pampiniform venous plexus may also be readily identified on the MR images.

PATHOLOGIC CHANGE

Prostate

Benign Prostatic Hypertrophy

Both benign and malignant conditions can cause focal alterations in the signal intensities of the prostate.[5–7, 9] Benign prostatic hypertrophy (BPH), which is common in men over the age of 40, includes several pathologic entities that occur in the central gland (mixed, sclerotic, fibromuscular, and glandular types). In addition to generalized glandular enlargement, a wide variation in the signal intensity of benign prostatic hypertrophy can be seen.[9] On long TR/TE spin-echo (SE) images, central foci of increased signal intensity, as well as foci of decreased signal intensity, may be identified. In addition, in some patients, particularly those with very enlarged glands, the distinction between central and peripheral zones of the prostate may be lost (Fig. 32–2).

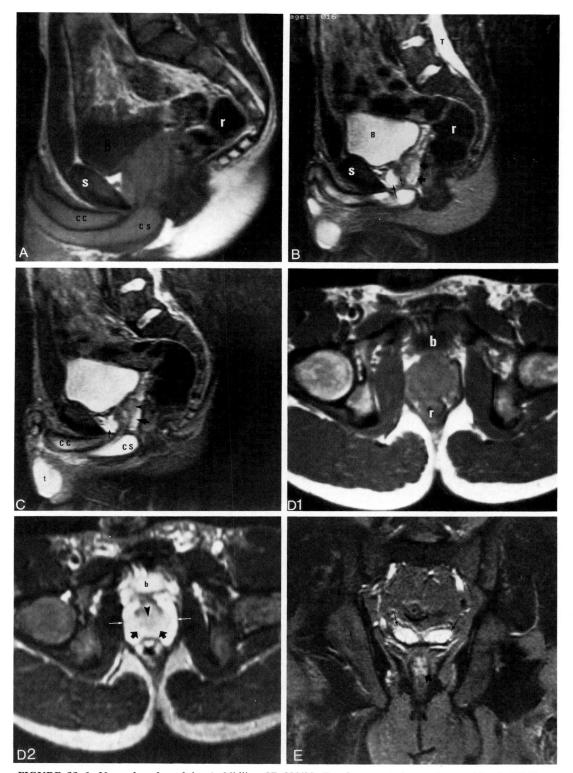

FIGURE 32–1. Normal male pelvis. *A*, Midline SE 600/20. Zonal anatomy is not descernible. *B*, Midline sagittal view 2500/80. *C*, Paramedian sagittal view 2500/80. The periprostatic venous plexus *(thin arrow)* and central *(short thin arrow)*, transitional *(arrowhead)*, and peripheral *(thick arrows)* zones of the prostate are seen. The prostatic portion of the urethra can be identified in its course through the gland. B = Bladder; CC = corporus cavernosum; CS = corpora spongiosa; r = rectum; S = symphysis pubis, T = CSF of thecal sac; t = testes. *D*, Axial view. (i) 600/20 and (ii) 2500/80. The zonal anatomy of the prostate is seen *(arrowhead—transitional; thick arrows—peripheral)* on long TR/TE, in addition to the periprostatic venous plexus *(thin arrows)*. b = bladder; r = rectum. *E*, Coronal SE 2500/80. The seminal vesicles *(thin arrows)* are readily identified on this sequence *(thick arrow = posterior portion of prostate)*. I = Ischium; S = sacrum.

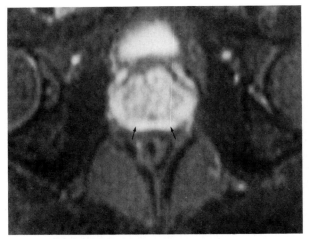

FIGURE 32–2. Benign prostatic hypertrophy—axial SE 2500/80. Foci of high signal are seen in the low-signal central zone of the gland with normal high-signal peripheral zone discernible *(arrows).*

Although microcalcifications of the gland are generally not identified, large calcifications may be delineated as regions of signal void in the relatively high-signal prostate on long TR/TE images.

The tremendous range of variation of signal pattern seen with benign prostatic hypertrophy has limited the utility of magnetic resonance imaging in the identification of prostatic carcinoma that is purely intraglandular.[9] Nodules of mixed or fibromuscular BPH are not easily distinguished from carcinoma by their signal intensity.[9a] Similarly, the coexistence of chronic prostatitis limits detection of intraglandular prostatic carcinoma, also owing to the associated heterogeneity of signal and peripheral zone localization.

Prostatic Cancer

Ninety-five per cent of carcinoma of the prostate is adenocarcinoma, the remaining 5 per cent being

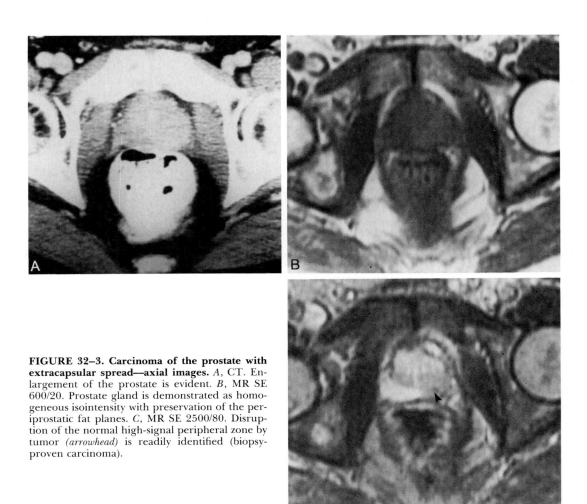

FIGURE 32–3. Carcinoma of the prostate with extracapsular spread—axial images. *A,* CT. Enlargement of the prostate is evident. *B,* MR SE 600/20. Prostate gland is demonstrated as homogeneous isointensity with preservation of the periprostatic fat planes. *C,* MR SE 2500/80. Disruption of the normal high-signal peripheral zone by tumor *(arrowhead)* is readily identified (biopsy-proven carcinoma).

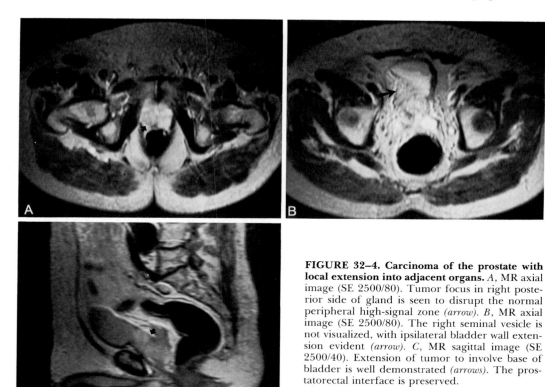

FIGURE 32–4. Carcinoma of the prostate with local extension into adjacent organs. *A*, MR axial image (SE 2500/80). Tumor focus in right posterior side of gland is seen to disrupt the normal peripheral high-signal zone *(arrow)*. *B*, MR axial image (SE 2500/80). The right seminal vesicle is not visualized, with ipsilateral bladder wall extension evident *(arrow)*. *C*, MR sagittal image (SE 2500/40). Extension of tumor to involve base of bladder is well demonstrated *(arrows)*. The prostatorectal interface is preserved.

either transitional or squamous carcinoma. In general, carcinomas arise from the peripheral zone of the prostate and as such may be delineated as focal areas of signal decrease within the normal high-signal peripheral zone of the prostate in T_2-weighted images (Fig. 32–3C). In our experience, peripheral zone defects larger than 1 cm tend to be associated with extracapsular spread of tumor.

MR imaging may also be of use in identifying extracapsular extension of carcinoma to contiguous organs[6, 7] (Fig. 32–4). Asymmetry of the seminal vesicles, particularly on the long TR/TE images, should suggest the possibility of tumor invasion. While hemorrhage in the seminal vesicles due to prior biopsy may present a confusing appearance, in general this appears as high signal in both the short and long TR/TE images and should not present a problem.

The long TR/TE images are useful in identifying contiguous spread to the bladder and rectum.[6, 7] Sagittal long TR/TE images are particularly helpful in this regard. Focal thickening of the bladder wall and/or alteration in bladder wall signal intensity suggests contiguous spread of tumor. Obliteration of the low signal from the rectal fascial interface also suggests direct extension into the rectum.

More distant spread of tumor to lymph nodes and bone may also be delineated with magnetic resonance imaging. Axial short TR/TE images are useful in identifying the presence of enlarged lymph nodes.[10]

On long TR/TE images these involved nodes are typically of high signal intensity on the long TR/TE images. However, increased signal on the long TR/TE images is nonspecific.[10, 11] Bony metastases may also be identified on MR imaging. As these tend to be sclerotic in nature, they typically appear as low signal on both the short and long TR/TE pulse sequences.

In comparing MR imaging to other imaging modalities in defining intra- and extraglandular involvement, it must be emphasized that a multisequence, multiplanar approach for MR imaging is essential. Coronal and sagittal planes are necessary for accurately defining extracapsular extent (levator ani, seminal vesicles, and bladder base). Short and long TR/TE sequences in the axial plane should be performed to assess zonal anatomy, particularly the peripheral zone. CT has been found to have accuracy of 61 to 75 per cent,[33, 34, 41] with better results in advanced disease. The emerging modality of transrectal ultrasonography has not yet yielded enough data for defining true accuracy. Operator dependence and limited field of view are considerations. Sonography appears to be very sensitive in delineating intraglandular lesions but lacks specificity, with extensive overlap between hypertrophy, malignancy, and prostatitis.[41] In staging carcinoma proven by subsequent biopsy, transrectal ultrasonography has an accuracy of 63 per cent with regard to capsular involvement.[38] However, as a guide for biopsy, transrectal ultrasonography is a superb imaging adjunct. Its role as a screening tool is suggested but not yet substantiated.[40] MR imaging had a demonstrated staging accuracy of 83 per cent in defining intra- versus extracapsular spread in a recent series.[41] In defining nodal involvement, neither CT nor MR imaging is completely definitive, the former lacking sensitivity and the latter specificity.[41]

Current recommendations for screening are inde- terminate. Clinical examination is probably still the method of choice, but state-of-the-art transrectal so- nography may be considered a triage modality. Prior to staging by imaging, histologic confirmation is re- quired. MR imaging should be used for postbiopsy preoperative staging in assessing both local extent and presence of adenopathy.

MR imaging appears to be particularly effective in identifying extent of disease into the seminal vesicles and is also a promising technique for identifying local extracapsular spread.[33] While MR imaging can detect macroscopic tumor spread beyond the capsule, present techniques do not allow demonstration of microscopic capsular invasion, and postbiopsy hem- orrhage may be a source of both over- and under- staging.[33]

Bladder

Adequate bladder distention is essential for the evaluation of bladder wall abnormalities. Staging of bladder carcinoma is based on the determination of the layers of involvement of the wall from the mucosa through the serosa. MR imaging has not yet been of value in identifying intravesicular extent of tumor. However, extension into the perivesicular fat may be readily identified on both the short and long TR/TE pulse sequences.[12, 13] As in prostate carcinoma, re-

gional nodal involvement (the external, internal, and common iliac nodal chains) may be identified on the short TR/TE pulse sequences, which typically also demonstrate increased signal on the long TR/TE pulse sequences.[11]

Intravesicular tumor detection is facilitated by the multiplanar approach of MR imaging, with improved visualization of the dome and base, which are not as readily demonstrated on CT (Fig. 32–5). Neither MR imaging nor CT is able to determine degree of involvement by tumor confined to the wall.[12, 33]

Extravesicular extension can be evaluated on CT by utilizing asymmetry of adjacent soft-tissue struc- tures and effacement of perivesicular fat planes. However, direct assessment of local tumor extension is best demonstrated by MR imaging, which enables evaluation of retrovesicular space, including the sem- inal vesicles, prostate, and rectum, by disruption of normal signal intensities of these structures (Fig. 32– 6). Loss of fascial planes is well demonstrated with di- rect sagittal and coronal planar imaging (Fig. 32–7).

The accuracy rate for pelvic lymph node involve- ment as assessed by CT was 79 per cent in one series.[33] CT is limited to determining size changes, however. MR imaging is able to utilize signal intensity changes in addition to size, but signal changes are nonspecific. Neoplastic and inflammatory changes both yield high signal on long TR/TE SE sequences.[10, 11]

Bladder wall thickening may also be seen in a number of inflammatory conditions. The signal fea- tures and morphology of inflammatory bladder le- sions may be difficult to distinguish from neoplasm, although focal involvement does tend to suggest neoplasm.[12–14]

In the bladder as in the prostate, postbiopsy edema and hemorrhage may result in bladder wall thicken- ing and perivesicular reaction, which may simulate the primary neoplasm.

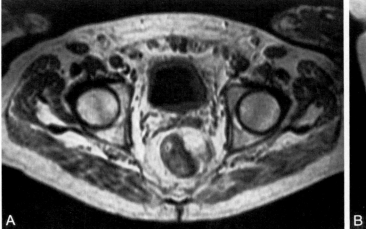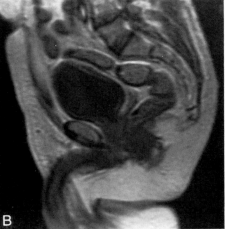

FIGURE 32–5. A 75-year-old male with transitional cell carcinoma of the bladder confined to the wall. *A,* Axial SE 800/25. *B,* Sagittal SE 800/25. Irregular thickening of the bladder wall is evident involving superior and left lateral portions. Perivesicular fat is preserved.

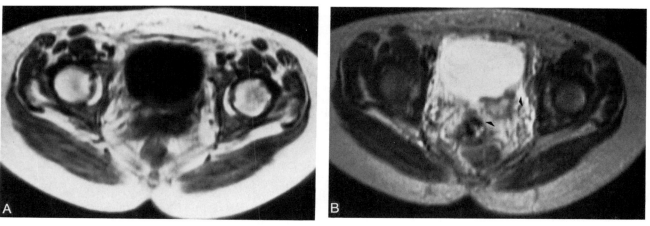

FIGURE 32–6. Middle-aged female with transitional cell carcinoma of the bladder—extramural extension. *A,* Axial SE 600/20. Note left posterolateral irregular mural thickening with effacement of posterior high-intensity perivesicular fat. *B,* Axial SE 2500/80. High-intensity fluid content of the bladder outlines the moderate-intensity tumor mass *(arrowheads),* which is poorly marginated and extends into the perivesicular tissues.

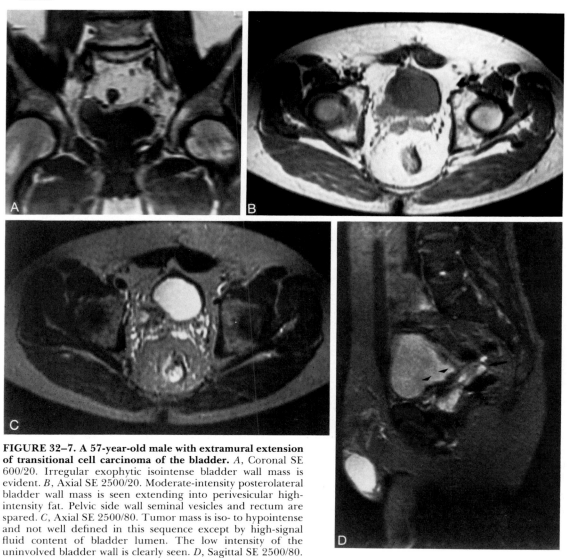

FIGURE 32–7. A 57-year-old male with extramural extension of transitional cell carcinoma of the bladder. *A,* Coronal SE 600/20. Irregular exophytic isointense bladder wall mass is evident. *B,* Axial SE 2500/20. Moderate-intensity posterolateral bladder wall mass is seen extending into perivesicular high-intensity fat. Pelvic side wall seminal vesicles and rectum are spared. *C,* Axial SE 2500/80. Tumor mass is iso- to hypointense and not well defined in this sequence except by high-signal fluid content of bladder lumen. The low intensity of the uninvolved bladder wall is clearly seen. *D,* Sagittal SE 2500/80. Irregular tumor mass can be seen involving posterosuperior wall of bladder *(short arrowheads).* High intensity of seminal vesicle *(arrow)* and prostate *(long arrowhead)* can be appreciated, confirming tumor sparing.

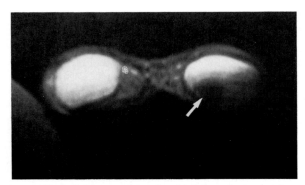

FIGURE 32–8. A 21-year-old male with left testicular seminoma. Axial SE 2500/80 utilizing surface coil. Note focal rounded low-intensity focus in left testis *(arrow)*.

Testes

The examination of the testes is facilitated by the use of surface coils. We have employed a round 5-inch coil for this purpose. The high signal of the normal testes on the long TR/TE pulse sequences may be useful in localizing undescended testes, as is the ability to image in a variety of planes. In general, neoplastic involvement of the testes is delineated as a focal or diffuse decrease in the normal high signal of the testes on the long TR/TE pulse sequence (Fig. 32–8). Associated nodal involvement may also be detected. MR imaging may be useful in identifying other scrotal abnormalities, including hydrocele, varicocele, and inguinal hernia(s) (Fig. 32–9). This subject is considered in greater depth in Chapter 34.

Rectum and Colon

MR imaging can aid in determining the local extent of rectal tumor. Air insufflation of the rectum with glucagon (1 mg intramuscularly) immediately prior to the examination is essential to obtain adequate distention and optimize the visualization of the rectal walls. The high contrast with surrounding perirectal fat is useful in visualizing extraserosal spread of disease. In addition, on long TR/TE images rectal tumors typically have signal intensities greater than that of fat, which is also useful in identifying extraserosal spread of disease (Fig. 32–9).

FEMALE PELVIS

Normal Anatomy

The uterus is well demonstrated on magnetic resonance images.[15] On long TR/TE images, increased parenchymal detail is appreciated (Fig. 32–10*F* and *G*). On the long TR/TE images, a zone of intermediate signal, the peripheral myometrium, surrounds a ring of low signal. This dark ring surrounds a

central area of high signal that is derived from the endometrium. The low-signal junctional zone, originally believed to represent stratum basale, is now thought to represent a more central high-flow vascular zone of myometrium.[16, 20]

The thickness of the high-signal endometrial zone varies with the patient's age, menstrual status, and exogenous hormonal stimulation.[17, 18] Typically, in menstruating women, the endometrium is 1 to 3 mm thick during the proliferative phase and increases to 5 to 7 mm during the midsecretory phase of the cycle. Demas et al.[19] have noted that this increase in the endometrium during the midsecretory phase of the cycle is also accompanied by a slight increase in uterine volume, prominence of the junctional zone, and some increase in myometrial signal on the long TR/TE sequences. The high-signal endometrial zone is typically less than 3 mm thick and is not visualized in women on oral contraceptives. In addition, the cyclic alterations are less pronounced in these women.[17–19] The premenarchal and postmenopausal uterus typically demonstrates decrease in size, thinning of the endometrium, and indistinct junctional zone.

The cervix demonstrates relatively decreased signal

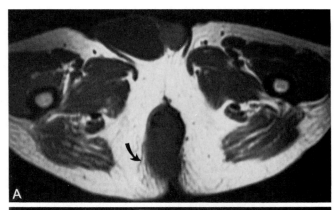

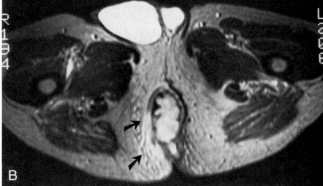

FIGURE 32–9. Rectal carcinoma. *A,* MR axial image (SE 600/20). Isointense exfoliative mass is seen in the rectum. The adjacent fat planes are asymmetric, suggesting right-sided extension *(arrow).* Of note is an incidental right hydrocele with hypointensity in the scrotum. *B,* MR axial image (SE 2500/80). Tumor mass demonstrates high signal, with local extension into adjacent fat evident. The right hydrocele shows fluid high-signal intensity.

on all pulse sequences, presumably related to the increased fibrous tissue present in the cervix. The cervical canal demonstrates increased signal on long TR/TE pulse sequences, presumably related to cervical mucus[19, 20] (Fig. 32–10*F*, *G*, and *J*).

The supporting structures of the uterus—the cardinal ligament, sacral ligament, and broad ligament—may be visualized with MR imaging (Fig. 32–10*A* to *C*). The broad ligament is most readily identified on coronal images, whereas on parasagittal images it may be recognized because of its characteristic triangular appearance (Fig. 32–10*C*).

On short TR/TE images, the ovaries typically are intermediate in signal intensity[15, 25, 27] (Fig. 32–10*D*). Although they are commonly homogeneous in nature, normal ovaries may contain small areas of focal decreased or increased signal. These areas represent small follicular cysts or hemorrhagic corpus luteum cysts. On long TR/TE images, there is generalized increased signal intensity from the ovaries (Fig. 32–10*E*). In the coronal plane, the ovaries may be recognized by identifying the broad ligaments and fallopian tubes and tracing these structures laterally (Fig. 32–10*D* and *E*). The ovaries are located on the posterior surface of the broad ligament, with the fallopian tubes typically located superiorly and somewhat medially. The support to the ovaries is provided by two ligamentous structures, the infundibulopelvic ligament and the ovarian ligament.[21] The infundibulopelvic ligament has on occasion been identified on MR images, originating in the fascia overlying the external iliac vessels and psoas muscles and attaching to the upper pole of the ovary.[16]

The vagina can be demonstrated on both the long and short TR/TE images. As noted previously, placement of a vaginal tampon facilitates the evaluation of this structure. The vaginal vault and body may be recognized. On both long and short TR/TE, the signal intensity of the vagina generally approximates that of adjacent striated muscle. On occasion, high signal may be identified in the vaginal canal on the long TR/TE images, presumably secondary to secretions.[16]

PATHOLOGIC CHANGE

Leiomyoma

Leiomyomas are the most common tumors of the uterus and may be identified in 20 per cent of women over 35 years of age.[22] Generally, these are asymptomatic; however, they may be responsible for a variety of symptoms, including menorrhagia, pain, dysuria, constipation, and infertility. As many as 22 per cent of patients with leiomyomas will have normal sonograms.[28a] MRI can provide a more precise assessment of the number and size of the lesions. The submucosal, myometrial, or subserosal location is well shown by multiplanar imaging. Body habitus is not a limiting factor. Leiomyomas have a variable appear-

ance on magnetic resonance imaging.[16, 20] Typically, uncomplicated leiomyomas are low-signal masses on the long TR/TE images (Figs. 32–11 and 32–12). On short TR/TE images they may be identified as a distortion of the uterine contour, but they have signal features similar to those of the uterus. Cystic degeneration of the fibroid typically results in an area of increased signal intensity on the long TR/TE images. Hyaline degeneration may be associated with variable signal intensity within the low-signal mass.[20]

Endometrial Carcinoma

Endometrial carcinoma is now more common than cervical carcinoma in the U.S.[23] Three quarters of the cases occur in postmenopausal women. These patients often complain of abnormal bleeding or menorrhagia. With its superior soft-tissue contrast resolution, MR imaging readily demonstrates changes in normal uterine zonal anatomy. Endometrial carcinoma has a variable appearance on T_2-weighted images (Figs. 32–13 and 32–14). Blood clots, adenomatous hyperplasia, and endometrial carcinoma are not readily differentiated from each other.[24] All demonstrate high signal on long TR/TE SE sequences. Histologic diagnosis is necessary. With uterine obstruction by tumor, the uterine cavity may be fluid-filled.

Once the diagnosis was established, the overall accuracy in staging of endometrial carcinoma was 92 per cent in a recent study.[24] Long TR/TE SE sequences are essential for evaluation. Correlation with the patient's endocrine status is also necessary, as the presence of a junctional myometrial zone surrounding the endometrial cavity is used for differentiating tumor confined to endometrium from tumor superficially invading myometrium. In the healthy postmenopausal female, the junctional zone is not identified, making this assessment difficult.

Defining extent of the carcinoma beyond the uterus into the cervix and vagina and into the parametrium is facilitated by the superior soft-tissue discrimination afforded by MR imaging. Proper patient preparation with use of a vaginal tampon, rectal air insufflation, mild bladder distention, and prone positioning is essential. Omental and mesenteric involvement, and microscopic invasion, have been difficult to ascertain.[24] If small bowel loops are present in the pelvis owing to decompression of the bladder, assessment of extrauterine extent will be difficult because of peristaltic motion artifact and high-signal fluid contents of bowel on long TR/TE SE sequences. The evaluation of nodal involvement is similar to that of other pelvic neoplasms, with nonspecificity being the major limiting factor. However, as a guide to surgical biopsy, the detection of abnormal nodes is useful.

Sonographic assessment of the depth of myometrial invasion has been shown to be accurate in 70 per cent of patients.[37] This contrasts with 82 per cent accuracy on MR imaging.[24] Ultrasonography is insensitive in detection of cervical involvement and degree

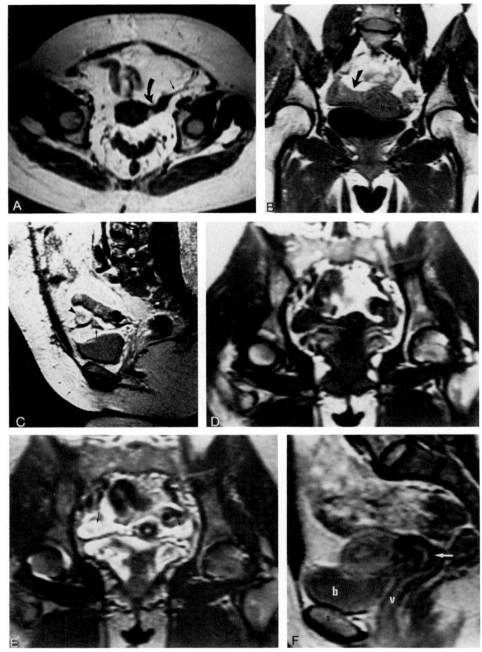

FIGURE 32–10. Normal female pelvis. Normal ovary and broad ligament. *A,* Axial SE 600/25. The left ovary and broad ligament are seen *(curved arrow).* In addition, the round ligament *(straight arrow)* is seen in its course toward the inguinal canal. *B,* Coronal SE 800/25. The right broad ligament, ovary, and fallopian tube are readily identified *(arrow). C,* Sagittal SE 2000/35. The right ovary is seen *(arrowhead)* anterior to the triangular broad ligament *(arrow). D,* Coronal SE 600/25. *E,* Coronal SE 2500/80. The normal ovaries *(arrows)* are identified as dark structures on T_1-weighted and bright on T_2-weighted images. *F,* Sagittal SE 2500/20.

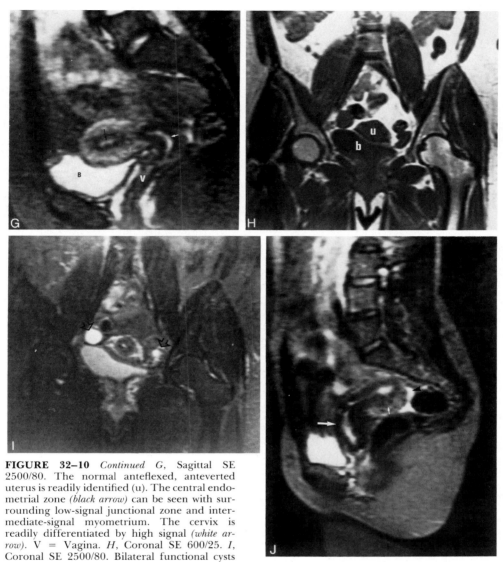

FIGURE 32–10 *Continued G*, Sagittal SE 2500/80. The normal anteflexed, anteverted uterus is readily identified (u). The central endometrial zone *(black arrow)* can be seen with surrounding low-signal junctional zone and intermediate-signal myometrium. The cervix is readily differentiated by high signal *(white arrow)*. V = Vagina. *H*, Coronal SE 600/25. *I*, Coronal SE 2500/80. Bilateral functional cysts of the ovaries *(arrows)* are seen with high signal on long TR/TE. U = Uterus; b = bladder. *J*, Sagittal SE 2500/80. Retroverted uterus is seen with high-signal endometrial and endocervical canals *(large arrow)*. Multiple small areas of low signal in the fundus represent fibroids *(open arrow)*. High-signal free fluid is incidentally noted in the cul-de-sac *(arrowhead)*. (Parts *A-C, F,* and *G* from Spritzer CE, Kressel HY, Mitchell D: Magnetic Resonance Imaging of the Female Pelvis. New York, Raven Press, 1987, pp 208, 211, 212; with permission.)

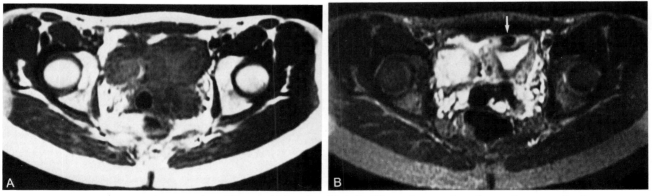

FIGURE 32–11. Leiomyoma in a 27-year-old female with infertility and a question of a uterine anomaly. *A*, Axial SE 600/20. *B*, Axial SE 2500/80. Leiomyoma *(arrow)* is identified in fundus of uterus with isointensity in *A* and hypointensity in *B*. Adjacent loops of small bowel are seen on right side of pelvis as a pseudomass. (From Spritzer CE, Kressel HY, Mitchell D: Magnetic Resonance Imaging of the Female Pelvis. New York, Raven Press, 1987, p 218; with permission.)

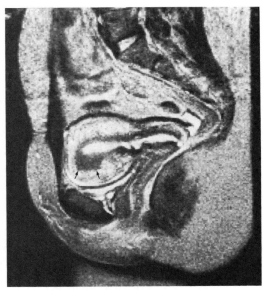

FIGURE 32–12. Submucosal fibroid. Sagittal T$_2$-weighted SE image shows a dark lesion *(arrows)* contiguous with the junctional zone of the uterus.

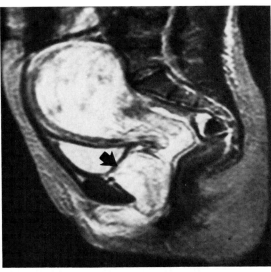

FIGURE 32–14. Uterine sarcoma. Sagittal SE image (TR/TE = 2000 msec/100 msec). A local metastasis *(arrow)* posterior to the bladder and pubic symphysis has obstructed the vagina and trapped blood within it around the cervix. The endometrial cavity is distended and filled with tumor, which appears inhomogeneously bright. (Courtesy of J. Newhouse, M.D.)

of extrauterine extent in advanced disease.[36] MR imaging is more readily suited to this assessment, with its inherent soft-tissue resolution and multiplanar capabilities.

CT is only able to define change in overall uterine size and shape in evaluating disease confined to the myometrium. Loss of normal tissue fat planes can be used in defining tumor extension beyond the uterus, but limited soft-tissue resolution makes accurate assessment difficult.

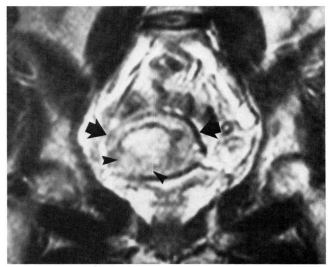

FIGURE 32–13. Endometrial carcinoma. Axial T$_2$-weighted SE image (TR/TE = 2000 msec/100 msec) shows that the uterus *(arrows)* is enlarged. The endometrial cavity is distended by tumor and blood, and the tumor has invaded the myometrium inferiorly *(arrowheads)*. (Courtesy of J. Newhouse, M.D.)

Cervical Carcinoma

Cervical carcinoma continues to be a significant health problem in the United States, the incidence approximating 15 cases per 100,000 per year. Precise staging is important for therapy. Patients with parametrial involvement (FIGO Stage IIB) or more advanced disease are generally treated by radiation. Radical hysterectomy may be used for invasive but less severe disease (Stages IB, IIA), and less extensive surgery is used for lower stages.[37a] The importance of proper patient preparation cannot be overemphasized for proper staging evaluation. Rectal air insufflation, vaginal tampon insertion, and prone positioning are essential to localize and define pelvic structures and their relationships. In our experience, cervical carcinoma has appeared isointense with skeletal muscle on the short TR/TE images. On T$_2$-weighted images, cervical cancer usually appears as a high intensity mass or less commonly as a disruption of the architecture of the normally dark cervix.[37b, 37c] In one study, MR had a staging accuracy of 76 per cent, and accuracy for parametrial status was 89 per cent. Once again, short TR/TE images are useful in identifying extension into surrounding fat, whereas spread into the uterus may be best visualized on the long TR/TE images. Sagittal scanning (Figs. 32–15 through 32–18) is particularly useful in assessing direct extension into bladder or rectum. Axial and coronal long TR/TE SE sequences define lateral extension and pelvic side wall involvement.

CT with its poor soft-tissue differentiation and abdominal sonography with the limited window provided by the bladder are not able to yield the same

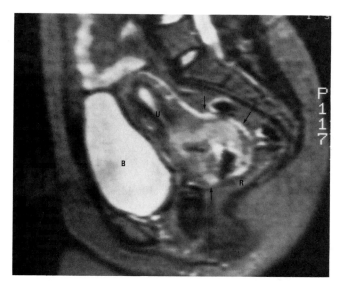

FIGURE 32–15. Carcinoma of cervix with extension into the uterus. Sagittal SE 2500/80. The large tumor mass with moderate intensity is seen to extend into the lower uterine segment. The normal endometrial, junctional, and myometrial zones are seen in the uninvolved body of the uterus. Air is present in the tumor mass, secondary to either rectal fistula formation or tumor necrosis, and is seen as areas of signal void.

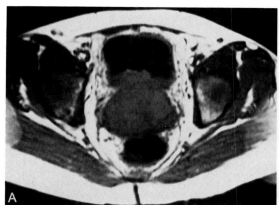

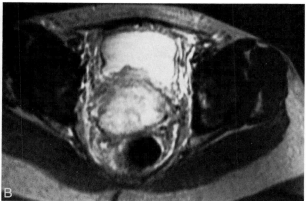

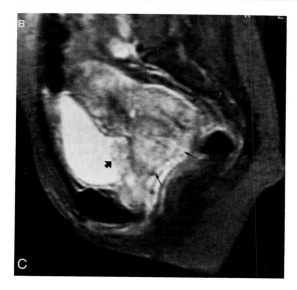

FIGURE 32–16. Carcinoma of the cervix with anterior extension into the bladder. *A*, Axial SE 600/20. *B*, Axial SE 2500/80. Cervical mass of isointensity in *A* and inhomogeneous hyperintensity in *B* is demonstrated to extend through the bladder wall and project into the bladder lumen as an irregular mass. *C*, Sagittal SE 2500/80. The large tumor mass *(small arrows)* is seen to extend into the bladder base *(large arrow)* as well as superiorly. (From Spritzer CE, Kressel HY, Mitchell D: Magnetic Resonance Imaging of the Female Pelvis. New York, Raven Press, 1987, pp 220–221; with permission.)

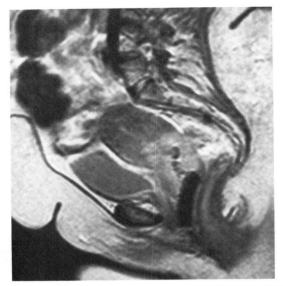

FIGURE 32—17. Cervical carcinoma. Sagittal SE image (TR/TE = 2000 msec/50 msec). The patient has a vaginal tampon. The myometrium of the uterine fundus appears normal, whereas that of the cervix and distal uterine body has been replaced by tumor, which appears brighter. The small dark spots in the center of the tumor are air in the cervical canal introduced by a recent surgical procedure.

delineation as is MR imaging. Transvaginal sonography may prove very useful for defining local extent, but this remains to be confirmed in a large multimodality series.

Adnexa

Cystic Lesions

Adnexal abnormalities may be identified and characterized to some extent on MR imaging.[25, 27] Adjacent bowel loops do not usually pose a problem with the use of orthogonal planes in imaging. Simple cysts and cystic lesions of the adnexa appear as they do elsewhere in the body—low signal on the short TR/TE and high signal on the long TR/TE images (Fig. 32–10I). Patients with polycystic ovaries demonstrate a characteristic appearance on long TR/TE images.[26] In these patients a peripheral rim of small, high-signal cysts and a central region of relatively decreased signal intensity may be observed (Fig. 32–19). The region of decreased signal relates to the central thecal stroma.[16, 26]

The appearance of a teratoma varies with its composition. As might be expected, signal intensities may approximate those of fatty tissue, fluid, blood, or proteinaceous debris (Figs. 32–20 through 32–22). In general, these lesions appear adipose, as in nature, with high signal intensity on the short TR/TE images and intermediate signal intensity on the long TR/TE images.

Hemorrhagic Lesions

The appearance of hemorrhagic collections on MR has been described in the central nervous system and body.[29-31] Pelvic inflammatory disease (PID), carcinoma, and endometriosis may all present as hemor-

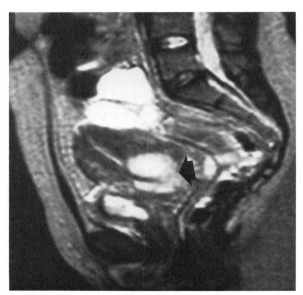

FIGURE 32–18. Cervical carcinoma in a patient undergoing radiotherapy. Sagittal SE image (TR/TE = 2000 msec/100 msec). The tumor (arrow) appears moderately intense; the bright line anterior to it is the endometrial cavity. The intense fluid collections superior to the uterine fundus represent adnexal abscesses that had been exacerbated by radiation therapy.

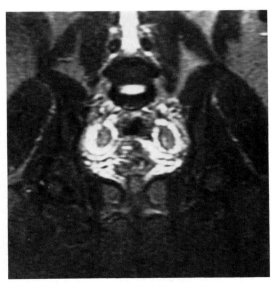

FIGURE 32–19. Polycystic ovarian disease. Coronal SE 2500/80. Note the peripheral ring of high-signal cysts surrounding the central stroma. (From Spritzer CE, Kressel HY, Mitchell D: Magnetic Resonance Imaging of the Female Pelvis. New York, Raven Press, 1987, p 228; with permission.)

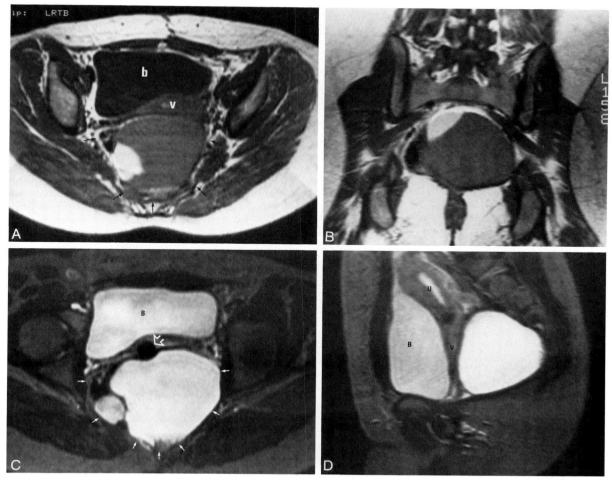

FIGURE 32–20. Presacral dermoid, extraovarian in origin (proven surgically). *A,* Axial SE 600/20. *B,* Coronal SE 600/20. A large mass with distinct components of differing signal intensities is demonstrated to be positioned posterior to the vagina (V) and bladder (b). *C,* Axial SE 2500/80. A vaginal tampon is present *(open arrow).* The fluid, hemorrhagic fat, and calcific components of the mass can be differentiated on the basis of their signal characteristics. *D,* Sagittal SE 2500/80. The relationship of the dermoid to adjacent pelvic structures is well demonstrated. B = Bladder; U = uterus; V = vagina.

rhagic masses. The appearance of a hemorrhagic mass varies with the age of the hemorrhagic collection. Most commonly, these lesions demonstrate high signal intensity on both short and long TR/TE im-

ages, as would be expected in the subacute stage of a hematoma with free methemoglobin. However, more acute appearances of hemorrhage, that is, intermediate signal on the short TR/TE images and

FIGURE 32–21. Dermoid of left ovary. *A,* Sagittal SE 600/20. *B,* Sagittal SE 2500/80. Rounded tumor mass above uterus *(arrows)* shows slight homogeneous hyperintensity in *A* and moderate hyperintensity in *B.* Pathologically this tumor contained primarily hair, accounting for its relatively uniform intensity.

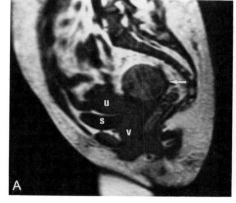

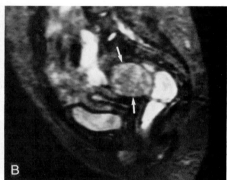

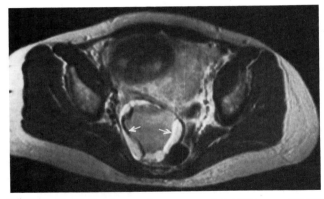

FIGURE 32–22. Benign cystic teratoma. Axial SE image (TR/TE = 2500 msec/20 msec). The presence of chemical shift artifact *(arrows)* within the lesion may be diagnostic for a fat-containing tumor. (Courtesy of R. Edelman, M.D.)

decreased signal on the long TR/TE images (consistent with intracellular deoxyhemoglobin), as well as high signal on the short TR/TE images and low signal on the long TR/TE images consistent with intracellular methemoglobin, have also been identified.[28–31] Although hemorrhage can be recognized on an MR image, and this may help in differential diagnosis, the recognition of a hemorrhagic adnexal mass is in itself nonspecific (Fig. 32–23).

Ovarian Carcinoma

The appearance of ovarian carcinoma is variable, depending on the protein and mucin content of cyst fluid and whether the tumor is cystic or solid (Figs. 32–24 through 32–27). In view of this nonspecificity, with the possible exception of teratomas, MR imaging

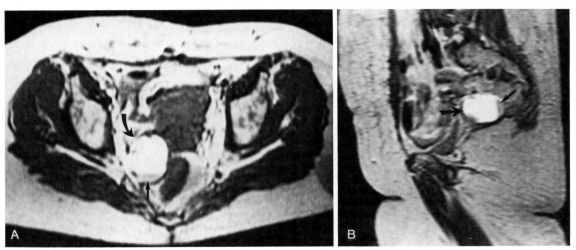

FIGURE 32–23. Cystadenocarcinoma, recurrent. *A*, Axial SE 600/25. *B*, Sagittal SE 2500/80. The area is circumscribed with primarily high-signal contents *(large arrow)*. Intermediate-intensity solid component is identified posteriorly *(small arrow)*. Note the similarity to Figure 32–29—endometrioma.

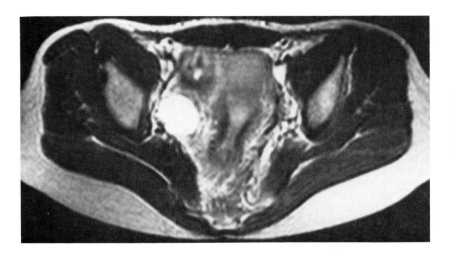

FIGURE 32–24. Carcinoma of the ovary. SE image (TR/TE = 2000 msec/50 msec). The uterus lies in the transverse plane of section with the cervix posterior and fundus anterior. The tumor is seen as an intense ovoid, fluid-filled structure to the right of the uterus.

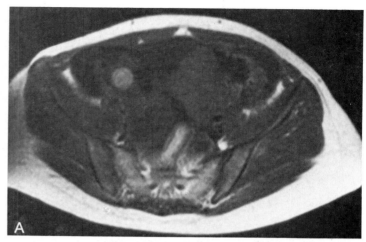

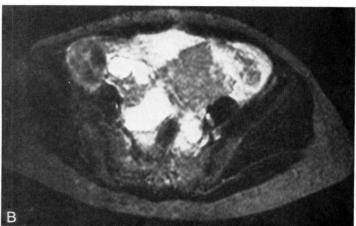

FIGURE 32–25. Ovarian carcinoma. *A*, T₁-weighted SE image (TR/TE = 700 msec/20 msec). *B*, T₂-weighted SE image (TR/TE = 2000 msec/100 msec). In this extensive multilobular tumor, the T₁-weighted image reveals solid portions of the tumor to be of approximately the same intensity as muscle and the fluid portions to be of low intensity. A circular hemorrhagic region appears of intermediate intensity. On the T₂-weighted image, the fluid-containing portions of the tumor appear relatively bright.

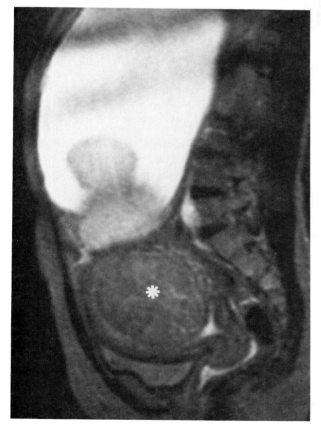

FIGURE 32–26. Fibroid and ovarian carcinoma. SE image (TR/TE = 2000 msec/50 msec). The ovarian tumor is very large and is primarily filled with intense fluid. The bilobed portion of the tumor superior to the uterus is solid tissue. The submucosal fibroid *(asterisk)* is heterogeneous; it distends the myometrium and distorts the endometrial cavity, which is seen as a bright three-pointed region proximal to the cervix.

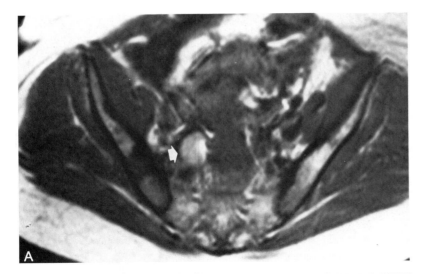

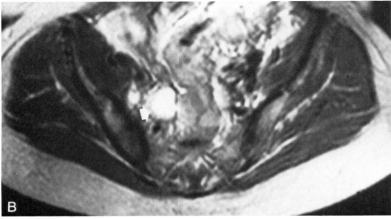

FIGURE 32–27. Recurrent ovarian carcinoma. *A*, T₁-weighted image. *B*, T₂-weighted image. This patient has had a hysterectomy and bilateral salpingo-oophorectomy. The recurrent tumor *(arrow)*, which has a hemorrhagic portion, is seen as a circular region on the right side of the pelvis; it appears predominantly intermediate in intensity on the T₁-weighted image and quite intense on the T₂-weighted image. The patient also has bony metastases from breast carcinoma.

is unable to differentiate among various types of ovarian tumors. Nor can a distinction between benign and malignant tumors be made on the basis of any tissue signal characteristics defined on MR imaging (Fig. 32–28). Therefore, at present MR imaging cannot be recommended as a primary modality in the initial diagnosis of ovarian carcinoma.

Endometriosis

Endometriosis can be divided into two entities: internal (adenomyosis) and external.[38] With its highly specific appearance on high-field MR imaging, hemorrhage is readily detected using short and long TR/TE SE sequences.[29] The diagnosis of endometriosis is suggested by the presence of more than one hemorrhagic cystic focus in the pelvis, frequently not in contiguity with the adnexa (often involving the cul-de-sac), with or without associated free fluid. Loss of clear margination of the uterine body and adhesive tethering of the rectum are also seen as sequelae of diffuse involvement.[28] The high-signal cystic collections demonstrate multilocularity, a low-signal rim (attributed either to hemosiderin-laden macrophages[29, 30] or a fibrous capsule),[28] and internal lower

signal intensity shading, possibly related to hemorrhage in evolution[29] (Figs. 32–29 and 32–30). To date, MR has shown insufficient sensitivity and specificity to substitute for laparoscopy, but might prove useful in monitoring treatment once a diagnosis has been established.[29a, 29b]

Adenomyosis, the presence of endometrial glands and stroma within the myometrium, can be divided into focal and diffuse forms. It rarely demonstrates hemorrhage, unlike endometriosis. Instead, adenomyosis demonstrates low signal relative to normal myometrium on long TR/TE SE sequences, with occasional bright spots. In diffuse disease there is widening of the normal low-signal junctional zone surrounding the high-signal endometrium. When this is irregular or greater than 5 mm in thickness, the diagnosis is clear[38] (Fig. 32–31). However, if it is 3 to 5 mm in thickness, this low-signal zone can represent a normal junctional zone. Repeating the study at a different phase of the menstrual cycle should differentiate the two, as the normal junctional zone changes during the cycle, whereas adenomyosis is resistant to hormonal fluctuations and remains unchanged[38] (Fig. 32–30). Focal adenomyosis may be separated from leiomyomas by the ill-defined mar-

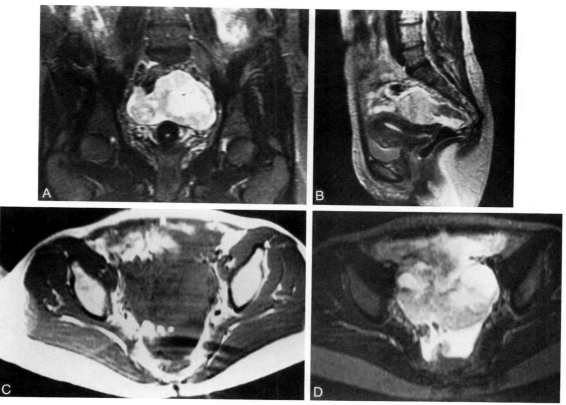

FIGURE 32–28. Bilateral cystadenocarcinoma of the ovary. *A,* Coronal SE 2500/80. *B,* Sagittal SE 2500/80. Note solid moderate-intensity and cystic high-intensity components of the confluent tumor mass above the uterus. *C,* Axial SE 600/20. *D,* Axial SE 2500/80. Free fluid in the cul-de-sac can be seen as high signal posterior to the large tumor mass in *D.*

gins and oval shape of the adenomyosis relative to the clear definition and round shape of leiomyomas.[38, 38a] These appearances on MR imaging are made possible by the superior soft-tissue resolution and multiplanar capability this modality offers. MR imaging provides definite clinical utility not available with CT and increased specificity relative to ultrasonography.

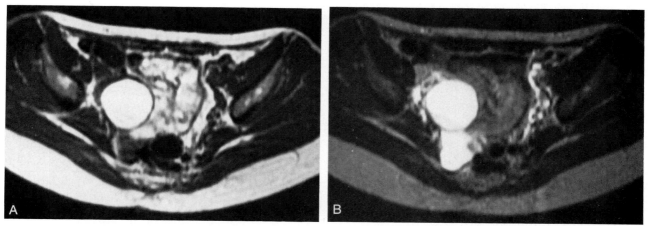

FIGURE 32–29. Endometrioma of right adnexa. *A,* Axial SE 600/20. *B,* Axial SE 2500/80. Well-circumscribed subacute hemorrhagic lesion with low-signal rim is present in the right adnexal region. The presence of subacute blood accounts for the high signal intensity on short and long TR/TE sequences. (From Spritzer CE, Kressel HY, Mitchell D: Magnetic Resonance Imaging of the Female Pelvis. New York, Raven Press, 1987, p 227; with permission.)

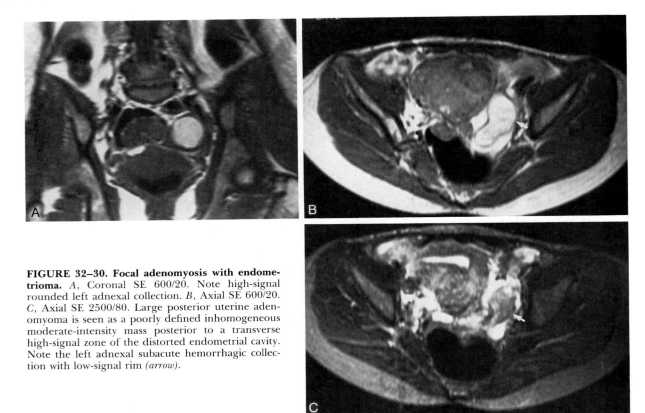

FIGURE 32–30. Focal adenomyosis with endometrioma. *A,* Coronal SE 600/20. Note high-signal rounded left adnexal collection. *B,* Axial SE 600/20. *C,* Axial SE 2500/80. Large posterior uterine adenomyoma is seen as a poorly defined inhomogeneous moderate-intensity mass posterior to a transverse high-signal zone of the distorted endometrial cavity. Note the left adnexal subacute hemorrhagic collection with low-signal rim *(arrow).*

Recurrence and Postoperative Appearances

MR imaging shows great promise in the diagnosis of local recurrence of gynecologic tumors following

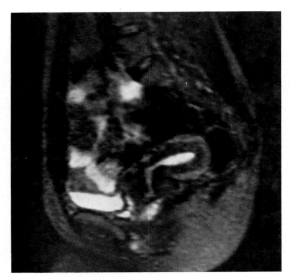

FIGURE 32–31. Diffuse adenomyosis. Sagittal SE 1500/80. Note markedly thickened low-signal junctional zone of the myometrium surrounding high-signal endometrial cavity. The uterus is retroverted.

therapy. Surgical clips create local signal voids but do not distort the overall resolution or contrast of the image. The detection of surgical complications and local neoplastic recurrences is facilitated by this property and also by multiplanar imaging capability. Glazer et al[32] reported that the differentiation of fibrosis from recurrent tumor is possible on MR imaging owing to the relatively short T_2 of fibrotic tissue, which demonstrates decreased signal on both short and long TR/TE pulse sequences. Tumor recurrence demonstrates relatively increased signal on long TR/TE images and thus may be reliably distinguished from mature fibrosis (fibrosis more than 1 year after treatment). Within the first year following therapy, immature fibrosis may simulate the signal intensities of recurrent tumor on long TR/TE images and may present a diagnostic problem.[34] By suggesting the presence of recurrent disease in patients followed for at least 1 year after treatment, MR may be useful in localizing the site of recurrence and directing needle aspiration biopsy in patients who have coexistent fibrotic change and recurrent tumor (Figs. 32–32 and 32–33).

Fluid collections may be difficult to characterize. In the immediate postoperative period, hematomas are potentially difficult to define, as acute blood is isointense on short TR/TE sequences; on long TR/TE sequences, acute blood may appear relatively bright. However, subacute hematomas frequently show high

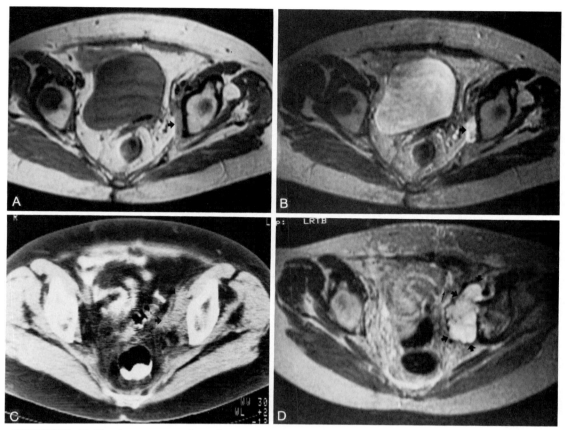

FIGURE 32–32. Focal recurrence of ovarian carcinoma. *A*, Axial SE 600/20. *B*, Axial SE 2500/80. Left pelvic side wall involvement with increased signal and thickening of the obturator internus. *C*, CT. *D*, Axial SE 2500/80 at same level. Excellent soft-tissue delineation of left pelvic wall tumoral involvement adjacent to bone *(arrows)*.

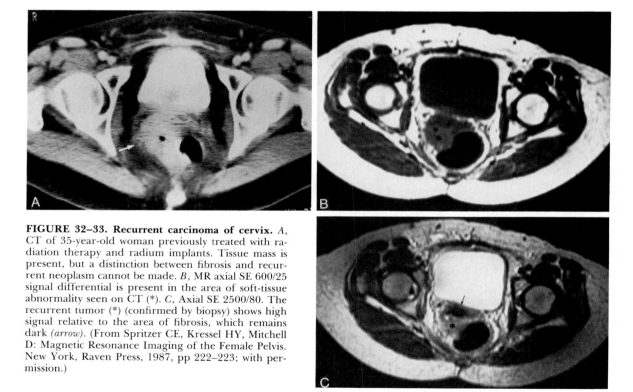

FIGURE 32–33. Recurrent carcinoma of cervix. *A*, CT of 35-year-old woman previously treated with radiation therapy and radium implants. Tissue mass is present, but a distinction between fibrosis and recurrent neoplasm cannot be made. *B*, MR axial SE 600/25 signal differential is present in the area of soft-tissue abnormality seen on CT (*). *C*, Axial SE 2500/80. The recurrent tumor (*) (confirmed by biopsy) shows high signal relative to the area of fibrosis, which remains dark *(arrow)*. (From Spritzer CE, Kressel HY, Mitchell D: Magnetic Resonance Imaging of the Female Pelvis. New York, Raven Press, 1987, pp 222–223; with permission.)

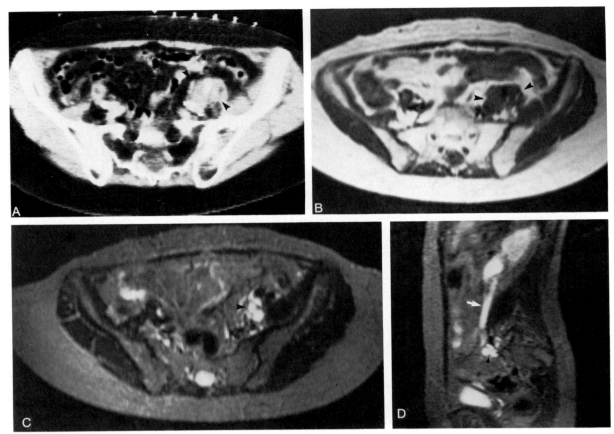

FIGURE 32–34. Nodal recurrence of cervical carcinoma. *A*, CT with enhancement. Left-sided pelvic brim soft-tissue mass encasing left ureter *(arrowheads)*. *B*, Axial MR SE 600/20. *C*, Axial MR SE 2500/80. Mass of enlarged nodes surrounding ureter demonstrates high signal on long TR/TE sequence. *D*, Sagittal SE 2500/80. The course of the involved left ureter *(arrow)* can be traced to the area of lymphadenopathy at the pelvic inlet *(arrowhead)*.

signal on both sequences.[29–31] Urinomas and lymphoceles show the characteristics of simple fluid with low signal intensity on short TR/TE and high signal intensity on long TR/TE.

Adenopathy can, as previously discussed, also be evaluated on the basis of signal characteristics and not on the basis of size only (Figs. 32–34 and 32–35).

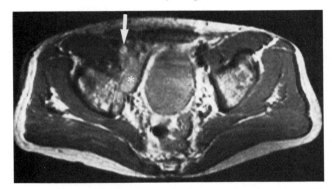

FIGURE 32–35. Lymphadenopathy in a young male patient with lymphogranuloma venereum. Axial SE image (TR/TE = 2500 msec/20 msec). A large lymph node mass *(asterisk)* compresses the right common femoral vein *(arrow)*. The increased signal intensity in the vein is due to slow flow.

REFERENCES

1. McNeal JE: The anatomic heterogeneity of the prostate. In: Murphy GP (ed). Models for Prostate Cancer. New York: Alan R. Liss, Inc, 1980, pp 149–160.
1a. Schnall MD, Lenkinski RE, Pollack HM, et al: Prostate: MR imaging with an endorectal surface coil. Radiology 172:570–574, 1989.
2. McNeal JE: The prostate gland: Morphology and pathology. Monogr Urol 4:3–33, 1983.
3. Hricak H, Dooms GC, McNeal JE, et al: MR imaging of the prostate gland: Normal anatomy. AJR 148:51, 1987.
4. Phillips ME, Kressel HY, Spritzer CE, et al: Normal prostate and adjacent structures: MR imaging at 1.5 Tesla. Radiology 164:381–385, 1987.
5. Phillips ME, Kressel HY, Spritzer CE, et al: Prostate pathology: MR imaging at 1.5 Tesla. Radiology 164:386–392, 1987.
6. Biondetti PR, Lee JKT, Ling D, Catalona WJ: Clinical stage B prostate carcinoma: Staging with MR imaging. Radiology 162:325, 1987.
7. Hricak H, Dooms GC, Jeffrey RB, et al: Prostatic carcinoma: Staging by clinical assessment, CT, and MR imaging. Radiology 162:331, 1987.
8. Babcock EE, Brateman L, Weinreb JC, et al: Edge artifacts in MR images: Chemical shift effect. J Comput Assist Tomogr 9:252–257, 1985.
9. Ling D, Lee JKT, Heiken JP, et al: Prostatic carcinoma and benign prostatic hyperplasia: Inability of MR imaging to

distinguish between the two diseases. Radiology 158:103, 1986.

9a. Schiebler ML, Tomaszewski JE, Pollack HM, et al: Prostatic carcinoma and benign prostatic hyperplasia: Correlation of high-resolution MR and histopathologic findings. Radiology 172:131–137, 1989.

10. Lee JKT, Heiken JP, Ling D, et al: Magnetic resonance imaging of abdominal and pelvic lymphadenopathy. Radiology 153:181, 1984.

11. Dooms GC, Hricak H, Crooks LE, Higgins CB: Magnetic resonance imaging of the lymph nodes: Comparison with CT. Radiology 153:719–728, 1984.

12. Amendola MA, Glazer GM, Grossman HB, et al: Staging of bladder carcinoma: MRI-CT-surgical correlation. AJR 146:1179–1183, 1986.

13. Fisher MR, Hricak H, Tanagho EA: Urinary bladder MR imaging. Part II. Neoplasm. Radiology 157:471, 1985.

14. Fisher MR, Hricak H, Crooks LE: Urinary bladder MR imaging. Part I. Normal and benign conditions. Radiology 157:467, 1985.

15. Hricak H: MRI of the female pelvis: Review. AJR 146:1115, 1986.

16. Spritzer CE, Kressel HY, Mitchell D: Magnetic resonance imaging of the female pelvis. In Kressel HY (ed): Magnetic Resonance Annual 1987. New York: Raven Press, 1987, pp 203–235.

17. Haynor DR, Mack LA, Soules MR, et al: Changing appearance of normal uterus during the menstrual cycle: MR studies. Radiology 161:459, 1986.

18. McCarthy S, Tauber C, Gore J: Female pelvic anatomy: MR assessment of variations during the menstrual cycle and with use of oral contraceptives. Radiology 160:119, 1986.

19. Demas BE, Hricak H, Jaffe RB: Uterine MR imaging: Effects of hormonal stimulation. Radiology 159:123, 1986.

20. Lee JKT, Gersell DJ, Balfe DM, et al: The uterus: In vitro MR anatomic correlation of normal and abnormal specimens. Radiology 157:175–179, 1985.

21. Wagner M, Lawson TL: Segmental Anatomy—Applications to Clinical Medicine. New York, Macmillan Publishing Co, 1982.

22. Jones HW, Jones GS (eds): Novak's Textbook of Gynecology. 10th ed. London, Williams & Wilkins, 1981, pp 427–441.

23. Jones HW, Jones GS (eds): Novak's Textbook of Gynecology. 10th ed. London, Williams & Wilkins, 1981, pp 410–422.

24. Hricak H, Stern JL, Fisher MR, et al: Endometrial carcinoma staging by MR imaging. Radiology 297:162, 1987.

25. Mitchell DG, Mintz MC, Spritzer CE, et al: Adnexal masses: MR imaging observations at 1.5 T with US and CT correlation. Radiology 162:319–324, 1987.

26. Mitchell DG, Gefter WB, Spritzer CE, et al: Polycystic ovaries: MR imaging. Radiology 160:425–429, 1986.

27. Dooms GC, Hricak H, Tscholakoff D: Adnexal structures: MR imaging. Radiology 158:639, 1986.

28. Nishimura K, Togashi K, Itoh K, et al: Endometrial cysts of the ovary: MR imaging. Radiology 162:315, 1987.

28a. Gross BM, Silver TM, Jaffe MH: Sonographic features of uterine leiomyomas. J Ultrasound Med 2:401–406, 1983.

29. Gomori JM, Grossman RI, Goldberg HI, et al: Intracranial hematomas: Imaging by high-field MR. Radiology 157:87–93, 1985.

29a. Arrive L, Hricak H, Martin MC: Pelvic endometriosis: MR imaging. Radiology 171:687–692, 1989.

29b. Zawin M, McCarthy S, Scoutt L, Comite F: Endometriosis: Appearance and detection at MR imaging. Radiology 171:693–696, 1989.

30. Hahn PF, Saini S, Stark DD, et al: Intraabdominal hematoma: The concentric-ring sign in MR imaging. AJR 148:115–119, 1987.

31. Rubin JI, Gomori JM, Grossman RI, et al: High field MR imaging of extracranial hematomas. AJR 148:813, 1987.

32. Glazer HS, Lee JKT, Levitt RG, et al: Radiation fibrosis: Differentiation from recurrent tumor by MR imaging. Radiology 156:721–726, 1985.

33. Bezzi M, Kressel HY, Allen KS, et al: Prostatic carcinoma: Staging with MR imaging at 1.5 T. Radiology 169:339–346, 1988.

34. Ebner F, Kressel HY, Mintz MC, et al: Tumor recurrence versus fibrosis in the female pelvis: Differentiation with MR imaging at 1.5 T. Radiology 166:333–340, 1988.

35. Emory Th, Reinke DB, Hill AL, Lange PH: Use of CT to reduce under-staging in prostatic cancer: Comparison with conventional staging techniques. AJR 141:351–354, 1983.

36. Requard CK, Wicks JD, Mettler FA: Ultrasonography in the staging of endometrial adenocarcinoma. Radiology 140:781–785, 1981.

37. Fleischer AC, Dudley BS, Entman SS, et al: Myometrial invasion by endometrial carcinoma: Sonographic assessment. Radiology 162:307–310, 1987.

37a. Stafl A, Mattingly RF: Cervical intraepithelial neoplasia: Invasive carcinoma of the cervix. In Mattingly RF, Thompson JD (eds): Te Linde's Operative Gynecology. 6th ed. Philadelphia, JB Lippincott Co., 1985.

37b. Togashi K, Nishimura K, Sagah T, et al: Carcinoma of the cervix: Staging with MR imaging. Radiology 171:245–251, 1989.

37c. Hricak H, Lacey CG, Sandles LG, et al: Invasive cervical carcinoma: Comparison of MR imaging and surgical findings. Radiology 166:623–631, 1987.

38. Mark AS, Hricak H, Heinrichs LW, et al: Adenomyosis and leiomyoma: Differential diagnosis with MR imaging. Radiology 163:527–529, 1987.

38.a Togashi K, Ozasa H, Konishi I, et al: Enlarged uterus: Differentiation between adenomyosis and leiomyoma with MR imaging. Radiology 171:531–534, 1989.

39. Ebner R, Kressel HY, Mintz MC, et al: Tumor recurrence versus fibrosis in the female pelvis: Differentiation by MR imaging at 1.5 Tesla. Radiology 166:333–340, 1988.

40. Rifkin MD: Endorectal sonography of the prostate: Clinical implications. AJR 148:1137–1142, 1987.

41. Hricak H, Dooms GC, Jeffrey RB, et al: Prostatic carcinoma: Staging by clinical assessment, CT, and MR imaging. Radiology 162:331–336, 1987.

33

OBSTETRICAL MR IMAGING

BERNARD A. BIRNBAUM and JEFFREY C. WEINREB

MATERNAL ANATOMY
   UTERUS AND CERVIX
   PLACENTA
   ADNEXA
   PELVIC VASCULATURE
   MATERNAL SPINE
   PELVIMETRY

FETAL IMAGING
   IMAGING TECHNIQUE
   THORAX
   ABDOMEN
   MUSCULOSKELETAL SYSTEM
   CENTRAL NERVOUS SYSTEM
   AMNIOTIC FLUID
   INTRAUTERINE GROWTH RETARDATION

With the knowledge that prenatal exposure to low-dose ionizing radiation is associated with increased risks of childhood cancer,[1] alternative modalities to diagnostic x-ray imaging for evaluating the fetus have become necessary. The introduction of diagnostic ultrasound has revolutionized antenatal care, making placentography, fetography, and amniography obsolete. At this time, high-resolution, state-of-the-art, real-time sonography is the premier obstetrical imaging technique. Ultrasound offers safety, accuracy, and availability, as well as an inexpensive flexible way to visualize the fetus in multiple planes under real-time. Unfortunately, it also has its limitations, and an alternative method for imaging the fetus and gravid mother would be advantageous and complementary.

MRI is such a technique. Similar to ultrasound, it involves no ionizing radiation, is noninvasive, and can provide images in multiple orthogonal planes. However, unlike ultrasound, it is not operator dependent, and MR images are not limited by interference from intervening skeletal, fatty, and air-filled structures. Furthermore, imaging of deep pelvic organs is not dependent on the presence of an overlying acoustic window, such as the urinary bladder or amniotic fluid. Whereas ultrasound image contrast is based upon the differences in acoustical impedance between tissues, MRI produces excellent contrast resolution between soft tissues, with contrast depen-

dent on such tissue characteristics as T_1 and T_2 relaxation times, proton density, and flow. As a result, MRI may demonstrate both normal and pathologic features not detectable with ultrasound.

The Food and Drug Administration (FDA) guidelines for acceptable exposure levels to MRI do not specifically address the risks for pregnant patients or operators.[2] Potential adverse effects from obstetrical MRI may arise from exposure to pulsed radiofrequency radiation, static magnetic fields, and rapidly changing time/varying electromagnetic fields. Although no short-term adverse effects have been reported from MRI patient exposure,[3] it is too soon for long-term follow-up. Moreover, while MRI is thought by many to be safe, a thorough evaluation of potential adverse bioeffects on the fetus has not yet been performed. The FDA requires labeling of MRI devices to indicate that the safety of MRI, when used to image fetuses and infants, has not been established. As a result, it is wise to exclude pregnant women during the first trimester when rapid organogenesis occurs (unless subsequent abortion is planned). This policy has been adopted by the National Radiation Protection Board of Great Britain[4] as well as by numerous institutional review boards in the United States. The National Institutes of Health Consensus Development Conference on MRI has recommended that "MRI as with all interventions in pregnancy, should be used during the first trimester only when there are clear medical indications and when it offers a definite advantage over other tests."[5]

MATERNAL ANATOMY

UTERUS AND CERVIX

Female pelvic anatomy is particularly well demonstrated with MR imaging, and usually maternal respiration does not create significant motion artifact.[6–8] The uterus is visible above the bladder, often compressing its dome. With increasing gestational age, the uterus changes in both shape and size, becoming progressively more round or oval and often attaining lengths greater than 20 cm at term.[9] The uterine myometrium is composed of smooth muscle, which has a relatively long T_1 relaxation time.[6] This wall may become so stretched and thinned by the gestational sac that it may not be appreciated in its entire circumference. While there is an increase in collagen content and smooth muscle hypertrophy within the uterine corpus during pregnancy,[10] no consistent or significant alterations of myometrial signal characteristics have been noted. In the early gestational period, the high signal intensity endometrium and low intensity "junctional zone" are occasionally visible as in the nongravid state. Later, however, these regions are no longer detected.

Uterine leiomyomas may have a significant impact on obstetrical management. The predominant view in the obstetrical literature is that leiomyomas, known to be estrogen responsive, tend to enlarge during pregnancy and involute during the puerperium.[11] A recent sonographic study refuted this, demonstrating that leiomyomas may remain stable or may either increase or decrease in size depending on the trimes-

ter and initial size of the leiomyoma.[12] Rapid growth may lead to infarction and pain. Depending on their numbers and locations, leiomyomas may adversely affect the course of pregnancy. Multiple leiomyomas increase the frequency of malpresentation, retained placenta, and premature uterine contractions, and, if located in the lower uterine segment, may preclude vaginal delivery. Therefore, knowledge about their extent in pregnancy may be useful in determining the type of delivery, as well as for providing prognostic information with regard to possible complications.

Ultrasound evaluation of the gravid uterus for leiomyomas may be limited secondary to technical factors, unusual size and location, or because the conceptus may obscure parts of the myometrium.[13] With MRI, leiomyomas, whether simple or degenerated, may be clearly depicted in both the gravid and nongravid uterus[14–16] (Fig. 33–1). As in a nonpregnant patient, MRI appears to be more accurate than ultrasound for precise sizing and localization of leiomyomas.

A significant contribution provided by MR is the consistent definition of the cervix and lower uterine segment in the obstetrical patient. Sagittal images readily depict the internal and external os, as well as their relationship to the lower uterine segment, placenta, the presenting fetal parts superiorly, and the vagina inferiorly.[8] While cervical length and orientation may vary with the degree of bladder distention, MR visualization of the cervix does not require a significant degree of bladder filling, as with ultrasound, to image adequately this anatomy transabdominally.[8] Overdistention of the urinary bladder may compress the lower uterine walls, leading to overestimation of cervical length.[17] This may also result in the false sonographic diagnosis of placenta previa, as well as the missed diagnosis of a shortened, incompetent cervix.[8, 18]

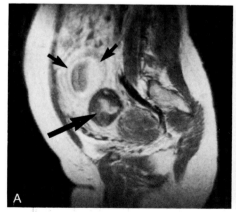 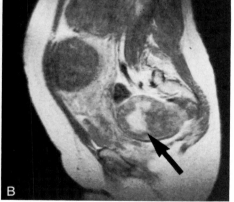

FIGURE 33–1. *A* and *B*, Fourteen-week pregnancy associated with multiple uterine leiomyomas. SE 2000/30. Multiple low-intensity round masses are identified, some of which contain high-intensity regions, representing areas of degeneration *(long black arrows)*. The conceptus is present superiorly *(short black arrows)*. (Reproduced by permission from Weinreb JC: Obstetrics. *In* Stark D, Bradley WG Jr [eds]: Magnetic Resonance Imaging. St. Louis, 1988, The C.V. Mosby Company.)

As in the nonpregnant patient, the noneffaced, gravid cervix has a characteristic laminar configuration, particularly on T_2-weighted images.[6, 8, 18, 19] The peripheral zone appears as a low intensity stripe, demonstrating decreased signal on both T_1- and T_2-weighted images. This zone, thought to represent cervical stroma rich in collagen, has been noted to become wider and more prominent with pregnancy.[19] The central zone, possessing the highest signal intensity, represents both cervical mucous and glandular tissue. This tissue has high signal on both T_1- and T_2-weighted studies, reflecting its relatively short T_1 and long T_2 relaxation times. Toward the latter stages of pregnancy, proliferation of endocervical mucosa and the formation of a viscous mucous plug both contribute to thickening of this central high intensity zone.

As term approaches, fibroblast proliferation within the cervical stroma increases collagen and proteoglycan content as the surrounding tissues become progressively hydrated. The cervix softens and dilates as effacement occurs. MR imaging of a "ripened" preterm cervix demonstrates these changes, as the cervical lumen appears shortened and widened with loss of distinction of the fibrous stroma.[8] Because MR is able to assess such morphologic and physiologic cervical changes, it may be possible to evaluate such abnormalities of cervical function as dystocia, slow cervimetric progress, failure of ripening, and cervical incompetence.

PLACENTA

The placenta is first identified as a focal area of thickening at the periphery of the gestational sac (Fig. 33–2). Representing the decidua basalis and chorion frondosum, these early findings may be seen

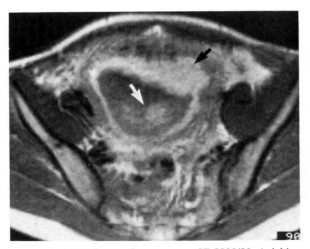

FIGURE 33–2. Twelve-week pregnancy. SE 2000/30. Axial image demonstrates focal thickening *(black arrow)* along the gestational sac, representing the developing placenta. Fetus *(white arrow)*. (Reproduced by permission from Weinreb JC: Obstetrics. *In* Stark D, Bradley WG Jr [eds]: Magnetic Resonance Imaging. St. Louis, 1988, The C.V. Mosby Company.)

between 10 and 12 weeks. As gestation progresses, the placenta enlarges and thickens. While full thickness may be attained by four months, circumferential growth may continue into the final trimester.[20, 21] Placental tissue tends to demonstrate a fairly homogeneous appearance on MR images. Neither internal architecture (i.e., basal plate, chorionic plate, and septations) nor physiologic calcifications have yet been seen. Occasionally, vascular channels (representing spiral arterioles and draining endometrial veins) may be appreciated as multiple, serpentine signal void structures visible at the placental-myometrial interface.

On both T_1-weighted spin-echo and inversion recovery images, the moderately long T_1 relaxation time of placental tissue manifests itself as low signal intensity, slightly greater than that of myometrium. The placenta is bright on T_2-weighted spin-echo images, with its relative signal intensity increasing substantially as a result of its relatively long T_2. As a result of excellent soft tissue contrast, MR easily depicts placental tissue. This may facilitate the diagnosis of placental enlargement (as seen with RH incompatibility, maternal anemia, and diabetes) as well as those conditions in which placental tissue is smaller than normal (e.g., preeclampsia).[22] MR may also provide a complementary technique to ultrasound in the detection of succenturiate lobes.[23] If not diagnosed antenatally, this condition may be complicated by retained products or rupture during labor, with the threat of associated hemorrhage.[22]

Placenta previa usually presents as painless third trimester bleeding. It represents the most significant condition affecting the lower uterine segment, with an incidence of 0.5 per cent.[24] Recently, ultrasound has replaced other modalities as the procedure of choice to diagnose this entity. Unfortunately, ultrasound is operator dependent and may be inaccurate. False-positive diagnoses occur in 5 to 7 per cent of cases, usually secondary to overdistention of the urinary bladder, lower uterine segment focal contractions, or early detection prior to "placental migration."[25-27] False-negative diagnoses, seen in less than 2 per cent of instances, are more significant because of the associated increased fetal and maternal morbidity and mortality.[25] Sonographic diagnosis is especially problematic when the fetal head obscures a posterior previa or when a low-lying placenta is laterally located.[28] Sagittal MRI can precisely delineate the relationship of the inferior aspect of the placenta to the internal cervical os (Fig. 33–3). Because it does not suffer from the limitations affecting sonography, MRI may be used as an alternative modality to visualize the lower uterine segment when ultrasound is indefinite. This was recently shown in a study which demonstrated that MRI is equal to ultrasound for localization of placental site, but more accurate in the precise definition of the degree of placenta previa.[18] In 15 of 25 cases, the two modalities produced discrepant results, and in 7 cases the MR findings led to alterations in patient management.

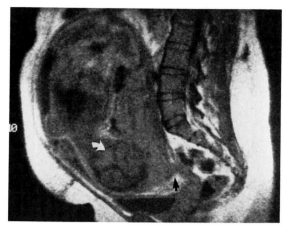

FIGURE 33–3. Thirty-week pregnancy with complete placenta previa. SE 500/28. The placenta is seen to completely cover the internal cervical os *(black arrow)*. Fetal head *(white arrow)*.

Retroplacental hemorrhage may occur as early as the first trimester. The sonographic characteristics of abruptio placentae have been well described.[29] These hematomas most often appear as retroplacental or marginal, sonolucent, or complex sonographic collections. This condition has now been detected by MRI, and while the MR signal characteristics of hematomas may be quite complex, it is hoped that MR will provide an alternative means to diagnose this entity.[19]

Placental masses may be of trophoblastic or nontrophoblastic origin. The gestational trophoblastic diseases may be classified clinically into benign and malignant disorders. Using this scheme, both complete and partial molar pregnancies are considered benign, while invasive moles (chorioadenoma destruens) and choriocarcinoma are thought to represent malignant nonmetastatic and malignant metastatic diseases, respectively.[30] Clinically, the diagnosis is suspected in a patient who presents with a uterus large for dates, severe preeclampsia prior to 24 weeks' gestation, or first trimester bleeding. The passage of grape-like vesicles per vaginum as well as having markedly elevated serum beta human chorionic gonadotropin (HCG) levels are usually considered diagnostic.[30, 31]

Sonography can adequately identify this neoplasm within the uterus, assess response to chemotherapy, and evaluate the remainder of the abdomen and pelvis for evidence of metastatic disease.[30, 32, 33] It now appears that MRI may do the same. Several case reports of the MR diagnosis of hydatidiform moles have now been published[14, 34, 35] (Fig. 33–4). In some, the "cluster of grapes" vesicular nature of the mass was appreciated, as were areas of high signal on T_1-weighted images thought to represent hemorrhage. MR was able to clearly separate molar tissue from the uterine wall, which may help demonstrate macroscopic myometrial invasion. Furthermore, changes in myometrial signal intensity following molar evacuation may help confirm recurrence of disease. When present, associated adnexal theca-lutein cysts are well demonstrated.[34] MRI should prove useful in staging patients with gestational trophoblastic neoplasia, and its eventual role in this interesting spectrum of disease remains to be defined.

The most common primary, nontrophoblastic placental tumor is the chorioangioma, a vascular malformation seen in about 1 per cent of placentas.[36] Whereas small tumors are incidental without clinical significance, larger lesions protrude from the fetal surface of the placenta. These may be associated with fetal hydrops, low birth weight, premature labor, and fetal demise.[22, 37] When visualized by MRI, this malformation appears to exhibit signal intensity greater than that of surrounding placenta on both T_1- and T_2-weighted spin-echo images.[14] In one case report, it appeared well demarcated from surrounding placental tissue by a low-intensity rim, which histologically represented a thin fibrous capsule. Other placental neoplasms, such as the relatively rare teratoma or metastasis, have not yet been reported with MRI.

Preliminary research involving placental contrast enhancement has now been performed. Nontoxic, intravenous doses of manganese sulfate and manganese chloride given to laboratory animals produced measured decreases in placental T_1 relaxation times.[38] In another study, dose-dependent decreases in both T_1 and T_2 values were achieved following incubation of human placentas with varying concentrations of manganese chloride.[39] Uteroplacental insufficiency is

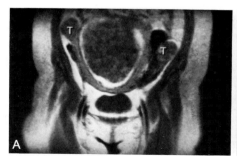
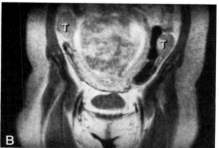

FIGURE 33–4. Hydatidiform mole. *A,* SE 1000/28; *B,* SE 2000/28. Coronal pelvic images demonstrate a vesicular intrauterine mass. Areas within and around the mass, which demonstrate high signal intensity, are hemorrhage. Also seen are bilateral theca-lutein cysts (T). (Reproduced by permission from Weinreb JC, Lowe TW, Santos-Ramos R, et al: Magnetic resonance imaging in obstetric diagnosis. Radiology 154:157–161, 1985.)

a known cause of fetal intrauterine growth retardation (IUGR). It is hoped that these and similar MRI studies may lead to an increased understanding of placental perfusion and metabolism and how these may relate to IUGR.

ADNEXA

While often an incidental finding, the detection of an adnexal mass in the obstetrical patient creates a diagnostic problem for the clinician. If malignant, therapeutic intervention may need to be taken.. If benign, ovarian masses may become increasingly symptomatic as a result of torsion around a pedicle, internal hemorrhage, rupture, or from compression of adjacent pelvic organs. Because physical examination is often inaccurate in determining the size, origin, and etiology of such masses, sonography has become widely accepted as a means to obtain this information. Ultrasound is an innocuous test, which, unlike invasive diagnostic procedures, does not have the risk of inducing premature labor. Unfortunately, sonography may not always determine the origin or entire extent of such masses, and the examination may be suboptimal secondary to overlying bowel gas, obesity, or the enlarged gravid uterus. MRI is not subject to such limitations and, like ultrasound, involves no ionizing radiation and is noninvasive. Because of its ability to visualize the entire anatomy of the pelvis, it serves as a viable alternative to ultrasound for the evaluation of adnexal masses in the pregnant patient.

Normal-sized ovaries are not routinely visualized by MRI in pregnant women. If large enough, physiologic cysts may be seen if their signal characteristics differ from those of surrounding pelvic structures. Corpus luteum cysts are among the most common encountered. Their diagnosis becomes important when they persist beyond 16 weeks' gestation or when they enlarge to greater than 6 cm. Once reaching this size, an enlarging mass during pregnancy may represent an indication for surgical intervention.[40] At times, conservative management may be practiced if sonography demonstrates an anechoic, smooth, thin-walled cystic mass with appropriate through transmission for the size of the mass. However, not all corpus luteum cysts display such ideal characteristics. The MRI appearance of these physiologic cysts has now been described.[14] "Simple" corpus luteum cysts appear as homogeneous, round, smooth-walled masses with signal intensities similar to pure fluid (i.e., long T_1 and T_2 relaxation times) (Fig. 33–5). This should permit nonhemorrhagic corpus luteum cysts to be distinguished from hemorrhagic cysts, endometriomas, and solid tumors, but unfortunately, this appearance is nonspecific. Malignant adenocarcinomas and serous cystadenomas may look identical. Similarly, "complex" hemorrhagic corpus luteum cysts will have signal characteristics altered by blood or clot, and MRI may have trouble separating such

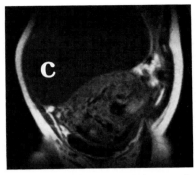

FIGURE 33–5. Twenty-seven-week gestation associated with giant corpus luteum cyst. SE 500/28. Coronal image demonstrates a 33-cm, low-intensity mass superior to the uterus which proved to be a corpus luteum cyst (C). (Reproduced by permission from Weinreb JC: Obstetrics. *In* Stark DD, Bradley WG Jr [eds]: Magnetic Resonance Imaging. St. Louis, 1988, The C. V. Mosby Company.)

masses from other adnexal lesions. In these instances, clinical history and multiple imaging modalities will be needed to help narrow the differential diagnosis.

Dermoid cysts may present for the first time during pregnancy, as the enlarged gravid uterus displaces the mass from the pelvis. Sonographically, dermoids demonstrate a spectrum of sonographic presentations, ranging from a totally sonolucent mass to a complex structure with echogenic components.[41] At times, the echogenic sebum within a teratoma may mimic a gas-filled bowel loop, and the diagnosis may be missed sonographically.[42] MRI may be useful in such situations, as well as when fluid- or gas-filled bowel loops simulate pelvic masses on ultrasound.[14] As with ultrasound, the MRI characteristics of ovarian dermoids are extremely variable, with the T_1 and T_2 relaxation times differing depending on the variable constitution of the internal architecture of these lesions.[43]

At present, the diagnosis of ectopic pregnancy is based on a combination of clinical findings, correlation with serum beta HCG levels, and sonographic imaging using either transabdominal or endovaginal techniques. While MRI has no defined role in this clinical setting, it has proven useful in at least one instance. In a reported case of a viable, full-term abdominal pregnancy, MRI was helpful in prenatally confirming the exact relationship of the fetus, uterus, and placenta.[44] MRI will most likely play only an ancillary role in such situations, however, since it will probably be difficult to reliably image a small ectopic gestation located within the fallopian tube. A secondary finding in some ectopic pregnancies is the presence of fluid within the cul-de-sac. MRI, unlike ultrasound, may specifically identify the hemorrhagic nature of this fluid (Fig. 33–6). While this may be occasionally helpful, it should be remembered that such a finding is nonspecific and may result from rupture of hemorrhagic ovarian cysts or from other pelvic pathology.

Currently, ultrasound should continue to be the

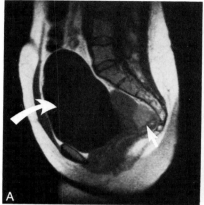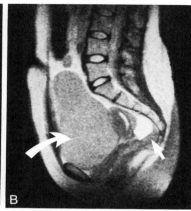

FIGURE 33–6. Blood in the cul-de-sac from ectopic pregnancy. *A,* SE 500/28; *B,* SE 2000/56. Whereas the ectopic gestational sac was not identified, these sagittal images depict fluid in the cul-de-sac *(straight arrows),* with signal characteristics consistent with the presence of hemorrhage. Distended bladder *(curved arrows).* (Reproduced by permission from Weinreb JC: Obstetrics. *In* Stark DD, Bradley WG Jr [eds]: Magnetic Resonance Imaging. St. Louis, 1988, The C.V. Mosby Company.)

initial imaging technique for the evaluation of pelvic masses in obstetrical patients. MRI may be useful in those situations in which sonographic evaluation is limited, its results are equivocal, or when additional data provided by MRI will influence the therapeutic approach toward treating the patient.

PELVIC VASCULATURE

Previous contrast studies have demonstrated that when pregnant patients are lying in the supine position, the inferior vena cava may appear virtually occluded and venous return occurs via collateral vessels.[45] These changes have now also been seen with MRI.[8] In addition, the ovarian veins have been noted to be enlarged bilaterally, and the common iliac and femoral veins have been seen to be 2 to 3 times the diameter of their arterial companions.[8] MR has already proven useful in identifying a case of puerperal ovarian vein thrombosis.[46] In the future, it is possible that MRI may help monitor the degree of venous stasis occurring during pregnancy. This may help prevent such sequelae as thrombophlebitis and pulmonary emboli.

MATERNAL SPINE

Low back pain is a relatively common complaint during pregnancy. Relaxin, a hormone secreted by the corpus luteum during pregnancy, softens the ligaments of the sacroiliac joints and pubic symphysis. A preliminary MRI study of women in late gestation suggested that these patients had a higher-than-expected prevalence of lumbosacral disc herniations and disc bulges.[8] The authors suggested that this may be secondary to relaxation of the posterior longitudinal ligament as well, allowing these abnormalities to occur. This study supported the claim that parity is a predisposing factor for lumbosacral disc disease.[47] This belief has recently been challenged, an alternative explanation being that there is a much higher incidence of degenerative disc disease in younger populations than previously suspected.[19] A more recent MR investigation supports this latter hypothesis.[48] In this study, a group of 45 pregnant subjects and 41 asymptomatic nonpregnant women of childbearing age had a similar incidence of lumbosacral disc abnormalities on sagittal MR images. Thus, while MRI may be used to evaluate the maternal spine during pregnancy, the presence of disc abnormalities should be cautiously evaluated and interpreted in the proper context of the patient's specific clinical findings and complaints before therapy is contemplated.

PELVIMETRY

Pelvimetry represents the single major source of ionizing radiation to the fetus.[49] Following the signing of the pelvimetry policy statement, national rates of its utilization fell from 7 per cent in 1980 to 2 per cent in 1984 within the United States.[50] This statement, agreed upon by the American College of Radiology, American Roentgen Ray Society, and the American College of Obstetricians and Gynecologists, affirmed that pelvimetry generally provides only limited additional information to physicians involved in the management of labor and delivery while exposing the fetus to a not insignificant amount of radiation.[50] Despite this, the examination continues to be performed by those who support its usefulness in determining the adequacy of the maternal pelvis to accommodate the passage of the fetus when vaginal breech delivery is contemplated.[51]

In an effort to decrease the radiation dose to the fetus, some institutions have instituted CT pelvimetry as a means to assess cephalopelvic disproportion.[52] It is now possible that MRI may provide the same information without the use of ionizing radiation.[19, 53, 54] MRI clearly demonstrates the necessary bony landmarks used to determine maternal pelvic dimensions. Midline sagittal images are utilized to measure the anteroposterior diameter of the pelvic inlet, while axial images allow the interspinous diameter to be calculated.[53] Furthermore, a comparative study of both conventional and MR pelvimetry has now been performed which established excellent concordance between the measurements obtained by the two techniques.[55] While widespread use of MR pelvimetry is not advocated, it is possible for it to become the procedure of choice in the future in those select clinical settings where pelvimetry measurements may be of use to the clinician.

FETAL IMAGING

IMAGING TECHNIQUE

The accurate diagnosis of fetal anomalies is important because certain defects may warrant in utero intervention or early delivery, while others may be so serious as to suggest termination of pregnancy by abortion. Ultrasound has been revolutionary in this regard, allowing both an assessment of fetal anatomy as well as real-time evaluation of fetal motion. MRI is an alternative technique to image the fetus and may be useful when sonographic findings are questionable, the diagnosis is uncertain, or when ultrasound evaluation is limited for technical reasons.

A limitation of MR fetal imaging is the lack of image sharpness caused by fetal motion. Fetal movement becomes progressively more frequent and complex throughout gestation, gradually increasing up to a short time prior to labor.[56] Because most conventional spin-echo pulse sequences are time consuming, it is quite likely that the fetus will move during data acquisition, leading to a loss of anatomic detail. This problem is most severe during the first half of pregnancy; however, it may still lead to image degradation during the third trimester. Apparently, while fetal movement increases toward term, the decrease in relative amniotic fluid volume in the last trimester limits the potential motion of the fetus, and hence motion artifacts are less severe at this time. Nevertheless, in order to overcome this limitation, it will be necessary either to immobilize the fetus in some way or to shorten the scanning time.

Some investigators have advocated that fetal motion may be minimized, and image quality improved, if pregnant patients are imaged in a left lateral decubitus position.[57] While this position is more comfortable for the mother, it is difficult to maintain without moving for the time required for a thorough obstetrical evaluation. As an alternative, others have achieved satisfactory results with their patients lying in the supine position, knees flexed and supported by pillows.[58] Evidence exists that fetal activity increases following elevation of maternal serum glucose levels.[59] This suggests that fetal motion may be minimized if the mother were to refrain from eating for several hours prior to imaging. Other reports suggest that fetal movement occurs more in the evening than in the morning, and that fetal activity increases in response to changes in maternal posture.[60] Thus, it may be possible to minimize motion artifact by imaging the mother in the morning, after she has remained recumbent for a period of time.

In order to limit the time during which fetal activity can occur, it has been suggested that imaging sequences with short pulse repetition times be used.[58] Other investigators have reported that either short or long repetition times may be selected without serious motion degradation by fetal movement.[19, 61] To date, no significant experience with fast MR pulse sequences using small flip angles has been reported. The only way to ensure that excessive fetal motion will not occur during data acquisition is to sedate the fetus. Diazepam is a sedative that has been safely prescribed as a uterine muscle relaxant[62] and as an anticonvulsant for preeclampsia in pregnant patients.[63] In a study in which MR images were obtained both before and after use of intravenous diazepam, anatomic fetal detail was universally improved following sedation.[58] Because its use may entail minimal risk, the authors suggest that such sedation be used selectively in those instances in which demonstration of fetal detail is imperative. Nevertheless, until high-resolution rapid imaging sequences become available, it is likely that fetal motion will remain problematic.

The selection of imaging planes, scanning parameters, and pulse sequences will be influenced by both the particular indications for the examination as well as the individual capabilities of the magnet being used. Early research performed on a 0.08-T resistive magnet found that the pulse sequences of choice varied with the length of gestation.[64] After 26 weeks, decreases in the amount of amniotic fluid as well as in fetal motion allowed improved imaging of the fetus on both inversion recovery and calculated T_1 images. During the first two trimesters, however, the fetus was seen best on proton density and "difference images" (produced by subtracting inversion recovery from proton density signals). This same group demonstrated that short T_1 inversion recovery images with TI values of less than 200 msec were useful in identifying the placenta, heart, and lungs.[65] Imaging with medium length inversion recovery sequences, with TIs ranging from 300 to 500 msec, allowed better visualization of fetal fat.[65] Others have found inversion recovery sequences to be of only limited use. Using a 0.15-T resistive unit, these investigators successfully used spin-echo techniques (TE 40 to 80 msec) with both short and long repetition times to provide good spatial resolution and tissue discrimination in the fetus.[19]

Additional experience using 0.35-T superconducting magnets confirmed the value of imaging the fetus with both T_1- and T_2-weighted spin-echo sequences.[58, 61] T_1-weighted sequences provided excellent definition of the fetus, with high signal fetal fat (short T_1) outlined against the surrounding low signal amniotic fluid (long T_1)[58, 66] (Fig. 33–7). T_2-weighted images allowed visualization of the brain[58] and lung,[61] but as TR values increased, contrast was lost between the amniotic fluid, placenta, and subcutaneous fetal fat.[58, 66] In addition, other significant imaging "trade-

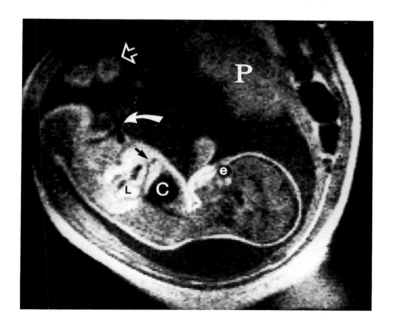

FIGURE 33–7. Thirty-four-week normal fetus and polyhydramnios. SE 500/28. The eye (e), cardiac chambers (c), liver (L), intrahepatic vessels *(black arrow)*, and umbilical vessels *(curved white arrow)* are well depicted. With this pulse sequence, the bright signal originating from subcutaneous fat is easily outlined against the surrounding amniotic fluid. The placenta is seen superiorly (P), and the lower extremities are only partially visualized in cross-section *(open arrow)*. (Reproduced by permission from Weinreb JC, Lowe T, Cohen JM, et al: Human fetal anatomy: MR imaging. Radiology 157:715–720, 1985.)

offs" were noted. For instance, spin-echo sequences using long TRs allowed investigators to acquire multiple images in a single imaging sequence. While this allowed the entire fetus to be studied at once, there was often more image degradation from fetal motion.[58, 61]

In general, fetal anatomy is better visualized as pregnancy progresses, fetal motion decreases, and organ size and inherent tissue contrast increase.[58] Several studies have now shown that fetal anatomy is best displayed on sagittal images of the maternal pelvis, as the fetal axis is most often parallel to the midsagittal plane of the mother.[19, 61] In those instances in which this is not the case, off-axis imaging in planes other than the standard orthogonal views will be necessary to adequately study the fetus.[58]

THORAX

The fetal lungs are fluid-filled, allowing them to be well visualized by MRI. Pulmonary tissue is easily contrasted from the liver inferiorly and from the cardiovascular structures centrally.[61] Typical of tissues containing large amounts of "simple" fluid (long T_1 and long T_2 relaxation times), the pulmonary parenchyma demonstrates low signal intensity on T_1-weighted images and high signal intensity with progressive T_2 weighting (Fig. 33–8).

Currently, research is underway to determine how fetal pulmonary signal characteristics vary throughout gestation. As fetal lung matures, lipid-containing surfactant is produced in increasing concentration toward term.[67] If it is found that the changing con-

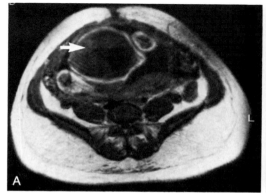
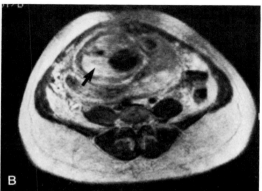

FIGURE 33–8. Forty-week pregnancy. *A,* SE 500/30; *B,* SE 2000/60. The fetal lungs *(arrow)* have low signal intensity on the T_1-weighted image and become brighter with T_2 weighting. The central low-intensity structure present on the images represents the fetal heart. (Reproduced by permission from Weinreb JC: Obstetrics. *In* Stark DD, Bradley WG Jr [eds]: Magnetic Resonance Imaging. St. Louis, 1988, The C.V. Mosby Company.)

centrations of surfactant alter the signal characteristics of pulmonary tissue, MR may play a role in the noninvasive assessment of fetal lung maturity. Furthermore, the MR characteristics of fetal pulmonary hypoplasia have now been described.[34] In a fetus with urethral atresia, the lungs displayed the typical compressed, concave appearance that one expects to see in this condition.

The fetal heart may be seen as early as 15 weeks and always after 25 weeks of gestation.[58] Because of both flow void and dephasing phenomena, the rapidly flowing blood causes the cardiac chambers to appear dark, silhouetted by the surrounding lungs.[68] The internal architecture of the heart is rarely discernible until the third trimester, and even then the atria, ventricles and interventricular septum are only occasionally seen[58] (Fig. 33–9). The individual cardiac chambers may be displayed without electrocardiographic gating, probably because of the small amplitude of ventricular contractions in the rapidly beating fetal heart.[68] Similarly, major vessels such as the thoracoabdominal aorta, inferior vena cava, and pulmonary vessels may be depicted, but unreliably so and always late in pregnancy.[58]

ABDOMEN

The fetal liver, occupying most of the upper abdomen, is usually visible in the third trimester of pregnancy.[58] Because the lungs have a longer T_2 relaxation time than liver, the two adjacent organs are well demarcated on T_2-weighted spin-echo pulse sequences.[61] In addition, measurements of liver T_1 values demonstrate a steady decline throughout pregnancy.[57] It would, therefore, be expected that T_1-weighted images should show a relative increase in hepatic signal intensity toward term. The portal vessels are only occasionally seen and must be traced on contiguous anatomic sections.[58]

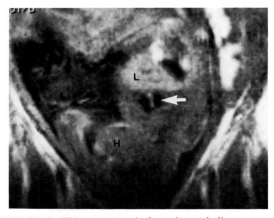

FIGURE 33–9. Thirty-one-week fetus in cephalic presentation. SE 500/28. This sagittal image demonstrates the interventricular septum within the heart *(white arrow)*. Liver (L); head (H). (Reproduced by permission from Weinreb JC: Obstetrics. *In* Stark DD, Bradley WG Jr [eds]: Magnetic Resonance Imaging. St. Louis, 1988, The C. V. Mosby Company.)

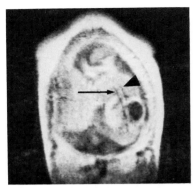

FIGURE 33–10. Thirty-week fetus. SE 500/28. Coronal image of fetal abdomen demonstrates an oval-shaped low-intensity structure in the right renal fossa representing a hydronephrotic right kidney. Aorta *(long arrow)*; inferior vena cava *(arrowhead)*. Image purposely inverted. (Reproduced by permission from Weinreb JC, Lowe T, Cohen JM, et al: Human fetal anatomy: MR imaging. Radiology 157:715–720, 1985.)

On T_1-weighted images, the fluid-filled fetal stomach may occasionally be depicted as a low-intensity structure in the left upper quadrant.[61] Individual bowel loops are only sometimes seen. Portions of the umbilical cord, including the cord insertion, may also be identified (see Fig. 33–7). At this time, the fetal pancreas, spleen, and adrenals have not yet been resolved with MRI. In addition, the normal fetal kidneys have rarely been depicted. This is thought to be secondary to their small size, as well as due to a scarcity of adjacent contrasting retroperitoneal fat.[58, 61] Nevertheless, both renal cysts and hydronephrosis have been noted[54] (Fig. 33–10). As with ultrasound, the fetal bladder will be seen if distended with urine. The bladder will be seen as a round or oval low-intensity organ in the pelvis on T_1-weighted images, with increasing signal intensity seen with longer TR and TE pulse sequences[61] (Fig. 33–11). Fetal genitalia, specifically the testes and penis, have also been reported in one study.[61]

Many third trimester fetuses demonstrate a thin, low-intensity rim that surrounds the abdomen within the subcutaneous fat layer. While this may simulate ascites on T_1-weighted images, this region has MR signal characteristics similar to muscle (relatively long T_1 and short T_2) rather than fluid (long T_1 and long T_2) and will remain low intensity on T_2-weighted sequences[58] (Fig. 33–12). In addition, abdominal wall defects such as omphaloceles have now been detected (Fig. 33–13).

An interesting finding is that fetuses studied after 31 weeks often have multiple, 3- to 10-mm, high signal intensity areas within the abdomen and pelvis on both T_1- and T_2-weighted spin-echo images[58] (Fig. 33–12). The etiology of these findings is unknown; however, an appearance toward the end of pregnancy and a signal intensity similar to fat suggest that this may represent deposition of normal adipose tissue within the fetal abdomen. An alternative ex-

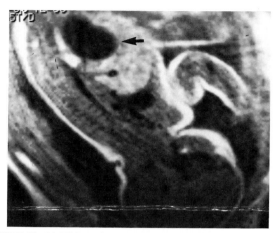

FIGURE 33–11. Thirty-six-week pregnancy. SE 500/30. The fetus, present in cephalic position, is well outlined by low-intensity amniotic fluid on this T_1-weighted image. The distended, low-intensity fetal bladder *(black arrow)* is easily seen. (Reproduced by permission from Weinreb JC: Obstetrics. *In* Stark DD, Bradley WG Jr [eds]: Magnetic Resonance Imaging. St. Louis, 1988, The C. V. Mosby Company.)

planation is that these regions are manifestations of normal gastrointestinal tract accumulations of mucin-containing meconium.

MUSCULOSKELETAL SYSTEM

MR imaging of the fetal musculoskeletal structures appears to be limited, with detail varying considerably and only parts of extremities able to be identified, even in the last trimester[58, 61] (Fig. 33–14). In general,

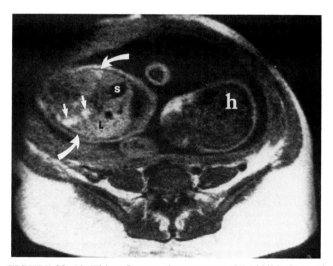

FIGURE 33–12. Thirty-four-week pregnancy. SE 500/28. Coronal image of fetal abdomen depicts fluid-filled stomach (S), liver (L), high-intensity areas *(short white arrows)*, and low-intensity muscle *(curved white arrows)*, surrounded by high-intensity subcutaneous fat. Within the amniotic fluid, portions of the upper extremities are seen in cross-section. Fetal head (h). (Reproduced by permission from Weinreb JC, Lowe T, Cohen JM, et al: Human fetal anatomy: MR imaging. Radiology 157:715–720, 1985.)

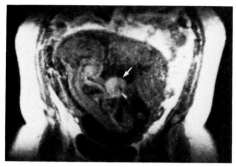

FIGURE 33–13. Twenty-nine-week fetus with omphalocele. SE 500/30. Sagittal image depicts midline herniation of liver *(arrow)* protruding through anterior abdominal wall. (Reproduced by permission from Weinreb JC: Obstetrics. *In* Stark DD, Bradley WG Jr [eds]: Magnetic Resonance Imaging. St. Louis, 1988, The C. V. Mosby Company.)

fetal muscle, subcutaneous fat, epiphyseal cartilage, and osseous structures display similar MR signal characteristics as in the adult. Unfortunately, the combination of fetal motion and the scarcity of tissue fat planes usually prevents the adequate depiction of individual muscle groups and detailed anatomy.

CENTRAL NERVOUS SYSTEM

The fetal head may be identified in utero after 20 weeks' gestation, and brain architecture can be seen in the final trimester.[58] The cerebral hemispheres, ventricles, and eyes are usually visualized. The cerebellum, midbrain, brain stem, cervicomedullary junction, tentorium, falx, and cisterns have been displayed less commonly[58, 61] (Fig. 33–15). The fetal brain appears featureless on inversion recovery images.[19, 61] With spin-echo techniques, the brain parenchyma demonstrates low to intermediate signal intensity on T_1-weighted images and higher signal intensity as T_2 weighting increases.[19] This is a reflection of the increased water content of the immature brain, manifested by prolongation of T_1 and T_2

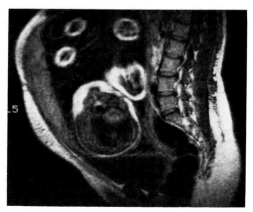

FIGURE 33–14. Sagittal SE 500/40 image demonstrates how the extremities are often visualized only segmentally and in cross-section.

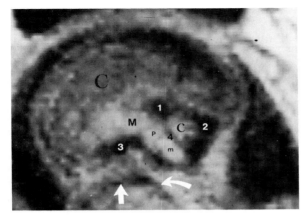

FIGURE 33–15. Fetal head, twenty-eight-week gestational age. Parasagittal SE 500/28 image. Cerebrum (C), cerebellum (c), midbrain (M), pons (P), medulla (m), superior cerebellar cistern (1), cisterna magna (2), suprasellar cistern (3), fourth ventricle (4), nasopharynx *(straight arrow)*, oropharynx *(curved arrow)*. (Reproduced by permission from Weinreb JC, Lowe T, Cohen JM, et al: Human fetal anatomy: MR imaging. Radiology 157:715–720, 1985.)

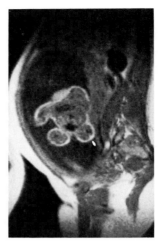

FIGURE 33–17. Twenty-nine-week fetus with anencephaly and polyhydramnios. SE 500/28. No fetal head is visualized above the neck. (Reproduced by permission from Weinreb JC, Lowe TW, Santos-Ramos R, et al: Magnetic resonance imaging in obstetric diagnosis. Radiology 154:157–161, 1985.)

relaxation times.[61] Images of the fetal brain exhibit little gray matter/white matter differentiation.[19, 61] This is consistent with the fact that most myelination tends to occur in the first year of life.[69, 70] As in the adult, the intensity of cerebrospinal fluid within the ventricles is low on T_1-weighted images and increases with a longer TR or TE[61] (Fig. 33–16).

Several fetal CNS abnormalities have been depicted by MRI. These include anencephaly[54] (Fig. 33–17), holoprosencephaly,[71] hydrocephalus,[34, 71] cystic hygroma,[34] and parenchymal autolysis.[71]

The MR signal characteristics of the fetal spinal cord have been found to be similar to those of fetal brain[61] (Fig. 33–18). Imaging techniques currently used are limited, however, because a major portion of the spinal cord is only occasionally visualized on a single, sagittal image of the fetus (Fig. 33–19). While some segments of the spinal cord and vertebral column may be depicted, the clinical usefulness of such information remains uncertain, as it is often difficult to mentally reconstruct the anatomy from pieces of structures seen on nonorthogonal cross-sections.[58]

AMNIOTIC FLUID

Amniotic fluid possesses relatively long T_1 and T_2 relaxation times, similar to other "simple" biologic fluids. It therefore acts as a natural contrast agent to outline the placenta and fetus on T_1-weighted images.[58, 61, 72] This property permits an excellent quan-

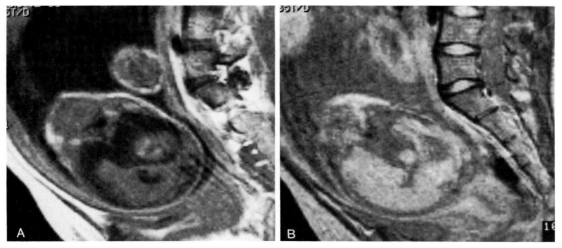

FIGURE 33–16. Thirty-six-week fetus with hydrocephalus. A, SE 500/30; B, SE 2000/40. Similar to amniotic fluid, the enlarged CSF-filled ventricles appear dark on *A* and demonstrate increased signal intensity with progressive T_2 weighting *(B)*. (Reproduced by permission from Weinreb JC: Obstetrics. *In* Stark DD, Bradley WG Jr [eds]: Magnetic Resonance Imaging. St. Louis, 1988, The C. V. Mosby Company.)

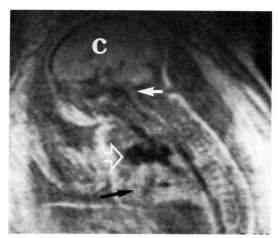

FIGURE 33–18. Third-trimester pregnancy in cephalic presentation. SE 2000/30. Sagittal image demonstrates cerebrum (C), cervicomedullary junction *(white arrow)*, heart *(open arrow)*, and liver *(black arrow)*. (Image purposely inverted.)

titative assessment of the amount of amniotic fluid present, and, as a result, polyhydramnios and oligohydramnios are readily apparent. With progressive T_2 weighting, both the placenta and amniotic fluid will increase in signal intensity. As this occurs, it becomes increasingly difficult to distinguish these two structures from each other, as well as from the fetus itself.[58, 66]

Thus far, the qualitative evaluation of amniotic fluid has been limited. Utilizing amniotic fluid obtained by amniocentesis, several physiologically relevant compounds related to fetal acidosis and CNS disorders have been identified by high-resolution proton NMR spectroscopy.[73] MRI may furnish information regarding fetal distress, as other researchers have been able to reliably estimate the concentration

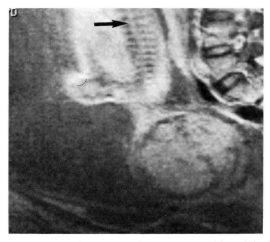

FIGURE 33–19. Thirty-one-week pregnancy with polyhydramnios. SE 2000/30. A considerable segment of the thoracic spine and spinal cord *(black arrow)* is demonstrated. (Reproduced by permission from Weinreb JC: Obstetrics. *In* Stark DD, Bradley WG Jr [eds]: Magnetic Resonance Imaging. St. Louis, 1988, The C. V. Mosby Company.)

of meconium in amniocentesis specimens by demonstrating that T_2 values are sensitive to the presence of meconium.[74] Because amniotic fluid is known to reflect fetal metabolic and renal functions, it is possible that future, in vivo, spectroscopic evaluation of this fluid may provide an understanding of fetal biologic status.

INTRAUTERINE GROWTH RETARDATION

Intrauterine growth retardation (IUGR) is known to be associated with increased perinatal morbidity and mortality, as well as long-term neurologic impairment.[75] While ultrasonography has been the most useful test for the diagnosis of this condition, it may be difficult to distinguish IUGR fetuses from low birth weight normals, and overdiagnosis is relatively common. To predict IUGR more reliably, a multiparameter approach that uses both sonographic and clinical data has now been developed. By analyzing amniotic fluid volume, estimated fetal weight, and maternal blood pressure, researchers established a scoring system that was found to more confidently diagnose or exclude IUGR in third trimester fetuses.[76] It has been proposed that the quantitation of subcutaneous fat by MRI may provide an alternative method of diagnosing IUGR.[66, 77] Subcutaneous fat deposition is first thought to occur around 27 weeks.[78] It is easily seen on either inversion recovery or T_1-weighted spin-echo images, as its high signal intensity contrasts with the surrounding low intensity amniotic fluid.[58, 66] In a series of 11 high-risk third trimester fetuses, MR prospective estimates of fetal fat stores were found to correlate with neonatal outcome better than sonographic measurements of fetal growth parameters or actual birth weight.[66] In addition, the authors pointed out that, while oligohydramnios associated with IUGR may hinder the sonographic examination of the fetus, it tends to limit fetal movement and may therefore improve the quality of MR examinations. In a related case report, MRI was able to demonstrate a relative difference in the degree of subcutaneous fat in a pair of twins, who after delivery were found to demonstrate birth weight discordancy.[79]

While a noninvasive means of accurately diagnosing IUGR in utero is needed, the use of MRI in this setting may, nevertheless, prove very difficult in clinical practice. IUGR may manifest itself not only as a decrease in weight, but also as a decrease in length, subcutaneous fat, muscle mass, head circumference, chest circumference, and abdominal circumference (either singly or in various combinations).[75] Thus, even if a reliable and consistent method of quantifying fetal subcutaneous fat thickness could be developed, this method would not be able to detect IUGR in all of its various presentations.

In a similar fashion, MRI has been able to depict the increased subcutaneous fat found in macrosomic fetuses of diabetic mothers.[57] Because measurements of fetal fat thickness are reported to correlate with weight, this information may allow the clinician to determine the optimal time to deliver the child of a diabetic patient.[64]

Future prospective studies are needed to determine if MRI measurements of fetal fat are able to truly correlate with other established growth parameters and with neonatal outcome. If so, this modality may ultimately prove useful in the clinical evaluation of fetal growth abnormalities and, in doing so, may aid in the management of the obstetrical patient.

CONCLUSION AND OVERALL ASSESSMENT

MRI is a promising technique that represents a complementary imaging modality to ultrasound for the evaluation of the fetus and the gravid pelvis. Its use is advocated when the sonographic findings are equivocal or when sonography is nondiagnostic secondary to technical limitations. MR has proven to be of value in determining the nature and extent of both uterine and adnexal masses and may be helpful in the diagnosis of both placenta previa and potential pelvic outlet obstruction, for which pelvimetric measurements may be performed without the use of ionizing radiation. In addition, it provides an alternative method of imaging fetal anatomy, which may prove beneficial in the assessment of fetal anomalies and possibly intrauterine growth retardation.

REFERENCES

1. Harvey EB, Boice JD, Honeyman M, et al: Prenatal x-ray exposure and childhood cancer in twins. N Engl J Med 312(9):541–545, 1985.
2. United States Food and Drug Administration Guidelines for Evaluating Electromagnetic Exposure Risk for Trials of Clinical NMR Systems. Rockville, MD, Food and Drug Administration, Bureau of Radiological Health, 1982.
3. Reid A, Smith FW, Hutchison JM: NMR imaging and its safety implications: Follow-up of 181 patients. Br J Radiol 55:784–786, 1982.
4. Smith H: Revised guidance on acceptable limits of exposure during nuclear magnetic resonance clinical imaging. The National Radiological Protection Board Ad Hoc Advisory Group on Nuclear Magnetic Resonance Clinical Imaging. Br J Radiol 56:974–977, 1983.
5. Consensus Conference: Magnetic resonance imaging. JAMA 259(14):2132–2138, 1988.
6. Hricak H, Alpers C, Crooks LE, et al: Magnetic resonance imaging of the female pelvis: Initial experience. AJR 141:1119–1128, 1983.
7. Bryan PJ, Butler HE, Lipuma JP, et al: NMR scanning of the pelvis: Initial experience with a 0.3T system. AJR 141:1111–1118, 1983.
8. McCarthy SM, Stark DD, Filly RA, et al: Obstetrical magnetic resonance imaging: Maternal anatomy. Radiology 154:421–425, 1985.
9. Harrison RG: The urogenital system. In Romanes GF (ed): Cunningham's Textbook of Anatomy. London, Oxford University Press, 1984, p 514.
10. Harkness MLR, Harkness RD: The collagen content of the reproductive tract of the rat during pregnancy and lactation. J Physiol 123:492–500, 1954.
11. Pritchard JA, MacDonald PC, Gant NF (eds): Williams Obstetrics. 17th ed. New York, Appleton-Century-Crofts, 1985.
12. Lev-Toaff AS, Coleman BG, Arger PH, et al: Leiomyomas in pregnancy: Sonographic study. Radiology 164:375–380, 1987.
13. O'Brien WF, Buck DR, Nash JD: Evaluation of sonography in the initial assessment of the gynecologic patient. Gynecol Obstet Invest 149:598–602, 1984.
14. Weinreb JC, Brown C: Pelvic masses in pregnant patients: MR and US imaging. Radiology 159:717–724, 1986.
15. Hamlin DJ, Petterson H, Fitzsimmons J, et al: MR imaging of uterine leiomyomas and their complications. J Comput Assist Tomogr 9(5):902–907, 1985.
16. Hricak H, Lacey C, Shriock E: Gynecologic masses: Value of magnetic resonance imaging. Am J Obstet Gynecol 153(1):31–37, 1985.
17. Zemlyn S: The length of the cervix and its significance. J Clin Ultrasound 9:267, 1981.
18. Powell MC, Buckley J, Price H, et al: Magnetic resonance imaging and placenta previa. Am J Obstet Gynecol 154:565–569, 1986.
19. Powell MC, Worthington BS: MRI: A new milestone in modern OB care. Diagn Imaging April 86–91, 1986.
20. Hoddick WK, Mahony BS, Callen PW, et al: Placental thickness. J Ultrasound Med 4:479–482, 1985.
21. Yiu-Chiu Y, Chiu L: Sonographic features of placental complications of pregnancy. AJR 138:879, 1982.
22. Spirit BA, Gordon LP, Kagan EH: Sonography of the placenta. In Sanders RC, James AE (eds): The Principles and Practice of Ultrasonography in Obstetrics and Gynecology. 3rd ed. Norwalk, CT, Appleton-Century-Crofts, 1985, pp 333–354.
23. Spirit BA, Kagan EH, Gordon LP, et al: Antepartum diagnosis of a succenturiate lobe. Sonographic and pathologic correlation. J Clin Ultrasound 9:139, 1981.
24. Goplerud CP: Bleeding in late pregnancy. In Danforth DN (ed): Obstetrics and Gynecology. 3rd ed. Hagerstown, MD, Harper and Row, 1987, pp 378–384.
25. Bowie JD, Rochester D, Cadkin AV, et al: Accuracy of placental localization by ultrasound. Radiology 128:177, 1978.
26. Rizos N, Doran TA, Miskin M, et al: Natural history of placenta previa ascertained by diagnostic ultrasound. Am J Obstet Gynecol 133:287, 1979.
27. Wexler P, Gottesfeld KR: Early diagnosis of placenta previa. Obstet Gynecol 54:231, 1979.
28. Laing FC: Ultrasound evaluation of obstetric problems relating to the lower uterine segment and cervix. In Sanders RC, James AE (eds): The Principles and Practice of Ultrasonography in Obstetrics and Gynecology. 3rd ed. Norwalk, CT, Appleton-Century-Crofts, 1985, pp 355–367.
29. Spirit BA, Kagan EH, Rozanski RM: Abruptio placentae: Sonographic and pathologic correlation. AJR 133:877, 1979.
30. Fleischer AC, Jones HW, James AE: Sonography of trophoblastic diseases. In Sanders RC, James AE (eds): The Principles and Practice of Ultrasonography in Obstetrics and Gynecology. 3rd ed. Norwalk CT, Appleton-Century-Crofts, 1985, pp 387–398.
31. Yuen BH, Cannon W, Benedet JL, et al: Plasma beta-subunit human chorionic gonadotrophin assay in molar pregnancy and choriocarcinoma. Am J Obstet Gynecol 127:711–712, 1977.
32. Fleischer AC, James AE, Krause D, et al: Sonographic patterns in trophoblastic disease. Radiology 126:215, 1978.
33. Requard CK, Mettler FA: The use of ultrasound in the evaluation of trophoblastic disease and its response to therapy. Radiology 135:419–422, 1980.
34. McCarthy SM, Filly RA, Stark DD, et al: Magnetic resonance imaging of fetal anomalies in utero: Early experience. AJR 145:677–682, 1985.
35. Powell MC, Buckley J, Worthington BS, et al: The features of molar pregnancy as shown by magnetic resonance imaging. Book of Abstracts for Fourth Annual Meeting of

Society of Magnetic Resonance in Medicine. London, August, 1985, p 241.

36. Fox H: Pathology of the placenta. *In* Bennington JL (ed): Major Problems in Pathology. Philadelphia, WB Saunders Company, 1978.

37. Battaglia MC, Woolever CA: Fetal and neonatal complications associated with recurrent chorioangiomas. Pediatrics 41:62, 1967.

38. Knop RH, Mattison DR, Kay HH, et al: MR placental and fetal imaging: Placental contrast enhancement following manganese infusion in primates and rats. RSNA Scientific Program, Washington DC, November, 1984, p 31.

39. Angtuaco T, Littlerock AR, Thomford PJ, et al: Effect of manganese on human placental spin lattice (T1) and spin-spin (T2) relaxation times. RSNA Scientific Program, Chicago, November, 1985, p 310.

40. Fleischer AC, Boehm FH, James AE: Sonographic evaluation of pelvic masses and maternal disorders occurring during pregnancy. *In* Sanders RC, James AE (eds): The Principles and Practice of Ultrasonography in Obstetrics and Gynecology. 3rd ed. Norwalk, CT, Appleton-Century-Crofts, 1985, pp 435–447.

41. Fleischer AC, James AE, Mills J, et al: Differential diagnosis of pelvic masses by gray scale sonography. AJR 131:469, 1978.

42. Guttman P: In search of the elusive benign cystic teratoma: "Tip of the iceberg sign." J Clin Ultrasound 5:403, 1977.

43. Lupetin AR, Dash N, Ja-Ja C, et al: MRI diagnosis of the pelvic dermoid. Presented at the Annual Meeting of the Society of Magnetic Resonance Imaging, Philadelphia, 1986.

44. Cohen JM, Weinreb JC, Lowe TW, Brown C: MR imaging of a viable full-term abdominal pregnancy. AJR 145:407–408, 1985.

45. Kerr MG, Scott DB, Samuel E: Studies of the inferior vena cava in late pregnancy. Br Med J 1:532–533, 1964.

46. Savader SJ, Otero RR, Savader BL: Puerperal ovarian vein thrombosis: Evaluation with CT, US and MR imaging. Radiology 167:637–639, 1988.

47. Kelsey JL: An epidemiological study of acute herniated lumbar intervertebral discs. Rheumatol Rehabil 14:144–159, 1975.

48. Weinreb JC, Wolarsht LB, Cohen JM, et al: Prevalence of lumbosacral intervertebral disc abnormalities on MRI in pregnant and asymptomatic nonpregnant women. (Presented at the RSNA annual meeting, Chicago, November, 1986.) Radiology 170:125–128, 1989.

49. Cefalo RC, Moseley RD, Villforth JC: The selection of patients for x-ray examinations: The pelvimetry examination. Washington DC, US Department of Health and Human Services, 1980 (HHS Publ[FDA] 80–8128).

50. Villforth JC: Medical radiation protection: A long view. AJR 145:1114–1118, 1985.

51. Varner MW, Cruikshank DP, Laube DW: X-ray pelvimetry in clinical obstetrics. Obstet Gynecol 56:296–300, 1980.

52. Federle M, Cohen H, Brant-Zawadzki M, et al: Pelvimetry by digital radiography: A low dose examination. Radiology 14:733–736, 1982.

53. Stark DD, McCarthy SM, Filly RA, et al: Pelvimetry by magnetic resonance imaging. AJR 144:947–950, 1985.

54. Weinreb JC, Lowe TW, Santos-Ramos R, et al: Magnetic resonance imaging in obstetric diagnosis. Radiology 154:157–161, 1985.

55. Powell MC, Buckley J, Worthington BS, et al: Comparative study of conventional and MR pelvimetry. RSNA Scientific Program, Chicago, November, 1985, p 83.

56. Sadovsky E, Polishuk WZ: Fetal movements in utero: Nature, assessment, prognostic value, timing of delivery. Obstet Gynecol 50:49–55, 1977.

57. Smith FW: Magnetic resonance imaging of human pregnancy.

Book of Abstracts from Fourth Annual Meeting of Society of Magnetic Resonance in Medicine. London, August, 1985, pp 214–215.

58. Weinreb JC, Lowe T, Cohen JM, et al: Human fetal anatomy: MR imaging. Radiology 157:715–720, 1985.

59. Miller FC, Skiba H, Klapholz H: The effect of maternal blood sugar levels on fetal activity. Obstet Gynecol 52:662–665, 1978.

60. Minors DS, Waterhouse JM: The effect of maternal posture, meals, and time of day on fetal movements. Br J Obstet Gynecol 86:717–723, 1979.

61. McCarthy SM, Filly RA, Stark DD, et al: Obstetrical magnetic resonance imaging: Fetal anatomy. Radiology 154:427–432, 1985.

62. Yeh SY, Paul RH, Cordero L, Hon EH: A study of diazepam during labor. Obstet Gynecol 43:363–373, 1974.

63. Lean TH, Rafnam SS, Sivamboo R: Use of benzodiazapines in the management of eclampsia. J Obstet Gynecol Br Cwlth 75:856–862, 1968.

64. Smith FW: The potential use of nuclear magnetic resonance imaging in pregnancy. J Perinat Med 13:265–276, 1985.

65. Smith FW, Sutherland HW: Short TI inversion recovery (STIR) imaging in human pregnancy. Magn Res Imaging 4:137, 1986.

66. Stark DD, McCarthy SM, Filly RA, et al: Intrauterine growth retardation: Evaluation by magnetic resonance. Radiology 155:425–427, 1985.

67. Possmayer F: The perinatal lung. *In* Jones E (ed): The Biochemical Development of the Fetus and Neonate. Amsterdam, Elsevier Biomedical Press, 1982, pp 287–328.

68. McCarthy S, Stark DD, Higgins CB: Case report: Demonstration of the fetal cardiovascular system by MR imaging. J Comput Assist Tomogr 8(6):1168–1169, 1984.

69. Davidson AM, Peters A: Myelination. Springfield, IL, Charles C Thomas, 1970.

70. Dobbing J, Sands J: Quantitative growth and development of the human brain. Arch Dis Child 48:757–767, 1973.

71. Thickman D, Mintz M, Menhuti M, et al: MR imaging of cerebral abnormalities in utero. J Comput Assist Tomogr 8(6):1058–1061, 1984.

72. Foster MA, Knight CH, Rimington JE, et al: Fetal imaging by nuclear magnetic resonance: A study in goats. Radiology 149:193–195, 1983.

73. Gillies RJ, Powell DA, Nelson TR, et al: High resolution proton NMR spectroscopy of human amniotic fluid. Book of Abstracts for Society of Magnetic Resonance in Medicine Fourth Annual Meeting, London, 1985, pp 789–790.

74. Borcard B, Hiltbrand E, Magnin P, et al: Estimating meconium (fetal feces) concentration in human amniotic fluid by nuclear magnetic resonance. Physiol Chem Phys 14:181–191, 1982.

75. Deter RL, Hadlock FP, Harrist RB: Evaluation of normal fetal growth and the detection of intrauterine growth retardation. *In* Callen PW (ed): Ultrasonography in Obstetrics and Gynecology. Philadelphia, WB Saunders Company, 1988, pp 113–140.

76. Benson CB, Boswell SB, Brown DC, et al: Improved prediction of intrauterine growth retardation with use of multiple parameters. Radiology 168:7–12, 1988.

77. Smith FW, Kent C, Abramovich DR, et al: Nuclear magnetic resonance imaging—A new look at the fetus. Br J Obstet Gynecol 92:1024–1033, 1985.

78. England MA: Color Atlas of Life Before Birth: Normal Fetal Development. Chicago, Year Book Medical Publishers, 1983.

79. Brown CE, Weinreb JC: Magnetic resonance imaging appearance of growth retardation in a twin pregnancy. Obstet Gynecol 71:987–988, 1988.

34

MR IMAGING OF THE SCROTUM AND TESTES

ROBERT MATTREY and MICHAEL TRAMBERT

IMAGING TECHNIQUE
  PATIENT POSITIONING AND PREPARATION
  PULSING SEQUENCE
  IMAGING PLANES

NORMAL ANATOMY

PATHOLOGY
  NEOPLASMS
  General Comments
  Seminoma
  Nonseminomatous Tumors
  Stromal Tumors
  Other Tumors
  INFLAMMATION
  Epididymitis
  Orchitis
  TRAUMA
  TORSION

Intravaginal Spermatic Cord Torsion
Extravaginal Torsion
Torsion of Testicular Appendix
Torsion of Epididymal Appendix
  EXTRATESTICULAR LESIONS
Spermatocele
Hydrocele
Varicocele
UNDESCENDED TESTIS
  IMAGING TECHNIQUES
  ROLE OF MRI IN CRYPTORCHIDISM
  INTRAABDOMINAL TESTES
  INTRACANALICULAR TESTES
  TESTICULAR ATROPHY
DIFFERENTIAL DIAGNOSIS
  TUMOR VERSUS INFECTION
  TORSION VERSUS INFECTION
CONCLUSION

A variety of imaging techniques have been utilized to supplement physical examination in the evaluation of scrotal disease. At present, high-resolution sonography is the imaging modality of choice. Its contribution has been widely documented.[1-5] The success of sonography is based upon its excellent depiction of scrotal anatomy, its display of testicular disease, its low cost, and its lack of ionizing radiation. However, high-resolution sonography is limited by its small field of view, its high dependence on technical expertise, and its lack of specificity in many disease conditions.

Magnetic resonance imaging provides outstanding contrast resolution and, with the use of high field strengths and surface coils, satisfactory spatial reso-

lution.[6-10] MRI, like sonography, is nonionizing and has, as yet, no known harmful effects. With its wide field of view, MRI is well suited to image and evaluate the scrotum. Since our first reports,[6,7] our experience and that of others has increased.[8-10] Over 120 cases with a variety of scrotal diseases have been studied at our institution. The ability of MRI to characterize scrotal disease, as had been described,[7] has been substantiated with our added experience (data not yet published) and that of others.[8,9] While many disease processes have a characteristic appearance to allow their recognition with sufficient specificity, the exact specificity is not yet clear. In a recent report in which 14 tumors were imaged by both sonography and MRI, sonography missed four tumors and MRI missed none.[10] The ability to recognize each intra-scrotal structure because of its signal intensity, appearance, and location separate from any other structure, the ability to view the right and left hemiscrotum along with the inguinal region, and the high contrast afforded by MRI make MRI less subjective than ultrasound. MRI has changed the sonographic diagnosis of testicular disease from normal to cancer in 4 of 23 subjects (17 per cent),[10] and from malignant to benign disease in nearly 6 per cent of our cases (data not yet published). The proven efficacy of sonography established during several years of experience, its unlimited access, and its low cost have hindered the advance of this new application to assess the impact of MRI. At our institution, we have been able to decrease examination time to less than 30 minutes in the majority of patients, without compromising diagnostic quality, and have reduced the charge to $500, which is 1.8 times that of scrotal sonography. It is by decreasing cost and providing fast turnaround time that MRI could compete with well-established sonography. Given the limited experience with scrotal MRI, it is difficult at this time to assess its true clinical impact. However, it seems inevitable, given its sensitivity and convincing display of disease to the referring physician, that if the cost and access are improved, MRI would become the imaging modality of choice.

This chapter is intended to describe the imaging techniques found to be most optimal, present the normal appearance of the scrotum on MRI, and demonstrate some common pathologic conditions to provide the reader with the necessary data to perform and interpret scrotal MR scans. While this chapter is intended to present in an objective manner the current state of this application, it is unavoidable that its content reflects the bias of the authors.

IMAGING TECHNIQUE

PATIENT POSITIONING AND PREPARATION

The patient is positioned supine on the scan table and the scrotum elevated by means of a rolled towel placed between the thighs and another towel draped over the thighs. The penis is angled to the side and the whole region draped. To improve spatial and contrast resolution and signal homogeneity, a 12.5-cm standard equipment circular surface coil is centered over the scrotum and placed horizontally on a 1-cm standoff. The coil is positioned such that the bottom of the coil is over the caudal tip of the scrotal sac. In infants and toddlers the diaper serves as the standoff. The entire area is then wrapped with a 14-inch strap that is attached to the table to minimize patient motion. The isocenter is positioned at mid-scrotum. In infants, the standard 9-cm circular coil is used in lieu of the 12.5-cm coil.

PULSING SEQUENCE

Multislice imaging is obtained in the coronal and sagittal planes. A spin-echo pulsing sequence is used in the sagittal plane with a repetition time (TR) of 600 msec and an echo time (TE) of 20 msec. This series is acquired with 256 x 128 matrix, a 20-cm field of view, and two excitations. The center of the field of view is shifted anteriorly by 5 cm to ensure that the scrotum is properly centered. This sequence, requiring approximately 2.5 minutes to acquire, provides T_1-weighted contrast for tissue characterization and serves as a localizer to plan the longer and most important sequence.

The next sequence is obtained in the coronal plane starting from the posterior aspect of the scrotum and proceeding anteriorly to include the anterior aspect of the external inguinal ring. This series is obtained with a field-of-view of 16 cm and a slice thickness of 3 mm, with a 1.5-mm interslice gap to ensure proper T_2-weighting. Thinner interslice gaps may produce cross-talk, increasing T_1 contrast, which is undesirable in T_2-weighted images. This spin-echo sequence is acquired with TR = 2000 and TE = 20/70 msec. The data acquisition matrix of 256 × 256 obtained with two excitations results in an imaging time of 17.5 minutes. These two series are sufficient for better than 80 per cent of cases. Axial series are reserved for patients with complex findings requiring further definition or for patients with suspected mass whose coronal series was normal. Axial images allow right and left comparison and provide optimal visualization of the anterior and posterior aspect of the testis and scrotum. When axial images are needed, they are obtained with longer TR set at 3000 and two echoes, one at 20 and the other at 70 msec. All other parameters are kept constant except for reduction of the number of excitations to one, resulting in a 13.5-minute acquisition time. The loss in signal-to-noise ratio due to the one excitation is partly recovered by lengthening the TR.

IMAGING PLANES

The coronal plane is the ideal plane to image the scrotum.[6, 7] It allows complete visualization of all important anatomic structures and demonstrates the epididymis and the spermatic cord optimally. It also allows comparison of the right and left hemiscrotal and inguinal regions. Since the coronal plane is parallel to the plane of the surface coil, coronal images are the most pleasing to view; the signal across the field is homogeneous and can be photographed with optimal window and center settings. The sagittal plane defines the full anteroposterior dimension of the scrotum and ensures that the coronal plane covers the entire area of interest. Occasionally, the "bare area" of the testes and cord is best seen in this plane. However, sagittal images offer limited recognition of

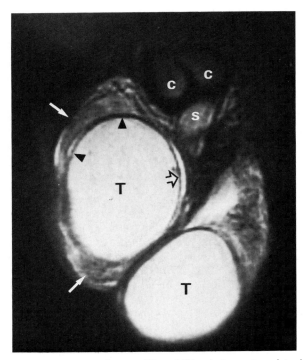

FIGURE 34–1. Normal testes (T), epididymis *(arrows)*, and tunica albuginea *(arrowheads)* shown in the coronal plane on a T₂-weighted image. Small amount of fluid *(open arrow)* between the tunical layers, shown best on T₂-weighted images, is frequently seen. A cross-section of the penis is seen superior to the scrotum, demonstrating the corpus cavernosa (c) and corpus spongiosa (s). The corpus cavernosa is surrounded by a thick dark band, the tunica albuginea of the penis. (From Baker LL, Hajek PC, Burkhard TK, et al: Magnetic resonance imaging of the scrotum: Normal anatomy. Radiology 163:89, 1987; with permission.)

the epididymis, epididymis–scrotal wall interface, and epididymis–testis interface and do not allow right and left comparison on the same image. While the axial plane allows comparison of right and left structures, it does not offer any advantages over the coronal plane. It is reserved for cases in whom pathology is suspected along the anterior or posterior testicular surface or to further define complex findings.

NORMAL ANATOMY

The normal testis is a sharply demarcated oval structure of homogeneous signal intensity, slightly brighter than water and darker than fat on T₁-weighted images. Its signal becomes equal to or slightly brighter than water but darker than fat on hydrogen density–weighted images. Testes become slightly darker than water but much brighter than fat on T₂-weighted images (Fig. 34–1). The intensity of the testis on T₂-weighted images is contrasted with that of the fluid frequently present between the layers of the tunica vaginalis, allowing the assessment of its signal behavior. The testis is completely surrounded

by the tunica albuginea, a thin layer of dense fibrous tissue. This layer is thin and of very low signal intensity on T₂-weighted images. It can adopt a slightly brighter signal due to partial volume when the slice plane is near tangential to the testicular surface. The tunica vaginalis, an extension of peritoneum, is fused to the tunica albuginea except along the bare area of the testis, which becomes highlighted by hydrocele (Fig. 34–2). The testis is therefore analogous to a retroperitoneal structure. Along the bare area, the tunica albuginea invaginates the testis to produce the mediastinum testis, through which the testis receives its blood supply, nerves, lymphatics, and tubules. The mediastinum testis is recognized on hydrogen density–weighted images as a region of lower signal intensity than testis, ranging in length from 1 to 3 cm (dependent upon the plane of section) and becoming of yet lower signal than testis on T₂-weighted images (Fig. 34–2). Intrinsic testicular signal, while homogeneous, displays in some patients internal texture outlining lobules and rete testes. Intratesticular vessels are infrequently seen in normal testes.

On hydrogen density–weighted images, the epididymis is inhomogeneous with intermediate intensity less than or equal to the signal of normal testicular tissue. On T₂-weighted images, the normal epididymis is moderately less intense than normal testis. The head, body, and at times tail of the normal epididymis are easily delineated (Fig. 34–1). The head of the epididymis, lying lateral to the upper pole of the testis, drapes the tunical signal (Fig. 34–1). The normal tail, best seen when highlighted by fluid, is smaller than the epididymal head. The body of the epididymis lies alongside the mediastinum testis and is extravaginal in location. It can be easily recognized from testis because it has a darker signal on T₂-weighted images, and it is separated from testicular tissue by the dark band of the tunica albuginea.

The outer parietal and inner visceral layers of the tunica vaginalis are frequently separated by a small amount of fluid (Fig. 34–1). On T₂-weighted images and in the presence of hydrocele, the fluid completely surrounds the testes except posteromedially, the bare area where the testis is attached to the scrotal wall (Fig. 34–2). The scrotal sac structures such as fat and dartos muscle can at times be seen (Fig. 34–3).

The spermatic cord is easily imaged in all cases. Tortuous tubular structures of low signal intensity located at the posterosuperior aspect of the scrotal sac represent the pampiniform plexus which can be followed into the inguinal canal (Fig. 34–4). Serpiginous high signal intensity areas within the cord on hydrogen density and T₂-weighted images are presumed to represent phase shift artifact due to slow flow in the venous plexus. At times, the cremasteric reflex causes foreshortening of the cord, which may give the cord a nodular appearance on a coronal section (Fig. 34–4). Mild tortuosity of the cord is acceptable. The deferent duct can be seen in some patients. When seen, it is a smooth undulating tu-

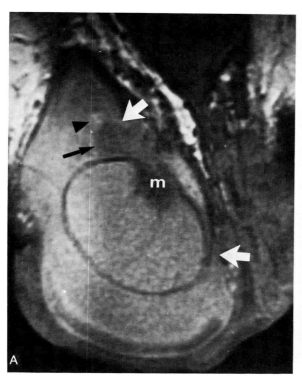
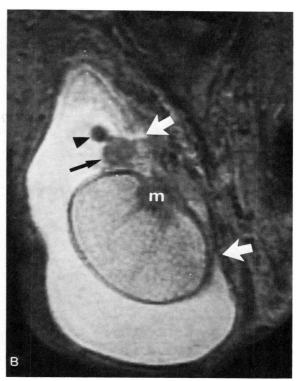

FIGURE 34–2. Acute simple hydrocele (H) is shown on hydrogen density *(A)* and T$_2$-weighted images *(B)*. Note that the signal of hydrocele is consistent with water signal (intermediate on hydrogen density and bright on T$_2$ weighting). This sympathetic hydrocele is thought to be due to torsion of the epididymal appendix, shown to be hemorrhagic on MRI *(arrowhead)* (slightly bright on hydrogen density and dark on T$_2$ weighting) and attached to the normal epididymis *(black arrow)*. In this example, the lobular septae can be seen on T$_2$ weighting *(B)* emanating from the mediastinum testes (m). Note that the presence of sizable hydrocele demonstrates the "bare area" of the testis, the edges of which are marked by large white arrows. (From Baker LL, Hajek PC, Burkhard TK, et al: Magnetic resonance imaging of the scrotum: Pathologic conditions. Radiology 163:98, 1987; with permission.)

FIGURE 34–3. Sagittal T$_2$-weighted image *(A)* shows clear delineation of tunica albuginea *(arrowheads)*, epididymal head and tail *(arrows)*, and the various layers of the scrotal wall, including the dartos muscle *(open arrow)*. Cadaveric specimen *(B)* shows similar anatomy. Note that the mediastinum testis *(open arrow)* and the vas deferens *(curved arrow)* can be seen on this particular section of the specimen. (From Baker LL, Hajek PC, Burkhard TK, et al: Magnetic resonance imaging of the scrotum: Normal anatomy. Radiology 163:90, 1987; with permission.)

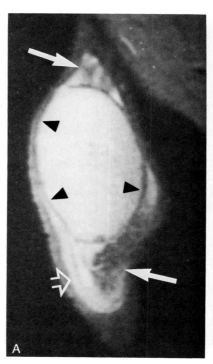
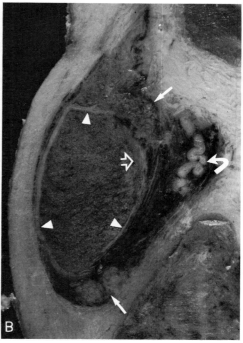

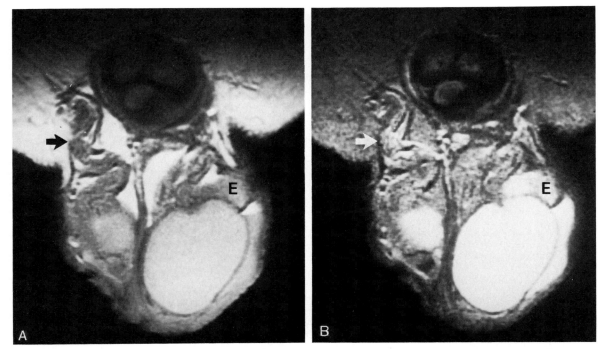

FIGURE 34–4. Hydrogen density *(A)* and T_2-weighted *(B)* images in the coronal plane show the accordion-shaped spermatic cord *(arrow)* entering the base of the right hemiscrotum. Note that small hydrocele on the left outlines the epididymal head (E). (From Baker LL, Hajek PC, Burkhard TK, et al: Magnetic resonance imaging of the scrotum: Normal anatomy. Radiology 163:91, 1987; with permission.)

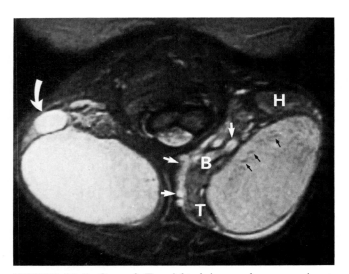

FIGURE 34–5. Coronal T_2-weighted image shows prominent serpentine structure in the body of the epididymis *(white arrows)*. Its signal was similar to testis on all sequences (not shown). This is presumed to represent the vas deferens, but could represent a dilated vein with stagnant blood. Note that the entire epididymis can be seen: head (H), body (B), and tail (T). Also note the clear delineation of testis from epididymis by the dark tunica albuginea. Small linear dark signals *(small arrows)* within the testis are interlobular septae converging toward the mediastinum, seen on the following slice (not shown). Also note the presence of an epididymal cyst *(curved arrow)* on the right. Since it was dark on hydrogen density (not shown), it behaved similar to water.

bular structure similar in signal intensity to that of testis (Fig. 34–5). It is not clear yet whether only ectatic ducts are seen, since the deferent duct is not visualized in most patients. Further experience and clinical correlation are required to resolve this question.

PATHOLOGY

The homogeneous high signal intensity of the normal testes on T_2-weighted images provides an excellent background for visualizing intratesticular pathology. Except for old hematoma, all intratesticular pathology has been less intense than normal testicular tissue on T_2-weighted images. The integrity of the tunica albuginea can be assessed; however, beware of partial volume which may assign the tunica a brighter signal. If the integrity of the tunica albuginea must be assessed, ensure that the slice is perpendicular to the area of interest.

The majority of pathologic conditions of the scrotum are best visualized on T_2-weighted (TR 2000 msec, TE 70 msec) images. Coronal hydrogen density–weighted and sagittal T_1-weighted images provide tissue characterization potential. Complete assessment of the scrotum is possible in most cases with coronal sections only. Sagittal and axial T₂-weighted images add confidence and demonstrate to a better advantage small lesions abutting the anterior or posterior surfaces.

NEOPLASMS

General Comments

All tumors are of inhomogeneous signal intensity consistently equal to or lower than that of normal testis on hydrogen density–weighted images and moderately lower on T₂-weighted images. Their margination and extent, as well as influence on normal testicular size and shape, are well demonstrated on MR images. Extension of mass into extratesticular locations such as epididymis or cord is clearly shown.[7] Whereas MRI has been shown to incorrectly stage 4 of 11 cases and sonography 6 of 11,[10] this seeming handicap is irrelevant preoperatively, since testicular cancer, regardless of the stage of disease, requires orchiectomy for pathologic staging.

Cancer typically leaves a rim of normal testicular tissue, even when large (Fig. 34–6). Of the more than 25 cancers reported in the literature,[7–10] and of an additional nine at our institution (data not yet published), primary cancers totally replace normal testicular tissue in only one case. It is possible in infiltrative disorders (lymphoma/leukemia) for the testis to become totally replaced.[10] In such instances, the signal of the affected testis can be compared with that of the contralateral testis or surrounding structures and hydrocele. When a fibrous tumor capsule is seen

histologically around the tumor, which is typical for nonseminomatous lesions, it is also seen on MR (Fig. 34–6).[11] Hemorrhage in lesions is clearly depicted and is assigned signals dependent upon its age (Fig. 34–6).

Whereas MR has not missed any lesion seen sonographically and has detected all 14 cancers, including the four missed by sonography,[10] it is not clear what would be the minimum consistently detectable lesion size. It is possible, given the long imaging time, that owing to the continuous contraction of the dartos muscle producing wormian motion of the scrotal wall and constant motion of the testes, that small lesions may be of partial volume, with the bright testicular background significantly decreasing their contrast and detectability. The smallest lesion detected by MRI prospectively and proven surgically was a 3-mm germ cell tumor (not shown). Given that partial volume effect is increased by testicular motion, any study compromised by motion aimed at detecting testicular neoplasm should be repeated if no lesions are found. On the other hand, when clear depiction of the interlobular septae or intratesticular morphology is achieved, it should be regarded as evidence for sufficient quality to negate the presence of disease (see Fig. 34–2). Further clinical experience is, however, required to define the true sensitivity of MRI.

Testicular neoplasms can be primary or metastatic. Primary cancers can take origin from any cell type present in normal testes and account for 5000 new cases and 1000 deaths per year in the United States.[12] Testicular neoplasms are most frequently detected in males below 10 years of age, between 20 and 40 years of age, and then over 60. They have peak incidence

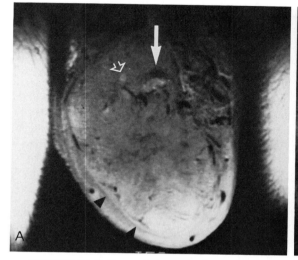 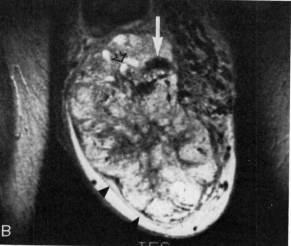

FIGURE 34–6. Coronal views of a large (7 × 10 cm), mixed, nonseminomatous tumor. Note that even with this very large lesion, a rim of normal testicular tissue is still seen *(arrowheads)* separated from the tumor by a thick fibrous tumor capsule proven pathologically. Note the region of high signal on hydrogen density–weighted image *(A)*, which remains high signal on T₂ weighting *(B) (open arrow)*. Also note areas of intermediate signal on hydrogen density *(A)*, which become darker on T₂ weighting *(B) (arrow)*. These are areas of hemorrhage characteristic of this tumor type. Note the hypervascularity observed along the scrotal wall and cord. (From Johnson JO, Mattrey RF, Philpson J: Differentiation of seminomatous from nonseminomatous testicular tumors with MR imaging. AJR [in press] with permission.)

and are the most common solid tumors detected between the ages of 20 and 34. Primary testicular neoplasms, from the imaging as well as treatment perspective, are grouped into germ cell and nongerm cell or stromal tumors. Germ cell tumors account for 90 to 95 per cent of all primary testicular malignancies, while nongerm cell or stromal tumors account for 5 to 10 per cent. Germ cell lesions are in turn grouped into seminomatous and nonseminomatous lesions. Pure seminoma account for nearly 40 per cent of all primary tumors; nonseminomatous form the remaining 55 per cent. Tumors of mixed cellularity, seminomatous and nonseminomatous, occur in 10 to 15 per cent of cases. When seminoma is mixed with nonseminomatous elements, the lesion is regarded and treated as a nonseminomatous tumor. Germ cell tumors of yolk sac origin are the predominant lesions of infancy. Testicular lymphoma is the most common neoplasm affecting the testes of men over 50 years of age.

Testicular tumors are bilateral, either at the time of diagnosis or on follow-up, in 1 to 3 per cent of cases.[13] Therefore, careful examination of the contralateral testis at the time of diagnosis and close follow-up are mandatory.

The differentiation of seminomatous from nonseminomatous lesions is critical, in that patients with pure seminomatous lesions are irradiated and those with nonseminomatous lesions undergo retroperitoneal dissection and chemotherapy. While these modes of therapy remain controversial,[12] they are standard practice at this time. Since seminomatous lesions may harbor small islands of nonseminomatous histology in 10 to 15 per cent of cases,[12] treatment is planned following detailed histologic analysis of the resected testis. This is particularly true when there is elevation of beta–human chorionic gonadotropin (HCG) or alpha-fetoprotein, findings suggesting the presence of nonseminomatous elements. While treatment cannot be determined preoperatively in seminomatous lesions, if nonseminomatous lesions are consistently diagnosed with 100 per cent specificity it is possible that the retroperitoneal dissection could be performed along with the orchiectomy at the same sitting, saving one operative procedure. From our data[11] and that presented in the literature to date,[8–10] it appears that MRI may offer such differentiation.

In this section, the characteristics of each lesion type will be presented. While the preoperative histologic diagnosis is less critical for patient management at this time, there are some characteristic findings for seminomatous and nonseminomatous cancers emerging which may allow their specific diagnosis.

Seminoma

Seminoma is rare in patients below the age of 10 and above 60, but it is the most common cell type accounting for 40 per cent of all testicular neoplasms with peak incidence in the late 30s. Spermatocystic seminoma, a subtype accounting for 10 per cent of all detected seminomas, occurs most frequently in men over the age of 50. Nearly 10 to 15 per cent of seminomatous lesions are not pure seminomas. They have islands of nonseminomatous cells which change their classification to nonseminomatous lesions. Thus, seminomatous lesions mandate careful pathologic search to ensure their pure cell types to allow for proper treatment planning. Elevation of beta-HCG or alpha-fetoprotein suggests mixed cellularity. Seminomatous lesions are sheets of cells intermixed with fibrous strands presenting a homogeneous histologic pattern. They rarely bleed or necrose centrally.

The MR appearance of this tumor type, like its histology, has been consistent for all seminomatous lesions imaged. Its signal is mildly inhomogeneous, and its intensity is consistently lower than that of normal testicular tissue or hydrocele fluid on T_2-weighted images. The tumors may contain well-defined regions of low signal (Fig. 34–7) thought to be due to regions with increased fibrosis. While atypical, some seminomatous lesions may bleed internally, resulting in a focus of different signal dependent on the age of the bleed. This was seen in one of the six seminomas imaged to date (not shown). Metastases to the epididymis and cord in one of the cases were clearly demonstrated (Fig. 34–7).[7] The signal of these deposits was similar to that of the intratesticular mass.

A small rim of normal testicular tissue was always visible and was clearly demarcated from lesion (Fig. 34–8). The appearance of the mass suggested coalescence of multiple nodules (Fig. 34–7). Indeed, when smaller lesions were imaged, daughter nodules could be detected (not shown). While seminomatous lesions present darker signal than testis, similar to infection or infarction, there are characteristic features that allow their distinction (see "Differential Diagnosis").

Nonseminomatous Tumors

Lumped in this category and listed in order of occurrence are teratocarcinomas, embryonal cell, teratomas, and choriocarcinomas. Nearly 40 per cent of nonseminomatous lesions are a mixture of two or three elements. They all carry similar prognosis and are treated in a similar fashion. Therefore, preoperative distinction of the cell type is not necessary. These lesions account for nearly 50 per cent of all primary testicular neoplasms with peak incidence in the 20s and early 30s. They therefore afflict slightly younger males than do seminomatous lesions. These lesions present heterogeneous histology owing to their mixed cellularity, their attempt at tubular formation, and their high propensity to invade vessels, causing internal hemorrhage and necrosis.

These tumors, given their histologic patterns, are markedly inhomogeneous on MRI, which represents their most distinctive feature when compared with seminomatous lesions. Over the background that is

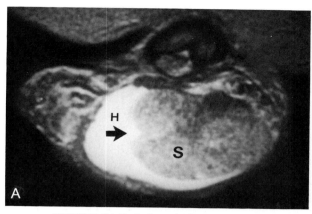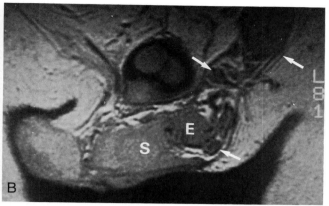

FIGURE 34–7. Left testicular seminoma (S) is mildly inhomogeneous on T_2-weighted image *(A)* and is of markedly lower signal than the remaining normal testicular tissue *(arrow)* and hydrocele (H). Hydrogen density image *(B)*, obtained at a different level than *(A)*, demonstrates the upper aspect of testicular tumor (S) along with epididymal (E) and spermatic cord involvement *(arrows)*. Extratesticular nodules had similar signals as intratesticular lesion on hydrogen density *(B)* and T_2-weighted images (not shown). (From Baker LL, Hajek PC, Burkhard TK, et al: Magnetic resonance imaging of the scrotum: Pathologic conditions. Radiology 163:94, 1987; with permission.)

isointense or slightly brighter than normal testis on T_2-weighted images, multiple areas of high and low signal intensities on both hydrogen density and T_2-weighted images are seen. These areas represent hemorrhage of various ages within the mass, very characteristic of these lesions (see Fig. 34–6). The degree of heterogeneity and the overall signal intensity are much greater than are seen with seminoma. A band of low signal intensity is visible, circumscribing the mass in most cases. This has been shown

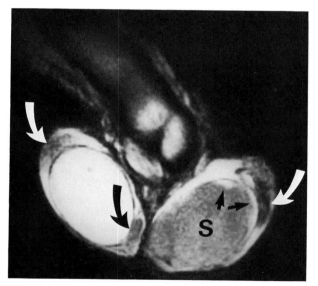

FIGURE 34–8. Left testicular seminoma (S) is of significantly darker signal than normal testis on a T_2-weighted image. It was mildly inhomogeneous and of slightly lower signal on hydrogen density (not shown). Note well-marginated small rim of normal testicular tissue near the upper pole of testis *(arrows)*. Also note small ipsilateral hydrocele and normal epididymal head *(curved arrow)*. Normal epididymal head and tail are seen on the normal contralateral side *(curved arrows)*. (From Johnson JO, Mattrey RF, Philpson J: The ability of MR imaging to differentiate seminomatous from non-seminomatous testicular tumors. AJR [in press]; with permission.)

histologically to represent the fibrous tumor capsule, also typical for these lesions. Remaining normal testicular tissue is easily differentiated from tumor by its homogeneous and characteristic intensity, even when the lesion is very large (Fig. 34–6). One nonseminomatous lesion has appeared darker than testis (not shown). Its signal was much darker than is typically seen with seminoma and was markedly heterogeneous.

In a recent study, the ability of MRI to differentiate seminomatous from nonseminomatous lesions was assessed prospectively.[11] It was found that of the 12 patients with sizable lesions that could be characterized, MRI allowed the correct classification of 11 of them. The degree of heterogeneity of signals was the most discriminating factor, nonseminomatous lesions being more heterogeneous than seminomatous ones.[11] The only error was in a patient whose lesion was characteristic for seminoma; the tumor had a central region of higher signal which misled the reader to believe that it was an island of nonseminomatous tissue in an otherwise pure seminoma. This high signal region proved histologically to be hemorrhage in a pure seminoma. This error could have been avoided since the mix of nonseminomatous elements in seminoma is a heterogeneous distribution of many small microscopic islands rather than a single large focus as was seen in this case. In the literature,[7–10] tumor signals also match the above description, suggesting that MRI may indeed be able to differentiate these two tumor types. Though sonography demonstrates characteristic echographic findings for seminomatous and nonseminomatous lesions, there is significant overlap in their appearance.[14]

Stromal Tumors

Stromal tumors account for nearly 5 per cent of all primary testicular tumors. They occur in males

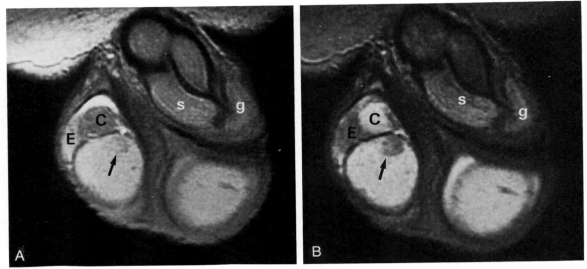

FIGURE 34–9. Mildly inhomogeneous well-marginated testicular tumor *(arrow)*, which proved histologically to be a Leydig cell tumor, is better seen on the T_2-weighted image *(B)* than on the hydrogen density image *(A)*. Epididymal cyst (C) within the normal epididymal head (E) has MRI characteristics similar to water. Oblique section through the penis shows the paired corpora cavernosa each surrounded by a dark signal and the brighter corpora spongiosa (s) and glans (g). (From Baker LL, Hajek PC, Burkhard TK, et al: Magnetic resonance imaging of the scrotum: Pathologic conditions. Radiology 163:95, 1987; with permission.)

20 to 60 years of age. They are well circumscribed and rarely exhibit hemorrhage or necrosis. Since these lesions generally produce hormones, prepubertal boys can present with precocious puberty and adults with gynecomastia. The cell types include Leydig and Sertoli cells. These lesions are malignant in 10 per cent of cases. Malignancy is suspected histologically when lesions are large, necrotic, infiltrative, or have invaded blood vessels. Malignancy is clearly established when there are metastases. One could hypothesize that, given their homogeneous histology and lack of hemorrhage and necrosis, their appearance on MRI would mimic seminomatous lesions.[7, 10] However, when malignant, the hemorrhage and necrosis would change their appearance to mimic nonseminomatous lesions. The experience with these lesions is limited to test this hypothesis.

Two published proven cases of Leydig cell tumor show the mass on T_2-weighted images to be of moderately darker signal intensity than normal testis.[7, 10] One was small, well-circumscribed, and homogeneous as would be expected from the histology (Fig. 34–9).[7] The other tumor totally infiltrated the testis on MRI in a prepubertal boy, causing sonography to miss the lesion. It is not yet clear that these lesions could be differentiated from seminomatous lesions.

Other Tumors

Lymphomatous or leukemic infiltration of the testis is common. Lymphoma accounts for nearly 5 per cent of all testicular neoplasms.[12] It may be primary in the testis, the manifestation of occult disease seated elsewhere, or the late manifestation of disseminated lymphoma. Lymphomatous lesions are the most common testicular lesions in males over 50 years of age.[12] The majority of these lesions are infiltrative and may extend into or originate in the epididymis (Fig. 34–10). The major cell type is histiocytic lymphoma.

The testis is the prime site of relapse of leukemia

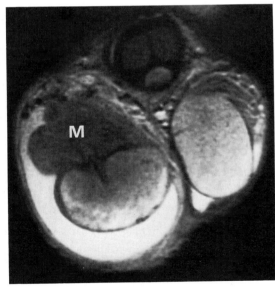

FIGURE 34–10. Scrotal lymphoma involving the right epididymis and testis is shown on a T_2-weighted image. Note that the center of the mass (M) is in the epididymis and infiltrates the testis from the hilum. The mass, located along the "bare area" of the testis, rotated the testis into a horizontal position. Note that the mass within the testis is patchy and that its margins with normal testicular tissue are generally poorly defined. There is mild hypervascularity and moderate ipsilateral hydrocele.

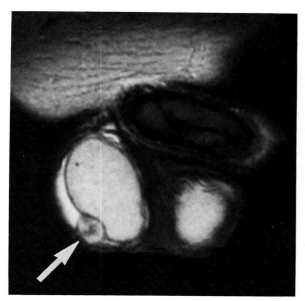

FIGURE 34–11. Adenomatoid tumor *(arrow)*, proven surgically, has similar signals as testis on a T_2-weighted image. Its signal was also similar to testis on hydrogen density (not shown). Note its extratesticular location as it deviates the tunica albuginea medially. Indentation of testis suggested that the lesion was between the layers of tunica albuginea and tunica vaginalis, confirmed at surgery.

in children. A blood-testis barrier exists, similar to the blood-brain barrier, which prevents chemotherapeutics from eradicating disease in the testes. Testicular evaluation and biopsy are commonly performed at the end of chemotherapy to exclude testicular involvement. Although ultrasound can detect leukemic infiltration,[15] it has poor sensitivity.[10] While we have not evaluated the role of MRI in this setting to determine sensitivity, four cases have been detected by MRI that were missed by sonography.[10] Leukemia in these cases affected the entire testis diffusely and decreased its signal.[10]

Adenomatoid tumors are benign lesions characteristic of the genital tract consisting of fibrous stroma and epithelial cells. These lesions are benign and usually occur in the epididymis but may rarely occur in the testis. We have imaged two such tumors; one was surgically proven (Fig. 34–11). Dependent upon the degree of fibrosis, their signal may vary from being similar to testis to being darker than testis. Since the testicular appendix may have similar appearance, particularly if fibrotic, it might be difficult to differentiate these two entities. This differentiation is not important since neither condition requires surgical intervention.

INFLAMMATION

Epididymitis

Epididymitis is the most common intrascrotal infection. It may be diffuse or focal and is frequently

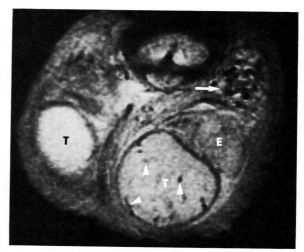

FIGURE 34–12. Patient with acute epididymitis shown on a T_2-weighted image in the coronal plane. Testis (T) is of slightly lower signal than the contralateral side and is hypervascular *(arrowheads)*. The epididymis (E) is enlarged and assumes a higher signal on T_2 weighting than is normally observed. Note the hypervascularity in the cord typical of this condition *(arrow)*. (From Trambert MA, Mattrey RF, Levine D, Berthoty D: The role of MRI in subacute scrotal pain: Torsion versus epididymitis. Radiology [in press]; with permission.)

secondary to prostatitis. Most cases of epididymitis are treated conservatively. Surgery is reserved for complications such as abscess formation. Therefore, diagnostic follow-up in patients with poor response to therapy may be warranted.

Patients with clinical evidence of acute epididymitis consistently show epididymal enlargement (Fig. 34–12). The epididymis, which is normally of lower signal intensity than testis on T_2-weighted images, maintains a higher signal that could be nearly equal

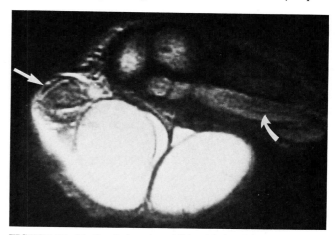

FIGURE 34–13. Focal chronic epididymitis involving the head of the right epididymis shown on a T_2-weighted image. Note the enlarged dark epididymis *(arrow)*. Patient, known to have chronic epididymitis, presented with acute exacerbation. There is mild reactive ipsilateral hydrocele. Acute exacerbations may be difficult to diagnose in the setting of chronic changes. Oblique view of the penis shows urethra *(curved arrow)* traveling through corpus spongiosa. (From Baker LL, Hajek PC, Burkhard TK: Magnetic resonance imaging of the scrotum: Pathologic conditions. Radiology 163:98, 1987; with permission.)

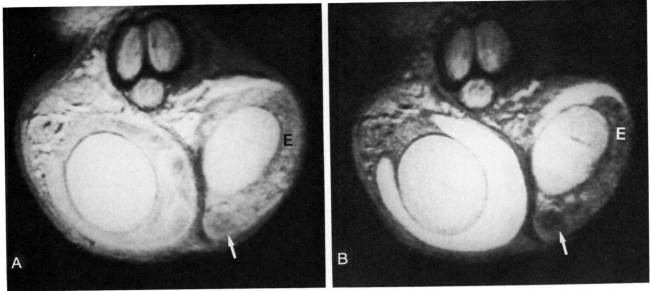

FIGURE 34–14. Diffuse chronic epididymitis involving the entire epididymis on the left and shown in the coronal plane on hydrogen density *(A)* and T$_2$-weighted *(B)* images. Note diffuse enlargement of the entire epididymis (E) with possible hemorrhage in the tail *(arrow)*. Mild ipsilateral and moderate contralateral hydrocele are present. The right hydrocele outlines the "bare area" in its transverse direction *(B)*. Note motion-related signal loss in the right hydrocele, better appreciated on hydrogen density *(A)*.

to that of testis. In chronic epididymitis, the epididymis is enlarged in a focal (Fig. 34–13) or diffuse manner (Fig. 34–14) and assumes darker signals than normal on T$_2$-weighting, becoming moderately darker than testis. In the setting of chronic epididymitis, acute exacerbation may not affect signal (Fig. 34–13). Therefore, when the epididymis is enlarged and assumes a dark signal, acute epididymitis cannot be excluded.

Acute epididymitis, particularly when severe, may be associated with hemorrhage within the epididymis (Fig. 34–15). If hemorrhage is present, MR signal follows its resorptive stages. The most common appearance has been signals associated with subacute bleeding (intermediate on hydrogen density and dark on T$_2$ weighting). We have not seen hematomas secondary to infection in the epididymis with signals associated with old blood (bright on T$_1$ and T$_2$ weighting). Whereas it is possible that we have fortuitously imaged all these individuals in their subacute state, it is tempting to hypothesize that, since changes of old blood have been seen in the epididymis in cases with torsion, extravasated blood in the epididymis may be resorbed prior to lysis and methemoglobin formation in patients with epididymitis.

In acute epididymitis, hypervascularity and thick-

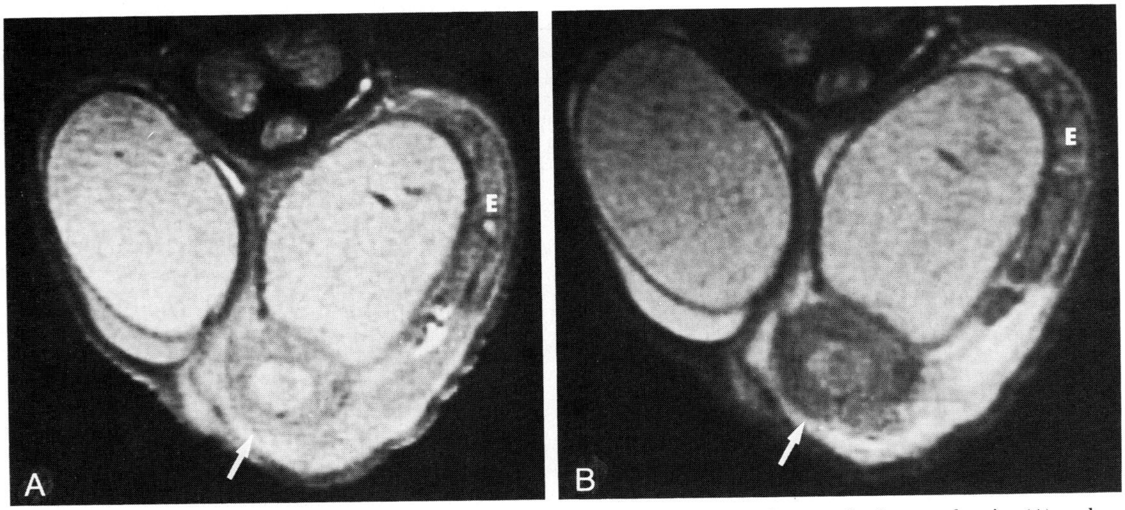

FIGURE 34–15. Focal epididymitis involving the tail shown in the coronal plane on hydrogen density *(A)* and T$_2$-weighted *(B)* images. Note focal enlargement of the tail *(arrow)* with hemorrhage and associated ipsilateral hydrocele. Upper epididymis (E) is darker than normal but is not enlarged.

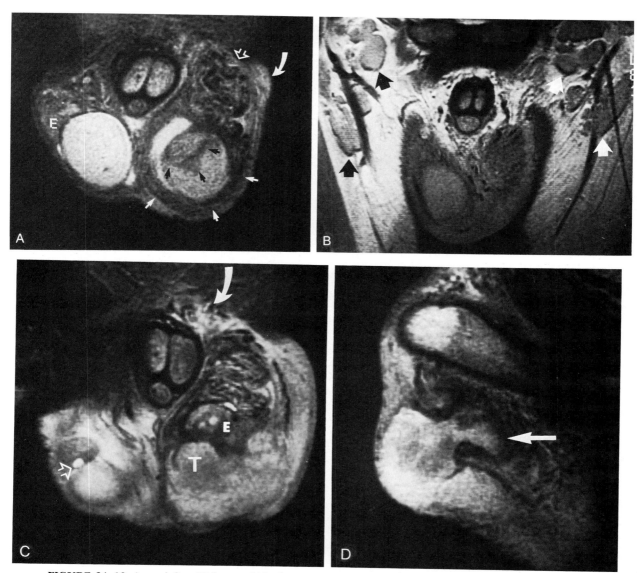

FIGURE 34–16. Acute left epididymoorchitis shown in the coronal plane on a T₂-weighted image *(A)*. Note diffuse loss of signal of the affected testis, the hypervascular cord *(open arrow)* at the base of the scrotum, associated skin thickening including scrotal septum *(arrows)*, and edema *(curved arrow)*. While the focus of orchitis *(black arrows)* could be confused for tumor at first, note the associated diffuse loss of testicular signal and the changes in the scrotal wall and cord. These, in conjunction with the clinical history, should eliminate such confusion. Note on *(A)* the enlarged contralateral darkened epididymis (E), suggesting the occurrence of previous episodes. Note associated bilateral inguinal adenopathy *(arrows)* on a hydrogen density–weighted image *(B)* obtained few levels posterior to *(A)*. A T₂-weighted image *(c)* obtained 10 days after *(A)* at nearly the same level shows complete destruction of the testis (T) and loss of intrascrotal anatomic detail. Note the cephalic extension of scrotal wall involvement and the spread of edema to the base of the penis *(curved arrow)* compared with *(A)*. At this time, the changes were due to an epididymal abscess *(D)* *(arrow)* that involved the testis and pointed along the anterior scrotal wall. Incidental note of a small hemorrhagic cyst *(open arrow)* in the right epididymis *(C)*; this cyst was bright on hydrogen density (not shown). (From Baker LL, Hajek PC, Burkhard TK: Magnetic resonance imaging of the scrotum: Pathologic conditions. Radiology 163:98, 1987; with permission.)

ening and swelling of the spermatic cord—increasing its signal on T₂-weighted images—are observed (see Figs. 34–12 and 34–16). While the degree of hypervascularity has been variable, it has been consistently present in all patients. Hypervascularity is seen as multiple serpiginous vessels with signal void due to

high flow. This is in contradistinction to normal vessels that are usually thinner and lack the very dark signal due to their slower flow (see Fig. 34–4). Hypervascularity of the testis associated with epididymitis has also been observed in some patients (see Fig. 34–12). Scrotal skin thickening and swelling can be easily seen and are detected in most but not all patients (Fig. 34–16); however, this finding is not specific to infection. Sympathetic hydrocele is present in most patients and assumes signals identical to those of water (dark on T_1, isointense on hydrogen density, and brighter than testis on T_2-weighted images) (see Fig. 34–15). Extensive inguinal adenopathy is frequently seen in these patients (Fig. 34–16). However, it is also frequently seen in normal patients or in those with a variety of conditions; therefore the presence of inguinal adenopathy adds no specificity.

Orchitis

Orchitis is often the sequel of epididymitis. Pure orchitis without epididymitis suggests viral etiology. When orchitis accompanies epididymitis, treatment is extended over a longer period of time due to the blood-testis barrier. Even when appropriately treated, orchitis can develop into an abscess requiring surgical intervention. Therefore, when a focus of orchitis is found, follow-up is necessary to ensure its resolution.

We have imaged two patients with acute bacterial orchitis. Both were associated with epididymitis. While on antibiotic therapy, one patient progressed to an epididymotesticular abscess 10 days later (Fig. 34–16).

Tuberculous orchitis is usually associated with tuberculous epididymitis. We have imaged three such patients with proven tuberculous scrotal infection. All had epididymal and testicular involvement. Testicular changes were patchy, poorly marginated areas of slightly lower signal than testis (Fig. 34–17). Epididymal changes were less severe than bacterial epididymitis, and the degree of hypervascularity was less prominent. In one patient with surgically proven diffuse chronic tuberculous orchitis, the testis was diffusely inhomogeneous with low signal intensity on T_2-weighted images but without mass effect (Fig. 34–18).

In some patients with fulminant epididymitis, epididymal swelling may be so severe that it can compromise the blood supply to the testis, resulting in infarction.[16] We have not imaged such patients. However, it would be expected that such ischemia would be on the basis of venous occlusion followed by arterial occlusion. Such infarction would more likely be hemorrhagic and should present different signals than the patchy ill-defined diminished signal of orchitis. This hypothesis requires further clinical testing.

TRAUMA

Surgical intervention in scrotal trauma is generally reserved for patients with testicular fracture or rupture or when the intratesticular hematoma is extensive, causing severe pain. MRI is well suited to assess

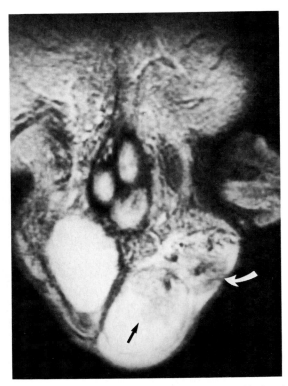

FIGURE 34–17. Acute tuberculous epididymoorchitis involving the upper pole of the left testis *(arrow)* and epididymal head *(curved arrow)* shown in the coronal plane on a T_2-weighted image. Note patchy involvement of the testis, which was seen only on T_2 weighting, and the enlarged epididymis that failed to darken on this T_2-weighted image. Note the mild degree of hypervascularity suggesting subacute inflammation.

both the integrity of the tunica albuginea and the degree of intratesticular hematoma. Because the normal tunica is well visualized as a band of low signal intensity surrounding the testes on both hydrogen density and T_2-weighted images, clear assessment of its integrity is possible. In this setting multiple imaging planes may be required to ensure that all surfaces are optimally imaged without partial volume effect. When it is known that multiple planes are required, T_2-weighted sequences, which are required for proper diagnosis, are obtained with TR = 3000, TE = 20/70, 256 × 256 matrix, and one excitation. This sequence requires 13.5 minutes to acquire in lieu of the 17.5 minutes of the typical sequence. It also yields adequate signal-to-noise ratio to evaluate scrotal pathology.

Overall, the traumatized testes are highly inhomogeneous with regions of high and low signal intensity compared with normal testicular tissue on both hydrogen density and T_2-weighted images. This is due to hemorrhage of different ages and degrees of organization (Fig. 34–19). Hematocele frequently accompanies trauma and assumes signals commensurate with the age of hemorrhage (Fig. 34–19). The classic signals described for hematoma are observed when hematoceles develop, since hemorrhage in this

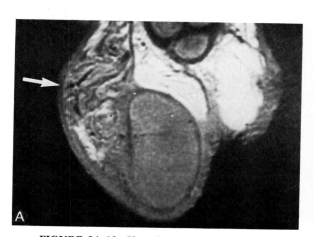
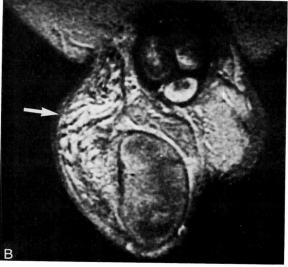

FIGURE 34–18. Chronic tuberculous orchitis shown in the coronal plane on hydrogen density *(A)* and T$_2$-weighted *(B)* images. Note the diffuse, poorly defined process involving the entire testis poorly seen on hydrogen density. Note the prominent cord at the base of the scrotum *(arrow)* compatible with varicocele. The left testis had been removed because of a tuberculous infection. (From Baker LL, Hajek PC, Burkhard TK, et al: Magnetic resonance imaging of the scrotum: Pathologic conditions. Radiology 163:96, 1987; with permission.)

space, as in the CNS, is reasonably well isolated. Intratesticular trauma causes more linear than spherical changes (Fig. 34–20), decreasing its confusion with mass lesions. Furthermore, associated clinical and scrotal changes with trauma differ from those of tumors.

TORSION

Intravaginal Spermatic Cord Torsion

The testis, like other abdominal organs, is retroperitoneal. When descended into the scrotum, the

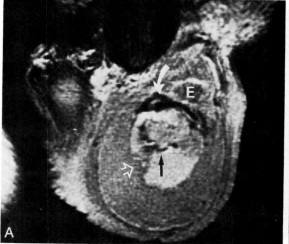
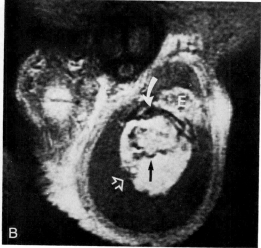

FIGURE 34–19. Three-day-old scrotal trauma is shown in the coronal plane on hydrogen density *(A)* and T$_2$-weighted (B) images. Note that the hematoma outlining the tunica along the upper pole of the testis is very dark *(curved arrow)* and that the intratesticular hematoma, although darker than testis, is brighter than upper pole collection *(arrow)*. The reason for the discrepancy of signals is not clear. The central hemorrhage is incompletely surrounded by a dark band. Given the age of these hematomas (3 days), these cannot represent hemosiderin-filled macrophages. Note that the tunica is interrupted along the medial lower pole *(open arrow)*. The tunical fluid, hematocele, has signals indicating subacute hemorrhage (intermediate on hydrogen density *[A]* and dark on T$_2$ weighting *[B]*). Also note that the epididymis (E) is enlarged, swollen, and inhomogeneous. (From Baker LL, Hajek PC, Burkhard TK: Magnetic resonance imaging of the scrotum: Pathologic conditions. Radiology 163:97, 1987; with permission.)

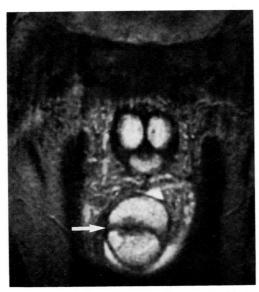

FIGURE 34–20. Seven-day-old trauma that resulted in testicular fracture is shown on a T$_2$-weighted image. Note that the intratesticular abnormality is a linear process that presumably follows the fracture line (arrow). Note the presence of hydrocele rather than hematocele.

testis is accompanied by peritoneum called the vaginal process. The vaginal process, upon testicular descent into the scrotum, becomes fused to the scrotal wall and a significant portion of the tunica albuginea. When fused, the vaginal process is called the tunica vaginalis. The tunica vaginalis invests the entire contour of the testis except for a strip that extends from the upper to lower pole leaving the region of the mediastinum testis uncovered (see Fig. 34–2). The transverse dimension of the bare area is variable but typically extends for at least one third of the perimeter of the testis (see Fig. 34–14). This bare area not only serves as a passage for support structures, but more importantly it anchors the testis to the posteromedial scrotal wall. This broad attachment prevents the testis from twisting. The surface area of this attachment can be variable depending upon the degree to which the tunica vaginalis invests the testis. The tunica vaginalis can undermine the support structures and epididymis to a degree that only a thin stalk remains allowing the passage of vessels and

other support structures. This anomalous condition, called the "bell-clapper" deformity, predisposes the affected testis to twist and strangulate. When the testis rotates upon its stalk, the veins become occluded. The intratesticular veins dilate and the testis swells. When intratesticular pressure exceeds arterial pressure, blood flow ceases and the testis undergoes hemorrhagic necrosis. The bell-clapper deformity is thought to occur bilaterally in a large percentage of patients who present with torsion, since subsequent contralateral torsion, if the condition is not corrected, has been observed in as many as 40 per cent in one series.[17]

Spermatic cord torsion typically occurs in the teens and twenties and affects 1 in 4000 males younger than 25 years.[17] The classic presentation is waking up with testicular pain radiating to the abdomen and/or groin which gradually worsens. Torsion may, however, present with acute onset of pain that can be so severe as to cause nausea and vomiting.[18] The affected hemiscrotum appears indurated, enlarged, and tender, mimicking epididymitis and leading to clinical misdiagnosis in a large percentage of cases. If torsion is suspected, immediate surgery is required, since salvage of testicular function decreases with time. While nearly all testes can be salvaged if ischemic for 5 hours or less, the salvage rate decreases to 20 per cent if surgery is done at or beyond 12 hours.[19] When patients present in the subacute phase (24 hours or later), surgery is still required to remove the twisted testis and fix the contralateral testis to the scrotum. The twisted testis should be removed to establish the diagnosis, to stop the pain which would otherwise last for 3 to 4 weeks, and to prevent the development of infertility in the contralateral testis due to the possible development of antisperm antibodies, although the latter is controversial.[20, 21] The contralateral orchiopexy is necessary since it prevents the remaining testis from twisting, rendering the patient infertile, and since the bell-clapper deformity is bilateral in a significant percentage of patients.[17]

We have imaged six patients with subacute torsion 5 to 30 days following their events. They presented several characteristic findings, three of which have been specific for torsion, allowing the prospective differentiation of torsion from epididymitis with 100 per cent accuracy in this small series.[22]

FIGURE 34–21. Five-day-old torsion. A, B, and D are hydrogen density–weighted coronal images. C is a T$_1$-weighted axial image. E is a T$_2$-weighted coronal image (second echo of [D]). This case demonstrates all the constellation of findings seen in torsion: (1) Torsion knot (A) (arrow) is a dark region that represents the point of twist. It is thought to be due to the wringing out of water from the cord at the point of twist. (2) "Whirlpool" pattern (B) (small arrows) represents the twisted fascial planes of the cord emanating from the point of twist seen just anterior to (A). (3) The swollen hypovascular cord (B) (large white arrows) compared with the normal contralateral cord seen on (D) (arrow). (4) The "bell clapper" deformity seen because of the hematocele (C) highlighting the stalk (arrow), proven surgically, perpendicular to which images A and B were obtained (dashed line is level of image A). (5) The hematocele (h) is seen as bright fluid on T$_1$ weighting (C), on hydrogen density (A, B, and D), and on T$_2$ weighting (E). (6) The enlarged hemorrhagic epididymis (E) is shown on coronal images obtained with hydrogen density (D) and T$_2$ weighting (E). (7) The superior and transverse position of the epididymis (D and E). (8) The testis with overall signal loss (D and E). Note that the intratesticular changes are oriented in the direction of the interlobular septae emanating from the region of the mediastinum (E) (arrows). (From Trambert MA, Mattrey RF, Levine D, Berthoty D: The role of MRI in subacute scrotal pain: Torsion versus epididymitis. Radiology [in press]; with permission.)

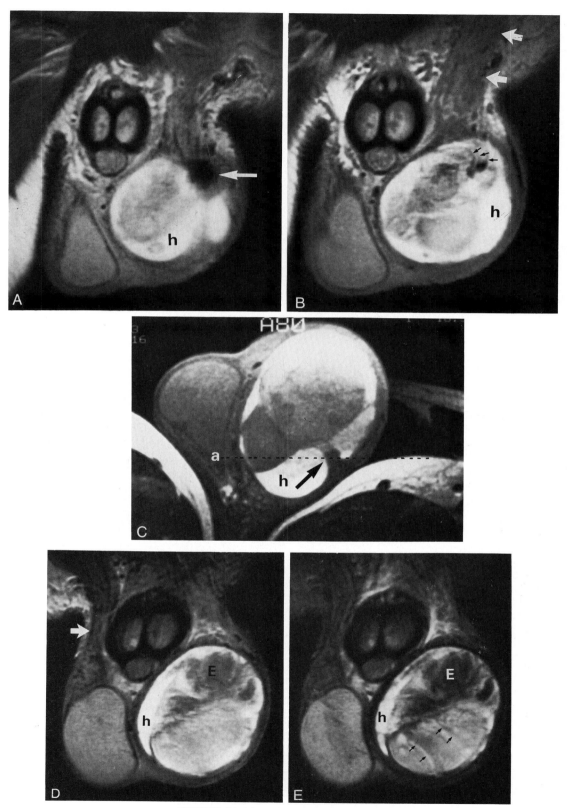

FIGURE 34–21 *See legend on opposite page*

The first finding is the appearance of the point of twist itself. The twisted stalk, which contains vessels, lymphatics, tubules, and fat, is usually near the posterosuperior aspect of the scrotum. The point of twist is very dark, presumably due to the water being squeezed out of the tissues, similar to the wringing of a wet towel (Figs. 34–21, 34–22, and 34–23). From this dark point (point of twist) emanates several curvilinear dark lines, presumably representing the spiraling fascial planes, resembling a whirlpool. To best demonstrate the point of twist, the stalk must be imaged perpendicular to its axis. In one series, the whirlpool sign was clearly seen in three of the six cases. The absence of this sign in the other three is presumably due to a suboptimal imaging plane. In an experiment conducted in rats with surgically in-

duced unilateral torsion, the whirlpool sign was the single most accurate finding, allowing the distinction of torsion in all twisted testes from sham controls.[23] In the rat study, the whirlpool sign was seen in one of the sham controls, presumably due to the surgical manipulation in these small animals, and disappeared two weeks after torsion due to necrosis and resorption of tissues.[23] In man the whirlpool pattern was seen in a patient in whom the acute episode occurred approximately three weeks prior to imaging.

The second finding is the appearance of the testis and epididymis. In all cases, the epididymis was markedly thickened with areas of swelling and subacute hemorrhage (intermediate signal intensity on hydrogen density and darker on T_2-weighted images) (Figs. 34–21 and 34–22). The epididymis was in an

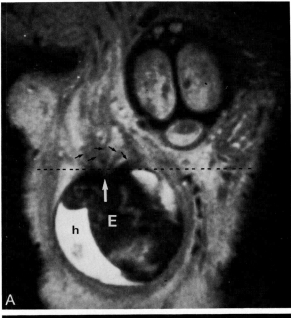

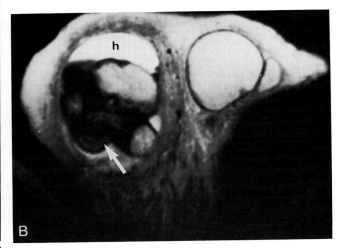

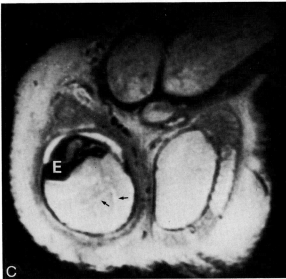

FIGURE 34–22. Three-day-old torsion demonstrating the torsion knot and "whirlpool" pattern on a T_2-weighted coronal image (A) (arrow). Transverse view obtained at the level of the dashed lines showed the spirals (B). Note the convergence of the fascial planes of the swollen hypovascular cord (small arrows) toward the point of twist (arrow in [A]). A and C, also T_2-weighted coronal images, show the hemorrhagic black epididymis (E). Note the mild loss of testicular signal and the appearance of the white branching lines (arrows in [C]), possibly representing thrombosed intratesticular vessels. Also note the presence of a hematocele (h). The hematocele was also bright on hydrogen density (not shown). (From Trambert MA, Mattrey RF, Levine D, Berthoty D: The role of MRI in subacute scrotal pain: Torsion versus epididymitis. Radiology [in press]; with permission).

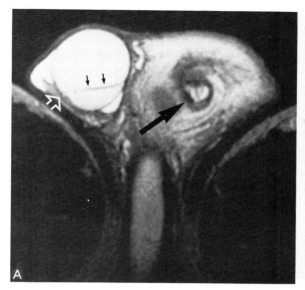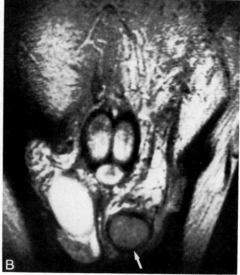

FIGURE 34–23. A "whirlpool" pattern was seen in this 3-week-old torsion on a transverse T_2-weighted image *(A)*. Note the thickened hypovascular cord seen on a coronal T_2-weighted image *(B)*. Also note the testicular changes *(arrow)* seen three weeks following torsion on the T_2-weighted *(B)* image. There is loss of testicular volume, thickening of the tunica albuginea, and complete darkening of the testis with no remaining normal testicular tissue. A thick septum *(small arrows)* is seen emanating from the mediastinum *(open arrow)* of the normal contralateral testis *(A)*. This septum is seen in a small percentage of normal testes.

abnormal position in most patients (superoanterior and in a transverse orientation rather than postero-medial and longitudinal). The position of the epidid-ymis was, however, not specific, especially since this orientation can be altered by patient positioning. The testis in the subacute phase (greater than 5 days) was slightly smaller than the contralateral testis (Figs. 34–21, 34–22, and 34–23). Its signal was generally di-minished and inhomogeneous. The inhomogeneity was due to linear bands of slightly diminished signals separated by thin lines of increased signal emanating from the mediastinum testis, possibly representing the affected lobules (Fig. 34–21). In some cases branching lines of higher signal than background could be seen, possibly representing thrombosed ves-sels (Fig. 34–22). A finding seen in some cases was thickening of the tunica albuginea. This is possibly related to the fact that the testis had lost volume, since these patients were imaged in the subacute setting. When imaged beyond three weeks from the episode, the loss of testicular volume and tunical thickening become striking (Fig. 34–23). Of interest, the testis becomes exceedingly dark on T_2-weighted images probably due to the hemorrhagic necrosis leaving behind significant accumulation of hemosid-erin and fibrosis. The entire testis becomes dark with no residual normal signal, unlike the dark signal of testicular masses leaving residual normal tissue (Fig. 34–23). The combination of tunical thickening, loss of testicular volume, and loss of signal of the entire testis is characteristic of old torsion.

The third finding is the appearance of the proxi-mal cord, which was thickened in all cases. All cords had absent or diminished vascularity (Figs. 34–21, 34–22, and 34–23). This is in contradistinction to the hypervascular cord associated with epididymitis (see Figs. 34–12 and 34–16). If the marked swelling and hemorrhage of the epididymis was due to infection, the infection would have to be severe to account for the epididymal changes. Severe infection should pro-duce marked hypervascularity. It is the discrepancy between epididymal and spermatic cord changes which is so striking in torsion.

Other associated findings that are helpful include a hematocele, which may be seen in torsion (Figs. 34–21 and 34–22), in lieu of a hydrocele, which was present in epididymitis. When these fluid collections are large, they could demonstrate the bell-clapper deformity (Fig. 34–21) or the testicular bare area (see Fig. 34–2), ruling in or out testicular torsion.

At this time with the high competition for MR time and limited accessibility, MRI is not advocated in the acute setting where delay in surgery is not appropri-ate. In the acute setting, the combination of sonog-raphy and scintigraphy is the most accurate.[24] MRI is, however, indicated in the subacute setting (greater than 24 hours) where it is very accurate.[22] Because of the hyperemic response in torsion, scintigraphy is less specific. MRI can confirm the diagnosis of torsion and differentiate torsion from epididymitis, which is the typical clinical question, one to two days after the episode. MRI should be able to diagnose torsion in the acute setting. Findings should be similar to those described above except the epididymal and testicular changes may be less severe. However, when P-31 testicular spectroscopy is performed, the absence of high energy phosphates should be diagnostic without exception.[25]

Extravaginal Torsion

Torsion in this setting is a spontaneous event that occurs perinatally. It occurs during testicular descent and involves the testis, its support structures, and the vaginal process.[17] The twisted vaginal process in the inguinal or spermatic canal can mimic strangulated intestinal hernia. Whereas the clinical presentation is clear in many cases, at times imaging is required to confirm the diagnosis. This condition is generally not treated surgically, since it is discovered too late to preserve testicular function, and is not associated with developmental anomaly such as the bell-clapper deformity to mandate contralateral orchiopexy.[17] Patients are usually followed until the testis is no longer palpable, usually for four to six months. If the testis does not regress, imaging or exploration is performed to exclude tumor.

We have imaged three infants with this condition, all of whom were late in their course. All testes were small, dark, and associated with thickened tunica albuginea, similar to changes seen in chronic torsion of adult males (Fig. 34–24). As in the adult, the entire testis was dark without any spared areas.

Torsion of Testicular Appendix

Testicular appendices can be found anywhere along the surface of the testis but are typically near the testicular poles.[17] They are located outside the tunica albuginea of the normal testis and have their own tunical covering. Like the normal testis, they are covered by the tunica vaginalis. They are therefore sandwiched between the tunica albuginea of the normal testis and the tunica vaginalis. When twisted, they instigate an inflammatory-like response in the epididymis and testis and can cause a sympathetic simple hydrocele. Torsion of the appendix is difficult to diagnose on imaging studies. Nuclear medicine techniques are rendered nonspecific secondary to the sympathetic epididymal reaction and the preserved normal flow to the testis.[26] They can, however, in the early stages exclude testicular torsion. Sonography can diagnose torsion of the appendix but is generally nonspecific.[24]

We have imaged one child with torsion of the appendix proven clinically and on follow-up (Fig. 34–25). The twisted appendix was hemorrhagic and was no longer present on follow-up MRI six weeks later. The images were sufficiently characteristic to exclude testicular torsion and allowed for conservative management. Surgery in this condition is performed to exclude testicular torsion when the diagnosis is not clear.[17]

Torsion of Epididymal Appendix

This anomaly is present in 30 to 40 per cent of males and rarely causes any symptoms.[17] These appendices can torse, producing acute hemiscrotal hydrocele and pain. While they can be visualized on ultrasound, other causes of pain or hydrocele cannot be excluded. On MRI, they appear spherical, are attached to the epididymis, and are filled with blood (see Fig. 34–2). The blood signal is commensurate with the time interval since the episode. In this setting, MRI can exclude with confidence testicular torsion, infection, or hemorrhage within a tumor,

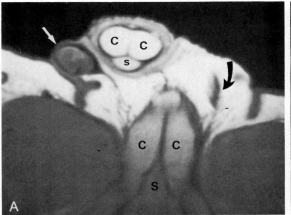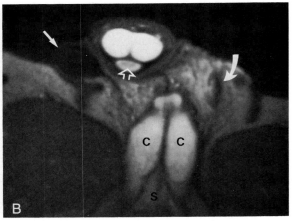

FIGURE 34–24. Axial hydrogen density *(A)* and T_2-weighted *(B)* images obtained in a 6-month-old infant with neonatal extravaginal torsion at the level of the affected testis *(arrow)*. Note the loss of testicular volume, the thickened tunica albuginea, and the complete darkening of the testis with no remaining normal testicular tissue, similar to the testis seen in Figure 34–23B. Also note that the testis is located in the spermatic canal at the level of the normal contralateral cord *(curved arrow)*. The penile anatomy is well seen: corpora cavernosa (C) and spongiosa (S) are bright on both images and are surrounded by the tunica albuginea of the penis. Note that the urethra is better seen on the T_2-weighted image *(open arrow)*. The lesser signal of the corpora at the base of the penis is due to increased distance from the surface coil.

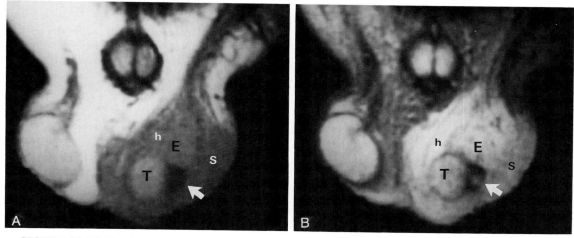

FIGURE 34–25. Torsion of the testicular appendix in a prepubertal boy shown on coronal hydrogen density *(A)* and T$_2$-weighted (B) images. Note the darkened testicular appendix *(arrow)* located between the slightly darkened testis (T) and the swollen epididymis (E). Also note the associated hemiscrotal swelling (s) and hydrocele (h). Because of MRI findings, the patient was treated conservatively. A repeat MR image 6 weeks later was normal (not shown). (From Semba et al, AJR [in press]; with permission.)

the three clinical conditions that can present with similar signs and symptoms.

EXTRATESTICULAR LESIONS

Spermatocele

On MRI, spermatoceles are easily identified within the epididymis, with the most frequent site of involvement being the globus major (head). They are round, well-circumscribed structures displaying signal intensity similar to that of hydrocele fluid (see Figs. 34–5

and 34–9). In a minority of cases, the spermatocele is brighter than water on hydrogen density–weighted images and remains bright on T$_2$-weighted images (see Fig. 34–16). We are uncertain whether the contents are old blood or high proteinaceous fluid. Indeed, the signal within these lesions reflects their contents (Fig. 34–26).

Hydrocele

Simple hydrocele has typical water signal characteristics on MRI which are intermediate on hydrogen density and high on T$_2$-weighted images relative to

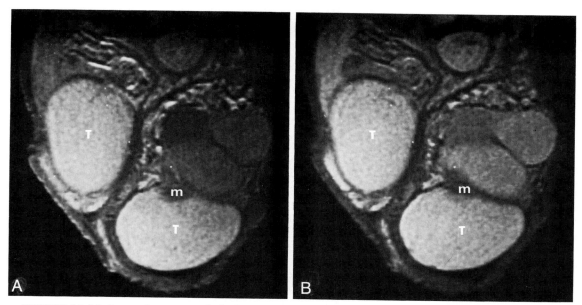

FIGURE 34–26. Septated spermatocele is shown on hydrogen density *(A)* and T$_2$-weighted *(B)* images. Note the rotation of the testis (T) by the multilocular spermatocele in the upper half of the epididymis (spermatocele reaches the mediastinum testis [m]). Also note the variable signals of each of the locules.

fat (see Fig. 34–2). Complicated hydroceles will demonstrate signals characteristic of their contents (see Figs. 34–21 and 34–22).

Varicocele

MRI clearly shows the entire spermatic cord from the inguinal ring to the mediastinum testis. Patients with varicocele had widening of the spermatic canal and prominence of the intrascrotal spermatic cord (see Fig. 34–18). The spermatic cord was more heterogeneous with greater number of serpiginous structures that had increased signal due to phase shift artifact from slow blood flow in these vessels. This was observed on both hydrogen density and T$_2$-weighted images. An insufficient number of patients have been studied with this condition to ascertain the role of MRI in this setting. In a prepubertal boy with varicocele, vessels with flow void in the cord as well as prominence of the distal cord at the base of the scrotum were evident (Fig. 34–27). In a recent study, abdominal compression, similar to that applied during intravenous urography, exaggerated the appearance of vessels in the cord in patients with varicoceles.[27] The degree of hypervascularity is not prominent as is seen in epididymitis. While clinically palpable varicoceles are easily depicted on MRI, it is not clear at this time whether MRI will be able to diagnose subclinical varicoceles with sufficient accuracy.

UNDESCENDED TESTIS

Cryptorchidism represents the most common disorder of sexual differentiation in man. It occurs in 2.7 to 6 per cent of full-term male neonates, with 0.8 per cent prevalence at one year of age. Spontaneous descent is unlikely after the first year.[28–30] Because of a significantly increased risk of malignancy[31, 32] and impaired spermatogenic function in the contralateral descended testis,[33] many techniques have been developed to aid in the diagnosis and treatment of the cryptorchid testis so as to monitor the testis for neoplasia and to diminish the incidence of infertility.

An undescended testis may be either intraabdominal, intracanalicular, ectopic, atrophic, or congenitally absent. Undescended testes may be located anywhere from the renal hilum to the superior scrotum. They may also be found in an ectopic location such as the perineum or superficial abdominal wall. Testes located proximal to the external inguinal ring are usually impalpable, as may be small or atrophic testes located distal to the external inguinal ring.

Surgical treatment consists of orchiopexy of a normal testis in children or orchiectomy in postpubertal patients. The standard surgical treatment of an undescended testis involves division of an associated patent vaginal process and straightening of the cord vessels to achieve sufficient length for the testis to easily reach the caudal extent of the scrotum. An intraabdominal testis is usually associated with insufficient vessel length to allow for a standard procedure to be performed. These testes are treated by ligating the testicular vessels at a point proximal to their junction with the vas deferens and relying on collateral revascularization from the artery supplying the vas deferens. Testicular autotransplantation is sometimes performed to improve upon the 60 to 70 per cent viability rate of the standard procedure. Autotransplantation involves the anastomosis of the distal testicular artery stump to the deep inferior epigastric artery, requiring microvascular surgical technique and longer operative procedure.

Neonatal extravaginal torsion results in complete

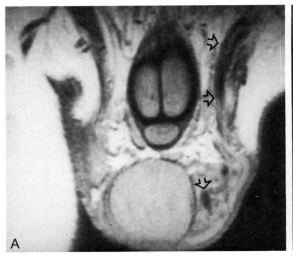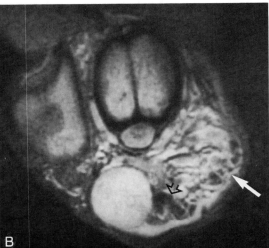

FIGURE 34–27. Left varicocele is seen on coronal hydrogen density *(A)* and T$_2$-weighted (B) images *(arrow)* obtained at different levels. Note the prominence of the cord at the base of the scrotum *(B) (arrow)* and the mild hypervascularity in the intracanalicular and intrascrotal cord *(A) (open arrows).*

replacement of testicular tissue with scar. If neonatal extravaginal torsion is missed at birth, the patient may present later in life with a nonpalpable undescended testis but possibly a palpable cord. Such a patient would require surgery for diagnosis. If the diagnosis of testicular atrophy could be reliably made preoperatively, surgery could be avoided or limited to those wanting prosthetic replacement.

Therefore, the adequate preoperative assessment and localization of the undescended testis are useful in guiding clinical management and surgical exploration, making a more limited operative procedure possible.

Various diagnostic modalities, such as ultrasound,[34, 35] computed tomography,[35–37] spermatic venography, and arteriography,[37–39] have been used to localize the cryptorchid testis. These modalities, however, have been accompanied by disadvantages such as invasiveness, technical difficulties, poor sensitivity and/or specificity, operator dependence, and exposure to ionizing radiation. Laparoscopy was introduced to evaluate the nonpalpable testis prior to exploration.[40] If testicular vessels and vas deferens end blindly in the abdomen, no exploration is performed. If tissue is present at the end of the vas deferens, exploration follows. However, if the vas deferens enters the internal inguinal ring, exploration of the inguinal canal is required to ensure the absence of testicular tissue. While laparoscopy is 100 per cent accurate in localizing the potential location of the testis and may obviate surgery in some patients, it is not useful if the cord enters the internal inguinal ring. Laparoscopy does not allow for preoperative planning. It also increases anesthesia and operating room time.

We have studied 35 patients with undescended testes at our institution. There were 48 total testes, with surgical proof available in 27 testes and clinical proof in 5.[44] MRI seems to be the most accurate noninvasive examination. These data are in concordance with other published reports.[41–43] The following discussion details the imaging technique used and presents the capabilities of MRI in this setting.

IMAGING TECHNIQUES

We use a high field system operated at 1.5 T. Lower fields could be used; however, thin slices, sufficient T_2 weighting, and adequate signal-to-noise ratio are required. Patients between 6 months and 6 years of age require sedation. Patients are placed directly in the head coil if they are small enough to fit. A standard 5-inch circular surface coil is centered approximately over the symphysis pubis to ensure that the base of the scrotum and lower pelvis are included in the field-of-view. The coil is placed on a 1-cm standoff to decrease the high near field signal. The diaper serves as a standoff in infants and toddlers. A 16-cm field-of-view, a 256×256 acquisition matrix, and a 3-mm slice thickness are used (voxel size = $0.63 \times 0.63 \times 3$ mm). In small infants, a 3-inch circular surface coil is used and the field of view is reduced to 12 cm while keeping other parameters constant.

Two series are sufficient in most cases, requiring a total examination time of 30 minutes. Keeping imaging time short is important since most cases require sedation. The first series is transaxial and is obtained with 3-, 5-, or 10-mm slice thickness and an interslice gap set at 50 per cent slice thickness. The TR and TE are set at 600/20. Slice thickness, gap, and TR are chosen relative to patient size to ensure that the imaging volume covers an area from the base of the scrotum to midbladder. This T_1-weighted series, which is obtained with two excitations and 256 phase encodes, requires approximately 5 minutes of data acquisition and serves to assess the entire spermatic cord to the level of the internal inguinal ring.

The axial series is then used to prescribe graphically the coronal multiecho and more time-consuming series, which covers the region from the posterior aspect of the scrotum to the anterior abdominal wall. Slice thickness for this series is set at 3 mm in all patients and is obtained with a 50 per cent interslice gap to ensure proper T_2 weighting. TR is set at 2000 msec, and the TEs are asymmetric and are set at 20 and 70 msec. All other parameters remain constant, resulting in an acquisition time of 17.5 minutes. This series allows further assessment of the cord within the spermatic canal and provides testicular tissue characterization. These two series are sufficient if the testes and cord are atrophic and are in the spermatic canal, or if the testis is located intracanalicular or more distal. This was true in 66 per cent of our cases. However, if testes are not seen or are intraabdominal, a third series is required.

If testes are seen and are intraabdominal in location near the internal inguinal ring, the third series is obtained in the transverse plane, utilizing the surface coil with all parameters unchanged from the coronal series except for a longer TR set at 3000 msec and one in lieu of two acquisitions requiring 13.5 minutes. This series helps to further characterize testicular tissue and to locate more precisely the position of the testis relative to the inguinal canal.

If, on the other hand, neither the cryptorchid testis nor its cord structures could be seen on the coronal series, the third series is obtained in the axial plane from the symphysis pubis to the upper pole of both kidneys utilizing either the head or body coil, dependent upon patient size. The pulsing sequence is set at TR = 2000 msec, TE = 20 and 70 msec, four excitations, 20 to 34 cm field-of-view, with either 10-mm slice thickness every 15 mm or 5-mm every 7.5 mm to ensure full coverage of the region of interest and proper T_2 weighting. This series obtained with a 256×128 matrix requires 17.5 minutes of data acquisition and allows the localization and characterization of the testis if present proximal to the internal inguinal ring.

MR data to be related to the surgeon should

describe the testis and the spermatic cord. If the testis is seen, its location, size, and signal behavior should be reported. If the testis is not visualized, the report should note whether the spermatic cord was visualized. If the spermatic cord is seen, then describe the location of its distal end, its thickness, and whether it enters the internal inguinal ring. These data allow the surgeon to assess whether surgery is necessary, to plan the surgical approach and treatment, and to determine if laparoscopy is required.

ROLE OF MRI IN CRYPTORCHIDISM

High-resolution MR imaging with surface coils clearly delineates the spermatic cord, inguinal canal, inguinal ring, pubic tubercle, testes, and regional lymph nodes.[6-10, 41-44] Both the coronal and axial planes are useful for imaging the spermatic cords. Undescended testes are best seen and recognized on coronal images.[41, 44] The axial plane provides an essential adjunct for more precisely locating the testis relative to the internal or external inguinal rings and femoral vessels and for increasing confidence. In most patients (23 of 34), two series (transaxial T_1 and coronal hydrogen density/T_2) were deemed sufficient for complete evaluation, requiring approximately 30 minutes of magnet time.[44] The remainder of cases required the transaxial multiecho long TR sequence since testes were intraabdominal or were not visualized on the previous series, increasing examination time by an additional 15 or 20 minutes.

The undescended testes in our series with surgical or clinical proof were found to be either intraabdominal in 19 per cent, intracanalicular in 37 per cent, or atrophic within the spermatic canal in 44 per cent. These relationships were nearly similar to the experience of others; however, they referred to the group with atrophic testes as absent.[42, 43] Four of the six intraabdominal testes were correctly located. Errors

made by others were also related to testes in intraabdominal locations.[42, 43] We believe that these errors should be avoidable with added experience. The overall accuracy of MRI in our prospective series was 93.8 per cent (30 of 32 testes),[44] which is comparable to previously published reports of 94 per cent (15 of 16)[42] and 93 per cent (retrospective data) (13 of 14).[43] Accuracy was lowest for intraabdominal testes.

Intraabdominal Testes

Intraabdominal testes located near or at the internal inguinal ring should be easily evaluated by MRI (Figs. 34–28 and 34–29). However, with lack of experience we missed two of six testes located near the internal inguinal ring which were easily seen in retrospect (Figs. 34–30 and 34–31). In both published reports each missed a high intraabdominal testis.[42, 43]

The task of locating intraabdominal testes is the most difficult on MRI. Confusion with lymph nodes and bowel higher in the abdomen becomes possible. With the advent of MR oral contrast and with added experience, this problem could be partially overcome. However, there will always be a degree of uncertainty when testes are not clearly depicted. In our series, there were six patients whose testes could not be localized. None of these six have had surgery to assess the role of MRI when testes are located proximal to the internal inguinal ring. Whereas it is important to visualize these high intraabdominal testes,[45] it is the author's belief that there will always be a degree of uncertainty concerning whether laparoscopy should precede exploration. Therefore, the inability to visualize the high intraabdominal testis is less critical for patient management, since patients with absent cord and testis would have to undergo surgical exploration that would be preceded by laparoscopy. When the testis, cord, or both are well evaluated, laparoscopy is not necessary. MRI in our

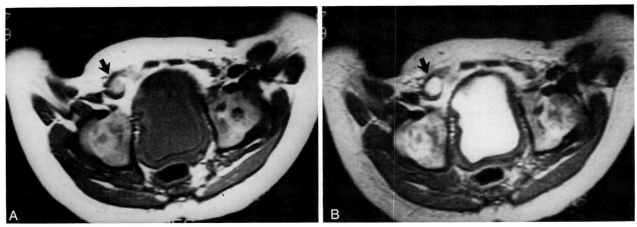

FIGURE 34–28. Right nonpalpable undescended testis located at the internal inguinal ring *(arrow)* shown on hydrogen density *(A)* and T_2-weighted *(B)* images. Note the normal testicular signal (intermediate on hydrogen density and bright on T_2 weighting).

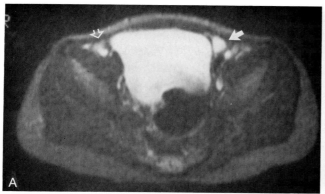
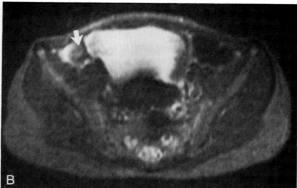

FIGURE 34–29. Bilaterally nonpalpable undescended testes shown on T_2-weighted images. The left testis is at the level of the internal inguinal ring *(arrow) (A)*. The left testis had normal signal, intermediate to bright on hydrogen density (not shown) and bright on T_2 weighting *(A)*. The bright area to the right of the bladder *(open arrow)* is not testis, since it was also bright on hydrogen density (not shown). The right testis *(arrow)* is best seen on the next cephalic slice near the level of the internal inguinal ring *(B)*. Note that testicular signal, while it was intermediate on hydrogen density (not shown), is dark on T_2 weighting *(B)*. Testicular biopsy showed normal left testis and moderately fibrotic right testis. (From Gylys-Morin VM, Landa HM, Mattrey RF, et al: MRI localization of the undescended testis and its potential impact on surgical management. AJR [submitted]; with permission.)

series could have potentially decreased laparoscopy from 100 per cent to only 13 per cent.

Assessment of the spermatic cord and testis together is essential for proper diagnosis. An empty spermatic canal is visible on MRI. It appears as a thin line extending from the inguinal canal to the base of the scrotum (Figs. 34–31 and 34–32) most likely representing the gubernaculum, which is a thin fi-

brous strand. This should not be mistaken for an atrophic cord. The latter has significant width but is thinner than the normal contralateral cord (Fig. 34–33). While an empty canal and an absent cord suggest the possibility of an intraabdominal testis, the presence of cord structures in the canal does not exclude this possibility (Fig. 34–31). Cord structures may precede the testis, or if attached to a long mesentery

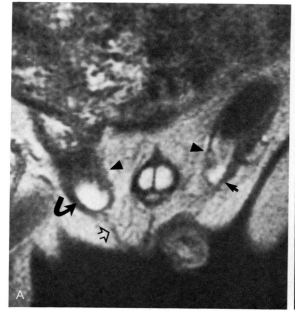
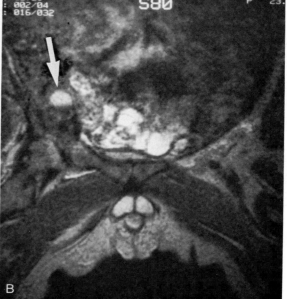

FIGURE 34–30. Newborn with bilateral hernias and bilateral undescended testes. The right and left hernia sacs shown on a T_2-weighted image *(A)* extend halfway into the spermatic canal *(arrowheads)*. Note that the gubernaculum continues into the base of the scrotum better seen on the right (open arrow). The right testis was thought to be at the distal end of the hernia sac *(curved arrow)*. This proved to be a loop of bowel at surgery. The right testis was located, in retrospect, 3 slices posterior to *(A)* in a typical intraabdominal location shown on a T_2-weighted image *(B) (arrow)*. The left testis was small and located at the distal end of its hernia sac *(A) (arrow)* proven surgically. (From Gylys-Morin VM, Landa HM, Mattrey RF, et al: MRI localization of the undescended testis and its potential impact on surgical management. AJR [submitted]; with permission.)

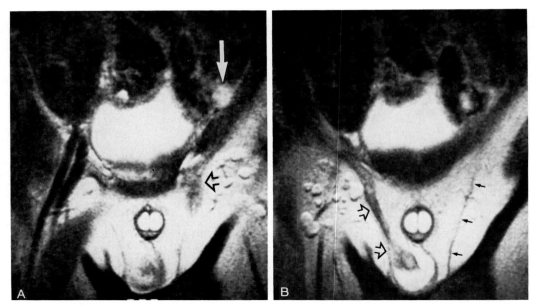

FIGURE 34–31. Left undescended and nonpalpable testis. *A,* A dark band thought to be a flattened end of the cord of an atrophic streak testis at the proximal spermatic canal is shown in a coronal plane on a T₂-weighted image *(open arrow). B,* The normal right cord and testis *(open arrows)* and the gubernaculum of the left testis *(small arrows)* are also shown on a T₂-weighted image. At surgery, the normal left undescended testis was intraabdominal, shown on *(A)* in a typical intraabdominal location just superior and lateral to the internal inguinal ring *(arrow),* clearly seen in retrospect. The dark region seen on MRI *(open arrow in A)* was cord structures preceding the testis. Note the presence of inguinal adenopathy lateral to the cords. (From Gylys-Morin VM, Landa HM, Mattrey RF, et al: MRI localization of the undescended testis and its potential impact on surgical management. AJR [submitted]; with permission.)

the testis may flip-flop between an intracanalicular and an intraabdominal location.

The majority of intraabdominal testes will be found near the internal inguinal ring where MRI should be reasonably accurate. Therefore, the goal of the imaging schemes should be to maximize the assessment of the internal inguinal ring. The technique described above would allow such assessment. The 5-

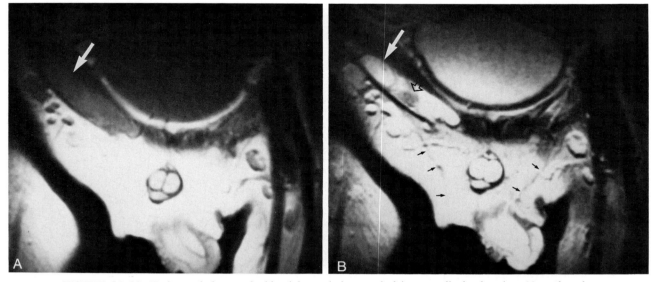

FIGURE 34–32. Undescended nonpalpable right testis in a typical intracanalicular location. Note that the testis has normal signal behavior when seen on hydrogen density *(A)* and T₂-weighted *(B)* images *(arrow)* and has an associated normal epididymis *(open arrow)* and ascites. In this location, fluid is technically ascitic since the vaginal process is patent. The other testis was intraabdominal (not shown here). Note the gubernaculum, best seen on the T₂-weighted image *(B),* bilaterally extends from the external inguinal ring to the base of the scrotum *(small arrows).* Note the presence of inguinal adenopathy lateral to the right and left canals. (From Gylys-Morin VM, Landa HM, Mattrey RF, et al: MRI localization of the undescended testis and its potential impact on surgical management. AJR [submitted]; with permission.)

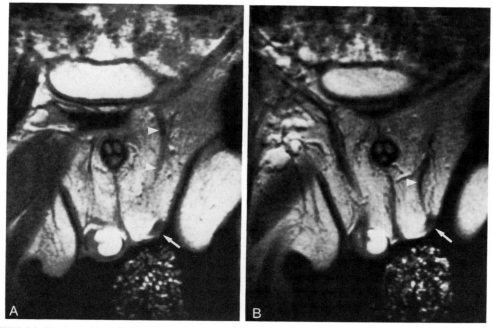

FIGURE 34–33. Atrophic left testis seen on T₂-weighted images *(A)* and *(B) (arrow)* on two coronal consecutive slices. Note the presence of an atrophic cord *(arrowheads)* that is thinner than the normal contralateral cord and thicker than the gubernaculum seen in Figure 34–31*B*. Also note that the atrophic cord reaches the base of the scrotum and does not end more proximal as is seen in Figure 34–31*A*. Note the presence of inguinal adenopathy lateral to the right cord. Heterogeneous signal seen below the scrotum is urine in a diaper. (From Gylys-Morin VM, Landa HM, Mattrey RF, et al: MRI localization of the undescended testis and its potential impact on surgical management. AJR [submitted]; with permission.)

inch surface coil should be centered over the pubic tubercle to place the testis at an optimal position in the field.

Intracanalicular Testes

MRI is extremely accurate in its ability to locate these testes. MR image interpretation is simple since these testes are contrasted with fat, are seen in association with intravaginal fluid in many cases, and are seen with their epididymis (Fig. 34–32). The testis has a normal ovoid shape with clear demonstration of the tunica albuginea. These testes assume three positions. They are either in the subcutaneous space anterior to the external inguinal ring (Fig. 34–34), in the spermatic canal, or in the inguinal canal (Fig. 34–32). When testes do not exit the inguinal canal, they frequently proceed laterally and insinuate themselves over the femoral vessels. In this location, they are frequently nonpalpable.

Intracanalicular testes are easily differentiated from lymph nodes, since their tunica albuginea can be discerned, they are associated with cord structures or epididymis, they are surrounded by fluid, and they are located in the path of the spermatic cord on axial scans. Lymph nodes, while of similar signal behavior, present different morphology and are lateral to the cord (Figs. 34–31, 34–32, and 34–34).

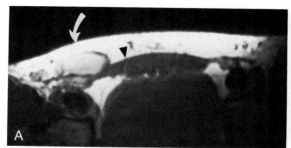
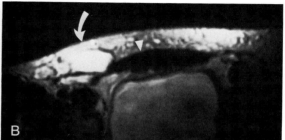

FIGURE 34–34. Undescended palpable right testis in a typical high spermatic canal location. Note that the testis *(curved arrow)* seen on hydrogen density *(A)* and T₂-weighted image *(B)* is external to the rectus muscle *(arrowheads)*. (From Landa HM, Gylys-Morin V, Mattrey RF, et al: MRI of the cryptorchid testis. Eur J Pediatr 146[Suppl]:S16–17, 1987; with permission.)

Testicular Atrophy

Testicular atrophy, most likely related to missed extravaginal torsion, is easily diagnosed. This non-invasive diagnosis, only possible with MRI, has far reaching clinical implication. This diagnosis must be reserved for those cases with an atrophic cord that reaches the base of the empty scrotum (Fig. 34–33). This finding has been specific for testicular atrophy proven surgically in nine of nine cases. Given the reliability of the MR diagnosis and given the proper clinical setting, the remaining cases with atrophy diagnosed by MRI in our series are being followed clinically.[44] Surgical resection to eliminate the potential for malignant degeneration is not required in these cases since viable testicular tissue is no longer present. If further clinical experience shows that MRI can indeed diagnose this entity with no false positives, surgical exploration in this subset of patients could be eliminated. This ability would have eliminated exploration in 14 of 35 cases in our series (40 per cent).

DIFFERENTIAL DIAGNOSIS

We have had limited experience to date to be able to extract sufficient differentiating features of each entity to truly assess the specificity of the findings observed on MR images. However, even with this limited experience, certain conditions have presented with such consistent constellation of findings that we believe MRI can at this time be used to differentiate them. MRI can distinguish torsion from epididymitis with very high accuracy, a diagnosis difficult to make 24 to 48 hours after the onset of pain by other methods. MRI can probably differentiate most tumors from infection. Indeed, in the acute scrotum, which can be caused by torsion, epididymitis, or tumor, MRI may prove to be the most specific of all scrotal imaging modalities. As experience increases, refinement would be possible and the efficacy of MRI in scrotal imaging will become better defined.

Tumor Versus Infection

It is possible at this time to distinguish most tumors from other intratesticular lesions. To diagnose disease one cannot rely solely on intratesticular signal intensity changes.[10] Signal changes allow the detection of disease, but these changes must be assessed in conjunction with clinical data and other associated changes. Tumors are generally well defined, and nonseminomatous lesions have a tumor capsule that defines their perimeter.

The differential diagnosis of intrinsic abnormalities includes tumor, infection, hemorrhage, fibrosis, or infarction. Infection of the testis is secondary to epididymitis, which has specific characteristic MR changes. Infection within the testis is poorly marginated, patchy in appearance, and does not produce mass effect. Though tumors may be poorly defined, patchy, and without mass effect, this pattern has not been seen in the 16 proven cases in our experience or in those reported by others.[8–10] It must be the unusual presentation. Furthermore, the associated epididymal changes and clinical setting would sway the diagnosis toward infection.

Hemorrhage within the testis on the basis of trauma is generally well marginated, homogeneous in signal within each intratesticular collection, and with signals characteristic of hemorrhage. Furthermore, hemorrhage in the setting of trauma would likely occur with other associated changes in the epididymis or possibly with hematocele. Nonseminomatous lesions are the only lesions that could possibly mimic trauma given their overall signal, which is comparable to normal testis, and their petechial hemorrhages. However, these lesions have a fibrous capsule, have an inhomogeneous background of high signal, and have patches of hemorrhage of various ages. Trauma, causing intratesticular hemorrhage that could potentially be confused with tumors, would have to be acute, making it easy to extract appropriate clinical history. If there is suspicion of underlying malignancy, follow-up scans should clarify the pathologic process.

Although fibrosis and focal infarction can in theory mimic lesions, we have not had sufficient experience with these entities to know whether they could be differentiated from mass lesions. However, in the setting of old torsion, the testis is small, diffusely dark, and has a thick tunical layer. Tumors, which may be dark, have left a small rim of unaffected normal testicular tissue and have not been associated with a thickened tunica.

Torsion Versus Infection

It is in this setting that MRI is clearly superior to any other imaging modality. The three characteristic findings of torsion described above (whirlpool pattern, hypovascular thick cord, and testicular and epididymal changes) have allowed us to differentiate epididymitis from torsion in 13 cases with 100 per cent accuracy.[22] While the combination of nuclear scanning and ultrasound is effective in differentiating these conditions acutely,[24] they are not as helpful in the subacute setting, where the hyperemic response and epididymal changes can mimic epididymitis.

CONCLUSION

MRI adds a new dimension to the assessment of scrotal disease. It demonstrates exquisite anatomic detail of the entire scrotum and inguinal region. It allows the recognition of each intrascrotal structure on the basis of its characteristic appearance and signal rather than strictly on the basis of its anatomic location. The interpretation of MR images is less subjective and less misleading than ultrasound, particularly when the normal relationship of scrotal contents is disturbed. Being less subjective, it is our belief that MRI is sufficiently specific to allow differentiation of the various pathologic processes, though this hypothesis requires proof. It also appears that MRI may be the most accurate noninvasive tool in localizing and guiding the management of patients with nonpalpable testes. In this setting, it can significantly decrease the number of laparoscopies performed and potentially eliminate the need for surgery in as many as 40 per cent of cases.[44]

REFERENCES

1. Leopold GR, Woo VL, Scheible FW, et al: High resolution ultrasonography of scrotal pathology. Radiology 131:719–722, 1979.
2. Leopold GR: Superficial organs. In Goldberg B (ed): Ultrasound in Cancer. New York, Churchill-Livingstone, 1981, pp 123–135.
3. Hricak H, Filly RA: Sonography of the scrotum. Invest Radiol 18:112–121, 1983.
4. Glazer HS, Lee JKT, Melson GL, McClennan BL: Sonographic detection of occult testicular neoplasms. AJR 138:673–675, 1982.
5. Carroll BA, Gross DM: High frequency scrotal sonography. AJR 140:511–515, 1983.
6. Baker LL, Hajek PC, Burkhard TK, et al: Magnetic resonance imaging of the scrotum: Normal anatomy. Radiology 163:89–92, 1987.
7. Baker LL, Hajek PC, Burkhard TK, et al: Magnetic resonance imaging of the scrotum: Pathologic conditions. Radiology 163:93–98, 1987.
8. Rholl KS, Lee JKT, Ling D, et al: MR imaging of the scrotum with a high resolution surface coil. Radiology 163:99–103, 1987.
9. Seidenwurm D, Smathers RL, Lo RK, et al: Testes and scrotum: MR imaging at 1.5T. Radiology 164:393–398, 1987.
10. Thurnher S, Hricak H, Carroll PR, et al: Imaging the testis: Comparison between MR imaging and US. Radiology 167:631–636, 1988.
11. Johnson JO, Mattrey RF, Philpson J: Differentiation of seminomatous from nonseminomatous testicular tumors with MR imaging. AJR (in press).
12. Morse MJ, Whitmore WF: Neoplasms of the testes. In Walsh PC, Gittes RF, Perlmutter AD, Stamey TA (eds): Campbell's Urology. Philadelphia, WB Saunders Company, 1986, pp 1535–1582.
13. Sokal M, Peckham MJ, Hendry WF: Bilateral germ cell tumours of the testis. Br J Urol 53:158, 1980.
14. Schwerk WB, Schwerk WN, Rodeck G: Testicular tumors: Prospective analysis of real-time ultrasound patterns and abdominal staging. Radiology 164:369–374, 1987.
15. Lupetin AR, King W III, Rich P, Lederman RB: Ultrasound diagnosis of testicular leukemia. Radiology 146:171–172, 1983.
16. Bird K, Rosenfield AT: Testicular infarction secondary to acute inflammatory disease: Demonstration by B-scan ultrasound. Radiology 152:785–788, 1984.
17. Gullenwater JY, Grayhack JT, Howards SS, Duckett JW: Adult and Pediatric Urology. Chicago, Year Book Medical Publishers, 1987, pp 1955–1962.
18. Finkelstein MS, Rosenberg HK, Snyder HM III, Duckett JW: Ultrasound evaluation of scrotum in pediatrics. Urology 27:1–9, 1986.
19. Hricak H, Jeffrey RB: Sonography of acute scrotal abnormalities. Radiol Clin North Am 21:595–603, 1983.
20. Williamson RCN, Anderson JB: The fate of the human testes following unilateral torsion. Br J Urol 58:698–704, 1986.
21. Ryan PC, Whelan CA, Gaffney EF, Fitzpatrick JM: The effect of unilateral experimental testicular torsion on spermatogenesis and fertility. Br J Urol 62:359–366, 1988.
22. Trambert MA, Mattrey RF, Levine D, Berthoty D: The role of MRI in subacute scrotal pain: Torsion versus epididymitis. Radiology (in press).
23. Landa HM, Gylys-Morin V, Mattrey RF, et al: Detection of testicular torsion by magnetic resonance imaging in a rat model. J Urol 140:1178–1180, 1988.
24. Mueller DL, Amundson GM, Rubin SZ, Wesenberg RL: Acute scrotal abnormalities in children: Diagnosis by combined sonography and scintigraphy. AJR 150:643–646, 1988.
25. Bretan PN Jr, Vigneron DB, Hricak H, et al: Assessment of testicular metabolic integrity with P-31 MR spectroscopy. Radiology 162:867–871, 1987.
26. Fischman AJ, Palmer EL, Scott JA: Radionuclide imaging of sequential torsions of the appendix testis. J Nucl Med 28:119–121, 1987.
27. Ziffer JA, Nelson RC, Chezmar JL, et al: Subclinical varicoceles: Detection with MRI. Presented at SMRI 1989, Los Angeles. Mag Res Imaging (abstr) 7(Suppl):78, 1989.
28. Scorer CG, Farrington GH: Congenital Deformities of the Testis and Epididymis. New York, Appleton-Century-Crofts, 1972.
29. Cour-Palar IJ: Spontaneous descent of the testicle. Lancet 1:403, 1966.
30. Hadziselimovic F: Cryptorchidism. Berlin, Springer-Verlag, 1983.
31. Batata MA, Whitmore WF Jr, Hilaris BS, et al: Cryptorchidism and testicular cancer. J Urol 124:382, 1980.
32. Pinch L, Aceto T Jr, Meyer-Bahlburg HFL: Cryptorchidism. A pediatric review. Urol Clin North Am 1:573–592, 1974.
33. Rajfer J: The testis and epididymis: Cryptorchidism. In Kaufmann JJ (ed): Current Urologic Therapy. Philadelphia, WB Saunders Company, 1986, pp 422–423.
34. Weiss RM, Carter AR, Rosenfield AT: High resolution real-time ultrasonography in the localization of the undescended testis. J Urol 135:936–938, 1986.
35. Wolverson MK, Houttin E, Heiberh E, et al: Comparison of CT with high resolution ultrasound in the localization of the undescended testis. Radiology 146:133–136, 1983.
36. Lee JKT, McClennan BL, Stanley RJ, Sagel SS: Utility of CT in the localization of the undescended testis. Radiology 135:121–125, 1980.
37. Green JR: Computerized axial tomography vs. spermatic venography in localization of the cryptorchid testis. Urology 26:513–517, 1985.
38. Glickman MF, Weiss RM, Itzchak Y: Testicular venography for undescended testes. AJR 129:67–70, 1977.
39. Diamond AB, Meng CH, Kodroff M, Goldman SM: Testicular venography in the non-palpable testis. AJR 129:71–75, 1977.
40. Lowe DH, Brock WA, Kaplan GW: Laparoscopy for localization of the nonpalpable testis. J Urol 131:728–729, 1984.
41. Landa HM, Gylys-Morin V, Mattrey RF, et al: MRI of the cryptorchid testis. Eur J Pediatr 146[Suppl]:S16–17, 1987.
42. Fritzsche PJ, Hricak H, Kogan BA, et al: Undescended testis: Value of MRI. Radiology 164:169–173, 1987.
43. Kier R, McCarthy S, Rosenfield AT, et al: Nonpalpable testes in young boys: Evaluation with MR imaging. Radiology 169:429–433, 1988.
44. Gylys-Morin VM, Landa HM, Mattrey RF, et al: MRI localization of the undescended testis and its potential impact on surgical management. AJR (submitted).
45. Friedland GW, Chang P: The role of imaging in the management of impalpable undescended testis. AJR 151:1107–1111, 1988.

35

MR IMAGING OF DEVELOPMENTAL ABNORMALITIES OF THE FEMALE PELVIS

KATHRYN GRUMBACH and WARREN B. GEFTER

EMBRYOLOGY AND CLASSIFICATION

TECHNIQUE OF EXAMINATION

MR FINDINGS

CONCLUSION

Although congenital anomalies of the female genital tract are rare, occurring in as few as one in 5000 women, they are responsible for morbidity in the form of infertility in a significant number.[1] As many as 9 per cent of women undergoing evaluation for infertility will prove to have a congenital anomaly involving the uterus or vagina.[2] As increasing numbers of women are being examined for reproductive failure, it has become necessary to develop safe and accurate methods for diagnosing genital tract anomalies. MRI is ideally suited to this purpose in that it is noninvasive, it provides superior anatomic detail of the female pelvis, and it allows imaging in multiple scan planes.[3–5] Thus, reliance upon sonography, hysterosalpingography (HSG), and diagnostic laparoscopy for the diagnosis of these anomalies may soon become outdated. However, since the transition to MRI is still in process, this section will review not only the salient MR features, but also the major ultrasound and HSG findings in each class of congenital anomalies.

EMBRYOLOGY AND CLASSIFICATION

In the sixth week of fetal development, both male and female embryos have two paired sets of genital ducts: (1) the mesonephric or wolffian ducts, and (2) the paramesonephric or müllerian ducts. If the fetus is genetically female, the müllerian ductal system develops into the fallopian tubes, uterine corpus, and cervix, whereas the wolffian ducts disappear except for minimal remnants.[2, 6]

During the first month of embryogenesis, the paired müllerian ducts descend from a superolateral position in the fetal abdominal cavity to fuse medially in the pelvis. The cranial and lateral portions of the ducts remain open to the peritoneal cavity and will become the fimbriated ends of the fallopian tubes. By the ninth week of fetal development, the caudal ends of the müllerian ducts reach the posterior aspect of the urogenital sinus and begin to fuse with two solid invaginations of the urogenital sinus (the sinovaginal bulbs). This solid core of tissue forms the vaginal plate and begins to canalize by the eleventh gestational week to form the vagina and its fornices. Full canalization of the vagina is complete by the fifth month of development, with only a thin membrane (the hymen) remaining to separate the vaginal tube from the remainder of the urogenital sinus. The müllerian ducts fuse in the midline to form the uterine corpus and cervix with complete resorption of the sagittal uterine septum by the ninth week of embryogenesis.[2, 6]

Female pelvic congenital anomalies are classified according to the stage of development at which the abnormality occurs.[2, 6, 7] Anomalies that result from arrested müllerian duct development include uterine aplasia (absence of the uterus) when the process is bilateral and unicornuate uterus (a uterus with a single horn and fallopian tube) when the process is unilateral. Partial failure of müllerian duct fusion results in arcuate uterus, which is caused by failure of fusion in the uterine fundal region only. A bicornuate uterus (one vagina, one cervix, and two separate uterine cornua) occurs when the two cornua and a variable portion of the uterine corpus fail to fuse normally. When complete failure of fusion occurs along the entire caudal portion of the müllerian ducts, uterus didelphys (two vaginas, two cervices, and two uterine corpora) is the result. Malformations resulting from nonresorption of the sagittal uterine septum may be partial, as in uterus subseptus, or complete, as in uterus septus (septate uterus). The septum is composed of only fibrous tissue and contains no myometrium. Congenital anomalies of the female genital organs may also result from decrease in or lack of hormonal stimulation during fetal development. Infantile uterus, uterine hypoplasia, and a variety of abnormalities in uterine configuration, such as T-shaped uterus, may result. Also, exposure to exogenous hormones in utero, such as diethylstilbesterol (DES), leads to the development of uterine malformations in approximately 15 per cent of fetuses so exposed.

Congenital anomalies of the vagina occur in only 0.027 per cent of women but are important to recognize due to their association with sexual dysfunction.[8, 9] Partial vaginal agenesis is usually associated with a normal functioning uterus and cervix and most commonly involves the lower two thirds of the vagina, which is derived from the urogenital sinus. Complete agenesis consists of absence of all vaginal tissue and may or may not be associated with agenesis of the uterus and cervix. Finally, vaginal septation or duplication may be seen and is commonly associated with duplication anomalies of the uterus and cervix such as uterus didelphys. When obstruction to the flow of menstrual secretions occurs, due either to partial vaginal agenesis or vaginal anomaly associated with imperforate hymen, hematometrocolpos may result, and can be seen in association with urinary

tract and skeletal anomalies (Mayer-Rokitansky-Küster-Hauser syndrome).[10]

TECHNIQUE OF EXAMINATION

The optimal MR techniques for imaging the female pelvis have been discussed in detail in previous chapters. T_2-weighted spin-echo (SE) pulse sequences, which demonstrate uterine zonal anatomy, most clearly delineate anomalies such as bicornuate uterus.[3–5] On a 1.5-T system, pulse sequences with a TR of 2000 to 2500 msec and a TE of 80 msec are utilized; septate uterus, however, is best imaged on long-TR, intermediate-TE (35 msec) pulse sequences. Likewise, similar T_2-weighted SE sequences are ideal for visualization of the vagina and of anomalies such as vaginal duplication or agenesis. Axial and coronal scan planes are complementary for demonstration of uterine and vaginal morphology. Sagittal images, which are important in evaluating acquired lesions of the uterus and cervix, are of less value in studying uterine anomalies but may contribute additional information in the evaluation of vaginal anomalies. Sections 5 mm in thickness with a 2.5-mm gap are utilized. Air insufflation of the rectum in conjunction with intramuscular administration of 1 mg glucagon, moderate distention of the bladder, and prone positioning enhance the quality of pelvic images and can be useful in depicting the pelvic anatomy.

MR FINDINGS

Bicornuate uterus is probably the most commonly encountered anomaly of the uterus. It is important to distinguish bicornuate uterus from other uterine anomalies, particularly septate uterus (Fig. 35–1). Septate uterus is the uterine anomaly most frequently associated with reproductive failure, and it is repaired by a different surgical procedure than is bicornuate uterus. Uterus didelphys is rarely associated with pregnancy loss, and patients with this anomaly are not surgical candidates.[7] The typical HSG findings in bicornuate uterus include (1) separation of the uterine cornua with a wide intercornual angle, (2) fusiform shape of each uterine horn, (3) discrepancy in size of the two cornua, and (4) elongation and widening of the cervical canal and isthmus.[2] The bilobed external uterine contour typical of bicornuate uterus is not visible on HSG, and ultrasound, although not diagnostic in all cases, may be superior in demonstrating external morphology (Fig. 35–2).[3] Not only is the bilobed fundal contour of a bicornuate uterus well demonstrated on MRI,[11, 12] but also the signal intensity of the different uterine zones may be utilized to distinguish it from septate uterus.[3–5] In bi-

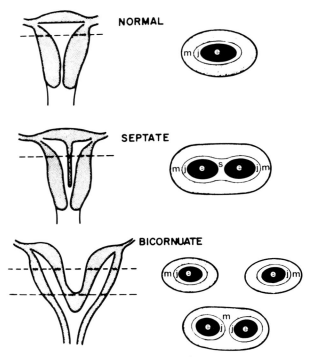

FIGURE 35–1. Schematic of coronal and axial sections of normal, septate, and bicornuate uteri. E = endometrial canal, j = junctional zone, m = myometrium, s = septum. (From Mintz MC, Thickman DI, Gussman D, Kressel HY: MR evaluation of uterine anomalies. AJR 148:287–290, 1987; © by American Roentgen Ray Society.)

cornuate uterus, the high signal–intensity endometrium is seen in each uterine horn surrounded by a low-signal junctional zone. The endometrial-junctional zone complexes of each horn are separated by a intermediate-signal band of myometrium. This is best demonstrated on transverse images (Figs. 35–1 and 35–3). On coronal images, the divergent endometrial cavities are seen to be most widely separated in the fundal region (Fig. 35–4A). Bicornuate uterus may be associated with a double cervix (uterus bicornis bicollis) and a septate vagina, which are also easily seen on MR. The fibrous band dividing the cervix or vagina appears low in signal intensity (Fig. 35–4B and C).

The HSG findings in complete or partial septate uterus are quite subtle and include a very acute angle between the two uterine cornua and functional interdependence of the two cavities in that they contract simultaneously.[2] The septum is generally quite thin and is usually impossible to resolve on ultrasound. Also in this anomaly the external uterine contour is normal, thus making ultrasound diagnosis difficult except during pregnancy. On T$_2$-weighted MR images, a uterine septum appears as a low-intensity zone separating the two endometrial cavities, and no low-signal junctional zone or intervening myometrium can be identified (Fig. 35–5). The fibrous composition of the septum is the primary factor contributing to its appearance on MR.[3–5] The septum

is very thin in complete septate uterus (Fig. 35–6), and it is thicker and forms a heart-shaped uterine cavity in uterus subseptus (Fig. 35–5B). Also, bicornuate uterus may occur with an inferior sagittal septum (Fig. 35–7), but this may be difficult to distinguish from bicornuate uterus alone, in which the junctional zones are in close proximity inferiorly.

Uterus didelphys consists of two separate uterine cavities, two cervices, and usually septate vagina. HSG requires injection of both cervices, and the typical findings are two entirely separate uterine cavities each arising from its own cervix.[2] The two uterine corpora may communicate at the base of the cornua forming an H-shaped uterus. On ultrasound it may be difficult to distinguish this anomaly from bicornuate uterus, as it may be impossible to distinguish two complete uterine corpora and cervices. On MRI the wide separation of the uterine cavities is clearly demonstrated, but a duplicated cervix may be difficult to distinguish from a low uterine septum. Correlation with pelvic examination findings, which should easily demonstrate two cervices, should allow a correct diagnosis to be made on MR.[3, 5]

Unicornuate uterus presents typical HSG findings of a solitary, fusiform uterine cavity that fails to taper

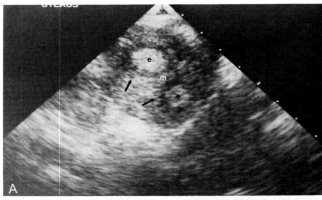

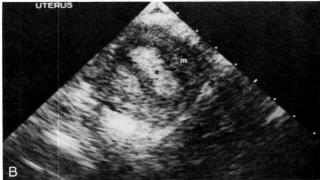

FIGURE 35–2. Ultrasound of a bicornuate uterus. *A,* Transverse sonogram through the fundus of a bicornuate uterus demonstrates the bilobed uterine contour and myometrium (m) intervening between the endometrial cavities of the two uterine cornua (e). Images were obtained using an endovaginal probe. *B,* At a more caudal level through the uterine corpus, the endometrial cavity (e) now has a bilobed shape and the myometrium (m) is a homogeneous, hypoechoic band surrounding the endometrium.

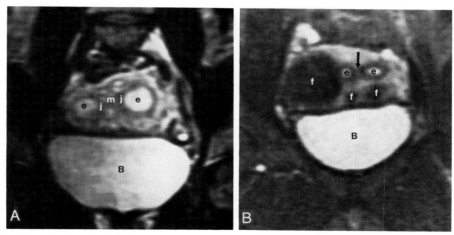

FIGURE 35–3. Bicornuate uteri. *A,* Coronal MR section (TR 2500 msec, TE 80 msec) showing a bicornuate uterus. The endometrial cavity (e) of each horn is separated by myometrium (m) of intermediate intensity. The junctional zones of the two cornua (j) are distinct and are low in signal intensity. B = bladder. *B,* Coronal MR image (TR 2500 msec, TE 80 msec) through a bicornuate uterus in another patient. Again the endometrial cavities (e) of the two cornua are distinct, with a small portion of myometrium *(arrow)* separating the two cavities. In addition, multiple low intensity masses (f) are seen within the myometrium, which proved to be fibroids. (From Mintz MC, Thickman DI, Gussman D, Kressel HY: MR evaluation of uterine anomalies. AJR 148:287–290, 1987; © by American Roentgen Ray Society.)

toward the uterine fundus and terminates in a single fallopian tube. The uterine cavity is laterally deviated in the pelvis.[2] Ultrasound often fails to demonstrate these findings. On MR, failure of a laterally deviated uterine cavity to taper as the scan plane approaches the fundus should suggest the diagnosis of unicornuate uterus (Fig. 35–8).[3, 4]

Arcuate uterus and hypoplastic uterus can also be distinguished on MR, although subtle abnormalities of cavitary shape, such as a T-shaped uterus, are best

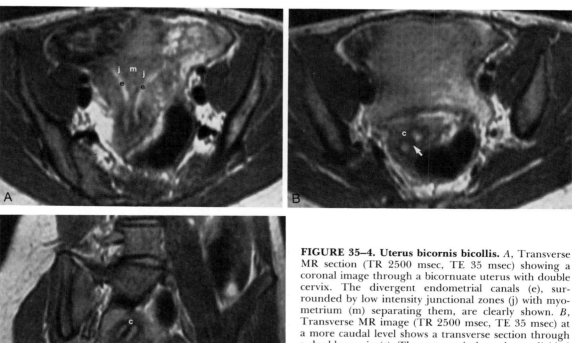

FIGURE 35–4. Uterus bicornis bicollis. *A,* Transverse MR section (TR 2500 msec, TE 35 msec) showing a coronal image through a bicornuate uterus with double cervix. The divergent endometrial canals (e), surrounded by low intensity junctional zones (j) with myometrium (m) separating them, are clearly shown. *B,* Transverse MR image (TR 2500 msec, TE 35 msec) at a more caudal level shows a transverse section through a double cervix (c). The two cervical canals are divided by a low intensity fibrous band *(arrow).* *C,* On a coronal MR image (TR 2500 msec, TE 40 msec), the double cervix (c) is again demonstrated just superior to the vagina demarcated by a tampon (t).

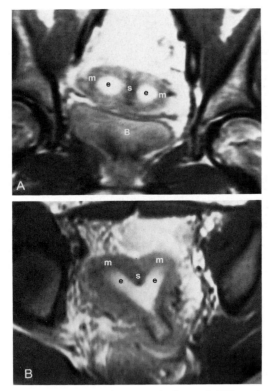

FIGURE 35–5. Uterus subseptus. *A*, Coronal MR section (TR 2000 msec, TE 35 msec) showing a transverse image through a septate uterus. The endometrial cavities (e) are separated by a low intensity septum (s) and no distinct junctional zones are detected. M = myometrium, B = bladder. *B*, Transverse MR section (TR 2000 msec, TE 35 msec) showing a coronal view of the uterus illustrating the heart-shaped endometrial cavity (e) caused by a partial sagittal septum (s). (*A* from Mintz MC, Thickman DI, Gussman D, Kressel HY: MR evaluation of uterine anomalies. AJR 148:287–290, 1987; © by American Roentgen Ray Society.)

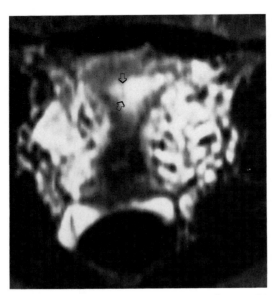

FIGURE 35–6. Septate uterus. Transverse MR image (TR 2500 msec, TE 30 msec) demonstrating a coronal section through the uterus. The complete sagittal septum *(arrows)* is very thin and divides the uterus into two endometrial cavities of unequal size.

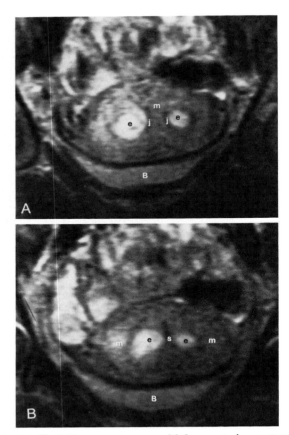

FIGURE 35–7. Bicornuate uterus with lower uterine septum. *A*, Coronal MR section (TR 2000 msec, TE 80 msec) through the uterine body reveals a typical configuration of bicornuate uterus. E = endometrium, j = junctional zone, m = myometrium, B = bladder. *B*, Coronal MR section (TR 2000 msec, TE 80 msec) through the lower uterine segment shows a septum (s) intervening between the two endometrial cavities (e). The septum is lower in signal intensity than is the surrounding myometrium (m). B = bladder. (From Mintz MC, Thickman DI, Gussman D, Kressel HY: MR evaluation of uterine anomalies. AJR 148:287–290, 1987; © by American Roentgen Ray Society.)

demonstrated on HSG.[2] Certainly, MR and ultrasound may be utilized to diagnose small uterine volumes as seen in DES-exposed women.[3]

Vaginal anomalies such as partial absence or septate vagina are not easily diagnosed on ultrasound or HSG, unless the vaginal pouch is distended with secretions or a water vaginogram is performed.[10] The easiest and least invasive method of studying vaginal anomalies is MR.[8, 9] In complete vaginal agenesis, no vaginal tissue can be seen between the rectum and urethra, and this is best demonstrated on T$_2$-weighted axial images of the perineum.[8] Partial vaginal agenesis usually affects only the lower two thirds and is commonly associated with a functioning uterus. In this case, hematometrocolpos may be seen after puberty, presenting as a uterus and upper vagina distended with high-intensity material on T$_1$-weighted and T$_2$-weighted images.[9] Also, in partial vaginal agenesis, the distance between the blind-

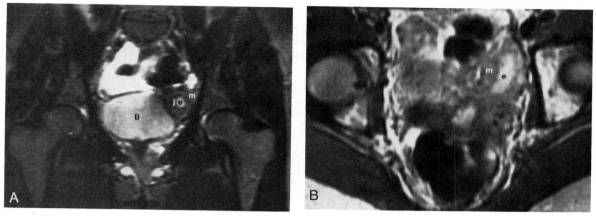

FIGURE 35–8. Unicornuate uterus. *A,* Coronal MR image (TR 2000 msec, TE 80 msec) shows a transverse section through a unicornuate uterus. Note that the uterine corpus is deviated far to the left side of the pelvis. E = endometrium, j = junctional zone, m = myometrium, B = bladder. *B,* Transverse MR view (TR 2000 msec, TE 80 msec) reveals the laterally deviated, fusiform-shaped uterine cavity. Note that the endometrial cavity (e) fails to taper toward the fundus. These findings are characteristic of unicornuate uterus. M = myometrium.

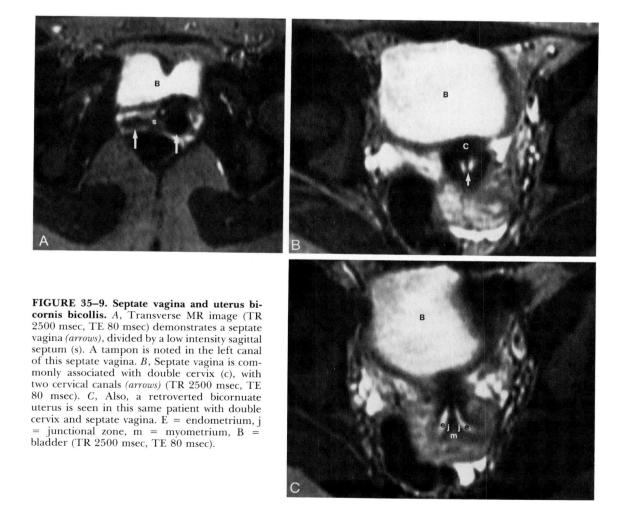

FIGURE 35–9. Septate vagina and uterus bicornis bicollis. *A,* Transverse MR image (TR 2500 msec, TE 80 msec) demonstrates a septate vagina *(arrows),* divided by a low intensity sagittal septum (s). A tampon is noted in the left canal of this septate vagina. *B,* Septate vagina is commonly associated with double cervix (c), with two cervical canals *(arrows)* (TR 2500 msec, TE 80 msec). *C,* Also, a retroverted bicornuate uterus is seen in this same patient with double cervix and septate vagina. E = endometrium, j = junctional zone, m = myometrium, B = bladder (TR 2500 msec, TE 80 msec).

ending vagina and the introitus can be measured on sagittal images to determine if vaginoplasty can be performed.[8] The presence or absence of a functioning uterus and cervix can also be readily identified on MR, and this will dictate whether hysterectomy must be performed to prevent endometriosis if normal egress of menstrual secretions cannot be established in complete vaginal agenesis.[9] Vaginal duplication or septation can also be demonstrated on MR as a low-intensity band dividing the vagina in the sagittal plane (Fig. 35–9). This anomaly almost always occurs with uterine and cervical duplication (uterus didelphys or uterus bicornis bicollis).[8] Optimal visualization of vaginal septae depends on axial sections and adequate vaginal distention, often with two tampons or water vaginography. Also, this anomaly may be associated with imperforate hymen and unilateral hydrometrocolpos, and a pelvic mass may be the result.

Finally, MRI provides a more global view of the abdomen than does HSG and may be used to diagnose associated urinary tract and skeletal anomalies without added cost or risk to the patient.[12] Approximately 20 to 25 per cent of patients with müllerian anomalies will have coexistent urinary tract anomalies such as unilateral renal agenesis, renal ectopia, or fusion abnormalities.[1] Skeletal anomalies, particularly of the spine, may also been seen as part of the Mayer-Rokitansky-Küster-Hauser syndrome.[10]

CONCLUSION

Congenital anomalies of the female genital tract may be classified by the stage of embryologic development at which the abnormality occurs. Although uncommon in the population as a whole, female pelvic anomalies are found in 9 per cent of women undergoing infertility evaluation. Traditionally, HSG, ultrasound, and laparoscopy have been important diagnostic tools for studying these abnormalities, but it is now clear that MRI provides detailed anatomic images in multiple scan planes and without the use of invasive techniques. The entire gamut of anomalies may be reliably imaged, from simple uterine, cervical, or vaginal agenesis to subtle anomalies of fusion or segmentation, such as bicornuate and septate uterus. MR images can be relied upon to supply sufficient information to guide surgical intervention, as in the cases of septate uterus or partial vaginal agenesis. Finally, MR can provide a global view of the abdomen and pelvis allowing accurate diagnosis of associated urinary tract or skeletal anomalies.

REFERENCES

1. Woolf RB, Allen WM: Concomitant malformations: The frequent simultaneous occurrence of congenital malformations of the reproductive and urinary tracts. Obstet Gynecol 2:236–265, 1953.
2. Zanetti E, Ferrari LR, Rossi G: Classification and radiographic features of uterine malformations: Hysterosalpingogram study. Br J Radiol 51:161–170, 1978.
3. Mintz MC, Grumbach K: Imaging of congenital uterine anomalies. Semin US, CT and MR 9(2):167–174, 1988.
4. Mintz MC, Thickman DI, Gussman D, Kressel HY: MR evaluation of uterine anomalies. AJR 148:287–290, 1987.
5. Hricak H, Chang YCF: The female pelvis. *In* Higgins CB, Hricak H (eds): Magnetic Resonance Imaging of the Body. New York, Raven Press, 1987, pp 403–431.
6. Langman J: Medical Embryology. Baltimore, Williams & Wilkins, 1975, pp 182–186.
7. Buttram VC, Gibbons WE: Müllerian anomalies: A proposed classification (an analysis of 144 cases). Fertil Steril 32:40–46, 1979.
8. Hricak H, Chang YCF, Thurnher S: Vagina: Evaluation with MR imaging. Part I. Normal anatomy and congenital anomalies. Radiology 169:169–174, 1988.
9. Togashi K, Nishimura K, Itoh K, et al: Vaginal agenesis: Classification by MR imaging. Radiology 162:675–677, 1987.
10. Rosenberg HK, Sherman NH, Tarry WF, et al: Mayer-Rokitansky-Küster-Hauser syndrome: US aid to diagnosis. Radiology 161:815–819, 1986.
11. Yuh WTC, DeMarino GB, Ludwig WD, et al: MR imaging of pregnancy in bicornuate uterus. J Comput Assist Tomogr 12(1):162–165, 1988.
12. Hamlin DJ, Petterson H, Ramey SL, Moazam F: Magnetic resonance imaging of bicornuate uterus with unilateral hematometrosalpinx and ipsilateral renal agenesis. Urol Radiol 8:52–55, 1986.

PART V

MUSCULOSKELETAL

36

MR IMAGING OF THE KNEE*

DAVID W. STOLLER, HARRY K. GENANT, and JOHN V. CRUES

GENERAL IMAGING PROTOCOLS
THE MENISCI
   IMAGING PROTOCOLS
   NORMAL MR IMAGING ANATOMY
   MENISCAL PATHOLOGY
   Degeneration and Tears
   PITFALLS IN THE INTERPRETATION OF
     MENISCAL TEARS
THE CRUCIATE LIGAMENTS
   ANTERIOR CRUCIATE LIGAMENT
   POSTERIOR CRUCIATE LIGAMENT
THE COLLATERAL LIGAMENTS
   MEDIAL COLLATERAL LIGAMENT
   LATERAL COLLATERAL LIGAMENT
THE PATELLOFEMORAL JOINT AND
EXTENSOR MECHANISM
   CHONDROMALACIA PATELLAE
   PATELLAR SUBLUXATION AND
     DISLOCATION
   RETINACULAR ATTACHMENTS
   PATELLAR TENDON ABNORMALITIES
   PATELLAR BURSA

GENERAL PATHOLOGIC
CONDITIONS AFFECTING THE KNEE
   ARTHRITIS
   Cartilage
   Synovium and the Irregular Infrapatellar
     Fat Pad Sign
   Juvenile Chronic Arthritis
   Rheumatoid Arthritis
   Pigmented Villonodular Synovitis
   Hemophilia
   Lyme Arthritis
   Osteoarthritis
   OSTEONECROSIS AND RELATED DISORDERS
   JOINT EFFUSIONS
   POPLITEAL CYSTS
   PLICAE
   FRACTURES
   INFECTION
   NEOPLASTIC CONDITIONS
   ARTIFACTS
SUMMARY

It has been demonstrated that MR imaging provides superior noninvasive imaging of the knee joint, and it is rapidly replacing arthrography as the radiographic imaging modality of choice in selected centers.[1–5] Multiplanar thin section sequences using surface coils produce optimal signal-to-noise (S/N) ratio and high spatial resolution.[6–15] Both pre- and postoperative assessments can be provided in an examination taking less than 20 minutes. Unlike arthrography and computed tomography (CT), which require ionizing radiation and injection of contrast material, MR imaging is not limited by anatomic restrictions to access imposed by the joint capsule and femoral condylar and tibial anatomy.[16–18] Correlative studies with arthrography, arthroscopy, and pathologic examination have demonstrated the accuracy of MR in imaging meniscal tears. Meniscal degeneration can be demonstrated earlier and more accurately than with techniques such as arthroscopy and arthrography that are limited to surface evaluation.[1, 2] Initial experience with MR imaging has also shown that this modality has the potential for imaging the effects of trauma and arthritis on the hyaline cartilage and collateral and cruciate ligaments.[1–3, 19–22]

GENERAL IMAGING PROTOCOLS

Protocols are designed so that the studies can be performed within a reasonable time frame (20 to 30 minutes) to facilitate subject cooperation, through-

---

*Portions of this chapter were previously published in Stoller DW (ed): MRI in Orthopedics and Rheumatology. Philadelphia, J.B. Lippincott, 1989.

put, and cost effectiveness and to provide images with high S/N and spatial resolution. A "routine knee" protocol can be modified to allow specific areas of clinical interest to be emphasized. Although orthopedic hardware produces local signal artifact, it does not interfere with the acquisition of diagnostic images from contiguous knee joint structures.

A circumferential extremity coil provides uniform S/N across the knee, without the posterior-to-anterior signal drop-off observed with flat-surface coils. The routine knee protocol for the evaluation of internal derangement uses T_1-weighted images in the axial, sagittal, and coronal planes. When a recovery time (TR) of 600 msec and an echo time (TE) of 20 msec are used, all three orthogonal planes can be imaged in approximately 10 minutes of acquisition time. High resolution is obtained with a 256 × 256 acquisition matrix and a 16-cm field-of-view (FOV) at one excitation (NEX). Spatial resolution is recorded at 0.6 mm in both the phase-encoded and the frequency-encoded directions. A 16-cm FOV provides adequate visualization of the quadriceps-patellar mechanism in the sagittal plane. A 12-cm FOV should be used for pediatric patients. The initial axial acquisition is used to evaluate the patellofemoral joint and serves as a localizer for subsequent sagittal and coronal plane images. The sagittal plane is most sensitive for identifying meniscal and cruciate pathology, and the coronal plane is best for displaying collateral ligament anatomy.

Patients are placed in the supine position, with the knee rotated 15 degrees externally (to realign the anterior cruciate ligament parallel to the sagittal imaging plane). The rotation of the knee does not need to be changed for imaging in either the axial or coronal plane. Thin (5-mm) sections with a 1-mm interslice gap are used for studies in the axial plane, 5-mm contiguous sections are used in the sagittal plane, and 5-mm sections without an interslice gap are used in the coronal plane. Three-millimeter slices are not necessary to accurately assess meniscal lesions in adults. In pediatric patients, however, a 3-mm slice thickness allows optimal medial-to-lateral joint coverage in the sagittal plane and anterior-to-posterior coverage in the coronal plane.

In selected cases of acute trauma, arthritis, infection, and neoplasia, T_2-weighted images are also acquired, using either conventional spin-echo (SE) or fast-scan techniques. Conventional T_2-weighted images are generated at a TR of 2000 msec and TE of 20 and 60 msec at a 256 × 128 acquisition matrix using 1 NEX. Fast-scan gradient-echo (refocused) images with less than a 90-degree flip angle can be used to give effective T_2 (or T_2^*) contrast. With this technique, studies can be performed in 3 minutes of imaging time using a TR of 400 msec, a TE of 30 msec, and a flip angle of 30 degrees at a 256 × 256 acquisition matrix using 2 NEX. With three-dimensional (3D) Fourier transform (3DFT) techniques, gradient-echo volumetric imaging reduces imaging

time and can reduce slice thickness to 0.7 mm. T_2-weighting is helpful in highlighting ligamentous edema in either the coronal (collateral ligaments) or the sagittal (cruciate ligaments) imaging planes. In arthritis, sagittal images provide the most information in early synovial reactions and cartilage erosions. Posterior femoral condylar defects, however, are best displayed on coronal images.

Neoplastic lesions, both benign and malignant, require both T_1- and T_2-weighted images in the axial plane. T_1-weighted sagittal or coronal images demonstrate the proximal and distal extent of a lesion in one section.

THE MENISCI

IMAGING PROTOCOLS

T_1-weighted or intermediate (proton density)–weighted protocols are most sensitive for the detection of meniscal lesions.[2] Additional images with conventional T_2-weighting using an SE sequence can be used to identify fluid, edema, or hemorrhage in acute ligamentous trauma or fracture. Gradient-echo T_2^* images offer the advantage of effective T_2-weighting without compromising the delineation of meniscal degenerations or tears.[23] (T_2^* images are acquired without a 180-degree refocusing pulse.) Gradient-recall techniques are also useful for demonstrating articular cartilage, which is imaged with high signal intensity using this sequence. Meniscal examinations should be performed with a dedicated extremity coil, as discussed above.

NORMAL MR IMAGING ANATOMY

The low signal intensity menisci can be visualized in coronal and sagittal orientations. The sagittal imaging plane is the most sensitive for detecting meniscal pathology, which may be confirmed in corresponding coronal sections. In sagittal sections (obtained most laterally and medially when viewing the lateral and medial menisci, respectively), the extreme peripheral concave surface of each meniscus (body segment) is imaged as a homogeneous dark band with a bow-tie appearance. The anterior and posterior horn segments of the meniscus are seen in profile as opposing dark triangles, analogous to the tangential view presented in arthrography (Figs. 36–1 to 36–3). The extreme anterior and posterior horn segments are thus imaged closest to the intercondylar notch in sagittal sectioning. The 2-mm-thick hyaline articular cartilage that covers the femoral condylar and tibial surfaces is imaged with a higher intensity signal than adjacent cortical bone and articular meniscal surfaces. The posterior horn of the normal medial meniscus is larger than the anterior and body segments.

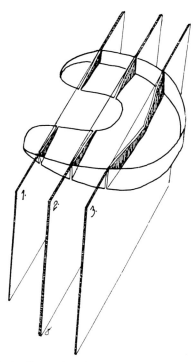

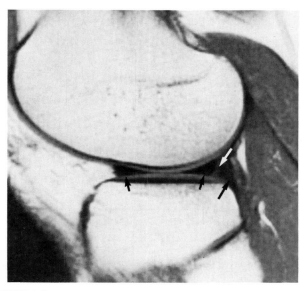

FIGURE 36–3. Intact anterior and posterior horns of the lateral meniscus (*small black arrows*). Intermediate signal intensity popliteus tendon sheath (*white arrow*) and low signal intensity popliteus tendon (*large black arrow*) are identified. (T$_1$-weighted sagittal image; TR = 600 msec, TE = 20 msec.)

FIGURE 36–1. Illustration demonstrates the planes of sagittal images through the anterior and posterior meniscal horns (1 and 2) and body of the meniscus (3).

Hoffa's infrapatellar fat pad is brightest on T$_1$-weighted sequences and can be seen posterior to the superficial dark patellar ligament on sagittal sections. The normal synovial membrane is not visualized on MR images and is reflected over the superior surface

of Hoffa's infrapatellar fat pad. The collapsed (3-mm) suprapatellar bursa does not show increased signal on T$_2$-weighting in the absence of joint effusion. Patellofemoral cartilage can be assessed in the sagittal or axial plane. The popliteal tendon and sheath are seen in their expected anatomic location between the capsule and periphery of the lateral meniscus (Fig. 36–3). Separate synovium-lined fascicles or struts of the meniscus allow intraarticular passage of the popliteal tendon as defined on MR images. These are usually best seen on T$_2$-weighted images, especially if an effusion is present.

MENISCAL PATHOLOGY (Fig. 36–4)

Degeneration and Tears

USEFULNESS OF MR. In comparison with arthroscopy, the sensitivity of MR imaging in the detection of meniscal tears has been reported to be between 75 per cent and 100 per cent.[5, 24, 25] In a large series by Mink et al.,[26] the accuracy rate of MR imaging in 600 menisci was 92 per cent, with 9 false negatives and 18 false positives. Fast 3D MR imaging of the meniscus produced a 95 per cent concurrence between MR imaging and arthroscopy in detection of meniscal tears and a 100 per cent correlation with meniscal degenerations.[27] The negative predictive value of MR approaches 100 per cent in exclusion of tears in normal MR imaging examinations of the meniscus. Further documentation with both arthrography and arthroscopy is needed to validate clinical efficacy. The variation in detection rates of meniscal lesions compared to arthroscopy may be due to

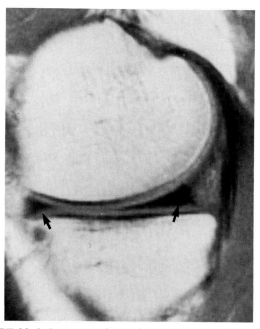

FIGURE 36–2. Intact anterior and posterior horns of the medial meniscus (*arrows*). (T$_1$-weighted sagittal image; TR = 600 msec, TE = 20 msec.)

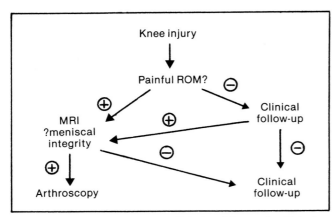

FIGURE 36–4. MR imaging as a clinical tool for meniscal injuries.

several factors, including (1) a learning curve on the part of the radiologist in interpreting MR imaging signal intensities, (2) the experience of several different arthroscopists participating in correlative studies, (3) incorrect interpretation of areas of fibrillation or fraying as meniscal tears, (4) the inability of arthroscopy to detect degenerative cleavage tears without probing, and (5) the variability in performing examinations with different imagers and surface coils at a variety of field strengths.

MR IMAGING APPEARANCE. Whereas the intact meniscus demonstrates homogenous low signal intensity regardless of the pulse sequence, degenerations and tears of the meniscus image with increased signal intensity, which is attributed to imbibed synovial fluid.[2] As synovial fluid diffuses through the meniscus, areas of degeneration and tears trap water molecules onto surface boundary layers, increasing the local spin density. T_1 and T_2 values are shortened as interaction of synovial fluid with large macromolecules in the meniscus slows the rotation rates of protons.[2] This explains the sensitivity of T_1-weighted and intermediate (proton density)–weighted images in visualizing meniscal degenerations and tears. Increased signal intensity in synovial fluid gaps has been confirmed in surgically induced tears in animal models.[28] In MR imaging studies performed after arthrography, increased signal intensity may be observed on T_2-weighted images. This change is related to the actions of joint fluid and a hyperosmolar contrast agent, which draw fluid into meniscal separations. This creates a motional narrowing effect (free water molecules in motion), allowing more mobile protons to be imaged separately from unbound water molecules.[29] In the absence of a joint effusion, meniscal degenerations and tears may actually decrease in signal intensity on T_2-weighted images. On T_2^* or gradient-refocused images, however, degenerations and tears generate increased signal intensities.[23]

The fibrocartilaginous meniscus provides added mechanical stability to femorotibial rotations and,

when injured, may accelerate the process of articular degeneration.[30–32] Detecting the extent and location of meniscal degeneration and tears is of clinical significance in pre- and postarthroscopic evaluations and therapeutic rehabilitation.

Early MR investigations reported increased signal intensities within normally low signal intensity menisci.[1, 14, 33] Initial false-positive results with MR imaging can be traced to interpretations of signal intensities without the use of a pathologic and histologic model for reference. We have developed a grading system for meniscal signals and an objective pathologic staging system for meniscal degeneration and tears.[2] Comparisons have been made with arthrography and arthroscopy, which both have sensitivities of less than 100 per cent for pathologically detectable tears. MR signal abnormalities may be seen in degenerative intrasubstance tears before progression through the meniscal surface makes them visible at arthroscopy or arthrography.

Grades of MR meniscal signal intensity are based on signal distribution relative to an articular surface (Fig. 36–5). The peripheral capsular margin of the meniscus is considered nonarticular. MR grade 1 is represented by one or several punctate areas of increased signal intensity not contiguous with an articular surface (Fig. 36–6). This corresponds to stage 1 pathology, in which there is histologic evidence of discrete foci of mucinous or mucoid degeneration in pale-staining hypocellular (chondrocyte-deficient) areas on hematoxylin and eosin–stained preparations. These changes are seen as part of a spectrum of degenerative meniscal responses in which mechanical loading leads to increased production of mucopolysaccharide ground substance.[31, 32, 34, 35]

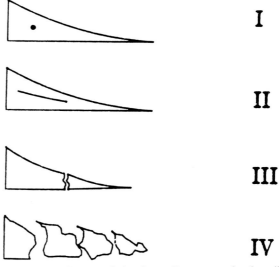

FIGURE 36–5. Diagram of simple grading system for describing meniscal tears. Grade 3 and 4 tears were recommended for arthroscopy. Grade 1 and 2 tears represent intrameniscal abnormalities not visible arthroscopically. Grade 4 abnormalities include meniscal capsular separation. In this chapter peripheral tears and meniscal macerations are classified as grade 3 abnormalities.

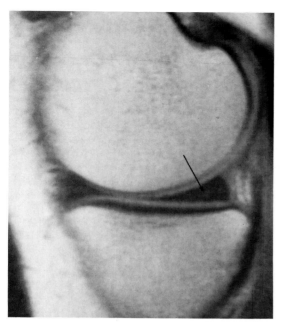

FIGURE 36–6. Focus of grade 1 signal intensity in the posterior horn of the medial meniscus *(arrow)*.

Grade 1 signal intensity may be seen in asymptomatic athletes and in young and elderly patients.

Grade 2 MR changes are linear, nonarticular, intrameniscal signal intensities usually oriented in a horizontal plane extending from the capsular periphery of the meniscus (Fig. 36–7). In corresponding

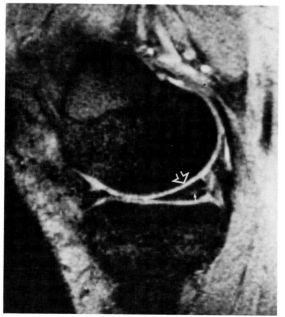

FIGURE 36–7. Grade 2 degeneration in the posterior horn of the medial meniscus *(solid white arrow)*. High signal intensity hyaline articular cartilage *(open arrow)* is indicated on this T_2^* gradient-echo image.

stage 2 pathology, histologic findings include distinct bands of mucinous degeneration with microscopic clefting in adjacent hypocellular regions of the fibrocartilaginous matrix.[35, 36] A distinct cleavage plane or tear is not observed in this stage. The midmeniscus functions as an interface, buffering superior femoral and inferior tibial frictional forces, and is the site for mucinous degeneration imaged as linear grade 2 signal intensity. Although patients with grade 2 MR signal may or may not present with knee pain, these lesions may progress to fibrocartilaginous tears.[2, 30, 34–36]

In MR grade 3, increased signal intensity extends to at least one articular surface (Fig. 36–8). This grade corresponds to stage 3 pathology, in which there is histologic evidence of fibrocartilaginous separation with or without visible extension to an articular surface. Thus, although all grade 3 MR signal represents fibrocartilaginous separation, in approximately 5 to 10 per cent of cases this disruption is confined to degenerative intrasubstance cleavage tears that may require surgical probing for diagnosis at arthroscopy and may escape arthrographic detection.[18, 31] This in part explains preliminary false-positive interpretations (6 per cent) of grade 3 signal when assessed by arthroscopy.[33] These lesions may rapidly extend to become complete tears.[10] The mechanical instability created by confined horizontal cleavage tears may be responsible for the clinical presentation of acute knee pain. Bucket handle tears manifest characteristic appearances on coronal and sagittal images (Fig. 36–9).

In stage 3, tears occur adjacent to areas of mucinous degeneration, supporting the theory that in sites subjected to increased mechanical loading, stage 1 and 2 degenerations progress to stage 3 fibrocartilaginous tears.

Fresh traumatic tears differ from degenerative horizontal cleavage tears. They have more vertical orientations and smaller areas of associated mucinous degenerations as sites for structural weakening.[31] The finding of lower histologic stages (stages 1 and 2) in conjunction with inferior surface tears (stage 3), especially in posteromedial horn segments, suggests a traumatic etiology for these tears. This is supported by observations of increased stress and strain generated on the undersurface of the meniscus with femorotibial rotations.[30, 31] Arthroscopic accuracy is reported to be as low as 45 to 69 per cent with inferior surface tears of the posteromedial meniscus, further illustrating the significant contribution of MR imaging to the study of this frequently injured site.

PITFALLS IN THE INTERPRETATION OF MENISCAL TEARS

Knowledge of pitfalls encountered in MR signal interpretation will improve the specificity and accuracy for reading MR imaging knee studies. The concave meniscal edge may pose a problem on sagittal

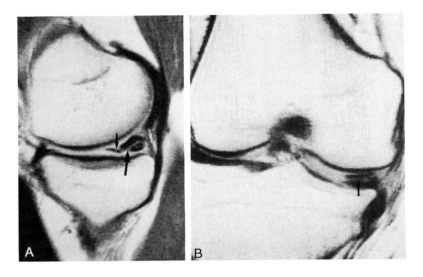

FIGURE 36–8. Meniscal tear. *A*, Grade 3 signal intensity in a meniscal tear in the posterior horn of the medial meniscus *(large black arrow)*. Fragmented apex of the posterior horn is shown *(small black arrow)*. *B*, Grade 3 meniscal tear demonstrated in the coronal plane.

sections (Fig. 36–10). Fibrillatory degeneration of the free concave edge of the meniscal surface may be missed on 5-mm MR sections. When seen, this fibrillation or fraying is visualized as increased signal intensity restricted to the apex of the meniscus. Rarely, degeneration perpendicular to the sagittal imaging plane may be undergraded; however, focal degeneration observed on contiguous images would indicate the true extent of degeneration. The transverse ligament of the knee, which connects the anterior horns of the medial and lateral menisci and courses adjacent to the anterior horn of the lateral meniscus, is a frequent cause (30 per cent) of false-positive identification of tears in the anterolateral

meniscus (Figs. 36–11 and 36–12).[37, 38] Prominent branch vessels of the lateral inferior geniculate artery may be associated with this ligament. The ligament can be recognized as a tubular structure of low signal

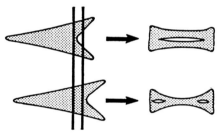

FIGURE 36–10. Schematic line drawing of the meniscus shows the concave meniscal edge. The upper figure demonstrates a sagittal section through the edge of the meniscus that produces a linear artifact in the image. A section located more medially in the meniscus *(lower diagram)* may produce a short artifact in the anterior or posterior horns of the meniscus when the curvature of the meniscus places the meniscal edge at the edge of the section.

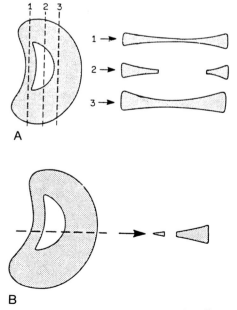

FIGURE 36–9. Schematic drawings of a bucket-handle tear show sagittal and coronal sections through a torn meniscus.

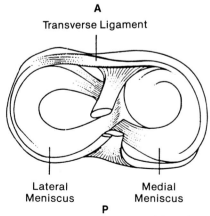

FIGURE 36–11. Line drawing of an axial section through the knee shows the transverse ligament arising from the medial meniscus and inserting along the anterior aspect of the lateral meniscus. A = anterior; P = posterior.

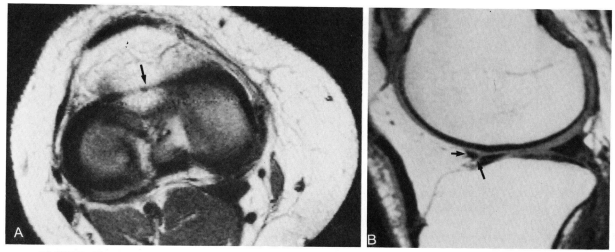

FIGURE 36–12. Transverse ligament. *A,* Axial image demonstrating transverse ligament of the knee connecting the anterior horns of the medial and lateral menisci *(arrow).* (T_1-weighted image; TR = 600 msec, TE = 20 msec.) *B,* Grade 3 pseudotear of the anterior horn of the lateral meniscus caused by the low signal intensity transverse ligament *(short black arrow)* surrounding fat *(long arrow).* (T_1-weighted sagittal image.)

intensity coursing through Hoffa's fat pad contiguous with this "pseudotear." The popliteal tendon sheath may mimic a grade 3 vertical tear, but its characteristic orientation and location in the posterior horn of the lateral meniscus distinguish this normal structure. The inability to visualize the body segment of the medial meniscus on medial sagittal images is a clue to the existence of a bucket handle tear (see Fig. 36–9).[39] MR imaging may not resolve the attenuated width of the torn meniscus, which may approximate the 5-mm resolution thickness in the sagittal plane. The converse is true for discoid lateral menisci, where

a continuous body segment is visualized on multiple sagittal sections. Postmeniscectomy menisci generate an intermediate signal intensity as a result of fibrous growth (Fig. 36–13).[40] The same criteria for interpreting meniscal tears in nonoperative knees is applied to postsurgical and meniscal remnants. Meniscocapsular separations may be detected when the periphery of the meniscus fails to approach the cortical edge of the tibial plateau (Fig. 36–14). Crystals of calcium pyrophosphate deposited on the surface of surgically excised menisci were not optimally imaged in either sagittal or coronal MR planes.

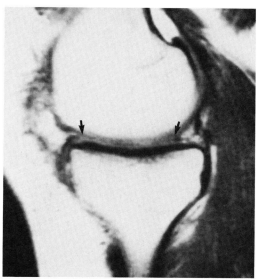

FIGURE 36–13. Absent fibrocartilage in total medial meniscectomy *(arrows).* (T_1-weighted sagittal image; TR = 600 msec, TE = 20 msec.)

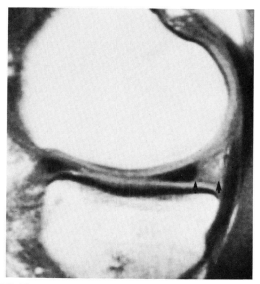

FIGURE 36–14. Meniscocapsular separation with exposed tibial articular cartilage *(arrows).* (T_1-weighted sagittal image.)

THE CRUCIATE LIGAMENTS

ANTERIOR CRUCIATE LIGAMENT
(Fig. 36–15)

On coronal and sagittal images the normal anterior cruciate ligament (ACL) is imaged as a band of low signal intensity with separate fiber striations visible near attachment points (Figs. 36–16 and 36–17). Independent of partial voluming, the ACL may be visualized with a minimally greater signal than that observed in the homogeneously dark posterior cruciate ligament.

In complete tears of the ACL there is discontinuity in the low signal intensity band, with or without loss of its normally taut parallel margins (Fig. 36–18).[11, 12] Partial or complete ligamentous disruptions may be associated with blurring of the cruciate ligament's fascicles from edema or hemorrhage. In acute tears or strains, fluid and edema image with high signal intensity on T_2-weighted images. On sagittal images, partial voluming of the ACL with the lateral femoral condyle may be mistaken for a tear. However, in partial voluming no increase in signal intensity is observed on T_2-weighting. Hemorrhagic joint effusions associated with tears of the anterior cruciate ligament may incite a synovitic reaction associated with irregularity of the infrapatellar fat pad.[41]

Accurate assessment of partial ligamentous tears is more difficult than detection of complete disruptions. Posterior bowing of the anterior cruciate ligament or buckling of the posterior cruciate ligament may be associated with increased laxity or with a chronic tear of the ACL. Absence of the ACL on both sagittal and coronal images is diagnostic of ACL disruption. Forward displacement of the tibia visualized on MR imaging is the equivalent of a positive anterior drawer test on physical examination seen in the injured or deficient ACL.

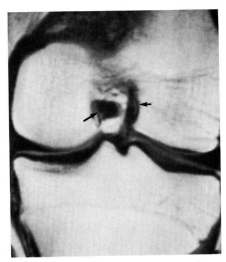

FIGURE 36–16. Intact anterior *(short arrow)* and posterior *(long arrow)* cruciate ligaments on T_1-weighted coronal image.

POSTERIOR CRUCIATE LIGAMENT

In the sagittal plane the posterior cruciate ligament (PCL) is visualized as a uniform dark band, usually displayed on a single sagittal image (Fig. 36–19). The anatomy of the PCL is not as sensitive to positioning as that of the ACL. In partial knee flexion, the PCL is taut on MR images (Fig. 36–20). An abnormally high arc or buckling in the PCL, however, may indicate a tear of the ACL with forward tibial displacement. Within this normally low signal intensity ligament, any increase in signal intensity on either T_1- or T_2-weighted images should be interpreted as abnormal (Figs. 36–21 and 36–22). Hemorrhage and edema, seen in acute injuries, are bright on T_2-weighted images and cause less distortion or mass effect than with tears of the ACL. Complete disruption of the PCL is imaged as a loss or "gap" in ligament continuity. Partial tears may be more diffi-

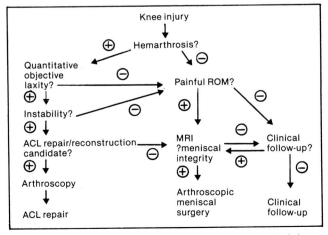

FIGURE 36–15. MR imaging as a clinical tool for ACL injury.

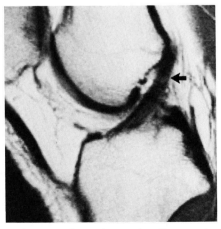

FIGURE 36–17. Normal anterior cruciate ligament *(arrow)* on T_1-weighted sagittal image.

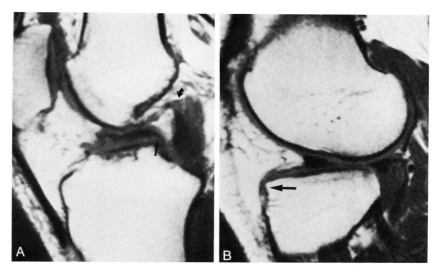

FIGURE 36–18. Anterior cruciate tear. *A*, Disrupted anterior cruciate ligament *(straight arrow)* and high-arched posterior cruciate ligament *(curved arrow)* on T$_1$-weighted sagittal image. *B*, Anterior translation of the tibia *(arrow)* imaged in the same patient.

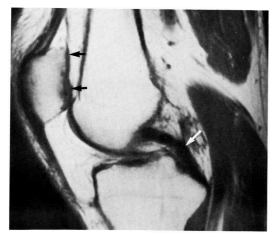

FIGURE 36–19. Intact posterior cruciate ligament *(white arrow)* on T$_1$-weighted sagittal image. Thinning of patellar facet cartilage is also shown *(black arrows)*.

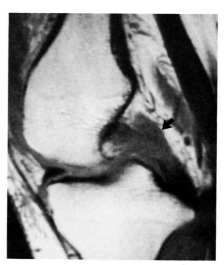

FIGURE 36–21. High signal intensity in disrupted posterior cruciate ligament *(arrow)*. (T$_1$-weighted sagittal image.)

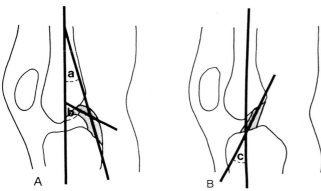

FIGURE 36–20. Straight sagittal MR images of the extended knee *(A)* and 50 degrees flexed knee *(B)* of the same subject. Note that the posterior cruciate ligament bows posteriorly in extension but is straight in flexion.

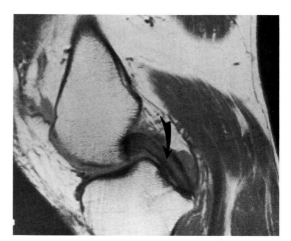

FIGURE 36–22. Torn posterior cruciate ligament. Sagittal T$_1$-weighted spin-echo image. High signal intensity is seen within the substance of the posterior cruciate ligament *(arrow)*.

cult to assess. Chronic tears with fibrous scarring do not show increased signal intensity on T_2-weighted images and show intermediate signal intensity on T_1-weighted images. Coronal images, with the PCL on cross-sectional display, are also helpful in identifying increased signal intensity.

THE COLLATERAL LIGAMENTS

MEDIAL COLLATERAL LIGAMENT

On MR imaging examination, partial tears or strains of the medial collateral ligament (MCL) are seen with increased distance between the subcutaneous tissue and cortical bone (Fig. 36–23). T_2-weighted images demonstrate edema and/or hemorrhage around low signal intensity ligamentous fibers. Compared with ligamentous strains, tears show loss of continuity of ligament fibers. Complete tears are associated with extensive joint effusions (hemarthrosis) and extravasation of joint fluid that tracks along the MCL. Focal hemorrhage can be visualized at the femoral epicondylar attachment in complete ligamentous avulsions. Subacute hemorrhage is visualized with increased signal intensity on T_1- and T_2-weighted images. Conventional T_2-weighted and gradient-echo T_2^* images have been useful in documenting interval healing with reattachment of the torn MCL ligament.

LATERAL COLLATERAL LIGAMENT

The lateral collateral ligament (LCL) is best seen on posterior coronal images and is visualized as a band of low signal intensity. Occasionally, peripheral sagittal images demonstrate LCL anatomy at the level

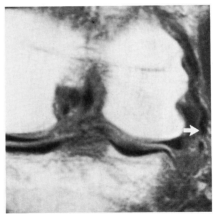

FIGURE 36–24. Disrupted lateral collateral ligament is imaged with wavy and lax contour *(arrow)*. (T_1-weighted coronal image.)

of the fibular head. Edema and hemorrhage, although less frequent in this location, are seen as ligamentous thickening with increased signal intensity on T_2-weighted images. The degree of increased signal in LCL injuries is less noticeable than that demonstrated in MCL disruptions. This may be related to the normal capsular separation of the LCL, which excludes the accumulation of extravasated joint fluid. In complete disruptions, the LCL images with a wavy contour and loss of ligamentous continuity (Fig. 36–24). Edema and hemorrhage in LCL tears may also be confirmed on peripheral sagittal images.

THE PATELLOFEMORAL JOINT AND EXTENSOR MECHANISM

Axial images are required to characterize the patellofemoral articulation accurately. The lateral and medial patellar facets are oblique and cannot be

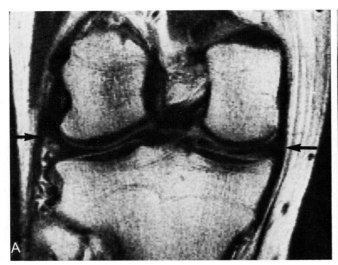
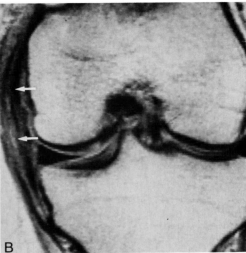

FIGURE 36–23. Collateral ligaments. *A,* Intact low signal intensity medial and lateral collateral ligaments *(arrows)*. *B,* Thickened and edematous medial collateral ligament images with increased signal intensity *(arrows)*. (TR = 1500 msec, TE = 40 msec.)

characterized precisely on sagittal or coronal images. Patellar cartilage and retinacular attachments are defined in axial sections through the patellofemoral joint. The quadriceps muscles and tendon can be visualized on sagittal or axial images. The patellar tendon is imaged *en face* in the coronal plane, in profile in the sagittal plane, and in cross-section on axial planar images.

CHONDROMALACIA PATELLAE

On axial MR images, early cartilage attenuation or erosions can be appreciated in either the medial or the lateral facets (Fig. 36–25).[42] Frequently, the opposing femoral cartilage also demonstrates thinning on sagittal images. Sagittal images, which are less sensitive to cartilage erosions, may show a straightening or loss of the normal convex curve seen in patellar hyaline cartilage when viewed in profile. T_2-weighted or gradient-echo sequences are useful for demonstrating inhomogeneity of the signal obtained from patellar cartilage in areas of focal edema. Subchondral low signal intensity, representing sclerosis, may be associated with irregular surface erosions. Low signal intensity patellar cysts are sometimes seen in early stages of patellar softening, preceding cartilage erosions.

PATELLAR SUBLUXATION AND DISLOCATION

Patellar subluxation sometimes presents with symptoms of joint locking and may be mistaken for

a torn meniscus.[43] The repetitive trauma caused by lateral displacements of the patella accelerates articular surface degeneration. Torn medial retinacular attachments can be identified on axial images subsequent to patellar dislocation and traumatic subluxations.

RETINACULAR ATTACHMENTS

The medial and lateral retinacula are fascial extensions of the vastus medialis and lateralis muscle groups, respectively (Fig. 36–26).[44] The retinacula reinforce and guide normal patellar tracking. On anterior coronal images, the retinacular attachments can be visualized as low signal intensity structures converging on the medial and lateral patellar facets.

The medial retinaculum is more frequently torn than the lateral, especially after patellar dislocation. Axial MR images may demonstrate a free-floating retinaculum, without patellar attachment, or a mass-like effect in compressed torn retinacular fibers or chondral fragments. Associated edema and hemorrhage produce increased signal intensity on T_2-weighted images.

PATELLAR TENDON ABNORMALITIES

Patellar tendon tears, resulting in loss of extension and a high-riding patella, can occur with avulsion injuries from the tibial tubercle or inferior pole of the patella (Fig. 36–27).[45] Bony fragments, which

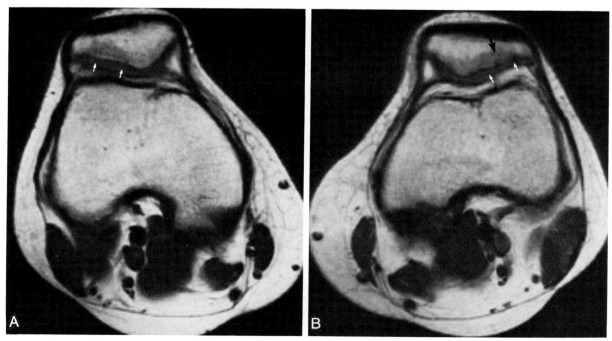

FIGURE 36–25. Chondromalacia patellae. *A,* Intact lateral facet cartilage in asymptomatic knee *(arrows). B,* Attenuated lateral facet articular cartilage *(white arrows)* and subchondral erosions *(black arrow)* in symptomatic knee.

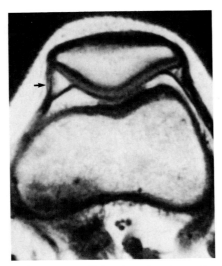

FIGURE 36–26. Intact medial retinaculum imaged as low signal intensity attachment.

image with the signal intensity of marrow, may be identified on sagittal MR images. Increased tendon laxity with a wavy contour can be visualized in acute or chronic tears. A thickened patellar tendon may be seen after arthroscopy or trauma.

PATELLAR BURSA

Prepatellar bursitis is visualized as a localized soft-tissue mass anterior to the patella. It shows low signal intensity on T_1-weighted images and high signal intensity on T_2-weighted images. Infrapatellar bursitis is identified posterior to the patellar tendon and inferior to Hoffa's fat pad.[44]

GENERAL PATHOLOGIC CONDITIONS AFFECTING THE KNEE

ARTHRITIS

Assessment of the extent, progression, and therapeutic response in adult arthritic disorders and in juvenile chronic arthritis is enhanced by MR imaging of articular cartilage.[41] Even in cases in which conventional radiographs are negative, joint effusions, synovial reactions, popliteal cysts, and osteonecrosis can be demonstrated and evaluated with MR studies.

Cartilage

Cartilage of the patellar, femoral, and tibial articular surfaces is best visualized on T_1-weighted images.[41] Because of its hydropic composition, normal hyaline cartilage is imaged with intermediate signal intensity compared to the low signal intensity of cortex and fibrocartilaginous menisci. On conventional T_2-weighted images, hyaline cartilage maintains an intermediate signal intensity. With gradient-echo, chemical shift, and fast low angle shot (FLASH) techniques, however, hyaline cartilage is imaged with high signal intensity (Fig. 36–28), and with these techniques it is possible to detect early stages of hyaline cartilage degeneration.[23]

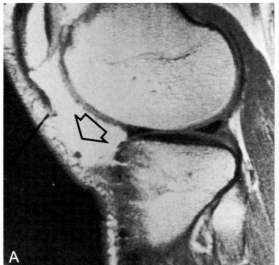
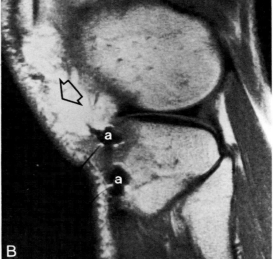

FIGURE 36–27. Unsuccessful patellar tendon repair with patellar tendon rupture. Sagittal T_1-weighted spin-echo images. Absence of the normal low intensity tendon is evident in the vicinity of Hoffa's fat pad *(arrows)*, in association with artifacts from surgical staples in the tibial tubercle (a).

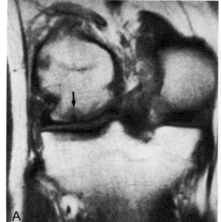
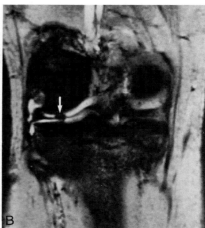

FIGURE 36–28. Osteochondral defect. *A,* Low signal intensity traumatic osteochondral lesion on T_1-weighted coronal image *(arrow). B,* Corresponding T_2^* gradient-echo coronal image identifying overlying articular cartilage defect *(arrow).*

Synovium and the Irregular Infrapatellar Fat Pad Sign

Synovial reaction and proliferations are imaged as changes in the contour of synovial reflections. Irregularity, with loss of the smooth posterior concave free border of the infrapatellar fat pad, can be observed with a variety of synovial reactions and is referred to as the irregular infrapatellar fat pad sign.[41] Although the synovium cannot be imaged directly in early synovitis, a corrugated surface along Hoffa's fat pad is evident in the initial stages of synovial irritation. This irregular fat pad sign has been seen in patients with hemophilia, rheumatoid arthritis, pigmented villonodular synovitis, Lyme arthritis, and hemorrhagic effusions (from arthritis or trauma) with reactive synovium. Synovial hypertrophy and pannus generally show low to intermediate signal intensity on T_1- and T_2-weighted sequences. Fluid associated with synovial masses generates increased signal intensity on T_2-weighted images.

Juvenile Chronic Arthritis

In juvenile rheumatoid (chronic) arthritis (JRA), MR imaging studies have characterized early synovitis with an irregular infrapatellar fat pad in the initial stages of clinical presentation.[46] Articular cartilage erosions and synovial hypertrophy can be identified before joint space narrowing is evident on plain film radiography. Posterior popliteal cysts of the gastrocnemius and semimembranosus bursa are commonly associated with JRA and show low signal intensity on T_1-weighted images and uniform high signal intensity on T_2-weighted images. Thickening of the synovium of the suprapatellar bursa can be visualized with low signal intensity on T_1- and T_2-weighted images. With MR imaging scans, subarticular cysts, subchondral sclerosis, and osteonecrosis can be detected on both femoral and tibial surfaces in more advanced disease, findings frequently not evident on conventional radiographs. Hypoplastic menisci with a small ante-

rior body and posterior horns have also been observed on MR imaging studies in JRA patients. This finding may be related to an alteration in the composition of synovial fluid, impairing normal fibrocartilage development.

Rheumatoid Arthritis

In adult patients with rheumatoid arthritis, bi- and tricompartmental disease is displayed on MR images through the medial and lateral femorotibial compartments and patellofemoral joint (Fig. 36–29).[41] Marginal and subcondral erosions with diffuse loss of hyaline articular cartilage are evident on both femoral and tibial surfaces. Large joint effusions with popliteal cysts are commonly seen and demonstrate uniform high signal intensity on T_2-weighted images.

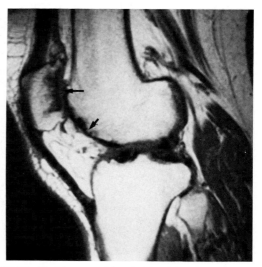

FIGURE 36–29. Rheumatoid arthritis with severe patellofemoral joint disease *(long arrow)* and articular cartilage erosions *(short arrow).* (T_1-weighted sagittal image.)

Pigmented Villonodular Synovitis

Pigmented villonodular synovitis (PVNS) is a monoarticular synovial proliferative disorder. It usually presents a a nonpainful soft-tissue mass, and the knee is a frequent site of involvement, especially with the diffuse form of the disease. Hemosiderin-laden macrophages are frequently deposited in hyperplastic synovial masses, and there may be associated sclerotic bone lesions.

In a series of 10 cases of PVNS of the knee, pathologic changes were correctly identified on MR imaging studies, with surgical confirmation in all cases.[47, 48] The hemosiderin-infiltrated synovial masses had low signal intensity on T_1- and T_2-weighted images because of the paramagnetic effect of iron (Fig. 36–30). Adjacent synovial fluid, however, was visualized with increased signal intensity on T_2-weighted images.

Hemophilia

In MR imaging studies of patients with hemophilic arthropathy, hemosiderin and fibrous tissue, formed

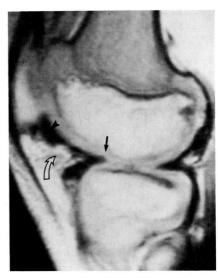

FIGURE 36–31. Hemophilia with dark hemosiderin deposits seen along an irregular infrapatellar fat pad *(arrows).* (T_1-weighted sagittal image.)

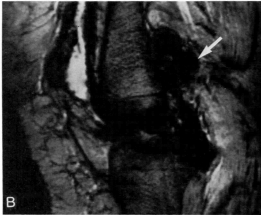
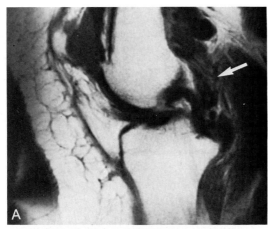

FIGURE 36–30. Pigmented villonodular synovitis. T_1-weighted *(A)* and T_2^*-weighted *(B)* sagittal images identifying low signal intensity masses of hyperplastic synovium with hemosiderin in the popliteal fossa *(arrows).*

from repeated episodes of joint hemorrhage, show low signal intensity on T_1- and T_2-weighted images (Fig. 36–31).[49, 50] Irregular fat pads and markedly thickened, hemosiderin-laden synovial reflections (of low signal intensity) were present in five of five separate cases we have studied.[41] Although conventional radiographs were normal, articular cartilage irregularities and erosions were detected on MR scans.

Subchondral and intraosseous cysts or hemorrhage can be identified on coronal and sagittal MR images. Fluid-filled cysts generate high signal intensity on T_2-weighted images. Areas of fibrous tissue remain low in signal intensity on T_1- and T_2-weighted images, and low signal intensity synovial effusions can be differentiated from adjacent hemosiderin and fibrous depositions on T_2-weighted sequences. In a study of the knees of 10 hemophiliacs, articular and subchondral abnormalities were found in 80 per cent.

Lyme Arthritis

Lyme disease and resultant arthritis are transmitted by the *Ixodes* tick and are characterized by the delayed appearance of an oligo- or polyarticular inflammatory arthritis.[51] The knee is most commonly affected, with development of inflammatory synovial effusions, synovial hypertrophy, infrapatellar fat pad edema, and (in severe chronic cases) cartilage erosions. In one patient, studied three months after a documented tick bite, MR studies revealed an extensive joint effusion and an irregular corrugated infrapatellar fat pad.[41]

Osteoarthritis

The MR imaging findings in degenerative arthrosis represent a spectrum varying from osteophytic spur-

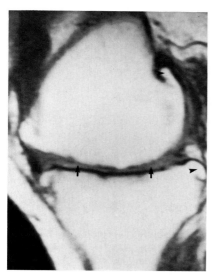

FIGURE 36–32. Osteoarthritis with denuded articular cartilage, joint space narrowing *(arrows)*, and osteophytes *(arrowheads)*.

ring (which has the bright signal intensity of marrow) to compartment collapse, denuded articular cartilage, torn and degenerative meniscal fibrocartilage, and diminished marrow signal intensity in areas of subchondral sclerosis (Fig. 36–32).[4, 10, 13] The ability to assess hyaline cartilage surfaces accurately gives MR imaging an advantage over plain film radiography in preoperative planning for joint arthroplasty procedures. Chondral fragments, of intermediate signal intensity, and loose bodies, with the high signal intensity of marrow fat, may be associated with more advanced degenerative disease.

In synovial chondromatosis, multiple synovium-based chondral fragments are visualized with low to intermediate signal intensity (Fig. 36–33). In primary chondromatosis these metaplastic fragments are usu-

ally similar to one another in size. In secondary chondromatosis they are visualized in a variety of sizes.

OSTEONECROSIS AND RELATED DISORDERS

Spontaneous osteonecrosis of the knee typically affects an older patient group, predominantly female, and presents with acute medial joint pain.[10, 52, 53] Most commonly, spontaneous osteonecrosis involves the weight-bearing surface of the medial femoral condyle (Fig. 36–34), although cases have been described in which the medial and lateral tibial plateaus and the lateral femoral condyle were involved.[54]

Conventional radiographic evaluation is not sensitive to identification of the osteonecrotic focus prior to the development of sclerosis and osseous collapse. However, a low signal intensity focus can be detected on T_1- and T_2-weighted images in patients with osteonecrosis who have no other demonstrable radiographic findings.

Osteochondritis dissecans differs from spontaneous osteonecrosis of the knee in that it affects primarily young male patients and involves the non–weight-bearing surface of the medial femoral condyle.[55-57] On MR imaging scans, the focus of osteochondritis shows low signal intensity on T_1- and T_2-weighted images even prior to detection on conventional radiographs.

Bone infarcts are usually metaphyseal in location but have also been imaged in more epiphyseal and diaphyseal locations (Fig. 36–35).[58] The MR appearance of a bone infarct is characteristic, with a serpiginous low signal intensity border of reactive bone

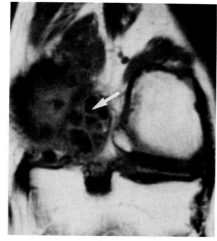

FIGURE 36–33. Synovial chondromatosis with multiple loose osteochondral fragments seen in the posterior capsule *(arrow)* on a posterior T_1-weighted coronal image.

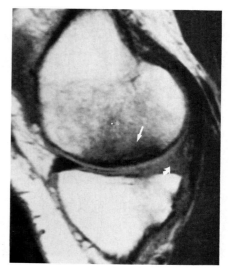

FIGURE 36–34. Spontaneous osteonecrosis of the knee visualized as low signal intensity focus *(straight arrow)* associated with a posterior horn meniscal tear *(curved arrow)*. (T_1-weighted sagittal image.)

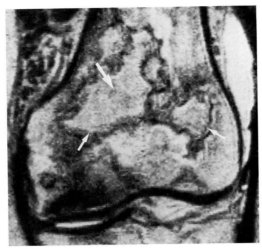

FIGURE 36–35. Characteristic appearance of bone infarct with low signal intensity periphery *(small arrows)* and higher signal intensity central portions *(large arrow)*. (TR = 1500 msec, TE = 40 msec.)

and a central compartment of high signal intensity equivalent to yellow marrow (Fig. 36–36). On T_2-weighted images a chemical shift artifact may be seen as a linear segment of high signal intensity paralleling the outline of the infarct. Bone infarcts can be differentiated from enchondromas on MR imaging; the latter lack a serpiginous border and have a central region of low signal intensity on T_1-weighted images, which increases with progressive T_2-weighting.

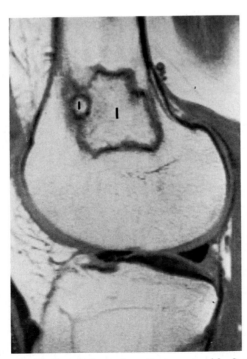

FIGURE 36–36. Bone infarcts in patient on steroids. Sagittal T_1-weighted spin-echo image. Well-marginated areas (I) with central fat and peripheral reactive bone formation are evident within the distal femoral marrow.

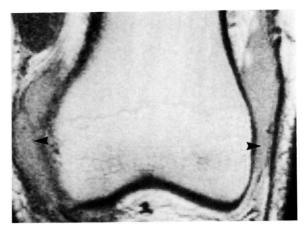

FIGURE 36–37. Saddle bag distribution of joint fluid on intermediate-weighted coronal image.

JOINT EFFUSIONS

Joint effusions image with low signal intensity on T_1-weighted images and with bright signal intensity on corresponding T_2-weighted images.[59] Our experience indicates that T_1-weighted sequences are adequate for detecting small effusions, and there is no need for longer TR settings. Coronal images are complementary, and the "saddle bag" distribution of fluid in the medial and lateral gutters extending into the suprapatellar bursa can be seen (Fig. 36–37).

POPLITEAL CYSTS

Classically, popliteal or Baker's cysts of the gastrocnemiosemimembranosus bursa arise between the medial head of the gastrocnemius muscle and the more lateral semimembranosus muscle (Fig. 36–38).[60, 61] These cysts show low signal intensity on T_1-weighted images and uniform increased signal intensity on T_2-weighted images.

PLICAE

Synovial plicae are embryonic remnants of the septal division of the knee joint into three compartments.[62] They may be found as a normal variant in 20 to 60 per cent of adult knees. The suprapatellar, mediopatellar, and infrapatellar are the common plicae. The mediopatellar and infrapatellar plicae are best visualized on axial images, whereas the suprapatellar plicae are best visualized on sagittal images traversing the suprapatellar bursae. Plica tissue has low signal intensity on T_1- and T_2-weighted images.[63] Infrapatellar plicae, the most common, may be confused with the anterior cruciate ligament on arthrography.

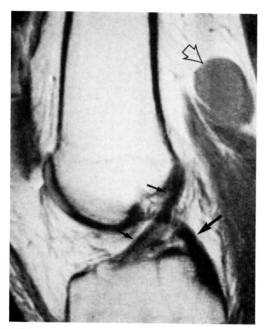

FIGURE 36–38. Popliteal cyst *(open arrow)* adjacent to the medial head of the gastrocnemius muscle. Anterior *(small solid arrows)* and posterior *(large solid arrow)* cruciate ligaments are indicated. (TR = 1500 msec, TE = 40 msec.)

FRACTURES

Fractures about the knee can be identified on MR scans in patients with acute or chronic knee pain and negative conventional radiographs. Subsequent radiography often shows areas of sclerosis or periosteal reaction at the fracture sites initially identified on MR imaging. The most frequent MR imaging pattern of fracture is sharp, well-defined linear segments of decreased signal intensity visualized in the distal femur or proximal tibia (Fig. 36–39). In an acute fracture, associated fluid or hemorrhage shows increased signal intensity on T_2-weighted images (Fig. 36–40). Fractures with diffuse areas of associated low signal intensity on T_1-weighted images demonstrate increased signal intensity with long TR and TE settings, reflecting the prolonged T_2 values in edematous marrow. Chronic fractures remain low in signal intensity with variable TR and TE parameters.

MR imaging is also useful in the differentiation of stress fractures, common in the proximal tibia, from neoplastic processes.[64] The linear segment of the stress fracture in the knee is usually accompanied by marrow edema. Lack of a soft-tissue mass, cortical destruction, or characteristic marrow extension effectively excludes a tumor from the differential consideration.

A diffuse or localized pattern of low signal intensity on T_1-weighted images without a defined fracture is seen with bone bruises or contusions at sites of impaction or repetitive trauma. In an acute or subacute setting, increased signal intensity is visualized on T_2-weighted images prior to the appearance of sclerosis on plain films.

INFECTION

Capsular distention and joint effusion are identified on MR scans of joint infection but are nonspecific.[65] A septic joint may be further characterized by intraarticular debris and synovitis from hematogenous seeding. In one child with staphylococcal osteomyelitis, a mottled pattern of the yellow marrow stores could be identified in the tibial epiphyseal center. This appearance should not be confused with the coarsened trabecular pattern seen in Paget's disease. In a case of osteomyelitis involving the distal femur, collections of infected fluid confined by elevated periosteum were demonstrated on MR scans

FIGURE 36–39. Plateau fracture. *A,* Anteroposterior radiograph showing depressed lateral plateau fracture *(arrow). B,* T_1-weighted axial image identifying depressed fracture site *(large arrow)* and radiating fracture segments *(curved arrow).*

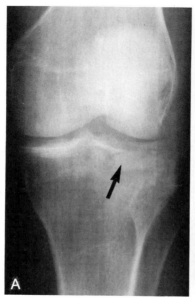
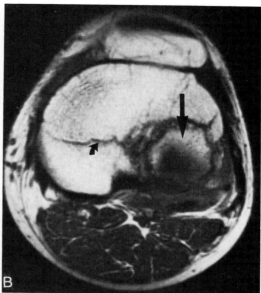

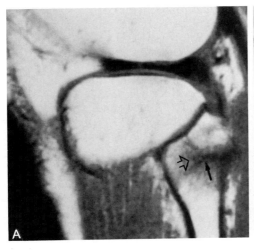
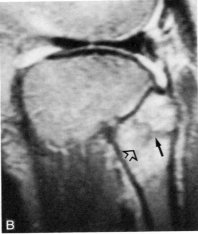

FIGURE 36–40. Fibular fracture. *A,* Low signal intensity marrow edema *(open arrow)* and linear fracture segments *(closed arrow)* are visualized on T_1-weighted sagittal image. *B,* Marrow edema and hemorrhage are displayed as bright signal intensity on T_2-weighted sagittal image *(open arrow).* Fracture segments maintain low signal intensity *(closed arrow).*

and surgically debrided. Plain film radiographs and nuclear bone scans were negative in this case.

An infectious tract with fluid may simulate a pathologic or stress fracture, and, when associated with extensive surrounding edema, can be confused with tumor. In a patient with multifocal osteomyelitis, seeding of the distal femur and proximal humerus was identified on MR scans as a central nidus of high signal intensity marrow and calcified sequestra of low signal intensity. Marrow infiltration and soft-tissue extension of osteomyelitis have also been demonstrated using short T_1 inversion recovery (STIR) sequences.

NEOPLASTIC CONDITIONS

Magnetic resonance has been used to image benign and primary malignant tumors for staging, to plan

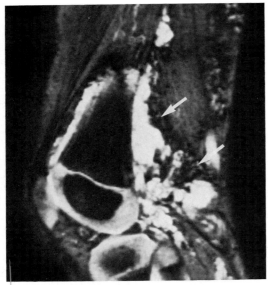

FIGURE 36–41. T_2^*-weighted gradient-refocused image displaying neurofibromatosis as bright signal intensity.

limb-salvage procedures, and to monitor chemotherapeutic response (Fig. 36–41).[66–70] The longitudinal extent of marrow and cortical involvement is displayed on coronal or sagittal images, facilitating preoperative planning for allograft salvage techniques (Fig. 36–42). T_1- and T_2-weighted axial images define intracompartmental extension and proximity to neurovascular structures. Interval response to preoperative chemotherapy can be assessed, and changes in tumor size; marrow infiltration; cortex, soft-tissue, and muscle invasion; hemorrhage; calcification; and necrosis can be recorded. It is important to perform MR imaging studies prior to biopsy in order to avoid postsurgical inflammation and edema, which may prolong the T_2 values of uninvolved tissues. Muscle edema is nonspecific and has also been imaged with trauma, infection, and vascular insults. High signal intensity on T_1-weighting in surrounding musculature can be seen in atrophy with fatty infiltration or neuromuscular disorders and should not be mistaken for tumor (Fig. 36–43).

Red to yellow marrow conversion in middle-aged female patients may be seen as low signal intensity in metaphyseal or diaphyseal locations without extension into the epiphysis. These regions become isointense with the adjacent marrow on heavily T_2-weighted images. Inhomogeneity of metaphyseal red and yellow marrow may also be observed in the immature skeleton. Marrow infiltrative disorders such as leukemia, lymphoma, and Gaucher's disease, however, do extend into the epiphysis or subchondral bone.[71, 72] Leukemic infiltrates have been detected on MR examination of the knee, prior to clinical diagnosis and even before peripheral blood smears become abnormal. Coarsened nonuniformity of marrow signal intensity is characteristically imaged in Paget's disease.

ARTIFACTS

The presence of orthopedic hardware (including plates, screws, pins, and prostheses) is not a contrain-

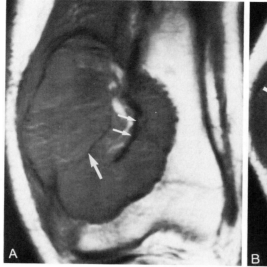 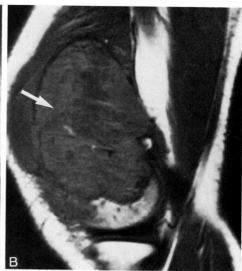

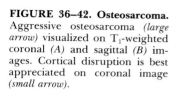

FIGURE 36–42. Osteosarcoma. Aggressive osteosarcoma *(large arrow)* visualized on T_1-weighted coronal *(A)* and sagittal *(B)* images. Cortical disruption is best appreciated on coronal image *(small arrow)*.

dication to MR imaging. Low signal intensity artifact is a function of the size, composition, orientation, and design of the device and of the number of devices present within the imaging field (see Fig. 36–27).[73-76] MR imaging has been successfully used to evaluate tumor recurrence in patients with limb salvage prostheses. A femoral rod or stem does not preclude evaluation of adjacent meniscal or ligamentous structures.

SUMMARY (Fig. 36–44)

For the diagnosis of meniscal and ligamentous injuries in internal knee derangements, MR imaging has gained substantial acceptance by radiologists and orthopedists as a replacement for the more traditional techniques of arthrography and CT scans.

Current indications for the use of MR imaging in internal knee derangements include acute hemarthrosis and tibial collateral ligament injuries, both of which may have associated meniscal tears. Patients under 15 years of age and over 50 years of age are better evaluated with MR imaging prior to arthroscopy. Negative arthroscopies should also be considered a basis for MR imaging referral.

In evaluating arthritis, fractures, infection, and neoplasia, noninvasive MR imaging provides superior tissue characterization, which is not possible with conventional radiographic techniques. Specificity in diagnostic interpretation of knee studies is also enhanced by direct multiplanar imaging with T_1, conventional T_2, and T_2 gradient-echo contrast. With improved surface coils and fast-scan techniques, routine knee examinations can be performed with 10 minutes of imaging time and have become more cost effective than arthrography.

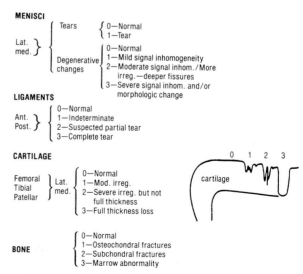

FIGURE 36–43. High signal intensity infiltrating lipoma *(arrow)* on T_1-weighted axial image.

MENISCI

Lat. med. }
- Tears { 0—Normal / 1—Tear
- Degenerative changes { 0—Normal / 1—Mild signal inhomogeneity / 2—Moderate signal inhom./More irreg.—deeper fissures / 3—Severe signal inhom. and/or morphologic change

LIGAMENTS

Ant. Post. }
- 0—Normal
- 1—Indeterminate
- 2—Suspected partial tear
- 3—Complete tear

CARTILAGE

Femoral Tibial Patellar } Lat. med. }
- 0—Normal
- 1—Mod. irreg.
- 2—Severe irreg. but not full thickness
- 3—Full thickness loss

BONE
- 0—Normal
- 1—Osteochondral fractures
- 2—Subchondral fractures
- 3—Marrow abnormality

FIGURE 36–44. Evaluation criteria for MR imaging.

REFERENCES

1. Reicher MA, Hartzmann S, Duckweiler GR, et al: Meniscal injuries: Detection using MR imaging. Radiology 159:753–757, 1986.
2. Stoller DW, Martin C, Crues JV, et al: Meniscal tears: Pathologic correlation with MR imaging. Radiology 163:452, 1987.
3. Lotysch M, Crues JV, Mink J: Scrutinizing knee joints: MRI offers new insight. Diagn Imag 7:80–94, 1986.
4. Hartzman MD, Reicher MA, Bassett LW, et al: MR imaging of the knee, Part II: Chronic disorders. Radiology 162:553, 1987.
5. Reicher MA, Hartzmann S, Bassett LW, et al: MR imaging of the knee, Part I: Traumatic disorders. Radiology 162:547, 1987.
6. Moon KL Jr, Genant HK, Helms CA, et al: Musculoskeletal applications of nuclear magnetic resonance. Radiology 147:161–171, 1983.
7. Li KC, Henkelman M, Poon PY, et al: MR imaging of the ligaments and menisci of the knee. J Comput Assist Tomogr 8:1147–1154, 1984.
8. Kean DM, Worthington BS, Preston BJ, et al: NMR imaging of the knee: Example of normal anatomy and pathology. Br J Radiol 56:355–364, 1984.
9. Gallimore GW, Harms SE: Knee injuries: High-resolution MR imaging. Radiology 160:457–461, 1986.
10. Burk DL, Kanal E, Burnberg JA, et al: 1.5T surface-coil MRI of the knee. AJR 147:293–300, 1986.
11. Li DKB, Adams ME, McConkey JP: Magnetic resonance imaging of the ligaments and menisci of the knee. Radiol Clin North Am 24:209–228, 1986.
12. Turner DA, Prodomos CC, Petasnick JP, et al: Acute injury of the ligaments of the knee: Magnetic resonance evaluation. Radiology 154:717–772, 1985.
13. Beltran J, Noto AM, Mosure JC, et al: The knee: Surface-coil MR imaging at 1.5T. Radiology 159:747–751, 1986.
14. Reicher MA, Rauschning W, Gold RH, et al: High resolution magnetic resonance imaging of the knee joint: Normal anatomy. AJR 145:895–902, 1985.
15. Reicher MA, Bassett IW, Gold RH, et al: High resolution magnetic resonance imaging of the knee joint: Pathologic correlations. AJR 145:903–909, 1985.
16. Ghelman B: Meniscal tears of the knee: Evaluation by high-resolution CT combined with arthrography. Radiology 157:23–27, 1985.
17. Thijn CJP: Accuracy of double-contrast arthrography and arthroscopy of the knee joint. Skeletal Radiol 8:187–192, 1982.
18. Watts I, Tasker T: Pitfalls in double contrast knee arthrography. Br J Radiol 53:754–759, 1980.
19. Gillies H, Seligson D: Precision in the diagnosis of meniscal lesions: A comparison of clinical evaluation, arthrography and arthroscopy. J Bone Joint Surg 61A:343–346, 1979.
20. Ireland J, Trickey EL, Stoker DJ: Arthroscopy and arthrography of the knee: A critical review. J Bone Joint Surg 62B:3–6, 1980.
21. Jackson RW, DeHaven KE: Arthroscopy of the knee. Clin Orthop 107:87–93, 1975.
22. Levinsohn ME, Baker BE: Prearthrotomy diagnostic evaluation of the knee: Review of 100 cases diagnosed by arthrography and arthroscopy. AJR 134:107–111, 1980.
23. Stoller DW, Helms CA, Genant HK: Gradient echo MR imaging of the knee. Radiology 165(P), 1987.
24. Crues JV III, Mink J, Levy TL, et al: Meniscal tears of the knee: Accuracy of MR imaging. Radiology 164:445, 1987.
25. Mandelbaum BR, Magid D, Fishman EK, et al: Magnetic resonance imaging as a tool for evaluation of traumatic knee injuries: Anatomical and pathoanatomical correlations. Am J Sports Med 14:361, 1986.
26. Mink JH, Levy T, Crues JV III: MR imaging of the knee: Technical factors, diagnostic accuracy, and further pitfalls. Radiology 165(P):175, 1987.
27. Tyrrell R, et al: Fast three-dimensional MR imaging of the knee: A comparison with arthroscopy. Radiology 165(P), 1987.
28. Beltran J, Noto AM, Mosure JC, et al: Meniscal tears: MR demonstration of experimentally produced injuries. Radiology 158:691–693, 1986.
29. Koenig SH, Brown RD: The importance of the motion of water for magnetic resonance imaging. Invest Radiol 20:297–306, 1985.
30. Smillie LS: Diseases of the Knee Joint. 2nd ed. London, Livingstone, pp 340–347.
31. Ricklin P, Ruttimann A, Del Buono MS: Meniscus Lesions: Diagnosis, Differential Diagnosis, and Therapy. 2nd ed. New York, Thieme Stratton, 1983.
32. Noble J, Hamblen PL: The pathology of the degenerate meniscus lesion. J Bone Joint Surg 57B:180–186, 1975.
33. Lotysch M, Mink J, Crues JV, et al: Magnetic resonance in the detection of meniscal injuries. Magn Reson Imaging 4:94, 1986.
34. Tobler TH: Makroskopische und histologische Befund am kniegelenk Meniscus in verschiedenen Lebensaitern. Schweiz Med Wochenschr 56:1359, 1926.
35. Roca FO, Vilalta A: Lesions of the meniscus, I: Macroscopic and histologic findings. Clin Orthop 146:289–300, 1980.
36. Roca FO, Vilalta A: Lesions of the meniscus, II: Horizontal cleavages and lateral cysts. Clin Orthop 146:301–307, 1980.
37. Arnoczky SP, Warren RF: Microvasculature of the human meniscus. Am J Sports Med 10:90–95, 1982.
38. Mink JR, Stoller DW, Martin C, et al: MR imaging of the knee: Pitfalls in interpretation. Radiology 165(P):239, 1987.
39. Shakespeare DT, Rigby HS: The bucket handle tear of the meniscus. J Bone Joint Surg 65B:383–386, 1983.
40. Debnam JW, Stablet W: Arthrography of knee after meniscectomy. Radiology 113:67–71, 1974.
41. Stoller DW, Genant HK: MR imaging of knee arthritides. Radiology 165(P):233, 1987.
42. Stoller DW: MRI of the patella and patellofemoral joint. Presented to the American Roentgen Ray Society, San Francisco, CA, May 8–13, 1988.
43. Resnick D, Niwayama G: Diagnosis of Bone and Joint Disorders. 2nd ed. Philadelphia, WB Saunders Company, 1988, Vol 5, pp 2896–2897.
44. Mink JH, Reicher MA, Crues JV III: Magnetic Resonance Imaging of the Knee. New York, Raven Press, 1987.
45. Rockwood CA, Green CP: Fractures. Philadelphia, JB Lippincott, 1975.
46. Stoller DW: MRI in juvenile rheumatoid (chronic) arthritis. Presented to Association of University Radiologists, Charleston, SC, March 22–27, 1987.
47. Stoller DW, Genant HK: MRI of pigmented villonodular synovitis. Presented to the American Roentgen Ray Society, San Francisco, CA, May 8–13, 1988.
48. Kottal RA, Vogler JB III, Matamoros A, et al: Pigmented villonodular synovitis: Report of MR imaging in two cases. Radiology 163:551, 1987.
49. Kulkarni MV, Drolshagen LP, Kaye JJ, et al: MR imaging of hemophiliac arthropathy. J Comput Assist Tomogr 10:445–449, 1986.
50. Yulish BS, Lieberman JM, Newman AJ, et al: Hemophilic arthropathy: Assessment with MR imaging. Radiology 164:759, 1987.
51. Johnston YE, Duray PH, Steere AC, et al: Lyme arthritis: Spirochetes found in synovial microangiopathic lesions. Am J Pathol 118:26, 1985.
52. Ahlback S, Bauer GC, Bohne WH: Spontaneous osteonecrosis of the knee. Arthritis Rheum 11:705, 1968.
53. Williams JL, Cliff MM, Bonakdarpour A: Spontaneous osteonecrosis of the knee. Radiology 107:15, 1973.
54. Lotke PA, Ecker ML: Osteonecrosis-like syndrome of the medial tibial plateau. Clin Orthop 176:148, 1983.
55. Linden B: The incidence of osteochondritis dissecans in the condyles of the femur. Acta Orthop Scand 47:664, 1976.
56. Mesgarzadeh M, Sagega AA, Bonakdarpour A, et al: MR imaging of osteochondritis dissecans. Radiology 161(P):24, 1986.

57. Mesgarzadeh M, Sapega AA, Bonakdarpour A, et al: Osteochondritis dissecans: Analysis of mechanical stability with radiography, scintigraphy, and MR imaging. Radiology 165:775, 1987.

58. Ehman RL, Berquist TH, McLeod RA: MR imaging of the musculoskeletal system: A 5-year appraisal. Radiology 166:313, 1988.

59. Beltran J, Noto AM, Herman JH, et al: Joint effusions: MR imaging. Radiology 158:133–137, 1986.

60. Guerra J, Newell JD, Resnick D, et al: Gastrocnemio-semimembranosus bursal region of the knee. AJR 136:593, 1981.

61. Lindgreen PG, Willen R: Gastrocnemius-semimembranosus bursa and its relation to the knee joint: Anatomy and histology. Acta Radiol (Diagn) 18:497, 1977.

62. Apple JS, Martinez S, Hardaker WT, et al: Synovial plicae of the knee. Skeletal Radiol 7:251, 1982.

63. Passariello R, Trecco F, DePaulis F, et al: CT and MR imaging of the knee joint in the "plica syndrome." Radiology 161(P):240, 1986.

64. Stafford SA, Rosenthal DI, Gebhardt MC, et al: MRI in stress fracture. AJR 147:553, 1986.

65. Resnick D, Niwayama G: Diagnosis of Bone and Joint Disorders. 2nd ed. Philadelphia, WB Saunders Company, 1988, Vol 1, Chap 18.

66. Stoller DW, Waxman A, Rosen J: Comparison of T$_1$-201, GA-67, Tc-99m MDP and MR imaging of musculoskeletal sarcoma. Radiology 165(P):223, 1987.

67. Bloem JL, Bloemm RG, Taminiau AHM, et al: Magnetic resonance imaging of primary malignant bone tumors. RadioGraphics 7:425, 1987.

68. Wetzel LH, Levine E, Murphey MD: A comparison of MR imaging and CT in the evaluation of musculoskeletal masses. RadioGraphics 7:851, 1987.

69. Petasnick JP, Turner DA, Charters JR, et al: Soft-tissue masses of the locomotor system: Comparison of MR imaging with CT. Radiology 160:125, 1986.

70. Totty WG, Murphy WA, Lee JKT: Soft-tissue tumors: MR imaging. Radiology 160:135, 1986.

71. Lanir A, Hadar H, Cohen I, et al: Gaucher disease: Assessment with MR imaging. Radiology 161:239, 1986.

72. Olson DO, Shields AF, Scheurich CJ, et al: Magnetic resonance imaging of the bone marrow in patients with leukemia, aplastic anemia, and lymphoma. Invest Radiol 21:540, 1986.

73. Porter BA, Hastrup W, Richardson ML, et al: Classification and investigation of artifacts in magnetic resonance imaging. RadioGraphics 7:271, 1987.

74. Pusey E, Lupkin RB, Brown RKJ, et al: Magnetic resonance imaging artifacts: Mechanism and clinical significance. RadioGraphics 6:891, 1986.

75. Augustiny N, von Schulthess GK, Meier D, Bösiger P: MR imaging of large nonferromagnetic metallic implants at 1.5T. J Comput Assist Tomogr 11:678, 1987.

76. James R, Bartlett CR, Renicker J, Orchard K: Unusual MR metallic artifact due to steel threads. J Comput Assist Tomogr 11:722, 1987.

37

MR IMAGING OF THE GLENOHUMERAL JOINT

MICHAEL B. ZLATKIN and J. BRUCE KNEELAND

TECHNIQUE

ANATOMY
  RELEVANT GENERAL ANATOMY
  MR IMAGING ANATOMY

ROTATOR CUFF ABNORMALITIES

CAPSULAR ABNORMALITIES

OTHER GLENOHUMERAL JOINT ABNORMALITIES
  TRAUMA
  SYNOVIAL INFLAMMATORY DISEASE
  OSTEONECROSIS
  CRYSTAL DEPOSITION DISEASE
  LOOSE BODIES
  NEOPLASMS

The shoulder is an extremely mobile joint that is prone to injury from trauma and to degeneration from overuse. Therefore, shoulder pain is a very common clinical problem. As there are many different causes whose clinical symptoms and signs often overlap, radiologic evaluation has been a necessary and valuable adjunct to the clinical examination in patients with this clinical problem. Noninvasive imaging modalities, including plain radiography, radionuclide studies, tomography, and computed tomography (CT), are utilized but are often nonspecific. Invasive examinations such as arthrography[1, 2] and conventional and computed arthrotomography[3-6] may yield a more specific diagnosis but are not without morbidity.[7] Ultrasonography has been reported to be a useful technique in evaluating the shoulder for rotator cuff abnormalities[8] but is limited in the scope of diseases it can assess and is highly dependent on the experience of the examiner.

Recent technical advances have allowed significant improvement in our ability to obtain diagnostic images of the shoulder with MR imaging. Included among these are off-center field-of-view and oblique imaging, as well as improvements in surface coils.

We have utilized MR imaging to evaluate a large number of patients with shoulder pain. MR imaging has performed well in noninvasively diagnosing many shoulder disorders, particularly those due to rotator cuff disease, and we believe that, in conjunction with plain radiographs, it can replace most of the other techniques used to evaluate the shoulder. This chapter reviews current experience with this modality and discusses relevant technical, anatomic, and pathologic issues.

TECHNIQUE

The patient is placed in a supine position in the magnet. A dual surface coil array employing two 5½-inch general purpose surface coils is used. One coil is placed anterior and one posterior to the shoulder (Fig. 37–1A) in a Helmholtz configuration.[9] In this configuration the signal detected from the imaging volume of each coil should be additive. The patient's arm is left by his or her side at rest, usually in neutral or mild internal rotation, whichever is more comfortable, to minimize patient motion.

For patients with suspected rotator cuff tears, a coronal localizing image is performed first, utilizing a spin-echo (SE) 600/20 sequence and a field-of-view

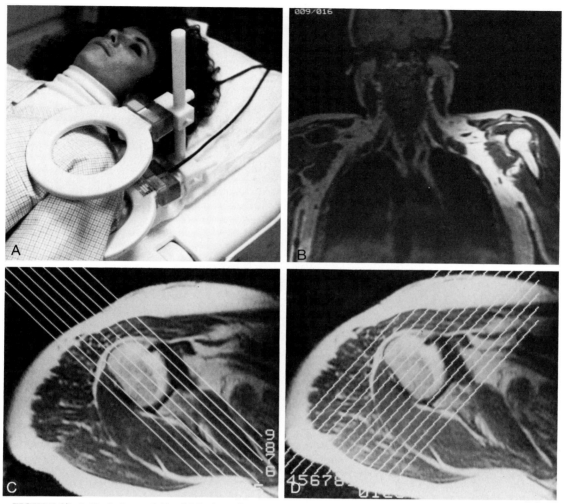

FIGURE 37–1. Technique. *A*, Dual 5-inch surface coil array with adjustable plastic holder in place on normal volunteer showing typical patient positioning. *B*, Coronal localizer image in body coil to set off center field-of-view and identify levels for axial images. *C*, Graphic localizer illustrating slice orientation perpendicular to the glenoid margin for coronal oblique images. *D*, Localizer parallel to glenoid margin for sagittal obliques.

of 40 to 48 cm in the body coil. This sequence determines the location of the off-center field of view (Fig. 37–1*B*). After the appropriate coordinates are determined, an axial SE 600/20 pulse sequence is obtained with 5-mm slice thickness from below the level of the acromion to the inferior glenoid margin. The axial images are beneficial in assessing the capsular mechanism of the shoulder, including the glenoid labrum. They are also used as a localizing image to determine the correct plane for the oblique coronal and sagittal images[10, 11] (Fig. 37–1*C* and *D*). The oblique coronal images are oriented perpendicular to the glenoid margin, parallel to the supraspinatus muscle and tendon. The continuity of the supraspinatus muscle and tendon is easily identified in this plane. The relationship of the anteroinferior acromion and acromioclavicular joint to the supraspinatus muscle and tendon can also be discerned. Two pulse sequences are performed in the coronal oblique

plane, one with a variable-echo SE 2500/20/70 with a 5-mm slice thickness, the second with a relatively T_1-weighted interleaved sequence SE 1000/20 with a 3-mm slice thickness. The anatomy is best demonstrated on the proton density and T_1-weighted images, which define the detail of the muscles and tendon. The T_2-weighted images are more helpful in outlining any intra- or extraarticular fluid or edema. Sagittal oblique images, which are parallel to the glenoid margin and perpendicular to the supraspinatus muscle and tendon, are obtained with an SE 800/20 sequence at 5-mm intervals. The authors utilize a field-of-view of 14 cm for the axial imaging plane and 16 cm for the oblique imaging planes. The matrix size is 256 × 128, utilizing two signal excitations. In patients with a history of recurrent dislocations or suspected glenoid labral tears, a T_2-weighted axial series is performed and the sagittal oblique series is omitted. In addition, the axial T_1 sequence previously outlined for patients with rotator cuff problems is replaced by an SE 800/20 interleaved sequence performed at 3-mm intervals.

ANATOMY

RELEVANT GENERAL ANATOMY[12]

The glenohumeral joint is a multiaxial ball-and-socket joint lying between the roughly hemispheric humeral head and the shallow glenoid fossa of the scapula. Although this anatomy permits a wide range of motion, the joint is relatively unstable owing to the small size of the glenoid fossa compared to the humeral head and also because of the redundancy of the joint capsule.

The proximal end of the humerus consists of the head and greater and lesser tuberosities. The anatomic neck of the humerus lies at the base of the articular surface of the proximal end of the bone. The neck is the site of attachment of the inferior aspect of the capsule. The greater tuberosity is located on the lateral aspect of the proximal humerus and serves as the site of insertion of the supraspinatus, infraspinatus, and teres minor muscles. The supraspinatus muscle inserts on the promontory, or highest point, of the greater tuberosity. The infraspinatus and teres minor tendons localize, respectively, to the middle and lower thirds of the greater tuberosity and lie somewhat more posteriorly than the supraspinatus insertion. The lesser tuberosity is situated on the anterior portion of the proximal humerus, and the subscapularis tendon inserts here. The intertubercular (bicipital) groove is located between the greater and lesser tuberosities. The tendon of the long head of the biceps brachii muscle passes through here, surrounded by a synovial sheath. The tendon is secured within the groove by the transverse humeral ligament, which passes between the tuberosities over the synovial sheath of the tendon.

The glenoid cavity is situated on the superolateral aspect of the scapula. The articular surface of this cavity is very shallow, but the cavity is deepened and enlarged by the fibrocartilaginous glenoid labrum and by the thin cartilaginous lining in the center of the cavity. The supraglenoid tubercle is immediately above the cavity, and the long head of the biceps tendon is attached here. Hyaline articular cartilage lines the surfaces of the glenoid and the humeral head. The cartilage on the humeral head is thickest at its center; the reverse is true of the glenoid cavity. A loose fibrous capsule envelops the joint. It is lined by a synovial membrane. The synovium is prolonged distally to line the bicipital groove. Superiorly, the capsule encroaches on the root of the coracoid process and inserts in the supraglenoid region, thus including the long head of the biceps muscle within the joint. Laterally, the capsule inserts into the anatomic neck of the humerus and, medially, into the periosteum of the humeral shaft. With the arm at the side, the lower part of the capsule is lax and redundant, forming the axillary recess. Medially, the capsular insertion is variable.[13] It may insert directly into the labrum or more medially along the scapular neck. The fibrous capsule is strengthened in several areas. The coracohumeral ligament is a strong fibrous band that arises proximally from the lateral edge of the coracoid process, extending over the head of the humerus to attach to the greater tuberosity. Anteriorly, the capsule may thicken to form the superior, middle, and inferior glenohumeral ligaments.[14] In addition, the tendons of the supraspinatus, infraspinatus, teres minor, and subscapularis muscles all blend with the fibrous capsule to form the rotator cuff.

There are a number of bursae about the glenohumeral joint, the most important of which are the subscapularis bursa and the subacromial bursa. The subacromial bursa is the largest bursa in the human body. It is composed primarily of the subacromial and subdeltoid portions and is found between the acromion and deltoid muscle and the rotator cuff. The bursa is lined by fine filmy areolar tissue and acts as a gliding mechanism between the deltoid and teres major muscles and the rotator cuff muscles. It communicates with the joint cavity only if a tear involving the full thickness of the musculotendinous rotator cuff opens into the floor of the bursa. The subscapularis bursa or recess is situated anteriorly, lying between the posterior aspect of the subscapularis tendon and the scapula. It communicates with the joint cavity through an opening that forms between the middle and superior glenohumeral ligaments.

The acromioclavicular joint is a small synovial articulation between the medial aspect of the acromion and the lateral portion of the clavicle. The articular surfaces of the acromion and clavicle are covered with fibrocartilage. In the central portion of the joint there is an articular disk that partially divides the joint. An articular capsule surrounds the joint, attaching at the joint margins. The coracoclavicular ligament is the major source of stability of the acromioclavicular joint, extending from the clavicle to the coracoid process, thus anchoring the clavicle to the scapula. It consists of the posteromedial conoid and anterolateral trapezoid ligaments. The coracoacromial arch consists primarily of the acromion and the acromioclavicular joint, the coracoid process, and the coracoacromial ligament. The coracoacromial ligament is a strong triangular structure that joins the coracoid and acromial processes. This unyielding, strong bony and ligamentous arch protects the humeral head and rotator cuff tendons from direct trauma. However, because of its unyielding nature and close approximation to the humeral head during abduction, it limits the space available to the rotator cuff tendons during abduction. Chronic impingement and attrition of these tendons are therefore produced.

MR Imaging Anatomy

A number of recent articles have illustrated the anatomy of the glenohumeral joint as it appears on MR imaging.[15–18] Figures 37–2 to 37–4 are a series of short TR/TE SE images of a normal shoulder in the axial, coronal oblique, and sagittal oblique planes. Subcutaneous fat, intermuscular fat planes, and bone marrow have the high signal on T_1-weighted images owing to their relatively short T_1. Muscles and hyaline articular cartilage have an intermediate signal intensity. Owing to a relative lack of mobile protons, certain structures have essentially no MR signal and are therefore identified by anatomic location and contrast with surrounding tissues. These structures include cortical bone, the fibrocartilaginous glenoid labrum, the articular capsule, and tendinous and ligamentous structures such as the tendinous insertions of the rotator cuff musculature and the long head of biceps as it courses in the bicipital groove.

Axial images demonstrate the relationship between the humeral head and glenoid cavity. The hyaline articular cartilage and the glenoid labrum are well depicted. The anterior glenoid labrum most commonly has a triangular configuration in this plane, although there may be considerable variability in its normal appearance.[19] The posterior labrum is more commonly rounded in appearance.[20] Intermediate signal is normally present at the base of the glenoid labrum. This represents hyaline articular cartilage and should not be confused with a labral tear. The subscapularis muscle and its tendon insertion into the lesser tuberosity are well visualized in this plane.

The long head of the biceps tendon is also best seen on axial sections. It appears as a round area of signal void in the bicipital groove. Its sheath is seen as a fine surrounding ring of moderate signal intensity.[15] The subscapularis bursa may not be identified as a separate structure except in the presence of synovial fluid. The anterior capsule and its insertion into the glenoid margin and the glenohumeral ligaments are usually evident on routine axial images but are most easily identified when an intraarticular effusion is present.

The tendons of the rotator cuff muscles are best identified on serial coronal oblique images. As previously stated, this plane courses parallel to the supraspinatus muscle and tendon; therefore, these structures can be seen in continuity. The subacromial-subdeltoid bursa is a potential space and hence is not visualized as a separate structure. However, in the normal shoulder a high signal intensity fat plane is identified separating the rotator cuff tendons from the acromioclavicular joint, acromion, and overlying deltoid muscle. This most likely conforms to the fat located within and beneath the synovial lining of the subacromial-subdeltoid bursa.[18] This has been termed the subacromial-subdeltoid fat plane.[21] On the most anterior coronal oblique images, the coracoclavicular and coracohumeral ligaments, subscapularis muscle, and long head of biceps tendon may be identified. The superior and inferior labra can also be identified in this plane.

The sagittal oblique plane also demonstrates the rotator cuff muscles. The anteroposterior extent of the rotator cuff tendons can be identified. The rela-

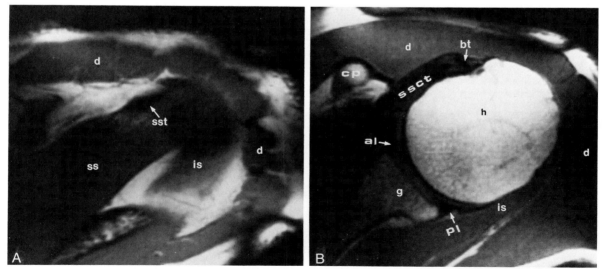

FIGURE 37–2. Axial MR images of the normal shoulder. *A,* Superior shoulder. *B,* Midshoulder. Key to Figures 37–2 to 37–4 (cap and lower case abbreviations have the same meaning): ACR = acromion process; AL = anterior labrum; AR = axillary recess; BT = biceps tendon; CAL = coracoacromial ligament; CCL = coracoclavicular ligament; CL = clavicle; CP = coracoid process; D = deltoid muscle; G = glenoid; H = humerus; IS = infraspinatus muscle; IST = infraspinatus tendon; PL = posterior labrum; PMN = pectoralis minor; SAF = subacromial fat plane; SDF = subdeltoid fat plane; SS = supraspinatus muscle; SSCM = subscapularis muscle; SSCT = subscapularis tendon; SST = supraspinatus tendon; TM = teres minor muscle; TR = trapezius muscle; cb = coracobrachial muscles; tmt = teres minor tendon.

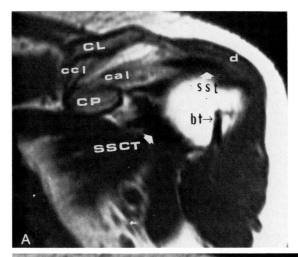

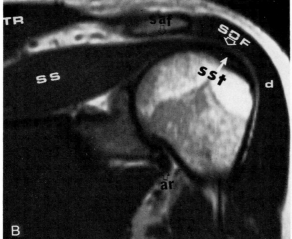

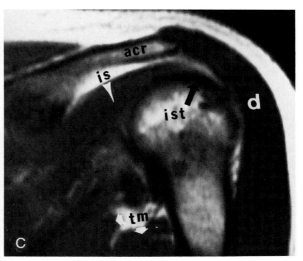

FIGURE 37–3. Coronal oblique MR images of the normal shoulder. *A*, Anterior shoulder. *B*, Midshoulder. *C*, Posterior shoulder.

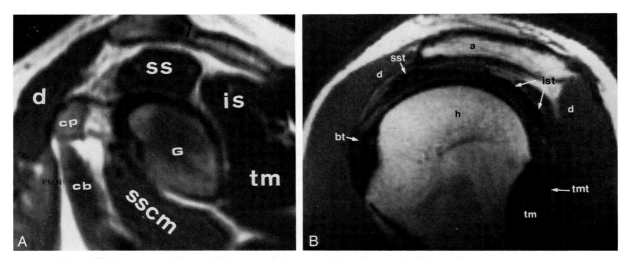

FIGURE 37–4. Sagittal oblique MR images of the normal shoulder. *A*, Medial shoulder. *B*, Lateral shoulder.

tionship of the acromion process and the acromioclavicular joint to the supraspinatus tendon is also well depicted in this plane.

ROTATOR CUFF ABNORMALITIES

Injury to the rotator cuff tendons is usually chronic. It is recognized that normal tendons do not tear, as 30 per cent or more of the tendon must be damaged to produce a substantial reduction in its strength.[22] Therefore, trauma may enlarge a preexisting tear but would rarely be the initiating event.

It has been postulated that 95 per cent of rotator cuff lesions result from chronic impingement of the supraspinatus tendon against the undersurface of the anterior third of the acromion, the coracoacromial ligament, and the acromioclavicular joint. Injury to the rotator cuff represents a continuum of disease that is classified into three progressive pathologic stages.[23, 24] In the first stage, reversible edema and hemorrhage are observed within the supraspinatus tendon. This generally occurs in patients less than 25 years of age. Clinically these patients present with a history of acute overuse. This is most often seen in athletes who are active in swimming, tennis, and baseball. The second stage is one of fibrosis and tendinitis. The symptoms are generally more chronic in nature, and the patients tend to be somewhat older. In the third or final stage, tendon degeneration and rupture occur, often in association with bony changes. These patients are usually older than 40 years.

Microangiographic studies have revealed that the rotator cuff tendons have abundant vascular supply, except for a 1-cm area adjacent to the tendinous insertion of the supraspinatus into the greater tuberosity. This area of relative avascularity has been called the "critical zone"[25] and is the region where the majority of tendon ruptures occur. Mechanical impingement on this relatively avascular area leads to an inflammatory tendinitis, the first stage in the degenerative process. These reversible inflammatory changes may subsequently involve the acromioclavicular joint, subacromial bursa, and biceps tendon.[26] Continued impingement leads to fibrosis and weakening of the tendon. If the process continues, further attrition of the tendon results in tears of the rotator cuff. Associated osseous changes consist of acromioclavicular joint osteoarthritis, spur formation on the undersurface of the anterior aspect of the acromion, and irregularity, sclerosis, and cyst formation on the posterolateral surface of the humeral head.

The clinical signs and symptoms of rotator cuff impingement can be nonspecific, and thus the diagnosis may be delayed prior to the development of a full-thickness tear of the rotator cuff. Conventional radiography plays little or no role in the early diagnosis, as plain radiographic changes generally occur late in the course of the disease. Arthrography is also usually of little value in the early diagnosis of impingement syndrome. Findings will not usually be evident until a rotator cuff tear is present (stage III).[21, 27, 28] Some authors have utilized subacromial bursography in an attempt to diagnose impingement syndrome.[29, 30] It may reveal difficulty in filling of the bursa owing to soft-tissue edema or thickening; however, bursography is invasive, painful, and not highly accurate.

Our experience and that of others[21, 28, 31] indicate that MR imaging can demonstrate abnormalities in patients with rotator cuff impingement syndrome. It can demonstrate rotator cuff tears but also tendon abnormalities (tendinitis) in patients with intact cuffs.

In patients with tendinitis the rotator cuff tendons are intact, but there is high signal intensity seen in the distal tendon (Fig. 37–5). This probably reflects the presence of increased free water within the tendon secondary to edema and inflammation. This abnormal signal is usually best seen on T_1 and proton density images owing to better contrast and signal-to-noise ratio on these sequences. The subacromial-subdeltoid fat plane is intact, and fluid is not seen in the subacromial or subdeltoid bursa. In these patients arthrography is normal,[21] but patients with this abnormality who have come to surgery showed inflammation and mucoid degenerative changes[31] within the tendon. Thus these MR imaging findings probably correspond to the stage I and II pathologic changes described by Neer.

Secondary osseous changes of chronic impingement may be identified in these patients, including subacromial spurs, degenerative changes of the acromioclavicular joint, and hypertrophy of its capsule (Fig. 37–6). Small subacromial spurs are characterized by foci of signal void that project from the acromion tip. Large spurs frequently contain marrow and are seen as regions of bright signal continuous with the acromion, which may be surrounded by a rim of signal void representing cortical bone.[27] A low-lying anterior acromion may also be identified. Bony impingement on the supraspinatus musculotendinous junction may also be evident (Fig. 37–6).

The ability to detect changes noninvasively within the rotator cuff tendons in patients without complete or partial tears is a distinct advantage of MR imaging. It presents the surgeon with objective criteria on which to base a treatment plan, which usually begins with conservative management. Based on these findings and the presence of persistent symptoms refractory to conservative management, the orthopedic surgeon may then utilize MR imaging to plan surgery, such as acromioplasty and coracoacromial ligament excision.

MR imaging findings of complete rotator cuff tears (Figs. 37–7 to 37–10) include increased signal within the rotator cuff tendons associated with changes in morphology such as thinning, irregularity, or discontinuity of the rotator cuff tendons, usually the supraspinatus. In the majority of cases with discontinuity

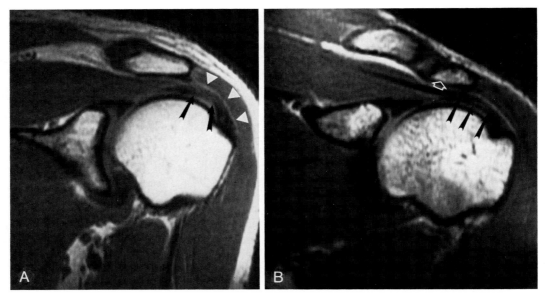

FIGURE 37–5. Tendinitis. Grade 1 tendon. *A,* Coronal oblique section (TR/TE 1000/20). Diffuse increased signal is identified in the distal supraspinatus tendon *(arrows).* The subdeltoid fat plane is normal *(arrowheads).* Also note the small subacromial spur. *B,* Similar signal intensity changes in another patient *(arrows).* Also note the low-lying anterior acromion *(open arrow).*

identified in the tendon, increased signal consistent with fluid is identified within the area of disruption on T$_2$-weighted images. Associated signs include loss of the subacromial and subdeltoid fat on T$_1$ and proton density images. On T$_2$-weighted images, increased signal consistent with fluid is usually seen in the subacromial-subdeltoid bursa. This is thought to represent extension of intraarticular fluid through the tear into the bursa.[21] In chronic tears atrophy of the rotator cuff musculature is often apparent. This is manifested by decrease in the muscle bulk and size

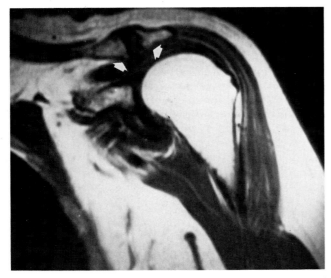

FIGURE 37–6. Bony impingement. Anterior coronal section (TR/TE 800/20) reveals osteophytes projecting inferiorly from the acromioclavicular joint, impinging upon the proximal supraspinatus tendon *(arrows).*

and the presence of high-signal linear bands within the muscle belly, indicative of fatty replacement.[21] In patients with moderate and large tears there is often retraction of the supraspinatus tendon. Secondary osseous changes of chronic impingement are often present in these patients.

Kneeland and coworkers[32] studied 25 patients with known or suspected tears of the rotator cuff. MR visualized the tears in 20 of the 22 tears diagnosed by arthrography or surgery. In most cases the tears were identified as a region of increased signal within the cuff on long TR sequences. Kieft and coworkers[31] and others correlated the severity of tendon signal changes at MR to arthrographic and surgical findings. They found that the tendons with the most severe distortion of shape and the greatest amount of increased signal were most likely to have tears.

Based on our observations of patients with rotator cuff disease, we have developed distinct MR imaging criteria for diagnosis.[28] These criteria are based on a grading system for changes within the rotator cuff tendons, which we consider primary signs, as well as for abnormalities involving the subacromial-subdeltoid fat plane and bursa, which we consider secondary signs. The grading system for changes of the rotator cuff tendons is as follows: Grade 0 is a tendon with normal signal and morphology. Grade 1 is defined as a tendon with increased signal but normal morphology (see Fig. 37–5). Grade 2 is a tendon with increased signal intensity with change in morphology (see Fig. 37–7). Abnormal morphology is defined as distinct tendon thinning and/or irregularity. Grade 3 is a tendon with a distinct area of discontinuity in the normal signal void of the tendon (Figs. 37–8 to 37–10). As previously noted, these areas of disconti-

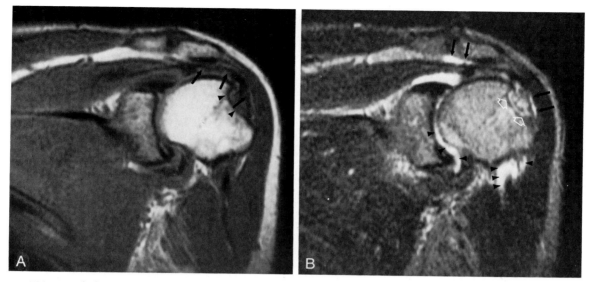

FIGURE 37–7. Rotator cuff tear. Grade 2 tendon. *A,* Coronal oblique image (TR/TE 1000/20) demonstrating increased signal, irregularity, and thinning of the distal supraspinatus tendon *(arrows).* The subdeltoid fat plane is lost. Note also the decreased signal in the marrow in the region of the greater tuberosity from an associated fracture *(arrowheads). B,* Long TR/TE image (2500/70) demonstrates fluid in the subacromial-subdeltoid bursa *(arrows).* High signal intensity fluid is also present in the glenohumeral joint and in the biceps tendon sheath *(arrowheads).* There is increased signal consistent with marrow edema in the region of the greater tuberosity fracture *(open arrows).*

nuity usually demonstrate increase in signal on T$_2$-weighted images. Therefore, a normal cuff is one with a grade 0 tendon and a normal subacromial-subdeltoid fat plane. A diagnosis of tendinitis or tendon degeneration is made in the presence of a grade 1 or 2 tendon with a normal fat plane. A rotator cuff tear is diagnosed in the presence of a grade 2 or grade 3 tendon with loss of the subacromial-subdeltoid fat on T$_1$- and proton density–weighted images and/or fluid in the subacromial-subdeltoid bursa on T$_2$-weighted images.

These criteria were tested in a recent study[28] of 32 surgically confirmed cases. Utilizing the criteria outlined above, sensitivity, specificity, and accuracy of

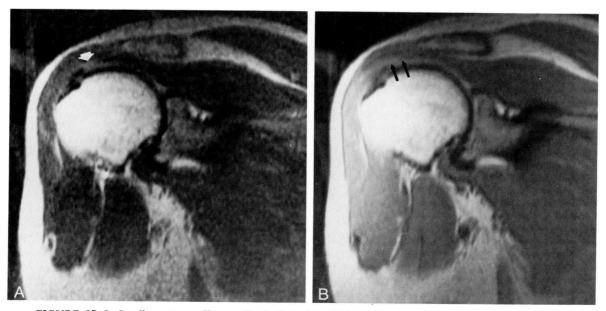

FIGURE 37–8. Small rotator cuff tear. Grade 3 tendon. *A,* Midcoronal oblique image (TR/TE 2500/20) demonstrating a small region of discontinuity in the midsupraspinatus tendon *(arrow)* with loss of the overlying subdeltoid fat plane. *B,* The second echo (TR/TE 2500/80) demonstrates further increase in signal intensity within the tendon defect *(arrows).*

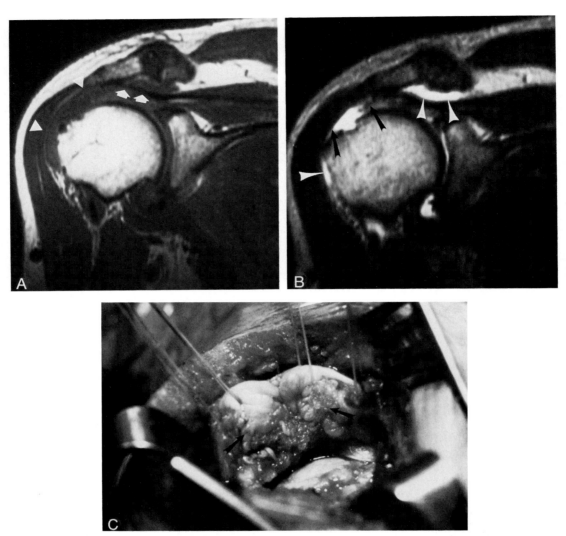

FIGURE 37–9. Large rotator cuff tear. Grade 3 tendon. *A,* Coronal oblique image (TR/TE 1000/20) demonstrating loss of the signal void of the supraspinatus tendon with retraction of the irregular torn tendon edges to the level of the acromioclavicular joint *(arrows).* The subacromial-subdeltoid fat plane is disrupted *(arrowheads). B,* T$_2$-weighted coronal oblique image (TR/TE 2500/70) demonstrates high signal intensity fluid outlining the large area of discontinuity in the supraspinatus tendon *(arrows).* Note the excellent visualization of the retracted tendon edges. Fluid is also identified in the subacromial-subdeltoid bursa *(arrowheads). C,* Intraoperative photograph demonstrating the large tear. Note the absence of the supraspinatus tendon over the humeral head and the retracted torn tendon edges *(arrows).*

91 per cent, 88 per cent, and 89 per cent for all tears (partial and complete), respectively, were found. In this series[28] MR imaging was also found to be more sensitive than arthrography, particularly in the diagnosis of small tears in the anterior aspect of the supraspinatus tendon, less than 1.5 cm in size, in which arthrography may be negative (Fig. 37–10). In this same study there was excellent correlation with the size of the tears, the site of the tear, and the specific tendons involved (i.e., supraspinatus and infraspinatus), as well as the quality of the torn tendon edges. This information can be very helpful to the surgeon in preoperative planning.

In another recent study by Evancho and coworkers of 31 patients who had MR imaging examinations confirmed by arthroscopy or arthrography,[33] sensitivity, specificity, and accuracy of 80 per cent, 94 per cent, and 89 per cent for complete rotator cuff tears and 69 per cent, 94 per cent, and 84 per cent for all tears (partial and complete), respectively, were found.

Currently there are no definitively established criteria to distinguish partial from small full-thickness tears. In Kneeland's study[32] the MR imaging appearance of two surgically confirmed partial-thickness tears was similar to that seen with full-thickness tears. In our experience with a small number of surgically confirmed cases[21, 28] (MBZ, unpublished data), partial tears of the inferior surface may appear as areas of increased signal within the affected tendon, with some associated irregularity in outline or thinning of

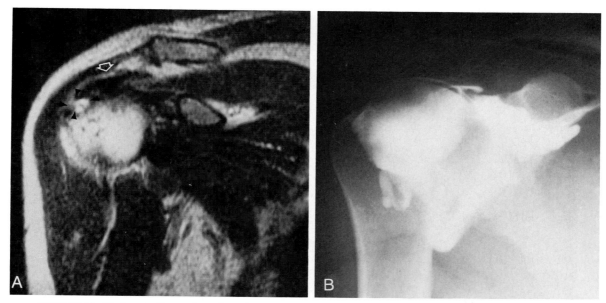

FIGURE 37–10. Surgically confirmed small tear, grade 3 tendon, negative arthrogram. *A,* T$_2$-weighted (2500/70) coronal oblique image at the anterior leading edge of the supraspinatus tendon demonstrates a small region of discontinuity in the tendon outlined by fluid *(arrowheads).* A tiny amount of fluid is identified in the subdeltoid bursa *(open arrow). B,* A single contrast arthrogram performed that day was negative.

the tendon (Fig. 37–11). Definite areas of discontinuity (grade 3 tendon) with retraction of tendon edges have not been observed. The overlying subacromial-subdeltoid fat plane is decreased in signal intensity or lost in the region of the tendinous abnormality, likely owing to associated inflammation. Fluid in the subacromial-subdeltoid bursa has not been observed. Two surgically confirmed partial tears

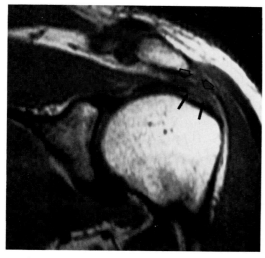

FIGURE 37–11. Coronal oblique image at the level of the acromioclavicular joint reveals a small area of increased signal, irregularity, and thinning of the distal supraspinatus tendon (grade 2) *(arrows).* The subacromial-subdeltoid fat is lost in the region of the tendon abnormality *(arrowheads).* No fluid was seen in the subdeltoid bursa or within the abnormal region of the tendon on T$_2$-weighted images. These findings are indicative of a small, partial-thickness tear.

of the superior surface of the tendon had similar findings, but these were evident only in retrospect. The necessity of distinguishing between severe changes of tendinitis and tendon degeneration, partial tears, and small full-thickness tears in many cases depends on the treating orthopedic surgeon's philosophy of management. There are some data to show that patients may do as well with conservative therapy,[34, 35] and the decision to perform surgery would then depend more on whether the patient has persistent severe symptoms. Other studies[22] have shown that as many as 50 per cent of patients with small tears do not respond to conservative management, and hence early surgery may be indicated in this group. Preliminary results indicate, however, that MR imaging can make these distinctions with some accuracy. Further closely monitored prospective studies with careful clinical correlation, currently under way at our hospital, may help form a more ordered approach to the management of these patients, using MR imaging as a predictor of clinical outcome.

The MR imaging evaluation of the rotator cuff in the postoperative patient can be divided into two categories. The first involves patients following acromioplasty. In these patients, prior resection of the anterior acromion can be identified. Imaging in the sagittal plane may be most useful to assess the adequacy of the resection. Evaluation of the integrity of the cuff itself may be more difficult in these patients, as the subacromial-subdeltoid fat plane is usually distorted by the surgery, making the secondary signs of rotator cuff tears unreliable in this setting.

The second category involves patients following rotator cuff repair. In general, arthrography may be

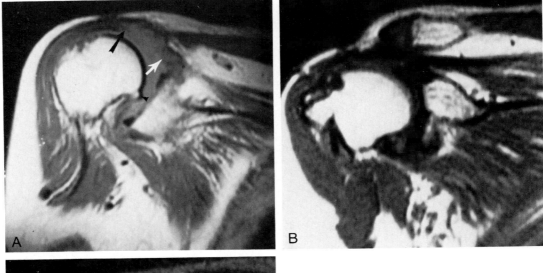

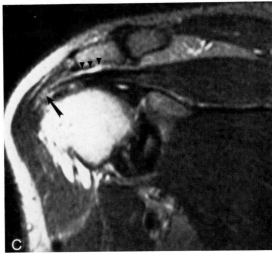

FIGURE 37–12. MR image of post–rotator cuff repair. *A,* Long TR/TE image (2500/80) illustrating a disrupted cuff at the site of a previous repair *(arrows).* There is also severe atrophy present in the surrounding musculature. Note the small osteophyte projecting from the humeral head *(arrowhead). B,* Note the marked irregularity of the subcutaneous tissues and loss of the fat planes in this patient with an irregular-appearing but essentially intact tendon following cuff repair. *C,* Long TR/TE image (2500/70) delineates a small region of discontinuity in the distal supraspinatus tendon *(arrow)* with fluid in the subacromial bursa *(arrowheads)* in this patient following primary cuff repair.

misleading in these cases, as many of the arthrograms performed in these patients show a leak following injection of contrast, often in spite of adequate repair, relief of symptoms, and return of good function.[36] MR imaging can directly visualize the cuff following repair (Fig. 37–12). It can demonstrate recurrent tears or evidence of inadequate repair; however, in the absence of a baseline postoperative study it may be difficult in some cases to separate out changes in signal and morphology in the tendon due to recurrent tear from those due to previous surgery.

In summary, MR imaging can diagnose rotator cuff abnormalities due to chronic impingement. Tendon abnormalities can be seen in patients without cuff tears. Complete cuff tears can be reliably identified. The size and extent of rotator cuff tears can also be depicted. It may not be possible to distinguish between tendinitis and tendon degeneration and between partial and small full-thickness tears in all cases; however, disease of the rotator cuff represents a continuum and no doubt there will be some overlap of the MR imaging appearance of these entities. This,

of course, awaits further experience with larger numbers of cases.

CAPSULAR ABNORMALITIES

Anterior dislocations of the glenohumeral joint account for approximately 50 per cent of all dislocations.[37] In the vast majority of cases with recurrent dislocation, the initial dislocation is caused by trauma. When the initial event occurs between the ages of 15 and 35, the dislocations are more likely to become recurrent or habitual.

The anterior capsular mechanism of the shoulder consists of the synovial membrane, the capsule and glenohumeral ligaments, the glenoid labrum, the subscapularis bursa and related recesses, and the subscapularis muscle and tendon (Fig. 37–13). The capsular mechanism is important as a barrier, preventing anterior displacement of the humeral head

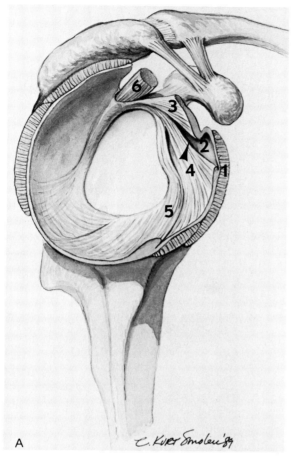

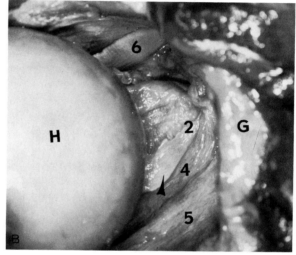

FIGURE 37–13. Artist's diagram *(A)* and shoulder specimen dissected from posterior *(B)* demonstrate the anatomy of the anterior capsular mechanism. Key to Figure 37–13: 1 = Subscapularis muscle; 2 = fibrous capsule; 3 = superior glenohumeral ligament; 4 = middle glenohumeral ligament; 5 = inferior glenohumeral ligament; 6 = biceps tendon, long head; G = glenoid; H = humeral head; arrowhead = opening into subscapularis bursa. (From Zlatkin MB, Bjorkengren A, Gylys-Morin V, et al: Cross sectional imaging of the capsular mechanism of the glenohumeral joint. AJR 150:151–158, 1988; with permission.)

in abduction and external rotation, which is the most common position at the time of dislocation. These structures have been visualized with MR imaging after intraarticular injection of gadolinium diethylene triamine pentaacetic acid (Gd-DTPA) or saline in cadaveric specimens with an efficacy equal or superior to CT arthrography.[20] Most of these structures can also be depicted noninvasively on conventional MR images.[15–18] We have found that the structures making up the capsular mechanism are best identified with images in the axial plane. They are also best seen on long TR/TE images when an effusion is present.

Abnormalities of the capsular mechanism and associated structures occur predominantly in patients with a history of recurrent subluxations and dislocations. The spectrum of abnormalities that have been observed clinically and experimentally in association with recurrent glenohumeral joint subluxations and dislocations includes capsular and labral tears and detachments, formation of a large anterior pouch,

and laxity of the subscapularis muscle and tendon.[38–42] Bony defects, particularly the Hill-Sachs lesion, may be identified as well.

Bankart believed that the essential lesion of recurrent dislocation consisted of a torn or detached glenoid labrum.[42] More recent reports, however, dispute the concept of the glenoid labrum alone as an important stabilizing factor. Currently lesions of the entire capsular mechanism are believed to be the most important factor in the development of instability, and labral lesions are thought to be the result rather than the cause of this instability.

Although the role of the glenoid labrum is in dispute, the frequent association of labral lesions with shoulder instability is proven and is a reliable sign of instability. Labral abnormalities have been demonstrated with both arthrotomography and CT arthrography.[5, 6] The normal glenoid labrum on MR images has a homogeneous dark signal. On axial images the anterior labrum generally has a triangular configuration,[5] although a recent study with CT arthrography stated that the normal anterior labrum may occasionally appear rounded.[19] There is normally intermediate signal intensity seen at the base of the labrum, which represents hyaline articular cartilage.

In a study of cadaveric shoulder specimens subjected to recurrent shoulder subluxations and dislocations, MR imaging with the injection of Gd-DTPA or saline proved capable of demonstrating tears of the glenoid labrum.[20] Three recent studies have, however, demonstrated the efficacy of conventional MR imaging in depicting labral pathology in patients.[21, 43, 44] MR imaging findings associated with labral tears include linearly increased signal within the low signal intensity labrum extending to the surface (Fig. 37–14A), or diffusely increased signal (Fig. 37–14B).[20, 21, 43] The abnormal signal in labral tears is intermediate on T_1-weighted images and may become bright on T_2-weighted images (Fig. 37–14). Changes in morphology including blunting, fraying, or attenuation may be identified as well (Fig. 37–16).

The normal anterior capsule and glenohumeral ligaments appear as a homogeneous dark band adjacent to and at times difficult to separate from the subscapularis tendon. The subscapularis bursa is usually not seen unless an effusion is present. Particularly in the presence of joint fluid, these glenohumeral ligaments as well as other folds of capsular tissue may be seen as separate structures and should not be confused with pathologic lesions.[20]

Three types of anterior capsules have been described (Fig. 37–15).[13] MR imaging can define the particular type of capsule depending on its insertion site: Type 1 inserts in or near the labrum, and types 2 and 3 insert more broadly along the scapular neck. The normal posterior capsule inserts directly into the labrum. The type 3 capsule, often in association with an enlarged subscapularis bursa, forms an "anterior pouch." It is not clear whether this occurs as a result of the first or subsequent dislocation (i.e., from capsular stripping), or whether it is developmental in

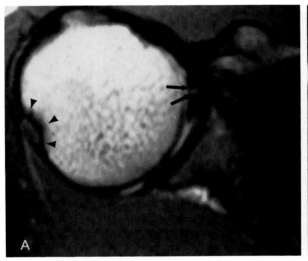

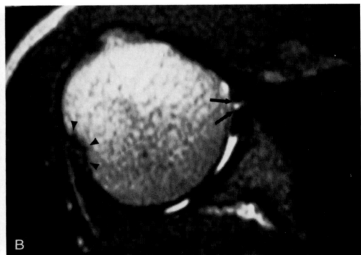

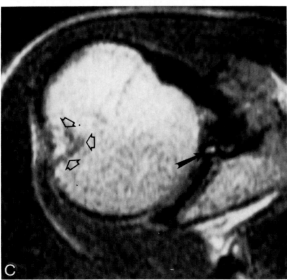

FIGURE 37–14. Anterior instability. Glenoid labral tears. Axial image (TR/TE 800/20) *(A)* at the midglenoid level demonstrates a linear focus of increased signal intensity at the base of the anterior labrum extending to the surface, which increases in signal intensity on the T_2-weighted images (TR/TE 2500/70) *(B) (arrows)*. Note the Hill-Sachs deformity on the posterolateral humeral head *(arrowheads)*. *C,* Axial long TR/TE image (2500/70) in another patient at a similar level demonstrates diffuse increased signal in the anterior labrum *(arrow)*. Note the Hill-Sachs deformity on the humeral head *(open arrows)* also present in this patient.

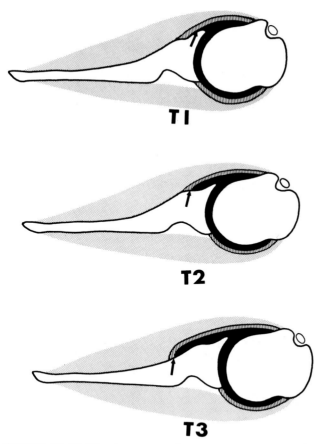

FIGURE 37–15. The three types of capsular insertions. Type 1 inserts adjacent to the glenoid labrum. Types 2 and 3 insert more medially along the scapular neck. Arrows indicate sites of capsular insertion. (From Zlatkin MB, Bjorkengren A, Gylys-Morin V, et al: Cross sectional imaging of the capsular mechanism of the glenohumeral joint. AJR 150:151–158, 1988; with permission.)

origin[38–41]; nonetheless, it creates a potential space for the humeral head to sublux or dislocate into. This "anterior pouch" has been identified with CT arthrography and can be depicted with MR imaging but is best seen in the presence of joint fluid, particularly on T_2-weighted images (Fig. 37–16). A distorted appearance of the capsular insertion into the glenoid, with either loss or thickening of the intervening soft-tissue layer over the scapular margin, may be seen as well (Fig. 37–16C). Seeger and coworkers[43] have also found that these patients may show evidence of retraction or atrophy of the subscapularis muscle.

Bony lesions that can be identified include fractures of the glenoid rim (the so-called bony Bankart lesion), as well as regions of abnormally low signal intensity in the marrow at the glenoid margin (Fig. 37–17). Hill-Sachs lesions are identified as large wedge-shaped defects on the posterolateral surface of the humeral head (Figs. 37–14 and 37–16).

Although at the present time CT arthrography is considered the procedure of choice in patients with a history of recurrent subluxations and dislocations, the ability of MR imaging to define many of the structural changes seen in patients with clinically significant shoulder instability may eventually allow MR imaging to replace CT arthrography in studying such patients, as it is noninvasive. This, of course, awaits the results of further comparative studies of these two modalities.

OTHER GLENOHUMERAL JOINT ABNORMALITIES

TRAUMA

MR imaging has also proven useful in a number of other post-traumatic disorders. Occasionally patients who present with shoulder pain after trauma are found to have hematomas or edema in muscles outside the rotator cuff, such as the trapezius or the deltoid (Fig. 37–18A and B).[21]

Dislocation of the acromioclavicular joint is a common injury that can be classified into three types.[45] Type 1 represents a minor strain of the fibers of the acromioclavicular ligaments. In type 2 injuries, there is disruption of the ligaments of the acromioclavicular joint. The coracoclavicular ligaments may be stretched but remain intact. In type 3 injuries, there is disruption of both the acromioclavicular and coracoclavicular ligaments. In patients with acromioclavicular joint dislocations MR imaging can assess the degree and severity of separation, the presence of intracapsular fluid and debris can be seen, and in many instances actual disruption of the acromioclavicular and coracoclavicular ligaments can be identified (Fig. 37–18C). In most cases, however, an MR imaging study is not required in these patients unless they are being considered for surgery, in which case the integrity of the rotator cuff can be evaluated at the same time.

Fractures about the glenohumeral joint are quite common. Most cases are well assessed with the use of conventional radiography and CT. MR imaging is most helpful in assessing the surrounding soft tissues. In the presence of complicated fractures, or in fractures in areas difficult to see well with conventional radiographs such as the scapula, the multiplanar capability of MR imaging can be useful in assessing the extent and location of the abnormalities and may be useful in depicting involvement of the glenohumeral joint (Fig. 37–18D and E). In addition, MR imaging can also demonstrate occult fractures or bony contusions not evident on the radiographs.

SYNOVIAL INFLAMMATORY DISEASE

The glenohumeral joint is commonly involved in patients with synovial inflammatory processes, partic-

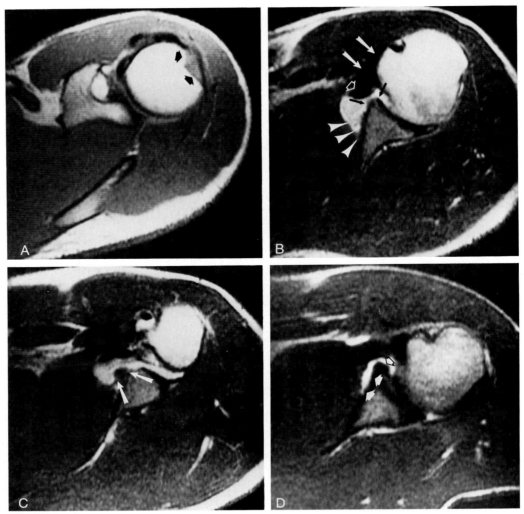

FIGURE 37–16. Anterior instability. Capsular abnormalities. *A,* Axial image at the level of the coracoid process demonstrates a large wedge-shaped defect on the humeral head indicative of a Hill-Sachs deformity *(arrows). B,* Long TR/TE image (2500/70) at the midglenoid level illustrates complete absence of the anterior labrum *(black arrows)* and a very medial capsular insertion that forms a large anterior pouch filled with synovial fluid *(arrowheads).* Note the markedly thickened appearance of the middle glenohumeral ligament *(open arrow)* and subscapularis tendon *(white arrows)* which is in part related to the patient's prior capsular repair. *C,* Axial image (TR/TE 2500/80) at the inferior glenoid reveals thickening of the soft tissues at the inferior capsular insertion *(arrows). D,* Axial image (TR/TE 2500/80) at the midglenoid in another patient also demonstrates a very medial capsular insertion (type 3) outlined by synovial fluid *(closed arrows).* Also note the blunted, rounded, anterior labrum *(open arrow).* A discrete labral tear was present at a higher level in this patient.

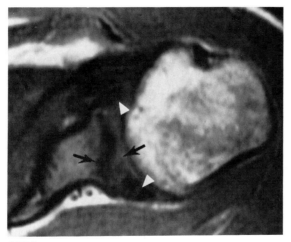

FIGURE 37–17. Anterior and posterior instability. Axial image at the midglenoid level depicts linear tears in the anterior and posterior labra *(arrowheads).* Diffuse decrease in signal intensity is identified in the mid-posterior bony glenoid *(arrows).*

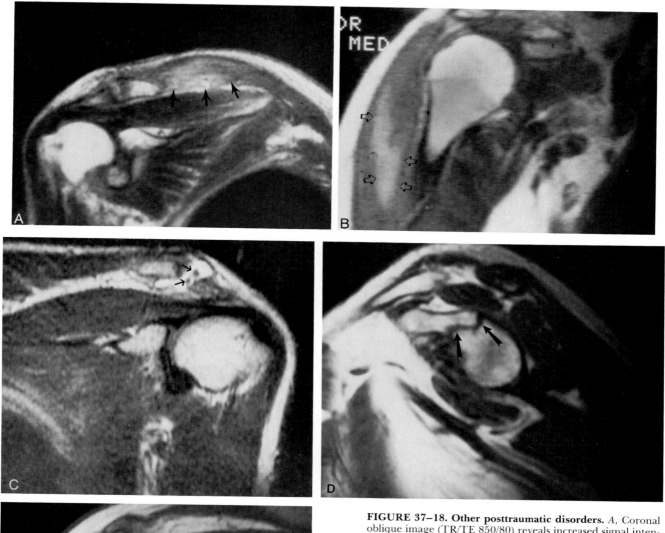

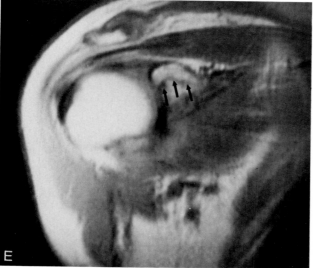

FIGURE 37–18. Other posttraumatic disorders. *A,* Coronal oblique image (TR/TE 850/80) reveals increased signal intensity and swelling of the trapezius muscle *(arrows).* The first echo of this sequence showed similar but less extensive areas of increased signal intensity. These findings are due to hemorrhage and edema in this muscle. This patient was clinically suspected of having a rotator cuff tear. *B,* Similar findings in the deltoid muscle in another patient *(arrows)* (TR/TE 850/30). *C,* Coronal oblique image (TR/TE 2500/80) depicting acromioclavicular joint separation with fluid in the joint capsule and disruption of the joint ligaments *(arrows).* The MR imaging was performed to assess the rotator cuff, which is intact. *D,* Sagittal oblique image (TR/TE 800/20) demonstrates a low signal intensity fracture line at the base of the coracoid process *(arrows).* This patient had persistent pain after trauma, and multiple plain films did not reveal this fracture. *E,* Image in the coronal oblique plane shows the fracture extending to the articular surface of the glenoid *(arrows).* (*B* from Zlatkin MB, Reicher MA, Kellerhouse L, et al: The painful shoulder. MR imaging of the glenohumeral joint. J Comput Assist Tomogr 12:995–1001, 1988; with permission.)

ularly rheumatoid arthritis and ankylosing spondylitis.[12] In the early stages of disease, synovitis may lead to soft-tissue edema and effusion. With progression and persistent inflammation a proliferative synovitis develops, which destroys the articular cartilage, erodes the underlying bone, and may disrupt the ligaments, tendons (including those of the rotator cuff), and joint capsule (Fig. 37–19A and B). With disruption of the capsule, synovial cysts may develop (Fig. 37–19C), which can increase in size, dissect through soft-tissue planes, or rupture. MR imaging can demonstrate all of the above findings in a noninvasive manner. Although loss of articular cartilage and osseous erosions may be visualized with conventional radiography, they may be visualized at an earlier stage with MR imaging, and their extent may be better assessed.[46]

In septic arthritis, intraarticular effusions, exudate, and destruction of articular cartilage, with or without subchondral bone involvement, are the major pathologic changes. MR imaging can depict the intraarticular fluid, the loss of signal from the articular cartilage, and any associated medullary bone destruction.[47] Other synovial inflammatory processes such as pigmented villonodular synovitis (PVNS) or synovial osteochondromatosis may be visualized as well. In PVNS MR imaging can demonstrate the presence of synovial effusions, osseous erosions, and hemosiderin, which will appear as nodules of low signal intensity on both short and long TR/TE sequences.[48] Owing to greater sensitivity to magnetic susceptibility effects, these nodular areas of hemosiderin will be highlighted on scans performed with gradient-echo techniques. These changes are somewhat nonspecific,

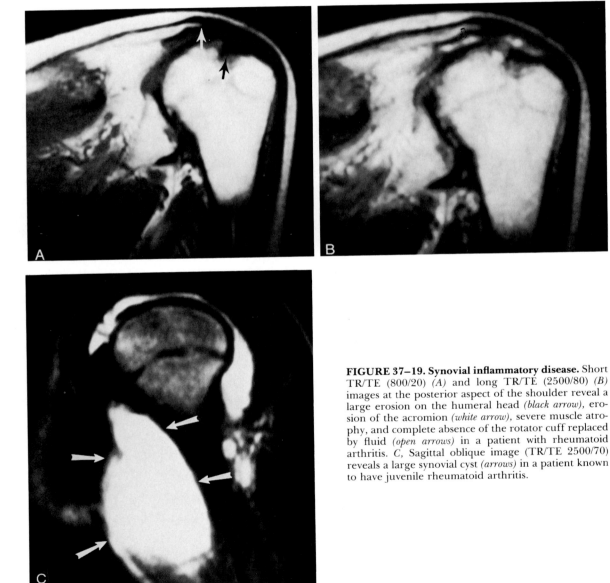

FIGURE 37–19. Synovial inflammatory disease. Short TR/TE (800/20) *(A)* and long TR/TE (2500/80) *(B)* images at the posterior aspect of the shoulder reveal a large erosion on the humeral head *(black arrow)*, erosion of the acromion *(white arrow)*, severe muscle atrophy, and complete absence of the rotator cuff replaced by fluid *(open arrows)* in a patient with rheumatoid arthritis. *C*, Sagittal oblique image (TR/TE 2500/70) reveals a large synovial cyst *(arrows)* in a patient known to have juvenile rheumatoid arthritis.

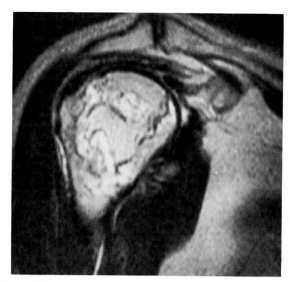

FIGURE 37–20. Avascular necrosis. Midcoronal image (TR/TE 2500/70) demonstrating linear and circular areas of low signal intensity within the humeral head with high signal intensity at their margins, consistent with avascular necrosis and bone infarction.

as similar changes may be seen in patients with hemophilia or rheumatoid arthritis.[48]

OSTEONECROSIS

Ischemic necrosis of the humeral head often follows trauma, particularly fractures of the anatomic neck. The vessels that supply the humeral head pierce the bony cortex just distal to the anatomic neck, and fractures proximal to this level may result in ischemic necrosis of the articular segment of the humeral head. Osteonecrosis of the humerus also occurs commonly in patients who are receiving exogenous steroid preparations, in alcoholics, and in patients with sickle cell disease or caisson disease, or it may be idiopathic.[12]

Early diagnosis of osteonecrosis with imaging techniques in the past has been difficult despite the use of radionuclide studies and CT. Plain radiographs and tomography are useful in assessing the extent and severity of disease but are not helpful in early detection, as changes tend to occur late in the course of the disease.

MR imaging has achieved wide clinical acceptance for the evaluation of osteonecrosis, particularly in the hip.[49] It has now been well accepted that MR imaging is more sensitive than radionuclide imaging in the detection of osteonecrosis.[50] Although there are no specific reports studying the efficacy of MR imaging in the diagnosis of osteonecrosis of the shoulder, it should have a utility similar to that in other joints. The appearance of osteonecrosis in the shoulder in our experience is similar to that in other joints, with evidence of decreased signal intensity in the humeral head at the articular surface owing to disruption of the signal intensity from fatty marrow (Fig. 37–20). In addition, with the use of high-resolution studies with surface coils one can assess the presence of articular collapse and the status of the overlying glenohumeral articular cartilage.

CRYSTAL DEPOSITION DISEASE

The shoulder is the most common site of involvement with calcium hydroxyapatite crystal deposition

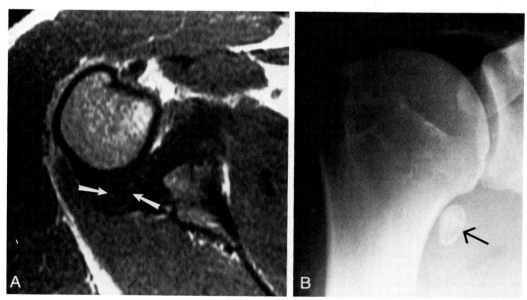

FIGURE 37–21. *A,* Axial short TR/TE image (800/20) demonstrates a large low signal intensity loose body at the posterior inferior glenoid margin *(arrows). B,* Correlative plain radiograph.

disease (HADD). The pathogenesis of hydroxyapatite crystal deposition is unknown, although trauma, ischemia, or other systemic factors may induce abnormalities in the connective tissue leading to crystal deposition.[12] Crystal deposition most commonly occurs in the tendinous and bursal structures about the shoulder, particularly the supraspinatus tendon. These crystals incite a synovitis, tendinitis, or bursitis and periarticular inflammation. The nodular calcific deposits in this disease can usually be easily seen with plain radiographs. We have observed three patients with this disease on MR imaging. In two patients nodular areas of signal void could be outlined at the insertion site of the rotator cuff tendon corresponding to the calcific deposit on the plain film. Increased signal intensity was seen within the tendon, presumably owing to tendinitis. In another patient with calcific deposits in the subacromial bursa, fluid within this bursa was identified.

LOOSE BODIES

In general, loose bodies are best assessed with the use of CT arthrography. Loose bodies that are small and lack mature marrow within may be difficult to localize on MR images. Calcified loose bodies appear as low signal intensity, generally round structures, in

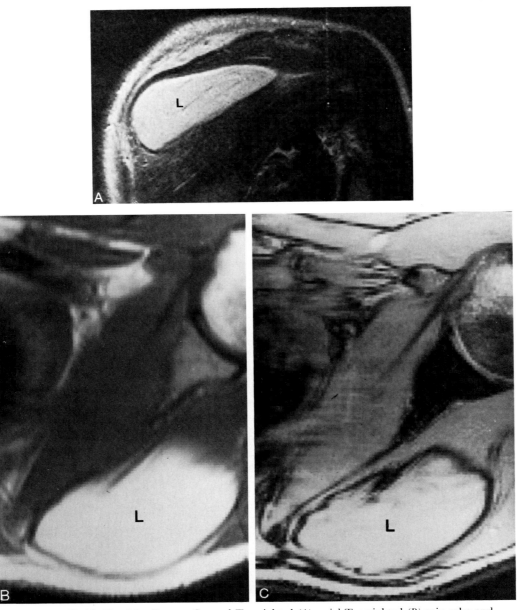

FIGURE 37–22. Shoulder lipoma. Coronal T_2-weighted *(A)*, axial T_1-weighted *(B)* spin-echo and axial GRASS with 15-degree FLIP angle *(C)*. A well-defined mass (L) with signal behavior identical to that of subcutaneous fat is seen.

the joint space (Fig. 37–21). They may develop mature marrow within and in this situation have a signal intensity similar to that of fatty marrow.

NEOPLASMS

The vast majority of tumors occurring in the scapula and the proximal end of the humerus are either metastases or myeloma. Although less common, primary osseous lesions, such as osteosarcoma, chondrosarcoma, osteochondroma, and Ewing's sarcoma, may be found at this site.

MR imaging is proving to be a valuable technique in the evaluation of patients with neoplasms of the bone and soft tissues, particularly because of the high contrast between tumors and normal tissues found with MR imaging (Fig. 37–22). Although a specific diagnosis is still best made with the use of plain radiographs, MR imaging is very useful in assessing the extent of disease in these cases and has proven superior to CT in this regard.[51] Short TR/TE sequences are best for maximal contrast between the lesion and fat, including bone marrow fat, and long TR/TE sequences are best for optimal contrast between the lesion and adjacent muscle. In the shoulder girdle the ability of MR to image in multiple planes and its good soft-tissue contrast allow one to evaluate involvement of adjacent vascular and neurogenic structures such as the axillary vessels and nerves and the brachial plexus without the use of contrast material. Transgression of the epiphyseal plate and spread into the joint capsule may also be visualized best with MR imaging; it is therefore the most useful modality currently available for preoperative staging, planning the surgical approach, and determining the potential for limb salvage.[51] Problems associated with MR imaging include difficulty in distinguishing reactive edema from neoplastic tissue,[52] although recent reports with the use of Gd-DTPA[53] hold promise in this area. In addition, calcification, ossification, and periosteal reaction are somewhat more difficult to evaluate with MR imaging than with CT, although MR imaging in combination with plain films usually suffices to evaluate these findings.

In conclusion, MR imaging is an excellent technique that performs well in the evaluation of patients with shoulder pain. Abnormalities of the rotator cuff in patients with impingement syndrome are well depicted with MR imaging, which should be the procedure of choice in this evaluation. In the assessment of patients with shoulder instability, MR imaging also performs well. Whether it will completely replace CT arthrography awaits the results of further comparative studies. MR imaging is also excellent in evaluating patients with soft-tissue trauma, complicated fractures, osteonecrosis, and bone or soft-tissue tumors. Finally, a distinct advantage of MR imaging over other modalities is its ability to evaluate a wide spectrum of abnormalities, particularly in patients who present with nonspecific clinical findings, thus often obviating the need to use multiple imaging modalities. It is our belief, therefore, that in combination with plain radiographs, MR imaging is the procedure of choice in the evaluation of the shoulder.

REFERENCES

1. Goldman AB, Ghelman B: The double contrast shoulder arthrogram: A review of 158 studies. Radiology 127:655–663, 1978.
2. Mink JH, Harris E, Rappaport M: Rotator cuff tears: Evaluation using double-contrast shoulder arthrography. Radiology 157:621–623, 1985.
3. Beltran J, Gray LA, Bools JC, et al: Rotator cuff lesions of the shoulder: Evaluation by direct sagittal CT arthrography. Radiology 160:161–165, 1986.
4. Deutsch AZ, Resnick D, Mink JH, et al: Computed and conventional arthrotomography of the glenohumeral joint: Normal anatomy and clinical experience. Radiology 153:603–609, 1984.
5. Rafii M, Firooznia H, Bonamo JJ, et al: Athlete shoulder injuries: CT arthrographic findings. Radiology 162:559–564, 1987.
6. Rafii M, Firooznia H, Golimbu C, et al: CT arthrography of the capsular structures of the shoulder. AJR 146:361–367, 1986.
7. Hall FM, Rosenthal DI, Goldberg RP, Wyshak G: Morbidity from shoulder arthrography: Etiology, incidence, and prevention. AJR 136:56–62, 1981.
8. Harcke AT, Grissom LE, Finkelstein MS: Evaluation of the musculoskeletal system with sonography. AJR 150:1253–1261, 1988.
9. Hoult D: The NMR receiver: A description and analysis of design. Prog NMR Spectrosc 12:41–47, 1978.
10. Edelman RR, Stark DD, Sairi S, et al: Oblique planes of section in MR imaging. Radiology 159:807–810, 1986.
11. Huber DJ, Mueller E, Heribes A: Oblique magnetic resonance imaging of normal structures. AJR 145:843–846, 1985.
12. Greenway GD, Danzig LA, Resnick D, Haghighi P: The painful shoulder. Med Radiogr Photgr 58:22–67, 1982.
13. Rothman RH, Marvel JP, Heppenstall RB: Anatomic considerations in the glenohumeral joint. Orthop Clin North Am 6:341–352, 1975.
14. Depalma AF: Surgery of the Shoulder. Philadelphia, JB Lippincott, 1983, pp 47–64.
15. Huber DJ, Sauter R, Mueller E, et al: MR imaging of the normal shoulder. Radiology 158:405–408, 1986.
16. Kieft GJ, Bloem JL, Obermann WR, et al: Normal shoulder: MR imaging. Radiology 159:741–745, 1986.
17. Middleton WD, Kneeland JB, Carrera GF, et al: High resolution MR imaging of the normal rotator cuff. AJR 148:559–564, 1987.
18. Seeger LL, Ruszkowski JT, Bassett LW, et al: MR imaging of the normal shoulder: Anatomic correlation. AJR 148:83–91, 1987.
19. McNiesh LM, Callaghan JJ: CT arthrography of the shoulder; variations of the glenoid labrum. AJR 149:963–966, 1987.
20. Zlatkin MB, Bjorkengran AG, Gylys-Morin V, et al: Cross-sectional imaging of the capsular mechanism of the glenohumeral joint. AJR 150:151–158, 1988.
21. Zlatkin MB, Reicher MA, Kellerhouse LE, et al: The painful shoulder: MR imaging of the glenohumeral joint. J Comput Assist Tomogr 12:995–1001, 1988.
22. Cofield RH: Rotator cuff disease of the shoulder. J Bone Joint Surg 67A:974–979, 1985.
23. Neer CS III: Impingement lesions. Clin Orthop 173:70–77, 1983.
24. Neer CS III: Anterior acromioplasty for the chronic impingement syndrome of the shoulder: A preliminary report. J Bone Joint Surg 54A:41–50, 1972.

25. MacNab I, Hastings D: Rotator cuff tendonitis. Can Med Assoc J 99:91–98, 1968.

26. Hawkins RJ: The rotator cuff and biceps tendon. *In* Evarts CM (ed): Surgery of the Musculoskeletal System. New York, Churchill Livingstone, 1983, pp 5–35.

27. Seeger LL, Gold RH, Bassett LW, Ellman H: Shoulder impingement syndrome: MR findings in 53 shoulders. AJR 150:343–347, 1988.

28. Zlatkin MB, Iannotti JP, Roberts MC, et al: Rotator cuff disease. Diagnostic performance of high resolution MR imaging. Radiology 172:223–229, 1989.

29. Lie S, Mast WA: Subacromial bursography: Techniques and clinical application. Radiology 144:626–630, 1982.

30. Strizak AM, Danzig L, Jackson DW, et al: Subacromial bursography. J Bone Joint Surg 64A:196–201, 1982.

31. Kieft GH, Bloem JL, Rosing PM, Oberman WR: Rotator cuff impingement syndrome: MR imaging. Radiology 166:211–214, 1988.

32. Kneeland JB, Middleton WD, Carrera GF, et al: MR imaging of the shoulder: Diagnosis of rotator cuff tears. AJR 149:333–337, 1987.

33. Evancho AM, Stiles RG, Fajman WA, et al: MR imaging diagnosis of rotator cuff tears. AJR 151:751–754, 1988.

34. Rowe CR: Ruptures of the rotator cuff: Selection of cases for conservative treatment. Surg Clin North Am 43:1531, 1963.

35. Takagishi N: Conservative treatment of the ruptures of the rotator cuff. J Jpn Orthop Assoc 52:781–787, 1978.

36. Calvert PT, Pacher NP, Stoker DJ, et al: Arthrography of the shoulder after operative repair of the torn rotator cuff. J Bone Joint Surg (Br) 68:147–150, 1986.

37. Neer CS III, Rockwood CA Jr: Fractures and dislocations of the shoulder. *In* Rockwood CA Jr, Green GP (eds): Fractures. Philadelphia, JB Lippincott, 1975, pp 585–815.

38. Moseley HG, Overgaard B: The anterior capsular mechanism in recurrent anterior dislocation of the shoulder: Morphological and clinical studies with special reference to the glenoid labrum and the glenohumeral ligaments. J Bone Joint Surg (Br) 44:913–927, 1962.

39. Turkel SJ, Panio MW, Marshall JL, Girgis FG: Stabilizing mechanisms prevent anterior dislocation of the glenohumeral joint. J Bone Joint Surg (Am) 63:1208–1217, 1981.

40. Oveson J, Sojbjerg JO: Lesions in different types of anterior glenohumeral joint dislocations. Arch Orthop Trauma Surg 105:216–218, 1986.

41. Townley CO: The capsular mechanism in recurrent dislocation of the shoulder. J Bone Joint Surg (Am) 32:370–380, 1950.

42. Rose CO, Patel D, Southnayd WW: The Bankart procedure. J Bone Joint Surg (Am) 60:1–16, 1978.

43. Seeger LL, Gold RH, Bassett LW: Shoulder instability: Evaluation with MR imaging. Radiology 168:695–697, 1988.

44. Kieft GJ, Bloem JL, Rosing PM, Obermann WR: MR imaging of recurrent anterior dislocation of the shoulder: Comparison with CT arthrography. AJR 150:1083–1087, 1988.

45. Pavlov M, Freiberger RH: Fractures and dislocations about the shoulders. Semin Roentgenol 13:85–96, 1978.

46. Kieft GH, Sartoris DJ, Bloem JL, et al: Magnetic resonance imaging of glenohumeral joint disease. Skeletal Radiol 16:285–290, 1987.

47. Tang JS, Gold RH, Bassett LW, Seeger LL: Musculoskeletal infection of the extremities: Evaluation with MR imaging. Radiology 166:205–209, 1988.

48. Spritzer CE, Dalinka MK, Kressel HY, et al: Magnetic resonance imaging of pigmented villonodular synovitis: A report of two cases. AJR 147:67–71, 1986.

49. Mitchell DG, Kundel JL, Steinberg ME, Kressel HY: Avascular necrosis of the hip: Comparison of MR, CT and scintigraphy. AJR 147:67–71, 1986.

50. Mitchell DG, Kressel HY, Arger PH, Dalinka MK: Avascular necrosis of the femoral head: Morphologic evaluation with MRI and CT correlation. Radiology 161:739–742, 1986.

51. Aisen AM, Martel W, Braunstein EM, et al: MRI and CT evaluation of primary bone and soft tissue tumors. AJR 146:749–756, 1986.

52. Beltran J, Simon DC, Katz W, Weis LD: Increased MR signal intensity in skeletal muscle adjacent to malignant tumors: Pathologic correlation and clinical relevance. Radiology 162:251–255, 1987.

53. Imhof H, Hajek PC, Kramer J, Ritschl P: GdDTPA: Help in diagnosis of malignant bone lesions? Presented at the 73rd Scientific Assembly and Annual Meeting of the Radiological Society of North America. Chicago, Nov. 27–Dec. 2, 1988.

38

MR IMAGING OF THE TEMPOROMANDIBULAR JOINT

STEVEN E. HARMS

TECHNICAL CONSIDERATIONS
   SURFACE COILS
   PULSE SEQUENCES
   ACQUISITION METHODS
ANATOMY AND PHYSIOLOGY

PATHOLOGY

ETIOLOGY
DISK DISEASE
OTHER INTERNAL DERANGEMENTS
ARTHRITIS
SURGICAL COMPLICATIONS
OTHER DISEASES
PROBLEMS

The use of magnetic resonance (MR) for temporomandibular joint (TMJ) imaging is a good example of how new technology can dramatically change medical and dental practice.[1-8] MR imaging has replaced conventional TMJ diagnostic methods at many centers. Before MR, a patient with suspected TMJ disease by clinical examination who required confirmation by imaging could undergo radiography, tomography, arthrography, and/or computed tomography (CT). However, CT scans, radiographs, and tomograms often could not provide sufficient information for complete diagnosis and treatment. Radiographs and tomograms can demonstrate bony abnormalities but cannot provide adequate soft-tissue contrast for the visualization of the soft-tissue anatomy of the joint that is most important for TMJ diagnosis.[9-11] CT provides better soft-tissue contrast, but direct sagittal views are difficult to produce.[12-22] Reformatted CT planes cannot provide adequate resolution for quality anatomic descriptions of joint pathology. Arthrography provides more information, since the disk can be indirectly visualized with the addition of contrast medium.[23-33] Arthrography, however, is an invasive examination. A recent study of morbidity associated with TMJ arthrography revealed pain lasting longer than one week following

the examination in 10 of 31 previously asymptomatic individuals.[34] With the injection of contrast into the joint, there is also potential for contamination and infection. TMJ arthrograms are technically difficult to perform and interpret, and the diagnostic quality is largely dependent upon the individual performing the examination. All of the examinations discussed utilize x-rays, and ionizing radiation produces well-known side effects that ideally should be avoided in the predominantly young female population typically encountered in TMJ disease.

A number of factors have led to the popularity of MR in the diagnosis and treatment of TMJ disease. MR imaging provides excellent soft-tissue contrast and can directly acquire tomographic images in any desired plane. MR can directly visualize the disk and does not rely on the use of contrast media. MR is a very flexible modality. Technique can be tailored to specific applications. High-resolution MR techniques have been developed that can produce images equalling or surpassing the resolution of current CT scanners. Several MR methods can now yield very thin slices that exceed the thinnest slice of any commercially available CT scanner. There are no known biologic hazards for exposure related to an MR examination.[35-39]

TMJ disease is a significant health problem. An estimated 4 to 28 per cent of the population of the United States have some form of TMJ abnormality.[40-42] Young females are particularly prone to develop TMJ disease.[43] With the development of MR, an effective, nonhazardous diagnostic technique, diagnostic imaging departments can expect a new group of TMJ referrals that previously would not have been evaluated. Increased public awareness of the disease and the use of MR as a diagnostic tool could further increase the caseload for TMJ disease. At Baylor University Medical Center, clinical TMJ imaging with MR has been active since September of 1984. TMJ examinations now rank third in frequency at Baylor, following cranial and spinal studies. With the availability of specialized surface coils, the use of MR for evaluation of the TMJ is becoming more popular at other institutions.

TMJ imaging differs significantly from other MR applications in the spectrum of pathology that is seen as well as in the methods needed for imaging these abnormalities. In this chapter, the anatomy of the normal joint and the various technical considerations involved in producing quality TMJ images are discussed. The commonly encountered pathologic entities of the joint are reviewed with examples of MR images.

TECHNICAL CONSIDERATIONS

SURFACE COILS

Surface coils are essential in obtaining adequate signal-to-noise ratios (S/N) for TMJ imaging.[2-5] A variety of surface coils for TMJ imaging are shown in Figure 38–1. In general, the smallest diameter coil that will cover the area of interest is most desirable. A 3-inch diameter coil is nearly ideal for TMJ im-

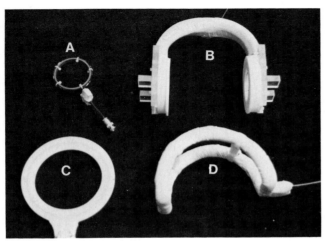

FIGURE 38–1. Surface coils. Various surface coils have been used for TMJ imaging: (A) 3-inch diameter flat coil, (B) bilateral CRC loop coil, (C) 5-inch diameter flat coil, and (D) saddle coil.

aging. Coils for bilateral TMJ imaging are advantageous. Simultaneous imaging of both joints allows comparison between sides utilizing the same degree of mouth opening. Differences in translation can be assessed that are not possible if separate acquisitions are used. A variety of bilateral coil arrangements are possible. The first bilateral TMJ coil had a saddle configuration.[5] A counterrotating loop coil with a single loop for each joint has the advantage of being internally decoupled from the transmit coil as well as having separate fields-of-view.[35] If loop gap resonators are used for each side, then the coils can vary in position for small or large faces without interacting.[46]

Quadrature detection can be used for an improvement equal to the square root of 2 in S/N. Another way to improve the S/N is to totally isolate the receiver functions of both sides. This objective is achieved by separate receivers for each side or by switching the receiver between the coils during the active phases.[46]

Surface coil technology is very important in TMJ imaging. Perhaps more can be achieved in this area to improve imaging capability than in any other single technical factor.

PULSE SEQUENCES

The spin-echo (SE) sequence has been the workhorse of most TMJ imaging protocols. Because of the short T_2 values encountered in the normal TMJ tissues (muscle, fibrocartilage, and fat), a short echo time (TE) is the primary concern in choosing timing parameters for SE imaging of the TMJ.[8, 35, 43] A TE of 20 msec or less is preferred for the imaging of joint anatomy. If, for some reason, visualization of joint fluid, edema, tumor, or infection is desired, a more T_2-weighted sequence may be necessary. The main objective in T_2-weighting is to enhance tissues of increased water content relative to fat. Sufficiently long TE values should be employed to reduce the signal of fat compared to fluid. At 0.6 tesla, a TE 120, TR 2000 scan can produce this effect.

Most of the T_1 values encountered in the normal constituents of the TMJ are in the moderate range. Heavily T_1-weighted images enhance contrast by increasing the relative signal of fat compared to muscle. T_1-weighting is achieved with a short repetition time (TR). Because of the shorter T_1 values of these tissues when compared to tissues of higher water content such as brain, a lengthening of the TR does not provide as great an improvement in S/N as in head imaging. If the S/N is not adequate, signal averaging is preferred instead of lengthening the TR, as a longer TR reduces T_1 contrast. Signal averaging improves the S/N by the square root of the number of excitations. Using a short TR and signal averaging improves the S/N, reduces motion artifacts, and maintains T_1 contrast.

Gradient-echo sequences (FLASH, FISP, GRASS) have shown promise for TMJ imaging.[47-49] These sequences employ small tip angle radiofrequency (RF) pulses and a gradient-refocused echo. Inherent joint contrast is adequate to display the disk, even on proton density–weighted gradient-echo sequences. Other joint features, however, are not well seen when compared to a T_1-weighted SE sequence. T_1-weighted gradient-echo sequences are limited by the contribution of higher signal from the slice edges compared to the center of the slice owing to relative saturation of the center. This feature makes T_1-weighted thin two-dimensional (2D) sections difficult to achieve.

Very efficient acquisitions are possible using gradient-echo sequences. Multiple views can be obtained at various phases of opening and closing and played back in a cine loop for visualization of joint dynamics. This feature produced some of the initial excitement concerning the use of gradient-echo sequences in TMJ imaging. In practice, a short TE/short TR SE sequence can produce images of both joints when used with a bilateral TMJ coil with almost the same efficiency as a 2D single slice fast scan of both joints. The T_1-weighted SE sequence has far better image quality than the proton density–weighted fast scan sequence. For these reasons, SE sequences are preferred even when acquiring cine data (see Fig. 38–7B and C). Improvements in fast scan sequences and the use of three-dimensional (3D) imaging may make these methods a feasible alternative to SE imaging.

The use of stimulated echoes (STEAM) also has promise for reducing the imaging time needed for TMJ examinations.[50, 51] Stimulated echoes are not limited by susceptibility effects as are gradient echoes. Slab selection for 3D imaging is facilitated by the three RF pulses of stimulated-echo sequences. It is expected that the availability of fast imaging sequences will substantially improve the speed and quality of TMJ examinations.

ACQUISITION METHODS

Most commercial imagers use the 2D multislice acquisition method (Fig. 38–2A). This method is well suited to brain imaging, in which long TR values are useful. However, 2D multislice is less efficient when short TR values are needed. Because slices are defined by a selective excitation, the thinness of the slice is limited by the band width narrowness of the RF pulse and the strength of the slice-selective gradient. As no RF slice excitation is perfectly square, gaps are left between slices. Square-shaped pulses have reduced but not totally eliminated the interslice gap. To reduce the RF band width for thinner slices, longer pulses may be necessary, which increases the TE and signal losses due to T_2.[52]

The selective 3D method solves some of the problems encountered with 2D multislice (Fig. 38–2B). Because slices are not excited individually by a selective excitation, the thinness of the slice is not limited by the RF band width or the gradient strength. A thick slab is selected, and very thin slices can be phase-encoded and reconstructed from the 3D array. No interslice gaps are present. The RF band width can be widened and the pulse length shortened for a shorter TE. The number of available slices per scan is not TR limited, so very short TR scans are possible. The S/N of a 3D scan improves with the square root of the number of slices.[35–37, 53]

If 3D imaging of both joints is needed, then the 3D multislab method has many advantages (Fig. 38–2C). Two slabs are selectively excited at different times during the TR cycle, similar to 2D multislice. Slice definition within each selected slab is achieved by phase-encoding, as in a conventional selective 3D. Using this method, 3D images of both joints are possible in the same acquisition time as a single joint examination.[38, 39, 54] As in the single-slab method, thin slices without interslice gaps are produced with a short TR, T_1-weighted sequence.

The short TR and short TE capability of 3D methods is particularly well suited for the TMJ. As fast imaging methods emerge, the use of very short TR sequences will further enhance the value of the 3D techniques.

ANATOMY AND PHYSIOLOGY

The TMJ is a complex joint having both sliding and rotating movements.[44] The basic joint anatomy is summarized in Figures 38–3 and 38–4. The bony portions of the joint are composed of the mandibular condyle and the articular fossa and eminence of the temporal bone. Cortical bone has a very low proton density and a very short T_2, resulting in low signal intensity on all images. The condyle and eminence normally have marrow fat that has high signal on T_1- and proton density–weighted images and moderate signal on T_2-weighted images. The fossa is a very thin bony structure that usually has no underlying marrow fat. The temporal lobe of the brain lies just adjacent to the cortex of the fossa. Traumatic injuries to the TMJ can result in a break in the thin cortex, with penetration into the middle cranial fossa. Surgical complications have also led to involvement of the temporal lobe owing to its close proximity to the joint. The disk has a very short T_2, resulting in a low signal structure on all images. Muscle has moderate signal on T_1- and proton density–weighted images and low signal on T_2-weighted images.

The bony structures are separated from each other by the articular disk, a lens-shaped structure composed of fibrous connective tissue (Fig. 38–5). The disk is devoid of any blood vessels or nerve fibers. The thickened anterior and posterior portions of the disk are called the anterior and posterior bands, respectively. The posterior band normally is thicker than the anterior band, but the precise morphology is determined by the shape of the condyle and fossa

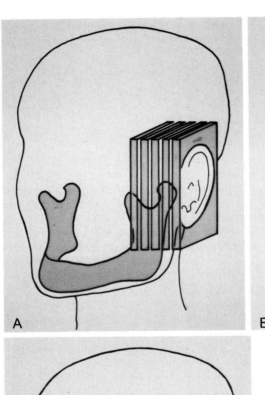

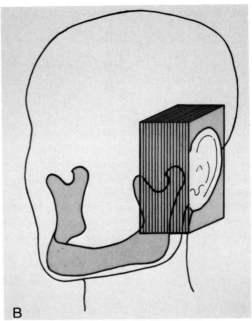

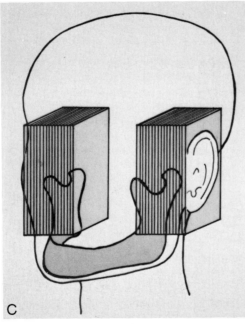

FIGURE 38–2. Acquisition methods. The *(A)* 2D multislice, *(B)* selective 3D, and *(C)* 3D multislab acquisition methods are diagrammed. In the 2D multislice method, the thinness of the slices is limited by the TR. In selective 3D, very thin slices without interslice gaps are possible, but the acquisition time increases with the number of slices. Both 2D multislice and selective 3D are practically limited by unilateral imaging by the TR limiting the number of slices in 2D and a very long acquisition time in 3D. The 3D multislab combines the attributes of both methods. Separate 3D slabs can be obtained in the same acquisition for reduced imaging time and thin slices without gaps.

along with physiologic forces. The middle portion of the disk, called the thin zone or intermediate zone, is the articular portion of the disk. The joint is divided into superior and inferior spaces by the disk and the ligaments. The disk is firmly attached medially and laterally to the mandibular condyle by the highly innervated discal or collateral ligaments (Fig. 38–6). Because of the attachment of the disk to the condyle, translatory movements can occur only between the condyle-disk complex and the articular fossa. The only movement that is possible between the condyle and disk is rotation. Anteriorly, the disk is attached to the superior belly of the lateral ptery-

goid muscle, which originates anteromedial to the joint from the infratemporal surface of the greater sphenoid wing. Posteriorly, the disk is attached to two thin bands of elastic tissue that connect the posterior band of the disk with the posterior portion of the fossa. These elastic bands are called the retrodiscal lamina. The posterior portion of the joint is thus called the bilaminar zone, or retrodiscal pad. The retrodiscal pad is highly innervated and contains many blood-filled endothelium-lined spaces. The anteromedial pull of the superior belly of the lateral pterygoid muscle is opposed by elastic tissue of the bilaminar zone (Fig. 38–7). Therefore, the loss of

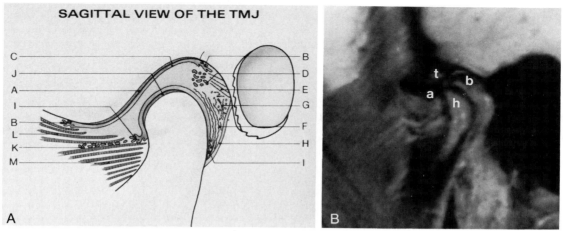

FIGURE 38–3. TMJ anatomy. *A*, A sagittal diagram of the TMJ shows the following structures: (A) articular surface of eminence and fossa, (B) synovial membrane of superior joint cavity, (C) superior cavity, (D) vascular knee, (E) superior retrodiscal lamina, (F) interior retrodiscal lamina of the bilaminar zone, (G) loose areolar connective tissue, (H) posterior capsule, (I) synovial membrane of interior cavity, (J) articular surface of condyle, (K) blood vessels, (L) superior belly of the lateral pterygoid muscle, and (M) inferior belly of the lateral pterygoid muscle. *B*, corresponding T_1-weighted image. t = Temporal eminence; h = condylar head; a = anterior band; b = bilaminar zone.

the elastic integrity of the bilaminar zone commonly results in anteromedial displacement of the disk due to the unopposed pull of the superior belly of the lateral pterygoid muscle. The entire joint is encompassed by the capsular ligament. The capsular ligament is well innervated and provides proprioceptive feedback regarding joint position.

Several other anatomic structures of importance can be seen on TMJ images. The inferior belly of the lateral pterygoid muscle originates at the lateral pterygoid plate and inserts on the anteromedial surface of the condylar neck. The medial pterygoid can be seen on medial sections running from the origin at the medial pterygoid plate to the medial surface

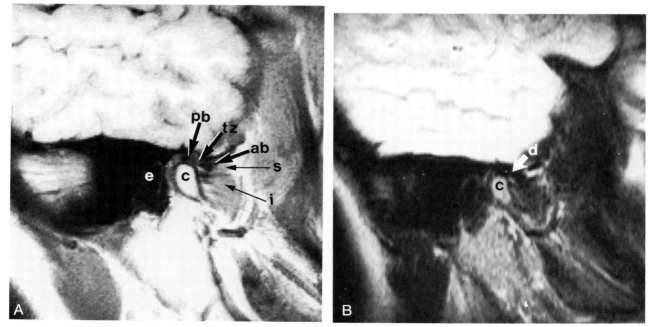

FIGURE 38–4. MR anatomy. *A*, T_1-weighted sagittal view of the TMJ in the closed-mouth position demonstrates a normally positioned posterior band (pb), thin zone (tz), and anterior band (ab) of the disk. The superior belly (s) and inferior belly (i) of the lateral pterygoid muscle, the external auditory meatus (e), and the condyle (c) are labeled. *B*, T_2-weighted image has poor definition of normal structures due to the very short T_2 of these tissues. Normally there is no high signal within the joint on T_2-weighted images. A TE of 120 is chosen to reduce the fat signal relative to fluid. The condyle (c) and disk (d) are labeled.

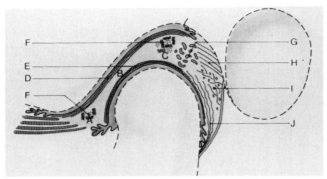

FIGURE 38–5. Disk anatomy. A sagittal diagram of disk anatomy shows (A) anterior band, (B) thin zone or intermediate zone, (C) posterior band, (D) superior joint space, (E) inferior joint space, (F) collagen oriented in all three directions, (G) attachment of superior retrodiscal lamina to disk, (H) elastic tissue of the superior retrodiscal lamina of the bilaminar zone, (I) loose areolar connective tissue of the bilaminar zone, and (J) inferior retrodiscal lamina of the bilaminar zone.

inferior joint cavity (the condyle and articular disk). Since the disk is tightly bound to the condyle by the lateral and medial discal ligaments, the only physiologic movement that can occur between these surfaces is rotation of the disk on the articular surface of the condyle. The initial motion on opening the mouth is rotation. The second joint system is the condyle-disk complex, which functions as a unit articulating with the surface of the mandibular fossa and eminence of the superior joint cavity. Since the disk is not firmly bound to the fossa, free sliding movement or translation can occur. Translation is the second motion of mouth opening.

The articular surfaces of the joint have no structural union. Stability is maintained by the constant activity of the muscles across the joint. The width of the disk space varies with the interarticular pressure. With increased pressure, the joint space narrows and the condyle seats itself on the thin zone of the disk. The primary mechanisms changing disk position with opening are the morphology of the disk and the interarticular pressure. The elastic tissues of the retrodiscal lamina passively restrict anterior movement of the disk. The superior belly of the lateral pterygoid opposes the force of the retrodiscal lamina. The superior belly of the lateral pterygoid is constantly maintained in a mild state of contraction. This muscle is primarily activated during the power stroke when pressure is applied with chewing and interarticular pressure is decreased. With decreased joint pressure, the pull of the retrodiscal lamina tends to retract the disk posteriorly. To avoid this situation, the superior belly of the lateral pterygoid contracts to maintain articular contact. In the closed-mouth position, the posterior band of the disk normally lies at 12 o'clock relative to the mandibular condyle. Recent studies indicate that this position can vary by 10 per cent.[45] With opening, there is rotation of the

of the mandibular angle. The masseter muscle can be seen on lateral sections and extends from an origin on the zygomatic arch to its insertion on the lateral aspect of the mandibular ramus. The temporalis muscle extends from a broad insertion on the temporal fossa through the zygomatic arch to form a tendon that inserts on the coronoid process of the mandible. The external auditory canal is seen posterior to the joint. The facial nerve canal is identified posterior to the external auditory canal. The internal maxillary artery can be seen running medially, often between the two bellies of the lateral pterygoid muscle. Inferior and medial to the joint is the styloid process.

As mentioned previously, the TMJ is functionally divided into two separate joints (Fig. 38–8). One joint system is composed of the tissues that surround the

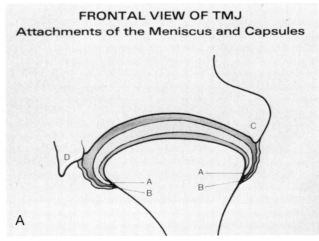

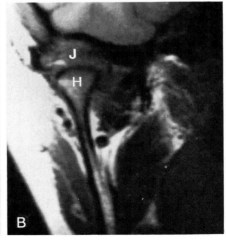

FIGURE 38–6. Coronal TMJ anatomy. *A,* The following structures are labeled: (A) discal or collateral ligaments, (B) capsule, (C) lateral lip of fossa, and (D) spinous portions of the sphenoid bone. *B,* Corresponding T$_1$-weighted image. H = Condylar head; J = joint space containing disk.

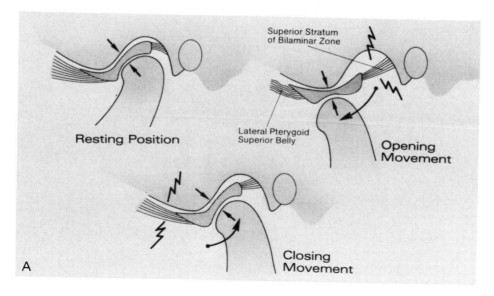

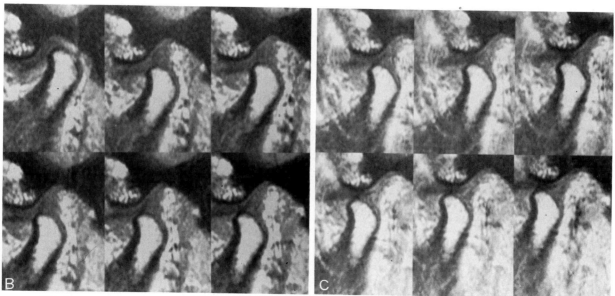

FIGURE 38–7. Joint physiology. *A,* At rest, the joint is held into position by the slight tonus of the muscles. The thin zone lies between the weight-bearing portions of the condyle and fossa. With opening, the weight-bearing portion of the joint moves anteriorly, resulting in an anterior translation of the disk that is opposed by the elastic tissues of the bilaminar zone. The superior retrodiscal lamina is opposed by the superior belly of the lateral pterygoid. *B* and *C,* Sequential T_1-weighted images depicting normal meniscocondylar dynamics in a cine mode.

condyle on the disk and translation of the condyle-disk complex under the eminence. The posterior band thickens, and the thin zone rotates posteriorly.

PATHOLOGY

ETIOLOGY

Epidemiologic studies indicate that symptoms of TMJ disorder could be present in one of four patients in the general population, yet only 5 per cent of the population have problems severe enough to seek treatment.[44] In a recent TMJ imaging study of 454 joints, 90 per cent of patients were female, with a mean age of 32 years. Because young females of childbearing age most commonly encounter TMJ disease, the use of a nonhazardous imaging technique is particularly advantageous.[55]

A variety of factors predispose to TMJ disease. Jaw trauma immediately prior to the onset of the problem was cited in 25 per cent of patients with internal derangements diagnosed by arthrography.[24] Of these patients, 32 per cent had a history of iatrogenic trauma such as third molar removal, endoscopy, or

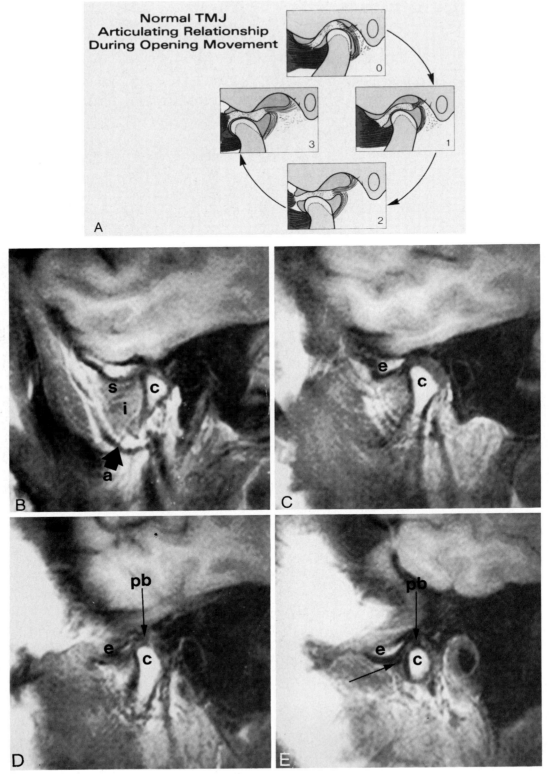

FIGURE 38–8 *See legend on opposite page*

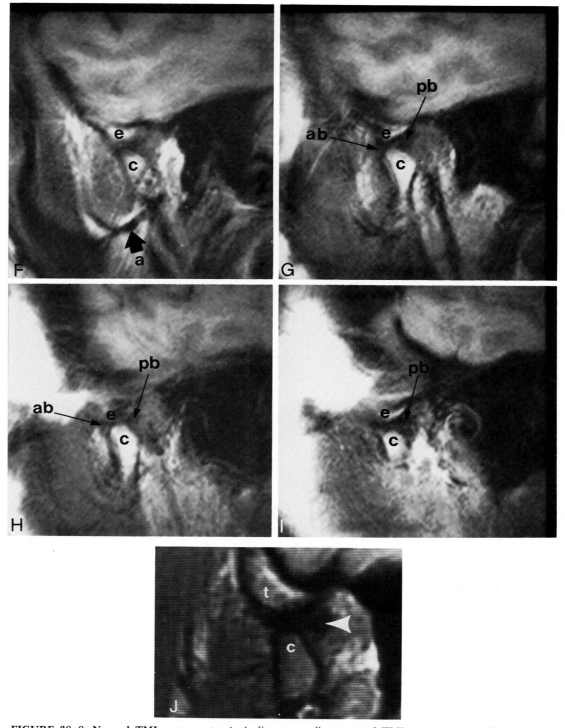

FIGURE 38–8. Normal TMJ movements. *A,* A diagram outlines normal TMJ movements. In the closed-mouth position, the posterior band of the disk lies directly superior to the condyle. With opening, the condyle rotates on the disk. Further opening results in the anterior translation of the disk-condyle complex. With closing, these relationships reverse. T_1-weighted closed- (*B* to *E* from medial to lateral) and open- (*F* to *I* from medial to lateral) mouth views provide information on TMJ dynamics. The eminence (e), condyle (c), anterior band (ab), posterior band (pb), superior belly of the lateral pterygoid muscle (s), inferior belly of the lateral pterygoid muscle (i), and the internal maxillary artery (a) are labeled. *J,* T_1-weighted image in position 2-3. The posterior band is clearly identified *(arrowhead)* and contributes to the characteristic "bow-tie" or "bat-wing" appearance of normalcy. t = Temporal eminence; c = condyle. (From Harms SE, Wilk RW: Magnetic resonance of the temporomandibular joint. RadioGraphics 7:521–542, 1987; with permission.)

tonsillectomy. Malocclusions are cited as a frequent cause of TMJ symptoms. Orthodontic treatment has also been implicated as a possible predisposing factor. Bruxism and emotional stress are often found in patients with TMJ symptoms.[33]

Anatomic defects in the joint may increase the risk of joint disease. A steep articular eminence requires a greater degree of rotation for opening and predisposes to TMJ disease. Hypermobile joints in which the condyle translates far past the eminence are also associated with a greater frequency of TMJ symptoms.[33, 44]

Systemic diseases can predispose to TMJ disease. Rheumatoid arthritis, psoriatic arthritis, calcium pyrophosphate deposition disease, and gout have affected the TMJ.[44]

Patients having unilateral symptoms and an internal derangement on one side may also have disease on the asymptomatic side. It is estimated that 50 to 80 per cent of internal derangements are bilateral.[39, 56, 57] This factor emphasizes the importance of imaging both joints, especially if unilateral surgery is contemplated. Accurate staging of the disease should avoid the development of contralateral symptoms from an undiagnosed internal derangement soon after surgical correction of a supposedly unilateral problem.

DISK DISEASE

Internal derangements of the TMJ encompass a spectrum of abnormalities ranging from minimal disk displacement to end-stage degenerative joint disease.

A mild internal derangement is depicted in Figure 38–9. In the closed-mouth position, the disk is anteriorly displaced. With opening, the condyle slides under the posterior band of the disk. A normal position of the disk and condyle is seen at maximum opening, and the disk is described as reduced. An opening click may be present on physical examination. With closing, the condyle slides back across the posterior band and a displaced disk is again seen. An example of the MR imaging findings in anterior displacement with reduction is shown in Figure 38–10. In Figure 38–11, the posterior band is within normal limits in position but is quite thinned. This is the first step in the development of an internal derangement. This patient also has a steep eminence, a predisposing factor in TMJ disease. In the absence of morphologic disk abnormality or other joint disease, most mild internal derangements are treated conservatively, at least in the initial phases of treatment.[2, 4, 5, 7, 8]

A diagram of a more severe internal derangement is shown in Figure 38–12. In this example, the disk is markedly displaced anteriorly. With opening, anterior translation of the condyle is impaired by the anteriorly displaced disk (Fig. 38–13). On physical examination, a locked joint is seen. No reduction of the disk can be demonstrated at maximum opening. An MR image of a patient having an anteriorly displaced disk without reduction is shown in Figure 38–14. Anterior displacements are the most common internal derangement. Tears or stretching in the retrodiscal lamina result in an anterior displacement due to the unopposed pull of the superior belly of the lateral pterygoid muscle. Tears of the retrodiscal tissues are commonly associated with severe internal derangements. Perforations of the retrodiscal tissues are not typically demonstrated by MR imaging.[2–8, 58] Medial and lateral displacements also can occur (Figs. 38–15 to 38–17). Posterior displacements are rare.

Disk morphology is of considerable importance in the treatment evaluation. A severely thickened or distorted disk may be difficult to manage by conservative treatment. A simple plication procedure may be a good surgical treatment for a morphologically normal disk but would not be possible for a fragmented disk. An example of a perforated disk is

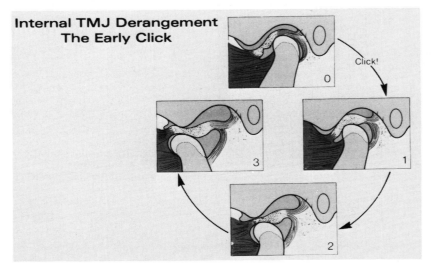

**Internal TMJ Derangement
The Early Click**

Click!

0

3

1

2

FIGURE 38–9. Mild internal derangement. In the closed-mouth position, the disk is anteriorly displaced. With opening, the condyle translates under the posterior band of the displaced disk, and a click may be heard on physical exam. At maximum opening, the condyle and disk are in a normal position. With closing, the condyle returns to the fossa, but the disk remains anteriorly displaced. (From Harms SE, Wilk RW: Magnetic resonance of the temporomandibular joint. RadioGraphics 7:521–542, 1987; with permission.)

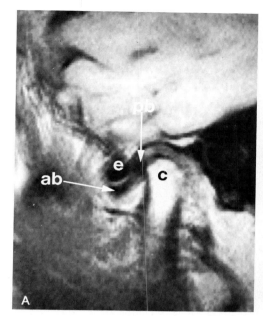
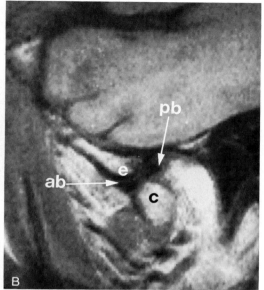

FIGURE 38–10. Anterior displacement with reduction. Closed-mouth T₁-weighted image *(A)* shows an anteriorly displaced disk that reduces on the *(B)* closed-mouth view. The anterior band (ab) and posterior band (pb) of the disk, the condyle (c), and the eminence (e) are labeled.

shown in Figure 38–18.² Disk perforations are far less common than retrodiscal perforations.

Chronic internal derangements result in additional joint abnormalities. Osteophytes and anterior "beaking" of the condyle are often seen (Figure 38–18). Adhesions between the disk and condyle, disk and eminence, or both can severely impair movement between the disk and either the eminence or the condyle. Lack of movement of the disk relative to the adherent structure can be demonstrated on the open-mouth view. Lysing of joint adhesions is currently the basis of arthroscopic treatment of TMJ disease.²,⁸

Long-term severe internal derangements result in further joint destruction and degenerative arthritis. In these cases, the disk is severely fragmented or degenerated. The joint space is narrowed, and the eminence and condyle are often flattened. An example of end-stage TMJ disease is shown in Figure 38–19.⁸

OTHER INTERNAL DERANGEMENTS

Because of the highly innervated retrodiscal area, inflammatory disease in this region results in severe joint pain. A patient with a normally positioned disk and severe symptoms due to retrodiscitis is shown in Figure 38–20. A hypertrophic retrodiscal pad is demonstrated on the T₁-weighted images. This situation provides a useful role for T₂-weighted imaging. With T₂-weighting, the retrodiscal tissues enhance dramatically in retrodiscitis. Occasionally this condition may be confused with a condyle displaced out

of the fossa owing to chronic retrodiscal hyperplasia such as that seen with splint therapy. In this situation, the changes are chronic and no enhancement can be appreciated on T₂-weighted images.²,⁸

Joint sepsis can be well demonstrated on T₂-weighted images owing to the high water content of the pus and edema. Septic joints may be associated with either a penetrating wound, spreading infections from adjacent structures, or bacteremia.

ARTHRITIS

Rheumatoid arthritis predisposes to TMJ disease. Erosions commonly occur along the articular surfaces of the condyle. Joint destruction and fibrous ankylosis are typical findings.⁴⁴

Other arthritides can involve the TMJ. Hyperuricemia can rarely lead to gout of the TMJ. Calcium pyrophosphate deposition has been reported.⁵⁹ In psoriatic arthritis, bony sclerosis and internal derangements are commonly demonstrated. Recent evidence indicates internal derangements in 50 per cent of patients with psoriatic arthritis (Fig. 38–21).⁶⁰

SURGICAL COMPLICATIONS

Adhesions (Fig. 38–22) are commonly demonstrated in patients who have had previous surgery. Plication surgery is infrequently complicated by joint adhesions. In plication surgery, the disk is repositioned within the joint and secured. Patients sometimes return following surgery with new clicks or

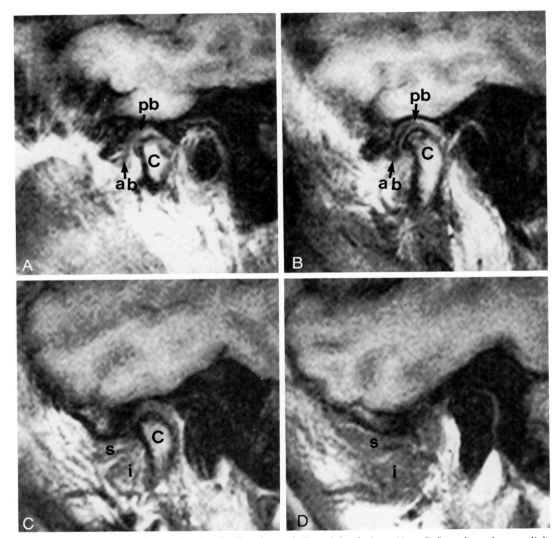

FIGURE 38–11. Thinned posterior band. Closed-mouth T_1-weighted views (*A* to *D* from lateral to medial) demonstrate a normally positioned but thinned posterior band (pb). The condyle (C), anterior band (ab), superior belly of the lateral pterygoid muscle (s), and inferior belly of the lateral pterygoid muscle (i) are labeled. Thinning of the posterior band is thought by some workers to represent stress on the disk in a patient who may eventually develop an internal derangement.

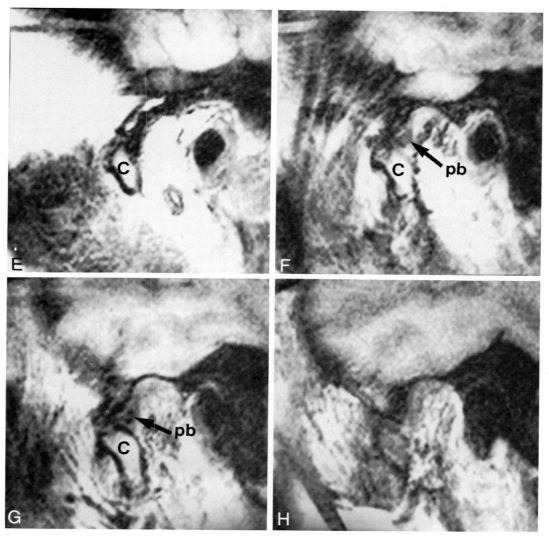

FIGURE 38–11 *Continued* Open-mouth views (*E* to *H* from lateral to medial) show good translation of the condyle and normal disk position.

FIGURE 38–12. Severe internal derangement. The disk is anteriorly displaced on the closed-mouth view. Translation of the condyle is impaired by the anteriorly displaced disk, and a locked joint is observed on physical examination. (From Harms SE, Wilk RW: Magnetic resonance of the temporomandibular joint. RadioGraphics 7:521–542, 1987; with permission.)

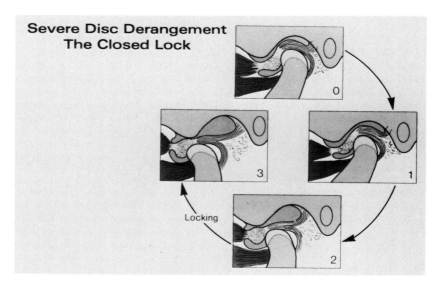

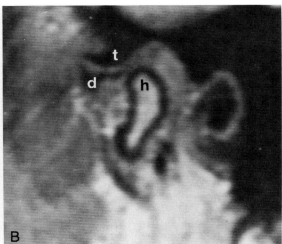

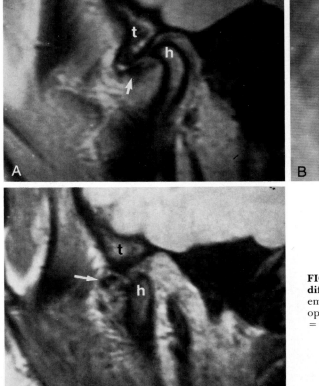

FIGURE 38–13. Anterior disk displacement in three different patients. *A*, Closed position. t = Temporal eminence; h = condylar head; arrow = disk. *B*, Semi-open position. d = disk. *C*, Semi-open position. Arrow = disk.

impaired motion due to adhesions. Adhesions are best demonstrated by lack of motion of the disk relative to surroundings, as shown on the open-mouth view compared to the closed-mouth view. The disk may be adherent to either the condyle or the eminence or both. Low-signal fibrous connecting bands can sometimes be seen.

Joint prostheses are used when the disk is too distorted for a plication (Fig. 38–23). Because many of these implants are not radiopaque, the exact position cannot be ascertained by radiographic methods. MR is useful in evaluating implants suspected of migration (Fig. 38–24) or fracture (Fig. 38–25).[2] Giant cell reactions are sometimes seen in patients with Proplast prostheses (Fig. 38–26).[61–63]

Total joint replacements are reserved for the most severe joints. These metallic devices resemble total hip prostheses in design. Because there is metal involved, these devices cannot be demonstrated by MR imaging.

OTHER DISEASES

A variety of illnesses can present with TMJ symptoms. On MR examination, it is important to be alert to the possibility of skeletal metastases, meningioma in the middle cranial fossa, and mastoiditis. Clinically, migraine headaches, arthritis, trigeminal neuralgia, and glossopharyngeal neuralgia may produce similar symptoms.

PROBLEMS

Because TMJ symptoms commonly occur in young females, orthodontic appliances are often encountered in patients referred for MR imaging of the TMJ. Orthodontic treatment itself has been cited as a potential cause of TMJ disease.[44] Artifacts due to the metal of the orthodontic appliance interacting

Text continued on page 1055

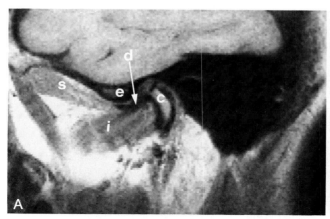

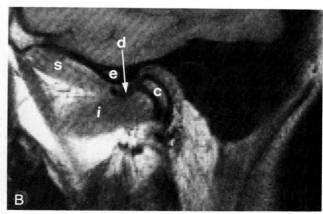

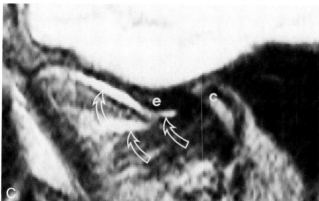

FIGURE 38–14. Anterior displacement without reduction. *A,* Open-mouth T₁-weighted view demonstrates an anteriorly displaced disk (d) with poor translation of the condyle (c) and continued anterior displacement of the disk (d) on the *(B)* closed-mouth view. A locked joint was noted on physical examination. *C,* T₂-weighted image shows abnormally high signal *(arrows)* around the pterygoid muscles and disk as evidence of fluid or edema. The superior belly of the lateral pterygoid muscle (s), inferior belly of the lateral pterygoid muscle (i), and eminence (e) are labeled. (From Harms SE, Wilk RW: Magnetic resonance of the temporomandibular joint. RadioGraphics 7:521–542, 1987; with permission.)

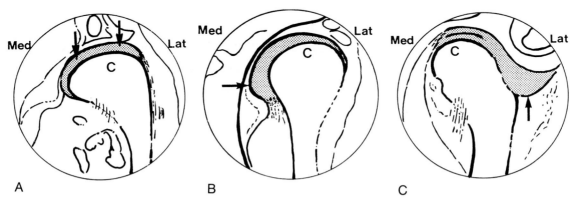

FIGURE 38–15. Diagrams in the coronal plane depicting *(A)* normal, *(B)* medially displaced, and *(C)* laterally displaced disks *(arrows).* C = Condyle.

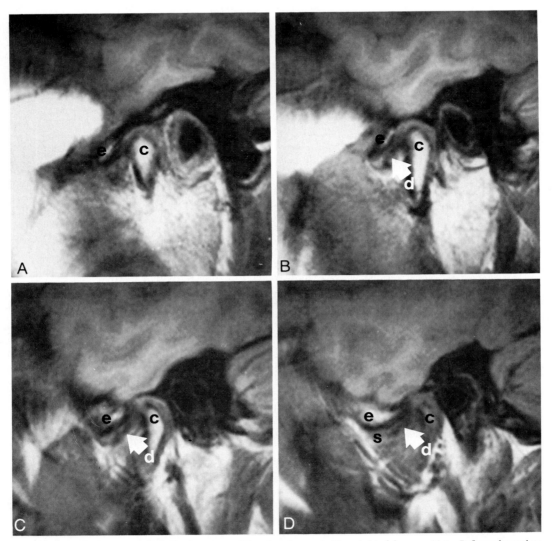

FIGURE 38–16. Anteromedial displacement. The closed-mouth T_1-weighted images (*A* to *D* from lateral to medial) demonstrate an anteriorly displaced disk (d) that is better demonstrated on the medial sections near the superior belly of the lateral pterygoid muscle (s). The eminence (e) and condyle (c) are identified for orientation.

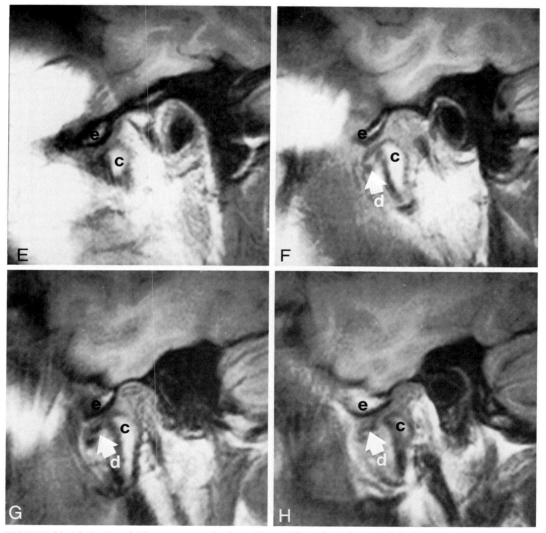

FIGURE 38–16 *Continued* The open-mouth views (*E* to *H* from lateral to medial) show no reduction of the anteromedial displacement. Because of the anteromedial pull of the superior belly of the lateral pterygoid muscle, this is the most common form of disk displacement.

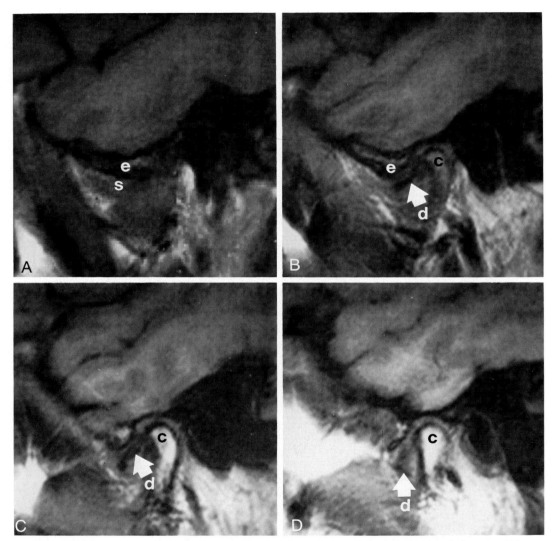

FIGURE 38–17. Anterolateral displacement. The closed-mouth T_1-weighted views (*A* to *D* from medial to lateral) show a displaced disk (d) that is better seen on the lateral than on the medial sections. The disk can be seen wrapping around the anterolateral aspect of the condyle (c). The eminence (e) and superior belly of the lateral pterygoid muscle (s) are labeled.

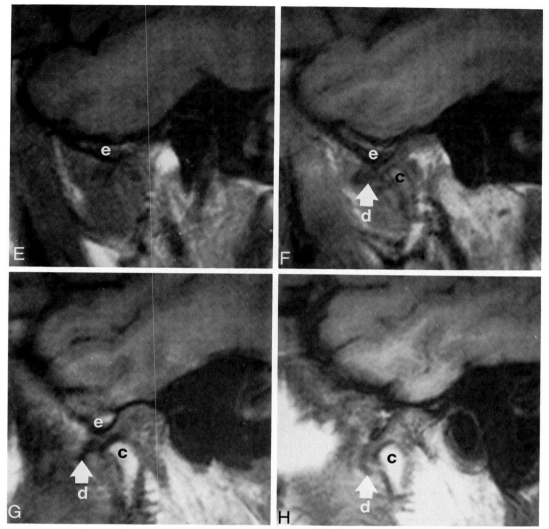

FIGURE 38–17 *Continued* With opening (*E* to *H* from medial to lateral), the disk (d) remains anterolaterally displaced.

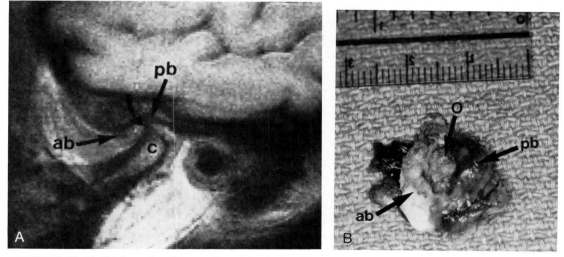

FIGURE 38–18. Disk perforation. *A*, T$_1$-weighted closed-mouth view demonstrates an osteophyte *(curved arrow)* extending superiorly from the condylar (c) surface through the disk separating the anterior (ab) and posterior (pb) bands of the disk. The surgical specimen *(B)* shows the osteophyte (o) of the condyle protruding through the disk.

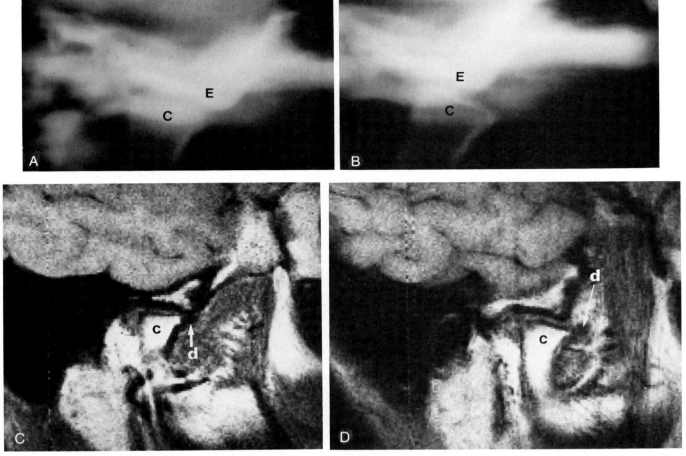

FIGURE 38–19. Degenerative joint disease. *A,* Closed- and *(B)* open-mouth tomograms demonstrate flattened mandibular condyle (C) and eminence (E). *C,* Closed- and *(D)* open-mouth T_1-weighted images better show the bony abnormality and disk fragments (d) anterior to the condyle (c) on both views. (From Harms SE, Wilk RW: Magnetic resonance of the temporomandibular joint. RadioGraphics 7:521–542, 1987; with permission.)

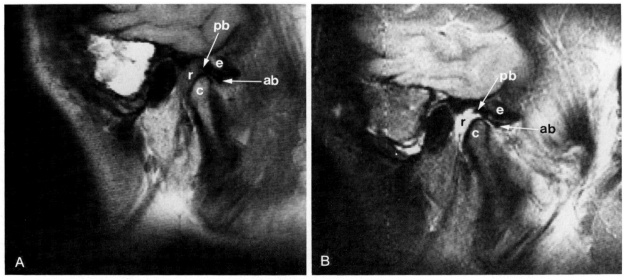

FIGURE 38–20. Hyperplastic retrodiscal tissues. *A,* T_1-weighted closed-mouth view demonstrates a condyle (c) displaced inferiorly out of the fossa by a thickened retrodiscal (r) pad. *B,* with T_2-weighting, marked enhancement of the retrodiscal (r) area is seen as evidence of edema or inflammation. A normal disk is noted. The anterior band (ab) and posterior band (pb) of the disk and the eminence (e) are labeled. (From Harms SE, Wilk RW: Magnetic resonance of the temporomandibular joint. RadioGraphics 7:521–542, 1987; with permission.)

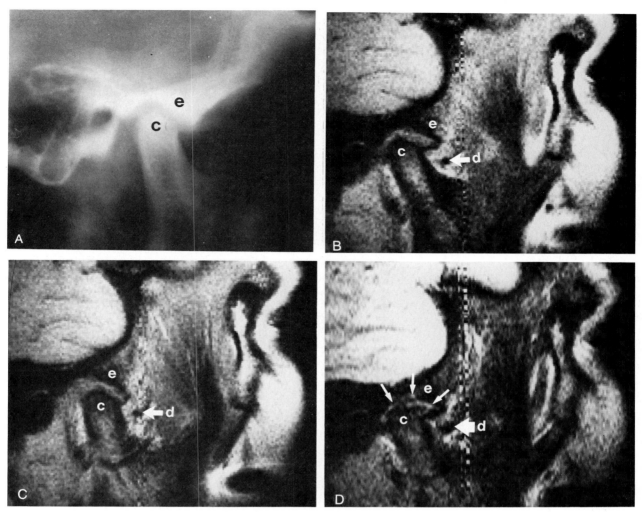

FIGURE 38–21. Psoriatic arthritis. *A,* Tomogram shows an irregular articular surface and sclerosis of the condyle (c) and eminence (e). *B,* T₁-weighted open-mouth view demonstrates a low signal intensity sclerotic condyle (c) with a very irregular articular surface and a narrowed joint space. Disk fragments (d) are markedly displaced. There is poor translation of the condyle (c) on the *(C)* open view, with continued anterior displacement of the disk fragments (d). *D,* T₂-weighted image shows an extensive amount of high signal fluid or edema in the joint *(arrows)* that extends into the defects in the articular surfaces. (From Harms SE, Wilk RW: Magnetic resonance of the temporomandibular joint. RadioGraphics 7:521–542, 1987; with permission.)

FIGURE 38–22. Adhesion. Closed-mouth T₁-weighted image shows a sclerotic condyle (c) with a thickened cortex and decreased marrow fat continuous with the low-signal, anteriorly displaced disk (d) owing to a thick adhesion *(open arrow).* Another sign of adhesion is the lack of positional change with opening. (From Harms SE, Wilk RW: Magnetic resonance of the temporomandibular joint. RadioGraphics 7:521–542, 1987; with permission.)

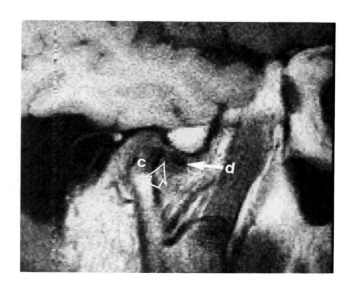

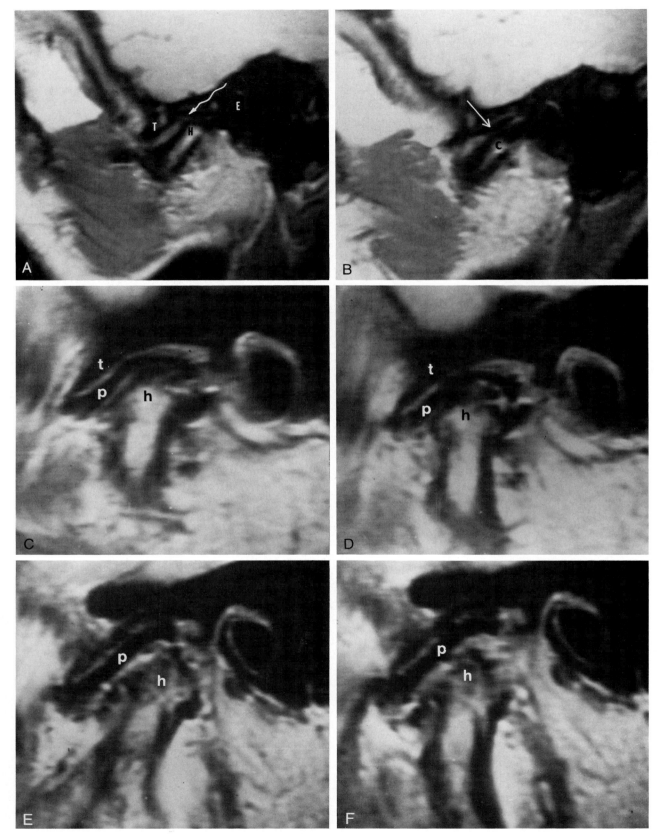

FIGURE 38–23 *See legend on opposite page*

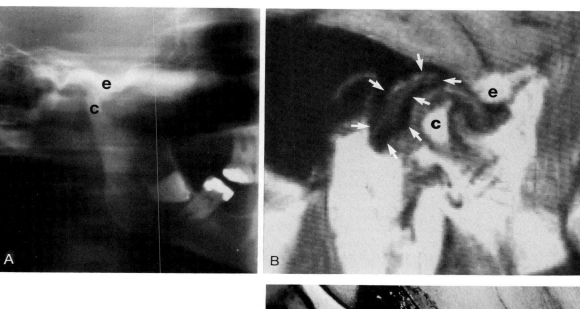

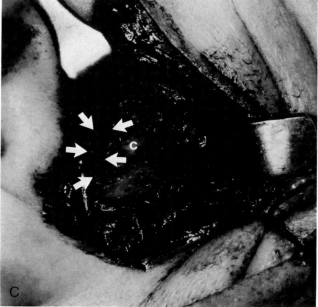

FIGURE 38–24. Displaced prosthesis. *A,* Tomogram in a postoperative patient shows an anteriorly displaced condyle (c). *B,* Closed-mouth T_1-weighted image demonstrates a posteriorly dislocated Proplast prosthesis *(arrows)*. *C,* At surgery the displaced prosthesis is noted *(arrows)*. The condyle (c) and eminence (e) are labeled. (From Harms SE, Wilk RW: Magnetic resonance of the temporomandibular joint. RadioGraphics 7:521–542, 1987; with permission.)

FIGURE 38–23. Normally positioned prostheses with limited condylar excursion in three different patients. *A, C,* and *E,* Closed position; *B, D,* and *F,* open position. *A,* T = Temporal eminence; H = condylar head; E = external auditory canal; arrow = prosthesis. *B,* C = Condyle; arrow = prosthesis. *C* and *D,* t = Temporal eminence; h = condylar head; p = prosthesis. *E* and *F,* h = Condylar head; p = prosthesis.

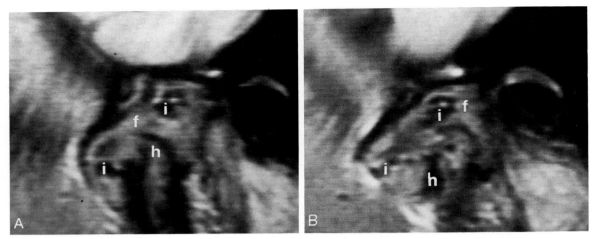

FIGURE 38–25. Failed prosthesis with fragmentation. h = Condylar head; i = implant fragments; f = reactive fibrosis/granulation tissue. (From Harms SE, Wilk RW: Magnetic resonance of the temporomandibular joint. RadioGraphics 7:521–542, 1987; with permission.)

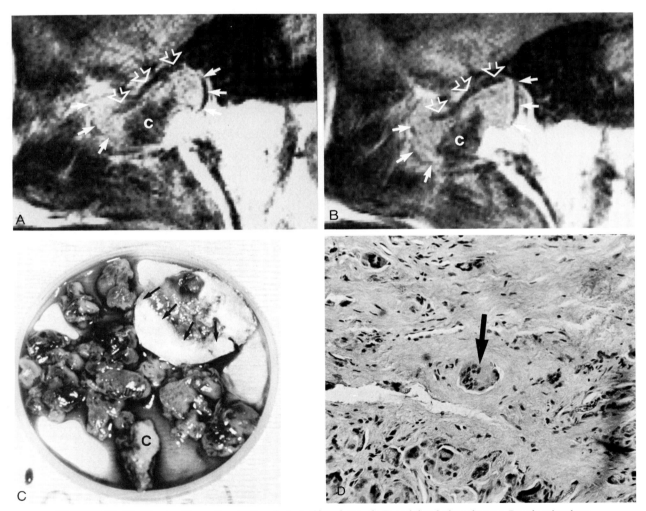

FIGURE 38–26. Giant cell reaction to Proplast. *A,* Closed-mouth T_1-weighted view shows a Proplast implant *(open arrows),* a severely eroded mandibular condyle (c), and a soft-tissue mass distending the entire intracapsular space *(closed arrows). B,* Open-mouth T_2-weighted view shows very poor translation of the condyle; however, no high signal is present to indicate a joint effusion or edema. *C,* Surgical specimen shows the Proplast *(arrows)* and the condyle (c) surrounded by the soft-tissue mass. *D,* Photomicrograph in which a giant cell *(arrow)* reaction to the Proplast is identified as the cause of joint destruction.

with the magnetic field have not been a problem. In a series of over 1200 cases at 0.6 tesla, we have seen no artifacts that prevented adequate visualization of the joint owing to these appliances, and no complications due to the magnetic field have been determined to date.

There is an association between TMJ disease and emotional stress.[44] Perhaps for this reason a greater number of patients with claustrophobia are encountered than in the general patient population. Oral diazepam or, occasionally, intravenous Versed (midazolam) has been used with excellent success in these cases. Knowledge of claustrophobia prior to scanning is helpful, as the patient and MR staff can prepare prior to the patient's arrival.

REFERENCES

1. Helms CA, Richardson ML, Moon KL, Ware WH: Nuclear magnetic resonance imaging of the temporomandibular joint; preliminary observations. J Craniomand Pract 2:219–224, 1984.
2. Harms SE, Wilk RM, Wolford LM, et al: The temporomandibular joint: Magnetic resonance imaging using surface coils. Radiology 157:133–136, 1985.
3. Roberts D, Schenk J, Joseph P, et al: Magnetic resonance imaging of the temporomandibular joint tissues. Radiology 155:829–830, 1985.
4. Katzberg RW, Schenck J, Roberts D, et al: Magnetic resonance imaging of the temporomandibular joint meniscus. Oral Surg Oral Med Oral Pathol 59:332–335, 1985.
5. Wilk RM, Harms SE, Wolford LM: Magnetic resonance imaging of the temporomandibular joint with a surface coil. J Oral Maxillofac Surg 44:935–943, 1986.
6. Chiles DG, Wilk RM, Harms SE: MRI in the diagnosis of temporomandibular joint disorders with a report of two cases. J Craniomand Pract 4:306–312, 1986.
7. Katzberg RW, Bessette RW, Tallents RH, et al: Normal and abnormal temporomandibular joint: MR imaging with surface coil. Radiology 158:183–189, 1986.
8. Harms SE, Wilk RW: Magnetic resonance of the temporomandibular joint. RadioGraphics 7:521–542, 1987.
9. Campbell W: Clinical radiological investigations of the mandibular joints. Br J Radiol 38:401–420, 1964.
10. Katzberg RW, Keith DA, Guralnick WC, et al: Internal derangements and arthritis of the temporomandibular joint. Radiology 146:107–112, 1983.
11. Stanson AW, Baker HL: Routine tomography of the temporomandibular joint. Radiol Clin North Am 14:105–127, 1983.
12. Helms CA, Morrish R, Kircos L, et al: Computed tomography of the meniscus of the temporomandibular joint: Preliminary observations. Radiology 145:719–722, 1982.
13. Helms CA, Katzberg RW, Morrish R, Dolwick MF: Computed tomography of the temporomandibular joint meniscus. J Oral Maxillofac Surg 41:512–517, 1983.
14. Manzione JV, Seltzer SE, Katzberg RW, et al: Direct sagittal computed tomography of the temporomandibular joint. AJR 140:165–167, 1983.
15. Manzione JV, Katzberg RW, Brodsky GL, et al: Internal derangements of the temporomandibular joint. Diagnosis by direct sagittal computed tomography. Radiology 150:111–115, 1984.
16. Helms CA, Katzberg RW, Morrish R, Dolwick MF: Computed tomography of the temporomandibular joint meniscus. J Oral Maxillofac Surg 41:512–517, 1983.
17. Katzberg RW, Dolwick MF, Keith DA, et al: New observations with routine and CT-assisted arthrography in suspected internal derangements of the temporomandibular joint. Oral Surg 51:569–574, 1981.
18. Manzione JV, Katzberg RW, Brodsky GL, et al: Internal derangements of the temporomandibular joint: Diagnosis by direct sagittal computed tomography. Radiology 150:111–115, 1984.
19. Kaplan PA: Computed tomography vs. arthrography in the evaluation of the temporomandibular joint. Radiology 152:825–827, 1984.
20. Helms CA, Vogler JB III, Morrish RB Jr, et al: Temporomandibular joint internal derangements: CT diagnosis. Radiology 152:459–462, 1984.
21. Thompson JR, Christiansen E, Sauser D, et al: Dislocation of the temporomandibular joint meniscus: Contrast arthrography vs. computed tomography. AJNR 5:747–750, 1984.
22. Sartoris DJ, Neumann CH, Riley RW: Temporomandibular joint: True sagittal computed tomography with meniscus visualization. Radiology 150:250–254, 1984.
23. Bronstein SL, Tomasetti BJ, Ryan DE: Internal derangements of the temporomandibular joint: Correlation of arthrography with surgical findings. J Oral Surg 39:572–584, 1981.
24. Katzberg RW, Dolwick MF, Helms CA, et al: Arthrotomography of the temporomandibular joint. AJR 134:995–1003, 1980.
25. Dolwick MF, Katzberg RW, Helms CA, Bales DJ: Arthrotomographic evaluation of the temporomandibular joint. J Oral Surg 37:793–799, 1979.
26. Westesson P: Double-contrast arthrotomography of the temporomandibular joint. J Oral Maxillofac Surg 41:163–172, 1983.
27. Blaschke DD, Solbert WK, Sanders B: Arthrography of the temporomandibular joint: Review of current status. J Am Dent Assoc 100:388, 1980.
28. Lynch TP, Chase DC: Arthrography in the evaluation of the temporomandibular joint. Radiology 126:667–672, 1978.
29. Katzberg RW, Dolwick MF, Bales DJ, Helms CA: Arthrotomography of the TMJ: New technique and preliminary observations. AJR 132:949–955, 1979.
30. Farrar WB, McCarty WL: Inferior joint space arthrography and characteristics of the condylar paths in internal derangements of the TMJ. J Prosthet Dent 41:548–555, 1979.
31. Katzberg RW, Dolwick MF, Helms CA, et al: Arthrotomography of the temporomandibular joint. AJR 134:995–1003, 1980.
32. Murphy WA: Arthrography of the temporomandibular joint. Radiol Clin North Am 51:569–574, 1981.
33. Helms CA, Katzberg RW, Dolwick MF (eds): Internal Derangements of the Temporomandibular Joint. San Francisco, Radiology Research and Education Foundation, 1983.
34. Lydiatt D, Kaplan P, Tu H, Sleder P: Morbidity associated with temporomandibular joint arthrography in clinically normal joints. J Oral Maxillofac Surg 44:8–10, 1986.
35. Wilk RM, Harms SE: Three-dimensional FT magnetic resonance imaging of the temporomandibular joint. Abstract 1060. J Dent Res 65:287, 1986.
36. Harms SE, Muschler G: Three-dimensional MR imaging of the knee using surface coils. J Comput Assist Tomogr 10:773–777, 1986.
37. Gallimore G, Harms SE: Selective three-dimensional MR imaging of the spine. J Comput Assist Tomogr 11:124–128, 1987.
38. Harms SE, Wilk RM: Thin slice, high resolution MRI of the temporomandibular joint with surgical and pathologic correlation. Book of Abstracts. Society of Magnetic Resonance in Medicine, 1986, pp 273–274.
39. Wilk RM, Harms SE: Temporomandibular joint: multislab three-dimensional Fourier transformation MR imaging. Radiology 167:861–863, 1988.
40. Guralnick W, Kaban LB, Merril RG: Temporomandibular joint afflictions. N Engl J Med 229:123–129, 1978.
41. Solberg WK, Woo MW, Houston JB: Prevalence of mandibular dysfunction in young adults. J Am Dent Assoc 98:25–34, 1979.
42. Bush FM, Butler JH, Abbott DM, Carter WH: Prevalence of mandibular dysfunction: Subjective signs and symptoms. In

Little MA (ed): Occlusion: Diagnosis and Treatment. Publishing Sciences Group, 1981.

43. Harms SE, Wilk RM: Magnetic Resonance of the Temporomandibular Joint. MRI Update Series. Vol 2, Book 5, 1986.

44. Okeson JP: Fundamentals of Occlusion and Temporomandibular Disorders. St. Louis, CV Mosby, 1985.

45. Drace S, Enzmann DR: MR imaging of the temporomandibular joint (TMJ). Part I: Closed-, partially open-, and open-mouthed views of the normal TMJ. Radiology 161(P):193, 1986.

46. Hyde JS, Froncisz W, Jesmanowicz A, et al: Parallel image acquisition from non-interacting local coils. Book of Abstracts. Society of Magnetic Resonance in Medicine, 1986, pp 43–44.

47. Frahm J, Hasse A, Matthari W: Rapid three-dimensional MR imaging using the FLASH technique. J Comput Assist Tomogr 10:363–368, 1986.

48. Hasse A, Frahm J, Matthari W, Hanicke KD: Rapid images and NMR movies. Program. Society of Magnetic Resonance in Medicine, 1985, pp 980–981.

49. Burnett KR, Davis CL, Read J: Dynamic display of the temporomandibular joint meniscus by using "fast-scan" MR imaging. AJR 149:959–962, 1987.

50. Frahm J, Merboldt KD, Hanicke W, Hasse A: Stimulated echo imaging. J Magn Reson 64:81–93, 1985.

51. Hasse A, Frahm J: NMR imaging of spin-lattice relaxation using stimulated echoes. J Magn Reson 65:481–490, 1985.

52. Crooks LE, Ortendahl PA, Kaufman L, et al: Clinical efficiency of nuclear magnetic resonance imaging. Radiology 146:123–128, 1983.

53. Harms SE, Kramer DM: Fundamentals of magnetic resonance imaging. CRC Crit Rev Diagn Imaging 25:79–111, 1985.

54. Kramer DM, Compton RA, Yeung HN: A volume (3D) analog of 2D multislice or "multislab" MR imaging. In Proceedings of the Society of Magnetic Resonance, 1985, pp 162–163.

55. Hall EJ: Radiobiology for the Radiologist. Hagerstown, MD, Harper and Row, 1978.

56. Katzberg RW, Tallents RH, Hayakawa K, et al: Internal derangements of the temporomandibular joint: Findings in the pediatric age group. Radiology 154:125–127, 1985.

57. Miller TL, Katzberg RW, Tallents RH: Temporomandibular joint clicking with nonreducing anterior displacement of the meniscus. Radiology 154:121–124, 1985.

58. Schellhas KP, Wilkes CH, Omlie MR, et al: The diagnosis of temporomandibular joint disease: Two-compartment arthrography and MR. AJR 151:341–350, 1988.

59. Wyngaarden JB: Etiology and pathogenesis of gout. In Hollander JL: Arthritis and Allied Conditions. Philadelphia, Lea and Febiger, 1966, p 899.

60. Harms SE, Menter A: Unpublished observation.

61. Timmis DP, Aragon SB, Van Sickels JE, Aufdemorte TB: Comparative study of alloplastic materials for temporomandibular joint disk replacement in rabbits. J Oral Maxillofac Surg 44:541–554, 1986.

62. Kaplan PA, Ruskin JD, Tu HK, Knibbe MA: Erosive arthritis of the temporomandibular joint caused by Teflon-Proplast implants: Plain film features. AJR 151:337–339, 1988.

63. Schellhas KP, Wilkes CH, El Deeb M, et al: Permanent Proplast temporomandibular joint implants: MR imaging of destructive complications. AJR 151:731–735, 1988.

39

MR IMAGING OF THE WRIST

LELAND E. KELLERHOUSE, MURRAY A. REICHER,
SEVIL KURSUNOGLU-BRAHME, and MARK S. SLONIM

MRI WRIST TECHNIQUE
CARPAL TUNNEL SYNDROME
  VOLUMETRIC INCREASE WITHIN THE
    CARPAL TUNNEL
  DECREASED CROSS-SECTIONAL AREA OF
    THE CARPAL TUNNEL
  MRI FOLLOWING CARPAL TUNNEL
    RELEASE
  MRI EVALUATION OF THE FAILED
    CARPAL TUNNEL RELEASE
EXTENSOR TENDON
  ABNORMALITIES
CARPAL INSTABILITY
  NORMAL ANATOMY AND BIOMECHANICS
  WRIST PATHOMECHANICS

DORSAL INTERCALATED SEGMENTAL
  INSTABILITY (DISI) AND
  SCAPHOLUNATE DISSOCIATION (SLD)
KIENBÖCK'S DISEASE
THE ULNAR ASPECT OF THE WRIST
  ANATOMY OF THE DISTAL RADIOULNAR
    JOINT
  BIOMECHANICS OF THE ULNAR ASPECT OF
    THE WRIST
  PATHOMECHANICS OF THE ULNAR ASPECT
    OF THE WRIST
  VOLAR INTERCALATED SEGMENTAL
    INSTABILITY (VISI)
GANGLIONS OF THE HAND AND
  WRIST
CONCLUSION

Standard radiography, tomography, fluoroscopy, scintigraphy, arthrography, and computed tomography have all been previously employed to image the wrist. Although these methods are all capable of providing valuable information about the carpal bones, none of these techniques enables simultaneous direct visualization of the periarticular and intraarticular soft tissues. Recently, MR imaging has proved valuable in delineating both osseous and soft tissue disorders of the wrist. MR imaging offers several fundamental advantages: (1) the capability of depicting the complex wrist anatomy in multiple planes; (2) direct depiction of ligaments, tendons, articular cartilage, and fibrocartilage; (3) extreme sensitivity in detecting disease involving both soft tissues and bone marrow; and (4) the ability to study the wrist in multiple anatomic positions. MR imaging is also, of course, painless and without biologic risk. It often provides diagnostic information that would require a costly battery of other examinations.

In this chapter, we review a spectrum of clinical wrist disorders and demonstrate the value of MR imaging for investigating these pathologic states. The topics include MR imaging techniques, carpal tunnel evaluation, tendon and triangular fibrocartilaginous abnormalities, carpal instability syndromes, and ulnar wrist pain. Normal and pathologic anatomy on MR imaging is reviewed, as well as MR imaging applications in evaluating the postsurgical patient.

MRI WRIST TECHNIQUE

Optimal wrist positioning and use of a surface coil are critical for obtaining reproducible diagnostic images of the wrist. The hand and wrist must be placed in neutral alignment so that the third metacarpal and radius are co-linear. By taking great care in positioning the wrist and obtaining scans in true sagittal, axial, and coronal planes, images of consistently high quality can be reproducibly obtained. The ability to interpret wrist MR imaging reliably depends on avoiding random variations in wrist posture and obliquity of imaging planes. The fingers are held in extension with no radial or ulnar deviation. Rigid stabilization of the wrist in the neutral position is achieved with a dorsal splint applied to the hand, wrist, and distal forearm.

To maximize the patient's comfort, we now image the wrist utilizing a dedicated send-receive surface coil (Medical Advances, Milwaukee, WI), which allows imaging with the patient supine and the arm at his or her side. The precise technique we now employ is as follows:

1. An axial localizer spin-echo (SE) scan is performed first (repetition time [TR]/echo time [TE] = 300/20, 5-mm slice, 2-mm gap between slices, 128 × 256 matrix, 14-cm field-of-view [FOV], one excitation). The technologist manually measures the distance from the center frequency to the patient's wrist when the patient is placed in the scanner to program the proper offset and thereby accurately spatially localize the wrist within the FOV of the scan.

2. Using the axial images as a guide, we next obtain true coronal SE images of the wrist (TR/TE = 500/20, 3-mm slices, 1-mm gap, 256 × 256 matrix, 12-cm FOV, one excitation). The sequence is repeated twice, with the second set of coronal scans located within the gaps of the first set.

3. True sagittal scans of the wrist are performed next (TR/TE = 500/20, 3-mm slices, 1-mm gap, 256 × 256 matrix, 12-cm FOV, one excitation).

4. Next, a multiecho sequence is utilized to obtain axial images of the wrist (TR/TE = 1500/30,80, 5-mm slices, 1-mm gap, 128 × 256 matrix, 10-cm FOV, one excitation). This yields intermediate and T$_2$-weighted images.

5. A gradient recalled acquisition in the steady state (GRASS) series is then obtained in the coronal plane (TR/TE = 250/20, flip angle = 30 degrees, 3-mm slices, 1-mm gap, 256 × 256 matrix, 12-cm FOV, one excitation). This yields T$_2^*$-weighted images, which facilitate visualization of the intercarpal ligaments and triangular fibrocartilage complex (TFCC).

6. If the clinical history indicates ulnar wrist pain, the axial multiecho sequence described previously is repeated with the wrist pronated to evaluate subluxation of the distal ulna or extensor carpi ulnaris tendon or both.

This imaging technique results in a highly detailed, reliable, reproducible, and comprehensive evaluation of the wrist. The technique described previously should be used as a general guideline and will undoubtedly change as new software and hardware become available. We anticipate, for example, that multislice gradient-echo (GRE) imaging and three-dimensional Fourier transform (3DFT) techniques will play an increasingly prominent role in wrist MR imaging.

CARPAL TUNNEL SYNDROME

The carpal tunnel is a confined anatomic structure encasing the flexor tendons and median nerve of the hand and wrist. The tunnel is bounded medially, dorsally, and laterally by an arch of tightly linked carpal bones.[1-3] The volar boundary of the carpal tunnel is formed by the transverse carpal ligament. The transverse carpal ligament primarily attaches to the distal carpal row, coursing between the tubercle of the trapezium and the hook of the hamate, with secondary attachments bridging from the tuberosity of the scaphoid to the pisiform. The anatomy of the carpal tunnel is best demonstrated in axial sections, where the deep and superficial flexor tendons, the median nerve, the arching carpal bones, and the transverse carpal ligament can all be separately identified (Fig. 39–1).

Carpal tunnel syndrome is the most common compression neuropathy in the upper extremity.[1] Common symptoms include weakness and clumsiness, as well as paresthesias in the distribution of the median nerve, often aggravated by grasping. Compression of the median nerve can be caused by a decrease in the cross-sectional area of the carpal canal. More commonly, an increase in the volume of the structures within the carpal canal results in compression of the median nerve within this restricted space.

Diagnosis of carpal tunnel syndrome depends on the presence of typical physical signs and clinical symptoms. MR imaging may play a valuable role in delineating the anatomic cause of median nerve com-

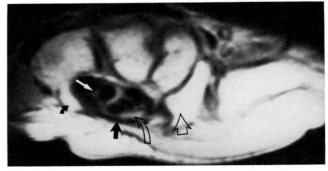

FIGURE 39–1. Axial MR image of normal carpal tunnel. The normal flexor tendons are demonstrated as tightly packed, homogeneous structures of low signal intensity *(small white arrow)*. The volar carpal ligament is a thin, flatly configured structure of low signal intensity *(black arrow)* coursing between the hook of the hamate *(curved arrow)* and the trapezium *(open arrow)*. The normal dorsally arched configuration of the bony carpus is demonstrated. The median nerve *(curved open arrow)* is elliptical in shape and yields moderate signal intensity on this intermediate-weighted scan.

pression, documenting the severity of median nerve compression, and evaluating the cause of a failed surgical release of the carpal tunnel.

VOLUMETRIC INCREASE WITHIN THE CARPAL TUNNEL

The most common cause of carpal tunnel syndrome is tenosynovitis of the flexor tendons. This condition usually occurs because of occupation-related repetitive flexion of fingers or wrists or both. Keyboard punch operators, typists, grocery store checkers, and tradesmen who frequently use hand tools may develop tenosynovitis.[1, 4] The volumetric increase of the flexor tendon sheaths resulting from tenosynovitis causes median nerve compression, since the arched bony carpus and transverse carpal ligament form relatively unyielding borders of the carpal tunnel. Work-related tenosynovitis may subside when the activity is discontinued, resulting in relief of the nerve compression symptoms (RM Braun, K Davidson, and S Doehr, unpublished results). Other conditions producing increased volume of the carpal tunnel contents include synovitis, ganglions, lipomas, calcium deposits, hematomas, fluid retention, amyloid, aberrant artery, increased growth of connective tissue, acromegaly, venous distention, anomalous proximal origin of the lumbrical muscles, and hormonal changes associated with pregnancy and menopause.[1, 4]

Flexor tendon tenosynovitis is manifested on MR imaging by the presence of variably sized effusions within the flexor tendon sheaths. This may be accompanied by volar bowing of the transverse carpal ligament (Fig. 39–2). The median nerve is often visibly compressed in the carpal tunnel but is often paradoxically enlarged immediately proximal and distal to the transverse carpal ligament. As the flexor

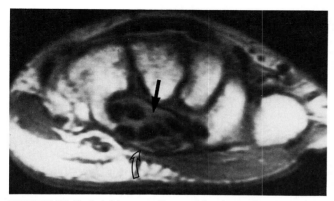

FIGURE 39–2. Axial intermediate-weighted scan in patient with carpal tunnel syndrome secondary to flexor tendon tenosynovitis. Effusions within flexor tendon sheaths (*black arrow*) yield moderate signal intensity on this intermediate-weighted pulse sequence. As a result, flexor tendons appear to be separated rather than tightly packed. The volar carpal ligament (*open arrow*) is bowed in a volar direction.

tendon sheaths enlarge, the fat within the carpal canal may also be compressed and virtually obliterated. Finally, the median nerve may manifest increased signal intensity on T_2-weighted images, representing demyelination or edema.

DECREASED CROSS-SECTIONAL AREA OF THE CARPAL TUNNEL

Carpal tunnel syndrome is often primarily attributable to or aggravated by conditions that cause a decrease in the cross-sectional area of the carpal canal.[1, 5–8] The carpal tunnel may be relatively small on a congenital basis or may diminish in size owing to a variety of acquired conditions. The most common cause of acquired reduction in the cross-sectional area of the carpal tunnel is degenerative arthritis or deformity resulting from trauma.

Carpal tunnel narrowing may also result from shortening of the wrist (Fig. 39–3) (J Taleisnik, personal communication). Shortening of the wrist refers to proximal migration of the capitate toward the distal radius. Since the transverse carpal ligament is primarily attached to the distal carpal row, any process that results in wrist shortening allows the ligament to migrate proximally toward the radiocarpal joint, where the carpal canal is significantly less commodious. Compared with the markedly dorsally arched contour of the distal carpal canal, the dorsal contour of the proximal carpal canal is flattened; thus, proximal migration of the transverse carpal ligament results in functional narrowing of the carpal tunnel.

Many diverse conditions may result in shortening of the wrist, including Kienböck's disease with lunate collapse, dorsal intercalated segmental instability (DISI), scapholunate dissociation (SLD), rheumatoid arthritis, and scaphoid osteonecrosis with collapse.

MRI FOLLOWING CARPAL TUNNEL RELEASE

During operative treatment of carpal tunnel syndrome, the surgeon normally divides the ulnar aspect of the transverse carpal ligament near its insertion on the hook of the hamate.[1] The entire breadth of the ligament is divided after good exposure of the neurovascular bundle on the ulnar aspect of the wrist.

Axial MR images after successful carpal tunnel release reveal the transverse carpal ligament displaced volarly from the hook of the hamate (Fig. 39–4). The contents of the carpal canal typically also migrate volarly, since they are no longer restrained by the transverse carpal ligament.[9] The fat stripe normally interposed between the deep flexor tendons and proximal carpal row often appears thickened owing to volar subluxation of the flexor tendons. The median nerve no longer appears compressed

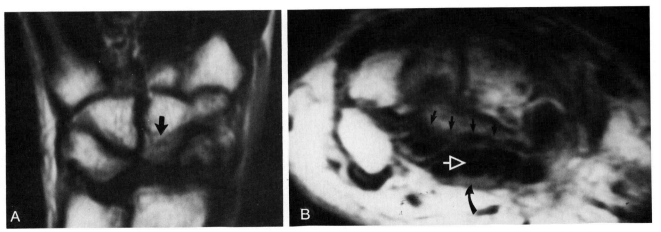

FIGURE 39–3. Median nerve compression secondary to shortening of the wrist. *A,* Coronal T_1-weighted scan demonstrates proximal migration of the capitate *(arrow)* relative to the radius. The lunate is completely collapsed and no longer visible as a separate structure on this image. *B,* Axial scan reveals loss of the normally dorsally arched configuration of the carpus. Hypertrophied bony elements *(small black arrows)* now compress the dorsal aspect of the flexor tendons *(open arrow).* As a result, the median nerve *(curved black arrow)* is markedly flattened.

and may, in fact, enlarge. Although flexor tendon tenosynovitis may remain, the area of the carpal canal is no longer restricted.

MRI EVALUATION OF THE FAILED CARPAL TUNNEL RELEASE

The most common cause of recurrent carpal tunnel syndrome is inadequate or incomplete release of the transverse carpal ligament. Sometimes, however, despite adequate surgical division, the transverse carpal

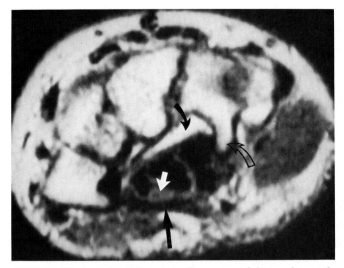

FIGURE 39–4. Axial MR image after successful carpal tunnel release. The remaining radial portion of the volar carpal ligament *(solid black arrow)* is no longer attached to the hook of the hamate *(open curved arrow).* The flexor tendons are volarly subluxated, and, as a result, the fat stripe interposed between the bony carpus and flexor tendons is widened *(solid curved arrow).* The median nerve *(white arrow)* is normal in shape.

ligament may reattach to the hook of the hamate and adjacent pisiform, resulting in reentrapment of the median nerve. In addition, shortening of the transverse carpal ligament caused by scarring may worsen median nerve compression. In advanced postoperative scarring, the shortened transverse carpal ligament may appear contracted into the carpal canal, resulting in a V-shaped cleft along the volar aspect of the wrist (Fig. 39–5A). The retracted ligament, median nerve, and flexor tendons may be scarred into a tightly contracted mass. MR imaging, in cases of failed carpal tunnel release, may also reveal persistent flexor tendon tenosynovitis (Fig. 39–5B). It should also be recognized that median nerve entrapment may occur proximal to the wrist, as in the pronator syndrome and the anterior interosseous syndrome.[1]

EXTENSOR TENDON ABNORMALITIES

The extensor tendons can be subdivided into six compartments as they course along the dorsal aspect of the wrist (Fig. 39–6). Of the six extensor compartments, the first and sixth are most commonly diseased.[10] A combination of tendinitis and tenosynovitis of the first compartment is known as de Quervain's syndrome (Fig. 39–7). In this disorder, the abductor pollicis longus and extensor pollicis brevis tendons become inflamed as they pass through the fibroosseous tunnel of the first dorsal compartment at the level of the radial styloid. These two tendons, restrained within the first dorsal compartment, tend to angulate at the wrist, especially during wrist ulnar deviation. Ordinarily, the diagnosis of de Quervain's

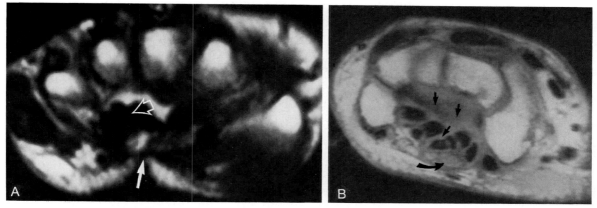

FIGURE 39–5. Examples of failed carpal tunnel release. *A,* Retraction and scarring result in V-shaped palmar cleft *(white arrow)* and clumping of flexor tendons *(open white arrow). B,* In a different patient, despite very adequate release of volar carpal ligament, there is massive deep and superficial tenosynovitis *(small black arrows)* and resultant marked volar displacement of median nerve *(curved arrow).* Although median nerve is not flattened, clinical signs and symptoms of carpal tunnel syndrome persisted.

FIGURE 39–6. Diagrammatic depiction of six extensor tendon compartments. ECU = extensor carpi ulnaris; EDQ = extensor digiti quinti; EDC = extensor digitorum communis; EIP = extensor indicis proprius; EPL = extensor pollicis longus; ECRL = extensor carpi radialis longus; ECRB = extensor carpi radialis brevis; APL = abductor pollicis longus; EPB = extensor pollicis brevis.

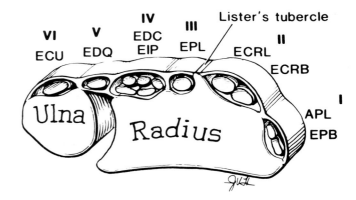

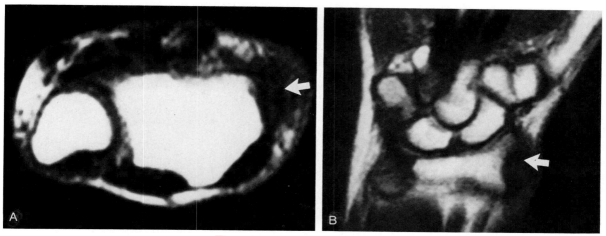

FIGURE 39–7. Coronal *(A)* and axial *(B)* T_1-weighted images demonstrate marked soft tissue swelling both within and surrounding the first extensor compartment *(arrow),* a condition referred to as de Quervain's syndrome.

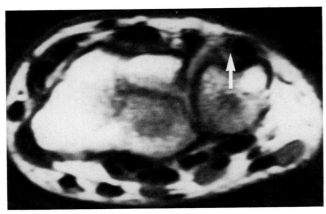

FIGURE 39–8. Extensor carpi ulnaris tenosynovitis. Axial intermediate-weighted scan demonstrates effusion within extensor carpi ulnaris tendon sheath *(arrow).*

syndrome is easily made on a clinical basis, but MR imaging may be valuable in diagnosing clinically equivocal cases, documenting multicompartmented tendons, and determining severity of disease. Tenosynovitis is manifested on MR images by swelling of the tendon sheath. In contrast, tendinitis is exhibited by enlargement and increased signal intensity of the tendon itself.

Tenosynovitis frequently also affects the sixth dorsal compartment, which contains the extensor carpi ulnaris tendon (Fig. 39–8). The extensor carpi ulnaris tendon normally courses through a rather unyielding fibrous canal as it passes along a groove on the dorsomedial aspect of the distal ulna. Disease of the extensor carpi ulnaris tendon is a relatively frequent cause of ulnar wrist pain, a topic addressed separately later in this chapter.

CARPAL INSTABILITY

NORMAL ANATOMY AND BIOMECHANICS

The wrist is composed of the distal surfaces of the radius and ulna; four proximal carpal bones (lunate, scaphoid, triquetrum, pisiform); four distal carpal bones (trapezium, trapezoid, capitate, hamate); and intercarpal, capsular, and intracapsular ligaments. The scaphoid is unique, as it links the proximal and distal carpal bones. Alignment of the carpus is maintained principally by the volar carpal ligaments. The volar carpal ligaments form a confluent network. Depending on how the wrist is dissected, identification of specific ligaments varies among authors[11–18] (Fig. 39–9A). However, most authors agree that the most important proximal volar carpal ligaments include the radioscapholunate ligament and the radioscaphocapite ligament. The radioscapholunate ligament can be further divided into the radiolunate ligament (ligament of Testut) and the radioscaphoid ligament (ligament of Kuenz). The radiolunate ligament courses from the distal volar margin of the radius to the distal volar margin of the lunate. This ligament plays a critical role in restraining dorsal angulation of the lunate. The radioscaphocapitate ligament, or "sling ligament," courses from the volar aspect of the distal radius along the volar margin of the midscaphoid to insert upon the volar aspect of the capitate. This ligament plays a critical role in restraining volar angulation or rotatory subluxation of the necessarily mobile scaphoid, which links the distal carpal bones to the proximal carpal row. Some authors describe the existence of ulnar and radial collateral ligaments on the medial and lateral aspects

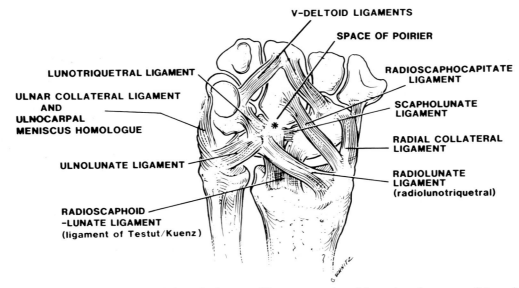

FIGURE 39–9. Diagrammatic depiction of volar carpal ligaments as viewed from the solar aspect of the wrist.

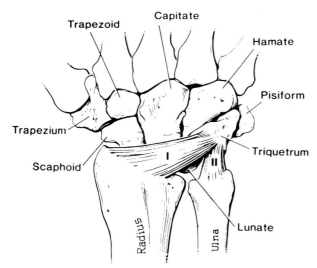

FIGURE 39–10. Diagrammatic depiction of the most important dorsal carpal ligaments as viewed from the dorsum of the wrist. I = radiolunotriquetral ligament; II = dorsal ulnotriquetral ligament.

of the wrist, although others dispute that these exist as separate structures.

The volar aspect of the distal carpal row is also stabilized by the deltoid ligament. This ligament has two components that merge from separate origins upon the scaphoid and triquetrum to a common insertion upon the volar aspect of the capitate.

The interosseous ligaments include the scapholunate and lunotriquetral ligaments. The interosseous ligaments are significantly less important as stabilizing structures of the carpus and, in fact, are frequently degenerated by the third decade of life.

On the dorsal surface of the carpus, the two primary ligaments are the radiolunotriquetral ligament and the dorsal ulnotriquetral ligament (Fig. 39–10). Most authors agree that the dorsal wrist ligaments are not as critical as the volar carpal ligaments in maintaining carpal stability.

On MR images, ligaments appear as thin black structures. On sagittal MR images, the radioscapholunate and radioscaphocapitate ligaments are routinely identified (Fig. 39–11). The deep and superficial flexor tendons are identified volar to these ligaments. With the wrist in neutral position, sagittal images normally demonstrate the radius, lunate, and capitate in co-linear alignment. Sagittal images also normally demonstrate the scaphoid to be tilted approximately 47 degrees volar to the longitudinal axis of the wrist.[16] When present, the scapholunate and lunotriquetral interosseous ligaments are also readily identified on SE or GRE coronal MR images (Fig.

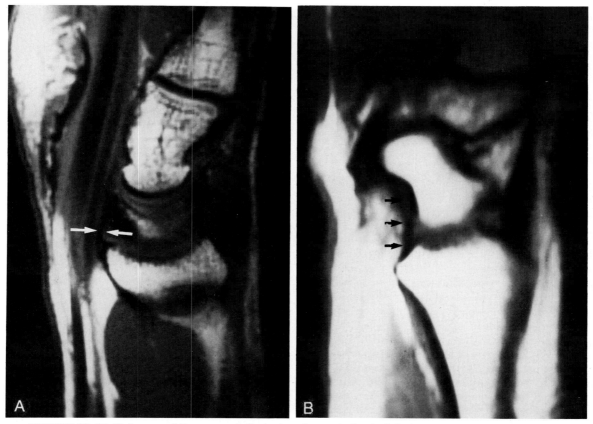

FIGURE 39–11. Volar carpal ligaments. *A,* Sagittal section at the level of the lunate clearly demonstrates the radiolunate portion of the radioscapholunate ligament *(white arrows). B,* Sagittal section at the level of the scaphoid clearly depicts the sling ligament or radioscaphocapitate ligament *(arrows).*

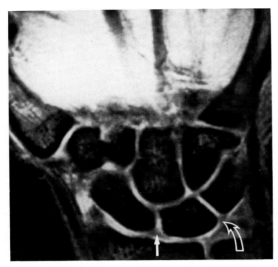

FIGURE 39–12. Gradient-echo (GRE) coronal MR image demonstrates the scapholunate (*solid white arrow*) and lunotriquetral (*curved white arrow*) interosseous ligaments as structures of moderately low signal intensity.

39–12). These ligaments are seen as thin structures of low signal intensity bridging the proximal scapholunate and lunotriquetral intervals.

MR imaging offers considerable advantage over wrist arthrography, since the latter technique allows evaluation of only the less important intercarpal ligaments and not the volar carpal ligaments. It is important to recognize that radial and ulnar deviation of the wrist normally alters the relationship of the carpal bones. With ulnar deviation, the normal volar tilt of the mobile scaphoid is reduced, and the lunate tends to tilt dorsally. With radial deviation, the volar tilt of the scaphoid is accentuated, and the lunate tends also to tilt volarly.[16] Positioning of the wrist in neutral posture is therefore critical in yielding MR images of reliable interpretive quality.

Wrist Pathomechanics

The relationship of the carpal bones and ligaments is complex, and the pathogenesis of carpal injuries, although extensively studied by many, remains controversial. The following is a simplified explanation of wrist pathomechanics that we believe accurately reflects a compromise of several authors' views.

Regardless of what activity the hand or wrist is engaged in, the resultant forces are distributed along the longitudinal axis of the wrist. Most of these axial loading forces are borne along the axis of the capitate, lunate, and radius. The remaining carpal bones and ligaments help balance the axial or longitudinal loading forces through the capitate, lunate, and radius when the wrist is deviated in either the radial or the ulnar direction.[16] In particular, the scaphoid is necessarily mobile because it is long relative to the

other carpal bones and it is the main link between the distal and proximal carpal rows. As mentioned previously, the alignment of the carpus is maintained principally by the volar carpal ligaments. The dorsal ligaments and the interosseous ligaments are considerably less important in maintaining carpal stability. In addition, the collateral ligaments probably do not act as collateral stabilizers of the wrist and may not, in fact, exist as distinct structures.

The dominant axial loading forces that occur at the wrist tend to result pathologically in wrist shortening (proximal migration of the capitate). Wrist shortening can occur gradually over time or secondary to severe, acute trauma. Acute fractures and dislocations may, of course, result from severe, acute axial loading forces, such as those caused by a fall on an outstretched hand. More subtle chronic or acute injuries may also affect the proximal carpal row and volar carpal ligaments. Depending on the precise derangement, the resultant wrist shortening may be associated with DISI, volar intercalated segmental instability (VISI), SLD, scaphoid osteonecrosis, lunate osteonecrosis, or scapholunate advanced collapse.[11–18]

In addition to understanding the axial loading forces in the sagittal plane of the wrist, it is also important to understand how these forces are distributed in the coronal plane. In the average individual, the articular surfaces of the ulna and radius extend distally to virtually an identical level.[19, 20] This condition is referred to as *neutral ulnar variance*. In patients with neutral ulnar variance, 80 per cent of the axial loading forces are transmitted through the lunate to the radius. The remaining 20 per cent of the axial loading forces are transmitted through the lunate to the ulna.

Variations in radial and ulnar length will significantly alter the relative forces borne by the distal radius and ulna (Fig. 39–13). For example, reduction in the length of the ulna in relation to the radius (*negative ulnar variance*) by as little as 2.5 mm may result in the buttressing by the radius of nearly 96 per cent of the axial loading forces. On the other hand, increasing the ulnar length by 2.5 mm (*positive ulnar variance*) reduces the relative force borne by the radius to 58 per cent.

Congenital or posttraumatic differences in ulnar variance therefore markedly influence the biomechanics of the wrist. Negative variance, for example, is associated with Kienböck's disease. Positive ulnar variance may predispose to early degeneration of the triangular fibrocartilage (TFC) and ulnolunate impingement syndrome.

Dorsal Intercalated Segmental Instability (DISI) and Scapholunate Dissociation (SLD)

Of the aforementioned forms of wrist shortening, DISI and SLD are the most commonly observed.[13, 16]

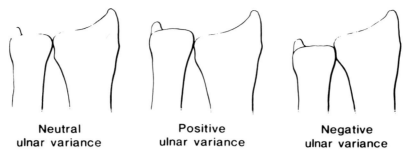

| Neutral | Positive | Negative |
| ulnar variance | ulnar variance | ulnar variance |

FIGURE 39–13. Diagrammatic demonstration of neutral ulnar variance, positive ulnar variance, and negative ulnar variance.

These two conditions frequently, in fact, coexist. How does DISI occur? As a patient falls on an outstretched hand, the forces generated may be sufficient to fracture the radius or produce a lunate or perilunate dislocation or fracture the scaphoid. However, less severe forces may result in stretching or frank tearing of the volar radioscapholunate and radioscaphocapitate ligaments. When the radioscapholunate ligament is stretched or torn, the volar aspect of the

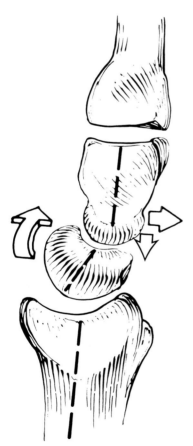

FIGURE 39–14. Dorsal intercalated segmental instability (DISI). When the radioscapholunate ligament is stretched or torn, the lunate is free to tilt dorsally. The dorsal tilt of the lunate also secondarily allows the capitate to migrate proximally, producing wrist shortening (anterior is on reader's left).

lunate is no longer properly tethered to the volar margin of the radius, and the lunate is therefore free to tilt dorsally (Figs. 39–14 and 39–15). The dorsal rotation of the lunate allows the capitate to migrate proximally, producing wrist shortening.

As viewed on sagittal MR images, the relationship of the radius, lunate, and capitate is no longer co-linear, but rather shortened in a Z-like configuration (Fig. 39–16A). The scaphoid commonly also rotates forward to an accentuated volar tilt (Fig. 39–16B). The constellation of these pathologic findings is referred to as DISI.

When great care is taken to position the wrist properly, marked DISI deformity can be reliably diagnosed on routine radiographs. However, even excellent radiographs may fail to detect subtle DISI, which, in our experience, is a relatively common condition and more dramatically depicted on MR images. MR imaging simultaneously provides a precise sagittal tomographic view of the bony structures and defines pathology of the radiolunate and radioscaphocapitate ligaments. Tears of these ligaments are easily detected, particularly when there is retraction or associated synovitis (Fig. 39–17). In most cases, however, MR imaging demonstrates the radiolunate and radioscaphocapitate ligaments to be stretched and redundant rather than frankly torn. As incompetence of the radioscapholunate and radioscaphocapitate ligaments allows the wrist to foreshorten into DISI malalignment, the transverse carpal ligament migrates proximally along with the distal carpal row. This situation places the patient at risk for developing carpal tunnel syndrome, since proximal migration of the transverse carpal ligament functionally narrows the carpal tunnel. As mentioned earlier in this chapter, the dorsal border of the carpal tunnel at the level of the radiocarpal joint is considerably flatter than the commodious dorsal arch of the distal carpal row.

Aside from the aforementioned ligaments, the interosseous scapholunate ligament is also easily identified by MR imaging (see Fig. 29–12). Tears of the scapholunate ligament may occur normally as one ages without associated DISI deformity or rotatory subluxation of the scaphoid. T_1-weighted coronal SE images usually demonstrate the scapholunate interosseous ligament tear (Fig. 39–18), but recently we

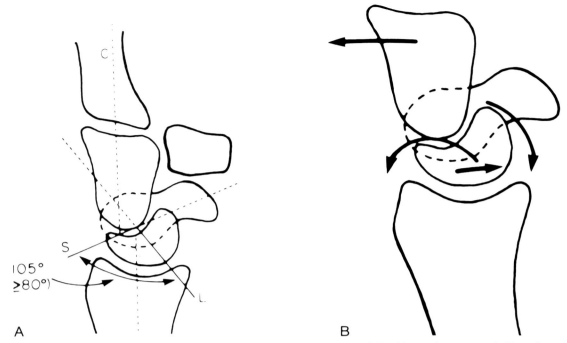

FIGURE 39–15. Dorsal intercalated segmental instability (DISI). Dorsal tilt of lunate is accompanied by volar rotation of scaphoid in this disorder (anterior is on reader's right).

have found T_2^*-weighted GRE images to be even more effective. Tears of the scapholunate interosseous ligament allow the scaphoid and lunate to separate, a condition known as SLD. The wrist then further shortens as the capitate migrates proximally into the gap between the scaphoid and the lunate. The end stage of this pathologic process is known as *scapholunate advanced collapse* (the SLAC wrist) (see Fig. 29–3).[21]

KIENBÖCK'S DISEASE

In addition to shortening of the carpal length due to laxity or tears of the volar carpal ligaments or interosseous ligaments, the wrist may also shorten when there is collapse of the lunate caused by avascular necrosis.[16, 22] As previously described, if the distal ulnar articular surface is proximal to the adjacent aspect of the distal radial articular surface, this

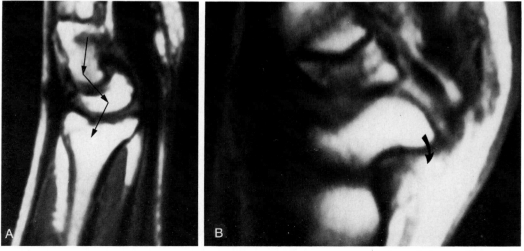

FIGURE 39–16. DISI depicted on adjacent sagittal MR sections. *A,* Section through lunate demonstrates shortening of wrist in Z-like configuration. *B,* Section through scaphoid demonstrates volar rotation of scaphoid (anterior is on reader's right).

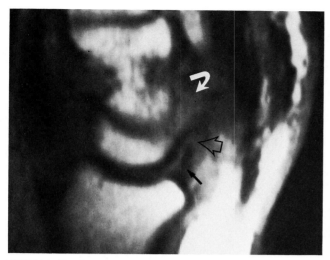

FIGURE 39–17. T$_1$-weighted sagittal MR scan reveals tear of radiolunate ligament. Proximal stump of radiolunate ligament is demonstrated *(arrow)*, but distal attachment is obliterated *(open arrow)*. Synovitis and edema *(curved arrow)* are seen volar to capitate (anterior is on reader's right).

condition is referred to as negative ulnar variance, or ulnar-minus variance (see Fig. 39–13). Subtle variations of ulnar length cause huge variations in axial loading. For example, in patients with 2- to 3-mm ulnar-minus variance, the radius bears nearly 100 per cent of the axial loading forces transmitted through the lunate.[19, 20] In addition, degeneration of the TFCC in patients with ulnar neutral variance

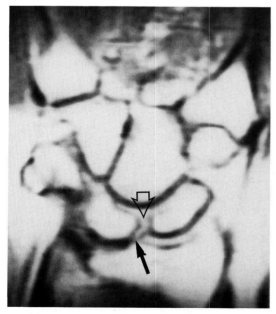

FIGURE 39–18. Scapholunate dissociation with scapholunate interosseous ligament tear. Coronal T$_1$-weighted scan demonstrates widening of the scapholunate interosseous interval *(open arrow)*. The lunate attachment of the scapholunate interosseous ligament is torn *(solid arrow)*.

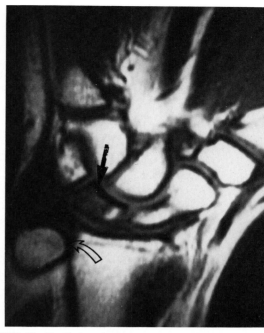

FIGURE 39–19. Early Kienböck's disease. Coronal T$_1$-weighted image reveals a broad area of diminished signal intensity within the medullary bone of the lunate *(solid arrow)*. There is associated ulnar-minus variance *(open arrow)*. Although the signal intensity of the lunate is abnormal, structural collapse has not yet occurred.

diminishes the normal buttressing height of the triangular fibrocartilage (TFC), resulting in functional ulnar-minus variance. It is well accepted that ulnar-minus variance predisposes to the development of avascular necrosis of the lunate, also known as Kienböck's disease.

MR imaging is capable of depicting Kienböck's disease with exquisite sensitivity (Fig. 39–19). The hallmark of osteonecrosis on MR imaging is diminished signal intensity on T$_1$-weighted SE images. Discovery of Kienböck's disease before structural collapse of the lunate has occurred may permit the surgeon to perform an ulnar lengthening procedure to achieve ulnar neutral variance and relief of pain.[23]

We have observed an interesting pattern on sagittal MR scans in which the central portion of the lunate is diminished in signal intensity and sometimes collapsed, but the volar and dorsal thirds of the lunate are relatively spared (Fig. 39–20). This pattern supports the proposed etiology that Kienböck's disease is, in fact, related to axial loading forces transmitted along the capitate-lunate-radius axis.

When the osteonecrotic lunate collapses, the capitate migrates proximally toward the radius. Consequential shortening of the wrist resulting from lunate collapse is analogous to DISI. Both rotatory subluxation of the scaphoid and carpal tunnel syndrome may occur. In fact, median nerve compression is compounded by migration of the volar pole of the lunate into the carpal tunnel (Fig. 39–21). It has been reported that release of the transverse carpal

FIGURE 39–20. Coronal *(A)* and sagittal *(B)* scans demonstrate advanced collapse of an osteonecrotic lunate *(arrow)*. On the sagittal scan *(B)*, the central third of the lunate is diminished in signal intensity *(solid arrow)*, but the volar and dorsal poles of the lunate *(open arrows)* yield normal high signal intensity.

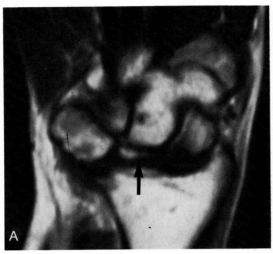

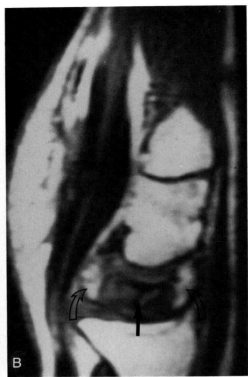

ligament in these patients not only will relieve the median nerve compression but also may alleviate the pain that was clinically attributed to lunate osteonecrosis.

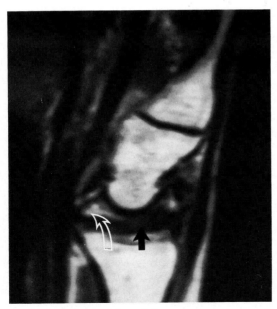

FIGURE 39–21. Compromise of the carpal canal secondary to Kienböck's disease. Sagittal MR image demonstrates advanced collapse of the lunate *(solid arrow)*. In addition, the volar pole of the lunate has subluxated into the carpal canal *(open arrow)*, bowing the flexor tendons forward.

THE ULNAR ASPECT OF THE WRIST

ANATOMY OF THE DISTAL RADIOULNAR JOINT

An appreciation of potential sources of ulnar wrist pain depends on an understanding of the anatomy and biomechanics of the distal radioulnar joint. The distal ulna is normally covered with articular cartilage over most of its circumference and articulates with the concave sigmoid notch on the ulnar aspect of the distal radius (Fig. 39–22A).

The distal radioulnar joint is primarily stabilized by the TFCC.[19, 20] The TFCC includes the TFC, the ulnocarpal ligaments, and the extensor carpi ulnaris tendon subsheath (Fig. 39–23). As its name implies, the TFC is composed of a central portion of fibrocartilage. This central portion may be quite thin and is sometimes fenestrated. Whereas the central zone is thin, the peripheral margins are composed of thick lamellar collagen and are often referred to as the dorsal and volar radioulnar ligaments.[19, 20, 24] The TFC is anchored laterally to the ulnar aspect of the distal radius and medially to the fovea at the base of the ulnar styloid. It is joined by longitudinally oriented ligamentous fibers arising from the ulnar aspect of the ulnar styloid process, which are often referred to as the ulnar collateral ligament. The longitudinally oriented longitudinal fibers frequently thicken just distal to the TFC to form a structure

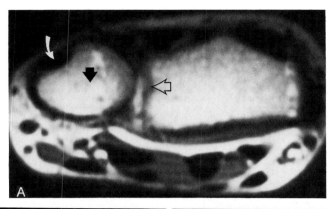

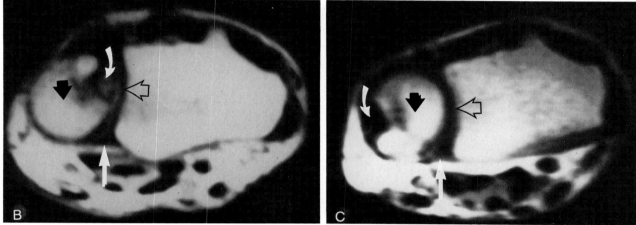

FIGURE 39–22. Axial MR images of normal distal radioulnar joint in neutral position *(A)*, extreme supination *(B)*, and extreme pronation *(C)*. Note that in all three positions the distal ulna *(solid arrow)* remains articulated with the sigmoid notch of the distal radius *(open arrow)*. The extensor carpi ulnaris tendon *(curved white arrow)* remains within its ulnar groove. The volar margin of the TFCC is well seen *(solid white arrow)*. Some authors refer to this structure as the volar radioulnar ligament.

known as the meniscus homologue (Fig. 39–23). Ultimately, these ulnar ligamentous fibers insert upon the lunate, triquetrum, hamate, and base of the fifth metacarpal. Dorsomedially, the TFCC is attached to the subsheath of the extensor carpi ulnaris tendon. Volarly, it is attached to the ulnocarpal ligaments. Just as the volar radioscapholunate ligament is composed of two components, the volar ulnocarpal ligament can be divided into the ulnolunate and ulnotriquetral ligaments.

Coronal and sagittal MR images depict the TFCC in exquisite detail. The TFC is generally triangular on coronal images and discoid on sagittal scans. In young individuals, the TFC is homogeneously devoid of signal (Fig. 39–24). Above age 50, the TFC commonly degenerates and may therefore yield some signal intensity. Both the ulnar and the radial attachments of the TFC are well seen on coronal images. T$_2^*$-weighted GRE images are particularly valuable in assessing the TFCC. On T$_2^*$-weighted GRE images, the meniscus homologue usually yields higher signal intensity compared with the TFC (Fig. 39–25).

Axial images normally depict the distal ulna artic-

ulating with the sigmoid notch of the distal radius (see Fig. 39–22). The extensor carpi ulnaris tendon is also well seen as a structure of homogeneous low signal intensity coursing along its groove in the distal ulna.

BIOMECHANICS OF THE ULNAR ASPECT OF THE WRIST

The TFCC has two primary functions: One is to cushion the compressive longitudinal forces generated between the ulnar carpal bones and the ulna; the second function is to stabilize the distal radioulnar joint. As previously discussed in this chapter, under normal circumstances, approximately 80 per cent of the longitudinal forces that are transmitted through the lunate are borne by the radius, and 20 per cent are borne by the distal ulna. Removal of the TFCC has been shown to decrease the axial loading forces borne by the distal ulna by approximately 12 per cent, and removal of the distal ulna obviously shifts all of the axial loading forces to the radius. In

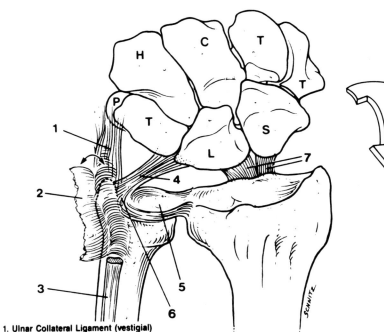

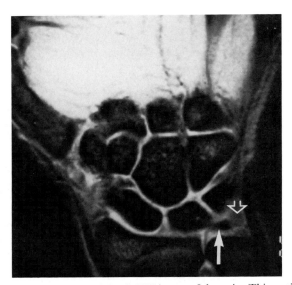

FIGURE 39–23. Diagrammatic depiction of the distal radioulnar joint. The TFCC includes the TFC, the ulnocarpal ligaments, the extensor carpi ulnaris tendon subsheath, and the ulnomeniscal homologue.

1. Ulnar Collateral Ligament (vestigial)
2. Retinacular Sheath
3. Tendon of Extensor Carpi Ulnaris
4. Ulnolunate Ligament
5. Triangular Fibrocartilage (articular disc)
6. Ulnocarpal Meniscus Homologue
7. Volar Radioscaphoid Lunate Ligament

DORSAL VIEW OF FLEXED WRIST JOINT

addition, radial deviation of the wrist decreases, and ulnar deviation increases, the forces borne by the ulna.

The TFCC also stabilizes the distal radioulnar joint by restraining the normal tendency for the ulna to subluxate dorsally when the wrist is pronated or volarly when the wrist is supinated.[25] In young individuals, the integrity of the TFCC maintains remarkable stability of the distal radioulnar joint through the extremes of pronation and supination (see Fig.

39–22). However, as individuals age, normal degeneration of the TFCC leads to greater mobility of the distal radioulnar joint (Fig. 39–26). A tear of the volar margin of the TFCC allows dorsal displacement of the ulna when the forearm is pronated (Fig. 39–

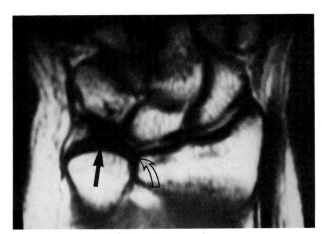

FIGURE 39–24. Coronal T_1-weighted image of the TFC *(solid arrow)* demonstrates its normal homogeneously low signal intensity and its attachment to the distal radius *(open arrow)*.

FIGURE 39–25. T_2^*-weighted GRE image of the wrist. This section reveals only a portion of the volume of the TFC *(solid white arrow)*. On this pulse sequence, the ulnomeniscal homologue *(open white arrow)* yields higher signal intensity than the remainder of the TFC.

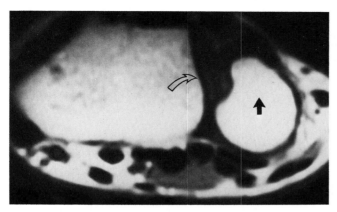

FIGURE 39–26. Axial MR image of the wrist obtained with maximal wrist pronation demonstrates mild volar displacement of the distal ulna *(solid arrow)* relative to the sigmoid notch of the distal radius *(open arrow).*

27A and B). Conversely, a tear of the dorsal margin of the TFCC allows volar displacement of the ulna when the forearm is supinated.

PATHOMECHANICS OF THE ULNAR ASPECT OF THE WRIST

It is well demonstrated that positive ulnar variance leads to premature degeneration of the TFC. On MR images, the TFC may be clearly stretched over the distal end of a positive variance ulna. The radial attachment often appears strained, and the entire articular disk may appear stretched between the radius and ulnar styloid, as well as draped over the end of the distal ulna (Fig. 39–28). In more severe cases, the TFC may be avulsed off its radial attachment (Fig. 39–29) but usually remains attached to the ulnar styloid. In addition, linear increased signal intensity through the TFC is frequently demonstrated, representing a tear of the cartilage. Understanding the concept of positive ulnar variance is important, as shortening the length of the ulna may prevent premature degeneration of the TFCC.[20, 23, 24]

Positive ulnar variance may also result in the ulnolunate impingement syndrome (Figs. 39–28 and 39–29). This syndrome of ulnar wrist pain results from impaction of the elongated distal ulna against the proximal-ulnar aspect of the lunate. As a result, the TFC is often thinned or torn. The articular cartilage of the distal ulna and the proximal lunate prematurely degenerates. Frequently, a degenerative cyst forms within the ulnar aspect of the lunate.

As stated previously, the TFCC performs two main functions. In addition to absorbing the axial loading forces between the ulnar carpus and the ulnar head, the TFC is the main structure stabilizing the distal radioulnar joint. During both pronation and supi-

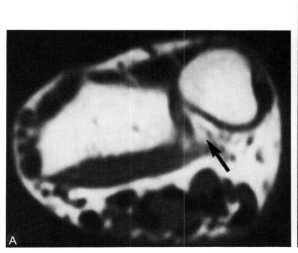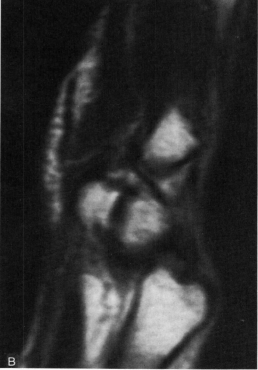

FIGURE 39–27. Both axial *(A)* and sagittal *(B)* images reveal dorsal subluxation of the distal ulna relative to the radius. The volar component of the TFCC, sometimes referred to as the volar radioulnar ligament, is not seen in its normal position *(arrow)* and is presumably chronically torn. See Figure 39–22 for comparison with normal.

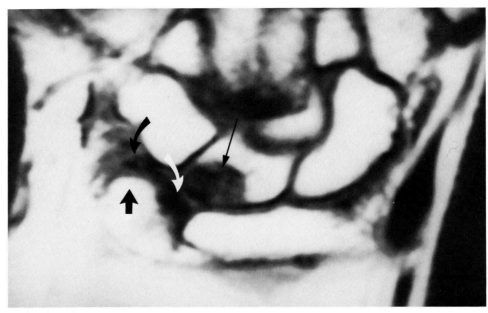

FIGURE 39–28. Pathologic changes associated with ulnar-positive variance. The distal ulna *(black arrow)* extends well beyond the distal radial articular surface. The TFC *(curved white arrow)* is thinned, stretched, and draped over the distal ulna, but not avulsed from its radial attachment. The ulnar aspect of the TFCC *(curved black arrow)* is elevated in signal intensity, thinned, and degenerated. The diminished signal intensity within the proximal ulnar aspect of the lunate *(long, thin arrow)* represents either cystic degeneration or early osteonecrosis. This constellation of findings is referred to as ulnolunate impingement syndrome.

nation, the distal ulna rotates within the sigmoid notch of the distal radius. Upon pronation, the distal ulna may normally slightly subluxate dorsally, and, conversely, upon supination, the distal ulna often slightly volarly subluxates. During supination, therefore, the dorsal aspect of the TFCC is maximally taut, and during pronation, the volar aspect of the TFCC is maximally taut.

Tears of the dorsal or volar aspect of the TFCC may therefore predispose to volar or dorsal subluxation of the distal ulna, respectively. In our experi-

ence, volar subluxation of the distal ulna is less common. Dorsal subluxation of the ulna, with the forearm in either the neutral or the pronated position, is much more common (Figs. 39–26 and 39–27). Thus, axial images must be obtained in the neutral position and with both pronation and supination when ulnar subluxation is suspected.

Although the TFCC is the most important anatomic structure on the ulnar aspect of the wrist, it is important not to overemphasize abnormalities of the TFCC to the point where one fails to recognize other

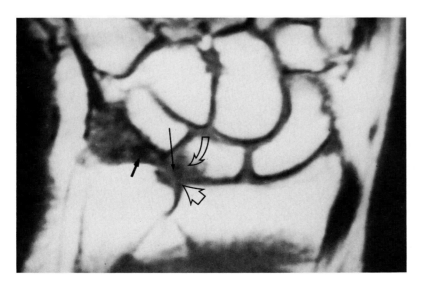

FIGURE 39–29. Advanced ulnolunate impingement syndrome. The TFC *(black arrow)* is severely attenuated, degenerated, and avulsed off its radial attachment *(open arrow)*. The positive-variance ulna directly impinges upon the proximal ulnar aspect of the lunate *(thin black arrow)*. Cystic degeneration or early osteonecrosis is seen involving a portion of the lunate *(open curved arrow)*.

potential causes of ulnar wrist pain. In particular, we must keep in mind that the TFCC commonly degenerates in patients over 50, even in those individuals with neutral ulnar variance. In fact, one should be cautious about incriminating degenerative changes of the TFCC demonstrated on MR examinations or wrist arthrography if there is no associated positive ulnar variance. Even in those cases in which there is marked positive ulnar variance and marked degeneration or tears of the TFCC, one should still address other potential causes of ulnar wrist pain and, simultaneously, carefully scrutinize the radial aspect of the wrist for additional abnormalities.

A relatively common cause of ulnar wrist pain is tendinitis or tenosynovitis of the extensor carpi ulnaris tendon (see Fig. 39–8). This condition may be associated with subluxation of the extensor carpi ulnaris tendon. Axial MR imaging best demonstrates these disorders. Extensor carpi ulnaris subluxation may be elicited on axial MR images when the wrist is supinated and deviated in an ulnar direction.

VOLAR INTERCALATED SEGMENTAL INSTABILITY (VISI)

VISI is an uncommon form of carpal instability associated with pain on the ulnar side of the wrist. In this disorder, the lunate tends to tilt forward in a volar direction. The Z-like foreshortening of the wrist that is seen in sagittal images forms a virtual mirror image to that seen with DISI (Fig. 39–30). VISI is a consequence of lunotriquetral dissociation resulting from tears of the lunotriquetral interosseous ligament. Although we have observed multiple tears of the lunotriquetral interosseous ligament on wrist arthrograms, in our experience, VISI has not been associated with this disorder.

Although it has not been extensively discussed in the surgical literature, it appears that ulnar-minus variance can also lead to dramatic changes in the TFCC (Fig. 39–31). We have observed individuals with marked ulnar-minus variance in whom the lunate and scaphoid are markedly translated in the ulnar direction. As the lunate translates ulnarly, it appears to impinge upon the TFCC and sever the TFCC off its radial attachment. This disorder certainly requires further study.

GANGLIONS OF THE HAND AND WRIST

Ganglions represent 50 to 70 per cent of all soft tissue tumors of the hand and wrist.[26, 27] The mucin-filled cystic structures are usually attached to an underlying joint capsule tendon or tendon sheath. They are more prevalent in women, and more than 70 per cent occur between the second and fourth decades of life.

A visible protrusion under the skin, pain, and a complaint of weakness are the usual presenting symptoms. Clearly defined etiologic factors are unknown.

Most ganglions arise on the dorsal aspect of the wrist. However, there are volar wrist ganglions, flexor tendon sheath ganglions, distal interphalangeal joint and proximal interphalangeal joint ganglions; extensor tendon ganglions, first extensor compartment ganglions, carpal tunnel ganglions, ulnar canal ganglions, and interosseous ganglions.

MR examination usually reveals a smooth, marginated, cystic-appearing lesion of intermediate signal intensity on T_1-weighted images. T_2-weighted images usually reveal a high-signal lesion. Accordingly, these lesions are not usually distinguished from neurofibromas based on their signal characteristics when only SE images are obtained. The diagnosis, however, is usually easily made based on the location of the lesion.

Although the surgical literature indicates that ganglions are usually solitary, it has been our experience that they are often multiple and frequently located in compartments that are relatively remote from each other. MR imaging has been particularly helpful in identifying ganglions located in deep compartments where they are not easily palpable and may be producing only vague pain.

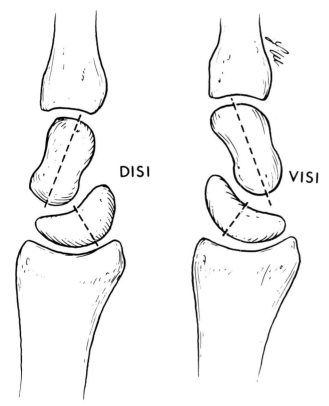

FIGURE 39–30. Diagrammatic depiction of DISI versus VISI (anterior is on reader's right).

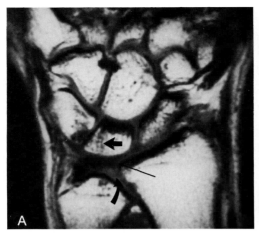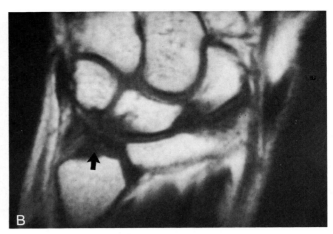

FIGURE 39–31. Consequences of ulnar-minus variance. *A,* There is ulnar translocation of the lunate *(arrow)* associated with an effusion in the distal radioulnar joint *(curved arrow)* and thinning of the radial attachment of the TFCC *(thin black arrow)*. *B,* Ulnar-minus variance in a different patient is associated with severe degeneration of the TFCC *(arrow)*.

On the dorsal aspect of the wrist, they are frequently multiloculated, which probably accounts for the high incidence of recurrence (approximately 50 per cent). We have frequently discovered multiple loculated lesions in patients who continued to have pain after being operated on. Although clinicians usually identify these as "recurrent," it is possible that the surgeon has removed only one of several original lesions. The purported high recurrence rate would seem to support this hypothesis.

CONCLUSION

Accurate diagnosis of wrist disorders is of paramount value in planning treatment, particularly now that wrist arthroscopy is gaining in popularity among orthopedists. Prior to the advent of MR imaging, radiologic evaluation of the wrist was primarily limited to osseous structures and the interosseous ligaments. With MR imaging, it is now possible to visualize the finest detail of soft tissue anatomy of this complex joint, allowing diagnosis of previously undetected pathology. Future applications, such as cine MR imaging, may allow better evaluation of abnormal carpal motion. New techniques, such as 3DFT image construction, also hold great promise.

MR imaging now allows for earlier and more accurate detection of bone and soft tissue abnormalities of the wrist, which, it is hoped, will lead to more appropriate and effective treatment. At our institution, MR imaging has become the imaging procedure of choice in diagnosing clinical wrist dilemmas.

ACKNOWLEDGMENTS: Thanks to the technologists at the Mercy Magnetic Resonance Imaging Center for their dedicated efforts and intelligent contributions. Thanks also to the forbearance of our colleagues and families during the preparation of this chapter.

REFERENCES

1. Eversmann WW Jr: Entrapment and compression neuropathies. *In* Green DP (ed): Operative Hand Surgery. 2nd ed. New York, Churchill Livingstone, 1988, pp 1423–1441.
2. Weiss KL, Beltran J, Shamam OM, et al: High-field MR surface-coil imaging of the hand and wrist. Part I. Normal anatomy. Radiology 160:143–146, 1986.
3. Baker LL, Hajek PC, Bjorkengren A, et al: High-resolution magnetic resonance imaging of the wrist: Normal anatomy. Skeletal Radiol 16:128–132, 1987.
4. Bleecker ML: Medical surveillance for carpal tunnel syndrome in workers. J Hand Surg [Am] 12A:845–848, 1987.
5. Weiss KL, Beltran J, Lubbers LM: High-field MR surface-coil imaging of the hand and wrist. Part II. Pathologic correlation and clinical relevance. Radiology 160:147–152, 1986.
6. Richman JA, Gelberman RH, Rydevik BL, et al: Carpal tunnel volume determination by magnetic resonance imaging three-dimensional reconstruction. J Hand Surg [Am] 12A:712–717, 1987.
7. Zucker-Pinchoff B, Hermann G, Srinivasan R: Computed tomography of the carpal tunnel: A radioanatomical study. J Comput Assist Tomogr 5:525–528, 1981.
8. Bleecker ML, Bohlman M, Moreland R, Tipton A: Carpal tunnel syndrome: Role of carpal canal size. Neurology 35:1599–1604, 1985.
9. Jessurun W, Hillen B, Huffstadt AJC: Carpal tunnel release: Postoperative care. Handchir Mikrochir Plast Chir 20:30–40, 1988.
10. Wood MB, Dobyns JH: Sports-related extraarticular wrist syndromes. Clin Orthop 202:93–102, 1986.
11. Mayfield JK: Patterns of injury to carpal ligaments: A spectrum. Clin Orthop 187:36–42, 1984.
12. Linscheid RL, Dobyns JH, Beabout JW, Bryan RS: Traumatic instability of the wrist. J Bone Joint Surg 8:1612–1632, 1972.
13. Green DP: Carpal dislocations and instabilities. *In* Green DP (ed): Operative Hand Surgery. 2nd ed. New York, Churchill Livingstone, 1988, pp 875–938.
14. Kauer JMG, de Lange A: The carpal joint. *In* Taleisnik J (ed):

Management of Wrist Problems. Hand Clin III:23–29, 1987.

15. Watson HK, Black DM: Instabilities of the wrist. *In* Taleisnik J (ed): Management of Wrist Problems. Hand Clin III:103–111, 1987.

16. Taleisnik J: The Wrist. New York, Churchill Livingstone, 1985, pp 1–442.

17. Mayfield JK: Pathogenesis of wrist ligament instability. *In* Lichtman DM (ed): The Wrist and Its Disorders. Philadelphia, WB Saunders, 1988, pp 53–73.

18. Lichtman DM, Martin RA: Introduction to the carpal instabilities. *In* Lichtman DM (ed): The Wrist and Its Disorders. Philadelphia, WB Saunders, 1988, pp 244–250.

19. Palmer AK: The distal radioulnar joint. *In* Lichtman DM (ed): The Wrist and Its Disorders. Philadelphia, WB Saunders, 1988, pp 220–231.

20. Taleisnik J: Pain on the ulnar side of the wrist. *In* Taleisnik J (ed): Management of Wrist Problems. Hand Clin III:51–69, 1987.

21. Wat HK, Ballet FL: The SLAC wrist: Scapholunate advanced collapse pattern of degenerative arthritis. J Hand Surg [Am] 9A(3):358–365, 1984.

22. Alexander AH, Lichtman DM: Kienböck's disease. *In* Lichtman DM (ed): The Wrist and Its Disorders. Philadelphia, WB Saunders, 1988, pp 329–343.

23. Linscheid RL: Ulnar lengthening and shortening. *In* Taleisnik J (ed): Management of Wrist Problems. Hand Clin III:69–79, 1987.

24. Bowers WH: The distal radioulnar joint. *In* Green DP (ed): Operative Hand Surgery. 2nd ed. New York, Churchill Livingstone, 1988, pp 939–989.

25. Hagert C-G: The distal radioulnar joint. *In* Taleisnik J (ed): Management of Wrist Problems. Hand Clin III:41–50, 1987.

26. Angelides AC: Ganglions of the hand and wrist. *In* Green DP (ed): Operative Hand Surgery. 2nd ed. New York, Churchill Livingstone, 1988, pp 2281–2299.

27. Bogumill GP: Tumors of the wrist. *In* Lichtman DM (ed): The Wrist and Its Disorders. Philadelphia, WB Saunders, 1988, pp 373–375.

40

MR IMAGING OF THE FOOT AND ANKLE

DAVID J. SARTORIS, MICHAEL J. MITCHELL, and DONALD RESNICK

TECHNIQUE
NORMAL ANATOMY
    BONES AND LIGAMENTS
    MUSCLES AND TENDONS
    VESSELS AND NERVES
APPLICATIONS

TENDON ABNORMALITIES
CARTILAGE DISORDERS
NEOPLASMS
INFECTION
MISCELLANEOUS POSTTRAUMATIC
    ABNORMALITIES
CONCLUSION

Cross-sectional imaging of the foot and ankle had its inception with the development of high-resolution CT equipment. During recent years, CT has been successfully applied to a wide variety of podiatric disorders, including calcaneal fractures, subtalar coalition, tarsometatarsal fracture-dislocations, and primary soft tissue pathology. The advent of high-resolution proton MR imaging has provided an alternative means for noninvasive evaluation of foot and ankle disease. In this pictorial review, representative cases illustrating the diagnostic utility of MR imaging are discussed, with comparative reference to CT in selected instances. The goal of this chapter is to provide the practicing radiologist with insight into the relative merits of the two techniques, as a guide to the appropriate selection of MR imaging in specific clinical circumstances.

TECHNIQUE

MR imaging has become an extremely important noninvasive diagnostic tool for the evaluation of a variety of disorders affecting the foot and ankle. This section is intended to provide practicing radiologists with the specific technical guidelines for optimal imaging of podiatric disease using this method. Although details may vary according to scanner differences and imaging time considerations, the information provided herein should, at the minimum, serve as a baseline from which to develop acceptable site-specific protocols. The majority of the images depicted in this chapter were acquired on a 1.5-T superconducting system (Signa, General Electric, Milwaukee, WI).

The patient is positioned prone with the feet together and parallel to each other. Their dorsal aspects are thus in contact with and stabilized by the table top, resulting in a lesser tendency for undesired movement by the patient during the examination than occurs with supine scanning. In the latter position, unconscious muscular twitches can result in slight excursion of the toes with secondary image degradation. The feet are secured with adhesive tape, and appropriate steps are taken to maximize the overall comfort of the patient during the study (pillow, foam pad, blanket, and so forth). Careful attention to symmetric positioning of the feet will ensure that comparable anatomic levels are depicted on individual images, greatly facilitating interpretation. Claustrophobic and pediatric patients may require sedation, because motion must be avoided for up to 20 minutes at a time and, if present, results in degradation of an entire series of images rather than only one, as with CT.

The authors have found, in general, that satisfactory image quality is afforded by use of the same coil used routinely for MR imaging studies of the head. This approach eliminates the problem of signal intensity fall-off inherent in the application of surface coils and produces images of uniform homogeneity. A 20-cm field-of-view (FOV) with a 256×256 data acquisition matrix results in a pixel size of 0.78×0.78 mm, which is equivalent to the spatial resolution of the images acquired. A single signal average with a slice thickness of 5 mm and an interslice gap of 2.5 mm creates practical imaging times and adequate coverage of the tissue volume under evaluation. Contiguous imaging may be required in certain situations involving subtle pathology but is not routinely indicated, as it necessitates an objectionably longer total examination time.

Initially, a T_1-weighted localization sequence should be performed in the plantar plane, using the shortest available imaging time. This generally involves a pulse repetition time (TR) on the order of 600 msec and a time to echo (TE) of approximately 25 msec (partial saturation spin-echo [SE] technique). This sequence can be completed in 5 minutes, and the resulting images (which may in themselves be beneficial in planning operative approaches) are then used to delineate the specific region to be evaluated subsequently in the coronal plane of the body (transverse plane of the foot). Alternatively, a gradient-echo (GRE) sequence, also accomplished in a relatively short time, can be utilized for localization images. This imaging plane is generally of greatest value for most foot and ankle disorders, owing to anatomic consideration and facilitation of comparison between the two sides.

The pulse sequences selected for imaging in the transverse plane will depend upon the specific type of pathology suspected on the basis of prior clinical assessment or diagnostic imaging studies or both. For the detection of bone marrow disease (ischemic necrosis, osteomyelitis, malignancy), a T_1-weighted imaging sequence using a TR and TE comparable to those of the localization scans usually suffices and translates to an extremely short total imaging time of approximately 10 minutes. All such processes generally produce decreased signal intensity in marrow-bearing areas regardless of image weighting, although recent preliminary evidence suggests that T_2-weighted sequences may have merit in identifying acute areas of infarction or infection by virtue of their bright signal. Conversely, in the evaluation of soft tissue disorders affecting the foot and ankle (neurogenic and other neoplasms, abscesses, cellulitis, tendinitis, traumatic injury) by MR imaging, several different pulse sequences are usually required for optimal delineation and characterization of pathology. This is true because (1) the specific signal behavior of the abnormal tissue cannot be predicted before imaging and (2) the type or types of normal tissue (fat, muscle, tendon, fascia) with which it interfaces are similarly unknown in advance. Thus, because it is usually unclear regarding which specific pulse sequence will produce optimal contrast discrimination between normal and abnormal tissue, multiple TR/TE combinations must be used. This combination is most conveniently achieved by initially performing a T_1-weighted sequence identical with that recommended for bone marrow disease, followed by a multiple SE sequence, which results in two sets of images, weighted, respectively, toward proton density and T_2. The latter imaging strategy generally involves a TR on the order of 2000 msec, a first-echo TE of about 25 msec for proton density–weighted images, and a second-echo TE of approximately 70 msec for T_2-weighted images. The typical multiple SE sequence can be completed in about 17 minutes. Thus, the total examination time for adequate evaluation of a soft tissue disorder in the foot or ankle is approximately 27 minutes $(5 + 5 + 17)$, not including positioning of the patient and scan set-up time. As a time-saving alternative or supplement to T_2-weighted images, a GRE sequence using short TR and TE with a low flip angle can be employed to yield a T_2 effect.

The importance of multiple pulse sequences for optimal imaging of the soft tissues in the foot and ankle cannot be overemphasized. Several cases are shown in this chapter, including a TR-TE combination that renders significant pathology occult.

Images in the sagittal plane of the foot are readily obtained without moving the patient, but they contribute significant additional information only in rare instances and hence are seldom necessary. However, this imaging plane may be optimal for disease processes oriented along the axis of one or several rays. In specific cases, obliquely oriented images can be helpful, particularly for visualizing the course of a certain tendon or muscle group, such as the peroneal tendons. Imaging in nonroutine planes always increases the total examination time and thus is usually performed using the single pulse sequence that is deemed likely to provide the greatest information based upon preliminary screening of the transverse images.

Upon completion of an MR imaging examination of the foot or ankle, all images acquired should be photographed on radiographic film for permanent records of the patient. It is imperative, however, that the radiologist view the entire study on the scanner console, which allows for image optimization via window (contrast) and level (brightness) manipulation. The technologist cannot always be relied upon to select the most diagnostic image display settings for photography. As a final technical consideration, because the method exhibits high sensitivity but only moderate specificity, it is mandatory that all MR imaging examinations of the foot and ankle be interpreted in conjunction with any available prior diagnostic imaging studies as well as with complete knowledge of the clinical history and physical examination findings.

Two technical problems may be encountered. Imaging in oblique orientations may not be available at this time with certain systems. This capability is particularly important for imaging joints where tendons and ligaments may not align with the x-, y-, or z-axes. In the ankle, we have encountered similar difficulties; misinterpretation can thus occur in evaluating ligament integrity after acute trauma. Even with the use only of conventional planes, however, acute ligamentous ruptures can be clearly detected in certain cases.[1]

Dedicated surface coils for joint studies may yield images superior to those obtained with planar coils. Both patients and healthy volunteers have been studied with a 3- or 5-inch circular transmit-receive surface coil. These particular coils provide very superficial signal detection, and although structures close to the coil are well depicted, deeper lesions cannot be accurately studied unless the coil is repositioned (encountered with marked soft tissue swelling or a cast). A rectangular, receive-only surface coil designed for spinal imaging provides a more uniform signal throughout the joint.[1]

NORMAL ANATOMY

Multiplanar MR imaging is advantageous when evaluating the complex three-dimensional (3D) anatomy of the ankle joint. Direct coronal and sagittal imaging is especially helpful in demonstrating the tibiotalar joint and the three facets of the subtalar joint. The soft tissue structures of the foot are also well demonstrated on MR imaging. All of the tendons and many of the ligaments can be identified.[2]

Beltran and associates have discussed the normal MR anatomy of the foot and ankle. The tendons and many of the ligaments are well demonstrated, as are the neurovascular bundles.[1]

BONES AND LIGAMENTS

The term "ankle joint," strictly speaking, refers to the talocrural joint, which is formed by the talus and the lower ends of the tibia and fibula. The articular surfaces are covered with hyaline cartilage, seen as the medium-intensity layer external to the low-intensity cortical bone. On the medial aspect of the talus is a projection called the sustentaculum tali.

The anterior and posterior tibiofibular ligaments are flat, broad bands on the anterior and posterior surfaces of the tibiofibular syndesmosis that course obliquely downward. The anterior and posterior talofibular ligaments pass from the anterior and posterior surfaces of the fibula to the talus. The calcaneo-fibular ligament runs posteriorly from the fibular malleolus to the lateral surface of the calcaneus. On the medial surface lies the triangle-shaped deltoid ligament, which extends from the medial malleolus to the navicular, talus, and calcaneus, as indicated by the names of its divisions.

There are posterior and anterior articulations between the talus and underlying calcaneus. The posterior articulation is the subtalar joint proper, and the more anterior articulation is a part of the talocalcaneonavicular joint. The bones of the subtalar joint are connected by the interosseous talocalcaneal ligament. On the medial aspect, there is a deep depression between the talus and calcaneus, called the tarsal sinus. The talocalcaneonavicular joint consists of the anterior head of the talus, the posterior surface of the navicular, and the middle and anterior facets of the calcaneus. On the plantar surface, several ligaments are present, including the plantar calcaneonavicular ("spring") ligament, which passes from the sustentaculum tali of the calcaneus to the plantar surface of the navicular; the calcaneocuboid (short plantar) ligament, which passes from the calcaneus to the cuboid; and the long plantar ligament, which passes from the calcaneus to the bases of the metatarsals.

MUSCLES AND TENDONS

The muscles on the lateral surface of the ankle include the peroneus longus and brevis. Both muscles originate from the lateral surface of the fibula. The tendons of both muscles pass beneath the superior and inferior peroneal retinacula, with the brevis tendon lying superior and anterior to the longus tendon. The peroneus longus and brevis tendons insert on the medial and lateral aspects of the foot, respectively.

Anteriorly lie four muscles: the tibialis anterior, extensor hallucis longus, extensor digitorum longus, and peroneus tertius. All four muscles originate from the anterior surfaces of the tibia, fibula, and/or interosseous membrane. The tendons of all these muscles pass deep to the superior and inferior portions of the extensor retinaculum on the anterior surface of the ankle, with the tibialis anterior most medial, the extensor hallucis longus tendon just lateral to the tibialis anterior, and the conjoined extensor digitorum longus and peroneus tertius tendons lying most lateral.

Three muscles are present on the medial surface of the ankle: the tibialis posterior, flexor digitorum longus, and flexor hallucis longus. All three muscles arise from the posterior aspect of the tibia, fibula, and/or interosseous membrane. The tendons of all three muscles pass beneath the flexor retinaculum prior to insertion on the plantar surface of the foot. Beneath the flexor retinaculum, the posterior tibial tendon lies in the most anteromedial position, the flexor hallucis longus lies in the most posteroinferior position, and the flexor digitorum lies between them.

Superficial to the tibialis posterior, flexor digitorum longus, and flexor hallucis muscles in the calf lie the soleus and gastrocnemius muscles. The tendons from both muscles unite to form the Achilles tendon, which inserts on the back of the calcaneus.

On the plantar surface, the most superficial layer is the plantar aponeurosis, which attaches to the undersurface of the calcaneus and extends forward to the toes. Deep to the plantar fascia is the first layer of muscles, which includes, running medial to lateral, the abductor hallucis, the flexor digitorum brevis, and the abductor digiti minimi. All three muscles originate on the calcaneus and the adjacent fibrous tissues and proceed distally to insert on the toes. Deep to the first layer of muscles lie the tendons of the flexor digitorum longus and flexor hallucis longus, which, after passing through the flexor retinaculum, traverse the foot, with the digitorum longus superficial to the hallucis longus, and insert on the toes. Also in this layer lies the quadratus plantae muscle, which arises by two heads from the medial and lateral sides of the plantar surface of the calcaneus and inserts on the tendon of the flexor digitorum longus.

The muscles of the deeper layers arise distal to the ankle.

VESSELS AND NERVES

The terminal branch of the peroneal artery is present along the lateral aspect of the ankle, where it divides into multiple small calcaneal branches. The lesser saphenous vein arises on the lateral surface of the foot and passes behind the lateral malleolus and then up the calf. The sural nerve, a branch of the tibial nerve, accompanies the lesser saphenous vein in its course along the lateral aspect of the ankle.

The deep peroneal nerve and the anterior tibial artery and its accompanying veins course together along most of the lower leg and pass beneath the extensor retinaculum on the anterior surface of the ankle, deep to the extensor hallucis longus tendon. At the level of the ankle, the anterior artery becomes the dorsalis pedis.

The tibial nerve and posterior tibial artery and its accompanying veins travel together down the lower leg on the surface of the tibialis posterior muscle (the posterior tibial neurovascular bundle). At the ankle they pass beneath the flexor retinaculum, between the flexor hallucis and the flexor digitorum longus. The tibial nerve divides into the lateral and medial plantar nerves at the level of the flexor retinaculum; these course laterally and medially, as their names indicate, accompanied by the similarly named terminal branches of the posterior tibial artery.

Also running along the medial surface of the ankle is the great saphenous vein, which originates on the medial aspect of the foot and passes upward in front of the medial malleolus and runs up the medial side of the leg.

APPLICATIONS

TENDON ABNORMALITIES

Although MR imaging of tendons using surface coils is a relatively recent innovation, early experience indicates that the improved soft tissue contrast and resolution represent significant advantages over CT and ultrasound in evaluating traumatic, inflammatory (Fig. 40–1), and infectious tendon abnormalities.[3]

High-resolution MR imaging of the tendons of the feet and ankles of six healthy volunteers and six cadavers was performed using receive-only surface coils and reduced field-of-view (FOV) imaging in one investigation. Normal anatomy was identified and compared with gross anatomic sections of the six cadavers. Experimentally produced tears of the Achilles tendon in domestic swine were identified on MR images. The hands and feet of 11 patients were examined, and a variety of pathologic lesions were identified, including acute posttraumatic rupture, acute tenosynovitis, chronic tendinitis, and postsurgical complications. MR imaging provides inherently greater soft tissue contrast than any other currently available imaging modality. With the use of surface coils and reduced FOV imaging to enhance spatial resolution, MR imaging has become a valuable tool for imaging tendons. Advantages over other available methods include excellent depiction of anatomic detail, superior contrast resolution, and the potential for multiplanar imaging.[3]

Experimentally produced ruptures are seen as gaps of high signal intensity without surrounding edema or hemorrhage; however, it should be noted that the applicability of postmortem animal studies to in vivo human pathologic conditions has limitations. Posttraumatic tendon ruptures and postsurgical reruptures are seen on MR images as larger gaps within the substance of the tendon. Posttraumatic ruptures and postsurgical reruptures are surrounded by soft tissue edema and hemorrhage. In one reported case of calcaneal tendon rupture, the distal end of the tendon was shown to be irregular, and the adjacent small plantaris tendon was correctly shown to be intact.[3]

Nontraumatic causes of tendon disorders include several diseases that produce inflammatory changes in the tissues, such as infection, rheumatoid arthritis, syphilis, systemic lupus erythematosus, diabetes mellitus, and gout. Both acute and chronic inflammatory changes are clearly demonstrated on MR images. Localized nodular thickening of the calcaneal tendon and a thin stripe of high signal intensity within the substance of the tendon were seen on both transaxial and sagittal images of a runner with chronic pain in

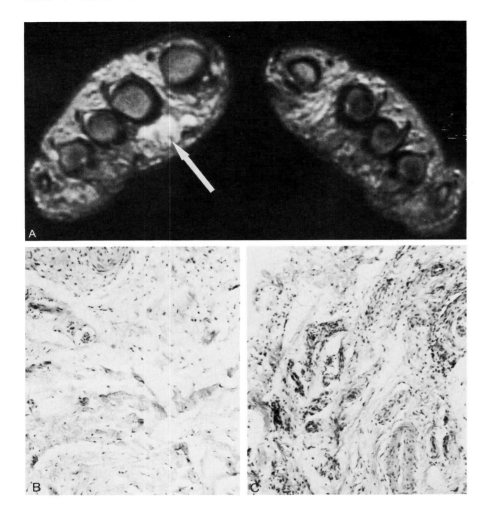

FIGURE 40–1. Plantar tenosynovitis. *A,* Coronal T$_2$-weighted image discloses a lobulated fluid collection of high signal intensity plantar to the second metatarsal and flexor digitorum longus *(arrow)*, consistent with tenosynovitis. *B* and *C,* Nonspecific inflammation was confirmed by biopsy, which excluded neoplasm.

one study. These findings were thought to indicate chronic tendinitis and possibly a partial tear of the calcaneal tendon, although surgical proof was not obtained. Acute inflammatory tenosynovitis is seen as fluid distending the tendon sheath. The fluid is identified as collections of low signal intensity around a well-demarcated tendon on short TR–short TE sequences. The fluid collections are more easily seen on long TR–long TE sequences, in which the fluid has a higher signal intensity than the surrounding fat. The distended tendon sheaths are seen as lines of low signal intensity separating the inflammatory fluid from the surrounding fat. Distinction between serous and purulent tenosynovitis has not been possible with current techniques.[3]

Until recently, noninvasive tendon imaging has been limited to the depiction of the silhouette of the tendon using low-kilovoltage techniques and xeroradiography; however, internal defects and fluid collections can be difficult to evaluate with these methods. Ultrasound has been used to demonstrate normal and pathologic anatomy of the tendons of the hand, calcaneal tendon, and rotator cuff. Ultrasound evaluation of the tendons has the advantages of widespread availability and low cost. The disadvantages include limited anatomic detail, the ability to image only superficially located tendons, and the inability to image bone. The depiction of an entire anatomic area, including osseous structures, is a significant advantage of MR imaging over ultrasound. In some patients referred for evaluation of possible tendon lesions, MR imaging can exclude a tendon abnormality and demonstrate other unsuspected pathology, including stress fractures.[3]

In addition to the potential for displaying tendons surrounded by inflammation, hemorrhage, and scar tissue, MR imaging has a significant advantage in its ability to image in the sagittal and coronal planes. With software improvements, it is expected to be feasible to image tendons along their long axes without having to align them with the orthogonal planes in the magnet, a technique that is time consuming and subject to errors.[3]

The Achilles tendon remains low in signal intensity on T$_1$-, T$_2$-, and T$_2^*$-weighted images, while the pre-Achilles fat manifests a gray signal on GRE images (Fig. 40–2). Transaxial and sagittal assessment of Achilles tendon injuries with effective T$_2$ weighting is possible in less than 5 minutes of imaging time using this approach.[4]

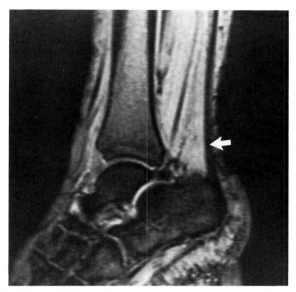

FIGURE 40–2. Normal Achilles tendon. Sagittal GRE image depicts normal tendinous width *(arrowhead)*.

MR imaging provides several advantages in the imaging of acute injury. The definition of the soft tissue planes, muscular bundles, and tendons is much better than with any other imaging modality. Sagittal imaging allows direct visualization of the ends of an injured tendon. The weak signal of the tendon contrasts sharply with the greater intensity of the tissue occupying the gap, probably edema and hemorrhage. It is likely that MR imaging can provide definition of soft tissue injuries that has never been achieved before by other imaging modalities.[5]

MR images show complete tears as complete disruption of the tendons, usually in the midst of edema and hemorrhage. The degree of tendon injury or healing sometimes is difficult to determine from sagittal images because it may be seen only partially. The transaxial plane is helpful in determining the degree of a tear or healing because it is at right angles to the long axis of the tendon.[6]

The diagnosis of acute tendon ruptures of the extensor mechanism of the Achilles tendon at the ankle can usually be made by clinical means. Massive soft tissue swelling accompanying these injuries often obscures the findings, however. MR imaging can rapidly demonstrate these tendon ruptures. Numerous examples of the use of MR imaging for Achilles tendon rupture have been presented.[7] Tears of the calcaneofibular and talocalcaneal interosseous ligaments and the flexor hallucis longus tendon have also been demonstrated.

MR imaging has been shown to be effective in demonstrating muscles and tendons around the ankle. Imaging with T_1 weighting (TR = 0.6 second, TE = 35 msec) has been shown to be effective in demonstrating not only the normal anatomy but also the site of rupture and associated soft tissue swelling. The procedure is easy to perform and may be accom-

plished rapidly with no discomfort to the patient. Three patients with Achilles tendon rupture have been examined by MR imaging, with the results confirmed surgically. Although experience is limited at the present time, this procedure is valuable and may become the most useful diagnostic study for evaluating patients with these types of tendon ruptures as well as similar injuries in other parts of the body.[7]

It appears that MR imaging will be able to facilitate the determination of the degree of tendinous or fibrous union occurring with healing, which could help in the pacing of rehabilitation. The rate of rerupture in conservatively treated cases is approximately 10 per cent and in the surgically treated group, 4 per cent. These figures could very well be changed by a more specific schedule for mobilization. The periods of immobilization have been dictated in the past by trial and error, but MR imaging could enable this decision to be made precisely and on an individual basis.[6]

Achilles tendinitis can be a difficult therapeutic and diagnostic problem, but MR imaging readily demonstrates fluid around the tendon in the acute situation (Fig. 40–3). With chronic tendinitis, there may be appreciable thickening of the tendon, with or without abnormal intratendinous signal (Fig. 40–4). MR imaging may help indicate supportive evidence in difficult cases of Achilles tendinitis.[6]

Thirty MR examinations of the Achilles tendon were performed in one study: 20 from patients without suspected tendon abnormalities and 10 from patients with suspected tendon abnormalities. The appearance of the normal Achilles tendon is hypoin-

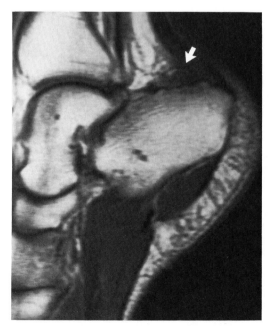

FIGURE 40–3. Acute Achilles tendinitis. Parasagittal T_1-weighted image reveals thickening of the Achilles tendon near its calcaneal insertion and diminished signal within the pre-Achilles fat pad *(arrow)*, consistent with edema.

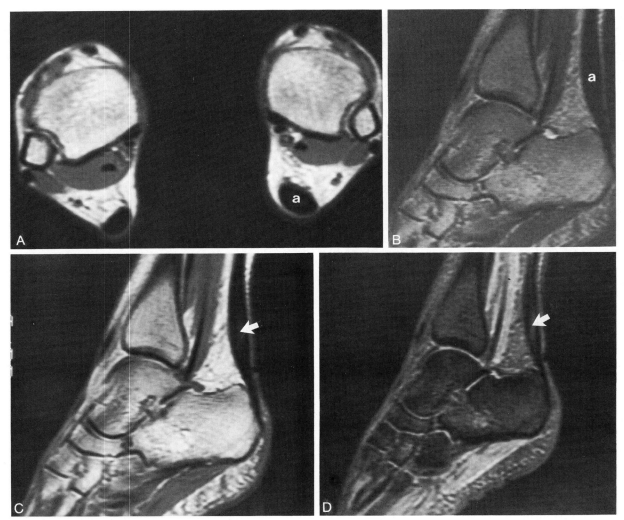

FIGURE 40–4. Chronic Achilles tendinitis. *A,* Axial T_1-weighted image obtained just above the ankle joint demonstrates thickening of the tendon with a rounded configuration (a). The opposite extremity reveals the normal flattened appearance of the tendon. *B–D,* Parasagittal T_2-weighted, proton density–weighted, and GRE images, respectively, through the ankle region confirm diffuse tendinous thickening (a). The abnormal central linear pattern of increased signal intensity within the tendon *(arrows)* is compatible with inflammation.

tense and flattened. Partial tears appear as high-signal intratendinous collections, complete acute ruptures appear as tendinous discontinuity, and uncomplicated surgical repairs appear as areas of tendinous continuity with inhomogeneous signal in the operative site. Chronic tendinitis appears as a diffuse thickening of the tendon. MR imaging of the Achilles tendon at 1.5 T enables the determination of the degree of tendinous continuity, which may help with diagnosis, treatment, and the planning of rehabilitation.[6]

The results of this study demonstrated that at 1.5 T the Achilles tendon can be routinely identified with confidence. Except for minor variations, the normal tendon has a typical hypointense, flattened appearance. The anatomic hallmark of the abnormal Achilles tendon is thickening of the tendon complex. In the regions of injury, there are foci of intermediate

T_1 and prolonged T_2 relaxation times that are consistent with fluid but not hemorrhage. In one patient who underwent an 8-week follow-up MR examination, the foci demonstrated a slight shortening of the T_2 relaxation time. The natural history of these foci is uncertain, and sequential studies will be necessary to evaluate their evolution.[6]

In summary, the Achilles tendon is easily imaged with MR at 1.5 T. The normal tendon is hypointense and flattened. Chronic tendinitis shows tendinous thickening, partial tears have intratendinous collections, and complete tears show total tendinous discontinuity.[6]

In acute peroneal tendinitis, oblique intermediate (TR 2000/TE 25) and T_2-weighted (TR 2000/TE 70) SE images of the lateral aspect of the ankle optimally demonstrate the peroneus longus and brevis tendons as they course distally around the lateral malleolus.

An abnormal linear pattern of increased signal intensity is noted within their sheaths, indicative of fluid accumulation and compatible with inflammation.

In the normal situation, the spatial resolution capabilities of MR imaging as well as CT are insufficient to delineate tendons and the synovial sheaths that surround them as separate structures. MR imaging affords extreme sensitivity in the detection of small fluid collections in the foot and ankle, including intraarticular effusions and others related to inflammatory disease. T_2-weighted imaging sequences are of particular importance in this regard. A comparable CT image would reveal only apparent thickening of the affected tendons, owing to isodensity between the latter and fluid within their sheaths.

CARTILAGE DISORDERS

The joints have been of particular interest to MR imaging researchers because their various components cannot otherwise be thoroughly evaluated by noninvasive means. Preliminary results in the foot and ankle have been encouraging. Effusions are clearly depicted, even when small and in joints difficult to evaluate clinically. Cartilage integrity can be clearly assessed because of the relatively high signal intensity of the hyaline cartilage compared with that of fibrocartilage or subchondral cortical bone. Inflammatory conditions such as juvenile rheumatoid arthritis have been demonstrated in the ankle. On the basis of preliminary experience, MR imaging of the ankle in acute and chronic trauma has proved to be clinically valuable. The method allows direct visualization of soft tissue lesions in all patients, with excellent demonstration of ligamentous and articular cartilage damage.[1]

In one investigation, high-field surface-coil MR images were obtained of 12 ankles: 2 from healthy volunteers, 7 from patients, and 3 from fresh cadavers. The cadaver ankles were sectioned in the coronal, sagittal, and transaxial planes for direct comparison with the MR images. Plain film confirmation of pathologic conditions was obtained in all patients, and five underwent arthroscopy or surgery, or both. MR imaging provided excellent delineation of ligamentous and cartilaginous structures in all cases.[1]

In many cases, MR imaging can yield clinically relevant information for the referring physician. Cartilage is well delineated in all ankles, and severe chondromalacia has been clearly demonstrated in patients with hemophilic arthropathy. Conversely, intact cartilage thickness can be delineated in individuals with unsuspected osteochondral fractures. In such patients, although loose bodies may be seen at arthroscopy, the cartilage thickness may not be amenable to assessment.[1]

Osteochondral lesions of the dome of the talus are seen as regions of decreased signal intensity on T_1-weighted images and varying appearance on T_2-weighted images (Fig. 40–5). In their series, Yulish and colleagues[8] found that MR imaging accurately depicted the condition of the overlying cartilage.

In addition to the secondary degenerative changes seen in hemophilic arthropathy, MR imaging reveals hypertrophy of the synovium, with low-intensity signal, presumably caused by the paramagnetic effect of the hemosiderin deposits. Pigmented villonodular synovitis may have a similar appearance on MR images.[5]

MR imaging, because of its inherent soft tissue contrast, is well suited to the differentiation between the various components of a joint and its surrounding structures (e.g., cortical and cancellous bone, hyaline articular cartilage and fibrocartilage, fluid, abnormal synovium, ligaments, and muscle), and it has been used in the evaluation of hemophilic arthropathy of the ankle. Advantages include the fact that it does not use ionizing radiation and allows multiplanar imaging.[8]

Despite absence of surgical correlation with MR imaging results in one study, findings implied that the method can be used to image hemophilic arthropathy, including abnormal articular cartilage, synovial hypertrophy, and bone lesions.[8]

Abnormal articular cartilage is shown as focal or diffuse thinning or cartilage loss. Synovial hypertrophy is seen as areas of low to intermediate signal intensity on T_1- and T_2-weighted images, with areas of increased signal intensity in some joints on T_2-weighted images. The low-intensity areas on T_1- and T_2-weighted images are consistent with hemosiderin-laden synovium, and those areas that increase in intensity on T_2-weighted images are presumed to be fluid collections or inflammation. It is not possible to distinguish between the viscous joint field normally found in hemophilic arthropathy and areas of fresh blood, although no patients with clinically proved acute hemarthroses were studied in this investigation. End-stage joints (disorganized, contracted, and fibrotic with exposure of subchondral bone) had less synovium and fluid visible.[3]

Bone lesions (erosions and subchondral cysts) are seen on T_1-weighted images as areas of low signal intensity containing occasional foci of intermediate signal intensity that increase in intensity with T_2-weighted pulse sequences. These foci are thought to represent fluid.[8]

Because MR imaging appears to allow the evaluation of synovial hypertrophy and articular cartilage, it may prove useful in selecting patients for synovectomy and in monitoring response to factor therapy. Although factor replacement aborts acute hemarthrosis and relieves its symptoms, the treatment may not prevent the arthropathy of hemophilia that occurs secondary to repeated hemarthroses. MR imaging should not replace clinical evaluation of patients with hemophilic arthropathy, but it seems reasonable to suggest that intermittent evaluation of patients with severe hemophilia by MR imaging may identify candidates for synovectomy or patients who

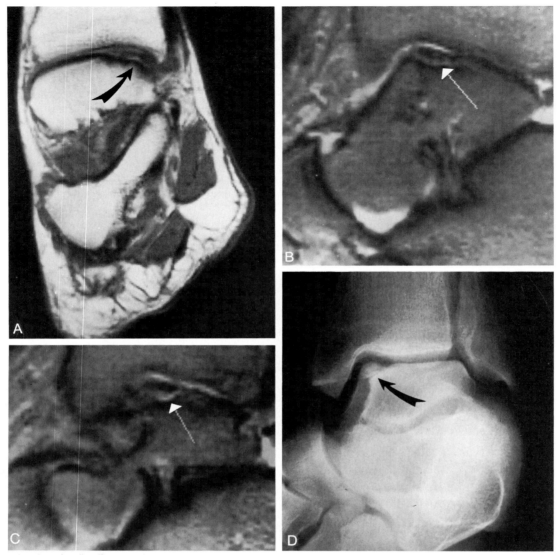

FIGURE 40–5. Osteochondritis dissecans of the talar dome. T_1- and T_2-weighted images in the coronal *(A)* and sagittal *(B and C)* planes, respectively, confirm the conventional radiographic findings *(D)* of a medial osteochondral defect *(arrows)*, which demonstrates a margin of high signal intensity.

may require more intense medical treatment before their cartilage is destroyed.[8]

In cases of talar body fracture, MR imaging can reveal fragment displacement and joint incongruity. Moreover, the fatty bone marrow displays a homogeneous high signal intensity. This finding indicates viability and effectively excludes ischemic necrosis. Osteochondral fractures are also clearly demonstrated on MR images in patients.[1]

Thirty-three joints of the appendicular skeleton in 15 children with juvenile rheumatoid arthritis were examined with MR imaging to determine if it could demonstrate synovial hypertrophy and the status of the articular cartilage. Presumed synovial hypertrophy was seen in 13 joints as masses of varying sizes of low to intermediate signal intensity on T_1- and T_2-weighted images; sometimes foci of increased signal

intensity, most likely due to fluid or inflammation, were seen on T_2-weighted images. Probably abnormal articular cartilage was detected in 10 joints, and MR imaging also demonstrated epiphyseal overgrowth, bone erosions, joint effusions, and joint space narrowing. Because MR imaging appears to provide an objective method of evaluating both synovial hypertrophy and the status of articular cartilage, it may prove to be useful in monitoring the progression of juvenile rheumatoid arthritis and the response to therapy.[9]

GRE T_2-weighted images of the ankle have defined capsular distention in coronal, sagittal, and transaxial planes, with fluid appearing as areas of higher signal intensity than intertarsal, subtalar, and tibiotalar cartilages. Thin-section, fast scan sequences have distinguished fluid in areas of devitalized cortex found in osteochondritis dissecans (transchondral fractures). In three of six patients evaluated in one study, unattached cartilage and osteochondral fragments were identified that were not detected by either conventional T_1- or T_2-weighted images. The subchondral focus of low signal intensity, as demonstrated on conventional T_1- or T_2-weighted sequences, was, however, masked, in contrast to surrounding yellow or fatty marrow of low signal intensity on T_2-weighted images.[4]

Subarticular and juxtaarticular cysts show uniform increases in signal intensity using GRE techniques. Sagittal images allow visualization of tendinous structures in their long axis as bands of low signal intensity, whereas adjacent vascular structures generate high signal intensities.[4]

Overall, MR imaging allows excellent assessment of the ligaments and cartilaginous components of the ankle joint. More research is needed to compare the sensitivity and specificity of this relatively new non-invasive method with the sensitivity and specificity of clinical, CT, and arthroscopic evaluation.[1]

NEOPLASMS

MR imaging has proved useful in defining separate compartments and fascial divisions, important in the evaluation and staging of neoplasms affecting the foot and ankle (Fig. 40–6).[4]

In the early experience with neurofibromatosis and synovial sarcoma involving the foot and ankle, T_2-weighted images (TR 2000/TE 60 msec) have provided superior contrast resolution, compared with the shorter SE T_1 acquisitions (Figs. 40–7 and 40–8). In patients with fibrous dysplasia, involved cortex may demonstrate high signal intensity on conventional T_2-weighted images.[4]

MR imaging of the painful ankle of a 15-year-old boy has revealed the nidus of a subarticular osteoid osteoma of the talus, along with markedly abnormal signal intensity in the neighboring bone marrow, documented by histopathologic examination. In this report, MR imaging of the talus was performed on a 1.5-T superconducting system. A transmit-receive extremity coil was used with a 16-cm FOV. SE images

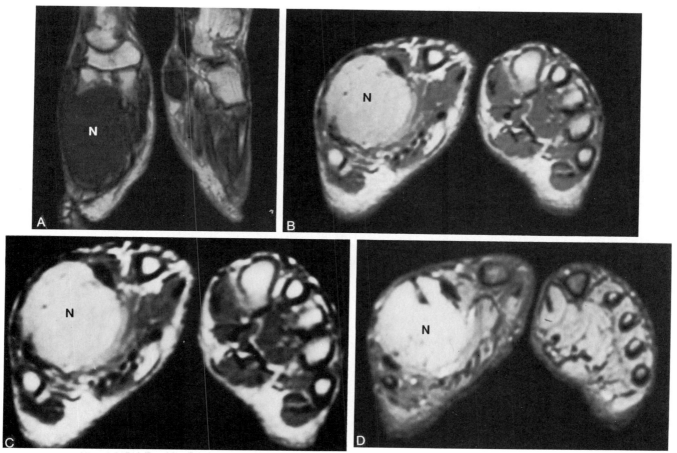

FIGURE 40–6. Chondromyxoid fibroma. *A*, Axial T_1-weighted image reveals replacement of the third metatarsal by a large, well-circumscribed mass (N) that is isointense with muscle. *B*, Coronal balanced SE image at the level of the metatarsal shafts shows a homogeneous tumor mass splaying the adjacent metatarsals (N). Serpiginous areas of signal void are present within the tumor dorsally, consistent with tumor vascularity. *C* and *D*, Coronal T_2-weighted and GRE images at the same location document striking tumor hyperintensity (N).

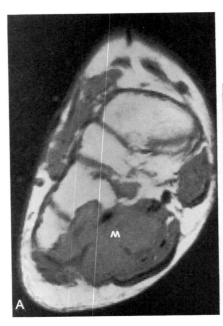

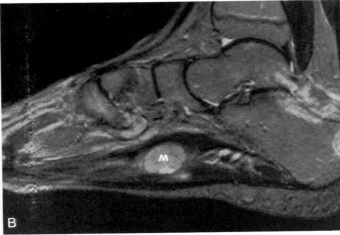

FIGURE 40–7. Synovial sarcoma. *A*, Axial T₁-weighted image depicts a soft tissue mass (M) within the plantar aspect of the foot that is isointense with normal muscle. *B*, Contrast between the lesion (M) and adjacent tissue is optimized on a T₂-weighted image (sagittal plane).

(TR 600/TE 20 msec, TR 2800/TE 40 and 80) were obtained in the coronal and sagittal planes; section thickness was 5 mm with a 2.5-mm intersection gap. On the SE 600/20 images, there was a dramatic decrease in signal intensity involving all but the most anterior portion of the talus. The same area showed markedly increased signal intensity on the SE 2500/80 images.[10]

In the setting of plantar cavernous hemangiomas of the foot, transaxial MR imaging (SE 500/30) may fail to show areas of signal void within the lesion because of the small size of the phleboliths. Symmet-

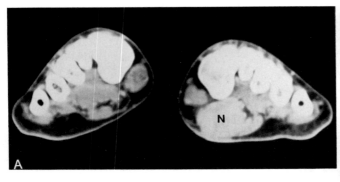

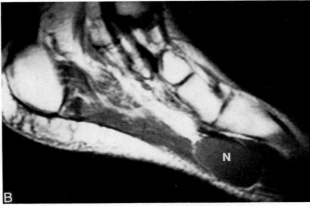

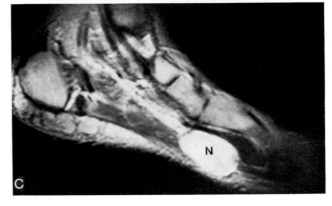

FIGURE 40–8. Synovial sarcoma. *A*, Coronal CT image (soft tissue window) reveals a plantar mass (N) of slightly higher density than normal muscle. *B* and *C*, Sagittal T₁- and T₂-weighted images demonstrate the lesion (N), which is well defined and of intermediate to high signal intensity.

ric signal void areas in the soft tissues of both feet are due to vessels and tendons. Plantar cavernous hemangiomas have very high signal intensity on SE 2100/90 MR images. The lesion-to-muscle signal intensity ratio can be as high as 11.6:1. Sharp demarcation of lesion margins on MR images is characteristic.[11]

MR imaging usually defines the extent of soft tissue masses better than CT. This is particularly true in areas such as the foot and ankle, where fat planes are poorly identified by CT. The extent of intramedullary masses is usually easier to determine by MR imaging than by CT. MR imaging is often more useful than CT for evaluating vascular and joint involvement by tumor (Fig. 40–9). CT is superior to MR imaging for detecting small areas of calcification or ossification and early cortical bone erosion. Visibility of small mineralized areas by MR imaging is dependent on the specific imaging sequence. Occasionally, MR imaging in nontransaxial planes helps to solve specific diagnostic problems. Simple fluid masses and benign lipomatous masses are equally well identified by CT and MR imaging. The latter is more useful in characterizing fibrous and angiomatous lesions.[11]

Extrahepatic cavernous hemangiomas of the foot and ankle have been evaluated by MR imaging and CT. In this study, MR imaging was done with a 1-T superconducting magnet and SE imaging. MR imaging detected all hemangiomas and was more accurate than CT in determining their true extent in some cases. At a pulse-repetition interval of 2000 msec and an echo delay time of 90 msec, all hemangiomas were markedly hyperintense compared with skeletal muscle. Quantitatively, at this pulse sequence, intensity ratios of hemangiomas to skeletal muscle were all 7:1 or greater (mean = 9.89), while the ratios for other tumors were usually less than 7:1 (mean = 5.14). Small cavernous hemangiomas were homogeneous, well-defined round or oval lesions, while large hemangiomas consisted of dilated, tortuous vascular channels. In contrast, other tumors are usually heterogeneous owing to hemorrhage and necrosis and have irregular margins. MR imaging may thus be useful for distinguishing cavernous hemangiomas from other soft tissue tumors, particularly sarcomas.[12]

TR 2000/TE 30 MR images reveal that cavernous hemangiomas are significantly more intense than muscle, but only slightly less intense than fat. TR 2000/TE 90 images reveal a markedly hyperintense appearance of hemangiomas. Lesions are more intense than both fat and muscle and have high signal intensity similar to that of superficial veins. The true extent of hemangiomas is well displayed using T_2 weighting because of high contrast. Lesion extent is also well demonstrated on sagittal TR 2000/TE 90 MR images, in which large, tortuous vascular structures separated by low-intensity fibrous connective tissue stroma are seen.[12]

Hemangiomas of the foot and ankle region are common congenital lesions that may have devastating sequelae. The extent and location of a lesion determine the therapeutic approach. In one investigation, 11 patients with mucocutaneous or peripheral soft tissue hemangiomas were studied to illustrate the ability of MR imaging to define clearly and noninvasively the extent and anatomic relationships of these lesions. The major advantage of MR imaging over CT or angiography is the exquisite difference in contrast between hemangiomas and the surrounding structures on T_2-weighted sequences, in which hemangiomas have a relatively intense signal. Hemangiomas demonstrate relatively low signal intensity (similar to muscle) on T_1-weighted images, which are markedly inferior to T_2-weighted images in defining their extent. Phleboliths and feeding or draining vessels are rarely visible. The information obtained with MR imaging may be valuable clinically in planning surgical resection or laser therapy of aggressive lesions, in evaluating effectiveness of medical or embolic therapy, and in defining recurrence.[13] Following surgery for hemangioma, in the setting of recurrent pain, T_2-weighted MR images (2000/70) may show recurrent hemangioma of high signal intensity within low-intensity scar.[13]

Aggressive juvenile fibromatosis can be accurately staged for extent by MR imaging (Fig. 40–10). An infiltrative soft tissue mass is typically identified. The lesion exhibits slightly higher signal intensity than the adjacent musculature on T_1-weighted images but is much brighter than the latter if a T_2-weighted sequence is used. The process demonstrates lower signal intensity than subcutaneous and bone marrow fat on both sequences. On CT images using a soft tissue window, the abnormality is frequently isodense with normal muscle and difficult to distinguish from postoperative fibrosis in the setting of suspected recurrence. Definite evidence of osseous invasion is difficult to appreciate by MR imaging. On CT images using a soft tissue window, dorsal lesions are readily delineated, owing to their obliteration of the normal subcutaneous fat, infiltration of the extensor tendons, and deformity of the skin. The interface between plantar lesions and the adjacent musculature cannot be accurately determined, however, because of near isodensity between these two types of tissue. Despite this limitation, bone window renditions of CT images readily document early osseous invasion. By MR imaging, dorsal lesions are best delineated on T_1-weighted sequences, in which their relatively low signal intensity contrasts sharply with the bright subcutaneous fat. On T_2-weighted images, the process is only slightly less intense than the adjacent adipose tissue. The superior soft tissue contrast discrimination capabilities of MR imaging, compared with CT, render it the preferred method for staging this neoplasm, although several different pulse sequences are needed to optimize this advantage. Alternatively, the ability of CT to demonstrate subtle abnormalities

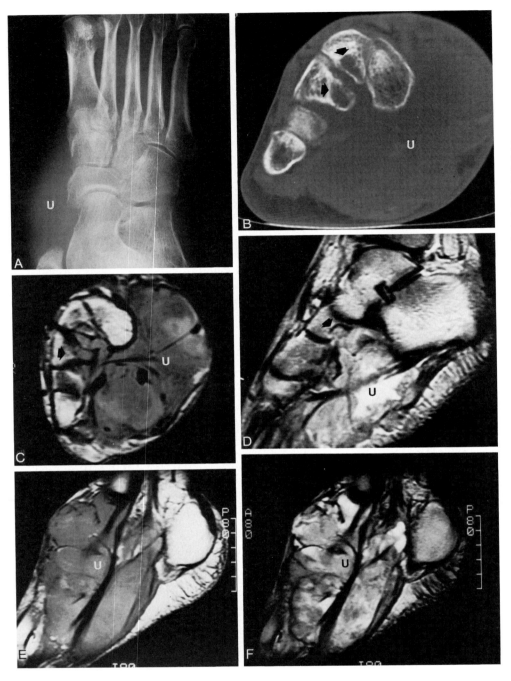

FIGURE 40–9. Undifferentiated soft tissue sarcoma. *A,* An oblique radiograph of the right foot reveals a large, medially located soft tissue mass (U). No tumor matrix or osseous destruction is identified. *B,* Coronal CT (bone window) image demonstrates encasement and displacement of the plantar tendons by tumor mass (U) and osseous destruction with cortical breakthrough of the bases of the second and third cuneiforms *(black arrows). C,* Coronal balanced SE image at the same level as the CT section reveals signal heterogeneity within the mass (U). Encasement of low-signal tendinous structures is more optimally demonstrated. Tumor extension to involve the plantar aspect of the second and third cuneiforms is again identified *(arrow). D,* Sagittal T_2-weighted image shows osseous invasion *(arrow)* and increased signal within portions of the tumor, representing either fluid collections or tumor necroses (U). *E* and *F,* Sagittal balanced and T_2-weighted images demonstrate replacement of plantar tissues and encasement of linear tendinous structures by tumor mass (U).

affecting cortical bone more readily than MR imaging may also render it useful in the management of patients with aggressive juvenile fibromatosis.

True plantar neuromas have characteristic behavior on MR images (Figs. 40–11 and 40–12). On relatively T_1-weighted SE images (TR 600/TE 20), no definite abnormalities may be appreciated, as the lesion often exhibits a signal intensity identical with that of the plantar musculature. An unusually circular zone may, however, be detectable with the muscle. Because neuromatous tissue and normal muscle exhibit similar degrees of attenuation on

radiographs, the abnormality would be comparably subtle on a CT image. On SE images with intermediate weighting (TR 2000/TE 25), the lesion is identified by virtue of its higher signal intensity compared with the adjacent musculature. The abnormality remains less bright than fat within the bone marrow and subcutaneous region by a slight degree. On relatively T_2-weighted SE images (TR 2000/TE 70), the lesion is demonstrated as a well-encapsulated area manifesting a signal intensity much greater than that of fat or muscle. Through the application of several different pulse sequences, the full contrast discrimi-

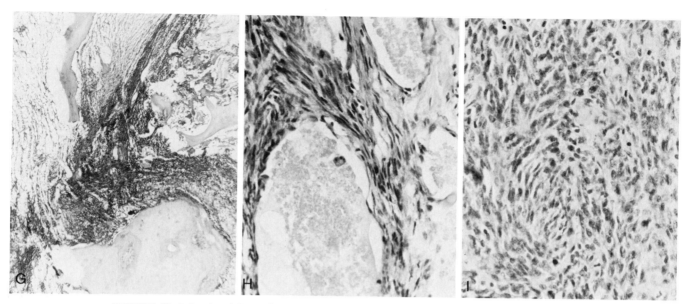

FIGURE 40–9 *Continued G–I,* Histologic features are those of an undifferentiated malignancy.

nation capabilities of MR imaging, which exceed those of CT, are optimally used in the setting of clinically suspected plantar neuroma.

Interdigital (Morton's) neuroma, a lesion that represents thickening of a plantar digital nerve as opposed to a true neuroma, can be detected by high-

resolution MR imaging (Fig. 40–13). On T_1-weighted partial saturation images (TR 600/TE 25), in the region of the metatarsophalangeal articulations, a well-encapsulated plantar soft tissue mass of relatively low signal intensity can be identified. The classic lesion lies immediately plantar to the third interdigital space and manifests a signal intensity compara-

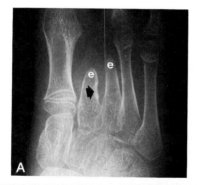

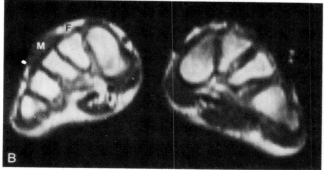

FIGURE 40–10. Aggressive juvenile fibromatosis. *A,* Conventional radiograph following earlier resection demonstrates tapering of the metatarsal stumps (e) and associated cortical erosion *(arrow). B,* Coronal T_1-weighted image at the level of the metatarsal bases demonstrates an infiltrative soft tissue mass of intermediate signal intensity dorsal to the second and third metatarsals (M), delineated by fat (F).

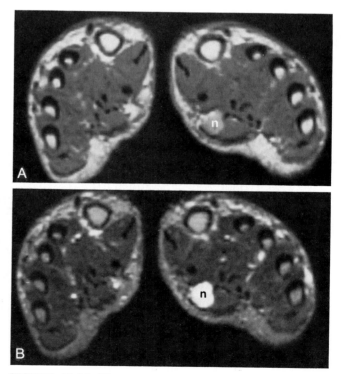

FIGURE 40–11. Plantar neuroma. *A* and *B,* Proton density–weighted and T_2-weighted coronal images reveal a well-defined mass of moderate to high signal intensity (n) within the flexor digitorum brevis muscle.

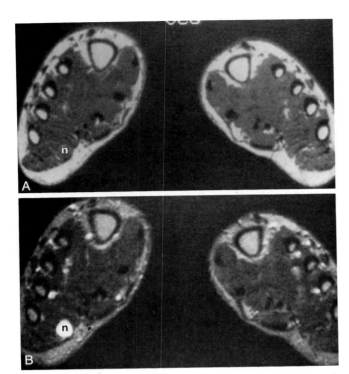

FIGURE 40–12. Neuroma of the lateral plantar nerve. *A,* Coronal T₁-weighted image reveals a well-circumscribed, homogeneous mass, isointense with muscle, within the abductor digiti minimi (n). *B,* The lesion (n) brightens significantly with T₂ weighting. This case emphasizes the need for utilizing several different pulse sequences to optimize soft tissue contrast discrimination.

ble with that of the adjacent flexor tendon sheaths but far below that of the subcutaneous fat. On intermediate (TR 2000/TE 25) and T₂-weighted (TR 2000/TE 70) SE images, progressively poorer discrimination from adipose tissue is noted with increasing T₂ weighting. The lesion is less well delineated on the intermediate-weighted image than on the T₁-weighted series and is difficult to recognize using the T₂-weighted pulse sequence. On all pulse sequences, the mass maintains close apposition to the medial plantar aspect of the bones of the fourth toe, without evidence of secondary osseous abnormalities.

Recurrent multifocal schwannoma behaves similarly to true plantar neuromas on MR imaging (Fig. 40–14). On relatively T₁-weighted partial saturation images (TR 600/TE 25), discrete rounded zones with signal intensity comparable to that of normal muscle are observed. On intermediate-weighted SE images (TR 2000/TE 25), the signal intensity of the lesion is much higher than that of muscle and only slightly less bright than that of subcutaneous and bone marrow fat. Contrast between the abnormal masses and adjacent tissue is optimized on T₂-weighted SE images (TR 2000/TE 50), in which their signal intensity exceeds that of muscle and both intraosseous and extraosseous fat. On corresponding CT images using a soft tissue window, distally located masses are readily identified owing to their delineation by adjacent subcutaneous fat of lower density. Lesions po-

sitioned more proximally, however, cannot be unequivocally visualized, as they are surrounded by isodense muscle. Nevertheless, using bone window settings, CT may demonstrate reactive periostitis involving the adjacent bones, which is depicted indirectly and thus potentially detectable only in retrospect by MR images. For surgical planning purposes, localization of such lesions on T₁-weighted partial saturation images (TR 600/TE 25) obtained in the coronal plane without repositioning of the patient can be extremely useful. MR imaging offers superior soft tissue contrast discrimination capabilities compared with CT but requires multiple variable pulse sequences to optimize this advantage. Although multiplanar imaging of the foot and ankle is more practical using MR imaging than CT, the latter is generally superior in demonstrating abnormalities of cortical bone.

INFECTION

Bone scans are highly sensitive for the diagnosis of acute osteomyelitis, but the difficulty of distinguishing bone marrow processes from soft tissue disease limits the specificity and accuracy. A technique capable of distinguishing bone marrow processes from soft tissue disease would improve the diagnostic accuracy of osteomyelitis. To evaluate the use of MR imaging in the diagnosis of osteomyelitis, examinations have been performed in patients with suspected acute osteomyelitis of the foot and ankle,

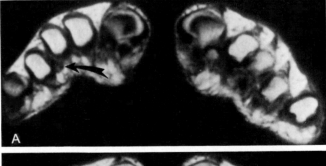

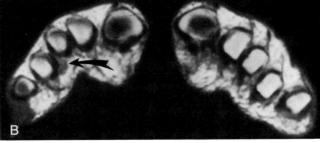

FIGURE 40–13. Interdigital (Morton) neuroma. *A* and *B,* Coronal balanced SE images in the region of the metatarsophalangeal joints reveal a well-circumscribed plantar soft tissue mass of low signal intensity *(arrows).* The lesion lies immediately plantar and medial to the fourth metatarsal and is well delineated by adjacent adipose tissue of high signal intensity. No osseous alterations are identified.

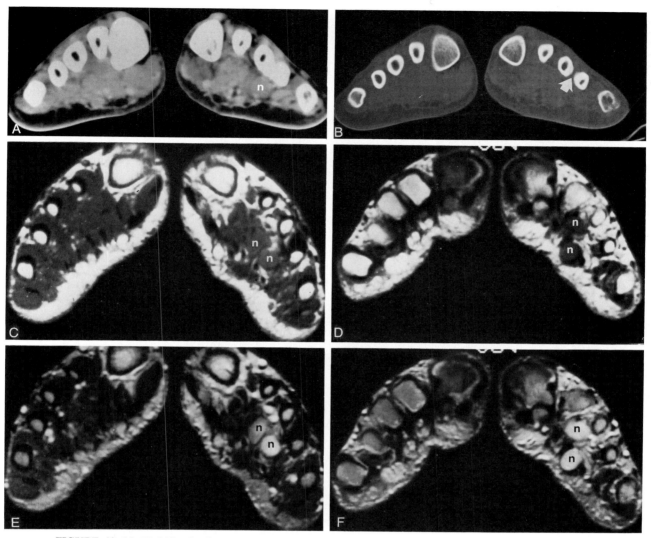

FIGURE 40–14. Multifocal schwannoma. *A,* Coronal CT image (soft tissue window) reveals a well-defined mass (n) that is isodense with muscle. *B,* Coronal CT image (bone window) reveals reactive periostitis *(arrow).* Coronal balanced (*C* and *D*) and T$_2$-weighted (*E* and *F*) images demonstrate well-circumscribed masses plantar to the second and third metatarsals. The masses are homogeneous and of intermediate to high signal intensity.

some of whom were proved to have osteomyelitis either by surgery or by clinical follow-up. In the remainder, osteomyelitis was excluded by surgery or the clinical course. Evidence of osteomyelitis on MR imaging consisted of abnormalities of the bone marrow with decreased signal intensity on the T$_1$-weighted images and increased signal intensity on the T$_2$-weighted or short T$_1$ inversion recovery (STIR) images (Fig. 40–15). The sensitivities of MR imaging and static bone scan were 100 per cent for bone marrow abnormality. Because bone marrow abnormality in osteomyelitis associated with healing fractures was incorrectly diagnosed by MR imaging and bone scintigraphy in a few instances, their respective sensitivities for the diagnosis of osteomyelitis were 92 per cent and 82 per cent. The specificities of MR imaging and scintigraphy were 96 per cent and 65 per cent respectively. The overall accuracy

for the diagnosis of osteomyelitis was 94 per cent for MR imaging and 71 per cent for bone scan.[14]

MR imaging has been performed after CT in the setting of calcaneal osteomyelitis, using a 0.3-T magnet. Transaxial scans were obtained, using SE 28/500 and a pulse sequence of SE 28/2000 for sagittal scans. Abnormalities in the calcaneus were detected more readily with a T$_1$ SE 28/500 sequence. Markedly decreased signal was obtained from the calcaneus and adjacent edematous soft tissue. The extent of abnormality of the calcaneus shown by MR imaging was much greater than the bone destruction demonstrated on CT. With the T$_2$-weighted SE 56/2000 sequence, the signal from the calcaneus was only minimally greater than normal, so that the lesion was hardly detectable with this technique.[15]

In the setting of osteomyelitis, the extent of edema, as shown by decreased signal from the entire tarsal

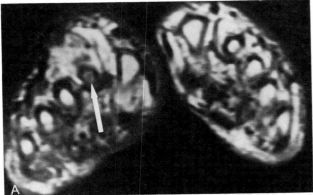

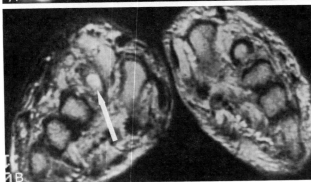

FIGURE 40–15. Osteomyelitis in a patient with diabetes mellitus.
A, Coronal balanced SE image at the level of the metatarsal shafts demonstrates diminished signal intensity within the medullary canal of the second metatarsal. *(arrow).* No cortical erosion is identified. *B,* Coronal T₂-weighted image at the same level reveals relative increased signal intensity within the second metatarsal *(arrows),* suggesting osteomyelitis.

bone on MR imaging, can be much larger than the limited area of bone destruction depicted by plain films or CT. The extent of the inflammation and edema of the marrow in osteomyelitis is greater than recognized in the past (before MR imaging) and not limited to the areas of bone destruction shown on plain films or CT. In cases of Brodie's abscess or in more extensive instances of chronic osteomyelitis, the infection is confined by osteoblastic reaction, so that plain films and CT may approximate the extent of involvement. The relatively considerable involvement demonstrated by MR imaging, compared with the limited changes shown by roentgenograms or CT, may have diagnostic value, favoring acute infection rather than other disorders, although this statement must be proven by further studies.[15]

In the foot and ankle, MR imaging has permitted successful identification of osteomyelitis (acute, sub-acute with Brodie's abscess, chronic, and acute with septic arthritis) and of cellulitis in the absence of osteomyelitis, including soft tissue abscess. Active osteomyelitis can also be excluded; both T₁- and T₂-weighted images are needed to identify such foci. MR images provide more accurate and detailed information regarding the extent of involvement than do radionuclide bone scans, CT scans, or standard radiographs. MR imaging also permits the differentiation of septic arthritis or cellulitis from osteomyelitis. In limited experience to date, MR imaging has been particularly useful for identifying foci of active infection in areas of chronic osteomyelitis complicated by surgical intervention or fracture.[16]

In the setting of soft tissue infection, the underlying medullary signal appears normal. The signal intensity of areas of cellulitis is similar to that of the inflamed soft tissue adjacent to foci of osteomyelitis (low intensity on T₁-weighted images and high intensity on T₂-weighted images), and the margins of the lesions are similarly ill defined (Fig. 40–16). Soft tissue abscesses are well marginated in contrast.[16]

Transaxial MR images of soft tissue abscess of the ankle (SE 500/28) depict a fairly well defined area of intermediate signal intensity. Diffuse areas of intermediate signal intensity may be seen in adjacent skin. On SE 2000/84 images, soft tissue abscesses are very bright, well demarcated, and covered by bright, edematous subcutaneous fat and skin. Underlying bone may or may not be normal.[16]

Patients with clinical findings consistent with osteomyelitis, soft tissue infection, or both, were studied with MR imaging at 1.5 T in one investigation. Another group of patients with joint effusion, but no clinical or laboratory signs of infection, served as control subjects. Soft tissue abscesses, osteomyelitis, joint and tendon sheath effusion, and cellulitis were well depicted by MR imaging, allowing the correct diagnosis of the presence and extent of infection in most cases. MR imaging was as sensitive as technetium-99m methylene diphosphonate bone scintigraphy in demonstrating osteomyelitis and was more specific and more sensitive than other scintigraphic techniques in demonstrating soft tissue infections, primarily because of its superior spatial resolution. CT, performed in some cases, was as accurate as MR imaging in revealing bone and soft tissue infections. Infected and noninfected synovial effusions had the same signal intensity, but associated findings such as soft tissue fluid collections or osteomyelitis made the distinction possible.[17]

In the diabetic foot, sagittal and coronal MR images (SE 2000/80) may demonstrate hyperintensity of the bone marrow space or multiple well-demarcated areas of increased signal intensity in the soft tissues of the foot, representing abscesses (Fig. 40–17).[17]

The diabetic foot with cellulitis shows ill-defined areas of increased signal intensity in the soft tissues on sagittal MR images of the ankle and tarsal region (SE 2000/80). Associated small joint effusions in the tarsal joints may be noted.[17] Distinction from postoperative fibrosis (Fig. 40–18) is readily accomplished.

Infected tenosynovitis in the diabetic foot is seen on transaxial MR images (SE 2000/80) as marked distention of the tendon sheaths by infected synovial fluid. No difference in signal intensity is noted between noninfected and infected collections.[17]

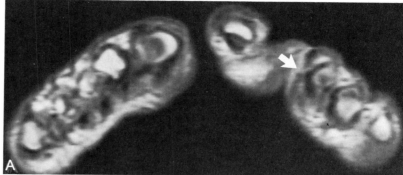

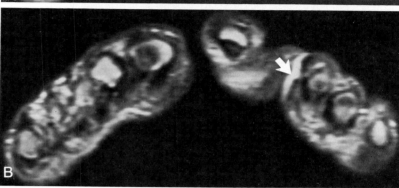

FIGURE 40–16. Cellulitis in the diabetic foot. *A* and *B*, Balanced and T$_2$-weighted coronal images reveal the superficial area of infection *(arrows)*.

MR imaging is a sensitive technique for identifying pathology in the soft tissues of children, and it consistently shows more abnormality than does CT. MR images are not histologically specific, but with careful attention to the location of the abnormality, to the definition of its margins, and to the evaluation of involvement of adjacent muscle, bone, subcutaneous fat, and skin, the correct diagnosis can be strongly predicted in most cases. The ability of MR imaging to demonstrate anatomy in multiple planes aids in the evaluation of the extent of lesions and their relationship to adjacent structures. MR imaging can accurately predict the extent of abnormality and has great potential for the study of disease of soft tissues in the foot and ankle.[18]

On T$_1$-weighted images, osteomyelitis of the calcaneus may exhibit marked swelling of soft tissues and marked reduction of signal from fat, with loss of the normal sharply defined interface between subcutaneous fat and adjacent muscle. Soft tissue

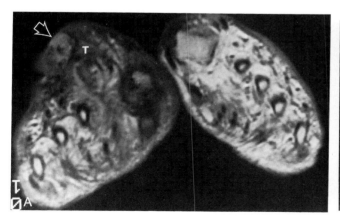

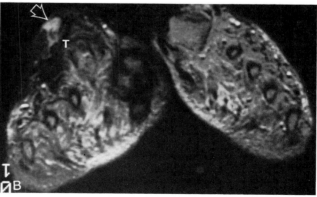

FIGURE 40–17. Soft tissue abscess in a patient with diabetes mellitus. *A*, Coronal balanced SE image at the level of the metatarsal shafts shows marked dorsal soft tissue swelling (T) and a large dorsal ulcer. A prominent region of heterogeneous signal intensity is evident dorsally *(arrow)*, with regions of intermediate signal intensity and areas of low signal intensity. *B*, Coronal T$_2$-weighted image at the same location indicates signal increase dorsally *(arrow)*, consistent with a purulent fluid collection. The region of low signal intensity deep to the fluid collection (T) shows further decrease in signal, indicative of fibrous or scar tissue.

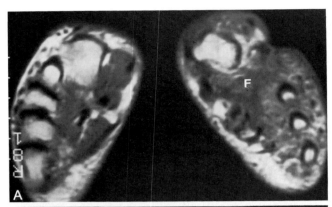

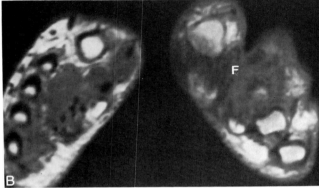

FIGURE 40–18. Postoperative fibrosis in the diabetic foot. *A* and *B,* Balanced coronal images depict abnormal soft tissue (F) that is isointense with muscle within the second metatarsal resection bed.

abnormality between fat and bone is identified as ill-defined regions of swelling of intermediate intensity. The margins of the calcaneus may be poorly defined, in association with marked reduction in signal intensity from its marrow space.[18]

MR imaging has been performed in children with acute, subacute, chronic, and recurrent osteomyelitis of the foot and ankle. Saturation recovery, T_2-weighted SE, and inversion recovery pulse sequences were employed in one study. A reduction in the normally bright image of bone marrow corresponded to abnormalities seen on radiographs, CT scans, and radionuclide studies. Saturation recovery images produced the best signal-to-noise (S/N) ratios. Contrast between normal and abnormal marrow was most pronounced on inversion recovery sequences, which suggested an increase in the water content of inflamed marrow. Abnormalities were sometimes seen on MR images before they could be detected on radiographs. Some MR abnormalities were present when CT and radionuclide studies were normal or equivocal.[19]

Saturation recovery images in the coronal plane (recovery time, 0.5 second) show areas of diminished intensity in the medullary cavity corresponding to lytic lesions seen radiographically. Adjacent soft tissue swelling and disruption of the bright signal of subcutaneous fat may be observed. Inversion recovery transaxial sections reveal areas of reduced intensity in infected bones, with adjacent soft tissue swelling. Less marked diminution in signal from the involved area is observed on saturation recovery pulse sequences (recovery time, 1.0 second). T_2-weighted images may show no difference in contrast between involved and normal marrow.[19]

MISCELLANEOUS POSTTRAUMATIC ABNORMALITIES

MR imaging is capable of demonstrating a variety of alterations in both bone and soft tissue after trauma to the foot and ankle, including stress fractures (Figs. 40–19 and 40–20), reflex sympathetic dystrophy syndrome (Fig. 40–21), and muscular atrophy related to disuse.

CONCLUSION

This chapter has endeavored to enlighten the practicing radiologist with regard to the indications for cross-sectional imaging by MR in the evaluation of specific clinical problems affecting the foot and ankle. In most instances, MR imaging will answer the diagnostic questions posed, although CT may provide complementary information and thus both may be required in certain instances. Direct multiplanar images of the foot and ankle can be obtained with both methods, although positioning of the patient is more easily achieved with MR imaging. As a general rule, MR imaging is preferred to CT in the setting of suspected soft tissue pathology or disorders with early involvement of bone marrow, because of its superior contrast discrimination capabilities and exquisite sensitivity. Because cortical bone contains a relative paucity of mobile protons and generates a weak MR signal, however, CT is preferred in the assessment of osseous alterations that do not begin in the marrow space. For younger patients, MR imaging should be the procedure of choice because it delivers no ionizing radiation and involves no known biologic hazard.

The disadvantages of MR imaging are not inconsequential. It is an expensive test and not yet widely available. MR imaging at low magnetic field strength is not capable of producing high-resolution images such as those obtained with a 1.5-T magnet. Dedicated surface coils are useful to achieve high-quality images, and commercial production of such coils is still limited. The absence of signal from calcified soft tissue is another disadvantage, although cortical and trabecular bone can be seen, owing to the contrast of fat in the surrounding subcutaneous tissue and marrow. The characterization of different types of fluid is not possible with current techniques. For example, MR imaging is unable to distinguish between purulent and serous fluid collections. Finally, claustropho-

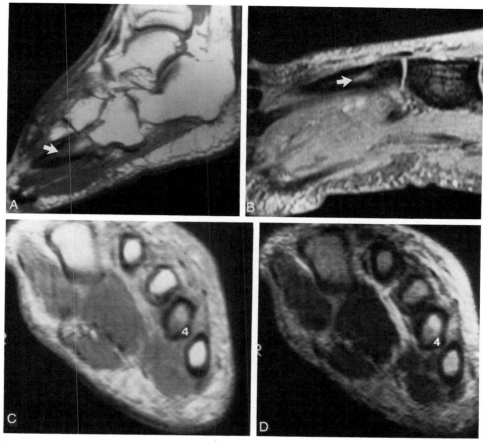

FIGURE 40–19. Stress fracture. *A*, Parasagittal T_1-weighted image through the lateral aspect of the foot shows a focal linear area of decreased signal intensity within the base of the fourth metatarsal *(arrow)*, consistent with a stress fracture. *B*, Parasagittal GRE image through the base of the fourth metatarsal and cuboid reveals focal increased signal intensity of the bone marrow *(arrow)*, representing edema within the marrow. *C*, Coronal balanced SE image at the level of the metatarsal shafts shows cortical irregularity and diminished signal within the fourth metatarsal (4). *D*, Coronal T_2-weighted image at the same level demonstrates increased bone marrow signal intensity (4), indicating areas of increased water content.

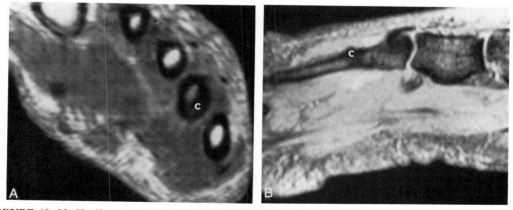

FIGURE 40–20. Healing stress fracture. *A*, Coronal T_1-weighted image at the level of the metatarsal shafts documents a curvilinear band of decreased signal intensity along the plantar aspect of the fourth metatarsal (c), representing periosteal new bone formation. *B*, Parasagittal GRE image through the base of the fourth metatarsal and cuboid shows callus formation dorsally (c) as a region of decreased signal intensity contiguous with the metatarsal cortex. The inhomogeneous region of increased signal intensity in the soft tissues plantar to the metatarsal indicates adjacent soft tissue edema.

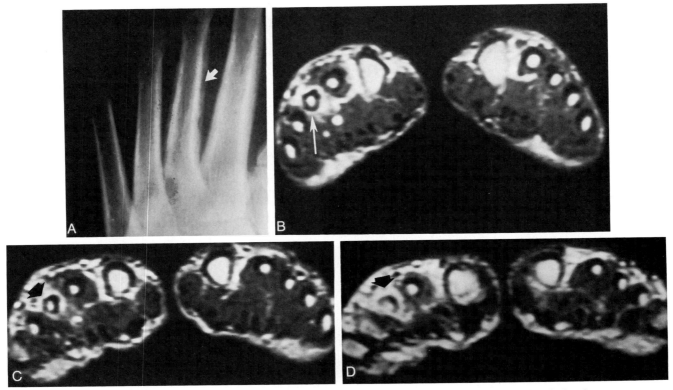

FIGURE 40–21. Reflex sympathetic dystrophy syndrome. *A,* Anteroposterior radiograph of the foot demonstrates intracortical bone resorption *(arrow)* along the third metatarsal diaphysis, resulting in a striated appearance of the cortex. *B,* Coronal T₂-weighted image at the metatarsal shaft level reveals a striking region of increased signal intensity surrounding the metatarsal diaphysis *(arrow),* representing soft tissue edema. *C* and *D,* Coronal T₂-weighted images obtained distal to *B* reveal similar soft tissue findings *(arrows).*

bia and motion are occasional problems; patients may be unable to hold their feet rigid for the entire series of images because of uncomfortable positioning.[3]

REFERENCES

1. Beltran J, Noto AM, Mosure JC, et al: Ankle: Surface coil MR imaging at 1.5 T. Radiology 161:203–210, 1986.
2. Middleton WD, Macrander S, Lawson TL, et al: High resolution surface coil magnetic resonance imaging of the joints: Anatomic correlation. RadioGraphics 7:645–683, 1987.
3. Beltran J, Noto AM, Herman LJ, Lubbers LM: Tendons: High-field-strength, surface coil MR imaging. Radiology 162:735–740, 1987.
4. Stoller DW, Genant HK, Goumas CG, et al: Fast MR improves imaging of musculoskeletal system. Diagn Imag 10:98–198, 1988.
5. Reinig JW, Dorwart RH, Roden WC: MRI of a Ruptured Achilles Tendon. Bethesda, MD, National Institutes of Health, and Washington, DC, Department of Orthopedic Surgery, Walter Reed Army Medical Center.
6. Quinn SF, Murray WT, Clark RA, Cochran CF: Achilles tendon: MR imaging at 1.5 T. Radiology 164:767–770, 1987.
7. Daffner RH, Reimer BL, Lupetin ARE, Dash N: Magnetic resonance imaging in acute tendon ruptures. Skeletal Radiol 15:619–621, 1986.
8. Yulish BS, Lieberman JM, Strandjord SE, et al: Hemophilic arthropathy: Assessment with MR imaging. Radiology 164:759–752, 1987.
9. Yulish BS, Lieberman JM, Newman AJ, et al: Juvenile rheumatoid arthritis: Assessment with MR imaging. Radiology 165:149–152, 1987.
10. Yeager BA, Schiebler ML, Wertheim SB, et al: Case report—MR imaging of osteoid osteoma of the talus. J Comput Assist Tomogr 11:916–917, 1987.
11. Wetzel LH, Levine E, Murphey MD: A comparison of MR imaging and CT in the evaluation of musculoskeletal masses. RadioGraphics 7:851–874, 1987.
12. Levine E, Wetzel LH, Neff JR: MR imaging and CT of extrahepatic cavernous hemangiomas. AJR 147:1299–1304, 1986.
13. Kaplan PA, Williams SM: Mucocutaneous and peripheral soft-tissue hemangiomas: MR imaging. Radiology 163:163–166, 1987.
14. Unger E, Moldofsky P, Gatenby R, et al: Diagnosis of osteomyelitis by MR imaging. AJR 1509:605–610, 1988.
15. Mesgarzadeh M, Bonkdarpour A, Redecki PD: Case Report 395. Skeletal Radiol 15:584–588, 1986.
16. Tang JSH, Gold RH, Bassett LW, Seeger LL: Musculoskeletal infection of the extremities: Evaluation with MR imaging. Radiology 166:205–209, 1988.
17. Beltran J, Noto AM, McGhee RB, et al: Infections of the musculoskeletal system: High-field-strength MR imaging. Radiology 164:449–454, 1987.
18. Cohen MD, DeRosa GP, Kleimann M, et al: Magnetic resonance evaluation of disease of the soft tissues in children. Pediatrics 79:696–701, 1987.
19. Fletcher BD, Scoles PV, Nelson AD: Osteomyelitis in children: Detection by magnetic resonance—work in progress. Pediatr Radiol 150:57–60, 1984.

41

MR IMAGING OF THE MUSCULOSKELETAL SYSTEM

MARK W. RAGOZZINO, R. CHISIN, and DANIEL I. ROSENTHAL

TECHNIQUE

SOURCES OF ERROR

NEOPLASM

MARROW DISORDERS

NORMAL BONE MARROW

MALIGNANT INFILTRATION

AVASCULAR NECROSIS (AVN), LEGG-
CALVÉ-PERTHES (LCP) DISEASE, AND
OSTEOCHONDRITIS DISSECANS

HYPERPLASTIC AND APLASTIC ANEMIAS

GAUCHER'S DISEASE

TRANSIENT OSTEOPOROSIS (TP)

JOINT DISORDERS

CONGENITAL HIP DISLOCATION (CDH)

INFLAMMATORY ARTHRITIDES

MISCELLANEOUS JOINT DISORDERS

THE WRIST

THE ANKLE

INFECTION

TRAUMA

MISCELLANEOUS MUSCLE
DISORDERS

MR imaging is well suited for the musculoskeletal system.[1-4] Inherent contrast between muscle, adipose tissue, ligament, and tendon is great. Vascular structures, marrow, fascial planes, hyaline cartilage, and joint effusions can be identified. Pathologic processes contrast greatly with normal structures with the appropriate selection of pulse sequence. No intravenous or intraarticular contrast needs to be administered. There is freedom in selection of imaging plane. Reconstruction artifacts from cortical bone, casts, or hardware are minimal compared with those of CT.[5] No ionizing radiation is employed.

MR imaging appears more sensitive than other imaging modalities for musculoskeletal tumor staging,[6-18] osteomyelitis,[19-25] avascular necrosis,[26-33] malignant infiltration of marrow,[10, 34, 35] joint disorders,[36, 37] and muscle abnormalities.[38-41] Furthermore, MR imaging promises to be useful for evaluation of scoliosis,[42] pediatric hip disorders,[43, 44] and inflammatory arthritis.[45-50]

In this chapter, we discuss the technical considerations, demonstrate the clinical applications, and review the available literature on MR imaging of the musculoskeletal system.

TECHNIQUE

The wide variety of imaging tasks within the musculoskeletal system defies the establishment of universally applicable protocols; however, certain principles should be applied to all imaging plans. The relevant clinical issues must be known for optimal planning of the MR examination. The MR imaging characteristics (T_1, T_2, proton density, flow, susceptibility) of the tissues of interest should also be known so that pulse sequences can be optimized.

Two-dimensional (2D) spin-echo (SE) imaging is most often used in clinical imaging at this time. Optimal T_1 contrast-weighted images are obtained with short echo time (TE) (less than 30 msec) and short repetition time (TR) (approximately equal to 0.5 to 1.0 times the average T_1 relaxation time of the tissues of interest). Optimal T_2 contrast-weighted images are achieved with long TE (approximately equal to the average T_2 relaxation time of the tissues of interest) and long TR (>3 to 4 times the average T_1 relaxation time of the tissues of interest). T_1 contrast-weighted images are most time efficient for demonstrating anatomic detail. In addition, T_1 contrast-weighted images are usually most sensitive for marrow and adipose tissue disorders. T_2 contrast-weighted sequences are usually most sensitive for identification of pathologic processes in muscle. Recently, gradient-echo (GRE) imaging techniques have shown great promise for the evaluation of a variety of specific musculoskeletal disorders.

Signal contrast within marrow can often be improved using phase-contrast imaging or chemical shift imaging, which exploits the small difference in resonance frequency of protons in water and adipose tissue.[51] Inversion recovery sequences with short inversion time (TI), called STIR, can be designed so that marrow generates little signal (inversion time: $TI = 0.693\,T_1$), creating a background against which hematopoietic tissue and pathologic tissue are clearly seen.[52, 53]

Imaging planes should be perpendicular to the tissue interface of interest. For staging neoplasms of the extremities, we obtain T_2 contrast-weighted images in the axial plane to demonstrate muscle involvement and compartmental relationships, along with T_1 contrast-weighted images in either the coronal or the sagittal plane to demonstrate intraosseous and extraosseous longitudinal extent.

Field-of-view (FOV) and receiver coil should be the smallest that will resolve the clinical issue, thereby maximizing the spatial resolution and signal-to-noise (S/N) ratio of the image. The number of phase-encoding steps per image should be the smallest that will provide adequate spatial resolution for the clinical problem. Spatial resolution along the phase-encoding direction is proportional to the FOV divided by the number of phase-encoding steps. The patient's motion is reduced by making the patient physically and emotionally comfortable as well as gently restraining the patient in the desired position. Motion suppression pulse sequences, described in Chapter 10, may be chosen to improve image quality further.

SOURCES OF ERROR

Potential sources of error in MR imaging include physical phenomena of MR imaging, instrument artifacts, and patient-related variations.[54, 55] Chemical shift artifact results in apparent thinning of the bone cortex on one side and thickening on the opposite side of a particular bone along the direction of the frequency-encoding gradient. There are numerous flow effects that produce signal voids and signal

enhancement, as discussed in Chapter 4. Pulsatile motion generates an artifact along the phase-encoding direction. Improper selection of pulse sequence can result in little or no contrast between normal and pathologic structures owing to the counteracting effects of T_1- and T_2-related contrast. Aliasing occurs when the FOV is smaller than the area producing detectable signal, resulting in "fold-over" of signal arising outside the FOV into the image. Partial volume averaging of signal can result in errors of interpretation. Generally, the above artifacts can be clarified by imaging in several projections, switching the direction of the frequency- and phase-encoding gradients, and using both T_1 and T_2 contrast-weighted images.

Ferromagnetic implants usually produce discrete distortions of the image, which are easily identified. Nonferrous metals may result in very subtle artifacts, which may cause confusion.

There are numerous anatomic variants that are well known to the practicing radiologist. However, several common, normal MR imaging findings within marrow may cause confusion. Children and young adults may have patchy, symmetric areas of decreased signal intensity within marrow because of active hematopoietic tissue. Focal areas of increased signal are seen in the vertebra of adults as a result of focal deposits of yellow marrow. The normal physis appears as a linear signal void on both T_1 and T_2 contrast-weighted images.

NEOPLASM

Several studies have concluded that MR imaging is often superior to other imaging methods for staging of musculoskeletal tumors.[2, 6–18] Staging requires adequate demonstration of tumor margins. The proximal and distal ends of the lesion as well as affected muscle compartments must be identified. The relationship of the lesion to vital nerves and arteries must be delineated. Furthermore, identification of joint involvement is critical.

MR imaging provides detailed assessment of soft tissue involvement (Fig. 41–1). Fascial planes defining anatomic compartments are well visualized because dense connective tissue gives little signal and the adjacent adipose tissue gives high signal. Patent arteries and veins demonstrate flow voids or enhancement, depending upon pulse sequence, allowing for noninvasive assessment of the vascular system without administration of contrast. Neurovascular bundles are often surrounded by fat. Obliteration of the fat interface between neurovascular bundle and neoplasm is a sensitive but not specific indicator of invasion. The intrinsic contrast and multiplanar capability of MR imaging is advantageous for determination of joint involvement by tumor. In addition, these unique capabilities of MR imaging make it ideal

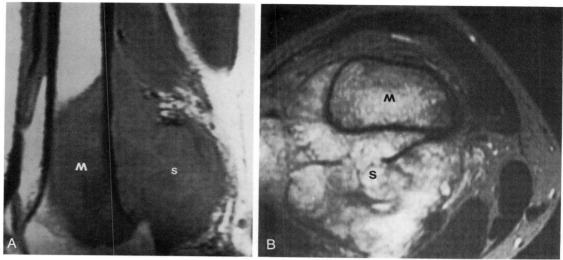

FIGURE 41–1. Osteosarcoma. Sagittal T_1 (A) and axial T_2 (B) contrast-weighted images, spin echo. A mass involves the distal femoral marrow (M) as well as the adjacent soft tissues posteriorly (S).

for assessing tumors in areas of complex anatomy, such as the osseous spine[17] (see Chapters 23 and 24) as well as the head and neck[56] (see Chapter 21). Invasion of cortical bone may be seen as signal within the normally sharp signal void of cortex[7, 8] (Figs. 41–2 to 41–19).

Primary and secondary neoplasms can be made to contrast strongly with surrounding tissues on appropriately selected pulse sequences (Fig. 41–20). T_1 relaxation time of most neoplasms is long compared with that of adipose tissue, so that neoplasms contrast strongly with adipose tissue and fatty bone marrow on T_1-weighted images (Figs. 41–7, 41–9, 41–10, 41–13, and 41–14). The T_2 relaxation time of neoplasms tends to be long compared with that of muscle, and thus neoplasms contrast strongly on T_2 contrast-weighted images[41] (Figs. 41–7 to 41–10). It has been suggested that T_2 prolongation is proportional to tumor aggressivity; however, there are many exceptions to this rule.[6] The appearance of neoplasms on

T_2-weighted images also depends, in part, upon the relative cellularity and collagen content of the lesion.[57]

Marrow signal abnormality on T_1 contrast-weighted images generally correlates well with tumor extent on pathologic examination.[7, 10, 13, 58] Occasionally, the extent of signal abnormality on T_1-weighted images exceeds the margins of the lesions.[59]

Prolongation of T_2 relaxation time within muscle adjacent to malignant soft tissue neoplasm occurs with and without tumor invasion of the muscle. Thickened muscle with indistinct fat planes implies invasion; hence morphology, rather than MR imaging signal characteristics, appears more valuable in predicting muscle invasion. Benign and malignant bone tumors confined to bone without invasion of adjacent muscle generally do not result in signal abnormality in adjacent muscle.[16]

There are no entirely reliable MR imaging criteria for distinguishing benign and malignant tumors. In

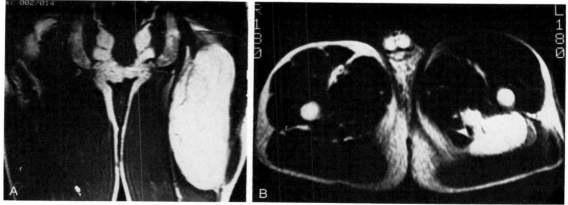

FIGURE 41–2. Lipoma. Coronal T_1 (A) and axial T_2 (B) contrast-weighted sequences of large, homogeneous, well-defined thigh mass with MR characteristics of adipose tissue. Note the fine internal septations.

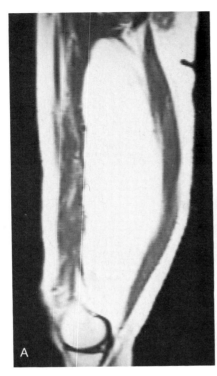

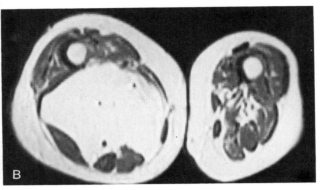

FIGURE 41–3. Well-differentiated liposarcoma. Sagittal *(A)* and axial *(B)* T_1 contrast-weighted images of thigh demonstrating large homogeneous mass with short T_1 relaxation time. The mass extends below the knee. Note chemical shift artifact causing apparent thinning of medial cortex of right femur and lateral cortex of left femur.

fact, similar changes in signal may be seen with nonneoplastic conditions, such as edema, radiation myositis, myositis ossificans, and trauma (Fig. 41–21). In general, soft tissue invasion, permeation of cortex, ill-defined borders, heterogeneity of signal, and prolonged T_2 relaxation times suggest malignancy, whereas absence of these features implies a benign process (Fig. 41–22). Differentiation of benign and malignant tumors by T_1 and T_2 relaxation times has not been successful owing to the great overlap in values.[8, 9, 60] Rarely, tumor histology can be deduced from MR imaging signal characteristics. Lipomas and liposarcomas generally have high signal on T_1- and T_2-weighted sequences. Lipomas are well marginated and internally uniform except for fine septations caused by fibrous strands. Liposarcomas have mixed signal. Occasionally, a very poorly differentiated liposarcoma will have no fat characteristics

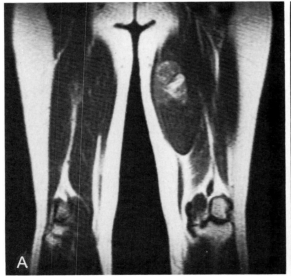

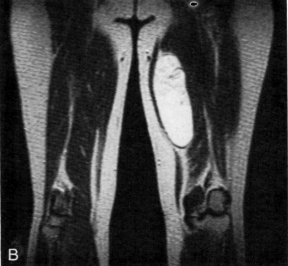

FIGURE 41–4. Liposarcoma. Coronal T_1 *(A)* and T_2 *(B)* contrast-weighted sequences demonstrating a heterogeneous mass with a short T_1, long T_2 component (fat) and long T_1, long T_2 component (high water content) within medial compartment of thigh.

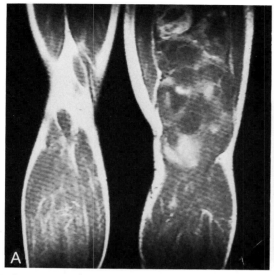
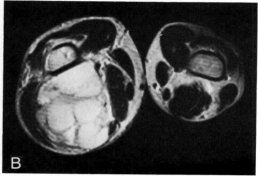

FIGURE 41–5. Liposarcoma. Coronal T_1 *(A)* and axial T_2 *(B)* contrast-weighted sequences demonstrating lobulated, heterogeneous mass, with short T_1 relaxation time regions within posterior fascial compartment of thigh and popliteal fossa, displacing but not encasing the popliteal artery. Note chemical shift artifact causing apparent thinning of lateral cortex of right femur and medial cortex of left femur.

and will be indistinguishable from other malignant soft tissue tumors (Figs. 41–2 to 41–6). Cysts are recognized by well-defined margins with low signal on T_1-weighted images and high signal on T_2-weighted images (see Fig. 41–37). Aneurysmal bone cysts have regions of hemorrhage with short T_1 relaxation time, internal septations, and characteristic fluid-fluid levels[61] (Fig. 41–16). Hypervascular tumors and arteriovenous malformations may contrast

with surrounding normal structures owing to MR imaging flow effects, which can be enhanced with GRE sequences.[62] Hemophilic pseudotumors demonstrate areas of hemorrhage of varying age[63] (Fig. 41–17). Bone and soft tissue neoplasms arising from hyaline cartilage have a distinctive appearance of homogeneous high signal intensity in a defined lobulated configuration on T_2 contrast-weighted images[64] (Fig. 41–18). Soft tissue hemangiomas have

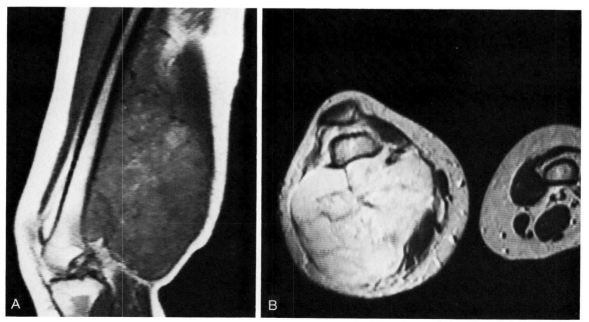

FIGURE 41–6. Poorly differentiated liposarcoma. Sagittal T_1 *(A)* and axial T_2 *(B)* contrast-weighted sequences of distal thigh demonstrating mass of posterior thigh and popliteal fossa that encases popliteal artery and vein and spares marrow and knee joint.

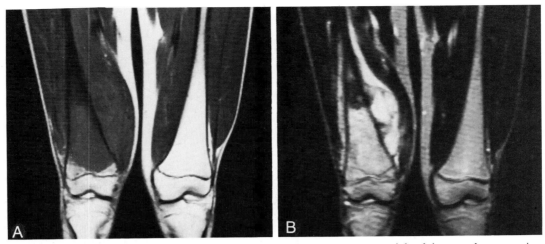

FIGURE 41–7. Osteogenic sarcoma. Coronal T_1 *(A)* and T_2 *(B)* contrast-weighted images demonstrating marrow replacement, muscle invasion, and mass effect.

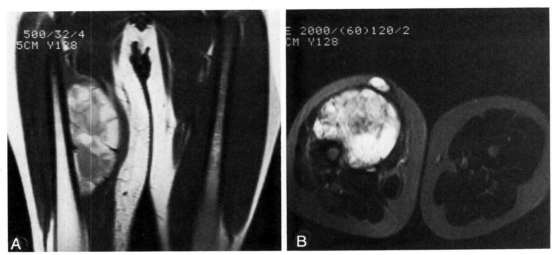

FIGURE 41–8. Fibrosarcoma. Coronal T_1 *(A)* and axial T_2 *(B)* contrast-weighted images demonstrate a heterogeneous mass with short T_1 relaxation time regions similar to the liposarcoma. Mass is in the anterior compartment of thigh and is similar to the liposarcoma. Note sparing of marrow and localized seeding of adipose tissue by tumor.

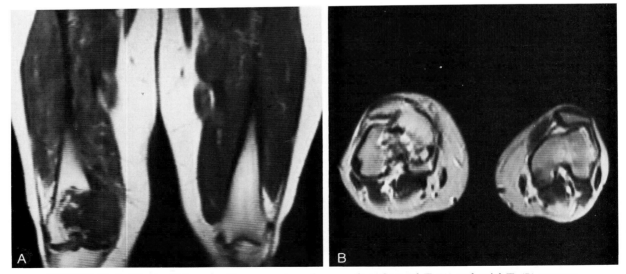

FIGURE 41–9. Giant cell tumor with sarcomatous degeneration. Coronal T_1 *(A)* and axial T_2 *(B)* contrast-weighted sequences demonstrating marrow replacement, cortical breakthrough, and muscle invasion by mass originating near distal growth plate of femur.

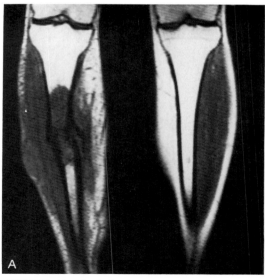

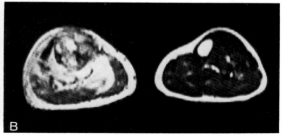

FIGURE 41–10. Ewing's tumor. Coronal T_1 *(A)* and axial T_2 *(B)* contrast-weighted images demonstrating marrow replacement, cortical breakthrough, muscle invasion, and pathologic fracture.

FIGURE 41–11. Fibromatosis. T_2 contrast-weighted sequences, 2000/60 *(A)* and 2000/120 *(B),* demonstrating plexiform masses invading adipose tissue and muscle of the arm.

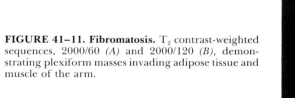

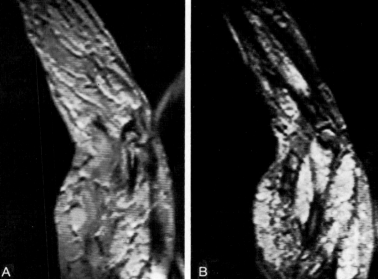

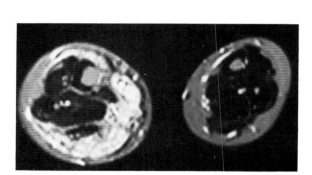

FIGURE 41–12. Neurofibromatosis. Axial T_2 contrast-weighted sequence demonstrating large mass infiltrating muscle and adipose tissue of thigh and sparing bone marrow.

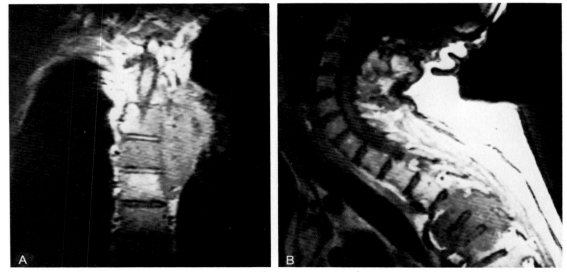

FIGURE 41–13. Bronchogenic carcinoma. Coronal *(A)* and sagittal *(B)* T_1 contrast-weighted sequences demonstrating direct invasion of thoracic spine by bronchogenic carcinoma, with characteristic sparing of the disk by invading tumor, replacement of marrow by tumor, and extension into multiple neural foramina.

a high-signal septated-striated configuration on T_2 contrast-weighted images, with peripheral areas of high signal on T_1 contrast-weighted images and absence of flow-related phenomena.[65] The intraosseous portion of vertebral hemangiomas has high signal intensity on both T_1 and T_2 contrast-weighted images.[66]

MR imaging is useful for following patients after therapy. Nonferromagnetic prostheses, fixation devices, and clips generally result in little artifact on MR images compared with CT,[5, 7] making MR imaging superior to CT for evaluation of patients in the postoperative period (Fig. 41–18). Radiation ef-

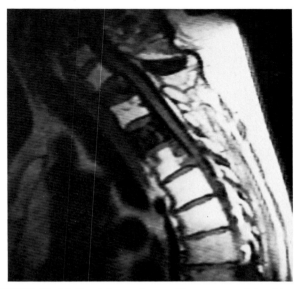

FIGURE 41–14. Prostate carcinoma. T_1 contrast-weighted image demonstrating multiple metastases to thoracic vertebral bodies and a thoracic spinous process with cord compression.

fects upon the marrow following therapy can be demonstrated by MR imaging.[67, 68] Shortening of T_1 relaxation time, presumably due to replacement of hematopoietic marrow by adipose tissue, is seen 2 months to 10 years following an absorbed dose greater than 401 Gy. Residual tumor is distinguished from post-therapy marrow in adults because of the prolonged T_1 relaxation time of tumor.[67] Differentiation between tumor and fibrosis following therapy is sometimes possible because of the low signal of fibrosis on both T_1 and T_2-weighted images.[6, 69] However, in the early stages of fibrotic reactions or in radiation-induced inflammation, relatively high signal may be observed, mimicking residual or recurrent tumor. High signal present 1 or more years after surgery without adjuvant radiation therapy indicates active tumor.[69]

MARROW DISORDERS

MR imaging has three important advantages in imaging diseases of bone marrow. First, inherent contrast between normal marrow components and pathologic processes is great. Second, there are negligible reconstruction artifacts from cortical bone. Third, true coronal and sagittal images can be obtained, allowing evaluation of the longitudinal extent of disease.

NORMAL BONE MARROW

Bone marrow is a dynamic organ that changes with time, so familiarity with the normal MR imaging appearance of marrow at various stages in life is mandatory. Marrow consists of varying proportions

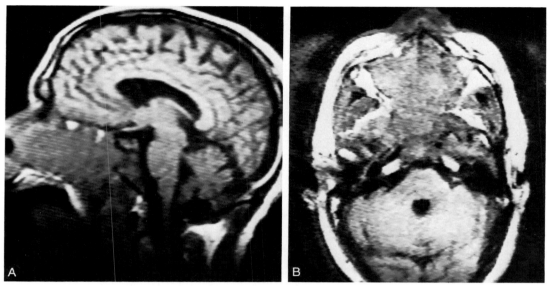

FIGURE 41–15. Rhabdomyosarcoma. Axial *(A)* and sagittal *(B)* T_1 contrast-weighted images demonstrating large nasopharyngeal mass with complete replacement of clival marrow by tumor and loss of bony cortex of anterior aspect of clivus.

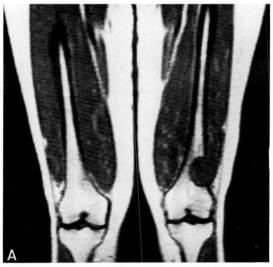

FIGURE 41–16. Aneurysmal bone cyst. Coronal T_1 *(A)*, axial T_1 *(B)*, and axial T_2 *(C)* contrast-weighted sequences demonstrate a cystic mass with prolonged T_2 relaxation time. Note the relatively short T_1 relaxation time compared with that of most fluids, suggesting methemoglobin or other dilute protein solution.

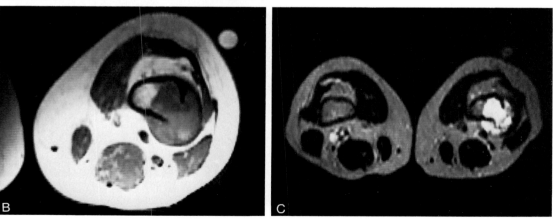

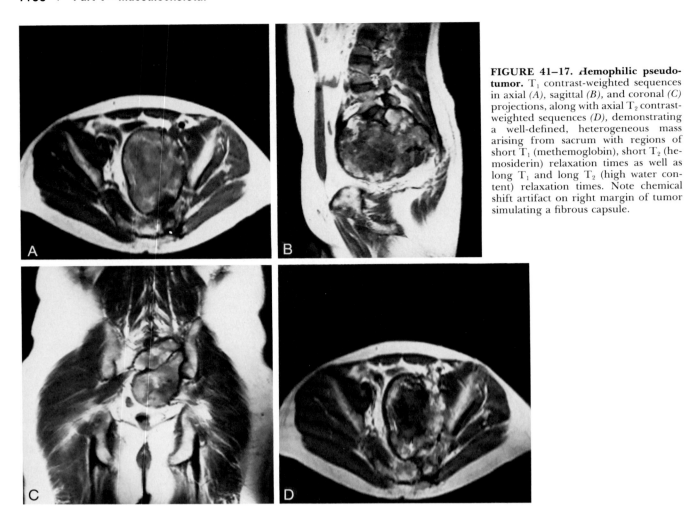

FIGURE 41–17. Hemophilic pseudo-tumor. T_1 contrast-weighted sequences in axial *(A)*, sagittal *(B)*, and coronal *(C)* projections, along with axial T_2 contrast-weighted sequences *(D)*, demonstrating a well-defined, heterogeneous mass arising from sacrum with regions of short T_1 (methemoglobin), short T_2 (hemosiderin) relaxation times as well as long T_1 and long T_2 (high water content) relaxation times. Note chemical shift artifact on right margin of tumor simulating a fibrous capsule.

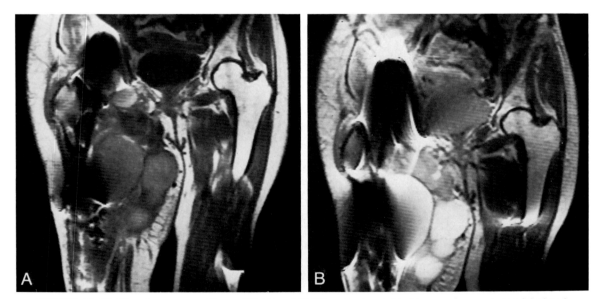

FIGURE 41–18. Chondrosarcoma. Coronal T_1 *(A)* and T_2 *(B)* contrast-weighted images demonstrate a lobulated mass invading thigh with intermediate T_1 and long T_2 relaxation time. Metal artifact from intramedullary rod obscured the mass on CT to a greater degree than on MR image.

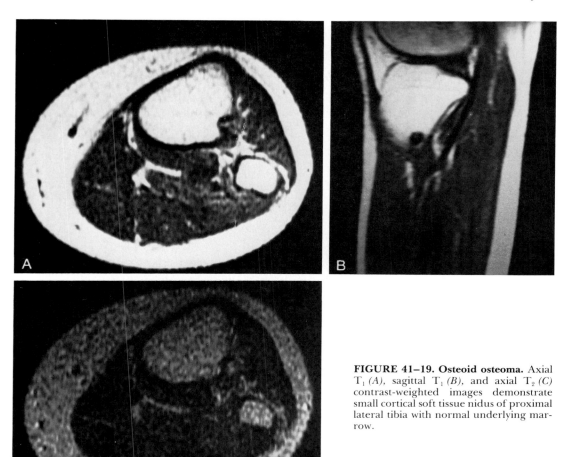

FIGURE 41–19. Osteoid osteoma. Axial T_1 *(A)*, sagittal T_1 *(B)*, and axial T_2 *(C)* contrast-weighted images demonstrate small cortical soft tissue nidus of proximal lateral tibia with normal underlying marrow.

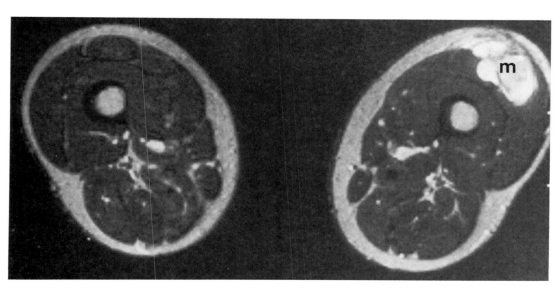

FIGURE 41–20. Synovial cell sarcoma. Axial T_2 weighted, spin echo. A lobulated, well-defined soft tissue mass of high signal intensity (m) involves the quadriceps musculature and adjacent subcutaneous fat.

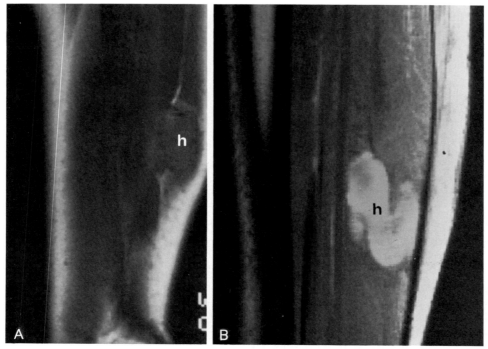

FIGURE 41–21. Calf hematoma (h) following motor vehicle accident. Coronal T_1 *(A)* and T_2 *(B)* contrast-weighted images, spin echo.

of hematopoietic tissue (red marrow), adipose tissue (yellow marrow), and trabecular bone.[70–72] The MR imaging characteristics of these components are very different. Bone has very low signal on T_1 and T_2 contrast-weighted images owing to its low mobile proton density. Adipose tissue (short T_1, long T_2) has high signal on T_1 and T_2 contrast-weighted images. Hematopoietic tissue (intermediate T_1 and T_2) has intermediate signal on T_1 and T_2 contrast-weighted images. The resultant MR imaging appearance of marrow is the summation of signal from the adipose tissue, hematopoietic tissue, and bone. Magnetic sus-

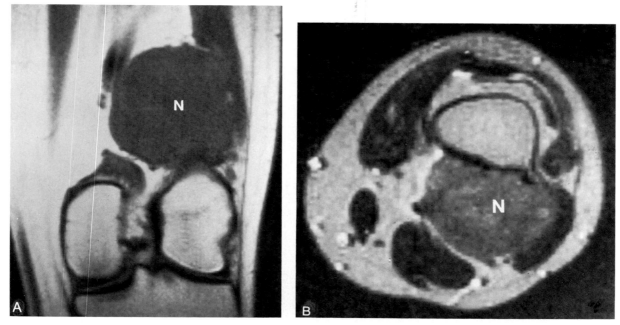

FIGURE 41–22. Benign spindle cell tumor. Coronal T_1 *(A)* and axial T_2 *(B)* contrast-weighted images, spin echo. A well-defined mass (N) of relatively low signal intensity on both pulse sequences is evident posterior to the distal femur.

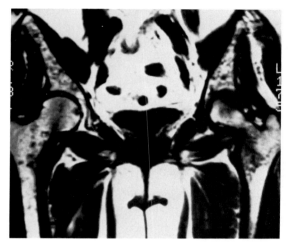

FIGURE 41–23. Chronic microcytic anemia mimicking myeloma. Coronal T_1 contrast-weighted image of pelvis and proximal femurs demonstrating focal areas of red marrow in this elderly woman. Two marrow biopsies showed no malignancy.

ceptibility effects and partial volume effects due to the relatively small dimensions of the marrow cavity[34, 54, 70] also influence the images.

At birth, functioning hematopoietic tissue is widely distributed throughout the skeleton. With increasing age, there is progressive involution of hematopoietic tissue with fatty replacement. Involution begins first in the most peripheral skeleton and progresses centrally. Within the long bones, involution of hematopoietic tissue begins first in the diaphyses and epiphyses, with relative preservation of metaphyseal hematopoiesis. At the end of adolescence, active hematopoietic tissue remains in the proximal metaphyses of the femur and humerus as well as in the vertebral bodies, sternum, ribs, and skull. With further aging, there is continued involution of hemato-

poietic tissue. The residual red marrow may simulate pathology, particularly in the femoral metaphysis;[34, 52, 54] however, residual hematopoietic tissue is usually symmetric, and bone scans are normal.[54] Islands of focal fatty replacement are seen with increasing age and are particularly evident in vertebral marrow.

MALIGNANT INFILTRATION

MR imaging is a sensitive method for detection of focal and diffuse neoplastic infiltration of bone marrow[10, 34, 35, 51, 68, 73–75] and is increasingly used for staging of hematopoietic and neoplastic disorders.[52] Replacement of the normal marrow adipose tissue by tumor cells results in low signal intensity on T_1 contrast-weighted images (Figs. 41–6 to 41–8 and 41–11). The effect upon signal intensity in T_2 contrast-weighted sequences is variable. A variety of processes, including osteomyelitis, ischemia, hyperplastic anemias, and marrow packing disorders, may have signal characteristics similar to those of neoplastic disorders (Fig. 41–23); hence MR imaging must be interpreted in light of the morphology of the lesion or lesions and the clinical setting.[68] However, bone islands, healed fractures, and areas of fibrosis or sclerosis that have low mobile proton density and short T_2 relaxation time can be differentiated from tumor, infection, and edema—processes with relatively high proton density and long T_2 relaxation time.[52]

Metastasis and primary bone tumors tend to be focal lesions, whereas leukemias tend to be patchy and diffuse. Myeloma and lymphoma may be either focal or diffuse (Fig. 41–24). Malignant processes of marrow tend to involve areas of active hematopoiesis, that is, red marrow.[52, 68, 75] In highly selected groups of patients with myeloma (30 patients) or other malignancy with suspected bone metastasis (50 pa-

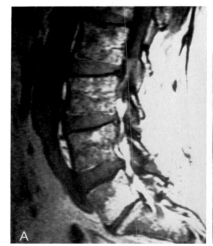
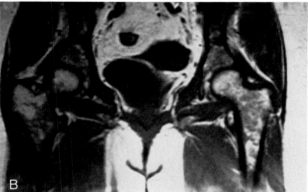

FIGURE 41–24. Multiple myeloma. Sagittal T_1 contrast-weighted image of the spine (A) and coronal T_1 contrast-weighted image of proximal femurs (B) in different patients demonstrate replacement of normal yellow marrow by myeloma.

tients), MR imaging resulted in no false-positive or false-negative interpretations.[34] Radionuclide imaging resulted in an 80 per cent false-negative rate for myeloma and a 20 per cent false-positive rate for nonmyelomatous malignancies.[34] The improved sensitivity of MR imaging for detection of marrow involvement should have great clinical impact upon staging and therapy of myeloma, lymphoma, and other secondary marrow neoplasms.

MR imaging is useful in the diagnosis and monitoring of leukemias. It has even been suggested that MR imaging may be more sensitive to diffuse bone marrow abnormalities than bone marrow aspiration because of the problems of sampling.[73] T_1 relaxation times of marrow of children with newly diagnosed, untreated acute lymphoblastic leukemia (ALL) are significantly longer than those of normal marrow. The marrow of children with ALL in relapse has intermediate values of T_1, while the T_1 relaxation times in children with ALL in remission have short T_1 comparable to normal control subjects.[73] No consistent change in appearance of marrow on T_2-weighted sequences was noted following therapy.[73] T_1-weighted MR imaging is therefore an attractive method for noninvasive monitoring and staging of ALL.

Unusual patterns of red marrow hyperplasia in the setting of anemia may mimic myeloma, leukemia, and other infiltrative marrow processes (Fig. 41–23). Clinical data and sometimes biopsy are necessary for accurate evaluation.

AVASCULAR NECROSIS (AVN), LEGG-CALVÉ-PERTHES (LCP) DISEASE, AND OSTEOCHONDRITIS DISSECANS

The numerous causes and associations of AVN include corticosteroids, trauma, alcohol, sickle cell anemia, Gaucher's disease, and pancreatitis, among others.[76, 77] Serious sequelae result when epiphyses are affected, leading to deformity of the articular surface. Early detection of ischemia allows a variety of interventions that may prevent subsequent necrosis and articular deformity.[33, 78, 79] Although the value of surgical decompression is being debated, if it is to be effective, it must be performed prior to the development of deformity, making early diagnosis essential.[78–81]

MR imaging is more sensitive than plain film, radionuclide imaging, or CT for detection of early marrow necrosis.[26–33] Mitchell and colleagues[26, 28] found MR imaging to be significantly better than radionuclide bone scanning and CT for detection of AVN of the femoral head. Totty and associates[29] observed several patients with known or suspected hip necrosis who had abnormal MR findings but false-negative scintigrams. However, false-negative MR imaging examinations do occur. Three false-negative MR imaging studies in surgically proved AVN of the femoral head were observed in a large series of 110 hips.[31] The pathology of the false-negative examinations showed minimal marrow degeneration with maintenance of intramedullary lipid spaces. Plain films and radionuclide studies of these patients were also normal. Beltran and coworkers[82] also found MR imaging to be more sensitive than other imaging modalities but did report five cases of AVN of the femoral head with normal MR imaging findings and positive radionuclide scan. MR imaging appears both sensitive and specific for detection of AVN of the carpal and tarsal bones.[83–85]

The evolution of MR imaging findings of AVN of the femoral head reflects the pathophysiology (Figs. 41–25 and 41–26). AVN of the femoral head usually first occurs in the superior, anterior, lateral aspect of the femoral head, where weight bearing occurs.[26, 28] Focal abnormalities in the anterosuperior aspect of the femoral head were observed in 96 per cent (54 of 56) of patients in one series.[26] Ninety-one per cent (51 of 56) of hips with AVN had a characteristic low-signal margin around the lesion. Furthermore, 80 per cent of cases of AVN of the femoral head (45 of 56) demonstrated a low-intensity margin with an

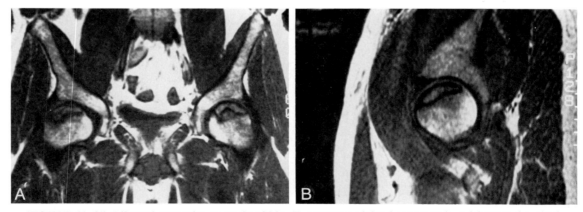

FIGURE 41–25. Bilateral avascular necrosis of hip. T_1 contrast-weighted sequence in axial (A) and sagittal (B) projection demonstrating characteristic signal abnormality in anterosuperior aspect of the femoral heads with surrounding low-signal line.

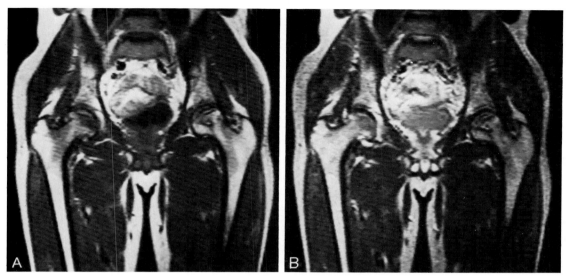

FIGURE 41–26. Bilateral avascular necrosis of the hip. T_1 *(A)* and T_2 *(B)* contrast-weighted images. *Right,* class B. *Left,* class D.

inner rim of high intensity on T_2 contrast-weighted images, a finding that may be pathognomonic for AVN.[26] The double line corresponds to a rim of peripheral bony sclerosis with an inner zone of granulation tissue.[26]

Four patterns of MR imaging findings have been recognized and correlated with radiographic, radionuclide, and clinical findings.[26] All have a low-signal outer ring on both T_1 and T_2 contrast-weighted images, corresponding to the sclerotic rim. In the center of class A lesions, there is high signal on T_1 images and intermediate signal on T_2 images. These lesions are found predominantly in patients with early AVN, and the MR imaging findings reflect preservation of normal fat signal within the marrow with a sclerotic reactive margin. Class B (high signal on T_1 and T_2 images) and class C (low signal on T_1 images and high signal on T_2 images) do not correlate well with radiographic or clinical findings. However, in a cohort with sickle cell anemia and bone marrow infarction, the pattern of low signal on T_1 and bright signal on T_2 contrast-weighted images correlated well with pain.[86] Class B and class C lesions are thought to represent a heterogeneous group of lesions with variable amounts of inflammation, hemorrhage, hyperemia, lipid, and fibrous tissue. Class D signal characteristics (low signal on T_1 and T_2 images) correspond to advanced AVN by clinical and radiographic criteria. Deformation of the articular surface may be seen. The MR imaging findings reflect fibrosis and compression of trabecular bone. Joint effusions produce a crescent of high signal intensity on T_2-weighted images[87] and are seen in the majority of cases of AVN.[27]

Mitchell and colleagues[88] made the intriguing observation that patients with AVN had early conversion of hematopoietic marrow to fatty marrow within the intertrochanteric region of the femur compared with control subjects. In normal subjects, no women and 17 per cent of men younger than 50 years had fatty marrow in the intertrochanteric region, compared with 54 per cent of women and 79 per cent of men with AVN, therefore possibly providing a marker for individuals at increased risk of developing AVN.

Coleman and associates[33] confirmed previous findings that MR imaging is more sensitive than plain radiography, CT, or radionuclide bone scanning in identifying early AVN and that early conversion to fatty marrow is a useful marker for AVN. More important, they observed that core decompression stopped progression of AVN in 17 of 18 hips with abnormal MR imaging findings but negative plain film studies of AVN.

We have found MR imaging valuable in the evaluation of AVN of the femoral condyles (Figs. 41–27 and 41–28), lunate (Fig. 41–29), medial malleolus (Fig. 41–30), and radial head (see Fig. 41–47). In addition, we have observed atypical patterns in biopsy-proven AVN (see Figs. 41–28 and 41–44).

In LCP disease, MR imaging is a useful noninvasive method for evaluating articular cartilage, the shape of the femoral head, and containment of the femoral head within the acetabulum without use of ionizing radiation.[44, 89, 90] Staging of LCP disease is critical for determining if and what surgical intervention is necessary.[44, 91] In the past, some authors have recommended hip arthrography for accurate staging of incompletely ossified hips. MR imaging should supplant arthrography for this purpose because of its ability to image cartilaginous portions of the hip noninvasively. Although radionuclide imaging can detect LCP disease, its poor spatial resolution does not permit staging. Plain films are insensitive.

Osteochondritis dissecans, presumably a subset of AVN, is well delineated by MR imaging,[92] and the

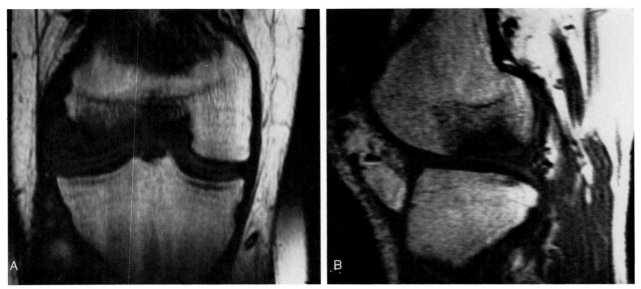

FIGURE 41–27. Avascular necrosis of lateral femoral condyle. Coronal (A) and sagittal (B) T₁ contrast-weighted images demonstrate deformity and decreased signal of subchondral marrow.

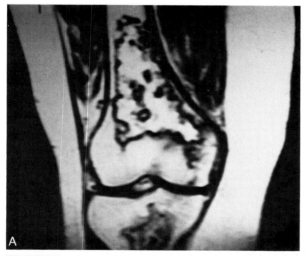

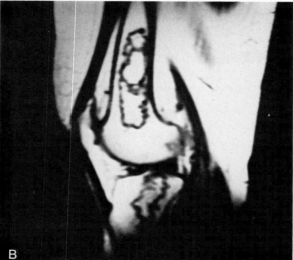

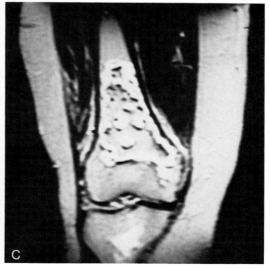

FIGURE 41–28. Avascular necrosis of femoral metaphysis. Sagittal (A) and coronal (B) T₁ and coronal T₂ (C) contrast-weighted images demonstrating class A pattern in female patient with Crohn's disease taking prednisone and experiencing recent onset of knee pain. Note that the line delineating the area of necrosis has the MR characteristics of high water content and not sclerosis or fibrosis. MR also demonstrated AVN of femoral heads, although she had no hip pain.

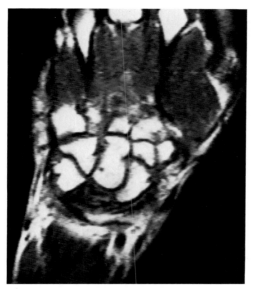

FIGURE 41–29. Avascular necrosis of lunate. T_1 contrast-weighted image demonstrating decreased signal of lunate marrow.

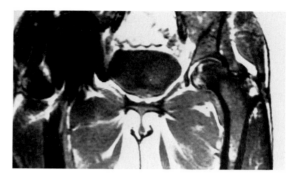

FIGURE 41–31. Sickle cell anemia. Coronal T_1 contrast-weighted image demonstrating hyperplastic marrow with negligible yellow marrow, medullary bone infarction of left femur, and right hip arthroplasty.

stability of the fragment can be accurately assessed. Fluid between fragment and parent bone and discontinuity of hyaline cartilage overlying the fragment indicate a loose fragment that requires surgical removal or internal fixation.[92]

HYPERPLASTIC AND APLASTIC ANEMIAS

Expansion of the hematopoietic system in response to chronic anemia may be diffuse throughout the skeleton or found in focal deposits. Increased hematopoiesis results in areas of decreased signal intensity of marrow on T_1 and variable signal on T_2 contrast-weighted images, compared with images in normal individuals of the same age (Figs. 41–23 and 41–31). Hemosiderin deposition within marrow may cause marked loss of signal intensity owing to susceptibility effects.[86] Gradient-refocused images are more sensitive than SE images for detection of hemosiderin deposition.[93] Marrow infarction is a common sequela of sickle cell anemia and is discussed in detail in the previous section. MR imaging may enable the differentiation of patients undergoing acute infarctive crisis from patients with old infarcts experiencing pain from other causes.[86]

The MR imaging findings of the hyperplastic anemias are mimicked by other diffuse abnormalities of marrow, including neoplasm, infection, and metabolic disorders; hence, clinical correlation is important.

Aplastic anemias by definition have a paucity of hematopoietic tissue. Replacement by fat results in higher marrow signal than normal on T_1 contrast-weighted images.[52, 68] In myelofibrosis, hematopoietic

FIGURE 41–30. Presumed necrosis of medial malleolus. Coronal T_1 *(A)* and T_2 *(B)* contrast-weighted images demonstrate sharp low-signal line on both images, with prolongation of T_1 and T_2 relaxation times of marrow of malleolus.

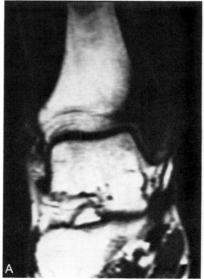
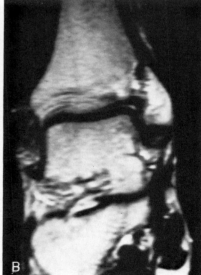

tissue is replaced by fat and fibrous tissue,[52, 68] resulting in areas of high signal on both T_1- and T_2-weighted images and low signal on both T_1- and T_2-weighted images, respectively.

GAUCHER'S DISEASE

Gaucher's disease, a metabolic disorder characterized by deposition of glucocerebrosides within various organs, including bone marrow, has been studied by MR imaging.[94, 95] Features of this disease include widening of the medullary cavity, coarsening and reduction of trabecular bone, undertubulation of long bones, and thinning of cortical bone. The Erlenmeyer flask appearance characteristic of marrow packing disorders may be observed by MR imaging in patients with Gaucher's disease[94] (Figs. 41–32 to 41–34).

In patients with Gaucher's disease, there is decreased signal from femoral and tibial diaphyseal and metaphyseal marrow, compared with normal patients, owing to the longer T_1 and shorter T_2 relaxation times[94, 95] of the abnormal marrow. The short T_2 relaxation time helps differentiate Gaucher's disease from edematous processes of marrow, such as infection or neoplasm. Patients with Gaucher's disease are at high risk for bone infarctions in diaphyseal, metaphyseal, and epiphyseal regions. As in sickle cell anemia, acute crisis is seen on MR imaging as areas of prolonged T_1 and T_2 relaxation time, resembling osteomyelitis. The replacement of normal marrow by glucocerebrosides limits detection of early AVN of the femoral heads on T_1 contrast-weighted sequences, as both processes may have low intensity.

TRANSIENT OSTEOPOROSIS (TP)

TP is a poorly understood, self-limited disorder most commonly affecting the femoral heads of pregnant women and middle-aged men.[96, 97] MR imaging demonstrates ill-defined decreased signal on T_1 contrast-weighted images and matching increased signal on T_2 contrast-weighted images, presumably representing transient bone marrow edema. Absence of signal abnormality in adjacent soft tissues helps differentiate TP from infection or neoplasm. The ill-defined borders seen in TP are atypical of AVN.

JOINT DISORDERS

MR imaging has proved to be very useful in the evaluation of the knee, shoulder, and temporomandibular joint, and separate chapters address each joint. In this chapter, we discuss other specific areas in which MR imaging shows particular utility.

CONGENITAL DISLOCATION OF THE HIP (CDH)

Congenital hip dislocation (CDH) is a common disorder (13 of 1000) of neonates thought to be due to lax ligamentous structures of the hip.[98] Other factors, such as shape of the femoral head and acetabulum, position of the labrum, and iliopsoas tendon invagination of the capsule, also contribute to the disorder.[99] Diagnosis is by physical examination and plain film radiography. Incomplete ossification of the femoral head and acetabulum, however, limits

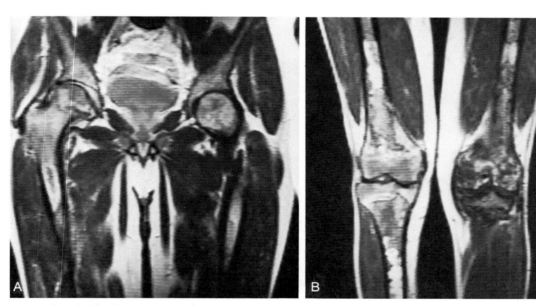

FIGURE 41–32. Gaucher's disease. Proton density–weighted image of hips *(A)* and T_1 contrast-weighted image of knees *(B)* demonstrating AVN of right femoral head, with joint effusion, multiple bone infarcts, and marrow replacement by Gaucher's cells.

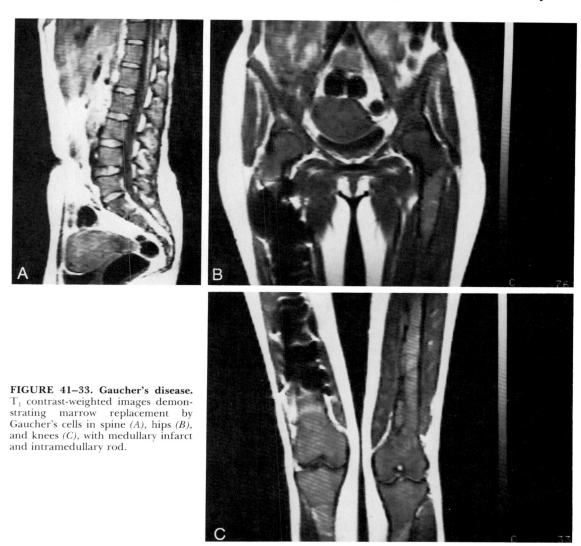

FIGURE 41–33. Gaucher's disease. T_1 contrast-weighted images demonstrating marrow replacement by Gaucher's cells in spine *(A)*, hips *(B)*, and knees *(C)*, with medullary infarct and intramedullary rod.

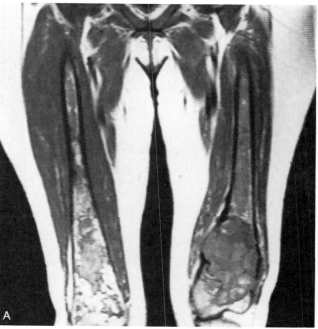

FIGURE 41–34. Gaucher's disease. Coronal T_1 *(A)* and axial T_2 *(B)* contrast-weighted images demonstrating marrow replacement, medullary infarction, and tumorous collection of Gaucher's cells that has broken through cortex.

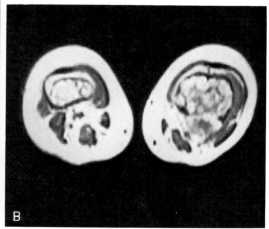

plain film assessment of the adequacy of reduction, sometimes requiring use of arthrography.[98] MR imaging enables direct visualization of the cartilaginous and osseous portions of the hip in coronal and axial projections, making possible the accurate assessment of the hip before and after reduction without the use of ionizing radiation or intraarticular contrast.[37, 43, 44, 99] Imaging can be performed with the patient in a plaster cast without significant image degradation. Rapid imaging of hips in neonates is performed using very short TR and TE sequences, small FOV, a small number of phase-encoding steps, and a small number of repetitions per phase-encoding step.

INFLAMMATORY ARTHRITIDES

There is no established role for MR imaging in the routine evaluation of inflammatory arthritides. However, the ability of MR imaging to detect early arthritic changes suggests an increasing role in the future as a sensitive and objective method for monitoring therapy.[47, 48] MR imaging demonstrates joint and tendon sheath effusions, hyaline and fibrocartilage destruction, and pannus better than plain radiography[47] (Fig. 41–35). Early identification of the changes of inflammatory arthritis made possible by MR imaging may lead to an earlier alteration in the medical regimen to minimize destruction.[46–48]

The MR imaging appearance can be predicted from the pathophysiology.[36, 37, 45–50] Effusions produce little signal on T_1 contrast-weighted images and high signal on T_2-weighted images (Fig. 41–36). Inflamed, edematous synovium generally has low signal intensity on T_1 and relatively high signal on

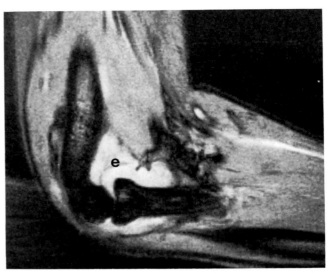

FIGURE 41–36. Monoarticular synovitis of uncertain etiology. Sagittal GRASS with 15-degree flip angle. A nonspecific high signal intensity effusion (e) is present with the elbow joint.

T_2 contrast-weighted images; however, it may have low signal on both T_1 and T_2 contrast-weighted images, presumably because of hemosiderin deposition.[46, 47] Destruction of the hyaline cartilage may be seen as the disappearance of the high-signal line on T_1-weighted images. Early marginal erosions are evident on T_1-weighted images by replacement of the normal marrow signal by the low signal of the eroding edematous pannus.

MR imaging is particularly valuable for evaluation of rheumatoid cervical spine disease: odontoid and facet erosions, synovial hypertrophy, subluxation,

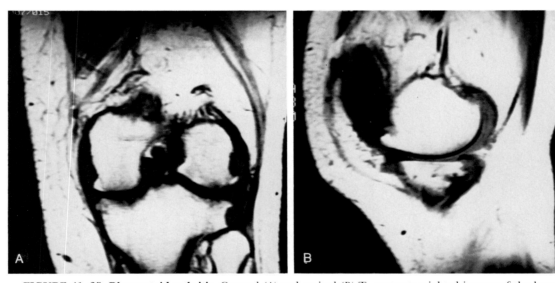

FIGURE 41–35. Rheumatoid arthritis. Coronal *(A)* and sagittal *(B)* T_1 contrast-weighted images of the knee demonstrating marginal erosions, joint effusion, thinning of articular cartilage, and secondary degenerative changes.

craniovertebral settling, and resultant cord compression.[50]

MISCELLANEOUS JOINT DISORDERS

Pigmented villonodular synovitis (PVNS) may produce a tumor mass of either high or low signal on T_2 contrast-weighted images. It may destroy areas of cartilage and underlying bone. Narrowing and irregularity of hyaline cartilage and fibrocartilage resulting from degenerative and traumatic processes can be visualized with MR imaging.[37] MR imaging may be useful in the evaluation of patients with transient synovitis of the hip. Patients with the clinical diagnosis of transient synovitis have normal signal within the epiphyseal marrow, differentiating transient synovitis from LCP disease, osteomyelitis, fracture, and dislocation.[44] Acute tenosynovitis and chronic tendinitis have been examined with MR imaging.[100] Fluid identified by its long T_1 and T_2 relaxation times distends tendon sheaths in tenosynovitis. Synovial cysts (Fig. 41–37), enlarged bursae (Fig. 41–38), and meniscal cysts are well demonstrated on MR imaging, enabling differentiation from other bone and soft tissue masses.[101]

THE WRIST

High resolution and soft tissue contrast, combined with flexibility of imaging plane, make MR imaging useful for imaging the wrist.[36, 84, 102] Ganglion cysts, carpal fractures, tendon ruptures, arteriovenous malformations, AVN (Fig. 41–29), and rheumatoid arthritis have been delineated with MR imaging. Detailed imaging of the carpal tunnel has been described.[36, 84, 102] MR imaging observations in patients with carpal tunnel syndrome (CTS) include swelling, thinning of the median nerve and/or edema of the median nerve (bright signal on T_2-weighted images), thickening of tendon sheaths, postoperative scarring, and a fibrolipoma.[84, 102] MR imaging is capable of delineating several normal variants, including persistent median artery and anomalous lumbrical muscles within the tunnel,[102] which may contribute

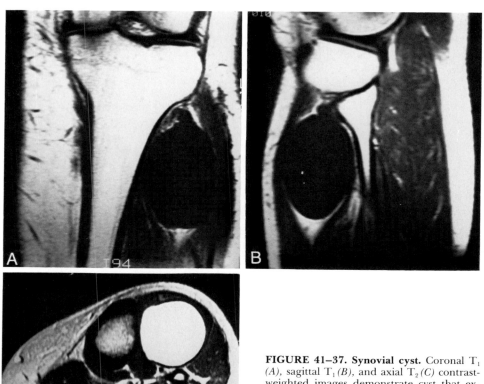

FIGURE 41–37. Synovial cyst. Coronal T_1 *(A),* sagittal T_1 *(B),* and axial T_2 *(C)* contrast-weighted images demonstrate cyst that extends into tibiofibular joint.

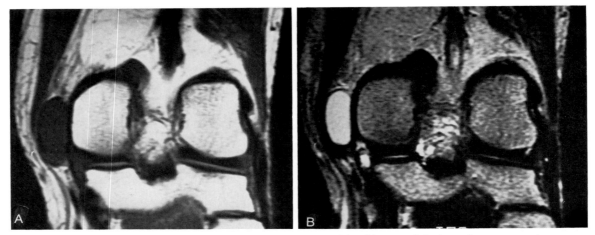

FIGURE 41–38. Bursitis. Coronal $T_1 (A)$ and $T_2 (B)$ contrast-weighted images of the knee demonstrate a bursa distended with fluid.

to the development of CTS. The detailed anatomic information should be useful for medical and surgical management of CTS.

THE ANKLE

MR imaging has been used to reveal tears of the talocalcaneal and calcaneofibular ligaments, directly visualizing trapping of the calcaneofibular ligament in the subtalar joint.[85] The cartilage of the tibiotalar joint was well evaluated for traumatic, inflammatory, and degenerative disorders. MR imaging detected unsuspected osteochondral fractures.[85] Marrow abnormalities adjacent to the ankle joint, such as AVN, are well demonstrated by MR imaging (Fig. 41–30).

INFECTION

Clinical and experimental studies have shown that MR imaging is valuable for the evaluation of musculoskeletal infections.[19–25] MR imaging is at least as sensitive as gallium-67 citrate and technetium-99m methylene diphosphonate imaging for detection of osteomyelitis[20, 22–25] and more sensitive for detection of soft tissue infections without associated osteomyelitis.[22–23] Indium-labeled leukocyte imaging may be more sensitive than MR imaging but is limited by complicated radiopharmaceutical preparation, high radiation dose, and prolonged study duration. CT appears superior to MR imaging for detection of air bubbles,[40] an important finding in the diagnosis of abscess.

The advantage of MR imaging over radionuclide imaging is its higher spatial resolution, enabling differentiation among soft tissue cellulitis, soft tissue abscess, and osteomyelitis. The greatest utility of MR imaging in our clinical practice is the evaluation of the diabetic foot, in which the MR imaging scan supplants the various radionuclide imaging examinations. MR imaging is useful in the assessment of regions adjacent to open growth plates, where the normal high activity on technetium-diphosphonate bone scan may obscure abnormalities.[20] MR imaging is useful when recent surgery or fracture decreases the utility of radionuclide imaging.[103, 104]

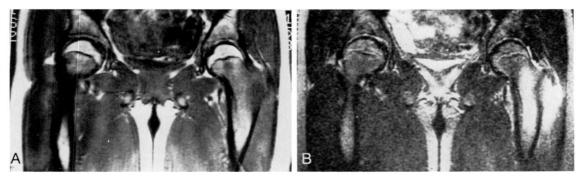

FIGURE 41–39. Acute osteomyelitis. Coronal $T_1 (A)$ and $T_2 (B)$ contrast-weighted images demonstrate diffuse edema within femoral metaphyseal marrow and surrounding muscle. No abnormality was evident on T_1 contrast-weighted images (A) owing to the similar T_1 relaxation times and spin densities of normal and infected red marrow. Bone biopsy revealed *Staphylococcus aureus*.

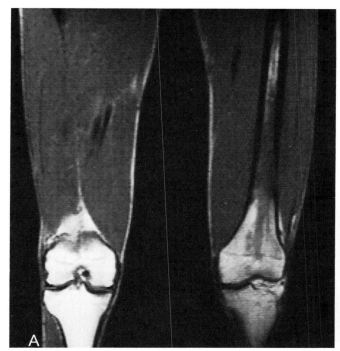

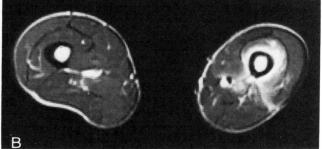

FIGURE 41–40. Acute osteomyelitis. T_1 contrast-weighted coronal *(A)* and T_2 axial *(B)* images demonstrate replacement of normal fat signal of femoral metaphyseal marrow by inflammatory process and diffuse edema within surrounding muscle.

T_1 and T_2 relaxation times of infected soft tissue and marrow increase as a result of the edema and inflammatory response. Thus, areas of active inflammation or edema or both generally have low signal on T_1-weighted images and high signal on T_2 contrast-weighted images (Figs. 41–39 to 41–43). Although MR is relatively specific for osteomyelitis, an unusual case of AVN caused confusion (Fig. 41–44). Osteomyelitis can be differentiated from soft tissue infection without osteomyelitis, the latter having normal marrow signal[20, 21, 25] (Fig. 41–45). Soft tissue abscess appears as a well-defined area of long T_1 and long T_2 relaxation times, compared with an ill-defined area of signal abnormality seen in cellulitis (Figs. 41–45 and 41–46). Chronic infection with fibrosis may have low signal intensity on both T_1 and T_2 contrast-weighted images.[21]

After successful therapy, the signal within marrow slowly returns to its normal appearance over a period of months.[19] In some cases, marrow signal intensity will be greater than normal on T_1 contrast-weighted images owing to lack of hematopoietic tissue in recovered marrow.[25] There is rapid resolution of the signal abnormality in soft tissues following successful therapy. Findings of osteomyelitis on MR imaging are not obscured by short-term antibiotic administration or leukopenia, as sometimes occurs with gallium imaging[19] and indium-labeled leukocyte imaging.

Spinal osteomyelitis can be detected by MR imaging with greater accuracy than by technetium diphosphonate imaging alone, and MR imaging is as accurate as combined gallium citrate and technetium diphosphonate imaging.[19] MR imaging yields positive findings early in the course of the illness, at approxi-

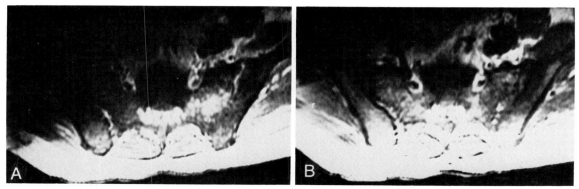

FIGURE 41–41. Osteomyelitis. T_2 contrast-weighted image *(A)* of sacrum demonstrates edematous, inflamed marrow on only one side of the sacroiliac joint, suggesting hematogenous spread instead of extension from the adjacent sacroiliac joint. T_1 contrast-weighted image *(B)* is normal.

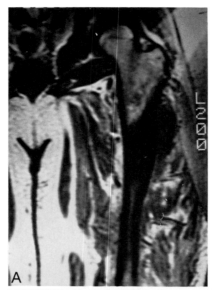

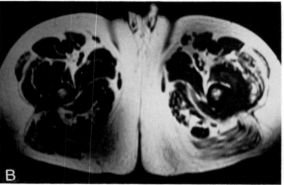

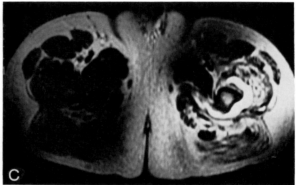

FIGURE 41–42. Chronic osteomyelitis. Coronal T_1 *(A)*, axial T_1 *(B)*, and axial T_2 *(C)* contrast-weighted images of femur demonstrate edematous marrow, abscess adjacent to bone, edematous adjacent muscle, and periosteal reaction.

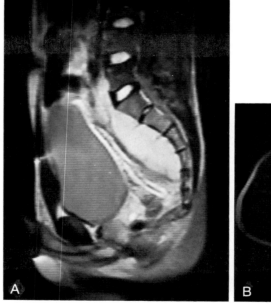

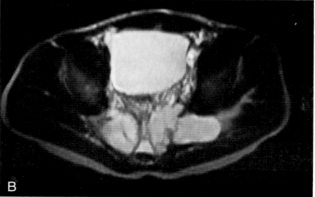

FIGURE 41–43. Pelvic abscess. Sagittal *(A)* and axial *(B)* T_2 contrast-weighted sequences demonstrating large abscess within retrorectal space, perirectal region, and greater sciatic notch.

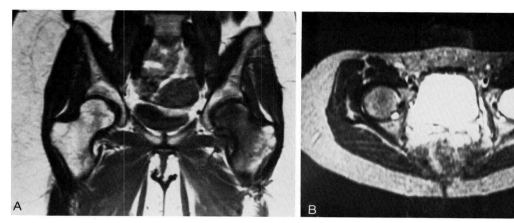

FIGURE 41–44. Unusual appearance of avascular necrosis mimicking osteomyelitis. Coronal T_1 *(A)* and axial T_2 *(B)* contrast-weighted images of proximal femurs demonstrating very high water content within epiphyseal and metaphyseal marrow of left femur, with small joint effusion, in 37-year-old woman with 1 month of worsening hip pain. Note absence of edema in adjacent muscle. Two biopsies demonstrated marked trabecular thickening and some necrotic, xanthomatous cells compatible with AVN. Cultures were negative.

mately the same time as does radionuclide scanning.[19] MR imaging enables assessment of the spinal canal in cases of vertebral osteomyelitis, a clear advantage over radionuclide scanning. The greater spatial resolution of MR imaging, compared with radionuclide imaging, provides greater specificity and more accu-

rate staging of the infection. Thecal sac, neural structures, and paravertebral regions can be evaluated in great detail. Nearly all (96 per cent) patients with spinal osteomyelitis have an abnormal adjacent disk, which helps to differentiate infection from malignancy, the latter rarely destroying disk. Signal

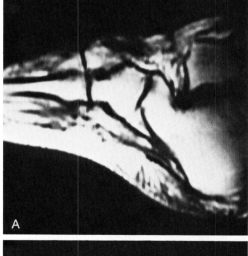

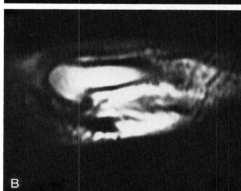

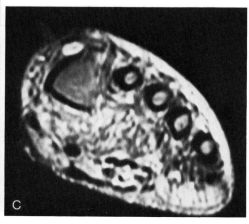

FIGURE 41–45. Cellulitis without osteomyelitis. Sagittal T_1 contrast-weighted image of the ankle *(A)* demonstrates normal calcaneal marrow in a diabetic with a chronic decubitus ulcer and cellulitis of the heel. Sagittal *(B)* T_1 and coronal *(C)* T_2 contrast-weighted images of the toes of this same patient demonstrate normal marrow of metatarsal bone adjacent to a soft tissue abscess characterized by a well-defined area of prolonged T_2 relaxation time. Radionuclide studies suggested osteomyelitis.

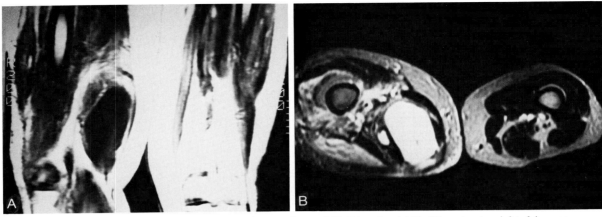

FIGURE 41–46. Soft tissue cellulitis and abscess. Coronal T_1 *(A)* and axial T_2 *(B)* contrast-weighted images of right femur demonstrating extensive multicompartmental cellulitis and large posterior compartment abscess without osteomyelitis.

changes similar to those of osteomyelitis are noted within vertebral bodies adjacent to disks treated with chymopapain.[19]

TRAUMA

There is little role for MR imaging of long bone trauma as yet. However, in certain instances, the high spatial and contrast resolution of MR imaging and its multiplanar capability are most useful (Fig. 41–47). MR imaging may be helpful in spine trauma, in which it is nearly as sensitive as CT in the detection of vertebral body fractures and enables evaluation of the ligamentous and neural elements.[105] MR imaging may be useful in differentiating benign from malignant vertebral compression fractures and in assessing neural impingement. Vertebrae with old, benign compression fractures have marrow signal similar to that of adjacent vertebral bodies.[52] Acute, benign compression fractures may be difficult to differentiate from pathologic fractures owing to the admixture of edematous tissue, hemorrhage, and marrow found in both situations. The natural evolution of MR imaging characteristics of healing, benign vertebral compression fractures needs to be further explored. Benign, discogenic sclerosis may result in false-positive diagnosis on radionuclide bone scan. However, the MR imaging appearance of low signal on both T_1 and T_2 contrast-weighted images adjacent to and parallel to the end plate is characteristic. Bandlike or focal areas of variable signal intensity are observed in vertebral marrow adjacent to degenerative disks on both T_1 and T_2 contrast-weighted images and are thought to result from varying

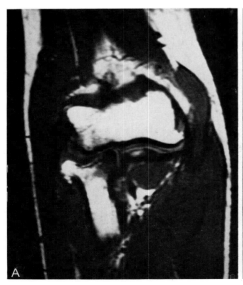
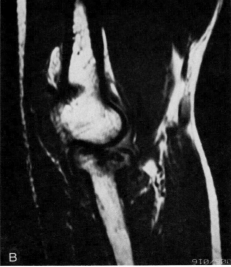

FIGURE 41–47. Radial head fracture with posttraumatic necrosis. Coronal *(A)* and sagittal *(B)* T_1 contrast-weighted images demonstrate posttraumatic deformity of radial head with resulting necrosis 6 months following the injury.

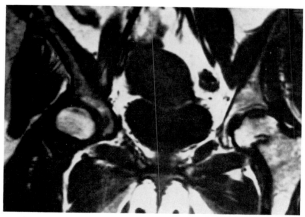

FIGURE 41–48. Incomplete subcapital stress fracture. Coronal T_1 contrast-weighted image in patient with bilateral hip pain demonstrates AVN and linear, low-signal region corresponding to an incomplete fracture.

amounts of fatty conversion of hematopoietic marrow, marrow edema, sclerosis or compression of trabecular bone, or fibrosis of marrow spaces.[106]

MR imaging of stress fractures has been described by several authors, with disparate findings.[15, 107, 108] Marrow may appear normal or may show extensive low-signal region on T_1 contrast-weighted images. The cortex may appear normal or disrupted on the images (Fig. 41–48). MR imaging may identify occult intraosseous fractures or microfractures about the knee, seen as a subchondral region of prolonged T_1 and T_2 relaxation times,[109] an important observation in symptomatic patients following an acute traumatic event with otherwise normal radiologic evaluation.

MR imaging is a valuable method for noninvasive imaging of tendon and ligament trauma.[100, 108] The low number of mobile protons within these structures results in minimal signal on both T_1 and T_2 images. Injury may cause swelling, thinning, or gross disruption of the tendon or ligament. Edema, inflammatory response, or hemorrhage, or any combination within tendon or ligament results in high signal on T_2-weighted images, contrasting strongly with surrounding normal tendon or ligament. Chronic and repetitive injuries to tendon and ligament cause thickening of the tendons, which is best appreciated by compar-

FIGURE 41–49. Soleus hematoma after motorcycle accident. Sagittal T_1 *(A)*, sagittal T_2 *(B)*, and axial T_2 *(C)* contrast-weighted images, spin echo. The well-marginated, lobulated mass (h) exhibits central low and peripheral high signal intensity on the T_1 contrast-weighted image and a more homogeneous high signal intensity on the T_2 contrast-weighted scans.

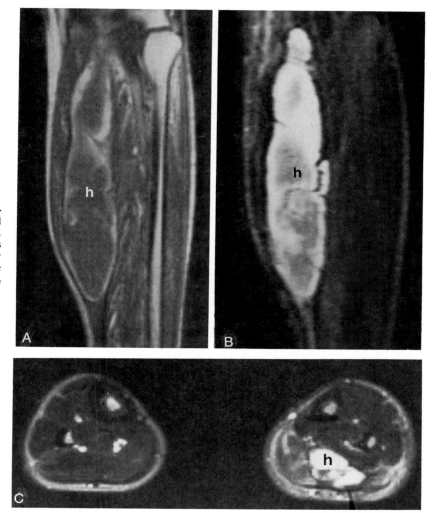

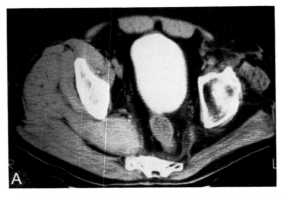

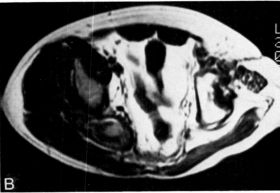

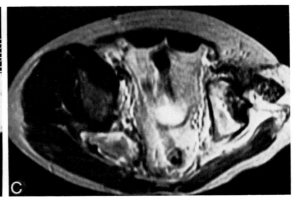

FIGURE 41–50. Disuse muscle atrophy and contralateral hematoma. CT *(A)*, axial T_1 *(B)* and T_2 *(C)* contrast-weighted images. The patient with amputated left leg at the hip joint noticed the right buttock mass, which showed high density on CT and was typical of hematoma on MR.

ison with the opposite side.[108] The Achilles tendon, patellar tendon, and cruciate ligaments are easily imaged. Smaller tendons require clever use of surface coils and imaging planes to obtain diagnostic information.

Muscles can be contused or lacerated, resulting in an admixture of muscle fiber, fluid of variable protein content, and hemorrhage. Detailed anatomic imaging of the muscles and adjacent anatomy is possible with T_1 contrast-weighted images in appropriate planes. In an acute situation, T_2 contrast-weighted images will accurately define the extent of edema and fluid collections. Posttraumatic rhabdomyolysis has been imaged with MR,[110] demonstrating prolongation of T_2 relaxation time. Hemorrhage has variable char-

acteristics, as discussed in Chapter 8. Subacute hematomas (>3 days) generally have a rim of high signal on T_1 contrast-weighted images[40] (Figs. 41–49 and 41–50). Early myositis ossificans appears as an area of long T_1 and long T_2 relaxation times before calcifications are visible on plain film (MW Ragozzino, R Chisin, and D Rosenthal, unpublished observations) (Fig. 41–51).

Trauma to the extremity may result in increased pressure within a closed fascial compartment due to edema and hemorrhage, which is detectable with MR imaging (Fig. 41–52). Early diagnosis and treatment are mandatory to minimize ischemic damage to the compartment itself and the extremity distal to the compartment. Compartment syndromes are often

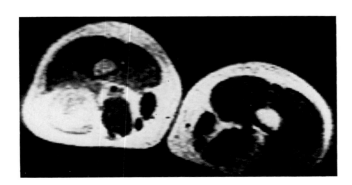

FIGURE 41–51. Myositis ossificans. Axial T_2 contrast-weighted image demonstrates marked T_2 prolongation and swelling in region of biceps femoris.

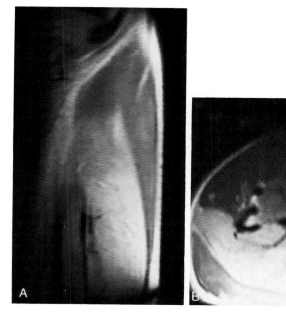

FIGURE 41–52. Compartment syndrome of deep compartment of calf. Sagittal *(A)* and axial *(B)* T_2 contrast-weighted images of calf demonstrating T_2 prolongation within calf confined to deep compartment.

difficult to diagnose on physical examination and may require invasive measurement of pressure. The volar compartment of the forearm and anterior compartment of the leg are most often affected. Although MR imaging and magnetic resonance spectroscopy (MRS) can demonstrate tissue changes in compartment syndromes,[111] we have not been able to quantify increases in pressure with MR imaging (MW Ragozzino and colleagues, unpublished observations).

Acute denervation or recent orthopedic surgical procedures may result in prolonged T_1 and T_2 relaxation times of affected muscles[38, 111] (MW Ragozzino, R Chisin, and D Rosenthal, unpublished observations). The chronic sequelae of trauma are well imaged with MR imaging.[108] Muscle atrophy is evident by asymmetry of muscle dimensions with variable degrees of fatty infiltration and edema (Figs. 41–50, 41–53, and 41–54). Scarred, fibrotic muscle has low signal intensity on both T_1 and T_2 contrast-weighted images.

Exercise results in transient (less than 1 hour) prolongation of T_1 and T_2 relaxation time and increased spin density of the affected skeletal muscle or muscles, with resultant changes in signal intensity on MR imaging.[112] These changes are due to increased extracellular and total water content of skeletal muscle. Conceivably, exercise-induced signal changes or those changes resulting from nonvoluntary muscle contractions could be confused with the above-mentioned pathologic conditions.

Trauma to subcutaneous adipose tissue is well visualized by MR imaging (Fig. 41–55). The short T_1 relaxation time of fat contrasts greatly with the long T_1 relaxation time of edematous tissue.

MISCELLANEOUS MUSCLE DISORDERS

Denervation of muscle results in atrophy of muscle, fatty infiltration, and edema[38, 108] (MW Ragozzino, R Chisin, and D Rosenthal, unpublished observations). Muscular dystrophy shows varying degrees of atrophy, pseudohypertrophy, and fatty replacement on T_1 contrast-weighted images.[38] Cerebral palsy, amyotrophic lateral sclerosis, and hereditary sensorimotor neuropathy demonstrated atrophy with little, if any, fatty replacement, while poliomyelitis showed atrophy with marked fatty replacement. Direct assessment of the metabolic status of muscle at various levels of activity can be made using the spectroscopic capabilities of MR.[113, 117] Noninvasive measurement of pH, adenosine monophosphate (AMP), adenosine diphosphate (ADP), adenosine triphosphate (ATP),

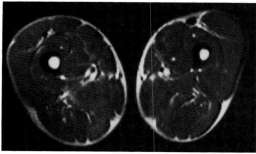

FIGURE 41–53. Old rupture of left rectus femoris muscle. T_1 contrast-weighted image demonstrating atrophy without evidence of edema or fatty infiltration.

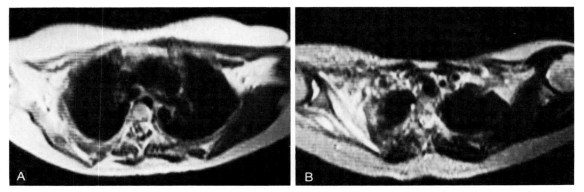

FIGURE 41–54. Brachial plexus injury. T_1 *(A)* and T_2 *(B)* contrast-weighted images demonstrate atrophy of pectoralis and trapezius muscles, with fatty replacement and edema.

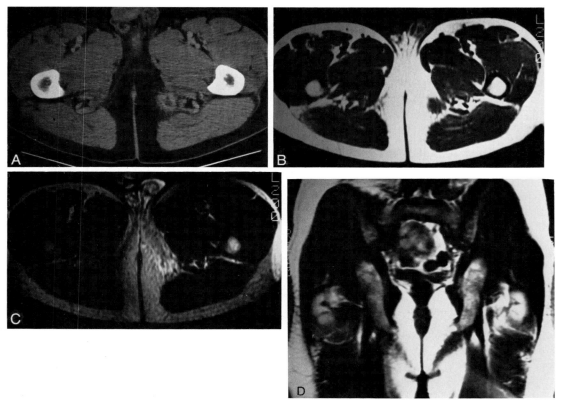

FIGURE 41–55. Traumatic fat necrosis. CT *(A)*, axial T_1 *(B)*, axial T_2 *(C)*, and coronal T_1 *(D)* contrast-weighted images demonstrate ill-defined mass within subcutaneous fat in a linear and symmetric distribution. The patient was a competitive cyclist who had recently replaced the seat on his bicycle.

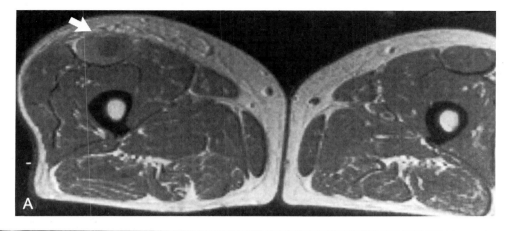

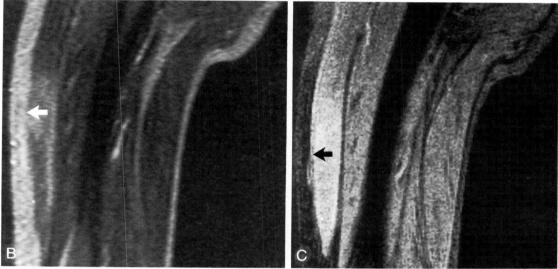

FIGURE 41–56. Myositis in diabetic patient. Axial proton density–weighted spin echo *(A)*, sagittal T$_2$-weighted spin echo *(B)*, sagittal GRASS with 15-degree flip angle *(C)*. Thickening with increased signal intensity *(arrows)* is noted within the affected quadriceps muscle.

phosphocreatine, and lactate is possible. MR imaging and MRS have been used to evaluate numerous primary muscle disorders[38, 39] in addition to muscle changes secondary to exercise,[117, 118] heart failure,[115] and ischemia[116] (Fig. 41–56).

REFERENCES

1. Murphy W, Totty W: Musculoskeletal magnetic resonance imaging 1986. *In* Kressel H (ed): Magnetic Resonance Annual. New York, Raven Press, 1986, pp 1–35.
2. Easton E, Powers J: Musculoskeletal Magnetic Resonance Imaging. Thorofare, NJ, Charles B Slack, 1986.
3. Berquist T, Ehman R, Richardson M: Magnetic Resonance Imaging of the Musculoskeletal System. New York, Raven Press, 1987.
4. Ehman R, Berquist T, McLeod R: MR imaging of the musculoskeletal system: A 5-year appraisal. Radiology 166:313–320, 1988.
5. Mechlin M, Thickman D, Kressel H, et al: Magnetic resonance imaging of postoperative patients with metallic implants. AJR 143:1281–1284, 1984.
6. Vanel D, Di Paola R, Contesso G: Magnetic resonance imaging in musculoskeletal primary malignant tumors. *In* Kressel H (ed): Magnetic Resonance Annual. New York, Raven Press, 1987, pp 237–261.
7. Zimmer W, Berquist T, McLeod R, et al: Magnetic resonance imaging of osteosarcomas: Comparison with computed tomography. Clin Orthop 208:289–299, 1986.
8. Zimmer W, Berquist T, McLeod R, et al: Bone tumors: Magnetic resonance imaging versus computed tomography. Radiology 155:709–718, 1985.
9. Petasnick J, Turner D, Charters J, et al: Soft-tissue masses of the locomotor system: Comparison of MR imaging with CT. Radiology 160:125–133, 1986.
10. Gillesby T, Manfrini M, Ruggieri P, et al: Staging of intraosseous extent of osteosarcoma: Correlation of preoperative CT and MR imaging with pathologic macroslides. Radiology 167:765–767, 1988.
11. Demas B, Heelan R, Lane J, et al: Soft-tissue sarcomas of the extremities: Comparison of MR and CT in determining the extent of the disease. AJR 150:615–620, 1988.
12. Aisen A, Martel W, Braunstein E, et al: MRI and CT evaluation of primary bone and soft-tissue tumors. AJR 146:749–756, 1986.
13. Reiser M, Rupp N, Biehl T: MR in the diagnosis of bone tumors. Eur J Radiol 5:1–7, 1985.

14. Boyko O, Cory D, Cohen D, et al: MR imaging of osteogenic and Ewing's sarcoma. AJR 148:317–322, 1987.

15. Atlan H, Sigal R, Hadar R, et al: Nuclear magnetic resonance proton imaging of bone pathology. J Nucl Med 27:207–215, 1986.

16. Beltran J, Simon D, Katz W, Weis L: Increased MR signal intensity in skeletal muscle adjacent to malignant tumors: Pathologic correlation and clinical relevance. Radiology 162:251–255, 1987.

17. Beltran J, Noto A, Chakeres D, et al: Tumors of the osseous spine: Staging with MR imaging versus CT. Radiology 162:565–569, 1987.

18. Totty W, Murphy W, Lee J: Soft-tissue tumors: MR imaging. Radiology 160:135–141, 1986.

19. Modic M, Feiglin D, Piraino D, et al: Vertebral osteomyelitis: Assessment using MR. Radiology 157:157–166, 1985.

20. Fletcher B, Scoles P, Nelson A: Osteomyelitis in children: Detection by magnetic resonance. Radiology 150:57–60, 1984.

21. Modic M, Pflanze W, Feiglin D, Belhobek G: Magnetic resonance imaging of musculoskeletal infections. Radiol Clin North Am 24:246–258, 1986.

22. Beltran J, McGhee R, Shaffer P, et al: Experimental infections of the musculoskeletal system: Evaluation with MR imaging and Tc-99m MDP and Ga-67 scintigraphy. Radiology 167:167–172, 1988.

23. Tang J, Gold R, Bassett L, et al: Musculoskeletal infection of the extremities: Evaluation with MR imaging. Radiology 166:205–209, 1988.

24. Beltran J, Noto A, McGhee R, et al: Infections of the musculoskeletal system: High-field-strength MR imaging. Radiology 164:449–454, 1987.

25. Unger E, Moldofsky P, Gatenby R, et al: Diagnosis of osteomyelitis by MR imaging. AJR 150:605–610, 1988.

26. Mitchell D, Roa V, Dalinka M, et al: Femoral head avascular necrosis: Correlation of MR imaging, radiographic staging, radionuclide imaging and clinical findings. Radiology 162:709–715, 1987.

27. Gillespy T, Genant H, Helms C: Magnetic resonance imaging of osteonecrosis. Radiol Clin North Am 24:193–207, 1986.

28. Mitchell M, Kundel H, Steinberg M, et al: Avascular necrosis of the hip: Comparison of MR, CT and scintigraphy. AJR 147:67–81, 1986.

29. Totty W, Murphy W, Ganz W, et al: Magnetic resonance imaging of the normal and ischemic femoral head. AJR 143:1273–1280, 1984.

30. Markisz J, Knowles R, Altchek D, et al: Segmental pattern of avascular necrosis of the femoral heads: Early detection with MR imaging. Radiology 162:717–720, 1987.

31. Cohen J, Weinreb J, Muschler G, et al: MR imaging of avascular necrosis of the femoral head. *In* Abstracts of the Fifth Annual Meeting of Society for Magnetic Resonance Imaging, San Antonio, TX, February 28–March 4, 1987. New York, Pergamon Press.

32. Burk J, Beltram J, Herman L, et al: MRI of avascular necrosis of the femoral heads. Part I: Clinical-pathological correlation. *In* Abstracts of the Fifth Annual Meeting of Society for Magnetic Resonance Imaging, San Antonio, TX, February 28–March 4, 1987. New York, Pergamon Press.

33. Coleman B, Kressel H, Dalinka M, et al: Radiographically negative avascular necrosis: Detection with MR imaging. Radiology 168:525–528, 1988.

34. Daffner R, Lupetin A, Dash N, et al: MRI in the detection of malignant infiltration of bone marrow. AJR 146:353–358, 1986.

35. Cohen M, Klatte E, Baehner R, et al: Magnetic resonance imaging of bone marrow disease in children. Radiology 151:715–718, 1984.

36. Weiss K, Beltran J, Lubbers L: High-field MR surface coil imaging of the hand and wrist. Part II. Pathological correlation and clinical relevance. Radiology 160:147–152, 1986.

37. Sims R, Genant H: Magnetic resonance imaging of joint diseases. Radiol Clin North Am 24:179–187, 1986.

38. Murphy W, Totty W, Carroll J: MRI of normal and pathological skeletal muscle. AJR 146:565–574, 1986.

39. Vock P, Hoeppeler H, Hartl W: Combined use of magnetic resonance imaging (MRI) and spectroscopy (MRS) by whole body magnets in studying skeletal muscle morphology. Invest Radiol 20:486–491, 1985.

40. Lee J, Glaser H: Psoas muscle disorders: MR imaging. Radiology 160:683–687, 1986.

41. Weinreb J, Cohen J, Maravilla K: Iliopsoas muscles: MR study of normal anatomy and disease. Radiology 156:435–440, 1985.

42. Nokes S, Murtagh F, Jones J, et al: Childhood scoliosis: MR imaging. Radiology 164:791–797, 1988.

43. Johnson N, Wood B, Jackman K: Complex infantile and congenital hip dislocation: Assessment with MR imaging. Radiology 168:151–156, 1988.

44. Toby E, Koman L, Bechtold R: Magnetic resonance imaging of pediatric hip disease. J Pediatr Orthop 5:665–671, 1985.

45. Yulish B, Lieberman J, Mulopulos G, et al: MR imaging of arthropathies of juvenile arthritis and hemophilia. Presented at 72nd Session of the Radiological Society of North America, Chicago, 1986.

46. Baker D, Schumacher H, Wolf G: Nuclear magnetic resonance evaluation of synovial fluid and articular tissues. J Rheumatol 12:1062–1065, 1985.

47. Beltran J, Caudill J, Herman L, et al: Rheumatoid arthritis: MR imaging manifestations. Radiology 165:153–157, 1987.

48. Yulish B, Lieberman J, Newman A, et al: Juvenile rheumatoid arthritis: Assessment with MR imaging. Radiology 165:149–152, 1987.

49. Senac M, Deutsch D, Bernstein B, et al: MR imaging in juvenile rheumatoid arthritis. AJR 150:873–878, 1988.

50. Aisen A, Martel W, Ellis J, et al: Cervical spine involvement in rheumatoid arthritis: MR imaging. Radiology 165:159–163, 1987.

51. Wismer G, Rosen B, Buxton B, et al: Chemical shift imaging of bone marrow: Preliminary experience. AJR 145:1031–1037, 1985.

52. Porter B: MR may become routine for imaging bone marrow. Diagn Imag Feb 104–108, 1987.

53. Bydder G, Pennock J, Steiner R, et al: The short TI inversion recovery sequence—an approach to MR imaging of the abdomen. Magn Reson Imaging 3:251–254, 1985.

54. Richardson M, Helms C: Artifacts, normal variants and imaging pitfalls of musculoskeletal magnetic resonance imaging. Radiol Clin North Am 24:145, 1986.

55. Knowles J, Markisz J: Quality Assurance and Image Artifacts in Magnetic Resonance Imaging. Boston, Little, Brown and Company, 1988.

56. Dietrich R, Lufkin R, Kangarloo H, et al: Head and neck MR imaging in the pediatric patient. Radiology 159:769–776, 1986.

57. Sundaram M, McGuire M, Schajowicz F: Soft-tissue masses: Histologic basis for decreased signal (short T_2) on T_2-weighted images. AJR 148:1247–1250, 1987.

58. Sundaram M, McGuire M, Herbold D, et al: Magnetic resonance imaging in planning limb-salvage surgery for primary malignant tumors of bone. J Bone Joint Surg 68:809–819, 1986.

59. Milgrom C, Sigal R, Robin G, et al: MRI and CT compared with microscopic histopathology. Orthop Rev 15:91–95, 1986.

60. Pettersson H, Slone R, Spanier S, et al: Musculoskeletal tumors: T_1 and T_2 relaxation times. Radiology 167:783–785, 1988.

61. Beltran J, Simon D, Levy M, et al: Aneurysmal bone cysts: MR imaging at 1.5 T. Radiology 158:689–690, 1986.

62. Cohen J, Weinreb J, Redman H: Arteriovenous malforma-

tions of the extremities: MR imaging. Radiology 158:475–479, 1986.

63. Wilson D, Prince J: MR imaging of hemophiliac pseudotumors. AJR 150:349–350, 1988.

64. Cohen E, Kressel H, Frank T, et al: Hyaline cartilage—origin bone and soft-tissue neoplasms: MR appearance and histologic correlation. Radiology 167:477–481, 1988.

65. Cohen E, Kressel H, Perosio T, et al: MR imaging of soft-tissue hemangiomas: Correlation with pathologic findings. AJR 150:1079–1081, 1988.

66. Ross J, Masaryk T, Modic M, et al: Vertebral hemangiomas: MR imaging. Radiology 167:165–169, 1987.

67. Ramsey R, Zacharias C: MR imaging of the spine after radiation therapy: Easily recognizable effects. AJR 144:1131–1135, 1985.

68. Porter B, Shields A, Olson D: Magnetic resonance imaging of bone marrow disorders. Radiol Clin North Am 24:269–289, 1986.

69. Vanel D, Lacombe M, Couanet D, et al: Musculoskeletal tumors: Follow-up with MR imaging after treatment with surgery and radiation therapy. Radiology 164:243–245, 1987.

70. Dooms G, Fisher M, Hricak H, et al: Bone marrow imaging: Magnetic resonance studies related to age and sex. Radiology 155:429–432, 1985.

71. Crisy M: Active bone marrow distribution as a function of age in humans. Phys Med Biol 26:389–400, 1981.

72. Trabowitz S, Davis S: The bone marrow matrix. *In* The Human Bone Marrow: Anatomy, Physiology and Pathophysiology. Boca Raton, FL, CRC, 1982, pp 43–76.

73. Moore S, Gooding C, Brasch R, et al: Bone marrow in children with acute lymphocytic leukemia: MR relaxation times. Radiology 160:237–240, 1986.

74. McKinstry C, Steiner R, Young A, et al: Bone marrow in leukemia and aplastic anemia: MR imaging before, during and after treatment. Radiology 162:701–707, 1987.

75. Kricun M: Red-yellow marrow conversion: Its effect on the location of some solitary bone lesions. Skeletal Radiol 14:10–19, 1985.

76. Norman A: Osteonecrosis of bone. *In* Taveras J, Ferrucci J (eds): Radiology: Diagnosis-Imaging-Intervention. Philadelphia, JB Lippincott, 1986.

77. Sweet D, Madewell J: Pathogenesis of osteonecrosis. *In* Resnick D, Niwayama G (eds): Diagnosis of Bone and Joint Disorders. Philadelphia, WB Saunders Company, 1981, pp 2780–2831.

78. Hungerford D, Lenox D: The importance of intraosseous pressure in the development of osteonecrosis of the femoral head: Implications for treatment. Orthop Clin North Am 16:635–654, 1985.

79. Steinberg M, Brighton C, Steinberg D, et al: Treatment of avascular necrosis of the femoral head by a combination of bone grafting, decompression and electrical stimulation. Orthop Clin North Am 15:163–175, 1984.

80. Camp J, Colwell C: Core decompression of the femoral head for osteonecrosis. J Bone Joint Surg 68:1313–1319, 1986.

81. Ficat RF: Idiopathic bone necrosis of the femoral head: Early diagnosis and treatment. J Bone Joint Surg [Br] 67:3–9, 1985.

82. Beltran J, Herman L, Burk J, et al: Femoral head avascular necrosis: MR imaging with clinical-pathologic and radionuclide correlation. Radiology 166:215–220, 1988.

83. Reinus W, Conway W, Totty W, et al: Carpal avascular necrosis: MR imaging. Radiology 160:689–693, 1986.

84. Koenig H, Lucas D, Meissner R: The wrist: A preliminary report on high-resolution MR imaging. Radiology 160:463–467, 1986.

85. Beltran J, Noto A, Mosure J, et al: Ankle: Surface coil MR imaging at 1.5 T. Radiology 161:203–209, 1986.

86. Rao V, Fishman M, Mitchell DG, et al: Painful sickle cell crisis: Bone marrow patterns observed with MR imaging. Radiology 161:211–215, 1986.

87. Beltran J, Noto A, Herman L, et al: Joint effusions: MR imaging. Radiology 158:133–137, 1986.

88. Mitchell D, Rao V, Dalinka M, et al: Hematopoietic and fatty bone marrow distribution in the normal and ischemic hip: New observations with 1.5 T MR imaging. Radiology 161:199–202, 1986.

89. Rush B, Bramson R, Ogden J: Legg-Calvé-Perthes disease: Detection of cartilaginous and synovial changes with MR imaging. Radiology 167:473–476, 1988.

90. Hodge B, Bramson R, Ogden J: Legg-Calvé-Perthes disease: Detection of cartilaginous changes by MR imaging. Presented at 72nd Session of the Radiological Society of North America, Chicago, 1986.

91. Lehman W: Legg-Calvé-Perthes disease. *In* Taveras J, Ferrucci J (eds): Radiology: Diagnosis-Imaging-Intervention. Philadelphia, JB Lippincott, 1986.

92. Mesgarzadeh M, Sapega A, Bonakdarpour A, et al: Osteochondritis dissecans: Analysis of mechanical stability with radiography, scintigraphy and MR imaging. Radiology 165:775–780, 1987.

93. Edelman R, Johnson K, Buxton R, et al: MR of hemorrhage: A new approach. AJNR 7:751–756, 1986.

94. Lanir A, Hadar H, Cohen I, et al: Gaucher disease: Assessment with MR imaging. Radiology 161:239–244, 1986.

95. Rosenthal D, Scott J, Barranger J, et al: Evaluation of Gaucher's disease using magnetic resonance imaging. J Bone Joint Surg 68:802–808, 1986.

96. Bloem J: Transient osteoporosis of the hip: MR imaging. Radiology 167:753–755, 1988.

97. Wilson A, Murphy W, Hardy D, et al: Transient osteoporosis: Transient bone marrow edema? Radiology 167:757–760, 1988.

98. Freiberger R: Congenital dislocation of the hip and other skeletal abnormalities of the lower extremities. Vol 5. *In* Taveras J, Ferrucci J (eds): Radiology: Diagnosis-Imaging-Intervention. Philadelphia, JB Lippincott, 1986.

99. Johnson N, Wood B, Jackman K: Complex infantile and congenital hip dislocation: Assessment with MR imaging. Radiology 168:151–156, 1988.

100. Beltran J, Noto A, Herman L, et al: Tendons: High-field-strength surface coil MR imaging. Radiology 162:735–740, 1987.

101. Burk D, Dalinka M, Kanal E, et al: Meniscal and ganglion cysts of the knee: MR evaluation. AJR 150:331–336, 1989.

102. Middelton W, Kneeland J, Kellman G, et al: MR imaging of the carpal tunnel: Normal anatomy and preliminary findings in the carpal tunnel syndrome. AJR 148:307–316, 1987.

103. Berquist T, Brown M, Fitzgerald R, May G: Magnetic resonance imaging: Application in musculoskeletal infection. Magn Res Imaging 3:219–229, 1985.

104. Van Nostrand D, Abreu S, Callaghan J, et al: In-111 white blood cell uptake in noninfected closed fracture in humans: Prospective study. Radiology 167:495–498, 1988.

105. McArdle C, Crofford M, Mirfakhraee M, et al: Surface coil MR of spinal trauma: Preliminary experience. AJNR 7:885–893, 1986.

106. DeRoos A, Kressel H, Spritzer C, Dalinka M: MR imaging of marrow changes adjacent to end plates in degenerative lumbar disk disease. AJR 149:531–534, 1987.

107. Stafford S, Rosenthal D, Gebhardt M, et al: MRI in stress fracture. AJR 147:553–556, 1986.

108. Ehman R, Berquist T: Magnetic resonance imaging of musculoskeletal trauma. Radiol Clin North Am 24:292–318, 1986.

109. Yao L, Lee J: Occult intraosseous fracture: Detection with MR imaging. Radiology 167:749–751, 1987.

110. Zagoria R, Karstaedt N, Koubek T: MR imaging of rhabdomyolysis. J Comput Assist Tomogr 10:268–270, 1986.

111. Heppenstall R, Scott R, Sapega A, et al: A comparison study of the tolerance of skeletal muscle to ischemia. J Bone Joint Surg 68A:820–828, 1986.

112. Fleckenstein J, Canby R, Parkey R, et al: Acute effects of exercise on skeletal muscle in normal volunteers. AJR 151:231–238, 1988.

113. Rodiek S, Kuther G, Juretschke H, et al: MR-tomography and -spectroscopy of skeletal muscles using high magnetic field strengths. ROFO 144:89–95, 1986.

114. Wiener D, Fink L, Maris J, et al: Abnormal skeletal muscle bioenergetics during exercise in patients with heart failure: Role of reduced muscle blood flow. Circulation 73:1127–1136, 1986.

115. Keller U, Oberhansli R, Huber P, et al: Phosphocreatine content and intracellular pH of calf muscle measured by phosphorus NMR spectroscopy in occlusive arterial disease of the legs. Eur J Clin Invest 15:382–388, 1985.

116. Mole P, Coulson R, Caton J, et al: In vivo 31P-NMR in human muscle: Transient patterns with exercise. J Appl Physiol 59:101–104, 1985.

117. Wiener D, Maris J, Chance B, et al: Detection of skeletal muscle hypoperfusion during exercise using phosphorus-31 nuclear magnetic resonance spectroscopy. J Am Coll Cardiol 7:793–799, 1986.

APPENDIX I
MR Imaging Scan Protocols

APPENDIX II
Staging Systems of Primary Malignancies

GLOSSARY OF MR TERMS

APPENDIX I

MR IMAGING SCAN PROTOCOLS*

See p. 1152 for key to terms and abbreviations

We freely admit that there are numerous ways to obtain MR images that are of diagnostic quality. In many cases, it is the preference of the radiologist that determines the most appropriate pulse sequences. Included herein are pulse sequences that have been used on the General Electric (GE) Signa, 1.5-T superconducting magnet, software version 3.2 with the performance plus package. The performance plus package provides the ability to acquire three-dimensional (3D)/volume images, multiplanar gradient-echo (GRE) images, and 192 phase-encoding step images, as well as to utilize fractional number of excitations (NEX), and a rectangular field-of-view (FOV).

Criteria used in developing these pulse sequences included the following:
1. Being able to cover the area of interest with appropriate slice thicknesses
2. Optimizing tissue contrast
3. Optimizing the trade-offs between signal-to-noise (S/N) ratios, spatial resolution, and scan time
4. Minimizing patient-induced artifact
5. Maximizing patient safety
6. Maximizing patient throughout

---

*Compiled by Henry George Adams, M.D., and Thomas J. Riccio, M.D., MRI Fellows, 1988–89, UCSD/AMI Magnetic Resonance Institute, San Diego, CA.

Examination	Indication	Coil	Plane	Options	TR	TE
Brain	Screen	Head	Sagittal		200	20
			Axial	FC	3000	30/80
Brain	Demyelinating disease (e.g., multiple sclerosis [MS])	Head	Axial	FC	3000	30/80
			*Choice		800	20
			†Choice		800	20
	References AJR 149:357–363, 1987 Radiology 165:497–504, 1987 Radiology 166:173–180, 1988					
Brain	1. Tumor	Head	Axial	FC	3000	30/80
	2. Infection		Choice		800	20
	3. Meningitis		Choice		800	20
	References AJR 151:449–454, 1988 Radiology 165:619–624, 1987 AJR 151:583–588, 1988					
Brain	1. Delayed development	Head	Axial	FC	2000	30/80
	2. Congenital anomaly		Sagittal		600	20
			*Coronal	MPIR, TI 708 Nonsequential	1500	25
	Reference AJR 152:583–590, 1989					

Although there is great utility in an appendix such as this, one soon realizes that these pulse sequences may not be suitable under all clinical situations or imaging settings. Most radiologists agree that the best imaging tool available is a thorough understanding of MR imaging principles. With a well-founded knowledge of MR imaging, the radiologist will be able to select pulse sequences and adjust timing intervals that will best display the tissue characteristics of the region of interest efficiently and effectively. Diagnostically, a thorough understanding will give the radiologist the ability to explain pathologic tissue intensity changes as a result of a particular pulse sequence selection.

Sequences that follow may be used to supplement the chapters of this textbook. Variations on these protocols should be encouraged, so that the sequences that work best under a given clinical setting may be found. Abbreviations are adopted from the GE Signa software to maintain continuity for Signa users. The abbreviations and options key is found at the end of this appendix.

FOV	SLTHK	SLSPACE	Matrix	NEX	Freq	Contrast	Comments
20	5	2.5	128	0.5	SI		Base to vertex; if normal, follow
20	5	2.5	192	1.0	AP	—	protocols below

FOV	SLTHK	SLSPACE	Matrix	NEX	Freq	Contrast	Comments
20	5	2.5	192	1	AP		*If axial scans abnormal
20	5	2.5	128	1			†Optional
20	5	2.5	192	2		Gd	

FOV	SLTHK	SLSPACE	Matrix	NEX	Freq	Contrast	Comments
20	5	2.5	192	1	AP		*Choose imaging plane most ap-
20	5	2.5	128	1	AP		propriate for abnormality
20	5	2.5	192	2	SI	Gd	

FOV	SLTHK	SLSPACE	Matrix	NEX	Freq	Contrast	Comments
20	5	2.0	192	1.0	AP	—	*For age < 6 mo; BW = 16 K
20	5	1.5	192	2.0	SI		
20	5	1.5	192	2.0	SI		

Table continued on following page

APPENDIX I

MR IMAGING SCAN PROTOCOLS *Continued*

Examination	Indication	Coil	Plane	Options	TR	TE
Brain	1. Stroke 2. Trauma 3. Hemorrhage	Head	Axial *Choice	FC	3000 800	30/80 20
	References Radiology 168:803–807, 1988 Radiology 165:625–629, 1987 AJR 149:351–356, 1987					
Brain	1. AVM 2. Aneurysm	Head	Axial Choice Choice	FC ST-I GRE/60, FC	3000 800 33	30/80 20 13
Brain	Quick: postoperative, uncooperative, and so on	Head	Axial	FC	3000	30/80
Brain	Seizures	Head	Coronal Axial *Choice	FC FC	3000 3000 800	30/80 30/80 20
	References AJR 149:1231–1239, 1987 Radiology 166:181–185, 1988					
Internal Auditory Canal	1. Neurosensory hearing loss 2. Dizziness 3. Rule out cerebellopontile angle tumor	Head	Axial Coronal *Axial	FC CS, NP CS, NP	3000 800 800	30/80 25 25
	References AJR 150:1371–1381, 1988 Radiology 161:761–765, 1986 Radiology 168:213–214, 1988 Radiology 165:481–485, 1987					
Sella	1. Pituitary dysfunction 2. Enlarged sella 3. Suprasellar mass effect	Head	Coronal *Coronal Sagittal	CS, NF/NP CS, NF/NP CS, NF/NP	800 800 800	25 25 25
	References Radiology 161:761–765, 1986 Radiology 165:481–485, 1987 Radiology 165:487–489, 1987 Radiology 165:491–495, 1987 AJR 149:383–388, 1987					

FOV	SLTHK	SLSPACE	Matrix	NEX	Freq	Contrast	Comments
20	5	2.5	192	1	AP	—	*If axial scan abnormal
20	5	2.5	192	2			Choose imaging plane appropriate for lesion

FOV	SLTHK	SLSPACE	Matrix	NEX	Freq	Contrast	Comments
20	5	2.5	192	1	AP	—	Choose imaging plane appropriate for lesion
20	5	1.0	192	2			
24	5	0	192	4			

FOV	SLTHK	SLSPACE	Matrix	NEX	Freq	Contrast	Comments
20	5	2.5	128	1	AP	—	Base to vertex; use other appropriate protocols for abnormalities

FOV	SLTHK	SLSPACE	Matrix	NEX	Freq	Contrast	Comments
20	5	2.5	256	1	SI		Position head to slice temporal lobes in coronal
20	5	2.5	128	1	AP		
20	5	2.5	192	2		Gd	*Use optional contrast if abnormality observed

FOV	SLTHK	SLSPACE	Matrix	NEX	Freq	Contrast	Comments
20	5	2.5	128	1	AP		*Optional
16–18	3	0	128	4	SI	Gd	
18	3	0	128	4	AP	Gd	

FOV	SLTHK	SLSPACE	Matrix	NEX	Freq	Contrast	Comments
16	3	0	128	4	RL		*For macroadenomas use SLTHK = 3; SLSPACE = 1–2 and MEMP to cover mass
16	3	0	256	2	RL	Gd	
16	3	0	256	2	AP		

Table continued on following page

APPENDIX I

MR IMAGING SCAN PROTOCOLS *Continued*

Examination	Indication	Coil	Plane	Options	TR	TE
Orbits	1. Proptosis	5-inch	*Axial-oblique	NP, FC	2000	20/60
	2. Pain		Coronal	NP	600	20
	3. Mass		†Axial	NP, IR, TI 140	1800	25
	4. Optic neuropathy					
	References Radiology 168:875–876, 1988 Radiology 168:773–779, 1988 Radiology 168:781–786, 1988					
Eye	Abnormality in globe	3-inch	Axial	ST-P	2000	20/70
			Sagittal	ST-P	600	20
			*Coronal	ST-P	600	20
Sinuses	1. Suspected mass	Head	Axial	ST-I	800	20
	2. Chronic sinus disease		Coronal	ST-I	2000	20/70
			*Choice	ST-I	800	20
	Reference Radiology 167:803–808, 1988					
Facial Glands	1. Mass	Head	Axial	ST-I	2000	20/70
	2. Pain		Coronal-oblique	ST-I, NP	800	20
Thyroid/ Para- thyroid	1. Substernal thyroid	5-inch	Coronal	EG, NP, NF,	R-R	20
	2. High parathyroid hormone levels		Axial	ST-I for all	2–3 R-R	20/70
	3. Thyroid cancer or recurrence					
	References Radiology 168:753–757, 1988 Radiology 168:759–764, 1988 AJR 147:1255–1261, 1986 AJR 151:1095–1106, 1988					
Neck	1. Suspected anterior mass	Neck	Coronal	ST-I, NF	6000	20
	2. Vascular anomaly		Axial	EG, ST-I, NP	2–3 R-R	20/70
			*Sagittal	ST-I, NF	600	20
			†Axial	GRASS/25, FC	35	min
	Reference Radiology 166:199–206, 1987					
Brachial Plexus	1. Brachial plexus injury	Body	Coronal	EG, NP, ST-I	R-R	20
	2. Plexus nerve deficit or pain		Axial	EG, NP, ST-I	R-R	20
			Axial	EG, NP, ST-I	2–3 R-R	20/70
	References Radiology 167:161–167, 1988 AJR 149:1219–1222, 1987 Radiology 165:763–767, 1987 AJR 148:1149–1151, 1987					

FOV	SLTHK	SLSPACE	Matrix	NEX	Freq	Contrast	Comments
16	3	1.0	128	2	—		*Parallel to optic nerves from sag-
16	5	1.5	256	2	SI		ittal localizer
16	3	1.0	128	2			†Optional; BW = 12 K

FOV	SLTHK	SLSPACE	Matrix	NEX	Freq	Contrast	Comments
8	3	1.5	192	2	AP	—	*Optional
8	3	0.5	192	2	AP		
8	3	1.5	192	42	SI		

FOV	SLTHK	SLSPACE	Matrix	NEX	Freq	Contrast	Comments
20	5	1.0	192	2	AP		*Optional for sinus masses; center
20	5	1.0	192	2	SI		to area of interest
20	5	1.0	192	2	SI	Gd	

FOV	SLTHK	SLSPACE	Matrix	NEX	Freq	Contrast	Comments
20	5	2.5	128	2	RL	—	Cushion shoulders and extend
20	3	1.0	192	4	SI		neck to raise chin in coil; offset
							approximately 70 mm anterior

FOV	SLTHK	SLSPACE	Matrix	NEX	Freq	Contrast	Comments
16	5	0.5	128	4	RL	—	Secure coil off chest to prevent
16	4	2.0	128	2	AP		breathing artifact
					AP		

FOV	SLTHK	SLSPACE	Matrix	NEX	Freq	Contrast	Comments
20	5	0.5	128	4	SI	—	*Do for midline lesions
16	5	2.0	128	2	RL		†Do GRASS for vascular occlusion
20	5	0.5	128	4	SI		
16	5	0.0	128	6	AP		

FOV	SLTHK	SLSPACE	Matrix	NEX	Freq	Contrast	Comments
36–40	5	2.0	128	4	SI	—	C5 to sternum; use FOV = dis-
32–38	10	2.5	128	4	RL		tance between shoulders
32–38	5	2.5	128	4	RL		*Offset center to include appro-
							priate shoulder and show con-
							tralateral jugular
							Use cross–R-R acquisition

Table continued on following page

APPENDIX I

MR IMAGING SCAN PROTOCOLS *Continued*

Examination	Indication	Coil	Plane	Options	TR	TE
Cervical Spine	1. Trauma	5-inch	Sagittal	RT, ST-AP	600	20
	2. Radiculopathy		Sagittal	MPGR, RT, ST-AP	450	17
	3. Pain			MPGR, ST-I,		
	4. Rule out disk			FC for MPGRs		
			Axial		600	17
	References					
	AJR 149:149–157, 1987					
	AJR 149:159–164, 1987					
	AJNR 9:145–151, 1988					
Cervical Spine	1. Cord tumor	5-inch	Sagittal	RT, ST-AP	600	20
	2. Syrinx		Sagittal	RT, ST-AP	600	20
			Axial	ST-I, NP	600	20
	References					
	AJR 149:149–157, 1987					
	AJR 149:159–164, 1987					
Cervical Spine	MS	5-inch	Sagittal	RT, ST-AP, EG	R-R	20
			Sagittal	EG, FC, RT, ST-AP	2–3 R-R	35/70
			Axial	FC, ST-I, EG	2–3 R-R	35/70
Thoracic Spine	1. Radiculopathy	License	Sagittal	ST-A, RC	600	20
	2. Pain		Axial	ST-A, NP, RC	600	20
			*Axial	MPGR/25, ST-A, FC	600	17
	References					
	AJR 149:1241–1248, 1987					
	Radiology 165:541–544, 1987					
	Radiology 165:511–515, 1987					
	Radiology 165:635–637, 1987					
Thoracic Spine	1. Cord tumor	License	Sagittal	ST-A	600	20
	2. Syrinx		Sagittal	ST-A	600	20
			Axial	NP, ST-A	600	20
	References					
	AJR 149:1241–1248, 1987					
	Radiology 165:541–544, 1987					
	Radiology 165:511–515, 1987					
	Radiology 165:635–637, 1987					
Thoracic Spine	1. MS	License	Sagittal	RC, ST-A	600	20
	2. Trauma		Sagittal	FC, ST-A, RC	2000	35/70
	3. Cord infarct		Axial	FC, ST-A, NP	2000	35/70
	References					
	AJR 149:1241–1248, 1987					
	Radiology 165:541–544, 1987					
	Radiology 165:511–515, 1987					
	Radiology 165:635–637, 1987					

FOV	SLTHK	SLSPACE	Matrix	NEX	Freq	Contrast	Comments
24	3	0.5	256	4	SI	—	Flip angle 25 for MPGRs
24	3	0	256	4	SI		
20	3	0	128	2	AP		

FOV	SLTHK	SLSPACE	Matrix	NEX	Freq	Contrast
24	3	0.5	256	4	SI	
24	3	0.5	256	2	SI	Gd
16	5	1.0	192	2	AP	Gd

FOV	SLTHK	SLSPACE	Matrix	NEX	Freq	Contrast	Comments
24	3	0.5	256	2	SI	—	Use cross–R-R acquisition for R-Rs greater than 1
24	3	1.5	256	1	SI		
16	5	1.0	192	2	RL		

FOV	SLTHK	SLSPACE	Matrix	NEX	Freq	Contrast	Comments
28–36	3	0.5	128	4	SI	—	Axial scans to area of interest
16	5	1.0	128	4	AP		*Optional for epidural disease
20	3	0.0	128	2	AP		SATGAPY for sagittal

FOV	SLTHK	SLSPACE	Matrix	NEX	Freq	Contrast	Comments
28–36	3	0.5	192	4	SI		Mod CVs: SATGAPY for sagittal;
28–36	3	0.5	192	4	SI	Gd	axial scans through area of in-
16	5	1.0	128	4	AP	Gd	terest

FOV	SLTHK	SLSPACE	Matrix	NEX	Freq	Contrast	Comments
28–36	3	0.5	192	4	SI	—	Mod CVs: SATGAPY on sagittal;
28–36	3	0.5	192	2	SI		axial scans to area of interest
16	5	1.0	128	2	AP		

Table continued on following page

APPENDIX I

MR IMAGING SCAN PROTOCOLS *Continued*

Examination	Indication	Coil	Plane	Options	TR	TE
Lumbar	1. Trauma	License	Sagittal	RT, ST-AP	600	20
Spine	2. Radiculopathy		Sagittal	MPGR/25, RT,	450	17
	3. Pain			ST-AP, FC		
	4. Possible conus lesions		Axial-oblique	ST-S, NP	2000	20/70

References
Radiology 168:469–472, 1988
Radiology 165:517–525, 1987
AJR 149:1249–1254, 1987
AJR 149:1025–1032, 1987

Examination	Indication	Coil	Plane	Options	TR	TE
Lumbar	1. Postoperative follow-up	License	Sagittal	RT, ST-AP	600	20
Spine	2. Intradural lesion		Axial-oblique	ST-S, NP	800	20
			Axial-oblique	ST-S, NP	800	20

References
Radiology 168:469–472, 1988
Radiology 167:817–824, 1988
Radiology 165:517–525, 1987
AJR 149:1249–1253, 1987
AJR 149:1025–1032, 1987
AJR 149:531–534, 1987

Examination	Indication	Coil	Plane	Options	TR	TE
Lumbar	Tethered cord	License	Sagittal	RT, ST-AP	600	20
Spine			Axial	ST-S, NP	800	20

Reference
Radiology 166:679–685, 1988

Examination	Indication	Coil	Plane	Options	TR	TE
Spine Me-	1. Primary with suspected epi-	License	Sagittal-C	RT, ST-AP	600	20
tastases	dural disease		Sagittal-T	RT, ST-AP	600	20
Screening	2. Possible drop metastases*		Sagittal-L	RT, ST-AP	600	20
			†Axial	ST-SI, NP	600	20

Reference
Radiology 167:217–223, 1988

Examination	Indication	Coil	Plane	Options	TR	TE
Medias-	1. Mass on other modality	Body	Coronal	EG, ST-SI, RC	R-R	20
tinum	2. Node follow-up		Axial	EG, ST-SI, RC	2–4 R-R	20/70
				NP, NF for all		

References
AJR 140:251–256, 1987
Radiology 165:691–695, 1987

FOV	SLTHK	SLSPACE	Matrix	NEX	Freq	Contrast	Comments
24	5	0.5	256	4	SI	—	Angle axial scans to disk spaces;
24	5	0	256	2	SI		for conus lesions, center to in-
							clude conus
16	5	1.0	128	4	AP		

FOV	SLTHK	SLSPACE	Matrix	NEX	Freq	Contrast	Comments
24	5	0.5	256	4	SI		Axial scans angled through disk
16	5	1.0	128	4			spaces
16	5	1.0	128	4		Gd	

FOV	SLTHK	SLSPACE	Matrix	NEX	Freq	Contrast	Comments
24–28	5	0.5	256	4	SI	—	Open FOV to include conus and
16	5	2.5	128	4	AP		cauda equina; for infants reduce
							FOV and SLTHK accordingly

FOV	SLTHK	SLSPACE	Matrix	NEX	Freq	Contrast	Comments
24	3	0.5	256	4	SI	Gd*	*Use gadolinium only for sus-
28–36	3	0.5	256	4	SI		pected intradural drop metas-
20	5	1.0	256	4	SI		tases
16	5	1.0	128	4	AP		†Optional axial scans through area
							of interest on sagittal scans

FOV	SLTHK	SLSPACE	Matrix	NEX	Freq	Contrast	Comments
32–40	10	1.0	128	4	SI	—	2–4 R-R to yield TR near 2000;
32–40	5	2.5	128	2	RL		cardiac phase [OTHER], 1, to
							yield cross–R-R slices

Table continued on following page

APPENDIX I

MR IMAGING SCAN PROTOCOLS *Continued*

Examination	Indication	Coil	Plane	Options	TR	TE
Heart *(Adult)*	1. Valvular insufficiency 2. Congenital anomalies	Body	Coronal Axial-oblique Sagittal-oblique Choice	EG, ST-SI, RC EG, ST-SI, RC EG, ST-SI, RC CINE/30, FC	R-R R-R R-R 21	25 25 25 12
	References AJR 151:239–248, 1988 Radiology 155:671–679, 1985 Circulation 69:523–531, 1984					
Heart *(Adult)*	1. Pericardial disease or mass 2. Intracardiac masses 3. Ventricular aneurysm	Body	Coronal Axial Choice	EG, ST-SI, RC EG, ST-SI, RC CINE/30, FC	R-R 2–3 R-R 25	25 25/70 13
	References AJR 151:239–248, 1988 AJR 147:245–256, 1986 Radiology 165:117–122, 1987					
Heart *(Child)*	1. Congenital heart disease (CHD) 2. Pericardial disease	Body	Coronal Axial-oblique Sagittal-oblique Choice	EG, ST-SI, RC, CS EG, ST-SI, RC, CS EG, ST-SI, RC, CS CINE/30, FC	R-R R-R R-R 50	20 20 20 13
	References Dyn Cardiac Imag 1:133–138, 1987 Circulation 77:104–109, 1987 Circulation 77:736–744, 1987					
Heart *(Infant)*	CHD	Head	Coronal Axial Sagittal Choice	EG, ST-SI, RC, CS EG, ST-SI, RC, CS EG, ST-SI, RC, CS CINE/30, FC	R-R R-R R-R 25–33	20 20 20 13–17
	References Dyn Cardiac Imag 1:133–138, 1987 Circulation 77:104–109, 1987 Circulation 77:736–744, 1987					
Thoracic Aorta	1. Dissection 2. Aneurysm	Body	Axial Sagittal-oblique *Axial Sagittal-oblique	EG, ST-SI, RC EG, ST-SI, RC EG, ST-SI, RC CINE/30, FC	R-R R-R 2–3 R-R 33	25 25 20/70 17
	References Radiology 168:347–352, 1988 Radiology 166:651–655, 1988 Radiology 155:399–406, 1985 Radiology 157:149–155, 1985 Radiology 155:407–412, 1985 AJR 146:309–314, 1986 AJR 146:1286–1288, 1986					
Aorta	Coarctation	Body/head	Sagittal Sagittal-oblique Choice	EG, ST-SI, RC, CS EG, ST-SI, RC, CS CINE/30, FC	R-R R-R 33	20 20 17
	References Circulation 78:142–148, 1988 AJR 149:251–256, 1987 Radiology 165:691–695, 1987					

FOV	SLTHK	SLSPACE	Matrix	NEX	Freq	Contrast	Comments
32	5	1.0	128	2	SI	—	Heart, long axis
32	5	1.0	128	2			Heart, short axis
32	5	1.0	128	2			
32	5	1.0	128	2			

FOV	SLTHK	SLSPACE	Matrix	NEX	Freq	Contrast	Comments
32	5	1.5	128	2	SI	—	Cardiac phases [OTHER], 1
32	5	2.5	128	2	AP		
32	5	1.5	128	2	SI		

FOV	SLTHK	SLSPACE	Matrix	NEX	Freq	Contrast	Comments
24	5	0.0	128	2	SI	—	For pericardial disease may choose
24	5	0.0	128	2			variable-echo 3–4 R-R, as with
24	5	0.0	128	2			adult
24	5	0.0	128	2			

FOV	SLTHK	SLSPACE	Matrix	NEX	Freq	Contrast	Comments
24	5	0.0	128	2	SI	—	Oblique scans parallel and per-
24	5	0.0	128	2	AP		pendicular to long axis of heart
24	5	0.0	128	2	SI		may be necessary
24	5	0.0	128	2			

FOV	SLTHK	SLSPACE	Matrix	NEX	Freq	Contrast	Comments
32–36	10	5.0	128	4	AP	—	*Do only if path expected behind
32–36	5	2.0	128	4			heart
32–36	10	5.0	128	4	AP		Do cine in plane to best visualize
32–36	5	0	128	2			abnormality

FOV	SLTHK	SLSPACE	Matrix	NEX	Freq	Contrast	Comments
24–40	5	0.0	128	2	SI	—	Use head coil for infants, TR =
24–40	5	0.0	128	2			22, TE = 13
24–40	5	0.0	128	2			

Table continued on following page

APPENDIX I

MR IMAGING SCAN PROTOCOLS *Continued*

Examination	Indication	Coil	Plane	Options	TR	TE
Abdominal Aorta	1. Dissection 2. Aneurysm	Body	Coronal Sagittal Axial Choice	EG, ST-SI, RC EG, ST-SI, RC EG, ST-SI, RC CINE/30, FC	R-R R-R 2–4 R-R 33	25 25 20/70 13
	Reference Radiology 166:651–655, 1988					
Liver	1. Masses by other modality 2. Follow-up masses 3. Portal/hepatic vein thrombosis	Body	Coronal Axial *Axial	EG, ST-SI, RC EG, ST-SI, RC GRASS/8, FC	R-R 2–4 R-R 29	20 20/80 20
	References AJR 151:79–84, 1988 Radiology 164:21–25, 1987 Radiology 168:319–338, 1988 Radiology 168:621–623, 1988					
Kidneys	Renal mass by other mode–rule out vein involvement or extension	Body	Coronal Axial *Choice	EG, ST-SI, RC EG, ST-SI, RC CINE/30, FC	R-R 2–4 R-R 29	20 20/70 17
	References Radiology 165:837–842, 1987 AJR 147:949–953, 1986					
Inferior Vena Cava	1. Obstruction 2. Invasion 3. Anomaly	Body	Coronal Sagittal Axial Coronal-axial	EG, ST-SI, RC EG, ST-SI, RC EG, ST-SI, RC CINE/15, FC	R-R R-R 2–3 R-R 59	25 25 20/70 17
	Reference Radiology 166:371–375, 1988					
Pancreas	Artifact on CT	Body	Coronal Axial Sagittal	RC, ST-SI, NP RC, ST-SI, NP RC, ST-SI, NP	600 2000 800	25 20/70 20
	Reference AJR 148:703–709, 1987					
Adrenals	1. Suprarenal mass by other modality 2. Abnormal chemistries	Body	Coronal Axial	RC, ST-SI, NP RC, ST-SI, NP	600 2000	25 20/70
	Reference AJR 147:493–496, 1986					

FOV	SLTHK	SLSPACE	Matrix	NEX	Freq	Contrast	Comments
36	10	1.0	128	4	SI	—	Graphics to visualize aorta; cine in
36	5	0.5	128	4	SI		plane to visualize pathology best
34–38	10	5.0	128	2	AP		
40	10	0	128	2	SI		

FOV	SLTHK	SLSPACE	Matrix	NEX	Freq	Contrast	Comments
40	10	1.0	128	4	SI	—	Glucagon, binder, bellows, for left
36–40	5	2.5	128	4	RL		lobe lesions use anteroposterior
40	10	0	128	6			frequency direction on axial
							scans
							*Breath hold; EG optional

FOV	SLTHK	SLSPACE	Matrix	NEX	Freq	Contrast	Comments
40	10	1.0	128	4	SI	—	Bellows, binder, glucagon
36	5	2.5	128	4	RL		*Breath hold for renal veins; car-
40	5	0	128	6	SI		diac phase [OTHER], 1, for
							cross–R-R scan; EG optional

FOV	SLTHK	SLSPACE	Matrix	NEX	Freq	Contrast	Comments
40	10	1.0	128	4	SI	—	Bellows, glucagon, EG optional
40	10	1.0	128	4	SI		
32–40	10	1.0	128	2	RL		
30	5	0	128	2	SI/RL		

FOV	SLTHK	SLSPACE	Matrix	NEX	Freq	Contrast	Comments
40	10	1.0	128	4	SI	Oral Fe	Bellows, glucagon, binder
32–40	5	1.0	128	4	RL		
32	5	1.0	128	4	SI		

FOV	SLTHK	SLSPACE	Matrix	NEX	Freq	Contrast	Comments
36	10	1.0	128	4	SI	—	Bellows, glucagon, axial scans cen-
36	5	1.0	128	4	RL		tered to region of interest

Table continued on following page

APPENDIX I

MR IMAGING SCAN PROTOCOLS *Continued*

Examination	Indication	Coil	Plane	Options	TR	TE
Bladder	1. Mass by other modality	Body	Sagittal	ST-SI, RC, NF	600	20
	2. Unexplained hematuria		Sagittal	ST-SI, RC, NF	2000	20/70
			Coronal	ST-SI, RC, NF	2000	20/70
			*Axial	ST-SI, RC, NP	3000	20/70
	Reference Radiology 166:11–16, 1988					
Pelvis *(Male)*	1. Screen	Body	Coronal	RC, ST-SI, NF	600	20
	2. Tumor		Sagittal	RC, ST-SI, NF	2000	20/70
	3. Postoperative follow-up		Axial	RC, ST-SI, NF	1000	20/70
	References Radiology 168:307–311, 1988 AJR 148:51–58, 1987 Radiology 162:325–329, 1987 Radiology 162:331–336, 1987					
Prostate	Prostate cancer	Rectal	Sagittal		800	20
			Axial-oblique	NP	2200	20/70
			90-degree	NP	2200	20/70
			oblique	NP	3000	20/70
	References Radiology 167:268–270, 1988 AJR 148:51–58, 1987 Radiology 162:325–329, 1987 Radiology 162:331–336, 1987 Radiology 163:521–525, 1987					
Ovaries	Adnexal mass found by an- other modality	Body	Coronal	RC, ST-SI, NF	800	20
			Axial	RC, ST-SI	2000	20/70
			Coronal	RC, ST-SI, NF	1200	20/70
	References Radiology 166:11–16, 1988					
Uterus/ *Cervix*	1. Abnormal bleeding	Body	Coronal	RC, ST-SI, NF	800	20
	2. Mass on other modality		Sagittal	RC, ST-SI, NF	2000	20/70
			Coronal-oblique	RC, ST-SI, NP	2000	20/70
	References Radiology 166:11–16, 1988 Radiology 166:895–896, 1988 Radiology 166:333–340, 1988 Radiology 166:111–114, 1988 Radiology 167:627–630, 1988 Radiology 166:623–631, 1988 Radiology 167:233–237, 1988					
Fetus	Fetal abnormality	Body	Sagittal	RC, ST-SI, NF	600	20
			Fetal sagittal	RC, NP, NF	600	20
			Fetal axial	RC, NP, NF	600	20
			Fetal coronal	RC, NP	600	20

FOV	SLTHK	SLSPACE	Matrix	NEX	Freq	Contrast	Comments
30	10	1.0	128	4	SI	—	*Do if needed
30	5	2.5	128	4	SI		Center at umbilicus; bellows,
30	5	2.5	128	4	SI		binder, glucagon
34	5	2.5	128	2	RL		

FOV	SLTHK	SLSPACE	Matrix	NEX	Freq	Contrast	Comments
36	10	1.0	128	4	SI	—	Glucagon, bellows, binder; center
36	5	2.5	128	4	SI		at umbilicus
36	5	2.5	128	4	RL		

FOV	SLTHK	SLSPACE	Matrix	NEX	Freq	Contrast	Comments
34	5	2.0	128	4	SI	—	Empty bladder; do fourth acquisi-
16	3	1.5	128	4			tion only on failure of 2 or 3;
16	3	1.5	128	4			center at anterosuperior iliac
16	3	1.5	128	2			spine for sagittal

FOV	SLTHK	SLSPACE	Matrix	NEX	Freq	Contrast	Comments
36–40	10	1.0	128	4	SI	—	Center at iliac crests; glucagon,
34–44	5	2.5	128	4	RL		bellows, binder
34–36	5	2.5	128	4	SI		

FOV	SLTHK	SLSPACE	Matrix	NEX	Freq	Contrast	Comments
36	10	1.0	128	4	SI	—	Center at anterosuperior iliac
36	5	2.5	128	4	SI		spine; bellows, binder, glucagon,
36	5	2.5	128	4			coronal-oblique angled to plane
							of uterus or cervix

FOV	SLTHK	SLSPACE	Matrix	NEX	Freq	Contrast
36	10	1.0	128	4	SI	—
36	10	1.0	128	4		
36	10	1.0	128	4		
36	10	1.0	128	4		

Table continued on following page

APPENDIX I

MR IMAGING SCAN PROTOCOLS *Continued*

Examination	Indication	Coil	Plane	Options	TR	TE
Testes	1. Torsion	5-inch	Sagittal	ST-PS, NP	800	20
	2. Tumor		Coronal	ST-PS, NP	2000	20/70
			*Axial	ST-PS, NP	3000	20/70

References
Radiology 167:631–636, 1988
Radiology 168:19–23, 1988
Radiology 163:89–92, 1987
Radiology 163:93–98, 1987

Examination	Indication	Coil	Plane	Options	TR	TE
Testes	Undescended testicles	Select	Axial	ST-SIP, NP	600	20
			Coronal	ST-IP, NP	2000	20/70
			*Axial	ST-SI, NP	3000	20/70
			†Axial	ST-SI, NP	2000	20/70

Reference
AJR 151:1107–111, 1988

Examination	Indication	Coil	Plane	Options	TR	TE
Knee	1. Rule out tear	Extremity	Axial	MPGR/25	450	17
	2. Mass seen on other modality		Coronal	NP, CS	800	25
	3. Acute ligament injury		Sagittal	NF, ST-SI, CS	2000	25/60
			*Coronal-oblique	NP, ST-SI, CS	2000	25/60

References
Radiology 167:775–581, 1988
Radiology 159:753–757, 1986
Radiology 162:547–551, 1987
Radiology 162:553–557, 1987
Radiology 165:775–780, 1987
Radiology 159:747–752, 1986

Examination	Indication	Coil	Plane	Options	TR	TE
Shoulder	1. Rotator cuff tear	5-inch	Axial	NP, NF	2000	20/60
	2. Impingement syndrome	pair	Sagittal-oblique	NP, NF	2000	20/60
	3. Instability		Coronal-oblique	NP, NF	2000	20/60

References
AJR 150:151–158, 1988
Radiology 168:695–697, 1988
Radiology 168:699–704, 1988
AJR 150:1083–1087, 1988

Examination	Indication	Coil	Plane	Options	TR	TE
Temporo-mandibu-lar Joint (TMJ)	TMJ dysfunction	3-inch	Coronal	NP, ST-I	600	20
			Sagittal-oblique	NP, ST-I	700	20
			Sagittal-oblique	NP, ST-I	700	20

References
AJR 150:381–389, 1988
AJR 151:341–350, 1988
AJR 149:959–962, 1987

FOV	SLTHK	SLSPACE	Matrix	NEX	Freq	Contrast	Comments
16	5	1.0	192	2	SI	—	*Do only if necessary
16	3	1.5	192	2	SI		Place penis to side; raise testes off
16	3	1.5	192	1	RL		legs; coil 1 inch from testes; center 60 mm anterior; 3-inch coil < 9 months

FOV	SLTHK	SLSPACE	Matrix	NEX	Freq	Contrast	Comments
16–20	3–10	50%	192	2	AP	—	3-inch coil <9 months, 5-inch in others
16	3–10	50%	192	2	SI		
16	3–10	50%	192	1	RL		*For testes at abdominal wall
20–23	5–10	7.5–10	192	2	RL		†For testes not seen on first two sequences (body coil)

FOV	SLTHK	SLSPACE	Matrix	NEX	Freq	Contrast	Comments
18	5	0.5	128	2	AP	—	*Do for acute anterior cruciate ligament (ACL) injury along ACL axis
16	5	0.0	128	2	RL		
16	5	0.5	128	1	SI		
16	5	0.5	128	1			

FOV	SLTHK	SLSPACE	Matrix	NEX	Freq	Contrast	Comments
14	3	1.5	128	2	RL	—	Hand alongside with palm to thigh; image top of acromioclavicular (AC) joint through glenoid; include infraspinatus and coronid
14	5	2.0	128	2			
14	3	1.5	128	2			

FOV	SLTHK	SLSPACE	Matrix	NEX	Freq	Contrast	Comments
10	3	0.5	128	2	RL	—	Coronal scans with closed mouth; sagittal scans open with bite block and closed
10	3	0.5	128	2			
10	3	0.5	128	2			

Table continued on following page

APPENDIX I

MR IMAGING SCAN PROTOCOLS *Continued*

Examination	Indication	Coil	Plane	Options	TR	TE
Wrist	1. Carpal tunnel syndrome (CTS)	3-inch pair	Coronal	NP, NF, ST-S	600	20
			Sagittal	NF, RT, ST-S	800	20
	2. Arthritis preoperatively		Choice	NP, NF, ST-S	2000	20/70
	3. Internal derangement		*Axial	NF, RT, ST-S	800	20
Elbow	Mass not demonstrated by other modality	5-inch	Coronal	ST-I, NP	600	20
			Axial	ST-I, NP	2500	20/70
			Sagittal	ST-I, NP	600	20

References
AJR 149:543–547, 1987
Radiology 165:527–531, 1987

Examination	Indication	Coil	Plane	Options	TR	TE
Hips	1. Avascular necrosis (AVN)	Body	Coronal	NP, NF	600	20
	2. Occult fracture		Coronal	NP, NF	2500	20/70
	3. Effusion		Sagittal	NP, NF	850	20

References
AJR 148:1159–1164, 1987
Radiology 162:709–715, 1987
AJR 150:1073–1078, 1988
Radiology 168:525–528, 1988
Radiology 162:717–720, 1987
Radiology 168:521–524, 1988

Examination	Indication	Coil	Plane	Options	TR	TE
Foot	1. Unexplained pain	Head or extremity	Sagittal	ST-S	600	20
	2. Mass on other modality		Axial-oblique	ST-S	600	20
			Coronal-oblique	ST-S	2000	20/60
Ankle	1. Unexplained pain	Head or extremity	Sagittal	ST-S, NP	600	20
	2. Mass on other modality		Axial	ST-S	2000	20/60
			Coronal	ST-S, NP	2000	20/60

References
AJR 151:117–123, 1988
Radiology 166:221–226, 1988
Radiology 167:489–493, 1988

FOV	SLTHK	SLSPACE	Matrix	NEX	Freq	Contrast	Comments
10	3	0.5	128	2	SI	—	Arm at patient's side built up to
10	3	0.5	256	2	SI		isocenter
10	3	1.5	128	2	SI		*Axial scans for CTS; ST-I for
10	5	0.5	256	2	RL		prone patient

FOV	SLTHK	SLSPACE	Matrix	NEX	Freq	Contrast	Comments
16	5	1.0	128	2	SI	—	Do GRASS if vascularity involved;
12	5	2.5	128	2	SI		patient supine with elbow ex-
12	5	1.0	128	2	RL		tended alongside; coil to symp-
							tomatic side

FOV	SLTHK	SLSPACE	Matrix	NEX	Freq	Contrast	Comments
34	5	1.0	128	2	SI	—	Do sagittal scans on affected side
36	5	1.0	128	2	SI		only
34	5	1.0	128	2	SI		

FOV	SLTHK	SLSPACE	Matrix	NEX	Freq	Contrast	Comments
24	5	1.0	128	2	SI	—	Use head coil and foot holder for
16	3	3.0	192	2			bilateral examination and fore-
20	5	2.5	128	2			foot; axial scans obliqued to
							plane of affected forefoot

FOV	SLTHK	SLSPACE	Matrix	NEX	Freq	Contrast	Comments
20	3	0.5	256	2	SI	—	Head coil and foot holder for bi-
16	5	0.5	128	2	AP		lateral examination
16	5	1.0	128	2	RL		

APPENDIX I

MR IMAGING SCAN PROTOCOLS *Continued*

Key: Scan protocols are designed for the 1.5-T Signa System of General Electric Company with Signa software version 3.2. These current protocols are continuing to evolve as clinical experience and new software capabilities are developed. The following are definitions of headings and abbreviations used in the preceding protocols:

MPGR: Multiplanar gradient recalled (multiplanar GRASS)
MPIR: Multiplanar inversion recovery
CS: CSMEMP—contiguous-slice multiecho, multiplanar

Contrast: Gd–gadolinium diethylenetriaminepentaacetate (DTPA), 0.2 ml/kg, intravenously administered to a maximum of 20 ml. Other contrast agents such as perfluorocarbons and ferrite have not been approved for use by the Food and Drug Administration (FDA) at time of publication.

FOV: Field of view for the acquisition.

RT: Rectangular field of view. Acquires only the middle half of the phase-direction FOV. Long axis is in frequency direction.

Freq: Frequency-encoding selection; superoinferior (SI), right to left (RL), anteroposterior (AP).

GRASS: Gradient-recalled acquisition in the steady state; also known as fast scan and gradient (recalled) echo.

Matrix: Number of data points acquired in the phase direction, program selectable at 128, 192, and 256. The frequency direction is fixed at 256 data points.

NEX: Number of excitations. The number of times the acquisition sequence is repeated to increase S/N ratio.

Options: Refers to motion artifact reduction techniques, as follows:
EG: Gates the acquisition of the image to the R wave of the electrocardiogram (ECG). Reduces cardiac motion artifact. Cross–R-R imaging increases the number of slices when gating a TR of greater than 2 R-R by acquiring slices during each R-R interval.
CINE: Dynamic imaging of moving organs utilizing high-speed gradient echo (GRASS) technique.
FC: Flow compensation technique that utilizes additional gradients to refocus protons out of phase as a result of flow.
RC: Respiratory compensation database. This technique reorders the phase encodings into a nonsequential acquisition by monitoring the respiratory cycle with the bellows pressure transducer. This reordering reduces respiratory motion artifacts, or ghosts, in the phase-encoding direction.
ST: Saturation subroutine that utilizes additional radiofrequenty (RF) pulses to saturate spins outside the imaging volume immediately prior to each slide-selection gradient to reduce artifacts. Pulses can be applied in one or all of six planes: S = superior, I = inferior, A = anterior, P = posterior, R = right, L = left.
NP: No phase wrap—eliminates wraparound artifact, or aliasing, in the phase-encoding direction.
NF: No frequency wrap—eliminates wraparound artifact, or aliasing, in the frequency-encoding direction.

Plane: Anatomic plane of imaging desired.

SATGAPY: Anterior RF saturation pulse.

SLSPACE: Interslice spacing (mm). INTERLV: Interleaving results in a 100 per cent slice gap between images with an automatic second acquisition that images the slice gaps. Results in images with no slice gaps but without cross-talk artifact.

SLTHK: Slice thickness (mm).

TE: Echo time.

TR: Pulse repetition time.

STAGING SYSTEMS OF PRIMARY MALIGNANCIES

Compiled by Jeffrey Siegel, M.D., Department of Radiology, Beth Israel Hospital, Boston, MA.

LUNG CARCINOMA: DEFINITION OF TNM CATEGORIES

Primary Tumor (T)*

T0   No evidence of primary tumor

TX   Tumor proven by the presence of malignant cells in bronchopulmonary secretions but not visualized roentgenographically or bronchoscopically, or any tumor that cannot be assessed (i.e., a retreatment staging)

T1S   Carcinoma in situ

T1   Tumor that is 3 cm or less in greatest diameter, surrounded by lung or visceral pleura, and without evidence of invasion proximal to a lobar bronchus at bronchoscopy

T2   Tumor more than 3 cm in greatest diameter, or a tumor of any size that either invades visceral pleural or has associated atelectasis or obstructive pneumonitis extending to the hilar region. At bronchoscopy, the proximal extent of demonstrable tumor must be within a lobar bronchus or at least 2 cm distal to the carina. Any associated atelectasis or obstructive pneumonitis must involve less than an entire lung, and there must be no pleural effusion.

T3   Tumor of any size with direct extension into an adjacent structure, such as the parietal pleura or chest wall, the diaphragm, or the mediastinum and its contents, or a tumor demonstrable bronchoscopically to involve a main bronchus, less than 2 cm distal to the carina, or any tumor associated with atelectasis or obstructive pneumonitis of an entire lung or pleural effusion (whether or not malignant cells are found)

Regional Lymph Nodes (N)*

N0   No demonstrable metastasis to regional lymph nodes

N1   Metastasis to lymph nodes in the peribronchial or the ipsilateral hilar region, or both, including direct extension

N2†   Metastasis to lymph nodes in the mediastinum

Distant Metastasis (M)*

MX   Not assessed

M0   No known distant metastasis

M1   Distant metastasis present with site specified (i.e., scalene, cervical, or contralateral hilar lymph nodes; or metastasis to brain, bone, liver, soft tissue, or contralateral lung)

*In all cases, the designation of the T, N, or M category should be for the greatest extent of disease, providing the evidence of this extent is reasonable.

†Vocal cord paralysis, superior vena cava obstruction, and compression of the trachea or esophagus are scored as N2.

From Mountain CF (chairman): Staging of lung cancer, 1979. American Joint Committee for Cancer Staging and End-Results Reporting. Task Force on Lung Cancer; with permission.

LUNG CARCINOMA: STAGE GROUPING FOR LUNG CANCER

Occult Carcinoma

TX N0 M0   An occult carcinoma with bronchopulmonary secretions containing malignant cells but without other evidence of the primary tumor or evidence of metastasis to the regional lymph nodes or distant metastasis

Stage I*

T1S N0 M0   Carcinoma in situ

T1 N0 M0

T1 N1 M0   Tumor that can be classified T1 without any metastasis or with metastasis to the lymph nodes in the peribronchial or ipsilateral hilar region only, or a tumor that can be classified T2 without any metastasis to nodes or distant metastasis*

T2 N0 M0

Stage II

T2 N1 M0   A tumor classified as T2 with metastasis to the lymph nodes in the peribronchial or ipsilateral hilar region only

Stage III

T3 with any N or M

N2 with any T or M   Any tumor more extensive than T2, or any tumor with metastasis to the lymph nodes in the mediastinum, or any tumor with distant metastasis

M1 with any T or N

*TX N1 M0 and T0 N1 M0 are also theoretically possible, but such a clinical diagnosis would be difficult, if not impossible, to make.

From Mountain CF (chairman): Staging of lung cancer, 1979. American Joint Committee for Cancer Staging and End-Results Reporting. Task Force on Lung Cancer; with permission.

RENAL CELL CARCINOMA: COMPARISON OF THE TWO CLASSIFICATION SYSTEMS

	TNM (1978)	ROBSON
Small tumor, no enlargement of kidney	T1	A
Large tumor, cortex not broken	T2	A
Perinephric or hilar extension	T3	B
Extension to neighboring organs	T4	D
Nodal invasion	N_+	C
Renal vein involved	V_1	C
Vena cava involved	V_2	C
Distant metastasis	M_+	D

From Selli C, Hinshaw WM, Woodard BH, Paulson DF: Stratification of risk factors in renal cell carcinoma. Cancer 52:899, 1983; with permission.

TNM CLASSIFICATION: KIDNEY

Primary Tumor (T)

TX	Minimum requirements cannot be met
T0	No evidence of primary tumor
T1	Small tumor, minimal renal and calyceal distortion or deformity; circumscribed neovasculature surrounded by normal parenchyma
T2	Large tumor with deformity or enlargement of kidney or collecting system
T3a	Tumor involving perinephric tissues
T3b	Tumor involving renal vein
T3c	Tumor involving renal vein and infradiaphragmatic vena cava. *Note:* Under T3, tumor may extend into the perinephric tissues, into renal vein, and into vena cava, as shown on cavography; in these instances, the T classification may be shown as T3a, b, and c, or some appropriate combination, depending on extension, e.g., T3a, b is a tumor in perinephric fat and extending into renal vein
T4a	Tumor invasion of neighboring structures (e.g., muscle, bowel)
T4b	Tumor involving supradiaphragmatic vena cava

Nodal Involvement (N)

The regional lymph nodes are the paraaortic and paracaval nodes. The juxtaregional lymph nodes are the pelvic nodes and the mediastinal nodes.

NX	Minimum requirement cannot be met
N0	No evidence of involvement of regional nodes
N1	Single, homolateral regional nodal involvement
N2	Involvement of multiple regional or contralateral or bilateral nodes
N3	Fixed regional nodes (assessable only at surgical exploration)
N4	Involvement of juxtaregional nodes

Note: If lymphography is a source of staging, add "1" between "N" and designator number; if histologic proof is provided, "+" if positive, and "−" if negative; thus, N1+ indicates multiple positive nodes seen on lymphography and proved at operation by biopsy

Distant Metastasis (M)

MX	Not assessed
M0	No (known) distant metastasis
M1	Distant metastasis present

Specify site according to the following notations

Pulmonary—PUL	Bone marrow—MAR
Osseous—OSS	Pleura—PLE
Hepatic—HEP	Skin—SKI
Brain—BRA	Eye—EYE
Lymph nodes—LYM	Other—OTH

Note: Add "+" to the abbreviated notation to indicate that the pathology (p) is proved.

From DeVita VT Jr, Hellman S, Rosenberg SA: Cancer: Principles and Practice of Oncology. 2nd ed. Philadelphia, JB Lippincott Co, 1985, p 899.

CARCINOMA OF THE PANCREAS

Surgical Staging System

Stage I	Localized within pancreatic capsule
Stage II	Invasion of duodenum or peripancreatic tissues
Stage III	Involvement of lymph nodes
Stage IV	Distant spread

TNM Classification

T1	No direct extension of the primary tumor beyond the pancreas
T2	Limited direct extension to duodenum, bile duct, or stomach
T3	Advanced direct extension, incompatible with surgical resection
TX	Direct extension not assessed
N0	Regional lymph nodes not involved
N1	Regional lymph nodes involved
NX	Regional lymph nodes not assessed
M0	No distant metastasis
M1	Distant metastasis present
MX	Distant metastasis not assessed

TNM Staging System

Stage I	T1–2, N0, M0
	No direct extension with no regional nodal involvement
Stage II	T3, N0, M0
	Direct extension into adjacent tissue with no lymph node involvement
Stage III	T1–3, N1, Mo
	Regional lymph node involvement with or without direct tumor extension
Stage IV	T1–3, N0–1, M1
	Distant metastatic disease present

From DeVita VT Jr, Hellman S, Rosenberg SA: Cancer: Principles and Practice of Oncology. 2nd ed. Philadelphia, JB Lippincott Co, 1985, p 707.

PROSTATE CARCINOMA: TNM CLASSIFICATION

Primary Tumor (T)

TX		Minimum requirement to assess the primary tumor cannot be met
T0		No tumor present
	T1a	No palpable tumor; on histological sections no more than three high-power fields of carcinoma found
	T1b	No palpable tumor; histological sections revealing more than three high-power fields of prostatic carcinoma
	T2a	Palpable nodule less than 1.5 cm in diameter with compressible, normal-feeling tissue on at least three sides
	T2b	Palpable nodule more than 1.5 cm in diameter or nodule or induration in both lobes
T3		Palpable tumor extending into or beyond the prostatic capsule
	T3a	Palpable tumor extending into the periprostatic tissues, or involving one seminal vesicle
	T3b	Palpable tumor extending into the periprostatic tissues, involving one or both seminal vesicles; tumor size more than 6 cm in diameter
T4		Tumor fixed or involving neighboring structures

Nodal Involvement (N)

The regional nodes are those within the true pelvis; all others are distant nodes. Histologic examination is required for stages N0 through N3, except subset "c."

NX	Minimum requirements to assess the regional nodes cannot be met
N0	No involvement of regional lymph nodes
N1	Involvement of a single homolateral regional lymph node
N2	Involvement of contralateral, bilateral, or multiple regional lymph nodes
N3	A fixed mass on the pelvic wall with a free space between this and the tumor

Distant Metastasis (M)

MX	Minimum requirements to assess the presence of distant metastasis cannot be met
M0	No (known) distant metastasis
M1	Distant metastasis present—specify

Specify site according to the following notations:

Distant Lymph Nodes—LYM	Pleura—PLE
Pulmonary—PUL	Skin—SKI
Osseous—OSS	Eye—EYE
Hepatic—HEP	Other—OTH
Brain—BRA	

From Beahrs OH, Myers MH (eds.): Manual for Staging Cancer, American Joint Committee on Cancer. Philadelphia, JB Lippincott, 1983.

TESTICULAR CARCINOMA: STAGE GROUPINGS

Stage I	Disease confined to the testis
Stage II	Positive nodal metastatic disease in the node-bearing area of the periaortic or caval zone, but with no demonstrable metastases above the diaphragm or in visceral organs
Stage III	Clinical or radiographic evidence of metastases above the diaphragm or in other visceral organs

From DeVita VT Jr, Hellman S, Rosenberg SA: Cancer: Principles and Practice of Oncology. 2nd ed. Philadelphia, JB Lippincott Co, 1985, p 980.

PATHOLOGIC CLASSIFICATION OF TESTICULAR CARCINOMA

I. Primary Neoplasms
  A. Germinal neoplasms (may demonstrate one or more of the following components)
    1. Seminoma
      a. Classic (typical) seminoma
      b. Anaplastic seminoma
      c. Spermatocytic seminoma
    2. Embryonal carcinoma
    3. Teratoma
      a. Mature
      b. Immature
    4. Choriocarcinoma
    5. Yolk sac tumor (endodermal sinus tumor; embryonal adenocarcinoma of the prepubertal testis)
  B. Nongerminal neoplasms
    1. Specialized gonadal stromal neoplasms
      a. Leydig cell tumors
      b. Other gonadal stromal tumors
    2. Gonadoblastomas*
      a. Adenocarcinoma of the rete testis
      b. Neoplasms of mesenchymal origin
      c. Adrenal rest "tumors"
      d. Adenomatoid tumor

II. Secondary Neoplasms
  A. Reticuloendothelial neoplasms
  B. Metastatic carcinomas

*Gonadoblastomas show both germ cell and gonadal stromal elements and, strictly speaking, should not be considered nongerminal. They are included under this heading for convenience, since they differ from germ cells tumors.

From DeVita VT Jr, Hellman S, Rosenberg SA: Cancer: Principles and Practice of Oncology. 2nd ed. Philadelphia, JB Lippincott Co, 1985, p 980.

PROSTATE CARCINOMA: STAGE GROUPING

AUS Stage*	Stage	AJC-UICC† Classification	Local Lesion	Prostatic Acid Phosphatase	Bone Metastases by Bone Radiograph
A₁-focal	IA	$T_0 N_x M_0$	Not palpable, focal	Not elevated	No
A₂-diffuse	IB	$T_0 N_x M_0$	Not palpable, diffuse	Not elevated	No
B	II	$T_1 T_2 N_x M_0$	Confined to prostate	Not elevated	No
C	III	$T_3 N_x M_0$	Local extension	Not elevated	No
D₁	IVA	$T_{any} N_x M_0$	Any	Elevated	No
D₁	IVB‡	$T_{any} N_{1-4} M_0$	Any	Any	No
D₂	IVC	$T_{any} N_{any} M_1$	Any	Any	Yes

*American Urological Society
†American Joint Commission–International Union Against Cancer (French)
‡IVB patients cannot be assigned a stage classification until after node dissection because this category is reserved for patients with lymph node extension.

From DeVita VT Jr, Hellman S, Rosenberg SA: Cancer: Principles and Practice of Oncology. 2nd ed. Philadelphia, JB Lippincott Co, 1985, p 939.

OVARIAN CARCINOMA: FIGO STAGE GROUPING FOR PRIMARY CARCINOMAS OF THE OVARY (1976)

Stage I	Growth limited to the ovaries
Stage IA	Growth limited to one ovary; no ascites
Stage IAi	No tumor on the external surface; capsule intact
Stage IAii	Tumor present on the external surface, or capsule ruptured, or both
Stage IB	Growth limited to both ovaries; no ascites
Stage IBi	No tumor on the external surface; capsule intact
Stage IBii	Tumor present on the external surface, or capsule ruptured, or both
Stage IC	Tumor either stage IA or IB but with ascites present or with positive peritoneal washings
Stage II	Growth involving one or both ovaries with pelvic extension
Stage IIA	Extension or metastases to the uterus or tubes
Stage IIC	Tumor either Stage IIA or IIB but with ascites present or with positive peritoneal washings
Stage III	Growth involving one or both ovaries with intraperitoneal metastases outside the pelvis or positive retroperitoneal nodes. Tumor limited to the true pelvis with histologically proved malignant extension to small bowel or omentum
Stage IV	Growth involving one or both ovaries with distant metastases. If pleural effusion is present, there must be positive cytology to allot a case to stage IV. Parenchymal liver metastases indicate stage IV.

From Uldfelder H (chairman): Staging system for cancer at gynecologic sites. *In* Manual for Staging of Cancer. Philadelphia, JB Lippincott, 1978, pp 94–97.

FIGO = International Federation of Gynecology and Obstetrics.

CARCINOMA OF THE CERVIX UTERI

Preinvasive Carcinoma

Stage 0	Carcinoma in situ, intraepithelial carcinoma

Invasive Carcinoma

Stage I	Carcinoma strictly confined to the cervix (extension to the corpus should be disregarded)
Stage Ia	Microinvasive carcinoma (early stromal invasion)
Stage Ib	All other cases of stage I; occult cancer should be marked "occ"
Stage II	The carcinoma extends beyond the cervix but has not extended onto the pelvic wall; the carcinoma involves the vagina but not the lower third
Stage IIa	No obvious parametrial involvement
Stage IIb	Obvious parametrial involvement
Stage III	The carcinoma has extended onto the pelvic wall; on rectal examination there is no cancer-free space between the tumor and the pelvic wall; the tumor involves the lower third of the vagina; all cases with a hydronephrosis or nonfunctioning kidney should be included, unless they are known to be due to other cause
Stage IIIa	No extension onto the pelvic wall
Stage IIIB	Extension onto the pelvic wall and hydronephrosis or nonfunctioning kidney
Stage IV	The carcinoma has extended beyond the true pelvis or has clinically involved the mucosa of the bladder or rectum; a bullous edema as such does not permit a case to be allocated to stage IV
Stage IVa	Spread of the growth to adjacent organs
Stage IVb	Spread to distant organs

Adopted in 1976 by the International Federation of Gynecology and Obstetrics (FIGO).

ENDOMETRIAL CARCINOMA

Stage 0		(TIS)	Carcinoma in situ
Stage I		(T1)	Carcinoma confined to the corpus
	IA	(T1a)	Uterine cavity 8 cm or less in length
	IB	(T1b)	Uterine cavity greater than 8 cm in length. Stage I should be subgrouped as follows: G1: highly differentiated G2: moderately differentiated G3: undifferentiated
Stage II		(T2)	Extension to cervix only
Stage III		(T3)	Extension outside the uterus but confined to the true pelvis
Stage IV		(T4)	Extension beyond true pelvis or invading bladder or rectum

From Rubin P (ed): Clinical Oncology for Medical Students. 5th ed. American Cancer Society, 1978, p 109; with permission.

CLASSIFICATION OF FIBRILLARY ASTROCYTIC NEOPLASMS

Bailey and Cushing	Kernohan	World Health Organization (WHO)
Astrocytoma	Astrocytoma grade 1	Astrocytoma (grade 2)*
Astroblastoma	Astrocytoma grade 2	Anaplastic astrocytoma (grade 3)
Spongioblastoma multiforme	Astrocytoma grade 3 Astrocytoma grade 4	Glioblastoma multiform (poorly differentiated glioma, grade 4)†

*Lesions considered grade 1 include the optic nerve glioma, pilocytic astrocytoma, and cerebellar astrocytoma.

†Not classified as an astrocytic neoplasm.

HODGKIN'S DISEASE: ANN ARBOR STAGING CLASSIFICATION

Stage I	Involvement of a single lymph node region (I) or a single extralymphatic organ or site (I$_E$)
Stage II	Involvement of two or more lymph node regions on the same side of the diaphragm (II) or localized involvement of an extralymphatic organ or site (II$_E$)
Stage III	Involvement of a lymph node region on both sides of the diaphragm (III) or localized involvement of an extralymphatic organ or site (III$_E$) or spleen (III$_S$) or both (III$_{SE}$)
Stage IV	Diffuse or disseminated involvement of one or more extralymphatic organs with or without associated lymph node involvement. The organ(s) involved should be identified by a symbol:
	A: Asymptomatic
	B: Fever, sweats, weight loss >10% of body weight

From DeVita VT Jr, Hellman S, Rosenberg SA: Cancer: Principles and Practice of Oncology. 2nd ed. Philadelphia, JB Lippincott Co, 1985, p 1648.

NON-HODGKIN'S LYMPHOMA: LYMPHOMA CLASSIFICATION

Working Formulation	Rappaport Terminology
Low-Grade	
A. Malignant lymphoma, small lymphocytic consistent with chronic lymphocytic leukemia, plasmacytoid	Diffuse, well-differentiated, lymphocytic
B. Malignant lymphoma, follicular, predominantly small cleaved cell, diffuse areas, sclerosis	Nodular, poorly differentiated lymphocytic
C. Malignant lymphoma, follicular mixed, small cleaved and large cell, diffuse areas, sclerosis	Nodular, mixed lymphocytic-histiocytic
Intermediate-Grade	
D. Malignant lymphoma, follicular, predominantly large cell, diffuse areas, sclerosis	Nodular histiocytic
E. Malignant lymphoma, diffuse, small cleaved cell	Diffuse, poorly differentiated lymphocytic
F. Malignant lymphoma, diffuse, mixed small and large cell, sclerosis, epithelioid cell component	Diffuse, mixed lymphocytic-histiocytic
G. Malignant lymphoma, diffuse large cell, cleaved cell, noncleaved cell, sclerosis	Diffuse histiocytic
High-Grade	
H. Malignant lymphoma, large cell immunoblastic, plasmacytoid, clear cell, polymorphous, epithelioid cell component	Diffuse histiocytic
I. Malignant lymphoma, lymphoblastic, convoluted cell, nonconvoluted cell	Diffuse lymphoblastic
J. Malignant lymphoma, small noncleaved cell, Burkitt's, follicular areas	Diffuse undifferentiated

From DeVita VT Jr, Hellman S, Rosenberg SA: Cancer: Principles and Practice of Oncology. 2nd ed. Philadelphia, JB Lippincott Co, 1985, p 1634.

GLOSSARY OF MR TERMS

ROBERT R. EDELMAN, DENNIS J. ATKINSON,
and J. PAUL FINN

Acquisition matrix: Designation of the number of pixels spanning the field-of-view along each in-plane dimension.

  Rectangular matrix: Having an unequal number of pixels along the two dimensions, e.g., 256×192.

  Square acquisition matrix: Having the same number of pixels along both dimensions, e.g., 256×256.

Acquisition (imaging, scan) time: Time for acquiring an image, expressed as:

$$TR \times N_y \times NEX \text{ for 2D acquisitions, or}$$
$$TR \times N_y \times N_z \times NEX \text{ for 3D acquisitions}$$

where N_y = number of y phase-encoding steps and N_z = number of z phase-encoding steps or *partitions*.

Adiabatic fast passage (AFP): A method, usually used for inversion of the spins, that produces reorientation of the macroscopic magnetization vector by sweeping the frequency of the RF irradiation through resonance quickly enough that the excitation time is short compared with the relaxation times.

Aliasing: Spurious appearance of high frequency signals at lower frequencies, due to sampling at a rate less than the Nyquist limit. Manifested as several types of artifacts in MR images (e.g., truncation artifact, wraparound artifact).

Alpha (α) pulse: RF pulse having a flip angle usually ≤ 90 degrees used in gradient-echo sequences.

Analog-to-digital converter (ADC): Device that samples an analog signal (voltage) into a digital form that can be read by the computer. The ADC is activated during the read-out period in order to measure the MR signal.

Angular frequency (ω): Frequency of rotation, measured in radians per second. $\omega = 2\pi f$, where f = frequency in Hertz (Hz) or cycles per second.

Angular momentum: A vector quantity possessed by spinning objects which is equal to the product of the object's position and momentum vectors. A force, called *torque*, applied at an angle to the axis of rotation causes the object (e.g., a spinning nucleus) to *precess* or wobble about its axis of rotation.

Anisotropic resolution: Spatial resolution in which voxel dimensions are unequal. Images acquired by 2D techniques are generally anisotropic, since they have reduced spatial resolution along the slice-selection axis compared with the other two axes.

Artifacts: Spurious features in an image relating to the imaging process (see Chapter 3). Examples of MR artifacts:

  Center line artifact: Line that appears in the middle of the image, oriented perpendicular to the phase-encoding axis. Etiologies include instrument instabilities and stimulated echoes.

  Chemical shift artifact: Artifactual bright or dark bands that appear along the frequency-encoding axis between a fat-containing tissue and a water-containing tissue. The artifact represents spatial mispositioning of the fat signal due to the difference in resonance frequencies (approximately 3.5 ppm) between fat and water.

  Ferromagnetic artifact: Geometric and signal distortions due to local magnetic field inhomogeneity caused by a ferromagnetic object. This artifact is usually worse in gradient-echo images.

  Ghost artifact: False images of a tissue which propagate along the phase-encoding axis, usually due to periodic motion.

  Stimulated echo artifact: Artifact due to the production of stimulated echoes, which is manifested as a spurious image of a tissue and/or center line artifact. Etiologies include inadequate spoiling of transverse magnetization after signal read-out.

  Susceptibility artifact: Signal loss and geometric distortion similar to, but less severe than, ferromagnetic artifact. May appear at the boundary of two tissues with differing magnetic susceptibility (e.g., brain and air-containing paranasal sinus).

Portions modified from the *ACR Glossary of MRI Terms,* 2nd ed, by S. Koenig, R. Brown, R. Price, and R. Tarr.

Truncation (Gibbs, ringing) artifact: Multiple bands of alternating high and low intensity which appear parallel to a boundary between two tissues with markedly different signal intensities. Caused by sampling at a rate less than the Nyquist limit, the artifact is worsened as the acquisition matrix is reduced (e.g., 256×128 is worse than 256×256).

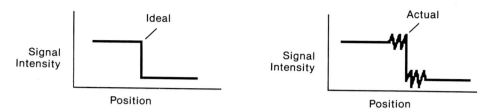

Wraparound artifact: Image of a tissue, located outside the field-of-view, appears within the field-of-view on the opposite side of the image. Represents aliasing due to inadequate number of phase-encoding steps or frequency-encoding samples.

Asymmetric sampling: Miscentering of the read-out period with respect to the echo. This method can be used to shorten the echo time, although when the echo is miscentered too far there will be truncation artifacts along the frequency-encoding direction.

Attenuation: Reduction of power or signal, commonly expressed in dB.

Bandwidth: Range of frequencies.

Low bandwidth pulse sequence: Sequence that employs long read-out period and weak frequency-encoding gradient in order to maximize signal-to-noise, at the expense of increased chemical shift and magnetic susceptibility artifacts and the possibility of an increased minimum echo time.

Bloch equations: Basic equations that describe the motion of the macroscopic magnetization vector, including the effects of the static and radiofrequency magnetic fields and the T_1 and T_2 relaxation times.

Boltzmann distribution: Description of relative population of two energy states for particles in thermal equilibrium.

$$N_1/N_2 = \exp\left[-\Delta E/kT\right]$$

where k is Boltzmann's constant, ΔE is the energy difference between the two states (proportional to field strength), and T is absolute temperature. Describes the ratio of protons aligned with and against the static magnetic field for fully magnetized spins.

Carr-Purcell-Meiboom-Gill (CPMG) sequence: Pulse sequence consisting of a 90-degree radiofrequency pulse followed by multiple 180-degree radiofrequency pulses to produce a train of spin echoes. There is a 90-degree phase shift in the rotating frame between the 90-degree pulse and the 180-degree pulses to reduce effects of imperfections in the 180-degree pulses; the phases of the 180-degree pulses are alternated to reduce accumulation of phase errors. Useful for measuring T_2 relaxation times.

CE-FAST (contrast-enhanced fast acquisition steady-state, PSIF): Gradient-echo sequence that produces, in conjunction with very short repetition times (e.g., 20 to 40 msec), more T_2 contrast than FISP or GRASS sequences. The effective echo time is approximately twice the repetition time.

Chemical shift (σ): Change in resonance frequency due to shielding of a nucleus from the applied magnetic field by electron orbitals. In spectroscopy, chemical shift produces different spectral peaks for different molecules. In imaging, it is responsible for chemical shift artifacts and phase-contrast effects between fat and water.

Chemical shift imaging (CSI): Method for producing an image showing the concentration and spatial distribution of one or more selected chemical species (e.g., lactate). CSI of fat/water is also called *phase-contrast imaging* (see entry).

CHESS (chemical shift selective) pulses: Method for either producing or eliminating signal from a particular species of nucleus. Accomplished by applying a radiofrequency pulse with very narrow bandwidth (i.e., of long duration), it is typically used to produce selective fat or water images.

Cineangiography (cine): Method for acquiring multiple images at one or more levels through the heart, blood vessels, or cerebrospinal fluid. The acquisitions are gated to the cardiac cycle, and when the cine images are replayed in a closed loop, they demonstrate cardiac pulsation and blood and cerebrospinal fluid flow.

Circularly polarized (CP, quadrature) coil: Radiofrequency coil that detects two orthogonal components of the precessing magnetization, resulting in a theoretical 40 per cent signal-to-noise improvement and a 50 per cent reduction in power deposition compared with a linear coil.

Coil: Loops of wire designed to produce a magnetic field from current flowing in the wire, or to detect a voltage induced in the wire by a changing magnetic field.

Continuous wave (CW): Spectroscopic technique for studying samples by measuring radiofrequency absorption as the radiofrequency irradiation is swept through a range of frequencies. Now superceded by pulsed Fourier techniques.

Contrast: Difference in signal intensities of two objects. Can be altered in MRI by changing the pulse sequence or by administering a contrast agent.

Contrast-to-noise ratio (CNR or C/N): Ratio of the signal difference between two tissues relative to the standard deviation of the background noise, expressed as:

$$C/N = (S_1 - S_2)/\sigma_{noise}$$

Useful for comparing performance of different pulse sequences with respect to lesion detection.

Contrast agent: Substance that alters tissue contrast.

T_1 **active:** Contrast agent that predominantly alters tissue contrast in T_1-weighted images (e.g., gadolinium-DTPA, a paramagnetic substance).

T_2 **active:** Contrast agent that predominantly alters tissue contrast in T_2-weighted images (e.g., a superparamagnetic iron oxide particle).

Nonproton: Contrast agent that produces a signal void with all pulse sequences because it lacks hydrogen (e.g., perfluorocytlbromide).

Counter-rotating current (CRC) coil: Pair of coils with currents in opposite directions. With proper design, these coils are intrinsically decoupled from the transmitter coil and can therefore be placed in arbitrary orientations with respect to the transmitter.

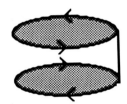

Crossed-coil: Coil pair arranged so that their magnetic fields are perpendicular so as to minimize their electromagnetic interaction.

Cross-talk: Radiofrequency interference between adjacent slices due to nonrectangular slice profiles. This results in a reduced signal-to-noise ratio and, particularly in T_2-weighted images, a loss of contrast. Cross-talk can be reduced by use of large slice gaps and/or computer-optimized radiofrequency pulses.

Cryogens: Cold liquids, typically liquid helium and liquid nitrogen, used to maintain the magnet coils at superconducting temperatures.

Cryostat: The insulating dewar in superconducting magnets used to maintain the magnet coils and liquid helium bath at very low temperatures.

Cryoshield: Lining of the cryostat. Magnetic interactions between the cryoshield and gradient coils are largely responsible for the production of eddy currents, which can degrade image quality.

dB/dt: Rate of change of a magnetic field with time. There is potential concern for patient safety with rapidly changing magnetic field gradients, since changing magnetic fields induce electrical currents.

Decibel (dB): Index of relative power or voltage, expressed as:

$$dB = 20 \log_{10} (V_1/V_2) \text{ or } 10 \log_{10} (P_1/P_2)$$

For instance, a reduction in power by a factor of two corresponds to -3 dB attenutation.

Decoupling: Spectroscopic technique of irradiating one resonance in order to reduce its effects on the spectrum of interest. Particularly useful in carbon-13 spectroscopy.

Diamagnetic: Property of most substances with paired orbital electrons such that they weakly repel an applied magnetic field. Has only minimal effect on MR signal intensities except where there are large gradients of magnetic susceptibility (e.g., near the paranasal sinuses).

Diffusion: Random motion of molecules due to thermal energy. Diffusion-sensitive pulse sequences rely on the fact that diffusion produces signal loss—the magnitude of which depends on the echo time, on local field gradients due to susceptibility differences, and on the applied magnetic field gradients, in order to measure the diffusion constant **D.** Diffusion measurements may provide information about the tissue, such as microscopic structure, the temperature, and so forth.

Dipole: Having a north and south magnetic pole, similar to a bar magnet or compass needle. The proton, with spin of ½, is a dipole and can have only two possible alignments in an applied magnetic field.

Dipole-dipole interactions: Magnetic interactions of two spins in which the magnetic field produced by one influences another. Proton dipole-dipole interactions, which require close-range interactions, are important contributors to T_1 and T_2 relaxation.

Dispersion: Variation of relaxation rates with static magnetic field strength.

Display matrix: Number of picture elements displayed on the monitor, typically 512×512 or 1024×1024.

Echo: MR signal produced after the FID has decayed, owing to rephasing of the transverse magnetization.

> **Gradient echo (GRE, gradient-refocused echo, field echo):** Echo produced by single radiofrequency pulse (alpha, usually ≤ 90 degrees) followed by a gradient reversal. It is useful for fast and flow imaging but is sensitive to magnetic field inhomogeneities and chemical shift differences.

> **Spin echo (SE):** Echo produced by 90-degree radiofrequency pulse followed by one or more 180-degree radiofrequency pulses. The spin echo, used for most clinical imaging, is relatively insensitive to the effects of magnetic field inhomogeneities and chemical shift differences.

Echo-planar imaging (EPI): Rapid acquisition of a train of separately phase-encoded gradient echoes to produce a fully resolved image after a single excitation (e.g., 90 degrees --- 180 degrees --- [gradient echoes] or alpha pulse --- [gradient echoes]). Total acquisition time is typically ≤ 60 msec. Requires large peak gradient amplitudes, rapid oscillation of the phase-encoding gradient, and minimal eddy currents. At present, EPI produces images having lower spatial resolution than conventional techniques and is sensitive to magnetic susceptibility effects. It may be useful for cardiac imaging and for the study of dynamic processes.

Echo time (TE): Time between center of radiofrequency excitation pulse and center of read-out period. Typically short (e.g., 15 to 30 msec) for proton density- and T_1-weighted sequences and long (e.g., 60 to 90 msec) for T_2-weighted sequences.

Eddy currents: Electrical currents induced in a conductor by a changing magnetic field. Changing gradient magnetic fields induce undesirable currents in the cryoshield and other conducting structures, resulting in distortion of the gradient waveform and image artifacts.

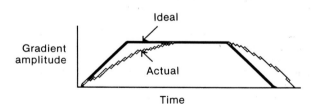

> **Actively shielded gradients:** An extra set of current-carrying coils is placed around the gradient coils to generate an opposing time-varying magnetic field, to eliminate the induction of eddy currents in the cryoshield.

> **Eddy current compensation:** The voltages driving the gradient coils are modified to anticipate and, therefore, compensate for the effects of eddy currents, so that the desired gradient waveform is achieved.

Excitation: Application of radiofrequency energy to a spin system to produce a net transverse magnetization or an inversion of the population.

Exorcist: See *ROPE*.

Even-echo rephasing: Signal enhancement of blood flowing at constant velocity within a slice, which occurs in even-echo images due to elimination of flow-related phase shifts. Can be produced by spin-echo imaging as well as by gradient-echo (e.g., field-echo even-echo rephasing—FEER) imaging. Most commonly occurs when: (1) the echoes are symmetric (e.g., TE_1/TE_2 = 30 msec/60 msec) rather than asymmetric (e.g., TE_1/TE_2 = 20 msec/80 msec), and (2) in a spin-echo sequence, when the gradients are symmetric about the 180-degree radiofrequency pulses.

Faraday shield: Electrical conductor sometimes interposed between a radiofrequency coil and the patient in order to minimize electrical interactions that would reduce the performance of the coil.

Ferromagnetic: Substance with large positive magnetic susceptibility that becomes magnetized within a magnetic field and remains magnetized after being removed from the field. Causes large magnetic field distortions and signal loss.

Field-echo: See *gradient-echo.*

Fourier transform (FT): Mathematical method for converting a time-varying signal into its frequency and/or phase components, or vice-versa. Used to obtain position information from the MR signal.

Fast Fourier transform (FFT): An efficient digital implementation of the Fourier transform, used in most MR systems.

Field-of-view (FOV): Area spanned by the image, defined as (horizontal distance across the image) × (vertical distance across the image). Large fields-of-view (e.g., 42 cm × 42 cm) are typically used for body imaging, whereas smaller fields-of-view (e.g., 16 cm × 16 cm) are often used for higher resolution imaging (e.g., joint studies).

  Asymmetric (rectangular) field-of-view: Having unequal horizontal and vertical distances across the image (e.g., 50 cm × 25 cm).

Filling factor: Index of the geometric relationship between a radiofrequency coil and the body. A high filling factor is desirable for maximizing the signal-to-noise ratio and can be achieved by matching the size and shape of the coil to the body part of interest (e.g., a small head coil provides a better filling factor for brain imaging than a body coil).

FISP (fast imaging with steady-state free precession): Gradient-echo sequence containing an inverted phase-encoding gradient after read-out to rephase residual transverse magnetization. In conjunction with very short repetition times and a phase-alternated radiofrequency pulse with a relatively large flip angle (e.g., 90 degrees), it produces strong signal from tissues with a large T_2/T_1 ratio, such as cerebrospinal fluid. Primarily a single slice acquisition technique, but well suited to 3D imaging. Essentially same as *GRASS* technique.

FLASH (fast low angle shot): Gradient-echo sequence containing spoiler gradient after read-out to disperse residual transverse magnetization. Produces T_1-weighted images with large flip angle (e.g., 75 degrees) and proton density–weighted images with low flip angle (e.g., 10 degrees). Can be used as single or multislice acquisition technique.

Flip angle: The amount by which the macroscopic magnetization vector **M** is rotated by a radiofrequency pulse with respect to the direction of the static magnetic field. Typically, 90-degree and 180-degree radiofrequency pulses are used for spin-echo sequences, and flip angles ≤ 90 degrees are used for gradient-echo sequences.

Flow compensation (gradient motion rephasing [GMR], gradient motion nulling [GMN], motion artifact suppression technique [MAST]): Method for minimizing phase dispersion and associated signal loss due to flow or other types of motion. Employs one or more extra gradient pulses incorporated into the pulse sequence, pulses that may rephase spins along one or more axes. In general, prolongs the minimum echo time and/or requires larger gradient amplitudes.

Flow displacement artifact: Apparent displacement of obliquely flowing spins from their true positions due to the time delays between excitation, phase-encoding, and read-out and to nonlinear phase shifts occuring during the application of the phase-encoding gradient.

Flow-related enhancement (FRE or paradoxical enhancement): Bright signal from flowing blood or cerebrospinal fluid relative to stationary tissues. Inflow of fresh, unsaturated spins into the slice produces more signal than partially saturated stationary spins within the slice.

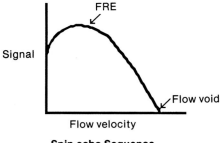

Spin-echo Sequence

Flow void (washout): Loss of vascular signal observed in spin-echo images when moving spins are displaced out of the slice during the time interval TE/2 between the 90-degree and 180-degree radiofrequency pulses.

Free induction decay (FID): Signal produced immediately following a radiofrequency pulse. Not usually directly used for imaging.

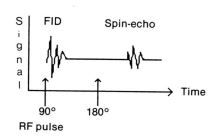

Frequency-encoding: Spatial encoding along one in-plane dimension, done by applying the frequency-encoding (read-out) gradient for a period of time before and after the echo time.

Full width–half maximum (FWHM): Width of spectral peak at one half the maximal height. Proportional to $1/T_2^*$. FWHM is also used in other MR contexts, such as defining the effective slice thickness.

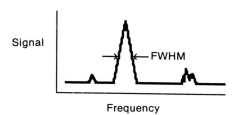

Gating: Method for synchronizing data acquisition to periodic physiologic motion.

ECG gating: A generic term describing the synchronization of data acquisition to patient's ECG signal.

Prospective ECG gating (triggering): Method of collecting data used for both standard and cine acquisitions. Data are collected at defined intervals after each R wave.

Retrospective ECG gating: Method of collecting data which is primarily used for cine studies. Data are collected at constant time intervals, independent of the cardiac cycle. The data are then sorted during postprocessing according to the phase of the cardiac cycle in order to produce cine images. The method is generally preferred over prospective gating for cine studies, due to its lesser sensitivity to arrhythmias.

Respiratory gating: Synchronization of data acquisition to a specific period during respiration (e.g., end expiration). Respiration is typically monitored using a bellows-type device placed about the chest or abdomen.

Physiologic (in vivo) gating: Synchronization of data acquisition to physiologic motion, done with a modified pulse sequence. The modified sequence uses an extra echo that is not phase-encoded and therefore represents a full-thickness projection through the patient. Motion-dependent changes in the signal intensity of the echo vary with different phases of the cardiac and/or respiratory cycle. These periodic changes can be used to simulate, in effect, an ECG or respiratory tracing. They permit retrospective gating to the cardiac and/or respiratory cycle without the need for ECG leads or respiratory monitors.

Gauss (G): A unit of magnetic induction, where $1\ G = 10^{-4}\ T$. The earth's magnetic field strength is approximately 0.6 G.

Golay coil: Typical design for a gradient coil used to produce a magnetic field perpendicular to the static magnetic field.

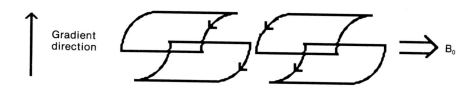

Gradient coil: Current-carrying coils designed to produce a linear magnetic field gradient along a particular direction. Typically, MR systems contain three sets of gradient coils.

Gradient-echo: See *echo.*

Gradient reversal: Combination of a negative *dephasing* gradient and a positive *rephasing* gradient, used to ensure that stationary spins have the same phase at the echo time. Applied along the slice-selection and frequency-encoding directions in gradient-echo sequences.

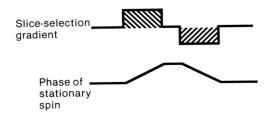

GRASS (gradient-recalled acquisition steady-state): See *FISP*.

Gyromagnetic ratio (γ): Constant for a given nucleus which represents the ratio of magnetic moment to the angular momentum. For protons, this may be expressed as 42.56 MHz/ Tesla.

Half-Fourier: Method for acquiring the data using approximately half the usual number of phase-encoding steps. Half-Fourier images can be acquired in about half the time of a conventional image, at the expense of a 40 per cent reduction in signal-to-noise and increased sensitivity to some artifacts.

Helmholtz coil: Pair of parallel coils with current in same direction having relatively uniform sensitivity for signals from tissues located between them.

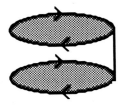

Hertz (Hz): Unit of frequency, equal to cycles per second.

Homogeneity: Uniformity of the magnetic field, usually expressed in ppm over a defined volume (e.g., over a 50-cm sphere). Good static field homogeneity is required for imaging, and homogeneity an order of magnitude better is needed for high-resolution spectroscopy.

Hybrid scanning: Similar to echo-planar imaging but with less rapid oscillation of the phase-encoding gradient and therefore fewer gradient echoes per read-out period. Unlike echo-planar imaging, hybrid scanning requires multiple excitations and typically improves acquisition time by a factor of only two to eight when compared with conventional 2DFT methods.

Inversion recovery (IR) pulse sequence: Sequence consisting of an initial 180-degree radio-frequency pulse to invert the magnetization, followed by a spin-echo (90 to 180 degrees) or gradient-echo sequence. Useful for producing strongly T_1-weighted images.

STIR (short tau inversion recovery): IR sequence using short inversion time to minimize signal from fat, thereby reducing respiratory motion artifacts. Typical parameters are: TR/TI/TE = 2000 msec/150 msec/20 msec. Particularly useful for suppressing fat signal in the orbital cone and bone marrow; also used to enhance lesion conspicuity in the liver, pelvis, and other areas.

Inversion time (TI): Time between the 180-degree inversion pulse and the 90-degree pulse in an inversion recovery sequence.

Isochromat: Group of spins that have identical phase.

Isotope: Species of an element with same atomic number but different atomic mass (same number of protons but different number of neutrons). Isotopes have similar chemical properties (e.g., H-1 [hydrogen] vs. H-2 [deuterium]) but may have very different properties with regard to MR (e.g., 42.56 vs. 6.53 MHz/T gyromagnetic ratios).

Isotropic resolution: Having equal spatial resolution along all three dimensions. Most readily achieved with three-dimensional acquisitions, isotropic acquisitions permit images of equal resolution to be reconstructed along any plane of section.

K-space: Representation of data from image acquisition (raw data) as a two-dimensional matrix of points. The coordinates of each point represent a unique combination of frequency (k_x) and phase (k_y) corresponding to the time-integral of the frequency- and phase-encoding gradients, respectively. Acquisition trajectories in k-space are particularly useful for understanding fast imaging methods.

Laminar flow: Flow profile, usually seen in veins and small arteries, with maximal velocity (v_{max}) occurring in center of vessel; velocity is slower near edge of vessel due to friction between flowing blood and the wall of the vessel. The average velocity in a vessel with fully developed laminar (parabolic) flow is $\frac{1}{2} v_{max}$.

Larmor equation: Relationship between field strength and resonance frequency, expressed as:

$$f_L = \gamma B_0$$

where γ is expressed in MHz/Tesla and B_0 is expressed in Tesla.

Linearly polarized coil: Radiofrequency coil that detects a single component of the precessing transverse magnetization. Used for most surface coil designs, but is less efficient than circularly polarized coil for head and body imaging.

Linewidth: Broadness of a spectral peak, which has an inverse dependence on the T_2^* relaxation time. Usually defined at full width–half maximum.

Longitudinal magnetization (M_z): Component of macroscopic magnetization **M** oriented along the direction of the static magnetic field.

Lorentzian: Typical shape of a peak in an MR spectrum, with a central peak and broad tails. A Lorentzian shape in the frequency domain is equivalent to an exponential decay in the time domain.

Magnetic dipole moment: A measure of the magnetic properties of a dipolar nucleus, which interacts with an applied magnetic field like a bar magnet.

Magnetic field (H): Property of the space surrounding a magnet; a dipole within a magnetic field will experience a torque that causes it to align with the field. Excludes the effect of magnetization.

Magnetic induction (B): Net magnetic effect from an applied magnetic field. Differs from **H** in that it includes the effect of magnetization. **B** and **H** are identical in a vacuum and are often used interchangeably to represent magnetic fields. However, these terms differ significantly in materials with large magnetic susceptibilities.

B_0: Term for the highly homogeneous static main field.

B_1: Term for the oscillating magnetic field produced by the radiofrequency coil.

Magnetic resonance (MR): The enhanced absorption of radiofrequency energy by nuclei or electrons in a static magnetic field when the energy is applied at the resonance frequency. In clinical applications, the term is assumed to represent interactions with nuclei, also called nuclear magnetic resonance (NMR). When applied to electrons, the method is called electron spin resonance (ESR) or electron paramagnetic resonance (EPR).

MRI: Magnetic resonance imaging.

Magnetic resonance signal: Voltage induced in a receiver coil by precession of the transverse magnetization of a sample.

Magnetic susceptibility (χ): Tendency of a substance to become magnetized or to distort an applied magnetic field. Includes the contributions from diamagnetic, paramagnetic, and ferromagnetic components.

Magnetic shielding: Method for containing the stray (fringe) magnetic field from an MR system.

Active magnetic shielding: An extra set of current-carrying coils surround the main magnet coils and create an opposing magnetic field.

Passive magnetic shielding: Iron plates are applied directly to the magnet (self-shielding) or are placed in strategic locations on the walls of the magnet enclosure.

Magnitude image: Form of image presentation, reconstructed from magnitude data:

$$\text{Magnitude data} = ([\text{real data}]^2 + [\text{imaginary data}]^2)^{1/2}$$

The magnitude image is generally used instead of the real or imaginary image because of its insensitivity to phase errors.

Maximum intensity projection (MIP): Method for producing MR angiograms. A series of slices are processed along a user-selected angle, and the pixel with highest signal intensity is extracted. When the method is applied to a series of images acquired by two- or three-dimensional flow-compensated gradient-echo sequences, the result is an angiographic image in which flowing blood appears bright.

Maxwell coil: Coil design that produces a gradient in the direction of the static magnetic field.

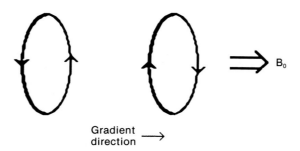

Gradient direction $\longrightarrow$

Minimum intensity projection (MIN): Technique similar to maximum intensity projection method but using pixels with the lowest intensity. Permits reconstruction of MR angiograms from images in which flowing blood appears dark.

MRS: Magnetic resonance spectroscopy. A group of methods for investigating tissue metabolism by using magnetic resonance to determine the concentrations and kinetics of various metabolites. In conjunction with magnetic field gradients and/or profiled static or radiofrequency magnetic fields, MRS can be used to produce *in vivo* spectra that are spatially localized.

Multifrequency excitation: Simultaneous excitation of more than one slice simultaneously by a radiofrequency pulse containing multiple frequencies. The method is commonly used to produce two presaturation volumes simultaneously for flow presaturation. It can also be used to increase the number of slices that can be acquired for a given repetition time (e.g., POMP).

Net (macroscopic) magnetization vector (M): Net sum of all the individual magnetic moments in a sample. M_z represents the vector along the longitudinal axis, and M_{xy} represents the vector in the transverse direction.

NEX (number of excitations): Number of times that the spins are excited in a given view (i.e., for a given amplitude of the phase-encoding gradient). The signals from these excitations are averaged together. Same as *number of acquisitions* (NAQ).

NMR (nuclear magnetic resonance spectroscopy): MR spectroscopy, specifically of nuclei rather than electrons.

Nuclear spin: Property of certain nuclei with an odd number of nucleons (protons or neutrons) which results in an intrinsic angular momentum and magnetic moment.

Nutation: Displacement of the axis of a spinning body from the simple cone shape produced by precession; used to describe, in the rotating frame, the rotation of the macroscopic magnetization vector caused by a radiofrequency pulse.

Nyquist limit: Sampling frequency for a signal which must be equalled or exceeded in order to avoid aliasing of high frequencies into lower frequencies. For example, to properly represent a 11-kHz sine wave, sampling must be done at 22 kHz or higher.

Oversampling: Method for overcoming the Nyquist limit in order to eliminate wraparound (aliasing) artifact. Done by acquiring extra frequency-encoding samples (with no increase in acquisition time) or by oversampling along the phase-encoding direction (with an attendant increase in acquisition time) and increasing the field-of-view.

Paramagnetic: Substance with positive magnetic susceptibility. These substances (e.g., gadolinium) usually contain one or more unpaired electrons and produce marked reductions in the T_1 and T_2 relaxation times. In vivo, the dominant effect is usually increased signal due to T_1 shortening. Examples of paramagnetic substances include gadolinium-DTPA, methemoglobin, and free radicals.

Partition: Thin slice created from a thick slab excitation with three-dimensional acquisitions by phase-encoding along the slice-selection direction.

Perfusion: Tissue blood flow at the capillary level. One method for studying tissue perfusion by MR is to administer a contrast agent intravascularly and observe the kinetics of tissue enhancement.

Permanent magnet: Magnet composed of large quantities of a ferromagnetic material with high magnetic remanence, used to produce field strengths ≤ 0.3 T. Typically have a vertical static field orientation and minimal stray magnetic fields.

Phase: Relative position of peaks and troughs of a signal with respect to those of a reference signal.

Phase coherent (in-phase): Peak of one signal within a voxel occurs simultaneously with peak of another signal in the same voxel, resulting in maximum constructive interference.

Phase incoherent (out-of-phase, phase dispersion, dephased): Peak of one signal in a voxel occurs in opposition to another signal in the same voxel, resulting in a weak net signal. Causes of phase dispersion include T_2 decay, static field inhomogeneity, flow and other kinds of motion, and, in a phase-contrast image, presence of fat and water within the same voxel.

Phase-contrast image (out-of-phase image): Image in which signal cancellation occurs in voxels containing both fat and water protons. Can be produced with a spin-echo sequence by shifting the 180-degree radiofrequency pulse from the middle of the sequence by an appropriate field strength–dependent time interval, so that the spin echo and gradient echo do not occur at the same time. Alternatively, the image can be produced with a gradient-echo sequence by choosing an appropriate echo time for the field strength. Useful for demonstrating abnormal changes in the fat/water content of a tissue (e.g., leukemic infiltration of red bone marrow).

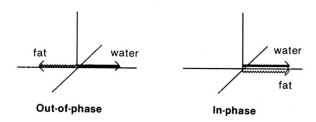

Out-of-phase　　　　　**In-phase**

Phase-encoding: Technique for spatially encoding the position along one in-plane dimension by applying a series of unique phase-encoding gradient integrals (i.e., gradient amplitude × duration).

Phase/frequency swap: Interchange of the phase-encoding and frequency-encoding axes so as to keep ghost artifacts, which propagate along the phase-encoding direction, off the region of interest.

Phase image: Image produced from the arctangent of the ratio of the imaginary and real data. Typically, the brightness of each pixel is mapped in proportion to the phase. Sometimes used for evaluating flow and hemorrhage since flowing spins or local field inhomogeneities will produce phase shifts.

Pixel: Two-dimensional picture element. The dimensions of a pixel are equal to (field-of-view)/(number of pixels in acquisition matrix along that dimension).

Precession: Cone-shaped motion of the rotation axis of a spinning body which occurs when a torque is applied (e.g., precession of a spinning top or precession of a nucleus in a magnetic field). Precession of the transverse magnetization generates a measurable MR signal.

Presaturation (Presat, Sat, FLAK, FRODO): Method for reducing flow or motion artifacts which involves application of extra radiofrequency pulses to user-specified regions, so as to eliminate signal from those regions.

Projection acquisition: A two-dimensional imaging method, typically used for MR angiography, by which data from a large thickness of the body are acquired simultaneously. It is similar to a conventional angiogram in that there is no discrimination of depth. Projection acquisition methods use either a weak or no slice-selection gradient.

Proton density: Number of MR-visible protons in a unit volume of tissue. Generally has minor effect on image contrast compared with T_1 and T_2. Provides a small positive contribution to tissue contrast on T_2-weighted images and opposes contrast on T_1-weighted images.

Proton density–weighted pulse sequence: Sequence that emphasizes the effect of differences in proton density on tissue contrast, that is, spin-echo sequence with long TR and short TE (e.g., TR/TE = 2500 msec/20 msec), or gradient-echo sequence with small flip angle and short TE (e.g., TR/TE/flip angle = 100 msec/10 msec/10 degrees).

Plug flow: Flow profile in which all spins flow at approximately the same velocity. Characteristic of some large arteries with highly pulsatile flow, such as the ascending aorta.

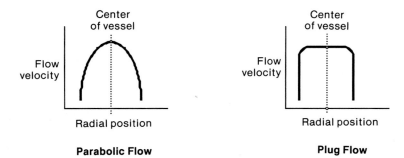

Parabolic Flow   **Plug Flow**

Proton: The nucleus of a hydrogen-1 atom.

Pulse Fourier NMR: Generally used MRI and MRS method that applies radiofrequency pulses of relatively short duration to excite the spins.

Pulse programmer (sequence controller): A computer system that controls timing, shape, and strength of the radiofrequency and gradient pulses.

Pulse sequence: Series of radiofrequency and gradient pulses used to excite the spins and measure the MR signal.

Gradient-echo (GRE) sequence: Pulse sequence having a single radiofrequency (alpha) pulse. The echo is produced by reversal of the magnetic field gradients.

Spin-echo (SE) sequence: Pulse sequence consisting of an initial 90-degree radiofrequency pulse, followed after a time interval equal to TE/2 by a 180-degree pulse. A spin-echo sequence results in the production of both a spin echo, refocused by the 180-degree radiofrequency pulse, and a gradient echo, resulting from the reversal of the magnetic field gradients. These echoes normally occur at the same time (i.e., the echo time), and the result is an image that is insensitive to chemical shift differences and magnetic field inhomogeneities. However, the spin echo can be offset in time relative to the gradient echo and center of the read-out period, resulting in destructive interference between fat and water signals (see *phase-contrast imaging*).

Quadrature coil: See *circularly polarized coil*.

Quadrature detector: Standard method for detecting MR signal. It consists of a phase-sensitive detector (demodulator) that detects two components of the signal: one in-phase *(real component)* and the other 90 degrees out-of-phase *(imaginary component)* with respect to a reference signal.

Quality (Q): Quantity inversely related to the fraction of energy lost each cycle in an oscillating system; also, inversely related to the range of frequencies over which the coil will resonate. Quality is a measure of the performance of a coil: signal-to-noise (S/N) is proportional to $\sqrt{Q}$, so a high Q is generally desirable. The Q of a loaded coil (with patient) is less than the Q of an unloaded coil (no patient).

Quench: Sudden loss of superconductivity, typically causing rapid evaporation of cryogens. May be spontaneous or due to inadequate levels of liquid helium.

RARE (rapid acquisition with relaxation enhancement): A research method (not in general use) for rapidly producing an image with strong T_2 contrast, consisting of a train of individually phase-encoded spin echoes.

Radiofrequency (RF) coil: Current-carrying coil used to excite the spins *(transmitter coil)* or to detect the MR signal *(receiver coil)*.

Radiofrequency (RF) pulse: Oscillating magnetic field (B_1), typically of relatively short duration (e.g., 1 to 10 msec), produced by an RF coil. In MR imaging, RF pulses are applied to excite a selected slice of tissue.

Computer-optimized RF pulse: RF pulse modulated by a computer-optimized series of numbers not representing a simple mathematical function, which produces a highly rectangular slice profile even when the pulse is of relatively short duration (e.g., 3 msec). Computer-optimized pulses are useful for minimizing cross-talk and reducing RF power deposition.

Gaussian pulse: RF pulse modulated by an exponential function which produces a nonrectangular slice profile having a broad peak and tails.

Sinc pulse: RF pulse modulated by a sinc function: sin(x)/x. For a given amplitude of the selection gradient, the slice profile becomes more rectangular as the pulse duration is increased (more zero crossings). Sinc pulses of short duration produce nonrectangular (essentially Gaussian) slice profiles, resulting in cross-talk if small slice gaps are used.

Ramp time: Time required for the field strength of a superconducting magnet to increase from zero to its operating strength.

Gradient ramp (rise) time: Time for a magnetic field gradient to increase from zero to a selected amplitude. Ramp times are typically on the order of a few hundred microseconds to 1 millisecond.

Raw data: Data acquired from the image acquisition, organized as a two-dimensional matrix with points along one axis representing individual frequency-encoded samples and points along the other axis representing individual phase-encoding steps.

Relaxation rate (R_1, R_2): The inverse of the T_1 or T_2 relaxation time, expressed in sec^{-1}. Relaxation rates are a useful concept for discussions of relaxation mechanisms and contrast agent effects because, unlike relaxation times, relaxation rates from different sources can be directly added to assess their cumulative effect.

Repetition time (TR): Time between successive excitations of the spins. For a spin-echo sequence, the time between successive 90-degree radiofrequency pulses; for a gradient-echo sequence, the time between successive alpha pulses.

Resistive magnet: Magnet composed of current-carrying coils which requires continuous input of electrical current; used to produce field strengths $\leq$ 0.4 T. May have horizontal or vertical field orientation depending on magnet design.

Resonator coil: Radiofrequency coil typically having symmetrical geometry, often used at high field strengths.

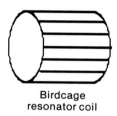

Birdcage
resonator coil

ROPE (respiratory ordered phase encoding): Method for reducing ghost artifacts by reordering application of phase-encoding steps according to the phase of the respiratory cycle.

Rotating frame: Frame of reference as if the observer is precessing at the same rate as the magnetization vector. Useful for providing a simplified description of the relative motions of the magnetization vectors.

Saddle coil: Coil geometry, often used in medium or lower field systems, consisting of two opposed curved coils.

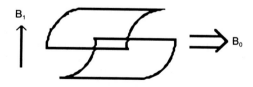

Half-saddle coil: Surface coil having only a single curved coil, often used for imaging of the neck.

Sampling interval: Time used to measure signal for each data point during the read-out period. There are typically from 5 to 30 microseconds per sampling interval, and 256 to 512 sampling intervals per read-out period.

Sampling time (read-out period): Duration over which the signal is measured. Signal-to-noise improves approximately in proportion to the (sampling time)$^{1/2}$. The sampling time is equal to (number of sampling intervals) $\times$ (duration of the sampling interval).

Saturation: Incomplete realignment of the net magnetization with the static magnetic field, due to repeated application of radiofrequency pulses in a time that is short compared with

T_1. The term saturation has a different meaning when applied to a material placed within a magnetic field. In this latter context, saturation means that the material is fully magnetized.

Selective excitation (selective irradiation): Application of a radiofrequency pulse with a defined frequency range (bandwidth) which, in conjunction with a magnetic field gradient, excites a plane of nuclei oriented perpendicular to the gradient.

Shimming: Process of maximizing the homogeneity of the static magnetic field using one or more of the following methods.

Active shimming: Shimming by adjusting the current flow through one or more coils positioned within the magnet bore.

Passive shimming: Shimming by placing sheets of iron at various locations around the magnet.

Skin effect: Attenuation of high frequency radiofrequency energy with increasing depth due to dissipation by conductive media (e.g., superficial tissues). Can become a significant problem at high field strengths (high RF frequencies), resulting in depth-dependent variations in signal intensity.

Signal averaging: Use of multiple radiofrequency excitations with averaging of the resultant signals. Improves signal-to-noise in proportion to $(NEX)^{1/2}$ also reduces ghost artifacts due to pulsatile flow and other kinds of motion.

Signal-to-noise ratio (SNR or S/N): Measure of graininess of image, defined as

$$S/N = S_1/\sigma_{noise}$$

where S_1 is tissue signal, and σ_{noise} is the standard deviation of background noise. SNR depends on many factors, including magnetic field strength, radiofrequency coil, pulse sequence parameters, size and shape of the body part being imaged.

Slice gap: Distance between the centers of adjacent slices. When the slice profile is not rectangular, a large slice gap (e.g., 50 to 100 per cent of the slice thickness) is needed to prevent cross-talk.

Solenoidal coil: Radiofrequency coil consisting of wire wrapped around a cylinder, having relatively uniform sensitivity within the coil. Often used in conjunction with permanent or resistive magnet systems that have a vertical static field orientation.

Solomon-Bloembergen equations: Set of equations that relate certain types of molecular motion and effects of interactions with electron magnetic moments to the T_1 and T_2 relaxation times. Useful for analyzing sources of tissue relaxation and contrast agent effects.

Solvent suppression: Techniques for suppressing the large signal from the solvent which would otherwise limit detection of smaller signals from other molecules. Commonly used in proton spectroscopy to reduce undesirable signals from bulk water and fat, which obscure signals from metabolites of interest such as lactate.

Spectrum: Display of signal amplitude versus frequency. Since nuclei in different chemical environments have different resonance frequencies, MR spectra provide information about chemical structure and metabolism.

Spectrometer: Apparatus for exciting the spins and measuring the MR signal; includes the magnet, shims, radiofrequency coils, transmitter, receiver, controlling circuitry, and so forth, but does not include the gradient systems.

Spin: See *nuclear spin*. Also used synonymously for a nucleus possessing spin (e.g., hydrogen-1).

Spoiler: Gradient pulse or table of gradient amplitudes applied to eliminate transverse magnetization that persists after the read-out period.

Steady-state free precession (SSFP): Method for producing large signal from tissues with large T_2/T_1 ratio (e.g., cerebrospinal fluid). Radiofrequency pulses are applied at intervals that are short compared with T_1 and T_2. See *FISP*.

Stimulated echo: Spurious echo that can be a source of image artifacts. The echo results from the application of three radiofrequency pulses, e.g., 90 degrees - - TS - - 90 degrees - - - - *wait* - - - - 90 degrees - - TS - - (stimulated echo). T_1 decay occurs during the *wait* interval.

STEAM (stimulated echo acquisition method): Method for producing an image or spectrum from stimulated echoes. Suffers from reduced signal-to-noise compared with standard spin-echo or gradient-echo sequences, but has novel contrast properties. Particularly useful for localized spectroscopy.

Subtraction angiography: MR angiography performed by acquiring a pair of images in which flowing blood has different signal intensities (e.g., flow compensated/uncompensated). Pairwise subtraction of the images produces a pure flow image, analogous to digital subtraction angiography.

Superconducting magnet: Magnet consisting of miles of a superconducting material. Once ramped up to full field, it requires no additional input of electrical current. Typically used to produce field strengths ≥ 0.35 T, these magnets have a horizontal static field orientation, and stray magnetic fields extend for large distances from the magnet unless magnetic shielding is used.

Superconductivity: Property of certain materials, such as titanium-niobium, which loses all electrical resistance when maintained at a temperature lower than the critical temperature of the material.

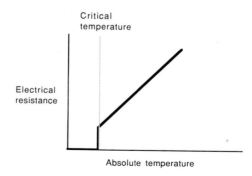

Superparamagnetic: Substance with large positive magnetic susceptibility. These substances (e.g., certain iron oxide compounds) have a single magnetic domain and become transiently magnetized in a magnetic field.

T_1 (longitudinal or spin-lattice relaxation time): Time constant for spins to realign with the static magnetic field. There is 63 per cent realignment in one T_1 interval.

   T_1-weighted image: Sequence that emphasizes the effect of differences in T_1 on tissue contrast, that is, spin-echo sequence with short TR, short TE (e.g., TR/TE = 500 msec/ 20 msec); inversion recovery sequence (e.g., TR/TI/TE = 2000 msec/500 msec/20 msec); or gradient-echo sequence with large flip angle and short TE (e.g., TR/TE/flip angle = 100 msec/10 msec/75 degrees.)

T_2 (transverse or spin-spin relaxation time): Time constant for loss of phase coherence among a group of spins, which results in loss of the MR signal. Excludes the effects of static magnetic field inhomogeneities.

   T_2-weighted image: Sequence that emphasizes the effect of differences in T_2 on tissue contrast, that is, spin-echo sequence with long TR, long TE (e.g., TR/TE = 2500 msec/ 80 msec).

   T_2^*: Same as T_2, but includes the effects of static magnetic field inhomogeneities, expressed as:

$$1/T_2^* = 1/T_2 + \gamma\Delta B/2$$

where ΔB is the local magnetic field inhomogeneity. T_2^* effects are seen in gradient-echo images, particularly when acquired with long TE (e.g., TR/TE/flip angle = 100 msec/30 msec/10 degrees), but not in spin-echo images.

Tesla (T): Unit of magnetic induction (B) equal to 10,000 Gauss.

Three-dimensional (3DFT or volume) acquisition: Method for data acquisition by which a relatively thick slice is excited, then thin slices are resolved by phase-encoding along the slice-selection direction. The two in-plane dimensions are spatially resolved by frequency-encoding and by phase-encoding. A three-dimensional Fourier transform is then applied to the data, analogous to the 2DFT used for two-dimensional single or multislice imaging. The method is advantageous, particular in conjunction with short repetition times and gradient-echo pulse sequences, for producing thin ($\leq$ 1 mm) contiguous slices, for multi-planar and surface reconstructions, and for MR angiography.

Tuning: Process of adjusting the circuit resonance of a radiofrequency coil so that the coil resonates at the Larmor frequency of the tissue protons. Radiofrequency coils are commonly retuned every time a different patient or body part is imaged.

Turbulent flow: Chaotic flow pattern that typically occurs with rapid flow through a stenosis or valvular regurgitation. In MR imaging, turbulent flow produces signal loss due to phase dispersion.

Two-dimensional (2DFT) acquisition: Method for data acquisition by which a relatively thin slice is excited, followed by frequency- and phase-encoding to spatially resolve the two in-plane dimensions. Most commonly used acquisition method.

Vector: Quantity having a magnitude and direction, often represented by an arrow whose length is proportional to the magnitude and with an arrowhead at one end to show direction.

Voxel: Volume element, defined as (pixel area) $\times$ (slice thickness). Signal-to-noise is directly proportional to the voxel volume.

INDEX

Note: Page numbers in *italics* refer to illustrations; page numbers followed by t refer to tables.

Abdomen, angiography in, *158*, 160–162, *160–165*
  fetal, *946*, 946–947, *947*
  imaging of, gradient-echo, 200, *201, 202*
    technique of, 845–852, *846–852*
  undescended testes in, *974–976, 974–977*
Abdominal aorta. See *Aorta.*
Abscess, epididymotesticular, *963*, 964
  of brain, AIDS-related, 584, *586–588*
    bacterial, 576–577, *576–578*
    fungal, 577, *579*
    parasitic, 577–580, *580, 581*
  of foot, in diabetes, 1092, *1093*
  of liver, amebic, 875, *878*
  orbital, 614, *616*
  paravertebral, 695, *696*
  pelvic, *1120*
  retroperitoneal, 909
  vs. osteomyelitis, 1119, *1120, 1122*
Absorption mode spectra, 298
Absorption rate, specific, 48–49
N-Acetylaspartate, in proton spectroscopy, 279, 281, *281*
Achilles tendon, disorders of, 1080–1082, *1081, 1082*
Aciduria, spectroscopy of, 277
Acoustic nerve, anatomy of, 623
  axial view of, *386*
  meningioma of, in neurofibromatosis, 431, *434*
  neuroma of, 470–473, *472, 473*, 625, *625*
    in neurofibromatosis, 431, *433*
  sagittal view of, *407–409*
Acquired immunodeficiency syndrome, and brain infection, 583–589, *586–590*
  primary malignant lymphoma in, 452, *453*
Acquisition, projection, definition of, 1167
  in angiography, 152–155, *152–155*
Acquisition matrix, definition of, 1158
Acquisition time, definition of, 1158
Acromioclavicular joint, anatomy of, 1012
  bony impingement from, in rotator cuff injury, 1015, *1016*
  dislocation of, 1023, *1025*
Acute disseminated encephalomyelitis, 552
Acute lymphocytic leukemia, marrow changes in, spinal, 692–693
Acute tubular necrosis, 902–903
Adenoid cystic carcinoma, orbital, 612, *613*
  palatal, 635, *636*
  tracheal, 738, *740*
Adenoid tissue, of brain, axial view of, *384, 385*
  sagittal view of, *404, 406*
Adenoma, adrenal, *890*, 891–893
  hepatic, 869, *871*
  parathyroid, 647–649, *648*
  pituitary, 460–463, *461–463*
    and hemorrhage, *462*, 463, 511, *511*
    as indication for brain imaging, 380
  pleomorphic, of parapharyngeal space, *632*, 633
Adenomatoid tumor, testicular, 961, *961*
Adenomyosis, 932–933, *934*
Adenosine diphosphate, in spectroscopy, 273, *273*
Adenosine triphosphate, in spectroscopy, 272–278, *273–275*
  ratio of, to phosphocreatine, 764–766, *765*
  myocardial level of, during induced ischemia, 760, *761*

Adenylate kinase, in spectroscopy, 273, *273*
Adhesions, postoperative, of temporomandibular joint, 1041–1044, *1051*
Adiabatic fast passage, definition of, 1158
  in angiography, 153
  in spectroscopy, 295
Adnexa uteri, carcinoma of, 930–932, *930–933*
  recurrent, 934, *935*
  staging of, 1156
  cysts of, 928, *928–930*
  hemorrhage of, 928–930, *930*
  imaging of, protocols for, 1146–1147
    technical aspects of, 916, 916t
  in pregnancy, 942, *942–943, 943*
ADP, in spectroscopy, 273, *273*
Adrenal glands, 888–894, *890–894*
  anatomy of, *890*, 890–891, *891*
  imaging of, gadolinium-DTPA in, 250
    protocols for, 1144–1145
  mass lesions in, *890*, 891–894, *892–894*
Adrenocorticotropic hormone, hypersecretion of, pituitary adenoma and, 460
Adrenoleukodystrophy, 552, 595, *595*
AIDS, and brain infection, 583–589, *586–590*
  primary malignant lymphoma in, 452, *453*
Air cells, ethmoid, *400*
Aliasing, *94–96*, 94–97, 329, *329*, 1158
Alpha pulse, definition of, 1158
Alzheimer's disease, 592, *592*
Ambient cistern, *391, 407*
Amebic abscess, of liver, 875, *878*
AMI-25, in cardiac perfusion studies, 751
Amniotic fluid, 944, *945*, 948–949, *949*
Amygdala, *390, 408*
Amyloid, in heart disease, 800, *801*
Amyloid angiopathy, and brain hemorrhage, 503–504, *505*
Amyotrophic lateral sclerosis, 679
Analog-to-digital converter, 324, 1158
Anemia, aplastic, 1113–1114
  marrow changes in, spinal, 693
  hyperplastic, 1113, *1113*
  microcytic, vs. myeloma, 1109, *1109*
  sickle cell, *1113*
Anencephaly, 948, *948*
Aneurysm(s), and lobar hemorrhage, 501–502
  aortic, *137*, 780–783, *781–782*
    angiography of, *165*
    imaging protocols for, 1142–1145
    arteriosclerotic, 542–543
    basilar artery, angiography of, *171*
  brain, 536–543, *537–542*
    imaging protocols for, 1134–1135
    carotid artery, 541, *541*, 649, *650*
    clips for, and artifacts, 77, *77*
      precautions for, 41, 70
    false, 132, *132*
    giant, *541*, 541–542, *542*
    hemorrhage of, and hydrocephalus, 540
      and vasospasm, 540
    miliary, 496
  ventricular, cineangiography of, *130*
Aneurysmal bone cysts, 1101, *1105*
Angiofibroma, nasopharyngeal, *631*, 632–633
Angiography, 147–172
  abdominal, *158*, 160–162, *160–165*

Angiography *(Continued)*
  cerebrospinal fluid flow in, 138, *139*
  cine. See *Cineangiography.*
  contrast agents in, 156–157, *157*
  conventional, limitations of, 147–148, *148*, 149t
    in aortography, 780, *780*
  display methods in, 156, *156*
  fast imaging in, 206–207
  of cerebrovascular disease, 162–169, *165–172*
  of coronary arteries, 169–172
  of lung, *159*
  of peripheral vessels, *157*, 157–160
  one-dimensional, 155–156, *156*
  projection acquisition in, 152–155, *152–155*
  sequential two-dimensional, 151–152
  subtraction, *152–155*, 153–155, 1170
  three-dimensional, 148–150, 149t, *150*
    maximum intensity projection in, *150*, 150–151, *151*
Angioma. See also *Hemangioma.*
  cavernous, 532, *534*
  venous, of brain, 535, *535–536, 536*
Angiomatosis, encephalotrigeminal, 432–434, *435, 436*
Angiomyolipoma, of kidney, 907, *907*
Angiopathy, amyloid, and brain hemorrhage, 503–504, *505*
Angular frequency, definition of, 1158
Angular gyrus, *396, 397*
Angular momentum, definition of, 1158
Anisotropic resolution, definition of, 1158
Anisotropic three-dimensional imaging, 23
Ankle, 1076–1096, *1118*
  anatomy of, *1078–1079*
  cartilage disorders in, 1083–1085, *1084*
  imaging of, protocols for, 1150–1151
    technical aspects of, 1076–1078
  infection of, 1090–1094, *1092, 1093*
  tendon disorders in, 1079–1083, *1080–1082*
  tumors of, *1085*, 1085–1088, *1086, 1088, 1089*
Antennas, adjustment of, subject-dependent, 372
  in radiofrequency system, 366–368, *366–369*
Anterior capsule, of shoulder, 1020–1023, *1021–1024*
Anterior cerebral artery, axial view of, *390, 391, 393*
  feeding arteriovenous malformation, angiography of, *169*
Anterior clinoid process, *401*
Anterior commissure, *393, 405*
Anterior communicating artery, aneurysm of, 537, *537, 538*
  cross-flow through, in carotid occlusion, *168*
Anterior cruciate ligament, of knee, 996, *996, 997*
Anterior scalene muscle, anatomy of, 655–656, *656, 657*
Anticoagulants, and brain hemorrhage, 504, *506*
Antiferromagnetism, 240
  in biologic tissue, 265
Antrochoanal polyp, 636, *637*
Anulus fibrosus, lumbar, 708, *709*
  degeneration of, 710–711, *711, 712*
Aorta, abdominal, aneurysms of, *137, 165*
  angiography of, *158, 161, 165*
  aneurysms of, 780–783, *781–782*
  ascending, anatomy of, 732, *733*
  cineangiography of, *819*, 820, *820*

Aorta *(Continued)*
  coarctation of, 786–787, *788, 789*
    cineangiography of, 820, *820, 826,* 837–840, *839, 840*
    imaging protocols for, 1142–1143
  computed tomography of, 780, *780*
  hematoma of, dissecting, 782–785, *784–787*
  hemodynamics in, 111t, 112, *113*
  imaging of, electrocardiographic gating in, 56
    protocols for, 1142–1145
    technical aspects of, 779, 780, *780*
  in tetralogy of Fallot, 832, *833*
  inflammation of, giant cell, 782, *783*
  regurgitation from, cineangiography of, *130*
    echo-planar imaging of, 747, *747*
  stenosis of, congenital, 792, *794*
  transposition of, with pulmonary artery, 788–792, *794*
    cineangiography of, 835–836, *838, 839*
Aplastic anemia, 1113–1114
  marrow changes in, spinal, 693
Apoplexy, pituitary, 461, *462*
Appendix, epididymal, torsion of, 970–971
  testicular, torsion of, 970, *971*
Appliances, orthodontic, and artifacts, *79, 80,* 1044–1055
  precautions for, 71
Aqueduct of Sylvius, axial view of, *390, 392*
  coronal view of, *403*
  sagittal view of, *404*
Arachnoid cyst, 466–468, *467*
  of cerebellopontine angle, 625, *626*
  retrocerebellar, 429, *429, 430*
Arachnoid diverticula, and lumbar nerve root compression, 712, *716*
Arachnoiditis, of lumbar spine, 724, *724*
Archival, of magnetic resonance images, 63
Arcuate foramen, *408*
Arnold-Chiari malformation, 424–426, *425, 426*
Arteries. See specific arteries, e.g., *Middle cerebral artery.*
Arteriosclerosis, and aneurysms, 542–543
Arteriovenous malformations, in brain, 528–532, *530–534*
  and hemorrhage, 502–503, *503, 504*
  angiography of, *169*
  imaging protocols for, 1134–1135
  in neck, 649, *650*
  in spinal cord, *680,* 680–681
Arteritis, cerebral, 523–524, *529*
  Takayasu's, 781–782
Arthritis, *1116,* 1116–1117
  juvenile rheumatoid, synovial hypertrophy in, of ankle, 1084
  of knee, 1000–1003, *1001–1003*
  of shoulder, 1023–1026, *1026*
  of temporomandibular joint, 1041, *1051*
  of wrist, imaging protocols for, 1150–1151
  psoriatic, spinal, 701, *701*
  spinal, cervicothoracic, 700–701, *701*
Arthrography, temporomandibular, 1031
Artifacts, 75, *75,* 76t
  aliasing, *94–96,* 94–97, 329, *329,* 1158
  central point, 76t, 84, *85*
  chemical shift, 34, 92–94, *93,* 1158
    field gradient for, 361, *361*
    pulse sequence–related, 106–107
  contact, 84
  data clipping, 89, *90*
  definitions of, 1158–1159
  displacement, blood flow and, 130–132, *131*
  eddy currents and, 97
  ferromagnetic, 76–80, *77–80,* 1158
  flow, 104, *105, 106,* 110t. See also *Blood flow; Cerebrospinal fluid; Flow.*
  ghost, 98–104, *98–104,* 99t, 100t. See also *Ghost artifacts.*
  gradients and, 86–97, *88–91, 93–97*
  in brain imaging, 382
  in echo-planar imaging, 215–217
  in knee imaging, *1000,* 1006–1007
  in musculoskeletal imaging, 1098
  in myelography, 138–143, *140–143*
  in spinal imaging, *668,* 668–669, 672
  in static magnetic field, 75–81, *77–82*

Artifacts *(Continued)*
  lightening, in cineangiography, of heart, 813–814, *814*
  motion, 98–104, *98–105,* 99t, 100t
    gradient motion rephasing for, 332–334, *333, 334*
    in abdominal imaging, 847–848, *848, 849*
    suppression technique for, 1162
  orthodontic appliances and, 1044–1055
  pulsation, in brain imaging, *389*
  pulse sequences and, 105–107, *107*
  radiofrequency field, 82–86, *82–87*
  reduction of, saturation pulses in, *331,* 331–332, *332*
    in brain imaging, 382
  ringing, 91, *91–92,* 1159
  snowstorm, 65, *65*
  stimulated echo, 85, *86,* 1158
  susceptibility, 80–81, *81, 82,* 1158
  telescoping and, 97, *98*
  truncation, *91,* 91–92, 328–329, *329,* 1159
    in spinal imaging, 672
  wraparound, 76t, 95, *95,* 1159
Aspartate, in carbon-13 spectroscopy, of heart, 762
Aspergillosis, of brain, 577
Astrocytoma, cerebellar, 476, *476*
  cerebral, 449, 450, *450–452*
  in tuberous sclerosis, 436
  of spinal cord, 673, *675*
  phosphorus spectroscopy of, 277, 278t
  staging of, 1156
Asymmetric sampling, 325t, 329–330, *330,* 1159
Atherosclerosis, and aortic aneurysm, 781, *781, 782*
Atlas vertebra, *402*
ATP, in spectroscopy, 272–278, *273–275*
  ratio of, to phosphocreatine, 764–766, *765*
  myocardial level of, during induced ischemia, 760, *761*
Atrium, myxoma of, with myocardial infarction, cineangiography of, *822*
  septum of, congenital defect of, 787–788, *790, 791*
  lipomatous hypertrophy of, 803, *805*
Attenuation, definition of, 1159
Auditory canal, imaging of, protocols for, 1134–1135
Avascular necrosis, 1110–1111, *1110–1113, 1121*
  imaging of, protocols for, 1150–1151
  of lunate, 1066–1068, *1067, 1068,* 1111, *1113*
Axilla, hematoma of, *658,* 659
Azygos vein, anatomy of, *732,* 733

Bacterial abscess, of brain, 576–577, *576–578*
Bacterial infection, and diskitis, 695
Bacterial meningitis, 580–581
Baker's cyst, 1004, *1005*
Bandwidth, and signal-to-noise ratio, *327,* 327–328, *328*
  low, 57–58, 325t
  definition of, 1159
Basal cell carcinoma, of eyelid, 614, *618*
Basal ganglia, calcified, vs. brain hemorrhage, 495
  in brain development, 415, *416*
Basal vein of Rosenthal, axial view of, *392–395*
Basilar artery, aneurysm of, angiography of, *171*
  giant, 542
  axial view of, *388, 389*
Basis pontis, axial view of, *388, 389*
  coronal view of, *402*
Becker's muscular dystrophy, spectroscopy of, 275
Behçet's disease, vs. multiple sclerosis, 561
Bell clapper deformity, and testicular torsion, 966, *967*
Bentonite, as contrast agent, 252–253
Berry aneurysms, congenital, 536–538, *537–539*
Biliary tract, 882–884, *882–884*
Binomial suppression, in spectroscopy, 307, *308*
Black blood sequence, 54–55, 119–122, *120, 121.* See also *Presaturation.*

Bladder, carcinoma of, 920, *920, 921*
  extending from cervix, *927*
  fetal, 946, *947*
  imaging of, protocols for, 1146–1147
    technical aspects of, 915, 916t
  tumors of, and ureteral dilatation, *909*
  imaging of, ferioxamine methane sulfonate in, 251–252, *253*
Blake's pouch, of cisterna magna, 428, 429, *429*
Bloch equations, 1159
Blood, arterial, in cerebral hemorrhage, iron in, 257, *257*
  bright, imaging sequence for, 53–54, 122–129, *122–130.* See also *Flow compensation.*
  coagulation of, in cerebral hemorrhage, 259, 504
  dark, imaging sequence for, 54–55, 119–122, *120, 121.* See also *Presaturation.*
  relaxation time in, 110–111
  tissue characteristics of, 110–111
Blood cells, red, lysis of, in cerebral hemorrhage, 257–258, 261t, 262–263
Blood flow, and artifacts, 104, *105*
  displacement, 130–132, *131*
  ghost, 132, *132*
  and saturation effects, *115,* 115–116, *116*
  compensation for, 53–55
  cutaneous, monitoring of, during imaging, 40, 73
  dynamics of, *111,* 111t, 111–114, 112t, *113, 114*
  effect of, on fast gradient-echo imaging, 198–199, *199*
  laminar profile of, 112, *113*
  measurement of, 172–177, *172–178*
  phase effects of, 116–119, *117, 118*
  plug profile of, 112–114, *113*
  signal intensity in, 16t
  signal of, vs. thrombosis, 132–137, *133–137*
  velocity of, 111t, 111–112, 112t
  vs. thrombosis, even-echo rephasing for, 124, *125*
Blood pressure, elevated, and brain hemorrhage, 494
  portal, 877–878, *880, 881*
  pulmonary, 792
  monitoring of, during imaging, 40, 73
Blood vessels, coincidental phase cancellation of, 128–129
  contrast agents in, 233
  hepatic, diseases of, 875–878, *878–881*
  implanted devices in, imaging of, 137, *137*
    precautions for, 41, 71
  of brain, diseases of, 516–543
    occlusive, 516–525, *517–530*
    malformations of, 525–536, *530–536*
  overlap of, in angiography, *154,* 155
  peripheral, angiography of, *157,* 157–160
Blood-brain barrier, impairment of, in cerebral hemorrhage, 259
  in cerebrovascular infarction, 517, 521, *524*
Blurring, motion and, 76t, 98, 100t
Bohr effect, in cerebral hemorrhage, 257
Boltzmann distribution, 1159
Bolus, tracking of, in flow measurement, 172–173, *172–174*
Bone. See also specific bones, e.g., *Lunate.*
  aneurysmal cysts of, 1101, *1105*
  avascular necrosis, imaging protocols for, 1150–1151
  avascular necrosis of, 1066–1068, *1067, 1068,* 1110–1111, *1110–1113, 1121*
  cortical, signal intensity in, 16t, 17
  infarction of, in knee, 1003–1004, *1004*
  tumors of, 1098–1104, *1099–1108*
Bone marrow, abnormalities of, in anemia, *1113,* 1113–1114
  in Gaucher's disease, 1114, *1114, 1115*
  in knee, 1006
  in osteomyelitis, of foot and ankle, 1091–1092
  fat in, in anterior clinoid process, *401*
  in crista galli, *400*
  FLASH imaging of, 197–198, *198*

Bone marrow *(Continued)*
  malignant infiltration of, 692–693, *1102, 1109,*
    1109–1110
  normal, 1104–1109
  proton spectroscopy of, 278, *280*
  radiation injury of, 693, 1104
  signal intensity in, 15t, 16t
  vertebral, *670, 673, 673*
    diseases of, 691–693, *693*
Boundary effect, in imaging of brain hemorrhage,
    489, *491*
Bowel, gadolinium-DTPA imaging of, 248, *249*
  motion of, in abdominal imaging, 158, 848–
    852, *850–852*
Brachial plexus, 653–663, *654–665*
  anatomy of, 655–658, *656, 657*
  computed tomography of, 653
  imaging of, protocols for, 1136–1137
    technical aspects of, 653–655, *654, 655*
  nontraumatic lesions of, 659–663, *661–665*
  trauma to, 658–659, *658–660*
    and muscular atrophy, *1126*
Brachium pontis, *389*
Brain. See also specific structures, e.g., *Pons,* and
    disorders, e.g., *Aneurysm(s).*
  abscess of, 576–580, *576–581*
    AIDS-related, 584, *586–588*
  anatomy of, atlas of, *384–411*
  atrophy of, hydrocephalus and, 557, *558*
    in multiple sclerosis, 551
  blood flow separation from, impairment of, in
      hemorrhage, 259
    in infarction, 517
  computed tomography of, 379–380, *382*
  concussion of, 563–564
  congenital malformations of, 413–446
    classification of, 413, 414t
  contusion of, *564,* 565–570, *566, 569–574*
  cysts of, benign, 466–470, *467–469, 471*
  degenerative diseases of, 590–592, *590–593*
  development of, 414–420, 415t, *416–422*
  fetal, 947–948, *948, 949*
  glioma of, 449–450, *450–452*
  hemorrhage into, 255–267, 483–512
    and infarction, 507–508, *508–510,* 518, *520*
    blood-brain barrier in, 259
    causes of, 494, 495, 495t, 496t
    clinical signs of, 495–496
    coagulation disorders and, 504
    computed tomography of, 483–484, 487t
    differential diagnosis of, 493–494, *494, 495*
    evolution of, *262, 263,* 263–264
    extracerebral, 491–493
      traumatic, 564–565, *564–569*
    gradient-echo imaging of, 489, *490, 491*
    hypertensive, 494, 496–499, *497–501*
    imaging of, pulse sequences in, 259–260, *260*
      relaxivity in, 259
    iron in, *256–258,* 256–259, 261t, 261–263
    lobar, 501–510, *502–510*
    of undetermined cause, 511
    primary intraventricular, 510–511
    prognosis of, 512
    spontaneous, 483–512
    subarachnoid, aneurysms and, *537,* 538–540,
      539–541
    oxygenation in, 489–491, *492*
    time course of, *486,* 487t, 487–489, *488,* 488t,
      494–495
  tumors and, 505–507, *507*
    metastatic, 454–455
  imaging of, indications for, 380–381
    magnetic resonance in, vs. computed tomog-
      raphy, 379–380, *382*
    photography of, *63*
    protocols for, 1132–1135
    techniques of, 381–382
  infarction in, and infection, 575–576
  inflammation of, 575–589, *576–590*
    AIDS-related, 583–589, *586–590*
  lymphoma of, 451–452, *453*
  meningioma of, 455–458, *456–458*
  metabolic disorders of, 592–595, *594, 595*
  metastatic tumors of, 452–455, *453–455*
  oxygen in, fluorine spectroscopy of, 286, *286*

Brain *(Continued)*
  radiation injury of, 554–555, *555, 556*
  shear injury of, 570–574, *574, 575*
  signal intensity in, 15t, 16t
  spectroscopy of, phosphorus, 275–277, *276*
    proton, 279–282, *281*
  trauma to, 563–575, *564–575*
  tumors of, 448–480
    and hemorrhage, 454–455, 505–507, *507*
    imaging of, fast three-dimensional, *211*
      gadolinium-DTPA in, *238*
      proton spectroscopy of, 281–282
    metastatic, 452–455, *453–455*
    nerve sheath, 470–474, *472, 473*
    pineal, 458–460, *459, 460*
    sellar, 460–465, *461–466*
  vascular diseases of, 516–543
    angiography of, 162–169, *165–172*
    cineangiography of, 543, *543*
    occlusive, 516–525, *517–530*
  vascular malformations in, 525–536, *530–536*
  white matter of, abnormalities of, 545–561
    ischemia of, 546–549, *547–549*
    differential diagnosis of, 560
Brain stem, contusion of, 568–570, *573*
  glioma of, *474,* 474–475
  hemorrhage of, 499, *499–501*
    in Arnold-Chiari malformation, 425, *426*
  infarction of, *518*
Breast, carcinoma of, gadolinium-DTPA imaging
    of, 249–250
  metastasis from, to brain, *453*
    to spine, *699*
  tumors of, proton spectroscopy of, 282
Breath-holding, during imaging, 62
  abdominal, 848
Bright blood sequence, 53–54, 122–129, *122–130*
Broad ligament, anatomy of, 923, *924*
Bronchi, anatomy of, *732,* 733
Brown's syndrome, 612, *612,* 612t
Budd-Chiari syndrome, angiography of, *162*
  hepatic thrombosis in, 877, *879*
Bursa(e), of shoulder, anatomy of, 1012, *1013*
  in rotator cuff injury, 1016, 1017, *1017*
    prepatellar, inflammation of, 1000
Bypass graft, coronary, 752, 752–753, *753,* 807,
    807
  cineangiography of, 824
  for coarctation of aorta, 786–787, *789*

Calcaneus, osteomyelitis of, 1091, *1093*
Calcarine sulcus, axial view of, *394, 395*
  sagittal view of, *404, 405*
Calcification, in pericarditis, 800, *801*
  in Sturge-Weber syndrome, 433, *435*
  of mediastinal masses, 735
  of meningioma, 458, *458*
    vs. brain hemorrhage, 493–494, *494, 495*
Callosomarginal artery, axial view of, *393, 394*
  coronal view of, *401*
Cancellation, coincidental phase, 128–129
Cancer. See also *Carcinoma, Lymphoma,* and
    Sarcoma.
  liver. See *Liver.*
  marrow abnormalities in, *1102, 1109,* 1109–
    1110
  staging of, 1153–1157
Capillaries, cerebral, telangiectasia of, 535
Carbohydrates, metabolism of, spectroscopy of,
    273
Carbon, magnetic resonance characteristics of, 5t
Carbon-13, in spectroscopy, 282–283
  for cardiac imaging, 761–762, *762, 763*
Carcinoma, adrenal, 892, *893*
  bladder, 920, *920, 921,* 927
  brachial plexus, metastatic, 659–660, *661–663*
  brain, metastatic, 452–455, *453–455*
    and hemorrhage, 505–507, *507*
  breast, gadolinium-DTPA imaging of, 249–250
    metastasis from, to brain, *453*
      to spine, 699
  cardiac invasion by, *804*
  cervical, 926–928, *927, 928*

Carcinoma *(Continued)*
  metastasis of, to liver, 857
    recurrent, 934, *935, 936*
  colonic, carbon-13 spectroscopy of, 283
  endometrial, 923–926, *926*
  eyelid, 614, *618*
  gallbladder, 883–884, *884, 885*
  liver. See *Liver.*
  lung. See *Lung(s).*
  mediastinal, metastatic, *738*
  nasopharyngeal, *630,* 632
  ocular, metastatic, vs. choroidal melanoma, 604
  orbital, extraconal, 612, *613,* 613t
  ovarian, 930–932, *930–933*
    recurrent, 934, *935*
  palatal, 635, *636*
  pancreatic, 886, *886–888*
    imaging of, bowel motion in, *851, 852*
  paranasal sinus, 634, *635,* 636
  parotid, 638, *641, 642*
  prostatic. See *Prostate.*
  rectal, 922, *922*
  renal, metastatic, 907
  renal cell, 905–906, *906,* 908
    metastasis of, to lung, 743, *743*
    thrombosis in, 901, *902*
  spinal cord, metastatic, 673, *676,* 688–690, *688–*
    690
      extramedullary, intradural, 698–699, *699*
      gadolinium-DTPA imaging of, 243, *244*
  spine, metastatic, 688–690, *688–690, 1104*
    imaging protocols for, 1140–1141
  staging of, 739–740, *741, 742,* 1153–1156
  supraglottic, *646*
  testicular, *957, 957–961, 959–961*
  thyroid, imaging protocols for, 1136–1137
    metastasis from, *689*
  tracheal, 738–739, *740*
Cardiac gating, 55–57, *55–57,* 773–774
  definition of, 1163
  for myelographic artifacts, *141,* 143
  in subtraction angiography, 153, *154*
  indications for, 732
  vs. cineangiography, *812,* 812–813
Cardiography, electromagnetic effects in, 114, *114*
Cardiomyopathy, cineangiography of, 824, *825*
  congestive, 800
  hypertrophic, 800–801, *802*
  in hemochromatosis, 873
  phosphorus spectroscopy of, 277
    in congenital disease, 764, *765*
  restrictive, with pericarditis, 799–800, *800, 801*
Cardiopulmonary resuscitation, magnetic interfer-
    ence with, 354
Carotid artery, aneurysm of, giant, 541, *541*
  traumatic, 649, *650*
  angiography of, 162–169, *165–168, 170, 172*
  bifurcation of, cineangiography of, 543, *543*
  dissection of, *134,* 526
  flow velocity in, 112t
  internal, axial view of, *384–389, 391*
    coronal view of, *401*
    sagittal view of, *406–409*
  occlusion of, *526*
  ulceration of, angiography of, *172*
  ultrasonography of, 162–163
Carpal tunnel syndrome, 1058–1060, *1058–1061,*
    1117–1118
  imaging protocols for, 1150–1151
  in Kienböck's disease, 1067–1068, *1068*
Carr-Purcell sequence, 1159
  rotational axis in, 321
Cartilage, of ankle, disorders of, 1083–1085, *1084*
  of knee, defects of, 1000, *1001*
  of skull base, sarcoma of, 478–479
  of thigh, sarcoma of, *1106*
  of wrist, 1068–1073, *1069–1074*
  signal intensity in, 16t
Cataracts, sodium spectroscopy of, 284–285
Caudate nucleus, axial view of, *393, 395, 397*
  hemorrhage of, *497,* 497–498
  infarction of, *519*
  sagittal view of, *406, 407*
  shear injury of, *566*
Cavernous angioma, 532, *534*

Cavernous sinus, dural margin of, axial view of, *388, 389*
CE-FAST imaging, 49, 50, 195, *196,* 1159
Cellulitis, of foot, in diabetes, 1092, *1093, 1121*
  orbital, 613–614, *616*
  vs. osteomyelitis, 1119, *1121, 1122*
Central line artifact, 76t, 85, *85–87,* 1158
Central nervous system, fetal, 947–948, *948, 949*
  imaging of, 377–728
    gadolinium-DTPA in, *238,* 243–244, *244, 245*
Central point artifact, 76t, 84, *85*
Central pontine myelinolysis, 592–593, *594*
Central sulcus, axial view of, *394, 396–399*
  coronal view of, *402*
  sagittal view of, *407, 409, 410*
Centrum ovale, shear injury of, 570
Centrum semiovale, axial view of, *396–399*
  coronal view of, *401*
  in brain development, *417, 419–421*
Cephaloceles, 420–422, *423*
Cerebellar artery, posterior inferior, axial view of, *384–387*
  infarction of, *509*
  superior, *388*
Cerebellar cistern, superior, axial view of, *392, 395*
  sagittal view of, *406, 410*
Cerebellar peduncle, in brain development, *418*
  middle, coronal view of, *402*
  sagittal view of, *406*
Cerebellar tonsil, axial view of, *384–386, 388*
  coronal view of, *403*
  sagittal view of, *404–406*
Cerebellar vein, *404*
Cerebellopontine angle, arachnoid cyst of, 625, *626*
  cistern of, axial view of, *387*
  sagittal view of, *407*
  tumors of, imaging protocols for, 1134–1135
Cerebellum, agenesis of, 429–430
  astrocytoma of, 476, *476*
  dysplasia of, 428–431, *428–431*
  encephalomyelitis in, *585*
  folia of, *391, 392*
  hemispheres of, axial view of, *384, 387, 391*
    in brain development, *419*
    sagittal view of, *409, 411*
  hemorrhage of, 499, *501, 503*
    and infarction, *509*
  hypoplasia of, *430,* 430–431, *431*
  infarction of, *509, 519, 520*
  semilunar lobules of, *403*
Cerebral aqueduct, axial view of, *390, 392*
  coronal view of, *403*
  sagittal view of, *404*
Cerebral artery (arteries), anterior, axial view of, *390, 391, 393*
    feeding arteriovenous malformation, *169*
  dissection of, 521, *526*
  flow velocity in, 112t
  middle, aneurysm of, *539*
    angiography of, in carotid occlusion, *168*
    axial view of, *390–393, 397*
    infarction of, *517*
    sagittal view of, *407, 409*
  occlusion of, 521, *525*
  posterior, axial view of, *391*
    sagittal view of, *408*
Cerebral hemorrhage. See *Brain, hemorrhage into.*
Cerebral peduncle, axial view of, *390*
  coronal view of, *402*
Cerebral vein, internal, axial view of, *394, 395*
  coronal view of, *403*
  sagittal view of, *404*
Cerebritis, bacterial infection and, *576,* 576–577, *577*
Cerebrospinal fluid, flow of, 138, *139*
  and artifacts, 104, *106*
    in brain imaging, 382
    in myelography, 138–146, *140–145*
  and void signal, in syringohydromyelia, 677, *677, 678*
  compensation for, 53–54

Cerebrospinal fluid *(Continued)*
    in spinal imaging, 126, *127*
    in hydrocephalus, 555–560, *557–560*
    in imaging of spinal cysts, *145,* 145–146
  signal intensity in, 15t, 16t
Cerebrum. See *Brain.*
Cervical rib, and thoracic outlet syndrome, 661, *665*
Cervix uteri, anatomy of, 922–923, *924, 925*
  carcinoma of, 926–928, *927, 928*
    metastasis of, to liver, *857*
    recurrent, 934, *935, 936*
    staging of, 1156
  imaging of, protocols for, 1146–1147
    technical aspects of, 916, 916t
  in pregnancy, 939–940
Chemical exchange, in spectroscopy, *302,* 302–303
Chemical shift, 34
  and artifacts, 34, 92–94, *93,* 1158
    field gradient for, 361, *361*
    pulse sequence–related, 106–107
  definition of, 1159
  in fast gradient-echo imaging, 197–198, *198*
  in pulse sequence design, *326,* 326–327
  in spectroscopy, 270, *271,* 300–301, *301*
    localized, *289,* 289–290, *290*
Chemical shift imaging, three-dimensional, of heart, 766, *766*
Chemical shift selective saturation technique, 336, 337, *338,* 1159
Chemodectoma, *479,* 479–480
CHESS technique, 336, 337, *338,* 1159
Chiari malformation, 422–426, *424–426,* 701, *701*
  with syringohydromyelia, 677, *677*
Chloral hydrate, before imaging, of brain malformations, 413
  of congenital heart disease, 832
Cholelithiasis, *883,* 883–884, *884*
Cholesteatoma, of tympanic cavity, *628*
Cholesterol cyst, of brain, 469
Chondroma, 478–479
Chondromalacia patellae, *999, 999*
Chondromatosis, synovial, of knee, *1003, 1003*
Chondrosarcoma, intracranial, 478–479
  of thigh, *1106*
Chordoma, 477–479, *478*
  nasopharyngeal, *631,* 632
  sacral, 720–721, *723*
Chorea, Huntington's, 592, *593*
Chorioadenoma destruens, 941
Chorioangioma, 941
Choriocarcinoma, 941
  pineal, 458
  testicular, 958–959
Choroid, melanoma of, 603t, *604, 606*
Choroid plexus, axial view of, *394*
  papilloma of, 475
Choroidal fissure, *402*
Chromium, in contrast agents, relaxivity of, 225t
  magnetic moment of, 222t, 240t
Ciliary body, *386*
Cineangiography, 128, *129,* 130
  definition of, 1159
  fast imaging in, 206–207
  of cardiac thrombosis, 823–824, *825*
  of cardiac tumors, 816t, *822, 823, 824*
  of cardiomyopathy, 824, *825*
  of cerebrovascular disease, 543, *543*
  of coarctation of aorta, 820, *820, 826,* 837–840, *839, 840*
  of dissecting hematoma, aortic, 785, *786*
  of great artery transposition, 835–837, *838, 839*
  of heart, 810–844
    future of, 826–828, *827*
    methods of, 816–821, *818–820*
    technical aspects of, *811,* 811–815, *812, 814–816,* 816t
    vs. echocardiography, 842–844, 843t
  of heart disease, congenital, 830–844
    method of, 830–832, *832*
  of hypoplastic right heart syndrome, 833–834, *835–838*
  of left heart lesions, 841, *842*
  of myocardial infarction, 822, *822*

Cineangiography *(Continued)*
  of pulmonary artery banding, 840–841, *841, 842*
  of tetralogy of Fallot, 832–833, *833–835*
  of valvular regurgitation, 822–823, *823*
  of valvular stenosis, 815, *815,* 816t
  of ventricular function, 821–822
Cingulate gyrus, axial view of, *392, 394, 396, 397*
  sagittal view of, *405, 407*
Cingulate herniation, with subdural hematoma, *565*
Cingulate sulcus, axial view of, *396*
  coronal view of, *402*
  sagittal view of, *406*
Circumesencephalic cistern, *391*
Cirrhosis, hepatic, angiography of, 160, *163*
  of liver, 875, *877*
Cisterna magna, Blake's pouch of, 428, 429, *429*
Cisterns. See specific cisterns, e.g., *Quadrigeminal cistern.*
Claustrophobia, management of, before imaging, 40
  with temporomandibular joint dysfunction, 1055
Claustrum, *392*
Clay, as contrast agent, 252–253
Clinoid process, anterior, *401*
Clipping artifact, 89, *90*
Clivus, axial view of, *384, 385, 387*
  coronal view of, *401*
  sagittal view of, *405, 406*
Coagulation, in cerebral hemorrhage, 259, 504
Coarctation, of aorta, 786–787, *788, 789*
  cineangiography of, 820, *820, 826,* 837–840, *839, 840*
  imaging protocols for, 1142–1143
Coats' disease, 603, 603t, *605*
Cobalt, effect of, on imaging, 33
  magnetic moment of, 240t
Coccidioidomycosis, of brain, 577, *579*
Cochlea, axial view of, *386, 387*
  implants in, precautions for, 41, 71
Cochlear nerve, anatomy of, 623
Coil(s), for cineangiography, of heart, 816–817
  Gianturco, and artifact, *78*
  Golay, 1163
  gradient, 322–323, 1163
  Helmholtz, 43, *43,* 1164
  linearly polarized, definition of, 1165
  Maxwell, 1166
  quadrature, 37, 368
    definition of, 1160
    positioning of, *45,* 45–46
  radiofrequency, 36, *36–37,* 366–369, *366–369*
    definition of, 1168
    in orbital imaging, 600
    shielding from, 83
  receiver, 36, *36–37*
    centering of, with magnet, *46, 46*
    design restrictions in, 44–45
    positioning of, *45,* 45–46
    selection of, *43,* 43–44, *44*
    tuning of, 46, *47*
  resonator, 1169
  saddle, 1169
  solenoidal, definition of, 1170
    positioning of, *45, 45*
  surface. See *Surface coils.*
  transmitter, 7, 37
  tuning of, subject-dependent, 372
Coincidental phase cancellation, 128–129
Collateral ligament(s), of knee, *998, 998*
  radial, anatomy of, *1062,* 1062–1063
Colliculus, inferior, axial view of, *392*
  coronal view of, *403*
  sagittal view of, *405*
  superior, axial view of, *392*
  coronal view of, *403*
  sagittal view of, *405*
Colloid cyst, 470, *471*
Colon, carcinoma of, carbon-13 spectroscopy of, 283
  metastasis of, to brain, *455*
    to liver, *855, 860, 861, 870*

Communicating artery, anterior, aneurysm of, 537, *537, 538*
posterior, *390*
Compartment syndromes, 1124–1125, *1125*
Compression syndrome, of median nerve, 1058–1060, *1058–1061*, 1117–1118
imaging protocols for, 1150–1151
in Kienböck's disease, 1067–1068, *1068*
Computed tomography, of aorta, 780, *780*
of brachial plexus, 653
of brain, 379–380, 382
in hemorrhage, 483–484, 487t
of head, 622–623, 626–629, 629t
after trauma, 574–575
of liver, 853, 854, 878–882
of spine, 667–668
of trachea, 738–739, *740*
Concussion, cerebral, 563–564
Congestive heart failure, skeletal muscle metabolism in, spectroscopy of, 766–767
Conjoint root, lumbar, 712, *716*
Conjugate synthesis, *186, 186–188, 187,* 336
Contact artifacts, 84
Continuous wave, definition of, 1160
Contrast, definition of, 1160
enhancement of, in FLASH imaging, 191, *191,* 195, *196,* 219
in echo-planar imaging, 217
in fast gradient-echo imaging, 191–199, *192–196, 198, 199,* 1159
in optimal imaging, 43
in spin-echo images, 29–31, *30, 31*
Contrast agents, 33, 60–61, 221–253. See also specific agents, e.g., *Gadolinium-DTPA.*
definition of, 1160
distribution of, in vivo, 223
excretability of, 223
historical aspects of, 222
in angiography, 156–157, *157*
in fast gradient-echo imaging, 207, *207*
magnetism of, 238–241, *239,* 240t
nonproton, 33
oral, 60–61
paramagnetic, effect of, on bowel signal, 849
in cardiac perfusion studies, 751
relaxivity of, 223
T_1, *224–227,* 224–228, 225t
stability of, in vivo, 223
T_1, 33, 60, *224–227,* 224–233, 225t, *229, 231–233*
intravascular distribution of, 233
vs. T_2 agents, 223
T_2, 33, 61, 233–235, *234*
vs. T_1 agents, 223
targeting of, in vivo, *229,* 229–233, *231–233*
toxicity of, 223
T_1, 228t, 228–229
Contrast-enhanced fast imaging, 49, 50, 195, *196,* 1159
Contrast resolution, in abdominal imaging, *846,* 846–847, *847*
Contrast-to-noise ratio, definition of, 1160
echo time and, 365, *365, 366*
Control systems, 337
Contusion, of brain, *564,* 565–570, *566, 569–574*
of spinal cord, 700, *700*
COPE method, to reduce ghost artifacts, 101, *101*
Copper, for shielding, against radiofrequency interference, 345–346, *346, 347*
in contrast agents, relaxivity of, 225t
magnetic moment of, 240t
metabolism of, Wilson's disease of, 593–595, 875
Coracoid process, anatomy of, 1012
Corona radiata, *396, 397*
Coronal suture, axial view of, *398*
sagittal view of, *406, 409*
Coronary arteries, angiography of, 169–172
bypass graft of, *752,* 752–753, *753, 807, 807*
cineangiography of, 824
disease of, *806,* 806–807, *807*
ventricular motion abnormality with, 796, *797*
imaging of, *753,* 753–754, *754*

Coronary arteries *(Continued)*
stenosis of, echo-planar imaging of, 747–748, *749*
Coronoid process, of mandible, *384*
Corpus callosum, agenesis of, with meningoencephalocele, *423*
anomalies of, *442,* 442–444, *443*
axial view of, *393–396*
coronal view of, *401*
in brain development, *419, 420*
multiple sclerosis plaques in, *550,* 551
sagittal view of, *404–406*
shear injury of, 570, *575*
thinning of, in hydrocephalus, 557, *559*
Corpus luteum, cysts of, 942, *942*
Correlation spectroscopy, 305, *306*
Correlation time, and molecular effect on relaxation time, 13–15, *14*
Cortical veins, axial view of, *398, 399*
sagittal view of, *409*
thrombosis of, and infarction, *510*
Coumadin, and brain hemorrhage, 504
Counter-rotating current coil, definition of, 1160
Coupling, in radiofrequency system, 369
in spectroscopy, 270, *272*
Crafted radiofrequency pulses, 320, *320*
Cranial nerve(s), eighth. See *Vestibulocochlear nerve.*
fifth, axial view of, *388*
coronal view of, *402*
in Sturge-Weber syndrome, 432
neuroma of, 473, *473*
fourth, *391*
ninth, axial view of, *386*
coronal view of, *402*
sagittal view of, *408, 409*
second. See *Optic nerve.*
seventh, anatomy of, 623–625
axial view of, *386*
neuroma of, 473–474
sagittal view of, *407–409, 411*
tenth, axial view of, *386*
coronal view of, *402*
sagittal view of, *408, 409*
third, *405*
twelfth, *384*
Craniopharyngioma, 464–465, *465*
Craniovertebral junction, abnormalities of, *701,* 701–702, *702*
Creatine kinase, in spectroscopy, 273, *273*
Crista falciformis, *409*
Crista galli, axial view of, *391*
coronal view of, *400*
Crossed coil, definition of, 1160
Cross-over, 30–31, *31*
Cross-talk, definition of, 1160
reduction of, interslice gap for, 51, *51–53*
Cruciate ligaments, of knee, *996,* 996–998, *997*
Crural cistern, *390*
Cryogens, definition of, 1160
for superconductive magnets, in site planning, 342
Cryoshield, definition of, 1160
Cryostat, definition of, 1160
in superconductive magnet, 358
Cryptococcosis, of brain, AIDS-related, 584, *588*
Cryptorchidism, 972–978, *974–977*
imaging protocols for, 1148–1149
Crystal deposition disease, of shoulder, 1027–1028
Culmen, *404*
Cuneus, *405*
Cushing's disease, 460
Cyst(s), adrenal, 891, 892, *892*
aneurysmal, of bone, 1101, *1105*
arachnoid, 466–468, *467*
of cerebellopontine angle, 625, *626*
retrocerebellar, 429, *429, 430*
bronchogenic, 733, *734*
cholesterol, 469
colloid, 470, *471*
Dandy-Walker, 428, 428–429
dermoid, in pregnancy, 942, *942*
of brain, 469, *469*
orbital, 612, 613t, *614*

Cyst(s) *(Continued)*
epidermoid, of brain, 468, 468–469
ganglion, of wrist, 1073–1074
hepatic, *856, 865, 866*
vs. malignancy, 860, 862
maxillary, 637, *638*
mucous retention, *400*
odontogenic, 637, *637*
of ankle, 1085
of brain, benign, 466–470, *467–469, 471*
of uterine adnexa, 928, *928–930*
in pregnancy, 942, *942*
pericardial, 801, *802*
pharyngeal, 649, *649*
pineal, 458–460, *460*
popliteal, 1004, *1005*
porencephalic, vs. arachnoid cyst, 466–468
renal, 903–904, *904,* 907–908
fetal, 946, *946*
signal intensity in, 16t
spinal, and lumbar nerve root compression, 712, *716*
cerebrospinal fluid flow effects in, *145,* 145–146
extramedullary, intradural, 697
intramedullary, 674–675, *677,* 677–678, *678*
synovial, 1101, 1117, *1117*
of shoulder, 1026, *1026*
thymic, 733, *735*
thyroglossal duct, *648,* 649
Cystic carcinoma, adenoid, orbital, 612, *613*
palatal, 635, *636*
tracheal, 738, *740*
Cystic medial necrosis, and aortic aneurysm, in Marfan's syndrome, 782, *783*
Cysticercosis, of brain, 577–580, *580, 581*
Cytomegalovirus, and encephalitis, AIDS-related, 586–589

Dacryocystitis, 614–620, *618*
Dandy-Walker malformation, *428,* 428–429
Dark blood sequence, 54–55, 119–122, *120, 121.* See also *Presaturation.*
Dartos muscle, 954, *955*
Data, clipping of, and artifact, 89, *90*
loss of, and artifact, 89–90, *90*
De Morsier's syndrome, 428, *428*
de Quervain's syndrome, 1060, *1061*
Deafness, imaging protocols for, 1134–1135
Decibels, definition of, 1160
Declive, *404*
Decoupling, definition of, 1160
in radiofrequency system, 369
in spectroscopy, 270, *272*
Deferent duct, 954–956, *956*
Deltoid ligament, of wrist, anatomy of, *1062,* 1063
Demodulator, quadrature, 371
mathematical principles of, *375,* 375–376
Demyelination, imaging protocols in, 1132–1133, 1138–1139
in multiple sclerosis, 549–552*550, 551, 553*
in spinal cord, 678, 678–679
Dental materials, and artifacts, 79, 80, 1044–1045
precautions for, 71
Deoxyhemoglobin, in brain hemorrhage, 489
water accessibility in, *258*
Dephasing, and artifact, 107
definition of, 9, *10*
gradient, in subtraction angiography, 153–155, *154, 155*
to reduce flow artifacts, *121,* 121–122
DEPTH pulses, in localized spectroscopy, 291
Depth resolved surface coil spectroscopy, 291
Dermoid cysts, of brain, 469, *469*
orbital, 612, 613t, *614*
ovarian, in pregnancy, 942
Dermoid tumors, of spinal cord, 673, *676*
ovarian, 928, *929*
Deuterium, magnetic resonance characteristics of, 5t
Diabetes, foot disorders in, 1092, *1092–1094, 1121*

Diabetes *(Continued)*
  maternal, and fetal macrosomia, 949–950
  myositis with, *1127*
Diamagnetism, 238–239, *239*, 240t, 1160
  and static field artifacts, 76–77
  and T_1 relaxation time, 241
  effect of, on imaging, 32
    fast gradient-echo, 197
  in biologic tissue, 265
Diaphragm, precautions for, 72
Diastematomyelia, with tethered cord, 727, *727–728*
Diastole, pseudogating in, 122–123
Diazepam, for claustrophobia, 40
  use of, before fetal imaging, 944
Diencephalon, in Arnold-Chiari malformation, 425
Diethylenetriaminepentaacetic acid. See *Gadolinium-DTPA.*
Diethylstilbestrol, as teratogen, 981
Diffusion, definition of, 1161
  in imaging of brain hemorrhage, 489
  in spectroscopy, 304–305
  of water, phase effects of, 177–179, *179*
Diploë, *406, 408*
Diploic space, *398, 399*
Diploomyelia, with tethered cord, 727–728
Dipole, definition of, 1161
Dipole-dipole interactions, 1161
Dipyridamole, and coronary vasodilation, 747, *748, 749*
Direct current, interference by, and artifacts, 84, *85*
Disk(s), intervertebral, degenerative disease of, cervicothoracic, 681, *682–684*
    fast imaging of, 200, *203, 204*
    lumbar, 709–714, *710–716*
    recurrent postoperative, 719–720, *720, 721, 723*
  infection of, cervicothoracic, 694–696, *695, 696*
  lumbar, anatomy of, *707–709*, 708–709
    sagittal view of, *405*
    signal intensity in, 16t
  of temporomandibular joint, anatomy of, 1033–1035, *1035, 1036*
    degeneration of, 1040–1041, *1049, 1050*
    displacement of, 1040, *1040, 1042–1049*
Dispersion, definition of, 1161
Dispersion mode, in spectroscopy, 298
Displacement artifacts, blood flow and, 130–132, *131*
Display matrix, definition of, 1161
Dixon technique, *336*, 336–337
Dizziness, ear lesions and, imaging protocols for, 1134–1135
Donut sign, *121*, 121–122
Doppler ultrasonography, of carotid artery, 162–163
Dorsal dermal sinus, 725
Dorsal induction, in brain development, 414
  disorders of, 414t, 420–426, *423–426*
Dorsal intercalated segmental instability, 1064–1065, *1065–1067*
DOTA, structure of, *225*
  with gadolinium contrast agent, 227, 250
Doughnut sign, *121*, 121–122
Driven-equilibrium methods, in fast imaging, 210–214, *212, 213*
Drug abuse, and brain hemorrhage, 504–505
DTPA. See *Gadolinium-DTPA.*
Duchenne's muscular dystrophy, spectroscopy of, 275
Duodenum, gadolinium-DTPA imaging of, 248, *249*
Dysprosium, in contrast agents, relaxivity of, 225t
  T_2, *234*, 235
  magnetic moment of, 222t, 240t
Dysprosium-DTPA, in angiography, 157
  in echo-planar imaging, of heart, 747–748, *749*

Ear, imaging of, protocols for, 1134–1135
  implants in, precautions for, 41, 71

Echo, definition of, 1161
  gradient. See *Gradient-echo.*
  spin. See *Spin echo.*
  stimulated. See *Stimulated echo.*
Echo time, alignment of sampling with, 325t, 329–330, *330*
  and contrast-to-noise ratio, 365, *365, 366*
  definition of, 1161
  in pulse sequence design, 314t
  in T_2 relaxation, 11, *12*
Echocardiography, of congenital heart disease, 785–786
  of tumors, 801–803
  vs. cineangiography, 842–844, 843t
  vs. magnetic resonance imaging, of aorta, 780, *780*
Echo-planar imaging, 214–215, *216*
  artifacts in, 215–217
  contrast in, 217
  definition of, 1161
  of heart, 745–748, *746–749*
  signal-to-noise ratio in, 217
Ectopic pregnancy, 942, *943*
Eddy currents, 38, 1161
  and artifacts, 97
  compensation for, 364, 1161
  effect of, on gradient dephasing, in angiography, *154*, 155
  gradient-induced, *363*, 363–364, *364*
Edema, as indication for brain imaging, 380
  in brachial plexus injury, 659, *660*
  in brain hematoma, 488
  in osteomyelitis, *1118–1120*, 1119
  loss of blood-brain barrier and, in cerebral hemorrhage, 259
  with brain contusion, 566, 568, *570*
Edge-ringing artifacts, *91*, 91–92
EDTA, in contrast agents, 225, 226, *227*
Effervescent agents, in contrast imaging, 252
Effusion, pericardial, 799, *800*
Elbow, imaging of, protocols for, 1150–1151
  synovitis of, *1116*
Electrocardiography, 114, *114*. See also *Cardiac gating.*
  in cineangiography, 814, 817
  magnetic interference with, 354
Electromagnetic spectrum, 4, *4*
Electron cloud, effect of, on magnetic field, 34
Electrons, orbital shells of, and energy levels, 238, *239*
  in paramagnetism, 222
Embolism, pulmonary, 743, *743*
  cineangiography of, 816t, 823–824, *825*
Embryonal carcinoma, pineal, 458
  testicular, 958–959
Empty sella syndrome, 461, *463*
Encephalitis, 582–583, *583–585*
  human immunodeficiency virus and, 586–589, *590*
  of white matter, 552–553
Encephalocele, 420–422, *423*
  orbital, 613, 613t
Encephalomalacia, infarction and, 521, *521*
  vs. arachnoid cyst, 468
Encephalomyelitis, acute disseminated, 583, *585*
Encephalomyelopathy, necrotizing, subacute, 593, *594*
Encephalopathy, of white matter, 552, *554*
Encephalotrigeminal angiomatosis, 432–434, *435, 436*
Endocrine ophthalmopathy, 610, *612*, 612t
Endometriosis, 932–933, *933, 934*
Endometrium, anatomy of, 922, *925*
  carcinoma of, 923–926, *926*
  staging of, 1156
Endophthalmitis, *Toxocara canis* infection and, 603, 603t
Enhancement, flow-related, 115, *115*
  definition of, 1162
  presaturation for, 119–121, *120*
Entrance slice phenomenon, 122, *122, 123*
Entrapment syndrome, of median nerve, 1058–1060, *1058–1061*, 1117–1118
  imaging protocols for, 1150–1151

Entrapment syndrome *(Continued)*
  in Kienböck's disease, 1067–1068, *1068*
Eosinophilic granuloma, of spine, 691, *692*
Ependyma, porous, in hydrocephalus, 559
Ependymitis, streptococcal abscess and, 578
Ependymoma, 475, *475*
  imaging of, surface receiver coil in, *44*
  of spinal cord, 673, *674*
Epidermoid cyst, of brain, 468, *468–469*
Epidermoid tumor, of cerebellopontine angle, 625, *626*
  orbital, 612, 613t, *615*
Epididymis, anatomy of, 954, *954, 956*
  appendix of, torsion of, 970–971
  in testicular torsion, 968, *968–969*
  seminoma involving, 958, *959*
Epididymitis, *961–963*, 961–964
Epididymoorchitis, *963*, 964, *964*
Epidural hematoma, 564, *564–565*
Epiglottis, *404*
Epilepsy, as indication for brain imaging, 380
  imaging protocols for, 1134–1135
Erythrocytes, lysis of, in cerebral hemorrhage, 257–258, 261t, 262–263
Esophagus, anatomy of, *732, 733*
  carcinoma of, extension of, to heart, *804*
Ethmoid air cells, coronal view of, *400*
Ethmoid sinus, axial view of, *386, 387*
  mucocele of, 633, *635*
  sagittal view of, *406*
Ethylenediamine tetraacetic acid, in contrast agents, 225, 226, 227
Even-echo rephasing, *124*, 124–125, *125*
  definition of, 1161
  for myelographic artifacts, *141*, 143–144
  in portal vein imaging, 853
Ewing's sarcoma, *1103*
  metastasis of, to thorax, 739
Excitation(s), definition of, 1161
  multifrequency, definition of, 1166
  number of, in fast imaging, 183–186, *185*
  selection of, 50, 54t
  variation of, to reduce ghost artifacts, 101
  selective, definition of, 1170
EXORCIST method, to reduce ghost artifacts, 98, 101
Extensor carpi ulnaris tendon, inflammation of, 1062, *1062*, 1073
Extensor tendons, of wrist, abnormalities of, 1060–1062, *1061, 1062*
External capsule, *392, 393*
Eye. See also *Optic* and *Orbit.*
  anatomy of, 598–599, *599–601*
  axial view of, *387, 389*
  coronal view of, *400*
  imaging of, protocols for, 1136–1137
    technical aspects of, 599–603
  lesions of, 603t, 603–606, *604–606*
  oblique muscles of, coronal view of, *400*
  sagittal view of, *409, 410*
  superior, Brown's syndrome of, 612, *612*, 612t
  shrapnel injury of, precautions for, 42
  sodium spectroscopy of, 284–285
Eyelid, basal cell carcinoma of, 614, *618*

Facet joint disease, lumbar, 715–717, *717*
Facial colliculus, of fourth ventricle, *388*
Facial glands, imaging of, protocols for, 1136–1137
Facial nerve, anatomy of, 623–625
  axial view of, *386*
  neuroma of, 473–474
  sagittal view of, *407–409, 411*
Fallot's tetralogy, 792, *795*
  cineangiography of, 832–833, *833–835*
Falx cerebri, axial view of, *391, 392, 399*
  ossification of, vs. meningioma, 458
Faraday shield, definition of, 1162
Fast imaging, 128, *129, 130*
  contrast-enhanced, 49, 50, 195, *196*, 1159
  data collection in, *185–188*, 185–189

Fast imaging (Continued)
driven-equilibrium methods of, 210–214, 212, 213
echo-planar, 214–217, 216
gradient-echo sequences in, 189–196, 189–199, 190t, 198, 199. See also Gradient-echo sequences.
clinical applications of, 199t, 199–210, 200t, 201–211, 206t
hybrid, 216, 217, 218
in cineangiography, 206–207
of heart, 745–749, 746–751
single-shot, 214–215, 216
stimulated-echo method in, 214
types of, 183–184, 184t
vs. spin-echo imaging, 183–185
Fast low angle shot imaging. See FLASH imaging.
Fast passage, adiabatic, definition of, 1158
in angiography, 153
in spectroscopy, 295
Fast rotating gradient spectroscopy, 291, 292
Fast scan pulse sequence, in cineangiography, of heart, 812
Fast-imaging steady-state precession, 49, 50, 190–191
contrast in, 192–195, 193–195
definition of, 1162
in myelography, 145
Fat, imaging of, chemical shift effects on, 197–198, 198
in plasma, malignancy and, proton spectroscopy of, 282, 282
interhemispheric, 443, 443–444
liver infiltration by, 873, 874, 875
marrow, in anterior clinoid process, 401
in crista galli, 400
necrosis of, after trauma, 1125, 1126
orbital, 599, 599
axial view of, 384, 385
sagittal view of, 407
periorbital, coronal view of, 400
resonance of, in chemical shift effect, 326, 326–327
separation of, from water, in pulse sequence design, 336, 336–337, 338
in spectroscopy, 292–293, 293
proton, 278, 280
signal intensity in, 15t, 16, 16t
subcutaneous, in axial brain images, 398, 399
in fetal macrosomia, 949–950
T_1 relaxation time in, 12, 16
vs. brain hemorrhage, 493
Fat pad, infrapatellar, anatomy of, 991
FATE pulse sequence, 212, 212
Fatty acids, metabolism of, in spectroscopy, 273
Femoral artery, hemodynamics in, 111t
Femoral vein, hemodynamics in, 111t
Femur, avascular necrosis of, 1110–1111, 1110–1112, 1121
osteomyelitis of, 1118–1120
osteosarcoma of, 1099
Ferioxamine methane sulfonate, as contrast agent, 251–252, 252, 253
Ferrimagnetic materials, 240–241
Ferrites, 240–241, 250–251, 251, 252
Ferritin, intracellular storage of, 258–259
magnetism of, 485, 487t
Ferromagnetism, 239, 240, 240t
and artifact, 1158
static field, 76–80, 77–80
definition of, 1162
effect of, on imaging, 33
fast gradient-echo, 196
in biologic tissue, 265–266
in fringe fields, 349–353
Fetus, abdomen of, 946, 946–947, 947
brain of, 947–948, 948, 949
effect of magnetic resonance imaging on, 42
growth retardation in, 941–942, 949–950
imaging of, protocols for, 1146–1147
technical aspects of, 944–945, 945
injury to, diethylstilbestrol and, 981
musculoskeletal system of, 947, 947
nervous system of, 947–948, 948, 949

Fetus (Continued)
thorax of, 945, 945–946, 946
Fibrocartilage complex, triangular, anatomy of, 1068–1070, 1069, 1070
disorders of, 1070–1073, 1071–1074
Fibroid tumors, uterine, 923, 925, 926, 931
Fibromatosis, 1103
juvenile, of ankle, 1087–1088, 1089
Fibrosarcoma, 1102
Fibrosis, retroperitoneal, 909, 909
Fibrous dysplasia, orbital, 613t, 620
Field gradient, 17–18, 18
Field strength, and relaxation time, 15, 15t, 16
in cerebral hemorrhage, 261
and signal-to-noise ratio, 35, 36
in spectroscopy, 294, 295
Field-of-view, and aliasing artifact, 329, 329
asymmetric, in fast imaging, 188, 188–189
definition of, 28–29, 1162
in pulse sequence design, 314t
selection of, 51, 54t
in brachial plexus imaging, 654
with single excitation, 186
Filling factor, definition, 1162
Filter, low pass, and artifact, 89
quantum, in spectroscopy, 309
umbrella, vena caval, precautions for, 41, 71
FISP imaging, 49, 50, 190–191
contrast in, 192–195, 193–195
definition of, 1162
in myelography, 145
FLAME pulse sequence, 212, 212, 213
FLASH imaging, 49, 127–128, 128
contrast-enhanced, 191, 191, 195, 196, 219
definition, 1162
in myelography, 200, 203, 204
to reduce artifacts, 144, 145
of abdomen, 200, 201, 202
of bone marrow, 197–198, 198
spoiled, 190, 190
contrast in, 192, 193–195
steady-state, 190–191, 191
contrast in, 192–195, 195
zebra stripes in, 196, 196
three-dimensional, angiographic, 149, 150
Flexor tendons, in carpal tunnel syndrome, 1058–1060, 1058–1061
Flip angle, 7, 8
definition of, 1162
reduced, in fast gradient-echo imaging, 189, 189
in steady-state FLASH imaging, 194, 194
Flocculus, axial view of, 386
coronal view of, 402
sagittal view of, 408
Flow. See also Blood flow and Cerebrospinal fluid, flow of.
and signal intensity, 34
artifacts from, 104, 105, 106
elimination of, 110t
effect of, on fast gradient-echo imaging, 198–199, 199
enhancement of, selection of, 50
fast imaging of, 128, 129, 130, 206, 206–207
measurement of, 172–177, 172–178
vs. thrombosis, 132–137, 133–137
even-echo rephasing for, 124, 125
Flow compensation, 53–54, 125–127, 125–127
definition of, 1162
for myelographic artifacts, 142, 143–144, 144
in subtraction angiography, 153–155, 154, 155
pseudogating in, 122–124, 124
Flow displacement artifact, definition of, 1162
Flow enhancement, gradient-echo imaging in, 128, 128
Flow void, definition of, 1162
Flow-encoding gradients, 176–177, 178
Fluorine, in spectroscopy, 285, 285–286, 286
magnetic resonance characteristics of, 5t
5-Fluorouracil, in spectroscopy, 285, 285
Fluosol, signal intensity in, 16t
Fontan operation, for hypoplastic right heart, 834, 837, 838
Foot, anatomy of, 1078–1079
disorders of, in diabetes, 1092, 1092–1094, 1121

Foot (Continued)
imaging of, protocols for, 1150–1151
technical aspects of, 1076–1078
infection of, 1090–1094, 1092, 1093
posttraumatic abnormalities of, 1094, 1095, 1096
tumors of, 1085, 1085–1090, 1086, 1088–1091
Foramen, arcuate, 408
stylomastoid, 411
Foramen magnum, 404, 405
Foramen of Luschka, 387
Foramen of Monro, axial view of, 395
coronal view of, 402
Forceps major, axial view of, 397
in brain development, 419
Forceps minor, axial view of, 393, 395
in brain development, 416, 419
Fornix, axial view of, 392–394
coronal view of, 401, 402
sagittal view of, 404–407
Fourier series window technique, in phosphorus spectroscopy, of myocardial ischemia, 757–758, 757–759
Fourier transform, 21, 22, 23
definition of, 1162
in spectroscopy, 299–300, 300
two-dimensional, 305, 305–306, 306
in spin-echo imaging, 314t, 314–316, 314–316
modified, in half-Fourier imaging, 53, 54t, 186, 186–188, 187, 325t, 336, 1164
three-dimensional, 317
Fourth ventricle, axial view of, 386–389, 391
coronal view of, 403
ependymoma of, 475, 475
facial colliculus of, 388
sagittal view of, 404, 405
Fracture(s), of hip, 1123
imaging of, protocols for, 1150–1151
of knee, 1005, 1005, 1006
of radius, 1122
of shoulder, 1023, 1025
of spine, 1122
of talus, 1084
orbital, 619, 620
stress, 1123, 1123
of foot, 1094, 1095
Free fatty acids, metabolism of, in spectroscopy, 273
Free induction decay, 24, 24t
and artifact, 85, 87
definition of, 1163
Frequency. See Radiofrequency.
Fringe fields, in site planning, 349–353, 350
of superconductive magnets, 359–360, 360
Frontal gyrus, inferior, axial view of, 396
coronal view of, 400
middle, axial view of, 396, 398, 399
coronal view of, 400
superior, axial view of, 396, 398, 399
coronal view of, 400, 402
sagittal view of, 404
Frontal horn, of lateral ventricle, 394
Frontal lobe, axial view of, 391, 393
sagittal view of, 406, 408, 410
Frontal sinus, axial view of, 390, 392
sagittal view of, 406
Full width–half maximum, definition of, 1163
Fungal infection, of brain, 576, 577, 579
Fusiform gyrus, 401, 402

Gadolinium, in contrast agents, relaxivity of, 225t, 225–227, 226, 227
magnetic moment of, 222, 222t, 240t
Gadolinium-DOTA, 227, 250
Gadolinium-DTPA, 33, 33, 60
as T_2 contrast agent, 234, 235
dosage of, 242–243, 1152
effect of, on presaturation, 121
in angiography, 156–157, 157
in cardiac perfusion studies, 749–752
in imaging, instant inversion recovery, 748–749, 750, 751
of acoustic neuroma, 472, 472

Gadolinium-DTPA *(Continued)*
  of adrenal gland, 250
  of brain, 381–382
  of brain abscess, 576–577, *578*
  of brain tumor, *238*
  of breast cancer, 249–250
  of central nervous system, *238*, 243–244, *244, 245*
  of cerebrovascular infarction, 521, *524*
  of gastrointestinal tract, 248, *249*
  of heart, 249
    echo-planar, 747, *748*
  of kidney, 250
  of liver, 200, 244–248, *246–248*, 882
  of lumbar spine, postoperative, 720, *722, 723*
  of lung cancer, 249
  of multiple sclerosis, 552, *553*
  of musculoskeletal system, 250
  of pelvis, 250
  of pituitary adenoma, *461, 462*, 463
  of spinal cord tumors, 673, *674, 675*
  of spinal nerve sheath tumors, 697, *697*
  of syringohydromyelia, 677
  side effects of, 242–243
  signal intensity of, 16t
  structure of, 225, *225–227*
  toxicity of, 228t, 228–229
Galen's vein, axial view of, *395, 397*
  malformation of, *530,* 531
  sagittal view of, *404*
Gallbladder, 882–884, *882–885*
  carcinoma of, 883–884, *884, 885*
  imaging of, contrast agents in, 230–232, *232*
Gallstones, 883, 883–884, *884*
Ganglion cyst, 1073–1074
Gastrointestinal tract, gadolinium-DTPA imaging of, 248, *249*
  motion of, in abdominal imaging, 848–852, *850–852*
Gas-water interface, intestinal, magnetic susceptibility effect of, 849, *851*
Gating, cardiac. See *Cardiac gating*.
  physiologic, 814, 1163
  respiratory, 1163
    for motion artifacts, 732
    in abdominal imaging, 848
    to reduce ghost artifacts, *100*, 100t, 100–101
Gaucher's disease, 1114, *1114, 1115*
Gauss, definition of, 1163
Gaussian pulse, definition of, 1168
Genioglossus muscle, coronal view of, *400*
  sagittal view of, *405*
Genitalia. See *Pelvis* and specific structures, e.g., *Testes.*
Germinoma, pineal, 458–459, *459*
Ghost artifacts, 32, 76t, 98–104, *98–104*, 99t, 100t
  definition of, 1158
  flow compensation for, 126, *126, 127*
  gating for, *100*, 100t, 100–101
  in abdominal imaging, 847, *848*
  in brachial plexus imaging, 654–655
  presaturation for, 119–121, *120*
  vascular pulsation and, 132, *132*
  with single excitation, 185
Giant cell aortitis, 782, *783*
Giant cell arteritis, 524, *529*
Giant cell reactions, to Proplast, in temporomandibular prostheses, 1044, *1054*
Giant cell tumor, sarcomatous degeneration of, *1102*
Gianturco coil, and artifact, *78*
Gibbs artifact, *91*, 91–92, 328–329, *329*, 1159
  in spinal imaging, 672
Glenohumeral joint, 1010–1029
  anatomy of, 1012–1015, *1013, 1014*
  capsular injury of, 1020–1023, *1021–1024*
  crystal deposition disease of, 1027–1028
  imaging of, protocols for, 1148–1149
    technical aspects of, 1010–1012, *1011*
  loose bodies in, *1027*, 1028–1029
  osteonecrosis of, 1027, *1027*
  synovitis of, 1023–1027, *1026*
  trauma to, 1023, *1025*
  tumors of, *1028*, 1029
Glenoid cavity, anatomy of, 1012

Glenoid labrum, in shoulder stability, 1021–1022, *1022–1024*
Glioblastoma, phosphorus spectroscopy of, 277, *278*, 278t
  spin-echo imaging of, *26*
Glioma, cerebral, 449–450, *450–452*
  fast imaging of, contrast agents with, *207*
  FLASH imaging of, contrast-enhanced, *196*
  hypothalamic, 463–464, *464*
  in neurofibromatosis, 431
  of brain stem, 474, *474–475*
  of optic chiasm, 431, 463, *464*
  of optic nerve, 431, 609, 609t, *610*
  parenchymal, 431
  phosphorus spectroscopy of, 277, *278*, 278t
  pineal, 459, *460*
Globe, optic, anatomy of, 598, *599–601*
  axial view of, *387, 389*
  coronal view of, *400*
  imaging of, protocols for, 1136–1137
Globoid cell leukodystrophy, Krabbe's, 552
Globus pallidus, axial view of, *393*
  iron deposition in, *590*, 590–591, *591*
Glomerulonephritis, 901
Glomus, in atrium of lateral ventricle, *408*
Glomus jugulare, 626, *627*
Glomus tumor, *479*, 479–480
  of parapharyngeal space, 633
Glomus tympanicum, 626, *627*
Glossopharyngeal nerve, axial view of, *386*
  coronal view of, *402*
  sagittal view of, *408, 409*
Glucagon, for suppression of peristalsis, 158, 849, *850*, 852
Glucose, brain storage of, and response to stroke, 276–277
  metabolism of, in spectroscopy, 273
Glutamate, in carbon-13 spectroscopy, of heart, 761–762, *762*
Glycogen, metabolism of, in spectroscopy, 273
Glycogen storage disease, Type IX, spectroscopy of, 274–275
Goiter, 735, *737*
  multinodular, *647*
Golay coil, definition of, 1163
Gradient, *37*, 37–38. See also *Pulse sequences.*
  actively shielded, to reduce eddy currents, 364, 1161
  and artifacts, 86–97, *88–91, 93–97*
  fast rotating, in spectroscopy, 291, *292*
  field, 17–18, *18*
  flow-encoding, 176–177, *178*
  instrumentation for, 363–366, *363–366*
  magnetic field, 17–18, *18*, 322–324, *323*
  refocusing of, 325
  reorientation of, to reduce ghost artifacts, 102, *103*
  rephasing of, to reduce ghost artifacts, 103, *104*
  spoiler, 330, 1170
  strength of, 323–324
  waveforms of, 323, *323*
Gradient coils, 322–323, 1163
Gradient dephasing, in subtraction angiography, 153–155, *154, 155*
Gradient echo, definition of, 1161
Gradient motion rephasing, 125–127, *125–127*, 317, 1162
  to reduce artifacts, 332–334, *333, 334*
Gradient ramp time, definition of, 1169
Gradient reversal, 317, 1164
Gradient rotation, 55
  for myelographic artifacts, 143
Gradient-echo sequences, 24t, 25–26, *27*, 127–129, *128–130*, 317, *317*
  definition of, 1168
  for myelographic artifacts, *144*, 144–145
  in brain hemorrhage, 260, 489, *490, 491*
  in imaging, fast, 184, 189–210
    clinical applications of, 199t, 199–210, 200t, *201–211*, 206t
    contrast agents in, 207, *207*
    contrast in, 191–199, *192–196, 198, 199*, 1159
    flow effects on, 198–199, *199*

Gradient-echo sequences *(Continued)*
  low intensity in, causes of, 206t
    three-dimensional, 208–210, *210, 211*
    types of, *190*, 190t, 190–191, *191*
  fat-water, in spectroscopy, 293, *293*
  of temporomandibular joint, 1032–1033
  spinal, 669, *670, 671*
  three-dimensional, *58*, 58–60, *59*
    for susceptibility artifact, 81
  selection of, 49–50
Gradient-recalled acquisition steady-state (GRASS) imaging, 49, 50, 190–191
  contrast in, 192–195, *193, 194*
  definition of, 1162
  in myelography, 145
Graft, bypass, coronary, 752, *752–753, 753*, 807, *807*
  cineangiography of, 824
  for coarctation of aorta, 786–787, *789*
Granulation tissue, postoperative, and thoracic outlet syndrome, 661, *665*
Granuloma, cholesterol, of brain, 469
  eosinophilic, of spine, 691, *692*
  in pyelonephritis, 905
GRASS imaging, 49, 50, 190–191
  contrast in, 192–195, *193, 194*
  definition of, 1162
  in myelography, 145
Graves' disease, ophthalmopathy in, 610
Growth, retardation of, intrauterine, 941–942, 949–950
Growth hormone, hypersecretion of, pituitary adenoma and, 460
Gyromagnetic ratio, 4, 1164
Gyrus. See also specific gyri, e.g., *Precentral gyrus.*
Gyrus rectus, axial view of, *390*
  coronal view of, *400*
  sagittal view of, *404, 406*

Habenular commissure, *403*
Haemophilus influenzae infection, and meningitis, 580–581
Half-Fourier imaging, 53, 54t, *186*, 186–188, *187*, 325t, 336
  definition of, 1164
Half-saddle coil, 1169
Hallervorden-Spatz disease, 595
Hand, ganglion cyst of, 1073–1074
Hard palate, *404*
Harrington rod, and magnetic field distortion, 41–42
Head. See also specific structures, e.g., *Brain; Temporomandibular joint.*
  computed tomography of, 622–623, 626–629, 629t
    after trauma, 574–575
  imaging of, 622–651
    trauma to, and brain injury, 563–575, *564–575*
      as indication for brain imaging, 380
Headache, migraine, 524–525, *530*
  vs. multiple sclerosis, 561
Heart, 745–844
  cineangiography of, 810–844
    future of, 826–828, *827*
    methods of, 816–821, *818–820*
    technical aspects of, *811*, 811–815, *812*, 814–816, 816t
    vs. echocardiography, 842–844, 843t
  congenital diseases of, 785–792, *788–795*
    cineangiography of, 830–844
      method of, 830–832, *831*
      right ventricular, 832–837, *833–839*
  fetal, 946, *946*
  imaging of, electrocardiographic gating in. See *Cardiac gating.*
    gadolinium-DTPA in, 249
    planes for, 774–779, *774–779*
    protocols for, 1142–1143
    three-dimensional, chemical shift in, 766, *766*
    ultrafast, 745–749, *746–751*
  left, cineangiography of, 841, *842*

Heart *(Continued)*
  pacemaker for, as contraindication to imaging, 41, 354
  perfusion studies of, 749–752, *750, 751*
  spectroscopy of, carbon-13, 761–762, *762, 763*
    hydrogen, 766, *767*
    phosphorus, 277
      after transplantation, *756,* 756–757, *757,* 761
      in workload assessment, 759–760, *760*
  thrombosis of, cineangiography of, 823–824, *825*
  tumors of, 801–803, *803, 804*
    cineangiography of, 816t, *822,* 823, *824*
  valves of, implants in, precautions for, 41, 70–71
    insufficiency of, imaging protocols for, 1142–1143
    regurgitation through, cineangiography of, 822–823, *823*
    stenosis of, cineangiography of, 815, *815,* 816t
Heart rate, monitoring of, during imaging, 40, 73
Helium, liquid, for superconductive magnets, in site planning, 342
  in quenches, 343–344
Helmholtz coils, 43, *43,* 1164
Hemangioblastoma, 476–477, *478*
  in Hippel-Lindau disease, 436–437, *438, 439*
  of spinal cord, 673, *675*
Hemangioendothelioma, hepatic, 869, *872*
Hemangioma, of foot and ankle, cavernous, 1086–1087
  of liver, 865–869, *866–869, 871*
    fast imaging of, *201, 202*
    gadolinium-DTPA imaging of, 248, *248*
  of masseter muscle, *640*
  of portal vein, imaging of, even-echo rephasing in, *853*
  of spinal cord, cavernous, 680–681
  orbital, cavernous, 606t, 606–608, *607*
  soft tissue, 1101–1104
  vertebral, 690–691, *691*
Hematocele, in testicular torsion, *967, 968,* 969
  traumatic, 964–965, *965*
Hematoma. See also *Hemorrhage.*
  brain. See *Brain, hemorrhage into.*
    dissecting, of aorta, 782–785, *784–787*
    epidural, *564,* 564–565
    in brachial plexus injury, *658,* 659
    in lumbar spine, postoperative, 719, *719*
    mediastinal, 733–735, *736*
    of liver, *857*
      imaging of, effect of respiration on, *850*
    perinephric, 900–901, *901*
    signal intensity in, 16t
    subdural, 564–565, *564–568*
    traumatic, *1108, 1123,* 1124, *1124*
Hematuria, imaging protocols for, 1146–1147
Hemochromatosis, 873–875, *876*
Hemodynamics, *111,* 111t, 111–114, 112t, *113, 114*
Hemoglobin, deoxygenated, in cerebral hemorrhage, 257, 261, 261t
  paramagnetic breakdown products of, 133, 135, *485,* 485–487
Hemoglobinuria, paroxysmal, 901–902
Hemophilia, and arthritis, of knee, 1002, *1002*
  and arthropathy, of ankle, 1083–1084
  pseudotumor in, 1101, *1105*
Hemorrhage. See also *Hematoma.*
  and spinal cord infarction, 679, *680*
  brain. See *Brain, hemorrhage into.*
    imaging of, 33
      fast, *205,* 205–206, 206t
    in brachial plexus tumors, 660, *663*
    in epididymitis, 962, *962*
    in pituitary adenoma, *462,* 463, 511, *511*
    in renal cysts, 904, *904*
    in testicular trauma, 978
    ocular, 603, 603t, *605,* 605–606
    of brain stem, 499, *499–501*
    of liver, 869–873, *873*
      in hepatoblastoma, *859,* 864, *865*
    of uterine adnexa, 928–930, *930*

Hemorrhage *(Continued)*
  retroplacental, 941
  with testicular tumor, 957, *957*
Hemosiderin, magnetism of, 485, 487t
  in subarachnoid hemorrhage, 540, *541*
  in vascular malformation, 502–503, *504*
Hemostasis, clips for, precautions for, 41, 70
Heparin, and brain hemorrhage, 504
Hepatic veins, angiography of, *158,* 160, *160, 161*
Hepatitis, 875, *877*
Hepatoblastoma, *859,* 864, *865*
Hepatolenticular degeneration, 593–595
Hepatoma, 861–862, *864*
Herniation, cingulate, with subdural hematoma, *565*
  inguinal, with cryptorchidism, *975*
  of intervertebral disks, cervicothoracic, 681, *682–684*
    lumbar, 710–714, *712–715*
  transtentorial, 512
    aneurysmal hemorrhage and, 540–541
Herpes simplex infection, and encephalitis, 583, *583, 584*
Hertz, definition of, 1164
Heterotopia, in neurofibromatosis, 431, *432*
  in tuberous sclerosis, 436
  of gray matter, 440, *441*
Hill-Sachs deformity, of humerus, 1021, *1022,* 1023, *1024*
Hilum, pulmonary, 740–743, *742*
  renal, 901, *902*
Hip, avascular necrosis of, *1110,* 1110–1111, *1111, 1121*
  dislocation of, congenital, 1114–1116
  imaging of, protocols for, 1150–1151
  stress fracture of, *1123*
Hippel-Lindau disease, 436–437, *438, 439*
Hippocampal formation, *391, 393*
Hippocampal gyrus, *402*
Hippocampus, *402*
Histoplasmosis, adrenal, 893, *894*
Hodgkin's lymphoma, ferrite-enhanced imaging of, 251, *252*
  mediastinal, 735–737
  staging of, 1157
Hoffa's infrapatellar fat pad, anatomy of, 991
Holmium, magnetic moment of, 222t
Holoprosencephaly, *426,* 426–427, *427*
Homogeneity, definition of, 1164
  of magnetic field, antennas for, 367–368, *367–369*
Horizontal fissure, *403*
Human immunodeficiency virus, and brain infection, 583–589, *586–590*
  and primary malignant lymphoma, 452, *453*
Humerus. See also *Glenohumeral joint.*
  Hill-Sachs deformity of, 1021, *1022,* 1023, *1024*
  proximal, anatomy of, 1012, *1013*
Huntington's chorea, 592, *593*
Hyaline cartilage, tumors of, 1101, *1106*
Hybrid imaging, 216, 217, *218,* 1164
Hydatidiform mole, 941, *941*
Hydrocele, 922, *922,* 954, *955,* 971–972
  in epididymitis, *961, 962,* 964
  traumatic, 966
Hydrocephalus, 555–560, *557–560*
  aneurysmal hemorrhage and, 540
  fetal, 948, *948*
  in bacterial meningitis, 581
  in tuberous sclerosis, 436
Hydrogen, in spectroscopy, of heart, 766, *767*
  magnetic resonance characteristics of, 4, 5, 5t
  spectra of, resolution of, solvent suppression for, 307–309, *308*
Hydronephrosis, 900, *900*
  fetal, 946, *946*
Hygroma, subdural, 565, *569*
Hyperadrenocorticism, pituitary adenoma and, 460
Hyperglycinemia, and myelination disorders, 444–446, *444–446*
Hyperplastic anemia, 1113, *1113*
Hypertension, and brain hemorrhage, 494, 496–499, *497–501*
  portal, 877–878, *880, 881*

Hypertension *(Continued)*
  pulmonary, 792
Hypoglossal canal, *385*
Hypoglossal nerve, *384*
Hypoplastic right heart syndrome, 833–834, *835–838*
Hypothalamus, displacement of, in hydrocephalus, 557, *558–559*
  glioma of, 463–464, *464*

Image selected in vivo spectroscopy, 288, *288*
  in cardiac imaging, 766, *766*
Implants, metallic, and artifacts, 76–80, *77–80*
  in knee imaging, *1000,* 1006–1007
  cardiac, cineangiography of, 816t, *826,* 826
  precautions for, 41t, 41–42, 70–72
Induction, magnetic, definition of, 1165
Infarction, cerebrovascular, 507–508, *508–510,* 516–521, *517–524*
  and infection, 575–576
  brain glucose stores in, 276–277
  hemorrhagic, 518, *520*
  trauma and, *573*
  imaging protocols in, 1134–1135
  lacunar, and white matter ischemia, 548, *549*
  myocardial, 806, 806–807, *807*
    cineangiography of, 822, *822*
  of bone, in knee, 1003–1004, *1004*
  of spinal cord, 679–680, *680*
    imaging protocols for, 1138–1139
    perfusion imaging of, *179*
    sodium spectroscopy of, 284
Inferior colliculus, axial view of, *392*
  coronal view of, *403*
  sagittal view of, *405*
Inferior frontal gyrus, axial view of, *396*
  coronal view of, *400*
Inferior nasal turbinate, coronal view of, *400*
  sagittal view of, *406*
Inferior oblique muscle, of eyeball, *409, 410*
Inferior rectus muscle, axial view of, *386*
  coronal view of, *400*
  sagittal view of, *408, 409*
Inferior semilunar lobule, of cerebellum, *403*
Inferior temporal gyrus, axial view of, *386*
  coronal view of, *401*
  sagittal view of, *411*
Inferior vena cava, anatomy of, 859–860, *860*
  imaging of, protocols for, 1144–1145
  leiomyosarcoma of, blood flow measurement in, *177*
  thrombus of, in renal cell carcinoma, 901, *902*
Infrapatellar fat pad, Hoffa's, anatomy of, 991
Infratemporal fossa, 630, *630*
Infundibulum, axial view of, *390*
  coronal view of, *401*
Inhomogeneity, main field, 361
  and artifacts, 75–76, *77*
Innominate artery, anatomy of, *732*
Innominate vein, anatomy of, *733*
Instant inversion recovery imaging, 748–749, *749–751*
Insula, axial view of, *392, 394, 395*
  coronal view of, *401*
Insular cistern, *410*
Insular gyri, *410*
Interference, radiofrequency, in site planning, 344, *346–349*
Interhemispheric fissure, axial view of, *397–399*
  coronal view of, *400*
Internal capsule, axial view of, *393, 395*
  coronal view of, *401*
  in brain development, 415t, *417, 419–421*
  infarction of, *509*
Internal carotid artery, axial view of, *384–389, 391*
  coronal view of, *401*
  sagittal view of, *406–409*
Internal cerebral vein, axial view of, *394, 395*
  coronal view of, *403*
  sagittal view of, *404*
Internal jugular vein, axial view of, *384, 385*
  sagittal view of, *409, 410*

Internal occipital protuberance, *387*
Interpeduncular cistern, axial view of, *391*
    coronal view of, *402*
Intervertebral disks. See *Disk(s), intervertebral.*
Intestine, gadolinium-DTPA imaging of, 248, *249*
    motion of, in abdominal imaging, 158, 848–852, *850–852*
Intracranial pressure, increased, in hydrocephalus, 555–560
Intravascular devices, imaging of, 137, *137*
    precautions for, in imaging, 41, 71
Inversion recovery sequence, 26–28, *27, 28, 334,* 334–335
    bounce point of, and artifacts, 105–106, *107*
    definition of, 1164
    instant, 748–749, *749–751*
    short time, 28, *28*
        definition of, 1164
        in orbital imaging, 601
        to reduce ghost artifacts, 102
Inversion time, definition of, 1164
Inversion transfer, in spectroscopy, 304
Iophendylate (Pantopaque), in lumbar spine, 724, *725*
Iris, axial view of, *386*
Iron, deposition of, hepatic, 873–875, *876*
    in degenerative brain disease, 590, *590–591, 591*
    effect of, on imaging, 33
    in cerebral hemorrhage, effect of, on imaging, 261t, 261–263
    metabolism of, *256–258, 256–259*
    in contrast agents, hepatobiliary excretion of, 231–232, *232*
        relaxivity of, 225t
        toxicity of, 228t
    magnetic moment of, 222t, 240t
Iron ethylene-bis-(2-hydroxyphenylglycine), as contrast agent, 252
Ischemia, and osteonecrosis, of shoulder, 1027, *1027*
    cardiac, cineangiography of, 816t
    myocardial, induction of, for operation, 760, *761*
        phosphorus spectroscopy of, 755–758, *755–759*
    of spinal cord, 679–680, *680*
    of white matter, 546–549, *547–549*
        differential diagnosis of, 560
    sodium spectroscopy of, 284
ISIS sequence, 288, *288*
    in cardiac imaging, 766, *766*
Isochromat, definition of, 1164
    in phase effect, 117
Isotope, definition of, 1164
Isotropic resolution, definition of, 1164
Isotropic three-dimensional imaging, 23

Jatene operation, for transposition of great arteries, 835–836
J-coupling, in spectroscopy, 270, *301,* 301–302
Jugular vein, internal, axial view of, *384, 385*
    sagittal view of, *409, 410*
    thrombosis of, vs. donut sign, *121*
Juvenile fibromatosis, of ankle, 1087–1088, *1089*
Juvenile rheumatoid arthritis, of knee, 1001
    synovial hypertrophy in, of ankle, 1084

Kaolin, as contrast agent, 252–253
Kidney, *899–907,* 899–908
    anatomy of, *899,* 899–900
    angiography of, *158,* 160, 160–162, *163–165*
    carcinoma of, metastatic, 907
        renal cell, 905–906, *906,* 908
            metastasis of, to lung, 743, *743*
            thrombosis in, 901, *902*
        staging of, 1153, *1154*
    cysts of, 903–904, *904,* 907–908
    excretion of contrast agents by, 230, *231*
    fast imaging of, contrast agents with, *207*

Kidney *(Continued)*
    fetal, 946, *946*
    imaging of, chemical shift artifact in, 93, *94*
        gadolinium-DTPA in, 250
        protocols for, 1144–1145
    inflammation of, 901, 905, *905*
    lymphoma of, 906–907, *907*
    parenchymal disease of, diffuse, 901–902
    transplantation of, 902–903, *903*
    tumors of, 905–908, *906, 907*
Kienböck's disease, 1066–1068, *1067, 1068*
Knee, 989–1007
    angiography of, *157,* 158
    arthritis of, 1000–1003, *1001–1003*
    bone infarcts in, 1003–1004, *1004*
    cartilage defects of, 1000, *1001*
    cysts of, 1004
    fast imaging of, 207–208, *208, 209*
    fractures of, 1005, *1005, 1006*
    imaging of, artifacts in, *1000,* 1006–1007
        evaluation criteria for, 1007, *1007*
        photography of, 62, *64, 65*
        protocols for, 1148–1149
        technical aspects of, 989–990
    infection of, 1005–1006
    joint effusions in, 1004, *1004*
    ligaments of, 996–998, *996–998*
    menisci of, 990–995, *991–995*
    osteitis dissecans in, 1003
    osteochondrosis of, 1003, *1003*
    synovial plicae of, 1004
    tumors of, 1006, *1006, 1007*
Krabbe's globoid cell leukodystrophy, 552
K-space, definition of, 1165
    in data measurement, 214–215, *215*

Labrum, glenoid, in shoulder stability, 1021–1022, *1022–1024*
Lacrimal duct, *384, 386*
Lacrimal gland, *388, 390*
Lacrimal sac, dacryocystitis of, 614–620, *618*
Lactate, in spectroscopy, of heart, 762–763, *763, 764*
Lacunar infarction, 521, *522*
    and white matter ischemia, 548, *549*
Lamina terminalis, *392*
Laminar flow, definition of, 1165
Laminar profile, of blood flow, 112, *113*
Laparoscopy, in cryptorchidism, 973
Larmor equation, definition of, 1165
Larmor frequency, 4, 7, *7*
    adjustment of transmitted pulse frequency to, 46–47
    definition of, 1165
Larynx, anatomy of, *644,* 645
    tumors of, *646,* 647
Laser cameras, for photography of images, 63
Lateral collateral ligament, of knee, 998, *998*
Lateral pterygoid muscle, axial view of, *384*
    coronal view of, *401*
    physiology of, 1034–1037, *1035, 1037*
    sagittal view of, *410, 411*
Lateral pterygoid plate, sagittal view of, *408*
Lateral recess syndrome, 717
Lateral rectus muscle, axial view of, *388*
    sagittal view of, *411*
Lateral ventricle, atrium of, glomus in, *408*
    body of, *396, 397*
    coronal view of, *401–403*
    frontal horn of, *394*
    sagittal view of, *406–410*
    temporal horn of, axial view of, *388, 391, 393*
        sagittal view of, *408–410*
    trigone of, *395*
Leg. See also specific structures, e.g., *Femur.*
    angiography in, 159–160
Legg-Calvé-Perthes disease, 1111
Leigh's disease, 593, *594*
Leiomyoma, uterine, 923, *925, 926*
    in pregnancy, 939, *939*
Leiomyosarcoma, metastasis from, to liver, fast imaging of, *202*

Leiomyosarcoma *(Continued)*
    of inferior vena cava, blood flow measurement in, *177*
    of liver, hemorrhage in, *873*
Lemniscus, medial, *388*
Lens, axial view of, *386, 387*
Lentiform nucleus, *393, 395*
Leukemia, hepatic infiltration in, 864
    lymphocytic, 692–693
    marrow abnormalities in, 692–693, *1110*
    metastasis of, to spleen, 895
    testicular infiltration by, 957, 960–961
Leukodystrophy, 552
    with adrenal dysfunction, 595, *595*
Leukoencephalitis, 552–553
Leukoencephalopathy, progressive multifocal, 552, *554*
    AIDS-related, 584–586, *589*
Leydig cell tumors, 960, *960*
Ligament(s), broad, anatomy of, 923, *924*
    carpal, anatomy of, 1062–1064, *1062–1064*
    of ankle, anatomy of, 1078
    of knee, 996–998, *996–998*
        imaging of, protocols for, 1148–1149
        transverse, vs. meniscal tear, 994, 994–995, *995*
    radioulnar, tears of, 1070–1071, *1071*
    signal intensity in, 16t
    trauma to, 1123–1124
Lightening artifact, in cineangiography, of heart, 813–814, *814*
Line scan angiography, 155–156, *156*
Linewidth, definition of, 1165
    in spectroscopy, 271, *272,* 299–300, *300*
Lingual gyrus, *407*
Lipid. See *Fat.*
Lipohyalinosis, and brain hemorrhage, 496
Lipoma, *1099,* 1100
    adrenal, 891, *892*
    cardiac, 803, *805*
    intraspinal, in dysraphism, 725, *726*
    of brain, 469
        interhemispheric, *443,* 443–444
    of heart, ventricular, echo-planar imaging of, 746, *746–747*
    of kidney, 907, *907*
    of knee, 1006, *1007*
    of parotid gland, *640*
    of shoulder, *1028,* 1029
Lipomyelomeningocele, 725
Lipomyeloschisis, 724, *725, 726*
Liposarcoma, *1100,* 1100–1101, *1101*
Lissencephaly, 438–439, *440*
Lithium, in spectroscopy, 286
Liver, 852–882
    adenoma of, 869, *871*
    anatomy of, 858–860, *860*
    angiography of, *158,* 160, *160–163*
    blastoma of, 869–873, *873*
    cancer of, extension of, to heart, *804*
        hemorrhage in, 872, *873*
        metastatic, *855, 857,* 860–861, *861–863*
            fatty infiltration with, 873, *874, 875*
            imaging of, contrast agents in, 232, *232,* 244–246, *246, 247*
                fast, *202*
                receiver adjustment for, *48*
            venography of, 160, *162*
        primary, 861–864, *864, 865*
            vs. hemangioma, 866–869, *867–870*
    cirrhosis of, 875, *877*
        angiography of, 160, *163*
    computed tomography of, 853, 854, 878–882
    cysts of, 856, 865, *866*
        vs. malignancy, 860, *862*
    excretion of contrast agents by, 230–233, *232, 233*
    fatty infiltration of, 873, *874, 875*
    ferrite-enhanced imaging of, 250–251, *251*
    focal nodular hyperplasia of, 869, *871*
    hemangioendothelioma of, 869, *872*
    hemangioma of, 865–869, *866–869, 871*
        fast imaging of, *201,* 202
        gadolinium-DTPA imaging of, 248, *248*
    hematoma of, *857*

Liver *(Continued)*
    imaging of, effect of respiration on, *850*
    hemorrhage of, 869–873, *873*
    imaging of, gadolinium-DTPA in, 200, 244–248, *246–248,* 882
    left lobe in, vs. stomach, 849, *851*
    protocols for, 1144–1145
    technical aspects of, 852–860, *855–860*
    inflammation of, 875, *877, 878*
    iron deposition in, 873–875, *876*
    regenerating nodules in, 875
    signal intensity in, 15t, 16t
    vascular diseases of, 875–878, *878–881*
Lobar hemorrhage, *502–510, 510–510*
Localization, in spectroscopy, 286–292, *287–292*
    spatial, of signal, 17–23, *18–23*
Longitudinal ligament, posterior, *405*
Longitudinal magnetization, definition of, 1165
    effect of repetition time on, 12, *14*
Longus capitis muscle, axial view of, *384, 385*
    sagittal view of, *406*
Longus colli muscle, *406*
Lorentzian shape, definition of, 1165
Lower extremity. See also specific structures,
    e.g., *Knee.*
    angiography in, 159–160
Lunate, avascular necrosis of, 1066–1068, *1067, 1068,* 1111, *1113*
Lung(s). See also *Pulmonary.*
    carcinoma of, angiography of, *159*
        carbon-13 spectroscopy of, 283
        extension of, to spine, *1104*
        gadolinium-DTPA imaging of, 249
        metastasis of, to brain, *454*
            to mediastinum, *738*
            to spine, *688*
        staging of, 739–740, *741, 742,* 1153–1156
    cysts of, 733, *734*
    fetal, 945, *945–946*
    imaging of, 743, *743*
    Pancoast tumor of, extension of, to brachial plexus, 660, *663*
    signal intensity in, 16t
Lunotriquetral dissociation, 1073, *1073*
Lunotriquetral ligament, anatomy of, 1063–1064, *1064*
Lupus erythematosus, systemic, vs. multiple sclerosis, 561
Luschka's foramen, *387*
Lyme arthritis, of knee, 1002
Lymph nodes, metastases to, in cancer staging, 1153–1155
Lymphadenopathy, in lymphogranuloma venereum, *936*
    mediastinal, 735, *738*
    retroperitoneal, 909–911, *911*
Lymphangioma, orbital, *607,* 608
Lymphocele, retroperitoneal, 909, *910*
Lymphocytic leukemia, acute, marrow changes in, spinal, 692–693
Lymphogranuloma venereum, *936*
Lymphoma, cardiac invasion by, *804*
    classification of, 1157
    ferrite-enhanced imaging of, 251, *251, 252*
    marrow changes in, 693, 1109
    mediastinal, 735–737
    metastasis of, to spine, *689*
        to spleen, 895
    of liver, 862–863, *864*
    of parotid gland, 638, *642*
    orbital, 606t, 608, *608,* 610–612, 612t
    paraspinal, 694, *694*
    phosphorus spectroscopy of, 277–278, *279*
    primary malignant, of brain, 451–452, *453*
    renal, 906–907, *907*
    testicular infiltration by, 922, *922,* 957, 960, *960*

Macrosomia, fetal, maternal diabetes and, 949–950
Magnet(s), fringe fields of, in site planning, 349–353, *350*
    in imaging systems, 34, 34–35, *35*
    permanent, definition of, 1167

Magnet(s) *(Continued)*
    in imaging systems, 35, *35*
        site planning for, 343
    receiver coil centered with, 46, *46*
    resistive, definition of, 1169
        site planning for, 342–343
    role of, in imaging, 5–7, *6*
    superconductive, *357,* 357t, 358–361, *359–361*
        definition of, 1170
        in imaging systems, 34–35, *35*
        safety of, 362t, 362–363, 363t
        site planning for, 341–342
            fringe fields in, 349–353, *350*
            quenches in, 343–344
Magnetic field, definition of, 1165
    homogeneity of, 357–358
        antennas for, 367–368, *367–369*
    in fast gradient-echo imaging, 195–198, *196, 198*
    inhomogeneity in, 361
        and artifacts, 75–76, *77*
        in fast gradient-echo imaging, 195–197, *196*
        in imaging of brain hemorrhage, 489, *491*
    shimming of, *360,* 360–361, *361*
        mathematical principles of, 374
    stability of, 358
    static, artifacts in, 75–81, *77–82*
    strength of, 357
        selection of, *361,* 361t–363t, 361–363, *362*
        with superconductive magnets, 358
Magnetic induction, definition of, 1165
Magnetic moment, 222, 222t, 240t, 1165
Magnetic resonance, definition of, 1165
    topical, 287
Magnetic resonance imaging. See also specific technical aspects, e.g., *Pulse sequences,* bodily structures, e.g., *Knee,* and disorders, e.g., *Multiple sclerosis.*
    contraindications to, 41, 41t, 68–72
    patient preparation for, 40, 40–42, 68–73
    photography in, 62–63, *63–65*
    procedure of, *61,* 61–63, *63–65*
    quality control in, 63–66, *65*
Magnetic shielding. See *Shielding.*
Magnetic susceptibility, 32–33. See also *Diamagnetism, Ferromagnetism, Paramagnetism,* and *Superparamagnetism.*
    and artifact, 80–81, *81, 82*
    definition of, 1165
    in biologic tissue, 266
    of intestinal water-gas interface, 849, *851*
Magnetism, of contrast agents, 238–241, *239,* 240t
    of hemoglobin, *484,* 484–485, 487t
Magnetite, in angiography, 157
    signal intensity of, 16t
Magnetization, in fast gradient-echo imaging, vs. spin-echo, 189, *189*
    longitudinal, definition of, 1165
        effect of repetition time on, 12, *14*
    net, 5, 1166
    residual, in two-dimensional imaging, 316
    slice, rephasing of, 321
    transverse, 8, *9*
        reduction of, with T_2 relaxation, 9–10, *10, 11*
        refocusing of, 320–321
Magnetization transfer, in spectroscopy, 271–272, 303–304, *304*
Magnevist. See *Gadolinium-DTPA.*
Magnitude image, definition of, 1165
Magnitude reconstruction, 27–28
Malleolus, medial, avascular necrosis of, 1111, *1113*
Mamillary bodies, axial view of, *391*
    sagittal view of, *405*
Mamillothalamic tract, *393*
Mandible. See also *Temporomandibular joint.*
    coronal view of, *400*
    coronoid process of, *384*
    osteosarcoma of, *646*
    ramus of, *411*
    sagittal view of, *405, 411*
Mandibular condyle, anatomy of, 1033, 1034, *1035*
    axial view of, *384*
    coronal view of, *401*

Manganese, in contrast agents, 222, 222t
    relaxivity of, 225t, 227, 227–228
    toxicity of, 228t
    magnetic moment of, 222t, 240t
Marfan's syndrome, aortic aneurysm in, 782, *783*
    blood flow measurement in, *177*
Marrow. See *Bone marrow.*
Mascara, and artifact, 79
Masseter muscle, axial view of, *384*
    coronal view of, *400*
    hemangioma of, *640*
    sagittal view of, *411*
Mastoid sinus, *384*
Matrix, acquisition, definition of, 1158
    display, definition of, 1161
Matrix size, definition of, 29
    reduced, in fast imaging, 186
    selection of, 51–52, *53,* 54t
Maxillary antrum, coronal view of, *400*
Maxillary sinus, axial view of, *384*
    carcinoma of, 634, *635*
    cyst of, 637, *638*
    sagittal view of, *407–409*
Maximum intensity projection, definition of, 1165–1166
    in angiography, *150,* 150–151, *151*
Maxwell coil, 1166
McArdle's syndrome, spectroscopy of, 274, *275, 276*
Measurement, of image, *61,* 61–62
Medial collateral ligament, of knee, 998, *998*
Medial lemniscus, *388*
Medial malleolus, avascular necrosis of, 1111, *1113*
Medial pterygoid muscle, coronal view of, *401*
    sagittal view of, *410*
Medial rectus muscle, axial view of, *386, 388*
    coronal view of, *400*
Median nerve, compression of, in carpal tunnel, 1058–1060, *1058–1061,* 1117–1118
    imaging protocols for, 1150–1151
    in Kienböck's disease, 1067–1068, *1068*
Mediastinum, 733–739, *734–740*
    imaging of, protocols for, 1140–1141
Medulla, axial view of, *385, 387*
    sagittal view of, *405*
Medullary cistern, *384, 387*
Medullary pyramid, *402*
Medulloblastoma, 476, *477*
    hydrocephalus with, *557*
Melanin, vs. brain hemorrhage, 493
Melanoma, choroidal, 603t, 604, *606*
Meningioma, 455–458, *456–458*
    acoustic, in neurofibromatosis, 431, *434*
    calcified, 458, *458*
        vs. brain hemorrhage, *494*
    gadolinium-DTPA imaging of, 243, *244*
    of optic nerve sheath, 609, 609t, *611*
    parasellar, 465, *466*
    phosphorus spectroscopy of, 277, 278t
    pineal, 459
    thoracic, 698, *698*
    vs. acoustic neuroma, 473
Meningitis, bacterial, 580–581
    coccidioidal infection and, 579
    cryptococcal, AIDS-related, 584, *588*
    of brain, imaging protocols in, 1132–1133
    phosphorus spectroscopy of, 276
    sarcoidosis and, 581–582, *582*
    syphilitic, 582
    tuberculous, 581
Meningocele, 420
    with tethered cord, 725–727
Meningoencephalocele, 420–422, *423*
Menisci, anatomy of, 990–991, *991*
    degeneration of, 991–993, *992, 993*
    tears of, 991–995, *992–995*
        fast imaging of, 207, *208, 209*
Meniscus homologue, 1068–1069, *1070*
Mesencephalon, hemorrhage of, 499, *500, 501*
    in Arnold-Chiari malformation, 425
Mesenteric vein, varices of, angiography of, *163*
Mesoderm, in Arnold-Chiari malformation, 426

Mesothelioma, pericardial, cineangiography of, *824*

Metabolism, disorders of, effect of, on brain, 592–595, *594, 595*

in skeletal muscle, in congestive heart failure, 766–767

myocardial, phosphorus spectroscopy of, 757–760, *757–760*

of carbohydrates, spectroscopy of, 273

of copper, Wilson's disease of, 593–595, 875

of fatty acids, spectroscopy of, 273

of iron, in cerebral hemorrhage, *256–258, 256–259*

Metachromatic leukodystrophy, 552

Metallic implants, and artifacts, 76–80, *77–80*

in knee imaging, *1000*, 1006–1007

cardiac, cineangiography of, 816t, 826, *826*

precautions for, 41t, 41–42, 70–72

Metallic shrapnel injury, precautions for, 42

Metalloporphyrins, in tumor localization, 233

Metastasis. See also *Carcinoma.*

in cancer staging, 1153–1156

of Ewing's sarcoma, to thorax, *739*

Metencephalon, 415

Methemoglobin, magnetism of, 485–487

water accessibility in, *258*

Microadenoma, pituitary, 460, 461, *461, 462*

gadolinium-DTPA imaging of, 243–244, *245*

Microcytic anemia, vs. myeloma, 1109, *1109*

Microglioma, 451

Microgyria, 439–440

Midbrain tegmentum, axial view of, *390*

sagittal view of, *405*

Middle cerebellar peduncle, coronal view of, *402*

sagittal view of, *406*

Middle cerebral artery, aneurysm of, *539*

angiography of, in carotid occlusion, *168*

axial view of, *390–393, 397*

infarction, *517*

sagittal view of, *407, 409*

Middle frontal gyrus, axial view of, *396, 398, 399*

coronal view of, *400*

Middle nasal turbinate, axial view of, *385*

coronal view of, *400*

sagittal view of, *406*

Middle scalene muscle, anatomy of, 656, *656, 657*

Middle temporal gyrus, axial view of, *389*

coronal view of, *401*

sagittal view of, *411*

Migraine, 524–525, *530*

vs. multiple sclerosis, 561

Migration, in brain development, 415, 415t

disorders of, 414t, 437–444, *440–443*

Minimum intensity projection, definition of, 1166

Mitral regurgitation, cineangiography of, 815, *816, 816t, 819*, 822–823, *823*

Modulator, in radiofrequency transmission, 370, *370*

mathematical principles of, 375, *375*

Mole, hydatidiform, 941, *941*

Molecules, effect of, on relaxation time, 12–16, *15, 16*, 16t

Monitoring, compatibility of, with magnetic resonance imaging, 40, 73

Monro's foramen, axial view of, *395*

coronal view of, *402*

Morton's neuroma, 1089–1090, *1090*

Motion artifacts, 98–104, *98–105*, 99t, 100t

gradient motion rephasing for, 332–334, *333, 334*

in abdominal imaging, 847–848, *848, 849*

respiratory gating for, 732

suppression technique for, 1162

Motion-interface etching, 107

Mucocele, of ethmoid sinus, 633, *635*

orbital, 613, 613t, *615*

Mucormycosis, of brain, 577

Mucous retention cyst, *400*

Mullerian ducts, 980–981

Multifrequency excitation, definition of, 1166

Multiple myeloma, spinal, 692, *693*

Multiple quantum filtering, in spectroscopy, 309

Multiple sclerosis, 549–552, *550, 551, 553*

as indication for brain imaging, 380

Multiple sclerosis *(Continued)*

differential diagnosis of, 560–561

imaging of, cross-over in, 30–31, *31*

gadolinium-DTPA in, 244, *245*

protocols for, 1132–1133, 1138–1139

in spinal cord, *678*, 678–679

Multislab three-dimensional acquisition, 59–60

Muscle(s). See also specific muscle(s), e.g., *Masseter muscle.*

atrophy of, after trauma, *1124–1126*, 1125

proton spectroscopy of, 279

signal intensity in, 15t, 16t

skeletal, metabolism in, in congestive heart failure, spectroscopy of, 766–767

Muscular dystrophy, spectroscopy of, 275, *276*

Musculoskeletal system, 987–1130. See also specific structures, e.g., *Knee.*

fetal, 947, *947*

imaging of, gadolinium-DTPA in, 250

phosphorus spectroscopy in, 274–275, *274–276*

technical aspects of, 1097–1098

trauma to, 1122–1125, *1122–1126*

tumors of, 1098–1104, *1099–1108*

Mustard operation, for transposition of great arteries, 835, *838, 839*

Myelination, accelerated, in Sturge-Weber syndrome, 434, *436*

in brain development, 415t, 415–420, *416–422*

disorders of, 414t, 444–446, *444–446*

loss of, imaging protocols in, 1132–1133, 1138–1139

in multiple sclerosis, 549–552, *550, 551, 553*

in spinal cord, *678*, 678–679

Myelinolysis, pontine, central, 592–593, *594*

Myelography, 138–146, *140–145*

fast imaging in, 200, *203, 204*

of brachial plexus, 653

Pantopaque residue after, 724, *725*

selection of, 50

Myelolipoma, adrenal, 891, *892*

Myeloma, multiple, *1109*, 1109–1110

spinal, 692, *693*

Myelopathy, cord compression and, 669

Myocardial infarction, *806*, 806–807, *807*

cineangiography of, 822, *822*

Myocardial ischemia, induction of, for operation, 760, *761*

phosphorus spectroscopy of, 755–758, *755–759*

Myocardium, hypertrophy of, cineangiography of, 824, *825*

metabolism in, phosphorus spectroscopy of, 757–760, *757–760*

Myolipoma, of kidney, 907, *907*

Myometrium, anatomy of, 922, *925*

in endometriosis, 932–933, *934*

Myopathy, hereditary, spectroscopy of, 274–275, *274–276*

Myositis, in diabetes, *1127*

Myositis ossificans, 1124, *1124*

Myxoma, atrial, with myocardial infarction, cineangiography of, *822*

cardiac, *803*

N-acetylaspartate, in proton spectroscopy, 279, 281, *281*

NADH-CoQ reductase, deficiency of, spectroscopy of, 275

Nasal cavity, 633–638, *634–638*

axial view of, *386, 387*

Nasal septum, *385, 387*

Nasal turbinate, inferior, coronal view of, *400*

sagittal view of, *406*

middle, axial view of, *385*

coronal view of, *400*

sagittal view of, *406*

superior, coronal view of, *400*

Nasolacrimal duct, *384, 386*

Nasolacrimal sac, dacryocystitis of, 614–620, *618*

Nasopharynx, 629–633, *630–632*

rhabdomyosarcoma of, *1105*

sagittal view of, *404*

Neck. See also *Spine, cervical.*

Neck *(Continued)*

imaging of, protocols for, 1136–1137

lesions of, 647–650, *647–650*

Necrosis, avascular, 1110–1111, *1110–1113*

imaging of, protocols for, 1150–1151

of lunate, 1066–1068, *1067, 1068*, 1111, *1113*

Necrotizing encephalomyelopathy, subacute, 593, *594*

Nembutal, before imaging, of brain malformations, 414

Nephritis, 901, 905, *905*

Nerve(s), cranial. See *Cranial nerve(s).*

median, compression of, in carpal tunnel, 1058–1060, *1058–1061*, 1117–1118

imaging protocols for, 1150–1151

in Kienböck's disease, 1067–1068, *1068*

myelination of. See *Myelination.*

Nerve roots, avulsion of, in brachial plexus injury, 659, *659*

edema of, in brachial plexus injury, 659, *660*

spinal, compression of, 671–672

cervicothoracic, disk degeneration and, *682*

disk degeneration and, lumbar, 712, *712, 714–716*

imaging of, fast, 200, *203, 204*

protocols for, 1138–1141

Nerve sheath, optic, lesions of, 609, 609t, *611*

tumors of, 470–474, *472, 473*

spinal, 696, *696–697, 697*

Nervous system, central, fetal, 947–948, *948, 949*

imaging of, 377–728

gadolinium-DTPA in, *238*, 243–244, *244, 245*

Net magnetization, 5, 1166

Neural tube, in brain development, 414

Neurilemmoma, spinal, 696–697

Neurinoma, in neurofibromatosis, 431–432, *433*

Neuritis, optic, 609, 609t

Neuroblastoma, paraspinal, 693–694, *694*

phosphorus spectroscopy of, 278, *279*

Neurofibroma, intracranial, 470

spinal, 696, *696–697, 697*

Neurofibromatosis, 431–432, *432–434, 1103*

of knee, *1006*

Neuroma, acoustic, 470–473, *472, 473, 625, 625*

in neurofibromatosis, 431, *433*

facial nerve, 473–474

Morton's, 1089–1090, *1090*

plantar, 1088–1089, *1089, 1090*

trigeminal, 473, *473*

Neurons, proliferation of, in brain development, 415

Nickel, magnetic moment of, 222t

Nitrogen, liquid, for superconductive magnets, 342

magnetic resonance characteristics of, 5t

Nitrogen-15, in spectroscopy, 286

Nocardia, in brain abscess, *576*

Nodulus cerebelli, axial view of, *388*

coronal view of, *403*

sagittal view of, *404*

Noise, external, and radiofrequency field artifacts, 82, *82–83*

ratio of contrast to, definition of, 1160

echo time and, 365, *365, 366*

ratio of signal to. See *Signal-to-noise ratio.*

sources of, 76t, 366–367

thermal, and artifact, 84

Nuclear magnetic relaxation dispersion, 261

Nuclear magnetic resonance. See *Magnetic resonance.*

Nuclear spin, definition of, 1166

Nucleus pulposus, in lumbar disk, 708, *709*

degeneration of, 710, 711, *711*

Nutation, definition of, 1166

Nyquist frequency, in aliasing, 94, *94*

in spectroscopy, 297

Nyquist limit, definition of, 1166

Oblique imaging, 331, *331*

Oblique muscles, of eyeball, coronal view of, *400*

sagittal view of, *409, 410*

Oblique muscles *(Continued)*
    superior, Brown's syndrome and, 612, *612,*
      612t
Oblique stripes, data loss and, 89–90, *90*
Obstetrics, 938–950, *939–943, 943–949*
Occipital horn, of lateral ventricle, *408, 409*
Occipital lobe, axial view of, *391–393, 395, 397*
    hemorrhage of, *486, 508*
    infarction of, *508, 518*
    sagittal view of, *406–408, 410*
Occipital protuberance, internal, *387*
Occipitotemporal gyrus, axial view of, *386*
    coronal view of, *401, 402*
Oculomotor nerve, *405*
Odontogenic cyst, 637, *637*
Off-center imaging, 331, *331*
Olfactory sulcus, axial view of, *390*
    coronal view of, *400*
Oligodendroglioma, cerebral, 449
Olive, axial view of, *384, 386*
Omohyoid muscle, anatomy of, 656, *657*
Omphalocele, 946, *947*
Ophthalmic artery, anatomy of, 599, *600, 601*
    axial view of, *388*
Ophthalmic vein, superior, coronal view of, *400*
    sagittal view of, *408*
Ophthalmitis, *Toxocara canis* infection and, 603,
    603t
Ophthalmopathy, endocrine, 610, *612,* 612t
Optic canal, axial view of, *389*
Optic chiasm, axial view of, *390*
    coronal view of, *401*
    glioma of, 463, *464*
      in neurofibromatosis, 431
    sagittal view of, *404, 405*
Optic nerve, anatomy of, 598–599, *599–601*
    axial view of, *388*
    coronal view of, *400*
    glioma of, in neurofibromatosis, 431
    inflammation of, 609, 609t
    lesions of, 609, 609t, *610, 611*
      imaging protocols for, 1136–1137
    sagittal view of, *409*
Optic tract, axial view of, *390, 391*
    coronal view of, *402*
    sagittal view of, *406*
Orbit, 598–620
    adenoid cystic carcinoma in, 612, *613*
    anatomy of, 598–599, *599–601*
    cavernous hemangioma in, 606t, 606–608, *607*
    cellulitis in, 613–614, *616*
    Coats' disease of, 603, 603t, *605*
    dacryocystitis in, 614–620, *618*
    dermoid cyst of, 612, 613t, *614*
    epidermoid tumor of, 612, 613t, *615*
    fat in, 599, *599*
      axial view of, *384, 385*
      coronal view of, *400*
      sagittal view of, *407*
    fracture of, *619,* 620
    hemorrhage in, 603, 603t, *605,* 605–606
    imaging of, protocols for, 1136–1137
      technical aspects of, 599–603
    lymphangioma in, *607,* 608
    lymphoma in, 606t, 608, *608,* 610–612, 612t
    melanoma in, 603t, 604, *606*
    mucocele in, 613, 613t, *615*
    muscle lesions in, 610–612, *612,* 612t
    nerve lesions in, 609, 609t, *610, 611*
    ocular lesions in, 603t, 603–606, *604–606*
    osteoma of, 613t, *619,* 620
    persistent hyperplastic primary vitreous in, 603,
      603t, *605*
    pseudotumor in, 608, *608,* 610
    retinoblastoma of, 603, 603t, *604*
    shrapnel injury in, precautions for, 42
    Tolosa-Hunt syndrome of, 613t, 614, *617*
    Toxocara canis infection in, 603, 603t
    vascular lesions of, 606–609, *607, 609*
Orbital gyri, axial view of, *390*
    sagittal view of, *409, 410*
Orbitals, and energy levels, 238, *239*
    in paramagnetism, 222
Orchiopexy, for testicular torsion, 966
    for undescended testes, 972

Orchitis, *963–965,* 964
Oropharynx, anatomy of, *639,* 640–645
    tumors of, *645, 646,* 647
Orthodontic appliances, and artifacts, 79, 80,
    1044–1055
    precautions for, 71
Orthopedic implants, precautions for, 71
Osteitis deformans, sacral, 722–724
Osteitis dissecans, of knee, 1003
Osteoarthritis, of knee, 1002–1003, *1003*
Osteoblastoma, vertebral, 691, *692*
Osteochondral defect, of knee, 1000, *1001*
Osteochondritis dissecans, 1111–1113
    of knee, 1003
Osteochondrosis, of ankle, 1083–1085, *1084*
Osteoid osteoma, *1107*
Osteoma, orbital, 613t, *619,* 620
    osteoid, *1107*
    talar, 1085–1086
Osteomyelitis, *1118–1120,* 1118–1122
    of foot and ankle, 1090–1094, *1092*
    of skull base, 629
    vertebral, 694–696, *695*
Osteonecrosis, of knee, 1003, *1003*
    of lunate, 1066–1068, *1067, 1068*
    of shoulder, 1027, *1027*
Osteophytes, in lumbar spondylosis, 717, *718*
    in spondylosis, 681–683, *685, 686*
    in temporomandibular disk degeneration, 1041,
      1049
    signal intensity in, 16t
Osteoporosis, transient, 1114
Osteosarcoma, *1099, 1102*
    of femur, *1099*
    of knee, *1007*
    of mandible, *646*
Otitis externa, 627, *629*
Ovary, anatomy of, 923, *924*
    carcinoma of, 930–932, *930–933*
      recurrent, 934, *935*
      staging of, 1156
    cysts of, 928, *928, 929*
    in pregnancy, 942, *942*
Oversampling, definition of, 1166
    to eliminate wraparound, 55
Oxygen, in brain, fluorine spectroscopy of, 286,
    286
    loss of, in cerebral hemorrhage, 257, *257, 258,*
      261t
    magnetic resonance characteristics of, 5t
Oxygen-17, in spectroscopy, 286
Oxygenation, in brain hemorrhage, 489–491, *492*
Oxyhemoglobin, in brain hemorrhage, 261, 261t

Pacemaker, as contraindication to imaging, 41,
    354
Pachygyria, 439, *440*
Paget's disease, sacral, 722–724
Palate, adenoid cystic carcinoma of, 635, *636*
    hard, *404*
    soft, *406*
Pancoast tumor, of brachial plexus, 660, *663*
Pancreas, *882,* 883–888, *885–889*
    carcinoma of, 886, *886–888*
      staging of, 1154
    imaging of, bowel motion in, *851, 852*
      protocols for, 1144–1145
    signal intensity in, 15t, 16t
Pancreatitis, 886–888, *888, 889*
Pantopaque, in lumbar spine, 724, *725*
Papillary muscles, imaging planes through, *774,*
    776, 777
Papilloma, of choroid plexus, 475
Parabolic flow, 1168
Paracentral lobule, *404, 405*
Paraganglioma, *479,* 479–480, 626, *627*
    of parapharyngeal space, 633
Parahippocampal gyrus, *401, 402*
Paramagnetism, *239,* 239–240, 240t
    and nuclear relaxation, 222, 222t, 224
    and static field artifacts, 77
    and T_1 relaxation time, 241

Paramagnetism *(Continued)*
    definition of, 1166
    effect of, on imaging, 32
      fast gradient-echo, 197
    in biologic tissue, 265
    in contrast agents, effect of, on bowel signal,
      849
    in hemorrhage, *485,* 485–487
      and exclusion of water, 257, *258*
      hemoglobin breakdown products and, 133,
        135
Paramesonephric ducts, 980–981
Paranasal sinuses, 633–638, *634–638*
Parapharyngeal space, *630,* 630–633, *633*
Parasitic abscess, of brain, 577–580, *580, 581*
    AIDS-related, 584, *586–588*
Parasitic endophthalmitis, 603, 603t
Parathyroid gland, adenoma of, 647–649, *648*
    imaging of, protocols for, 1136–1137
Parietal bone, sagittal view of, *406, 408*
Parietal lobe, hemorrhage of, *486, 502*
Parietal lobule, superior, *408*
Parietal visual radiations, in sagittal imaging, *410*
Parietooccipital fissure, *405*
Parietooccipital sulcus, *394, 397*
Parkinsonism, *591,* 591–592
Parotid gland, anatomy of, 638, *639*
    coronal view of, *401*
    tumors of, *632, 633,* 638, *640–642*
Partial volume averaging, 87–89, *88, 89*
Partition, definition of, 1166
Pascal's triangle, in peak intensity prediction, in
    spectroscopy, 302, *302*
Patella, chondromalacia of, 999, *999*
    dislocation of, 999
    subluxation of, 999
Patellar bursa, 1000
Patellar tendon, lesions of, 999–1000, *1000*
Patellofemoral joint, 998–1000, *999, 1000*
Patient, preparation of, for imaging, 40, 40–42,
    68–73
Pectoralis minor muscle, anatomy of, 656
Pelvis, abscess of, *1120*
    female, 916, 916t, 922–936, *924–936*
      anatomy of, 922–923, *924, 925*
      in pregnancy, 938–944, *939–943*
      blood supply of, in pregnancy, 943
      developmental abnormalities of, 980–986,
        982–985
      imaging of, protocols for, 1146–1147
      measurement of, in pregnancy, 943–944
    imaging of, gadolinium-DTPA in, 250
      technical aspects of, 915–916, 916t
    male, 916t, 916–922, *917–922*
      anatomy of, 916, *917*
      imaging of, protocols for, 1146–1147
Penile implants, precautions for, 41, 71
Pentobarbital, before imaging, of brain malforma-
    tions, 413–414
Perfluorooctylbromide, in contrast imaging, of
    bowel, 849–852, *852*
    in pancreatic imaging, 884, *885*
Perfusion, brain, *179*
    cardiac, 749–752, *750, 751*
    definition of, 1167
Periaqueductal gray matter, *393*
Pericallosal artery, axial view of, *392, 394, 395*
    coronal view of, *401*
Pericardium, 797–800, *799–801*
    cineangiography of, 816t, *824*
    cyst of, 801, *802*
    imaging of, protocols for, 1142–1143
    inflammation of, 799–800, *800, 801*
    motion of, and artifact, 122
Perinephric space, 900, 900–901, *901*
Peripheral blood vessels, angiography of, *157,*
    157–160
Peristalsis, effect of, on imaging, 848–852, *850–*
    852
    suppression of, glucagon for, 158
Permanent magnets, definition of, 1167
    in imaging systems, 35, *35*
    site planning for, 343
Peroneal tendons, inflammation of, 1082–1083

Persistent hyperplastic primary vitreous, 603, 603t, *605*
Petrooccipital fissure, *386*
Petrous bone, *409*
Pharyngobasilar fascia, *384, 385*
Pharynx. See also *Nasopharynx.*
  anatomy of, *639,* 640–645
  cyst of, 649, *649*
Phase, definition of, 1167
  in T₂ relaxation, 9, *10*
Phase dispersion, definition of, 9, *10*
  to reduce flow artifacts, *121,* 121–122
Phase dispersion artifact, 107
Phase effects, of blood flow, 116–119, *117, 118*
  of water diffusion, 177–179, *179*
Phase encoding, definition of, 1167
  in two-dimensional imaging, 20–21, *21, 22,* 315–316, *316*
    reordering of, for respiratory movement, 55
    to reduce ghost artifacts, *98,* 99, 100t, 101, *101*
Phase imaging, definition of, 1167
  in thrombosis, 136, *136*
Phase mapping, in flow measurement, *175,* 175–176
Phase reordering, in abdominal imaging, 848
Phase-contrast image, definition of, 1167
Phase-frequency swap, definition of, 1167
Phase-sensitive reconstruction, 27, *27–28*
Phase shift, in flow measurement, 173–177, *175–177*
Pheochromocytoma, 892, *894*
Phosphocreatine, in spectroscopy, 272–278, *273–276*
  as reference, 300, 301, *301*
  ratio of, to adenosine triphosphate, 764–766, *765*
Phosphofructokinase, deficiency of, spectroscopy of, 274–275
Phosphorus, in spectroscopy, 272–278, *273–276, 278, 279.* See also *Spectroscopy.*
  magnetic resonance characteristics of, 5t
Photography, of magnetic resonance images, 62–63, *63–65*
Phthisis bulbi, 603, 603t
Physiologic gating, 814
Pia mater, siderosis of, 540, *541*
Pick's disease, 593
Pigmented villonodular synovitis, 1117
  of knee, 1002, *1002*
  of shoulder, 1026–1027
Pineal body, coronal view of, *403*
Pineal tumors, 458–460, *459, 460*
Pineocytoma, 458
Pituitary gland, adenoma of, 460–463, *461–463*
  and hemorrhage, 511, *511*
  as indication for brain imaging, 380
  gadolinium-DTPA imaging of, 243–244, *245, 461, 462,* 463
  axial view of, *388, 389*
  coronal view of, *401*
  imaging of, protocols for, 1134–1135
  microadenoma of, 460, 461, *461, 462*
    gadolinium-DTPA imaging of, 243–244, *245*
  sagittal view of, *404*
Pixel, definition of, 1167
  size of, and spatial resolution, 28–29
Placenta, *940,* 940–942, *941*
Placenta previa, 940, *941*
Plantar neuroma, 1088–1089, *1089, 1090*
Plasma, lipids in, malignancy and, proton spectroscopy of, 282, *282*
Plasmacytoma, 478, *479*
  spinal, 692
Pleomorphic adenoma, of parapharyngeal space, *632,* 633
  of parotid gland, 638, *640*
Plicae, synovial, of knee, 1004
Plug flow, 1168
Plug profile, of blood flow, 112–114, *113*
Polycystic disease, of kidney, 904, *904*
  of ovaries, 928, *928*
Polycythemia vera, marrow changes in, spinal, 693

Polyhydramnios, *945,* 948, *948, 949*
Polymicrogyria, 439–440
Polyp, antrochoanal, *636,* 637
Pons, axial view of, *387*
  hemorrhage of, *486,* 499, *499*
  in brain development, *417, 418*
  infarction of, *518*
  metastatic tumor of, *455*
  sagittal view of, *405, 406*
Pontine cistern, *387, 389*
Pontine myelinolysis, central, 592–593, *594*
Pontine tegmentum, axial view of, *388, 389*
Popliteal cyst, 1004, *1005*
Popliteal tendon, anatomy of, 991, *991*
  sheath of, vs. meniscal tear, 995
Porencephalic cyst, vs. arachnoid cyst, 466–468
Porphyrins, in tumor localization, 233
Porta hepatis, gallbladder cancer in, 883–884, *884, 885*
Portal vein, anatomy of, 859
  angiography of, *158,* 160, *160, 161, 163*
  disease of, 877–878, *880, 881*
  imaging of, even-echo rephasing in, *853*
Positioning, for magnetic resonance imaging, 41
Postcentral gyrus, axial view of, *394, 396–399*
  coronal view of, *402*
  sagittal view of, *408, 411*
Posterior cerebral artery, axial view of, *391*
  sagittal view of, *408*
Posterior communicating artery, *390*
Posterior cruciate ligament, of knee, 996–998, *997*
Posterior fossa, anatomy of, 623–625, *624*
  cystic malformation of, 428–429, *428–430*
  hemorrhage of, 499, *501*
  lesions of, 623–629, *625–629*
    as indication for brain imaging, 380
Posterior inferior cerebellar artery, axial view of, *384–387*
  infarction of, *509*
Posterior longitudinal ligament, *405*
Posterior scleritis, 603, 603t
Posterosuperior fissure, *403*
Potassium, in spectroscopy, 286
  in cardiac imaging, 763–764
  magnetic resonance characteristics of, 5t
Potassium chloride, cardiac arrest induced with, for operation, 760
Potts shunt, for pulmonic valve stenosis, *793*
Praseodymium, in contrast agents, T₂, *234,* 235
  magnetic moment of, 222t
Precentral cerebellar vein, *404*
Precentral gyrus, axial view of, *394, 396–399*
  coronal view of, *402*
  sagittal view of, *408, 411*
Precentral lobule, *404*
Precession, definition of, 1167
  steady-state free, definition of, 1170
Precuneus, *405*
Pregnancy, diethylstilbestrol use in, as teratogen, 981
  ectopic, 942, *943*
  imaging in, fetal, 944–950, *945–949*
    protocols for, 1146–1147
  maternal, 938–944, *939–943*
  safety of, 42
Preinversion, in subtraction angiography, 153
Preparation scans, 61, *61*
Prepatellar bursitis, 1000
Prepontine cistern, *406*
Presaturation, 54–55, 119–121, *120*
  definition of, 1167
  for abdominal angiography, *158,* 160, *160, 161, 163*
  for aliasing, *95, 96*
  in flow measurement, 173, *173, 174*
  in subtraction angiography, 153, *153*
  in thrombosis, 135
  to reduce ghost artifacts, *96,* 103–104, *104*
Progressive multifocal leukoencephalopathy, 552, *554*
  AIDS-related, 584–586, *589*
Progressive supranuclear palsy, *591,* 591–592
Projection acquisition, definition of, 1167

Projection acquisition *(Continued)*
  in angiography, 152–155, *152–155*
Projection reconstruction, 335–336
Prolactinoma, 460
Proplast, in temporomandibular prostheses, 1044, *1053, 1054*
Proptosis, imaging protocols for, 1136–1137
Prosencephalon, 415
  developmental disorders of, *426,* 426–427, *427*
Prostate, anatomy of, 916, *917*
  benign hypertrophy of, 916–918, *918*
  carcinoma of, *918,* 918–920, *919*
    and lymphadenopathy, *911*
    and lymphocele, *910*
    carbon-13 spectroscopy of, 283
    metastasis from, *689,* 919, *1104*
    staging of, 1155
  imaging of, protocols for, 1146–1147
  technical aspects of, 916, 916t
Prostheses, of temporomandibular joint, 1044, *1052–1054*
Proteinaceous fluid, vs. brain hemorrhage, 493
Proton density, 17, *17*
  definition of, 1167
  field strength and, 15t
Proton density–weighted images, contrast in, 29
Proton spectroscopy, 278–282, *280–282*
  in cardiac imaging, 762–763, *764*
Protons, alignment of, with magnetic fields, 6, *6*
Pseudoaneurysm, 132, *132*
Pseudogating, in flow compensation, 122–124, *124*
Pseudomeningocele, in brachial plexus injury, *659, 660*
Pseudotumor, hemophilic, 1101, *1105*
  orbital, 608, *608,* 610
PSIF imaging, 49, 50, 195, *196,* 1159
Psoriatic arthritis, of temporomandibular joint, 1041, *1051*
  spinal, 701, *701*
Pterygoid muscle, lateral, axial view of, *384*
  coronal view of, *401*
  physiology of, 1034–1037, *1035, 1037*
  sagittal view of, *410, 411*
  medial, coronal view of, *401*
  sagittal view of, *410*
Pterygoid plate, lateral, *408*
Pterygomaxillary fissure, *408*
Pulmonary arteries, anatomy of, 732, *733*
  angiography of, *159*
  atresia of, in hypoplastic right heart syndrome, 833–834, *835–838*
    Rastelli shunt for, *793*
  banding of, cineangiography of, 840–841, *841, 842*
  hemodynamics in, 111t
  imaging of, cardiac gating in, 56
  in congenital transposition disorders, 788–792, *794*
    cineangiography of, 835–836, *838, 839*
  in tetralogy of Fallot, 832, *833*
Pulmonary embolism, 743, *743*
  cineangiography of, 816t, 823–824, *825*
Pulmonary hilum, 740–743, *742*
Pulmonary hypertension, 792
Pulmonary veins, hemodynamics in, 111t
  in atrial septal defect, 788, *790, 791*
  in transposition of great arteries, 835–836, *838, 839*
Pulmonic valve, stenosis of, Potts shunt for, *793*
Pulsation artifact, in brain imaging, *389*
Pulse amplitude, calibration of, subject-dependent, 372–373, *373*
Pulse Fourier imaging, definition of, 1168
Pulse programmer, definition of, 1168
Pulse sequences, 23–28, 24t, *24–28.* See also specific types, e.g., *Spin-echo sequences.*
  and artifacts, 105–107, *107*
  Carr-Purcell, 1159
    rotational axis in, 321
  definitions of, 1168
  design of, 313–339
    calibration in, 335
    data acquisition in, *324,* 324–325
    data read-out in, 325t, 325–330, *325–330*

Pulse sequences *(Continued)*
 fat-water separation in, *336,* 336–337
 gradients in, 317, *317,* 322–324, *323.* See also
  Gradient.
 half-Fourier reconstruction in, 336
 inversion recovery in, *334,* 334–335
 off-center imaging in, 331, *331*
 projection reconstruction in, 335–336
 radiofrequency pulses in, 318–322, *319, 320,*
  322. See also *Radiofrequency pulses.*
 saturation pulses in, *331,* 331–332, *332*
 three-dimensional Fourier transform in, 317
 to reduce artifacts, 85–86, *87*
 two-dimensional Fourier transform in, 314t,
  314–316, *314–316*
 diffusion-sensitive, 177–179, *179*
 editing of, 337–339, *339*
 fast scan, in cineangiography, of heart, 812
 in imaging, of adrenal glands, 889–890, *890,*
  891
  of liver, 854–858, *855–859*
  of orbit, 600–601
  of scrotum, 953
  of spine, cervicothoracic, 669
   lumbar, 706, *706–709*
  of temporomandibular joint, 1032–1033
  of thrombosis, 136–137, *137*
 low bandwidth, 57–58
 proton density–weighted, definition of, 1167
 selection of, 49–50
Pulvinar, of thalamus, *407*
Putamen, axial view of, *393, 395*
 hemorrhage of, 497
  gradient-echo imaging of, *490*
 infarction of, *519*
  and white matter ischemia, *549*
 iron deposition in, 591, *591*
Pyelocalyceal system, hydronephrosis in, *900,* 901
Pyelonephritis, 905, *905*
Pyramid, medullary, axial view of, *384, 386*
 coronal view of, *402*
 sagittal view of, *404*

Quadrature, in flow measurement, 175, *175*
Quadrature coils, 37, 368
 definition, 1160
 positioning of, *45,* 45–46
Quadrature demodulator, 371
 mathematical principles of, *375,* 375–376
Quadrature detector, definition of, 1168
Quadrigeminal cistern, axial view of, *390, 392*
 sagittal view of, *404*
Quadrupolar nuclei, in spectroscopy, 306–307
Quality, definition of, 1168
 of radiofrequency coils, 37
 receiver coil tuning for, 46, *47*
Quality control, in imaging, 63–66, *65*
Quantum filtering, in spectroscopy, 309
Quenches, definition of, 1168
 in superconductive magnets, 358
 site planning for, 343–344
Quervain's syndrome, 1060, *1061*

Radial collateral ligament, anatomy of, *1062,*
 1062–1063
Radiation injury, of bone marrow, 1104
 spinal, 693
 of brachial plexus, 660–661, *664*
 of brain, 554–555, *555, 556*
 optic, 609, 609t
Radiculopathy, cervical, 671–672
 disk degeneration and, cervicothoracic, *682*
  lumbar, 712, *712, 714–716*
 imaging of, fast, 200, *203, 204*
 protocols for, 1138–1141
Radiofrequency, adjustment of, subject-dependent, 372
 in signal, Fourier transform for, 21, *22, 23*
 of transmitted pulse, adjustment of, to nuclear
  Larmor frequency, 46–47
 refocusing of, 325

Radiofrequency coils, *36,* 36–37, 366–369, *366–*
 369
 definition of, 1168
 in orbital imaging, 600
 shielding from, 83
Radiofrequency encoding, definition of, 1163
 in two-dimensional imaging, 20, 316, *316*
Radiofrequency field artifacts, 82–86, *82–87*
Radiofrequency interference, in site planning,
 344–349, *346–349*
Radiofrequency power, transmitter adjustment
 for, 47
Radiofrequency pulses. See also *Pulse sequences.*
 crafted, 320, *320*
 definition of, 1168–1169
 in imaging, 7–8, *7–9*
  two-dimensional, 314–315, *315*
 instrumentation for, 318
 nonselective, 83–84, 318
 penetration of, 362
 power of, deposition of, 362
 selective, 83–84, 318–319, *319, 321*
  for fat-water imaging, in spectroscopy, 293
 sinc, 50–51, *51,* 319
 spoiler, 330, 1170
  in FLASH imaging, 190, *190*
   contrast in, 192, *193–195*
 synthesis of, 320
Radiofrequency system, instrumentation for, *366–*
 370, 366–372
Radiolunotriquetral ligament, anatomy of, 1063,
 1063
Radioscaphocapitate ligament, anatomy of, 1062,
 1062, 1063
Radioscapholunate ligament, anatomy of, 1062,
 1062, 1063
Radioulnar joint, anatomy of, 1068–1071, *1069–*
 1071
Radioulnar ligament, volar, tears of, 1070–1071,
 1071
Radius, fracture of, *1122*
 length of, vs. ulnar length, 1064, *1065,* 1071–
  1073, *1072, 1074*
Ramp time, definition of, 1169
Ramping, of superconductive magnets, 357–358,
 358
Ranula, 640, *643*
Rapid acquisition with relaxation enhancement
 (RARE) sequence, 217, 1168
Rastelli shunt, for pulmonary atresia, *793*
Receiver, adjustment of, 47–48, *48*
 subject-dependent, 373
Receiver coil, *36,* 36–37
 centering of, with magnet, 46, *46*
 design restrictions in, 44–45
 positioning of, *45,* 45–46
 selection of, *43,* 43–44, *44*
 tuning of, 46, *47*
Receiver gain adjustment, and artifact, 89, *90*
Receiver low pass filter adjustment, 89
Reconstruction time, 62
Rectum, carcinoma of, 922, *922*
 imaging of, technical aspects of, 915, 916t
Rectus muscle, inferior, axial view of, *386*
 coronal view of, *400*
 sagittal view of, *408, 409*
 lateral, axial view of, *388*
 sagittal view of, *411*
 medial, axial view of, *386, 388*
 coronal view of, *400*
 superior, axial view of, *390*
 coronal view of, *400*
 sagittal view of, *409, 410*
Red blood cells, lysis of, in cerebral hemorrhage,
 257–258, 261t, 262–263
Red nucleus, axial view of, *390, 393*
 coronal view of, *402*
 iron deposition in, 590, *590*
Reflex sympathetic dystrophy, of foot, 1094, *1096*
Relaxation dispersion, nuclear magnetic, 261
Relaxation rate, definition of, 1169
Relaxation time, field strength and, 15, 15t, 16
 in tissue imaging, 222–223
 measurement of, in spectroscopy, 303

Relaxation time *(Continued)*
 molecular effect on, 12–16, *15, 16,* 16t
 of whole blood, 110–111
 T_1, 11–12, *13, 14,* 241, 1171
  and signal-to-noise ratio, 362, *362*
  correlation of, with T_2, 16–17, *17*
  field strength and, 15t, 16
 T_2, 9–11, *10–12,* 241, 1171
  correlation of, with T_1, 16–17, *17*
  field strength and, 15t
 T_2^*, 10–11, *11*
Relaxivity, in biologic tissue, 266–267
 in cerebral hemorrhage, 259, 266–267
 of contrast agents, 223
 T_1, 224–227, *224–228,* 225t
Renal. See also *Kidney.*
Renal arteries, angiography of, 160–162, *163–165*
 hemodynamics in, 111t
Renal cell carcinoma, 905–906, *906,* 908
 metastasis of, to lung, 743, *743*
 staging of, 1153
 thrombosis in, 901, *902*
Renal cysts, 903–904, *904,* 907–908
 fetal, 946, *946*
Renal hilum, 901, *902*
Renal parenchyma, diffuse disease of, 901–902
Renal transplantation, 902–903, *903*
Renal tubules, acute necrosis of, 902–903
Repetition time, definition of, 1169
 effect of, on longitudinal magnetization, 12, *14*
 in fast imaging, 183–184
  gradient-echo, 189
 in pulse sequence design, 314t
 variation of, to reduce ghost artifacts, 101
Rephasing, even-echo, *124,* 124–125, *125*
 definition of, 1161
  for myelographic artifacts, *141,* 143–144
  in portal vein imaging, *853*
 gradient motion, 125–127, *125–127,* 317, 1162
  to reduce artifacts, 332–334, *333, 334*
 of slice magnetization, 321
Reproductive system. See *Pelvis* and specific
 structures, e.g., *Ovary.*
Resistive magnets, definition of, 1169
 site planning for, 342–343
Resolution, spatial. See *Spatial resolution.*
Resonance frequency, 4, 7, *7*
 in spectroscopy, 294
Resonator coil, 1169
Respiration, and bowel motion, effect of, on imaging, 848–852, *850–852*
 mechanical, during imaging, 73
 monitoring of, during imaging, 40, 73
 movement in, compensation for, 54–55. See
  also *Presaturation.*
 suspension of, during imaging, 62
Respiratory gating, definition of, 1163
 for motion artifacts, 732
 in abdominal imaging, 848
Retention cyst, mucous, coronal view of, *400*
Reticulum cell sarcoma, 451
Retinacula, of knee, 999, *1000*
Retinoblastoma, 603, 603t, *604*
 imaging of, surface receiver coil in, *44*
Retroperitoneum, 908–911, *909–911*
Reynolds number, 111t, 114
Rhabdomyosarcoma, nasopharyngeal, *1105*
 orbital, 610–612, 612t
Rheumatoid arthritis, *1116,* 1116–1117
 juvenile, synovial hypertrophy in, of ankle,
  1084
 of knee, 1001, *1001*
 of shoulder, 1023–1026, *1026*
 of temporomandibular joint, 1041
Rhombencephalon, 415
 in Arnold-Chiari malformation, 424–425
Rib, cervical, and thoracic outlet syndrome, 661,
 665
Ringing artifacts, *91,* 91–92, 1159
ROPE method, to reduce ghost artifacts, 101,
 101, 1169
Rosenthal's basal vein, axial view of, *392–395*
Rotating frame, definition of, 1169
 in zeugmatography, 290–291, *291*
Rotator cuff, anatomy of, 1013–1015

Rotator cuff (Continued)
    imaging of, protocols for, 1148–1149
    injury to, 1015–1020, 1016–1020

Sacroiliac joint, osteomyelitis of, 1119
Saddle coil, 1169
Sagittal sinus, superior, axial view of, 394–399
    coronal view of, 401
    occlusion of, 523, 527, 528
    sagittal view of, 404
    thrombosis of, angiography of, 171
Salivary glands, anatomy of, 638, 639
    inflammation of, 640, 643
    tumors of, 632, 633, 638, 640–642
Sampling, asymmetric, 325t, 329–330, 330, 1159
Sampling interval, definition of, 1169
Sampling time, definition of, 1169
Sarcoidosis, and meningitis, 581–582, 582
Sarcoma, Ewing's, 1103
    metastasis of, to thorax, 739
    giant cell tumor in, 1102
    lipomatous, 1100, 1100–1101, 1101
    of ankle, 1085, 1086, 1087, 1088, 1089
    of cartilage, of skull base, 478–479
        of thigh, 1106
    of femur, 1099
    of foot, 1085, 1086
    of knee, 1007
    of mandible, 646
    of nasopharynx, 1105
    of orbit, 610–612, 612t
    of uterus, 926
    osteogenic, 1099, 1102
    reticulum cell, 451
    synovial cell, 1107
Saturation. See also Presaturation.
    definition of, 1169–1170
    in flow measurement, 172–173, 172–174
Saturation effects, of blood flow, 115, 115–116, 116
Saturation pulses, artifacts reduced by, 331, 331–332, 332
    in brain imaging, 382
Saturation transfer, in spectroscopy, 304, 304
Scalar coupling, in spectroscopy, 270
Scalene muscles, anatomy of, 655–656, 656, 657
Scalp, sagittal view of, 406
Scapholunate dissociation, 1064–1066, 1067
Scapholunate ligament, anatomy of, 1062, 1063–1064, 1064
Scarring, epidural, after lumbar spinal operation, 720, 721, 722
Schizencephaly, 440, 441
Schwannoma, intracranial, 470, 625–627, 627, 628
    of brachial plexus, 661, 664
    of foot, 1090, 1091
    of parapharyngeal space, 632, 633
    spinal, 696–697
        drop metastasis of, 699, 699
Scleritis, posterior, 603, 603t
Scrotum, 952–979
    anatomy of, 954–956, 954–956
    imaging of, protocols for, 1148–1149
        technical aspects of, 952–954
    trauma to, 964–965, 965, 966
    tumors of, 957, 957–961, 959–961
Sedation, before imaging, fetal, 944
    of congenital heart disease, 832
    for claustrophobia, 40
        in temporomandibular joint dysfunction, 1056
Seizures, as indication for brain imaging, 380
    imaging protocols for, 1134–1135
Selective excitation, definition of, 1170
Sella turcica, imaging of, protocols for, 1134–1135
    lesions of, as indication for brain imaging, 380
    sagittal view of, 404
    tumors of, 460–465, 461–466
Semilunar lobules, of cerebellum, 403
Seminal vesicles, anatomy of, 916, 917
    imaging of, technical aspects of, 916, 916t
    in prostatic cancer, 919

Seminoma, 922, 922, 958, 959
Senning operation, for transposition of great arteries, 794
Sepsis, of temporomandibular joint, 1041
Septal vein, 394
Septooptic dysplasia, 428, 428
Septum, atrial, congenital defect of, 787–788, 790, 791
        lipomatous hypertrophy of, 803, 805
    nasal, 385, 387
    of sphenoid sinus, axial view of, 386
    ventricular, defect of, 788, 792
        in tetralogy of Fallot, 832, 833
        pulmonary banding for, cineangiography of, 840–841, 841, 842
Septum pellucidum, axial view of, 394, 396
    coronal view of, 401
Sequence calibration, 335
Serratus anterior muscle, anatomy of, 656, 657
Sertoli cell tumors, 960
Shear artifact, 107
Shear injury, of brain, 570–574, 574, 575
    of caudate nucleus, 566
Shielding, definition of, 1165
    for fringe fields, 352, 359–360, 360
    from radiofrequency coil, 83
    of radiofrequency room, 345–349, 346–349, 372
    to reduce eddy currents, 364, 1161
Shimming, definition of, 1170
    in spectroscopy, 271, 272, 294–295
    of magnetic fields, 35, 360, 360–361, 361
        mathematical principles of, 374
Short tau, inversion recovery sequence, 28, 28
    definition of, 1164
    in orbital imaging, 601
    to reduce ghost artifacts, 102
Shoulder, 1010–1029. See also Glenohumeral joint.
Shrapnel injury, precautions for, 42
Shunts, and artifact, 78
    cardiac, cineangiography of, 841
    cerebral ventricular, precautions for, 72
    systemic-pulmonary, 788, 792, 793
Sickle cell anemia, 1113
Sickle cell nephropathy, 901
Siderosis, pial, 540, 541
Sigmoid sinus, 410
Signal, Fourier transform of, for frequency content, 21, 22, 23
    intensity of, 15t, 15–17, 16t
        flow and, 34
        in tumors, 237
    localization of, 17–23, 18–23
    loss of, with T_2 relaxation, 9–11, 10, 11
Signal averaging, 21–22
    definition of, 1170
    in abdominal imaging, 848
    to reduce ghost artifacts, 99t, 101–102, 102
Signal-to-noise ratio, 31–32
    bandwidth and, 327, 327–328, 328
    definition of, 1170
    effect of scan parameters on, 54t
    field strength and, 35, 36
    in echo-planar imaging, 217
    in optimal imaging, 42
    in spectroscopy, 294–295
    T_1 relaxation time and, 362, 362
    with asymmetric field of view, in fast imaging, 188
    with reduced matrix size, in fast imaging, 186
    with single excitation, 185, 185
Simon-Nitinol filter, imaging of, 137, 137
Sinc pulses, 50–51, 51, 319
    definition of, 1169
Single-shot imaging, 214–215, 216
Sinus venosus, in atrial septal defect, 791
Sinuses. See also specific sinuses, e.g., Ethmoid sinus.
    confluence of, axial view of, 391, 397
    imaging of, protocols for, 1136–1137
Sinusitis, paranasal, 633, 634
Site planning, 341t, 341–354, 346–350
    for magnets, 341–343
    for quenches, 343–344

Site planning (Continued)
    fringe fields in, 349–353, 350
    radiofrequency interference in, 344–349, 346–349
    safety issues in, 353–354
Sjögren's syndrome, salivary glands in, 640, 643
Skin, blood flow in, monitoring of, during imaging, 40, 73
Skin effect, definition of, 1170
Skull, base of, tumors of, 477–480, 479
    fracture of, 563, 569
Slice(s), gap between, 1170
    in abdominal imaging, 846, 846
    selection of, 50–51, 51–53
        magnetization of, rephasing of, 321
        offset frequency for, 321–322, 322
        profile of, and tissue contrast, in fast gradient-echo imaging, 192
        selection of, in two-dimensional imaging, 18–20, 19, 20, 314t
        thickness of, in gradient-echo three-dimensional imaging, 58, 58–59, 59
            in pulse sequence design, 314t
            selection of, 50, 54t
Slit hemorrhage, 504
Snowstorm artifacts, 65, 65
Sodium, in contrast agents, toxicity of, 228t
    in spectroscopy, 283–285, 283–285
        in cardiac imaging, 763–764
    magnetic resonance characteristics of, 5t
Soft palate, 406
Solenoidal coils, definition of, 1170
    positioning of, 45, 45
Soleus, hematoma of, traumatic, 1123
Solomon-Bloembergen equations, 1170
Solvent suppression, definition of, 1170
    for resolving hydrogen spectra, 307–309, 308
Sonography, in pregnancy, 938, 939
    of carotid artery, 162–163
    of liver, 853
Spatial localization, of signal, 17–23, 18–23
Spatial resolution, adjustment of, for partial volume averaging, 87–89
    determinants of, 28–29
    effect of scan parameters on, 54t
    in abdominal imaging, 846, 846–847, 847, 849
    in optimal imaging, 43
    in spectroscopy, 288–289
Specific absorption rate, 48–49
Spectral leakage artifacts, 91, 91–92
Spectrometer, definition of, 1170
Spectroscopy, 269–309
    carbon-13, 282–283
        in cardiac imaging, 761–762, 762, 763
    chemical exchange in, 302, 302–303
    chemical shift in, 270, 271, 300–301, 301
        localized, 289, 289–290, 290
    correlation, 305, 306
    data acquisition in, 297
    data postprocessing in, 297–298
    definition of, 270, 1166
    diffusion in, 304–305
    fat-water separation in, 278, 280, 292–293, 293
    fluorine, 285, 285–286, 286
    Fourier transform in, 299–300, 300
        two-dimensional, 305, 305–306, 306
    hydrogen, in cardiac imaging, 766, 767
    image selected in vivo, 288, 288
        in cardiac imaging, 766, 766
    instruments for, 294–296, 295
    J-coupling in, 270, 301, 301–302
    lithium, 286
    localized, 286–292, 287–292
    magnetic resonance effect in, 298–299, 299
    magnetization transfer in, 271–272, 303–304, 304
    nitrogen-15 in, 286
    oxygen-17 in, 286
    patient preparation for, 296–297
    phosphorus, 272–278, 273–276, 278, 279
        in cardiac imaging, 277, 754–761, 755–761, 764–767, 765–767
        of brain, 275–277, 276
        of musculoskeletal system, 274–275, 274–276

Spectroscopy (Continued)
  of skeletal muscle metabolism, in congestive heart failure, 766–767
  of tumors, 277–278, 278, 278t, 279
  potassium, 286
  in cardiac imaging, 763–764
  proton, 278–282, 280–282
  in cardiac imaging, 762–763, 764
  quadrupolar nuclei in, 306–307
  relaxation time in, 303
  sodium, 283–285, 283–285
  in cardiac imaging, 763–764
  solvent suppression in, 307–309, 308
  spatially resolved, 288–289
  temperature measurement in, 305
Spectrum, definition of, 1170
Spermatic cord, anatomy of, 954, 956
  hypervascularity of, in epididymitis, 961, 963, 963–964
  in cryptorchidism, 974–977, 975–977
  seminoma involving, 958, 959
  torsion of, 965–970, 967–970
Spermatocele, 971, 971
Sphenoid bone, sagittal view of, 410, 411
Sphenoid sinus, axial view of, 387
  coronal view of, 401
  sagittal view of, 405, 406
  septum of, axial view of, 386
Spin, in spectroscopy, 270, 271
  nuclear, definition of, 1166
Spin echo, definition of, 1161
Spin warp, 18, 214
Spin-echo imaging, contrast in, 29–31, 30, 31
  magnetization in, vs. fast gradient-echo imaging, 189, 189
  vs. fast imaging, 183–185
Spin-echo sequences, 24t, 24–25, 24–26
  asymmetric, in cerebral hemorrhage, 260, 260
  definition of, 1168
  for fat-water imaging, in spectroscopy, 292–293
  in cerebral hemorrhage, 259–260, 260
  in two-dimensional imaging, 314t, 314–316, 314–316
  selection of, 49
  sensitivity of, to T_2 relaxation, 11, 12
Spin-lattice relaxation. See Relaxation time, T_1.
Spin-spin relaxation. See Relaxation time, T_2.
Spinal cord, cervicothoracic, trauma to, 700, 700–701, 701
  compression of, 669
    metastatic tumors and, 688
  degenerative disease of, 678, 678–679
  in Arnold-Chiari malformation, 425
  injury to, disk herniation and, 684
  intramedullary disease of, 673–681, 674–678, 680
  ischemia of, 679–680, 680
  meningioma of, 698, 698
  multiple sclerosis in, 678, 678–679
  sagittal view of, 405
  syringohydromyelia of, 677, 677–678, 678
  tethered, 724–728, 725–727
    imaging protocols for, 1140–1141
  tumors of, intramedullary, 673–677, 674–676
  vascular malformations of, 680, 680–681
Spindle cell tumor, 1108
Spine, 667–728
  cervical, degenerative disease of, fast imaging of, 203, 204
  imaging of, cerebrospinal fluid in, flow compensation for, 126, 127
    photography of, 62, 63, 64
    protocols for, 1138–1139
  junction of, with cranium, abnormalities of, 701, 701–702, 702
  sagittal view of, 405
  three-dimensional imaging of, 59, 59
  cervicothoracic, anatomy of, 670, 671, 673–674, 674
  bone marrow disease in, 691–693, 693
  degenerative disease of, 681–687, 682–687
  imaging of, technical aspects of, 668, 668–672
  infection of, 694–696, 695, 696
  stenosis of, 685–687, 687

Spine (Continued)
  trauma to, 699–701, 700, 701
  tumors of, metastatic, 688–690, 688–690
    nerve sheath, 696, 696–697, 697
    primary, 690–691, 691, 692
  computed tomography of, 667–668
  cysts in, cerebrospinal fluid flow effects in, 145, 145–146
  degenerative disease of, cervicothoracic, 681–687, 682–687
    fast imaging of, 200, 203, 204
    lumbar, 709–714, 710–716
    recurrent postoperative, 719–720, 720, 721, 723
  dysraphism of, 724–728, 725–727
  Harrington rod in, and magnetic field distortion, 41–42
  imaging of, positioning for, 41
    surface receiver coil in, 44, 44
  lumbar, anatomy of, 707–709, 708–709
    arachnoiditis of, 724, 724
    degenerative disease of, 709–714, 710–716
      fast imaging of, 204
    imaging of, protocols for, 1140–1141
      technical aspects of, 705–706, 706–709
    pain in, in pregnancy, 943
    Pantopaque in, 724, 725
    postoperative complications in, 719–720, 719–723
    spondylosis of, 715–717, 717–719
    stenosis of, 717–718, 718, 719
  osteomyelitis of, 1119–1121
  sacral, lesions of, 720–724, 723
  thoracic, carcinoma of, bronchogenic, 1104
    metastatic, 1104
    imaging of, protocols for, 1138–1139
    trauma to, 699–701, 700, 701, 1122–1123
Spleen, 895
  lymphoma of, ferrite-enhanced imaging of, 251, 251, 252
  signal intensity in, 15t, 16t
Splinting, to reduce ghost artifacts, 102
Spoiler pulses, 330, 1170
  in FLASH imaging, 190, 190
  contrast in, 192, 193–195
Spondylolisthesis, lumbar, 718, 719
Spondylosis, cervicothoracic, 681–685, 685, 686
  lumbar, 715–717, 717–719
Staphylococcus aureus infection, and diskitis, 695
Stapling, surgical, and artifact, 80
Starr-Edwards cardiac valves, precautions for, 41, 70–71
Static magnetic field, artifacts in, 75–81, 77–82
Steady-state free precession, definition of, 1170
Steady-state imaging, FLASH, 190–191, 191
  contrast in, 192–195, 195
  zebra stripes in, 196, 196
  gradient-recalled, 49, 50, 190–191
  contrast in, 192–195, 193, 194
  definition of, 1162
  in myelography, 145
STEAM. See Stimulated-echo acquisition method.
Stewart-Hamilton equation, in cardiac perfusion studies, 749–751
Stimulated echo, definition of, 1170
Stimulated-echo acquisition method, definition of, 1170
  in fast imaging, 214
  in localized spectroscopy, 287, 287–288
  in proton spectroscopy, 279–281, 281
  in temporomandibular joint imaging, 1033
Stimulated-echo artifact, 85, 86, 1158
STIR sequence, 28, 28
  definition of, 1164
  in orbital imaging, 601
  to reduce ghost artifacts, 102
Stomach, gadolinium-DTPA imaging of, 248, 249
  signal in, effect of, on hepatic imaging, 849, 851
Straight sinus, axial view of, 392–395
  sagittal view of, 404
Streptococcus, in brain abscess, 578
Stress fractures, 1123, 1123
  of foot, 1094, 1095
Stria terminalis, 406

Stripes, oblique, data loss and, 89–90, 90
  zebra, in flow measurement, 176, 176, 177
  in steady-state FLASH imaging, 196, 196
Stroke, 516–521, 517–524. See also Infarction, cerebrovascular.
Sturge-Weber syndrome, 432–434, 435, 436
Stylomastoid foramen, 411
Subacromial-subdeltoid bursa, anatomy of, 1013
  in rotator cuff injury, 1016, 1017, 1017
Subaortic stenosis, hypertrophic, idiopathic, 802
Subarachnoid hemorrhage, aneurysms and, 537, 538–541, 539–541
  oxygenation in, 489–491, 492
Subclavian artery, anatomy of, 732
Subclavian vein, anatomy of, 732, 732–733
Subdeltoid bursa, in rotator cuff injury, 1019, 1019
Subdural hematoma, 564–565, 564–567
Subdural hygroma, 565, 569
Subependymoma, 475
Sublingual glands, anatomy of, 638, 639
  obstruction of, and ranula, 640, 643
Submandibular gland, anatomy of, 638, 639
  obstruction of, 640, 643
Substantia nigra, axial view of, 390, 393
  iron deposition in, 590, 590
Subtraction angiography, 152–155, 153–155, 1170
Sulci. See also specific sulci, e.g., Calcarine sulcus.
  in brain development, 415, 415t
Sulfur, magnetic resonance characteristics of, 5t
Superconductivity. See also Magnet(s), superconductive.
  definition of, 1171
Superior cerebellar artery, 388
Superior cerebellar cistern, axial view of, 392, 395
  sagittal view of, 406, 410
Superior colliculus, axial view of, 392
  coronal view of, 403
  sagittal view of, 405
Superior frontal gyrus, axial view of, 396, 398, 399
  coronal view of, 400, 402
  sagittal view of, 404
Superior nasal turbinate, 400
Superior oblique muscle, of orbit, Brown's syndrome of, 612, 612, 612t
Superior ophthalmic vein, coronal view of, 400
  sagittal view of, 408
Superior parietal lobule, 408
Superior rectus muscle, axial view of, 390
  coronal view of, 400
  sagittal view of, 409, 410
Superior sagittal sinus, axial view of, 394–399
  coronal view of, 401
  occlusion of, 523, 527, 528
  sagittal view of, 404
Superior semilunar lobule, of cerebellum, 403
Superior sulcus, carcinoma of, 739–740, 741
Superior temporal artery, 388
Superior temporal gyrus, axial view of, 389
  coronal view of, 401
  sagittal view of, 411
Superior vena cava, anatomy of, 732
  in transposition of great arteries, 835–836, 838, 839
  persistent left, 788, 791
Superparamagnetism, 239, 240t, 241
  and T_2 relaxation time, 241–242, 242
  definition of, 1171
  in imaging, effect of, 32–33
  of hemorrhage, 485
  of contrast agents, for cardiac perfusion studies, 751
Suppression, solvent, definition of, 1170
  for resolving hydrogen spectra, 307–309, 308
Supramarginal gyrus, 396, 397
Supranuclear palsy, progressive, 591, 591–592
Suprasellar cistern, axial view of, 390, 391
  coronal view of, 401
Supraspinatus tendon, injury to, 1015–1019, 1016–1020
Surface coils, in abdominal imaging, 848, 849
  in imaging, of brachial plexus, 654, 654, 655

Surface coils *(Continued)*
   of coronary artery bypass graft, 807, *807*
   of retinoblastoma, *44*
   of shoulder, 1010, *1011*
   of spinal metastasis, 688
   of temporomandibular joint, 1032, *1032*
   in phosphorus spectroscopy, of myocardial ischemia, 757–758, *757–759*
   localization with, in spectroscopy, 290, *290,* 291
   placement of, in spectroscopy, 296
   sensitivity to, and artifacts, 83, *83*
Susceptibility, magnetic, 32–33. See also *Diamagnetism, Ferromagnetism, Paramagnetism,* and *Superparamagnetism.*
   and artifact, 80–81, *81, 82*
   definition of, 1165
   in biologic tissue, 266
   of intestinal water-gas interface, 849, *851*
Sylvian aqueduct, axial view of, *390, 392*
   coronal view of, *403*
Sylvian cistern, axial view of, *390, 392, 393, 397*
   sagittal view of, *409, 411*
Sylvian fissure, axial view of, *396, 397*
   coronal view of, *401*
   sagittal view of, *407, 408*
Sympathetic dystrophy, reflex, of foot, 1094, *1096*
Synovial cell sarcoma, *1107*
Synovial chondromatosis, of knee, 1003, *1003*
Synovial cyst, 1101, 1117, *1117*
   of shoulder, 1026, *1026*
Synovial plicae, of knee, 1004
Synovitis, in carpal tunnel syndrome, 1059, *1059, 1061*
   of elbow, *1116*
   of knee, 1001, 1002, *1002*
   of shoulder, 1023–1027, *1026*
   pigmented villonodular, 1117
Synovium, hypertrophy of, in ankle, 1083, 1084
   of foot, sarcoma of, 1085, *1086*
Syphilis, and meningitis, 582
Syringohydromyelia, 677, 677–678, *678*
Syrinx, imaging protocols for, 1138–1139
   spinal cord, posttraumatic, 701, *701*
   with tethered cord, 727
Systemic lupus erythematosus, vs. multiple sclerosis, 561

T₁ contrast agents, in vivo targeting of, 229, *229–233, 231–233*
   intravascular distribution of, 233
   relaxivity of, *224–227,* 224–228, 225t
   toxicity of, 228t, 228–229
   vs. T₂ agents, 223
T₁ relaxation, definition of, 11–12, *13, 14*
T₁ relaxation time. See *Relaxation time, T₁.*
T₁ weighting. See *Weighting.*
T₂ contrast agents, 233–235, *234*
   vs. T₁ agents, 223
T₂ relaxation, definition of, 9–11, *10–12*
T₂ relaxation time. See *Relaxation time, T₂.*
T₂ weighting. See *Weighting.*
T₂* relaxation time, 10–11, *11*
Taenia solium infestation, and brain abscess, 577–580, *580, 581*
Takayasu's arteritis, 781–782
Talocrural joint, anatomy of, 1078
Talus, fracture of, 1084
   osteoid osteoma of, 1085–1086
Tapeworm infestation, and brain abscess, 577–580, *580, 581*
Tarlov's cyst, and lumbar nerve root compression, 712, *716*
Teeth, sagittal view of, *407*
Tegmentum, midbrain, axial view of, *390*
   sagittal view of, *405*
Telangiectasia, capillary, 535
Telencephalon, 415
   in Arnold-Chiari malformation, 425
Telescoping, and artifacts, 97, *98*
Temperature, blood flow in, monitoring of, during imaging, 40, 73
   effect of radiofrequency pulses on, 48–49
   measurement of, in spectroscopy, 305

Temporal artery, superior, *388*
Temporal bone, sagittal view of, *410*
   tumors of, 627–629, *628, 629*
Temporal gyrus, inferior, axial view of, *386*
   coronal view of, *401*
   sagittal view of, *411*
   middle, axial view of, *389*
   coronal view of, *401*
   sagittal view of, *411*
   superior, axial view of, *389*
   coronal view of, *401*
   sagittal view of, *411*
Temporal horn, of lateral ventricle, axial view of, *388, 391, 393*
   sagittal view of, *408–410*
Temporal lobe, axial view of, *392*
   bacterial abscess of, *577*
   herpes encephalitis in, 583, *583, 584*
   infarction of, encephalomalacia in, *521*
    gadolinium-DTPA imaging of, *524*
   metastatic tumor of, and hemorrhage, *507*
   sagittal view of, *409*
Temporal vessels, superficial, *385, 387, 389*
Temporalis muscle, axial view of, *384, 386, 388*
   coronal view of, *400*
   sagittal view of, *411*
Temporomandibular joint, 1031–1055
   anatomy of, 1033–1036, *1035, 1036*
   dysfunction of, 650–651
    claustrophobia with, 1055
    disk disease in, 1040–1041, *1040–1050*
    etiology of, 1037–1040
   imaging of, protocols for, 1148–1149
    technical aspects of, *1032,* 1032–1033, *1034*
   inflammation of, 1041, *1050, 1051*
   physiology of, 1036–1037, *1037–1039*
   prostheses for, 1044, *1052–1054*
   surgical complications in, 1041–1044, *1051–1054*
Tendinitis, of rotator cuff, 1015, *1016*
   of wrist, 1060–1062, *1061,* 1073
Tendon(s), of foot and ankle, anatomy of, 1078–1079
   disorders of, 1079–1083, *1080–1082*
   of rotator cuff, tears of, 1015–1020, *1017–1020*
   of wrist, extensor, abnormalities of, 1060–1062, *1061, 1062*
    flexor, in carpal tunnel syndrome, 1058–1060, *1058–1061*
   patellar, lesions of, 999–1000, *1000*
   signal intensity in, 16t
   trauma to, 1123–1124
Tenosynovitis, in carpal tunnel syndrome, 1059, *1059, 1061*
   of extensor tendons, of wrist, 1060–1062, *1061, 1062,* 1073
   of foot, 1080, *1080*
Tentorial incisura, axial view of, *392*
Tentorium cerebelli, coronal view of, *403*
   herniation through, aneurysmal hemorrhage and, 540–541
   sagittal view of, *406*
Teratocarcinoma, testicular, 958–959
Teratoma, ovarian, 928, *930*
   pineal, 458, 459
   sacral, 722
   testicular, 958–959
Tesla, definition of, 1171
Testes, anatomy of, 916, *917,* 954, *954, 955*
   atrophy of, 978
   imaging of, 922, *922*
    protocols for, 1148–1149
   infection of, differential diagnosis of, 978
   inflammation of, 963–965, 964
   torsion of, 965–971, *967–971*
    vs. infection, 978
   trauma to, 964–965, *965, 966*
   tumors of, *957,* 957–961, *959–961*
    staging of, 1155
    vs. infection, 978
   undescended, 972–978, *974–977*
Tethered cord syndrome, 724–728, *725–727*
   imaging protocols for, 1140–1141

1,4,7,10–Tetraazacyclododecane tetraacetate (DOTA), structure of, *225*
   with gadolinium contrast agent, 227, 250
Tetralogy of Fallot, 792, *795*
   cineangiography of, 832–833, *833–835*
Tetramethylsilane, as reference, in spectroscopy, 300, *301*
Thalamostriate vein, 395
Thalamus, axial view of, *393, 394*
   coronal view of, *402*
   hemorrhage of, *486, 498,* 498–499
    with contusion, *572, 574*
   sagittal view of, *405–407*
   ventrolateral, in brain development, *416, 17*
Thalassemia major, 901
Thermal noise, and artifact, 84
Thigh, chondrosarcoma of, *1106*
   lipoma of, *1099*
   liposarcoma of, *1100*
Third ventricle, axial view of, *390, 392, 395*
   coronal view of, *401, 402*
Thoracic outlet syndromes, 661, *665*
Thorax, anatomy of, *732,* 732–733, *733*
   fetal, 945, 945–946, *946*
   imaging of, 731–743
    technical aspects of, 731–732
Three-dimensional imaging, *19,* 22–23
   definition of, 1171
   fast gradient-echo technique in, 197, 208–210, *210, 211*
   Fourier transform, 317
   gradient-echo methods in, *58,* 58–60, *59*
    for susceptibility artifact, 81
   in angiography, 148–150, 149t, *150*
    maximum intensity projection in, *150,* 150–151, *151*
   of heart, chemical shift in, *766, 766*
   of orbit, *600, 601,* 602–603
   of temporomandibular joint, 1033, *1034*
Thrombosis, cardiac, 801, 803, *805*
   cineangiography of, 816t, 823–824, *825*
   cortical venous, and infarction, *510*
   deep venous, venography of, 146–147, *146–148*
   in aortic aneurysm, 781, *781, 782*
   jugular vein, vs. donut sign, *121*
   of hepatic veins, in Budd-Chiari syndrome, 877, *879*
   of inferior vena cava, in renal cell carcinoma, 901, *902*
   sagittal sinus, angiography of, *171*
   venous, cerebral, 522–523, *527, 528*
    vs. flow signal, 110t, 132–137, *133–137*
    even-echo rephasing for, 124, *125*
Thymus, 737
   cyst of, 733, *735*
Thyroglossal duct cyst, 648, 649
Thyroid gland, carcinoma of, metastasis of, to spine, 689
   imaging of, protocols for, 1136–1137
   lesions of, *647,* 647–649, *648,* 735, *737*
Timing, parameters for, selection of, 49–52, *51–53*
Tip angle, in orbital imaging, 601–602
   variation of, and artifacts, 83, *84*
TNM system, in cancer staging, 1153–1155
Tolosa-Hunt syndrome, 613t, 614, *617*
Tomography, computed. See *Computed tomography.*
Tongue, anatomy of, *639,* 640–645
Tonsil, cerebellar, axial view of, *384–386, 388*
   coronal view of, *403*
   sagittal view of, *404–406*
Topical magnetic resonance, 287
Torcular Herophili, *390*
Toxocara canis endophthalmitis, 603, 603t
Toxoplasmosis, of brain, AIDS-related, 584, *586–588*
Trachea, 737–739, *740*
Transmitter, adjustment of, 47
Transmitter coils, 7, 37
Transplantation, of heart, phosphorus spectroscopy of, *756,* 756–757, *757,* 761
   of kidney, 902–903, *903*
Transtentorial herniation, 512

Transtentorial herniation (Continued)
  aneurysmal hemorrhage and, 540–541
Transverse ligament, of knee, vs. meniscal tear, 994, 994–995, 995
Transverse magnetization, 8, 9
  reduction of, with T₂ relaxation, 9–10, 10, 11
  refocusing of, 320–321
Transverse sinus, axial view of, 390
  sagittal view of, 407, 408
  thrombosis in, 136
Trauma, and carotid artery aneurysm, 649, 650
  as indication for brain imaging, 380
  musculoskeletal, 1122–1125, 1122–1126
  to brachial plexus, 658–659, 658–660
  to brain, 563–575, 564–575
    and extracerebral hemorrhage, 564–565, 564–568
    imaging protocols in, 1134–1135
  to foot, 1094, 1095, 1096
  to scrotum, 964–965, 965, 966, 978
  to shoulder, 1023, 1025
  to spine, 1122–1123
    cervicothoracic, 699–701, 700, 701
    imaging protocols for, 1138–1141
Triangular fibrocartilage complex, anatomy of, 1068–1070, 1069, 1070
  disorders of, 1070–1073, 1071–1074
Tricarboxylic acid cycle, in carbon-13 spectroscopy, of heart, 761–762
Tricuspid valve, atresia of, in hypoplastic right heart syndrome, 833–834, 835
  Waterston shunt for, 792
Trigeminal nerve, axial view of, 388
  coronal view of, 402
  in Sturge-Weber syndrome, 432
  neuroma of, 473, 473
Triggering, electrocardiographic, 55–57, 55–57. See also Cardiac gating.
Trigone, of lateral ventricle, 395
Trochlear nerve, 391
Trophoblastic disease, 941, 941
Truncation artifacts, 91, 91–92, 328–329, 329, 1159
  in spinal imaging, 672
Tuberculosis, and meningitis, 581
  and orchitis, 964, 964, 965
Tuberous sclerosis, 434–436, 437
Tumor(s). See also specific neoplasms, e.g., Sarcoma.
  glomus, 479, 479–480
    of carotid sheath, angiography of, 170
    of parapharyngeal space, 633
  laryngeal, 646, 647
  localization of, T₁ contrast agents in, 233
  marrow infiltration by, 1102, 1109, 1109–1110
  mediastinal, 733–737, 734, 738–740
  musculoskeletal, 1098–1104, 1099–1108
  nerve sheath, 470–474, 472, 473
    spinal, 696, 696–697, 697
  of ankle, 1085, 1085–1088, 1086, 1088, 1089
  of bladder, and ureteral dilatation, 909
    imaging of, ferioxamine methane sulfonate in, 251–252, 253
  of brachial plexus, 659–661, 661–664
  of brain, 448–480. See also Brain, tumors of.
  of breast, proton spectroscopy of, 282
  of foot, 1085, 1085–1090, 1086, 1088–1091
  of heart, 801–803, 803, 804
    cineangiography of, 816t, 822, 823, 824
    imaging protocols for, 1142–1143
  of kidney, 905–908, 906, 907
  of knee, 1006, 1006, 1007
  of orbit, 602–620
  of oropharynx, 645, 646, 647
  of ovary, dermoid, 928, 929
  of salivary glands, 632, 633, 638, 640–642
  of scrotum, 957, 957–961, 959–961
  of shoulder, 1028, 1029
  of temporal bone, 627–629, 628, 629
  of uterus, fibroid, 923, 925, 926, 931
  phosphorus spectroscopy of, 277–278, 278, 278t, 279
  plasma lipids with, proton spectroscopy of, 282, 282
  signal intensity in, 237

Tumor(s) (Continued)
  spinal, imaging protocols for, 1138–1141
    spinal cord, 673–677, 674–676
    T₁ relaxation time in, 12
Tumor-node-metastasis system, in cancer staging, 1153–1155
Tunica albuginea, anatomy of, 954, 954–956
Tunica vaginalis, anatomy of, 954, 954
  in testicular torsion, 966
Tuning, definition of, 1171
  of receiver coil, 46, 47
Turbinate, inferior, coronal view of, 400
    sagittal view of, 406
  middle, axial view of, 385
    coronal view of, 400
    sagittal view of, 406
  superior, coronal view of, 400
Turbulence, definition of, 1171
  in blood flow, 113, 114
Two-dimensional imaging, 18–22, 19–23
  definition of, 1171
  in spectroscopy, 305, 305–306, 306
  sequential, in angiography, 151–152
    in venography, 151–152
  spin-echo sequence in, 314t, 314–316, 314–316
Tympanic cavity, cholesteatoma of, 628

U fibers, subcortical, 399
Ulceration, carotid artery, angiography of, 172
Ulna, displacement of, 1070, 1071, 1072
Ulnar collateral ligament, anatomy of, 1062, 1062–1063
Ulnar variance, 1064, 1065, 1071–1073, 1072, 1074
Ulnolunate impingement syndrome, 1071, 1072
Ulnotriquetral ligament, anatomy of, 1063, 1063
Ultrasonography, in pregnancy, 938, 939
  of carotid artery, 162–163
  of liver, 853
Umbilical vein, patent, in Budd-Chiari syndrome, angiography of, 162
Umbrella filters, vena caval, precautions for, 41, 71
Uncinate process, of pancreas, 884, 885
Uncus, axial view of, 388, 390
  sagittal view of, 407
Undersampling (Gibbs) artifacts, 91, 91–92, 328–329, 329, 1159
  in spinal imaging, 672
Ureter, dilatation of, 908–909, 909
Urinary tract, bleeding in, imaging protocols for, 1146–1147
  imaging of, ferioxamine methane sulfonate in, 251–252, 252, 253
Urinoma, perinephric, 900, 901
Uterus, anatomy of, 922, 924, 925
  arcuate, 983–984
  bicornuate, 981–982, 982–985
  cervical carcinoma extending to, 927
  developmental abnormalities of, 981–984, 982–985
  embryology of, 981
  fibroid tumors of, 923, 925, 926, 931
  hypoplastic, 983–984
  imaging of, protocols for, 1146–1147
    technical aspects of, 915, 916t
  in pregnancy, 939, 939
  leiomyoma of, 923, 925, 926, 939, 939
  sarcoma of, 926
  septate, 981–982, 982, 985
  unicornuate, 982–983, 985
Uterus didelphys, 981, 982
Uvula vermis, axial view of, 386
  sagittal view of, 404

Vagina, agenesis of, 984–986
  anatomy of, 923, 925
  developmental abnormalities of, 984–986, 985
  embryology of, 980–981
  imaging of, technical aspects of, 915, 916, 916t
  septate, 985, 986

Vagus nerve, axial view of, 386
  coronal view of, 402
  sagittal view of, 408, 409
Valium (diazepam), for claustrophobia, 40
  use of, before fetal imaging, 944
Vallecula, axial view of, 384
  sagittal view of, 404
Valvular implants, precautions for, 41, 70–71
Valvular insufficiency, imaging protocols for, 1142–1143
Valvular regurgitation, cineangiography of, 822–823, 823
Valvular stenosis, cineangiography of, 815, 815, 816t
Varicocele, 972, 972
Varix, of mesenteric vein, angiography of, 163
  orbital, 609, 609
Vas deferens, anatomy of, 954–956, 956
Vasculitis, cerebral, 523–524, 529
  vs. multiple sclerosis, 561
Vasospasm, aneurysmal hemorrhage and, 540
Vector, definition of, 1171
Vein. See also specific veins, e.g., Cerebral vein.
Vein of Galen, axial view of, 395, 397
  malformation of, 530, 531
  sagittal view of, 404
Velocity, of blood flow, 111t, 111–114, 112t
Velum interpositum cistern, 394–397
Vena cava, anatomy of, 732
  hemodynamics in, 111t
  inferior, anatomy of, 859–860, 860
    imaging of, protocols for, 1144–1145
    leiomyosarcoma of, blood flow measurement in, 177
    thrombus of, in renal cell carcinoma, 901, 902
  superior, in transposition of great arteries, 835–836, 838, 839
    persistent left, 788, 791
  umbrella filters in, precautions for, 41, 71
Venography, 146–147, 146–148
  of hepatic cancer, 160, 162
  sequential two-dimensional, 151–152
Venous plexus, periprostatic, 916, 917
Ventral induction, in brain development, 415
  disorders of, 414t, 426–431, 426–431
Ventricle(s), cerebral, enlargement of, in hydrocephalus, 555–560, 557, 558
  fourth, axial view of, 386–389, 391
    coronal view of, 403
    ependymoma of, 475, 475
    facial colliculus of, 388
    sagittal view of, 404, 405
  hemorrhage of, primary, 510–511
  lateral, atrium of, glomus in, 408
    body of, 396, 397
    coronal view of, 401–403
    frontal horn of, 394
    sagittal view of, 406–410
    temporal horn of, axial view of, 388, 391, 393
      sagittal view of, 408–410
    trigone of, 395
  third, axial view of, 390, 392, 395
    coronal view of, 401, 402
  of heart, left, dimensions of, 796–797, 797t, 798
    function studies of, 796–797, 796–799
      cineangiography in, 821
      imaging planes through, 774–779, 774–779
    lipoma of, 803, 805
    right, congenital lesions of, 832–834, 833–838
      function of, cineangiography of, 821–822
      hypertrophy of, vs. tumor, 803
      outflow obstruction from, 792, 795
    single, pulmonary banding for, cineangiography of, 840–841, 841, 842
Ventricular septal defect, 788, 792
  in tetralogy of Fallot, 832, 833
  pulmonary banding for, 840–841, 841, 842
Vermian vein, inferior, 388, 389
Vermis cerebelli, axial view of, 388, 389, 392
  medulloblastoma of, 476, 477
  nodulus of, axial view of, 388

Vermis cerebelli *(Continued)*
  coronal view of, *403*
    sagittal view of, *404*
  sagittal view of, *405*
  uvula of, axial view of, *386*
    sagittal view of, *404*
Versed, before imaging, of congenital heart disease, 832
Vertebra(e). See also *Spine*.
  atlas, coronal view of, *402*
  cervical, sagittal view of, *405*
  cervicothoracic, bone marrow in, *670*, 673, *673*
    diseases of, 691–693, *693*
    tumors of, primary, 690–691, *691*, *692*
Vertebral artery, aneurysm of, and subarachnoid hemorrhage, *540*
  axial view of, *385*, *387*
  malformation of, in neck, *650*
  sagittal view of, *407–409*
Vestibular nerve, anatomy of, 623
Vestibule, axial view of, *386*, *387*
Vestibulocochlear nerve, anatomy of, 623
  axial view of, *386*
  meningioma of, in neurofibromatosis, 431, *434*
  neuroma of, 470–473, *472*, *473*, 625, *625*
    in neurofibromatosis, 431, *433*
  sagittal view of, *407–409*
Villonodular synovitis, pigmented, 1117
  of knee, 1002, *1002*
  of shoulder, 1026–1027
Virchow-Robin spaces, 545–546, *546*
  dilation of, 521, *523*
Virus(es), and brain infection, 576
  herpes simplex, and brain infection, 583, *583*, *584*
  human immunodeficiency, and brain infection, 583–589, *586–590*
    and primary malignant lymphoma, 452, *453*
Viscosity, of blood, effect of, on velocity, 112–114

Vitreous, persistent hyperplastic primary, 603, 603t, *605*
Volar intercalated segmental instability, 1073, *1073*
Volar radioulnar ligament, tears of, 1070–1071, *1071*
Volume acquisition, 317
von Hippel-Lindau disease, 436–437, *438*, *439*
Voxel, definition of, 1171
  volume of, and signal-to-noise ratio, 32

Warfarin (Coumadin), and brain hemorrhage, 504
Washout, blood flow and, 115–116, *116*
  definition of, 1162
Water, diffusion of, phase effects of, 177–179, *179*
  paramagnetic exclusion of, in cerebral hemorrhage, 257, *258*
  resonance of, in chemical shift effect, *326*, 326–327
Water-fat separation, in pulse sequence design, *336*, 336–337, *338*
  in spectroscopy, 292–293, *293*
  proton, 278, *280*
Water-gas interface, intestinal, magnetic susceptibility effect of, 849, *851*
Waterson shunt, for tricuspid atresia, *792*
Waveforms, gradient, 323, *323*
Weighting, definition of, 11, 12, 16t, 16–17, *17*
  in orbital imaging, 601–602
  spin-echo sequences in, 24–25
  T_1, contrast in, 29–30, *30*
    definition of, 1171
    in brain imaging, 381
    selection of, 49
  T_2, contrast in, 30, *30*
    definition of, 1171

Weighting *(Continued)*
  in brain imaging, 381
  selection of, 49
  with gadolinium-DTPA contrast, 60
Wharton's duct, obstruction of, 640, *643*
Wilms' tumor, 906
Wilson's disease, 593–595, 875
Wraparound artifact, 76t, 95, *95*, 1159
  elimination of, oversampling for, 55
Wrist, 1057–1074, 1117–1118
  anatomy of, 1062–1064, *1062–1064*, 1068–1071, *1069–1071*
  avascular necrosis of, 1066–1068, *1067*, *1068*, 1111, *1113*
  extensor tendon abnormalities of, 1060–1062, *1061*, *1062*
  ganglion cyst of, 1073–1074
  imaging of, protocols for, 1150–1151
    technical aspects of, 1057–1058
  instability of, 1064–1068, *1065–1068*
    ulnar, 1071–1073, *1072–1074*
  Kienböck's disease of, 1067–1068, *1068*
  median nerve compression in, 1058–1060, *1058–1061*, 1117–1118

Xanthogranuloma, in pyelonephritis, 905

Yolk-sac tumor, pineal, 458

Zebra stripes, in flow measurement, 176, *176*, *177*
  in steady-state FLASH imaging, 196, *196*
Zero frequency artifact, 85, *85*
Zero phase artifact, 85–86, *86*, *87*
Zeugmatography, 335–336
  rotating frame, 290–291, *291*
Zygomatic arch, *384*